Litt's

DRUG
ERUPTION
REFERENCE MANUAL
INCLUDING DRUG INTERACTIONS
15th EDITION

Litt's DRUG ERUPTION

REFERENCE MANUAL

INCLUDING DRUG INTERACTIONS

15TH EDITION

Jerome Z. Litt, MD

Assistant Clinical Professor of Dermatology
Case Western Reserve University School of Medicine
Cleveland, Ohio, USA

informa
healthcare

New York   London

Informa Healthcare USA, Inc.
52 Vanderbilt Avenue
New York, NY 10017

© 2009 by Informa Healthcare USA, Inc.
Informa Healthcare is an Informa business

No claim to original U.S. Government works
Printed in the United States of America on acid-free paper
10 9 8 7 6 5 4 3 2 1

International Standard Book Number-10: 1-8418-4690-2 (Hardcover)
International Standard Book Number-13: 978-1-8418-4690-3 (Hardcover)

Visit the Informa Web site at
www.informa.com

and the Informa Healthcare Web site at
www.informahealthcare.com

CONTENTS

To Vel – my Muse

Introduction

Any drug has the potential to cause a rash or other adverse effect.

An adverse effect, be it an adverse drug reaction (ADR) or an adverse drug event (ADE), is an unwanted, unpleasant, noxious, or harmful consequence associated with the use of a medication that has been administered in a standard dose by the proper route, for the purpose of prophylaxis, diagnosis, or treatment. This definition does not apply to effects resulting from medication abuse, overdose or withdrawal, or error of administration. It appears that most ADRs are related to the dose. Death is the ultimate adverse drug event.

Adverse drug reactions are the most common iatrogenic illness, complicating five to 15 percent of therapeutic drug courses. Some examples of these include:*

Immunologic Drug Reactions

1. IgE-mediated	Anaphylaxis from B-lactam antibiotics
2. Cytotoxic	Hemolytic anemia from penicillin
3. Immune complex	Serum sickness from tetanus antitoxin
4. Cell-mediated, delayed	Contact dermatitis from nickel
5. Specific T-cell activation	Exanthem from sulfonamides
6. Fas/Fas ligand induced	Stevens-Johnson syndrome; Toxic epidermal necrolysis
7. Miscellaneous	Anticonvulsant hypersensitivity syndrome; Lupus-like syndrome

Nonimmunologic Drug Reactions

1. Pharmacologic side effect	Dry mouth from antihistamine
2. Secondary pharmacologic side effects	Candidiasis from oral antibiotics
3. Toxicity	Hepatotoxicity from methotrexate
4. Drug-drug interactions	Seizure from theophylline while taking erythromycin
5. Overdose	Excessive lidocaine
6. Pseudoallergic	Anaphylactoid reactions from radiocontrast media
7. Idiosyncratic	Hemolytic anemia from primaquine, dapsone, etc.
8. Intolerance	Tinnitus from aspirin

A growing problem

Clearly, ADRs are a major problem in drug therapy. They are a leading cause of morbidity and mortality in healthcare and they should therefore be considered in the differential diagnosis of a wide variety of medical disorders. Indeed, they are a growing cause for concern. More and more people – particularly the elderly – are taking more and more prescription and over-the-counter medications. In addition, new drugs are appearing in the medical marketplace on an almost daily basis.

It is unsurprising that, at the same time, more and more drug reactions – especially in the form of cutaneous eruptions – are emerging. It has been reported that in 1999 more than 100,000 hospitalized people in the United States died as a result of medications. About 5% of hospital admissions in the United States are estimated to be for the treatment of adverse drug reactions. Moreover, as many as one-third of all emergency department and urgent care center visits are drug related. Between 1% and 3% of hospitalized patients suffer some sort of cutaneous adverse drug reaction. Anti-infective and anticonvulsant agents are among the drugs most frequently associated with adverse reactions on the skin.

Fortunately, most adverse drug reactions are relatively mild, and many disappear when the drug is either stopped or when the dose has changed. However, other adverse drug reactions are more serious and longer lasting. Severe and life-threatening eruptions do occur, such as Stevens-Johnson syndrome and toxic epidermal necrolysis. Despite the frequency and sometimes life-threatening nature of ADRs, they remain underreported and thus are an underestimated cause of morbidity and mortality.

Increasing complexity

The incidence and severity of ADRs can be influenced by patient-related factors (age, sex, disease, genetics, geography). They can also be influenced by drug-related factors (type of drug, route of administration – intramuscular, intravenous and topical administrations are more likely to cause hypersensitivity reactions; oral medications are less likely to result in drug hypersensitivity – duration of therapy, dosage, and bioavailability) as well as by interactions with other drugs. Furthermore, the prevention, diagnosis and treatment of ADRs are becoming more and more complex. More drugs – and more combinations of drugs – are being used to treat patients than ever before.

The situation is further complicated by the variety of ways in which we talk about adverse drug reactions. The terms 'drug allergy,' 'drug hypersensitivity,' and 'drug reaction' are used interchangeably. Drug **allergy** specifically refers to a reaction mediated by IgE; drug **hypersensitivity** is an immune-mediated response to a drug agent in a sensitized patient; and drug **reactions** comprise all adverse events related to drug administration, regardless of etiology. Factors associated with an increased risk for hypersensitivity drug reactions include asthma, lupus erythematosus, or use of beta-blockers. Atopic patients are at increased risk for serious allergic reactions.

Adverse drug reactions have been arbitrarily classified into six types:

1. Dose-related (e.g. digoxin toxicity)
2. Non-dose-related (e.g. immunological reactions)
3. Dose-related and time-related (e.g. corticosteroids)
4. Time-related (e.g. tardive dyskinesia)
5. Withdrawal (e.g. opiate or beta-blocker withdrawal)
6. Unexpected failure of therapy (e.g. inadequate dosage of an oral contraceptive)

It is to be expected that physicians in all specialties often are perplexed by the nature of ADRs. Just one of the problems hindering them in finding out more about drug reactions is that the few sources that are available to identify the causes of many of drug side effects cannot be accessed by proprietary (Trade, Brand) names.

Enter Litt's Drug Eruption Reference Manual

This manual is a drug eruption reference work that describes and catalogues the adverse cutaneous side effects of more than **1,250** commonly prescribed and over-the-counter **Generic Drugs** (more than **60** of which are new to this edition). All drugs have been listed and indexed by both their **Generic** and **Trade (Brand)** names for easy accessibility.

Because of space constraints, several of the **Generic Drugs** from earlier editions have been extirpated because either they have been withdrawn from the marketplace or they are rarely if ever prescribed today. These, please note, are still available – and always will be – on our website – www.drugeruptiondata.com.

In addition to adverse cutaneous reactions, the manual contains details of many severe, hazardous interactions known to occur between two or more drugs. I have incorporated only the highly clinically significant drug interactions that can trigger potential harm, and that could be life-threatening. These interactions are predictable and well documented in controlled studies; they should be avoided. This subdivision denoting hazardous interactions has been omitted from those drugs where no such interactions have been reported.

For each drug, I have listed the known adverse side effects – in the form of drug reactions – that can result from the use of the matching drug, focusing particularly on dermatological reactions. I have cited appropriate references (author, journal or book, volume, date and page) for each side effect of every drug. Where there is more than one reference to a specific side effect, I have employed the most illustrative and recent citation(s) in the literature.

In this, the 15th edition of the Drug Eruption Reference Manual, I have cited more than **32,000** references and

sources: from journal articles and books along with observations from dermatologists from all over the world. These references date back to 1980. You will find over **41,000** references on our website, from as far back as 1922 (visit www.drugeruptiondata.com).

The first part of the manual is an index of **1,254 Generic Drugs** and their corresponding **Trade Names** (almost 6,000), so that you can easily find the product you are looking for in the **A-Z** section, which is the main body of the manual.

Next comes a listing of the various **Classes** of drugs, and those **Generic Drugs** that belong to each class. The major portion of the manual – the body of the work – lists in A-Z order the **1,254** Generic Drugs, herbals and supplements and the adverse reactions that can arise from their use, along with the appropriate references.

The latter parts of the manual include a **description** of the 41 most common **Reaction Patterns**; a **listing** of those drugs that can occasion more than 100 different reaction patterns, including, among others, **Acne, Acute generalized exanthematous pustulosis, Alopecia, Aphthous stomatitis, Bullous eruptions, Erythema multiforme, Erythema nodosum, Exanthems, Exfoliative dermatitis, Fixed eruptions, Lichenoid eruptions, Lupus erythematosus, Onycholysis, Pemphigus, Photosensitivity, Pityriasis rosea, Pruritus, Psoriasis, Purpura, Toxic epidermal necrolysis, Urticaria,** and **Vasculitis**.

USAGE, STYLE & CONVENTIONS EMPLOYED IN THIS MANUAL

The **Generic Drug** name is at the top of each page.

A category for **Synonyms** (where applicable) follows.

The **Trade (Brand) Name(s)** are then listed alphabetically.

When there are many **Trade Names**, the ten (or so) most commonly recognized ones are listed. This compilation lists and cross-references both the **Trade *and* Generic** names of all the catalogued drugs. Following the more common **Trade Name** drugs are recorded – in parentheses – the latest name of the pharmaceutical company that is marketing the drug. Many of the names of the companies have changed from earlier editions of this manual because of acquisitions, mergers, and other factors in the pharmaceutical industry.

Beneath the **Trade Name** listing is a list of **Other Common Trade Names**, those drugs from other countries.

Then appears the **Indication(s)**, the **Class** in which the drug belongs and the **Half-Life** of each drug, when known. On occasion, an important or pertinent **Note** will follow.

Reactions: These are the **Adverse Reactions** to the particular **Generic Drug**. They are classified in six **Categories: Skin, Hair, Nails, Eyes, Mucosal** (which include ear, nose and throat reactions), and **Other**. Other refers to the reactions available in Litt's Drug Eruption Database www.drugeruptiondata.com; in particular, these include cardiovascular, central nervous system and musculoskeletal reactions. **Reactions** are listed alphabetically in each **Category**.

Under each **Reaction Pattern** are listed the **References** (the sources of the information). These are arranged in reverse chronological order – the most recent reference appearing first on the list.

References in the English language predominate. For the few foreign references, we have resorted to the summary or abstract. The majority of the citations come from the *J Am Acad Dermatol, Arch Dermatol, Cutis, Int J Dermatol, Contact Dermatitis, Br J Dermatol, JAMA, Lancet, BMJ, Aust J Dermatol, N Engl J Med, Ann Intern Med*, and other prominent and easily accessible journals.

As a function of space limitations, the list of **References** has been restricted mainly to those after 1980. As already mentioned, all **References** going as far back as 1922 can still be accessed on our website.

Many reference works have been consulted in the course of compiling this manual. These include:

(2002): Stockley IH, STOCKLEY'S DRUG INTERACTIONS, Pharmaceutical Press, London and Chicago

(1998): Kauppinen K et al, SKIN REACTIONS TO DRUGS, CRC Press, Boca Raton

(1996): Bruinsma W, A GUIDE TO DRUG ERUPTIONS, The File of Medicines, PO Box 21, 1474 HJ Oosthuizen, Netherlands.

(1994): Goldstein S & Wintroub BU, ADVERSE CUTANEOUS REACTIONS TO MEDICATION, CoMedica, New York.

(1992): Zürcher K & Krebs A, CUTANEOUS DRUG REACTIONS, Karger, Basel.

(1992): Breathnach SM & Hintner H, ADVERSE DRUG REACTIONS and the SKIN, Blackwell, Oxford.

(1988): Bork K, CUTANEOUS SIDE EFFECTS OF DRUGS, WB Saunders, Philadelphia.

There are occasions when there are very few or no adverse reactions to a specific drug. These drugs are still included in the manual since there is often a **positive significance in negative findings**.

As a departure from the official, conventional and established style guide, the order of each **Reference** will appear as follows:

- The year in parentheses. The most recent citation appears first. This approach seems to be much more logical.

- Last name and initial(s) of the principal author.

- A plus sign (+) after the author's name represents one or more co-authors.

- Journal name (standard abbreviation where possible), in italics.

- Volume Number (often followed by a parenthetical Part or Supplemental Number).

- First page of the article

- Books when cited are italicized, followed by the publisher and page number.

Other notes:

- (sic) means **just so**. This is how the authors designated the REACTION.

- For example, **Rash** (sic); **Dermatitis** (sic); **Skin Rash** (sic)

- I have used the term **passim** to mean 'in passing'.

There are occasional allusions to the incidence of many of the listed **Reactions**. Percentages – which for the most part are essentially vague and meaningless – are obtained from articles, from Zürcher & Krebs, and from Bork.

I have simplified the references to the many **Reaction Patterns** by eliminating, for the most part, tags such as '–like' as in '–Psoriasis-like' '–reactivation' '–syndrome' '–dissemination' '–iform', etc.

Observation means just that. **Observations** (read **Anecdotes**) are derived from information obtained via the Internet from more than 1,500 reliable dermatologists worldwide, and via personal correspondence.

If you send me your observations at support@ drugeruptiondata.com they will be catalogued and you will be given appropriate attribution and recognition in the next edition.

Enjoy!
Jerome Z. Litt, M.D.
January, 2009

* Table adapted from American Family Physician, November 1, 2003, M. Riedel and A. Casillas

INDEX OF GENERIC AND TRADE NAMES

Generic drug names are in **bold**

2-amino-2-deoxyglucose hydrochloride	**glucosamine**
2-amino-deoxyglucose sulfate	**glucosamine**
5-FC	**flucytosine**
8-MOP	**methoxsalen, psoralens**
A-Acido	**tretinoin**
A-Gram	**amoxicillin**
abacavir	Trizivir, Ziagen
Abaprim	**trimethoprim**
abarelix	Plenaxis
abatacept	Orencia
Abbocillin	**penicillin V**
Abbokinase	**urokinase**
abciximab	ReoPro
Abelcet	**amphotericin B**
Abemin	**tolbutamide**
Abenol	**acetaminophen**
Aberal	**tretinoin**
Aberela	**tretinoin**
Abetol	**labetalol**
Abilify	**aripiprazole**
Abilitat	**aripiprazole**
Abitrate	**clofibrate**
Abraxane	**paclitaxel**
Abreva	**docosanol**
Abrifam	**rifampin**
ABZ	**albendazole**
Ac-De	**dactinomycin**
Acadione	**tiopronin**
Acamed	**trihexyphenidyl**
acamprosate	Aotal, Campral
acarbose	Glucobay, Glumida, Prandase, Precose
Acaren	**vitamin A**
Accenon	**ethotoin**
Accolate	**zafirlukast**
AccuNeb	**albuterol**
Accupril	**quinapril**
Accuprin	**quinapril**
Accupro	**quinapril**
Accuretic	**hydrochlorothiazide**
Accutane	**isotretinoin**
acebutolol	Acecor, Acetanol, Alol, Apo-Acebutolol, Monitan, Neptal, Novo-Acebutolol, Nu-Acebutolol, Prent, Rhodiasectral, Rhotral, Sectral
aceclofenac	Aflamin, Arrestin, Beofenac, Preservex
Acecor	**acebutolol**
acenocoumarol	Acenox, Acitrom, Sinthrome, Sintrom
Acenor-M	**fosinopril**
Acenorm	**captopril**
Acenox	**acenocoumarol**
Aceon	**perindopril**
Acepril	**captopril**
Acerbon	**lisinopril**
Acertil	**perindopril**
acetaminophen	Abenol, Anacin-3, Anaflon, Ben-U-Ron, Bromo-Seltzer, Darvocet-N, Datril, Doliprane, Excedrin, Geluprane, Liquiprin, Lorcet, Mapap, Neopap, Panadol, Percocet, Percogesic, Phenaphen, Sinutab, Tylenol, Valadol, Vicodin
Acetanol	**acebutolol**
Acetazolam	**acetazolamide**
acetazolamide	Acetazolam, Ak-Zol, Dazamide, Defiltran, Diamox, Diuramid, Novo-Zolamide
acetohexamide	Dimelin, Dimelor, Dymelor
Acetyl-L-carnitine	**l-carnitine**
acetylcysteine	Agisolvan, Alveolex, Ecomucyl, Encore, Exomuc, Fabrol, Fluimicil, Mucofillin, Mucolit, Mucolitico, Mucoloid, Mucomiste, Mucomyst, Mucomyst-10, Mucosil-10, Parvolex, Siran
Acfol	**folic acid**
Acid A Vit	**tretinoin**
Acidulated phosphate fluoride	**fluorides**
Acifol	**propranolol**
Acifur	**acyclovir**
Acimox	**amoxicillin**
Aciphex	**rabeprazole**
acitretin	Neotigason, Soriatane
Acitrom	**acenocoumarol**
Aclinda	**clindamycin**
Aclovate	**alclometasone**
Acnavit	**tretinoin**
Acomplia	**rimonabant**
Acon	**vitamin A**
Acova	**argatroban**
Act-3	**ibuprofen**
Acta	**tretinoin**
Actacode	**codeine**
Actagen	**triprolidine**
Actamin	**thiamine**
Actemra	**tocilizumab**
ActHIB	**hemophilus b vaccine**
Actidil	**triprolidine**
Actidilon	**triprolidine**
Actidose-Aqua	**charcoal**
Actifed	**triprolidine**
Actifen	**dexibuprofen**
Actigall	**ursodiol**
Actilyse	**alteplase**
Actin-N	**nitrofurazone**
Actiprofen	**ibuprofen**
Actiq	**fentanyl**
Activacin	**alteplase**
Activase	**alteplase**
Actonel	**risedronate**
Actos	**pioglitazone**
Acuitel	**quinapril**
Acular	**ketorolac**
Acupril	**quinapril**
Acutrim	**phenylpropanolamine**
Acyclo-V	**acyclovir**
acyclovir	Acifur, Acyclo-V, Acyvir, Avirax, Herpefug, Zovirax, Zyclir
Acyvir	**acyclovir**
Adaferin	**adapalene**
Adalat	**nifedipine**
Adalate	**nifedipine**
adalimumab	Humira
Adancor	**nicorandil**

INDEX OF GENERIC AND TRADE NAMES

Brietal Sodium	**methohexital**	**butorphanol**	Biforal, Busphen, Stadol, Stadol NS
brimonidine	Alphagan	Byclomine	**dicyclomine**
brinzolamide	Azopt		
Brisfirina	**cephapirin**	**cabergoline**	Dostinex
Brispen	**dicloxacillin**	Calagualine	**polypodium leucotomos**
Bristopen	**oxacillin**	Calagula	**polypodium leucotomos**
Britiazem	**diltiazem**	Calamine	**zinc**
Brocadopa	**levodopa**	Calan	**verapamil**
Bromed	**bromocriptine**	Calcicard	**diltiazem**
Bromfed	**pseudoephedrine, brompheniramine**	Calcidrine	**codeine**
bromfenac	Xibrom	Calcilat	**nifedipine**
Bromine	**brompheniramine**	Calcilean	**heparin**
Brommine	**brompheniramine**	Calcimar	**calcitonin**
Bromo-Seltzer	**acetaminophen**	Calciparin	**heparin**
bromocriptine	Apo-Bromocriptine, Bromed, Cryocriptina, Kripton, Parilac, Parlodel, Pravidel, Serocryptin	**calcipotriol**	Dovonex
		calcitonin	Calcimar, Caltine, Cibacalcine, Clasynar, Miacalcic, Miacalcin
Bromphen	**brompheniramine**	**calcium hydroxylapatite**	Radiesse
brompheniramine	Bromfed, Bromine, Brommine, Bromphen, Dimegan, Dimetane, Ilvin, Kinmedon, Nasahist, ND-Stat, Neo-Meton, Rondec	**calfactant**	Infasurf
		Calm-X	**dimenhydrinate**
Bromurex	**pancuronium**	Calmaril	**thioridazine**
Broncho-Spray	**albuterol**	Calmaxid	**nizatidine**
Bronitin	**epinephrine**	Calmazine	**trifluoperazine**
Bronkaid	**epinephrine**	Calte	**carteolol**
Bronkodyl	**aminophylline**	Caltine	**calcitonin**
Bronkomed	**isoetharine**	Calypsol	**ketamine**
Bropantil	**propantheline**	Camazole	**carbimazole**
Brothine	**terbutaline**	Campath	**alemtuzumab**
Brovana	**arformoterol**	Campral	**acamprosate**
Brufen	**ibuprofen**	Camptosar	**irinotecan**
Bucaril	**terbutaline**	Canasa	**mesalamine**
bucillamine	Rimatil	Cancidas	**caspofungin**
Bucladin-S	**buclizine**	**candesartan**	Amias, Atacand
Buclixin	**buclizine**	Candid	**clotrimazole**
buclizine	Aphilan, Bucladin-S, Buclixin, Longifene, Odetin, Postafeno, Vibazina, Vibazine	Candio-Hermal	**nystatin**
		Canestene	**clotrimazole**
budesonide	Pulmicort Turbuhaler, Rhinocort	Cantil	**mepenzolate**
Bufigen	**nalbuphine**	Capastat	**capreomycin**
Bumedyl	**bumetanide**	**capecitabine**	Xeloda
bumetanide	Bumedyl, Bumex, Burinex, Fondiuran, Fontego, Lunetoron, Miccil, Primex	Capex	**fluocinolone**
		Caplenal	**allopurinol**
Bumex	**bumetanide**	Capoten	**captopril**
Bunolgan	**levobunolol**	Capozide	**hydrochlorothiazide, captopril**
bupivacaine	Marcaine, Sensorcaine	Capramol	**aminocaproic acid**
buprenorphine	Suboxone, Subutex, Temgesic, Transtec	**capreomycin**	Capastat, Ogostal
bupropion	Wellbutrin, Zyban	Caprin	**aspirin, heparin**
Burinex	**bumetanide**	Caproamin	**aminocaproic acid**
Busetal	**disulfiram**	Caprolisin	**aminocaproic acid**
Busirone	**buspirone**	Captimer	**tiopronin**
BuSpar	**buspirone**	Captolane	**captopril**
Busphen	**butorphanol**	**captopril**	Acenorm, Acepril, Adocor, APO-Capto, Capoten, Capozide, Captolane, Captoril, Lopirin, Lopril, Nu-Capto, Precaptil
buspirone	Ansail, Apo-Buspirone, Bespar, Biron, Busirone, BuSpar, Bustab, Kallmiren, Narol, Neurosine, Nu-Buspirone		
		Captoril	**captopril**
Bustab	**buspirone**	Carac	**fluorouracil**
busulfan	Citosulfan, Leukosulfan, Mablin, Misulban, Myleran	Carace	**lisinopril**
butabarbital	Butalan, Buticaps, Butisol, Day-Barb	Carafate	**sucralfate**
Butace	**butalbital**	Carbac	**loracarbef**
Butalan	**butabarbital**	**carbachol**	Carbamann, Carbastat Ophthalmic, Carboptic Ophthalmic, Glaumarin, Isopto Carbachol Ophthalmic, Isopto Karbakolin, Karbakolin Isopto, Miostat Intraocular
butalbital	Amaphen, Anoquan, Axotal, Butace, Esgic, Fioricet, Fiorinal, Marnal, Medigesic, Phrenilin, Tecnal		
Butaline	**terbutaline**		
Butatab	**phenylbutazone**	Carbamann	**carbachol**
Butazolidine	**phenylbutazone**	**carbamazepine**	Apo-Carbamazepine, Atreol, Carbatrol, Epitol, Foxsalepsin, Kodapan, Lexin, Mazepine, Sirtal, Tegretol, Tegretol XR, Teril, Timonil
Butazone	**phenylbutazone**		
Butibel	**atropine sulfate**		
Buticaps	**butabarbital**		
Butisol	**butabarbital**	Carbametin	**methocarbamol**

chlorpheniramine	AL-R, Aller-Chlor, Chlo-Amine, Chlor-Pro, Chlor-Trimeton, Chlor-Tripolon, Chlorate, Ornade, Phenetron, Telachlor, Teldrin, Triaminic
Chlorpromanyl	**chlorpromazine**
chlorpromazine	Chloractil, Chlorazin, Chlorpromanyl, Esmino, Largactil, Novo-Chlorpromazine, Ormazine, Propaphenin, Prozin, Thorazine
chlorpropamide	Apo-Chlorpropamide, Arodoc C, Chlormide, Diabemide, Diabenese, Diabinese, Insogen, Melormin, Tesmel
Chlorquin	**chloroquine**
chlortetracycline	Aureomicina, Aureomycin
chlorthalidone	Combipres, Higroton, Hydro-Long, Hygroton, Hypertol, Igroton, Tenoretic, Thalidone, Thalitone, Uridon
chlorzoxazone	Escoflex, Flexaphen, Klorzoxazon, Muscol, Paraflex, Parafon Forte DSC, Prolax, Remular-S, Solaxin
Chlothin	**chlorothiazide**
Chlotride	**chlorothiazide**
Chol-Less	**cholestyramine**
Cholacid	**ursodiol**
Choledyl	**aminophylline**
Cholestabyl	**colestipol**
cholestyramine	Chol-Less, Colestrol, Lismol, PMS-Cholestyramine, Prevalite, Quantalan, Questran, Questran Lite
Cholit-Ursan	**ursodiol**
Cholofalk	**ursodiol**
Chronovera	**verapamil**
Cialis	**tadalafil**
Cibacalcine	**calcitonin**
Cibace	**benazepril**
Cibacen	**benazepril**
Cibacene	**benazepril**
ciclesonide	Alvesco, Omnaris
Ciclosporin	**cyclosporine**
cidofovir	Forvade, Vistide
Cidomycin	**gentamicin**
Ciflox	**ciprofloxacin**
cilazapril	Inhibase, Vascace
Cilecef	**ceftibuten**
Cillimicina	**lincomycin**
Cillimycin	**lincomycin**
cilostazol	Pletal
Ciloxan Ophthalmic	**ciprofloxacin**
Cimedine	**cimetidine**
Cimehexal	**cimetidine**
cimetidine	Apo-Cimetidine, Azucimet, Blocan, Cimedine, Cimehexal, Ciuk, Dyspamet, Novocimetine, Nu-Cimet, Peptol, Stomedine, Tagamet, Ulcedine, Zymerol
Cimogal	**ciprofloxacin**
Cimzia	**certolizumab pegol**
Cin-Quin	**quinidine**
cinacalcet	Sensipar
Cinarizins	**cinnarizine**
Cinazyn	**cinnarizine**
Cinlol	**propranolol**
Cinnabene	**cinnarizine**
Cinnacet	**cinnarizine**
Cinnageron	**cinnarizine**
Cinnarisine	**cinnarizine**
cinnarizine	Arlevert, Cerepar, Cinarizins, Cinazyn, Cinnabene, Cinnacet, Cinnageron, Cinnarisine, Cinnipirine, Clinadil, Derozin, Diclamina, Ederal, Libotacin, Medozine, Pericephal, Pervasum, Sepan, Stugeron, Surepil, Sureptil, Touristil, Vertizin
Cinnipirine	**cinnarizine**
Cinobac	**cinoxacin**
Cinobact	**cinoxacin**
Cinobactin	**cinoxacin**
cinoxacin	Cerexin, Cinobac, Cinobact, Cinobactin, Gugecin, Nossacin, Noxigram, Uronorm
Ciplactin	**cyproheptadine**
Ciplox	**ciprofloxacin**
Cipro	**ciprofloxacin**
Ciprobay Uro	**ciprofloxacin**
ciprofibrate	Lipanor, Modalim
ciprofloxacin	Ciflox, Ciloxan Ophthalmic, Cimogal, Ciplox, Cipro, Ciprobay Uro, Cipromycin, Ciproxin, Italnik, Kenzoflex, Uniflox
Cipromycin	**ciprofloxacin**
Ciproral	**cyproheptadine**
Ciproxin	**ciprofloxacin**
cisatracurium	Nimbex
cisplatin	Cisplatyl, Plasticin, Platiblastin, Platinex, Platinol, Platinol-AQ, Platistil
Cisplatyl	**cisplatin**
Cisticid	**praziquantel**
citalopram	Celexa
Citax	**immune globulin I.V.**
Citosulfan	**busulfan**
Citrec	**leucovorin**
Ciuk	**cimetidine**
Civeran	**loratadine**
Clacine	**clarithromycin**
cladribine	Leustatin
Claforan	**cefotaxime**
Clamoxyl	**amoxicillin**
Claragine	**aspirin**
Claratyne	**loratadine**
Clarinex	**desloratadine**
Claripex	**clofibrate**
Clarith	**clarithromycin**
clarithromycin	Biaxin, Biaxin HP, Clacine, Clarith, Klacid, Klaricid, Macladin, Veclam
Claritin	**loratadine**
Claritin-D	**loratadine**
Claritine	**loratadine**
Classen	**mercaptopurine**
Clasynar	**calcitonin**
Claversal	**mesalamine**
Clema	**clemastine**
clemastine	Aller-Eze, Antihist-1, Clema, Darvine, Tavegil, Tavegyl, Tavist
Cleocin	**clindamycin**
Cleocin-T	**clindamycin**
Cleridium	**dipyridamole**
clevidipine	Cleviprex
Cleviprex	**clevidipine**
Clexan	**enoxaparin**
Clexane 40	**enoxaparin**
clidinium	Bralix, Diporax, Epirax, Librax, Libraxin, Librocol, Nirvaxal, Quarzan, Spasmoten
Clinadil	**cinnarizine**
Clindacin	**clindamycin**
Clindagel	**clindamycin**
clindamycin	Aclinda, BB, Benzaclin, Cleocin, Cleocin-T, Clindacin, Clindagel, Clindets, Dalacin, Dalacin C, Dalacine, Galecin, Sobelin
Clindets	**clindamycin**
Clinofem	**medroxyprogesterone**
Clinoril	**sulindac**
clioquinol	Iodo Plain, Vioform
clobazam	Castillium, Frisium, Mystan, Odipam, Urbanil, Urbanyl
Cloben	**cyclobenzaprine**

INDEX OF HERBALS

MAIN CLASSES OF DRUGS

5-HT1 agonist
- almotriptan
- eletriptan
- frovatriptan
- naratriptan
- rizatriptan
- sumatriptan
- zolmitriptan

5-HT3 antagonist
- alosetron
- dolasetron
- granisetron
- ondansetron
- palonosetron

Adrenergic alpha-receptor agonist
- clonidine
- dexmedetomidine
- dopamine
- ephedrine
- guanabenz
- guanadrel
- guanethidine
- guanfacine
- methyldopa
- midodrine
- mirtazapine
- phenylephrine
- phenylpropanolamine
- polythiazide
- pseudoephedrine

Adrenergic alpha2-receptor agonist
- apraclonidine
- brimonidine
- tizanidine

Adrenergic alpha-receptor antagonist
- alfuzosin
- doxazosin
- phenoxybenzamine
- phentolamine
- prazosin
- tamsulosin
- terazosin
- urapidil

Adrenergic beta-receptor agonist
- albuterol
- arbutamine
- dobutamine
- isoetharine
- isoproterenol
- isoxsuprine
- levalbuterol
- metoprolol
- pirbuterol

Adrenergic beta2-receptor agonist
- formoterol
- ritodrine
- salmeterol
- terbutaline

Adrenergic beta-receptor antagonist
- acebutolol
- atenolol
- betaxolol
- bisoprolol
- carteolol
- carvedilol
- esmolol
- labetalol
- levobetaxolol
- levobunolol
- metipranolol
- nadolol
- nebivolol
- penbutolol
- pindolol
- propranolol
- sotalol
- timolol

Alkylating agent
- altretamine
- bendamustine
- busulfan
- carboplatin
- carmustine
- chlorambucil
- cisplatin
- cyclophosphamide
- dacarbazine
- estramustine
- ifosfamide
- lomustine
- mechlorethamine
- melphalan
- mitomycin
- oxaliplatin
- procarbazine
- streptozocin
- temozolomide
- thiotepa

Amphetamine
- benzphetamine
- dextroamphetamine
- diethylpropion
- MDMA

- methamphetamine
- methylphenidate
- pemoline
- phendimetrazine
- phentermine

Analgesic
- aceclofenac
- bromelain
- buprenorphine
- devil's claw
- oxymorphone
- peppermint
- **narcotic**
  - dextromethorphan
- **non-narcotic**
  - acetaminophen
- **non-opioid**
  - ketorolac
- **opioid**
  - alfentanil
  - fentanyl
- **urinary**
  - pentosan
  - phenazopyridine

Anesthetic
- alfentanil
- edrophonium
- fentanyl
- ketamine
- **general**
  - chloral hydrate
  - propofol
  - sodium oxybate
  - sufentanil
- **inhalation**
  - desflurane
  - enflurane
  - halothane
  - isoflurane
  - methoxyflurane
  - sevoflurane
- **local**
  - bupivacaine
  - cocaine
  - levobupivacaine
  - lidocaine

Angiotensin II receptor antagonist
- candesartan
- eprosartan
- irbesartan
- losartan
- olmesartan
- telmisartan
- valsartan

ACE inhibitor
- benazepril
- captopril
- cilazapril
- enalapril
- fosinopril
- imidapril
- lisinopril
- moexipril
- perindopril
- quinapril
- ramipril
- trandolapril

Anti-inflammatory
- aloe vera (gel, juice, leaf)
- amlexanox
- bloodroot
- boswellia
- bromelain
- butterbur
- caraway
- clofazimine
- colchicine
- devil's claw
- eucalyptus
- evening primrose
- fish oils
- henna
- horsetail
- juniper
- licorice
- linseed
- meadowsweet
- myrrh
- omega-3 fatty acids
- polypodium leucotomos
- sarsaparilla
- saw palmetto
- turmeric
- willow bark
- yarrow

Antiarrhythmic
class Ia
- disopyramide
- procainamide
- quinidine

class Ib
- diphenylhydantoin
- lidocaine
- mexiletine
- phenytoin
- tocainide

class Ic
- flecainide
- lorcainide
- moricizine
- propafenone

class II
- acebutolol
- atenolol
- esmolol
- labetalol
- metoprolol
- nadolol
- propranolol

class III
- amiodarone
- bretylium
- dofetilide
- ibutilide
- sotalol

class IV
- adenosine
- amlodipine
- bepridil
- digoxin
- diltiazem
- verapamil

Antibiotic
aminoglycoside
- amikacin
- gentamicin
- kanamycin
- neomycin
- paromomycin
- streptomycin
- tobramycin

anthracycline
- bleomycin
- dactinomycin
- daunorubicin
- doxorubicin
- epirubicin
- idarubicin
- mitomycin
- mitoxantrone
- peplomycin
- valrubicin

beta-lactam
- aztreonam
- ertapenem
- imipenem/cilastatin
- meropenem

glycopeptide
- daptomycin
- vancomycin

imidazole
- clotrimazole
- ketoconazole
- mebendazole
- miconazole
- sertaconazole
- thiabendazole

lincosamide
- clindamycin
- lincomycin

macrolide
- azithromycin
- clarithromycin
- dirithromycin
- erythromycin
- roxithromycin
- sirolimus
- telithromycin
- troleandomycin

nitrofuran
- furazolidone
- nitrofurazone

nitroimidazole
- metronidazole
- tinidazole

oxazolidinone
- linezolid

penicillin
- amoxicillin
- ampicillin
- bacampicillin
- carbenicillin
- cloxacillin
- dicloxacillin
- methicillin
- mezlocillin
- nafcillin
- oxacillin
- penicillin G
- penicillin V
- piperacillin
- ticarcillin

quinolone
- cinoxacin
- ciprofloxacin
- enoxacin
- gatifloxacin
- gemifloxacin
- grepafloxacin
- levofloxacin
- lomefloxacin
- moxifloxacin
- nalidixic acid
- norfloxacin
- ofloxacin
- sparfloxacin
- trovafloxacin

rifamycin
- rifabutin
- rifampin
- rifapentine
- rifaximin

streptogramin
- quinupristin/dalfopristin

sulfonamide
- co-trimoxazole
- sulfacetamide
- sulfadiazine
- sulfadoxine
- sulfamethoxazole
- sulfisoxazole

tetracycline
- chlortetracycline
- demeclocycline
- doxycycline
- minocycline
- oxytetracycline

tetracycline
tigecycline
topical
mupirocin
triazole
fluconazole
itraconazole
terconazole
voriconazole
miscellaneous
aminosalicylate sodium
bacitracin
capreomycin
chloramphenicol
cycloserine
dapsone
ethionamide
fosfomycin
INH
isoniazid
methenamine
nitrofurantoin
plicamycin
pyrazinamide
quinacrine
spectinomycin

Anticholinergic
benztropine
biperiden
dicyclomine
flavoxate
glycopyrrolate
hyoscyamine
ipratropium
oxybutynin
scopolamine
tiotropium
trospium

Anticoagulant
anisindione
ceprotin
danaparoid
fondaparinux
heparin
warfarin

Anticonvulsant
carbamazepine
divalproex
felbamate
gabapentin
lamotrigine
levetiracetam
oxcarbazepine
phenobarbital
phensuximide
pregabalin
primidone
tiagabine
topiramate

valproic acid
vigabatrin
hydantoin
ethotoin
fosphenytoin
mephenytoin
phenytoin
oxazolidinedione
paramethadione
trimethadione
succinimide
ethosuximide
methsuximide
sulfonamide
zonisamide

Antidepressant
bupropion
citalopram
duloxetine
escitalopram
fluoxetine
fluvoxamine
isocarboxazid
nefazodone
paroxetine
phenelzine
selegiline
sertraline
tranylcypromine
tryptophan
bicyclic
venlafaxine
tetracyclic
amoxapine
maprotiline
mirtazapine
tricyclic
amitriptyline
clomipramine
desipramine
doxepin
imipramine
nortriptyline
protriptyline
trazodone
trimipramine

Antifungal
posaconazole

Antihistamine
levocetirizine

Antimalarial
artemisia
atovaquone
chloroquine
hydroxychloroquine
mefloquine
primaquine
pyrimethamine

quinacrine
quinidine
quinine
sulfadoxine

Antimycobacterial
amphotericin B
clofazimine
dapsone
ethambutol
flucytosine
griseofulvin
INH
isoniazid
nystatin
potassium iodide
star anise (Chinese)
terbinafine
echinocandin
anidulafungin
caspofungin

Antineoplastic
asparaginase
azacitidine
capecitabine
carboplatin
cetuximab
cisplatin
cladribine
cytarabine
dacarbazine
decitabine
denileukin
floxuridine
fludarabine
fluorouracil
gemcitabine
gemtuzumab
hydroxyurea
ibritumomab
levamisole
mercaptopurine
mitotane
mitoxantrone
nelarabine
nilutamide
oxaliplatin
pegaspargase
pentostatin
porfimer
temozolomide
teniposide
testolactone
thioguanine
tositumomab & iodine[131]
trastuzumab

Antiplatelet
abciximab
aspirin
cilostazol

dipyridamole
eptifibatide
tirofiban
thienopyridine
clopidogrel
ticlopidine

Antiprotozoal
atovaquone
chloroquine
hydroxychloroquine
mefloquine
mepacrine
nitazoxanide
pentamidine
primaquine
pyrimethamine
quinidine
quinine

Antipsychotic
amisulpride
aripiprazole
carbamazepine
droperidol
lithium
molindone
olanzapine
pimozide
quetiapine
risperidone
thiothixene
trimeprazine
valproic acid
zuclopentixol acetate
zuclopentixol decanoate
zuclopentixol dihydrochloride
benzothiazolylpiperazine
ziprasidone
butyrophenone
haloperidol
phenothiazine
chlorpromazine
fluphenazine
mesoridazine
perphenazine
prochlorperazine
promazine
promethazine
thioridazine
trifluoperazine
tricyclic
clozapine
loxapine

Antiretroviral
abacavir
adefovir
amprenavir
atazanavir
darunavir
delavirdine

didanosine
efavirenz
emtricitabine
enfuvirtide
fosamprenavir
hydroxyurea
indinavir
lamivudine
maraviroc
nelfinavir
nevirapine
raltegravir
ritonavir
saquinavir
stavudine
tenofovir
zalcitabine
zidovudine

Antiviral
amantadine
cytarabine
entecavir
famciclovir
foscarnet
ganciclovir
imiquimod
oseltamivir
penciclovir
rimantadine
trifluridine
valacyclovir
valganciclovir
zanamivir
nucleoside analog
ribavirin
vidarabine
nucleotide analog
cidofovir
topical
acyclovir
docosanol

Anxiolytic
buspirone
chlormezanone
kava
lavender
meprobamate
valerian

Barbiturate
amobarbital
aprobarbital
butabarbital
butalbital
mephobarbital
methohexital
pentobarbital
phenobarbital
primidone
secobarbital

thiopental

Benzodiazepine
alprazolam
chlordiazepoxide
clobazam
clonazepam
clorazepate
diazepam
estazolam
flurazepam
lorazepam
midazolam
nitrazepam
oxazepam
prazepam
quazepam
temazepam
triazolam

Bisphosphonate
tiludronate

Calcium channel blocker
amlodipine
bepridil
clevidipine
diltiazem
felodipine
isradipine
nicardipine
nifedipine
nimodipine
nisoldipine
verapamil
ziconotide

Carbonic anhydrase inhibitor
acetazolamide
brinzolamide
dorzolamide
methazolamide

CB1 cannabinoid receptor antagonist
rimonabant

Central muscle relaxant
carisoprodol
chlormezanone
chlorzoxazone
cyclobenzaprine
meprobamate
metaxalone
methocarbamol
orphenadrine

Cephalosporin
1st generation
cefadroxil
cefazolin
cephalexin
cephalothin

cephapirin
cephradine
2nd generation
cefaclor
cefamandole
cefmetazole
cefonicid
cefotetan
cefoxitin
cefuroxime
loracarbef
3rd generation
cefdinir
cefditoren
cefixime
cefoperazone
cefotaxime
cefpodoxime
ceftazidime
ceftibuten
ceftizoxime
ceftriaxone
4th generation
cefepime

Cholinesterase inhibitor
donepezil
edrophonium
galantamine
physostigmine
rivastigmine
succinylcholine
tacrine

CNS stimulant
cocaine
dexmethylphenidate
lisdexamfetamine
modafinil

Corticosteroid
betamethasone
ciclesonide
cortisone
tixocortol
inhaled
beclomethasone
budesonide
cyclesonide
flunisolide
fluticasone
systemic
methylprednisolone
prednisolone
prednisone
triamcinolone
topical
alclometasone
amcinonide
clobetasol
desonide
desoximetasone

dexamethasone
difluprednate
flumetasone
fluocinolone
fluocinonide
fluticasone
halcinonide
halobetasol
halometasone
hydrocortisone
loteprednol
mometasone
prednicarbate
triamcinolone

COX-2 inhibitor
celecoxib
etodolac
etoricoxib
meloxicam
nimesulide
rofecoxib
valdecoxib

Dermal filler
calcium hydroxylapatite

Disease-modifying antirheumatic
auranofin
aurothioglucose
azathioprine
bucillamine
chloroquine
cyclosporine
gold and gold compounds
hydroxychloroquine
leflunomide
methotrexate
minocycline
penicillamine
sulfasalazine

Diuretic
acetazolamide
blue cohosh
boswellia
brinzolamide
caffeine
chicory
cranberry
dorzolamide
eplerenone
eucalyptus
horse chestnut (bark, flower, leaf, seed)
horsetail
isosorbide
meadowsweet
methazolamide
spironolactone
squill
theophylline

loop
bumetanide
ethacrynic acid
furosemide
torsemide
potassium-sparing
amiloride
triamterene
thiazide
bendroflumethiazide
benzthiazide
chlorothiazide
chlorthalidone
cyclothiazide
hydrochlorothiazide
hydroflumethiazide
indapamide
methyclothiazide
metolazone
polythiazide
quinethazone
trichlormethiazide

Dopamine receptor agonist
apomorphine
bromocriptine
cabergoline
fenoldopam
pergolide
pramipexole
ropinirole
rotigotine

Dopamine receptor antagonist
domperidone
metoclopramide

Endothelin receptor antagonist
ambrisentan
sitaxentan

Epidermal growth factor receptor (EGFR)
lapatinib

Eugeroic
armodafinil

Fibrinolytic
alteplase
anistreplase
reteplase
streptokinase
tenecteplase
urokinase

Gonadotropin-releasing hormone agonist
goserelin
histrelin
leuprolide
nafarelin

triptorelin

Gonadotropin-releasing hormone antagonist
abarelix
cetrorelix
ganirelix

Histamine
H1 receptor antagonist
astemizole
azatadine
azelastine
brompheniramine
buclizine
carbinoxamine
cetirizine
chlorpheniramine
cinnarizine
clemastine
cyproheptadine
desloratadine
dexchlorpheniramine
diphenhydramine
epinastine
fexofenadine
hydroxyzine
ketotifen
loratadine
meclizine
olopatadine
phenindamine
promethazine
pyrilamine
terfenadine
trimeprazine
tripelennamine
triprolidine
H2 receptor antagonist
cimetidine
famotidine
nizatidine
ranitidine
roxatidine

HMG-CoA reductase inhibitor
atorvastatin
fluvastatin
lovastatin
pravastatin
red rice yeast
rosuvastatin
simvastatin

Histone deacetylase (HDAC) inhibitor
vorinostat

Hormone
lanreotide
melatonin
oral contraceptives
sincalide

polypeptide
glucagon
insulin
mecasermin
nesiritide
secretin

Human insulin analog
insulin detemir
insulin glulisine

Immunomodulator
aldesleukin
aristolochia
arnica
bifidobacteria
brewer's yeast
cordyceps
dong quai
echinacea
efalizumab
garlic
ginseng
glatiramer
goldenseal
imiquimod
immune globulin IV
interferon alfa
interferon beta
lactobacillus
lemon balm
lenalidomide
levamisole
milk thistle
mistletoe
natalizumab
omalizumab
palivizumab
peg-interferon
pimecrolimus
propolis
resveratrol
sarsaparilla
Siberian ginseng
sinecatechins

Immunosuppressant
alefacept
alemtuzumab
cyclosporine
mizoribine
muromonab-CD3
mycophenolate
phellodendron
rituximab
tacrolimus
thalidomide

Mast cell stabilizer
cromolyn
lodoxamide
nedocromil

pemirolast

Monoamine oxidase (MAO) inhibitor
isocarboxazid
phenelzine
tranylcypromine

Monoclonal antibody
eculizumab
panitumumab

Muscarinic antagonist
amitriptyline
amoxapine
atropine sulfate
benactyzine
benztropine
biperiden
chlorpheniramine
chlorpromazine
cinnarizine
clidinium
clomipramine
darifenacin
dicyclomine
diphenhydramine
disopyramide
doxepin
flavoxate
glycopyrrolate
hydroxyzine
hyoscyamine
imipramine
ipratropium
maprotiline
mepenzolate
olanzapine
orphenadrine
oxybutynin
phenelzine
prochlorperazine
procyclidine
propantheline
scopolamine
solifenacin
tiotropium
tolterodine
trihexyphenidyl

Muscarinic cholinergic agonist
bethanechol
carbachol
cevimeline
methantheline
pilocarpine

mTOR inhibitor
everolimus
temsirolimus

Non-depolarizing neuromuscular blocker
atracurium
cisatracurium
doxacurium
pancuronium
pipecuronium
rapacuronium
rocuronium
vecuronium

Non-nucleoside reverse transcriptase inhibitor
delavirdine
efavirenz
nevirapine

Non-steroidal anti-inflammatory
aceclofenac
aspirin
bromfenac
celecoxib
dexibuprofen
diclofenac
diflunisal
etodolac
etoricoxib
fenbufen
fenoprofen
flurbiprofen
ibuprofen
indomethacin
ketoprofen
ketorolac
meclofenamate
mefenamic acid
meloxicam
metamizole
nabumetone
naproxen
nepafenac
nimesulide
oxaprozin
phenylbutazone
piroxicam
pranoprofen
rofecoxib
salsalate
sulindac
tolmetin
valdecoxib

Nucleoside analog reverse transcriptase inhibitor
telbivudine

Oligonucleotide
fomivirsen

Opiate agonist
codeine
heroin
hydrocodone
hydromorphone
loperamide
meperidine
methadone
morphine
nalbuphine
oxycodone
oxymorphone
pentazocine
propoxyphene
sufentanil
tramadol

Opioid antagonist
alvimopan
nalmefene
naloxone
naltrexone

Phosphodiesterase inhibitor
cilostazol
inamrinone
phosphodiesterase type 5 inhibitor
sildenafil
tadalafil
vardenafil

Pleuromutilin antibacterial
retapamulin

Prostaglandin
alprostadil
bimatoprost
dinoprostone
iloprost
latanoprost
travoprost
treprostinil
unoprostone

Proton pump inhibitor
esomeprazole
lansoprazole
omeprazole
pantoprazole
rabeprazole

Retinoid
acitretin
adapalene
alitretinoin
bexarotene
isotretinoin
tretinoin

Selective estrogen receptor modulator (SERM)
chlorotrianisene
clomiphene
raloxifene
tamoxifen
toremifene

Selective serotonin reuptake inhibitor (SSRIs)
citalopram
escitalopram
fluoxetine
fluvoxamine
paroxetine
sertraline

Serotonin antagonist
buspirone
sibutramine
serotonin receptor agonist
almotriptan
eletriptan
frovatriptan
rizatriptan
sumatriptan
zolmitriptan
serotonin receptor antagonist
naratriptan
serotonin reuptake inhibitor
duloxetine
trazodone
serotonin type 3 receptor antagonist
alosetron
dolasetron
granisetron
ondansetron
palonosetron
serotonin type 4 receptor agonist
tegaserod
serotonin-norepinephrine reuptake inhibitor
venlafaxine

Statin
atorvastatin
fluvastatin
lovastatin
pravastatin
rosuvastatin
simvastatin

Sulfonylurea
acetohexamide
chlorpropamide
glimepiride
glipizide
glyburide
tolazamide
tolazoline
tolbutamide

Topoisomerase I inhibitor
irinotecan
topotecan

Topoisomerase 2 inhibitor
- etoposide
- teniposide

Trace element
- arsenic
- selenium
- sulfites
- zinc

Vaccine
- anthrax vaccine
- BCG vaccine
- diphtheria antitoxin
- hemophilus B vaccine
- hepatitis A vaccine
- hepatitis B vaccine
- human papillomavirus vaccine
- influenza vaccines
- pneumococcal vaccine
- smallpox vaccine
- varicella vaccine
- zoster vaccine

Vasodilator
- ambrisentan
- amyl nitrite
- astragalus root
- bosentan
- diazoxide
- hydralazine
- iloprost
- isosorbide dinitrate
- isosorbide mononitrate
- minoxidil
- nitroglycerin
- nitroprusside

Vasodilator, peripheral
- cilostazol
- papaverine
- pentoxifylline
- peppermint

Vitamin
- ascorbic acid
- beta-carotene
- cyanocobalamin
- ergocalciferol
- folic acid
- niacin
- niacinamide
- pantothenic acid
- phytonadione
- pyridoxine
- riboflavin
- thiamine
- vitamin A
- vitamin E

Vitamin D receptor agonist
- dihydrotachysterol
- doxercalciferol
- paricalcitol

Xanthine alkaloid
- aminophylline
- caffeine
- green tea
- pentoxifylline

ABACAVIR

Trade names: Trizivir (GSK); Ziagen (GSK)
Indications: HIV infections in combination with other antiretrovirals
Category: Antiretroviral; Nucleoside analog reverse transcriptase inhibitor
Half-life: 1.5 hours
Clinically important, potentially hazardous interactions with: arbutamine, argatroban, arsenic

Reactions

Skin

Acute febrile neutrophilic dermatosis (Sweet's syndrome)
  (2004): Del Giudice P+, *J Am Acad Dermatol* 51(3), 474
Edema
  (1999): Spruance SL, *Skin and Allergy News* October, 37
Erythema multiforme
Erythroderma
  (2001): Shapiro M+, *The AIDS Reader* 11, 222
Exanthems
  (1999): Nathanson N (generalized) (from Internet) (observation)
  (1999): Spruance SL, *Skin and Allergy News* October, 37
  (1998): Saag M+, *AIDS* 12, F203
Pruritus
  (1998): Saag M+, *AIDS* 12, F203
Rash (sic) (10–69%)
  (2003): Lanzafame M+, *Infez Med* 11(1), 40
  (2002): Kessler HA+, *Clin Infect Dis* 34(4), 535
  (2001): Hetherington S+, *Clin Ther* 23(10), 1603
  (2000): Hervey PS+, *Drugs* 60, 447 (5%)
  (1999): Hughes W+, *Antimicrob Agents Chemother* 43, 609 (9%)
  (1999): Spruance SL, *Skin and Allergy News* October, 37 (69%)
  (1998): Foster RH+, *Drugs* 55, 729
  (1998): Kessler H+, *36th Meeting of the Infectious Disease Society of America, Denver* Abstract 453 (10–15%)
  (1998): Saag M+, *AIDS* 12, F203 (10–15%)
  (1998): Staszewski S+, *AIDS* 12, F197 (10–15%)
Stevens–Johnson syndrome
  (2002): Bossi P+, *Clin Infect Dis* 35(7), 902
Toxic epidermal necrolysis

Mucosal/ENT

Mucocutaneous lymph node syndrome (Kawasaki syndrome)
  (2002): Toerner JG+, *Clin Infect Dis* 34(1), 131
Oral ulceration
  (1999): Spruance SL, *Skin and Allergy News* October, 37
Oral vesiculation
  (2002): Fantry LE+, *AIDS Patient Care STDS* 16(1), 5

Other

Anaphylactoid reactions/Anaphylaxis (3%)
  (2001): Frissen PH+, *AIDS* 15, 289
  (1999): Spruance SL, *Skin and Allergy News* October, 37 (3–4%)
  (1999): Walensky RP+, *AIDS* 13, 999
Chills
  (1999): Escaut L+, *AIDS* 13, 1419
Cough
  (2002): Peyriere H+, *Allerg Immunol* (Paris) 34(10), 359
  (2001): Hetherington S+, *Clin Ther* 23(10), 1603 (10%)
Death
  (2003): Peyriere H+, *Ann Pharmacother* 37(10), 1392 (1.8%)
Fever
  (2003): Lanzafame M+, *Infez Med* 11(1), 40
Headache

  (2006): Castillo SA+, *Drug Saf* 29(9), 811 (16%) (with lamivudine)
Hypersensitivity (5%)
  (2007): Luther J+, *Am J Clin Dermatol* 8(4), 221
  (2006): James JS, *AIDS Treat News* 419, 6
  (2006): Moreno-Cuerda VJ+, *Med Clin* (Barc) 126(19), 744
  (2006): Rauch A+, *Clin Infect Dis* 43(1), 99 (8%)
  (2006): Stekler J+, *AIDS* 20(9), 1269
  (2003): Easterbrook PJ+, *HIV Med* 4(4), 321
  (2003): Lanzafame M+, *Infez Med* 11(1), 40
  (2003): Peyriere H+, *Ann Pharmacother* 37(10), 1392 (8.5%)
  (2002): *AIDS Patient Care STDS* 16(5), 242
  (2002): Clay PG, *Clin Ther* 24(10), 1502
  (2002): Dargere S+, *AIDS* 16(12), 1696
  (2002): Flexner C, *Hopkins HIV Rep* 14(3), 5
  (2002): Hetherington S+, *Lancet* 359(9312), 1121
  (2002): Hewitt RG, *Clin Infect Dis* 34(8), 1137 (3.7%)
  (2002): Kessler HA+, *Clin Infect Dis* 34(4), 535
  (2002): Mallal S+, *Lancet* 359, 727 (5%)
  (2002): Phillips EJ+, *AIDS* 16(16), 2223
  (2002): Symonds W+, *Clin Ther* 24(4), 565
  (2002): Toerner JG+, *Clin Infect Dis* 34(1), 131
  (2001): Cutrell A+, *International AIDS Society Conference on HIV Buenos Aires* Abstract 527
  (2001): Frissen PH+, *AIDS* 15, 289
  (2001): Hetherington S, *AIDS Read* 11(12), 620
  (2001): Hetherington S+, *Clin Ther* 23(10), 1603 (4.3%)
  (2001): Keiser P+, *8th Conferences on Retroviruses* (Chicago) Abstract 622
  (2001): Loeliger AE+, *AIDS* 15(10), 1325
  (2001): Peyriere H+, *Ann Pharmacother* 35(10), 1291
  (2001): Shapiro M+, *The AIDS Reader* 11, 222
  (2001): Wit FW+, *AIDS* 15(18), 2423
  (2000): *AIDS Read* 10, 525
  (2000): *AIDS Treat News* 337, 7
  (2000): *Prescrire Int* 9, 67
  (2000): Clay PG+, *Ann Pharmacother* 34, 247
  (2000): GlaxoWellcome, *Important Drug Warning* July (severe or fatal)
  (2000): Hervey PS+, *Drugs* 60, 447 (3–5%)
  (2000): Keiser P+, *Conference on Retroviruses & Opportunistic Infections* (Chicago) Abstract 622
  (1999): Escaut L+, *AIDS* 13, 1419
  (1999): Miller JL, *Am J Health Syst Pharm* 56, 304
  (1998): *AIDS Patient Care SDS* 12, 405
  (1998): *Newsline People AIDS Coalit N Y* Feb, 35
  (1998): Foster RH+, *Drugs* 55, 729 (2–3%)
  (1998): Saag M+, *AIDS* 12, F203 (2–5%)
  (1998): Staszewski S+, *AIDS* 12, F197
  (1997): James JS, *AIDS Treat News* 285, 1, 5
Lipoatrophy
  (2005): Nolan D+, *Sex Health* 2(3), 153
  (2004): McComsey GA+, *Clin Infect Dis* 38(2), 263
Lipodystrophy
  (2002): Bernasconi E+, *J Acquir Immune Defic Syndr* 31(1), 50
Myalgia/Myositis/Myopathy/Myotoxicity
  (1999): Escaut L+, *AIDS* 13, 1419
  (1999): Spruance SL, *Skin and Allergy News* October, 37
Nephrotoxicity
  (2006): Ahmad M, *J Postgrad Med* 52(4), 296 (Fanconi syndrome)
Paresthesias
Rhabdomyolysis
  (2005): Fontaine C+, *AIDS* 19(16), 1927 (with ciprofibrate)
Vertigo
  (2006): Castillo SA+, *Drug Saf* 29(9), 811 (27%) (with lamivudine)

ABARELIX

Trade name: Plenaxis (Praecis)
Indications: Prostate cancer (advanced)
Category: Gonadotropin-releasing hormone antagonist
Half-life: 13.2 days
**Clinically important, potentially hazardous interactions
with:** amiodarone, procainamide, quinidine, sotalol

Reactions

Skin
Allergic reactions (sic)
  (2006): Beer TM+, *Anticancer Drugs* 17(9), 1075
Cellulitis
Herpes simplex
Peripheral edema (15%)
Pruritus
Urticaria

Other
Asthenia (10%)
Gynecomastia (30%)
Headache (12%)
Hot flashes (79%)
Pain (31%)
Upper respiratory infection (12%)
Vertigo (12%)

ABATACEPT

Trade name: Orencia (Bristol-Myers Squibb)
Indications: Rheumatoid arthritis
Category: T-cell co-stimulation modulator
Half-life: 12–23 days
**Clinically important, potentially hazardous interactions
with:** certolizumab pegol. TNF antagonists

Reactions

Skin
Pruritus (<1%)
Rash (sic) (4%)
Urticaria (<1%)

Mucosal/ENT
Nasopharyngitis
  (2006): Nogid A+, *Clin Ther* 28(11), 1764

Other
Anaphylactoid reactions/Anaphylaxis
Cough (8%)
Headache
  (2006): Nogid A+, *Clin Ther* 28(11), 1764 (18.2%)
  (2005): Allison C, *Issues Emerg Health Technol* 73, 1 (18%)
Hypersensitivity (<1%)
Hypertension
  (2005): Allison C, *Issues Emerg Health Technol* 73, 1 (7%)
Hypotension (<1%)
Infections
  (2006): Nogid A+, *Clin Ther* 28(11), 1764 (53.8%)
Injection-site reactions
Upper respiratory infection
  (2006): Nogid A+, *Clin Ther* 28(11), 1764 (12.7%)
Vertigo (9%)

ABCIXIMAB

Synonym: C7E3
Trade name: ReoPro (Lilly) (Centocor)
Indications: Thrombotic arterial disease
Category: Antiplatelet; Glycoprotein IIb / IIIa inhibitor
Half-life: 10–30 minutes – given intravenously
**Clinically important, potentially hazardous interactions
with:** fondaparinux, reteplase

Reactions

Skin
Acute generalized exanthematous pustulosis (AGEP)
Allergic reactions
Cellulitis (0.3%)
Edema
  (2002): Pharand C+, *Pharmacotherapy* 22(3), 380
Hemorrhage
  (2002): Choi RK+, *Mayo Clin Proc* 77(12), 1340
Peripheral edema (1.6%)
Petechiae (0.3%)
Pruritus (0.3%)
  (2002): Pharand C+, *Pharmacotherapy* 22(3), 380

Mucosal/ENT
Gingival bleeding
  (2005): Lee DH+, *Acta Radiol* 46(5), 534 (2 cases)

Other
Anaphylactoid reactions/Anaphylaxis
  (2002): Pharand C+, *Pharmacotherapy* 22(3), 380
  (2001): Iakovou Y+, *Cardiology* 95(4), 215
  (1999): Guzzo JA+, *Catheter Cardiovasc Interv* 48, 71
Death
  (2006): McCorry RB+, *J Invasive Cardiol* 18(6), E173
  (2006): Usman MH+, *Heart Lung* 35(6), 423
Headache
Hypotension
  (2003): Hawkins C+, *Allergy* 58(7), 688
Injection-site reactions (3.6%)
  (2004): Dery JP+, *Am J Cardiol* 93(8), 979
Myalgia/Myositis/Myopathy/Myotoxicity (0.3%)

ACAMPROSATE

Trade names: Aotal; Campral (Forest) (Lipha)
Indications: Alcohol dependence
Category: Antialcoholism
Half-life: 20–33 hours
**Clinically important, potentially hazardous interactions
with:** None

Reactions

Skin
Abscess (<1%)
Acne (<1%)
Allergic reactions (sic) (<1%)
Dermatitis
  (2002): Soyka M+, *Drugs R D* 3(1), 1
Diaphoresis (2%)
Eczema (<1%)
Erythema

Erythema multiforme
  (1992): Fortier-Beaulieu M+, *Lancet* 339(8799), 991
Exanthems (<1%)
Exfoliative dermatitis (<1%)
Facial edema (<0.1%)
Peripheral edema (>1%)
Photosensitivity (<0.1%)
Pruritus (4%)
  (2003): Oscar MA+, *Therapie* 58(4), 371
  (2002): Soyka M+, *Drugs R D* 3(1), 1 (37 cases)
Rash (sic) (>1%)
Urticaria (<1%)
Vesiculobullous eruption (<1%)
Xerosis (<1%)

Mucosal/ENT
Dysgeusia (>1%)
Dysphagia (<1%)
Oral ulceration (<0.1%)
Rhinitis (>1%)
Sialorrhea (<0.1%)
Tinnitus (<1%)
Vaginitis (<1%)
Xerostomia (2%)

Hair
Hair – alopecia

Eyes
Amblyopia (<1%)
Diplopia (<1%)
Ophthalmitis (<0.1%)
Photophobia (<0.1%)

Other
Abdominal pain (>1%)
Asthenia (6%)
  (2002): Soyka M+, *Drugs R D* 3(1), 1 (16 cases)
Chest pain (>1%)
Chills (>1%)
Cough (>1%)
Death (<0.1%)
Depression (5%)
Fever (<1%)
Headache (>1%)
  (2002): Soyka M+, *Drugs R D* 3(1), 1 (28 cases)
Infections (sic) (>1%)
Myalgia/Myositis/Myopathy/Myotoxicity (>1%)
Pain (3%)
Paresthesias (2%)
Phlebitis (<1%)
Seizures (<1%)
Tremor (>1%)
Vertigo (3%)

ACARBOSE

Trade names: Glucobay; Glumida; Prandase; Precose (Bayer)
Indications: Non-insulin dependent diabetes type II
Category: Alpha-glucosidase inhibitor
Half-life: 2.7–9 hours

Reactions

Skin
Acute generalized exanthematous pustulosis (AGEP)
  (2003): Poszepczynska-Guigne E+, *Ann Dermatol Venereol* 130(4), 439
Erythema (<1%)
  (2000): Schmutz JL+, *Ann Dermatol Venereol* 127, 869 (polymorphous)
Erythema multiforme
  (1999): Kono T+, *Lancet* 354, 396 (generalized)
Rash (sic)
Urticaria (<1%)

Mucosal/ENT
Ageusia
  (1996): Martin Bun N+, *Med Clin* (Barc) (Spanish) 28, 399

Other
Hepatotoxicity
  (2006): Hsiao SH+, *Ann Pharmacother* 40(1), 151
  (2002): Chitturi S+, *Semin Liver Dis* 22(2), 169

ACEBUTOLOL

Trade names: Acecor; Acetanol; Alol; Apo-Acebutolol; Monitan; Neptal; Novo-Acebutolol; Nu-Acebutolol; Prent; Rhodiasectral; Rhotral; Sectral
Indications: Hypertension, angina, ventricular arrhythmias
Category: Adrenergic beta-receptor antagonist; Antiarrhythmic class II
Half-life: 3–7 hours
Clinically important, potentially hazardous interactions with: clonidine, verapamil

Note: Cutaneous side effects of beta-receptor blockaders are clinically polymorphous. They apparently appear after several months of continuous therapy. Atypical psoriasiform, lichen planus-like, and eczematous chronic rashes are mainly observed. (1983): Hödl St, *Z Hautkr* (German) 1:58, 17

Reactions

Skin
Dermatitis
Diaphoresis
  (1995): Schmutz JL+, *Dermatology* 190, 86
Edema (1–10%)
Erythema multiforme (<1%)
Exanthems (4%)
  (1985): Singh BN+, *Drugs* 29, 531
Exfoliative dermatitis
Facial edema (<1%)
Hyperkeratosis (palms and soles)
Lichenoid eruption
  (1982): Taylor AEM+, *Clin Exp Dermatol* 7, 219
Lupus erythematosus (<1%)
  (2005): Fenniche S+, *Skin Pharmacol Physiol* 18(5), 230
  (1997): Burlingame RW, *Clin Lab Med* 17, 367
  (1992): Rubin RL+, *J Clin Invest* 90, 165
  (1992): Stevens MB, *Hosp Pract* 27, 27
  (1987): Doktor D, *Rev Fr Allergol Immunol* (French) 27, 77
  (1985): Hourdebaight-Larrusse P+, *Ann Cardiol Angeiol* (Paris) (French) 34, 421
  (1985): Singh BN+, *Drugs* 29, 531
  (1984): Bigot MC+, *Therapie* (French) 39, 571

(1984): Meyer O+, *Rev Rhum Mal Osteoartic* (French) 51, 303
(1983): Homberg JC+, *J Pharmacol* (French) 14, 61
(1982): Taylor AE+, *Clin Exp Dermatol* 7, 219
(1981): Record NB, *Ann Intern Med* 95, 326
(1981): Simon P+, *Nouv Presse Med* (French) 10, 105
Pigmentation
Pityriasis rubra pilaris
Pruritus (<2%)
Psoriasis
  (1986): Czernielewski J+, *Lancet* 1, 808
  (1984): Arntzen N+, *Acta Derm Venereol* (Stockh) 64, 346
Rash (sic) (1–10%)
Raynaud's phenomenon
  (1984): Eliasson K+, *Acta Med Scand* 215, 333
Toxic epidermal necrolysis
Urticaria
  (2005): Chiffoleau A+, *Therapie* 60(6), 593
Vasculitis
  (1988): Bonnefoy M+, *Ann Dermatol Venereol* (French) 115, 27
Xerosis

Mucosal/ENT
Dysgeusia
Oral lichenoid eruption
Xerostomia (<1%)

Hair
Hair – alopecia

Nails
Nails – dystrophy
Nails – pigmentation
Nails – pincer (reverse transverse curvature of the nails)
  (1998): Greiner D+, *J Am Acad Dermatol* 39, 486

Eyes
Oculo-mucocutaneous syndrome
  (1982): Cocco G+, *Curr Ther Res* 31, 362

Other
Hypotension
  (2000): Joye F, *Presse Med* 29(18), 1027
Myalgia/Myositis/Myopathy/Myotoxicity (1–10%)
Peyronie's disease

ACECLOFENAC

Trade names: Aflamin; Arrestin; Beofenac; Preservex (UCB Pharma)
Indications: Ankylosing spondylitis, Osteoarthritis, inflammatory disease of the joints
Category: Analgesic; Non-steroidal anti-inflammatory
Half-life: 4 hours
Clinically important, potentially hazardous interactions with: lithium

Reactions

Skin
Contact dermatitis
  (2006): Pitarch Bort G+, *Contact Dermatitis* 55(6), 365
  (2001): Goday Bujan JJ+, *Contact Dermatitis* 45(3), 170
Fixed eruption
  (2007): Linares T+, *Contact Dermatitis* 56(5), 291
Photosensitivity
  (2007): Vargas F+, *Pharmazie* 62(5), 337
  (2001): Goday Bujan JJ+, *Contact Dermatitis* 45(3), 170

Pruritus
Psoriasis (Pustular) (Generalized)
  (2006): Vergara A+, *J Eur Acad Dermatol Venereol* 20(8), 1028
Purpura
Rash (sic)
Stevens–Johnson syndrome
  (2003): Ludwig C+, *Dtsch Med Wochenschr* 128(10), 487
Toxic epidermal necrolysis
  (2003): Ludwig C+, *Dtsch Med Wochenschr* 128(10), 487
Urticaria
Vasculitis
  (1997): Morros R+, *Br J Rheumatol* 36(4), 503
  (1995): Epelde F+, *Ann Pharmacother* 29(11), 1168
  (1993): Gomez Rodriguez N+, *Med Clin* (Barc) 101(6), 239

Mucosal/ENT
Dysgeusia
Stomatitis

Other
Abdominal pain
Anaphylactoid reactions/Anaphylaxis
  (2006): Rojas-Hijazo B+, *Allergy* 61(4), 511
Confusion
  (1994): Pallares Querol M, *Aten Primaria* 13(6), 331
Death
  (2003): Palop Larrea V+, *Aten Primaria* 32(2), 122 (following injection)
Headache
Hepatotoxicity
  (2006): Lapeyre-Mestre M+, *Fundam Clin Pharmacol* 20(4), 391
  (2001): Fernandez-Avala Novo M+, *Rev Clin Esp* 201(10), 616
  (1997): Prieto de Paula PM +, *Gastroenterol Hepatol* 20(3), 165
  (1996): Perez Moreno JM+, *Rev Esp Enferm Dig* 88(11), 815
  (1995): Hernandez Beriain J+, *Rev Esp Enferm Dig* 87(7), 550
  (1995): Zaragoza Marcet A+, *Rev Esp Enferm Dig* 87(6), 472
Hypersensitivity
  (1993): Gomez Rodriguez N+, *Med Clin* (Barc) 101(6), 239
Vertigo
  (1996): Kornasoff D+, *Rheumatol Int* 15(6), 225

ACENOCOUMAROL

Trade names: Acenox; Acitrom; Sinthrome (Alliance); Sintrom (Alliance)
Indications: Thromboembolic diseases
Category: Anticoagulant
Half-life: 8–11 hours
Clinically important, potentially hazardous interactions with: allopurinol, amiodarone, aspirin, cimetidine, danazol, disulfiram, heparin

Reactions

Skin
Allergic reactions (sic)
Blue toe syndrome
  (2001): Righini M+, *Thromb Haemost* 85(4), 744
Bullae
  (1993): Elis A+, *J Intern Med* 234(6), 615
Exanthems
  (1998): Kamm W+, *Rev Med Suisse Romande* 118(6), 565
Necrosis
  (2004): Muniesa C+, *Br J Dermatol* 151(2), 502
  (2004): Valdivielso M+, *J Eur Acad Dermatol Venereol* 18(2), 211
  (2001): Argaud L+, *Intensive Care Med* 27(9), 1555

Purpura
 (2007): Aouam K+, *Pharmacoepidemiol Drug Saf* 16(1), 113
 (2004): Borras-Blasco J+, *Ann Pharmacother* 38(2), 261
Rash (sic)
 (2007): Aouam K+, *Pharmacoepidemiol Drug Saf* 16(1), 113
Urticaria
Vasculitis
 (2007): Aouam K+, *Pharmacoepidemiol Drug Saf* 16(1), 113
 (1999): Jimenez-Gonzalo FJ+, *Haematologica* 84(5), 462

Hair

Hair – alopecia

Eyes

Vision blurred

Other

Abdominal pain
 (2006): Arnaiz Garcia AM+, *An Med Interna* 23(11), 558
Chest pain
Confusion
Fever
 (2007): Aouam K+, *Pharmacoepidemiol Drug Saf* 16(1), 113
 (1996): Renou C+, *Rev Med Interne* 17(1), 93
Headache
Hepatotoxicity
 (1997): Quintana MR+, *Haematologica* 82(6), 732
Hypersensitivity
Stroke
Vertigo

ACETAMINOPHEN

Synonyms: APAP; paracetamol
Trade names: Abenol; Anacin-3 (Wyeth); Anaflon; Ben-U-Ron; Bromo-Seltzer; Darvocet-N (aaiPharma); Datril; Doliprane; Excedrin (Bristol-Myers Squibb); Geluprane; Liquiprin; Lorcet (Forest); Mapap; Neopap; Panadol (GSK); Percocet (Endo); Percogesic; Phenaphen; Sinutab; Tylenol (Ortho-McNeil); Valadol; Vicodin (Abbott)
Indications: Pain, fever
Category: Analgesic, non-narcotic
Half-life: 1–3 hours
Clinically important, potentially hazardous interactions with: alcohol, cholestyramine, didanosine, **dong quai, melatonin**

Note: Acetaminophen is the active metabolite of phenacetin

Reactions

Skin

Acute generalized exanthematous pustulosis (AGEP)
 (2004): Wohl Y+, *Skinmed* 3(1), 47
 (2003): Mashiah J+, *Arch Dermatol* 139(9), 1181
 (2001): Cohen AD+, *Int J Dermatol* 40(7), 458
 (2000): Halevy S+, *Clin Exp Dermatol* 25(8), 652
 (1998): Leger F+, *Acta Derm Venereol* 78, 222
 (1996): DeConinck AL+, *Dermatology* 193, 338
 (1995): Moreau A+, *Int J Dermatol* 34, 263 (passim)
 (1991): Roujeau J-C+, *Arch Dermatol* 127, 1333
Allergic granulomatous angiitis (Churg–Strauss syndrome)
 (2005): Masuzawa A+, *Intern Med* 44(5), 496
Angioedema (<1%)
 (2002): Litt JZ, Beachwood, OH (personal case) (observation)
  (patient inadvertently re-challenged herself)
 (1997): de Almeida MA+, *Allergy Asthma Proc* 18, 313

 (1990): Van Diem L+, *Eur J Clin Pharmacol* 38, 389
 (1986): Idoko JA+, *Trans R Soc Trop Med Hyg* 80, 175
 (1985): Stricker BH+, *BMJ* 291, 938
Dermatitis
 (1997): Mathelier-Fusada P+, *Contact Dermatitis* 36, 267
 (1996): Szczurko C+, *Contact Dermatitis* 35, 299
 (1995): Barbaud A+, *Lancet* 346(8979), 902
Diaphoresis
Erythema
 (1985): Stricker BH+, *BMJ* 291, 938
Erythema multiforme
 (1995): Dubey NK+, *Indian Pediatr* 32, 1117
 (1984): Hurvitz H+, *Isr J Med Sci* 20, 145
Erythema nodosum (<1%)
Exanthems
 (1997): Foong H, Malaysia (from Internet) (observation)
 (1985): Matheson I+, *Pediatrics* 76, 651
 (1985): Stricker BH+, *BMJ* 291, 938
Exfoliative dermatitis
 (1984): Guerin C+, *Therapie* (French) 39, 47
Fixed eruption (<1%)
 (2006): Ayala F+, *Dermatitis* 17(3), 160 (bullous)
 (2006): Nnoruka EN+, *Int J Dermatol* 45(9), 1062 (3%)
 (2005): Daghfous R+, *Therapie* 60(5), 523 (13%)
 (2003): Hayashi H+, *Clin Exp Dermatol* 28, 455
 (2001): Silva A+, *Pediatr Dermatol* 18(2), 163
 (2000): Bernand S+, *Dermatology* 201, 184 (similar to ondansetron)
 (2000): Galindo PA+, *J Investig Allergol Clin Immunol* 9, 399
 (2000): Ko R+, *Clin Exp Dermatol* 25, 96
 (2000): Ozkaya-Bayazit E+, *Eur J Dermatol* 10, 288
 (1999): Sehgal VN, *Pediatr Dermatology* 16, 165 (multiple)
 (1998): Hern S+, *Br J Dermatol* 139, 1129,
 (1998): Litt JZ, Beachwood, OH (personal case) (observation)
 (1998): Mahboob A+, *Int J Dermatol* 37, 833
 (1996): Gomez-Martinez M+, *J Investig Allergol Clin Immunol* 6, 131
 (1996): Kawada A+, *Int J Dermatol* 35, 148
 (1996): Laude TA, *Cosmetic Dermatology* 9, 7
 (1995): Harris A+, *Br J Dermatol* 133, 790
 (1994): Rademaker M+, *N Z Med J* 107, 295
 (1992): Cohen HA+, *Ann Pharmacother* 26, 1596
 (1992): Zemtsov A+, *Cutis* 50, 281
 (1991): Thankappen TP+, *Int J Dermatol* 30, 867
 (1990): Duhra P+, *Clin Exp Dermatol* 15, 293
 (1990): Gaffoor PMA+, *Cutis* 45, 242 (passim)
 (1989): Valsecchi R, *Dermatologica* 179, 51
 (1988): Guin J+, *Cutis* 41, 107
 (1987): Bharija SC+, *Australas J Dermatol* 28, 85
 (1987): Guin J+, *J Am Acad Dermatol* 17, 399
 (1986): Meyrick-Thomas RH+, *Br J Dermatol* 115, 357
 (1985): Verbov J, *Dermatologica* 171, 60 (with chlormezanone)
Lichenoid keratoses (sic)
 (2007): Wohl Y+, *J Eur Acad Dermatol Venereol* 21(4), 548
Linear IgA dermatosis
 (2003): Avci O+, *J Am Acad Dermatol* 48(2), 299
Neutrophilic eccrine hidradenitis
 (2006): EL Sayed F+, *J Eur Acad Dermatol Venereol* 20(10), 1338
 (1988): Kuttner BJ+, *Cutis* 41, 403
Pemphigus
 (1990): Brenner S+, *Acta Derm Venereol* 70, 357
Penile edema
 (1997): Cabanes Higuero N+, *Med Clin* (Barc) (Spanish) 109, 685
Photosensitivity
 (1999): Popescu C, Bucharest, Romania (from Internet) (observation)
Pigmented purpuric eruption (Schamberg's disease)
 (1992): Abeck D+, *J Am Acad Dermatol* 27, 123

Pityriasis rosea
(1993): Yosipovitch G+, *Harefuah* (Israel) 124, 198; 247
Pruritus
(2001): Grant JA+, *Ann Allergy Asthma Immunol* 87(3), 227 (rare)
(1985): Stricker BH+, *BMJ* 291, 938
Purpura
(2006): Santoro D+, *Clin Nephrol* 66(2), 131 (with codeine)
(1998): Kwon SJ+, *J Dermatol* 25, 756
(1993): Guccione JL+, *Arch Dermatol* 129, 1267
(1992): Abeck D+, *J Am Acad Dermatol* 27, 123
(1980): Miescher PA+, *Clin Haematol* 9, 505
Purpura fulminans
(1993): Guccione JL+, *Arch Dermatol* 129, 1267
Pustules
(2005): Daghfous R+, *Therapie* 60(5), 523 (30%)
Rash (sic) (<1%)
Sensitivity (sic)
(1998): Mendizabal SL+, *Allergy* 53, 457
Stevens–Johnson syndrome
(1995): Kuper K+, *Ophthalmologue* (German) 92, 823
(1985): Ting HC+, *Int J Dermatol* 24, 587
Toxic epidermal necrolysis
(2004): Bygum A+, *Pediatr Dermatol* 21(3), 236
(2002): Cordova M, (Lima) (Peru) March AAD Poster
(2002): Thakker J+, *World Congress Dermatol* Poster, 0129 (with nimesulide)
(2000): Halevi A+, *Ann Pharmacother* 34, 32
(1991): Sakellariou G+, *Int J Artif Organs* 14, 634
(1986): Roupe G+, *Int Arch Allergy Appl Immunol* 80, 145
Urticaria
(2007): Tsujino Y+, *J Dermatol* 34(3), 224
(2006): Santoro D+, *Clin Nephrol* 66(2), 131 (with codeine)
(2005): Daghfous R+, *Therapie* 60(5), 523 (34%)
(2002): Bachmeyer C+, *South Med J* 95(7), 759
(2002): Litt JZ, Beachwood, OH (personal case) (observation) (patient inadvertently re-challenged herself)
(2001): Grant JA+, *Ann Allergy Asthma Immunol* 87(3), 227 (rare)
(2000): Samanta BB, *J Assoc Physicians India* 47, 464
(1997): de Almeida MA+, *Allergy Asthma Proc* 18, 313
(1997): Ownby DR, *J Allergy Clin Immunol* 99, 151
(1985): Cole TO, *Clin Exp Dermatol* 10, 404
(1985): Stricker BH+, *BMJ* 291, 938
Vasculitis
(1995): Harris A+, *Br J Dermatol* 133, 790
(1988): Dussarat GV+, *Presse Med* (French) 17, 1587
Xanthoderma
(2007): Haught JM+, *J Am Acad Dermatol* 57(6), 1051

Mucosal/ENT
Dysgeusia

Hair
Hair – alopecia
(1998): Litt JZ, Beachwood, OH (personal case) (observation)

Nails
Nails – changes (sic)

Other
Anaphylactoid reactions/Anaphylaxis
(2005): Daghfous R+, *Therapie* 60(5), 523
(2002): Bachmeyer C+, *South Med J* 95(7), 759
(2002): Liao CM+, *Acta Paediatr Taiwan* 43(3), 147
(2001): Verma S, Baroda, India (from Internet) (observation) (with ibuprofen)
(2000): Ayonrinde OT+, *Postgrad Med J.* 76, 501
(2000): de Paramo BJ+, *Ann Allergy Asthma Immunol* 85, 508 (4 patients)
(2000): Stephenson I+, *Postgrad Med* 76, 503
(1999): Kumar RK+, *Hosp Med* 60, 66

(1999): Spitz E, *Ann Allergy Asthma Immunol* 82, 591
(1998): Galindo PA+, *Allergol Immunopathol* (Madr) (Spanish) 26, 199
(1998): Huitema AD+, *Hum Exp Toxicol* 17, 406
(1990): Van Diem L+, *Eur J Clin Pharmacol* 38, 389
(1988): *Allergy Observer* (Janssen Pharmaceutica) 5(7), 1
(1985): Stricker BH+, *BMJ* 291, 938
Anticonvulsant hypersensitivity syndrome
(2006): Gaig P+, *J Investig Allergol Clin Immunol* 16(5), 321
Death
(2002): Sheen CL+, *Br J Clin Pharmacol* 54(4), 430
(2001): Stevenson R+, *Scott Med J* 46(3), 84 (overdose)
(1988): Minton NA+, *Hum Toxicol* 7(1), 33 (with phenytoin)
DRESS syndrome
(2006): Gaig P+, *J Investig Allergol Clin Immunol.* 16(5), 321
Headache
Hepatotoxicity
(2006): Antoniades CG+, *Hepatology* 44(1), 34
(2006): Holubek WJ+, *Hepatology* 43(4), 880
(2006): Lewis JH+, *Curr Opin Gastroenterol* 22(3), 223
(2006): Liu ZX+, *Expert Opin Drug Metab Toxicol* 2(4), 493
(2006): Mahadevan SB+, *Arch Dis Child* 91(7), 598
(2006): Moling O+, *Clin Ther* 28(5), 755
(2006): Patel KP, *N Engl J Med* 354(20), 2191
(2006): Perkins JD, *Liver Transpl* 12(4), 682
(2006): Schmidt LE+, *Crit Care Med* 34(2), 337
(2005): Jaeschke H, *Expert Opin Drug Metab Toxicol* 1(3), 389
(2005): Peters TS, *Toxicol Pathol* 33(1), 146
Hypersensitivity (<1%)
(2007): Kidon MI+, *Int Arch Allergy Immunol* 144(1), 51
(2001): Grant JA+, *Ann Allergy Asthma* 87(3), 227 (rare)
(1999): Kivity S+, *Allergy* 54, 187
(1997): Vidal C+, *Ann Allergy Asthma Immunol* 79, 320
(1996): Ibanez MD+, *Allergy* 51, 121
(1993): Martin JA+, *Med Clin* (Barc) (Spanish) 100, 158
Nephrotoxicity
(2006): Jochum E+, *Med Klin* (Munich) 101(10), 830
(2005): Mour G+, *Ren Fail* 27(4), 381
(1998): Gault MH+, *Am J Kidney Dis* 32(3), 351
Rhabdomyolysis
(2007): Nelson H+, *Pharmacotherapy* 27(4), 608 (overdose)
(2001): Yang CC+, *Vet Hum Toxicol* 43(6), 344 (overdose)
(1999): Moneret-Vautrin DA+, *Allergy* 54(10), 1115
(1996): Riggs JE+, *Mil Med* 161(11), 708 (with alcohol)

ACETAZOLAMIDE

Trade names: Acetazolam; Ak-Zol; Dazamide; Defiltran; Diamox (Wyeth); Diuramid; Novo-Zolamide
Indications: Epilepsy, glaucoma
Category: Carbonic anhydrase inhibitor; Diuretic
Half-life: 2–6 hours
Clinically important, potentially hazardous interactions with: ephedra, lithium

Note: Acetazolamide is a sulfonamide and can be absorbed systemically. Sulfonamides can produce severe, possibly fatal, reactions such as toxic epidermal necrolysis and Stevens–Johnson syndrome

Reactions

Skin
Acute generalized exanthematous pustulosis (AGEP)
(1995): Moreau A+, *Int J Dermatol* 34, 263 (passim)
(1992): Ogoshi M+, *Dermatology* 184, 142
Bullous dermatitis (<1%)

Erythema multiforme
Exanthems
Frostbite
(2001): Laemmle T, *Wilderness Environ Med* 12(4), 290
Lupus erythematosus
Photosensitivity
Pruritus
Psoriasis
(1995): Kuroda K+, *J Dermatol* 22, 784
Purpura
Pustules
(1992): Ogoshi M+, *Dermatology* 184, 142
Rash (sic) (<1%)
Rosacea
(1993): Shah P+, *Br J Dermatol* 129, 647
Stevens–Johnson syndrome
(2006): Ogasawara K+, *Neurol Med Chir (Tokyo)* 246(3), 161
(1981): Sud RN+, *Indian J Ophthalmol* 29(2), 101
Toxic epidermal necrolysis (<1%)
Urticaria

Mucosal/ENT
Ageusia
Anosmia
Dysgeusia (>10%) (metallic taste)
(1997): Martinez-Mir I+, *Ann Pharmacother* 31, 373
(1990): Miller LG+, *J Fam Pract* 31, 199
(1981): Lichter PR, *Ophthalmol* 88, 266
Tinnitus
Xerostomia (<1%)

Hair
Hair – hirsutism

Eyes
Glaucoma
(2007): Lee GC+, *Clin Experiment Ophthalmol* 35(1), 55

Other
Anaphylactoid reactions/Anaphylaxis
(2002): Gallerani M+, *Am J Emerg Med* 20(4), 371
(2000): Gerhards LJ+, *Ned Tijdschr Geneeskd* (Dutch) 144, 1228
(1998): Tzanakis N+, *Br J Ophthalmol* 82, 588
Extravasation
(1994): Callear A+, *Br J Ophthalmol* 78, 731
Headache
Myalgia/Myositis/Myopathy/Myotoxicity
(2002): Ikeda K+, *Intern Med* 41(9), 743
Paresthesias (<1%)
(1981): Lichter PR, *Ophthalmol* 88, 266

ACETOHEXAMIDE

Trade names: Dimelin; Dimelor; Dymelor (Barr)
Indications: Non-insulin dependent diabetes type II
Category: Sulfonylurea
Half-life: 1–6 hours
Clinically important, potentially hazardous interactions with: phenylbutazones

Note: Acetohexamide is a sulfonamide and can be absorbed systemically. Sulfonamides can produce severe, possibly fatal, reactions such as toxic epidermal necrolysis and Stevens–Johnson syndrome

Reactions

Skin
Diaphoresis
Eczema
Erythema (<1%)
Exanthems (<1%)
Jaundice
Lichenoid eruption
Photosensitivity (1–10%)
Pruritus (<1%)
Rash (sic) (1–10%)
Urticaria (1–10%)

Hair
Hair – alopecia

Other
Coma
Headache
Paresthesias
Porphyria cutanea tarda

ACETYLCYSTEINE

Synonyms: N-acetylcysteine; L-Cysteine; NAC
Trade names: Agisolvan; Alveolex; Ecomucyl; Encore; Exomuc; Fabrol; Fluimicil; Mucofillin; Mucolit; Mucolitico; Mucoloid; Mucomiste; Mucomyst (Bioniche); Mucomyst-10; Mucosil-10; Parvolex; Siran
Indications: Emphysema, bronchitis, tuberculosis, bronchiectasis, tracheostomy care, antidote for acetaminophen toxicity
Category: Antidote; Antioxidant
Half-life: N/A
Clinically important, potentially hazardous interactions with: carbamazepine, nitroglycerin

Reactions

Skin
Adverse effects (sic)
(2003): Kao LW+, *Ann Emerg Med* 42(6), 741
Angioedema
(2001): Tas S+, *Br J Dermatol* 145(5), 856
(1999): Schmidt LE+, *Ugeskr Laeger* 161(18), 2669
(1997): Mroz LS+, *Ann Emerg Med* 30(2), 240
(1984): Mant TG+, *Br Med J* 289(6439), 217
(1984): Tenenbein M, *Vet Hum Toxicol* 26(Suppl 2), 3
Clammy skin
Dermatitis
(2002): Davison SC+, *Contact Dermatitis* 47(4), 238
Diaphoresis
Pruritus
(1999): Schmidt LE+, *Ugeskr Laeger* 161(18), 2669
(1984): Tenenbein M, *Vet Hum Toxicol* 26(Suppl 2), 3
Rash (sic)
(1999): Schmidt LE+, *Ugeskr Laeger* 161(18), 2669
(1994): Chan TY+, *Hum Exp Toxicol* 13(8), 542
(1984): Mant TG+, *Br Med J* 289(6439), 217
Urticaria
(1984): Tenenbein M, *Vet Hum Toxicol* 26(Suppl 2), 3

Mucosal/ENT
Stomatitis

Other
Anaphylactoid reactions/Anaphylaxis
(2006): Kanter MZ, *Am J Health Syst Pharm* 63(19), 1821
(2002): Appelboam AV+, *Emerg Med J* 19(6), 594 (fatal)
(2001): Recasens M+, *Med Clin* (Barc) 117(14), 558
(1999): Schmidt LE+, *Ugeskr Laeger* 161(18), 2669
(1998): Bailey B+, *Ann Emerg Med* 31(6), 710
(1997): Stavem K, *Tidsskr Nor Laegeforen* 117(4), 2038
(1992): Bonfiglio MF+, *Ann Pharmacother* 26(1), 22
(1992): Sunman W+, *Lancet* 339(8803), 1231
(1984): Gervais S+, *Clin Pharm* 3(6), 586
(1982): Vale JA+, *Lancet* 2(8305), 988
Chills
Death
(1997): Ardissino D+, *J Am Coll Cardiol* 29(5), 941
Fever
(1994): Chan TY+, *Hum Exp Toxicol* 13(8), 542
Hypersensitivity
(1984): Tenenbein M, *Vet Hum Toxicol* 26, 3
Injection-site pain
(1984): Casola G+, *Radiology* 152(1), 233
Seizures
(1996): Hershkovitz E+, *Isr J Med Sci* 32(11), 1102

ACITRETIN

Trade names: Neotigason; Soriatane (Roche)
Indications: Psoriasis
Category: Retinoid
Half-life: 49 hours
Clinically important, potentially hazardous interactions with: alcohol, bexarotene, chloroquine, cholestyramine, corticosteroids, danazol, ethanolamine, isotretinoin, lithium, medroxyprogesterone, methotrexate, minocycline, progestins, tetracycline, vitamin A

Reactions

Skin
Atrophy (10–25%)
Bullous dermatitis (1–10%)
Clammy skin (1–10%)
Dermatitis (1–10%)
Diaphoresis (1–10%)
(1997): Buccheri L+, *Arch Dermatol* 133, 711 (18.2%)
(1988): Geiger J-M+, *Dermatologica* 176, 182 (9%)
Edema
(2006): Tey HL+, *J Dermatol* 33(5), 372
(2001): Liss WA, Pleasanton, CA (from Internet) (observation)
Erythema (18%)
(1997): Buccheri L+, *Arch Dermatol* 133, 711 (18.2%)
Erythema gyratum
(2003): Bryan ME+, *J Drugs Dermatol* 2(3), 315
Erythroderma
(2006): Mahe E+, *J Eur Acad Dermatol Venereol* 20(9), 1133
(2001): Liss WA, Pleasanton, CA (from Internet) (observation)
Exanthems (2–25%)
(1999): Katz HI+, *J Am Acad Dermatol* 41, S7
(1990): Ruzicka T+, *Arch Dermatol* 126, 482 (2%)
Exfoliative dermatitis (25–50%)
(2001): Blumenthal HL, Beachwood, OH (observation)
(1999): Katz HI+, *J Am Acad Dermatol* 41, S7 (25–50%)
(1997): Buccheri L+, *Arch Dermatol* 133, 711 (36.4%)
Fissures (1–10%)
Fragility

Hyperkeratosis
Milia
(1993): Chang A+, *Acta Derm Venereol* 73, 235
Palmar–plantar desquamation (20–80%)
(2001): Ami (from Internet) (observation) (severe)
(2001): Berbis P, *Ann Dermatol Venereol* 128(6), 737
(1991): Murray HE+, *J Am Acad Dermatol* 24, 598 (29%)
(1990): Ruzicka T+, *Arch Dermatol* 126, 482 (20–25%)
(1989): Gupta AK+, *J Am Acad Dermatol* 21, 1088 (50–80%)
(1988): Geiger J-M+, *Dermatologica* 176, 182 (26%)
Phototoxicity
(1999): Katz HI+, *J Am Acad Dermatol* 41, S7
Pruritus (10–50%)
(1999): Katz HI+, *J Am Acad Dermatol* 41, S7
(1997): Buccheri L+, *Arch Dermatol* 133, 711 (54.5%)
(1996): Lacour M+, *Br J Dermatol* 134, 1023
(1991): Murray HE+, *J Am Acad Dermatol* 24, 598 (32%)
(1990): Ruzicka T+, *Arch Dermatol* 126, 482 (37%)
(1989): Gupta AK+, *J Am Acad Dermatol* 21, 1088 (10–20%)
(1988): Geiger J-M+, *Dermatologica* 176, 182 (16%)
Psoriasis (1–10%)
Purpura (1–10%)
Pyogenic granuloma (1–10%)
(2002): Diederen PVMM+, *World Congress Dermatol* Poster, 0099
Rash (sic) (>10%)
Seborrhea (1–10%)
Stickiness (3–50%)
(1999): Katz HI+, *J Am Acad Dermatol* 41, S7
(1997): Buccheri L+, *Arch Dermatol* 133, 711 (18%)
(1991): Murray HE+, *J Am Acad Dermatol* 24, 598 (8%)
(1989): Schröder K+, *Acta Derm Venereol* (Stockh) 69, 111 (3%)
(1988): Geiger J-M+, *Dermatologica* 176, 182 (2.5%)
Sunburn (1–10%)
Ulcerations (1–10%)
Urticaria
Xerosis (25–50%)
(2001): Berbis P, *Ann Dermatol Venereol* 128(6), 737
(1999): Katz HI+, *J Am Acad Dermatol* 41, S7 (15–25%)
(1997): Buccheri L+, *Arch Dermatol* 133, 711 (45.5%)
(1991): Murray HE+, *J Am Acad Dermatol* 24, 598 (24%)
(1990): Ruzicka T+, *Arch Dermatol* 126, 482 (48%)
(1989): Gupta AK+, *J Am Acad Dermatol* 21, 1088 (10–20%)
(1989): Schröder K+, *Acta Derm Venereol* (Stockh) 69, 111 (65%)
(1988): Geiger J-M+, *Dermatologica* 176, 182 (30%)

Mucosal/ENT
Bromhidrosis (1–10%)
(2004): Goiham M, Caracas, Venezuela (from Internet) (observation)
(2001): Liss WA, Pleasanton, CA (from Internet) (observation)
(2000): Liss WA, Pleasanton, CA (from Internet) (observation)
Cheilitis (>75%)
(2001): Berbis P, *Ann Dermatol Venereol* 128(6), 737
(1999): Katz HI+, *J Am Acad Dermatol* 41, S7 (>75%)
(1997): Buccheri L+, *Arch Dermatol* 133, 711 (100%)
(1996): Lacour M+, *Br J Dermatol* 134, 1023
(1991): Murray HE+, *J Am Acad Dermatol* 24, 598 (49%)
(1990): Ruzicka T+, *Arch Dermatol* 126, 482 (80%)
(1989): Gupta AK+, *J Am Acad Dermatol* 21, 1088 (100%)
(1988): Geiger J-M+, *Dermatologica* 176, 182 (82%)
Dry mucous membranes
(2001): Berbis P, *Ann Dermatol Venereol* 128(6), 737
Gingivitis (1–10%)
Hearing loss
(2005): Mahasitthiwat V, *J Med Assoc Thai* 88(Suppl 1), S79
Oral lesions
(1988): Geiger J-M+, *Dermatologica* 176, 182 (6%)

Sialorrhea (1–10%)
Stomatitis (1–10%)
Ulcerative stomatitis (1–10%)
Vulvovaginal candidiasis
  (1995): Sturkenboom MC+, *J Clin Epidemiol* 48, 991
Xerostomia (10–60%)
  (1999): Katz HI+, *J Am Acad Dermatol* 41, S7
  (1997): Buccheri L+, *Arch Dermatol* 133, 711 (63.6%)
  (1989): Schröder K+, *Acta Derm Venereol* (Stockh) 69, 111
    (60%)
  (1988): Geiger J-M+, *Dermatologica* 176, 182 (30%)

Hair

Hair – alopecia (10–75%)
  (2001): Berbis P, *Ann Dermatol Venereol* 128(6), 737
  (2001): Popescu C, Bucharest, Romania (from Internet)
    (observation)
  (2001): Thaler D, Monona, WI (from Internet) (observation)
    (diffuse)
  (2001): Vedamurthy V, Chennai, India (from Internet)
    (observation) (scalp, mustache, eyebrows & beard)
  (1999): Katz HI+, *J Am Acad Dermatol* 41, S7 (10–25%)
  (1997): Buccheri L+, *Arch Dermatol* 133, 711 (45.5%)
  (1991): Murray HE+, *J Am Acad Dermatol* 24, 598 (33%)
  (1990): Ruzicka T+, *Arch Dermatol* 126, 482 (12%)
  (1989): Gupta AK+, *J Am Acad Dermatol* 21, 1088 (30–70%)
  (1989): Schröder K+, *Acta Derm Venereol* (Stockh) 69, 111
    (13%)
  (1988): Geiger J-M+, *Dermatologica* 176, 182 (20%)
Hair – alopecia totalis
  (2003): Chave TA+, *Br J Dermatol* 148(5), 1063
  (2002): Chave TA+, *World Congress Dermatol* Poster 0092
    (regrowth in 6 months)
Hair – alopecia universalis
  (1998): Haycox CL, Seattle, WA (from Internet) (observation)
  (1998): Nadel RS, Springfield, MA (from Internet) (observation)
Hair – pili torti
  (2001): Davidson DM, Groton, CT (from Internet) (observation)

Nails

Nails – brittle
  (1991): Murray HE+, *J Am Acad Dermatol* 24, 598 (27%)
  (1990): Ruzicka T+, *Arch Dermatol* 126, 482
  (1988): Geiger J-M+, *Dermatologica* 176, 182 (10%)
Nails – changes (sic) (25–50%)
Nails – paronychia (10–25%)
  (2002): Hirsch R, Brooklyn, NY (from Internet) (observation)
  (1999): Katz HI+, *J Am Acad Dermatol* 41, S7
  (1997): Buccheri L+, *Arch Dermatol* 133, 711 (18.2%)
  (1991): Murray HE+, *J Am Acad Dermatol* 24, 598 (7%)
Nails – periungual granuloma
  (1997): Buccheri L+, *Arch Dermatol* 133, 711 (9.1%)
Nails – pyogenic granulomas
  (1999): Guzick N, Houston, TX (from Internet) (observation)
Nails – subungual hemorrhages
  (2007): Aydogan K+, *Int J Dermatol* 46(5), 494

Eyes

Maculopathy
  (2004): Lois N+, *Arch Ophthalmol* 122(6), 928

Other

Chills
  (2001): Liss WA, Pleasanton, CA (from Internet) (observation)
Depression
  (2005): Starling J 3rd+, *J Drugs Dermatol* 4(6), 690
Hepatotoxicity
  (2002): Kreiss C+, *Am J Gastroenterol* 97(3), 775
Myalgia/Myositis/Myopathy/Myotoxicity
  (1996): Lister RK+, *Br J Dermatol* 134, 989

Neurotoxicity
  (2003): Tsambaos D+, *Skin Pharmacol Appl Skin Physiol* 16(1), 46
  (2002): Chroni E+, *Clin Neuropharmacol* 25(6), 310
Paresthesias (10–25%)
  (1999): Katz HI+, *J Am Acad Dermatol* 41, S7
Stroke
  (2002): Royer B+, *Ann Pharmacother* 36(12), 1879
Suicidal ideation
  (2006): Arican O+, *J Eur Acad Dermatol Venereol* 20(4), 464
Tremor

ACTINOMYCIN-D

(See DACTINOMYCIN)

ACYCLOVIR

Synonyms: aciclovir; ACV; acycloguanosine
Trade names: Acifur; Acyclo-V; Acyvir; Avirax; Herpefug; Zovirax (GSK); Zyclir
Indications: Herpes simplex, herpes zoster
Category: Antiviral; Antiviral, topical; Guanine nucleoside analog
Half-life: 3 hours (adults)
Clinically important, potentially hazardous interactions with: meperidine, tenofovir

Reactions

Skin

Acne (<3%)
Burning (topical)
Dermatitis
  (2001): Lammintausta K+, *Contact Dermatitis* 45(3), 181
  (2000): Serpentier-Daude A+, *Ann Dermatol Venereol* 127, 191
  (1996): Bourezane Y+, *Allergy* 51, 755
  (1995): Koch P, *Contact Dermatitis* 33, 255
  (1991): Goday J+, *Contact Dermatitis* 24, 381
  (1990): Baes H+, *Contact Dermatitis* 23, 200
  (1990): Valsecchi R+, *Contact Dermatitis* 23, 372
  (1989): Gola M+, *Contact Dermatitis* 20, 394
  (1989): O'Brien JJ+, *Drugs* 37, 233 (vesicular)
  (1988): Camarasa JG+, *Contact Dermatitis* 19, 235
  (1985): Robinson GE+, *Genitourin Med* 61, 62 (palms and soles)
Diaphoresis
Edema
  (1991): Medina S+, *Int J Dermatol* 30, 305
Erythema
  (2002): Carrasco L+, *Clin Exp Dermatol* 27(2), 132
Erythema nodosum
  (1983): Richards DM+, *Drugs* 26, 378
Exanthems (1–5%)
  (1991): Whitley R+, *N Engl J Med* 324, 444
  (1985): Robinson GE+, *Genitourin Med* 61, 62
  (1984): Strauss SE+, *N Engl J Med* 301, 1545
  (1983): Balfour HH+, *N Engl J Med* 308, 1448
  (1983): Richards DM+, *Drugs* 26, 378
Facial edema (3–5%)
  (2000): Colin J+, *Ophthalmology* 107, 1507
Fixed eruption
  (1997): Montoro J+, *Contact Dermatitis* 36, 225
Herpes zoster (recurrent)
  (1993): Murphy F, *The Schoch Letter* 43, 28, #104 (observation)
Lichenoid eruption
  (1985): Robinson GE+, *Genitourin Med* 61, 62

Peripheral edema
 (1991): Medina S+, *Int J Dermatol* 30, 305
 (1988): Hisler BM+, *J Am Acad Dermatol* 18, 1142
Photo-recall
 (2002): Carrasco L+, *Clin Exp Dermatol* 27(2), 132
 (2001): *Ann Dermatol Venereol* 128(2), 184
Photosensitivity
 (2001): Schmutz JL+, *Ann Dermatol Venereol* 128, 184
Pityriasis rosea
 (2007): Mavarkar L, *Indian J Dermatol Venereol Leprol* 73(3), 200
Pruritus (1–10%)
 (1993): Goldberg LH+, *Arch Dermatol* 129, 582 (passim)
Rash (sic) (<3%)
 (1985): Lundgren G+, *Scand J Infect Dis* Suppl 47, 137
 (1983): Balfour HH+, *N Engl J Med* 308, 1448
 (1983): Masaoka T+, *Gan To Kagaku Ryoho* (Japanese) 10, 944
Stevens–Johnson syndrome
 (1995): Fazal BA+, *Clin Infect Dis* 21, 1038
Stinging (topical)
Urticaria (1–5%)
 (1985): Robinson GE+, *Genitourin Med* 61, 62
 (1983): Richards DM+, *Drugs* 26, 378
 (1982): Smith CI+, *Am J Med* 73, 267
 (1981): Balfour HH+, *Minn Med* 64, 739
Vasculitis
 (1983): Richards DM+, *Drugs* 26, 378
Vesiculation
 (1993): Buck ML+, *Ann Pharmacother* 27, 1458

Mucosal/ENT
Auditory hallucinations
 (2007): Yang HH+, *Int J Dermatol* 46(8), 883
Dysgeusia (0.3%)
Vaginitis (candidal)
 (1993): Goldberg LH+, *Arch Dermatol* 129, 582 (passim)

Hair
Hair – alopecia (<3%)

Eyes
Periorbital edema (3–5%)
 (2000): Colin J+, *Ophthalmology* 107, 1507
Visual hallucinations
 (2007): Yang HH+, *Int J Dermatol* 46(8), 883

Other
Abdominal pain
 (2004): Sra KK+, *Skin Therapy Lett* 9(8), 1
Agitation
 (2007): Yang HH+, *Int J Dermatol* 46(8), 883
Anaphylactoid reactions/Anaphylaxis (<1%)
Delirium
 (2007): Yang HH+, *Int J Dermatol* 46(8), 883
Headache
 (2004): Sra KK+, *Skin Therapy Lett* 9(8), 1
Hypersensitivity
 (2001): Kawsar M+, *Sex Transm Infect* 77(3), 204
Injection-site inflammation (>10%)
 (1989): O'Brien JJ+, *Drugs* 37, 233
Injection-site necrosis
 (1987): Fayol J+, *Therapie* (French) 42(2), 249
Injection-site thrombophlebitis (9%)
 (1988): Arndt KA, *J Am Acad Dermatol* 18, 188
Injection-site vesicular eruption
 (1986): Sylvester RK+, *JAMA* 255, 385
Nephrotoxicity
 (2006): Bassioukas K+, *J Eur Acad Dermatol Venereol* 20(9), 1151
 (2006): De Deyne S+, *Rev Med Interne* 27(11), 892
 (2005): Izzedine H+, *Am J Kidney Dis* 45(5), 804

 (2005): Orion E+, *Clin Dermatol* 23(2), 182
 (2003): Sodhi PK+, *Scand J Infect Dis* 35(10), 770
 (1999): Da Conceicao M+, *Ann Fr Anesth Reanim* 18(9), 996
Neurotoxicity
 (2006): Chevret L+, *Pediatr Transplant* 10(5), 632
 (2005): Orion E+, *Clin Dermatol* 23(2), 182
Paresthesias (<1%)
 (1993): Goldberg LH+, *Arch Dermatol* 129, 582 (passim)
Tremor

ADALIMUMAB

Synonym: D2E7
Trade name: Humira (Abbott)
Indications: Rheumatoid arthritis
Category: Cytokine inhibitor; TNF inhibitor
Half-life: 10–20 days
Clinically important, potentially hazardous interactions with: None

Note: TNF blocking agents may lead to serious infections, lymphoma, or fatalities, particularly in patients receiving concomitant immunosuppressive therapy. Patients should be evaluated for latent tuberculosis prior to treatment with adalimumab.

Reactions

Skin
Acne
 (2008): Sun G+, *J Drugs Dermatol* 7(1), 69
Allergic reactions (sic) (1%)
Angioedema
 (2006): Sanchez-Cano D+, *Clin Exp Rheumatol* 24(5 Suppl 42), S128
Bacterial infections
 (2005): Botsios C, *Autoimmun Rev* 4(3), 162
Carcinoma
Cellulitis
 (2008): Van L+, *Arch Dermatol* 144(6), 804
Eosinophilic cellulitis
 (2006): Boura P+, *Ann Rheum Dis* 65(6), 839
Erysipelas
Erythema
 (2005): Sfikakis PP+, *Arthritis Rheum* 52(8), 2513 (1 case)
Erythema multiforme
 (2004): Beuthien W+, *Arthritis Rheum* 50(5), 1690
Fixed eruption
Fungal dermatitis
Herpes zoster
Lupus erythematosus (<0.1%)
 (2007): Ramos-Casals M+, *Medicine* (Baltimore) 86(4), 242 (15 cases)
 (2007): Sheth N+, *Clin Exp Dermatol* 32(5), 593
 (2006): van Rijthoven AW+, *Rheumatology* (Oxford) 45(10), 1317
 (2005): Scheinfeld N, *Expert Opin Drug Saf* 4(4), 637
Lupus syndrome
 (2005): Botsios C, *Autoimmun Rev* 4(3), 162
Lymphoma
 (2006): Moul DK+, *Arch Dermatol* 142(9), 1110
Malignancies
 (2006): Bongartz T+, *JAMA* 295(19), 2275
Melanoma
Peripheral edema
Pruritus
 (2004): Youdim A+, *Inflamm Bowel Dis* 10(4), 333

Psoriasis
  (2007): Heymann WR, *J Am Acad Dermatol* 56(2), 327 (pustular)
  (2007): Ubriani R+, *Arch Dermatol* 143(2), 270
  (2006): Kary S+, *Ann Rheum Dis* 65(3), 405
  (2006): Matthews C+, *Ann Rheum Dis* 65(11), 1529
  (2005): Sfikakis PP+, *Arthritis Rheum* 52(8), 2513
Rash (sic) (12%)
Side effects (sic)
  (2006): van der Heijde D+, *Arthritis Rheum* 54(7), 2136 (75%)
Squamous cell carcinoma
  (2008): Van L+, *Arch Dermatol* 144(6), 804
Urticaria
  (2006): George SJ+, *Dermatol Online J* 12(2), 4
  (2006): Sanchez-Cano D+, *Clin Exp Rheumatol* 24(5 Suppl 42), S128
Vasculitis
  (2007): Ramos-Casals M+, *Medicine* (Baltimore) 86(4), 242 (5 cases)
  (2006): Orpin SD+, *Br J Dermatol* 154(5), 998
  (2006): Saint Marcoux B+, *Joint Bone Spine* 73(6), 710
Vitiligo
  (2008): Smith DI+, *J Am Acad Dermatol* 58(2 Suppl), S50

Hair

Hair – alopecia areata
  (2006): Garcia Bartels N+, *Arch Dermatol* 142(12), 1654
Hair – alopecia universalis
  (2006): Garcia Bartels N+, *Arch Dermatol* 142(12), 1654
Hair – follicular mucinosis
  (2005): Dalle S+, *Br J Dermatol* 153(1), 207

Nails

Nails – onychocryptosis
  (2005): Sfikakis PP+, *Arthritis Rheum* 52(8), 2513 (3 cases)
Nails – subungual hyperkeratosis
  (2005): Sfikakis PP+, *Arthritis Rheum* 52(8), 2513 (3 cases)

Eyes

Optic neuritis
  (2006): Chung JH+, *J Neurol Sci* 244(1–2), 133

Other

Death
Headache
Infections (5%)
  (2006): Bongartz T+, *JAMA* 295(19), 2275
  (2006): Moul DK+, *Arch Dermatol* 142(9), 1110
  (2005): Efde MN+, *Neth J Med* 63(3), 112
  (2005): Scheinfeld N, *Expert Opin Drug Saf* 4(4), 637
  (2004): *Prescrire Int* 13(73), 171
  (2004): Scheinfeld N, *J Dermatolog Treat* 15(6), 348
Injection-site edema (15.2%)
Injection-site erythema (15.2%)
Injection-site pain (12%)
Injection-site reactions (sic)
  (2005): Papadakis KA+, *Am J Gastroenterol* 100(1), 75
  (2005): Scheinfeld N, *Expert Opin Drug Saf* 4(4), 637
  (2004): Moreland LW, *Pharmacoeconomics* 22(2 Suppl), 39 (20%)
  (2004): van de Putte LB+, *Ann Rheum Dis* 63(5), 508 (10%)
Nephrotoxicity
Neurotoxicity
  (2008): Van L+, *Arch Dermatol* 144(6), 804
Paresthesias
  (2005): Berthelot CN+, *J Am Acad Dermatol* 53(5 Suppl 1), S260
Tendinopathy/Tendon rupture
Tremor
Upper respiratory infection (17%)
  (2006): Moul DK+, *Arch Dermatol* 142(9), 1110

ADAPALENE

Trade names: Adaferin; Differin (Galderma)
Indications: Acne vulgaris
Category: Retinoid
Half-life: N/A
Clinically important, potentially hazardous interactions with: resorcinol, salicylates

Reactions

Skin

Acne (<1%)
Burning (<1%)
  (2001): Nyirady J+, *J Dermatolog Treat* 12(3), 149
  (2001): Tu P+, *J Eur Acad Dermatol Venereol* 15 (Suppl 3), 31
  (1998): Ellis CN+, *Br J Dermatol* 139, Suppl 52:41
Dermatitis (<1%)
Eczema (<1%)
Erythema (<1%)
  (2001): Leyden J+, *Cutis* 67(6 Suppl), 17
  (2001): Nyirady J+, *J Dermatolog Treat* 12(3), 149
  (2001): Tu P+, *J Eur Acad Dermatol Venereol* 15, (Suppl 3) 31
  (1998): Ellis CN+, *Br J Dermatol* 139, Suppl 52:41
Irritation (sic) (<1%)
  (2003): Brand B+, *Cutis* 72(6), 455
  (2003): Brand B+, *J Am Acad Dermatol* 49(3 Suppl), S227
  (2001): Queille-Roussel C+, *Clin Ther* 23(2), 205
  (1998): Bonardeaux C+, *Rev Med Liege* 53(2), 109 (mild)
Pruritus (<1%)
  (2001): Nyirady J+, *J Dermatolog Treat* 12(3), 149
  (2001): Tu P+, *J Eur Acad Dermatol Venereol* 15 (Suppl 3), 31
  (1998): Ellis CN+, *Br J Dermatol* 139, Suppl 52:41
Rash (sic) (<1%)
Scaling (<1%)
  (2001): Tu P+, *J Eur Acad Dermatol Venereol* 15 (Suppl 3), 31
  (1998): Ellis CN+, *Br J Dermatol* 139, Suppl 52:41
Xerosis (<1%)
  (2001): Leyden J+, *Cutis* 67(6 Suppl), 17
  (2001): Tu P+, *J Eur Acad Dermatol Venereol* 15 (Suppl 3), 31
  (1998): Dunlap FE+, *Br J Dermatol* 139 (Suppl 52), 17 (3 cases)
  (1998): Ellis CN+, *Br J Dermatol* 139, Suppl 52:41

Eyes

Conjunctivitis
Eyelid edema (<1%)

ADEFOVIR

Synonym: GS840
Trade names: Hepsera (Gilead); Preveon
Indications: HIV infection, Hepatitis B infection
Category: Antiretroviral; Nucleotide analog reverse transcriptase inhibitor
Half-life: 16–18 hours
Clinically important, potentially hazardous interactions with: amikacin, amphotericin B, delavirdine, drugs causing kidney toxicity, foscarnet, gentamicin, hydroxyurea, pentamidine, tobramycin

Reactions

Skin

Pruritus

Rash (sic)

Other

Asthenia
  (1998): *Treatment update* 10(1), 1
Headache
  (1998): *Treatment update* 10(1), 1
Hot flashes
Nephrotoxicity
  (2005): Izzedine H+, *Am J Kidney Dis* 45(5), 804
  (2004): Izzedine H+, *Kidney Int* 66(3), 1153 (mild)
  (2003): Perazella MA, *Am J Med Sci* 325(6), 349
  (2002): Bendele RA+, *Hum Pathol* 33(5), 574
  (2002): Skowron G+, *J Infect Dis* 186(7), 1028
  (2002): Verhelst D+, *Am J Kidney Dis* 40(6), 1331
  (2001): Tanji N+, *Hum Pathol* 32(7), 734
Pain
  (1998): *Treatment update* 10(1), 1

ADENOSINE

Trade names: Adenic; Adeno-Jec; Adenocard (Astellas); Adenocur; Adenoject; Adenoscan (King); Adrecar; Atp; Krenosin; Krenosine
Indications: Paroxysmal supraventricular tachycardia, varicose vein complications with stasis dermatitis
Category: Antiarrhythmic class IV; Neurotransmitter
Half-life: <10 seconds
Clinically important, potentially hazardous interactions with: carbamazepine, dipyridamole, theophylline

Reactions

Skin

Burning (<1%)
Diaphoresis (<1%)
Rash (sic)

Mucosal/ENT

Dysgeusia (<1%)

Other

Chest pain
  (2004): Sadigh-Lindell B+, *J Pain* 5(9), 469
  (1990): Parker RB+, *Clin Pharm* 9(4), 261
Headache
Paresthesias (1%)
Tendinopathy/Tendon rupture
Vertigo (1%)

AGALSIDASE

Trade name: Fabrazyme (Genzyme)
Indications: Fabry disease
Category: Enzyme
Half-life: 45–102 minutes
Clinically important, potentially hazardous interactions with: None

Reactions

Skin

Edema of lip
Pallor (14%)

Pruritus
Rash (sic)
Urticaria

Mucosal/ENT

Rhinitis (38%)
Sinusitis (7%)

Other

Abdominal pain
Anxiety
Application-site reactions (~50%)
Bronchospasm
Chest pain (17%)
Chills
Depression (10%)
Fever (48%)
Headache (45%)
Hypersensitivity
Hypertension
Hypotension
Injection-site reactions
  (2006): Ries M+, *Pediatrics* 118(3), 924
Myalgia/Myositis/Myopathy/Myotoxicity
Pain (21%)
Paresthesias (14%)
Vertigo (14%)

ALBENDAZOLE

Trade names: ABZ; Albenza (GSK); Albezole; Alzol; Bendex; Eskazole; Vermin; Zentel
Indications: Nematode infections, hydatid cyst disease
Category: Antihelmintic
Half-life: 8–12 hours
Clinically important, potentially hazardous interactions with: dexamethasone

Reactions

Skin

Adverse effects (sic)
  (2002): Supali T+, *Trop Med Int Health* 7(10), 894 (with diethylcarbamazine)
Allergic reactions (sic) (<1%)
Angioedema
  (2006): Olson BG+, *Pediatr Infect Dis J* 25(5), 466 (with ivermectin and praziquantel)
Dermatitis
  (1991): Macedo NA+, *Contact Dermatitis* 25, 73
Fixed eruption
  (1998): Mahboob A+, *Int J Dermatol* 37, 833
  (1998): Mahboob A+, *JPMA J Pak Med Assoc* 48, 316
Pruritus (<1%)
  (2002): Supali T+, *Trop Med Int Health* 7(10), 894 (with diethylcarbamazine)
Rash (sic) (<1%)
Stevens–Johnson syndrome
  (1997): Dewardt S+, *Acta Derm Venereol* 77, 411
Urticaria (<1%)
  (2006): Olson BG+, *Pediatr Infect Dis J* 25(5), 466 (with ivermectin and praziquantel)
  (1991): Macedo NA+, *Contact Dermatitis* 25, 73

Mucosal/ENT

Xerostomia (<1%)

Hair

Hair – alopecia (<1%)

(1993): Tomas S+, *Enferm Infecc Microbiol Clin* (Spanish) 11, 113

(1990): Pilar-Garcia-Muret M+, *Int J Dermatol* 29, 669

Other

Abdominal pain

(2006): Olson BG+, *Pediatr Infect Dis J* 25(5), 466 (with ivermectin and praziquantel)

(2004): Garcia HH+, *N Engl J Med* 350(3), 249 (with dexamethasone)

Fever

(2006): Olson BG+, *Pediatr Infect Dis J* 25(5), 466 (with ivermectin and praziquantel)

Myalgia/Myositis/Myopathy/Myotoxicity

(2002): Supali T+, *Trop Med Int Health* 7(10), 894 (with diethylcarbamazine)

ALBUTEROL

Synonym: salbutamol

Trade names: AccuNeb (DEY); Asmaven; Broncho-Spray; Cobutolin; Combivent (Boehringer Ingelheim); Duoneb (DEY); Proventil (Schering); Salbulin; Ventolin (GSK); Ventoline; Volmax (Muro)

Indications: Bronchospasm associated with asthma

Category: Adrenergic beta-receptor agonist; Tocolytic

Half-life: 3–6 hours

Clinically important, potentially hazardous interactions with: atomoxetine, epinephrine, insulin detemir, insulin glulisine

Note: Combivent is albuterol and ipratropium

Reactions

Skin

Angioedema

Dermatitis

(2006): Tsuruta D+, *Contact Dermatitis* 54(2), 121

(1994): Smeenk G+, *Contact Dermatitis* 31, 123

Diaphoresis (1–10%)

(1989): Price AH+, *Drugs* 38, 77

Erythema (palmar) (with infusion)

(1992): Lebre C+, *Ann Dermatol Venereol* (French) 119, 293

(1990): Morin Leport LRM+, *Br J Dermatol* 122, 116

Erythema multiforme

Exanthems

Lupus erythematosus (pseudo-lupus)

(1987): Lacour JP+, *Presse Med* (French) 16, 1599

Pallor

Palmar erythema

(2007): Serrao R+, *Am J Clin Dermatol* 8(6), 347

Pruritus

(1991): Hatton MQ+, *Lancet* 337, 1169

Rash (sic)

Stevens–Johnson syndrome

Urticaria

(1991): Hatton MQ+, *Lancet* 337, 1169

Mucosal/ENT

Dysgeusia (1–10%)

Tinnitus

Xerostomia (1–10%)

Other

Chills

Headache

Tremor

ALCLOMETASONE

Trade names: Aclovate (GSK); Modrasone (Pliva)

Indications: Dermatoses

Category: Corticosteroid, topical

Half-life: N/A

Clinically important, potentially hazardous interactions with: licorice, live vaccines

Reactions

Skin

Allergic reactions

(1995): Lepoittevin JP+, *Arch Dermatol* 131(1), 31

Bruising

Burning

Dermatitis

(1999): Iwakiri K+, *Contact Dermatitis* 41(4), 218

(1991): Reitamo S+, *Contact Dermatitis* 25(1), 78

(1990): Kabasawa Y+, *Contact Dermatitis* 23(5), 374

Edema

Photoallergic reaction

(1996): Stitt WZ+, *Am J Contact Dermat* 7(3), 166

Pruritus

Rash (sic)

Sensitivity

Side effects (sic)

(1985): Thornfeldt C+, *J Int Med Res* 13(5), 276

Thinning

Urticaria

(1987): Kuokkanen K+, *Clin Ther* 9(2), 223 (1 case)

Other

Infections

ALDESLEUKIN

Synonyms: IL-2; interleukin-2

Trade names: Aerovent; Atem; Atronase; Narilet; Proleukin (Chiron)

Indications: Metastatic renal cell carcinoma

Category: Immunomodulator; Interleukin-2

Half-life: 6–85 minutes

Clinically important, potentially hazardous interactions with: altretamine, amikacin, aminoglycosides, antineoplastics, bleomycin, busulfan, carboplatin, carmustine, chlorambucil, cisplatin, corticosteroids, cyclophosphamide, cytarabine, dacarbazine, dactinomycin, daunorubicin, docetaxel, doxorubicin, estramustine, etoposide, fludarabine, fluorouracil, gemcitabine, gentamicin, hydroxyurea, idarubicin, ifosfamide, indomethacin, kanamycin, levamisole, lomustine, mechlorethamine, melphalan, mercaptopurine, methotrexate, mitomycin, mitotane, mitoxantrone, neomycin, pentostatin, plicamycin, procarbazine, streptomycin, streptozocin, thioguanine, thiotepa, tobramycin, tretinoin, uracil, vinblastine, vincristine, vinorelbine

Reactions

Skin

Allergic granulomatous angiitis (Churg–Strauss syndrome)
  (1997): Shiota Y+, *Inren Med* 36, 709
Allergic reactions (sic) (<1%)
Angioedema
  (1992): Baars JW+, *Ann Oncol* 3, 243
Bullae
  (2005): Hofmann M+, *Dermatology* 210, 74
Bullous dermatitis
  (1991): Staunton MR, *J Natl Cancer Inst* 83, 56
Bullous pemphigoid
  (1993): Fellner MJ, *Clin Dermatol* 11, 515
Dermatitis
  (1989): Kerker BJ+, *Semin Dermatol* 8, 173
  (1987): Gaspari AA+, *JAMA* 258, 1624 (1–5%)
Desquamation
  (2001): Chi KH+, *Oncology* 60, 110
Edema (47%)
  (1994): Rosenberg SA+, *JAMA* 271, 907
  (1990): Chien CH+, *Pediatrics* 86, 937
Erythema (41%)
  (1993): Wolkenstein P+, *J Am Acad Dermatol* 28, 66
  (1992): Blessing K+, *J Pathol* 167, 313
  (1988): Lee RE+, *Arch Dermatol* 124, 1811
  (1987): Gaspari AA+, *JAMA* 258, 1624
Erythema multiforme
  (2003): Chodorowska G+, *Ann Univ Mariae Curie Sklodowska*
    [Med] 58(2), 7
Erythema nodosum
  (2003): Chodorowska G+, *Ann Univ Mariae Curie Sklodowska*
    [Med] 58(2), 7
  (1989): Kerker BJ+, *Semin Dermatol* 8, 173
  (1987): Weinstein A+, *JAMA* 258, 3120
Erythroderma
  (1992): Blessing K+, *J Pathol* 167, 313
  (1991): Siegel JP+, *J Clin Oncol* 9, 694 (>5%)
  (1989): Kerker BJ+, *Semin Dermatol* 8, 173
  (1987): Gaspari AA+, *JAMA* 258, 1624
Exanthems
  (2003): Chodorowska G+, *Ann Univ Mariae Curie Sklodowska*
    [Med] 58(2), 7
  (1991): Dummer R+, *Dermatologica* 183, 95
  (1991): Siegel JP+, *J Clin Oncol* 9, 694 (>5%)
  (1989): Jost LM+, *Schweiz Med Wochenschr* (German) 119, 137
  (1987): Gaspari AA+, *JAMA* 258, 1624
Exfoliative dermatitis (14%)
  (1993): Larbre B+, *Ann Dermatol Venereol* (French) 120, 528
Graft-versus-host reaction
  (1995): Costello R+, *Bone Marrow Transplant* 16, 199
Intertrigo
  (1996): Prussick R+, *J Am Acad Dermatol* 35, 705
Kaposi's sarcoma
  (1989): Krigel RL+, *J Biol Response Mod* 8, 359
Linear IgA dermatosis
  (2002): Cohen LM+, *J Am Acad Dermatol* 46, S32 (passim)
  (1996): Tranvan A+, *J Am Acad Dermatol* 35, 865
  (1993): Oeda E+, *Am J Hematol* 44, 213
  (1990): Guillaume JC+, *Ann Dermatol Venereol* (French) 117, 899
Necrosis
  (1993): Wolkenstein P+, *J Am Acad Dermatol* 28, 66
  (1988): Rosenberg SA+, *Ann Intern Med* 108, 853 (3%)
Pemphigus
  (1995): Wolkenstein P+, *Arch Dermatol* 130, 890
  (1994): Prussick R+, *Arch Dermatol* 130, 890
  (1989): Ramseur WL+, *Cancer* 63, 2005 (fatal)

Peripheral edema (1–10%)
Petechiae (4%)
Photosensitivity
  (1992): Blessing K+, *J Pathol* 167, 313
Pruritus (48%)
  (2001): Chi KH+, *Oncology* 60(2), 110
  (1995): Wahlgren CF+, *Arch Dermatol Res* 287, 572
  (1994): Rosenberg SA+, *JAMA* 271, 907
  (1993): Wolkenstein P+, *J Am Acad Dermatol* 28, 66
  (1988): Lee RE+, *Arch Dermatol* 124, 1811
  (1987): Gaspari AA+, *JAMA* 258, 1624
Psoriasis
  (1991): Siegel JP+, *J Clin Oncol* 9, 694 (>5%)
  (1989): Kerker BJ+, *Semin Dermatol* 8, 173
  (1988): Lee RE+, *Arch Dermatol* 124, 1811 (exacerbation)
  (1987): Gaspari AA+, *JAMA* 258, 1624
Purpura (4%)
  (1989): Kerker BJ+, *Semin Dermatol* 8, 173
Rash (sic) (26%)
Sarcoidosis
  (2000): Blanche P+, *Clin Infect Dis* 31, 1493
Scleroderma
  (1994): Boni R, *Dermatology* 189, 330
  (1994): Puett DW+, *J Rheumatol* 21, 752
Stevens–Johnson syndrome
  (2003): Chodorowska G+, *Ann Univ Mariae Curie Sklodowska*
    [Med] 58(2), 7
Toxic epidermal necrolysis
  (2003): Chodorowska G+, *Ann Univ Mariae Curie Sklodowska*
    [Med] 58(2), 7
  (1992): Wiener JS+, *South Med J* 85, 656
Urticaria (2%)
  (2003): Chodorowska G+, *Ann Univ Mariae Curie Sklodowska*
    [Med] 58(2), 7
  (1993): Wolkenstein P+, *J Am Acad Dermatol* 28, 66
  (1992): Baars JW+, *Ann Oncol* 3, 243
Vasculitis
  (2003): Chodorowska G+, *Ann Univ Mariae Curie Sklodowska*
    [Med] 58(2), 7
Vitiligo
  (1996): Rosenberg SA+, *J Immunother Emphasis Tumor Immunol*
    19, 81
  (1995): Wolkenstein P+, *Arch Dermatol* 130, 890
  (1994): Scheibenbogen C+, *Eur J Cancer* (30A) 8, 1209
Xerosis (15%)

Mucosal/ENT

Aphthous stomatitis
  (1987): Gaspari AA+, *JAMA* 258, 1624 (5%)
Dysgeusia (7%)
Glossitis
  (1987): Gaspari AA+, *JAMA* 258, 1624 (30%)
Oral mucosal eruption
  (1989): Kerker BJ+, *Semin Dermatol* 8, 173
  (1987): Gaspari AA+, *JAMA* 258, 1624
Oral ulceration
  (1990): Chien CH+, *Pediatrics* 86, 937
Stomatitis (32%)
Xerostomia
  (2001): Chi KH+, *Oncology* 60, 110

Hair

Hair – alopecia (<1%)
  (1989): Jost LM+, *Schweiz Med Wochenschr* (German) 119, 137
  (1987): Gaspari AA+, *JAMA* 258, 1624 (10%)

Other

Death
Depression

(2004): Capuron L+, *Brain Behav Immun* 18(3), 205
(2004): Patten SB+, *Psychother Psychosom* 73(4), 207
(2001): Maes M+, *Mol Psychiatry* 6(4), 475
Headache
Injection-site inflammation
  (2002): Assmann K+, *Hautarzt* 53(8), 554
  (1999): Asadullah K+, *Arch Dermatol* 135, 187
Injection-site nodules
  (2002): Assmann K+, *Hautarzt* 53(8), 554
  (1993): Klapholtz L+, *Bone Marrow Transplant* 11, 443
Injection-site panniculitis
  (1992): Baars JW+, *Br J Cancer* 66, 698
Injection-site reactions (sic) (3%)
  (2002): Assmann K+, *Hautarzt* 53(8), 554
Myalgia/Myositis/Myopathy/Myotoxicity (6%)
Rhabdomyolysis
  (1995): Anderlini P+, *Cancer* 76(4), 678

ALEFACEPT

Trade name: Amevive (Biogen)
Indications: Chronic plaque psoriasis (in adults)
Category: Immunosuppressant
Half-life: 270 hours
Clinically important, potentially hazardous interactions with: None

Reactions

Skin

Adverse effects (sic) (2.5%)
  (2002): Krueger GG+, *J Am Acad Dermatol* 47(6), 821
  (2001): Ellis CN+, *N Engl J Med* 345(4), 248
Allergic reactions
Angioedema
  (2002): Cather J+, *Am J Clin Dermatol* 3(3), 159
Herpes simplex
  (2002): Cather J+, *Am J Clin Dermatol* 3(3), 159
Lipodermatosclerosis
  (2005): Gribetz CH+, *J Am Acad Dermatol* 53(1), 73
Lymphoma (3 cases)
Malignancies (1.3%)
Necrotizing cellulitis
Nevi
  (2006): Bovenschen HJ+, *Br J Dermatol* 154(5), 880
Pruritus (2–5%)
  (2005): Scheinfeld N, *Expert Opin Drug Saf* 4(6), 975
Psoriasis
  (2004): Thaler D, Monona, WI (from Internet) (observation)
     (recurrence)
Urticaria (<1%)

Mucosal/ENT

Nasopharyngitis
  (2007): Strober BE+, *Dermatol Ther* 20(4), 270 (passim)
Rhinitis
  (2005): Scheinfeld N, *Expert Opin Drug Saf* 4(6), 975
Sinusitis
  (2006): Koo JY+, *J Drugs Dermatol* 5(7), 623

Other

Asthenia
  (2005): Gribetz CH+, *J Am Acad Dermatol* 53(1), 73
  (2005): Scheinfeld N, *Expert Opin Drug Saf* 4(6), 975
Chills (transient) (<2%)

(2003): Kimball AB+, *Poster, American Academy of Dermatology Meeting* San Francisco, CA
(2002): Krueger GG+, *J Am Acad Dermatol* 47(6), 821
(2001): Ellis CN+, *N Engl J Med* 345(4), 248
Cough (<2%)
  (2005): Gribetz CH+, *J Am Acad Dermatol* 53(1), 73
  (2001): Ellis CN+, *N Engl J Med* 345(4), 248
Headache
  (2007): Strober BE+, *Dermatol Ther* 20(4), 270 (passim)
  (2006): Koo JY+, *J Drugs Dermatol* 5(7), 623
  (2005): Gottlieb AB+, *J Drugs Dermatol* 4(6), 718
  (2005): Gribetz CH+, *J Am Acad Dermatol* 53(1), 73
  (2005): Scheinfeld N, *Expert Opin Drug Saf* 4(6), 975
Hepatotoxicity
  (2007): Strober BE+, *Dermatol Ther* 20(4), 270 (passim)
Hypersensitivity
Infections (0.7–1.5%)
  (2002): Krueger GG+, *J Am Acad Dermatol* 47(6), 821
  (2001): Ellis CN+, *N Engl J Med* 345(4), 248
Injection-site bleeding (4%)
Injection-site edema (2%)
Injection-site hypersensitivity
Injection-site inflammation (4%)
Injection-site pain (7%)
  (2005): Gribetz CH+, *J Am Acad Dermatol* 53(1), 73
Injection-site reactions
  (2007): Strober BE+, *Dermatol Ther* 20(4), 270 (passim)
Myalgia/Myositis/Myopathy/Myotoxicity (2–5%)
  (2005): Gribetz CH+, *J Am Acad Dermatol* 53(1), 73
Upper respiratory infection
  (2007): Strober BE+, *Dermatol Ther* 20(4), 270 (passim)
  (2006): Koo JY+, *J Drugs Dermatol* 5(7), 623
  (2005): Gribetz CH+, *J Am Acad Dermatol* 53(1), 73
  (2005): Scheinfeld N, *Expert Opin Drug Saf* 4(6), 975
Vertigo (<2%)
  (2001): Ellis CN+, *N Engl J Med* 345(4), 248

ALEMTUZUMAB

Synonyms: Campath-1H; DNA-derived Humanized Monoclonal Antibody; Humanized IgG1 Anti-CD52 Monoclonal Antibody
Trade names: Campath (Berlex); MabCampath (Schering)
Indications: B-cell chronic lymphcyotic leukemia, non-Hodgkin's lymphoma
Category: Immunosuppressant; Monoclonal antibody
Half-life: 12 days

Note: Prophylactic therapy against PCP pneumonia and herpes viral infections is recommended upon initiation of therapy and for at least 2 months following last dose

Reactions

Skin

Abscess
Allergic reactions (sic) (<1%)
Angioedema (<1%)
Bullous dermatitis (<1%)
Cellulitis (<1%)
Facial edema (<1%)
Hematomas (<1%)
Herpes simplex
  (2007): Laros-van Gorkom BA+, *Neth J Med* 65(9), 333 (6%)
  (2003): Lundin J+, *Blood* 101(11), 4267
Herpes zoster
  (2007): Laros-van Gorkom BA+, *Neth J Med* 65(9), 333 (9%)

(2004): Wendtner CM+, *Leukemia* 18(6), 1093
Peripheral edema (13%)
Pruritus
Purpura (8%)
Rash (sic)
(2003): Ferrajoli A+, *Cancer* 98(4), 773
Squamous cell carcinoma (<1%)
(2003): Lundin J+, *Blood* 101(11), 4267
Urticaria
(2000): Tang SC+, *Leuk Lymphoma* 24(1-2), 93

Mucosal/ENT
Dysgeusia (<1%)
Gingivitis (<1%)
Sinusitis
(2004): Wendtner CM+, *Leukemia* 18(6), 1093
Stomatitis (14%)
Stomatodynia

Other
Anaphylactoid reactions/Anaphylaxis (<1%)
Application-site reactions
(2003): Lynn A+, *Oncol Nurs Forum* 30(4), 689
(2002): Rai KR+, *J Clin Oncol* 20(18), 3891 (with fludarabine)
Asthenia
(2007): Laros-van Gorkom BA+, *Neth J Med* 65(9), 333 (22%)
Chills
(2000): Flynn JM+, *Curr Opin Oncol* 12(6), 574
Death
(2006): Martin SI+, *Clin Infect Dis* 43(1), 16
(2004): Enblad G+, *Blood* 103(8), 2920 (5 cases)
(2003): Lundin J+, *Blood* 101(11), 4267
(2002): Keating MJ+, *J Clin Oncol* 20(1), 205 (2 cases)
(1998): Lundin J+, *J Clin Oncol* 16(10), 3257
Depression (7%)
Fever
(2007): Laros-van Gorkom BA+, *Neth J Med* 65(9), 333 (72%)
(2003): Ferrajoli A+, *Cancer* 98(4), 773 (38%)
Headache
Inappropriate secretion of antidiuretic hormone (SIADH)
(2005): Kunz JS+, *Leuk Lymphoma* 46(4), 635
Infections
(2007): Lim Z+, *J Infect* 54(2), e83 (Opportunistic)
(Toxoplasmosis)
(2007): Peleg AY+, *Clin Infect Dis* 44(2), 204 (opportunistic)
(10%)
(2006): Martin SI+, *Clin Infect Dis* 43(1), 16 (opportunistic)
(2006): Osterborg A+, *Semin Oncol* 33(2 suppl 5), S29
(2006): Thursky KA+, *Br J Haematol* 132(1), 3
(2006): Tibes R+, *Cancer* 106(12), 2645
(2006): Wadhwa PD+, *Semin Oncol* 33(2), 240
(2004): Tan HP+, *Transplantation* 78(11), 1683
(2004): Wendtner CM+, *Leukemia* 18(6), 1093
(2003): Lundin J+, *Blood* 101(11), 4267
(2002): Keating MJ+, *J Clin Oncol* 20(1), 205
(2002): Lundin J+, *Blood* 100(3), 768
(2002): Rai KR+, *J Clin Oncol* 20(18), 3891 (with fludarabine)
(2001): Khorana A+, *Leuk Lymphoma* 41(1), 77
(2000): Tang SC+, *Leuk Lymphoma* 24(1-2), 93
(1998): Lundin J+, *J Clin Oncol* 16(10), 3257
Injection-site pruritus (30–40%)
Injection-site reactions (sic)
(2006): Osterborg A+, *Semin Oncol* 33(2 Suppl 5), S29
(2002): Keating MJ+, *Blood* 99(10), 3554
(2002): Keating MJ+, *J Clin Oncol* 20(1), 205
(2002): Lundin J+, *Blood* 100(3), 768 (90%)
(2001): Khorana A+, *Leuk Lymphoma* 41(1), 77
Lymphoproliferative disease (64% to 70%)
Myalgia/Myositis/Myopathy/Myotoxicity (<1%)

Phlebitis (<1%)
Polymyositis (<1%)
Thrombophlebitis (<1%)

ALENDRONATE

Trade names: Fosalan; Fosamax (Merck)
Indications: Osteoporosis in postmenopausal women, Paget's disease
Category: Bisphosphonate
Half-life: >10 years

Reactions

Skin
Angioedema
Erythema (<1%)
(1996): Keen RW+, *Br J Clin Pract* 50, 211
Erythema gyratum
(2003): High WA+, *J Am Acad Dermatol* 48(6), 945
Erythema multiforme
(2000): Madnani N, Mumbai, India (from Internet) (observation)
Exanthems
(2000): Madnani N, Mumbai, India (from Internet) (observation)
Fixed eruption
(1998): McCarthy J, Ft. Worth, TX (from Internet) (observation)
Peripheral edema
Petechiae
(1997): Berger R, St. George, UT (from Internet) (observation)
Photosensitivity
Pruritus (0.6%)
(2000): Madnani N, Mumbai, India (from Internet) (observation)
(1997): Kyriakidou-Himonas M+, *Advances in Therapy* 14, 281
Rash (sic) (<1%)
(1997): Berger R, St. George, UT (from Internet) (observation)
(1996): Freedholm D+, *Osteoporosis Int* 6, 261
(1996): Keen RW+, *Br J Clin Pract* 50, 211
(1996): Selby PL, *Osteoporosis Int* 6, S21
(1995): Chestnut CH+, *Am J Med* 99, 144
Stevens–Johnson syndrome
Toxic epidermal necrolysis
Urticaria

Mucosal/ENT
Dysgeusia (0.6%)
(1997): Kyriakidou-Himonas M+, *Advances in Therapy* 14, 281
Oral ulceration
(2004): Krasagakis K+, *J Am Acad Dermatol* 50(4), 651
(1999): Demerjian N+, *Clin Rheumatol* 18, 349
Stomatitis (Contact)
(2006): Rubegni P+, *N Engl J Med* 355(22), e25

Eyes
Conjunctivitis
(2003): Frauenfelder FW+, *N Engl J Med* 348, 1187
Ocular stinging
(2003): Frauenfelder FW+, *N Engl J Med* 348, 1187
Ophthalmitis
(1999): Mbekeani JN+, *Arch Ophthalmol* 117, 837
Uveitis
(2006): Richards JC+, *Cornea* 25(9), 1100
(2004): Asensio Sanchez VM+, *Arch Soc Esp Oftalmol* 79(2), 85
Visual disturbances
(2004): Coleman CI+, *Pharmacotherapy* 24(6), 799 (rare)

Other

Abdominal pain
  (2003): Segal E+, *Isr Med Assoc J* 5(12), 859 (42.8%)
Headache
Hypersensitivity
  (1996): Kirk JK+, *Am Fam Physician* 54, 2053
Seizures
  (2002): MacIsaac RJ+, *J R Soc Med* 95(12), 615

ALFENTANIL

Trade names: Alfenta (Akorn); Rapifen
Indications: General anesthesia, post-operative pain
Category: Analgesic, opioid; Anesthetic
Half-life: 83–97 minutes (adults)
Clinically important, potentially hazardous interactions with: erythromycin, ranitidine, ritonavir

Reactions

Skin

Clammy skin (<1%)
Pruritus (<1%)
  (1999): Kyriakides K+, *Br J Anaesth* 82, 439
Rash (sic) (<1%)
Shivering (3–9%)
  (2004): Crozier TA+, *Eur J Anaesthesiol* 21(1), 20 (41%)
Urticaria (<1%)

Other

Hypotension
  (2001): Maguire AM+, *Br J Anaesth* 86(1), 90 (4 cases)

ALFUZOSIN

Trade names: Uroxatral (Sanofi-Aventis); Xatral
Indications: Benign prostatic hyperplasia
Category: Adrenergic alpha-receptor antagonist
Half-life: 10 hours
Clinically important, potentially hazardous interactions with: atenolol, cimetidine, diltiazem, itraconazole, ketoconazole, ritonavir

Reactions

Skin

Allergic reactions (sic)
  (1997): Lopatkin NA+, *Urol Nefrol* (Mosk) 941(5), 14
Angioedema
Dermatomyositis
  (1998): Vela-Casasempere P+, *Br J Rheumatol* 37(10), 1135
Edema
Rash (sic)
Toxic epidermal necrolysis
  (2006): Wang YS+, *Arch Dermatol* 142(7), 938

Mucosal/ENT

Sinusitis (1–2%)

Other

Abdominal pain (1–2%)
Asthenia (3%)
Chest pain

Headache (3%)
Hypotension
  (2006): Hartung R+, *J Urol* 175(2), 624
Pain (1–2%)
Upper respiratory infection (3%)
Vertigo (6%)
  (2006): Elhilali M+, *BJU Int* 97(3), 513 (3%)
  (2006): Hartung R+, *J Urol* 175(2), 624 (5%)
  (2005): Nordling J, *BJU Int* 95(7), 1006 (6%)
  (2003): Marks LS+, *Urology* 62(5), 888
  (2003): Roehrborn CG+, *BJU Int* 92(3), 257
  (2000): Lukacs B+, *Urology* 55(4), 540 (6%)
  (2000): Sanchez-Chapado M+, *Eur Urol* 37(4), 421 (6%)
  (1996): Lukacs B+, *Eur Urol* 29(1), 29 (1.4%)
  (1994): Jardin A+, *Br J Urol* 74(5), 579 (4%)

ALGLUCERASE

Trade name: Ceredase (Genzyme)
Indications: Gaucher disease
Category: Enzyme, glucocerebrosidase
Half-life: 3.6–10.4 minutes
Clinically important, potentially hazardous interactions with: None

Reactions

Skin

Angioedema
Peripheral edema
Pruritus
  (1999): Rosenberg M+, *Blood* 93(6), 2081
Urticaria
  (1999): Rosenberg M+, *Blood* 93(6), 2081

Mucosal/ENT

Oral ulceration
Parosmia

Other

Asthenia
Chills
Fever
Headache
Hot flashes
Hypersensitivity
  (1999): Rosenberg M+, *Blood* 93(6), 2081
Hypertension
  (1997): Harats D+, *Acta Haematol* 98(1), 47
  (1996): Dawson A+, *Ann Intern Med* 125(11), 901
Injection-site burning
Injection-site edema

ALGLUCOSIDASE ALFA

Trade name: Myozyme (Genzyme)
Indications: Pompe disease (Glycogen storage disease Type II), GAA deficiency
Category: Alfa-glucosidase; Enzyme
Half-life: 2–3 hours
Clinically important, potentially hazardous interactions with: N/A

Note: Pompe disease is an autosomal recessive muscular disorder caused by the deficiency or lack of the enzyme acid alpha-glucosidase, which is essential for normal muscle development and function. The disease, which usually results in death from respiratory failure, is rapidly fatal in the newborn

Reactions

Skin
  Angioedema
  Dermatitis
  Hyperhidrosis
  Livedo reticularis
  Pallor
  Pruritus
  Rash (sic) (54%)
  Urticaria (21%)

Mucosal/ENT
  Oral candidiasis (31%)
  Otitis (44%)
  Rhinitis

Eyes
  Periorbital edema

Other
  Anaphylactoid reactions/Anaphylaxis
  Application-site reactions (51%)
  Asthenia
  Cough (46%)
  Fever (97%)
  Headache
  Hypersensitivity
  Upper respiratory infection (44%)

ALISKIREN

Trade name: Tekturna (Novartis)
Indications: Hypertension
Category: Antihypertensive; Renin inhibitor
Half-life: 24 hours
Clinically important, potentially hazardous interactions with: furosemide, ketoconazole

Reactions

Skin
  Angioedema
  Rash (sic) (1%)

Eyes
  Periorbital edema

Other
  Abdominal pain
  Cough
    (2006): Vaidyanathan S+, *Int J Clin Pract* 60(11), 1343
  Headache
    (2006): Vaidyanathan S+, *Int J Clin Pract* 60(11), 1343
  Vertigo

ALITRETINOIN

Trade name: Panretin (Ligand)
Indications: Kaposi's sarcoma cutaneous lesions
Category: Retinoid
Half-life: N/A

Reactions

Skin
  Abrasion
  Adverse effects (sic)
    (2000): Duvic M+, *Arch Dermatol* 136, 1461 (17%)
  Bullous dermatitis
  Burning
    (2002): Morganroth GS, *Arch Dermatol* 138, 542
  Edema (3–8%)
    (2000): Duvic M+, *Arch Dermatol* 136, 1461 (3%)
  Exfoliative dermatitis (3–9%)
  Photosensitivity
  Pigmentation (3%)
    (2000): Duvic M+, *Arch Dermatol* 136, 1461 (3%)
  Pruritus (8–11%)
  Rash (sic) (25–77%)
    (2000): Duvic M+, *Arch Dermatol* 136, 1461 (69%)
  Toxicity (sic)
    (2002): Miles SA+, *AIDS* 16(3), 421
  Ulcerations (2%)
    (2000): Duvic M+, *Arch Dermatol* 136, 1461
  Xerosis (10%)
    (2000): Duvic M+, *Arch Dermatol* 136, 1461 (10%)

Hair
  Hair – alopecia

Other
  Application-site dermatitis
    (2002): Morganroth GS, *Arch Dermatol* 138, 542
  Application-site reactions
    (1999): Walmsley S+, *J Acquir Immune Defic Syndr* 22, 325
  Headache
    (2002): Miles SA+, *AIDS* 16(3), 421 (13 cases)
  Myalgia/Myositis/Myopathy/Myotoxicity
  Pain
    (2000): Duvic M+, *Arch Dermatol* 136, 1461 (18%)
  Paresthesias (3–22%)

ALLOPURINOL

Trade names: Allo 300; Allo-Puren; Alloprin; Atisuril; Bleminol; Caplenal; Hamarin; Novo-Purol; Purinol; Unizuric; Zyloprim (Prometheus); Zyloric
Indications: Gouty arthritis
Category: Purine analog; Xanthine oxidase inhibitor
Half-life: 1–3 hours
Clinically important, potentially hazardous interactions with: acenocoumarol, amoxicillin, ampicillin, azathioprine, dicumarol, imidapril, mercaptopurine, pantoprazole, uracil/tegafur, vidarabine

Reactions

Skin
  Acute generalized exanthematous pustulosis (AGEP)

(2002): Lun K+, *Australas J Dermatol* 43(2), 140
(1995): Moreau A+, *Int J Dermatol* 34, 263 (passim)

Adverse effects (sic)
  (2006): Chandeclerc ML+, *Allergy* 61(12), 1492
  (2003): Chubar Y+, *Br J Haematol* 122(5), 768

Allergic reactions (sic) (severe)
  (1999): Tanna SB+, *Ann Pharmacother* 33, 1180

Angioedema
  (1996): Yale SH+, *Hosp Pract Off Ed* 31, 92

Diaphoresis (<1%)

Eosinophilic pustular folliculitis
  (2006): Ooi CG+, *Australas J Dermatol* 47(4), 270
  (2002): Maejima H+, *Acta Derm Venereol* 82(4), 316

Erythema multiforme (<1%)
  (2001): Perez A+, *Contact Dermatitis* 44, 113 (with amoxicillin)
  (1999): Fonseka MM+, *Ceylon Med J* 44, 190
  (1996): Kumar A+, *BMJ* 312, 173
  (1984): Pennell DJ+, *Lancet* 1, 463

Exanthems (1–5%)
  (2003): Masaki T+, *Acta Derm Venereol* 83(2), 128
  (2001): Fam AG+, *Arthritis Rheum* 44, 231
  (1998): Dintiman B, Fairfax, VA (from Internet) (observation)
  (1992): Fam AG+, *Am J Med* 93, 299
  (1989): Chan SH+, *Dermatologica* 179, 32
  (1987): Hoigné R+, *N Engl J Med* 316, 1217
  (1984): Hande KR+, *Am J Med* 76, 47
  (1981): Jick H+, *J Clin Pharmacol* 21, 456 (with ampicillin) (14%)
  (1981): McInnes GT+, *Ann Rheum Dis* 40, 245

Exfoliative dermatitis (>10%)
  (2004): Rodevand E+, *Tidsskr Nor Laegeforen* 21;124(20), 2618
  (2001): Dominguez Ortega J+, *An Med Intern* 18(1), 27
  (1996): Emmerson BT, *N Engl J Med* 334, 445
  (1996): Sigurdsson V+, *J Am Acad Dermatol* 35, 53
  (1989): Chan SH+, *Dermatologica* 179, 32
  (1984): Vinciullo C, *Aust J Dermatol* 25, 59

Fixed eruption (<1%)
  (2004): Teraki Y+, *Dermatology* 209(1), 29
  (2001): Dominguez Ortega J+, *An Med Intern* 18(1), 27
  (1999): Sehgal VN+, *J Dermatol* 26, 198 (transitory giant)
  (1998): Mahboob A+, *Int J Dermatol* 37, 833
  (1998): Umpierrez A+, *J Allergy Clin Immunol* 101, 286
  (1996): Gimbel Moral LF+, *Med Clin* (Barc) (Spanish) 106, 119
  (1996): Kelso JM+, *J Allergy Clin Immunol* 97, 1171
  (1990): Audicana M+, *Clin Exp Allergy* 20(Supp 1), 121

Graft-versus-host reaction
  (1998): Jappe U+, *Hautarzt* (German) 49, 126

Granuloma annulare (disseminated)
  (1996): Brechtel B+, *Hautarzt* 47(2), 143
  (1995): Becker D+, *Hautarzt* (German) 46, 343

Ichthyosis

Lichen planus (<1%)

Lupus erythematosus
  (1980): Condemi JJ, *Geriatrics* 35(3), 81

Lymphocytoma cutis
  (1988): Raymond JZ+, *Cutis* 41, 323

Necrotizing vasculitis

Perforating foot ulceration
  (1997): Bouloc A+, *Clin Exp Dermatol* 21, 351

Petechiae

Photosensitivity
  (1986): Lerman S, *Ophthalmology* 93, 304

Pityriasis rosea
  (2006): Atzori L+, *Dermatology Online Journal* 12(1), 1 (with hydrochlorothiazide)

Pruritus (<1%)
  (2003): Mete N+, *J Investig Allergol Clin Immunol* 13(4), 281
  (2002): Lun K+, *Australas J Dermatol* 43(2), 140
  (2001): Dominguez Ortega J+, *An Med Intern* 18(1), 27

(2001): Fam AG+, *Arthritis Rheum* 44, 231
(1998): Dintiman B, Fairfax, VA (from Internet) (observation)

Purpura (>10%)

Pustules
  (2002): Lun K+, *Australas J Dermatol* 43(2), 140

Pustuloderma
  (1994): Fitzgerald DA+, *Clin Exp Dermatol* 19, 243

Rash (sic) (>10%)
  (2005): Choi SH+, *Korean J Hepatol* 11(1), 80
  (2003): Mete N+, *J Investig Allergol Clin Immunol* 13(4), 281
  (2001): Dominguez Ortega J+, *An Med Intern* 18(1), 27
  (1996): Yale SH+, *Hosp Pract Off Ed* 31, 92

Sensitivity (sic)

Stevens–Johnson syndrome (>10%)
  (2008): Halevy S+, *J Am Acad Dermatol* 58(1), 25
  (2008): Lee HY+, *J Am Acad Dermatol* 59(2), 352
  (2007): Dainichi T+, *Dermatology* 215(1), 86
  (2005): Lin MS+, *Intern Med J* 35(3), 188
  (2003): Fine P+, *Optometry* 74(10), 659
  (2003): Yeung CK+, *Acta Derm Venereol* 83(3), 179 (8 cases)
  (1999): Halevy S+, *Int J Dermatol* 38(11), 835
  (1995): Gonzalez U+, *Rev Invest Clin* 47(5), 409
  (1995): Roujeau JC+, *N Engl J Med* 333(24), 1600
  (1993): Leenutaphong V+, *Int J Dermatol* 32, 428
  (1992): Goodglick TA+, *Ophthalmic Surg* 23, 557
  (1989): Chan SH+, *Dermatologica* 179, 32
  (1985): Edwards R+, *Dimens Crit Care Nurs* 4, 335
  (1985): Renwick IG, *BMJ* 291, 485
  (1985): Ting HC+, *Int J Dermatol* 24, 587
  (1984): Pennell DJ+, *Lancet* 1, 463 (fatal)

Toxic epidermal necrolysis
  (2008): Halevy S+, *J Am Acad Dermatol* 58(1), 25
  (2008): Lee HY+, *J Am Acad Dermatol* 59(2), 352
  (2007): Dainichi T+, *Dermatology* 215(1), 86
  (2007): Paquet P+, *Burns* 33(1), 100
  (2005): Kakeda M+, *J Dermatol* 32(8), 654
  (2005): Lin MS+, *Intern Med J* 35(3), 188
  (2005): Nasser M+, *Am J Med Sci* 329(2), 95
  (2003): Yeung CK+, *Acta Derm Venereol* 83(3), 179 (8 cases)
  (2002): Correia O+, *Arch Dermatol* 138, 29 (2 cases)
  (2001): Hammer B+, *Dtsch Med Wochenschr* 126(47), 1331
  (1999): Sorkin MJ, Denver, CO (from Internet) (observation)
  (1995): Roujeau JC+, *N Engl J Med* 333(24), 1600
  (1995): Wolkenstein P+, *Arch Dermatol* 131, 544
  (1994): Alfandari S+, *Infection* 22, 365
  (1993): Correia O+, *Dermatology* 186, 32
  (1993): Leenutaphong V+, *Int J Dermatol* 32, 428
  (1991): Sakellariou G+, *Int J Artif Organs* 14, 634
  (1987): Guillaume JC+, *Arch Dermatol* 123, 1166
  (1986): Kumar L, *Indian J Dermatol* 31, 53
  (1985): Auboeck J+, *BMJ* 290, 1969
  (1985): Renwick IG, *BMJ* 291, 485
  (1985): Zakraoui L+, *Tunis Med* (French) 63, 167
  (1984): Chan HL, *J Am Acad Dermatol* 10, 973
  (1984): Dan M+, *Int J Dermatol* 23, 142

Toxic erythema
  (1995): Rademaker M, *N Z Med J* 108, 165

Toxic pustuloderma
  (1994): Boffa MJ+, *Br J Dermatol* 131, 447
  (1994): Fitzgerald DA+, *Clin Exp Dermatol* 19, 243
  (1993): Yu RC+, *Br J Dermatol* 128, 95

Urticaria (>10%)
  (2001): Dominguez Ortega J+, *An Med Interna* 18(1), 27
  (1999): Litt JZ, Beachwood, OH (personal case) (observation)
  (1992): Breathnach SM+, *Adverse Drug Reactions and the Skin* Blackwell, Oxford, 193 (passim)
  (1991): Anderson MH+, *Ann Allergy* 66, 207

Vasculitis (<1%)
  (2001): Dominguez Ortega J+, *An Med Intern* 18(1), 27

(1998): Choi HK+, *Clin Exp Rheumatol* 16, 743
(1996): Emmerson BT, *N Engl J Med* 334, 445

Mucosal/ENT
Dysgeusia
Mucocutaneous eruption
Oral ulceration
  (1984): Chau NY+, *Oral Surg Oral Med Oral Pathol* 58, 397
    (lichenoid)
Stomatitis
  (1981): McInnes GT+, *Ann Rheum Dis* 40, 245
Tinnitus
Tongue edema (<1%)

Hair
Hair – alopecia (1–10%)

Eyes
Cataract
  (1985): Taylor F, *Aust Fam Physician* 14(8), 744
Corneal scarring
  (2003): Fine P+, *Optometry* 74(10), 659–64
Keratopathy
  (2003): Fine P+, *Optometry* 74(10), 659–64
Ocular xerosis
  (2003): Fine P+, *Optometry* 74(10), 659–64
Periorbital edema
  (1981): McInnes GT+, *Ann Rheum Dis* 40, 245
Symblepharon
  (2003): Fine P+, *Optometry* 74(10), 659–64

Other
Chills (1–10%)
Death
  (2005): Gutierrez-Macias A+, *BMJ* 331(7517), 623
  (2002): Correia O+, *Arch Dermatol* 138, 29 (1 case)
  (2001): Hammer B+, *Dtsch Med Wochenschr* 126(47), 1331
DRESS syndrome
  (2005): Markel A, *Isr Med Assoc J* 7(10), 656
  (2004): Cordel N+, *Ann Dermatol Venereol* 131(12), 1059 (2
    cases)
  (2004): Dia D+, *Dakar Med* 49(2), 114
  (2004): Marrakchi C+, *Rev Med Interne* 25(3), 252
  (2001): Descamps V+, *Arch Dermatol* 137, 301 (passim)
Fever
  (2005): Choi SH+, *Korean J Hepatol* 11(1), 80
  (2003): Mete N+, *J Investig Allergol Clin Immunol* 13(4), 281
Headache
Hypersensitivity
  (2007): Dainichi T+, *Dermatology* 215(1), 86
  (2006): Kano Y+, *J Am Acad Dermatol* 55(4), 727
  (2004): Rodevand E+, *Tidsskr Nor Laegeforen* 21;124(20), 2618
  (2003): Masaki T+, *Acta Derm Venereol* 83(2), 128
  (2003): Mete N+, *J Investig Allergol Clin Immunol* 13(4), 281
  (2002): Perez Pimiento AJ+, *Rev Clin Esp* 202(6), 339
  (2002): Sommers LM+, *Arch Intern Med* 162(10), 1190
  (2001): Arakawa M+, *Intern Med* 40(4), 331
  (2001): Benito-Leon J+, *Eur Neurol* 45, 186
  (2001): Dominguez Ortega J+, *An Med Interna* 18(1), 27
  (2001): Hammer B+, *Dtsch Med Wochenschr* 126(47), 1331
  (2001): Rivas Gonzalez P+, *Rev Clin Esp* 201(8), 493
  (1999): Gillott TJ+, *Rheumatology* (Oxford) 38, 85
  (1999): Melsom RD, *Rheumatology* 38, 1301 (familial)
  (1999): Morel D+, *Nephrol Dial Transplant* 14, 780
  (1998): Kluger E, *Ugeskr Laeger* (Danish) 160, 1179
  (1998): Pluim HJ+, *Neth J Med* 52, 107
  (1997): Carpenter C, *Tenn Med* 90, 151
  (1996): Kumar A+, *BMJ* 312, 173
  (1995): Elasy T+, *West J Med* 162, 360

(1994): Lee SS+, *Chung Hua Min Kuo Wei Sheng Wu Chi Mien I
  Hsueh Tsa Chih* 27, 140
(1994): Salinas Martin A+, *Aten Primaria* (Spanish) 14, 694
(1989): Puig JG+, *J Rheumatol* 16, 842
(1988): McDonald J+, *J Rheumatol* 15, 865
(1985): Stein CM, *S Afr Med J* 67, 935
(1984): Vinciullo C, *Aust J Dermatol* 25, 59
(1984): Vinciullo C, *Med J Aust* 141, 449
Myalgia/Myositis/Myopathy/Myotoxicity
  (2002): Terawaki H+, *Nippon Jinzo Gakkai Shi* 44, 50
  (1996): Ghanem BM+, *J Egypt Soc Parasitol* 26, 619
Paresthesias (<1%)
Polyarteritis nodosa
Pseudolymphoma
  (1993): Kerl H+, *Dermatology in General Medicine* McGraw-Hill
  New York
Thrombophlebitis (<1%)

ALMOTRIPTAN

Trade name: Axert (Ortho-McNeil)
Indications: Migraine headaches
Category: 5-HT1 agonist; Serotonin receptor agonist; Triptan
Half-life: 3–4 hours
**Clinically important, potentially hazardous interactions
with:** dihydroergotamine, ergotamine, ketoconazole,
methysergide

Reactions

Skin
Dermatitis
Diaphoresis (<1%)
Erythema (<1%)
Photosensitivity (<1%)
Pruritus (<1%)
Rash (sic) (<1%)

Mucosal/ENT
Dysgeusia (<1%)
Parosmia (<1%)
Sialorrhea (<1%)
Tinnitus (<1%)
Xerostomia (1%)
  (2002): Balbisi EA, *Am J Health Syst Pharm* 59(22), 2184

Other
Asthenia
  (2004): McEwen J+, *Biopharm Drug Dispos* 25(7), 303
  (2002): Balbisi EA, *Am J Health Syst Pharm* 59(22), 2184
Chest pain
  (2002): Mathew NT+, *Headache* 2002 Jan; 42(1), 32 (2%)
Chills (<1%)
Depression (<1%)
Headache
  (2005): Burstein R+, *Pain.* 2005 May; 115(1–2), 21 (transient)
  (2004): McEwen J+, *Biopharm Drug Dispos* 25(7), 303
Injection-site irritation
  (2001): Cabarrocas X, *Clin Ther* 23(11), 1867
Myalgia/Myositis/Myopathy/Myotoxicity (<1%)
Paresthesias (1%)
  (2002): Balbisi EA, *Am J Health Syst Pharm* 59(22), 2184
  (2002): Keam SJ+, *Drugs* 62(2), 387
  (2001): Dodick DW, *Headache* 41(5), 449
Upper respiratory infection (20%)
Vertigo

(2002): Balbisi EA, *Am J Health Syst Pharm* 59(22), 2184
(2002): Mathew NT+, *Headache 2002 Jan*; 42(1), 32 (2%)

ALOE VERA (GEL, JUICE, LEAF)

Scientific names: *Aloë africana; Aloë barbadensis; Aloë ferox; Aloë spicata*
Family: Liliaceae
Trade and other common names: Barbados aloe; Curacau aloe; Kumari; Lu Hui; SaliCept Patch (Carrington Labs)
Category: Anthroquinone glycoside; Anti-inflammatory
Purported indications and other uses: Oral: anesthetic, antiseptic, antipyretic, antipruritic, vasodilator, anti-inflammatory, vermifuge, antifungal. antiulcer, diabetes, asthma. **Topical:** promote healing, cold sores, ulceration, radiations injuries, psoriasis, frostbite. Also used in cosmetics and for its moisturizing and emollient properties
Half-life: N/A

Reactions

Skin
Allergic reactions (sic)
  (1999): Reynolds T+, *J Ethnopharmacol* 68(1–3), 3
Burning
  (1991): Hunter D+, *Cutis* 47(3), 193 (after dermabrasion)
Contact dermatitis
Dermatitis
  (1991): Hunter D+, *Cutis* 47(3), 193 (after dermabrasion)
Photosensitivity
  (1992): Dominguez-Soto, *Int J Dermatol* 31(5), 372

Other
Anaphylactoid reactions/Anaphylaxis
Hypersensitivity
  (1980): Morrow DM+, *Arch Dermatol* 116, 1064
Side effects (sic)
  (2000): Ernst E, *Br J Dermatol* 143(5), 923

ALOSETRON

Trade name: Lotronex (GSK)
Indications: Irritable bowel syndrome
Category: 5-HT3 antagonist; Serotonin type 3 receptor antagonist
Half-life: 1.5 hours

Note: This drug has been withdrawn
Only licensed for use in female patients

Reactions

Skin
Acne (<1%)
Allergic reactions (sic) (<1%)
Bacterial infections
Folliculitis (<1%)
Hematomas (<1%)
Jaundice
  (2005): Turgeon DK+, *J Clin Gastroenterol* 39(7), 641

Mucosal/ENT
Dysgeusia (<1%)
Parosmia (<1%)

Other
Abdominal pain
  (2005): Turgeon DK+, *J Clin Gastroenterol* 39(7), 641
Death
  (2004): Andresen V+, *Drug Saf* 27(5), 283

ALPHA-LIPOIC ACID

Synonyms: Lipoid acid; Thioctic acid; Dihydrothioctic acid
Indications: Diabetic neuropathy, vasodilation, photoaging
Half-life: N/A
Clinically important, potentially hazardous interactions with: N/A

Reactions

Skin
Dermatitis
  (2006): Bergqvist-Karlsson A+, *Contact Dermatitis* 55(1), 56
Pruritus
  (2005): Yadav V+, *Mult Scler* 11(2), 159
Rash (sic)
  (2005): Yadav V+, *Mult Scler* 11(2), 159
Urticaria
  (2005): Yadav V+, *Mult Scler* 11(2), 159

Other
Abdominal pain
  (2005): Yadav V+, *Mult Scler* 11(2), 159
Anaphylactoid reactions/Anaphylaxis
  (2004): Ziegler D, *Treat Endocrinol* 3(3), 173 (3 cases)
Vertigo
  (2006): Ziegler D+, *Diabetes Care* 29(11), 2365

ALPRAZOLAM

Trade names: Alprox; APO-Alpraz; Cassadan; Kalma; Nu-Alprax; Ralozam; Tafil; Xanax (Pfizer)
Indications: Anxiety, depression, panic attacks
Category: Benzodiazepine
Half-life: 11–16 hours
Clinically important, potentially hazardous interactions with: alcohol, aprepitant, clarithromycin, CNS depressants, delavirdine, digoxin, efavirenz, fluconazole, fluoxetine, fluvoxamine, **grapefruit juice**, indinavir, itraconazole, ivermectin, **kava**, ketoconazole, propoxyphene, ritonavir, saquinavir, **St John's wort**

Reactions

Skin
Acne
  (1985): Levy MH+, *Semin Oncol* 12, 411
Allergic reactions (sic)
  (1996): Bhatia MS, *Indian J Med Sci* 50, 285 (to tartrazine)
Dermatitis (3.8%)
  (1984): Elie R+, *J Clin Psychopharmacol* 4, 125
  (1982): Fawcett JA+, *Pharmacotherapy* 2, 243
  (1981): Evans RL, *Drug Intell Clin Pharm* 15, 633
  (1981): Kolin IS+, *J Clin Psychiatry* 42, 169
Diaphoresis (15.8%)
Edema (4.9%)
Exanthems

(1988): Warnock JK+, *Am J Psychiatry* 145, 425

Photosensitivity
  (1999): Watanabe Y+, *J Am Acad Dermatol* 40, 832
  (1998): Pazzagli L+, *Pharm World Sci* 20, 136 (with fluoxetine)
  (1994): Shelley WB+, *Cutis* 54, 70 (observation)
  (1990): Kanwar AJ+, *Dermatologica* 181, 75

Phototoxicity
  (1993): Litt JZ, Beachwood, OH (personal case) (observation)
  (1991): Shelley WB+, *Cutis* 48, 187 (observation)

Pruritus
  (1988): Islas JA+, *Curr Ther Res* 43, 384
  (1982): Chouinard G+, *Psychopharmacol* 77, 229

Purpura

Rash (sic) (10.8%)
  (1987): Fyer AJ+, *Am J Psychiatry* 144, 303
  (1985): Jerram TC, *Side Eff Drugs Annu* 9, 39
  (1985): Rush AJ+, *Arch Gen Psychiatry* 42, 1154
  (1983): Davison K+, *Psychopharmacol* 80, 308

Stevens–Johnson syndrome

Urticaria

Xerosis
  (1982): Chouinard G+, *Psychopharmacol* 77, 229

Mucosal/ENT

Angioedema (tongue)
  (2006): Sellas-Dupre G+, *Med Clin* (Barc) 127(10), 399

Dysgeusia (<1%)
  (1982): Chouinard G+, *Psychopharmacol* 77, 229

Oral ulceration

Sialopenia (32.8%)

Sialorrhea (4.2%)

Tinnitus

Xerostomia (14.7%)
  (1988): Islas JA+, *Curr Ther Res* 43, 384
  (1984): Elie R+, *J Clin Psychopharmacol* 4, 125
  (1982): Chouinard G+, *Psychopharmacol* 77, 229
  (1982): Fawcett JA+, *Pharmacotherapy* 2, 243
  (1981): Evans RL, *Drug Intell Clin Pharm* 15, 633

Other

Asthenia
  (2006): Glue P+, *Am J Ther* 13(5), 418

Death
  (2005): Wolf BC+, *J Forensic Sci* 50(1), 192 (with oxycodone)

Gynecomastia

Headache

Paresthesias (2.4%)

Pseudolymphoma
  (1995): Magro CM+, *J Am Acad Dermatol* 32, 419

Seizures
  (2002): Mena Martin FJ+, *Med Clin* (Barc) 119(20), 797
    (withdrawal)

ALPROSTADIL

Synonyms: PGE; prostaglandin E₁
Trade names: Caverject (Pfizer); Edex (Schwarz); Lyple;
Minprog; Muse (Vivus); Palux; Prostin VR (Pfizer); Prostine VR;
Prostivas
Indications: Impotence, to maintain patent ductus arteriosus
Category: Prostaglandin
Half-life: 5–10 minutes

Reactions

Skin

Diaphoresis (<1%)
Edema (1%)
Lichen sclerosus (penile shaft hypopigmentation)
  (1998): English JC+, *J Am Acad Dermatol* 39, 801
Penile edema (1%)
Penile pruritus (<1%)
Penile rash (1–10%)
Rash (sic) (<1%)
Toxic epidermal necrolysis
  (1996): Lecorvaisier-Pieto C+, *J Am Acad Dermatol* 35, 112
Urticaria
  (2000): Carter EL+, *Pediatr Dermatol* 17, 58

Mucosal/ENT

Balanitis (<1%)
Xerostomia (<1%)

Other

Application-site burning
  (2006): Kielbasa LA+, *Ann Pharmacother* 40(7-8), 1369
Application-site pruritus
  (2006): Kielbasa LA+, *Ann Pharmacother* 40(7-8), 1369
Injection-site ecchymoses (1–10%)
  (1996): Linet OI+, *N Engl J Med* 334, 873 (8%)
Injection-site hematoma (3%)
Injection-site inflammation (<1%)
Injection-site pain (2%)
  (1996): Hellstrom WJG, *Urology* 48, 851
Injection-site pruritus (<1%)
Thrombophlebitis
  (2002): Barthelmes L+, *Int J Impot Res* 14(3), 199

ALTEPLASE

Trade names: Actilyse; Activacin; Activase (Genentech);
Lysatec-rt-PA
Indications: Acute myocardial infarction, acute pulmonary
embolism
Category: Fibrinolytic; Plasminogen activator
Half-life: 30–45 minutes
**Clinically important, potentially hazardous interactions
with:** nitroglycerin, ticlopidine

Reactions

Skin

Allergic reactions
Angioedema
  (2002): Molinaro G+, *Stroke* 33(6), 1712
  (2001): Pechlaner C+, *Blood Coagul Fibrinolysis* 12(6), 491
  (2000): Hill MD+, *CMAJ* 162, 1281
  (2000): Rudolf J+, *Neurology* 55, 599
Purpura (<1%)
  (1990): De Trana+, *Arch Dermatol* 126, 690 (painful) (<1%)
Rash (sic) (<0.02%)
Urticaria (<1%)
  (1989): Collen D+, *Drugs* 38, 346

Mucosal/ENT

Gingivitis (<1%)
Orolingual angioedema
  (2005): Engelter ST+, *J Neurol* 252(10), 1167 (%)

Other
Anaphylactoid reactions/Anaphylaxis (<0.02%)
  (2001): Pechlaner C+, *Blood Coagul Fibrinolysis* 12(6), 491
  (2000): Hill MD+, *CMAJ* 162, 1281 (fatal)
  (1999): Rudolf J+, *Stroke* 30, 1142
Death
  (2003): Graham GD, *Stroke* 34(12), 2847 (13.4%)
Headache
Hypersensitivity
  (2001): Pechlaner C+, *Blood Coagul Fibrinolysis* 12(6), 491

ALTRETAMINE

Synonym: hexamethylmelamine
Trade names: Hexalen (MGI); Hexamethylmelamin; Hexastat; Hexinawas
Indications: Palliative treatment of recurrent ovarian cancer
Category: Alkylating agent
Half-life: 13 hours
Clinically important, potentially hazardous interactions with: aldesleukin

Reactions

Skin
Dermatitis
Exanthems
Pruritus (<1%)
Rash (sic) (<1%)

Mucosal/ENT
Mucocutaneous reactions (sic)

Hair
Hair – alopecia (<1%)

Other
Abdominal pain
  (1986): Foster BJ+, *Cancer Treat Rev* 13(4), 197
Asthenia
  (1986): Foster BJ+, *Cancer Treat Rev* 13(4), 197
Depression
  (1992): Vergote I+, *Gynecol Oncol* 47(3), 282
Neurotoxicity
  (1992): Vergote I+, *Gynecol Oncol* 47(3), 282
  (1991): Macdonald JS, *Cancer Treat Rev* 18 Suppl A, 99
  (1986): Foster BJ+, *Cancer Treat Rev* 13(4), 197
Paresthesias
  (2001): Rothenberg ML+, *Gynecol Oncol* 82(2), 317
Tremor (<1%)

ALVIMOPAN

Trade name: Entereg (Adolor)
Indications: Postoperative ileus
Category: Opioid antagonist
Half-life: 10–18 Hours
Clinically important, potentially hazardous interactions with: opioid receptor antagonist (for longer than 7 days)

Reactions

Skin
Purpura

Other
Abdominal pain
  (2001): Schmidt WK, *Am J Surg* 182(5A), 27S
Hypotension
  (2005): Delaney CP+, *Dis Colon Rectum* 48(6), 1114
Urinary retention (3%)

AMANTADINE

Trade names: Amixx; Endantadine; Grippin-Merz; Mantadix; PK-Merz; Protexin; Symmetrel (Endo); Tregor
Indications: Parkinsonism, influenza A viral infection
Category: Adamantane; Antiviral
Half-life: 10–28 hours
Clinically important, potentially hazardous interactions with: memantine

Note: Fifty to 90% of patients receiving amantadine for Parkinsonism develop 'a more or less livedo reticularis'

Reactions

Skin
Dermatitis (0.1%)
  (1997): Jauregui I+, *J Invest Allergol Clin Immunol* 7, 260
  (1990): Patruno C+, *Contact Dermatitis* 22, 187
  (1988): van Ketel WG, *Derm Beruf Umwelt* (German) 36, 23
  (1987): Angelini G+, *Contact Dermatitis* 15, 114
  (1987): Miranda A+, *Contact Dermatitis* 17, 55
  (1987): van Joost T+, *Ned Tijdschr Geneeskd* (Dutch) 131, 21
  (1987): van Ketel WG, *Ned Tijdschr Geneeskd* (Dutch) 131, 461
  (1985): Tosti A+, *Contact Dermatitis* 13, 339
  (1985): Valsecchi R+, *Contact Dermatitis* 13, 341
  (1984): Agathos M+, *Derm Beruf Umwelt* (German) 32, 157
  (1984): Lembo G+, *Contact Dermatitis* 10, 317
  (1984): Santucci B+, *Contact Dermatitis* 10, 317
  (1983): Przybilla B, *J Am Acad Dermatol* 9, 165
  (1982): Brandao FM+, *Contact Dermatitis* 8, 140
  (1982): van der Walle HB+, *Ned Tijdschr Geneeskd* (Dutch) 126, 1033
  (1982): van Ketel WG, *Contact Dermatitis* 8, 71
  (1980): Przybilla B+, *MMW Munch Med Wochenschr* (German) 122, 1195
Eczema
  (1983): Hellgren L+, *Dermatologica* 167, 267
Edema
Erythema multiforme
  (2000): Mitchell D, Thomasville, GA (from Internet) (observation)
Exanthems
Livedo reticularis (50–90%)
  (2006): Hayes BB+, *J Drugs Dermatol* 5(3), 288 (2 cases)
  (2005): Gibbs MB+, *J Am Acad Dermatol* 52(6), 1009
  (2003): Sladden MJ+, *Br J Dermatol* 149(3), 656
  (2002): Litt JZ, Beachwood, OH (observation)
  (2001): Vaughn K (from Internet) (observation)
  (2000): Litt JZ, Beachwood, OH (personal case) (observation)
  (1998): Loffler H+, *Hautarzt* (German) 49, 224
  (1996): Eisner J, Mount Vernon, WA (from Internet) (observation)
  (1995): Paulson GW+, *Clin Neuropharmacol* 18, 466
Peripheral edema
  (2002): Litt JZ, Beachwood, OH (observation)
Photosensitivity
  (1983): van den Berg WH+, *Contact Dermatitis* 9, 165
Pigmentation

Pruritus (<1%)
  (2002): Litt JZ, Beachwood, OH (observation)
Rash (sic) (<1%)
Urticaria

Mucosal/ENT
Xerostomia (1–10%)
  (2003): Stryjer R+, *Int Clin Psychopharmacol* 18(2), 93

Hair
Hair – alopecia
Hair – hypertrichosis

Nails
Nails – growth

Eyes
Eyelid edema

Other
Headache
Neurotoxicity
  (2006): Nakata M+, *Eur Neurol* 56(1), 59

AMBRISENTAN

Trade name: Letairis (Gilead)
Indications: Pulmonary arterial hypertension
Category: Endothelin receptor antagonist; Vasodilator
Half-life: 15 Hours
**Clinically important, potentially hazardous interactions
with:** CYP3A4-inhibitors such as ketoconazole, omeprazole etc.

Reactions

Skin
Peripheral edema (17%)

Mucosal/ENT
Nasopharyngitis (3%)
Sinusitis (3%)

Other
Abdominal pain (3%)
Headache (15%)
Hepatotoxicity
Teratogenicity

AMCINONIDE

Trade name: Cyclocort (Astellas)
Indications: Dermatoses
Category: Corticosteroid, topical
Half-life: N/A
**Clinically important, potentially hazardous interactions
with:** live vaccines

Reactions

Skin
Acne
Allergic reactions (sic)
  (1995): Lepoittevin JP+, *Arch Dermatol* 131(1), 31
Burning
  (1985): Huntley AC+, *Cutis* 35(5), 489

Dermatitis
  (2001): Sasseville D, *Contact Dermatitis* 45(4), 232
  (1993): Fedler R+, *Hautarzt* (German) 44, 91
  (1993): Hisa T+, *Contact Dermatitis* 28, 174 ([B, Bu, F, A, H])
  (1991): Dunkel FG+, *Contact Dermatitis* 25(2), 97 (2 cases)
  (1991): Gamboa PM+, *Contact Dermatitis* 24(3), 227 (with budesonide)
  (1989): Rivara G+, *Contact Dermatitis* 21(2), 83
  (1988): Sasaki E+, *Contact Dermatitis* 18(1), 61
  (1987): Hayakawa R+, *Contact Dermatitis* 16(1), 48
  (1986): Kubo Y+, *Contact Dermatitis* 15(2), 109
  (1985): Hayakawa R+, *Contact Dermatitis* 12, 213
  (1984): Boujnah-Khouadja A+, *Contact Dermatitis* 11(2), 83 (9 cases)
  (1984): Guin JD, *J Am Acad Dermatol* 10(5), 773
Eczema
  (1984): Guin JD, *J Am Acad Dermatol* 10(5), 773
Edema
Erythema
  (1993): Fedler R+, *Hautarzt* 44, 91 (diffuse and widespread)
Exanthems
  (2000): Bircher AJ+, *Dermatology* 200(4), 349
Irritation
Perioral dermatitis
  (1987): Edwards EK+, *Int J Dermatol* 26(10), 649
Pruritus
  (1985): Huntley AC+, *Cutis* 35(5), 489
Rash (sic)
  (1993): Hisa T+, *Contact Dermatitis* 28(3), 174
Thinning
  (1989): Lubach D+, *Dermatologica* 178(2), 93
Urticaria
  (1993): Fedler R+, *Hautarzt* 44, 91 ([A])

Eyes
Vision blurred
Visual halos

Other
Hypersensitivity
  (1984): Boujnah-Khouadja A+, *Contact Dermatitis* 11(2), 83 (3 cases)

AMIFOSTINE

Synonyms: ethiofos; gammaphos
Trade names: Ethyol (Medimmune); Ethyol 500
Indications: Nephrotoxicity prophylaxis
Category: Thiophosphate cytoprotective
Half-life: 9 minutes

Reactions

Skin
Allergic reactions (sic)
  (2007): Anne PR+, *Int J Radiat Oncol Biol Phys* 67(2), 445 (4%)
Bullous dermatitis
  (2004): Boccia R+, *Int J Radiat Oncol Biol Phys* 60(1), 302 (3 cases)
Erythema multiforme
  (2004): Boccia R+, *Int J Radiat Oncol Biol Phys* 60(1), 302 (8 cases)
Exfoliative dermatitis
Pruritus
Rash (sic) (<1%)
  (2007): Anne PR+, *Int J Radiat Oncol Biol Phys* 67(2), 445 (6%)

(2006): Koukourakis MI+, *Anticancer Res* 26(3B), 2437 (7%)
(2002): Koukourakis MI+, *Int J Radiat Oncol Biol Phys* 52(1), 144 (7%)
(1998): Buresh CM+, *J Pediatr Hematol Oncol* 20, 361
Stevens–Johnson syndrome
(2007): Zollo E+, *Tumori* 93(6), 634
(2004): Boccia R+, *Int J Radiat Oncol Biol Phys* 60(1), 302 (10 cases)
(2000): Lale Atahan I+, *Br J Dermatol* 143(5), 1072
Toxic epidermal necrolysis
(2004): Boccia R+, *Int J Radiat Oncol Biol Phys* 60(1), 302 (11 cases)
(2002): Demiral AN+, *Jpn J Clin Oncol* 32(11), 477
(2000): Lale Atahan I+, *Br J Dermatol* 143(5), 1072
Toxicoderma
(2004): Boccia R+, *Int J Radiat Oncol Biol Phys* 60(1), 302 (3 cases)
Urticaria

Mucosal/ENT
Dysgeusia
(2001): Genvresse I+, *Anticancer Drugs* 12(4), 345
(2000): Sriswasdi C+, *J Med Assoc Thai* 83, 374
Mucositis
(2007): Anne PR+, *Int J Radiat Oncol Biol Phys* 67(2), 445
(2006): Buentzel J+, *Int J Radiat Oncol Biol Phys* 64(3), 684 (39%)
Xerostomia
(2007): Anne PR+, *Int J Radiat Oncol Biol Phys* 67(2), 445
(2006): Buentzel J+, *Int J Radiat Oncol Biol Phys* 64(3), 684 (39%)
(2006): Jellema AP+, *Cancer* 107(3), 544
(2002): Anne PR+, *Semin Radiat Oncol* 12(1), 18
(2001): Genvresse I+, *Anticancer Drugs* 12(4), 345

Other
Anaphylactoid reactions/Anaphylaxis
(2007): Rolleman EJ+, *Radiother Oncol* 82(1), 110
(2006): Lin A+, *Radiother Oncol* 79(3), 352
(2002): Vardy J+, *Anticancer Drugs* 13(3), 327
Asthenia
(2006): Koukourakis MI+, *Anticancer Res* 26(3B), 2437
Chills (>10%)
(2000): Sriswasdi C+, *J Med Assoc Thai* 83, 374
Fever
(2006): Koukourakis MI+, *Anticancer Res* 26(3B), 2437 (7%)
(2002): Koukourakis MI+, *Int J Radiat Oncol Biol Phys* 52(1), 144 (7%)

AMIKACIN

Trade names: Amicacina; Amicasil; Amikacin Sulfate (Bedford); Amikan; Biclin; Biklin; Gamikal; Kanbine; Lukadin; Miacin; Yectamid
Indications: Short-term treatment of serious infections due to gram-negative bacteria
Category: Antibiotic, aminoglycoside
Half-life: 1.5–2.5 hours (adults)
Clinically important, potentially hazardous interactions with: adefovir, aldesleukin, aminoglycosides, atracurium, bumetanide, cephalexin, doxacurium, ethacrynic acid, furosemide, succinylcholine, torsemide

Reactions

Skin
Allergic reactions

Dermatitis
(1989): Rudzki E+, *Contact Dermatitis* 20, 391
(1985): Holdiness MR, *Int J Dermatol* 24, 280
Exanthems
Pruritus
(1985): Holdiness MR, *Int J Dermatol* 24, 280
Rash (sic) (<1%)
(1995): Rodriguez-Noriega E+, *J Chemother* 7, 155
Urticaria

Mucosal/ENT
Anosmia
(2003): Welge-Luessen A+, *Arch Otolaryngol Head Neck Surg* 129(12), 1331
Ototoxicity
(2004): Nagai J+, *Drug Metab Pharmacokinet* 19(3), 159
(2002): de Jager P+, *Int J Tuberc Lung Dis* 6(7), 622
Tinnitus

Eyes
Macular infarction
(2005): Venkatesh P+, *Indian J Ophthalmol* 53(4), 269
(2004): Galloway GD+, *Br J Ophthalmol* 88(9), 1228
Ocular toxicity
(2006): Widmer S+, *Klin Monatsbl Augenheilkd* 223(5), 456

Other
Injection-site induration
Injection-site necrosis
(1993): Plantin P+, *Presse Med* (French) 22, 1366
Injection-site pain
Nephrotoxicity
(2004): Nagai J+, *Drug Metab Pharmacokinet* 19(3), 159
(2003): Bartal C+, *Am J Med* 114(3), 194
(2003): Rougier F+, *Clin Pharmacokinet* 42(5), 493
(2002): de Jager P+, *Int J Tuberc Lung Dis* 6(7), 622
(1998): Karachalios GN+, *Int J Clin Pharmacol Ther* 36(10), 561
Paresthesias (<1%)
Tremor (<1%)

AMILORIDE

Trade names: Amikal; Kaluril; Medamor; Midamor (Merck); Midoride; Modamide; Moduretic (Merck); Nirulid; Ride
Indications: Prevention of hypokalemia associated with kaliuretic diuretics, management of edema in hypertension
Category: Diuretic, potassium-sparing
Half-life: 6–9 hours
Clinically important, potentially hazardous interactions with: ACE inhibitors, benazepril, captopril, cyclosporine, enalapril, fosinopril, lisinopril, magnesium, moexipril, potassium salts, quinapril, quinidine, ramipril, spironolactone, trandolapril

Note: Moduretic is amiloride and hydrochlorothiazide

Reactions

Skin
Diaphoresis
Exanthems
Photosensitivity
(1984): Ophir O+, *Harefuah* 107(1–2), 14
(1982): *Ugeskr Laeger* 144(15), 1101
(1981): *Aust Prescriber* 5, 23
(1980): Okrasinski H+, *Lakartidningen* 77(32–33), 2718
Pruritus (<1%)
Purpura

Rash (sic) (<1%)
Toxicity (sic)
  (1986): Dorevitch A+, *Am J Psychiatry* 143(2), 257
Urticaria
Vasculitis
Xerosis (<1%)

Mucosal/ENT
Dysgeusia (<1%)
Tinnitus
Xerostomia (<1%)

Hair
Hair – alopecia (<1%)

Other
Anaphylactoid reactions/Anaphylaxis
Gynecomastia (1–10%)
Headache
Paresthesias (<1%)
Seizures
  (1989): Johnston C+, *J R Soc Med* 82(8), 479
Tremor

AMINOCAPROIC ACID

Trade names: Amicar (Xanodyne); Capramol; Caproamin; Caprolisin; Ipron; Ipsilon; Resplamin
Indications: To provide hemostasis in the treatment of fibrinolysis
Category: Antifibrinolytic
Half-life: 1–2 hours

Reactions

Skin
Bullous dermatitis
  (1992): Brooke CP+, *J Am Acad Dermatol* 27, 880
Dermatitis
  (2000): Miyamoto H+, *Contact Dermatitis* 42, 50
  (1999): Villarreal O, *Contact Dermatitis* 40, 114 (systemic)
  (1989): Shono M, *Contact Dermatitis* 21, 106
Eczema
Edema
Exanthems
  (1995): Gonzalez-Gutierrez ML+, *Allergy* 50, 745
Kaposi's sarcoma
Pruritus
Purpura
  (1985): Verstraete M, *Drugs* 29, 236
  (1980): Chakrabarti A+, *BMJ* 281, 197
Purpura fulminans
  (2003): Culpeper KS+, *Lancet* 361(9355), 384
Rash (sic) (1–10%)
Urticaria

Mucosal/ENT
Tinnitus

Other
Anaphylactoid reactions/Anaphylaxis
Death
  (2001): Fanashawe MP+, *Anesthesiology* 95(6), 1525 (2 cases)
Headache
Injection-site erythema
Injection-site phlebitis

Injection-site reactions (sic)
Myalgia/Myositis/Myopathy/Myotoxicity (1–10%)
  (1988): Kane MJ+, *Am J Med* 85, 861
Rhabdomyolysis
  (1997): Seymour BD+, *Ann Pharmacother* 31(1), 56
  (1983): Luliri P+, *Haematologica* 68(5), 664 (2 cases)
  (1983): Morris CD+, *S Afr Med J* 64(10), 363
  (1982): Brown JA+, *J Neurosurg* 57(1), 130
  (1982): Vanneste JA+, *Eur Neurol* 21(4), 242
  (1980): Britt CW+, *Arch Neurol* 37(3), 187
  (1980): Brodkin HM+, *J Neurosurg* 53(5), 690
  (1980): Le Porrier M+, *Nouv Presse Med* 9(33), 2347
Thrombophlebitis

AMINOGLUTETHIMIDE

Trade names: Cytadren (Novartis); Orimeten; Orimetene; Rodazol
Indications: Suppression of adrenal function, metastatic carcinoma
Category: Aromatase inhibitor
Half-life: 7–15 hours
Clinically important, potentially hazardous interactions with: dexamethasone

Reactions

Skin
Angioedema
Erythema
  (1987): Williams DS+, *Br J Radiology* 60, 1226
Exanthems
  (1990): Vanek N+, *Med Pediatr Oncol* 18, 162
  (1987): Williams DS+, *Br J Radiology* 60, 1226
  (1986): Leloire O+, *Presse Med* (French) 15, 34
  (1984): Coltart RS, *Br J Radiol* 57, 531
  (1982): Naysmith A+, *N Engl J Med* 306, 45 (26%)
  (1982): Santen RJ+, *Ann Intern Med* 96, 94 (29%)
  (1980): Savaraj N+, *Med Pediatr Oncol* 8, 251
Exfoliative dermatitis
Lupus erythematosus (>10%)
  (1980): McCraken M+, *BMJ* 281, 1254
Pruritus (5%)
Psoriasis
  (1984): Coltart RS, *Br J Radiol* 57, 531
Purpura
  (1994): Stratakis CA+, *Am J Hosp Pharm* 51, 2589
Rash (sic) (>10%)
Urticaria

Mucosal/ENT
Oral mucosal eruption
  (1984): Coltart RS, *Br J Radiol* 57, 531
Oral ulceration
  (1984): Coltart RS, *Br J Radiol* 57, 531

Hair
Hair – hirsutism (1–10%)

Other
Anaphylactoid reactions/Anaphylaxis
  (1986): Leloire O+, *Presse Med* (French) 15, 34
Headache
Inappropriate secretion of antidiuretic hormone (SIADH)
  (1986): Box M+, *Br J Urol* 58(6), 724
Myalgia/Myositis/Myopathy/Myotoxicity (3%)

AMINOLEVULINIC ACID

Trade name: Levulan Kerastick (Dusa)
Indications: Non-hyperkeratotic actinic keratoses of face & scalp
Category: Photosensitizer; Protoporphyrin IX (PpIX)
Half-life: 30 ± 10 hours

Note: To be used in conjunction with the Blue Light Photodynamic Therapy Illuminator

Reactions

Skin
Burning (>50%)
  (2006): Schleyer V+, *J Eur Acad Dermatol Venereol* 20(7), 823
  (1997): Jeffes EW+, *Arch Dermatol* 133, 727
  (1996): Stender IM+, *Br J Dermatol* 135, 454
Contact dermatitis
  (2007): Hohwy T+, *Contact Dermatitis* 57(5), 321
Crusting (64–71%)
  (2000): Hongcharu W+, *J Invest Dermatol* 115, 183
  (1995): Lang S+, *Laryngorhinootologie* (German) 74, 85
Dermatitis
  (2004): Wulf HC+, *Br J Dermatol* 150(1), 143
  (1998): Gnaizdowska B+, *Contact Dermatitis* 38, 348
Edema (35%)
  (2004): Dragieva G+, *Transplantation* 77(1), 115
  (2004): Piacquadio DJ+, *Arch Dermatol* 140(1), 41
  (2003): Alster TS+, *J Drugs Dermatol* 2(5), 501
  (1997): Jeffes EW+, *Arch Dermatol* 133, 727
  (1995): Lang S+, *Laryngorhinootologie* (German) 74, 85
Erosions (14%)
Erythema (99%)
  (2006): Misra A+, *Plast Reconstr Surg* 117(7), 2522
  (2006): Wiegell SR+, *Br J Dermatol* 154(5), 969
  (2004): Dragieva G+, *Transplantation* 77(1), 115
  (2004): Piacquadio DJ+, *Arch Dermatol* 140(1), 41
  (2003): Alster TS+, *J Drugs Dermatol* 2(5), 501
  (2003): Wiegell SR+, *Arch Dermatol* 139(9), 1173
  (1997): Jeffes EW+, *Arch Dermatol* 133, 727
  (1995): Lang S+, *Laryngorhinootologie* 74, 85
Exfoliative dermatitis (when treated for acne)
  (2006): Wiegell SR+, *Br J Dermatol* 154(5), 969
  (2000): Hongcharu W+, *J Invest Dermatol* 115, 183
  (1996): Stender IM+, *Br J Dermatol* 135(3), 454
Hypomelanosis (22%)
Keratoacanthoma
  (2006): Maydan E+, *J Drugs Dermatol* 5(8), 804
Koebner phenomenon (psoriasis)
  (1996): Stender IM+, *Acta Derm Venereol* 76, 392
Melanoma
  (1997): Wolf P+, *Dermatology* 194, 53 (on scalp)
Photosensitivity
  (2007): Zeltser R+, *Cutis* 80(2), 124
  (2002): Hinnen P+, *J Photochem Photobiol B* 68(1), 8
  (1999): Ackroyd R+, *Photochem Photobiol* 70(4), 656
Phototoxicity
  (2007): Angell-Petersen E+, *Br J Dermatol* 156(2), 301
Pigmentation (when treated for acne) (22%)
  (2003): Clark C+, *Photodermatol Photoimmunol Photomed* 19(3), 134 (2%)
  (2002): Monfrecola G+, *J Photochem Photobiol B* 68(2-3), 147
  (2000): Hongcharu W+, *J Invest Dermatol* 115, 183
Pruritus (25%)
Pustules (<4%)
  (2006): Wiegell SR+, *Br J Dermatol* 154(5), 969
Scaling (64–71%)

Scar
  (2003): Clark C+, *Photodermatol Photoimmunol Photomed* 19(3), 134 (2%)
Stinging (>50%)
  (1997): Jeffes EW+, *Arch Dermatol* 133, 727
Ulcerations (4%)
Urticaria
  (2005): Yokoyama S+, *J Dermatol* 32(10), 843 (photocontact)
Vesiculation (4%)

Hair
Hair – alopecia
  (1999): Ackroyd R+, *Photochem Photobiol* 70(4), 656

Other
Asthenia
  (1999): Ackroyd R+, *Photochem Photobiol* 70(4), 656
Headache
  (1999): Ackroyd R+, *Photochem Photobiol* 70(4), 656
Pain
  (2006): Schleyer V+, *J Eur Acad Dermatol Venereol* 20(7), 823
  (2006): Wiegell SR+, *Br J Dermatol* 154(5), 969
  (2003): Clark C+, *Photodermatol Photoimmunol Photomed* 19(3), 134 (2%)
  (2003): Wiegell SR+, *Arch Dermatol* 139(9), 1173

AMINOPHYLLINE

Synonym: theophylline ethylenediamine
Trade names: Aerolate; Aminophyllin; Bronkodyl; Choledyl; Corophyllin; Elixophyllin (Forest); Euphyllin; Norphyl; Palaron; Phyllocontin (Napp); Phyllotemp; Planphylline; Quibron (Monarch); Slo-Bid; Somophyllin; Tefamin; Theo-Dur; Truphylline
Indications: Prevention or treatment of reversible bronchospasm
Category: Xanthine alkaloid
Half-life: 3–15 hours (in adult nonsmokers)
Clinically important, potentially hazardous interactions with: arformoterol, cimetidine, erythromycin, halothane, nilutamide, prednisone

Reactions

Skin
Adverse effects (sic)
  (1995): Simon PA+, *JAMA* 273(22), 1737
Allergic reactions (sic) (<1%)
  (1986): Cusano F+, *G Ital Dermatol Venereol* (Italian) 121, 443
  (1985): Editorial, *Lancet* 1, 289
  (1983): Gibb W+, *Br Med J* (Clin Res Ed) 13, 501
  (1983): Hardy C+, *Br Med J* (Clin Res Ed) 286, 2051
Baboon syndrome
  (1999): Guin JD+, *Contact Dermatitis* 40, 170
Bullous dermatitis
  (2002): Tsokos M+, *Am J Forensic Med Pathol* 23(3), 292
Dermatitis
  (1994): Corazza M+, *Contact Dermatitis* 31, 328
  (1984): Editorial, *Lancet* 2, 1192
  (1983): Berman BA+, *Cutis* 31, 594
  (1983): van den Berg WH+, *Ned Tijdschr Geneeskd* (Dutch) 127, 1801
  (1980): Vazquez Botet M, *Bol Asoc Med P R* (Spanish) 72, 14
Diaphoresis
Exanthems
  (1985): Editorial, *Lancet* 2, 1192
  (1984): Thompson PJ+, *Thorax* 39, 600

(1983): Hardy C+, *BMJ* 286, 2051
(1981): de Shazo RD+, *Ann Allergy* 46, 152
(1980): Lawyer CH+, *J Allergy Clin Immunol* 65, 353
Exfoliative dermatitis
  (1984): Thompson PJ+, *Thorax* 39, 600
  (1982): Nierenberg DW+, *West J Med* 137, 328
  (1981): Elias JA+, *Am Rev Respir Dis* 123, 550
Pruritus
  (1980): Lawyer CH+, *J Allergy Clin Immunol* 65, 353
Rash (sic) (<1%)
  (1983): Hardy C+, *BMJ* 286, 2051
Side effects (sic)
  (1995): Simon PA+, *JAMA* 273, 1737
Stevens–Johnson syndrome
  (1994): Brook U, *Int J Paediatr Dent* 4(2), 101
  (1989): Brook U+, *Pediatr Dermatol* 6(2), 126
  (1989): Hidalgo HA, *Pediatr Pulmonol* 6, 209 (theophylline)
Urticaria
  (1994): Urbani CE, *Contact Dermatitis* 31, 198
  (1985): Editorial, *Lancet* 2, 1192
  (1984): Thompson PJ+, *Thorax* 39, 600
  (1982): Neumann H, *Dtsch Med Wochenschr* (German) 107, 116

Mucosal/ENT
Parosmia

Hair
Hair – alopecia

Other
Death
  (2002): Tsokos M+, *Am J Forensic Med Pathol* 23(3), 292
Headache
Hypersensitivity
  (1999): Yoshizawa A+, *Arerugi* (Japanese) 48, 1206 (from
    ethylenediamine)
  (1985): Gibb WR, *Lancet* 1, 49
  (1981): Elias JA+, *Am Rev Respir Dis* 123, 550
Inappropriate secretion of antidiuretic hormone (SIADH)
  (2002): Liberopoulos EN+, *Ann Pharmacother* 36(7-8), 1180
  (1983): Tudehope D+, *Aust Paediatr J* 19(1), 55
Rhabdomyolysis
  (2001): Teweleit S+, *Med Klin* 96(1), 40
  (2000): Iwano J+, *J Med Invest* 47(1–2), 9
  (1999): Shimada N+, *Nippon Jinzo Gakkai Shi* 41(4), 460 (with
    clarithromycin)
  (1994): Tsai J+, *Hum Exp Toxicol* 13(10), 651 (4 cases)
  (1991): Aoshima M+, *Nihon Kyobu Shikkan Gakki Zasshi*
    29(8), 1064
Seizures
  (2007): Odajima Y+, *Arerugi* 56(7), 691
  (2003): Reuther LO+, *Ugeskr Laeger* 165(14), 1447
Tremor

AMINOSALICYLATE SODIUM

Synonyms: para-aminosalicylate sodium; PAS
Trade names: Aminox; Eupasal; Nemasol; Paser Granules
(Jacobus); Sodium P.A.S.; Tubasal
Indications: Tuberculosis
Category: Antibiotic; Salicylate
Half-life: 45–60 minutes

Reactions

Skin
Allergic reactions (sic)

(1988): Fardy JM+, *J Clin Gastroenterol* 10, 635
Angioedema
Bullous dermatitis
Eczema (<1%)
Erythema multiforme
Erythroderma
  (2006): Iemoli E+, *Inflamm Bowel Dis* 12(10), 1007
Exanthems
  (1988): Gron I+, *Ugeskr Laeger* (Danish) 150, 32
  (1982): Nagaratnam N, *Postgrad Med J* 58, 729
Exfoliative dermatitis
Fixed eruption
Lichenoid eruption
Lupus erythematosus
  (1985): Holdiness MR, *Int J Dermatol* 24, 280
  (1980): Agarwal MB+, *J Postgrad Med* 26(4), 263
Lymphoma (benign)
  (1982): Nagaratnam N, *Postgrad Med J* 58, 729
Photosensitivity
Pruritus
Purpura
  (1980): Miescher PA+, *Clin Haematol* 9, 505
Toxic epidermal necrolysis
  (2006): Iemoli E+, *Inflamm Bowel Dis* 12(10), 1007
Urticaria
Vasculitis (<1%)

Mucosal/ENT
Oral lichenoid eruption
Oral mucosal eruption

Hair
Hair – alopecia
  (1982): Kutty PK+, *Ann Intern Med* 97, 785

Eyes
Eyelid erythema
  (2004): Vodegel RM+, *Ned Tijdschr Geneeskd* 148(31), 1550
Periorbital edema
  (2004): Vodegel RM+, *Ned Tijdschr Geneeskd* 148(31), 1550
Rhinoconjunctivitis
  (2004): Vodegel RM+, *Ned Tijdschr Geneeskd* 148(31), 1550

Other
Hypersensitivity
Nephrotoxicity
  (2005): Muller AF+, *Aliment Pharmacol Ther* 21(10), 1217
  (1999): Agharazii M+, *Am J Nephrol* 19(3), 373

AMIODARONE

Trade names: Aratac; Corbionax; Cordarex; Cordarone
(Wyeth); Cordarone X; Pacerone (Upsher-Smith); Tachydaron
Indications: Ventricular fibrillation, ventricular tachycardia
Category: Antiarrhythmic class III
Half-life: 26–107 days
**Clinically important, potentially hazardous interactions
with:** abarelix, acenocoumarol, amisulpride, amprenavir,
anisindione, anticoagulants, arsenic, astemizole, carbimazole,
celiprolol, ciprofloxacin, dicumarol, digoxin, diltiazem, enoxacin,
fentanyl, fosamprenavir, gatifloxacin, **grapefruit juice**,
lomefloxacin, methotrexate, moxifloxacin, norfloxacin, ofloxacin,
quinidine, quinolones, rifabutin, rifampin, rifapentine, ritonavir,
simvastatin, sparfloxacin, tacrolimus, tipranavir, verapamil,
warfarin

Reactions

Skin

Allergic reactions (sic)
(1989): Reingardene DI, *Klin Med Mosk* (Russian) 67, 128
Angioedema
(2005): Lahiri K+, *Indian J Dermatol Venereol Leprol* 71(1), 46
(2000): Burches E+, *Allergy* 55, 1199
Basal cell carcinoma
(1995): Monk BE, *Br J Dermatol* 133, 148
Diaphoresis
(1985): Raeder EA+, *Am Heart J* 109, 979 (0.5%)
(1983): McGovern B+, *BMJ* 287, 175 (2.5%)
Edema (1–10%)
Erythema multiforme
(2002): Yung A+, *Australas J Dermatol* 43(1), 35
Erythema nodosum (<1%)
(1983): Fogoros RN+, *Circulation* 68, 88 (1%)
Exanthems
(1985): Raeder EA+, *Am Heart J* 109, 975 (0.9%)
(1984): Rotmensch HH+, *Ann Intern Med* 101, 462 (0.7%)
(1983): Fogoros RN+, *Circulation* 68, 88 (2%)
(1983): Harris L+, *Circulation* 67, 45
Exfoliative dermatitis
(1988): Moots RJ+, *BMJ* 296, 1332
Facial erythema (3.1%)
(1984): Rotmensch HH+, *Ann Intern Med* 101, 462
(1983): Harris L+, *Circulation* 67, 45
Iododerma
(1997): Ricci C+, *Ann Dermatol Venereol* (French) 124, 260
Keratosis pilaris
(1999): Capper N, Mobile, AL (from Internet) (observation)
Linear IgA dermatosis
(2003): Avci O+, *J Am Acad Dermatol* 48(2), 299 (passim)
(2002): Cohen LM+, *J Am Acad Dermatol* 46, S32 (passim)
(1996): Primka EJ+, *J Cutan Pathol* 23, 58
(1996): Tranvan A+, *J Am Acad Dermatol* 35, 865
(1994): Primka EJ+, *J Am Acad Dermatol* 31, 809
(1990): Espagne E+, *Ann Dermatol Venereol* (French) 117, 898
Lupus erythematosus
(2003): Kundu AK, *J Assoc Physicians India* 51, 216
(2002): Sheikhzadeh A+, *Arch Intern Med* 162(7), 834
(1999): Susano R+, *Ann Rheum Dis* 58, 655
(1985): Raeder EA+, *Am Heart J* 109, 979 (4.6%)
Myxedema
(2006): Raptis L+, *Eur J Dermatol* 16(5), 590
Necrosis
(2006): Russell SJ+, *Heart* 92(10), 1395
Palmar erythema
(2007): Serrao R+, *Am J Clin Dermatol* 8(6), 347
Photosensitivity (10–30%)
(2006): Bongard V+, *Am J Ther* 13(4), 315
(2005): Yones SS+, *Clin Exp Dermatol* 30(5), 500
(2004): Shah N+, *J Oral Pathol Med* 33(1), 56 (peri-oral)
(2000): Burns KE+, *Can Respir* 7, 193 (passim)
(1997): O'Reilly FM+, American Academy of Dermatology Meeting, Poster #14
(1995): Collins P+, *Br J Dermatol* 132, 956
(1995): Tisdale JE+, *J Clin Pharmacol* 35, 351
(1995): Zehender M, *Circulation* 92, 1665
(1993): Allen JE, *Clin Pharm* 12, 580
(1993): Ettler K+, *Sb Ved Pr Lek Fak Karlovy Univerzity Hradci Kralove* (Czech) 36, 305 (9.4%)
(1992): Editorial, *JAMA* 267, 3322
(1992): Gosselink AT+, *JAMA* 267, 3289
(1991): Feigl D+, *Harefuah* 121(10), 374
(1990): Monk B, *Clin Exp Dermatol* 15, 319
(1989): Rappersberger K+, *J Invest Dermatol* 93, 201

(1988): Hyatt RH+, *Age Aging* 17, 116 (10%)
(1988): Parodi A, *Photodermatol* 5, 146
(1987): Roupe G+, *Acta Derm Venereol* (Stockh) 67, 76
(1987): Waitzer S+, *J Am Acad Dermatol* 16, 779
(1986): Boyle J, *Br J Dermatol* 115, 253
(1986): Ferguson J, *Br J Clin Pract Symp* Suppl 44, 63
(1986): Ljunggren B+, *Photodermatol* 3, 26
(1986): Toback AC+, *Dermatol Clin* 4, 223
(1986): Török L+, *Hautarzt* (German) 37, 507 (24%)
(1985): Ferguson J+, *Br J Dermatol* 113, 537
(1985): Mulrow JP+, *Ann Int Med* 103, 68
(1985): Raeder EA+, *Am Heart J* 109, 979 (4.6%)
(1985): Stäubli M, *Postgrad Med J* 61, 245
(1985): Vila Serra MD+, *Med Clin* (Barc) (Spanish) 84, 379
(1984): Diffey BL+, *Clin Exp Dermatol* 9, 248
(1984): Ferguson J+, *Lancet* 2, 414
(1984): Guerciolini R+, *Lancet* 1, 962
(1984): Kaufmann G, *Lancet* 1, 51
(1984): Walter JF+, *Arch Dermatol* 120, 1591
(1984): Zachary CB+, *Br J Dermatol* 110, 451
(1983): Fogoros RN+, *Circulation* 68, 88 (11%)
(1983): Harris L+, *Circulation* 67, 45 (57%)
(1983): McGovern B+, *BMJ* 287, 175 (8.75%)
(1983): Nadamanee K+, *Ann Intern Med* 98, 577 (5.3%)
(1982): Chalmers RJ+, *Br Med J Clin Res Ed* 285, 341
Phototoxicity
(2006): *Prescrire Int* 15(82), 62
Pigmentation
(2008): Ammoury A+, *Arch Dermatol* 144(1), 92 (blue-gray)
(2007): Wiper A+, *Heart* 93(1), 15
(2006): Enseleit F+, *Circulation* 113(5), e63 (blue-gray)
(2006): Nikolidakis S+, *Heart* 92(4), 436 (blue-gray)
(2006): Raptis L+, *Eur J Dermatol* 16(5), 590
(2005): Yones SS+, *Clin Exp Dermatol* 30(5), 500 (slate-gray)
(2003): Dissemond J+, *Hautarzt* 54(10), 994
(2003): Ioannides MA+, *Int J Cardiol* 90(2-3), 345
(2002): Marko P+, *Acta Dermatoven* 11(3), 110 (3 cases)
(2001): Dereure O, *Am J Clin Dermatol* 2(4), 253
(2001): Haas N+, *Arch Dermatol* 137, 313 (blue-gray)
(2001): High WA+, *N Engl J Med* 345, 1464
(2001): Rubegni P+, *Am Fam Physician* 63, 1409
(2001): Wohlrab J+, *Internist* (Berl) 42(9), 1256
(2000): Burns KE+, *Can Respir* 7, 193 (passim)
(2000): Gutknecht DR, *Cutis* 66, 294 (blue-gray)
(1999): Karrer S+, *Arch Dermatol* 135, 251
(1997): Sivaram CA+, *N Engl J Med* 337, 1813
(1996): Ammann R+, *Hautarzt* (German) 47, 930
(1996): Kounis NG+, *Clin Cardiol* 19, 592
(1995): Tisdale JE+, *J Clin Pharmacol* 35, 351 (blue-gray)
(1993): Balslev E+, *Ugeskr Laeger* (Danish) 155, 4014 (blue-gray)
(1993): Colquhoun JP, *Aust Fam Physician* 22, 2168
(1993): Ettler K+, *Sb Ved Pr Lek Fak Karlovy Univerzity Hradci Kralove* (Czech) 36, 305 (9.4%)
(1992): Editorial, *JAMA* 267, 3322
(1992): Fitzpatrick JE, *Derm Clinics* 10, 19
(1992): Son En Ai+, *Klin Med Mosk* (Russian) 70, 46
(1991): Blackshear JL+, *Mayo Clin Proc* 66, 721
(1991): Fazekas T+, *Szent Gyorgyi Albert Orvostudomanyi Egyetem* (Hungarian) 132, 2157
(1991): Feigl D+, *Harefuah* 121(10), 374
(1990): Brazzelli V+, *G Ital Dermatol Venereol* (Italian) 125, 521
(1989): Klein AD+, *Arch Dermatol* 125, 417
(1989): Rappersberger K+, *J Invest Dermatol* 93, 201
(1989): Reingardene DI, *Kardiologiia* (Russian) 29, 112
(1988): Beukema WP+, *Am J Cardiol* 62, 1146
(1988): Zadionchenko VS+, *Klin Med Mosk* (Russian) 66, 126
(1987): Goldstein GD+, *Chest* 91, 772
(1987): Waitzer S+, *J Am Acad Dermatol* 16, 779
(1986): Dowson JH+, *Arch Dermatol* 122, 244
(1986): Rappersberger K+, *Br J Dermatol* 114, 189

(1986): Török L+, *Hautarzt* (German) 37, 507
(1985): Alinovi A+, *J Am Acad Dermatol* 12, 563
(1985): Lakatos A, *Orv Hetil* (Hungarian) 126, 1343
(1985): Varotti C+, *G Ital Dermatol Venereol* (Italian) 120, 183
(1984): Miller RAW+, *Arch Dermatol* 120, 646
(1984): Onofrey BE+, *J Am Optom Assoc* 55, 337
(1984): Rotmensch HH+, *Ann Intern Med* 101, 462 (4.6%)
(1984): Weiss SR+, *J Am Acad Dermatol* 11, 898
(1984): Zachary CB+, *Br J Dermatol* 110, 451
(1983): Harris L+, *Circulation* 67, 45 (1.4%)
(1983): McGovern B+, *BMJ* 287, 175
(1983): Trimble JW+, *Arch Dermatol* 119, 914
(1982): Ferrer I+, *Med Clin* (Barc) (Spanish) 79, 355
(1982): Quintanilla E+, *Med Cutan Ibero Lat Am* (Spanish) 10, 177
(1981): Granstein RD+, *J Am Acad Dermatol* 5, 1 (blue-gray)
(1981): Korting HC+, *Hautarzt* (German) 32, 301

Pruritus (1–5%)
Psoriasis
(1986): Abel EA+, *J Am Acad Dermatol* 15, 1007
(1982): Muir AD, *N Z Med J* 95, 711
Purpura (2%)
(1983): Fogoros RN+, *Circulation* 68, 88
Rash (sic) (<1%)
Rosacea
(1987): Reifler DM+, *Am J Ophthalmol* 103, 594
Side effects (sic) (12%)
(2006): Satomi K+, *Circ J* 70(8), 977
(1994): Shukla R+, *Postgrad Med J* 70, 492
Stevens–Johnson syndrome (<1%)
Toxic epidermal necrolysis
(2002): Yung A+, *Australas J Dermatol* 43(1), 35 (fatal)
(2000): Danby WF, Manchester, NH (from Internet) (observation)
(1985): Bencini PL+, *Arch Dermatol* 121, 838
Urticaria
(1983): McGovern B+, *BMJ* 287, 175 (1.25%)
Vasculitis (<1%)
(2001): Scharf C+, *Lancet* 358, 2045
(1994): Dootson G+, *Clin Exp Dermatol* 19, 422
(1994): Gutierrez R+, *Ann Pharmacother* 28, 537
(1985): Starke ID+, *BMJ* 291, 940
(1985): Stäubli M, *Postgrad Med J* 61, 245

Mucosal/ENT
Dysgeusia (1–10%)
(1983): McGovern B+, *BMJ* 287, 175
Parosmia (1–10%)
Sialorrhea (1–3%)

Hair
Hair – alopecia (<1%)
(2000): Litt JZ, Beachwood, OH (personal case) (observation) (after 2 weeks of therapy)
(1995): Ahmad S, *Arch Intern Med* 155, 1106
(1992): Samuel LM+, *Postgrad Med J* 68, 771
(1985): Raeder EA+, *Am Heart J* 109, 979 (4.1%)
(1984): Rotmensch HH+, *Ann Intern Med* 101, 462 (0.7%)
(1983): McGovern B+, *BMJ* 287, 175 (2.5%)
Hair – hypertrichosis
(1985): Ferguson J+, *Br J Dermatol* 113, 537

Eyes
Corneal edema
(2006): Dovie JM+, *Optometry* 77(2), 76
Dyschromatopsia
(2002): Ikaheimo K+, *Acta Ophthalmol Scand* 80(1), 59
Keratopathy
(2006): Dovie JM+, *Optometry* 77(2), 76

(2005): Bratulescu M+, *Oftalmologia* 49(4), 18
(2005): Chilov MN+, *Clin Experiment Ophthalmol* 33(6), 666
(2005): Every SG+, *Invest Ophthalmol Vis Sci* 46(10), 3616
Maculopathy
(2005): Bratulescu M+, *Oftalmologia* 49(4), 18
Ocular toxicity
(2006): *Prescrire Int* 15(82), 62
Optic edema
(2006): Shinder R+, *J Neuroophthalmol* 26(3), 192
Optic neuropathy
(2006): Purvin V+, *Arch Ophthalmol* 124(5), 696 (22 cases)
(2005): Murphy MA+, *J Neuroophthalmol* 25(3), 232
Vision blurred
(2006): Shinder R+, *J Neuroophthalmol* 26(3), 192
Visual halos
(2006): Dovie JM+, *Optometry* 77(2), 76

Other
Cardiotoxicity
(2006): *Prescrire Int* 15(82), 62
Cough
(2006): Azzam I+, *Postgrad Med J* 82(963), 73
Death
(2006): Fukumoto Y+, *Fukuoka Igaku Zasshi* 97(2), 37
(2002): Kharabsheh S+, *Am J Cardiol* 89(7), 896
(2002): Yung A+, *Australas J Dermatol* 43(1), 35
Headache
Hepatotoxicity
(2007): Coban S+, *J Gastroenterol Hepatol* 22(1), 140
(2006): *Prescrire Int* 15(82), 62
(2006): Kum LC+, *Clin Cardiol* 29(7), 295
(2006): Ricaurte B+, *Ann Pharmacother* 40(4), 753 (with simvastatin)
(2005): Oikawa H+, *World J Gastroenterol* 11(34), 5394
(2005): Puli SR+, *Am J Med Sci* 330(5), 257
Hypotension
(2006): Patel AA+, *Am J Health* 63(9), 829
(2005): Saul JP+, *Circulation* 112(22), 3470 (36%)
(2002): Zaidenstein R+, *Pharmacoepidemiol Drug Saf* 11(3), 235
Inappropriate secretion of antidiuretic hormone (SIADH)
(2006): Yoshikawa S+, *J Cardiol* 48(4), 215
(2004): Aslam MK+, *Pacing Clin Electrophysiol* 27(6 Pt 1), 831
(2002): Ikegami H+, *J Cardiovasc Pharmacol Ther* 7(1), 25 (2 cases)
(2002): Patel GP+, *Pharmacotherapy* 22(5), 649
(1999): Odeh M+, *Arch Intern Med* 159(21), 2599
(1996): Munoz Ruiz AI+, *An Med Interna* 13(3), 125
Myalgia/Myositis/Myopathy/Myotoxicity
(2005): Chouhan UM+, *Ann Pharmacother* 39(10), 1760 (with simvastatin and clarithromycin)
Neurotoxicity
(2006): Bongard V+, *Am J Ther* 13(4), 315
Paresthesias (4–9%)
Pseudoporphyria
(1988): Parodi A, *Photodermatology* 5, 146
Rhabdomyolysis
(2006): Ricaurte B+, *Ann Pharmacother* 40(4), 753 (with simvastatin)
(2004): Roten L+, *Ann Pharmacother* 38(6), 978 (with simvastatin)
(2003): de Denus S+, *Am J Health Syst Pharm* 60(17), 1791 (with amiodarone simvastatin)
Thrombophlebitis
(2006): Showkathali R+, *Emerg Med J* 23(8), 660
(2005): Aljitawi O+, *South Med J* 98(8), 814
Tremor
(2006): Bongard V+, *Am J Ther* 13(4), 315

AMISULPRIDE

Trade names: Deniban; Solian (Sanofi-Aventis)
Indications: Psychoses, schizophrenia
Category: Antipsychotic; Dopamine receptor antagonist
Half-life: 12 hours
**Clinically important, potentially hazardous interactions
with:** amiodarone, bepridil, cisapride, disopyramide, droperidol, erythromycin, flecainide, levodopa, pentamidine, procainamide, quinidine, sotalol, sparfloxacin, terfenadine, thioridazine

Reactions

Skin
Rash (sic)

Mucosal/ENT
Xerostomia

Other
Abdominal pain
Agitation
Anxiety
Asthenia
Gynecomastia
Hypertension
  (2001): Pedrosa Gil F+, *Pharmacopsychiatry* 34(6), 259
Hypotension
  (2001): Pedrosa Gil F+, *Pharmacopsychiatry* 34(6), 259
Insomnia
  (2001): Pedrosa Gil F+, *Pharmacopsychiatry* 34(6), 259
Mania
  (2003): Murphy BP, *Br J Psychiatry* 183, 172
Seizures
Somnolence
  (2001): Pedrosa Gil F+, *Pharmacopsychiatry* 34(6), 259
Tremor
Weight gain
  (2006): Gentile S, *Drug Saf* 29(4), 303
  (2006): Papadimitriou GN+, *Int Clin Psychopharmacol* 21(3), 181

AMITRIPTYLINE

Trade names: Amineurin; Domical; Elavil (AstraZeneca); Laroxyl; Lentizol; Levate; Limbitrol (Valeant); Novotriptyn; Saroten; Tryptanol; Tryptizol
Indications: Depression
Category: Antidepressant, tricyclic; Muscarinic antagonist
Half-life: 10–25 hours
**Clinically important, potentially hazardous interactions
with:** amprenavir, clonidine, **ephedra**, epinephrine, **eucalyptus**, guanethidine, isocarboxazid, linezolid, MAO inhibitors, paroxetine, phenelzine, quinolones, sparfloxacin, **St John's wort**, tranylcypromine

Note: Limbitrol is amitriptyline and chlordiazepoxide

Reactions

Skin
Acne
Allergic reactions (sic) (<1%)
Angioedema
  (1999): Garcia-Doval I+, *Cutis* 63, 35 (passim)
Bullous dermatitis (<1%)
Dermatitis
Dermatitis herpetiformis
Diaphoresis (1–10%)
  (1995): Feder R, *J Clin Psychiatry* 56, 35
Edema
  (2002): *Prescrire Int* 11(60), 111
Erythema
Erythema annulare centrifugum
  (1999): Garcia-Doval I+, *Cutis* 63, 35
Erythroderma
  (1999): Garcia-Doval I+, *Cutis* 63, 35 (passim)
Exanthems
Exfoliative dermatitis
Facial edema
Fixed eruption
  (2005): Dan Mitchel, Thomasville, GA (from Internet)
    (observation)
  (1998): McCarthy J, Ft. Worth, TX (from Internet) (observation)
Lichen planus
  (1999): Garcia-Doval I+, *Cutis* 63, 35 (passim)
Lupus erythematosus
  (1993): Dove FB, *Hosp Pract Off Ed* 28, 14
Necrosis
  (1999): Fogarty BJ+, *Burns* 25, 768
Petechiae
Photosensitivity (<1%)
  (1999): Garcia-Doval I+, *Cutis* 63, 35 (passim)
  (1996): Taniguchi S+, *Am J Hematol* 53, 49
Pigmentation
  (1999): Garcia-Doval I+, *Cutis* 63, 35 (passim)
  (1988): Warnock JK+, *Am J Psychiatry* 145, 425
  (1985): Basler RS+, *J Am Acad Dermatol* 12, 577
Pruritus
  (1999): Garcia-Doval I+, *Cutis* 63, 35 (passim)
  (1988): Larrey D+, *Gastroenterology* 94, 200
Purpura
  (1999): Garcia-Doval I+, *Cutis* 63, 35 (passim)
Rash (sic)
Urticaria
Vasculitis

Mucosal/ENT
Ageusia
Bromhidrosis
Dysgeusia (>10%)
Glossitis
Oral mucosal eruption
Sialopenia
  (1995): Loesche WJ+, *J Am Geriatr Soc* 43, 401
Sialorrhea
Stomatitis
  (1988): Larrey D+, *Gastroenterology* 94, 200
Stomatopyrosis
Tinnitus
  (1990): Feder R, *J Clin Psychiatry* 51(2), 85
  (1980): Miles SW, *N Z Med J* 92(664), 66
Tongue black
Tongue edema
Vaginitis
Xerostomia (>10%)
  (2002): Krymchantowski AV+, *Headache* 42(6), 510 (with
    fluoxetine)
  (1996): Rani PU+, *Anesth Analg* 83, 371
  (1995): Bremner JD, *J Clin Psychiatry* 56(11), 519
  (1995): Loesche WJ+, *J Am Geriatr Soc* 43, 401
  (1985): Feighner JP, *J Clin Psychiatry* 46(9), 369

(1984): Kerr TA+, *Acta Psychiatr Scand* 70(6), 573
(1981): Rafaelsen OJ+, *Acta Psychiatr Scand Suppl* 290, 364

Hair

Hair – alopecia (<1%)
(1992): Breathnach SM+, *Adverse Drug Reactions and the Skin* Blackwell, Oxford, 196 (passim)

Eyes

Nystagmus
(2004): Osborne SF+, *Eye* 18(1), 106

Other

Anaphylactoid reactions/Anaphylaxis
Anticonvulsant hypersensitivity syndrome
(2006): Gaig P+, *J Investig Allergol Clin Immunol* 16(5), 321
Congestive heart failure
(2003): Ansari A+, *Tex Heart Inst J* 30(1), 76
Depression
(2004): Jick H+, *JAMA* 292(3), 338
DRESS syndrome
(2006): Gaig P+, *J Investig Allergol* 16(5), 321
Gynecomastia (<1%)
Headache
Hypersensitivity
(2000): Milionis HJ, *Postgrad Med J* 76, 361
Inappropriate secretion of antidiuretic hormone (SIADH)
(2005): Miehle K+, *Pharmacopsychiatry* 38(4), 181
(1989): Henkin Y+, *Isr J Med Sci* 25(10), 587
(1986): Ananth J+, *Int J Psychiatry Med* 16(4), 401
Lymphoid hyperplasia
(1995): Crowson AN+, *Arch Dermatol* 131, 925
Neurotoxicity
(2006): Kitagawa N+, *Toxicol Appl Pharmacol* 217(1), 100
Paresthesias
Pseudolymphoma
(1995): Crowson AN+, *Arch Dermatol* 131, 925
(1995): Magro CM+, *J Am Acad Dermatol* 32, 419
Rhabdomyolysis
(1983): Caruana RJ+, *N C Med* 44(1), 18 (with lorazepam and perphenazine)
(1983): Lefkowitz D+, *J Neurol Neurosurg Psychiatry* 46(2), 183 (with perphenazine)
Seizures
(2002): Agelink MW+, *Eur J Med Res* 7(9), 415
Tremor
Weight gain
(2005): Ness-Abramof R+, *Drugs Today* 41(8), 547

AMLEXANOX

Trade names: Aphthasol (Discus); Aphtheal (Straken); Elics; OraDisc (Access); Solfa (Takeda)
Indications: Aphthous ulcers, Canker sores
Category: Anti-inflammatory
Half-life: ~3.5 hours
Clinically important, potentially hazardous interactions with: N/A

Reactions

Skin

Burning
Dermatitis
(1992): Hayakawa R+, *Contact Dermatitis* 27(2), 122 (systemic)
(1991): Kabasawa Y+, *Contact Dermatitis* 24(2), 148

(1991): Yamashita H+, *Contact Dermatitis* 25(4), 255
Erythema
(1998): Sugiura M+, *Contact Dermatitis* 38(2), 65
Fixed eruption
(1998): Sugiura M+, *Contact Dermatitis* 38(2), 65

Mucosal/ENT

Mucosal inflammation

Other

Application-site burning
Application-site pain
Application-site stinging

AMLODIPINE

Trade names: Amdepin; Amlodin; Amlogard; Amlopin; Amlor; Istin; Lotrel (Novartis); Norvas; Norvasc (Pfizer)
Indications: Hypertension, angina
Category: Antiarrhythmic class IV; Calcium channel blocker
Half-life: 30–50 hours
Clinically important, potentially hazardous interactions with: epirubicin, imatinib

Note: Lotrel is amlodipine and benazepril

Reactions

Skin

Angioedema
(2006): Piller LB+, *J Clin Hypertens* 8(9), 649 (Greenwich) (6%)
(2006): Shahzad G+, *Mt Sinai J Med* 73(8), 1123 (bowel) (with benazepril)
Dermatitis (1–10%)
Diaphoresis (<1%)
Edema (5–14%)
(2001): Chugh SK+, *J Cardiovasc Pharmacol* 38(3), 356
(2001): Maekawa Y+, *Nippon Ronen Igakkai Zasshi* 38(5), 696 (with candesartan)
(1996): Corea L+, *Clin Pharmacol Ther* 60, 341
(1992): DiBianco R+, *Clin Cardiol* 15, 519
(1992): Johnson BF+, *Am J Hypertens* 5, 727
(1991): Elliott HL+, *Postgrad Med J* 67, S20
(1991): Murdoch D+, *Drugs* 41, 478
(1989): Chahine RA+, *Am Heart J* 118, 1128
(1989): Doyle GD+, *Eur J Clin Pharmacol* 36, 205 (ankle)
(1989): Estrada JN+, *Am Heart J* 118, 1130
(1989): Osterloh I, *Am Heart J* 118, 1114
(1988): Glasser SP+, *Am J Cardiol* 62, 518
Erythema multiforme
(1993): Bewley AP+, *BMJ* 307, 241
Exanthems (2–4%)
(1989): Doyle GD+, *Eur J Clin Pharmacol* 36, 205
Exfoliative dermatitis
Granuloma annulare
(2002): Lim AC+, *Australas J Dermatol* 43(1), 24
Lichen planus
(2001): Swale VJ+, *Br J Dermatol* 144, 920
Lichenoid eruption
(1998): Silver B, Deerfield, IL (from Internet) (observation)
Lupus erythematosus
(2002): Boye T+, *World Congress Dermatol* Poster 0088
Peripheral edema (>10%)
(2006): Andersen J+, *Am J Ther* 13(3), 198
(2006): Hong SJ+, *Clin Ther* 28(4), 537 (4%)
(2004): Wu SC+, *Heart Vessels* 19(1), 13 (7.5%)
(2003): Franco RJ+, *Blood Press Suppl* Supp 2, 41

(2003): Malacco E+, *Clin Ther* 25(11), 2765 (27%)
(2002): Litt JZ, Beachwood, OH (personal case) (observation)
(2001): Lenz TL+, *Pharmacotherapy* 21(8), 898 (4 cases) (with nisoldipine)
(2001): Zanchetti A+, *J Cardiovasc Pharmacol* 38(4), 642
(1994): Clavijo GA+, *Am J Hosp Pharm* 51, 59
(1993): Ellis JS+, *Lancet* 341, 1102
Petechiae (<1%)
Pigmentation (<1%)
(2006): Enseleit F+, *Circulation* 113(5), e63
(2004): Erbagci Z, *Saudi Med J* 25(1), 103
Pruritus (2–4%)
(1998): Litt JZ, Beachwood, OH (personal case) (observation)
(1997): Orme S+, *BMJ* 315, 463
(1994): Baker BA+, *Ann Pharmacother* 28, 118
(1993): Ellis JS+, *Lancet* 341, 1102
Purpura (<1%)
(1994): Dacosta A+, *Therapie* (French) 49, 515
Rash (sic) (1–10%)
Stevens–Johnson syndrome
Telangiectasia (facial)
(2000): Grabczynska SA+, *Br J Dermatol* 142, 1255
(1999): van der Vleuten CJ+, *Acta Derm Venereol* 79, 323
(1997): Basarab T+, *Br J Dermatol* 136, 974 (photo-induced)
Urticaria (<1%)
Vasculitis
(1995): del Rio Fermandez MC+, *Rev Clin Esp* (Spanish) 195, 738
Xerosis (<0.1%)

Mucosal/ENT
Dysgeusia
(2007): Sadasivam B+, *Br J Clin Pharmacol* 63(2), 253
Gingival hyperplasia/hypertrophy
(2006): Yoon AJ+, *J Periodontol* 77(1), 119
(2003): Routray SN+, *J Assoc Physicians India* 51, 818
(2001): Morisaki I+, *Spec Care Dentist* 21(2), 60
(2000): James JA+, *J Clin Periodontol* 27, 109 (with cyclosporine)
(1999): Ellis JS+, *J Periodontol* 70, 63 (3.3%)
(1999): van der Vleuten CJ+, *Acta Derm Venereol* 79, 323
(1997): Infante-Cossio P+, *An Med Interna* (Spanish) 14, 83
(1997): Jorgensen MG, *J Periodontol* 68, 676
(1995): Salerno L+, *Clin Ter* (Italian) 146, 275
(1995): Wynn RL, *Gen Dent* 43, 218
(1994): Juncadella Garcia E+, *Med Clin* (Barc) (Spanish) 103, 358
(1994): Seymour RA+, *J Clin Periodontol* 21, 281
(1993): Ellis JS+, *Lancet* 341, 1102
(1993): Smith RG, *Br Dent J* 175, 279
(1991): Wynn RL, *Gen Dent* 39, 240
Oral pigmentation
(2004): Erbagci Z, *Saudi Med J* 25(1), 103
Parosmia (<0.1%)
Tinnitus
Xerostomia (<1%)

Hair
Hair – alopecia (<1%)

Nails
Nails – melanonychia
(2005): Sladden MJ+, *Br J Dermatol* 153(1), 219

Eyes
Keratopathy
(2006): Dovie JM+, *Optometry* 77(2), 76

Other
Asthenia
(2006): Andersen J+, *Am J Ther* 13(3), 198
Gynecomastia
(1994): Zochling J+, *Med J Aust* 160, 807

Headache
(2006): Hong SJ+, *Clin Ther* 28(4), 537 (2%)
Paresthesias (<1%)
Tendinopathy/Tendon rupture
(1999): Zambanini A+, *J Hum Hypertens* 13, 565 (Achilles)
Tremor
Upper respiratory infection
(2006): Hong SJ+, *Clin Ther* 28(4), 537 (7%)
Vertigo
(2006): Andersen J+, *Am J Ther* 13(3), 198

AMOBARBITAL

Trade names: Amytal; Amytal Sodium; Isoamitil Sedante; Neur-Amyl; Novambarb; Sodium Amytal
Indications: Insomnia, sedation
Category: Barbiturate
Half-life: initial: 40 minutes; terminal: 20 hours
Clinically important, potentially hazardous interactions with: alcohol, dicumarol, ethanolamine, warfarin

Reactions

Skin
Acne
Angioedema
Bullous dermatitis
Erythema
Exanthems
Exfoliative dermatitis (<1%)
Photosensitivity
Purpura
Rash (sic) (<1%)
Stevens–Johnson syndrome (<1%)
Toxic epidermal necrolysis
Urticaria (<1%)

Other
Headache
Hypersensitivity
Injection-site pain (>10%)
Rhabdomyolysis
(1990): Larpin R+, *Presse Med* 19(30), 1403
Serum sickness
Thrombophlebitis (<1%)

AMOXAPINE

Trade names: Amoxan; Amoxapine (Watson); Asendis; Defanyl; Demolox
Indications: Depression
Category: Antidepressant, tetracyclic; Muscarinic antagonist
Half-life: 11–30 hours
Clinically important, potentially hazardous interactions with: amprenavir, clonidine, epinephrine, guanethidine, isocarboxazid, linezolid, MAO inhibitors, phenelzine, quinolones, sparfloxacin, tranylcypromine

Reactions

Skin
Acne

Acute febrile neutrophilic dermatosis (Sweet's syndrome)
  (2004): Mecca P+, *J Cutan Pathol* 31(2), 189 (with citalopram
    and perphenazine) (photodistributed)
Acute generalized exanthematous pustulosis (AGEP)
  (2004): Mecca P+, *J Cutan Pathol* 31(2), 189
  (1998): Loche F+, *Acta Derm Venereol* 78, 224
  (1994): Larbre B+, *Ann Dermatol Venereol* (French) 121, 40
Allergic reactions (sic) (<1%)
Dermatitis
Diaphoresis (1–10%)
Edema (>1%)
Erythema multiforme (observation)
  (1982): Bishop L, *ADRRS* oral communication
Exanthems
  (1996): Nagayama H+, *J Dermatol* 23, 899
  (1982): Jue SG+, *Drugs* 24, 1
Neutrophilic dermatosis
  (2004): Mecca P+, *J Cutan Pathol* 31(2), 189
Petechiae
Photosensitivity (<1%)
Pruritus (<1%)
  (1988): Warnock JK+, *Am J Psychiatry* 145, 425
Purpura
Rash (sic) (>1%)
Side effects (sic) (5.1%)
  (1982): Jue SG+, *Drugs* 24, 1
Toxic epidermal necrolysis
  (1988): Warnock JK+, *Am J Psychiatry* 145, 425
  (1983): Camisa C+, *Arch Dermatol* 119, 709
Urticaria (<1%)
Vasculitis (<1%)
  (1988): Warnock JK+, *Am J Psychiatry* 145, 425
Xerosis

Mucosal/ENT
Bromhidrosis
Dysgeusia (>10%)
Glossitis
Sialorrhea
Stomatitis
Tinnitus
Tongue black
Vaginitis
Xerostomia (14%)
  (1982): Jue SG+, *Drugs* 24, 1

Hair
Hair – alopecia (<1%)

Other
Gynecomastia (<1%)
Headache
Paresthesias (<1%)
Tremor

AMOXICILLIN

Synonym: amoxycillin
Trade names: A-Gram; Acimox; Almodan; Amodex; Amoxil
(GSK); Apo-Amoxi; Augmentin (GSK); Clamoxyl; Eupen; Fisamox;
Lin-Amnox; Novamoxin; Nu-Amoxi; Prevpac (TAP); Pro-Amox;
Trimox (Bristol-Myers Squibb)
Indications: Infections of the respiratory tract, skin and urinary
tract
Category: Antibiotic, penicillin
Half-life: 0.7–1.4 hours
**Clinically important, potentially hazardous interactions
with:** allopurinol, **bromelain**, chloramphenicol, demeclocycline,
doxycycline, erythromycin, imipenem/cilastatin, methotrexate,
minocycline, oxytetracycline, sulfonamides, tetracycline

Note: Augmentin is amoxicillin and clavulanate

Reactions

Skin
Acute generalized exanthematous pustulosis (AGEP)
  (2008): Betto P+, *Int J Dermatol* 47(3), 295
  (2006): Harries MJ+, *Contact Dermatitis* 55(6), 372
  (2006): Reich A+, *Skinmed* 5(4), 197
  (2003): Saissi EH+, *Ann Dermatol Venereol* 130(6-7), 612
  (2002): Pattee SF+, *Arch Dermatol* 138(8), 1091
  (2001): de Thier F+, *Contact Dermatitis* 44, 114
  (2000): Meadows KP+, *Pediatric Dermatology* 17, 399
  (1997): Gibert-Agullo A+, *An Esp Pediatr* (Spanish) 46, 285
  (1997): Zabawski E, Dallas, TX (from Internet) (observation)
  (1996): Wolkenstein P+, *Contact Dermatitis* 35, 234
  (1995): Moreau A+, *Int J Dermatol* 34, 263 (passim)
  (1991): Roujeau J-C+, *Arch Dermatol* 127, 1333
  (1989): Epelbaum S+, *Pediatrie* (French) 44, 387
Angioedema (1–10%)
  (1998): Minguez MA+, *Allergol Immunopathol* (Madr) (Spanish)
    26, 43
  (1994): Galindo-Bonilla PA+, *Contact Dermatitis* 31, 319
  (1994): Vega JM+, *Allergy* 49, 317
  (1989): Chopra R+, *Can Med Assoc J* 140, 921 (in children)
Baboon syndrome
  (2004): Hausermann P+, *Contact Dermatitis* 51(5-6), 297
  (2003): Wolf R+, *Dermatol Online J* 9(3), 2 (4 cases) (with
    omeprazole and clarithromycin)
  (2002): Strub C+, *Schweiz Rundsch Med Prax* 91(6), 232
  (2000): Kick G+, *Contact Dermatitis* 43, 366
  (1999): Wakelin SH+, *Clin Exp Dermatol* 24(2), 71
  (1996): Kohler LD+, *Int J Dermatol* 35, 502
  (1994): Duve S+, *Acta Derm Venereol* 74, 480
  (1993): Herfs H+, *Hautarzt* (German) 44, 466
Bullous dermatitis
  (2007): Ho JC+, *Pediatr Dermatol* 24(5), E40 (Linear IgA)
Bullous pemphigoid
  (1997): Miralles J+, *Int J Dermatol* 36, 42
  (1988): Alcalay J+, *J Am Acad Dermatol* 18, 345
Dermatitis
  (2006): Dohar J+, *Pediatrics* 118(3), e561
  (2001): Petavy-Catala C+, *Contact Dermatitis* 44, 251 (consort)
  (1996): Garcia R+, *Contact Dermatitis* 35, 116
  (1995): Gamboa P+, *Contact Dermatitis* 32, 48 (occupational)
Diaper rash
  (1988): Honig PJ+, *J Am Acad Dermatol* 19, 275
Edema
  (1993): Echeverria-Arellano A+, *An Esp Pediatr* (Spanish) 39, 448
Erythema

(2005): Reig Rincon de Arellano I+, *Allergol Immunopathol (Madr)* 33(5), 282

Erythema multiforme
(2006): Gonzalez-Delgado P+, *Allergol Immunopathol (Madr)* 34(2), 76
(2006): Hernandez-Salazar A+, *Arch Med Res* 37(7), 899
(2001): Perez A+, *Contact Dermatitis* 44, 113 (with allopurinol)
(1999): Benjamin S+, *Ann Pharmacother* 33, 109
(1999): Wakelin SH+, *Clin Exp Dermatol* 24, 71
(1996): Webster GF, Philadelphia, PA (from Internet) (observation)
(1995): Wolkenstein P+, *Arch Dermatol* 131, 544
(1992): Gross AS+, *J Am Acad Dermatol* 27, 781
(1990): Chan HL+, *Arch Dermatol* 126, 43
(1990): Escallier F+, *Rev Med Interne* (French) 11, 73
(1989): Chopra R+, *Can Med Assoc J* 140, 921 (in children)
(1988): Massullo RE+, *J Am Acad Dermatol* 19, 358
(1988): Platt R, *J Infect Dis* 158, 474
(1986): Davidson NJ+, *BMJ* 292, 380
(1986): Dikland WJ+, *Pediatr Dermatol* 3, 135
(1982): Freeman T, *Can Med Assoc J* 127, 818

Exanthems (>5%)
(2007): Jappe U, *Allergy* 62(12), 1474
(2006): Hernandez-Salazar A+, *Arch Med Res* 37(7), 899
(2005): Reig Rincon de Arellano I+, *Allergol Immunopathol (Madr)* 33(5), 282
(2003): Leung AK+, *Int J Dermatol* 42(7), 553
(2003): Zhang YM+, *Zhonghua Er Ke Za Zhi* 41(2), 135 (2 cases)
(2002): Renn CN+, *Br J Dermatol* 147(6), 1166 (4 cases, all with infectious mononucleosis)
(1999): Wakelin SH+, *Clin Exp Dermatol* 24, 71 (flexural)
(1997): Barbaud AM+, *Arch Dermatol* 133, 481
(1997): Blumenthal HL, Beachwood, OH (personal case) (observation)
(1995): Romano A+, *Allergy* 50, 113
(1995): Wolkenstein P+, *Arch Dermatol* 131, 544
(1994): Litt JZ, Beachwood, OH (personal case) (observation)
(1993): Fellner MJ, *Int J Dermatol* 32, 308
(1993): Romano A+, *J Invest Allergol Clin Immunol* 3, 53
(1990): Pauszek ME, *Indiana Med* 83, 330
(1989): Battegay M+, *Lancet* 2, 1100
(1989): Chopra R+, *Can Med Assoc J* 140, 921 (in children)
(1989): Kennedy C+, *Contact Dermatitis* 20, 313
(1986): Bigby M+, *JAMA* 256, 3358 (5.14%)
(1986): de Haan P+, *Allergy* 41, 75
(1986): Sonntag MR+, *Schweiz Med Wochenschr* (German) 116, 142 (7%)
(1985): Levine LR, *Pediatr Infect Dis* 4, 358
(1981): Odegaard OR, *Tidsskr Nor Laegeforen* (Norwegian) 101, 1973

Exfoliative dermatitis

Fixed eruption
(2001): Agnew KL+, *Australas J Dermatol* 42(3), 200 (reproducible)
(2000): Brabek E+, *Dtsch Med Wochenschr* 125(42), 1260
(1998): Mahboob A+, *Int J Dermatol* 37, 833
(1997): Jimenez I+, *Allergol Immunopathol* (Madr) 25, 247 (glans penis)
(1997): Zabawski E, Dallas, TX (from Internet) (observation)
(1995): Arias J+, *Clin Exp Dermatol* 20, 339
(1995): Dhar S+, *Pediatr Dermatol* 12, 51 (tongue)
(1994): Gil-Garcia JF+, *Med Clin* (Barc) (Spanish) 102, 438
(1989): Shuttleworth D, *Clin Exp Dermatol* 14, 367 (pustular)
(1982): Chowdhury FH, *Practitioner* 226, 1450 (penile)

Fungal dermatitis
(2004): Leophonte P+, *Respir Med* 98(8), 708

Hematomas

Intertrigo
(1992): Wolf B+, *Acta Derm Venereol* (Stockh) 72, 441

Jarisch–Herxheimer reaction

(2003): Leblebicioglu H+, *Eur J Clin Microbiol Infect Dis* 22(10), 639
(1998): Maloy AL+, *J Emerg Med* 16, 437

Keratosis pilaris
(1997): Kay M, North Hollywood, CA (from Internet) (observation)

Linear IgA dermatosis
(2007): Ho JC+, *Pediatr Dermatol* 24(5), E40

Pemphigus
(1997): Brenner S+, *J Am Acad Dermatol* 36, 919
(1997): Landau M+, *Am J Dermatopathol* 19, 411
(1991): Escallier F+, *Ann Dermatol Venereol* (French) 118, 381
(1983): Toan ND+, *Ann Dermatol Venereol* (French) 110, 917

Perleche
(1982): Arata J+, *Jpn J Antibiot* (Japanese) 35, 394

Petechiae (Rumpel–Leede sign)
(1992): Gross AS+, *J Am Acad Dermatol* 27, 781

Pigmentation
(2003): Zhang YM+, *Zhonghua Er Ke Za Zhi* 41(2), 135 (2 cases)

Pruritus
(2005): Reig Rincon de Arellano I+, *Allergol Immunopathol (Madr)* 33(5), 282
(2000): Blumenthal HL, Beachwood, OH (personal case) (observation)
(1996): Drouet M+, *Allerg Immunol Paris* (French) 28, 311
(1995): Shelley WB+, *Cutis* 55, 202 (observation)
(1993): Fellner MJ, *Int J Dermatol* 32, 308
(1989): Battegay M+, *Lancet* 2, 1100

Psoriasis
(1993): Litt JZ, Beachwood, OH (from internet) (observation)
(1987): Katz M, *J Am Acad Dermatol* 17, 918

Purpura

Pustules
(2000): Whittam LR+, *Clin Exp Dermatol* 25, 122
(1995): Wolkenstein P+, *Arch Dermatol* 131, 544
(1992): Trueb R+, *Hautarzt* (German) 43, 595
(1991): Armster H+, *Hautarzt* (German) 42, 713
(1991): Roujeau J-C+, *Arch Dermatol* 127, 1333
(1990): Guy C+, *Nouv Dermatol* (French) 9, 540
(1989): Epelbaum S+, *Pédiatrie* (French) 44, 387
(1989): Shuttleworth D, *Clin Exp Dermatol* 14, 367

Rash (sic) (1–10%)
(1997): Van Buchem FL+, *Lancet* 349, 683
(1989): Battegay M+, *Lancet* 2, 1100
(1982): Arata J+, *Jpn J Antibiot* (Japanese) 35, 394
(1982): Millard G, *Scott Med J* 27, S35
(1980): Porter J+, *Lancet* 1, 1037

Side effects (sic)
(1994): Paparello SF+, *AIDS* 8, 276

Stevens–Johnson syndrome
(1999): Limauro DL+, *Ann Pharmacother* 33, 560
(1996): Cullimore KC, Westminster, CO (from Internet) (observation)
(1992): Martin Mateos MA+, *J Investig Allergol Clin Immunol* 2, 278
(1988): Platt R, *J Infect Dis* 158, 474

Toxic epidermal necrolysis
(2004): Najem JC+, *Middle East J Anesthesiol* 17(6), 1079
(2001): Spies M+, *Pediatrics* 108, 1162
(1996): Blum L+, *J Am Acad Dermatol* 34, 1088
(1996): Surbled M+, *Ann Fr Anesth Reanim* (French) 15, 1095
(1993): Correia O+, *Dermatology* 186, 32
(1993): Romano A+, *J Invest Allergol Clin Immunol* 3, 53
(1988): Massullo RE+, *J Am Acad Dermatol* 19, 358
(1984): Herman TE+, *Pediatr Radiol* 14, 439

Toxic pustuloderma
(1992): Trueb R+, *Hautarzt* (German) 43, 595
(1991): Armster H+, *Hautarzt* (German) 42, 713

Urticaria (1–5%)

(2006): Hernandez-Salazar A+, *Arch Med Res* 37(7), 899
(2005): Blumenthal H, Beachwood, OH (personal communication) (observation)
(2003): Zhang YM+, *Zhonghua Er Ke Za Zhi* 41(2), 135 (2 cases)
(2001): Torres MJ+, *Allergy* 56(9), 850
(2000): Blumenthal HL, Beachwood, OH (personal case) (observation)
(1998): Minguez MA+, *Allergol Immunopathol* (Madr) (Spanish) 26, 43
(1997): Delpre G+, *Dig Dis Sci* 42, 728
(1997): Thaler D, Monona, WI (from internet) (observation)
(1995): Litt JZ, Beachwood, OH (personal case) (observation)
(1994): Vega JM+, *Allergy* 49, 317
(1990): Fraj J+, *Clin Exp Allergy* 20, 121
(1989): Battegay M+, *Lancet* 2, 1100
(1989): Chopra R+, *Can Med Assoc J* 140, 921 (in children)
(1985): Goolamali SK, *Postgrad Med J* 61, 925

Vasculitis
(1999): Garcia-Porrua C+, *J Rheumatol* 26, 1942

Vesiculation

Mucosal/ENT

Dysgeusia
Glossitis
Glossodynia
Oral candidiasis
Stomatitis
(1996): Drouet M+, *Allerg Immunol Paris* (French) 28, 311
Stomatodynia
Tongue black
Vaginitis (1%)
(2004): Leophonte P+, *Respir Med* 98(8), 708
(1996): Drouet M+, *Allerg Immunol Paris* (French) 28, 311
Xerostomia
(1995): Hautekeete ML+, *J Hepatol* 22(1), 71

Eyes

Visual hallucinations
(1996): Stell IM+, *Br J Clin Pract* 50(5), 279

Other

Anaphylactoid reactions/Anaphylaxis
(2007): Del Furia F+, *Int J Cardiol* 117(1), e37
(2003): Gei AF+, *Obstet Gynecol* 102(6), 1332
(2001): Torres MJ+, *Allergy* 56(9), 850
(1999): Salgado Fernandez J+, *Rev Esp Cardiol* (Spanish) 52, 622
(1998): Rich MW, *Tex Heart Inst J* 25, 194
(1994): Vega JM+, *Allergy* 49, 317
(1993): van der Klauw MM+, *Br J Clin Pharmacol* 35, 400
(1990): Fraj J+, *Clin Exp Allergy* 20, 121
(1988): Blanca M+, *Allergy* 43, 508
Anticonvulsant hypersensitivity syndrome
(2006): Gaig P+, *J Investig Allergol Clin Immunol* 16(5), 321
Aseptic meningitis
(2003): Thaunat O+, *Allergy* 58(7), 687
DRESS syndrome
(2006): Gaig P+, *J Investig Allergol* 16(5), 321
Headache
Hepatotoxicity
(2007): Cundiff J+, *Am J Otolaryngol* 28(1), 28
(2006): Andrade RJ+, *Hepatology* 44(6), 1581
(2006): Lucena MI+, *Hepatology* 44(4), 850
(2005): Fontana RJ+, *Dig Dis Sci* 50(10), 1785
(2005): Solano Remirez M+, *An Med Interna* 22(7), 350
(2002): Jordan T+, *Gastroenterol Hepatol* 25(4), 240
(2001): Ersoz G+, *J Clin Pharm Ther* 26(3), 225
(1998): Julve R+, *Gastroenterol Hepatol* 21(2), 92
(1998): Nathani MG+, *Am J Gastroenterol* 93(8), 1363
(1995): Hautekeete ML+, *J Hepatol* 22(1), 71
Hypersensitivity

(2000): da Fonseca MA, *Pediatr Dent* 22(5), 401
(1995): Mokry C, *N Engl J Med* 333, 1151
(1993): Romano A+, *Contact Dermatitis* 28, 190
(1989): Kennedy C+, *Contact Dermatitis* 20, 313
Injection-site pain
Nephrotoxicity
(2006): Huang SF+, *Zhongguo Dang Dai Er Ke Za Zhi* 28(3), 254
Rhabdomyolysis
(2004): Bhatia V, *J Postgrad Med* 50(3), 234 (with simvastatin)
Serum sickness (1–10%)
(1995): Martin J+, *N Z Med J* 108, 123
(1992): Stricker BH+, *J Clin Epidemiol* 45, 1177
(1990): Heckbert SR+, *Am J Epidemiol* 132, 336
(1989): Chopra R+, *Can Med Assoc J* 140, 921 (in children)
(1988): Platt R+, *J Infect Dis* 158, 474

AMPHOTERICIN B

Trade names: Abelcet (Wyeth); AmBisome (Astellas); Ampho-Moronal; Amphocin (Pfizer); Fungilin; Fungizone
Indications: Potentially life-threatening fungal infections
Category: Antimycobacterial
Half-life: initial: 15–48 hours; terminal: 15 days
Clinically important, potentially hazardous interactions with: adefovir, aminoglycosides, astemizole, cephalothin, cidofovir, cyclosporine, digoxin, fluconazole, flucytosine, ganciclovir, griseofulvin, hydrocortisone, itraconazole, ketoconazole, probenecid, terbinafine

Reactions

Skin

Acute generalized exanthematous pustulosis (AGEP)
(2007): Heinemann C+, *J Am Acad* 57(2), S61
Angioedema
Burning (from topical)
Dermatitis
Diaphoresis
Erythema
Erythema multiforme
(2006): Hernandez-Salazar A+, *Arch Med Res* 37(7), 899
Exanthems (<1%)
(2006): Hernandez-Salazar A+, *Arch Med Res* 37(7), 899
(1999): Cesaro S+, *Support Care Cancer* 7, 284
Exfoliative dermatitis
Fixed eruption
Pigmentation
Pruritus
(1999): Cesaro S+, *Support Care Cancer* 7, 284
Purpura
Rash (sic)
(1995): Oppenheim BA+, *Clin Infect Dis* 21, 1145
Raynaud's phenomenon (cyanotic)
(1997): Zernikow B+, *Mycoses* 40, 359
Red man syndrome
(1990): Ellis ME+, *BMJ* 300, 1468
Toxicity (sic)
(2002): Bowden R+, *Clin Infect Dis* 35(4), 359
Ulcerations
Urticaria
(2006): Hernandez-Salazar A+, *Arch Med Res* 37(7), 899
Vasculitis
(2008): Cagatay AA+, *Mycoses* 51(1), 81
Vesiculation
Xerosis

Mucosal/ENT
Stomatitis
Tinnitus
Xerostomia

Hair
Hair – alopecia

Other
Anaphylactoid reactions/Anaphylaxis
(2002): Vaidya SJ+, *Ann Pharmacother* 36(9), 1480
(2001): Bishara J+, *Ann Pharmacother* 35, 308
(1999): Cronin JE+, *Clin Infect Dis* 28, 1342
(1998): Schneider P+, *Br J Haematol* 102, 1108
Chills
(2004): Martino R, *Curr Med Res Opin* 20(4), 485
(2002): Bowden R+, *Clin Infect Dis* 35(4), 359
(2000): Wingard JR+, *Clin Infect Dis* 31(5), 1155
Death
(2002): Johnson PC+, *Ann Intern Med* 137(2), 105
(2001): Collazos J+, *Clin Infect Dis* 33(7), E75
Fever
(2004): Martino R, *Curr Med Res Opin* 20(4), 485
Headache
Hepatotoxicity
(2002): Mohan UR+, *Pediatr Pulmonol* 33(6), 497
Hypertension
(2006): Rodrigues CA+, *Ren Fail* 28(2), 185
(2006): Wiwanitkit V, *J Hypertens* 24(7), 1445
(2005): Meaudre E+, *Ann Fr Anesth Reanim* 24(11-12), 1405
(1997): Ferreira E+, *Ann Pharmacother* 31(11), 1407
Injection-site pain
Injection-site reactions (sic)
(2004): Sundar S+, *Clin Infect Dis* 38(3), 377
(2003): Imhof A+, *Clin Infect Dis* 36(8), 943
(2002): Johnson PC+, *Ann Intern Med* 137(2), 105
(2000): Karthaus M+, *Chemotherapy* 46, 293
Injection-site thrombophlebitis
(1995): Goodwin SD+, *Clin Infect Dis* 20, 755
Myalgia/Myositis/Myopathy/Myotoxicity
Nephrotoxicity
(2006): Cesaro S+, *Pediatr Transplant* 10(2), 255
(2006): Chandrasekar P, *Int J Antimicrob Agents* 27 Suppl 1, 31
(2006): Jayasuriya NS+, *Oral Dis* 12(1), 67
(2006): Saliba F, *Int J Antimicrob Agents* 27 Suppl 1, 21
(2006): Ullmann AJ+, *Clin Infect Dis* 43(4), e29
(2006): Wasan KM+, *Cancer Chemother Pharmacol* 57(1), 120
(2005): Alexander BD+, *Clin Infect Dis* 40 Suppl 6, S414
(2005): Girmenia C+, *Support Care Cancer* 13(12), 987
(2005): Pai MP+, *Antimicrob Agents Chemother* 49(9), 3784
(2005): Uehara RP+, *Sao Paulo Med J* 123(5), 219 (30%)
(2005): Wegner B+, *Nephrol Dial Transplant* 20(10), 2071
(2004): Holler B+, *Pediatrics* 113(6), e608
(2004): Subira M+, *Eur J Haematol* 72(5), 342
(2004): Yokote T+, *Ann Hematol* 83(1), 64
(2002): Deray G, *J Antimicrob Chemother* 49 Suppl 1, 37
(2002): Deray G+, *Nephrologie* 23(3), 119
(2002): Furrer K+, *Swiss Med Wkly* 132(23–24), 316
(2002): Girmenia C+, *Am J Med* 113(4), 351
(2002): Gubbins PO+, *Pharmacotherapy* 22(8), 961
(2002): Harbarth S+, *Clin Infect Dis* 35(12), e120 (12%)
(2002): Mohan UR+, *Pediatr Pulmonol* 33(6), 497
(2002): Slain D+, *Clin Ther* 24(10), 1636 (6%)
(2002): Ural AU+, *Eur J Clin Pharmacol* 57(11), 771
(2001): Cannon JP+, *Pharmacotherapy* 21(9), 1107 (14%)
(2001): Costa S+, *Curr Opin Crit Care* 7(6), 379
(2001): Eriksson U+, *BMJ* 322(7286), 579
(2001): Girmenia C+, *Clin Infect Dis* 33(6), 915
(2001): Karthaus M+, *Wien Med Wochenschr* 151(3–4), 80

(2001): Razzaque MS+, *Nephron* 89(3), 251
(2000): Cagnoni PJ+, *J Clin Oncol* 18(12), 2476
(2000): Fanos V+, *J Chemother* 12(6), 463
(2000): Sandler ES+, *J Pediatr Hematol Oncol* 22(3), 242 (12%)
(2000): Wingard JR+, *Clin Infect Dis* 31(5), 1155
(1999): Hoffman-Terry ML+, *Am J Med* 106(1), 44 (8%)
(1999): Mayer J+, *Support Care Cancer* 7(1), 51
(1999): Rowles DM+, *Clin Infect Dis* 29(6), 1564
(1999): Wingard JR+, *Clin Infect Dis* 29(6), 1402
(1998): Camp MJ+, *Antimicrob Agents Chemother* 42(12), 3103
(1998): Coukell AJ+, *Drugs* 55(4), 585
(1997): Miano-Mason TM, *Cancer Pract* 5(3), 176
Paresthesias (1–10%)
Rhabdomyolysis
Thrombophlebitis (1–10%)
(1993): Dietze R+, *Clin Infect Dis* 17, 981

AMPICILLIN

Trade names: Amfipen; Ampicin; Binotal; D-Amp; Marcillin; Penbritin; Penstabil; Principen; Pro-Ampi; Sinaplin; Taro-Ampicillin Trihydrate; Totacillin (GSK); Totapen; Unasyn (Pfizer); Vidopen
Indications: Susceptible strains of gram-negative and gram-positive bacterial infections
Category: Antibiotic, penicillin
Half-life: 1–1.5 hours
Clinically important, potentially hazardous interactions with: allopurinol, anticoagulants, chloramphenicol, cyclosporine, demeclocycline, doxycycline, erythromycin, methotrexate, minocycline, oxytetracycline, sulfonamides, tetracycline

Note: Five to 10% of people taking ampicillin develop eruptions between the 5th and 14th day following initiation of therapy. Also, there is a 95% incidence of exanthematous eruptions in patients who are treated for infectious mononucleosis with ampicillin. The allergenicity of ampicillin appears to be enhanced by allopurinol or by hyperuricemia. Ampicillin is clearly the more allergenic of the two drugs when given alone

Reactions

Skin
Acute generalized exanthematous pustulosis (AGEP)
(2003): Saissi EH+, *Ann Dermatol Venereol* 130(6-7), 612
(1996): Campbell GAM+, *An bras derm* 71(1), 519
(1995): Moreau A+, *Int J Dermatol* 34, 263 (passim)
(1994): Manders SM+, *Cutis* 54, 194
(1991): Roujeau J-C+, *Arch Dermatol* 127, 1333
Allergic reactions (sic) (1–10%)
(2003): Medrala W+, *Pol Merkuriusz Lek* 14(79), 39
(1993): Grover JK+, *Indian J Physiol Pharmacol* 37, 247 (2.9%)
Angioedema (<1%)
(1982): Valsecchi R+, *Contact Dermatitis* 8, 278
(1980): Kraemer MJ+, *Pediatrics in Review* 1, 197
Baboon syndrome
(1993): Herfs H+, *Hautarzt* (German) 44, 466
(1985): Rasmussen LP+, *Ugeskr Laeger* (Danish) 147, 1341
(1984): Andersen KE+, *Contact Dermatitis* 10, 97
Bullous dermatitis (<1%)
(1982): Stepien B+, *Przegl Dermatol* (Polish) 69, 65
Bullous pemphigoid
(1990): Hodak E+, *Clin Exp Dermatol* 15, 50
Dermatitis
(2006): Kwon HJ+, *Contact Dermatitis* 54(3), 176
(1997): Romano A+, *Clin Exp Allergy* 27, 1425

(1995): Gamboa P+, *Contact Dermatitis* 32, 48
(1988): Andersen KE, *Acta Derm Venereol* Suppl (Stockh) 135, 62
    (systemic)
(1986): Pigatto PD+, *Contact Dermatitis* 14, 196
Diaper rash
Erythema annulare centrifugum
Erythema multiforme (<1%)
(1995): Dhar S+, *Dermatology* 191, 76
(1994): Garty BZ+, *Ann Pharmacother* 28, 730
(1990): Chan HL+, *Arch Dermatol* 126, 43
(1985): Konstantinidis AB+, *J Oral Med* 40, 168
(1984): Gebel K+, *Dermatologica* 168, 35
Exanthems (>10%)
(2006): Blumenthal HL, Beachwood, OH (personal
    communication) (observation)
(1997): Romano A+, *Clin Exp Allergy* 27, 1425
(1996): Adcock BB+, *Arch Fam Med* 5, 301
(1996): Marra CA+, *Ann Pharmacother* 30, 401
(1995): Romano A+, *Allergy* 50, 113
(1994): Grayson ML+, *Clin Infect Dis* 18, 683
(1994): Shelley WB+, *Cutis* 53, 40 (observation)
(1993): Romano A+, *J Invest Allergol Clin Immunol* 3, 53
(1993): Warrington RJ+, *J Allergy Clin Immunol* 92, 626
(1988): Hou SR, *Chung Hua Nei Ko Tsa Chih* (Chinese) 27, 36
(1987): Pavithran K, *Indian J Lepr* 59, 309
(1986): Cabo HA+, *Med Cutan Ibero Lat Am* (Spanish) 14, 177
(1986): de Haan P+, *Allergy* 41, 75
(1986): Sonntag MR+, *Schweiz Med Wochenschr* (German)
    116, 142 (8%)
(1985): Bruynzeel DP+, *Dermatologica* 171, 429
(1985): Hefelfinger DC, *Ala Med* 55, 16
(1983): Bianchi C+, *Med Cutan Ibero Lat Am* (Spanish) 11, 113
(1983): Scioli C+, *Boll Ist Sieroter Milan* (Italian) 62, 287
(1982): Dourmischev AL+, *Dermatol Monatsschr* (German)
    168, 469
(1982): Gatter KC+, *Clin Allergy* 12, 279
(1981): Jick H+, *J Clin Pharmacol* 21, 456 (5.9%)
(1981): Lin CS+, *Arch Dermatol* 117, 282
(1980): Kraemer MJ+, *Pediatrics in Review* 1, 197
(1980): Porter D+, *Lancet* 1, 1037
(1980): Scherzer W+, *Derm Beruf Umwelt* (German) 28, 175
Exfoliative dermatitis
(1985): Fong PH+, *Ann Acad Med Singapore* 14, 693
Fixed eruption
(2000): Brabek E+, *Dtsch Med Wochenschr* 125(42), 1260
(1998): Mahboob A+, *Int J Dermatol* 37, 833
(1990): Bharija SC+, *Dermatologica* 181, 237
(1990): Gaffoor PMA+, *Cutis* 45, 242
(1987): Sharma SN, *J Assoc Physicians India* 35, 608
(1986): Kanwar AJ+, *Dermatologica* 172, 315
(1986): Panagariya A, *J Ass Physicians India* 34, 458
(1984): Chan H-L, *Arch Dermatol* 120, 542
(1983): Chan H-L, *Int J Dermatol* 23, 607
Linear IgA dermatosis
(2004): Shimanovich I+, *J Am Acad Dermatol* 51(1), 95
(2002): Cohen LM+, *J Am Acad Dermatol* 46, S32 (passim)
(1996): Tranvan A+, *J Am Acad Dermatol* 35, 865
(1981): Boffety B+, *Journées Dermatologiques de Paris*
    (French), 53–53a
Pemphigus
(1997): Brenner S+, *J Am Acad Dermatol* 36, 919
(1996): Takizawa H+, *Am J Gastroenterol* 91, 1654
(1993): Brenner S+, *Isr J Med Sci* 29, 44
(1986): Brenner S+, *J Am Acad Dermatol* 14, 453
(1986): Wilson JP+, *Drug Intell Clin Pharm* 20, 219
(1980): Fellner MJ+, *Int J Dermatol* 19, 392
Photo-recall
(2002): Blanco J+, *J Investig Allergol Clin Immunol* 12(3), 215
Pityriasis rosea

(1987): Olumide Y, *Int J Dermatol* 26, 234
Pruritus (1–5%)
(2006): Blumenthal HL, Beachwood, OH (personal
    communication) (observation)
(2003): Gei AF+, *Obstet Gynecol* 102(6), 1332
(1996): Adcock BB+, *Arch Fam Med* 5, 301
(1982): Bernhard JD+, *Cutis* 29, 158
(1980): Kraemer MJ+, *Pediatrics in Review* 1, 197
Psoriasis
(1993): Litt JZ, Beachwood, OH (personal case) (observation)
(1992): Breathnach SM+, *Adverse Drug Reactions and the Skin*
    Blackwell, Oxford, 141 (passim)
(1990): Saito S+, *J Dermatol* 17, 677
(1988): Tsankov N+, *J Am Acad Dermatol* 19, 629
(1987): Katz M+, *J Am Acad Dermatol* 17, 918
(1986): Verner E+, *Harefuah* (Hebrew) 110, 132
Purpura
(1993): Pang BK+, *Ann Acad Med Singapore* 22, 870
(1990): Hannedouche T+, *J Antimicrob Chemother* 20, 3
(1982): Beeching NL+, *J Antimicrob Chemother* 10, 479
(1981): Valman HB, *Br Med J Clin Res Ed* 283, 970
Pustules
(1995): Lim JT+, *Cutis* 56, 163
(1994): Jay S+, *Arch Dermatol* 130, 787 (localized)
(1991): Roujeau J-C+, *Arch Dermatol* 127, 1333
(1990): Guy C+, *Nouv Dermatol* (French) 9, 540
Rash (sic) (1–10%)
Stevens–Johnson syndrome
(1990): Cavanzo FJ+, *Gastroenterology* 99, 854
(1990): Chan HL+, *Arch Dermatol* 126, 43
(1987): Howell CG+, *J Pediatr Surg* 22, 994
(1985): Ting HC+, *Int J Dermatol* 24, 587
(1985): Turck M, *Hosp Pract Off Ed* 20, 49
Toxic epidermal necrolysis (<1%)
(2003): Sogut A+, *Acta Neurol Belg* 103(2), 95
(2002): Zelenkova H+, *World Congress Dermatol* Poster, 0136
(1997): Rodrigues-Ares MT+, *Int Ophthalmol* 21, 39
(1993): Romano A+, *J Invest Allergol Clin Immunol* 3, 53
(1991): Heng MC+, *J Am Acad Dermatol* 25, 778
(1985): Robbens EJ+, *Acta Clin Belg* 40, 115
(1983): Tagami H+, *Arch Dermatol* 119, 910
(1981): Berkel AI+, *Turk J Pediatr* 23, 37
(1980): Giuffre L+, *Minerva Pediatr* (Italian) 32, 633
Urticaria
(2003): Gei AF+, *Obstet Gynecol* 102(6), 1332
(1997): Romano A+, *Clin Exp Allergy* 27, 1425
(1996): Adcock BB+, *Arch Fam Med* 5, 301
(1985): Goolamali SK, *Postgrad Med J* 61, 925
(1982): Valsecchi R+, *Contact Dermatitis* 8, 278
(1980): Kraemer MJ+, *Pediatrics in Review* 1, 197
Vasculitis
(1991): Estrada-Rodriguez JL+, *J Investig Allergol Clin Immunol*
    1, 69
(1990): Hannedouche T+, *J Antimicrob Chemother* 20, 3

Mucosal/ENT

Glossitis
Oral candidiasis
Oral mucosal eruption
(1984): Gebel K+, *Dermatologica* 168, 35
Stomatitis
Tongue black
Vulvovaginal candidiasis

Other

Anaphylactoid reactions/Anaphylaxis
(2003): Gei AF+, *Obstet Gynecol* 102(6), 1332
(1998): Rich MW, *Tex Heart Inst J* 25, 194
(1997): Romano A+, *Clin Exp Allergy* 27, 1425
(1996): Adcock BB+, *Arch Fam Med* 5, 301

Candidiasis
Congestive heart failure
  (1994): Garty BZ+, *Ann Pharmacother* 28(6), 730
Hypersensitivity
  (1996): Torricelli R+, *Hautarzt* (German) 47, 392
  (1993): Romano A+, *Contact Dermatitis* 28, 190
  (1987): Ackerman Z+, *Postgrad Med J* 63, 55
Injection-site pain (>10%)
Phlebitis
Pseudoporphyria
  (2004): Phung TL+, *J Am Acad Dermatol* 51(2), S80 (with cefepime)
Serum sickness
Thrombophlebitis

AMPRENAVIR

Trade name: Agenerase (GSK)
Indications: HIV infection
Category: Antiretroviral; Protease inhibitor, HIV
Half-life: N/A
Clinically important, potentially hazardous interactions with: amiodarone, amitriptyline, amoxapine, benzodiazepines, bepridil, clomipramine, clonazepam, clorazepate, delavirdine, desipramine, diazepam, dihydroergotamine, doxepin, ergotamine, fentanyl, flurazepam, imipramine, ixabepilone, lidocaine, lorazepam, methysergide, midazolam, nortriptyline, oxazepam, phenytoin, protriptyline, quazepam, quinidine, rifampin, ritonavir, sildenafil, **St John's wort**, temazepam, tricyclic antidepressants, trimipramine, vitamin E

Note: Protease inhibitors cause dyslipidemia which includes elevated triglycerides and cholesterol and redistribution of body fat centrally to produce the so-called 'protease paunch,' breast enlargement, facial atrophy, and 'buffalo hump'

Note: Amprenavir is a sulfonamide and can be absorbed systemically. Sulfonamides can produce severe, possibly fatal, reactions such as toxic epidermal necrolysis and Stevens–Johnson syndrome

Reactions

Skin
Acanthosis nigricans
  (2005): Mur A+, *Pediatr Infect Dis J* 24(8), 742
Exanthems
  (2006): Kohli-Pamnani A+, *Ann Allergy Asthma Immunol* 96(4), 620
Pruritus
Rash (sic) (25%)
  (2003): Justesen US+, *Br J Clin Pharmacol* 55(1), 100 (with delavirdine)
  (2001): Scott T+, *Clin Ther* 23(2), 252 (8%)
  (2000): Conway B+, *Expert Opin Investig Drugs* 9(2), 371
  (2000): Noble S+, *Drugs* 60(6), 1383
  (2000): Pedneault L+, *Clin Ther* 22(12), 1378 (3%)
Stevens–Johnson syndrome (4%)
  (2003): Rotunda A+, *Acta Derm Venereol* 83(1), 1

Mucosal/ENT
Dysgeusia (10%)

Other
Gynecomastia
Paresthesias (perioral) (26%)
  (2001): *Prescrire Int* 10(53), 70
  (2001): McMahon D+, *Antivir Ther* 6(2), 105

(2000): Conway B+, *Expert Opin Investig Drugs* 9(2), 371
(2000): Pedneault L+, *Clin Ther* 22(12), 1378

AMYL NITRITE

Synonym: isoamyl nitrite
Trade names: Amyl Nitrite; Nitrit
Indications: Angina pectoris
Category: Nitrate; Vasodilator
Half-life: N/A
Clinically important, potentially hazardous interactions with: furosemide, sildenafil

Reactions

Skin
Allergic reactions (sic)
  (1989): Dax EM+, *Am J Med* 86, 732
Dermatitis
  (1985): Bos JD+, *Contact Dermatitis* 12, 109
  (1984): Fisher AA, *Cutis* 34(2), 118
  (1982): Romaguera C+, *Contact Dermatitis* 8, 266
Diaphoresis
Edema
Pallor
Rash (sic) (<1%)

Other
Headache

ANAGRELIDE

Trade name: Agrylin (Shire)
Indications: Essential thrombocytopenia. To reduce elevated platelet count and the risk of thrombosis
Category: Phospholipase A2 inhibitor
Half-life: ~3 days
Clinically important, potentially hazardous interactions with: aspirin, fondaparinux

Reactions

Skin
Adverse effects (sic) (<5%)
Edema (19.8%)
  (2006): Birgegard G, *Semin Thromb Hemost* 32(3), 260
  (2004): Mazur G+, *Pol Arch Med Wewn* 112(6), 1445 (20%)
  (2002): Kornblihtt LI+, *Medicina* (B Aires) 62(3), 231
  (2000): James CW, *Pharmacotherapy* 20(10), 1224
  (1998): Oertel MD, *Am J Health Syst Pharm* 55(19), 1979
  (1998): Petrides PE+, *Eur J Haematol* 61(2), 71
  (1998): Trapp OM+, *Blood Cells Mol Dis* 24(1), 9
  (1997): Tefferi A+, *Semin Thromb Hemost* 23(4), 379
  (1992): Mazzucconi MG+, *Haematologica* 77(4), 315
Leg ulceration
  (2007): Rappoport L+, *Dtsch Med Wochenschr* 132(7), 319
Peripheral edema (7.1%)
  (1992): Mazzucconi MG+, *Haematologica* 77(4), 315
Photosensitivity (<5%)
Pruritus (<5%)
Rash (sic) (7.8%)
Urticaria (7.8%)

Mucosal/ENT

Aphthous stomatitis (<5%)

Tinnitus (<5%)

Hair

Hair – alopecia (<5%)

Eyes

Visual hallucinations

(2004): Swords R+, *Eur J Haematol* 73(3), 223

Other

Abdominal pain

(2006): *Prescrire Int* 15(83), 83

(2000): Pescatore SL+, *Expert Opin Pharmacother* 1(3), 537

(1998): Oertel MD, *Am J Health Syst Pharm* 55(19), 1979

Chills (<5%)

Congestive heart failure

(2006): *Prescrire Int* 15(83), 83

Death

(2006): *Prescrire Int* 15(83), 83

Depression (<5%)

Headache

(2006): *Prescrire Int* 15(83), 83

(2006): Birgegard G, *Semin Thromb Hemost* 32(3), 260

(2004): Mazur G+, *Pol Arch Med Wewn* 112(6), 1445 (25%)

(2001): Knutsen H+, *Tidsskr Nor Laegeforen* 121(12), 1478

(2000): Pescatore SL+, *Expert Opin Pharmacother* 1(3), 537

(1998): Oertel MD, *Am J Health Syst Pharm* 55(19), 1979

(1998): Petrides PE+, *Eur J Haematol* 61(2), 71

(1998): Trapp OM+, *Blood Cells Mol Dis* 24(1), 9

(1997): Tefferi A+, *Semin Thromb Hemost* 23(4), 379

Hypersensitivity

(2003): Raghavan M+, *Ann Pharmacother* 37(9), 1228

Hypotension

(2000): Pescatore SL+, *Expert Opin Pharmacother* 1(3), 537

Myalgia/Myositis/Myopathy/Myotoxicity (<5%)

Paresthesias (7.3%)

Stroke

(2006): *Prescrire Int* 15(83), 83

ANAKINRA

Synonym: IL-1RA

Trade name: Kineret (Amgen)

Indications: Rheumatoid arthritis

Category: Disease-modulating antirheumatoid drug; Interleukin-1 receptor antagonist (IL-1Ra)

Half-life: 4–6 hours

Clinically important, potentially hazardous interactions with: certolizumab pegol, etanercept

Reactions

Skin

Cellulitis

(2004): Riente L, *Reumatismo 2004 Jan–Mar* 56(1 Suppl 1), 74

Lichenoid eruption

(2005): Vila AT+, *Br J Dermatol* 153(2), 417

Mucosal/ENT

Sinusitis (7%)

Other

Headache

(2004): Riente L, *Reumatismo 2004 Jan–Mar* 56(1 Suppl 1), 74 (14%)

Hypersensitivity

Infections (40%)

(2004): *Prescrire Int* 13(70), 43

(2004): Turesson C+, *J Rheumatol* 31(9), 1876

(2003): Fleischmann RM+, *Arthritis Rheum* 48(4), 927 (2.1%)

(2003): Kary S+, *Int J Clin Pract* 57(3), 231

Injection-site ecchymoses

Injection-site edema

(2005): Vila AT+, *Br J Dermatol* 153(2), 417

Injection-site erythema

(2005): Vila AT+, *Br J Dermatol* 153(2), 417

Injection-site inflammation

Injection-site pain

Injection-site reactions (sic) (71%)

(2006): den Broeder AA+, *Ann Rheum Dis* 65(6), 760 (36%)

(2006): Fleischmann RM+, *Ann Rheum Dis* 65(8), 1006

(2005): Haibel H+, *Ann Rheum Dis* 64(2), 296

(2005): Vila AT+, *Br J Dermatol* 153(2), 417

(2004): *Prescrire Int* 13(70), 43 (75%)

(2004): Clark W+, *Health Technol Assess* 8(18), iii–iv, ix–x, 1

(2004): Cohen SB+, *Ann Rheum Dis* 63(9), 1062

(2004): Furst DE, *Clin Ther* 26(12), 1960

(2004): Riente L, *Reumatismo 2004 Jan–Mar* 56(1 Suppl 1), 74 (71%)

(2004): Schiff MH, *Drugs* 64(22), 2493

(2003): Fleischmann RM, *Rheumatology* (Oxford) 42(Suppl 2), ii29

(2003): Kary S+, *Int J Clin Pract* 57(3), 231

(2003): Langer HE+, *Int J Clin Pharmacol Res* 23(4), 119

(2002): Calabrese LH, *Ann Pharmacother* 36(7), 1204

(2002): Cohen S+, *Arthritis Rheum* 46(3), 614

(2001): Bresnihan B, *Semin Arthritis Rheum* 30(5 Suppl 2), 17

(2001): Garces K, *Issues Emerg Health Technol* May(16), 1

(1998): Bresnihan B+, *Arthritis Rheum* 41(12), 2196

Upper respiratory infection (4%)

(2006): Fleischmann RM+, *Ann Rheum Dis* 65(8), 1006

ANASTROZOLE

Trade name: Arimidex (AstraZeneca)

Indications: Breast carcinoma (localized-advanced or metastatic)

Category: Aromatase inhibitor

Half-life: 50 hours

Reactions

Skin

Angioedema

Diaphoresis

(1997): Jonat W, *Oncology* 54 (Suppl 2), 15

Erythema multiforme

Lupus erythematosus

(2007): Trancart M+, *Br J Dermatol*

Peripheral edema (10.1%)

Pruritus (2–5%)

Rash (sic) (7.5%)

Shivering

Stevens–Johnson syndrome

Urticaria

Mucosal/ENT

Vaginal dryness (1.7%)

Xerostomia

Hair

Hair – alopecia (2–5%)

Other

Asthenia
  (2003): del Carmen MG+, *Gynecol Oncol* 91(3), 596
Chills
Cough (10.9%)
Depression (4.5%)
Headache
Hepatotoxicity
  (2007): de la Cruz L+, *Lancet* 369(9555), 23 (with geftinib)
  (2006): Carlini P+, *J Clin Oncol* 24(35), e60
  (2006): Zapata E+, *Eur J Gastroenterol Hepatol* 18(11), 1233
Hot flashes (26.5%)
  (2005): *Prescrire Int* 14(76), 43 (30%)
  (2003): Baum M+, *Cancer* 98(9), 1802
  (2003): del Carmen MG+, *Gynecol Oncol* 91(3), 596
  (2002): Buzdar AU, *Expert Rev Anticancer Ther* 2(6), 623
  (1998): Higa GM+, *Am J Health* 55(5), 445
Infections (2–5%)
Myalgia/Myositis/Myopathy/Myotoxicity (2–5%)
Osteoporosis
  (2005): Mackey JR+, *Int J Cancer* 114(6), 1010
Pain (13.8%)
  (1998): Higa GM+, *Am J Health* 55(5), 445
Paresthesias
Thrombophlebitis (2–5%)
Tumor pain (>5%)

ANDROSTENEDIONE

Scientific names: *4-androstene-3,17-dione; Androst-4-ene-3,17-dione*
Family: N/A
Trade and other common names: Andro; Androstene
Category: Aromatase inhibitor
Purported indications and other uses: Enhanced athletic performance, increased energy, to keep red blood cells healthy
Half-life: N/A

Reactions

Skin

Acne
  (1999): Pheatt N, *Sports Supplements. Pharmacist's Letter* 99, 1
  (1998): *Med Lett Drugs Ther* 40, 105
Adverse effects (sic)
  (2003): Juhn M, *Sports Med* 33(12), 921
  (2003): Kicman AT+, *Clin Chem* 49(1), 167
  (2002): Leder BZ+, *J Clin Endocrinol Metab* 87(12), 5449
  (2001): Ahrendt DM, *Am Fam Physician* 63(5), 913
  (2001): Ayotte C+, *Can J Appl Physiol* 26(Suppl), S120
  (2000): Pecci MA+, *Phys Med Rehabil Clin N Am* 11(4), 949
Coarsening of skin
  (1998): *Med Lett Drugs Ther* 40, 105
Edema
Seborrhea

Hair

Hair – alopecia
  (1998): *Med Lett Drugs Ther* 40, 105
Hair – hirsutism (in women)
  (1999): Pheatt N, *Sports Supplements. Pharmacist's Letter* 99, 1

Other

Gynecomastia
Headache

Seizures
Side effects (sic)
  (2002): Lawrence ME+, *J Clin Gastroenterol* 35(4), 299

ANIDULAFUNGIN

Synonym: LY-303366
Trade name: Eraxis (Vicuron) (Roerig/Pfizer)
Indications: Candidemia, candidal esophagitis
Category: Antimycobacterial, echinocandin
Half-life: 40–50 hours
Clinically important, potentially hazardous interactions with: None

Reactions

Skin

Angioedema (<1%)
Diaphoresis (<1%)
Erythema
  (2006): Benjamin DK+, *Antimicrob Agents Chemother* 50(2), 632
Exanthems
  (2004): Krause DS+, *Clin Infect Dis* 39(6), 770
Peripheral edema (<1%)
Pruritus (<1%)
Rash (sic) (<1%)
Urticaria (<1%)

Eyes

Ocular pain (<1%)
Vision blurred (<1%)
Visual disturbances (<1%)

Other

Abdominal pain (<1%)
Cough (<1%)
Fever
  (2006): Benjamin DK+, *Antimicrob Agents Chemother* 50(2), 632
  (2004): Murdoch D+, *Drugs* 64(19), 2249
Headache
  (2004): Krause DS+, *Clin Infect Dis* 39(6), 770
  (2004): Murdoch D+, *Drugs* 64(19), 2249
Hypertension (<1%)
Hypotension (<1%)
Phlebitis
  (2004): Murdoch D+, *Drugs* 64(19), 2249
Seizures (<1%)
Thrombophlebitis
  (2004): Murdoch D+, *Drugs* 64(19), 2249
Vertigo

ANISINDIONE

Trade name: Miradon (Schering)
Indications: Adjunct in treatment of coronary occlusion, Atrial fibrillation
Category: Anticoagulant; Indanedione
Half-life: 3–5 days
Clinically important, potentially hazardous interactions with: amiodarone, anabolic steroids, antithyroid agents, barbiturates, bivalirudin, cimetidine, clofibrate, clopidogrel, cyclosporine, delavirdine, dextrothyroxine, disulfiram, fluconazole, glutethimide, imatinib, itraconazole, ketoconazole, metronidazole, miconazole, penicillins, phenylbutazones, piperacillin, quinidine, quinine, rifabutin, rifampin, rifapentine, rofecoxib, salicylates, sulfinpyrazone, sulfonamides, testosterone, thyroid, zileuton

Reactions

Skin
Dermatitis
Erythema
Erythema multiforme
Exanthems
Exfoliative dermatitis
Necrosis
Petechiae
Purple toe syndrome
Urticaria

Mucosal/ENT
Oral ulceration
Stomatitis
Stomatodynia

Hair
Hair – alopecia

Other
Chills
Death
Hypersensitivity

ANISTREPLASE

Synonym: APSAC
Trade names: Eminase; Iminase
Indications: Acute myocardial infarction
Category: Fibrinolytic
Half-life: 70–120 minutes

Reactions

Skin
Allergic reactions (sic)
Angioedema
Diaphoresis (<1%)
Exanthems
  (1995): Dykewicz MS+, *J Allergy Clin Immunol* 95, 1020
Livedo reticularis
  (1994): Gianni R+, *Ann Ital Med Int* (Italian) 9, 105
Purpura
Rash (sic)
  (1990): Burrows N+, *Br Heart J* 64(4), 289

Ulcerations
  (1994): Gianni R+, *Ann Ital Med Int* (Italian) 9, 105
Urticaria
  (1995): Dykewicz MS+, *J Allergy Clin Immunol* 95, 1020
Vasculitis
  (1994): Gianni R+, *Ann Ital Med Int* (Italian) 9, 105
  (1992): Burrows N+, *J Am Acad Dermatol* 26, 508
  (1990): Burrows N+, *Br Heart J* 64, 289
  (1988): Bucknall C+, *Br Heart J* 59, 9
  (1988): Gemmill JD+, *Br Heart J* 60, 361

Mucosal/ENT
Gingival bleeding

Other
Anaphylactoid reactions/Anaphylaxis (1–10%)
  (1997): Cannas S+, *G Ital Cardiol* (Italian) 27, 278
  (1992): Califf RM+, *Am J Cardiol* 69(2), 12A
Chills (<1%)
Hypersensitivity
  (1993): Lee HS+, *Eur Heart J* 14, 1640
Hypotension
  (1992): Califf RM+, *Am J Cardiol* 69(2), 12A
Myalgia/Myositis/Myopathy/Myotoxicity
  (1994): Gianni R+, *Ann Ital Med Int* (Italian) 9, 105
Serum sickness
  (1993): Lee HS+, *Eur Heart J* 14, 1640

ANTHRAX VACCINE

Trade names: Anthrax Vaccine Adsorbed [AVA] (BioPort); Carbosap
Indications: Anthrax prophylaxis
Category: Vaccine
Half-life: Requires 1 month to achieve immunity (92.5% efficient)

Note: Dr. Sue Bailey, Assistant Secretary for Health Affairs, released a statement on June 29, 1999 that 'almost one million shots given, the anthrax immunization is proving to be one of the safest vaccination programs on record.' The above reports occurred for '50 service members at one installation alone.' Note that no number of military personnel was mentioned at this installation, nor did it give any percentages of the above reaction patterns

Reactions

Skin
Allergic reactions (sic)
  (2000): Captain James Bishop, *Citizen Airman* (0.002%)
  (1999): Ellenberg SS, *Center for Biologics Evaluation & Research, FDA Statement* (widespread)
Angioedema
  (2004): Gilson RT+, *Cutis* 73, 319 (passim)
Bullous dermatitis
  (2004): Gilson RT+, *Cutis* 73, 319 (passim)
Cellulitis
  (2000): *MMWR* 49(RR15), 1
Diaphoresis
  (2006): Nasir JM+, *Mil Med* 171(4), 340
  (2001): Swanson-Biearman B+, *J Toxicol Clin Toxicol* 39(1), 81
  (1999): Dr. Sue Bailey, *Asst Sec Defense Health Affairs – Service Member #16* 21
Eczema
  (2006): Parker AL+, *Hum Vaccin* 2(3), 105
Edema (3%)

(2006): Vasudev M+, *Ann Allergy Asthma Immunol* 97(1), 110 (joint)

(2000): *MMWR* 49(RR15), 1

Erythema

(2000): *MMWR* 49(RR15), 1

Erythema multiforme

(2004): Gilson RT+, *Cutis* 73, 319

Exanthems

(2004): Gilson RT+, *Cutis* 73, 319 (passim)

Lupus erythematosus

(2000): *MMWR* 49(RR15), 1

(1999): Ellenberg SS, *Center for Biologics Evaluation & Research, FDA Statement*

Peripheral edema

Photosensitivity

(1999): Dr. Sue Bailey, *Asst Sec Defense Health Affairs – Service Member #1*

Pruritus

(2004): Gilson RT+, *Cutis* 73, 319 (passim)

(2000): *MMWR* 49(RR15), 1

(1999): Dr. Sue Bailey, *Asst Sec Defense Health Affairs – Service Member #5*

Purpura

Rash (sic)

(2004): Gilson RT+, *Cutis* 73, 319 (passim)

(1999): Dr. Sue Bailey, *Asst Sec Defense Health Affairs – Service Members #5, 9,14, 25, 44*

(1999): Ellenberg SS, *Center for Biologics Evaluation & Research, FDA Statement*

Scrotal edema

(1999): Dr. Sue Bailey, *Asst Sec Defense Health Affairs – Service Members #9*

Stevens–Johnson syndrome

(2004): Chopra A+, *Mayo Clin Proc* 79(9), 1193 (with smallpox and tetanus vaccines)

(2004): Gilson RT+, *Cutis* 73, 319 (passim)

Toxic epidermal necrolysis

(2004): Gilson RT+, *Cutis* 73, 319 (passim)

Urticaria

(2004): Gilson RT+, *Cutis* 73, 319

(2001): Swanson-Biearman B+, *J Toxicol Clin Toxicol* 39(1), 81

Vasculitis

(2003): Muniz AE, *J Emerg Med* 25(3), 271

Mucosal/ENT

Gingivitis

(1999): Dr. Sue Bailey, *Asst Sec Defense Health Affairs – Service Member #32*

Mucositis

(2004): Gilson RT+, *Cutis* 73, 319 (passim)

Oral pemphigus

(2004): Muellenhoff M+, *J Am Acad Dermatol* 50(1), 136

Tinnitus

(1999): Dr. Sue Bailey, *Asst Sec Defense Health Affairs – Service Members #1, 6, 7, 10, 11, 13, 14, 23, 24, 28, 29, 48, 49*

Hair

Hair – alopecia

Eyes

Chorioretinopathy

(2004): Foster BS+, *Retina* 24(4), 624

Eyelid edema

(1999): Dr. Sue Bailey, *Asst Sec Defense Health Affairs – Service Member #16 21*

Optic neuritis

(2006): Payne DC+, *Arch Neurol* 63(6), 871

Other

Anaphylactoid reactions/Anaphylaxis

(2004): Gilson RT+, *Cutis* 73(5), 319 (passim)

(1999): Dr. Sue Bailey, *Asst Sec Defense Health Affairs – Service Member #29*

Asthenia

(2000): *MMWR* 49(RR15), 1

Chills (<0.06%)

(2006): Vasudev M+, *Ann Allergy Asthma Immunol* 97(1), 110

(2000): *MMWR* 49(RR15), 1

Depression

(1999): Dr. Sue Bailey, *Asst Sec Defense Health Affairs – Service Member #23*

Fever (<1%)

(2006): Vasudev M+, *Ann Allergy Asthma Immunol* 97(1), 110

(2004): Gilson RT+, *Cutis* 73, 319 (passim)

(2000): *MMWR* 49(RR15), 1

Headache

(2006): Nasir JM+, *Mil Med* 171(4), 340

(2004): Gilson RT+, *Cutis* 73, 319 (passim)

Hot flashes

(1999): Dr. Sue Bailey, *Asst Sec Defense Health Affairs – Service Member #31 34, 37*

Hypersensitivity

(2001): Swanson-Biearman B+, *J Toxicol Clin Toxicol* 39(1), 81

(1999): Ellenberg SS, *Center for Biologics Evaluation & Research, FDA Statement* (2 cases)

(1996): Shlyakhov E+, *Med Trop (Mars)* 56(2), 148

(1996): Uhr JW, *Physiol Rev.* 46:359

(1994): Shlyakhov E+, *Med Trop (Mars)* 54(1):33

Injection-site burning

(1999): Dr. Sue Bailey, *Asst Sec Defense Health Affairs – Service Member #12,27*

Injection-site edema

(2000): *MMWR* 49(RR15), 1

(1999): Dr. Sue Bailey, *Asst Sec Defense Health Affairs – Service Member #4, 12, 32*

(1999): Ellenberg SS, *Center for Biologics Evaluation & Research, FDA Statement*

Injection-site erythema

(1999): Dr. Sue Bailey, *Asst Sec Defense Health Affairs – Service Member #21, 27, 47*

Injection-site hematoma

(1999): Dr. Sue Bailey, *Asst Sec Defense Health Affairs – Service Member #12*

Injection-site hypersensitivity

(2000): *MMWR* 49(RR15), 1

Injection-site induration

Injection-site inflammation

Injection-site nodules

(2006): Vasudev M+, *Ann Allergy Asthma Immunol* 97(1), 110

(1999): Dr. Sue Bailey, *Asst Sec Defense Health Affairs – Service Members #2, 24, 28, 37, 40, 47*

Injection-site numbness

(1999): Dr. Sue Bailey, *Asst Sec Defense Health Affairs – Service Members #6, 13, 15, 22, 26, 31, 39, 43*

Injection-site pain

(2001): Swanson-Biearman B+, *J Toxicol Clin Toxicol* 39(1), 81

(2000): *MMWR* 49(RR15), 1

(1999): Bailey S MD, *Asst Sec Defense Health Affairs – Service Members #1, 4, 8, 13, 18, 19, 20, 42, 45, 47, 49*

Injection-site pruritus

Injection-site reactions (sic)

(2001): Swanson-Biearman B+, *J Toxicol Clin Toxicol* 39(1), 81 (30%)

(2000): *MMWR* 49(RR15), 1

(2000): Hayes SC+, *J R Army Med Corps* 146(3), 191 (47%)

(1999): Ellenberg SS, *Center for Biologics Evaluation & Research, FDA Statement* (severe)

Myalgia/Myositis/Myopathy/Myotoxicity

(2006): Vasudev M+, *Ann Allergy Asthma Immunol* 97(1), 110
(2000): *MMWR* 49(RR15), 1
(1999): Dr. Sue Bailey, *Asst Sec Defense Health Affairs – Service Members #1, 6, 12, 22, 40, 41*

Pain
(2006): Vasudev M+, *Ann Allergy Asthma Immunol* 97(1), 110 (joint)
Paresthesias
(1999): Dr. Sue Bailey, *Asst Sec Defense Health Affairs – Service Members #3, 4, 11, 17, 28, 31, 34, 36, 37, 49*
Systemic reactions (sic)
(2000): Hayes SC+, *J R Army Med Corps* 146(3), 191 (47%)
Tremor
(1999): Dr. Sue Bailey, *Asst Sec Defense Health Affairs – Service Members #1*

APOMORPHINE

Trade names: Apokyn; Uprima (Abbott)
Indications: Parkinsonism, Erectile dysfunction
Category: Dopamine receptor agonist
Half-life: 40 minutes
Clinically important, potentially hazardous interactions with: alcohol, antihypertensives, vasodilators

Note: Apomorphine contains sodium metabisulfite which is capable of causing anaphylactoid reactions in patients with sulfite allergy

Reactions

Skin
Dermatitis
(1997): Carboni GP+, *Contact Dermatitis* 36(3), 177
Diaphoresis
(2002): *Prescrire Int* 11(59), 76 (severe)
Edema
(2007): Rudzinska M+, *Neurol Neurochir Pol* 41(2 Suppl 1), S40
Nodular eruption
(2004): Bowron A, *Neurology* 62(6), S32
Peripheral edema (10%)
Pigmentation
(2003): Loewe R+, *Hautarzt* 54(1), 58

Mucosal/ENT
Dysgeusia
(1999): Ondo W+, *Clin Neuropharmacol* 22(1), 1
Rhinorrhea (20%)

Other
Asthenia (>5%)
Chest pain (15%)
Congestive heart failure (>5%)
Depression (>5%)
Headache (>5%)
(2004): Caruso S+, *Urology* 63(5), 955
(2001): Bukofzer S+, *Int J Impot Res* 13(3), S40
Injection-site reactions (sic)
(2001): Dewey RB+, *Arch Neurol* 58(9), 1385
(1998): Pietz K+, *J Neurol Neurosurg Psychiatry* 65(5), 709
Panniculitis
(1998): Acland KM+, *Br J Dermatol* 138(3), 480
(1998): Acland KM+, *Hosp Med* 59(5), 413
Vertigo (20%)
(2004): Caruso S+, *Urology* 63(5), 955
(2002): *Prescrire Int* 11(59), 76

APRACLONIDINE

Trade name: Iopidine (Alcon)
Indications: Post-surgical intraocular pressure elevation
Category: Adrenergic alpha2-receptor agonist
Half-life: 8 hours

Reactions

Skin
Allergic reactions (sic) (<1%)
(2000): Geyer O+, *Graefes Arch Clin Exp Ophthalmol* 238, 149
(1999): Britt MT+, *Br J Ophthalmol* 83, 992 (progressing to ectropion)
(1998): Gordon RN+, *Eye* 12, 697
(1995): Butler P+, *Arch Ophthalmol* 113, 293
(1995): Feibel RM, *Arch Ophthalmol* 113, 1579
Burning
(1996): Stewart WC, *Klin Monatsbl Augenheilkd* (German) 209, A7
Dermatitis (<1%)
(2001): Holdiness MR, *Am J Contact Dermat* 12(4), 217
(2001): Silvestre JF+, *Contact Dermatitis* 45(4), 251
(1998): Armisen M+, *Contact Dermatitis* 39, 193
Facial edema (<1%)
Pruritus (10%)
(1996): Stewart WC, *Klin Monatsbl Augenheilkd* (German) 209, A7
Toxicity (sic)
(2005): Pekdemir M+, *Emerg Med J* 22(10), 753
Xerosis

Mucosal/ENT
Dysgeusia (3%)
Parosmia (0.2%)
Xerostomia (1–10%)
(1987): Abrams DA+, *Arch Ophthalmol* 105, 1205 (52%)

Eyes
Eyelid edema (<3%)
Ophthalmitis
(1999): Shin DH+, *Am J Ophthalmol* 127, 511
Periocular dermatitis
(2000): Williams GC+, *Glaucoma* 9, 235

Other
Headache
Myalgia/Myositis/Myopathy/Myotoxicity (0.2%)
Paresthesias (<1%)

APREPITANT

Synonyms: mk-869; l-754-030
Trade name: Emend (Merck)
Indications: Prevention of nausea and vomiting associated with cancer (cisplatin) chemotherapy
Category: Neurokinin 1 receptor antagonist
Half-life: 9–13 hours
Clinically important, potentially hazardous interactions with: alprazolam, astemizole, carbamazepine, cisapride, clarithromycin, dexamethasone, diltiazem, docetaxel, ifosfamide, imatinib, irinotecan, itraconazole, ketoconazole, methylprednisolone, midazolam, nefazodone, oral contraceptives, paroxetine, phenytoin, pimozide, rifampin, ritonavir, terfenadine, tolbutamide, troleandomycin, vinblastine, vincristine, warfarin

Note: Aprepitant treatment is given along with a 5-HT3-receptor antagonist and dexamethasone

Reactions

Skin
Acne
Angioedema
Diaphoresis (>0.5%)
Edema (>0.5%)
Rash (sic) (>0.5%)
Stevens–Johnson syndrome
Urticaria

Mucosal/ENT
Dysgeusia (>0.5%)
Mucocutaneous reactions (sic)
Sialorrhea (>0.5%)
Tinnitus (3.7%)

Hair
Hair – alopecia (>0.5%)

Other
Abdominal pain (>0.5%)
Asthenia (18%)
  (2005): Massaro AM+, *Ann Pharmacother* 39(1), 77
  (2004): Dando TM+, *Drugs* 64(7), 777
Cough (>0.5%)
Depression (>0.5%)
Fever
Headache
Infections
  (2004): Dando TM+, *Drugs* 64(7), 777
  (2003): Chawla SP+, *Cancer* 97(9), 2290 (13%)
Myalgia/Myositis/Myopathy/Myotoxicity (>0.5%)
Upper respiratory infection (>0.5%)
Vertigo (6.6%)

APROBARBITAL

Trade name: Alurate (Roche)
Indications: Short-term sedation, sleep induction
Category: Barbiturate
Half-life: 14–34 hours
Clinically important, potentially hazardous interactions with: alcohol, brompheniramine, buclizine, dicumarol, ethanolamine, warfarin

Reactions

Skin
Angioedema
Exanthems
Exfoliative dermatitis
Purpura
Rash (sic)
Stevens–Johnson syndrome
Urticaria

Other
Rhabdomyolysis
  (1990): Larpin R+, *Presse Med* 19(30), 1403
Serum sickness

APROTININ

Trade name: Trasylol (Bayer)
Indications: For prophylactic use to reduce blood loss in patients undergoing coronary artery bypass surgery
Category: Antifibrinolytic; Protease inhibitor
Half-life: 150 minutes

Note: This drug has been withdrawn from the market

Reactions

Skin
Allergic reactions (sic) (0.5%)
  (1994): Bayo M+, *Rev Esp Anestesiol Reanim* (Spanish) 41, 123
  (1983): Freeman JG+, *Curr Med Res Opin* 8, 559 (2 cases)
Angioedema
Erythema
Exanthems
  (2000): Beierlein W+, *Transfusion* 40, 302 (generalized)
Pruritus
Rash (sic)
Urticaria

Other
Anaphylactoid reactions/Anaphylaxis (0.5%)
  (2007): Kaddoum RN+, *J Cardiothorac Vasc Anesth* 21(2), 243
  (2007): Umeda Y+, *Kyobu Geka* 60(1), 69
  (2005): Shirai T+, *Intern Med* 44(10), 1088
  (2001): Dietrich W+, *Anesthesiology* 95(1), 64
  (2000): Beierlein W, *Ann Thorac Surg* 69, 1298
  (2000): Laxenaire MC+, *Ann Fr Anesth Reanim* (French) 19, 96
  (2000): Pecquet C+, *Ann Fr Anesth* 19(10), 755
  (1999): Cohen DM+, *Ann Thorac Surg* 67, 837
  (1999): Laxenaire MC, *Ann Fr Anesth Reanim* (French) 18, 796 (4 cases)
  (1999): Ong BC+, *Anaesth Intensive Care* 27, 538
  (1999): Ryckwaert Y+, *Ann Fr Anesth Reanim* (French) 18, 904
  (1998): Scheule AM+, *Gastrointest Endosc* 48, 83
  (1997): Dietrich W+, *J Thorac Cardiovasc Surg* 113, 194
  (1997): Orsel I+, *Ann Fr Anesth Reanim* (French) 16, 292
  (1997): Scheule AM+, *Ann Thorac Surg* 63, 242
  (1996): Martinelli L+, *Ann Thorac Surg* 61, 1288
  (1995): Ceriana P+, *J Cardiothorac Vasc Anesth* 9, 477
  (1995): Diefenbach C+, *Anesth Analg* 80, 830
  (1994): Kon NF+, *Masui* (Japanese) 43, 1606
  (1993): Cottineau C+, *Ann Fr Anesth Reanim* (French) 12, 590
  (1993): Schulze K+, *Eur J Cardiothorac Surg* 7, 495 (2 patients)
  (1984): *BMJ* 289, 1696
  (1984): LaFerla GA+, *BMJ* 289, 1176

Congestive heart failure
    (2006): Nasir JM+, *Mil Med* 171(4), 340
Hypersensitivity
    (2002): Jaquiss RD+, *Circulation* 106(12 Suppl 1), 190
    (2000): Beierlein W+, *Transfusion* 40, 302
    (1998): Dietrich W, *Ann Thoracic Surg* 65, S60 (1.8%)
Lipohypertrophy
    (1985): Boag F+, *N Engl J Med* 312, 245 (in a diabetic)
    (1985): Dandona P+, *Diabetes Res* 2, 213 (in a diabetic)
Nephrotoxicity
    (2006): Mangano DT+, *N Engl J Med* 354(4), 353
Phlebitis (1–10%)
Stroke
    (2006): Mangano DT+, *N Engl J Med* 354(4), 353
Thrombosis
    (2006): Cooper JR+, *J Thorac Cardiovasc Surg* 131(5), 963

ARBUTAMINE

Trade name: GenESA (Sicor)
Indications: Diagnostic aid for coronary artery disease
Category: Adrenergic beta-receptor agonist
Half-life: 1.8 hours
**Clinically important, potentially hazardous interactions
with:** abacavir, clidinium, clomipramine, desipramine,
dicyclomine, digoxin, doxepin, flavoxate, glycopyrrolate,
hyoscyamine, imipramine, mepenzolate, methantheline,
nortriptyline, oxybutynin, procyclidine, propantheline,
protriptyline, scopolamine, trihexyphenidyl, trimipramine

Reactions

Skin
Diaphoresis (1.5%)
Rash (sic)

Mucosal/ENT
Dysgeusia (1.3%)
    (2001): Wright DJ+, *Nucl Med Commun* 22(12), 1305 (23%)
Xerostomia (1.1%)

Other
Application-site reactions (0.1%)
Cough (0.2%)
Hot flashes (3%)
Pain (1.8%)
Paresthesias (2%)
Tremor (15%)
    (1997): Cohen A+, *Am J Cardiol* 79(6), 713 (5.6%)

ARFORMOTEROL

Trade name: Brovana (Sepracor)
Indications: Chronic obstructive pulmonary disease (COPD)
Category: Beta2-adreneric agonist
Half-life: 26 hours
**Clinically important, potentially hazardous interactions
with:** aminophylline, beta-blockers, MAO inhibitors,
theophylline, tricyclic antidepressants

Reactions

Skin
Abscess (<2%)
Allergic reactions (sic) (<2%)
Angioedema
Edema (<2%)
Herpes simplex (<2%)
Herpes zoster (<2%)
Neoplasms (<2%)
Peripheral edema (3%)
Pigmentation (<2%)
Rash (sic) (4%)
Urticaria
Xerosis (<2%)

Mucosal/ENT
Oral candidiasis (<2%)
Sinusitis (4%)

Eyes
Glaucoma (<2%)
Visual disturbances (<2%)

Other
Agitation (<2%)
Anaphylactoid reactions/Anaphylaxis
Chest pain (7%)
Cystitis (<2%)
Fever (<2%)
Headache
Hypersensitivity
Injection-site pain (<2%)
Insomnia
Pain (8%)
Paresthesias (<2%)
Somnolence (<2%)
Tremor (<2%)

ARGATROBAN

Trade name: Acova (GSK)
Indications: Heparin-induced thrombocytopenia
Category: Thrombin inhibitor
Half-life: 40–50 minutes
**Clinically important, potentially hazardous interactions
with:** abacavir, butabarbital

Reactions

Skin
Allergic reactions (sic)
Bullous dermatitis (<1%)
Rash (sic) (<1%)

Other
Headache
Infections (4%)
Injection-site bleeding (2–5%)

ARIPIPRAZOLE

Trade names: Abilify (Bristol-Myers Squibb); Abilitat
Indications: Schizophrenia
Category: Antipsychotic; Mood stabilizer
Half-life: 75–94 hours
**Clinically important, potentially hazardous interactions
with:** carbamazepine, ketoconazole, quinidine

Reactions

Skin

Acne
Angioedema
Diaphoresis
Eczema
Exanthems
Exfoliative dermatitis
Peripheral edema
Pruritus
Psoriasis
Purpura
Rash (sic) (6%)
Seborrhea
Stevens–Johnson syndrome
  (2007): Shen YC+, *Int Clin Psychopharmacol* 22(4), 247 (with
    lamotrigine)
Ulcerations
Urticaria
Vesiculobullous eruption
Xerosis

Mucosal/ENT

Auditory hallucinations
  (2006): Lee BH+, *Prog Neuropsychopharmacol Biol Psychiatry*
    30(4), 714
Cheilitis
Dysgeusia
Gingival bleeding
Gingivitis
Glossitis
Oral candidiasis
Oral ulceration
Oral vesiculation
Sialorrhea
Stomatitis
Tinnitus
Tongue edema
Vaginitis
  (2006): Keck PE Jr+, *J Clin Psychiatry* 67(4), 626
Vulvovaginal candidiasis
Xerostomia

Hair

Hair – alopecia

Eyes

Blepharitis
Epiphora
Xerophthalmia

Other

Anxiety
  (2006): Nickel MK+, *Am J Psychiatry* 163(5), 833
Candidiasis
Chills
Cough (3%)
Death
  (2005): *Prescrire Int* 14(77), 103
Depression
Fever (2%)
Gynecomastia
Headache
  (2007): Tran-Johnson TK+, *J Clin Psychiatry* 68(1), 111
  (2006): Nickel MK+, *Am J Psychiatry* 163(5), 833
  (2004): Swainston Harrison T+, *Drugs* 64(15), 1715
  (2003): Winans E, *Am J Health Syst Pharm* 60(23), 2437
Hypotension
  (2005): *Prescrire Int* 14(79), 163
Inappropriate secretion of antidiuretic hormone (SIADH)
  (2006): Bachu K+, *Am J Ther* 13(4), 370
Insomnia
  (2006): Nickel MK+, *Am J Psychiatry* 163(5), 833
  (2006): Tandon R+, *Schizophr Res* 84(1), 77 (24%)
Mania
  (2007): Padala PR+, *Am J Psychiatry* 164(1), 172
Myalgia/Myositis/Myopathy/Myotoxicity
Pain
  (2006): Keck PE Jr+, *J Clin Psychiatry* 67(4), 626
Paresthesias
  (2006): Nickel MK+, *Am J Psychiatry* 163(5), 833
Phlebitis
Rhabdomyolysis
Seizures
  (2005): Malik AR+, *Can J Psychiatry* 50(3), 186
Suicidal ideation
  (2006): Beers E+, *Ned Tijdschr Geneeskd* 150(7), 401
  (2006): Holzer L+, *Int Clin Psychopharmacol* 21(2), 125
  (2006): Slooff CJ+, *Ned Tijdschr Geneeskd* 150(7), 400
  (2005): Scholten MR+, *Ned Tijdschr Geneeskd* 149(41), 2296
Tendinopathy/Tendon rupture
Thrombophlebitis
Tremor (3%)
  (2006): Keck PE Jr+, *J Clin Psychiatry* 67(4), 626
Upper respiratory infection

ARISTOLOCHIA

Scientific names: *Aristolochia clematitis; Aristolochia serpentaria*
Family: Aristolochiaceae
Trade and other common names: Birthwort; Long Birthwort;
Pelican Flower; Red River Snakeroot; Sangree Root; Sangrel;
Serpentaria; Snakeweed; Virginia Serpentary
Category: Immunomodulator
Purported indications and other uses: Aphrodisiac, anti-
allergy, anticonvulsant, promotes menstruation
Half-life: N/A

Reactions

Other

Death
Nephrotoxicity
  (2007): Grollman AP+, *J Am Soc Nephrol* 18(11), 2817
  (2007): Grollman AP+, *Proc Natl Acad Sci U S A* 104(29), 12129
  (2007): Long DT+, *Croat Med J* 48(3), 300
  (2005): Hranjec T+, *Croat Med J* 46(1), 116
  (2003): Cosyns JP, *Drug Saf* 26(1), 33

ARMODAFINIL

Trade name: Nuvigil (Cephalon)
Indications: Narcolepsy, obstructive sleep apnea (OSA), shift work sleep disorder
Category: Eugeroic
Half-life: 12–15 Hours
Clinically important, potentially hazardous interactions with: cyclosporine

Reactions

Skin
Allergic reactions (sic)
Angioedema
Dermatitis (contact)
Hyperhidrosis
Rash (sic)
Stevens–Johnson syndrome
Toxic epidermal necrolysis

Mucosal/ENT
Dysphagia
Xerostomia

Eyes
Visual hallucinations

Other
Abdominal pain
Anaphylactoid reactions/Anaphylaxis
Anxiety
   (2006): Roth T+, *Clin Ther* 28(5), 689
Asthenia
Depression
DRESS syndrome
Fever
Headache
   (2007): Hirshkowitz M+, *Respir Med* 101(3), 616
   (2006): Harsh JR+, *Curr Med Res Opin* 22(4), 761
   (2006): Roth T+, *Clin Ther* 28(5), 689
Hypersensitivity
Insomnia
   (2006): Roth T+, *Clin Ther* 28(5), 689
Migraine
Pain
Paresthesias
Suicidal ideation
Tremor
Vertigo
   (2006): Harsh JR+, *Curr Med Res Opin* 22(4), 761
   (2006): Roth T+, *Clin Ther* 28(5), 689

ARNICA

Scientific names: *Arnica fulgens; Arnica montana; Arnica sororia*
Family: Asteraceae; Compositae
Trade and other common names: Leopard's Bane; Mountain snuff; Mountain tobacco; Wolf's Bane
Category: Immunomodulator
Purported indications and other uses: Bruising, aches and sprains, insect bites, superficial phlebitis, diuretic, flavoring agent, found in hair tonic and shampoo
Half-life: N/A
Clinically important, potentially hazardous interactions with: warfarin

Reactions

Skin
Acute febrile neutrophilic dermatosis (Sweet's syndrome)
Adverse effects (sic)
   (2002): Haller CA+, *Adverse Drug React Toxicol Rev* 21(3), 143
Allergic reactions (sic)
   (2002): Knuesel O+, *Adv Ther* 19(5), 209 (1 case)
Dermatitis
   (2002): Schempp CM+, *Hautarzt* 53(2), 93
   (2001): *Int J Toxicol* 20, 1
   (2001): Reider N+, *Contact Dermatitis* 45(5), 269
   (1980): Hausen BM, *Hautarzt* 31(1), 10
Irritation (sic)
Sensitization
   (2002): Paulsen E, *Contact Dermatitis* 47(4), 189

Mucosal/ENT
Mucosal irritation
Mucosal ulceration
   (1999): Moghadam BK+, *Cutis* 64(2), 131 (with alcohol and peppermint)

Other
Death
   (2001): *Int J Toxicol* 20, 1

ARSENIC

Trade names: Fowler's Solution (rarely employed; found in pesticides and herbal medicines); Trisonex (Cell Therapeutics)
Indications: Acute promyelocytic leukemia, psoriasis (in the early 1900s), devitalization of pulp in dental procedures
Category: Trace element
Half-life: N/A
Clinically important, potentially hazardous interactions with: abacavir, amiodarone, bretylium, chlorpromazine, ciprofloxacin, disopyramide, enoxacin, fluphenazine, gatifloxacin, lomefloxacin, mesoridazine, moxifloxacin, norfloxacin, ofloxacin, phenothiazines, procainamide, prochlorperazine, promethazine, quinidine, quinolones, sotalol, sparfloxacin, thioridazine, trifluoperazine

Reactions

Skin
Acral desquamation
   (2003): Uede K+, *Br J Dermatol* 149(4), 757 (11 cases)
Basal cell carcinoma
   (2005): Fumal I+, *Rev Med Liege* 60(4), 217

(1994): McNutt NS+, *Arch Dermatol* 130, 225
(1993): Alain G+, *Int J Dermatol* 32, 899 (passim)
(1993): Sass U+, *Dermatology* 186, 303
(1993): Ziegler A+, *Proc Natl Acad*
(1992): Breathnach SM+, *Adverse Drug Reactions and the Skin* Blackwell, Oxford, 236 (passim)
(1987): Chakraborty AK+, *Indian J Med Res* 85, 326
(1986): Munzberger H+, *Z Arztl Fortbild Jena* (German) 80, 985
(1985): Kastl J+, *Dermatol Monatsschr* (German) 171, 158
(1984): Schroeder P+, *Fortschr Med* (German) 102, 1128
(1980): Weiss J+, *Hautarzt* (German) 31, 654

Palmar–plantar erythema
Palmar–plantar hyperhidrosis
(2000): Gerdssn R+, *Acta Derm Venereol* 80, 292
Palmar–plantar hyperkeratosis
(2005): Fumal I+, *Rev Med Liege* 60(4), 217
(2002): Hall AH, *Toxicol Lett* 128(1), 69
(2000): Gerdsen R+, *Acta Derm Venereol* 80, 292
(1998): Tsuruta D+, *Br J Dermatol* 139, 291
(1997): Ohnishi Y+, *J Dermatol* 24, 310
(1996): Maloney ME, *Dermatol Surg* 22, 301 (passim)
(1996): Person JR, *Cutis* 58, 65
(1994): Hsieh LL+, *Cancer Lett* 86, 59
(1993): Alain G+, *Int J Dermatol* 32, 899 (passim)
(1992): Breathnach SM+, *Adverse Drug Reactions and the Skin* Blackwell, Oxford, 236 (passim)
(1989): Koh E+, *Eur Urol* 16, 398
(1989): Shannon RL+, *Hum Toxicol* 8, 99
(1988): Ismail R+, *J Dermatol* 15, 65
(1983): Heddle R+, *Chest* 84, 776
(1982): Ohyama K, *Dermatologica* 164, 161
(1982): Rosen T+, *J Am Acad Dermatol* 7, 364

Palmar–plantar punctate keratoses
(1996): Maloney ME, *Dermatol Surg* 22, 301 (passim)
(1992): Breathnach SM+, *Adverse Drug Reactions and the Skin* Blackwell, Oxford, 236 (passim)

Parapsoriasis
Photo-recall
(2003): Keung YK+, *Leukemia* 17(7), 1417
Photosensitivity
(1992): Breathnach SM+, *Adverse Drug Reactions and the Skin* Blackwell, Oxford, 236 (passim)
Pigmentation
(2004): Kwong YL, *Expert Opin Drug Saf* 3(6), 589
(2002): Hall AH, *Toxicol Lett* 128(1), 69
(2002): Liu J+, *Environ Health Perspect* 110(2), 119
(2002): Park JY+, *J Dermatol* 29(7), 446
(2001): Kurokawa M+, *Arch Dermatol* 137, 102
(2001): Yu HS+, *J Dermatol* 28(11), 628
(1999): Tondel M+, *Environmental Health Perspectives* 107, 727
(1998): Guha Mazumder DN+, *Int J Epidemiol* 27, 871
(1996): Maloney ME, *Dermatol Surg* 22, 301 (passim)
(1993): Alain G+, *Int J Dermatol* 32, 899 (passim)
(1992): Breathnach SM+, *Adverse Drug Reactions and the Skin* Blackwell, Oxford, 236 (passim)
(1989): Shannon RL+, *Hum Toxicol* 8, 99
(1981): Granstein RD+, *J Am Acad Dermatol* 5, 1 (bronze)
Pityriasis rosea (from organic arsenic)
(1988): Bork K, *Cutaneous Side Effects of Drugs* WB Saunders, 169
Pruritus
Psoriasis
Purpura
(1988): Bork K, *Cutaneous Side Effects of Drugs* WB Saunders, 191
Rash (sic)
(2004): Kwong YL, *Expert Opin Drug Saf* 3(6), 589
Raynaud's phenomenon
(2002): Hall AH, *Toxicol Lett* 128(1), 69

Squamous cell carcinoma
(2005): Fumal I+, *Rev Med Liege* 60(4), 217
(2002): Centeno JA+, *Environ Health Perspect* 110 Suppl 5, 883 (chronic exposure)
(2002): Park JY+, *J Dermatol* 29(7), 446
(2001): Guo HR+, *Cancer Causes Control* 12(10), 909
(1998): Wong SS+, *J Am Acad Dermatol* 38(2 Pt 1), 179
(1996): Maloney ME, *Dermatol Surg* 22, 301 (passim)
(1993): Alain G+, *Int J Dermatol* 32, 899 (passim)
(1992): Breathnach SM+, *Adverse Drug Reactions and the Skin* Blackwell, Oxford, 236 (passim)
(1989): Shannon RL+, *Hum Toxicol* 8, 99
(1988): Ismail R+, *J Dermatol* 15, 65
(1988): Scholz S+, *Z Arztl Fortbild Jena* (German) 82, 1201
Stevens–Johnson syndrome
(1990): Vassileva S+, *Int J Dermatol* 29, 381
Ulcerations
(2002): Liu J+, *Environ Health Perspect* 110(2), 119
Urticaria
Vitiligo
(1989): Bickley LK+, *N J Med* 86, 377
Xerosis

Mucosal/ENT

Dysgeusia
(2002): Hall AH, *Toxicol Lett* 128(1), 69
Oral mucosal eruption (8%)
Oral pigmentation
(1988): Bork K, *Cutaneous Side Effects of Drugs* WB Saunders, 288
Stomatitis

Hair

Hair – alopecia
(1993): Alain G+, *Int J Dermatol* 32, 899 (passim)
(1992): Breathnach SM+, *Adverse Drug Reactions and the Skin* Blackwell, Oxford, 236 (passim)
(1988): Bork K, *Cutaneous Side Effects of Drugs* WB Saunders, 249

Nails

Nails – leukonychia
(1988): Bork K, *Cutaneous Side Effects of Drugs* WB Saunders, 262
Nails – Mees' lines
(1993): Alain G+, *Int J Dermatol* 32, 899 (passim)
(1993): Sass U+, *Dermatology* 186, 303
Nails – pigmentation
(1988): Bork K, *Cutaneous Side Effects of Drugs* WB Saunders, 261

Other

Death
(2003): Uede K+, *Br J Dermatol* 149(4), 757
Gangrene
(2002): Alam MG+, *Int J Environ Health Res* 12(3), 235 (chronic exposure)
Gynecomastia
(1992): Breathnach SM+, *Adverse Drug Reactions and the Skin* Blackwell, Oxford, 237 (passim)
Headache
Hepatotoxicity
(2004): Kwong YL, *Expert Opin Drug Saf* 3(6), 589
Tumors (malignant)
(2001): Kurokawa M+, *Arch Dermatol* 137, 102

ARTEMISIA

Scientific names: *Artemisia annua; Benflumetol; Co-artemether; Coartem; Riamet (Novartis)*
Family: Asteraceae
Trade and other common names: Annual wormwood; Arsumax (Sanofi Synthelabo); Arteether; Artemether; Artemisinin; Artemisinine; Artesunate; Malarlife; Paluther (Rhone-Poulenc); Qinghao; Qinghaosu; Quinghao; Sweet Annie; Sweet wormwood; Thanh hao; Wormwood
Category: Antimalarial
Purported indications and other uses: Fever, multidrug-resistant malaria, parasitemia, leukemia, colon cancer, diarrhea, schistosomiasis, worms, insect bites (topical)
Half-life: 10 hours

Note: Derivatives of *Artemisia annua* are often used in combination with piperaquine, or mefloquine in treatment of malaria

Note: Benflumetol, Coartem and Co-artemether are a combination of artemether-lumefantrine

Reactions

Skin
Allergic reactions (sic)
  (1987): Leng X+, *Asian Pac J Allergy Immunol* 5(2), 125 (to pollen)
Pruritus
  (2000): Bakshi R+, *Trans R Soc Trop Med Hyg* 94(4), 419 (artemether-lumefantrine) (%)
Rash
  (2000): Bakshi R+, *Trans R Soc Trop Med Hyg* 94(4), 419 (artemether-lumefantrine) (%)

Mucosal/ENT
Ototoxicity
  (2004): Toovey S+, *Trans R Soc Trop Med Hyg* 98(5), 261
Sialorrhea
  (1999): Mishra SK+, *Ann Trop Med Parasitol* 93(4), 413
Tinnitus (with high doses)

Other
Abdominal pain
  (2000): Bakshi R+, *Trans R Soc Trop Med Hyg* 94(4), 419 (artemether-lumefantrine)
Fever (rare)
Headache
  (2000): Bakshi R+, *Trans R Soc Trop Med Hyg* 94(4), 419 (artemether-lumefantrine)
Injection-site pain
  (1994): Karbwang J+, *Southeast Asian J Trop Med Public Health* 25(4), 702
  (1991): Bunnag D+, *Southeast Asian J Trop Med Public Health* 22(3), 380
Side effects (sic) (<3%)
Vertigo
  (2000): Bakshi R+, *Trans R Soc Trop Med Hyg* 94(4), 419 (artemether-lumefantrine)

ARTICHOKE

Scientific names: *Cynara cardunculus; Cynara scolymus*
Family: Asteraceae; Compositae
Trade and other common names: Alcachofa; Alcaucil; ALE; Cardo; Cardon d'Espagne; Cardoon; Cynara (Lichtwer); Globe Kardone; HeparSL forte; Tyosen-Azami
Category: Antiemetic; Carminative
Purported indications and other uses: Dyspepsia, hyperlipidemia, nausea, hangover, irritable bowel syndrome (IBS), liver dysfunction, hypoglycemia. Flavoring, sweetener, prebiotic
Half-life: N/A

Note: Jerusalem artichoke (*Helianthus tuberosus*) is a completely different plant

Reactions

Skin
Dermatitis
  (1983): Meding B, *Contact Dermatitis* 9(4), 314
  (1980): Turner T, *Contact Dermatitis* 6(6), 444
Urticaria
  (1996): Quirce S+, *J Allergy Clin Immunol* 97(2), 710

Mucosal/ENT
Rhinitis
  (2003): Miralles JC+, *Ann Allergy Asthma Immunol* 91(1), 92

Other
Anaphylactoid reactions/Anaphylaxis
  (2005): Franck P+, *Int Arch Allergy Immunol* 136(2), 155 (to inulin)

ASCORBIC ACID

Synonym: vitamin C
Trade names: Apo-C; Ascorbicap; Ce-Vi-Sol; Cebid; Cebion; Cecon; Cemill; Cetane; Cetebe; Cevalin; Cevi-Bid; Dull-C; Laroscorbine; Potent C; Pro-C; Redoxon; Sunkist; Vita-C
Indications: Prevention of scurvy
Category: Vitamin
Half-life: N/A
Clinically important, potentially hazardous interactions with: deferoxamine, penicillamine

Reactions

Skin
Angioedema
  (1980): Bilyk MA+, *Vrach Delo* (Russian) May, 81
Eczema
  (1980): Metz J+, *Contact Dermatitis* 6, 172
Erythema
Side effects (sic)
  (1992): Breathnach SM+, *Adverse Drug Reactions and the Skin* Blackwell, Oxford, 265 (passim)
  (1980): Bilyk MA+, *Vrach Delo* (Russian) May, 81

Other
Injection-site irritation

ASPARAGINASE

Synonym: L-asparaginase
Trade names: Crasnitin; Elspar (Merck); Erwinase; Kidrolase; Laspar; Leunase
Indications: Acute lymphocytic leukemia, lymphoma
Category: Antineoplastic; Enzyme
Half-life: 8–30 hours (IV); 39–49 hours (IM)

Reactions

Skin
Allergic reactions (SIC)
  (2003): Obama K+, *Int J Hematol* 78(3), 248
Angioedema
  (1983): Bronner AK+, *J Am Acad Dermatol* 9, 645 (15%)
  (1981): Weiss RB+, *Ann Intern Med* 94, 66
Diaphoresis
Edema
Exanthems
Peripheral edema
Pruritus (<1%)
  (1981): Weiss RB+, *Ann Intern Med* 94, 66
Rash (sic) (<1%)
Toxic epidermal necrolysis
  (1989): Stern RS+, *J Am Acad Dermatol* 21, 317
  (1980): Rodriguez AR, *J Med Assoc Ga* 69, 355
Urticaria (1–15%)
  (1983): Bronner AK+, *J Am Acad Dermatol* 9, 645 (15%)
  (1981): Weiss RB+, *Ann Intern Med* 94, 66

Mucosal/ENT
Aphthous stomatitis (1–10%)
Oral lesions (26%)

Hair
Hair – alopecia

Other
Anaphylactoid reactions/Anaphylaxis (3–40%)
  (1983): Bronner AK+, *J Am Acad Dermatol* 9, 645 (15%)
  (1982): Dunagin WG, *Semin Oncol* 9, 14 (3%)
Chills
Headache
Hypersensitivity (6–40%)
  (2003): Rosen O+, *Br J Haematol* 123(5), 836
  (2001): Bryant R, *J Intraven Nurs* 24(3), 169
  (1998): Bonno M+, *J Allergy Clin Immunol* 101, 571
  (1998): Larson RA+, *Leukemia* 12, 660
  (1992): Weiss RB, *Semin Oncol* 19, 458
  (1982): Dunagin WG, *Semin Oncol* 9, 14 (33%)
  (1981): Weiss RB+, *Ann Intern Med* 94, 66 (6–43%)
Injection-site erythema
Neurotoxicity
  (2006): Nakajima D+, *No To Hattatsu* 38(3), 195
Serum sickness
  (1983): Bronner AK+, *J Am Acad Dermatol* 9, 645 (15%)
Thrombosis
  (2006): Ruud E+, *Pediatr Hematol Oncol* 23(3), 207

ASPARTAME

Trade names: Equal; Nutrasweet
Category: Sweetening agent
Half-life: N/A

Note: Aspartame can be found in instant breakfasts, breath mints, cereals, sugar-free chewing gum, cocoa mixes, coffee beverages, frozen desserts, gelatin desserts, juice beverages, laxatives, multivitamins, milk drinks, pharmaceuticals and supplements, shake mixes, soft drinks, tabletop sweeteners, tea beverages, instant teas and coffees, topping mixes, wine coolers, yogurt

Reactions

Skin
Allergic reactions (sic)
  (1998): Garriga MM+, *Ann Allergy* 61, 63
  (1996): Roberts HJ, *Arch Intern Med* 156, 1027
Angioedema
  (1992): Downham TF, *Clin Cases in Dermatol* 4, 12 (observation)
  (1988): Metcalfe DD, *Skin and Allergy News* 19, 52 (observation)
Dermatitis
  (1992): Downham TF, *Clin Cases in Dermatol* 4, 12 (observation)
Erythema nodosum
  (1997): Bohn S+, *Schweiz Med Wochenschr* 127(27-28), 1168
Exanthems
  (1986): *Arzneimittelinformation ATI Berlin GmbH* (German)
    12, 121
Pruritus
  (1994): Shelley WB+, *Cutis* 53, 77 (observation)
  (1988): Metcalfe DD, *Skin and Allergy News* 19, 52 (observation)
Pruritus ani et vulvae
  (1994): Shelley WB+, *Cutis* 53, 237 (observation)
Purpura
  (1999): Leal G, Fortaleza, Brazil (from Internet) (observation)
  (1992): Downham TF, *Clin Cases in Dermatol* 4, 12 (observation)
Rash (sic)
  (1988): Metcalfe DD, *Skin and Allergy News* 19, 52 (observation)
Urticaria
  (1995): Kulczycki A, *J Allergy Clin Immunol* 95, 639
  (1992): Downham TF, *Clin Cases in Dermatol* 4, 12 (observation)
  (1988): Metcalfe DD, *Skin and Allergy News* 19, 52 (observation)
  (1986): Kulczycki A, *Ann Intern Med* 104, 207
Vasculitis
  (1992): Downham TF, *Clin Cases in Dermatol* 4, 12 (observation)

Other
Anaphylactoid reactions/Anaphylaxis
  (1996): Roberts HJ, *Arch Intern Med* 156, 1027
Panniculitis
  (1992): Geha RS, *J Am Acad Dermatol* 26, 277 (lobular)
  (1991): McCauliffe DP+, *J Am Acad Dermatol* 24, 298 (lobular)
  (1985): Novick NL, *Ann Intern Med* 102, 206 (granulomatous)
Sjøgren's (Sicca) syndrome
  (2006): Robert HJ, *South Med J* 99(6), 631

ASPIRIN

Synonyms: acetylsalicylic acid; ASA
Trade names: Aggrenox (Boehringer Ingelheim); Alka-Seltzer; Anacin (Wyeth); ASA; Ascriptin (Novartis) (Wallace); Aspergum; Aspro; ASS; Bex; Caprin; Claragine; Coricidin D; Darvon Compound (aaiPharma); Disprin; Ecotrin (GSK); Empirin; Equagesic (Women First); Excedrin (Bristol-Myers Squibb); Fiorinal (Watson); Gelprin; Halfprin; Measurin; Norgesic (3M); Novasen; Rhonal; Robaxisal; Soma Compound (MedPointe); Talwin Compound (Sanofi-Aventis); Vanquish
Indications: Pain, fever, inflammation
Category: Antiplatelet; Non-steroidal anti-inflammatory; Salicylate
Half-life: 15–20 minutes
Clinically important, potentially hazardous interactions with: acenocoumarol, anagrelide, anticoagulants, bismuth, **boswellia**, calcium hydroxylapatite, **capsicum**, cholestyramine, desvenlafaxine, **devil's claw**, dexamethasone, dexibuprofen, dicumarol, etodolac, **evening primrose**, flunisolide, **ginkgo biloba**, **ginseng**, heparin, ibuprofen, indomethacin, ketoprofen, ketorolac, lumiracoxib, methotrexate, methylprednisolone, nilutamide, NSAIDs, **phellodendron**, prednisone, **resveratrol**, reteplase, sermorelin, **sulfites**, tirofiban, triamcinolone, urokinase, valdecoxib, valproic acid, verapamil, warfarin

Note: Aggrenox is aspirin and dipyridamole

Reactions

Skin

Acute generalized exanthematous pustulosis (AGEP)
　(1993)· Ballmer-Weber BK+, *Schweiz Med Wochenschr* (German) 123, 542
Allergic granulomatous angiitis (Churg–Strauss syndrome)
　(1982): Cozzutto C+, *Virchows Arch A Pathol Anat Histol* 397, 61
Allergic reactions (sic) (<1%) (with dipyridamole)
　(1991): VanArsdel PP Jr, *JAMA* 266, 3343
Angioedema (1–5%)
　(2006): Kaptanoglu AF+, *J Eur Acad Dermatol Venereol* 20(5), 617 (tongue)
　(2006): Kim SH+, *Curr Opin Allergy Clin Immunol* 6(4), 266
　(2006): Kim SH+, *Yonsei Med J* 47(1), 15
　(2004): Mastalerz L+, *J Allergy Clin Immunol* 113(4), 771
　(2003): Sanchez-Borges M+, *Clin Rev Allergy Immunol* 24(2), 125
　(2002): Higashi N+, *J Allergy Clin Immunol* 110(4), 666
　(2001): Nakamura T+, *Arerugi* 50(11), 1102
　(2000): Ghislain PD+, *Ann Med Interne* (Paris) 151, 227 (Nuchal scalp)
　(2000): Pradalier A+, *Rev Med Interne* (French) 21, 75
　(2000): Wong JT+, *J Allergy Clin Immunol* 105, 997
　(1998): Grzelewska-Rzymowska I, *Pol Merkuriusz Lek* (Polish) 4, 233
　(1997): Tomaz EM+, *Allergy Asthma Proc* 18, 319
　(1996): Chan TY, *Br J Clin Pract* 50, 412
　(1993): Grzelewska-Rzymowska I+, *Pneumonol Alergol Pol* (Polish) 61, 29
　(1988): Botey J+, *Allergol Immunopathol Madr* (Spanish) 16, 43
　(1984): Botey J+, *Ann Allergy* 53, 265
　(1981): Juhlin L, *Br J Dermatol* 104, 369
Baboon syndrome
　(2003): Wolf R+, *Dermatol Online J* 9(3), 2
Bullous dermatitis (<1%)
　(1989): Sfar Z +, *Tunis Med* 67, 805
Dermatitis herpetiformis
Dermatomyositis

Diaphoresis
Erythema multiforme (<1%)
　(1998): Lee SG+, *Eur J Dermatol* 8, 280
　(1985): Laurberg G+, *Ugeskr Laeger* 147, 1853
　(1985): Ting HC+, *Int J Dermatol* 24, 587
　(1982): Bailin PL+, *Clin Rheum Dis* 8, 493 (passim)
Erythema nodosum (<1%)
　(1996): Buckshee K+, *Int J Gynaecol Obstet* 55, 293
　(1996): Durden FM+, *Int J Dermatol* 35, 39
　(1994): Fernandes NC+, *Rev Inst Med Trop Sao Paulo* (Portuguese) 36, 507
　(1987): Blasetti P, *Clin Ter* 123(4), 303
　(1982): Bailin PL+, *Clin Rheum Dis* 8, 493 (passim)
　(1982): Ubogy Z+, *Acta Derm Venereol* 62, 265
Erythroderma
　(2006): Sugita K+, *Arch Dermatol* 142(6), 792
Exanthems
　(1993): Ballmer-Weber BK+, *Schweiz Med Wochenschr* 123, 542
　(1989): Hass WK+, *N Engl J Med* 321, 501 (5.2%)
　(1987): Castles JJ+, *Arch Intern Med* 138, 362 (2.8%)
　(1982): Morley PA+, *Drugs* 23, 250 (5%)
　(1980): Goerz G+, *Fortschr Med* 98, 726
Exfoliative dermatitis
Fixed eruption (<1%)
　(1999): Galindo PA+, *J Investig Allergol Clin Immunol* 9, 399
　(1998): Mahboob A+, *Int J Dermatol* 37, 833
　(1997): Bhargava P+, *Int J Dermatol* 36, 236
　(1992): Hatzis J+, *Cutis* 50, 50
　(1991): Thankappen TP+, *Int J Dermatol* 30, 867 (1.7%)
　(1990): Bharija SC+, *Dermatologica* 181, 237
　(1990): Gaffoor PMA+, *Cutis* 45, 242
　(1989): Shiohara T+, *Arch Dermatol* 125, 1371
　(1986): Kanwar AJ, *Dermatologica* 172, 315
　(1986): Kanwar AJ+, *J Dermatol* 11, 383
　(1985): Gomez B+, *Allergol Immunopathol Madr* (Spanish) 13, 87
　(1985): Kauppinen K+, *Br J Dermatol* 112, 575
　(1984): Boyle J+, *Br Med J Clin Res Ed* 289, 802
　(1984): Chan HL, *Int J Dermatol* 23, 607
　(1984): Pandhi RK+, *Sex Transm Dis* 11, 164
　(1982): Bailin PL+, *Clin Rheum Dis* 8, 493 (passim)
　(1981): Shukla SR, *Dermatologica* 163, 160
Graft-versus-host reaction
　(1998): Jappe U+, *Hautarzt* (German) 49, 126 (passim)
Herpes genitalis
Herpes simplex
　(1984): Boyle J, Moul B, *Br Med J* (Clin Res Ed) 289, 802
Lichenoid eruption
　(1988): Bharija SC+, *Dermatologica* 177, 19
Papuloerythroderma of Ofuji
　(2006): Sugita K+, *Arch Dermatol* 142(6), 792
Parapsoriasis
Pemphigus
　(1986): Pisani M+, *G Ital Dermatol Venereol* (Italian) 121, 39
Petechiae
　(1997): Blumenthal HL, Beachwood, OH (personal case) (observation)
Photo-recall
　(1998): Lee SG+, *Eur J Dermatol* 8, 280
Pigmented purpuric eruption
　(1999): Lipsker D+, *Ann Dermatol Venereol* (French) 126, 321
Pityriasis rosea
　(2006): Atzori L+, *Dermatology Online Journal* 12(1), 1 (with hydrochlorothiazide)
　(1993): Yosipovitch G+, *Harefuah* (Hebrew) 124, 198; 247
Pruritus
　(1981): Settipane GA, *Arch Intern Med* 141, 328
Psoriasis
Purpura

(2001): Tsuda T+, *J Int Med Res* 29(4), 374
(1997): Sola-Alberich R+, *Ann Intern Med* 126, 665
(1989): Hass WK+, *N Engl J Med* 321, 501 (2%)
(1980): Miescher PA+, *Clin Haematol* 9, 505

Rash (sic) (1–10%)

Stevens–Johnson syndrome
(1995): Kuper K+, *Ophthalmologe* 92(6), 823
(1993): Leenutaphong V+, *Int J Dermatol* 32, 428

Toxic epidermal necrolysis (<1%)
(2002): Correia O+, *Arch Dermatol* 138, 29
(1993): Leenutaphong V+, *Int J Dermatol* 32, 428
(1988): Dahle MG, *Tidsskr Nor Laegeforen* (Norwegian) 108, 1917
(1987): Guillaume JC+, *Arch Dermatol* 123, 1166

Ulcerations (<1%) (with dipyridamole)

Urticaria (1–10%)
(2006): Kim SH+, *Curr Opin Allergy Clin Immunol* 6(4), 266
(2006): Kim SH+, *Yonsei Med J* 47(1), 15
(2006): Padilla Serrato MT+, *Rev Alerg Mex* 53(5), 179
(2004): Mastalerz L+, *J Allergy Clin Immunol* 113(4), 771
(2003): Grattan CE, *Clin Exp Dermatol* 28(2), 123
(2003): Sanchez-Borges M+, *Clin Rev Allergy Immunol* 24(2), 125
(2002): Higashi N+, *J Allergy Clin Immunol* 110(4), 666
(2001): Cousin F+, *Ann Dermatol Venereol* 128(10), 1166
(2001): Harada S+, *Br J Dermatol* 145(2), 336
(2001): Nakamura T+, *Arerugi* 50(11), 1102
(2000): Pradalier A+, *Rev Med Interne* (French) 21, 75
(2000): Wong JT+, *J Allergy Clin Immunol* 105, 997
(1999): Asero R, *Ann Allergy Asthma Immunol* 82(6), 554 (19%)
(1999): Eseverri JL+, *Allergol Immunopathol* (Madr) (Spanish) 27, 104
(1998): Grzelewska-Rzymowska I, *Pol Merkuriusz Lek* (Polish) 4, 233
(1998): Ohnishi-Inoue Y+, *Br J Dermatol* 138, 483
(1997): Tomaz EM+, *Allergy Asthma Proc* 18, 319
(1995): Gebhardt M+, *Z Rheumatol* (German) 54, 405
(1995): Grzelewska-Rzymowska I+, *J Invest Allergol Clin Immunol* 5, 272
(1994): Paul E+, *Hautarzt* (German) 45, 12
(1994): Smith RJ+, *Br J Dermatol* 131, 583
(1993): Grzelewska-Rzymowska I+, *Pneumonol Alergol Pol* (Polish) 61, 29
(1992): Grzelewska-Rzymowska I+, *J Invest Alergol Clin Immunol* 2, 39
(1989): Alanko K+, *Acta Derm Venereol* (Stockh) 69, 223 (1–5%)
(1989): Grzelewska-Rzymowska I, *Allergol Immunopathol Madr* (Spanish) 16, 231
(1989): Hass WK+, *N Engl J Med* 321, 501 (0.3%)
(1988): Botey J+, *Allergol Immunopathol Madr* (Spanish) 16, 43
(1987): Asad SI+, *Ann Allergy* 59, 219
(1986): Dupont C, *Int J Dermatol* 25, 334
(1986): Finzi AF+, *Minerva Med* (Italian) 77, 1401
(1986): Nagy G+, *Dermatol Monatsschr* 72, 594
(1986): Wojnerowicz-Grajewska M+, *Przegl Dermatol* (Polish) 73, 115
(1984): Botey J+, *Ann Allergy* 53, 265
(1984): Kauppinen K+, *Allergy* 39, 469
(1983): Kaplan AP, *Postgrad Med* 74, 209
(1982): Kirchhof B+, *Dermatol Monatsschr* (German) 168, 513
(1981): Juhlin L, *Br J Dermatol* 104, 369
(1981): Settipane GA, *Arch Intern Med* 141, 328
(1980): Settipane RA+, *Allergy* 35, 149
(1980): Wuthrich B+, *Z Hautkr* (German) 55, 102

Vasculitis
(1999): Crutchfield CE+, *Skin and Aging* May, 84 (leukocytoclastic)
(1984): Ekenstam E+, *Arch Dermatol* 120, 484

Mucosal/ENT
Ageusia (<1%) (with dipyridamole)

Anosmia
(2003): Fahrenholz JM, *Clin Rev Allergy Immunol* 24(2), 113

Aphthous stomatitis
(2001): Vincent L+, *Ann Dermatol Venereol* 128, 57
(1982): Bailin PL+, *Clin Rheum Dis* 8, 493 (passim)

Dysgeusia

Gingivitis (<1%) (with dipyridamole)

Oral burn
(1998): Dellinger TM+, *Ann Pharmacother* 32, 1107

Oral lichen planus
(1989): Espana-Alonso A+, *An Med Interna* (Spanish) 6, 219

Oral mucosal eruption
(1988): Bork K, *Cutaneous Side Effects of Drugs* WB Saunders, 283

Oral ulceration

Rhinitis
(2003): Fahrenholz JM, *Clin Rev Allergy Immunol* 24(2), 113

Tinnitus
(2004): Wecker H+, *HNO* 52(4), 347
(2000): Cazals Y, *Prog Neurobiol* 62(6), 583
(1993): Brien JA, *Drug Saf* 9(2), 143
(1993): Jung TT+, *Otolaryngol Clin North Am* 26(5), 791
(1991): Boettcher FA+, *Am J Otolaryngol* 12(1), 33
(1991): Halla JT+, *Ann Rheum Dis* 50(10), 682 (30%)
(1988): Halla JT+, *Ann Rheum Dis* 47(2), 134 (40%)
(1988): Kolodny AL, *J Rheumatol* 15(8), 1205
(1985): Burch FX, *Am J Med* 79(4B), 28
(1984): Stevenson DD, *J Allergy Clin Immunol* 74(4 Pt 2), 617
(1983): Kahn SB+, *J Clin Pharmacol* 23(4), 139
(1981): Ekstrand R+, *Scand J Rheumatol* 10(2), 69 (with indomethacin)
(1981): Wolff F+, *Geburtshilfe Frauenheilkd* 41(2), 96
(1980): Lan JL+, *Zhonghua Min Guo Wei Sheng Wu Ji Mian Yi Xue Za Zhi* 13(1), 27

Hair
Hair – alopecia

Eyes
Ocular hemorrhage
(2004): Davies BR, *Br J Ophthalmol* 88(9), 1226 (with clopidogrel)

Periorbital edema
(1998): Quiralte J, *Ann Allergy Asthma Immunol* 81(5), 459
(1997): Price KS+, *Ann Allergy Asthma Immunol* 79, 420
(1993): Katz Y+, *Allergy* 48(5), 366 (2 cases)

Other
Anaphylactoid reactions/Anaphylaxis (1–10%)
(2003): Berkes EA, *Clin Rev Allergy Immunol* 24(2), 137
(2001): Harada S+, *Br J Dermatol* 145(2), 336
(2001): Morisset M+, *Allerg Immunol* (Paris) 33(3), 147
(1999): Kubota Y+, *Eur J Dermatol* 9, 559
(1984): Stevenson DD, *J Allergy Clin Immunol* 74, 617

Asthma
(2006): Kim SH+, *Yonsei Med J* 47(1), 15

Headache

Hypersensitivity
(2003): Kasper L+, *Allergy* 58(10), 1064 (30 cases)
(2001): Hinrichs R+, *Allergy* 56(8), 789
(2001): Rueff F+, *Allergy* 56, 258

Myalgia/Myositis/Myopathy/Myotoxicity (1.2%) (with dipyridamole)

Paresthesias (<1%) (with dipyridamole)

Pseudolymphoma
(1980): Olmos L+, *Rev Clin Esp* 157, 67

Pseudoporphyria
(1994): Hazen PG, *J Am Acad Dermatol* 31, 500

ASTEMIZOLE

Trade names: Adistan; Alestol; Astemina; Astimal; Astizol; Hismanal; Histeamen (Janssen); Pollon-Eze; Simprox; Stemiz
Indications: Urticaria, pruritus, allergic rhinitis
Category: Histamine H1 receptor antagonist
Half-life: 20 Hours
Clinically important, potentially hazardous interactions with: amiodarone, azithromycin, bepredil, bosentan, bretylium, cisapride, clarithromycin, disopyramide, erythromycin fluconazole, fluoxetine, fluvoxamine, **grapefruit juice**, indinavir, itraconazole, ketoconazole, metronidazole, miconazole, nefazodone, paroxetine, pimozide, probucol, procainamide, quinidine, quinine, ritonavir, saquinavir, sertraline, sotalol, SSRIs, terfenadine, troleandomycin, voriconazole, zileuton, ziprasidone

Note: Hismanal has been withdrawn in the USA as of 1999

Reactions

Skin
Angioedema
Dermatitis
   (1984): Richards DM+, *Drugs* f(1), 38
Exanthems
   (1984): Richards DM+, *Drugs* f(1), 38
Mucha–Habermann disease
   (1993): Stosiek N+, *Hautarzt* 44(4), 235
Photosensitivity
   (1996): Berkowitz RB+, *Ann Allergy Asthma* 76(4), 363
Pruritus
   (1983): Bateman DN+, *Eur J Clin Pharmacol* 25(4), 567
Rash
   (1989): Juniper EF+, *J Allergy Clin Immunol* TI(F), 627
Stevens–Johnson syndrome
   (1995): Cunliffe NA+, *Postgrad Med J* 71(836), 383
Urticaria
   (1989): Huerter CJ+, *Cleve Clin J Med* 56(3), 263
   (1983): Bateman DN+, *Eur J Clin Pharmacol* 25(4), 567

Mucosal/ENT
Dysgeusia
   (1987): Kailasam V+, *J Am Acad Dermatol* 16(4), 797
Oral mucosal eruption
   (1984): Richards DM+, *Drugs* f(1), 38
Xerostomia
   (1995): Breneman D+, *J Am Acad Dermatol* 33(2), 192
   (1991): Humphreys F+, *Br J Dermatol* 125(4), 364
   (1989): Juniper EF+, *J Allergy Clin Immunol* TI(F), 627
   (1984): Richards DM+, *Drugs* f(1), 38

Hair
Hair – alopecia
   (1987): Kailasam V+, *J Am Acad Dermatol* 16(4), 797
Hair – changes
   (1989): Huerter CJ+, *Cleve Clin J Med* 56(3), 263

Other
Anaphylactoid reactions/Anaphylaxis
   (1998): Highleyman L, *BETA* 113, 3
Cardiac arrest
   (1993): Broadhurst P+, *Br Heart J* 70(5), 469
Myalgia/Myositis/Myopathy/Myotoxicity
Paresthesias
   (1992): Bedi RS, *J Assoc Physicians India* 40(9), 642
   (1990): Kaufman HS+, *N Engl J Med* 323(10), 684
   (1988): Oei HD, *Ann Allergy* 61(ug), 436
Somnolence

   (1995): Breneman D+, *J Am Acad Dermatol* 33(2), 192
   (1995): Cudowska B+, *Rocz Akad Med Bialymst* 40(3), 613
   (1993): Miglior M+, *Acta Ophthalmol (Copenh)* 71(1), 73
Weight gain
   (1995): Cudowska B+, *Rocz Akad Med Bialymst* 40(3), 613

ASTRAGALUS ROOT

Scientific names: *Astragalus membranaceus; Astragalus mongholicus*
Family: Fabaceae; Leguminosae
Trade and other common names: Beg Kei; Buck Qi; Hwanggi; Mongolian Milk; Ogi; Radix Astragali
Category: Antioxidant; Immune stimulant; Vasodilator
Purported indications and other uses: arrhythmia, colds, upper respiratory infections, chronic fatigue syndrome, colitis, diabetes, hepatitis, hypotension, herpes simplex keratitis
Half-life: N/A
Clinically important, potentially hazardous interactions with: cyclophosphamide

Reactions

None

ATAZANAVIR

Trade name: Reyataz (Bristol-Myers Squibb)
Indications: HIV infection
Category: Antiretroviral; Protease inhibitor, HIV
Half-life: 7 hours
Clinically important, potentially hazardous interactions with: bepridil, cisapride, dasatinib, dofetilide, ergot derivatives, etravirine, fentanyl, **garlic**, indinavir, irinotecan, ixabepilone, lapatinib, lovastatin, marihuana, midazolam, pimozide, proton-pump inhibitors, raltegravir, rifampin, ritonavir, sildenafil, simvastatin, solifenacin, **St John's wort**, temsirolimus, triazolam

Reactions

Skin
Allergic reactions (sic)
Burning
Cellulitis
Diaphoresis
Eczema
Edema
Erythema multiforme
Exanthems
Fungal dermatitis
Jaundice
   (2003): Murphy RL+, *AIDS* 17(18), 2603
   (2003): Sanne I+, *J Acquir Immune Defic Syndr* 32(1), 18
Pallor
Peripheral edema
Photosensitivity
Pruritus
Purpura
Rash (sic) (20%)
   (2006): Ouagari Z+, *AIDS* 20(8), 1207
   (2004): Busti AJ+, *Pharmacotherapy* 24(12), 1732
Seborrhea

Stevens–Johnson syndrome
Urticaria
Vesiculobullous eruption
Xerosis

Mucosal/ENT
Aphthous stomatitis
Dysgeusia
Tinnitus

Hair
Hair – alopecia

Nails
Nails – changes (sic)

Other
Abdominal pain
  (2004): Busti AJ+, *Pharmacotherapy* 24(12), 1732
Asthenia (2%)
Cough
Fever
Gynecomastia
Headache (14%)
  (2004): Busti AJ+, *Pharmacotherapy* 24(12), 1732
Infections (~50%)
  (2004): Busti AJ+, *Pharmacotherapy* 24(12), 1732
Lipoatrophy
Myalgia/Myositis/Myopathy/Myotoxicity
Neurotoxicity
  (2004): Busti AJ+, *Pharmacotherapy* 24(12), 1732
Pain (3%)
Vertigo (3%)

ATENOLOL

Trade names: Antipressan; Apo-Atenol; AteHexal; Atendol;
Evitocor; Noten; Novo-Atenol; Nu-Atenol; Taro-Atenol; Tenolin;
Tenoretic (AstraZeneca); Tenormin (AstraZeneca); Tenormine
Indications: Angina, hypertension, acute myocardial infarction
Category: Adrenergic beta-receptor antagonist; Antiarrhythmic
class II
Half-life: 6–7 hours (adults)
**Clinically important, potentially hazardous interactions
with:** alfuzosin, cisplatin, clonidine, epinephrine, verapamil

Note: Tenoretic is atenolol and chlorthalidone

Note: Grinspan's syndrome: the triad of oral lichen planus, diabetes
mellitus, and hypertension

Reactions

Skin
Dermatitis
Diaphoresis
Edema
Erythema multiforme
Exanthems
Facial edema
Fixed eruption
  (1999): Palungwachira P+, *J Med Assoc Thai* 82, 1158
Grinspan's syndrome
  (1990): Lamey PJ+, *Oral Surg Oral Med Oral Pathol* 70, 184
Hyperkeratosis (palms and soles)
Lichenoid eruption

Lupus erythematosus
  (1997): McGuiness M+, *J Am Acad Dermatol* 37, 298
  (1986): Gouet D+, *J Rheumatol* 13, 446
Necrosis
Papulo-nodular lesions
  (1992): Shelley WB+, *Cutis* 50, 87 (observation)
Photosensitivity
Pityriasis rubra pilaris
Pruritus (1–5%)
Psoriasis
  (2002): Yilmaz MB+, *Angiology* 53(6), 737
  (1990): Wakefield PE+, *Arch Dermatol* 126, 968 (exacerbation)
  (1990): Wolf R, *Dermatologica* 181, 51
  (1988): Gold MH+, *J Am Acad Dermatol* 19, 837
  (1988): Heng MCY+, *Int J Dermatol* 27, 619
  (1986): Abel EA+, *J Am Acad Dermatol* 15, 1007
  (1984): Gawkrodger DJ+, *Clin Exp Dermatol* 9, 92
Purpura
Rash (sic)
  (1987): Bolzano K+, *J Cardiovasc Pharmacol* 9 (Suppl 3), S43
Raynaud's phenomenon
  (1987): Naeyaert JM+, *Br J Dermatol* 117, 371
Toxic epidermal necrolysis
Urticaria
  (1989): Wolf R+, *Cutis* 43, 231
  (1988): Howard PJ+, *Scott Med J* 33, 344
Vasculitis
  (1989): Wolf R+, *Cutis* 43, 231
Vitiligo
Xerosis

Mucosal/ENT
Oral lichenoid eruption
  (1990): Lamey PJ+, *Oral Surg Oral Med Oral Pathol* 70, 184

Hair
Hair – alopecia
  (1991): Shelley WB+, *Cutis* 48, 368 (observation)

Nails
Nails – dystrophy
Nails – pigmentation
Nails – splinter hemorrhages
  (1987): Naeyaert JM+, *Br J Dermatol* 117, 371

Eyes
Oculo-mucocutaneous syndrome
  (1982): Cocco G+, *Curr Ther Res* 31, 362

Other
Anaphylactoid reactions/Anaphylaxis
  (1988): Howard PJ+, *Scott Med J* 33, 344
Death
  (2001): Briggs GG+, *Ann Pharmacother* 35(7), 859
Hypotension
  (2000): Joye F, *Presse Med* 29(18), 1027
Peyronie's disease
Pseudolymphoma
  (1990): Henderson CA+, *Clin Exp Dermatol* 15, 119
Stroke
  (2004): Carlberg B+, *Lancet* 364(9446), 1684

ATOMOXETINE

Trade name: Strattera (Lilly)
Indications: Attention deficit hyperactivity disorder (ADHD)
Category: Norepinephrine reuptake inhibitor
Half-life: 5 hours
Clinically important, potentially hazardous interactions with: albuterol, MAO inhibitors

Reactions

Skin
Allergic reactions (sic)
Angioedema
Dermatitis
Diaphoresis
  (2004): Simpson D+, *Drugs* 64(2), 205
Pruritus (>2%)
Rash (sic)
Urticaria

Mucosal/ENT
Xerostomia (>5%)
  (2006): Adler L+, *Ann Clin Psychiatry* 18(2), 107
  (2004): Christman AK+, *Pharmacotherapy* 24(8), 1020
  (2004): Simpson D+, *Drugs* 64(2), 205

Other
Asthenia
  (2004): Kelsey DK+, *Pediatrics* 114(1), e1
Depression (>2%)
Headache
Hepatotoxicity
  (2006): Lim JR I , *J Pediatr* 148(6), 831
Suicidal ideation
  (2007): Reith DM+, *CNS Drugs* 21(6), 463
  (2005): Wooltorton E, *CMAJ* 173(12), 1447
Tremor (>2%)
Vertigo (>5%)
  (2004): Christman AK+, *Pharmacotherapy* 24(8), 1020
  (2004): Simpson D+, *Drugs* 64(2), 205

ATORVASTATIN

Trade name: Lipitor (Pfizer)
Indications: Hypercholesterolemia
Category: HMG-CoA reductase inhibitor; Statin
Half-life: 14 hours
Clinically important, potentially hazardous interactions with: azithromycin, bosentan, ciprofibrate, clarithromycin, clopidogrel, cyclosporine, erythromycin, fosamprenavir, fusidic acid, gemfibrozil, imatinib, itraconazole, niacin, quinine, **red rice yeast**, telithromycin, verapamil

Reactions

Skin
Acne (<2%)
Allergic reactions (sic) (<2%)
Angioedema
  (2005): Hampson JP+, *Pharm World Sci* 27(4), 279 (0.1%)
Bullae
Dermatitis (<2%)
Dermatomyositis

  (2001): Noel B+, *Am J Med* 110, 670
Dermographism
  (2001): Adcock BB+, *J Am Board Fam Prac* 14, 148
Diaphoresis (<2%)
Eczema (<2%)
Edema (<2%)
Eosinophilic fasciitis
  (2006): DeGiovanni C+, *Clin Exp Dermatol* 31(1), 131
Erythema multiforme
Exanthems
Facial edema (<2%)
Lichenoid eruption
  (1998): Silver B, Deerfield, IL (from Internet) (observation)
Linear IgA dermatosis
  (2003): Avci O+, *J Am Acad Dermatol* 48(2), 299 (passim)
  (2001): König C+, *J Am Acad Dermatol* 44, 689
Lymphocytic infiltration
  (2001): Faivre M+, *Ann Dermatol Venereol* 128, 67
Petechiae (<2%)
Photosensitivity (<2%)
Pruritus (<2%)
  (2004): Gershovich OE+, *Pharmacotherapy* 24(1), 150
Rash (sic) (>3%)
  (2001): Coverman M, *The Schoch Letter* 51, 23 (with simvastatin)
Seborrhea (<2%)
Stevens–Johnson syndrome
Toxic epidermal necrolysis
  (1998): Pfeiffer CM+, *JAMA* 279, 1613
Ulcerations (<2%)
Urticaria (<2%)
  (2002): Anliker MD+, *Allergy* 57(4), 366
Xerosis (<2%)

Mucosal/ENT
Ageusia (<2%)
Cheilitis (<2%)
Dysgeusia (<2%)
Glossitis (<2%)
Oral ulceration (<2%)
Parosmia (<2%)
Stomatitis (<2%)

Hair
Hair – alopecia (<2%)
  (2002): Burrow W, Jackson, MS (from Internet) (observation on himself)
  (2002): Litt JZ, Beachwood, OH (personal case)
  (2002): Segal AS, *Am J Med* 113(2), 171
  (2001): Altman E, West Orange, NJ (from Internet) (observation)
  (1999): Oakley A, Hamilton, New Zealand (from Internet) (observation)
  (1997): Litt JZ, Beachwood, OH (personal case) (observation)

Eyes
Glaucoma
  (2000): Kirschbaum J, San Francisco, CA (from Internet) (observation)

Other
Death
  (2003): Perger L+, *J Hepatol* 39(6), 1095
Gynecomastia (<2%)
Headache
  (2005): Holmberg B+, *Scand J Urol Nephro* 39(6), 503
Hepatotoxicity
  (2006): Andrade RJ+, *Hepatology* 44(6), 1581
  (2006): de Castro ML+, *Gastroenterol Hepatol* 29(1), 21
Hypotension

(2005): Hampson JP+, *Pharm World Sci* 27(4), 279 (0.1%)
Myalgia/Myositis/Myopathy/Myotoxicity
  (2007): Weffald LA+, *Pharmacotherapy* 27(2), 309 (with ezetimibe)
  (2006): Ertas FS+, *Ophthal Plast Reconstr Surg* 22(3), 222
  (2006): Hermann M+, *Clin Pharmacol Ther* 79(6), 532
  (2006): Newman C+, *Am J Cardiol* 97(1), 61 (1%)
  (2005): Wilke RA+, *Pharmacogenet Genomics* 15(6), 415
  (2003): Guis S+, *Arthritis Rheum* 49(2), 237
  (2003): Litt JZ, Beachwood, OH (personal case) (observation)
  (2003): Olsson AG+, *Clin Ther* 25(1), 119 (2.2%)
  (2002): Leon Vazquez F+, *Aten Primaria* 30(3), 188
  (2002): Litt JZ, Beachwood, OH (personal observation)
  (2002): Patel DN+, *J Heart Lung Transplant* 21(2), 204
  (2002): Phillips PS+, *Ann Intern Med* 137(7), 581
  (2002): Sinzinger H, *Wien Klin Wochenschr* 114(21–22), 943
  (2002): Sinzinger H, *Wien Klin Wochenschr* 114(21), 943
  (2001): Litt JZ, Beachwood, OH (2 personal cases)
  (2001): Rehbein H, Jacksonville, FL (from Internet) (observation)
  (2001): Sorkin M, Denver, CO (from Internet) (observation)
  (2001): Wright W, Castro Valley, CA (from Internet) (2 observations)
  (1998): Malinowski JM, *Am J Health Syst Pharm* 55, 2253
Neurotoxicity
  (2004): Jacobs MB, *Ann Intern Med* 141(1), 77
  (2003): Silverberg C+, *Ann Intern Med* 139(9), 792
Paresthesias (<2%)
Rhabdomyolysis
  (2007): Jose J+, *Am J Health Syst Pharm* 64(7), 726
  (2006): Law M+, *Am J Cardiol* 97(8A), 52C
  (2006): Silva MA+, *Clin Ther* 28(1), 26
  (2006): Tufan A+, *Ann Pharmacother* 40(7-8), 1466 (with colchinine)
  (2005): Andrejak M+, *Therapie* 60(3), 299
  (2005): Kahri J+, *Eur J Clin Pharmacol* 60(12), 905
  (2004): Graham DJ+, *JAMA* 292(21), 2585 (low risk)
  (2003): Guis S+, *Arthritis Rheum* 49(2), 237
  (2003): Mah Ming JB+, *AIDS Patient Care STDS* 17(5), 207 (with clarithromycin, and lopinavir/ritonavir)
  (2003): Sipe BE+, *Ann Pharmacother* 37(6), 808 (with clarithromycin and esomeprazole)
  (2002): Castro JG+, *Am J Med* 112(6), 505 (with delavirdine)
  (2002): Lewin JJ+, *Ann Pharmacother* 36(10), 1546 (with diltiazem)
  (2002): Patel DN+, *J Heart Lung Transplant* 21(2), 204
  (2000): Davidson MH, *Curr Atheroscler Rep* 2(1), 14
  (2000): Wenisch C+, *Am J Med* 109(1), 78 (with fusidic acid)
  (1999): Bottorff M, *Atherosclerosis* 147(Suppl 1), S23
  (1999): Maltz HC+, *Ann Pharmacother* 33(11), 1176 (with cyclosporine)
  (1998): Duell PB+, *Am J Cardiol* 81(3), 368 (with gemfibrozil)
Tendinopathy/Tendon rupture
  (2001): Chazerain P+, *Joint Bone Spine* 68(5), 430

ATOVAQUONE

Trade names: Malarone (GSK); Mepron (GSK); Wellvone
Indications: *Pneumocystis carinii* infection
Category: Antimalarial; Antiprotozoal
Half-life: 2.2–2.9 days
Clinically important, potentially hazardous interactions with: rifampin

Reactions

Skin
Diaphoresis (10%)

Erythema multiforme
Exanthems
  (1993): Haile LG+, *Ann Pharmacother* 27, 1488
Pruritus (11%)
  (1996): Radloff PD+, *Lancet* 347, 1511
Rash (sic) (23%)
  (1993): Artymowicz RJ+, *Clin Pharm* 12, 563
Stevens–Johnson syndrome
  (2003): Emberger M+, *Clin Infect Dis* 37(1), e5 (with proguanil)
  (1999): Smith HR+, *Clin Exp Dermatol* 24(4), 249
Toxic epidermal necrolysis
  (1999): Smith HR+, *Clin Exp Dermatol* 24(4), 249

Mucosal/ENT
Dysgeusia (3%)
Oral candidiasis (1–10%)

Other
Headache

ATOVAQUONE/PROGUANIL

Trade name: Malarone (GSK)
Indications: Malaria prophylaxis and treatment
Category: Antimalarial
Half-life: 24 hours
Clinically important, potentially hazardous interactions with: indinavir, metoclopramide, rifabutin, rifampicin

Reactions

Skin
Angioedema
Erythema multiforme
Exanthems
  (1991): Eriksson B+, *Scand J Infect Dis* 23(4), 489
Photosensitivity
Pruritus
Rash (sic)
Stevens–Johnson syndrome
  (2003): Emberger M+, *Clin Infect Dis* 37(1), e5
Urticaria
  (1991): Eriksson B+, *Scand J Infect Dis* 23(4), 489

Mucosal/ENT
Oral ulceration
  (1986): Daniels AM, *Lancet* 1(8475), 269
  (1986): Davidson NM, *Lancet* 1(8477), 384

Hair
Hair – alopecia
  (1989): Hanson SN+, *Lancet* 1(8631), 225

Other
Abdominal pain
  (2003): Overbosch D, *J Travel Med* 10 Suppl 1, S16 (2–5%)
  (2003): Paul MA+, *Aviat Space Environ Med* 74(7), 738
  (2003): Petersen E, *J Travel Med* 10 Suppl 1, S13
  (1999): Looareesuwan S+, *Am J Trop Med Hyg* 60(4), 533
  (1999): Sukwa TY+, *Am J Trop Med Hyg* 60(4), 521
Cough
  (2003): Paul MA+, *Aviat Space Environ Med* 74(7), 738
  (2003): Petersen E, *J Travel Med* 10 Suppl 1, S13
  (1999): Looareesuwan S+, *Am J Trop Med Hyg* 60(4), 533
Headache
  (2003): Overbosch D, *J Travel Med* 10 Suppl 1, S16 (1–4%)
  (2003): Paul MA+, *Aviat Space Environ Med* 74(7), 738

(2003): Petersen E, *J Travel Med* 10 Suppl 1, S13
(1999): Sukwa TY+, *Am J Trop Med Hyg* 60(4), 521
Hepatotoxicity
(2005): Grieshaber M+, *J Travel Med* 12(5), 289
Vertigo
(2003): Overbosch D, *J Travel Med* 10 Suppl 1, S16 (1–3%)
(2003): Paul MA+, *Aviat Space Environ Med* 74(7), 738
(1997): Hoebe C+, *Eur J Clin Pharmacol* 52(4), 269

ATRACURIUM

Trade name: Tracrium (Abbott)
Indications: Neuromuscular blockade, endotracheal intubation
Category: Non-depolarizing neuromuscular blocker
Half-life: initial: 2 minutes; terminal: 20 minutes
Clinically important, potentially hazardous interactions with: amikacin, aminoglycosides, anesthetics, antibiotics, gentamicin, halothane, kanamycin, neomycin, piperacillin, streptomycin, tobramycin

Reactions

Skin
Adverse effects (sic)
(1999): Fisher MM, *Anaesth Intensive Care* 27(4), 369
(1988): Lynas AG+, *Anaesthesia* 43(10), 825
Allergic reactions (sic)
(1985): Aldrete JA, *Br J Anaesth* 57, 929
(1983): Mirakhur RK+, *Anaesthesia* 38, 818
Edema
Erythema (<1%)
Pruritus (<1%)
Rash (sic)
(1994): Doenicke A+, *Anesth Analg* 78(5), 967
(1988): Beemer GH+, *Br J Anaesth* 61(6), 680 (3%)
Urticaria (<1%)

Eyes
Periorbital edema
(1987): Cohen AY+, *Anesthesiology* 66(3), 431
(1986): Nelson CC+, *J Ocul Pharmacol* 2(4), 379

Other
Anaphylactoid reactions/Anaphylaxis
(2005): Lafforgue E+, *Ann Fr Anesth Reanim* 24(5), 551
(2003): Rieder J+, *Anesth Analg* 96(1), 301
(2002): Soetens F+, *Anaesth Intensive Care* 30(5), 699
(1999): Barthelet Y+, *Ann Fr Anesth Reanim* 18(8), 896
(1993): Kumar AA+, *Anesth Analg* 76(2), 423
(1993): Ortalli GL+, *Minerva Anestesiol* 59(3), 133
(1992): Yu FK+, *Ma Zui Xue Za Zhi* 30(2), 131
(1991): Roy CA+, *AANA J* 59(5), 399
(1987): Haraldsted VY+, *Ugeskr Laeger* 149(44), 2983
(1986): Tetzlaff JE+, *Can Anaesth Soc J* 33(5), 647
Hypotension
(1994): Watkins J, *Acta Anaesthesiol Scand Suppl* 102, 6
(1988): Beemer GH+, *Br J Anaesth* 61(6), 680 (3%)
(1988): Lynas AG+, *Anaesthesia* 43(10), 825
Injection-site reactions (sic)

ATROPINE SULFATE

Trade names: Atropine Martinet; Atropt; Belladenal; Bellergal-S; Butibel; Chibro-Atropine; Donnagel; Donnatal; Donnazyme; Isopto; Isopto Atropine; Lofene; Logen; Lomanate; Lomotil (Pfizer); Tropyn Z; Urised; Vitatropine
Indications: Salivation, sinus bradycardia, uveitis, peptic ulcer
Category: Muscarinic antagonist
Half-life: 2–3 hours
Clinically important, potentially hazardous interactions with: anticholinergics

Note: Many of the above trade name drugs contain phenobarbital, scopolamine, hyoscyamine, hydrocodone, methenamine, etc.

Reactions

Skin
Adverse effects (sic)
(2002): Robenshtok E+, *Isr Med Assoc J* 4(7), 535
Allergic reactions (sic)
(2001): Decraene T+, *Contact Dermatitis* 45(5), 309
(1997): Moyano P+, *Rev Esp Anestesiol Reanim* (Spanish) 44, 290
Bullous dermatitis
Dermatitis
(2003): de Misa RF+, *Clin Exp Dermatol* 28(1), 97
(1988): Gutierrez-Ortega MC+, *Med Cutan Ibero Lat Am* (Spanish) 16, 430
(1985): Yoshikama K+, *Contact Dermatitis* 12, 56
Diaphoresis
Eccrine hidrocystomas
(1992): Masri-Fridling GD+, *J Am Acad Dermatol* 26, 780
Erythema (sheet-like)
Erythema multiforme (<1%)
Exanthems
Exfoliative dermatitis
Fixed eruption
(1998): Mahboob A+, *Int J Dermatol* 37(11), 833
Photosensitivity (1–10%)
Pruritus
Rash (sic) (<1%)
Stevens–Johnson syndrome
Urticaria
(1986): Bigby M+, *JAMA* 256, 3358
Xerosis

Mucosal/ENT
Dry mucous membranes
(1992): Amitai Y+, *JAMA* 268, 630
Dysgeusia
Xerostomia (>10%)
(1992): Kramer BA+, *Am J Psychiatry* 149(9), 1258
(1983): Rupreht J+, *Acta Anaesthesiol Belg* 34(4), 301

Eyes
Eyelid edema
Mydriasis
(2006): Schmidt J+, *Paediatr Anaesth* 16(3), 362
Ocular allergy (sic)
(2003): Ventura MT+, *Immunopharmacol Immunotoxicol* 25(4), 529
Periocular dermatitis
(2003): de Misa RF+, *Clin Exp Dermatol* 28(1), 97
(1987): van der Willigen AH+, *Contact Dermatitis* 17(1), 56
(1982): Gallasch G+, *Klin Monatsbl Augenheilkd* (German) 181, 96
Visual hallucinations

(2006): Jimenez-Jimenez FJ+, *Rev Neurol* 43(10), 603 (with scopolamine & phenylephrine)

Other
Anaphylactoid reactions/Anaphylaxis
  (2007): Coelho D+, *Eur J Anaesthesiol* 24(3), 289
  (2002): Robenshtok E+, *Isr Med Assoc J* 4(7), 535 (from eyedrops)
Anhidrosis
Headache
Injection-site irritation (>10%)
Tremor

AURANOFIN

(See GOLD and GOLD COMPOUNDS)

AUROTHIOGLUCOSE

(See GOLD and GOLD COMPOUNDS)

AZACITIDINE

Trade name: Vidaza (Pharmion)
Indications: Myelodysplastic syndromes, refractory anemia
Category: Antineoplastic; Cytosine analog
Half-life: 48 ± 8 min
Clinically important, potentially hazardous interactions with: None

Reactions

Skin
Adverse effects (sic)
  (1991): Goldsmith SM+, *Arch Dermatol* 127(12), 1847
Cellulitis (8%)
Diaphoresis (10.5%)
Edema (14.5%)
Erythema (17%)
Hematomas (9%)
Herpes simplex (9%)
Induration (<5%)
Nodular eruption (5%)
Pallor (15.5%)
Peripheral edema (19%)
Petechiae
  (2005): Kaminskas E+, *Oncologist* 10(3), 176
Pruritus (12%)
Purpura
Pyoderma gangrenosum (<5%)
Rash (sic) (14%)
  (1981): Saiki JH+, *Cancer* 47(7), 1739
Urticaria (6%)
Xerosis (5%)

Mucosal/ENT
Dysphagia (5%)
Gingival bleeding (9.5%)
Stomatitis (8%)
Tongue ulceration (5%)

Other
Abdominal pain (15.5%)

Anaphylactoid reactions/Anaphylaxis (<5%)
Asthenia (36%)
Chest pain (16%)
  (1997): Yogelzang NJ+, *Cancer* 79(11), 2237
  (1993): Creagan ET+, *Am J Clin Oncol* 16(3), 243
Coma
  (1981): Saiki JH+, *Cancer* 47(7), 1739
Cough (29.5%)
Depression (12%)
Fever
  (2005): Kaminskas E+, *Oncologist* 10(3), 176
Headache (22%)
  (2005): Kaminskas E+, *Oncologist* 10(3), 176
Hypersensitivity (<5%)
Hypotension
  (1981): Saiki JH+, *Cancer* 47(7), 1739
Injection-site edema (5%)
Injection-site erythema (35%)
Injection-site infection
Injection-site pain (23%)
Injection-site pigmentation (5%)
Injection-site pruritus (7%)
Injection-site purpura (14%)
Injection-site reactions (sic)
  (2005): Kaminskas E+, *Clin Cancer Res* 11(10), 3604
  (2005): Kaminskas E+, *Oncologist* 10(3), 176
  (2002): Gryn J+, *Leuk Res* 26(10), 893
Myalgia/Myositis/Myopathy/Myotoxicity (16%)
  (1981): Saiki JH+, *Cancer* 47(7), 1739
Nephrotoxicity
  (2001): Kintzel PE, *Drug Saf* 24(1), 19
Neurotoxicity
  (1985): Weisman SJ+, *Am J Pediatr Hematol Oncol* 7(1), 86
Pain (11%)
Phlebitis
  (1983): Gaynon PS+, *Oncology* 40(3), 192
Rhabdomyolysis
Seizures (<5%)
Upper respiratory infection (13%)
Vertigo (19%)
  (2005): Kaminskas E+, *Oncologist* 10(3), 176

AZATADINE

Trade names: Idulamine; Idulian; Lergocil; Nalomet; Optimine (Schering); Trinalin (Schering); Verben; Zadine
Indications: Allergic rhinitis, urticaria
Category: Histamine H1 receptor antagonist
Half-life: 9 hours
Clinically important, potentially hazardous interactions with: barbiturates, chloral hydrate, paraldehyde, phenylthiazines, zolpidem

Reactions

Skin
Angioedema (<1%)
Diaphoresis
Edema (<1%)
Exanthems
Photosensitivity (<1%)
Purpura
Rash (sic) (<1%)
Urticaria

Vasculitis
 (2005): Appelman M+, *Dermatology* 210, 366

Mucosal/ENT

Tinnitus
Xerostomia (1–10%)
 (1990): Small P+, *Ann Allergy* 64, 129

Other

Myalgia/Myositis/Myopathy/Myotoxicity (<1%)
Paresthesias (<1%)

AZATHIOPRINE

Trade names: Azamedac; Azamune; Azasan; Azatrilem; Imuprin; Imuran (Prometheus); Imurek; Imurel; Thioprine
Indications: Lupus nephritis, psoriatic arthritis, rheumatoid arthritis, autoimmune diseases, kidney transplant patients
Category: Antimetabolite; Disease-modifying antirheumatic; Purine anaolog
Half-life: 12 minutes
Clinically important, potentially hazardous interactions with: allopurinol, chlorambucil, cyclophosphamide, cyclosporine, **hemophilus B vaccine**, imidapril, mycophenolate, olsalazine, **vaccines**, warfarin

Reactions

Skin

Acanthosis nigricans
 (1980): L'Eplattenier JL+, *Schweiz Med Wochenschr* (German) 110, 1307 (0.5%)
Acne
 (1983): Schmoeckel C+, *Hautarzt* (German) 34, 413
Acute febrile neutrophilic dermatosis (Sweet's syndrome)
 (2007): Ammar D+, *Ann Dermatol Venereol* 134(2), 151
 (2004): Paoluzi OA+, *Dig Liver Dis* 36(5), 361
Acute generalized exanthematous pustulosis (AGEP)
 (2007): Elston GE+, *Clin Exp Dermatol* 32(1), 52
Allergic granulomatous angiitis (Churg–Strauss syndrome)
 (1998): Dietz A+, *Laryngorhinootologie* 77(2), 111
Allergic reactions (sic)
 (1996): Parnham AP+, *Lancet* 348, 542
Angioedema
 (1988): Saway PA+, *Am J Med* 84, 960 (passim)
Basal cell carcinoma
 (2001): Otley CC+, *Arch Dermatol* 137, 459
Carcinoma
 (2001): Austin AS+, *Eur J Gastroenterol Hepatol* 13, 193
 (1992): Taylor AE+, *Acta Derm Venereol* 72(2), 115
Cicatricial pemphigoid
 (2000): Burgess MJA+, *Arch Dermatol* 136, 1274
Dermatitis
 (2006): Patel AA+, *J Am Acad Dermatol* 55(3), 369
 (2001): Lauerma AI+, *Contact Dermatitis* 44, 129
 (1996): Soni BP+, *Am J Contact Dermat* 7, 116
 (1992): Burden AD+, *Contact Dermatitis* 27, 329
Erythema
 (2004): Mori H+, *J Dermatol* 31(9), 731
Erythema gyratum repens
 (2002): Gunther R+, *Med Klin* 97(7), 414
 (2002): von Rainer Gunther ZB+, *Med Klin* 97(12), 759
Erythema multiforme
 (1995): Knowles SR+, *Clin Exp Dermatol* 20, 353 (passim)
 (1988): Saway PA+, *Am J Med* 84, 960 (passim)
Erythema nodosum

 (2007): de Fonclare AL+, *Arch Dermatol* 143(6), 744
 (1995): Knowles SR+, *Clin Exp Dermatol* 20, 353 (passim)
 (1988): Saway PA+, *Am J Med* 84, 960 (passim)
Exanthems
 (1995): Knowles SR+, *Clin Exp Dermatol* 20, 353 (passim)
 (1990): Jeurissen ME+, *Ann Rheum Dis* 49, 25 (4%)
 (1988): Bergman SM+, *Ann Intern Med* 109, 83
 (1988): Saway PA+, *Am J Med* 84, 960
Exfoliative dermatitis
 (1997): Hermanns-Le T+, *Dermatology* 194, 175
Fixed eruption
 (1990): Black AK+, *Br J Dermatol* 123, 277 (observation)
Formication
 (1992): Shelley WB+, *Advanced Dermatologic Diagnosis* WB Saunders, 1042 (passim)
Fungal dermatitis
 (1980): L'Eplattenier JL+, *Schweiz Med Wochenschr* (German) 110, 1307 (42%)
Herpes simplex
 (1980): L'Eplattenier JL+, *Schweiz Med Wochenschr* (German) 110, 1307 (27%)
Herpes zoster
 (2006): Patel AA+, *J Am Acad Dermatol* 55(3), 369
 (2003): Lemyze M+, *Rev Mal Respir* 20(5), 773
 (2001): Vergara M+, *Gastroenterol Hepatol* 24, 47
 (1991): Callen JP+, *Arch Dermatol* 127, 515
 (1982): Speerstra F+, *Ann Rheum Dis* 41, Suppl 37
 (1980): L'Eplattenier JL+, *Schweiz Med Wochenschr* (German) 110, 1307 (27%)
Kaposi's sarcoma
 (2006): Patel AA+, *J Am Acad Dermatol* 55(3), 369
 (1997): Aebischer MC+, *Dermatology* 195, 91
 (1997): Halpern SM+, *Br J Dermatol* 137, 140
 (1997): Lesnoni-La-Parola I+, *Dermatology* 194, 229
 (1997): Vandercam B+, *Dermatology* 194, 180
 (1996): Ozen S+, *Nephrol Dial Transplant* 11, 1162
 (1991): Almog Y+, *Clin Exp Dermatol* 9, 285
 (1984): Luderschmidt C+, *Klin Wochenschr* (German) 62, 803
 (1982): Weiss VC+, *Arch Dermatol* 118, 183
 (1980): Iversen OH+, *Scand J Urol Nephrol* 14, 125
Keratoacanthoma
Lichenoid eruption
Lymphoma
 (2005): Hon C+, *Leuk Lymphoma* 46(2), 289
Neoplasms
 (2003): Li AC+, *Eur J Gastroenterol Hepatol* 15(2), 185
Nevi
 (2006): Bovenschen HJ+, *Br J Dermatol* 154(5), 880
Non-Hodgkin's lymphoma
 (2000): Lewis JD+, *Gastroenterology* 118, 1018
Pemphigus foliaceus
 (2000): Elston DM, *Cutis* 66(5), 332, 375
Peripheral edema
 (1996): Oakley A, Hamilton, New Zealand (from Internet) (observation)
Photosensitivity
Pigmentation (sun-exposed skin)
Porokeratosis
 (1997): Matsushita S+, *J Dermatol* 24, 110 (disseminated superficial actinic)
 (1988): Neumann RA+, *Br J Dermatol* 119, 375 (disseminated superficial actinic)
 (1987): Tatnall FM+, *J R Soc Med* 80, 180 (Mibelli)
Pruritus
 (2005): Appelman M+, *Dermatology* 210(4), 366
Purpura
Pyoderma gangrenosum
Rash (sic) (1–10%)

(2005): Bajaj JS+, *Am J Gastroenterol* 100(5), 1121
(2005): Heckmann JM+, *J Neurol Sci* 231(1-2), 71
(2004): Gearry RB+, *Pharmacogenetics* 14(11), 779
(1997): Lavaud F+, *Dig Dis Sci* 42, 823
(1990): Jeurissen ME+, *Ann Rheum Dis* 49, 25

Raynaud's phenomenon

Sarcoma
(1996): Csuka ME+, *Arch Intern Med* 156, 1573

Scabies
(2006): Patel AA+, *J Am Acad Dermatol* 55(3), 369
(1980): L'Eplattenier JL+, *Schweiz Med Wochenschr* (German) 110, 1307 (1%)

Scleroderma
(1993): Choy E+, *Br J Rheumatol* 32, 160

Squamous cell carcinoma
(2003): Li AC+, *Eur J Gastroenterol Hepatol* 15(2), 185
(2001): Otley CC+, *Arch Dermatol* 137, 459
(2001): Werth V, *Dermatology Times* 15
(1995): Bottomley WW+, *Br J Dermatol* 133, 460
(1993): Nachbar F+, *Acta Derm Venereol* 73, 217
(1992): McCain J, *Nurs Pract* 17, 13
(1988): Krickeberg H, *Z Hautkr* (German) 63, 773

Stevens–Johnson syndrome
(2004): Mori H+, *J Dermatol* 31(9), 731

Tinea
(1981): Burkhart CG+, *Cutis* 27(1), 56
(1980): L'Eplattenier JL+, *Schweiz Med Wochenschr* (German) 110, 1307 (3%)

Toxic epidermal necrolysis
(1990): Black AK+, *Br J Dermatol* 123, 277

Urticaria
(1995): Knowles SR+, *Clin Exp Dermatol* 20, 353 (passim)
(1990): Wijnands MJ+, *Scand J Rheumatol* 19, 167
(1988): Saway PA+, *Am J Med* 84, 960 (passim)

Vasculitis
(2005): Appelman M+, *Dermatology* 210(4), 366
(2003): Sinico RA+, *J Nephrol* 16(2), 272
(1995): Blanco R+, *Arthritis Rheum* 39, 1016
(1995): Knowles SR+, *Clin Exp Dermatol* 20, 353 (passim)
(1988): Bergman SM+, *Ann Intern Med* 109, 83

Verrucae
(2006): Patel AA+, *J Am Acad Dermatol* 55(3), 369
(1991): Callen JP+, *Arch Dermatol* 127, 515
(1980): L'Eplattenier JL+, *Schweiz Med Wochenschr* (German) 110, 1307 (21%)

Mucosal/ENT

Aphthous stomatitis (<1%)

Dysgeusia
(2007): Ellul P+, *Am J Gastroenterol* 102(3), 689

Oral ulceration
(2000): Madinier I+, *Ann Med Interne* (Paris) (French) 151, 248

Stomatitis
(1982): Bailin PL+, *Clin Rheum Dis* 8, 493 (passim)

Xerostomia

Hair

Hair – alopecia (<1%)
(2006): Patel AA+, *J Am Acad Dermatol* 55(3), 369
(1982): Bailin PL+, *Clin Rheum Dis* 8, 493 (passim)
(1980): L'Eplattenier JL+, *Schweiz Med Wochenschr* (German) 110, 1307 (27%)

Hair – curly
(1996): van der Pijl JW+, *Lancet* 348, 622 (with isotretinoin)

Nails

Nails – discoloration (red lunulae)
Nails – onychomycosis

(1980): L'Eplattenier JL+, *Schweiz Med Wochenschr* (German) 110, 1307 (1%)

Other

Anaphylactoid reactions/Anaphylaxis
(1993): Jones JJ+, *J Am Acad Dermatol* 29, 795

Asthenia
(2006): Patel AA+, *J Am Acad Dermatol* 55(3), 369

Chills (>10%)

Fever
(2006): Patel AA+, *J Am Acad Dermatol* 55(3), 369

Hepatotoxicity
(2007): Wise M+, *Dermatol Ther* 20(4), 206 (passim)
(2006): Patel AA+, *J Am Acad Dermatol* 55(3), 369
(2006): Seiderer J+, *Eur J Gastroenterol Hepatol* 18(5), 553
(2005): de Boer NK+, *Neth J Med* 63(11), 444
(2005): Eisenbach C+, *Immunopharmacol Immunotoxicol* 27(1), 77

Hypersensitivity (<1%)
(2007): Wise M+, *Dermatol Ther* 20(4), 206 (passim)
(2006): Bohannon-Grant J (from Internet) (observation)
(2006): Demirtas-Ertan+, *Neth J Med* 64(4), 124
(2006): Meggitt SJ+, *Lancet* 367(9513), 839
(2006): Mittal A, Udaipur (from Internet) (observation)
(2006): Patel AA+, *J Am Acad Dermatol* 55(3), 369
(2004): Mayo JM+, *Inflamm Bowel Dis* 10(5), 700
(2003): Sinico RA+, *J Nephrol* 16(2), 272
(2001): Corbett M+, *Intern Med J* 31(6), 366
(2001): Sofat N+, *Ann Rheum Dis* 60(7), 719
(2001): Werth V, *Dermatology Times* 15
(1999): Korelitz BI+, *J Clin Gastroenterol* 28, 341
(1998): Fields CL+, *South Med J* 91, 471
(1998): Garey KW+, *Ann Pharmacother* 32, 425
(1998): Schlienger RG+, *Epilepsia* 39, S3 (passim)
(1997): Caramaschi P+, *Lupus* 6, 616
(1997): Knowles S+, *Muscle Nerve* 20, 1467
(1996): Compton MR+, *Arch Dermatol* 132, 1254 (with rhabdomyolysis)
(1995): Knowles SR+, *Clin Exp Dermatol* 20, 353
(1982): Mosbech H+, *Ugeskr Laeger* (Danish) 144, 2424

Infections
(2003): Bernal I+, *Gastroenterol Hepatol* 26(1), 19

Lymphoproliferative disease
(1987): Phillips T+, *Clin Exp Dermatol* 12, 444
(1987): Pitt PI+, *J R Soc Med* 80, 428
(1982): Ulreich A+, *Z Rheumatol* (German) 41, 73

Myalgia/Myositis/Myopathy/Myotoxicity (<1%)

Nephrotoxicity
(2006): Bir K+, *J Rheumatol* 33(1), 185

Rhabdomyolysis
(1996): Compton MR+, *Arch Dermatol* 132, 1254

Serum sickness

Tumors
(1986): Gupta AK+, *Arch Dermatol* 122, 1288 (5.3%) (malignant)
(1982): Bailin PL+, *Clin Rheum Dis* 8, 493 (passim)
(1980): L'Eplattenier JL+, *Schweiz Med Wochenschr* (German) 110, 1307 (2.9%) (benign) (4.3%) (malignant)

AZELASTINE

Trade names: Allergodil; Astelin (MedPointe); Azeptin; Optivar (MedPointe)
Indications: Allergic rhinitis
Category: Histamine H1 receptor antagonist
Half-life: 22 hours
Clinically important, potentially hazardous interactions with: barbiturates, chloral hydrate, paraldehyde, phenothiazines, zolpidem

Reactions

Skin
Allergic reactions (sic) (<2%)
Dermatitis (<2%)
Eczema (<2%)
Exanthems
  (1989): McTavish D+, *Drugs* 38, 19
Facial edema
Folliculitis (<2%)
Furunculosis (<2%)
Herpes simplex (<2%)
Pruritus
Rash (sic)

Mucosal/ENT
Ageusia (<2%)
Aphthous stomatitis (<2%)
Dysgeusia (bitter taste)
  (2001): Banov CH+, *Ann Allergy Asthma Immunol* 86(1), 28
  (2001): Camarasa JM+, *Skin Pharmacol Appl Skin Physiol* 14(2), 77
  (1997): Lenhard G+, *Curr Med Res Opin* 14(1), 21 (14%)
  (1993): Davies RJ+, *Rhinology* 31, 159
  (1990): Tinkelman DG+, *Am Rev Respir Dis* 141, 569 (30–52%)
  (1988): Weiler JM+, *J Allergy Clin Immunology* 82, 801 (19.7%)
Glossitis (<2%)
Oral mucosal eruption
  (1989): McTavish D+, *Drugs* 38, 19
Stomatitis (ulcerative) (<2%)
Xerostomia
  (1990): Tinkelman DG+, *Am Rev Respir Dis* 141, 569 (4–6%)
  (1989): McTavish D+, *Drugs* 38, 19

Other
Headache
Myalgia/Myositis/Myopathy/Myotoxicity (1.5%)

AZITHROMYCIN

Trade names: Azenil; Azitrocin; Azitromax; Zeto; Zithromax (Pfizer); Zitromax
Indications: Infections of the upper and lower respiratory tract, skin infections, sexually transmitted diseases
Category: Antibiotic, macrolide
Half-life: 68 hours
Clinically important, potentially hazardous interactions with: astemizole, atorvastatin, cyclosporine, fluvastatin, lovastatin, pimozide, pravastatin, rifabutin, simvastatin, warfarin

Reactions

Skin
Allergic granulomatous angiitis (Churg–Strauss syndrome)

  (1998): Dietz A+, *Laryngorhinootologie* (German) 77, 111
  (1997): Kranke B+, *Lancet* 350, 1551
Allergic reactions (sic) (<1%)
  (1998): Salit IE+, *Infect Med* 15, 773 (0.4%)
Angioedema (<1%)
Dermatitis
  (2007): Milkovic-Kraus S+, *Contact Dermatitis* 56(2), 99 (contact)
  (2001): Milkovic-Kraus S+, *Contact Dermatitis* 45(3), 184
Diaper rash
  (1997): Arguedas A+, *Infections in Medicine* October, 807
Edema
Erythema
  (2003): Taylor WR+, *Antimicrob Agents Chemother* 47(7), 2199
  (1991): Felstead SJ+, *J Int Med Res* 19, 363
Erythema multiforme
Exanthems
  (2002): Dakdouki GK+, *Scand J Infect Dis* 34(12), 939
  (2000): Nakayama I, *Jpn J Antibiot* 53 Suppl B, 82 (1 case)
  (2000): Schissel DJ+, *Cutis* 65, 123 (in a patient with infectious mononucleosis)
Facial edema
Fixed eruption
  (1999): Smith KC, Niagara Falls, Ontario (from Internet) (observation)
Jarisch–Herxheimer reaction
  (2003): Taylor WR+, *Antimicrob Agents Chemother* 47(7), 2199
Photosensitivity (1%)
Pruritus
  (2003): Taylor WR+, *Antimicrob Agents Chemother* 47(7), 2199
  (2000): Schissel DJ+, *Cutis* 65, 123 (in a patient with infectious mononucleosis)
Pustules
  (1994): Trevis P+, *Clin Exp Dermatol* 19, 280
Rash (sic) (<1%)
  (2002): Dakdouki GK+, *Scand J Infect Dis* 34(12), 939
  (1991): Felstead SJ+, *J Int Med Res* 19, 363
  (1991): Hopkins S, *Am J Med* 91, 36s
Side effects (sic)
  (1993): Hopkins S, *J Antimicrob Chemother* 31 (Suppl E), 111
Stevens–Johnson syndrome
  (2006): Brkljacic N+, *Acta Dermatovenerol Croat* 14(1), 40
  (2005): Schmutz JL+, *Ann Dermatol Venereol* 132(8–9 Pt 1), 728
  (2004): Aihara Y+, *Allergy* 59(1), 118
  (2001): Brett AS+, *South Med J* 94, 342
  (1998): Smith KC, Niagara Falls, Ontario (from Internet) (observation)
Toxic pustuloderma
  (1994): Trevisi P+, *Clin Exp Dermatol* 19, 280
Urticaria
  (2001): Thaler D, Monana, WI (from Internet) (observation) (2-year-old child 3 hours after initiation of drug)
  (1991): Hopkins S, *Am J Med* 91, 36s
Vasculitis
  (2003): Odemis E+, *J Rheumatol* 30(10), 2292

Mucosal/ENT
Dysgeusia
  (2007): Drew H+, *J N J Dent Assoc* 78(2), 24
Tinnitus
  (2003): Taylor WR+, *Antimicrob Agents Chemother* 47(7), 2199
Vaginitis (2%)
  (1991): Hopkins S, *Am J Med* 91, 36s

Eyes
Uveitis
  (2005): Biuk D+, *Coll Antropol* 29 suppl 1, 127

Other

Anaphylactoid reactions/Anaphylaxis
Fever
  (2003): Taylor WR+, *Antimicrob Agents Chemother* 47(7), 2199
Headache
Hepatotoxicity
  (2005): Baciewicz AM+, *Am J Med* 118(12), 1438
Hypersensitivity (0.6%)
  (2001): Cascaval RI+, *Am J Med* 110, 330
  (1998): Salit IE+, *Infect Med* 15, 773
Inappropriate secretion of antidiuretic hormone (SIADH)
  (1997): Cadle RM+, *Ann Pharmacother* 31(11), 1308
Injection-site erythema
  (1997): Luke DR+, *Ann Pharmacother* 31, 965
Injection-site pain
  (2001): Zimmerman T+, *Clin Drug Invest* 21, 527 (67%)
  (1997): Luke DR+, *Ann Pharmacother* 31, 965
Myalgia/Myositis/Myopathy/Myotoxicity
  (2007): Desnica B+, *Scand J Infect* 39(2), 186
Paresthesias
  (2003): Taylor WR+, *Antimicrob Agents Chemother* 47(7), 2199

AZTREONAM

Synonym: azthreonam
Trade names: Azactam (Bristol-Myers Squibb); Primbactam; Urobactam
Indications: Aerobic gram-negative bacillary infections
Category: Antibiotic, beta-lactam
Half-life: 1.4–2.2 hours

Reactions

Skin

Angioedema
  (1990): Soto Alvarez J+, *Lancet* 335, 1094
Diaphoresis
Erythema multiforme
  (1997): Epstein ME+, *J Am Acad Dermatol* 37, 149 (passim)
Exanthems
  (1990): Adkinson NF, *Am J Med* 88 (Suppl 3C), 12S (1.6%)
  (1990): Fekete T+, *Drug Intell Clin Pharm* 24, 438 (1–5%)
  (1988): Pazmiño P, *Am J Nephrol* 8, 68
  (1986): Brogden RN+, *Drugs* 18, 241 (1.8%)
Exfoliative dermatitis
  (1997): Epstein ME+, *J Am Acad Dermatol* 37, 149 (passim)
Petechiae
  (1997): Epstein ME+, *J Am Acad Dermatol* 37, 149 (passim)
Pruritus
  (1997): Epstein ME+, *J Am Acad Dermatol* 37, 149 (passim)
  (1990): Adkinson NF, *Am J Med* 88 (Suppl 3C), 12S
  (1986): Brogden RN+, *Drugs* 18, 241 (1.8%)
Purpura
  (1997): Epstein ME+, *J Am Acad Dermatol* 37, 149 (passim)
  (1990): Adkinson NF, *Am J Med* 88 (Suppl 3C), 12S (0.1%)
Rash (sic) (1–10%)
  (1985): Newman TJ+, *Rev Infect Dis* 7, S648
Toxic epidermal necrolysis
  (1997): Epstein ME+, *J Am Acad Dermatol* 37, 149 (passim)
  (1992): McDonald BJ+, *Ann Pharmacother* 26, 34
Urticaria
  (1997): Epstein ME+, *J Am Acad Dermatol* 37, 149 (passim)
  (1993): de la Fuente-Prieto R+, *Allergy* 48, 634
  (1991): Hantson P+, *BMJ* 302, 294
  (1990): Adkinson NF, *Am J Med* 88 (Suppl 3C), 12S (0.2%)

  (1990): Soto Alvarez J+, *Lancet* 335, 1094

Mucosal/ENT

Aphthous stomatitis (<1%)
Dysgeusia (<1%)
Oral ulceration (<1%)
Tinnitus
Tongue numb (<1%)
Vaginitis (<1%)
Vulvovaginal candidiasis

Other

Anaphylactoid reactions/Anaphylaxis (<1%)
Hypersensitivity
Injection-site pain (1–10%)
Injection-site phlebitis (1–10%)
Injection-site reactions (sic)
  (1985): Newman TJ+, *Rev Infect Dis* 7, S648
Myalgia/Myositis/Myopathy/Myotoxicity (<1%)
Paresthesias
Thrombophlebitis (1–10%)

BACAMPICILLIN

Synonym: carampicillin
Trade names: Albaxin; Ambacamp; Ambaxin; Bacacil; Bacampicine; Penglobe; Spectrobid
Indications: Respiratory tract infections, urinary tract infections, gonorrhea
Category: Antibiotic, penicillin
Half-life: 65 minutes
Clinically important, potentially hazardous interactions with: anticoagulants, cyclosporine, demeclocycline, doxycycline, imipenem/cilastatin, methotrexate, minocycline, oxytetracycline, tetracycline

Reactions

Skin

Acute generalized exanthematous pustulosis (AGEP)
  (1990): Guy C+, *Nouv Dermatol* (French) 9, 540
Angioedema
Dermatitis
  (1986): Stejskal VD+, *J Allergy Clin Immunol* 77, 411
Edema
  (2002): Liccardi G+, *Lancet* 359, 1700 (lips) ("deep kissing" husband who had taken bacampicillin)
Erythema multiforme
Exanthems
  (1989): Alanko K+, *Acta Derm Venereol* (Stockh) 69, 223
  (1988): Kohl PK+, *Aktuel Dermatol* 14, 104
  (1986): Pauwels R+, *J Int Med Res* 14, 110
Exfoliative dermatitis
Fixed eruption
  (1984): Chan HL, *Arch Dermatol* 120, 542
Hematomas
Jarisch–Herxheimer reaction
Pruritus
  (2002): Liccardi G+, *Lancet* 359, 1700 (lips) ("deep kissing" husband who had taken bacampicillin)
Pustules
  (1998): Isogai Z+, *J Dermatol* 25, 612
Rash (sic) (<1%)
Stevens–Johnson syndrome
Urticaria

Mucosal/ENT
Dysgeusia
Glossitis
Glossodynia
Oral candidiasis
Stomatitis
Stomatodynia
Tongue black
Vaginitis
Xerostomia

Other
Anaphylactoid reactions/Anaphylaxis
Hypersensitivity (<1%)
Injection-site pain
Serum sickness

BACITRACIN

Trade names: Cortisporin; Neosporin; Polysporin
Indications: Bacterial infections
Category: Antibiotic
Half-life: N/A
**Clinically important, potentially hazardous interactions
with:** clioquinol. N/A

Note: Bacitracin is supplied in many forms and vehicles:
Intramuscular; topical, ophthalmic, otic, aerosols, for irrigations.
Many Bacitracin ointments are combinations with Neomycin and
Polymyxin B.

Reactions

Skin
Allergic reactions (sic)
(2005): Schalock PC+, *Cutis* 76(2), 105
Dermatitis
(2005): Sowa J+, *Contact Dermatitis* 53(3), 175
(2004): Jacob SE+, *Dermatol Surg* 30(4), 521
(2004): Mowad CM, *Adv Dermatol* 20, 237
(2003): Sood A+, *Am J Contact* 14(1), 3
(1994): Zaki I+, *Contact Dermatitis* 31(2), 92
(1990): Grandinetti PJ+, *J Am Acad Dermatol* 23(4), 646
(1987): Held JL+, *J Am Acad Dermatol* 17(4), 592
(1987): Katz BE+, *J Am Acad Dermatol* 17(6), 1016
(1983): Fisher AA, *Cutis* 32(6), 510
Urticaria
(1991): Palungwachira P, *J Med Assoc Thai* 74(1), 43

Other
Anaphylactoid reactions/Anaphylaxis
(2007): Greenberg K+, *Am J Emerg Med* 25(1), 95
(2005): Freiler JF+, *Ann Allergy Asthma Immunol* 95(4), 389
(2003): Antevil JL+, *J Bone Joint Surg Am* 85(2), 339
(2000): Blas M+, *Anesth Analg* 91(4), 1027
(2000): Carver ED+, *Anesthesiology* 93(2), 578
(1999): Gall R+, *Anesthesiology* 91(5), 1545
(1998): Lin FL+, *J Allergy Clin Allergy Immunol* 101(1), 136
(1998): Saryan JA+, *Am J Emerg Med* 16(5), 512
(1997): Dyck ED+, *Allergy* 52(8), 870
(1995): Knowles SR+, *Int J Dermatol* 34(8), 572
(1994): Fox KA, *J Emerg Nurs* 20(4), 262
(1990): Eedy DJ+, *Postgrad Med J* 66(780), 858
(1990): Sprung J+, *Anesth Analg* 71(4), 430
(1987): Netland PA+, *Neurosurgery* 21(6), 927
(1986): Goh CL, *Australas J Dermatol* 27(3), 125
(1984): Schechter JF+, *Arch Dermatol* 120(7), 909

Injection-site pain
Nephrotoxicity (from intramuscular injections)

BACLOFEN

Trade names: Alpha-Baclofen; Baclofen (Watson); Baclon;
Baclosal; Baklofen; Clofen; Dom-Baclofen; Gen-Baclofen; Lebic;
Lioresal (Medtronic); Nu-Baclo; Pacifen; PMS-Baclofen; Spinax
Indications: Spasticity resulting from multiple sclerosis
Category: GABA receptor agonist; Skeletal muscle relaxant
Half-life: 2.5–4 hours
**Clinically important, potentially hazardous interactions
with:** alcohol

Reactions

Skin
Allergic granulomatous angiitis (Churg–Strauss syndrome)
(2006): Murphy PM+, *Anesth Analg* 102(3), 848
Dermatitis
Diaphoresis
Exanthems
(1983): Lynde CW+, *Ann Neurol* 13, 216
Facial edema
Peripheral edema
(1993): Albright AL+, *JAMA* 270, 2475
Pruritus
(2005): Ben Smail D+, *Arch Phys Med Rehabil* 86(3), 494
(withdrawal)
Rash (sic) (1–10%)
Side effects (sic) (1–2%)
Toxicity (sic)
(1994): Aisen ML+, *Arch Phys Med Rehabil* 75(1), 109
Urticaria

Mucosal/ENT
Dysgeusia (<1%)
Tinnitus
Xerostomia (<1%)

Other
Abdominal pain
(1997): Chen KS+, *Ann Pharmacother* 31(11), 1315
Asthenia
(2004): Dario A+, *Drug Saf* 27(11), 799
(2001): Kroczak M+, *Przegl Lek* 58(4), 364
Coma
(2006): Tunali Y+, *J Spinal Cord Med* 29(3), 237
(1997): Stayer C+, *Neurology* 49(6), 1591
Fever
(2002): Wu SS+, *Anesthesiology* 96(5), 1270
Headache
Hypertension
(2005): Sein Anand J+, *Przegl Lek* 62(6), 462 (33%)
(2004): Chodorowski Z+, *Przegl Lek* 61(4), 389
Hypotension
(2005): Sein Anand J+, *Przegl Lek* 62(6), 462 (4%)
(2004): Chodorowski Z+, *Przegl Lek* 2004 61(4), 389
Paresthesias (<1%)
Rhabdomyolysis
(2004): Coco TJ+, *Curr Opin Pediatr* 16(2), 206
Seizures
(2006): Solaro C+, *Neurology* 66(5), 784
(2004): Dario A+, *Drug Saf* 27(11), 799
(2003): Hansel DE+, *Pediatr Neurol* 29(3), 203

(1997): Chen KS+, *Ann Pharmacother* 31(11), 1315
(1994): Kofler M+, *Neurology* 44(1), 25
Thrombosis
   (2002): Murphy NA, *Arch Phys Med Rehabil* 83(9), 1311
Vertigo
   (2004): Dario A+, *Drug Saf* 27(11), 799

BALSALAZIDE

Trade name: Colazal (Salix)
Indications: Mild to moderately active ulcerative colitis
Category: Aminosalicylate
Half-life: N/A
**Clinically important, potentially hazardous interactions
with:** azathioprine or 6-mercaptopurine

Reactions

Skin
Pruritus
Rash (sic)

Mucosal/ENT
Xerostomia (1%)

Hair
Hair – alopecia

Other
Headache
Hypersensitivity
   (2001): Adhiyaman V+, *BMJ* 323(7311), 489
   (2000): Adhiyaman V+, *BMJ* 320, 613
Myalgia/Myositis/Myopathy/Myotoxicity (1%)

BASILIXIMAB

Trade name: Simulect (Novartis)
Indications: Prophylaxis of organ rejection in renal
transplantation
Category: Interleukin-2 receptor antagonist; Monoclonal
antibody
Half-life: 7.2 days
**Clinically important, potentially hazardous interactions
with:** cyclosporine, **hemophilus B vaccine**, mycophenolate

Reactions

Skin
Acne (>10%)
Cyst (3–10%)
Edema (generalized) (3–10%)
Facial edema (3–10%)
Genital edema (3–10%)
Hematomas (3–10%)
Herpes simplex (3–10%)
Herpes zoster
Peripheral edema (>10%)
Pruritus (3–10%)
   (2002): Leonard PA+, *Transplantation* 74(12), 1697
Rash (sic) (3–10%)
   (2002): Leonard PA+, *Transplantation* 74(12), 1697
Ulcerations (3–10%)

Urticaria
Vasculitis
Wound complications (sic) (>10%)

Mucosal/ENT
Gingival hyperplasia/hypertrophy (3–10%)
Stomatitis (3–10%)
Tongue edema
   (2002): Leonard PA+, *Transplantation* 74(12), 1697
Ulcerative stomatitis

Hair
Hair – hypertrichosis (3–10%)

Other
Anaphylactoid reactions/Anaphylaxis
   (2002): Leonard PA+, *Transplantation* 74(12), 1697
Candidiasis (>10%)
Depression (3–10%)
Headache
Hypersensitivity (17 cases)
Infections (3–10%)
Myalgia/Myositis/Myopathy/Myotoxicity (3–10%)
Pain
Paresthesias (3–10%)
Tremor (>10%)

BCG VACCINE

Synonym: Bacille Calmette-Guerin
Trade names: Mycobax (Sanofi-Aventis); TICE BCG (Organon)
Indications: immunization against tuberculosis
Category: Vaccine
Half-life: N/A
**Clinically important, potentially hazardous interactions
with: monosodium glutamate**, theophylline

Note: Reactions to intravesical Bacillus-Calmette-Guerin instillation
therapy, as used in cancer therapy, are not included in this profile

Reactions

Skin
Abscess
   (2006): Bolger T+, *Arch Dis Child* 91(7), 594
   (2005): Bellet JS+, *Curr Opin Infect* 18(2), 97
   (2005): Deeks SL+, *Pediatr Infect Dis J* 24(6), 538 (with
      immunodeficiency)
   (2005): Schumacher HH+, *Plast Reconstr Surg* 115(7), 2172
   (2003): *Prescrire Int* 12(68), 220
   (2002): Szczuka I, *Przegl Epidemiol* 56(2), 205
   (1994): Taraszkiewicz F+, *Przegl Epidemiol* 48(4), 505
   (1993): Bonnlander H+, *Am J Public Health* 83(4), 583
   (1990): Kulkarni AG+, *East Afr Med J* 67(12), 922
   (1990): Praveen KN+, *Pediatr Infect Dis J* 9(12), 890
   (1989): Murphy PM+, *Rev Infect Dis* 11(2), 335
   (1988): Colebunders RL+, *JAMA* 259(3), 352
   (1988): Simila S+, *Tubercle* 69(1), 67
   (1984): Singh G+, *Lancet* 2(8409), 979
   (1981): Di Piramo D+, *Riv Med Aeronaut Spaz* 46(3-4), 190
Acute febrile neutrophilic dermatosis (Sweet's syndrome)
   (2002): Carpentier O+, *Acta Derm Venereol* 82(3), 221
   (1986): Radeff B+, *Acta Derm Venereol* 66(4), 357
Allergic granulomatous angiitis (Churg–Strauss syndrome)
   (2006): Chiu YK+, *J Am Acad Dermatol* 55(2), S1 (with
      monosodium glutamate)
   (2006): Seishima M+, *Arch Dermatol* 142(2), 249

(2005): Bellet JS+, *Curr Opin Infect Dis* 18(2), 97
(2002): Sataynarayana S+, *J Assoc Physicians India* 50, 788
(2002): Tan HH+, *Ann Acad Med Singapore* 31(5), 663
(2001): Cohen M+, *Diagn Cytopathol* 25(2), 134
(2001): Gasior-Chrzan B, *Acta Derm Venereol* 81(4), 302
(2001): Houcke-Bruge C+, *Ann Dermatol Venereol* 128(4), 541
(2001): Kakurai M+, *Int J Dermatol* 40(9), 579
(1997): Emile JF+, *J Pathol* 181(1), 25
(1997): Kuniyuki S+, *J Am Acad Dermatol* 37(2), 303
(1997): Pye RJ, *Clin Exp Dermatol* 22(2), 109
(1990): Torres GM+, *AJR Am J Roentgenol* 155(1), 195
(1984): Hodsagi M+, *Orv Hetil* 125(44), 2685
(1980): Martynova MI+, *Pediatriia* 741(8), 67

Carcinoma
(1981): Kendrick MA+, *J Natl Cancer Inst* 66(3), 431

Dermatitis
(1998): Dalton SJ+, *J R Soc Med* 91(3), 133
(1983): Sheikh M, *Contact Dermatitis* 9(5), 426

Eczema
(1990): Sadeghi E+, *Tubercle* 71(2), 145

Erythema
(2006): Inoue T+, *J Dermatol* 33(4), 268
(1994): Lee SM+, *J Dermatol* 21(2), 106
(1980): Dogliotti M, *S Afr Med J* 57(9), 332

Erythroderma
(2005): Bellet JS+, *Curr Opin Infect Dis* 18(2), 97

Fixed eruption
(2005): Bellet JS+, *Curr Opin Infect Dis* 18(2), 97
(1988): Kanwar AJ+, *Pediatr Dermatol* 5(4), 289

Keloid
(2005): Bellet JS+, *Curr Opin Infect Dis* 18(2), 97
(2004): Sagic L, *Med Pregl* 57, 41
(2003): Boran C+, *Pediatr Dermatol* 20(5), 460
(1985): Nikolaeva NV, *Probl Tuberk BTsZ*(7), 58

Lichenoid eruption
(1996): Hwang SM+, *Clin Exp Dermatol* 21(5), 393

Lupus vulgaris
(2007): Attia E, *Eur J Dermatol* 17(6), 547
(2005): Bellet JS+, *Curr Opin Infect* 18(2), 97
(2004): Senturk N+, *Pediatr Dermatol* 21(6), 660
(2002): Tan HH+, *Ann Acad Med Singapore* 31(5), 663
(2001): Handjani F+, *Br J Dermatol* 144(2), 444
(2001): Kokcam I+, *Australas J Dermatol* 42(4), 275
(2001): Sasmaz R+, *J Dermatol* 28(12), 762
(1998): Selimoglu MA+, *Turk J Pediatr* 40(3), 467
(1997): Hashimoto T, *Kekkaku* 72(11), 629
(1996): Stewart EJ+, *Clin Exp Dermatol* 21(3), 232
(1996): Vittori F+, *Arch Pediatr* 3(5), 457
(1993): Misery L+, *Dermatology* 186(4), 274
(1991): Marrak H+, *Tunis Med* 69(11), 651
(1990): Rodrigues A+, *Med Cutan Ibero Lat Am* 18(4), 224
(1988): Kanwar AJ+, *Int J Dermatol* 27(7), 525
(1986): Raj B+, *Indian J Chest Dis Allied Sci* 28(2), 84
(1986): Ramirez O+, *Med Cutan Ibero Lat Am* 14(2), 87
(1983): Lassale C+, *Arch Fr Pediatr* 40(8), 643
(1982): Izumi AK+, *Arch Dermatol* 118(3), 171
(1982): Ndiaye B+, *Dakar Med* 27(2), 187

Lymphadenopathy
(2006): Bolger T+, *Arch Dis Child* 91(7), 594
(2005): Nazir Z+, *J Ayub Med Coll Abbottabad* 17(4), 16 (60 cases)
(2005): Teo SS+, *Vaccine* 23(20), 2676
(2004): Barouni AS+, *Braz J Med Biol Res* 37(5), 697
(2004): Nieminen T+, *Duodecim* 120(18), 2247
(2004): Sagic L, *Med Pregl* 57, 41
(2004): Vieira AP+, *Pediatr Dermatol* 21(6), 646
(2003): *Prescrire Int* 12(68), 220
(2003): Cerda de Palou E+, *Ned Tijdschr Geneeskd* 147(12), 569
(2003): Salinas Sanz JA+, *An Pediatr* (Barc) 58(5), 507

(2002): Aribas OK+, *Eur J Cardiothorac Surg* 21(2), 352
(2002): Goraya JS+, *Postgrad Med J* 78(920), 327
(2002): Sataynarayana S+, *J Assoc Physicians India* 50, 788
(2002): Singla A+, *Pediatr Infect Dis J* 21(5), 446
(2002): Szczuka I, *Przegl Epidemiol* 56(2), 205
(2002): Torres-Rojas JR+, *Dermatol Online J* 8(2), 6
(2002): Turnbull FM+, *Clin Infect Dis* 34(4), 447
(2000): Lee TT+, *Aust N Z J Surg* 70(12), 902
(2000): Raos M+, *Lijec Vjesn* 122(7-8), 180
(1999): Karnak I+, *J Pediatr Surg* 34(10), 1534
(1999): Levi DT+, *Probl Tuberk* T(4), 4
(1999): Lin CJ+, *J Bone Joint Surg Am* 81(9), 1305
(1999): Szczuka I, *Pneumonol Alergol Pol* 67(5-6), 208 (%)
(1998): Grange JM, *Commun Dis Public Health* 1(2), 84
(1998): Hofstadler G+, *AIDS Patient Care STDS* 12(9), 677
(1998): Kuyucu N+, *Pediatr Infect Dis J* 17(6), 524
(1998): Lowry PW+, *J Infect Dis* 178(1), 138
(1998): Yan JJ+, *J Pathol* 184(1), 96
(1997): Banac S+, *Acta Paediatr* 86(8), 899
(1997): Castro-Rodriguez JA+, *Int J Tuberc Lung Dis* 1(5), 417
(1997): Hashimoto T, *Kekkaku* 72(11), 629
(1997): Hengster P+, *World J Surg* 21(5), 520
(1997): Karnak I+, *Pediatr Surg Int* 12(2-3), 220
(1997): Nishi J+, *Pediatr Infect Dis J* 16(3), 332
(1996): Fujimoto T+, *Int J Oral Maxillofac Surg* 25(2), 145
(1996): Jakubikova J+, *Int J Pediatr Otorhinolaryngol* 37(1), 85
(1996): Marcelino F+, *Acta Med Port* 9(10-1), 397
(1996): Mori T+, *Tuber Lung Dis* 77(3), 269
(1996): Rositto A+, *Pediatr Dermatol* 13(6), 451
(1995): Kroger L+, *J Infect Dis* 172(2), 574
(1995): Meijer PJ, *Ned Tijdschr Geneeskd* 139(52), 2759
(1995): Vitkova E+, *Cent Eur J Public Health* 3(3), 138
(1995): Withagen MI+, *Ned Tijdschr Geneeskd* 139(40), 2047
(1994): Hooi LN+, *Med J Malaysia* 49(4), 327
(1994): Kroger L+, *Pediatr Infect Dis J* 13(2), 113
(1994): Kumar PV+, *Acta Cytol* 38(2), 165
(1994): Olsztajn N+, *Arch Pediatr* 1(1), 101
(1994): Taraszkiewicz F+, *Przegl Epidemiol* 48(4), 505
(1994): Walter S+, *Klin Padiatr* 206(6), 433
(1993): Arya SC, *Lancet* 341(8858), 1482
(1993): Bonnlander H+, *Am J Public Health* 83(4), 583
(1993): Gocmen A+, *Turk J Pediatr* 35(3), 215
(1993): Romanus V+, *Acta Paediatr* 82(12), 1043
(1992): Hengster P+, *Arch Dis Child* 67(7), 952
(1992): Hoppe JE+, *Infection* 20(2), 94
(1992): Krepela V+, *Cesk Pediatr* 47(3), 134
(1991): Allerberger F, *Am Rev Respir Dis* 144(2), 469
(1991): Baki A+, *Infection* 19(6), 414
(1991): Caglayan S+, *Acta Paediatr Jpn* 33(6), 699 (50 cases)
(1991): Hengster P+, *Lancet* 337(8750), 1168
(1991): Spiess H, *Offentl Gesundheitswes* 53(8-9), 631
(1991): Stogmann W, *Wien Med Wochenschr* 141(12), 265
(1991): Teulieres L+, *Vaccine* 9(7), 521
(1990): Aggarwal NP+, *Indian J Pediatr* 57(4), 585
(1990): Gaitnietse Ria+, *Probl Tuberk* 227(9), 32
(1990): Heydolph F+, *Z Erkr Atmungsorgane* 175(2), 90
(1990): Newfield L+, *Harefuah - Harefuah* 119(7-8), 199
(1990): Praveen KN+, *Pediatr Infect Dis J* 9(12), 890
(1989): Burdeny DA+, *Can Assoc Radiol J* 40(2), 92
(1988): Ray CS+, *Cent Afr J Med* 34(12), 281
(1987): Caglayan S+, *Am J Dis Child* 141(11), 1213
(1986): Hanna JN, *Med J Aust* 145(11-1), 662
(1986): Helmick CG+, *West Indian Med J* 35(1), 12
(1986): Ivanenko OM, *Probl Tuberk diag*(4), 27
(1986): Loos T, *Dev Biol Stand* 58, 351
(1986): Nyerges G+, *Orv Hetil* 127(43), 2607
(1986): Quast U+, *Dev Biol Stand* 58, 321
(1986): Stephan U+, *Klin Padiatr* 198(4), 295 (0.3%)
(1985): Abdullah MA+, *Ann Trop Paediatr* 5(2), 77
(1985): Kasatkin VM, *Probl Tuberk* (7), 71

(1985): Victoria MS+, *Pediatr Infect Dis* 4(3), 295
(1984): Easton PA+, *Tubercle* 65(3), 205
(1984): Katzir Z+, *Eur J Pediatr* 141(3), 165
(1984): Kobayashi Y+, *Clin Pediatr* (Phila) 23(10), 586
(1983): Close GG+, *Arch Dis Child* 58(11), 939
(1983): de Souza+, *Tubercle* 64(1), 23
(1982): Tam PK+, *Arch Dis Child* 57(12), 952
(1980): Bhandari B+, *Indian J Pediatr* 47(388), 367
(1980): Mackay A+, *Lancet* 2(8208), 1332

Papular lesions
(2006): Muto J+, *Clin Exp Dermatol* 31(4), 611
(1998): Karte K+, *Pediatr Dermatol* 15(1), 73
(1996): Rositto A+, *Pediatr Dermatol* 13(6), 451
(1987): Figueiredo A+, *Int J Dermatol* 26(5), 291
(1984): Lorette G+, *Ann Dermatol Venereol* 111(5), 493
(1982): Lubbe D, *Dermatol Monatsschr* 168(3), 186

Pityriasis rosea
(1989): Kaplan B+, *Isr J Med Sci* 25(10), 570

Psoriasis
(2004): Koca R+, *J Trop Pediatr* 50(3), 178

Sarcoidosis
(2005): Bellet JS+, *Curr Opin Infect Dis* 18(2), 97
(2003): Osborne GE+, *J Am Acad Dermatol* 48(5), S99
(1989): Greally JF+, *Sarcoidosis* 6(2), 156
(1988): McLelland J+, *Arch Dermatol* 124(4), 496

Scar
(2005): Roth A+, *Vaccine* 23(30), 3991
(2005): Zhivotovskii BG+, *Probl Tuberk Bolezn Legk* L(1), 32
(2004): Gross S+, *Clin Infect Dis* 38(10), 1495
(1999): Guerin N+, *Vaccine* 17(2), 105
(1993): Fang JW+, *Child Care Health Dev* 19(1), 37
(1993): Kwamanga D+, *East Afr Med J* 70(9), 568
(1990): Sivarajah N+, *Ceylon Med J* 35(2), 75 (86%)
(1982): Sanders R+, *Br Med J (Clin Res Ed)* 285(6356), 1679

Scrofuloderma
(2005): Atasoy M+, *Pediatr Dermatol* 22(2), 179
(2005): Kumaran MS+, *Lepr Rev* 76(2), 170
(2003): Corrales IF+, *Biomedica* 23(2), 202
(2002): Tan H+, *Pediatr Dermatol* 19(4), 323
(1999): Park YM+, *J Am Acad Dermatol* 41(2), 262

Telangiectasia
(1994): Lee SM+, *J Dermatol* 21(2), 106

Toxic epidermal necrolysis
(2004): Zdziarski P+, *Pol Merkur Lekarski* 17(100), 382

Ulcerations
(2005): Bellet JS+, *Curr Opin Infect Dis* 18(2), 97
(2004): Cuchet E+, *Ann Dermatol Venereol* 131(12), 1077
(2003): *Prescrire Int* 12(68), 220
(2002): Fritz TM+, *Hautarzt - Der* 53(12), 816
(2002): Szczuka I, *Przegl Epidemiol* 56(2), 205
(1983): de Souza+, *Tubercle* 64(1), 23

Urticaria
(1993): Misery L+, *Ann Dermatol Venereol* 120(3), 233

Vasculitis
(1993): Misery L+, *Dermatology* 186(4), 274
(1992): Watson DA, *Tuber Lung Dis* 73(2), 126

Mucosal/ENT

Mucocutaneous lymph node syndrome (Kawaski syndrom)
(2005): Bellet JS+, *Curr Opin Infect Dis* 18(2), 97
(1996): Edelman K+, *Duodecim* 112(8), 698

Eyes

Iritis
(1995): Missioux D+, *J Rheumatol* 22(10), 2010

Optic neuritis
(2005): Hegde V+, *Acta Paediatr* 94(5), 635
(1991): Yen MY+, *J Clin Neuroophthalmol* 11(4), 246

Uveitis
(2005): Hegde V+, *Acta Paediatr* 94(5), 635

(1999): Chevrel G+, *J Rheumatol* 26(4), 1011

Other

Anaphylactoid reactions/Anaphylaxis
(2003): *Prescrire Int* 12(68), 220
(1991): Rudin C+, *Lancet* 337(8737), 377
(1986): van Assendelft AH+, *Tubercle* 67(3), 233
(1983): Tshabalala RT, *Lancet* 1(8325), 653
(1982): Harper JR, *Lancet* 1(8268), 403

Death
(2006): Hesseling AC+, *Clin Infect Dis* 42(4), 548 (with immunodeficiency)
(2005): Deeks SL+, *Pediatr Infect Dis J* 24(6), 538 (with immunodeficiency)
(2004): Sagic L, *Med Pregl* 57, 41
(2000): Doffinger R+, *J Infect Dis* 181(1), 379
(1997): Banac S+, *Acta Paediatr* 86(8), 899
(1997): Emile JF+, *J Pathol* 181(1), 25
(1997): Hashimoto T, *Kekkaku* 72(11), 629
(1996): Casanova JL+, *Pediatrics* 98(4), 774
(1996): Jouanguy E+, *N Engl J Med* 335(26), 1956
(1986): Fasth A, *Lakartidningen* 83(11), 969
(1982): Trevenen CL+, *Can Med Assoc J* 127(6), 502
(1980): Perelman R+, *Sem Hop* 56(9-10), 480

Hepatotoxicity
(1991): Simma B+, *Eur J Pediatr* 150(6), 423

Hypersensitivity
(1998): Grange JM, *Commun Dis Public Health* 1(2), 84
(1998): Lowry PW+, *J Infect Dis* 178(1), 138

Infections
(2004): Zwolska Z+, *Pneumonol Alergol Pol* 72(11-1), 505

Injection-site abscess
(2002): Turnbull FM+, *Clin Infect Dis* 34(4), 447
(1998): Grange JM, *Commun Dis Public Health* 1(2), 84

Injection-site ulceration
(1997): Pankowska A+, *Pneumonol Alergol Pol* 65(11-1), 761
(1991): Spiess H, *Offentl Gesundheitswes* 53(8-9), 631

Myalgia/Myositis/Myopathy/Myotoxicity
(2006): Franco-Paredes+, *Am J Med* 119(6), 470

Neurotoxicity
(1999): Wilmshurst JM+, *Eur J Paediatr Neurol* 3(6), 277
(1982): Katznelson D+, *Postgrad Med J* 58(682), 496

Tumors
(1993): Wolff M+, *Monatsschr Kinderheilkd* 141(5), 409

BECLOMETHASONE

Trade names: Beconase AQ (GSK); Qvar (3M); Vanceril (Schering)
Indications: Allergic rhinitis, Asthma
Category: Corticosteroid, inhaled
Half-life: N/A
Clinically important, potentially hazardous interactions with: diuretics, estrogens, ketoconazole, **live vaccines**, oral contraceptives, phenytoin, rifampin, warfarin

Reactions

Skin

Acne
Angioedema
Atrophy
(1999): Konietzko N, *Dtsch Med Wochenschr* 124(28-2), 882
Bruising
(2001): Berend N+, *Respirology* 6(3), 237
(1999): Lipworth BJ, *Arch Intern Med* 159(9), 941

(1999): Malo JL+, *Eur Respir J* 13(5), 993
Dermatitis
(2000): Tani A+, *Contact Dermatitis* 43(6), 363
Eczema
(2003): Kilpio K+, *Allergy* 58(11), 1131
Edema
Pruritus
Purpura
Rash (sic)
Striae
Urticaria

Mucosal/ENT
Oral candidiasis
(2003): Fukushima C+, *Ann Allergy Asthma Immunol* 90(6), 646
(1998): Reed CE+, *J Allergy Clin Immunol* 101, 14
Perianal ulcerations
(2002): Adams BB+, *Cutis* 69, 67
Stomatitis
(1990): Yamaguchi M+, *Kyobu Shikkan Gakkai Zasshi* (Japanese) 28, 1410

Eyes
Cataract
(2002): Dendukuri N+, *Br J Clin Pharmacol* 54(1), 59
(2001): Jick SS+, *Epidemiology* 12(2), 229
(1999): Lipworth BJ, *Arch Intern Med* 159(9), 941
Glaucoma
(2002): Dendukuri N+, *Br J Clin Pharmacol* 54(1), 59
(1999): Lipworth BJ, *Arch Intern Med* 159(9), 941
(1999): Mitchell P+, *Ophthalmology* 106(12), 2301

Other
Adverse effects (sic)
(2003): Coghlan D+, *Paediatr Drugs* 5(10), 685 (rare)
(2003): Delacourt C+, *Respir Med* 97, S27
(2003): Kunkel G+, *Respiration* 70(4), 399
(2003): Lumry W+, *Allergy Asthma Proc* 24(3), 203
(2003): Shah SS+, *Cochrane Database Syst Rev* LD(2), CD00
(2001): Reichel W+, *Int J Clin Pract* 55(2), 100
(2001): Terzano C+, *Eur Rev Med Pharmacol Sci* 5(1), 17
Candidiasis
(2003): Randell TL+, *Paediatr Drugs* 5(7), 481 (rare)
(2002): Prenner BM+, *Eur Rev Med Pharmacol Sci* 6(4), 61
Cough
(2003): Dubus JC+, *Fundam Clin Pharmacol* 17(5), 627
Headache
(1999): Berger WE+, *Ann Allergy Asthma Immunol* 82(6), 535 (6%)
Hypersensitivity
(2002): Sommer S+, *Br J Dermatol* 147(2), 266
Myalgia/Myositis/Myopathy/Myotoxicity
Osteoporosis
(2001): Fujita K+, *J Bone Miner Res* 16(4), 782
(2001): Sivri A+, *Respirology* 6(2), 131
(2000): Muratore M+, *Int J Clin Pharmacol Res* 20(3-4), 61
(2000): Saravi FD+, *Rev Panam Salud Publica* 7(4), 211
(1999): Lipworth BJ, *Arch Intern Med* 159(9), 941
Side effects (sic)
(2004): May C+, *Monaldi Arch Chest Dis* 61(3), 162

BENACTYZINE

Trade name: Deprol
Indications: Depression, anxiety
Category: Muscarinic antagonist
Half-life: N/A

Note: Deprol is benactyzine and meprobamate

Note: Most of the adverse reactions are due to meprobamate (which see)

Reactions

Skin
Angioedema
Bullous dermatitis
Edema
Erythema multiforme
Exanthems
Exfoliative dermatitis
Fixed eruption
Petechiae
Pruritus
Urticaria
Mucosal/ENT
Stomatitis
Xerostomia
Eyes
Visual disturbances
(1982): Brown B+, *Aviat Space Environ Med* 53(11), 1123
Other
Anaphylactoid reactions/Anaphylaxis
Paresthesias

BENAZEPRIL

Trade names: Cibace; Cibacen; Cibacene; Lotensin (Novartis); Lotensin-HCT (Novartis); Lotrel (Novartis)
Indications: Hypertension
Category: Angiotensin-converting enzyme inhibitor
Half-life: 11–12 hours
Clinically important, potentially hazardous interactions with: amiloride, spironolactone, triamterene

Note: Lotrel is benazepril and amlodipine; Lotensin-HCT is benazepril and hydrochlorothiazide

Reactions

Skin
Angioedema (<1%)
(2007): Khan MU+, *Int J Cardiol* 118(2), e68 (visceral)
(2006): Shahzad G+, *Mt Sinai J Med* 73(8), 1123 (bowel) (with amlodipine)
(2001): Cohen EG+, *Ann Otol Rhinol Laryngol* 110(8), 701 (64 cases)
(1996): O'Mara NB+, *Pharmacotherapy* 16, 675
(1992): Kuhn M, *Clin Issues Crit Care Nurs* 3, 461
(1991): Anon, *Med Lett Drugs Ther* 33, 83
(1991): Balfour JA+, *Drugs* 42, 511
(1991): MacNab M+, *Clin Cardiol* 14, IV33
Dermatitis
Diaphoresis (<1%)

(1991): Morant J+ (eds), *Arzneimittel-Kompendium der Schweiz*
    Basel (German), Documed, 1990
Exanthems
    (1991): Morant J+ (eds), *Arzneimittel-Kompendium der Schweiz*
    Basel (German), Documed, 1990
Linear IgA dermatosis
    (2003): Femiano F+, *Oral Surg Oral Med Oral Pathol Oral Radiol*
    Endod 95(2), 169
Lupus erythematosus
    (2002): Boye T+, *World Congress Dermatol* Poster 0088
Pemphigus foliaceus
    (2000): Ong CS+, *Australas J Dermatol* 41(4), 242
Peripheral edema
    (1990): Mirvis DM+, *Am J Med Sci* 300, 354
Photosensitivity (<1%)
Pruritus
    (1991): Morant J+ (eds), *Arzneimittel-Kompendium der Schweiz*
    Basel (German), Documed, 1990
Rash (sic) (<1%)
    (1991): MacNab M+, *Clin Cardiol* 14, IV33
Stevens–Johnson syndrome
Urticaria
    (1991): Moser M+, *Clin Pharmacol Ther* 49, 322
Vasculitis

Mucosal/ENT
Ageusia
Dysgeusia
    (1991): MacNab M+, *Clin Cardiol* 14, IV33
Tinnitus

Other
Cough
    (2004): Fuchs M+, *HNO* 52(11), 998
    (2004): Lu J+, *Zhonghua Liu Xing Bing Xue Za Zhi* 25(5), 412 (%)
    (2004): Ye RJ+, *Zhonghua Jie He He Hu Xi Za Zhi* 27(9), 581
    (2003): Lu J+, *Zhonghua Liu Xing Bing Xue Za Zhi* 24(5), 401
    (2001): Adigun AQ+, *West Afr J Med* 20(1), 46–7
    (2001): Lee SC+, *Hypertension* 38(2), 166
    (2000): Cao W+, *Zhonghua Liu Xing Bing Xue Za Zhi* 21(3), 190
    (1998): Karnik ND+, *J Assoc Physicians India* 46(3), 283
Headache
Hypersensitivity
Myalgia/Myositis/Myopathy/Myotoxicity (<1%)
Paresthesias (<1%)

BENDAMUSTINE

Trade names: Ribomustin (Mundipharma); Treanda (Cephalon)
Indications: Chronic lymphatic leukemia
Category: Alkylating agent
Half-life: 40 minutes
**Clinically important, potentially hazardous interactions
with:** none

Reactions

Skin
Allergic reactions (sic)
    (2001): Heider A+, *Anticancer Drugs* 12(9), 725
    (2001): Kath R+, *J Cancer Res Clin Oncol* 127(1), 48
    (1998): Reck M+, *Pneumologie* 52(10), 570
Bullae
Exanthems
Herpes simplex
Pruritus (8%)

Rash (sic) (12%)

Mucosal/ENT
Nasopharyngitis
Stomatitis
Xerostomia
    (2007): Schoppmeyer K+, *Anticancer Drugs* 18(6), 697
    (2000): Schoffski P+, *Ann Oncol* 11(6), 729
    (2000): Schoffski P+, *J Cancer Res Clin Oncol* 126(1), 41

Hair
Hair – alopecia
    (1998): Reck M+, *Pneumologie* 52(10), 570

Other
Asthenia
    (2008): Friedberg JW+, *J Clin Oncol* 26(2), 204
    (2007): Rasschaert M+, *Anticancer Drugs* 18(5), 587
    (2000): Schoffski P+, *Ann Oncol* 11(6), 729
Cardiotoxicity
    (2007): Rasschaert M+, *Anticancer Drugs* 18(5), 587
    (2000): Schoffski P+, *J Cancer Res Clin Oncol* 126(1), 41
Chills
    (2000): Schoffski P+, *J Cancer Res Clin Oncol* 126(1), 41
Cough
    (2008): Friedberg JW+, *J Clin Oncol* 26(2), 204
Fever (24%)
    (2008): Friedberg JW+, *J Clin Oncol* 26(2), 204
    (2000): Schoffski P+, *Ann Oncol* 11(6), 729
    (2000): Schoffski P+, *J Cancer Res Clin Oncol* 126(1), 41
    (1998): Reck M+, *Pneumologie* 52(10), 570
Headache
Hypersensitivity
Hypertension
Infections (sic)
    (2007): Bottke D+, *Strahlenther Onkol* 183(3), 128
    (2007): Koster W+, *J Thorac Oncol* 2(4), 312
Somnolence
Weight loss (11%)

BENDROFLUMETHIAZIDE

Trade names: Aprinox; Berkozide; Centyl; Corzide (Monarch);
Naturetin (Bristol-Myers Squibb); Naturine; Neo-Naclex; Pluryle
Indications: Edema, diabetes insipidus, hypertension
Category: Diuretic, thiazide
Half-life: 8.5 hours
**Clinically important, potentially hazardous interactions
with:** digoxin, lithium

Note: Corzide is bendroflumethiazide and nadolol

Note: Bendroflumethiazide is a sulfonamide and can be absorbed
systemically. Sulfonamides can produce severe, possibly fatal,
reactions such as toxic epidermal necrolysis and Stevens–Johnson
syndrome

Note: Grinspan's syndrome: the triad of oral lichen planus, diabetes
mellitus, and hypertension

Reactions

Skin
Allergic reactions (sic)
Dermatitis
    (1997): Pereira F+, *Contact Dermatitis* 35, 303
Diaphoresis
Exanthems

(1991): Morant J+ (eds), *Arzneimittel-Kompendium der Schweiz* Basel (German), Documed, 1990
Exfoliative dermatitis
Facial edema
Grinspan's syndrome
(1990): Lamey PG+, *Oral Surg Oral Med Oral Pathol* 70, 184
Pemphigus
Photosensitivity
(1989): Diffey BL+, *Arch Dermatol* 125, 1355
Phototoxicity
(1997): Selvaag E, *Arzneimittelforschung* (German) 47, 97
(1997): Selvaag E+, *In Vivo* 11, 103
Pruritus
(1991): Morant J+ (eds), *Arzneimittel-Kompendium der Schweiz* Basel (German), Documed, 1990
Purpura
Rash (sic)
Urticaria
Vasculitis

Mucosal/ENT
Tinnitus
Xerostomia
(2004): Nederfors T+, *Arch Oral Biol* 49(7), 507

Hair
Hair – alopecia

Eyes
Dyschromatopsia

Other
Anaphylactoid reactions/Anaphylaxis
Gynecomastia
Paresthesias

BENZALKONIUM

Synonyms: parasterol; drapolene; germitol; gesminol; rodalon; ammonyx; benirol; enuclene
Trade names: Benza; Mycocide; Ony-Clear; Zephrex (Sanofi-Aventis)
Indications: Antisepsis, Preoperative skin preparation, Wound treatment, vaginal douch
Category: Antiseptic
Half-life: N/A
Clinically important, potentially hazardous interactions with: None

Reactions

Skin
Allergic reactions (sic)
(1994): Cox NH, *Contact Dermatitis* 31(1), 50
(1991): Klein GF+, *Contact Dermatitis* 25(4), 269
Dermatitis
(2006): Haj-Younes L+, *Contact Dermatitis* 54(1), 69
(2001): Wong DA+, *Australas J Dermatol* 42(1), 33
(2000): Kanerva L+, *Contact Dermatitis* 42(6), 357
(2000): Park HJ+, *Contact Dermatitis* 42(5), 306
(1999): Diaz-Ramon L+, *Contact Dermatitis* 41(1), 53
(1997): Chiambaretta F+, *J Fr Ophtalmol* 20(1), 8 (2 cases)
(1997): Krogsrud NE+, *Contact Dermatitis* 36(2), 112 (airborne)
(1996): Ortiz-Frutos FJ+, *Contact Dermatitis* 35(5), 302
(1996): Placucci F+, *Contact Dermatitis* 35(5), 306
(1993): Corazza M+, *Contact Dermatitis* 28(3), 195 (airborne)
(1993): Cusano F+, *Contact Dermatitis* 28(2), 127

(1993): Fuchs T+, *Hautarzt* 44(11), 699 (225 cases)
(1988): Trevisan G+, *G Ital Dermatol Venereol* 123(10), 513

Eyes
Ocular adverse effects (sic)
(1997): Chiambaretta F+, *J Fr Ophtalmol* 20(1), 8 (2 cases)
Ocular allergy (sic)
(2003): Ventura MT+, *Immunopharmacol Immunotoxicol* 25(4), 529

Other
Anaphylactoid reactions/Anaphylaxis
(2004): Kim SH+, *J Korean Med Sci* 19(2), 289
Hypersensitivity
(1997): Chiambaretta F+, *J Fr Ophtalmol* 20(1), 8 (2 cases)

BENZONATATE

Trade names: Beknol; Benzonal; Pebegal; Tesalon; Tessalon (Forest); Tusehli
Indications: Symptomatic relief of cough
Category: Antitussive
Half-life: Duration: 3–8 hours
Clinically important, potentially hazardous interactions with: None

Note: Benzonatate is related to tetracaine and other anesthetics of the para-aminobenzoic acid class

Reactions

Skin
Pruritus
Rash (sic) (1–10%)

Eyes
Ocular burning (1–10%)

Other
Chills
Death
(1998): Crouch BI+, *J Toxicol Clin Toxicol* 36(7), 713 (2 cases)
(1986): Cohan JA+, *Vet Hum Toxicol* 28(6), 543
Headache
Hypersensitivity
Seizures
(1998): Crouch BI+, *J Toxicol Clin* 36(7), 713
Tremor (overdose)

BENZPHETAMINE

Trade names: Didrex (Pfizer); Inapetyl
Indications: Adjunct to diet plan to reduce weight
Category: Amphetamine
Half-life: N/A
Clinically important, potentially hazardous interactions with: furazolidone, guanethidine, MAO inhibitors, SSRIs

Reactions

Skin
Allergic reactions (sic)
Diaphoresis
Erythema
Rash (sic)

Urticaria
Mucosal/ENT
Xerostomia
Hair
Hair – alopecia
Other
Depression (following withdrawal)
Gynecomastia
Headache
Hypersensitivity
Myalgia/Myositis/Myopathy/Myotoxicity
Tremor
Vertigo

BENZTHIAZIDE

Trade names: Aquatag; Diurin; Exna; Fovane; Hydrex;
Marazide; Proaqua; Regulon
Indications: Hypertension
Category: Diuretic, thiazide
Half-life: N/A
**Clinically important, potentially hazardous interactions
with:** digoxin, lithium

Note: Benzthiazide is a sulfonamide and can be absorbed
systemically. Sulfonamides can produce severe, possibly fatal,
reactions such as toxic epidermal necrolysis and Stevens–Johnson
syndrome

Reactions

Skin
Allergic reactions (sic) (<1%)
Photosensitivity
Purpura
Rash (sic)
Urticaria
Vasculitis
Mucosal/ENT
Dysgeusia
Eyes
Dyschromatopsia
Other
Paresthesias (<1%)

BENZTROPINE

Trade names: Akitan; Apo-Benzthioprine; Cogentin (Merck);
Cogentine; Cogentinol; Phatropine; PMS-Benztropine
Indications: Parkinsonism
Category: Anticholinergic; Muscarinic antagonist
Half-life: 6–48 hours
**Clinically important, potentially hazardous interactions
with:** anticholinergics, haloperidol

Reactions

Skin
Exanthems

Photosensitivity (1–10%)
Pruritus
Rash (sic) (<1%)
Toxicity (sic)
(1998): Gjerden P+, *Tidsskr Nor Laegeforen* 118(1), 53
Urticaria
Xerosis (>10%)
Mucosal/ENT
Dysgeusia
(2000): Heymann WR, *Cutis* 66, 25
Glossodynia
Stomatodynia
Tinnitus
Tongue black
(2000): Heymann WR, *Cutis* 66, 25
Xerostomia (>10%)
(2000): Heymann WR, *Cutis* 66, 25
(1991): Goff DC+, *J Clin Psychopharmacol* 11(2), 106
(1989): Gelenberg AJ+, *J Clin Psychopharmacol* 9, 180
Other
Death
(2001): Lynch MJ+, *Med Sci Law* 41(2), 155
Paresthesias
Rhabdomyolysis
(1984): Thase ME+, *J Clin Psychopharmacol* 4(1), 46 (with
loxapine)
Somnambulism
(1986): Glassman JN+, *J Clin Psychiatry* 47(10), 523 (along with
chlorpromazine, lithium, and triazolam)

BEPRIDIL

Trade names: Bapadin; Bepricol; Cordium; Cruor; Vascor
(Ortho-McNeil)
Indications: Angina pectoris
Category: Antiarrhythmic class IV; Calcium channel blocker
Half-life: 24 hours
**Clinically important, potentially hazardous interactions
with:** amisulpride, amprenavir, atazanavir, celiprolol,
ciprofloxacin, enoxacin, epirubicin, fosamprenavir, gatifloxacin,
lomefloxacin, **mistletoe**, moxifloxacin, norfloxacin, ofloxacin,
quinolones, ritonavir, sparfloxacin, tipranavir

Reactions

Skin
Diaphoresis (<2%)
Edema (1–10%)
Irritation (sic)
Peripheral edema (<1%)
Rash (sic) (<2%)
(1988): Sharma MK+, *Am J Cardiol* 61, 1210
Mucosal/ENT
Dysgeusia (<1%)
Tinnitus
Xerostomia (1–10%)
(1988): Hasegawa GR, *Clin Pharm* 7, 97
(1988): Krusell LR+, *Eur J Clin Pharmacol* 34, 221
Other
Asthenia
(1991): Singh BN, *Am J Cardiol* 68(4), 306
Headache

(1991): Singh BN, *Am J Cardiol* 68(4), 306
Myalgia/Myositis/Myopathy/Myotoxicity (<1%)
Paresthesias (2.5%)
Tremor (<9%)
Vertigo
(1991): Singh BN, *Am J Cardiol* 68(4), 306

BERACTANT

Trade name: Survanta (Ross)
Indications: Respiratory distress syndrome (RDS), Hyaline membrane disease
Category: Pulmonary surfactant
Half-life: N/A
Clinically important, potentially hazardous interactions with: N/A

Reactions

Other
Hypertension (<1%)
Hypotension (<1%)

BERGAMOT

Scientific name: *Citrus aurantium ssp bergamia*
Family: Rutaceae
Trade and other common names: Bergamottin; Earl Grey tea; Florida Water; Kananga Water; Neroli oil; Oil of bergamot
Category: Stimulant, mild
Purported indications and other uses: Headache, bronchitis, vitiligo, mycosis fungoides, psoriasis (in conjunction with UVA), insecticide, essential oil in perfumery, cosmetics, flavoring
Half-life: N/A

Note: two distinct species are known by the common name of bergamot. This profile does not refer to *Monarda didyma*

Reactions

Skin
Adverse effects (sic)
(2001): Kaddu S+, *J Am Acad Dermatol* 45(3), 458
Berloque dermatitis
(2002): Gruson LM+, *Arch Pediatr Adolesc Med* 156(11), 1091
(2002): Wang L+, *Cutis* 70(1), 29
Bullous dermatitis
(2001): Kaddu S+, *J Am Acad Dermatol* 45(3), 458
Burning
(1998): Cocks H+, *Burns* 24(1), 82
Dermatitis
(1984): Zacher KD+, *Derm Beruf Umwelt* 32(3), 95
Erythema
(2002): Gruson LM+, *Arch Pediatr Adolesc Med* 156(11), 1091
Photosensitivity
(2001): Kaddu S+, *J Am Acad Dermatol* 45(3), 458
(1993): Moysan A+, *Skin Pharmacol* 6(4), 282
(1990): Morliere P+, *J Photochem Photobiol B* 7(2), 199
Phototoxicity
(2005): Weisenseel P+, *MMW Fortschr Med* 147(51-52), 53
(2001): Kaddu S+, *J Am Acad Dermatol* 45(3), 458
(1993): Moysan A+, *Skin Pharmacol* 6(4), 282
(1990): Dubertret L+, *J Photochem Photobiol B* 7(2), 251

(1986): Maibach HI+, *Dermatol Clin* 4(2), 217
Pigmentation
(2002): Gruson LM+, *Arch Pediatr Adolesc Med* 156(11), 1091
Vesiculation
(2002): Gruson LM+, *Arch Pediatr Adolesc Med* 156(11), 1091
Other
Tumors
(1990): Young AR+, *J Photochem Photobiol B* 7(2), 231

BETA-CAROTENE

Trade names: B-Tene; Betavin; Carotaben; Lumitene; Max-Caro; Solatene (Merck); Solvin
Indications: Photosensitivity reactions
Category: Vitamin
Half-life: N/A
Clinically important, potentially hazardous interactions with: bexarotene

Reactions

Skin
Carotenemia (>10%)
(2000): Frieling UM+, *Arch Dermatol* 136, 179 (15.9%)
Dermatitis
(1992): Zürcher K and Krebs A, *Cutaneous Drug Reactions* Karger, 280
Purpura (<1%)

BETAMETHASONE

Trade names: Alphatrex (Savage); Beta-Val (Teva); Betaderm (Roaco); Betatrex (Savage); Celestone (Schering); Diprolene (Schering); Luxiq (Connetics); Uticort; Valisone
Indications: Arthralgia, dermatoses, rhinitis (many others)
Category: Corticosteroid
Half-life: N/A
Clinically important, potentially hazardous interactions with: clotrimazole, diuretics, **live vaccines**, phenobarbital, tetracycline, vecuronium

Reactions

Skin
Acne
Adverse effects
(2003): Lumry W+, *Allergy Asthma Proc* 24(3), 203
Allergic reactions
(2003): Miguelez A+, *Br J Dermatol* 149(4), 894
(2002): Brazzini B+, *Am J Clin Dermatol* 3(1), 47
Atrophy
(1985): Serup J+, *Dermatologica* 170(4), 189
Baboon syndrome
(2005): Armingaud P+, *Ann Dermatol Venereol* 132(8–9 Pt 1), 675
Burning
(1985): Huntley AC+, *Cutis* 35(5), 489
Dermatitis
(1995): Bircher AJ+, *Acta Derm Venereol* 75, 490
(1993): Hisa T+, *Contact Dermatitis* 28, 174
(1991): Dunkel FG+, *Contact Dermatitis* 25(2), 97 (2 cases)
(1989): Rivara G+, *Contact Dermatitis* 21(2), 83

Edema
Exanthems
 (1987): Maucher OM+, *Hautarzt* (German) 38, 577
Facial edema
 (2005): Kobayashi M+, *Nippon Jibiinkoka Gakkai Kaiho*
  108(10), 986
Pigmentation
Psoriasis
 (2004): Augey F+, *Eur J Dermatol* 14(6), 415 (pustular)
  (generalized)
Rash (sic)
 (1993): Hisa T+, *Contact Dermatitis* 28(3), 174
Stinging
 (1985): Huntley AC+, *Cutis* 35(5), 489
Telangiectasia
 (1985): Serup J+, *Dermatologica* 170(4), 189

Eyes
Conjunctival hyperemia
 (2005): Gungor IU+, *Ophthalmic Surg Lasers Imaging* 36(4), 348
Glaucoma
 (1995): Katsushima H, *Nippon Ganka Gakkai Zasshi* 99(2), 238

Other
Anaphylactoid reactions/Anaphylaxis
 (1995): Jacqz-Aigrain E+, *Arch Pediatr* (French) 2, 353
Infections

BETAXOLOL

Trade names: Betoptic [Ophthalmic] (Alcon); Betoptic S;
Betoptima; Kerlon; Kerlone (Pfizer); Optipres
Indications: Open-angle glaucoma, hypertension
Category: Adrenergic beta-receptor antagonist
Half-life: 14–22 hours
**Clinically important, potentially hazardous interactions
with:** clonidine, verapamil

Note: Cutaneous side effects of beta-receptor blockaders are
clinically polymorphous. They apparently appear after several months
of continuous therapy. Atypical psoriasiform, lichen planus-like, and
eczematous chronic rashes are mainly observed. (1983): Hödl St, *Z
Hautkr* 1:58, 17

Reactions

Skin
Acne
Allergic reactions (sic) (<2%)
Angioedema
Cold extremities
Dermatitis
 (2001): Holdiness MR, *Am J Contact Dermat* 12(4), 217
 (1993): O'Donnell BF+, *Contact Dermatitis* 28, 121
Diaphoresis (<2%)
Edema (1.3%)
Erythema (1–10%)
Exanthems
Exfoliative dermatitis
Facial edema
Lupus erythematosus
 (1997): Hardee JT+, *West J Med* 167, 106
Photosensitivity
Pigmentation (palms)
 (1997): Adams DR+, *Am J Contact Dermat* 8, 183
Pruritus (1–10%)

Psoriasis
Purpura
Rash (sic) (1.2%)
 (1989): Burris JF+, *Arch Intern Med* 149, 2437
Raynaud's phenomenon
Toxic epidermal necrolysis
Urticaria
Xerosis

Mucosal/ENT
Ageusia (<2%)
Dysgeusia (<2%)
Glossitis (following topical use)
Oral ulceration (<2%)
Sialorrhea (<2%)
Tinnitus
Xerostomia (<2%)

Hair
Hair – alopecia (following topical use) (<2%)
 (1990): Buckley MMT+, *Drugs* 40, 75
Hair – hypertrichosis (<2%)

Nails
Nails – pigmentation (bluish)

Other
Anaphylactoid reactions/Anaphylaxis
Depression
 (2001): Schweitzer I+, *Aust NZ J Psychiatry* 35(5), 569
Headache
Myalgia/Myositis/Myopathy/Myotoxicity (3.2%)
Paresthesias (1.9%)
Peyronie's disease (<2%)

BETHANECHOL

Trade names: Muscaran; Myocholine-Glenwood; Myotonine
Chloride; Urecholine (Odyssey); Urocarb
Indications: Nonobstructive urinary retention
Category: Muscarinic cholinergic agonist
Half-life: up to 6 hours
**Clinically important, potentially hazardous interactions
with:** galantamine, physostigmine

Reactions

Skin
Diaphoresis (1–10%)
Miliaria

Mucosal/ENT
Sialorrhea (<1%)
 (2005): Boyce HW+, *J Clin Gastroenterol* 39(2), 89 (passim)
 (2003): Kunwar AR+, *Ann Pharmacother* 37(9), 1343

Other
Headache

BEVACIZUMAB

Trade name: Avastin (Genentech)
Indications: Colon cancer
Category: Monoclonal antibody; Vascular endothelial growth factor antagonist
Half-life: N/A
Clinically important, potentially hazardous interactions with: None

Reactions

Skin
Exfoliative dermatitis
Pigmentation
Ulcerations
Xerosis

Mucosal/ENT
Dysgeusia
Oral ulceration
Stomatitis
  (2006): Ramaswamy B+, *Clin Cancer Res* 12(10), 3124 (7%) (with docetaxel)
  (2005): Motl S, *Am J Health Syst Pharm* 62(10), 1021
Xerostomia

Hair
Hair – alopecia

Nails
Nails – changes

Eyes
Epiphora
Visual hallucinations
  (2007): Meyer CH+, *Am J Ophthalmol* 143(1), 169
  (2007): Tan CS+, *Am J Ophthalmol* 144(2), 330

Other
Abdominal pain
Asthenia
  (2006): Ramaswamy B+, *Clin Cancer Res* 12(10), 3124 (15%) (with docetaxel)
  (2006): Sanborn RE+, *Expert Opin Drug Saf* 5(2), 289
Headache
  (2005): Motl S, *Am J Health Syst Pharm* 62(10), 1021
Hypertension
  (2006): Kramer I+, *Med Monatsschr Pharm* 29(7), 249
  (2006): Ramaswamy B+, *Clin Cancer Res* 12(10), 3124 (with docetaxel)
  (2006): Sanborn RE+, *Expert Opin Drug Saf* 5(2), 289
  (2005): Gordon MS+, *Oncology* 69 Suppl 3, 25
  (2005): Hurwitz H+, *Oncology* 69 Suppl 3, 17
  (2005): Miller KD+, *J Clin Oncol* 23(4), 792
  (2005): Rosiak J+, *Clin J Oncol Nurs* 9(4), 407
  (2004): Hadj Tahar A, *Issues Emerg Health Technol* (63), 1
  (2004): Ignoffo RJ, *Am J Health Syst Pharm* 61(21 Suppl 5), S21
  (2004): Sandler AB+, *Clin Cancer Res* 10(12 Pt 2), 4258s
  (2004): Zondor SD+, *Ann Pharmacother* 38(7–8), 1258
  (2003): Yang JC+, *N Engl J Med* 349(5), 427
Infections
  (2006): Ramaswamy B+, *Clin Cancer Res* 12(10), 3124 (4%) (with docetaxel)
  (2006): Sanborn RE+, *Expert Opin Drug Saf* 5(2), 289
Myalgia/Myositis/Myopathy/Myotoxicity
Neurotoxicity

  (2006): Ramaswamy B+, *Clin Cancer Res* 12(10), 3124 (7%) (with docetaxel)
  (2006): Sanborn RE+, *Expert Opin Drug Saf* 5(2), 289
Pain
Thrombosis
  (2006): Kramer I+, *Med Monatsschr Pharm* 29(7), 249
  (2006): Ramaswamy B+, *Clin Cancer Res* 12(10), 3124 (with docetaxel)
  (2006): Sanborn RE+, *Expert Opin Drug Saf* 5(2), 289
  (2005): Gordon MS+, *Oncology* 69 Suppl 3, 25
  (2005): Hurwitz H+, *Oncology* 69 Suppl 3, 17
  (2004): Sandler AB+, *Clin Cancer Res* 10(12 Pt 2), 4258s
  (2004): Zondor SD+, *Ann Pharmacother* 38(7–8), 1258
Upper respiratory infection
Vertigo

BEXAROTENE

Trade name: Targretin (Ligand)
Indications: Cutaneous T-cell lymphoma (CTCL), mycosis fungoides
Category: Retinoid
Half-life: 7 hours
Clinically important, potentially hazardous interactions with: acitretin, beta-carotene, dexamethasone, gemfibrozil, isotretinoin, tretinoin, vitamin A

Reactions

Skin
Acne (<10%)
Adverse effects (sic)
  (2001): Duvic M+, *Arch Dermatol* 137, 581 (13%)
Allergic granulomatous angiitis (Churg–Strauss syndrome)
  (2006): Ruiz-de-Casas A+, *Br J Dermatol* 154(2), 372
Bacterial infections (1.2–13.2%)
Burning
  (2004): Hanifin JM+, *Br J Dermatol* 150(3), 545 (15%)
Cellulitis
Cold extremities
  (2000): Bedikian AY+, *Oncol Rep* 7, 883
Dermatitis
  (2004): Hanifin JM+, *Br J Dermatol* 150(3), 545 (16%)
Erythema
  (2002): Breneman D+, *Arch Dermatol* 138, 352
  (2002): Liu HL+, *Arch Dermatol* 138, 398
Exanthems (<10%)
Exfoliative dermatitis (10–28%)
  (2001): Duvic M+, *Arch Dermatol* 137, 581 (7%)
Facial edema
  (2002): Breneman D+, *Arch Dermatol* 138, 325
Irritation
  (2004): Hanifin JM+, *Br J Dermatol* 150(3), 545 (29%)
Necrosis
  (2002): Breneman D+, *Arch Dermatol* 138, 325
Nodular eruption (<10%)
Peripheral edema (13.1%)
Photosensitivity
Pruritus (20–30%)
  (2004): Singh F+, *J Am Acad Dermatol* 51(4), 570
  (2002): Breneman D+, *Arch Dermatol* 138, 325
  (2001): Duvic M+, *Arch Dermatol* 137, 581 (20%)
  (2000): Duvic M, *Dermatology Times,* August, 3 (25%)
Pustules
Rash (sic) (16.7%)

(2001): Duvic M+, *Arch Dermatol* 137, 581
Stinging
  (2004): Hanifin JM+, *Br J Dermatol* 150(3), 545 (15%)
Ulcerations (<10%)
  (2002): Breneman D+, *Arch Dermatol* 138, 325
Vasculitis
  (2002): Breneman D+, *Arch Dermatol* 138, 325
Vesiculobullous eruption (<10%)
  (2002): Breneman D+, *Arch Dermatol* 138, 325
Xerosis (10.7%)
  (2003): Esteva FJ+, *J Clin Oncol* 21(6), 999 (34%)

Mucosal/ENT
Cheilitis (<10%)
Gingivitis (<10%)
Xerostomia (<10%)

Hair
Hair – alopecia (4–11%)

Other
Asthenia
  (2003): Esteva FJ+, *J Clin Oncol* 21(6), 999 (30%)
Chills (9.5%)
  (2001): Duvic M+, *Arch Dermatol* 137, 581
Headache
Myalgia/Myositis/Myopathy/Myotoxicity (<10%)
  (2000): Bedikian AY+, *Oncol Rep* 7, 883
Pain
  (2002): Breneman D+, *Arch Dermatol* 138, 325

BICALUTAMIDE

Trade name: Casodex (AstraZeneca)
Indications: Metastatic prostatic carcinoma
Category: Androgen antagonist
Half-life: up to 10 days

Reactions

Skin
Angioedema
Carcinoma
Diaphoresis (6%)
Edema (2–5%)
Exanthems (<1%)
Herpes zoster
Peripheral edema (8%)
Pruritus (2–5%)
Rash (sic) (6%)
Urticaria
Xerosis (2–5%)

Mucosal/ENT
Xerostomia (2–5%)

Hair
Hair – alopecia (2–5%)

Other
Gynecomastia (38%)
  (2007): Abdah-Bortnyak R+, *Harefuah* 146(2), 126
  (2007): Di Lorenzo G+, *Eur Urol* 52(1), 5
  (2007): Fradet Y+, *Eur Urol* 52(1), 106
  (2007): Nuttall MC+, *BJU Int* 99(2), 243
  (2007): Sieber PR, *Expert Rev Anticancer Ther* 7(12), 1773
  (2007): Van Poppel H, *Eur Urol* 52(1), 115

(2006): Boccardo F+, *Int J Biol Markers* 21(2), 123
(2006): Haddad E, *Ann Urol* (Paris) 40(Suppl 2), S49
(2006): Nakabayashi M+, *J Clin Oncol* 24(18), 2958
(2005): Abrahamsson PA+, *Eur Urol* 48(6), 900
(2005): Boccardo F+, *J Clin Oncol* 23(4), 808 (73%)
(2005): Chianakwalam CI+, *Breast* 14(2), 163
(2005): Di Lorenzo G+, *J Urol* 174(6), 2197
(2005): Perdona S+, *Lancet Oncol* 6(5), 295
(2005): Saltzstein D+, *Prostate Cancer Prostatic Dis* 8(1), 75
(2005): Van Poppel H+, *Eur Urol* 47(5), 587
(2004): Tyrrell CJ+, *Int J Radiat Oncol Biol Phys* 60(2), 476
(2002): Iversen P, *Urology* 60(3 Suppl 1), 64
(2002): Mcleod DG, *Urology* 60(3 Suppl 1), 13
(2002): See WA+, *J Urol* 168(2), 429
(2001): Wirth M+, *Urology* 58(2), 146 (17.4%)
(1998): Goa KL+, *Drugs Aging* 12, 401
(1996): Bales GT+, *Urology* 47, 38
(1996): Kotake T+, *Hinyokika Kiyo* (Japanese) 42, 157
(1995): Lunglmayr G, *Anticancer Drugs* 6, 508
(1994): Eri LM+, *Eur Urol* 26, 219
(1990): Mahler C+, *J Steroid Biochem Mol Biol* 37, 921
Hepatotoxicity
  (2006): Manso G+, *Pharmacoepidemiol Drug Saf* 15(4), 253
Hot flashes (49%)
  (2002): Chuang CK+, *Chang Gung Med J* 25(9), 577 (5.4%)
  (2002): Gommersall LM+, *Expert Opin Pharmacother* 3(12), 1685
  (2001): Kucuk O+, *Urology* 58(1), 53 (23%)
  (1996): Bales GT+, *Urology* 47, 38
  (1995): Lunglmayr G, *Anticancer Drugs* 6, 508
  (1994): Eri LM+, *Eur Urol* 26, 219
  (1990): Mahler C+, *J Steroid Biochem Mol Biol* 37, 921
Injection-site reactions (sic) (2–5%)
Myalgia/Myositis/Myopathy/Myotoxicity (2–5%)
Paresthesias (6%)

BIFIDOBACTERIA

Scientific names: *Bifidobacterium adolescentis; Bifidobacterium animalis; Bifidobacterium bifidum; Bifidobacterium breve; Bifidobacterium infantis; Bifidobacterium lactis; Bifidobacterium longum*
Family: Actinomycetaceae
Trade and other common names: Bifantis (Proctor & Gamble); Bifido; Bifidum; DN-173 010; Probiotics; Yakult (Yakult)
Category: Immunomodulator; Probiotic
Purported indications and other uses: Diarrhea, atopic eczema, candidiasis, colds and flu, hepatitis, hypercholesterolemia, lactose intolerance, ulcerative colitis, pouchitis, irritable bowel syndrome
Half-life: N/A

Reactions

None

BIMATOPROST

Trade name: Lumigan (Allergan)
Indications: Open-angle glaucoma, ocular hypertension
Category: Prostaglandin analog
Half-life: 45 minutes

Reactions

Skin
Keratoses
  (2006): Kothari MT+, *Indian J Ophthalmol* 54(1), 47
Photoallergic reaction
  (2003): Packer M+, *J Cataract Refract Surg* 29(11), 2242

Hair
Hair – hirsutism (1–5%)
Hair – hypertrichosis
  (2004): Hart J+, *Am J Ophthalmol* 137(4), 756 (malar)

Eyes
Blepharitis (3–10%)
Conjunctival hyperemia (>10%)
  (2006): Brittain CJ+, *Adv Ther* 23(1), 68
  (2005): Arcieri ES+, *Arch Ophthalmol* 123(2), 186
  (2005): Chen J+, *Cardiovasc Drug Rev* 23(3), 231
  (2005): Konstas AG+, *Ophthalmology* 112(2), 262
  (2005): Vetrugno M+, *Eur J Ophthalmol* 15(4), 477
  (2005): Wanichwecha-Rungruang B+, *J Med Assoc Thai* 88(9), 1228 (20%)
  (2004): Leal BC+, *Am J Ophthalmol* 138(2), 310
  (2003): Abelson MB+, *Adv Ther* 20(1), 1
  (2003): Agarwal HC+, *J Ocul Pharmacol* 19(2), 105 (32%)
  (2003): Gandolfi SA+, *Ophthalmology* 110(3), 609
  (2003): Noecker RS+, *Am J Ophthalmol* 135(1), 55
  (2003): Stewart WC+, *Am J Ophthalmol* 135(3), 314
  (2002): Cantor LB, *Expert Opin Pharmacother* 3(12), 1753
  (2002): Easthope SE+, *Drugs Aging* 19(3), 231 (44%)
  (2002): Eisenberg DL+, *Surv Ophthalmol* 47 Suppl 1, S105
  (2002): Higginbotham EJ+, *Arch Ophthalmol* 120(10), 1286
  (2001): DuBiner H+, *Surv Ophthalmol* 45(Suppl 4), S353–60
  (2001): Gandolfi S+, *Adv Ther* 18(3), 110
  (2001): Laibovitz RA+, *Arch Ophthalmol* 119(7), 994
  (2001): Sherwood M+, *Surv Ophthalmol* 45(Suppl 4), S361–8
Eyelashes – hypertrichosis (>10%)
  (2005): Modschiedler K+, *J Dtsch Dermatol Ges* 3(4), 276
  (2005): Vetrugno M+, *Eur J Ophthalmol* 15(4), 477
  (2004): Jaffe P, Columbia, SC (from Internet) (observation)
  (2004): Manni G+, *Graefes Arch Clin Exp Ophthalmol* 242(9), 767
  (2004): Tosti A+, *J Am Acad Dermatol* 51(5), S149
  (2003): Herndon LW+, *Am J Ophthalmol* 135(5), 713
  (2003): Noecker RS+, *Am J Ophthalmol* 135(1), 55
  (2003): Whitcup SM+, *Br J Ophthalmol* 87(1), 57
  (2002): Cantor LB, *Expert Opin Pharmacother* 3(12), 1753
  (2002): Eisenberg DL+, *Surv Ophthalmol* 47(Suppl 1), S105
Eyelashes – pigmentation
  (2005): Modschiedler K+, *J Dtsch Dermatol Ges* 3(4), 276
  (2004): Jaffe P, Columbia, SC (from Internet) (observation)
Eyelid erythema (3–10%)
Eyelid irritation (3–10%)
Eyelid pain (3–10%)
Eyelid pigmentation (3–10%)
  (2005): Galloway GD+, *Arch Ophthalmol* 123(11), 1609
  (2005): Kapur R+, *Arch Ophthalmol* 123(11), 1541
  (2004): Manni G+, *Graefes Arch Clin Exp Ophthalmol* 242(9), 767
  (2003): Herndon LW+, *Am J Ophthalmol* 135(5), 713
Eyelid xerosis (3–10%)
Macular edema

  (2006): Kruse P+, *Klin Monatsbl Augenheilkd* 223(6), 534
Ocular edema
  (2005): Arcieri ES+, *Arch Ophthalmol* 123(2), 186
Ocular pain
  (2003): Packer M+, *J Cataract Refract Surg* 29(11), 2242
Ocular pigmentation (1–3%)
  (2004): Sodhi PK+, *Am J Ophthalmol* 137(4), 783
  (2003): Herndon LW+, *Am J Ophthalmol* 135(5), 713
  (2002): Novack GD+, *J Am Geriatr Soc* 50(5), 956
  (2002): Stjernschantz JW+, *Surv Ophthalmol* 47(Suppl 1), S162
  (2001): Sherwood M+, *Surv Ophthalmol* 45(Suppl 4), S361–8 (1.1%)
Ocular pruritus (>10%)
Uveitis
  (2005): Cano Parra J+, *Arch Soc Esp Oftalmol* 80(3), 137
  (2003): Packer M+, *J Cataract Refract Surg* 29(11), 2242

Other
Headache
Upper respiratory infection (10%)

BIPERIDEN

Trade names: Akineton (Par); Biperen; Bipiden; Dekinet; Desiperiden; Dyskinon
Indications: Parkinsonism
Category: Anticholinergic; Muscarinic antagonist
Half-life: 18–24 hours
Clinically important, potentially hazardous interactions with: anticholinergics

Reactions

Skin
Dermatitis
  (1995): Torinuki W, *Tohoku J Exp Med* 176, 249
Diaphoresis
  (2001): Richardson C+, *Am J Psychiatry* 158(8), 1329
Exanthems
Rash (sic)
Urticaria

Mucosal/ENT
Glossodynia
Stomatodynia
Xerostomia

Other
Paresthesias
Vertigo
  (1990): Povlsen UJ+, *Mov Disord* 5(1), 27

BISACODYL

Trade names: Apo-Bisacodyl; Biscolax; Carter's Little Pills; Dacodyl; Dulcagen; Dulcolan; Dulcolax (Boehringer Ingelheim); Fleet Laxative; Laxit
Indications: Constipation
Category: Stimulant laxative
Half-life: N/A
Onset of action: 6–10 hours
Clinically important, potentially hazardous interactions with: digoxin

Reactions

Skin
Diaphoresis
Exanthems
Fixed eruption
(1997): Burrow WH, Jackson, MS (from Internet) (observation)
Urticaria

BISMUTH

Trade names: Bismatrol; Bismuth subcitrate; Bismuth subgallate (colostomy deodorant); Bismuth subnitrate and Bismuth idoform paraffin paste (BIPP); Bismuth sucralfate; Caved-S; Colo-Fresh; De-Nol; Devrom; Diotame; Helidac (Prometheus); Pepto-Bismol (Procter & Gamble); Pink Bismuth
Indications: As part of 'triple therapy' (antibiotics + bismuth) for eradication of *H. pylori*. Bismuth subgallate initiates clotting via activation of factor XII, and is used for bleeding during tonsillectomy and adenoidectomy. BIPP impregnated ribbon gauze is used for packing following ear surgery. Bismuth subsalicylate is in OTC products for gastrointestinal complaints and peptic ulcer disease.
Category: Disinfectant; Heavy metal
Half-life: 21–72 days
Clinically important, potentially hazardous interactions with: aspirin, ciprofloxacin, doxycycline, hypoglycemics, lomefloxacin, methotrexate, minocycline, tetracycline, warfarin

Reactions

Skin
Adverse effects (sic) (triple therapy)
(2001): Danese S+, *Hepatogastroenterology* 48(38), 465
(2001): Sotudehmanesh R+, *J Gastroenterol Hepatol* 16(3), 264
(2000): de Boer WA+, *Am J Gastroenterol* 95(3), 641
(2000): Malekzadeh R+, *Aliment Pharmacol Ther* 14(3), 299
(2000): Spinzi GC+, *Aliment Pharmacol Ther* 14(3), 325
(1999): Monkemuller KE+, *Aliment Pharmacol Ther* 13(5), 661
(1999): Olafsson S+, *Aliment Pharmacol Ther* 13(5), 651
(1999): Xiao SD+, *Aliment Pharmacol Ther* 13(3), 311
(1998): Cammarota G+, *Aliment Pharmacol Ther* 12(6), 539
(1998): Cestari R, *Aliment Pharmacol Ther* 12(10), 991
(1998): Dobrucali A+, *Wien Med Wochenschr* (German) 148(20), 464
(1998): Lerang F+, *Am J Gastroenterol* 93(2), 212
(1998): Ricciardiello L+, *Aliment Pharmacol Ther* 12(6), 533
(1998): Spadaccini A+, *Aliment Pharmacol Ther* 12(10), 997
(1998): van der Wouden EJ+, *Am J Gastroenterol* 93(8), 1228
(1997): Henriksen M+, *Am J Gastroenterol* 92, 653
(1997): Huang JQ+, *J Gastroenterol Hepatol* 12(8), 590
(1997): Kolkman JJ+, *Aliment Pharmacol Ther* 11(6), 1123
(1997): Kung NN+, *Am J Gastroenterol* 92(3), 438
(1997): Laine L+, *Am J Gastroenterol* 92(12), 2213
(1996): Thijs JC+, *Am J Gastroenterol* 91(1), 93
(1996): van der Hulst RW+, *Helicobacter* 1(1), 6
(1996): Weldon MJ+, *Aliment Pharmacol Ther* 10(3), 279
(1995): al-Assi MT+, *Am J Gastroenterol* 90(3), 403
(1995): Hoffenberg P+, *Rev Med Chil* 123(2), 185
(1995): Rauws EA+, *Drugs* 50(6), 984
(1995): Webb DD+, *Am J Gastroenterol* 90(8), 1273
(1994): Borody TJ+, *Am J Gastroenterol* 89(1), 33
(1994): Hentschel E, *Wien Klin Wochenschr* (German) 106(17), 543
(1994): Park KN+, *Eur J Gastroenterol Hepatol* 6 (Suppl 1), S103

(1994): Reijers MH+, *Aliment Pharmacol Ther* 8(3), 351 (sucralfate)
(1994): Wilhelmsen I+, *Hepatogastroenterol* 41(1), 43
(1993): Malfertheiner P, *Scand J Gastroenterol* Suppl 196, 34
(1992): Berstad K+, *Scand J Gastroenterol* 27(12), 1006
(1992): Burgess E+, *Drug Saf* 7(4), 282
(1992): Wilhelmsen I+, *Tidsskr Nor Laegeforen* (Norwegian) 112(25), 3197
(1990): Steffen R, *Rev Infect Dis* 12(Suppl1), S80 (subsalicylate)
(1989): Bradley B+, *J Clin Pharm Ther* 14(6), 423 (subsalicylate and subcitrate)
(1988): Borsch G, *Med Klin* (German) 83(18), 605
(1988): Dipalma JR, *Am Fam Physician* 38(5), 244
(1988): Eskens GT, *Postgrad Med J* 64(755), 724
(1980): Fournier PE, *Therapie* (French) 35(3), 319
(1980): Henderson IW, *Can Med Assoc J* 123(9), 848
Allergic reactions (sic)
(1985): Jones PH, *J Laryngol Otol* 99(4), 389
(1981): Anchupane IS+, *Vestn Dermatol Venerol* (Russian) 11, 63
Angioedema (subcitrate)
(1994): Ottervanger JP+, *Ned Tijdschr Geneeskd* (Dutch) 138(3), 152
Dermatitis
(2001): Wictorin A+, *Contact Dermatitis* 45(5), 318 (ointment)
(1987): Goh CL+, *Contact Dermatitis* 16(2), 109 (subnitrate)
Erythema (subcitrate)
(1994): Ottervanger JP+, *Ned Tijdschr Geneeskd* (Dutch) 138(3), 152
Exanthems (subcitrate)
(1994): Ottervanger JP+, *Ned Tijdschr Geneeskd* (Dutch) 138(3), 152
Exfoliative dermatitis
Fixed eruption
(1981): Granstein RD+, *J Am Acad Dermatol* 5, 1
Livedo reticularis
(2005): Gibbs MB+, *J Am Acad Dermatol* 52(6), 1009
Pigmentation
(1997): Ruiz-Maldonado R+, *J Am Acad Dermatol* 37(3), 489
(1993): Zala L+, *Dermatology* 187(4), 288
(1981): Granstein RD+, *J Am Acad Dermatol* 5(1), 1
Pityriasis rosea
(2006): Hanjani NM+, *Cutis* 77(3), 166
Prurigo pigmentosa
(1987): Dijkstra JW+, *Int J Dermatol* 26(6), 379
Pruritus (triple therapy)
(1998): Pozzato P+, *Aliment Pharmacol Ther* 12(5), 447
Rash (sic)
(1990): Burnett JW, *Cutis* 45(4), 220
Vasculitis

Mucosal/ENT
Dysgeusia (46%) (triple therapy)
(2001): Gisbert JP+, *Helicobacter* 6(2), 157
(2001): Kaviani MJ+, *Eur J Gastroenterol Hepatol* 13(8), 915
(1998): Scott BB, *Aliment Pharmacol Ther* 12(3), 277 (10%)
(1997): Chey WD+, *Am J Gastroenterol* 92(9), 1483 (39%)
(1993): Ateshkadi A+, *Clin Pharm* 12(1), 34
(1993): Friedland RP+, *Clin Neuropharmacol* 16(2), 173 (subgallate)
Gingivitis
(1989): Slikkerveer A+, *Med Toxicol Adverse Drug Exp* 4(5), 303 (subnitrate, subcarbonate and subgallate)
Oral pigmentation
(1984): Sutak J+, *Prakt Zuban Lek* (Czech) 32(6), 166
(1983): Dayan D+, *Clin Prev Dent* 5(3), 25 (after root canal filling with AH-26)
Stomatitis
(1990): Burnett JW, *Cutis* 45(4), 220

(1989): Slikkerveer A+, *Med Toxicol Adverse rug Exp* 4(5), 303
   (subnitrate, subcarbonate and subgallate)
Tinnitus
   (1987): DuPont HL+, *JAMA* 257(10), 1347 (subsalicylate)
Tongue pigmentation (>10%)
   (2001): Ioffreda MD+, *Arch Dermatol* 137(7), 968 (black)
   (1987): DuPont HL+, *JAMA* 257(10), 1347 (black)
Xerostomia (41%) (triple therapy)
   (2001): Kaviani MJ+, *Eur J Gastroenterol Hepatol* 13(8), 915

Hair
Hair – alopecia
   (1990): Gollnick H+, *Z Haut* (German) 65, 1128

Other
Anaphylactoid reactions/Anaphylaxis
   (2002): More D+, *Allergy* 57(6), 558
Death
   (1991): Sainsbury SJ, *West J Med* 155(6), 637 (subsalicylate)
   (1990): Jones JA, *Oral Surg Oral Med Oral Pathol* 69(6), 668 (BIPP)
   (1989): Hudson M+, *BMJ* 299(6692), 159 (subcitrate)
   (1985): Sanz Gallen P+, *Med Clin* (Barc) (Spanish) 84(13), 538
   (1980): Allain P+, *Therapie* (French) 35(3), 303
Depression
Embolia cutis medicamentosa (Nicolau syndrome)
   (2001): Corazza M+, *J Eur Acad Dermatol Venereol* 15(6), 585
Headache
Hypersensitivity
   (1998): Lim PV+, *J Laryngol Otol* 112(4), 335 (impregnated tape)
   (1981): Anchupane IS+, *Vestn Dermatol Venerol* (Russian) Nov
      11, 63
Injection-site lymphoma
   (1984): Krivitzky A+, *Ann Med Interne* (Paris) (French)
      135(3), 205
Nephrotoxicity
   (2005): Cengiz N+, *Pediatr Nephrol* 20(9), 1355
Pain (10%) (triple therapy)
   (1998): Scott BB, *Aliment Pharmacol Ther* 12(3), 277 (10%)
Porphyria cutanea tarda
Tremor
   (1993): Kendel K+, *Dtsch Med Wochenschr* (German)
      118(7), 221 (subgallate)

BISOPROLOL

Trade names: Concor; Cordalin; Detensiel; Emcor; Fondril;
Monocor; Soprol; Zebeta (Barr); Ziac (Barr)
Indications: Hypertension
Category: Adrenergic beta-receptor antagonist
Half-life: 9–12 hours

Note: Ziac is bisoprolol and hydrochlorothiazide

Reactions

Skin
Acne
Angioedema
Diaphoresis (1%)
Eczema
Edema (3%)
Exanthems
Exfoliative dermatitis
Facial edema
Lupus erythematosus
Peripheral edema (1–10%)

Photosensitivity
Pigmentation
Pruritus
Psoriasis
Purpura
Rash (sic) (1–10%)
Raynaud's phenomenon (1–10%)
Urticaria
Vasculitis
Xerosis

Mucosal/ENT
Dysgeusia
Tinnitus
Xerostomia (1.3%)

Hair
Hair – alopecia

Nails
Nails – pigmentation

Other
Anaphylactoid reactions/Anaphylaxis
Headache
Hypotension
   (1999): Kanegae K+, *Int J Artif Organs* 22(12), 798
Myalgia/Myositis/Myopathy/Myotoxicity (1–10%)
Paresthesias
Peyronie's disease

BIVALIRUDIN

Synonym: Hirulog
Trade name: Angiomax (The Medicines Company)
Indications: Angioplasty adjunct
Category: Thrombin inhibitor
Half-life: 25 minutes
**Clinically important, potentially hazardous interactions
with:** anisindione, dicumarol, heparin, reteplase, streptokinase,
tenecteplase, urokinase, warfarin

Reactions

Skin
Allergic reactions

Other
Headache
Infections
Injection-site pain (8%)
Pain (15%)

BLACK COHOSH

Scientific names: *Actaea macrotys; Actaea racemosa; Cimicifuga racemosa*
Family: Ranunculaceae
Trade and other common names: Baneberry; Black Snake root; Bugbane; Bugwort; Macrotys; Rattletop; Rattleweed; Remifemin (PhytoPharmica/Enzymatic Therapy; Schaper & Brummer); Shengma; Squawroot
Category: Phytoestrogen
Purported indications and other uses: Anxiety, arthritis, asthma, cardiovascular and circulatory problems, climacteric, menstrual and premenstrual disorders, colds, cough, constipation, depression, kidney disorders, malaria, sore throat, tinnitus
Half-life: N/A
Clinically important, potentially hazardous interactions with: estrogens, salicylates, tamoxifen

Reactions

Skin
Diaphoresis
  (1996): Newell CA+, *Herbal Medicine: A Guide for Healthcare Professionals.* London: The Pharmaceutical Press
  (1985): Duke JA, *Handbook of Medicinal Herbs,* CRC Press, Boca Raton, FL (overdose)
Jaundice
  (2002): Whiting PW+, *Med J Aust* 177(8), 440
Petechiae (forearms)
Pruritus
  (2002): Whiting PW+, *Med J Aust* 177(8), 440
Rash (sic)
  (2003): Huntley A+, *Menopause* 10(1), 58

Other
Asthenia
  (2006): Minciullo PL+, *Phytomedicine* 13(1-2), 115
Myalgia/Myositis/Myopathy/Myotoxicity
  (2006): Minciullo PL+, *Phytomedicine* 13(1-2), 115
Seizures
  (1999): McFarlin BL+, *J Nurse Midwifery* 44, 295
  (1996): Shuster EA, *Mayo Clin Proc* 71(10), 991 (with *Vitex agnus-castus* and evening primrose) (reversible)
  (1996): Shuster J, *Hosp Pharm* 31, 1553
Tremor (overdose)
Vertigo
  (2002): Mahady GB+, *Nutr Clin Care* 5(6), 283

BLEOMYCIN

Synonyms: bleo; BLM
Trade names: Blenoxane (Mead Johnson); Bleo; Bleocin; Bleomycine; Bleomycinum; BLM
Indications: Melanomas, sarcomas, lymphomas, testicular carcinoma
Category: Antibiotic, anthracycline
Half-life: 1.3–9 hours
Clinically important, potentially hazardous interactions with: aldesleukin

Reactions

Skin
Acral erythema
  (2005): Tsuboi H+, *J Dermatol* 32(11), 921
  (1982): Burgdorf WHC+, *Ann Intern Med* 97, 61
Acral necrosis
  (1998): Reiser M+, *Eur J Clin Microbiol Infect Dis* 17, 58
  (1997): Hladunewich M+, *J Rheumatol* 24, 2371
Acral sclerosis
  (1984): Snauwaert J+, *Dermatologica* 169, 172
Allergic reactions (sic)
  (1998): Mullai N+, *J Clin Oncol* 16, 1625
  (1998): Yeo W+, *J Clin Oncol* 16, 1626
Angioedema
  (1984): Khansur T+, *Arch Intern Med* 144, 2267
Bullous dermatitis (1–5%)
Calcification
  (1983): Bork K+, *Hautarzt* (German) 34, 10
Dermatitis
Eccrine squamous syringometaplasia
  (2005): Tsuboi H+, *J Dermatol* 32(11), 921
Erythema
  (2005): Mseddi M+, *Rev Med Liege* 60(10), 772 (flagellate)
  (2003): Nayak N+, *Clin Exp Dermatol* 28(1), 105
  (2001): Robinson JB+, *Gynecol Oncol* 82(3), 550
  (1980): Lincke-Plewig H, *Hautarzt* (German) 31, 616
Erythema gyratum
  (1997): Polsky D+, New York, American Academy of Dermatology Meeting (SF), (gross and microscopic)
Exanthems
  (1993): Haerslev T+, *Cutis* 52, 45 (linear and symmetrical)
  (1980): Lincke-Plewig H, *Hautarzt* (German) 31, 616
Fixed eruption
  (1987): Lindae ML+, *Arch Dermatol* 123(3), 395
Flagellate erythema / pigmentation
  (2007): Chen YB+, *J Clin Oncol* 25(7), 898
  (2007): Vuerstaek JD+, *Int J Dermatol* 46, 3
  (2006): Kumar R+, *Indian Pediatr* 43(1), 74
  (2006): Yamamoto T+, *Int J Dermatol* 45(5), 627
  (2005): Mikhail M+, *J Drugs Dermatol* 4(1), 81
  (2005): Mseddi M+, *Rev Med Liege* 60(10), 772
  (2003): Abess A+, *Arch Dermatol* 139(3), 337
  (2003): Nayak N+, *Clin Exp Dermatol* 28(1), 105
  (2002): Gupta LK+, *Indian J Dermatol Venereol Leprol* 68(3), 158
  (2000): Spedini P+, *Haematologica* 85(8), 870
  (1999): Rubeiz NG+, *Int J Dermatol* 38(2), 140
  (1998): Yamamoto T+, *Dermatology* 197(4), 399
  (1994): Mowad CM+, *Br J Dermatol* 131(5), 700
  (1994): Templeton SF+, *Arch Dermatol* 130(5), 577
  (1994): Zaki I+, *Clin Exp Dermatol* 19(4), 366
  (1993): Tsuji T+, *J Am Acad Dermatol* 28(3), 503
  (1992): Albig J+, *Hautarzt* 43(6), 376
  (1992): Jolin Garijo L+, *An Med Interna* 9(10), 520
  (1991): Duhra P+, *Clin Exp Dermatol* 16(3), 216
  (1990): Cortina P+, *Dermatologica* 180(2), 106
  (1990): Miori L+, *Am J Dermatopathol* 12(6), 598
  (1990): Miori L+, *Dermatologica* 181(3), 238
  (1990): Vicente MA+, *Med Cutan Ibero Lat Am* 18(2), 148
  (1990): Wright AL+, *Dermatologica* 180(4), 255
  (1989): Vignini M+, *Clin Exp Dermatol* 14(3), 261
  (1988): Lazar AP+, *Cutis* 42(5), 397
  (1988): Massone L+, *G Ital Dermatol Venereol* 123(5), 225
  (1987): Lindae ML+, *Arch DermatolPG* 123(3), 395
  (1987): Rademaker M+, *Clin Exp Dermatol* 12(6), 457
  (1986): Polla BS+, *J Am Acad Dermatol* 14(4), 690
  (1985): Fernandez-Obregon AC+, *J Am Acad Dermatol* 13(3), 464
  (1984): Schuler G+, *Hautarzt - Der* 35(7), 383
Hand–foot syndrome
  (2005): Mikhail M+, *J Drugs Dermatol* 4(1), 81
Hyperkeratosis (palms and soles)
Ichthyosis

Intertrigo

Linear streaking
  (1989): Vignini M+, *Clin Exp Dermatol* 14, 261
  (1988): Lazar A+, *Cutis* 42, 397
  (1987): Rademaker M+, *Clin Exp Dermatol* 12, 457

Neutrophilic eccrine hidradenitis
  (1998): Wenzel FG+, *J Am Acad Dermatol* 38(1), 1
  (1988): Scallan PJ+, *Cancer* 62, 2532

Nodular eruption
  (2005): Mikhail M+, *J Drugs Dermatol* 4, 81

Palmar nodules
  (1993): Haerslev T+, *Cutis* 52, 45

Palmar–plantar erythema
  (1990): Pagliuca A+, *Postgrad Med J* 66, 242

Papulo-nodular lesions
  (1997): Polsky D+, New York, American Academy of
    Dermatology Meeting (SF), (gross and microscopic)

Photo-recall
  (1993): Stelzer KJ+, *Cancer* 71, 1322

Pigmentation (~50%)
  (2003): Abess A+, *Arch Dermatol* 139(3), 337
  (2003): Nayak N+, *Clin Exp Dermatol* 28(1), 105
  (2002): vonHilsheimer GE+, *J Am Acad Dermatol* 46(4), 642
  (2001): Mutafoglu-Uysal K+, *Turk J Pediatr* 43(2), 172
  (1999): Susser WS+, *J Am Acad Dermatol* 40(3), 367
  (1998): Behrens S+, *Hautarzt* (German) 49, 725
  (1993): Tsuji T+, *J Am Acad Dermatol* 28, 503 (in striae distensae)
  (1992): Gallais V+, *Ann Dermatol Venereol* (French) 119, 471
  (1990): Wright AL+, *Dermatologica* 181, 255 (reticulate)
  (1988): Massone L+, *G Ital Dermatol Venereol* (Italian) 123, 225
    (striae)
  (1986): Guillet G+, *Arch Dermatol* 122, 381 (in stripes)
  (1985): Polla L+, *Ann Dermatol Venereol* (French) 112, 821
  (1984): Schuler G+, *Hautarzt* (German) 35, 383 (linear)
  (1983): Bork K+, *Hautarzt* (German) 34, 10
  (1982): Kukla LJ+, *Cancer* 50, 2283
  (1981): Granstein RD+, *J Am Acad Dermatol* 5, 1 (brown-black)
  (1981): Nixon DW+, *Cutis* 27, 181

Pruritus (>5%)
  (2001): Robinson JB+, *Gynecol Oncol* 82(3), 550
  (1995): Watanabe T+, *Dermatology* 190(3), 230
  (1994): Templeton SF+, *Arch Dermatol* 130(5), 577 (generalized)
  (1990): Caumes E+, *Lancet* 336, 1593
  (1990): Cortina P+, *Dermatologica* 180(2), 106
  (1985): Fernandez-Obregon AC+, *J Am Acad Dermatol*
    13(3), 464

Rash (sic)

Raynaud's phenomenon (>10%)
  (2001): Vanhooteghem O+, *Pediatr Dermatol* 18(3), 249
  (1998): Reiser M+, *Eur J Clin Microbiol Infect Dis* 17, 58
  (1997): Emmerich J, *Presse Med* (French) 26, 1580
  (1997): Hladunewich M+, *J Rheumatol* 24, 2371
  (1997): Sibilia J+, *Presse Med* (French) 26, 1564 (12.6%)
  (1996): Epstein E, *The Schoch Letter* 46, 34 (observation)
  (1996): Munn SE+, *Br J Dermatol* 135, 969
  (1994): Toumbis-Ioannou E+, *Cleve Clin J Med* 61(3), 195
  (1993): von Gunten CF+, *Cancer* 72, 2004
  (1992): de Pablo P+, *Acta Derm Venereol* (Stockh) 72, 465
  (1992): Doll DC+, *Semin Oncol* 19(5), 580
  (1992): Gregg LJ, *J Am Acad Dermatol* 26, 279
  (1992): Hansen SW, *Dan Med Bull* 39(5), 391 (with cisplatin &
    vinblastine)
  (1991): Epstein E, *J Am Acad Dermatol* 24, 785
  (1990): Cortina P+, *Dermatologica* 180(2), 106
  (1990): Hansen SW+, *Ann Oncol* 1(4), 289
  (1989): Hansen SW+, *J Clin Oncol* 7(7), 940
  (1988): Stefenelli T+, *Eur Heart J* 9(5), 552 (with vinblastine, and
    cisplatin)
  (1987): Werquin S+, *Ann Cardiol Angeiol* (Paris) 36(8), 409

  (1986): Doll DC+, *J Clin Oncol* 4(9), 1405
  (1986): Dzieza-Lalowicz I+, *Pol Tyg Lek* 41(7), 218 (with
    vinblastine)
  (1985): Adoue D+, *Ann Dermatol Venereol* (French) 112, 151
  (1985): Bovenmyer DA, *J Am Acad Dermatol* 13, 470
  (1985): Epstein E, *J Am Acad Dermatol* 13, 468
  (1985): McGuire WA+, *Med Pediatr Oncol* 13(6), 392
  (1985): Smith EA+, *Arthritis Rheum* 28(4), 459
  (1985): Vogelzang NJ+, *Cancer* 56(12), 2765 (with vinblastine &
    cisplatin)
  (1984): Adoue D+, *Ann Intern Med* 100, 770
  (1984): Davis TE+, *Gynecol Oncol* 19(1), 46 (with vinblastine &
    cisplatin)
  (1984): Snauwaert J+, *Dermatologica* 169, 172
  (1983): Bork A+, *Hautarzt* (German) 34, 10
  (1982): Scheulen ME+, *Dtsch Med Wochenschr* 107(43), 1640
    (with vinblastine)
  (1981): Harvey HA+, *Ann Intern Med* 94(4 pt 1), 542 (with
    vinblastine)
  (1981): Kukla LJ+, *Arch Dermatol* 117, 604
  (1980): Paty JG+, *J Rheumatol* 7(6), 927 (with vinblastine)

Scleroderma
  (2005): Lahiri K, Kolkata, India (from Internet) (observation)
  (2004): Yamamoto T+, *J Invest Dermatol* 122(1), 44
  (2000): D'Cruz D, *Toxicol Lett* 112 and 421
  (1999): Passiu G+, *Clin Rheumatol* 18, 422
  (1998): Behrens S+, *Hautarzt* (German) 49, 725
    (pseudoscleroderma)
  (1997): Komosinska K+, *Postepy Hig Med Dosw* (Polish) 51, 285
  (1994): Marck Y+, *Ann Dermatol Venereol* (French) 121, 712,
  (1992): Kerr LD+, *J Rheumatol* 19, 294
  (1991): Bourgeois P+, *Baillieres Clin Rheumatol* 5, 13
  (1991): Guseva NG, *Revmatologiia Mosk* (Russian) 1, 33
  (1985): Haustein UF+, *Int J Dermatol* 24, 147
  (1984): Rush PJ+, *J Rheumatol* 11, 262
  (1983): Bork K+, *Hautarzt* (German) 34, 10
  (1980): Finch WR+, *J Rheumatol* 7, 651

Stevens–Johnson syndrome
  (1989): Brodsky A+, *J Clin Pharmacol* 29, 821
  (1986): Giaccone G+, *Tumori* 72, 331

Striae

Thickening

Urticaria

Vesiculation

Xerosis

Mucosal/ENT

Glossitis
  (1992): Breathnach SM+, *Adverse Drug Reactions and the Skin*
    Blackwell, Oxford, 292 (passim)

Oral papillomatosis

Oral ulceration
  (1992): Breathnach SM+, *Adverse Drug Reactions and the Skin*
    Blackwell, Oxford, 292 (passim)

Ototoxicity
  (1992): Hansen SW, *Dan Med Bull* 39(5), 391 (with cisplatin &
    vinblastine)

Stomatitis (>10%)
  (1999): Susser WS+, *J Am Acad Dermatol* 40(3), 367
  (1993): Haerslev T+, *Cutis* 52, 45
  (1990): Siegel RD+, *Chest* 98, 507
  (1983): Bronner AK+, *J Am Acad Dermatol* 9, 645

Tinnitus

Tongue erosions

Hair

Hair – alopecia (~50%)
  (1999): Susser WS+, *J Am Acad Dermatol* 40(3), 367
  (1992): Breathnach SM+, *Adverse Drug Reactions and the Skin*
    Blackwell, Oxford, 292 (passim)

(1990): Siegel RD+, *Chest* 98, 507
(1982): Kukla LJ+, *Cancer* 50, 2283
Hair – gray

Nails

Nails – Beau's lines (transverse nail bands)
(1994): Ben-Dyan D+, *Acta Haematol* 91, 89
Nails – dystrophy
(1984): Miller RAW, *Arch Dermatol* 120, 963
Nails – growth reduced
(1999): Susser WS+, *J Am Acad Dermatol* 40(3), 367
Nails – loss
(1999): Susser WS+, *J Am Acad Dermatol* 40(3), 367
(1986): Gonzalez FU+, *Arch Dermatol* 122, 974
Nails – onychodystrophy
(1999): Susser WS+, *J Am Acad Dermatol* 40(3), 367
(1985): Baran R, *Ann Dermatol Venereol* (French) 112, 463
Nails – pigmentation (banding)

Other

Anaphylactoid reactions/Anaphylaxis (<1%)
Chills (>10%)
Gangrene (digital)
(1998): Reiser M+, *Eur J Clin Microbiol Infect Dis* 17, 58
(1998): Surville-Barland J+, *Eur J Dermatol* 8, 221
(1993): Vayssairat M+, *J Rheumatol* 20, 921
Hypersensitivity (1–10%)
(2005): Lam MS, *Ann Pharmacother* 39(11), 1897 (1%)
(2001): Mutafoglu-Uysal K+, *Turk J Pediatr* 43(2), 172
(2001): Robinson JB+, *Gynecol Oncol* 82(3), 550
(1992): Weiss RB, *Semin Oncol* 19, 458
Inappropriate secretion of antidiuretic hormone (SIADH)
(1986): Hayes DF+, *J Surg Oncol* 32(3), 150
(1983): Ravikumar TS+, *J Surg Oncol* 24(3), 242
Induration
Injection-site phlebitis (1–10%)
Nephrotoxicity
(1992): Hansen SW, *Dan Med Bull* 39(5), 391 (with cisplatin & vinblastine)
Neurotoxicity
(1992): Hansen SW, *Dan Med Bull* 39(5), 391 (with cisplatin & vinblastine)
Paresthesias

BLOODROOT

Scientific name: *Sanguinaria canadensis*
Family: Papaveraceae
Trade and other common names: Coon Root; Indian Plant; Indian Red Paint; Red Puccoon; Red Root; Snakebite; Sweet Slumber; Tetterwort; Viadent
Category: Anti-inflammatory
Purported indications and other uses: Oral: emetic, cathartic, expectorant. **Topical:** debriding agent, bronchitis, asthma, croup, laryngitis, pharyngitis, scabies, eczema, athlete's foot, nasal polyps, rheumatism, fever, anemia
Half-life: N/A

Reactions

Skin

Dermatitis
(1998): Brinker F, *Contraindications and Drug Interactions* Eclectic Medical Publications
Irritation (sic)
Keratoses

(2000): Eversole LR+, *Oral Surg Oral Med Oral Pathol Oral Radiol Endod* 89(4), 455

Mucosal/ENT

Leukoplakia
(2001): Allen CL+, *Gen Dent* 49(6), 608
(2000): Eversole LR+, *Oral Surg Oral Med Oral Pathol Oral Radiol Endod* 89(4), 455

BLUE COHOSH

Scientific name: *Caulophyllum thalictroides*
Family: Berberidaceae
Trade and other common names: Beechdrops; Blue ginseng; Blueberry root; Papoose root; Squawroot; Yellow ginseng
Category: Diuretic; Oxytocic
Purported indications and other uses: Rheumatism, dropsy, epilepsy, hysteria, uterine inflammation, thrush, menopause, headache, sexual debility, aphthous stomatitis, laxative, colic, sore throat, hiccups
Half-life: N/A
Clinically important, potentially hazardous interactions with: cardioactive drugs

Reactions

Skin

Allergic reactions (sic)
Diaphoresis
(2002): Rao RB+, *Vet Hum Toxicol* 44(4), 221

Mucosal/ENT

Mucosal irritation

Other

Myalgia/Myositis/Myopathy/Myotoxicity
(2002): Rao RB+, *Vet Hum Toxicol* 44(4), 221

BORTEZOMIB

Synonyms: PS-341; LDP-341
Trade name: Velcade (Millennium)
Indications: Multiple myeloma
Category: Proteasome inhibitor
Half-life: 9–15 hours
Clinically important, potentially hazardous interactions with: None

Reactions

Skin

Acute febrile neutrophilic dermatosis (Sweet's syndrome)
(2005): Knoops L+, *Br J Haematol* 131(2), 142
(2005): Van Regenmortel N+, *Haematologica* 90(12 Suppl), ECR43
Allergic reactions
Angioedema
Edema (25%)
Erythema
(2006): Wu KL+, *J Am Acad Dermatol* 55(5), 897
Folliculitis
(2005): Pour L+, *Haematologica* 90(12 Suppl), ECR44
Herpes zoster (11%)
(2005): Wu KL+, *Clin Lymphoma Myeloma* 6(2), 96

(2003): Richardson PG, *Clin Adv Hematol Oncol* A(10), 596
Pruritus (11%)
  (2002): Aghajanian C+, *Clin Cancer Res* 8(8), 2505
Purpura
  (2005): Agterof MJ+, *N Engl J Med* 352(24), 2534
Rash (sic) (21%)
  (2007): Villarrubia B+, *Br J Dermatol* 156(4), 784
  (2005): Richardson PG+, *N Engl J Med* 352(24), 2487
  (2002): Aghajanian C+, *Clin Cancer Res* 8(8), 2505
Toxic epidermal necrolysis
Ulcerations
  (2006): Wu KL+, *J Am Acad Dermatol* 55(5), 897
Urticaria
Vasculitis
  (2007): Garcia-Navarro+, *Br J Dermatol* 157(4), 799
  (2006): Gerecitano J+, *Br J Haematol* 134(4), 391
  (2006): Min CK+, *Eur J Haematol* 76(3), 265
  (2005): Agterof MJ+, *N Engl J Med* 352(24), 2534

Mucosal/ENT
Dysgeusia (13%)
Dysphagia
Stomatitis

Other
Abdominal pain
  (2005): Richardson PG+, *N Engl J Med* 352(24), 2487
Anaphylactoid reactions/Anaphylaxis
Asthenia (65%)
  (2006): *Prescrire Int* 15(83), 98
  (2006): Kane RC+, *Clin Cancer Res* 12(10), 2955
  (2005): Dimopoulos MA+, *Haematologica* 90(12), 1655
  (2005): Goy A+, *J Clin Oncol* 23(4), 667 (13%)
  (2005): Richardson PG+, *N Engl J Med* 352(24), 2487
  (2004): Davis NB+, *J Clin Oncol* 22(1), 115
  (2003): Richardson PG+, *N Engl J Med* 348(26), 2609 (12%)
  (2002): Aghajanian C+, *Clin Cancer Res* 8(8), 2505
Congestive heart failure
  (2006): Voortman J+, *BMC Cancer* 6, 129
Cough (17%)
  (2005): Richardson PG+, *N Engl J Med* 352(24), 2487
Death
  (2006): Bang SM+, *Int J Hematol* 83(4), 309 (6%)
  (2005): Goy A+, *J Clin Oncol* 23(4), 667 (3 cases)
Fever (36%)
  (2006): Wu KL+, *J Am Acad Dermatol* 55(5), 897
  (2005): Dimopoulos MA+, *Haematologica* 90(12), 1655
  (2002): Aghajanian C+, *Clin Cancer Res* 8(8), 2505
Headache
  (2005): Richardson PG+, *N Engl J Med* 352(24), 2487
Hypersensitivity
Infections
  (2006): Kroger N+, *Exp Hematol* 34(6), 770
Injection-site irritation (5%)
Myalgia/Myositis/Myopathy/Myotoxicity (14%)
Neurotoxicity
  (2006): *Prescrire Int* 15(83), 98
  (2006): Bang SM+, *Int J Hematol* 83(4), 309
  (2006): Gupta S+, *Haematologica* 91(7), 1001
  (2006): Kane RC+, *Clin Cancer Res* 12(10), 2955
  (2006): Kroger N+, *Exp Hematol* 34(6), 770 (17%)
  (2006): Richardson PG+, *J Clin Oncol* 24(19), 3113
  (2006): San Miguel J+, *Oncologist* 11(1), 51
  (2005): Dimopoulos MA+, *Haematologica* 90(12), 1655
  (2005): Goy A+, *J Clin Oncol* 23(4), 667 (5%)
  (2005): Richardson PG+, *N Engl J Med* 352(24), 2487
  (2004): Kondagunta GV+, *J Clin Oncol* 22(18), 3720 (53%)
Pain
  (2004): Davis NB+, *J Clin Oncol* 22(1), 115

Paresthesias (26%)
  (2005): Richardson PG+, *N Engl J Med* 352(24), 2487
Seizures
Upper respiratory infection (18%)
Vertigo (21%)

BOSENTAN

Trade name: Tracleer (Actelion)
Indications: Pulmonary arterial hypertension
Category: Endothelin receptor antagonist; Vasodilator
Half-life: ~5 hours
**Clinically important, potentially hazardous interactions
with:** astemizole, atorvastatin, cyclosporine, fluvastatin,
glibenclamide, glyburide, itraconazole, ketoconazole, lovastatin,
oral contraceptives, reboxetine, simvastatin, **St John's wort**,
warfarin

Reactions

Skin
Angioedema
Edema (8%)
  (2004): Dingemanse J+, *Clin Pharmacokinet* 43(15), 1089
Necrotizing vasculitis
  (2004): Gasser S+, *BMJ* 329(7463), 430
Peripheral edema (8%)
Pruritus (4%)
Vasculitis

Other
Headache
  (2004): Dingemanse J+, *Clin Pharmacokinet* 43(15), 1089
  (2002): Prakash A+, *Am J Cardiovasc Drugs* 2(5), 335
Hepatotoxicity
  (2006): Suntharalingam J+, *Vascul Pharmacol* 44(6), 508
Vertigo
  (2002): Prakash A+, *Am J Cardiovasc Drugs* 2(5), 335

BOSWELLIA

Scientific names: *Boswellia carterii; Boswellia commiphora;
Boswellia ovalifoliolata; Boswellia serrata*
Family: Burseraceae
Trade and other common names: Boswellin; Frankincense;
Gum olibanum Ethiopia; Gum olibanum somalilands; Nopane;
Olibanum; Salai guggal; Shallaki
Category: Anti-inflammatory; Diuretic
Purported indications and other uses: Allergic rhinitis,
arthritis, asthma, atherosclerosis, chronic colitis, ulcerative colitis,
Crohn's disease, peritumoral brain edema, rheumatism,
trypanosomiasis, ulcers
Half-life: N/A
**Clinically important, potentially hazardous interactions
with:** aspirin, ibuprofen, montelukast, naproxen

Reactions

Skin
Irritation
  (1999): Buckle J, *Altern Ther Health Med* 5(5), 42
Rash (sic)

BOTULINUM TOXIN (A & B)

Trade names: Botox (Allergan); Dysport (Ipsen); Myobloc (Solstice)
Indications: Blepharospasm, hemifacial spasm, spasmodic torticollis, sialorrhea, hyperhidrosis, strabismus, oromandibular dystonia, cervical dystonia, spasmodic dysphonia. Cosmetic application for wrinkles
Category: Acetylcholine inhibitor; Neuromuscular blocker
Half-life: 3–6 months

Note: An antitoxin is available in the event of overdose or misinjection

Reactions

Skin
Acne
Allergic granulomatous angiitis (Churg–Strauss syndrome)
  (2006): Ahbib S+, *Ann Dermatol Venereol* 133(1), 43
Allergic reactions (sic)
Depigmentation
  (1999): Roehm PC+, *J Neuroophthalmol* 19(1), 7
Erythema multiforme
Hematomas
  (1997): Heinen F+, *Neuropediatrics* 28(6), 307 (local)
  (1997): Nussgens Z+, *Graefes Arch Clin Exp Opthalmol* 235(4), 197
Intertrigo
  (2002): Madalinski MH+, *Eur J Gastroenterol Hepatol* 14(8), 853 (1 case)
Peripheral edema (1–10%)
Pruritus (1–10%)
Psoriasis
Purpura (1–10%)
Rash (sic)
  (2005): Cote TR+, *J Am Acad Dermatol* 53(3), 407
Urticaria

Mucosal/ENT
Dysgeusia (1–10%)
  (2003): Murray C+, *Dermatol Surg* 29(5), 562
Dysphagia
  (2006): Dressler D+, *Neurotox Res* 9(2-3), 121
  (2004): Fishman LM+, *Am J Phys Med Rehabil* 83(1), 42 (50%)
Oral candidiasis
  (2003): Dressler D+, *Eur Neurol* 49(1), 34
Stomatitis (1–10%)
Tinnitus (1–10%)
  (2005): Cote TR+, *J Am Acad Dermatol* 53(3), 407
Vulvovaginal candidiasis (1–10%)
Xerostomia (3–34%)
  (2006): Dressler D+, *Neurotox Res* 9(2-3), 121
  (2005): Comella CL+, *Neurology* 65(9), 1423
  (2004): Brashear A+, *Arch Phys Med Rehabil* 85(5), 705
  (2004): Fishman LM+, *Am J Phys Med Rehabil* 83(1), 42 (50%)
  (2004): Ondo WG+, *Neurology* 62(1), 37 (3 cases)
  (2004): Schwerin A+, *Pediatr Neurol* 31(2), 109 (10%)
  (2003): Brashear A+, *Arch Phys Med Rehabil* 84(1), 103
  (2003): Dressler D+, *Eur Neurol* 49(1), 34

Eyes
Conjunctivitis
  (2006): Dressler D+, *Neurotox Res* 9(2-3), 121
Diplopia
  (2006): Aristodemou P+, *Ophthal Plast Reconstr Surg* 22(2), 134
Ectropion

(1990): *NIH Consensus Statement* 8(8), 1
Entropion
Eyelid edema
  (1990): NIH Consensus Statement 8(8), 1
Ptosis (14–20%)
  (2005): Cote TR+, *J Am Acad Dermatol* 53(3), 407 (2 cases)
  (2002): Molloy F, *eMedicine Journal* 3(2) (10%)
  (1997): Nussgens Z+, *Graefes Arch Clin Exp Ophthalmol* 235(4), 197
  (1990): *NIH Consensus Statement* 8(8), 1
Punctate keratitis
  (2004): Northington ME+, *Dermatol Surg* 30(12 Pt 2), 1515
Xerophthalmia (6.3%)
  (2004): Northington ME+, *Dermatol Surg* 30(12 Pt 2), 1515

Other
Anaphylactoid reactions/Anaphylaxis
  (2005): Li M+, *J Forensic Sci* 50(1), 169 (with lidocaine)
  (1997): LeWitt PA+, *Mov Disord* 12(6), 1064 (localized)
Death
  (2005): Li M+, *J Forensic Sci* 50(1), 169 (with lidocaine)
Depression
  (1999): Brenner R+, *South Med J* 92(7), 738
Headache
  (2005): Cote TR+, *J Am Acad Dermatol* 53(3), 407 (3 cases)
  (2004): Klein AW, *J Am Acad Dermatol* 50(1), 153
Infections (13–19%)
Injection-site bruising
  (2004): Klein AW, *J Am Acad Dermatol* 50(1), 153
  (2002): Molloy F, *eMedicine Journal* 3(2)
  (1998): Goodman G, *Australas J Dermatol* 39(3), 158
Injection-site burning
  (2000): Karamfilov T+, *Arch Dermatol* 136(4), 487
Injection-site ecchymoses
  (1997): Guerrissi J+, *Ann Plast Surg* 39(5), 447
  (1990): NIH, *Consensus Statement* 8(8), 1
Injection-site edema
  (2004): Klein AW, *J Am Acad Dermatol* 50(1), 153
  (2000): Ahn KY+, *Plast Reconstr Surg* 105(2), 778
  (2000): Wissel J+, *J Pain Symptom Manage* 20(1), 44
  (1997): Guerrissi J+, *Ann Plast Surg* 39(5), 447
Injection-site pain (2–10%)
  (2006): Kranz G+, *Dermatol Surg* 32(7), 886
  (2002): Madalinski MH+, *Eur J Gastroenterol Hepatol* 14(8), 853 (4 cases)
  (2002): Molloy F, *eMedicine Journal* 3(2)
  (2001): de Almeida+, *Dermatol Surg* 27(1), 34
  (2000): Karamfilov T+, *Arch Dermatol* 136(4), 487
  (2000): Wissel J+, *J Pain Symptom Manage* 20(1), 44
  (1990): *NIH Consensus Statement* 8(8), 1
Injection-site reactions
  (2005): Cote TR+, *J Am Acad Dermatol* 53(3), 407
Pain (6–13%)
  (2004): Ghazizadeh S+, *Obstet Gynecol* 104(5 Pt 1), 922 (mild)
  (2003): Yavuzer R+, *Plast Reconstr Surg* 111(1), 509
  (1997): Truong DD+, *Mov Disord* 12(5), 772
Seizures
  (2006): Turkel CC+, *Arch Phys Med Rehabil* 87(6), 786
  (2005): Cote TR+, *J Am Acad Dermatol* 53(3), 407
Tremor (1–10%)
  (1997): Truong DD+, *Mov Disord* 12(5), 772
Vertigo
  (2005): Cote TR+, *J Am Acad Dermatol* 53(3), 407

BRETYLIUM

Trade names: Bretylate; Critifib
Indications: Ventricular tachycardia and fibrillation
Category: Antiarrhythmic class III
Half-life: 4–17 hours
**Clinically important, potentially hazardous interactions
with:** arsenic, astemizole, ciprofloxacin, enoxacin, gatifloxacin,
lomefloxacin, moxifloxacin, norfloxacin, ofloxacin, quinolones,
sparfloxacin

Reactions

Skin
Diaphoresis (<1%)
Rash (sic) (<1%)
Side effects (sic)
 (2003): Kuczkowski KM, *Anaesthesia* 58(2), 201

Other
Abdominal pain
 (2002): Molyneux M+, *Eur J Anaesthesiol* 19(2), 147
Fever
 (1989): Perlman PE+, *Postgrad Med* 85(1), 111, 114
Hypotension
 (1995): Kowey PR+, *Circulation* 92(11), 3255
 (1985): Anderson JL, *Clin Ther* 7(2), 205
 (1983): Kron IL+, *Ann Thorac Surg* 35(3), 271
Injection-site atrophy (<1%)
Injection-site necrosis (<1%)

BREWER'S YEAST

Scientific names: *Saccharomyces boulardii; Saccharomyces
cerevisiae*
Family: Saccharomycetaceae
Trade and other common names: Baker's yeast; Faex
Medicinalis; Hansen CBS 5926; Levure De Biere; Perenterol (Cell
Tech Pharma); Probiotics; Ultra-Levura (Upsamedica)
Category: Immunomodulator; Probiotic
Purported indications and other uses: diarrhea, rotaviral
diarrhea, irritable bowel syndrome, Crohn's disease, ulcerative
colitis, urinary tract infections, vaginal infections, acne,
premenstrual syndrome, furunculosis
Half-life: N/A
**Clinically important, potentially hazardous interactions
with:** monoamine oxidase inhibitors (moias)

Reactions

Other
Headache
Hypersensitivity
 (1994): Kortekangas-Savolainen+, *Clin Exp Allergy* 24(9), 836

BRIMONIDINE

Trade name: Alphagan (Allergan)
Indications: Open-angle glaucoma, ocular hypertension
Category: Adrenergic alpha2-receptor agonist
Half-life: 12 hours

Note: The Teardrop sign is a laceration or deformity of the limbus of
the eye

Reactions

Skin
Allergic reactions (sic) (<1%)
 (1999): thoe Schwartzenberg GW+, *Ophthalmology* 106, 1616
 (1998): Gordon RN+, *Eye* 12, 697
Dermatitis
 (2003): Sodhi PK+, *J Dermatol* 30(9), 697 (topical)

Mucosal/ENT
Dysgeusia (1–10%)
Xerostomia (<10%)
 (2000): Detry-Morel M+, *J Fr Ophthalmol* 23, 763
 (1998): LeBlanc RP, *Ophthalmology* 105, 1960
 (1997): Derick RJ+, *Ophthalmology* 104, 131
 (1997): Schuman JS+, *Arch Ophthalmol* 115, 847 (33%)
 (1996): Schuman JS, *Surv Ophthalmol* 41, Suppl 1:S27
 (1996): Walters TR, *Surv Ophthalmol* 41, Suppl 1:S19

Nails
Nails – lichen planus
 (2003): Sodhi PK+, *J Dermatol* 30(9), 697 (topical)

Eyes
Blepharitis (1–10%)
Ectropion
 (2007): Hegde V+, *Ophthalmology* 114(2), 362 (23%)
Eyelid crusting (1–10%)
Eyelid edema (1–10%)
Eyelid erythema (1–10%)
Ocular allergy (sic) (4.2%)
 (2000): Melamed S+, *Clin Ther* 22, 103
 (1999): Shin DH+, *Am J Ophthalmol* 127, 511
 (1998): LeBlanc RP, *Ophthalmology* 105, 1960
 (1996): Schuman JS, *Surv Ophthalmol* 41, Suppl 1:S27
Ocular burning (<10%)
 (2005): Al-Shahwan+, *Ophthalmology* 112(12), 2143
 (2003): Hommer A+, *Br J Ophthalmol* 87(5), 592 (with timolol)
 (1998): LeBlanc RP, *Ophthalmology* 105, 1960
 (1997): Schuman JS+, *Arch Ophthalmol* 115, 847 (28.1%)
 (1996): Schuman JS, *Surv Ophthalmol* 41, Suppl 1:S27
Ocular erythema
 (2001): Stewart WC+, *Am J Ophthalmol* 131(5), 631
Ocular pruritus (<10%)
 (2005): Al-Shahwan S+, *Ophthalmology* 112(12), 2143
Ocular stinging (<10%)
 (2003): Hommer A+, *Br J Ophthalmol* 87(5), 592 (with timolol)
 (1998): LeBlanc RP, *Ophthalmology* 105, 1960
 (1997): Schuman JS+, *Arch Ophthalmol* 115, 847 (28.1%)
 (1996): Schuman JS, *Surv Ophthalmol* 41, Suppl 1:S27
Periocular dermatitis
 (2003): Sodhi PK+, *J Dermatol* 30(9), 697
 (2000): Williams GC+, *Glaucoma* 9, 235
Teardrop sign
 (2000): Scruggs JT+, *Br J Ophthalmol* 84, 671
Uveitis
 (2005): Cano Parra J+, *Arch Soc Esp Oftalmol* 80(3), 137
 (2000): Byles DB+, *Am J Ophthalmol* 130(3), 287
 (2000): Goyal R+, *Eye* 14(Pt 6), 908

Other
Depression
Headache
Hypersensitivity
(2003): Packer M+, *J Cataract Refract Surg* 29(11), 2242
(2002): Watts P+, *Eye* 16(2), 132
Upper respiratory infection (1–10%)

BRINZOLAMIDE

Trade name: Azopt (Alcon)
Indications: Open-angle glaucoma, ocular hypertension
Category: Carbonic anhydrase inhibitor; Diuretic
Half-life: 111 days
Clinically important, potentially hazardous interactions with: salicylates (high doses)

Note: Brinzolamide is a sulfonamide and can be absorbed systemically. Sulfonamides can produce severe, possibly fatal, reactions such as toxic epidermal necrolysis and Stevens–Johnson syndrome.

Reactions

Skin
Allergic reactions (sic) (<1%)
Dermatitis (1–5%)
Urticaria (<1%)

Mucosal/ENT
Dysgeusia (5–10%)
(2002): Novack GD+, *J Am Geriatr* 50(5), 956
(2000): Sall K, *Surv Ophthalmol* 44, S155
Xerostomia (<1%)
(2002): Novack GD+, *J Am Geriatr* 50(5), 956

Hair
Hair – alopecia (<1%)

Eyes
Blepharitis (1–5%)
Eyelid crusting (<1%)
Ocular burning
(2000): Barnebey H+, *Clin Ther* 22(10), 1204
(2000): Sall K, *Surv Ophthalmol* 44, S155
(1998): Silver LH, *Am J Ophthalmol* 126(3), 400 (1–5%)
Ocular pruritus (1–5%)
Ocular stinging
(2000): Barnebey H+, *Clin Ther* 22(10), 1204
(2000): Sall K, *Surv Ophthalmol* 44, S155
(1998): Silver LH, *Am J Ophthalmol* 126(3), 400 (1–5%)
Vision blurred (5–10%)
(2001): Seong GJ+, *Ophthalmologica* 215(3), 188
(2000): Sugrue MF, *Prog Retin Eye Res* 19(1), 87
Xerophthalmia (1–5%)
(2002): Novack GD+, *J Am Geriatr Soc* 50, 956

BROMELAIN

Scientific names: *Ananas comosus; Ananas duckei; Ananas sativus; Bromelia ananas; Bromelia comosa*
Family: Bromeliaceae
Trade and other common names: Bromelain-POS (Ursapharm); Bromelin; Debridase; Phlogenzym; Pineapple enzyme; Plant protease concentrate
Category: Analgesic; Anti-inflammatory
Purported indications and other uses: Oral: inflammation, mild ulcerative colitis, osteoarthritis, sinusitis, sprains. **Topical:** burn debridement
Half-life: N/A
Clinically important, potentially hazardous interactions with: amoxicillin, fluorouracil, tetracycline, vincristine

Note: Phlogenzym is rutoside, bromelain and trypsin

Reactions

Mucosal/ENT
Cheilitis
(2003): Raison-Peyron N+, *Contact Dermatitis* 49(4), 218
Rhinitis

Other
Adverse effects (sic)
(2005): Braun JM+, *In Vivo* 19(2), 417
(2001): Nettis E+, *Allergy* 56(3), 257
(1988): Gailhofer G+, *Clin Allergy* 18(5), 445
(1987): Gailhofer G+, *Derm Beruf Umwelt* 35(5), 174
(1985): Wuthrich B, *Hautarzt* 36(3), 123

BROMFENAC

Trade name: Xibrom (ISTA Pharma)
Indications: Postoperative ophthalmic inflammation
Category: Non-steroidal anti-inflammatory
Half-life: N/A
Clinically important, potentially hazardous interactions with: NSAIDs

Note: Bromfenac contains sodium sulfite, which may cause hypersensitivity in sensitive individuals

Reactions

Skin
Stevens–Johnson syndrome
(2007): Isawi H+, *J Cataract Refract Surg* 33(9), 1644

Eyes
Conjunctival hyperemia
Corneal melting
(2007): Isawi H+, *J Cataract Refract Surg* 33(9), 1644
(2006): Asai T+, *Cornea* 25(2), 224 (3 cases)
Iritis
Ocular burning
Ocular erythema
Ocular pain
Ocular stinging

Other
Headache

BROMOCRIPTINE

Trade names: Apo-Bromocriptine; Bromed; Cryocriptina; Kripton; Parilac; Parlodel (Novartis); Pravidel; Serocryptin
Indications: Amenorrhea, parkinsonism, infertility
Category: Dopamine receptor agonist
Half-life: initial: 6–8 hours; terminal: 50 hours
Clinically important, potentially hazardous interactions with: erythromycin, lanreotide, pseudoephedrine, sympathomimetics

Reactions

Skin
Diaphoresis
  (1998): Nakasu Y+, *Neurol Med Chir* (Tokyo) 38(10), 669
Exanthems
Livedo reticularis
  (1985): Hoehn MMM+, *Neurology* 35, 199
Morphea
  (1989): Leshin B+, *Int J Dermatol* 28, 177
Nodular eruption
Purpura
Rash (sic)
Raynaud's phenomenon (1–10%)
  (1996): Zenone T+, *Rev Med Interne* 17(11), 948
  (1987): Quagliarello J+, *Fertil Steril* 48(5), 877
Scleroderma
  (1989): Leshin B+, *Int J Dermatol* 28, 177
  (1983): Dupont E+, *Neurology* 33, 670
Urticaria
Vasculitis

Mucosal/ENT
Dysgeusia (metallic taste)
Stomatopyrosis
  (1985): Hoehn MMM+, *Neurology* 35, 199
Xerostomia (4–10%)
  (1985): Hoehn MMM+, *Neurology* 35, 199
  (1982): Gauthier G+, *Eur Neurol* 21, 217

Hair
Hair – alopecia
  (1993): Fabre N+, *Clin Neuropharmacol* 16, 266
  (1980): Blum I+, *N Engl J Med* 303, 1418

Eyes
Visual hallucinations
  (1980): Goodkin DA, *N Engl J Med* 302(26), 1479

Other
Anaphylactoid reactions/Anaphylaxis
  (1980): Parkes S, *N Engl J Med* 302, 750
Erythromelalgia
  (1983): Dupont E+, *Neurology* 33, 670
  (1981): Eisler T+, *Neurology* 31, 1368
Headache
  (2004): Barroso B+, *Rev Neurol* (Paris) 160(12), 1191
Hypertension
  (2004): Barroso B+, *Rev Neurol* (Paris) 160(12), 1191
Paresthesias
  (1985): Hoehn MMM+, *Neurology* 35, 199
Pseudolymphoma
  (2000): Wiesli P+, *Clin Endocrinol* (Oxford) 53(5), 656
Seizures
  (2004): Barroso B+, *Rev Neurol* (Paris) 160(12), 1191
  (2003): Burckard E+, *Ann Fr Anesth Reanim* 22(1), 46

BROMPHENIRAMINE

Trade names: Bromfed (Muro); Bromine; Brommine; Bromphen; Dimegan; Dimetane; Ilvin; Kinmedon; Nasahist; ND-Stat; Neo-Meton; Rondec (Biovail)
Indications: Allergic rhinitis, urticaria
Category: Histamine H1 receptor antagonist
Half-life: 12–48 hours
Clinically important, potentially hazardous interactions with: aprobarbital, butabarbital, chloral hydrate, ethchlorvynol, mephobarbital, pentobarbital, phenobarbital, phenothiazines, primidone, secobarbital, zolpidem

Reactions

Skin
Angioedema (<1%)
Exanthems (<1%)
Photosensitivity (<1%)
Rash (sic) (<1%)

Mucosal/ENT
Xerostomia (1–10%)

Other
Headache
Myalgia/Myositis/Myopathy/Myotoxicity (<1%)
Paresthesias (<1%)

BUCILLAMINE

Trade name: Rimatil (Santen)
Indications: Rheumatoid arthritis
Category: Disease-modifying antirheumatic
Half-life: N/A
Clinically important, potentially hazardous interactions with: N/A

Reactions

Skin
Allergic reactions (sic)
  (1998): Kimura M+, *Contact Dermatitis* 39(2), 98
Bullous pemphigoid
  (1989): Yamaguchi R+, *J Dermatol* 16(4), 308
Dermatomyositis
  (2005): Takeda T+, *Rinsho Shinkeigaku* 45(1), 45
Fixed eruption
  (2005): Izumi A+, *J Dermatol* 32(5), 397
Pemphigus
  (2006): Hur JW+, *J Korean Med Sci* 21(3), 585
  (1991): Amasaki Y+, *Ryumachi* 31(5), 528
Rash
  (2002): Kishimoto N+, *Nihon Kokyuki Gakkai Zasshi* 40(4), 321
Subcorneal pustular dermatosis (Sneddon-Wilkinson)
  (2001): Kishimoto K+, *Eur J Dermatol* 11(1), 41
Toxic epidermal necrolysis
  (2005): Izumi A+, *J Dermatol* 32(5), 397

Nails
Nails – dystrophy
  (1995): Ishizaki C+, *Int J Dermatol* 34(7), 493
  (1991): Ichikawa Y+, *Tokai J Exp Clin Med* T(5-6), 203

Other
Adverse effects
(2005): Nagashima M+, *Clin Exp Rheumatol* 23(1), 27 (23%)
(1993): Inokuma S+, *Ryumachi* 33(4), 316
Cough
(2001): Lee YH+, *Korean J Intern Med* 16(1), 36
(2001): Matsushima H+, *Nihon Kokyuki Gakkai Zasshi* 39(1), 55
(1995): Ogawa H+, *Respir Med* 89(3), 219
(1992): Hara A+, *Nihon Kyobu Shikkan Gakkai Zasshi* 30(9), 1743
Fever
(2002): Kishimoto N+, *Nihon Kokyuki Gakkai Zasshi* 40(4), 321
(2002): Miwa Y+, *Ryumachi* 42(1), 70
(2001): Matsushima H+, *Nihon Kokyuki Gakkai Zasshi* 39(1), 55
(1992): Hara A+, *Nihon Kyobu Shikkan Gakkai Zasshi* 30(9), 1743
Gynecomastia
(2002): Sakai Y+, *Ann Plast Surg* 49(2), 193
Nephrotoxicity
(2006): Hoshino J+, *Nephron Clin Pract* 104(1), c15
(2004): Ohno I+, *Nippon Rinsho* 62(10), 1919

BUCLIZINE

Trade names: Aphilan; Bucladin-S; Buclixin; Longifene; Odetin; Postafeno; Vibazina; Vibazine
Indications: Motion sickness, nausea/vomiting
Category: Histamine H1 receptor antagonist
Half-life: N/A
Clinically important, potentially hazardous interactions with: aprobarbital, butabarbital, chloral hydrate, ethchlorvynol, mephobarbital, pentobarbital, phenobarbital, phenothiazines, primidone, secobarbital, zolpidem

Reactions

Mucosal/ENT
Xerostomia

Other
Tremor

BUDESONIDE

Trade names: Pulmicort Turbuhaler (AstraZeneca); Rhinocort (AstraZeneca)
Indications: Asthma, rhinitis
Category: Corticosteroid, inhaled
Half-life: N/A
Clinically important, potentially hazardous interactions with: ketoconazole, **live vaccines**, oral contraceptives

Reactions

Skin
Acne
Adverse effects
(2003): Coghlan D+, *Paediatr Drugs* 5(10), 685 (rare)
(2003): Delacourt C+, *Respir Med* 97, S27
(2001): Reichel W+, *Int J Clin Pract* 55(2), 100
(2001): Terzano C+, *Eur Rev Med Pharmacol Sci* 5(1), 17
Allergic reactions (sic)
(2000): Bircher AJ+, *Dermatology* 200(4), 349
(1995): Lepoittevin JP+, *Arch Dermatol* 131(1), 31
(1993): Fedler R+, *Hautarzt* 44(2), 91

Angioedema
(2003): Pirker C+, *Contact Dermatitis* 49(2), 77
Bruising
(2001): Berend N+, *Respirology* 6(3), 237
Burning
Dermatitis
(1997): Vestergaard L+, *Ugeskr Laeger* (Danish) 159, 5662
(1993): Hisa T+, *Contact Dermatitis* 28, 174
(1993): Noda H+, *Contact Dermatitis* 28(4), 212 (5 cases)
(1991): Dunkel FG+, *Contact Dermatitis* 25(2), 97 (2 cases)
(1991): Gamboa PM+, *Contact Dermatitis* 24(3), 227
(1991): Piraccini BM+, *Contact Dermatitis* 24(1), 54
Eczema
Edema of lip
(2003): Pirker C+, *Contact Dermatitis* 49(2), 77
Exanthems
(2000): Bircher AJ+, *Dermatology* 200(4), 349
Pruritus
(2003): Pirker C+, *Contact Dermatitis* 49(2), 77
Pustules
Rash (sic)
(2003): Kilpio K+, *Allergy* 58(11), 1131
(1993): Hisa T+, *Contact Dermatitis* 28(3), 174
Striae

Mucosal/ENT
Dysphagia
(2003): Pirker C+, *Contact Dermatitis* 49(2), 77
Oral candidiasis
(1984): Clissold SP+, *Drugs* 28, 485

Eyes
Eyelid edema
(2003): Pirker C+, *Contact Dermatitis* 49(2), 77

Other
Anaphylactoid reactions/Anaphylaxis
(2000): Heeringa M+, *BMJ* 321(7266), 927
Asthenia
Cough
(2003): Dubus JC+, *Fundam Clin Pharmacol* 17(5), 627

BUMETANIDE

Trade names: Bumedyl; Bumex (Roche); Burinex; Fondiuran; Fontego; Lunetoron; Miccil; Primex
Indications: Edema associated with congestive heart failure
Category: Diuretic, loop
Half-life: 1–1.5 hours
Clinically important, potentially hazardous interactions with: amikacin, aminoglycosides, digoxin, gentamicin, kanamycin, neomycin, streptomycin, tobramycin

Note: Bumetanide is a sulfonamide and can be absorbed systemically. Sulfonamides can produce severe, possibly fatal, reactions such as toxic epidermal necrolysis and Stevens–Johnson syndrome

Reactions

Skin
Allergic reactions (sic)
Bullous dermatitis
(1990): Leitao EA+, *J Am Acad Dermatol* 23, 129
Bullous pemphigoid
(1998): Boulinguez S+, *Br J Dermatol* 138, 549
Dermatitis

(1989): Moller NE+, *Contact Dermatitis* 20, 393
Diaphoresis (0.1%)
Erythema multiforme (<1%)
Exanthems
Exfoliative dermatitis
  (1981): Handler B+, *J Clin Pharmacol* 21, 691
Photosensitivity
  (1990): Leitao EA+, *J Am Acad Dermatol* 23, 129
Pruritus (<1%)
  (1992): Shelley WB+, *Cutis* 50, 17 (observation)
  (1984): Ward A+, *Drugs* 28, 426 (1–5%)
Purpura
Rash (sic) (0.2%)
Side effects (sic) (1.1%)
  (1984): Ward A+, *Drugs* 28, 426 (1–5%)
Urticaria (0.2%)
  (1981): Handler B+, *J Clin Pharmacol* 21, 691
Vasculitis

Mucosal/ENT
Xerostomia (0.1%)

Eyes
Periorbital edema
  (1981): Handler B+, *J Clin Pharmacol* 21, 691

Other
Headache
Pseudoporphyria
  (1990): Leitao EA+, *J Am Acad Dermatol* 23, 129

BUPIVACAINE

Trade names: Marcaine (AstraZeneca); Sensorcaine (AstraZeneca)
Indications: Local or regional anesthesia or analgesia
Category: Anesthetic, local
Half-life: N/A
Clinically important, potentially hazardous interactions with: MAO inhibitors, oxytocic drugs, tricyclic antidepressants, vasopressor drugs

Reactions

Skin
Angioedema
Diaphoresis
Erythema
Pruritus
Urticaria

Mucosal/ENT
Tinnitus

Eyes
Vision blurred

Other
Anaphylactoid reactions/Anaphylaxis
Aseptic meningitis
  (2007): Besocke A+, *Neurologia*
Asthenia
Cardiac arrest
  (2006): Rosenblatt MA+, *Anesthesiology* 105(1), 217
  (2005): Levsky ME+, *Can J Clin Pharmacol* 12(3), e240
Chills
Depression

Fever
Headache
Hypotension
Paresthesias
Seizures
Tremor

BUPRENORPHINE

Trade names: Suboxone (Schering-Plough); Subutex (Schering-Plough); Temgesic; Transtec (Napp)
Indications: Opioid dependence, moderate to severe pain
Category: Analgesic; Mixed opioid agonist/antagonist; Narcotic
Half-life: 37 hours
Clinically important, potentially hazardous interactions with: antihistamines, azole antifungals, benzodiazepines, carbamazepine, delavirdine, diazepam, erythromycin, HIV protease inhibitors, ketorolac, macrolide antibiotics, neuroleptics, phenobarbital, phenytoin, rifampin, ritonavir

Note: Suboxone contains naloxone

Reactions

Skin
Allergic reactions
Dermatitis
  (2005): Callejo Melgosa+, *Allergy* 60(9), 1217
  (2005): Muriel C+, *Clin Ther* 27(4), 451 (1.3%)
Diaphoresis
Erythema
  (2006): Schmid-Grendelmeier P+, *Curr Med Res Opin* 22(3), 501 (patch)
  (2005): Muriel C+, *Clin Ther* 27(4), 451 (1.3%)
  (2003): Likar R+, *Wien Med Wochenschr* 153(13-1), 317 (from patch)
  (2003): Radbruch L+, *Int J Clin Pract Suppl* (133), 15
Hyperhidrosis
  (1993): Torres LM+, *Rev Esp Anestesiol Reanim* 40(4), 181
  (1989): Grill S+, *Cah Anesthesiol* 37(2), 89
  (1982): Taguchi T, *Gan To Kagaku Ryoho* 9(2), 250
Pruritus
  (2005): Muriel C+, *Clin Ther* 27(4), 451 (1.4%)
  (2003): Likar R+, *Wien Med Wochenschr* 153(13-1), 317 (from patch)
  (2003): Radbruch L+, *Int J Clin pract Suppl* (133), 15
  (2002): Khan FA+, *Paediatr Anaesth* 12(9), 786
  (1993): Torres LM+, *Rev Esp Anestesiol Reanim* 40(4), 181
  (1990): Abid A+, *Ann Fr Anesth Reanim* 9(3), 275 (sublingual)
  (1989): Ackerman WE+, *Can J Anaesth* 36(4), 388
  (1988): Simpson KH+, *Br J Anaesth* 60(6), 627
  (1988): Woodham M, *Anaesthesia* 43(9), 806 (sublingual)
Rash (sic)
Urticaria

Mucosal/ENT
Epistaxis
  (2004): Ray R+, *Pharmacoepidemiol Drug Saf* 13(9), 615 (sublingual)
Tinnitus
Xerostomia
  (1982): Taguchi T, *Gan To Kagaku Ryoho* 9(2), 250

Eyes
Diplopia
Vision blurred

Other

Abdominal pain
(2004): Herve S+, *Eur J Gastroenterol Hepatol* 16(10), 1033
(1993): Teoh SK+, *J Clin Psychopharmacol* 13(2), 87

Asthenia
(2006): Likar R+, *Clin Ther* 28(6), 943 (2.9%)
(2005): Lin YH+, *J Minim Invasive Gynecol* 12(4), 347
(2004): Ray R+, *Pharmacoepidemiol Drug Saf* 13(9), 615 (48.9%)

Death
(2006): Lai SH+, *Forensic Sci Int* 162(1-3), 80
(2004): Pirnay S+, *Addiction* 99(8), 978 (12%)
(2002): Kintz P, *Clin Biochem* 35(7), 513
(2001): Kintz P, *Forensic Sci Int* 121(1-2), 65
(1998): Tracqui A+, *J Anal Toxicol* 22(6), 430
(1998): Tracqui A+, *Presse Med* 27(12), 557 (with benzodiazepine)

Fever
(2004): Herve S+, *Eur J Gastroenterol Hepatol* 16(10), 1033

Headache
(1993): Teoh SK+, *J Clin Psychopharmacol* 13(2), 87
(1982): Taguchi T, *Gan To Kagaku Ryoho* 9(2), 250

Hepatotoxicity
(2006): *Prescrire Int* 15(82), 64
(2004): Herve S+, *Eur J Gastroenterol Hepatol* 16(10), 1033 (5 cases)
(2001): Wisniewski B+, *Gastroenterol Clin Biol* 25(3), 328
(2000): Petry NM+, *Am J Addict* 9(3), 265

Hypertension
(2004): Ray R+, *Pharmacoepidemiol Drug Saf* 13(9), 615 (5%)

Hypotension
(1995): Fukuda H+, *Masui* 44(1), 100
(1988): Weiss P+, *Anasth Intensivther Notfallmed* 23(6), 309

Injection-site erythema
(2006): Likar R+, *Clin Ther* 28(6), 943 (12.1%)

Injection-site exanthems
(2006): Likar R+, *Clin Ther* 28(6), 943 (8.8%)

Injection-site pain
(1993): Torres LM+, *Rev Esp Anestesiol Reanim* 40(4), 181

Injection-site pruritus
(2006): Likar R+, *Clin Ther* 28(6), 943

Myalgia/Myositis/Myopathy/Myotoxicity
(2004): Ray R+, *Pharmacoepidemiol Drug Saf* 13(9), 615 (39.5%)

Neurotoxicity
(2006): Seet RC+, *Ann Emerg Med* 47(4), 396

Rhabdomyolysis
(2006): Seet RC+, *Ann Emerg Med* 47(4), 396

Seizures
(2005): Schifano F+, *Hum Psychopharmacol* 20(5), 343
(2004): Ray R+, *Pharmacoepidemiol Drug Saf* 13(9), 615
(1994): Pathre AV+, *J Assoc Physicians India* 42(4), 327

Vertigo
(2006): Likar R+, *Clin Ther* 28(6), 943 (4.6%)
(2003): Radbruch L+, *Int J Clin Pract Suppl* (133), 15 (patch)
(1997): Wajima Z+, *Acta Anaesthesiol Scand* 41(8), 1061
(1993): Hayashi H+, *Masui* 42(12), 1763
(1988): Weiss P+, *Anasth Intensivther Notfallmed* 23(6), 309
(1982): Kjaer M+, *Br J Clin Pharmacol* 13(4), 487
(1982): Taguchi T, *Gan To Kagaku Ryoho* 9(2), 250
(1980): Cathelin M+, *Anesth Analg* (Paris) 37(5-6), 283

BUPROPION

Trade names: Wellbutrin (GSK); Zyban (GSK)
Indications: Depression, aid to smoking cessation
Category: Antidepressant; Dopamine reuptake inhibitor
Half-life: 14 hours
Clinically important, potentially hazardous interactions with: cyclosporine, erythromycin, escitalopram, isocarboxazid, methylphenidate, phenelzine, ritonavir, tranylcypromine, trimipramine

Reactions

Skin

Acne (1–10%)
Allergic reactions
Angioedema
Diaphoresis (5%)
(2001): Pederson KJ+, *Can J Cardiol* 17(5), 599
(1984): Feighner JP+, *Am J Psychiatry* 141(4), 525
(1983): Feighner JP, *J Clin Psychiatry* 44, 49
(1981): Halaris AE+, *Psychopharmacol Bull* 17, 140
Edema (>1%)
(1999): Peloso PM+, *JAMA* 282, 1817
Erythema multiforme
(2002): Drago F+, *Arch Intern Med* 162(7), 843
(2001): Carrillo-Jimenez R+, *Arch Intern Med* 161(12), 1556
(2001): Lineberry TW+, *Mayo Clin Proc* 76, 664
Exanthems (<0.1%)
(1983): Fabre LF+, *J Clin Psychiatry* 44, 88
(1981): Halaris AE+, *Psychopharmacol Bull* 17, 140
Exfoliative dermatitis
Lupus erythematosus
(2005): Cassis TB+, *Australas J Dermatol* 46(4), 266
(2004): Jumez N+, *Dermatology* 208(4), 362
Lupus panniculitis
(1986): Ottuso P, *The Schoch Letter*, 46, 37 (observation)
Peripheral edema
(1999): Peloso PM+, *JAMA* 282, 1817
Photosensitivity (<0.1%)
Pruritus (4%)
(2003): Litt JZ, Beachwood, OH (personal case) (observation)
(2002): Moreno Caballero+, *Aten Primaria* 30(10), 662
(1983): Cato AE+, *J Clin Psychiatry* 44, 187
Psoriasis
(2002): Cox NH+, *Br J Dermatol* 146(6), 1061
Rash (sic) (4%)
(2000): McCollom RA+, *Ann Pharmacother* 34, 471
(1985): Golden RN+, *Am J Psychiatry* 142, 1459 (vascular)
Stevens–Johnson syndrome
Urticaria
(2006): Litt JZ, Beachwood, OH (personal case) (observation)
(2004): Litt JZ, Beachwood, OH (personal case) (observation)
(2003): Chiaverini C+, *Ann Dermatol Venereol* 130(2), 208
(2003): Fays S+, *Br J Dermatol* 148(1), 177 (8 cases)
(2003): Litt JZ, Beachwood, OH (personal case) (observation) (generalized)
(2003): Loo WJ+, *Br J Dermatol* 149(3), 660 (generalized)
(1999): Peloso PM+, *JAMA* 282, 1817
(1983): Cato AE+, *J Clin Psychiatry* 44, 187
(1983): Fabre LF+, *J Clin Psychiatry* 44, 88
(1983): Feighner JP, *J Clin Psychiatry* 44, 49
(1983): Mendels J+, *J Clin Psychiatry* 44, 118
Xerosis (1–10%)

Mucosal/ENT
Bromhidrosis

Dysgeusia (4%)
   (1999): Berigan TR, *JAMA* 281, 233 (letter)
Gingivitis
Glossitis
Oral edema (<1%)
Sialorrhea
Stomatitis (>1%)
Tinnitus
   (1991): Settle EC, *J Clin Psychiatry* 52(8), 352
Tongue edema (0.1%)
   (2000): McCollom RA+, *Ann Pharmacother* 34, 471
Vaginitis
Xerostomia (up to 64%)
   (2003): Litt JZ, Beachwood, OH (personal case) (observation)
   (2003): West R, *Expert Opin Pharmacother* 4(4), 533
   (2002): Aubin HJ, *Drugs* 62 Suppl 2, 45
   (2002): George TP+, *Biol Psychiatry* 52(1), 53
   (2002): Tracey JA, *Expert Opin Drug* 1(4), 303
   (2002): Zwar N+, *Aust Fam Physician* 31(5), 443
   (2001): Johnston JA+, *Nicotine Tob Res* 3(2), 131
   (2000): Levine RS, *Br Dent J* 189(8), 412
   (1999): Settle EC+, *Clin Ther* 21, 454
   (1997): Hurd RD+, *N Engl J Med* 337, 1195
   (1991): James WA+, *South Med J* 84, 222
   (1986): Feighner JP+, *J Clin Psychopharmacol* 6, 27
   (1983): Chouinard G, *J Clin Psychiatry* 44, 121
   (1983): Feighner JP, *J Clin Psychiatry* 44, 49
   (1981): Halaris AE+, *Psychopharmacol Bull* 17, 140

Hair

Hair – alopecia (<1%)
   (2002): Klein AD, Statesboro, GA (from Internet) (observation)
Hair – hirsutism (1–10%)
Hair – pigmentation (<1%)

Eyes

Anisocoria
   (2007): Vleming EN+, *Arch Soc Esp Oftalmol* 82(8), 521
Visual hallucinations
   (2006): Charuvastra A+, *J Clin Psychiatry* 67(11), 1820 (tactile)
   (2005): Shepherd G, *Pharmacotherapy* 25(10), 1378
   (2002): Tracey JA+, *Ir Med J* 95(1), 23

Other

Anaphylactoid reactions/Anaphylaxis
   (2003): West R, *Expert Opin Pharmacother* 4(4), 533
Asthenia
   (2005): Shepherd G, *Pharmacotherapy* 25(10), 1378 (6%)
Cardiac arrest
   (2002): Tracey JA+, *Ir Med J* 95(1), 23
Chest pain
   (2003): de Graaf+, *Br J Clin Pharmacol* 56(4), 451
Death
   (2002): *Prescrire Int* 11(60), 117
   (2002): Wooltorton E, *CMAJ* 166(1), 68
Delirium
   (2006): Chan CH+, *J Clin Psychopharmacol* 26(6), 677 (with fluoxetine)
DRESS syndrome
   (2003): Bagshaw SM+, *Ann Allergy Asthma Immunol* 90(5), 572
Gynecomastia (<1%)
Headache
Hepatotoxicity
   (2000): Hu KQ+, *Dig Dis Sci* 45(9), 1872
Hot flashes
Hypersensitivity
   (2003): Ferry L+, *Int J Clin Pract* 57(3), 224 (0.12%)
   (2003): West R, *Expert Opin Pharmacother* 4(4), 533
   (2002): *Prescrire Int* 11(58), 49

(2002): Aubin HJ, *Drugs* 62 Suppl 2, 45 (0.1%)
   (2002): Zwar N+, *Aust Fam Physician* 31(5), 443
   (2001): Benson E, *Med J Aust* 174(12), 650
Inappropriate secretion of antidiuretic hormone (SIADH)
   (1984): Liskin B+, *J Clin Psychopharmacol* 4(3), 146
Mania
   (2000): Goren JL+, *Ann Pharmacother* 34(5), 619
Myalgia/Myositis/Myopathy/Myotoxicity (6%)
   (2003): Iskandar SB+, *Tenn Med* 96(10), 471
   (1999): Peloso PM+, *JAMA* 282, 1817
Paresthesias (2%)
Rhabdomyolysis
   (2004): Bobe F+, *Scand J Prim Health Care* 22(3), 191
   (1999): David D+, *J Clin Psychopharmacol* 19(2), 185
Seizures
   (2007): Rissmiller DJ+, *J Am Osteopath Assoc* 107(10), 441
   (2007): Vidal C+, *Ther Drug Monit* 29(3), 373
   (2005): *Prescrire Int* 14(78), 144 (in infant)
   (2005): Ross S+, *Expert Opin Drug Saf* 4(6), 995
   (2005): Shepherd G, *Pharmacotherapy* 25(10), 1378 (%)
   (2005): Solano Remirez M+, *An Med Interna* 22(8), 396
   (2004): Kuate C 1, *Rev Neurol* (Paris) 160(6-7), 701
   (2004): Shepherd G+, *J Emerg Med* 27(2), 147 (overdose) (11%)
   (2003): Balit CR+, *Med J Aust* 178(2), 61
   (2003): Ferry L+, *Int J Clin Pract* 57(3), 224 (0.1%)
   (2003): Gamarra M+, *Aten Primaria* 31(3), 202
   (2003): Hays JT+, *CNS Drugs* 17(2), 71
   (2003): Oncken CA+, *Nicotine Tob Res* 5(1), 131
   (2003): Reuther LO+, *Ugeskr Laeger* 165(14), 1447
   (2003): West R, *Expert Opin Pharmacother* 4(4), 533
   (2002): *Prescrire Int* 11(58), 49
   (2002): Aubin HJ, *Drugs* 62 Suppl 2, 45 (0.1%)
   (2002): Belson MG+, *J Emerg Med* 23(3), 223
   (2002): Bergmann F+, *J Clin Psychopharmacol* 22(6), 630
   (2002): Pesola GR+, *J Emerg Med* 22(3), 235
   (2002): Tracey JA, *Expert Opin Drug Saf* 1(4), 303
   (2002): Welsh CJ+, *N Engl J Med* 347(12), 951
   (2002): Wooltorton E, *CMAJ* 166(1), 68
   (2002): Zwar N+, *Aust Fam Physician* 31(5), 443
   (2001): Enns MW, *J Clin Psychiatry* 62(6), 476 (with trimipramine)
   (2001): Kwan AL+, *Ned Tijdschr Geneeskd* 145(6), 277
   (2001): Shah GD+, *Clin Neuropharmacol* 24(5), 304
   (1998): Dunner DL+, *J Clin Psychiatry* 59(7), 366
Serum sickness
   (2004): Hack S, *J Child Adolesc Psychopharmacol* 14(3), 478
   (2004): Ornetti P+, *Joint Bone Spine* 71(6), 583
   (2002): Wooltorton E, *CMAJ* 166(1), 68
   (2001): Davis JS+, *Med J Aust* 174, 479
   (2000): McCollom RA+, *Ann Pharmacother* 34, 471
   (1999): Peloso PM+, *JAMA* 282, 1817
   (1999): Tripathi A+, *Ann Allergy Asthma Immunol* 83, 165
   (1999): Yolles JC+, *Ann Pharmacother* 33, 931
Somnambulism
   (2003): Khazaal Y+, *Addict Biol* 8(3), 359
Somnolence
   (2005): Shepherd G, *Pharmacotherapy* 25(10), 1378
   (2002): Tracey JA+, *Ir Med J* 95(1), 23
Tremor (>10%)
   (2005): Shepherd G, *Pharmacotherapy* 25(10), 1378 (7%)
   (2003): Swan GE+, *Arch Intern Med* 163(19), 2337
   (1984): Feighner JP+, *Am J Psychiatry* 141(4), 525
Vertigo
   (2005): Shepherd G, *Pharmacotherapy* 25(10), 1378 (4%)

BUSPIRONE

Trade names: Ansail; Apo-Buspirone; Bespar; Biron; Busirone; BuSpar (Bristol-Myers Squibb); Bustab; Kallmiren; Narol; Neurosine; Nu-Buspirone
Indications: Anxiety
Category: Anxiolytic; Serotonin antagonist
Half-life: 2–3 hours
Clinically important, potentially hazardous interactions with: grapefruit juice, nefazodone, ritonavir, **St John's wort**

Reactions

Skin
Acne (<0.1%)
Allergic reactions
Bullous dermatitis (<1%)
Diaphoresis
 (1986): Newton RE+, *Am J Med* 3B:80, 17
Edema
Exanthems
Facial edema (1%)
Hypomelanosis
 (2002): Chapman MS+, *Am J Contact Dermat* 13(1), 46
Photo-recall
 (1989): Vassal G+, *Cancer Chemother Pharmacol* 23, 117
Pruritus (1%)
Purpura (1%)
Rash (sic) (<1%)
Seborrheic dermatitis
 (1993): Litt JZ, Beachwood, OH (personal case) (observation)
Urticaria (<1%)
Xerosis (1%)

Mucosal/ENT
Dysgeusia (<1%)
Glossodynia
Glossopyrosis
Parosmia (1%)
Sialorrhea
Tinnitus
Xerostomia (3%)

Hair
Hair – alopecia (1%)
 (2000): Mercke Y+, *Ann Clin Psychiatry* 12, 35
 (1995): Ljungman P+, *Bone Marrow Transplant* 15, 869

Nails
Nails – thinning (<0.1%)

Other
Chills
 (2004): Jagestedt M+, *Lakartidningen* 101(18), 1618 (with paroxetine)
Congestive heart failure
 (1988): Ritchie EC+, *J Clin Psychiatry* 49(6), 242
Fever
 (2004): Jagestedt M+, *Lakartidningen* 101(18), 1618 (with paroxetine)
Headache
Myalgia/Myositis/Myopathy/Myotoxicity
Paresthesias (1%)
 (1986): Newton RE+, *Am J Med* 3B:80, 17
Sjøgren's (Sicca) syndrome
Tremor
 (2004): Jagestedt M+, *Lakartidningen* 101(18), 1618 (with paroxetine)

BUSULFAN

Trade names: Citosulfan; Leukosulfan; Mablin; Misulban; Myleran (GSK)
Indications: Chronic myelogenous leukemia, bone marrow disorders
Category: Alkylating agent
Half-life: 3.4 hours (after first dose)
Clinically important, potentially hazardous interactions with: aldesleukin

Reactions

Skin
Allergic granulomatous angiitis (Churg–Strauss syndrome)
 (2002): Longo M+, *World Congress Dermatol* Poster, 0110
Bullous dermatitis
Eccrine squamous syringometaplasia
 (1997): Valks R+, *Arch Dermatol* 133, 873
Erythema (macular) (>10%)
 (1985): Hymes SR+, *J Cutan Pathol* 12, 125
Erythema multiforme (<1%)
 (1981): Weiss RB+, *Ann Intern Med* 94, 66
 (1980): Adrian RM+, *CA* 30, 143
Erythema nodosum (<1%)
Exanthems
 (1992): Fitzpatrick JE, *Derm Clinics* 10, 19 (passim)
Kaposi's sarcoma
 (1998): Roszkiewicz A+, *Cutis* 61, 137
Pigmentation (1–10%) ('busulfan tan')
 (1999): Simonart T+, *Ann Dermatol Venereol* (French) 126, 439
 (1992): Fitzpatrick JE, *Derm Clinics* 10, 19 (passim)
 (1985): Hymes SR+, *J Cutan Pathol* 12, 125
 (1983): Bronner AK+, *J Am Acad Dermatol* 9, 645
 (1981): Granstein RD+, *J Am Acad Dermatol* 5, 1 (brown-black)
 (1980): Adam BA+, *J Dermatol* 7, 405
Purpura
 (2001): Chuang C+, *Movement Disorders* 16, 990 (with cyclophosphamide)
Urticaria (>10%)
 (1981): Spiegel RJ, *Cancer Treat Rev* 8, 197
 (1981): Weiss RB+, *Ann Intern Med* 94, 66
Vasculitis
 (1992): Breathnach SM+, *Adverse Drug Reactions and the Skin* Blackwell, Oxford, 288 (passim)
 (1982): Weiss RB, *Sem Oncology* 9, 5
Xerosis

Mucosal/ENT
Cheilitis
 (1980): Wintroub B+, *Clinical Cancer Medicine* GK Hall and Company, 206
Dysgeusia
Oral mucositis
 (2006): Clopes A+, *Eur J Haematol* 77(1), 1
 (2000): Wardley AM+, *Br J Haematol* 110, 292
Oral pigmentation
Stomatitis

Hair
Hair – alopecia (>10%)
 (2005): Tosti A+, *Br J Dermatol* 152(5), 1056
 (2000): Tran D+, *Australas J Dermatology* 41, 106
 (1995): Ljungman P+, *Bone Marrow Transplant* 15, 869
 (1993): Vowels M+, *Bone Marrow Transplant* 12, 347

Nails
Nails – pigmentation

Other
Anhidrosis
Death
   (2004): Nakamae H+, *Chemotherapy* 50(4), 178
Gynecomastia (<1%)
Headache
Myoclonus
   (2006): Denison DJ+, *Saudi Med J* 27(4), 557
Porphyria cutanea tarda
   (1983): Bronner AK+, *J Am Acad Dermatol* 9, 645
Sjøgren's (Sicca) syndrome

BUTABARBITAL

Trade names: Butalan; Buticaps; Butisol (MedPointe); Day-Barb
Indications: Sedation
Category: Barbiturate
Half-life: 40–140 hours
Clinically important, potentially hazardous interactions with: alcohol, antihistamines, ardeparin, argatroban, brompheniramine, buclizine, chlorpheniramine, dalteparin, danaparoid, dicumarol, enoxaparin, ethanolamine, heparin, imatinib, tinzaparin, warfarin

Reactions

Skin
Acne
Angioedema (<1%)
Bullous dermatitis
Erythema multiforme
Exanthems
Exfoliative dermatitis (<1%)
Fixed eruption
Herpes simplex
Lupus erythematosus
Necrosis
Photosensitivity
Pruritus
Purpura
Rash (sic) (<1%)
Stevens–Johnson syndrome (<1%)
Toxic epidermal necrolysis
Urticaria
Vasculitis

Mucosal/ENT
Oral ulceration

Other
Porphyria variegata
Rhabdomyolysis
   (1990): Larpin R+, *Presse Med* 19(30), 1403
Thrombophlebitis (<1%)

BUTALBITAL

Trade names: Amaphen; Anoquan; Axotal; Butace; Esgic (Forest); Fioricet (Watson); Fiorinal (Watson); Marnal; Medigesic; Phrenilin; Tecnal
Indications: Tension headaches
Category: Barbiturate
Half-life: 35 hours
Clinically important, potentially hazardous interactions with: alcohol, dicumarol

Reactions

Skin
Bullous dermatitis
Erythema multiforme
   (1984): Gebel K+, *Dermatologica* 168, 35
Exanthems
Exfoliative dermatitis (<1%)
Fixed eruption
Herpes simplex
Lupus erythematosus
Necrosis
Photosensitivity
Pruritus
Purpura
Rash (sic) (1–10%)
Stevens–Johnson syndrome (<1%)
Toxic epidermal necrolysis
Urticaria
   (1993): Litt JZ, Beachwood, OH (personal case) (observation)
Vasculitis

Mucosal/ENT
Oral erythema multiforme
   (1984): Gebel K+, *Dermatologica* 168, 35
Oral ulceration

Other
Anaphylactoid reactions/Anaphylaxis (1–10%)
Headache
Porphyria variegata
Rhabdomyolysis
   (1990): Larpin R+, *Presse Med* 19(30), 1403

BUTORPHANOL

Trade names: Biforal; Busphen; Stadol (Bristol-Myers Squibb); Stadol NS
Indications: Pain, migraine
Category: Opiate agonist-antagonist
Half-life: 2.5–4 hours
Clinically important, potentially hazardous interactions with: cimetidine

Reactions

Skin
Clammy skin
Diaphoresis (1–10%)
Edema (<1%)
Exanthems
Gooseflesh

Pruritus (1–10%)
  (1989): Ackerman WE+, *Can J Anaesth* 36, 388
  (1981): Bernstein JE+, *J Am Acad Dermatol* 5, 227
Rash (sic) (<1%)
Urticaria (<1%)

Mucosal/ENT
Dysgeusia (3–9%)
Tinnitus
Xerostomia (3–9%)

Other
Headache
  (2005): Wermeling DP+, *Clin Ther* 27(4), 430 (17–46%)
Injection-site reactions (sic)
  (1986): Finucane BT+, *South Med J* 79(5), 548
Paresthesias
Vertigo
  (2005): Wermeling DP+, *Clin Ther* 27(4), 430 (46%)
  (2000): Desjardins PJ+, *J Oral Maxillofac Surg* 58(10 Suppl 2), 19
  (1995): Gora-Harper ML+, *Pharmacotherapy* 15(6), 798
  (1995): Hoffert MJ+, *Headache* 35(2), 65 (58%)

BUTTERBUR

Scientific names: *Petasites hybridus; Petasites officinalis*
Family: Asteraceae; Compositae
Trade and other common names: Blatterdock; bog rhubarb;
bogshorn; butterdock; butterfly dock; capdockin; flapperdock;
Petadolex (Weber & Weber)
Category: Anti-inflammatory
Purported indications and other uses: Allergic rhinitis,
asthma, bronchitis, chills, cough, dysmenorrhea, hay fever,
headache, heart tonic, migraine, peptic ulcer, appetite stimulant,
irritable bladder, poultice for wounds or skin ulcers
Half-life: N/A

Note: Petadolex formulation has had the potentially carcinogenic
pyrrolizidine alkaloids removed

Reactions

Skin
Edema (<0.1%)
  (2000): Grossmann WM+, *Int J Clin Pharmacol Ther* 38(9), 430
  (1996): Grossman W, *Der Freie Arzt* (German) 3, 44
Erythema (<0.1%)
  (2000): Grossmann WM+, *Int J Clin Pharmacol Ther* 38(9), 430
  (1996): Grossman W, *Der Freie Arzt* (German) 3, 44
Pruritus (<1%)
  (2002): Schapowal A, *Br Med J* 324(7330), 144
Rash (sic)
  (2000): Grossmann WM+, *Int J Clin Pharmacol Ther* 38(9), 430
  (1996): Grossman W, *Der Freie Arzt* (German) 3, 44

Eyes
Ocular pruritus (<1%)
  (2002): Schapowal A, *Br Med J* 324(733), 144

Other
Hypersensitivity (<0.1%)
  (2000): Grossmann WM+, *Int J Clin Pharmacol Ther* 38(9), 430
  (1996): Grossman W, *Der Freie Arzt* (German) 3, 44

CABERGOLINE

Trade name: Dostinex (Pfizer)
Indications: Hyperprolactinemia, parkinsonism
Category: Dopamine receptor agonist
Half-life: 63–69 hours

Reactions

Skin
Acne (1%)
  (1997): Rademaker M, New Zealand (from Internet)
    (observation)
Edema
  (1996): Inzelberg R+, *Neurology* 47(3), 785
Facial edema (1%)
Fixed eruption
  (1997): Rademaker M, New Zealand (from Internet)
    (observation)
Peripheral edema (1%)
  (2004): Bracco F+, *CNS Drugs* 18(11), 733 (16%)
Pruritus (1%)

Mucosal/ENT
Xerostomia (2%)

Hair
Hair – alopecia
  (2003): Miwa H+, *Parkinsonism Relat Disord* 10(1), 51

Eyes
Periorbital edema (1%)
Visual hallucinations
  (1993): Lera G+, *Neurology* 43(12), 2587 (5 cases)

Other
Asthenia
  (1993): Webster J+, *Clin Endocrinol (Oxf)* 39(3), 323 (10%)
  (1992): Webster J+, *Clin Endocrinol (Oxf)* 37(6), 534
  (1989): Ciccarelli E+, *J Clin Endocrinol Metab* 69(4), 725
Headache
  (2000): De Luis DA+, *J Endocrinol Invest* 23(7), 428
  (1993): Webster J+, *Clin Endocrinol (Oxf)* 39(3), 323 (13%)
  (1992): Webster J+, *Clin Endocrinol (Oxf)* 37(6), 534
  (1989): Ciccarelli E+, *J Clin Endocrinol Metab* 69(4), 725
Hot flashes (3%)
Hypotension
  (2004): Bracco F+, *CNS Drugs* 18(11), 733
  (1993): Webster J+, *Clin Endocrinol (Oxf)* 39(3), 323
  (1991): Cavallini A+, *Clin Neuropharmacol* 14(4), 343
  (1989): Ciccarelli E+, *J Clin Endocrinol Metab* 69(4), 725
Paresthesias (5%)
  (1996): Inzelberg R+, *Neurology* 47(3), 785
Vertigo
  (2004): Bracco F+, *CNS Drugs* 18(11), 733
  (2000): De Luis DA+, *J Endocrinol Invest* 23(7), 428
  (1993): Webster J+, *Clin Endocrinol (Oxf)* 39(3), 323 (13%)
  (1992): Webster J+, *Clin Endocrinol (Oxf)* 37(6), 534
  (1989): Ciccarelli E+, *J Clin Endocrinol Metab* 69(4), 725
  (1989): Ferrari C+, *J Clin Endocrinol Metab* 68(6), 1201

CAFFEINE

Scientific names: *Coffea arabica; Coffea canephora; Coffea robusta; Cola acuminata; guarana (Paullinia cupana); Thea sinensis; Theobroma cacao*
Family: Rubiales
Trade and other common names: 1, 3, 7 trimethylxanthine; Anacin; Aqua-Ban; Black tea; Cafergot; Cola; Coryban-D; Darvon Compound; Dexatrim; Dristan; Elsinore; Endolor; Esgic; Excedrin; Fioricet; Fiorinal; Midol; Migralam; NoDoz; Norgesic; Norgesic Forte; Synalgos-DC; Synalgos-DC-A; Triaminicin; Vanquish; Vivarin (GSK). Ingredient in: Adipokinetix
Category: Diuretic; Xanthine alkaloid
Purported indications and other uses: with ergotamine for migraine, with NSAIDs in analgesics, headache, respiratory depression in neonates, postprandial hypotension, enhances seizure duration in electroconvulsive therapy. Ingredient in cough and cold remedies
Half-life: 2–7 hours
Clinically important, potentially hazardous interactions with: carbamazepine, cimetidine, clozapine, **cocoa**, **ephedra**, fluorides, **ginseng**, **guarana**, idrocilamide, methoxsalen, mexiletine, phenylpropanolamine, zonisamide

Note: Caffeine is an addictive psychoactive substance. Spontaneous abortion and low birthweight babies have occurred in pregnant women consuming 150 mg caffeine per day. Abuse can lead to cardiac damage or death
Physical Dependence & Withdrawal of Caffeine
Common symptoms of caffeine withdrawal are headache; drowsiness; yawning, impaired concentration; lassitude; irritability; decreased contentedness, well-being and self-confidence; decreased sociability; flu-like symptoms; muscle aches and stiffness; hot or cold spells; nausea or vomiting; and blurred vision

Reactions

Skin
Angioedema
Bullous dermatitis
Burning (feet)
  (1982): Young JJ+, *Drug Intell Clin Pharm* 16(10), 779
Exfoliative dermatitis
Facial edema
Pemphigus
  (1990): Brenner S+, *Acta Derm Venereol* 70(4), 357
    (+paracetamol, chlorpheniramine, phenylephrine)
Pruritus
Purpura
Rash (sic)
Rosacea
  (2001): Goldman D, *J Am Acad Dermatol* 44(6), 995
Urticaria
  (2002): Fernandez-Nieto M+, *Allergy* 57(10), 967 (cola drink)
  (1999): Kubota Y+, *Eur J Dermatol* 9(7), 559 (+aspirin)
  (1993): Caballero T+, *J Investig Allergol Clin Immunol* 3(3), 160
  (1991): Quirce Gancedo+, *J Allergy Clin Immunol* 88(4), 680
  (1988): Pola J+, *Ann Allergy* 60(3), 207
Xanthoderma

Mucosal/ENT
Xerostomia
  (2002): Boozer CN+, *Int J Obes Relat Metab Disord* 26(5), 593
    (with ephedra)

Other
Anaphylactoid reactions/Anaphylaxis

  (2003): Infante S+, *Allergy* 58(7), 681
  (1999): Kubota Y+, *Eur J Dermatol* 9(7), 559 (+aspirin)
  (1983): Przybilla B+, *Hautarzt* (German) 34(2), 73
Chills
  (1988): Mattila M+, *Int Clin Psychopharmacol* 3(3), 215
Death (from abuse/overdose)
  (2003): Kanstrup MH+, *Ugeskr Laeger* 165(3), 239 (with ephedrine)
  (2001): Ahrendt DM, *Am Fam Physician* 63(5), 913
  (2000): Le Coz, *Presse Med* (French) 29(1), 33
  (2000): Tanskanen A+, *Eur J Epidemiol* 16(9), 789
  (2000): Zivkovic R, *Acta Med Croatica* 54(1), 33
  (1999): Zahn KA+, *J Emerg Med* 17(2), 289 (herbal ecstasy)
  (1998): Ferslew KE+, *J Forensic Sci* 43(5), 1082 (+clozapine, fluoxetine)
  (1997): Shum S+, *Vet Hum Toxicol* 39(4), 228
  (1990): Lake CR+, *Int J Obes* 14(7), 575 (+phenylpropanolamine)
  (1989): Mrvos RM+, *Vet Hum Toxicol* 31(6), 571 (diet pills)
  (1986): Hanzlick R+, *J Anal Toxicol* 10(3), 126
  (1985): Garriott JC+, *J Anal Toxicol* 9(3), 141
  (1985): Winek CL+, *Forensic Sci Int* 29(3–4), 207
  (1985): Zimmerman PM+, *Ann Emerg Med* 14(12), 1227
  (1981): Bryant J, *Arch Pathol Lab Med* 105, 685
  (1980): McGee MB, *J Forensic Sci* 25(1), 29
Depression
  (2002): Patten SB, *Expert Opin Pharmacother* 3(10), 1405
  (1996): Rapoport A+, *Headache* 36(1), 14 (+migraine medication)
Headache
Hypersensitivity
  (2002): Hinrichs R+, *Allergy* 57(9), 859
Paresthesias
  (2000): Yates KM+, *N Z Med* 113(1114), 315 (herbal ecstasy)
Rhabdomyolysis
  (1999): Kamijo Y+, *Vet Hum Toxicol* 41(6), 381 (oolong tea)
  (1998): Kasamatsu Y+, *Intern Med* 37(2), 169 (cold remedy)
  (1995): Dawson JK+, *J Accid Emerg Med* 12(1), 49 (+ephedrine, theophylline)
  (1991): Michaelis HC+, *J Toxicol Clin Toxicol* 29(4), 521 (overdose, +acetaminophen, phenazone)
  (1989): Wrenn KD+, *Ann Emerg Med* 18(1), 94 (overdose)
Seizures
  (2005): Haller CA+, *Clin Toxicol* (Phila) 43(1), 23
  (2001): Kockler DR+, *Pharmacotherapy* 21(5), 647 (with ephedra)
  (2000): Carrillo JA+, *Clin Pharmacokinet* 39(2), 127
Tremor
  (1992): Astrup A+, *Int J Obes Relat Metab Disord* 16(4), 269 (+ephedrine)
  (1991): Hughes JR+, *Arch Gen Psychiatry* 48(7), 611
  (1988): Mattila M+, *Int Clin Psychopharmacol* 3(3), 215 (+yohimbine)
  (1981): Malchow-Moller A+, *Int J Obes* 5(2), 183 (Elsinore[ephedrine])

CALCIPOTRIOL

Synonym: Calcipotriene
Trade name: Dovonex (Leo Pharma) (Galderma)
Indications: Psoriasis
Category: Antipsoriatic agent
Half-life: ~30 minutes

Reactions

Skin
Burning (sic) (>10%)
Contact dermatitis
  (2002): Park YK+, *Acta Derm Venereol* 82(1), 71
  (1999): Frosch PJ+, *Contact Dermatitis* 40(2), 66
  (1999): Krayenbuhl BH+, *Am J Contact Dermat* 10(2), 78
  (1996): Garcia-Bravo B+, *Am J Contact Dermat* 7(2), 118
  (1996): Molin L, *Acta Derm Venereol* 76(2), 163
  (1994): de Groot AC, *Contact Dermatitis* 30(4), 242 (2 cases)
  (1994): Steinkjer B, *Contact Dermatitis* 31(2), 122
  (1992): Bruynzeel DP+, *Br J Dermatol* 127(1), 66
Eczema
  (1996): Giordano-Labadie F+, *Ann Dermatol Venereol*
    123(3), 196
Erythema (1–10%)
Irritation (sic) (>10%)
  (1996): Darley CR+, *Br J Dermatol* 135(3), 390
Photosensitivity
  (1995): McKenna KE+, *Arch Dermatol* 131(11), 1305
Pigmentation
  (1998): Glaser R+, *Br J Dermatol* 139(1), 148
  (1996): Vazquez-Lopez F+, *Acta Derm Venereol* 76(5), 400
  (1995): Kokelj F+, *Acta Derm Venereol* 75(4), 307
Pruritus (>10%)
Psoriasis (1–10%)
  (2005): Tamiya H+, *Int J Dermatol* 44(9), 791 (aggravation)
Rash (sic)
Xerosis (1–10%)

CALCITONIN

Trade names: Calcimar (Sanofi-Aventis); Caltine; Cibacalcine;
Clasynar; Miacalcic; Miacalcin (Novartis)
Indications: Paget's disease of bone
Category: Parathyroid hormone antagonist
Half-life: 70–90 minutes

Reactions

Skin
Allergic reactions (sic)
  (2001): Rodriguez A+, *Allergy* 56(8), 801
Diaphoresis
Eczema
Exanthems
Granuloma annulare
  (1993): Goihman YM, *Int J Dermatol* 32, 150
Palmar–plantar tenderness
Peripheral edema
Pruritus
Rash (sic) (<1%)
Ulcerations
Urticaria (<1%)

Mucosal/ENT
Dysgeusia (metallic or salty)

Other
Anaphylactoid reactions/Anaphylaxis
  (2000): Porcel SL+, *Allergol Immunopathol* (Madr) 28(4), 243
Hypersensitivity
Injection-site edema (>10%)
Injection-site inflammation (>10%)

Injection-site pain
  (1988): Warrell RP+, *Ann Intern Med* 108, 669 (62%)
Paresthesias (<1%)

CALCIUM HYDROXYLAPATITE

Trade name: Radiesse (BioForm) (Radiance FM)
Indications: Correction of facial wrinkles and folds
Category: Dermal filler
Half-life: N/A
**Clinically important, potentially hazardous interactions
with:** anticoagulants, antiplatelet drugs, aspirin

Reactions

Skin
Edema
  (2006): Silvers SL+, *Plast Reconstr Surg* 118(3 Suppl), 34S
Erythema
  (2006): Silvers SL+, *Plast Reconstr Surg* 118(3 Suppl), 34S
Hematomas
  (2006): Jacovella PF+, *Plast Reconstr Surg* 118(3 Suppl), 15S
Nodular eruption
  (2006): Jansen DA+, *Plast Reconstr Surg* 118(3 Suppl), 22S
Pruritus
  (2006): Silvers SL+, *Plast Reconstr Surg* 118(3 Suppl), 34S

Other
Pain
  (2006): Silvers SL+, *Plast Reconstr Surg* 118(3 Suppl), 34S

CALFACTANT

Trade name: Infasurf (Forest)
Indications: Prevention of respiratory distress syndrome
Category: Pulmonary surfactant
Half-life: N/A

Reactions

Skin
Cyanosis 65%

CANDESARTAN

Trade names: Amias; Atacand (AstraZeneca)
Indications: Hypertension
Category: Angiotensin II receptor antagonist
Half-life: 9 hours

Reactions

Skin
Angioedema
  (2003): Hille K+, *Am J Ophthalmol* 135(2), 224
  (2002): Lo KS, *Pharmacotherapy* 22(9), 1176
Diaphoresis (>0.5%)
Edema
  (2001): Maekawa Y+, *Nippon Ronen Igakkai Zasshi* 38(5), 696
    (with amlodipine)
Erythema multiforme
  (2004): Ejaz AA+, *South Med J* 97(6), 614

Exanthems (<1%)
Jaundice
  (2003): Basile G+, *J Clin Gastroenterol* 36(3), 273
Linear IgA dermatosis
  (2003): Pena-Penabad C+, *Am J Med* 114(2), 163
Peripheral edema (>1%)
Perleche
  (2004): Chen C+, *Nephrologie* 25(3), 97
Pruritus
Psoriasis
  (2003): Kawamura A+, *Eur J Dermatol* 13(4), 406
Rash (sic) (>0.5%)
  (2004): Morton A+, *BMJ* 328(7430), 25
Urticaria

Mucosal/ENT
Ageusia
  (2004): Chen C+, *Nephrologie* 25(3), 97
Aphthous stomatitis
  (2004): Chen C+, *Nephrologie* 25(3), 97
Burning mouth syndrome
  (2004): Chen C+, *Nephrologie* 25(3), 97
Dysgeusia
  (2004): Chen C+, *Nephrologie* 25(3), 97
  (2004): Tsuruoka S+, *Br J Clin Pharmacol* 57(6), 807
Stomatitis
  (2004): Chen C+, *Nephrologie* 25(3), 97

Eyes
Glaucoma
  (2003): Hille K+, *Am J Ophthalmol* 135(2), 224

Other
Abdominal pain
  (2003): Basile G+, *J Clin Gastroenterol* 36(3), 273
Cough
  (2002): Cuspidi C+, *J Hypertens* 20(11), 2293
Headache
  (2004): Gleiter CH+, *Cardiovasc Drug Rev* 22(4), 263
  (2001): Neldam S+, *Drugs Aging* 18(3), 225
  (2000): See S+, *Am J Health Syst Pharm* 57(8), 739
Hypotension
  (2004): Young JB+, *Circulation* 110(17), 2618 (4%)
Myalgia/Myositis/Myopathy/Myotoxicity (>0.5%)
Paresthesias (>0.5%)
Upper respiratory infection
  (2004): Gleiter CH+, *Cardiovasc Drug Rev* 22(4), 263
Vertigo
  (2004): Gleiter CH+, *Cardiovasc Drug Rev* 22(4), 263
  (2001): Neldam S+, *Drugs Aging* 18(3), 225
  (2000): See S+, *Am J Health Syst Pharm* 57(8), 739

CAPECITABINE

Trade name: Xeloda (Roche)
Indications: Metastatic breast cancer
Category: Antimetabolite; Antineoplastic
Half-life: 0.5–1 hour

Reactions

Skin
Acral erythema
Dermatitis (37%)
  (2003): Wagstaff AJ+, *Drugs* 63(2), 217 (25%)
  (1999): Dooley M+, *Drugs* 58, 69

Diaphoresis (0.2%)
Edema (9%)
  (1996): Bajetta E+, *Tumori* 82, 450
Erythema
Exfoliative dermatitis (31–37%)
Hand–foot syndrome (7–58%)
  (2007): Bartsch R+, *J Clin Oncol* 25(25), 3853 (with trastuzumab)
  (2007): Kern E+, *Wien Med Wochenschr* 157(13-14), 337
  (2006): Blum JL+, *J Clin Oncol* 24(27), 4384 (with paclitaxel)
  (2006): Crane CH+, *J Clin Oncol* 24(7), 1145
  (2006): Gressett SM+, *J Oncol Pharm Pract* 12(3), 131
  (2006): Kara IO+, *Breast* 15(3), 414 (with docetaxel)
  (2006): Lin EH+, *Am J Clin Oncol* 29(3), 232
  (2006): Saif MW+, *Clin Colorectal Cancer* 6(3), 219
  (2006): Sharma R+, *Br J Cancer* 94(7), 964 (22%)
  (2006): Wolf JK+, *Gynecol Oncol* 102(3), 468
  (2006): Yamaguchi K+, *Gan To Kagaku Ryoho* 33(7), 891 (13%)
  (2006): Yerushalmi R+, *J Surg Oncol* 93(7), 529 (2%)
  (2005): Levy C+, *Cancer Treat Rev* 31 Suppl 4, S17
  (2005): Ramanathan RK+, *Cancer Chemother Pharmacol* 55(4), 354
  (2005): Rini BI+, *Cancer* 103(3), 553
  (2005): Walko CM+, *Clin Ther* 27(1), 23
  (2005): Wilkes GM+, *Clin J Oncol Nurs* 9(1), 103
  (2004): Guo L+, *Zhonghua Zhong Liu Za Zhi* 26(4), 250
  (2004): Heo YS+, *J Clin Pharmacol 2004 Oct* 44(10), 1166
  (2004): Hofheinz RD+, *Br J Cancer* 91(5), 834 (3%)
  (2004): Hong YS+, *Ann Oncol* 15(9), 1344 (9%)
  (2004): Lassere Y+, *Eur J Oncol Nurs* 8 Suppl 1, S31
  (2004): Lebowitz PF+, *Clin Cancer Res* 10(20), 6764
  (2004): Lee JJ+, *Jpn J Clin Oncol* 34(7), 400 (35%)
  (2004): Lokich J, *Cancer Invest* 22(5), 713 (8%)
  (2004): Mackey JR+, *Clin Breast Cancer* 5(4), 287 (30%)
  (2004): Marse H+, *Eur J Oncol Nurs* 8 Suppl, S16
  (2004): Morant R+, *Br J Cancer* 90(7), 1312
  (2004): Narasimhan P+, *Cutis* 73(2), 101 (3 cases)
  (2004): Park SH+, *Oncology* 66(5), 353
  (2004): Park YH+, *Br J Cancer* 90(7), 1329 (50%)
  (2004): Pierga JY+, *Breast Cancer Res Treat* 88(2), 117
  (2004): Rao S+, *Br J Cancer* 91(5), 839 (19.7%) (with mitomycin)
  (2004): Sakamoto J+, *Anticancer Drugs* 15(2), 137 (62%)
  (2004): Scheithauer W+, *Oncology (Williston Park)* 18(9), 1161
  (2004): Sternberg CN+, *Eur J Oncol Nurs* 8 Suppl, S4
  (2003): Chua DT+, *Oral Oncol* 39(4), 361 (58.8%)
  (2003): Gerbrecht BM, *Cancer Nurs* 26(2), 161
  (2003): Han JY+, *Cancer* 98(9), 1918 (33%) (with docetaxel)
  (2003): Jones KL+, *Pharmacotherapy* 23(8), 1076
  (2003): Kalbakis K+, *Int J Radiat Oncol Biol Phys* 56(5), 1284 (1 case)
  (2003): Makhnova EV+, *Vopr Onkol* 49(2), 193
  (2003): Risum S+, *Ugeskr Laeger* 165(33), 3161
  (2003): Scheithauer W+, *Ann Oncol* 14(12), 1735
  (2003): Vasey PA+, *Br J Cancer* 89(10), 1843
  (2003): Wagstaff AJ+, *Drugs* 63(2), 217 (25%)
  (2002): Abushullaih S+, *Cancer Invest* 20(1), 3 (68.3%)
  (2002): Dunst J+, *J Clin Oncol* 20(19), 3983
  (2002): Lin E+, *Oncology* 16(12 Suppl No 14), 31
  (2002): Liu X+, *Zhonghua Zhong Liu Za Zhi* 24(1), 71
  (2002): O'Shaughnessy J+, *J Clin Oncol* 20(12), 2812
  (2002): Rothenberg ML, *Oncology* 16(12), 16
  (2002): Scheithauer W+, *Ann Oncol* 13(10), 1583
  (2002): Wenzel C+, *Am J Kidney Dis* 39(1), 48 (7.7%)
  (2001): Chang DZ+, *Cancer Chemother Pharmacol* 48(6), 493 (67%)
  (2001): Elasmar SA+, *Jpn J Clin Oncol* 31(4), 172 (passim)
  (2001): Hoff PM+, *J Clin Oncol* 19(8), 2282
  (2001): McGavin JK+, *Drugs* 61(15), 2309
  (2001): O'Shaughnessy JA+, *Ann Oncol* 12(9), 1247
  (2001): Seitz JF, *Semin Oncol* 28(1 Suppl 1), 41

(1999): Blum JL, *Oncology* 57, 16
(1999): Blum JL+, *J Clin Oncol* 17, 485 (10%)
(1999): Dooley M+, *Drugs* 58, 69
(1999): Mrozek-Orlowski ME+, *Oncol Nurs Forum* 26, 753
(1999): Villalona-Calero MA+, *J Clin Oncol* 17(6), 1915 (with paclitaxel)
(1998): Budman DR+, *J Clin Oncol* 16, 1795

Lupus erythematosus
(2008): Weger W+, *J Am Acad Dermatol* 59(2), S4

Photo-recall (<1%)
(2006): Saif MW+, *Cancer Chemother Pharmacol* 58(6), 771
(2002): Camidge R+, *J Clin Oncol* 20(19), 4130
(2002): Ortmann E+, *J Clin Oncol* 20(13), 3029

Photosensitivity (<1%)
(2007): Hague JS+, *Clin Exp Dermatol* 32(1), 102 (lichenoid)
(2003): Phillips R, Melbourne, Australia (from Internet) (observation)
(2002): Willey A+, *J Am Acad Dermatol* 47(3), 453

Pigmentation
(2002): Liu X+, *Zhonghua Zhong Liu Za Zhi* 24(1), 71 (of vitiligo)
(2001): Schmid-Wendtner M-H+, *Lancet* 358, 1575

Pruritus

Purpura (0.2%)

Pyogenic granuloma
(2002): Piguet V+, *Br J Dermatol* 147(6), 1270

Rash (sic)

Ulcerations

Vesiculation

Vitiligo
(2001): Schmid-Wendtner MH+, *Lancet* 358(9293), 1575

Xerosis

Mucosal/ENT

Mucositis
(2004): Hofheinz RD+, *Br J Cancer* 91(5), 834 (3%) (with mitomycin)
(2001): Bell KA+, *J Am Acad Dermatol* 45(5), 790

Oral candidiasis (0.2%)

Oral ulceration

Stomatitis (24%)
(2006): Sharma R+, *Br J Cancer* 94(7), 964 (15%)
(2004): Hofheinz RD+, *Br J Cancer* 91(5), 834 (3%)
(2004): Pierga JY+, *Breast Cancer Res Treat* 88(2), 117
(2003): Han JY+, *Cancer* 98(9), 1918 (33%) (with docetaxel)
(2002): Liu X+, *Zhonghua Zhong Liu Za Zhi* 24(1), 71
(2002): Rothenberg ML, *Oncology (Huntingt)* 16(12), 16
(2001): Hoff PM+, *J Clin Oncol* 19(8), 2282
(2001): McGavin JK+, *Drugs* 61(15), 2309

Hair

Hair – alopecia (<1%)
(2003): Wagstaff AJ+, *Drugs* 63(2), 217
(2001): Hoff PM+, *J Clin Oncol* 19(8), 2282
(2001): McGavin JK+, *Drugs* 61(15), 2309
(2001): Oshaughnessy JA+, *Ann Oncol* 12(9), 1247

Nails

Nails – changes (sic) (7%)

Nails – hyponychial dermatitis
(2003): Chen GY+, *Br J Dermatol* 148, 1071 (with docetaxel)

Nails – loss
(2004): Mackey JR+, *Clin Breast Cancer* 5(4), 287 (45%)

Nails – onychomadesis
(2001): Chen G-Y+, *Br J Dermatol* 145(3), 521

Nails – paronychia
(2004): Guberman D, Jerusalem, Israel (fingers & toes) (from Internet) (observation)

Nails – subungual hyperkeratosis

(2006): Tejera A+, *Actas Dermosifiliogr* 97(8), 536 (with paclitaxel)

Other

Abdominal pain
(2006): Wolf JK+, *Gynecol Oncol* 102(3), 468
(2005): Walko CM+, *Clin Ther* 27(1), 23
(2003): Kalbakis K+, *Int J Radiat Oncol Biol Phys* 56(5), 1284 (1 case)

Asthenia
(2006): Blum JL+, *J Clin Oncol* 24(27), 4384
(2006): Sharma R+, *Br J Cancer* 94(7), 964 (27%)
(2006): Wolf JK+, *Gynecol Oncol* 102(3), 468
(2005): Walko CM+, *Clin Ther* 27(1), 23
(2004): Mackey JR+, *Clin Breast Cancer* 5(4), 287 (30%)
(2004): Pierga JY+, *Breast Cancer Res Treat* 88(2), 117
(2003): Han JY+, *Cancer* 98(9), 1918 (51%) (with docetaxel)
(2003): Wagstaff AJ+, *Drugs* 63(2), 217 (25%)
(2002): Liu X+, *Zhonghua Zhong Liu Za Zhi* 24(1), 71
(2002): Scheithauer W+, *Ann Oncol* 13(10), 1583

Cardiotoxicity
(2006): Wijesinghe N+, *Heart Lung Circ* 15(5), 337

Chest pain
(2006): Cardinale D+, *Can J Cardiol* 22(3), 251

Death
(2004): Pierga JY+, *Breast Cancer Res Treat* 88(2), 117
(2003): Han JY+, *Cancer* 98(9), 1918 (2 cases) (with docetaxel)

Fever
(2003): Kalbakis K+, *Int J Radiat Oncol Biol Phys* 56(5), 1284 (1 case)

Headache

Hypersensitivity (<1%)

Hypotension
(2006): Pagliaro LC+, *Urol Oncol* 24(6), 487

Infections (<1%)
(2004): Rao S+, *Br J Cancer* 91(5), 839 (2.3%) (with mitomycin)

Myalgia/Myositis/Myopathy/Myotoxicity (9%)
(1999): Villalona-Calero MA+, *J Clin Oncol* 17(6), 1915 (with paclitaxel)

Pain
(2006): Blum JL+, *J Clin Oncol* 24(27), 4384 (with paclitaxel)

Paresthesias (21%)

Thrombophlebitis (0.2%)

Vertigo
(2002): Liu X+, *Zhonghua Zhong Liu Za Zhi* 24(1), 71

CAPREOMYCIN

Trade names: Capastat (King); Ogostal
Indications: Tuberculosis
Category: Antibiotic
Half-life: 12 hours
Clinically important, potentially hazardous interactions with: aminoglycosides, non-depolarizing neuromuscular blocking agents

Reactions

Skin

Edema

Erythema

Exanthems

Pruritus

Rash (sic)

Urticaria

Mucosal/ENT
Tinnitus

Other
Hypersensitivity
Injection-site bleeding
Injection-site induration
Myalgia/Myositis/Myopathy/Myotoxicity
Pain
Vertigo

CAPSICUM

Scientific names: *Capsicum annuum; Capsicum baccatum; Capsicum chinense; Capsicum frutescens; Capsicum pubscens*
Family: Solanaceae
Trade and other common names: African chili; Bell pepper; Bird pepper; Capsaicin; Capsicool; Capsin; Capzasin-P; Cayenne; Cayenne Pepper; Chili; Dolorac; Goat's pod; Ici Fructus; Jalapeno; Louisiana long pepper; No Pain-HP; Oleoresin; Pain Doctor (with methyl-salicylate and menthol); Pain-X; Paprika; Pimento; R-Gel; Zanzibar pepper; Zostrix
Category: Rubefacient
Purported indications and other uses: nausea, neuropathic pain, osteoarthritis, fibromyalgia, anticarcinogen, rheumatoid arthritis, diabetic neuropathy, postherpetic neuralgia (shingles), psoriasis, pruritus, vitiligo, dyspepsia, flatulence, ulcers, stomach cramps, hypertension, improved circulation, weight-loss.
Half-life: N/A
Clinically important, potentially hazardous interactions with: ACE inhibitors, antiplatelet drugs, aspirin, disulfiram, heparin, latex, salicylic acid, theophylline, warfarin

Note: Pepper spray or gas contains 5% oleoresin capsicum (OC). It is used by police and in personal defense sprays

Reactions

Skin
Acute febrile neutrophilic dermatosis (Sweet's syndrome)
  (1993): Greer JM+, *Cutis* 51(2), 112
Adverse effects (sic)
  (2001): Keitel W+, *Arzneimittelforschung* 51(11), 896 (mild)
  (2001): Stam C+, *Br Homeopath J* 90(1), 21 (11%)
  (1991): Govindarajan VS+, *Crit Rev Food Sci Nutr* 29(6), 435
Allergic reactions (sic)
  (2002): Groenewoud GC+, *Clin Exp Allergy* 32(3), 434
  (1996): Sastre J+, *Allergy* 51(2), 117
Bullous dermatitis
  (1993): Greer JM+, *Cutis* 51(2), 112
Burning
  (2003): Fett DD, *Cutis* 72(1), 21
  (1998): Busker RW+, *Am J Forensic Med Pathol* 19(4), 309 (spray)
  (1990): Chan OY+, *J Soc Occup Med* 40(3), 111
  (1987): Jones LA+, *J Toxicol Clin Toxicol* 25(6), 483
Dermatitis
  (1996): Kanerva L+, *Contact Dermatitis* 35(3), 157
  (1995): Williams SR+, *Ann Emerg Med* 25(5), 713
  (1989): Burnett JW, *Cutis* 43(6), 534
Diaphoresis
  (1985): Locock, *Can Pharm J* 118, 517
Erosions
  (2000): Zollman TM+, *Ophthalmology* 107(12), 2186 (21%) (spray)

Erythema
  (1996): Watson WA+, *Ann Pharmacother* 30(7), 733
  (1993): Greer JM+, *Cutis* 51(2), 112
  (1987): Jones LA+, *J Toxicol Clin Toxicol* 25(6), 483
Erythema multiforme
  (1995): Raccagni AA+, *Contact Dermatitis* 33(5), 353
Inflammation
  (1998): Busker RW+, *Am J Forensic Med Pathol* 19(4), 309 (spray)
Irritation
  (2001): Babakhanian RV+, *Sud Med Ekspert* 44(1), 9 (spray)
Pustules
  (1993): Greer JM+, *Cutis* 51(2), 112
Sensitization
  (1997): Gallo R+, *Contact Dermatitis* 37(1), 36
Stinging
  (2003): Fett DD, *Cutis* 72(1), 21
Toxicoderma
  (1985): Rogov VD, *Vestn Dermatol Venerol* comp(5), 53
Urticaria
  (2003): Feldman H+, *Am J Emerg Med* 21(2), 159
  (1997): Foti C+, *Contact Dermatitis* 37(3), 135

Mucosal/ENT
Gingivitis
  (1991): Serio FG+, *J Periodontol* 62(6), 390
Mucosal bleeding
  (1987): Myers BM+, *Am J Gastroenterol* 82(3), 211

Eyes
Conjunctivitis
  (2003): Holopainen JM+, *Toxicol Appl Pharmacol* 186(3), 155 (spray)
  (1996): Lee RJ+, *J Am Optom Assoc* 67(9), 548 (spray)
  (1995): Steffee CH+, *Am J Forensic Med Pathol* 16(3), 185 (spray)
Epiphora
  (1996): Lee RJ+, *J Am Optom Assoc* 67(9), 548 (spray)
Ocular burning
  (1996): Watson WA+, *Ann Pharmacother* 30(7), 733 (spray)
Rhinoconjunctivitis
  (1998): Vega de la Osada F+, *Med Clin* (Barc) 111(7), 263

Other
Application-site burning
  (1992): Tandan R+, *Diabetes Care* 15(1), 8
Cough
  (1991): Blanc P+, *Chest* 99(1), 27
Death
  (2001): Olajos EJ+, *J Appl Toxicol* 21(5), 355 (spray)
  (1998): Pollanen MS+, *CMAJ* 158(12), 1603 (spray)
  (1995): Steffee CH+, *Am J Forensic Med Pathol* 16(3), 185 (spray)
  (1989): Mack RB, *N C Med J* 50(11), 627 (spray)
Fibrosis
  (1988): Escobar CH, *Rev ADM* 45(6), 369
Hypersensitivity
  (2002): Groenewoud GC+, *Clin Exp Allergy* 32(3), 434
  (1998): Busker RW+, *Am J Forensic Med Pathol* 19(4), 309 (spray)
Pain
  (2000): Zollman TM+, *Ophthalmology* 107(12), 2186 (spray)
  (1995): Steffee CH+, *Am J Forensic Med Pathol* 16(3), 185 (spray)
  (1992): Landau O+, *JAMA* 268(13), 1686
  (1991): Marabini S+, *Eur Arch Otorhinolaryngol* 248(4), 191
  (1987): Jones LA+, *J Toxicol Clin Toxicol* 25(6), 483

CAPTOPRIL

Synonym: ACE
Trade names: Acenorm; Acepril; Adocor; APO-Capto; Capoten (Par); Capozide (Par); Captolane; Captoril; Lopirin; Lopril; Nu-Capto; Precaptil
Indications: Hypertension
Category: Angiotensin-converting enzyme inhibitor
Half-life: <3 hours
Clinically important, potentially hazardous interactions with: amiloride, spironolactone, triamterene

Note: Capozide is captopril and hydrochlorothiazide

Reactions

Skin

Allergic granulomatous angiitis (Churg–Strauss syndrome)
    (1999): Winfred RI+, *South Med J* 92(9), 918
Allergic reactions (sic)
    (2001): Martinez JC+, *Allergol Immunopathol* (Madr) 29(6), 279
    (1998): Lluch-Bernal M+, *Contact Dermatitis* 39, 316
Angioedema (1–15%)
    (2002): Arzi H+, *Harefuah* 141(10), 869, 931 (tongue and oropharynax)
    (2001): Cohen EG+, *Ann Otol Rhinol Laryngol* 110(8), 701 (64 cases)
    (1998): Smoger SH+, *South Med J* 91, 1060
    (1997): Brown NJ+, *JAMA* 278, 232
    (1997): Tisch M+, *Anaesthesiol Intensivmed Notfallmed Schmerzther* (German) 32, 122
    (1996): Ekborn A+, *Lakartidningen* (Swedish) 93, 468
    (1996): Pillans PI+, *Eur J Clin Pharmacol* 51, 123
    (1995): Bauwens LJ+, *Ned Tijdschr Geneeskd* (Dutch) 139, 674
    (1995): Kozel MM+, *Clin Exp Dermatol* 20, 60
    (1993): Chu TJ+, *Ann Intern Med* 118, 314
    (1993): Thompson T+, *Laryngoscope* 103, 10
    (1992): Diehl KL+, *Dtsch Med Wochenschr* (German)117, 727
    (1992): Dobroschke B+, *Anasthesiol Intensivmed Notfallmed Schmerzther* (German) 27, 510
    (1992): Hedner T+, *BMJ* 304, 941
    (1992): Jason DR, *J Forensic Sci* 37, 1418 (fatal)
    (1992): Sanchez-Hernandez J+, *An Med Interna* (Spanish) 9, 572
    (1991): Pek F, *HNO* (German) 39, 410
    (1991): Roberts JR+, *Ann Emerg Med* 20, 555
    (1990): Cameron DI, *Can J Cardiol* 6, 265
    (1990): DiNardo LJ+, *Trans Pa Acad Ophthalmol Otolaryngol* 42, 998
    (1990): Gannon TH+, *Laryngoscope* 100, 1156
    (1990): McAreavey D+, *Drugs* 40, 326
    (1990): Motel PJ, *J Am Acad Dermatol* 23, 124
    (1990): Seidman MD+, *Otolaryngol Head Neck Surg* 102, 727
    (1990): Zech J+, *HNO* (German) 38, 143
    (1989): Barna JS+, *Va Med* 116, 147
    (1989): Werber JL+, *Otolaryngol Head Neck Surg* 101, 96
    (1988): Brogden RN+, *Drugs* 36, 540
    (1988): Slater EE+, *JAMA* 260, 967 (0.1%)
    (1988): Wernze H, *Z Kardiol* (German) 77, 61
    (1987): Edwards IR+, *Br J Clin Pharmacol* 23, 529
    (1987): Ferner RE+, *BMJ* 294, 1119
    (1987): No Author, *Am J Med* 82, 576
    (1987): Wood SM+, *BMJ* 294, 91
    (1986): Suarez M+, *Am J Med* 81, 336
    (1984): Jett GK, *Ann Emerg Med* 13, 489
    (1984): Materson BJ+, *Ann Intern Med* 144, 1947 (2.1%)
    (1984): Smit AJ+, *Clin Allergy* 14, 413 (2%)
    (1982): Vidt DG+, *N Engl J Med* 306, 214 (passim)
    (1980): Wilkin JK+, *Arch Dermatol* 116, 903 (15%)

Bullous dermatitis
    (1989): Klein LE+, *Cutis* 44, 393
Bullous pemphigoid
    (2000): Popescu C, Bucharest, Romania (from Internet) (observation)
    (1993): Fitzgerald DA, *Clin Exp Dermatol* 18, 196
    (1989): Mallet L+, *Drug Intell Clin Pharm* 23, 63
Dermatitis
    (2004): Pfutzner W+, *Acta Derm Venereol* 84(1), 91 (with fosinopril)
    (2001): Martinez JC+, *Allergol Immunopathol* (Madr) 29(6), 279 (positive patch test)
    (1990): Cnudde F+, *Contact Dermatitis* 23, 375
Erythema multiforme
Erythroderma
    (1989): Allegue F+, *Rev Clin Esp* (Spanish) 184, 210
    (1985): Goodfield MJ+, *BMJ* 290, 1111
Exanthems (4–7%)
    (1993): Fitzgerald DA, *Clin Exp Dermatol* 18, 196 (passim)
    (1990): Cnudde F+, *Contact Dermatitis* 23, 375
    (1990): McAreavey D+, *Drugs* 40, 326 (0.5–4%)
    (1990): Motel PJ, *J Am Acad Dermatol* 23, 124
    (1989): Clemens G+, *Verh Dtsch Ges Inn Med* (German) 95, 721
    (1989): Gomez-Martino-Arroyo JR+, *Rev Clin Esp* (Spanish) 184, 497
    (1988): Bretin N+, *Dermatologica* 177, 11
    (1988): Brogden RN+, *Drugs* 36, 540 (0.5–4%)
    (1988): Warner NJ+, *Drugs* 35 (Suppl 5), 89 (4–7%)
    (1985): Goodfield MJ+, *BMJ* 290, 1111
    (1985): Todd PA+, *Drugs* 31, 198
    (1984): Smit AJ+, *Clin Allergy* 14, 413 (7%)
    (1983): Romankiewicz JA+, *Drugs* 25, 6 (4.6%)
    (1983): Steinman TI+, *Am J Med* 75, 154
    (1982): Luderer JR+, *J Clin Pharm* 22, 151
    (1982): Vidt DG+, *N Engl J Med* 306, 214 (passim)
    (1980): Heel RC+, *Drugs* 20, 409 (8–14%)
    (1980): Wilkin JK+, *Arch Dermatol* 116, 903
Exfoliative dermatitis (<2%)
    (1990): Motel PJ, *J Am Acad Dermatol* 23, 124
    (1989): O'Neill PG+, *Tex Med* 85, 40
    (1988): Lai KN+, *Singapore Med J* 29, 526
    (1982): Solinger AM, *Cutis* 29, 437
Graft-versus-host reaction
    (1998): Jappe U+, *Hautarzt* (German) 49, 126 (passim)
Kaposi's sarcoma
    (1991): Larbre JP, *J Rheumatol* 18, 476
    (1990): Puppin D+, *Lancet* 336, 1251
Lichen planus (pemphigoides)
    (1986): Flageul B+, *Dermatologica* 173, 248
Lichenoid eruption
    (2002): Feijoo A+, *World Congress Dermatol* Poster, 0100 (generalized)
    (1996): Revenga-Arranz F+, *Rev Clin Esp* (Spanish) 196, 412
    (1994): Phillips WG+, *Clin Exp Dermatol* 19, 317
    (1992): Perez-Roldan E+, *Rev Clin Esp* (Spanish) 191, 501
    (1992): Wong SS+, *Acta Derm Venereol* (Stockh) 72, 358
    (1990): Pascual J+, *Nephron* 56, 110
    (1989): Cox NH+, *Br J Dermatol* 120, 319
    (1989): Rotstein E+, *Australas J Dermatol* 30, 9
    (1988): Bretin N+, *Dermatologica* 177, 11
    (1984): Smit AJ+, *Clin Allergy* 14, 413 (1%)
    (1983): Bravard P+, *Ann Dermatol Venereol* (French) 110, 433
    (1983): Bravard P+, *Presse Med* (French) 12, 577
    (1983): Reinhardt LA+, *Cutis* 31, 98
Linear IgA dermatosis
    (2003): Avci O+, *J Am Acad Dermatol* 48(2), 299 (passim)
    (2002): Cohen LM+, *J Am Acad Dermatol* 138, 29 (2 cases)
    (1998): Friedman IS+, *Int J Dermatol* 37, 608
    (1994): Kuechle MK+, *J Am Acad Dermatol* 30, 187

(1989): Klein LE+, *Cutis* 44, 393
Lupus erythematosus
  (2002): Ratliff NB 3rd, *J Rheumatol* 29(8), 1807
  (1995): Fernandez-Diaz ML+, *Lancet* 345, 398
  (1994): Yung RL+, *Rheum Dis Clin North Am* 20, 61
  (1993): Bertin P+, *Clin Exp Rheumatol* 11, 695
  (1993): Pelayo M+, *Ann Pharmacother* 27, 1541
  (1990): Sieber C+, *BMJ* 301, 669
  (1985): Patri P+, *Acta Derm Venereol* (Stockh) 65, 447
Mycosis fungoides
  (1995): Carroll J+, *Cutis* 56, 276 (pustular)
  (1986): Furness PN+, *J Clin Pathol* 39, 902
Palmar–plantar pustulosis
  (1995): Eriksen JG+, *Ugeskr Laeger* (Danish) 157, 3335
Pemphigus (<2%)
  (1995): Butt A+, *Br J Dermatol* 132, 315
  (1994): Kuechle MK+, *Mayo Clin Proc* 69, 1166
  (1994): Trinidad-Paz JM+, *Rev Clin Esp* (Spanish) 194, 999
  (1992): Kaplan RP+, *J Am Acad Dermatol* 26, 364
  (1992): Pinto GM+, *J Am Acad Dermatol* 27, 281 (vegetans)
  (1992): Ruocco V+, *Int J Dermatol* 31, 33
  (1991): Beaulieu P+, *Ann Dermatol Venereol* (French) 118, 547
  (1991): Korman NJ+, *J Invest Dermatol* 96, 273
  (1990): Black AK+, *Br J Dermatol* 123, 277
  (1990): Motel PJ, *J Am Acad Dermatol* 23, 124
  (1990): Ruocco V+, *Arch Dermatol* 126, 965
  (1988): Blanken R+, *Acta Derm Venereol* (Stockh) 68, 456
  (1988): Bretin N+, *Dermatologica* 177, 11
  (1987): Arnoux D+, *Ann Dermatol Venereol* (French) 114, 1241
  (1987): Katz RA+, *Arch Dermatol* 123, 20
  (1986): Ricci G+, *Recenti Prog Med* (Italian) 77, 321
  (1985): Bernard P+, *Ann Dermatol Venereol* (French) 112, 661
  (1982): Christeler A+, *Schweiz Med Wochenschr* (German) 112, 1483
  (1982): Ruocco V+, *Arch Dermatol Res* 274, 123
  (1981): Clement MI, *Arch Dermatol* 117, 525
  (1980): Parfrey PS+, *BMJ* 281, 194
Pemphigus foliaceus
  (2000): Ong CS+, *Australas J Dermatol* 41(4), 242
  (1981): Waeber B+, *J Clin Pharmacol* 21(11–12 Pt 1), 508
Penile ulcers
  (1983): Romankiewicz JA+, *Drugs* 25, 6 (4.6%)
  (1981): Nicholls MG+, *Ann Intern Med* 94, 695
Photosensitivity
  (2005): Perez-Ferriols A+, *Actas Dermosifiliogr* 96(3), 167
  (1994): Shelley WB+, *Cutis* 54, 70 (observation)
  (1990): Motel PJ, *J Am Acad Dermatol* 23, 124
  (1988): Mauduit G+, *Ann Dermatol Venereol* (French) 115, 167
Phototoxicity (<2%)
  (2005): Perez-Ferriols A+, *Actas Dermosifiliogr* 96(3), 167
Pigmentation
  (1990): Black AK+, *Br J Dermatol* 123, 277
  (1987): O'Neill MB+, *BMJ* 295, 33
Pityriasis rosea (<2%)
  (1990): Ghersetich I+, *G Ital Dermatol Venereol* (Italian) 125, 457
  (1990): Motel PJ, *J Am Acad Dermatol* 23, 124
  (1990): Wolf R+, *Dermatologica* 181, 51
  (1988): Bretin N+, *Dermatologica* 177, 11
  (1983): Reinhardt LA+, *Cutis* 31, 98
  (1982): Wilkin JK+, *Arch Dermatol* 118, 186
Pruritus (1–7%)
  (1992): Shelley WB+, *Cutis* 49, 391 (observation)
  (1990): Motel PJ, *J Am Acad Dermatol* 23, 124
  (1984): Materson BJ+, *Ann Intern Med* 144, 1947 (0.2%)
  (1983): Daniel F+, *Ann Dermatol Venereol* (French) 110, 441 (10%)
  (1983): Romankiewicz JA+, *Drugs* 25, 6 (4%)
  (1983): Steinman TI+, *Am J Med* 75, 154
  (1982): Liebau G, *Klin Wochenschr* (German) 60, 107

(1982): Vidt DG+, *N Engl J Med* 306, 214 (passim)
  (1980): Luderer JR+, *Clin Res* 28, 589A
Psoriasis
  (1995): Ikai K, *J Am Acad Dermatol* 32, 819
  (1993): Coulter DM+, *N Z Med J* 106, 392
  (1992): Shelley WB+, *Cutis* 50, 87 (observation)
  (1990): Sieber C+, *BMJ* 301, 669
  (1990): Wolf R+, *Dermatologica* 181, 51
  (1987): Hamlet DW+, *BMJ* 295, 1352
  (1987): Wolf R+, *Cutis* 40, 162
  (1986): Hauschild TT+, *Hautarzt* (German) 37, 274
Purpura
  (1989): Grosbois B+, *BMJ* 298, 189
Rash (sic) (4–7%)
  (2003): Pfeffer MA+, *N Engl J Med* 349(20), 1893
  (1990): Kahan A+, *Clin Pharmacol Ther* 47, 483
  (1985): Jenkins AC+, *J Cardiovasc Pharmacol* 7, S96
  (1984): Kubo SH+, *Ann Intern Med* 100, 616
  (1984): Martin MF+, *Lancet* 1, 1325
  (1983): Romankiewicz JA+, *Drugs* 25, 6
  (1983): Rotmensch HH+, *Pharmacotherapy* 3, 131
  (1983): Steinman TI+, *Am J Med* 75, 154
  (1982): Liebau G, *Klin Wochenschr* (German) 60, 107
  (1982): Rosendorff C, *S Afr Med J* 62, 593
  (1981): Luderer JR+, *Am J Med* 71, 493
Stevens–Johnson syndrome
  (1984): Pennell DJ+, *Lancet* 1, 463 (fatal)
Toxic epidermal necrolysis
  (2003): Alkurtass DA+, *Ann Pharmacother* 37(3), 380
  (1999): Winfred RI+, *South Med J* 92, 918
  (1983): Sala F+, *G Ital Dermatol Venereol* (Italian) 118, 89
Urticaria
  (1996): Pillans PI+, *Eur J Clin Pharmacol* 51, 123
  (1993): Fitzgerald DA, *Clin Exp Dermatol* 18, 196 (passim)
  (1988): Bretin N+, *Dermatologica* 177, 11
  (1988): Slater EE+, *JAMA* 260, 967
  (1987): Wood SM+, *BMJ* 294, 91
  (1985): Goodfield MJD+, *BMJ* 290, 1111
  (1984): Materson BJ+, *Ann Intern Med* 144, 1947 (1.4%)
  (1984): Smit AJ+, *Clin Allergy* 14, 413 (7%)
  (1980): Wilkin JK+, *Arch Dermatol* 116, 902
Vasculitis
  (1994): Dorman RL+, *AJR Am J Roentgenol* 163, 840
  (1990): Black AK+, *Br J Dermatol* 123, 277 (fatal)
  (1988): Lotti T+, *G Ital Dermatol Venereol* (Italian) 123, 657
  (1988): Miralles R+, *Ann Intern Med* 109, 514
  (1987): Laaban J+, *European Heart J* 8, 319
  (1984): Goodfield MJD+, *Lancet* 2, 517
  (1984): Smit AJ+, *Clin Allergy* 14, 413
Xerosis
  (1983): Smit AJ+, *Nephron* 34, 196

Mucosal/ENT

Ageusia (2–4%)
  (1997): Acanfora D+, *Am J Ther* 4, 181
  (1993): Fitzgerald DA, *Clin Exp Dermatol* 18, 196 (passim)
  (1988): Rumboldt Z+, *Int J Clin* 8(3), 181
  (1987): Edwards IR+, *Br J Clin Pharmacol* 23, 529
  (1987): O'Connor DT+, *J Clin Hypertens* 3(4), 405
  (1984): Martin MF+, *Lancet* 1, 1325
  (1983): Smit AJ+, *Nephron* 34, 196
  (1982): Liebau G, *Klin Wochenschr* (German) 60, 107
  (1982): Vidt DG+, *N Engl J Med* 306, 214 (passim)
Aphthous stomatitis (<2%)
  (1983): Daniel F+, *Ann Dermatol Venereol* (French) 110, 441
  (1982): Vidt DG+, *N Engl J Med* 306, 214 (passim)
  (1980): Heel RC+, *Drugs* 20, 409
Burning mouth syndrome
  (1992): Savino LB+, *Ann Pharmacother* 26(11), 1381
Dysgeusia (2–4%) (metallic or salty taste)

(2003): Pfeffer MA+, N Engl J Med 349(20), 1893
(2000): Zervakis J+, Physiol Behav 68, 405
(1993): Boyd I, Lancet 342, 304
(1993): Zazgornik J+, Lancet 341, 1542
(1990): Kahan A+, Clin Pharmacol Ther 47, 483
(1988): Jackson B+, Aust N Z J Med 18(1), 21
(1987): Robertson JI+, J Cardiovasc Pharmacol 10, S43
(1986): Packer M+, Ann Intern Med 104(2), 147
(1985): Jenkins AC+, J Cardiovasc Pharmacol 7, S96
(1985): Mauersberger H+, Lancet 1, 517
(1983): Kayanakis JG+, Arch Mal Coeur Vaiss (French) 76, 1065
(1983): Romankiewicz JA+, Drugs 25, 6
(1980): Atkinson AB+, Lancet 2(8186), 105

Glossitis
(1989): Drucker CR+, Arch Dermatol 125, 1437 (atrophic)
(1983): Romankiewicz JA+, Drugs 25, 6
(1981): Nicholls MG+, Ann Intern Med 94, 659

Glossopyrosis
(1989): Drucker CR+, Arch Dermatol 125, 1437

Oral burn
(1982): Vlasses PH+, BMJ 284, 1672

Oral mucosal eruption
(1989): Firth NA+, Oral Surg Oral Med Oral Pathol 67, 41 (lichenoid)
(1985): Todd PA+, Drugs 31, 198
(1980): Heel RC+, Drugs 20, 409

Oral ulceration
(2000): Madinier I+, Ann Med Interne (Paris) (French) 151, 248
(1993): Fitzgerald DA, Clin Exp Dermatol 18, 196 (passim)
(1987): Corone S+, Rev Med Interne 8(1), 73
(1982): Viraben R+, Arch Dermatol 118, 959

Sialorrhea
(1988): Biron P, Arch Intern Med 148(1), 245

Tongue ulceration
(1982): Viraben R+, Arch Dermatol 118, 959
(1982): Vlasses PH+, BMJ 284, 1672 (passim)
(1981): Nicholls MG+, Ann Intern Med 94, 659

Xerostomia (<2%)

Hair

Hair – alopecia (<2%)
(1994): Shelley WB+, Cutis 52, 264 (observation)
(1990): Motel PJ, J Am Acad Dermatol 23, 124
(1984): Leaker B+, Aust N Z J Med 14, 866
(1984): Smit AJ+, Clin Allergy 14, 413 (3%)
(1983): Smit AJ+, Nephron 34, 196

Hair – follicular mucinosis
(2005): Perez-Ferriols A+, Actas Dermosifiliogr 96(3), 167

Nails

Nails – dystrophy
(1984): Brueggemeyer CD+, Lancet 1, 1352
(1983): Smit AJ+, Nephron 34, 196

Other

Anaphylactoid reactions/Anaphylaxis (during hemodialysis)
(2002): Peces R, Nephrol Dial Transplant 17(10), 1859

Cough
(2005): Rodriguez-Moran M+, Clin Nephrol 64(2), 91
(2003): Pfeffer MA+, N Engl J Med 349(20), 1893
(2001): Adigun AQ+, West Afr J Med 20(1), 46–7
(2001): Huang PJ+, Cardiology 95(3), 146
(2001): Lee SC+, Hypertension 38(2), 166
(1998): Singh NP+, J Assoc Physicians India 46(5), 448
(1992): Lefebvre J+, Ann Pharmacother 26(2), 161
(1992): Reisin L+, Am J Cardiol 70(3), 398
(1992): Reisin L+, J Hum Hypertens 6(4), 333
(1991): Capella D+, Med Clin (Barc) 96(4), 126
(1991): Kaku T+, Nippon Ronen Igakkai Zasshi 28(3), 365
(1991): Katsumata U+, Tohoku J Exp Med 164(2), 103

(1991): Ogihara T+, Am J Hypertens 4(1 Pt 2), 46S
(1990): Bucca C+, Chest 98(5), 1133
(1990): Canessa PA+, Medicina (Firenze) 10(3), 296
(1990): Marcos Sanchez F+, Rev Clin Esp 186(7), 359
(1990): Nuss DW+, Ear Nose Throat J 69(9), 649
(1989): Katz A+, Harefuah 116(12), 632

Death

Gynecomastia
(2000): Hugues FC+, Ann Med Interne (Paris) (French) 151, 10 (passim)
(1990): Nakamura Y+, BMJ 300, 541
(1988): Markusse HM+, BMJ 296, 1262

Headache

Hepatotoxicity
(2006): Andrade RJ+, Hepatology 44(6), 1581

Inappropriate secretion of antidiuretic hormone (SIADH)
(1989): Inoue S+, Kokyu To Junkan 37(10), 1143

Myalgia/Myositis/Myopathy/Myotoxicity

Nephrotoxicity
(2006): Olowu WA+, Saudi J Kidney Dis Transpl 17(2), 216

Paresthesias (<2%)

Pseudolymphoma
(1986): Furness PN+, J Clin Pathol 39, 902
(1980): Wilkin JK+, Arch Dermatol 116, 902

CARAWAY

Scientific names: Apium carvi; Carum carvi
Family: Apiaceae Umbelliferae
Trade and other common names: Caraway seed; Carvene; Kummel
Category: Anti-inflammatory; Carminative
Purported indications and other uses: Hypotensive, dyspepsia, hysteria, tonic, stomachic, flatulent indigestion, flatulent colic of infants, fragrance, flavoring in foods, toothpaste, and cosmetics
Half-life: N/A

Reactions

Skin

Adverse effects (sic)
(1999): Madisch A+, Arzneimittelforschung 49(11), 925
(1996): May B+, Arzneimittelforschung 46(12), 1149

Allergic reactions (sic)
(1981): Niinimaki A+, Allergy 36(7), 487

Dermatitis
(2003): Ali BH+, Phytother Res 17(4), 299

Sensitivity
(2002): Moneret-Vautrin DA+, Allerg Immunol (Paris) 34(4), 135 (2%)

Urticaria
(1985): Wuthrich B+, Schweiz Med Wochenschr 115(11), 258

Eyes

Rhinoconjunctivitis
(2002): Garcia-Gonzalez JJ+, Ann Allergy Asthma Immunol 88(5), 518

Other

Anaphylactoid reactions/Anaphylaxis
(1985): Wuthrich B+, Schweiz Med Wochenschr 115(11), 258

Cough
(1988): Zuskin E+, Environ Res 47(1), 95 (occupational)

Hypersensitivity
(1984): Wuthrich B+, Dtsch Med Wochenschr 109(25), 981 (26%)

CARBACHOL

Trade names: Carbamann; Carbastat Ophthalmic (Novartis); Carboptic Ophthalmic (Miza; Optopics); Glaumarin; Isopto Carbachol Ophthalmic; Isopto Karbakolin; Karbakolin Isopto; Miostat Intraocular
Indications: Glaucoma
Category: Miotic; Muscarinic cholinergic agonist
Half-life: N/A
Clinically important, potentially hazardous interactions with: None

Reactions

Skin
Diaphoresis

Mucosal/ENT
Sialorrhea

Eyes
Conjunctivitis
Corneal edema
Eyelid twitching
Keratopathy
Miosis
  (1993): Roberts CW, *J Cataract Refract Surg* 19(6), 731
Ocular burning
Ocular stinging
Ophthalmitis

Other
Headache

CARBAMAZEPINE

Trade names: Apo-Carbamazepine; Atreol; Carbatrol; Epitol (Teva); Foxsalepsin; Kodapan; Lexin; Mazepine; Sirtal; Tegretol (Novartis); Tegretol XR; Teril; Timonil
Indications: Epilepsy, pain or trigeminal neuralgia
Category: Anticonvulsant; Antipsychotic; Mood stabilizer
Half-life: 18–55 hours
Clinically important, potentially hazardous interactions with: acetylcysteine, adenosine, aprepitant, aripiprazole, buprenorphine, **caffeine**, charcoal, clarithromycin, clobazam, clorazepate, clozapine, darunavir, dasatinib, delavirdine, dexamethasone, diltiazem, doxacurium, erythromycin, felodipine, fosamprenavir, imatinib, **influenza vaccines**, lapatinib, levetiracetam, lopinavir, methylprednisolone, midazolam, nelfinavir, prednisolone, propoxyphene, ritonavir, solifenacin, **St John's wort**, telithromycin, temsirolimus, terbinafine, troleandomycin, verapamil, voriconazole

Reactions

Skin
Acne keloid
  (1990): Grunwald MH+, *Int J Dermatol* 29, 559
Acute generalized exanthematous pustulosis (AGEP)
  (1999): Lachgar T, *Allerg Immunol* (Paris) (French) 31, 151
  (1999): Poster Exhibit #163, AAD Meeting, March 1999
    (Reported by ED and WB Shelley)
  (1996): Wolkenstein P+, *Contact Dermatitis* 35, 234
  (1995): Moreau A+, *Int J Dermatol* 34, 263 (passim)

  (1991): Roujeau J-C+, *Arch Dermatol* 127, 1333
Adverse effects (sic)
  (2003): Matthews R+, *Br Dent J* 194(3), 121
Allergic reactions (sic)
  (1999): Pasmans SG+, *Allergy* 54, 649
  (1995): Tijhuis GJ+, *Ned Tijdschr Geneeskd* (Dutch) 139, 2265
    (42 cases)
  (1993): Beran RG, *Epilepsia* 34, 163
  (1992): Dzianott A+, *Wiad Lek* (Polish) 45, 465
  (1985): Moore NC+, *Am J Psychiatry* 142, 974
Angioedema (<1%)
  (2006): Elias A+, *CNS Spectr* 11(5), 352
  (2001): Grieco A+, *Eur J Gastroenterol Hepatol* 13(8), 973
Bullous dermatitis (<1%)
  (2001): Grieco A+, *Eur J Gastroenterol Hepatol* 13(8), 973
  (1990): Gebauer K+, *Australas J Dermatol* 31, 89 (passim)
  (1988): Warnock JK+, *Am J Psychiatry* 145, 425
  (1983): Godden DJ+, *Postgrad Med J* 59, 336
Collagen disease
Dermatitis
  (1992): Duhra P+, *Contact Dermatitis* 27, 325
  (1991): Ljunggren B+, *Contact Dermatitis* 24, 259
  (1991): Rodriguez-Mosquera M+, *Contact Dermatitis* 25, 137
  (1989): Malanin G+, *Duodecim* (Finnish) 105, 784
  (1989): Terui T+, *Contact Dermatitis* 20, 260
  (1981): Roberts DL+, *Arch Dermatol* 117, 273
Diaphoresis (1–10%)
Eczema
  (1999): Ozkaya-Bayazit E+, *J Eur Acad Dermatol Venereol* 12, 182
  (1992): Duhra P+, *Contact Dermatitis* 27, 325
Edema
Eosinophilic pustular folliculitis (Ofuji's disease)
  (1998): Mizoguchi S+, *J Am Acad Dermatol* 38, 641
Epidermolysis bullosa
  (1992): Kong LN, *Chung Hua Hu Li Tsa Chih* (Chinese) 27, 495
Erythema (sheet-like)
  (2001): Gaida-Hommernick B+, *Epilepsia* 42(6), 793
Erythema multiforme
  (2004): Steinmann C+, *Psychiatr Prax* 31, S147
  (2003): Emmet SD, Solana Beach, CA (from Internet)
    (observation)
  (1999): Frederickson K (from Internet) (observation)
  (1994): Friedmann PS+, *Arch Dermatol* 130, 598
  (1993): Alanko K, *Contact Dermatitis* 29, 254
  (1993): Bruynzeel I+, *Br J Dermatol* 129, 45
  (1992): Chevenet C+, *Ann Dermatol Venereol* (French) 119, 929
  (1989): Alanko K+, *Acta Derm Venereol* (Stockh) 69, 223
  (1989): Busch RL, *N Engl J Med* 321, 692
  (1988): McDanal CE, *J Clin Psychiatr* 49, 369
  (1988): Warnock JK+, *Am J Psychiatry* 145, 425
  (1987): Fawcett RG, *J Clin Psychiatry* 48, 416
  (1986): Green ST, *Clin Neuropharmacol* 9, 561
  (1985): Delafuente JC, *Drug Intell Clin Pharm* 19, 114
  (1985): Patterson JF, *J Clin Psychopharmacol* 5, 185
  (1984): Meisel S+, *Clin Pharm* 3, 15
Erythema nodosum (<1%)
Erythroderma
  (2002): Kansky A+, *Acta Dermatoven* 11(3), 105
  (2000): Bugatti L, Italy (from Internet) (observation)
  (1998): Tayoro J+, *Therapie* 53, 513
  (1996): Okuyama R+, *J Dermatol* 23, 489
  (1995): Koga T+, *Contact Dermatitis* 33, 275
  (1993): Blasco-Sarramian A+, *An Med Interna* (Spanish) 10, 341
  (1990): Ruiz-Ezquerro JJ+, *An Med Interna* (Spanish) 31, 89
  (1989): Romaguera C+, *Contact Dermatitis* 20, 304
  (1987): Granier F+, *Rev Med Interne* (French) 8, 206
  (1986): Silva R+, *Contact Dermatitis* 15, 254
  (1982): Chennebault JM+, *Therapie* (French) 37, 106
  (1980): Gaulier A+, *Nouv Presse Med* (French) 9, 1388

Exanthems (>5%)
  (2006): Elias A+, *CNS Spectr* 11(5), 352
  (2006): Hung SI+, *Pharmacogenet Genomics* 16(4), 297
  (2003): Misra UK+, *Postgrad Med J* 79(938), 703 (with phenytoin)
  (2003): Warnock JK+, *Am J Clin Dermatol* 4(1), 21
  (2002): Kansky A+, *Acta Dermatoven* 11(3), 105
  (2002): Maradeix S+, *World Congress Dermatol* Poster, 0112
  (2000): Thaler D, Monona, WI (from Internet) (observation)
  (1999): Lombardi SM+, *Ann Pharmacother* 33, 571
  (1998): Nathan D+, *J Am Acad Dermatol* 38, 806
  (1997): Hyson C+, *Can J Neurol Sci* 24, 245
  (1995): Wolkenstein P+, *Arch Dermatol* 131, 544
  (1993): Alanko K, *Contact Dermatitis* 29, 254
  (1993): Hermle L+, *Nervenarzt* (German) 64, 208 (generalized)
  (1993): Konishi T+, *Eur J Pediatr* 152, 605
  (1990): Garavelli PL+, *Minerva Med* (Italian) 81, 115
  (1990): Gebauer K+, *Australas J Dermatol* 31, 89 (passim)
  (1989): Eames P, *Lancet* 1, 509
  (1988): Shear NH+, *J Clin Invest* 82, 1826
  (1988): Warnock JK+, *Am J Psychiatry* 145, 425
  (1984): Chadwick D+, *J Neurol Neurosurg Psychiatry* 47, 642 (17%)
  (1982): Breathnach SM+, *Clin Exp Dermatol* 7, 585 (4%)
  (1981): Sillanpää M, *Acta Neurol Scand* 64 (Suppl 88), 145
  (1981): Taylor MW+, *Practitioner* 225, 219
Exfoliative dermatitis
  (2001): Dintiman B, Fairfax, VA (from Internet) (observation)
  (1999): Lombardi SM+, *Ann Pharmacother* 33, 571
  (1996): Sigurdsson V+, *J Am Acad Dermatol* 35, 53
  (1996): Troost RJ+, *Pediatr Dermatol* 13, 316
  (1995): Bahamdan KA+, *Int J Dermatol* 34, 661
  (1995): Corazza M+, *Contact Dermatitis* 33, 447
  (1995): Koga T+, *Contact Dermatitis* 32, 181
  (1993): Alanko K, *Contact Dermatitis* 29, 254
  (1991): Blin O+, *Therapie* (French) 46, 91
  (1990): Gebauer K+, *Australas J Dermatol* 31, 89 (passim)
  (1989): Alanko K+, *Acta Derm Venereol* (Stockh) 69, 223
  (1989): Romaguera C+, *Contact Dermatitis* 20, 304
  (1989): Vaillant L+, *Arch Dermatol* 125, 299
  (1988): Cox NH+, *Postgrad Med J* 64, 249
  (1987): Gimenez Garcia RM+, *Rev Clin Esp* (Spanish) 181, 542
  (1987): Granier F+, *Rev Med Interne* 8, 206
  (1985): Camarasa JG, *Contact Dermatitis* 12, 49
  (1984): Shuttleworth D+, *Clin Exp Dermatol* 9, 421
  (1982): Reed MD+, *Clin Pharm* 1, 78
  (1981): Roberts DL+, *Arch Dermatol* 117, 273
Facial edema
  (2002): Kansky A+, *Acta Dermatoven* 11(3), 105
Fixed eruption (<1%)
  (2006): Alvarez VJ+, *Invest Clin* 47(1), 65
  (1997): Chan HL+, *J Am Acad Dermatol* 36, 259
  (1997): de Argila D+, *Allergy* 52, 1039
  (1993): Alanko K, *Contact Dermatitis* 29, 254
  (1990): Gaffoor PMA+, *Cutis* 45, 242 (passim)
  (1989): Stubb S+, *Br J Dermatol* 120, 583
  (1988): Bhariga JC+, *Sex Transm Dis* 15, 177
  (1988): Warnock JK+, *Am J Psychiatry* 145, 425
  (1985): Kauppinen K+, *Br J Dermatol* 112, 575
  (1984): Shuttleworth D+, *Clin Exp Dermatol* 9, 424
Lichenoid eruption
  (1994): Thompson DF+, *Pharmacotherapy* 14, 561
  (1990): Atkin SL+, *Clin Exp Dermatol* 15, 382
  (1990): Gebauer K+, *Australas J Dermatol* 31, 89 (passim)
  (1989): Ohtsuyama M+, *Nishinihon J Dermatol* (Japanese) 51, 958
  (1988): Yasuda S+, *Photodermatology* 5, 206 (photosensitive)
  (1981): Roberts DL+, *Arch Dermatol* 117, 273
Linear IgA dermatosis
  (2002): Cohen LM+, *J Am Acad Dermatol* 46(2), S32

Lupus erythematosus
  (2006): Amerio P+, *Eur J Dermatol* 16(3), 281
  (2006): Motta E+, *Neurol Neurochir Pol* 40(2), 151
  (2006): Pelizza L+, *Acta Biomed* 77(1), 17
  (2006): Wittchen F+, *Internist* (Berl) 47(1), 69
  (2006): You SL+, *Angew Chem Int Ed Engl* 45(32), 5246
  (2005): Capponi A+, *Arch Dermatol* 141(1), 103
  (1998): Bachmeyer C+, *Presse Med* (French) 27, 966
  (1998): Toepfer M+, *Eur J Clin Pharmacol* 54, 193 (late onset)
  (1997): Milesi-Lecat AM+, *Mayo Clin Proc* 72, 1145
  (1997): Reiffers-Mettelock J+, *Dermatology* 195, 306
  (1996): Ghorayeb I+, *Rev Med Interne* (French) 17, 503
  (1993): Drory VE+, *Clin Neuropharmacol* 16, 19 (passim)
  (1993): Ohashi T+, *Rinsho Shinkeigaku* (Japanese) 33, 1094
  (1992): Boon DM+, *Ned Tijdschr Geneeskd* (Dutch) 136, 2085 (disseminated)
  (1992): Kanno T+, *Intern Med* 31, 1303
  (1992): Schmidt S+, *Br J Psychiatry* 161, 560
  (1992): Yust I+, *Intern Med* 31, 1303
  (1991): De Giorgio CM+, *Epilepsia* 32, 128
  (1991): Jain KK, *Drug Saf* 6, 350
  (1990): Gebauer K+, *Australas J Dermatol* 31, 89 (passim)
  (1990): Oner A+, *Clin Neurol Neurosurg* 92, 261
  (1989): Drory VE+, *Clin Neuropharmacol* 12, 115
  (1987): Alballa S+, *J Rheumatol* 14, 599
  (1986): Leyh F+, *Z Haut* (German) 61, 611
  (1985): *Br Med J Clin Res Ed* 291, 1125
  (1985): Bateman DE, *Br Med J Clin Res Ed* 291, 632
  (1985): Lovisetto P+, *Recenti Prog Med* (Italian) 76, 84
  (1985): McNicholl B, *BMJ* 291, 1126
  (1983): Kolstee HJ, *Ned Tijdschr Geneeskd* (Dutch) 127, 1588
Lymphoma
  (2003): Cohen Y+, *Isr Med Assoc J* 5(6), 457
  (2001): Di Lernia V+, *Arch Dermatol* 137, 675
Mycosis fungoides
  (2003): Gul U+, *Ann Pharmacother* 37(10), 1441
  (1991): Rijlaarsdam U+, *J Am Acad Dermatol* 24(2 Pt 1), 219 (with phenytoin)
  (1990): Welykyi S+, *J Cutan Pathol* 17, 111
Pemphigus
  (2003): Patterson CR+, *Clin Exp Dermatol* 28(1), 98
Peripheral edema
  (2002): Valikhani M+, *World Congress Dermatol* Poster, 0131
  (1998): Heyer G+, *Hautarzt* (German) 49, 123
Petechiae
  (1993): Konishi T+, *Eur J Pediatr* 152, 605
Photosensitivity
  (2001): Hebert AA+, *J Clin Psychiatry* 62(suppl 14), 22
  (1991): Ljunggren B+, *Contact Dermatitis* 24, 259
  (1990): Gebauer K+, *Australas J Dermatol* 31, 89 (passim)
  (1989): Terui T+, *Contact Dermatitis* 20, 260
  (1988): Warnock JK+, *Am J Psychiatry* 145, 425
  (1988): Yasuda S+, *Photodermatology* 5, 206
  (1986): Silva R+, *Contact Dermatitis* 15, 54
  (1981): Sillanpää M, *Acta Neurol Scand* 64 (Suppl 88), 145
Pigmentation
Pruritus (<1%)
  (2003): Misra UK+, *Postgrad Med J* 79(938), 703 (with phenytoin)
  (2002): Kansky A+, *Acta Dermatoven* 11(3), 105
  (2001): Gaida-Hommernick B+, *Epilepsia* 42(6), 793
Psoriasis
  (1994): Brenner S+, *Isr J Med Sci* 30, 283
Purpura
  (2001): Hebert AA+, *J Clin Psychiatry* 62(suppl 14), 22
  (1988): Warnock JK+, *Am J Psychiatry* 145, 425
  (1984): Staughton RCD+, *J R Soc Med* 77 (Suppl 4), 6
Pustules
  (2002): Moreno-Ramirez D+, *Acta Derm Venereol* 82(5), 374

(1991): Kleier RS+, *Arch Dermatol* 127, 1361
(1990): Gebauer K+, *Australas J Dermatol* 31, 89 (passim)
(1988): Commens CA+, *Arch Dermatol* 124, 178
(1984): Staughton RCD+, *J R Soc Med* 77 (Suppl 4), 6
Rash (sic) (>10%)
(2007): Arif H+, *Neurology* 68(20), 1701
(2006): Dhand UK, *Muscle Nerve* 34(5), 646
(2003): Feliciani C+, *Int J Immunopathol Pharmacol* 16(1), 89 (8 cases)
(2003): Hogan RE+, *Clin Ther* 25(10), 2586 (3.4%)
(2003): Misra UK+, *Postgrad Med J* 79(938), 703
(1999): van Ginneken EE+, *Neth Med J* 54, 158
(1998): Cates M+, *Ann Pharmacother* 32, 884
(1996): Boyle N+, *Am J Psychiatry* 152, 1234
(1996): Puig L+, *Contact Dermatitis* 34, 435
(1994): Kramlinger KG+, *J Clin Psychopharmacol* 14, 408 (12%)
(1993): Hosoda N+, *Jpn J Psychiatry Neurol* 47, 300
(1993): Konishi T+, *Eur J Pediatr* 152, 605
(1991): Frederick TE, *Neurology* 41, 1328
(1991): Murphy JM+, *Neurology* 41, 144
(1990): Garavelli PL+, *Minerva Med* (Italian) 81, 115
(1983): Ponte CD, *Drug Intell Clin Pharm* 17, 642
(1983): Vick NA, *N Engl J Med* 309, 1193
Schamberg's disease
Side effects (sic)
(1994): Jones M+, *Dermatology* 188, 18 (4%)
Stevens–Johnson syndrome (1–10%)
(2007): Man CB+, *Epilepsia* 48(5), 1015
(2007): Yang CW+, *J Allergy Clin Immunol* 120(4), 870
(2006): Hung SI+, *Pharmacogenet Genomics* 16(4), 297
(2006): Lonjou C+, *Pharmacogenomics J* 6(4), 265
(2005): Devi K+, *Indian J Dermatol Venereol Leprol* 71(5), 325
(2005): Lin MS+, *Intern Med J* 35(3), 188
(2005): Mockenhaupt M+, *Neurology* 64(7), 1134
(2004): Chung WH+, *Nature* 428(6982), 486
(2004): Lam NS+, *J Microbiol Immunol Infect* 37(6), 366
(2003): Feliciani C+, *Int J Immunopathol Pharmacol* 16(1), 89
(2002): Garcia M+, *Dig Dis Sci* 47(1), 177
(2001): Duggal HS+, *J Assoc Physicians India* 49, 591
(2001): Hebert AA+, *J Clin Psychiatry* 62(suppl4), 22
(2000): Ramadasan P+, *J Assoc Physicians India* 48(7), 742
(2000): Straussberg R+, *Pediatr Neurol* 22, 231
(2000): Suarez Moro R+, *An Med Interna* (Spanish) 17, 105
(1999): DeToledo JC+, *Ther Drug Monit* 21(1), 137
(1999): Dhar S+, *Dermatology* 199, 194
(1999): Petter G+, *Hautarzt* (German) 50, 884
(1999): Ruble R+, *CNS Drugs* 12, 215
(1999): Rzany B+, *Lancet* 353, 2190
(1995): Huang SC+, *Gen Hosp Psychiatry* 17, 458
(1995): Hughes-Davies L, *N Engl J Med* 332, 959
(1995): Keating A+, *Ann Pharmacother* 29, 538
(1995): Wolkenstein P+, *Arch Dermatol* 131, 544
(1993): Konishi T+, *Eur J Pediatr* 152, 605
(1993): Leenutaphong V+, *Int J Dermatol* 32, 428
(1993): Pagliaro LA+, *Hosp Community Psychiatry* 44, 999
(1993): Server Climent M, *Aten Primaria* (Spanish) 11, 377
(1992): Chevenet C+, *Ann Dermatol Venereol* (French) 119, 929 (with brain irradiation)
(1990): Gebauer K+, *Australas J Dermatol* 31, 89 (passim)
(1990): Hoang-Xuan K+, *Neurology* 40, 1144 (with cranial irradiation)
(1990): Khe HX+, *Neurology* 40, 1144
(1990): Roustan G+, *Actas Dermosifiliogr* (Spanish) 81, 775
(1990): Wong KE, *Singapore Med J* 31, 432
(1989): Alanko K+, *Acta Derm Venereol* (Stockh) 69, 223
(1988): McDanal CE, *J Clin Psychiatr* 49, 369
(1988): Warnock JK+, *Am J Psychiatry* 145, 425
(1987): Fawcett RG, *J Clin Psychiatr* 48, 416
Toxic epidermal necrolysis (1–10%)
(2007): Huang LY+, *J Formos Med Assoc* 106(12), 1032 (fatal)

(2006): Hung SI+, *Pharmacogenet Genomics* 16(4), 297
(2006): Lonjou C+, *Pharmacogenomics J* 6(4), 265
(2005): Devi K+, *Indian J Dermatol Venereol Leprol* 71(5), 325
(2005): Lin MS+, *Intern Med J* 35(3), 188
(2005): Mansouri P+, *Arch Dermatol* 141(6), 788 (with lamotrigine)
(2004): Fischer M+, *Klin Padiatr* 216(5), 288
(2003): Feliciani C+, *Int J Immunopathol Pharmacol* 16(1), 89
(2002): Correia O+, *Arch Dermatol* 138, 29 (2 cases)
(2002): Jackel R+, *Anaesthesist* 51(10), 815
(2002): Kansky A+, *Acta Dermatoven* 11(3), 105
(2001): Udawat H+, *J Assoc Physicians India* 49, 918
(2000): Leyva L+, *J Allergy Clin Immunol* 105(1 Pt 1), 157
(1999): Dhar S+, *Dermatology* 199, 194
(1999): Egan CA+, *J Am Acad Dermatol* 40, 458
(1999): Petter G+, *Hautarzt* (German) 50, 884
(1999): Ruble R+, *CNS Drugs* 12, 215
(1999): Rzany B+, *Lancet* 353, 2190
(1997): Belgodere X+, *Arch Pediatr* (French) 4, 1020
(1997): Jarrett P+, *Clin Exp Dermatol* 22, 146
(1996): Blum L+, *J Am Acad Dermatol* 34, 1088
(1995): Sterker M+, *Int J Clin Pharmacol Ther* 33, 595
(1995): Urbanowski S+, *Wiad Lek* (Polish) 48, 154
(1995): Wolkenstein P+, *Arch Dermatol* 131, 544
(1994): Friedmann PS+, *Arch Dermatol* 130, 598
(1993): Correia O+, *Dermatology* 186, 32
(1993): Leenutaphong V+, *Int J Dermatol* 32, 428
(1993): Pagliaro LA+, *Hospital and Community Psychiatry* 44, 999
(1992): Park BK+, *Br J Clin Pharmacol* 34, 377
(1992): Weller M+, *Am J Psychiatry* 149, 1114
(1992): Weller M+, *Nervenarzt* (German) 63, 308
(1991): Sakellariou G+, *Int J Artif Organs* 14, 634
(1990): Gebauer K+, *Australas J Dermatol* 31, 89 (passim)
(1990): Roujeau JC+, *Arch Dermatol* 126, 37
(1988): Shear NH+, *J Clin Invest* 82, 1826
(1987): Guillaume JC I, *Arch Dermatol* 123, 1166
(1986): Rusciani L+, *G Ital Dermatol Venereol* (Italian) 121, 149
(1984): Husegaard HC+, *Ugeskr Laeger* (Danish) 146, 2784
(1984): Staughton RCD+, *J R Soc Med* 77 (Suppl 4), 6
(1982): Breathnach SM+, *Clin Exp Dermatol* 7, 585
Toxic pustuloderma (probably AGEP [ed])
(1990): Gebauer K+, *Australas J Dermatol* 31, 89
(1988): Commens CA+, *Arch Dermatol* 124, 178
(1984): Staughton RCD+, *J R Soc Med* 77 (Suppl 4), 6
Toxic-allergic shock
Toxicoderma
(1983): Rozov VD+, *Vestn Dermatol Venerol* (Russian) September, 48
Urticaria
(2001): Hebert AA+, *J Clin Psychiatry* 62(suppl 14), 22
(1993): Alanko K, *Contact Dermatitis* 29, 254
(1993): Konishi T+, *Eur J Pediatr* 152, 605
(1990): Gebauer K+, *Australas J Dermatol* 31, 89 (passim)
(1988): Warnock JK+, *Am J Psychiatry* 145, 425
(1987): Johannessen AC+, *Ugeskr Laeger* (Danish) 149, 376
(1984): Staughton RCD+, *J R Soc Med* 77 (Suppl 4), 6
Vasculitis
(1993): Drory VE+, *Clin Neuropharmacol* 16, 19 (passim)
(1990): Gebauer K+, *Australas J Dermatol* 31, 89 (passim)
(1987): Harats N+, *J Neurol Neurosurg Psychiatry* 50, 1241

Mucosal/ENT

Ageusia
(1996): Deguchi K+, *J Laryngol Otol* 110(6), 598
(1988): Barajas Garcia-Talavera F, *Neurologia* 3(3), 126
Auditory hallucinations
(2006): Beitinger PA+, *Pharmacopsychiatry* 39(5), 192
Dysgeusia
(1988): Barajas Garcia-Talavera F, *Neurologia* 3(3), 126
Glossitis

Mucocutaneous eruption
 (1999): Edwards SG+, *Postgrad Med J* 75, 680
 (1993): Konishi T+, *Eur J Pediatr* 152, 605
Mucocutaneous lymph node syndrome (Kawasaki syndrome)
 (1990): Gebauer K+, *Australas J Dermatol* 31, 89 (passim)
 (1987): Hicks RA+, *Pediatr Infect Dis J* 7, 525
Oral lichenoid eruption
 (1989): Ohtsuyama M+, *Nishinihon J Dermatol* (Japanese) 51, 958
Oral mucosal eruption
Oral ulceration
 (2003): Misra UK+, *Postgrad Med J* 79(938), 703 (with phenytoin)
 (2001): Hebert AA+, *J Clin Psychiatry* 62(suppl 14), 22
Stomatitis
Tinnitus
Tongue ulceration
 (1998): Melgarejo Moreno PJ+, *An Otorrinolaringol Ibero Am* (Spanish) 25, 167
Xerostomia

Hair

Hair – alopecia
 (2000): Mercke Y+, *Ann Clin Psychiatry* 12, 35 (~6%)
 (1997): Ikeda A+, *J Neurol Neurosurg Psychiatry* 63, 549
 (1996): McKinney PA+, *Ann Clin Psychiatry* 8, 183
 (1988): Warnock JK+, *Am J Psychiatry* 145, 425
 (1985): Shuper A+, *Drug Intell Clin Pharm* 19, 924
 (1982): Breathnach SM+, *Clin Exp Dermatol* 7, 585

Nails

Nails – discoloration (bluish-black)
 (1989): Mishra D+, *Int J Dermatol* 28, 460
Nails – hypoplasia
 (1985): Niesen M+, *Neuropediatrics* 16, 167
Nails – lichen planus
 (1989): Ohtsuyama M+, *Nishinihon J Dermatol* (Japanese) 51, 958
Nails – loss
 (1982): Breathnach SM+, *Clin Exp Dermatol* 7, 585
Nails – onychomadesis
 (1989): Mishra D+, *Int J Dermatol* 28, 460

Eyes

Dyschromatopsia
 (2000): Nousiainen I+, *Ophthalmology* 107, 884
Periorbital edema
 (2001): Dintiman B, Fairfax, VA (from Internet) (observation)
Visual hallucinations
 (2006): Beitinger PA+, *Pharmacopsychiatry* 39(5), 192

Other

Anticonvulsant hypersensitivity syndrome
 (2006): Beitinger PA+, *Pharmacopsychiatry* 39(5), 192
 (2006): Matsuda K+, *Prog Neuropsychopharmacol Biol Psychiatry* 30(4), 751
 (2006): So JS+, *Dermatology* 213(2), 166
 (2005): Hara H+, *Dermatology* 211(2), 159
 (2004): Duran-Ferreras E+, *Rev Neurol* 38(12), 1136
 (2004): Ogihara T+, *J Clin Psychopharmacol* 24(1), 105
 (2004): Papp Z+, *Orv Hetil* 145(32), 1665
 (2003): Bin-Nakhi HA+, *Med Princ Pract* 12(3), 197
 (2002): Galindo PA+, *J Investig Allergol Clin Immunol* 12(4), 299
 (2002): Kaur S+, *Pediatr Dermatol* 19(2), 142
 (2002): Metin A+, *World Congress Dermatol* Poster, 0116
 (2002): Romero Maldonado N+, *Eur J Dermatol* 12(5), 503
 (2000): Moore, SJ+, *J Med Genet* 37, 489
 (2000): Popescu C, Bucharest, Romania (from Internet) (observation)

 (1997): Morkunas AR+, *Crit Care Clin* 13(4), 727
 (1995): Vittorio CC+, *Arch Intern Med* 155(21), 2285
Chest pain
 (2006): Wittchen F+, *Internist (Berl)* 47(1), 69
Death
 (2006): Skopp G+, *Arch Kriminol* 217(5-6), 161 (with levetiracetam)
 (2002): Correia O+, *Arch Dermatol* 138, 29
Delirium
 (2001): Novakovic M+, *Psychiatr Prax* 28(1), 48
DRESS syndrome
 (2007): Reaud S+, *Gastroenterol Clin Biol* 31(2), 205
 (2006): Kim CW+, *J Korean Med Sci* 21(4), 768
 (2006): Obermoser G+, *J Am Acad Dermatol* 54(5), 913
 (2006): Yun SJ+, *Acta Derm Venereol* 86(3), 241 (with valproic acid)
 (2005): Syn WK+, *Int J Clin Pract* 59(8), 988
 (2004): Allam JP+, *Eur J Dermatol* 14(5), 339
 (2004): Valencak J+, *Int J Dermatol* 43(1), 51
 (2002): Maradeix S+, *World Congress Dermatol* Poster, 0112
 (2001): Descamps V+, *Arch Dermatol* 137, 301 (5 patients)
 (2001): Queyrel V+, *Rev Med Interne* 22(6), 582
Fetal hydantoin syndrome
 (2000): Moore SJ+, *J Med Genet* 37, 489
Headache
Hepatotoxicity
 (2006): Skopp G+, *Arch Kriminol* 217(5-6), 161 (with levetiracetam)
 (1999): Morales-Diaz M+, *Pharmacotherapy* 19(2), 252
 (1993): Martinez P+, *Rev Esp Enferm Dig* 84(2), 124
 (1989): Rodriguez Hernandez H+, *Rev Gastroenterol Mex* 54(4), 239
Hypersensitivity
 (2006): Alfirevic A+, *Pharmacogenet Genomics* 16(4), 287
 (2006): Beitinger PA+, *Pharmacopsychiatry* 39(5), 192
 (2006): Hung SI+, *Pharmacogenet Genomics* 16(4), 297
 (2006): Matsuda K+, *Prog Neuropsychopharmacol Biol Psychiatry* 30(4), 751
 (2006): Seitz CS+, *Ann Allergy Asthma Immunol* 97(5), 698
 (2005): Laad G+, *Indian J Dermatol Venereol Leprol* 71(1), 35
 (2003): Aihara Y+, *Br J Dermatol* 149(1), 165
 (2003): Feliciani C+, *Int J Immunopathol Pharmacol* 16(1), 89
 (2002): Kaur S+, *Pediatr Dermatol* 19(2), 142
 (2001): Bessmertny O+, *Ann Pharmacother* 35(5), 533
 (2001): Miranda-Romero A+, *Cutis* 67(1), 47
 (2001): Nashed MH+, *Pharmacotherapy* 21(4), 502
 (2001): Sekine N+, *JAMA* 285(9), 1153
 (2000): Bugatti L, Italy (from Internet) (observation)
 (2000): Elstner S+, *Fortschr Neurol Psychiatr* (German) 68, 188
 (2000): Ivry S+, *Harefuah* (Hebrew) 138, 545
 (2000): Straussberg R+, *Pediatr Neurol* 22, 231
 (2000): Verrotti A+, *Int J Immunopathol Pharmacol* 13(1), 49
 (1999): Balasubrananian S+, *Indian Pediatr* 36, 98
 (1999): Brown KL+, *Dev Med Child Neurol* 41, 267
 (1999): Eland IA+, *Epilepsia* 40(12), 1780
 (1999): Hamer HM+, *Seizure* 8, 190
 (1999): Lombardi SM+, *Ann Pharmacother* 33, 571
 (1999): Mesec A+, *J Neurol Neurosurg Psychiatry* 66, 249
 (1999): Moss DM+, *J Emerg Med* 17, 503
 (1999): Ronsdorf A+, *Schweiz Rundsch Med Prax* 88(41), 1660
 (1998): Dertinger S+, *J Hepatol* 28, 356
 (1998): Schlienger RG+, *Epilepsia* 39, S3 (passim)
 (1997): Morkunas AR+, *Crit Care Clin* 13, 727
 (1997): Pichler WJ+, *New Engl J Med* 336, 377
 (1997): Stein J+, *Dtsch Med Wochenschr* (German) 122, 314
 (1997): Tennis P+, *Neurology* 49, 542
 (1997): Waagner DC, *New Engl J Med* 336, 376
 (1996): *New Engl J Med* 335, 577
 (1996): Callot V+, *Arch Dermatol* 132, 1315
 (1996): Knowles SR+, *J Clin Psychopharmacol* 16, 263

(1996): Koopman R, Enschede, The Netherlands (from Internet) (observation)

(1996): Oakley A, Hamilton, New Zealand (from Internet) (observation)

(1995): Bellman B+, J Am Acad Child Adolesc Psychiatry 34, 1405

(1995): De Vriese AS+, Medicine Baltimore 74, 144

(1995): Periole B+, Ann Dermatol Venereol 122, 121

(1994): Alldredge BK+, Pediatr Neurol 10, 169

(1994): Gall H+, Hautarzt (German) 45, 494

(1994): Naranjo CA+, Clin Pharmacol Ther 56, 564

(1993): Handfield-Jones SE+, Br J Dermatol 129, 175

(1993): Parha S+, Eur J Pediatr 152, 1040

(1993): Scerri L+, Clin Exp Dermatol 18, 540

(1991): Baguena F+, Med Clin (Barc) (Spanish) 96, 237

(1991): Hosoda N+, Arch Dis Child 66, 722

(1989): Malanin G+, Duodecim (Finnish) 105, 784

(1983): Bernstein DI+, Clin Pediatr (Phila) 22, 524

Inappropriate secretion of antidiuretic hormone (SIADH)

(2005): Llinares-Tello F+, Rev Neurol 40(12), 768

(2001): Novakovic M+, Psychiatr Prax 28(1), 48

(1999): Inamura T+, No Shinkei Geka 27(1), 85

(1998): Perez-Camarero E+, Rev Neurol 27(157), 522

(1995): Boutros NN+, J Clin Psychiatry 56(8), 377

(1994): Van Amelsvoort T+, Epilepsia 35(1), 181

(1993): Atalay S+, Jpn Heart J 34(2), 239

(1992): Steelman R+, Spec Care Dentist 12(2), 79

(1990): Cooney JA, Am J Psychiatry 147(8), 1101

(1990): Emsley RA+, S Afr Med J 77(6), 307

(1989): Khan A+, Am J Psychiatry 146(12), 1639

(1985): Carranco E+, Arch Neurol 42(2), 187 (with erythromycin)

(1984): Appleby L, J Neurol Neurosurg Psychiatry 47(10), 1138

Lymphoproliferative disease

(1992): Schlaifer D+, Eur J Dermatol 48, 274

(1992): Sigal-Nahum M+, Br J Dermatol 127, 545

(1990): Katzin WE I, Arch Pathol Lab Med 114, 1244

(1987): Severson GS+, Am J Med 83, 597

(1984): Shuttleworth D+, Clin Exp Dermatol 9, 421

Nephrotoxicity

(2001): Mayan H+, Ann Pharmacother 35(5), 560

(1997): Eijgenraam JW+, Neth J Med 50(1), 25

Porphyria cutanea tarda

(1996): Leo RJ+, Am J Psychiatry 153, 443

Porphyria variegata

(2001): Grieco A+, Eur J Gastroenterol Hepatol 13(8), 973

Pseudolymphoma

(2006): Alvarez-Ruiz S+, Actas Dermosifiliogr 97(1), 43

(2001): Cogrel O+, Br J Dermatol 144(6), 1235

(2001): Miranda-Romero A+, Cutis 67(1), 47

(1999): Saeki H+, J Dermatol 26, 329

(1998): d'Incan M+, Ann Dermatol Venereol 125, 52

(1998): Nathan D+, J Am Acad Dermatol 38, 806

(1997): Kim ST+, Korea, American Academy of Dermatology Meeting (SF), Poster #82

(1997): Paramesh H+, Indian Pediatr 34, 829

(1996): Callot V+, Arch Dermatol 132, 1315

(1995): Magro CM+, J Am Acad Dermatol 32, 419

(1993): Rondas AA+, Ned Tijdschr Geneeskd (Dutch) 137, 1258

(1993): Sigal M+, Ann Dermatol Venereol (French) 120, 175

(1991): Rijlaarsdam U+, J Am Acad Dermatol 24(2), 216

(1990): Sinnige HAM+, J Intern Med 227, 355

(1986): Yates P+, J Clin Pathol 39, 1224

(1984): Shuttleworth D+, Clin Exp Dermatol 9, 424

Rhabdomyolysis

(1992): Zele I+, Minerva Med 83(12), 847

Seizures

(2006): Kikumoto K+, Epileptic Disord 8(1), 53

(2003): Yang MT+, Brain Dev 25(1), 51

(2002): Gansaeuer M+, Clin Electroencephalogr 33(4), 174

Serum sickness

(1993): Igarashi M+, Int Arch Allergy Immunol 100, 378

Thrombophlebitis

Vertigo

(2006): Bates DE+, Ann Pharmacother 40(6), 1190 (with antiretrovirals)

(2006): Owen RT, Drugs Today (Barc) 42(5), 283

Weight gain

(2007): Ben-Menachem, Epilepsia 48, 42

(2005): Ness-Abramof R+, Drugs Today (Barc) 41(8), 547

CARBENICILLIN

Trade names: Carbecin; Carbelin; Geocillin (Pfizer); Geopen; Pyopen

Indications: Urinary tract infections

Category: Antibiotic, penicillin

Half-life: 1.0–1.5 hours

Clinically important, potentially hazardous interactions with: anticoagulants, ceftobiprole, cyclosporine, demeclocycline, doxycycline, gentamicin, imipenem/cilastatin, methotrexate, minocycline, oxytetracycline, tetracycline

Reactions

Skin

Allergic reactions (sic)

(1994): Pleasants RA+, Chest 106, 1124 (in patients with cystic fibrosis)

Angioedema

Bullous dermatitis

Edema

Erythema multiforme

Erythema nodosum

Exanthems

Exfoliative dermatitis

Hematomas

Hemorrhage

Jarisch–Herxheimer reaction

Pruritus

Purpura

Rash (sic) (<1%)

(1991): Lang R+, Rev Infect Dis 13(1), 68

Stevens–Johnson syndrome

Toxic epidermal necrolysis

(1984): Westly ED+, Arch Dermatol 120, 721

Urticaria (<1%)

Vasculitis

Vesiculation

Mucosal/ENT

Dysgeusia (1–10%)

Glossitis (1–10%)

Glossodynia

Oral candidiasis

Stomatitis

Stomatodynia

Tongue black

Tongue furry

Vaginitis (<1%)

Xerostomia

Eyes

Punctate keratitis

(2003): Inoue K+, J Glaucoma 12(6), 480 (4%)

Vision blurred

Other
  Anaphylactoid reactions/Anaphylaxis
  Fever
    (1991): Lang R+, *Rev Infect Dis* 13(1), 68
  Headache
    (2003): Ozdemir M+, *Jpn J Ophthalmol* 47(1), 72
  Hypersensitivity
  Injection-site pain
  Seizures
  Serum sickness
  Thrombophlebitis (<1%)
    (1985): *Thorax* 40(5), 358
  Tremor
    (1988): Charak B+, *J Assoc Physicians India* 36(2), 184

CARBIDOPA

(See LEVODOPA)

CARBIMAZOLE

Trade names: Camazole; NeoMercazole (Amdipharm);
Thyrostat; Tyrazole
Indications: Hyperthyroidism
Category: Imidazole antithyroid agent
Half-life: 6–8 hours
**Clinically important, potentially hazardous interactions
with:** amiodarone, digoxin, theophylline

Note: Carbimazole is a pro-drug of Methimazole

Reactions

Skin
  Acute generalized exanthematous pustulosis (AGEP)
    (2006): Grange-Prunier A+, *Ann Dermatol Venereol* 133(8-9 Pt
    1), 708
  Dermatomyositis
    (2008): Alvarez F+, *Br J Dermatol* 158(1), 196
  Erythema nodosum
    (2002): Marazuela M+, *Endocr J* 49(3), 315
  Phototoxicity
    (1985): Goh CL+, *Contact Dermatitis* 12(1), 58
  Pruritus
  Rash (sic)
  Urticaria
  Vasculitis
    (2003): Day C+, *Nephrol Dial Transplant* 18(2), 429
    (1999): Yazbeck R+, *Rev Med Interne* 20(4), 350

Mucosal/ENT
  Hearing loss
    (1994): Hill D+, *BMJ* 309(6959), 929
  Sialadenitis
    (1996): Gaudouen Y+, *Ann Med Interne* (Paris) 147(6), 462
  Tinnitus
    (1994): Hill D+, *BMJ* 309(6959), 929

Hair
  Hair – alopecia

Other
  Abdominal pain
  Headache
  Hepatotoxicity

    (2006): Vilchez FJ+, *Ann Pharmacother* 40(11), 2059
    (2002): Woeber KA, *Endocr Pract* 8(3), 222
    (1996): Epeirier JM+, *Eur J Gastroenterol Hepatol* 8(3), 287
    (1993): Binder C+, *Dtsch Med Wochenschr* 118(42), 1515 (fatal)
    (1989): Ozenne G+, *J Clin Gastroenterol* 11(1), 95
    (1987): Cales P+, *Presse Med* 16(20), 1005
    (1986): Ayensa C+, *Arch Intern Med* 146(7), 1455
    (1981): Jenkins RM+, *Br J Clin Pract* 35(11-12), 415
  Hypersensitivity
    (2000): Vinzio S+, *Ann Endocrinol* (Paris) 61(2), 151
    (1993): Chena Alejandro JA+, *Rev Clin Esp* 193(8), 459
    (1981): Jenkins RM+, *Br J Clin Pract* 35(11-12), 415
  Myalgia/Myositis/Myopathy/Myotoxicity
    (1999): Marti J+, *Rev Neurol* 28(2), 217
    (1991): Pasquier E+, *Lancet* 338(8774), 1082
    (1989): Page SR+, *Lancet* 1(8644), 964
  Nephrotoxicity
    (2005): Calanas-Continente A+, *Thyroid* 15(3), 286
    (2003): Day C+, *Nephrol Dial Transplant* 18(2), 429

CARBINOXAMINE

Trade names: Allergefon; Andec; Biohist-LA; Carbic-D;
Carbiset; Cardec; Chemdec; Histex (TEAMM); Histin; Humex;
Lergefin; Maldec; Naldechol; Pediatex; Polistin T-caps;
Rondamine; Rondec; Sildec; Sinumine; Tuscal; Tussafed; Tylex;
Ziriton
Indications: Allergic rhinitis
Category: Histamine H1 receptor antagonist
Half-life: 10–20 hours

Reactions

Mucosal/ENT
  Xerostomia

Other
  Headache
  Vertigo

CARBOPLATIN

Trade names: Carboplat; Carbosin; Ercar; Oncocarbin;
Paraplatin (Bristol-Myers Squibb); Paraplatine
Indications: Various carcinomas and sarcomas
Category: Alkylating agent; Antineoplastic
Half-life: terminal: 22–40 hours
**Clinically important, potentially hazardous interactions
with:** aldesleukin

Reactions

Skin
  Allergic reactions (sic)
    (2001): Yu DY+, *J Pediatr Hematol Oncol* 23(6), 349 (11.1%)
  Depigmentation
    (1990): Costello SA+, *Clin Oncol R Coll Radiol* 2, 182
  Edema
    (2004): Furugen Y+, *Gan To Kagaku Ryoho* 31(8), 1205 (30%)
      (with docetaxel)
  Erythema (2%)
    (2001): Robinson JB+, *Gynecol Oncol* 82(3), 550
    (1995): Inbar M+, *Anticancer Drugs* 6, 775
  Exanthems

(1995): Inbar M+, *Anticancer Drugs* 6, 775
(1992): Beyer J+, *Bone Marrow Transplant* 10, 491
(1989): Wagstaff AJ+, *Drugs* 37, 162
Facial edema
(1992): Beyer J+, *Bone Marrow Transplant* 10, 491
Hand–foot syndrome
(2001): Verschraegen CF+, *Cancer* 92(9), 2327 (with doxorubicin)
Palmar fasciitis
(2006): Ollivier Y+, *Rev Med Interne* 27(4), 346
Photo-recall
(2006): Pinson PJ+, *Ned Tijdschr Geneeskd* 150(34), 1891 (myositis) (with gemcitabine)
(2004): Kundak I+, *Tumori* 90(2), 256 (with paclitaxel)
Pigmentation
(1992): Beyer J+, *Bone Marrow Transplant* 10, 491
(1991): Singal R+, *Pediatr Dermatology* 8, 231
Pruritus (2%)
(2001): Robinson JB+, *Gynecol Oncol* 82(3), 550
Rash (sic) (2%)
(2006): Winkeljohn D+, *Clin J Oncol Nurs* 10(5), 595
Raynaud's phenomenon
(2003): Clowse ME+, *J Rheumatol* 30(6), 1341 (with gemcitabine)
Scleroderma
(2002): Karim M+, *Clin Nephrol* 58(5), 384
Urticaria (2%)
(2004): Lee CW+, *Gynecol Oncol* 95(2), 370
(1996): Broome CB+, *Med Pediatr Oncol* 26, 105
(1995): Sredni B+, *J Clin Oncol* 13, 2342

Mucosal/ENT
Mucositis
(2002): Rein DT+, *Gynecol Oncol* 87(1), 98 (with docetaxel)
Oral lesions
(1989): Wagstaff AJ+, *Drugs* 37, 162
Ototoxicity
(2006): Buckner JC+, *J Clin Oncol* 24(24), 3871
(2006): Ozguroglu M+, *Int J Gynecol Cancer* 16 Suppl 1, 394 (with paclitaxel)
(2005): Knight KR+, *J Clin Oncol* 23(34), 8588
Stomatitis (>10%)
Tinnitus
(2005): Rybak LP, *Int Tinnitus J* 11(1), 23
(1988): Evans WK+, *Br J Cancer* 58(4), 464 (2 cases)

Hair
Hair – alopecia (3%)
(2002): *Lancet* 360(9332), 505 (with paclitaxel)
(2002): de Jonge ME+, *Bone Marrow Transplantation* 30, 593 (permanent) (with cyclophosphamide and thiotepa)
(2002): Rein DT+, *Gynecol Oncol* 87(1), 98 (with docetaxel)
(2002): Sehouli J+, *Gynecol Oncol* 85(2), 321 (with paclitaxel)
(1989): Wagstaff AJ+, *Drugs* 37, 162
Hair – alopecia areata
(2003): Motl SE+, *Pharmacotherapy* 23(1), 104 (recurrent) (with paclitaxel)
(2002): Rein DT+, *Gynecol Oncol* 87(1), 98
Hair – alopecia totalis
(2006): Pignata S+, *BMC Cancer* 6, 202 (with paclitaxel)

Nails
Nails – leukonychia
(2002): Lehoczky O+, *J Obstet Gynaecol* 22(6), 694 (with paclitaxel)

Eyes
Optic neuropathy
(2006): Schmack I+, *Am J Ophthalmol* 142(2), 310

Other
Anaphylactoid reactions/Anaphylaxis (<1%)
(2004): Choi J+, *Ann Allergy Asthma Immunol* 93(2), 137
(2003): Herzinger T+, *Dtsch Med Wochenschr* 128(30), 1595
(2003): Markman M+, *J Clin Oncol* 21(24), 4611
(2002): Ogle SK+, *J Pediatr Oncol Nurs* 19(4), 122
Asthenia
(2006): Buckner JC+, *J Clin Oncol* 24(24), 3871
(2006): Safra T+, *Isr Med Assoc J* 8(1), 27
Hepatotoxicity
(2006): Pignata S+, *BMC Cancer* 6, 202 (with paclitaxel)
Hypersensitivity (2%)
(2006): Gernez Y+, *Rev Mal Respir* 23(3 Pt 1), 269
(2006): Navo M+, *Gynecol Oncol* 103(2), 608 (3%)
(2006): Safra T+, *Isr Med Assoc J* 8(1), 27
(2004): Choi J+, *Ann Allergy Asthma Immunol* 93(2), 137 (30%)
(2004): Furugen Y+, *Gan To Kagaku Ryoho* 31(8), 1205 (25%) (with docetaxel)
(2004): Lee CW+, *Gynecol Oncol* 95(2), 370
(2003): Dizon DS+, *Gynecol Oncol* 91(3), 584
(2003): Jones R+, *Gynecol Oncol* 89(1), 112
(2003): Markman M+, *J Clin Oncol* 21(24), 4611
(2003): Moreno-Ancillo A+, *Allergol Immunopathol* (Madr) 31(6), 342
(2003): Rose PG+, *Gynecol Oncol* 89(3), 429 (4 cases, on rechallenge)
(2002): Chasen MR+, *Cancer Chemother Pharmacol* 50(5), 429
(2002): Markman M, *Gynecol Oncol* 84(2), 353
(2002): Porzio G+, *Eur J Gynaecol Oncol* 23(4), 335
(2001): Robinson JB+, *Gynecol Oncol* 82(3), 550 (with paclitaxel)
(1999): Menczer J+, *Eur J Gynaecol Oncol* 20, 214 (4 patients)
(1999): Schiavetti A+, *Med Pediatr Oncol* 32, 183 (9.2%)
(1999): Shukunami K+, *Gynecol Oncol* 72, 431
(1998): Kook H+, *Bone Marrow Transplant* 21, 727
(1996): Broome CB+, *Med Pediatr Oncol* 26, 105
Hypotension
(2006): Winkeljohn D+, *Clin J Oncol Nurs* 10(5), 595
Inappropriate secretion of antidiuretic hormone (SIADH)
(2005): Yokoyama Y+, *Eur J Gynaecol Oncol* 26(5), 531
Injection-site pain (>10%)
Nephrotoxicity
(2007): Stohr W+, *Pediatr Blood Cancer* 48(2), 140 (mild)
(2006): Ozguroglu M+, *Int J Gynecol Cancer* 16 Suppl 1, 394 (with paclitaxel)
(2003): Miyazaki J+, *Nippon Rinsho* 61(6), 973
(2001): Kintzel PE, *Drug Saf* 24(1), 19
(2000): Gerke P+, *J Cancer Res Clin Oncol* 126(3), 173
(1998): Agraharkar M+, *Am J Kidney Dis* 32(5), E5
(1997): Beyer J+, *Bone Marrow Transplant* 20(10), 813
Neurotoxicity
(2006): Bamias A+, *BMC Cancer* 6, 228 (with paclitaxel)
(2006): Bell J+, *Gynecol Oncol* 102(3), 432 (with paclitaxel)
(2006): Pignata S+, *BMC Cancer* 6, 202 (with paclitaxel)
(2004): Furugen Y+, *Gan To Kagaku Ryoho* 31(8), 1205 (6%) (with docetaxel)
Thrombosis
(2006): Yeung KK+, *Vascular* 14(1), 51

CARISOPRODOL

Synonyms: carisoprodate; isobamate
Trade names: Artifar; Carisoma; Myolax; Sanoma; Sodol; Soma (MedPointe); Somadril; Soridol
Indications: Painful musculoskeletal disorders
Category: Central muscle relaxant
Half-life: 4–6 hours
Clinically important, potentially hazardous interactions with: eucalyptus

Reactions

Skin
Angioedema (1–10%)
Dermatitis
Diaphoresis
(1983): Rollings HE+, *Curr Ther Res* 34, 926
Edema
(1983): Rollings HE+, *Curr Ther Res* 34, 926
Erythema multiforme (<1%)
Exanthems
Fixed eruption (<1%)
Photosensitivity
(1994): Hazen PG, *J Am Acad Dermatol* 31, 498
Pruritus (<1%)
Rash (sic) (<1%)
Urticaria (<1%)
(2002): Fernandez-Rivas M+, *Allergy* 57(1), 55

Mucosal/ENT
Tinnitus
Xerostomia
(1983): Rollings HE+, *Curr Ther Res* 34, 926

Other
Anaphylactoid reactions/Anaphylaxis
Headache
Paresthesias
(1983): Rollings HE+, *Curr Ther Res* 34, 926
Pseudoporphyria
(1994): Hazen PG, *J Am Acad Dermatol* 31, 498

CARMUSTINE

Synonym: BCNU
Trade names: Becenun; BiCNU (Bristol-Myers Squibb); Carmubris; Gliadel Wafer (Guilford); Nitrumon
Indications: Brain tumors, Hodgkin's disease, multiple myeloma
Category: Alkylating agent; Nitrosourea
Half-life: initial: 1.4 minutes; secondary: 20 minutes
Clinically important, potentially hazardous interactions with: aldesleukin, cimetidine, clorazepate

Reactions

Skin
Dermatitis (<1%)
(2000): Thomson KF+, *Contact Dermatitis* 42(2), 112
(1994): Zackheim HS, *Semin Dermatol* 13, 202
(1990): Zackheim HS+, *J Am Acad Dermatol* 22, 802
Eccrine squamous syringometaplasia
(1997): Valks R+, *Arch Dermatol* 133, 873
Erythema

(1992): Breathnach SM+, *Adverse Drug Reactions and the Skin* Blackwell, Oxford, 292
Exanthems
Pigmentation (on accidental contact)
(1982): Dunagin WG, *Semin Oncol* 9, 14
Telangiectasia
(1994): Zackheim HS, *Semin Dermatol* 13, 202
(1992): Breathnach SM+, *Adverse Drug Reactions and the Skin* Blackwell, Oxford, 292
Tenderness (sic)
(1992): Breathnach SM+, *Adverse Drug Reactions and the Skin* Blackwell, Oxford, 292

Mucosal/ENT
Oral mucositis
(2000): Wardley AM+, *Br J Haematol* 110, 292
Stomatitis (1–10%)

Hair
Hair – alopecia (1–10%)

Other
Gynecomastia
Headache
Injection-site burning (>10%)
Injection-site necrosis
(1987): Dufresne RG, *Cutis* 39, 197
Injection-site pain
Nephrotoxicity
(2001): Kintzel PE, *Drug Saf* 24(1), 19

CARTEOLOL

Trade names: Arteolol; Arteoptic; Calte; Carteol; Endak; Mikelan; Ocupress (ophthalmic) (Novartis); Teoptic
Indications: Glaucoma, hypertension
Category: Adrenergic beta-receptor antagonist
Half-life: 6 hours
Clinically important, potentially hazardous interactions with: clonidine, epinephrine, verapamil

Note: Cutaneous side effects of beta-receptor blockaders are clinically polymorphous. They apparently appear after several months of continuous therapy. Atypical psoriasiform, lichen planus-like, and eczematous chronic rashes are mainly observed. (1983): Hödl St, *Z Hautkr* (German) 1:58, 17

Reactions

Skin
Acne
Angioedema
Cold extremities
Dermatitis (eye-drops)
(2001): Holdiness MR, *Am J Contact Dermat* 12(4), 217
(2000): Quiralte J+, *Contact Dermatitis* 42, 245
(1999): Sanchez-Perez J+, *Contact Dermatitis* 41(5), 298
Diaphoresis (<1%)
(1997): Schmutz JL+, *Dermatology* 194, 197 (from topical)
Edema
Exanthems
Exfoliative dermatitis
Facial edema
Lupus erythematosus
Peripheral edema (<1%)
Photosensitivity

Pigmentation
Pruritus
Psoriasis
Purpura (<1%)
Rash (sic) (2.5%)
Raynaud's phenomenon (<1%)
Vesiculobullous eruption
Xerosis

Mucosal/ENT

Dysgeusia (from topical application)
Tinnitus
Xerostomia

Hair

Hair – alopecia

Nails

Nails – discoloration (bluish)

Eyes

Eyelid eczema
(1997): Giordano-Labadie F+, *Ann Dermatol Venereol*
124(4), 322

Other

Anaphylactoid reactions/Anaphylaxis
Headache
Myalgia/Myositis/Myopathy/Myotoxicity
Paresthesias (2%)
Peyronie's disease

CARVEDILOL

Trade names: Coreg (GSK); Dibloc; Dilatrend; Dimitone;
Kredex; Querto
Indications: Hypertension
Category: Adrenergic beta-receptor antagonist
Half-life: 7–10 hours

Reactions

Skin

Allergic reactions (sic) (<1%)
(1998): Simpson SH+, *Can J Cardiol* 14, 1277
Angioedema
(1988): Ogihara G+, *Drugs* 36, 75 (<1%)
Diaphoresis (2.9%)
Edema (generalized) (5.1%)
Erythema multiforme
Exanthems (<1%)
(2000): Litt JZ, Beachwood, OH (personal case) (observation)
(1988): Ogihara G+, *Drugs* 36, 75 (2%)
Exfoliative dermatitis (<1%)
Peripheral edema (1.4%)
Photosensitivity (<1%)
Pruritus (<1%)
(2000): Litt JZ, Beachwood, OH (personal case) (observation)
Psoriasis (<1%)
Purpura (1–10%)
Rash (sic) (<1%)
Stevens–Johnson syndrome
(1997): Kowalski BJ+, *Am J Cardiol* 80, 669
Toxic epidermal necrolysis

Mucosal/ENT

Xerostomia (<1%)

Hair

Hair – alopecia (<0.1%)

Other

Anaphylactoid reactions/Anaphylaxis (<1%)
Asthenia
(2005): Acharya NV+, *Int J Clin Pharmacol Ther* 43(1), 1
Congestive heart failure
(2004): Palloshi A+, *Am J Cardiol* 94(11), 1456
Headache
Hypotension
(2000): Brunner M+, *Am J Cardiol* 85(10), 1173
(2000): Joye F, *Presse Med* 29(18), 1027
Infections (2.2%)
Myalgia/Myositis/Myopathy/Myotoxicity (3.4%)
Pain (8.6%)
Paresthesias (2%)
Vertigo
(2005): Acharya NV+, *Int J Clin Pharmacol Ther* 43(1), 1

CASCARA

Scientific names: *Frangula purshianus; Rhamnus purshiana*
Family: Rhamnaceae
Trade and other common names: Bitter bark; Buckthorn;
Californian buckthorn; Cascara sagrada; Chittem bark; Pursh's
buckthorn; Yellow bark
Category: Stimulant laxative
Purported indications and other uses: Atonic constipation,
dyspepsia, colitis, diverticulitis, dyspepsia, gallstones, gout,
hemorrhoids, hypertension, indigestion, insomnia, jaundice, liver
disease, nervous disorders, parasites, stomach disorders
Half-life: N/A
**Clinically important, potentially hazardous interactions
with:** antiarrhythmics, cardiac glycosides, corticosteroids,
licorice, thiazide diuretics

Reactions

None

CASPOFUNGIN

Trade name: Cancidas (Merck)
Indications: Invasive Aspergillus infection
Category: Antimycobacterial, echinocandin
Half-life: Beta phase: 9–11 hours; terminal: 40–50 hours
**Clinically important, potentially hazardous interactions
with:** cyclosporine, rifampicin, tacrolimus

Reactions

Skin

Diaphoresis (<1%)
Edema (~3%)
Erythema (1–2%)
Facial edema (3%)
Pruritus (2–3%)
Rash (sic) (1–4%)
Vasculitis (2%)

Other

Anaphylactoid reactions/Anaphylaxis (<2%)
Chills (~3%)
Fever
  (2003): Denning DW, *Lancet* 362(9390), 1142
  (2003): Johnson MD+, *Expert Opin Pharmacother* 4(5), 807
  (2002): Stone EA+, *Clin Ther* 24(3), 351
  (2001): Keating GM+, *Drugs* 61(8), 1121
Headache
  (2003): Johnson MD+, *Expert Opin Pharmacother* 4(5), 807
  (2002): Stone EA+, *Clin Ther* 24(3), 351
Injection-site induration (~3%)
Injection-site reactions (sic) (2–12%)
  (2004): Walsh TJ+, *N Engl J Med* 351(14), 1391 (35.1%)
  (2002): *Prescrire Int* 11(61), 142
  (2002): Stone EA+, *Clin Ther* 24(3), 351
  (2001): Keating GM+, *Drugs* 61(8), 1121
Myalgia/Myositis/Myopathy/Myotoxicity (~3%)
Nephrotoxicity
  (2005): Wegner B+, *Nephrol Dial Transplant* 20(10), 2071
Pain (1–5%)
Paresthesias (1–3%)
Phlebitis (~16%)
  (2003): Denning DW, *Lancet* 362(9390), 1142
Thrombophlebitis
  (2003): Johnson MD+, *Expert Opin Pharmacother* 4(5), 807
Tremor (<2%)

CEFACLOR

Trade names: Alfatil; Apo-Cefaclor; CEC 500; Ceclor (Lilly); Cefabiocin; Distaclor; Kefolor; Panoral; Sigacefal
Indications: Various infections caused by susceptible organisms
Category: Cephalosporin, 2nd generation
Half-life: 0.6–0.9 hours

Note: Penicillin and cephalosporins share a common beta-lactam structure. People who are allergic to penicillin are approximately 4 times more likely to develop an allergic reaction to a cephalosporin than those people who have no penicillin allergy. (From 5 to 16% of patients allergic to penicillin develop reactions to cephalosporins)

Reactions

Skin

Acute generalized exanthematous pustulosis (AGEP)
  (1995): Moreau A+, *Int J Dermatol* 34, 263 (passim)
  (1992): Ogoshi M+, *Dermatology* 184, 142
Angioedema (<1%)
  (1998): Litt JZ, Beachwood, OH (personal case) (observation)
Dermatitis
  (1986): Hirata M+, *Kokyu To Junkan* (Japanese) 34, 791
Edema
  (1995): Dark DS+, *Infections in Medicine* October, 551
Erythema multiforme
  (2000): Ibia EO+, *Arch Dermatol* 136, 849
  (1999): Joubert GI+, *Can J Clin Pharmacol* 6, 197 (17 cases)
  (1988): Platt R+, *J Infect Dis* 158, 474 (0.6%)
  (1985): Levine LR, *Ped Infect Dis* 4, 358 (0.6%)
  (1982): Lovell SJ+, *Can Med Assoc J* 126, 1032
  (1980): Murray DL+, *N Engl J Med* 303, 1003
Exanthems
  (2000): Ibia EO+, *Arch Dermatol* 136, 849
  (1996): Nagayama H+, *J Dermatol* 23, 899
  (1994): Litt JZ, Beachwood, OH (personal case) (observation)
  (1994): Shelley WB+, *Cutis* 53, 40 (observation)

  (1987): Norrby SR, *Drugs* 34 (Suppl 2), 105 (1–5%)
  (1986): Ascher H, *Lakartidningen* (Swedish) 83, 411
  (1985): Murray DL+, *Pediatr Infect Dis* 4, 706
  (1983): Johnson T, *J Ark Med Soc* 80, 110
  (1982): Lovell SJ+, *Can Med Assoc J* 126, 1032
  (1981): Ackley AM+, *Southern Med J* 74, 1550
  (1980): Murray DL+, *N Engl J Med* 303, 1003
Fixed eruption
  (2005): Aihara Y+, *Pediatr Int* 47(6), 616
Pruritus (<1%)
  (1998): Litt JZ, Beachwood, OH (personal case) (observation)
  (1988): Platt R+, *J Infect Dis* 158, 474
  (1982): Lovell SJ+, *Can Med Assoc J* 126, 1032
  (1981): Ackley AM+, *Southern Med J* 74, 1550
  (1980): Murray DL+, *N Engl J Med* 303, 1003
Purpura
  (2002): Kurokawa I, *Int J Antimicrob Agents* 20(5), 393
  (1980): Murray DL+, *N Engl J Med* 303, 1003
Pustules
  (1992): Ogoshi M+, *Dermatology* 184, 142
Rash (sic) (1–1.5%)
  (2002): Siddiqui SJ+, *J Pak Med Assoc* 52(10), 451 (1 case)
Stevens–Johnson syndrome (<1%)
  (1988): Platt R+, *J Infect Dis* 158, 474
Toxic epidermal necrolysis
  (1987): Guillaume JC+, *Arch Dermatol* 123, 1166
Urticaria (<1%)
  (2000): Ibia EO+, *Arch Dermatol* 136, 849
  (1999): Joubert GI+, *Can J Clin Pharmacol* 6, 197 (26 cases)
  (1998): Litt JZ, Beachwood, OH (personal case) (observation)
  (1995): Blumenthal HL, Beachwood, OH (personal case) (observation)
  (1994): Litt JZ, Beachwood, OH (personal case) (observation)
  (1993): Litt JZ, Beachwood, OH (2 personal cases) (observation)
  (1991): Hebert AA+, *J Am Acad Dermatol* 25, 805
  (1985): Levine LR, *Pediatr Infect Dis* 4, 358 (1–5%)
  (1982): Lovell SJ+, *Can Med Assoc J* 126, 1032

Mucosal/ENT

Dysgeusia
  (1995): Dark DS+, *Infections in Medicine* October, 551
Glossitis
Oral candidiasis
Stomatitis
  (2002): Siddiqui SJ+, *J Pak Med Assoc* 52(10), 451 (1 case)
Vaginitis
  (1992): Stotka JL+, *Postgrad Med J* 68, S73 (candidiasis)

Other

Anaphylactoid reactions/Anaphylaxis (<1%)
  (2007): Shirai T+, *Intern Med* 46(6), 315
  (1999): Grouhi M+, *Pediatrics* 103, e50
  (1986): Nishioka K+, *J Dermatol* 13, 226
Hypersensitivity
Paresthesias
Serum sickness (<1%)
  (2002): Sanklecha MU, *Indian J Pediatr* 69(10), 921
  (2002): Yerushalmi J+, *Cutis* 69(5), 395
  (2000): Ibia EO+, *Arch Dermatol* 136, 849
  (1999): Joubert GI+, *Can J Clin Pharmacol* 6, 197 (31 cases)
  (1999): Parshuram CS+, *J Paediatr Child Health* 35, 223
  (1999): Phillips R, *Aust Fam Physician* 28, 539
  (1998): Boyd IW, *Med J Aust* 169, 443
  (1998): Kearns GL+, *Clin Pharmacol Ther* 63, 686 (10 patients)
  (1997): Szalai Z+, *Orv Hetil* (Hungarian) 138, 855
  (1996): *Can Med Assoc J* 155, 913
  (1996): Grammer LC, *JAMA* 275, 1152
  (1996): Reynolds RD, *JAMA* 276, 950
  (1995): Kearns GL+, *J Pediatr* 125, 805

(1995): Martin J+, *N Z Med J* 108, 123
(1992): Parra FM+, *Allergy* 47, 439
(1992): Stricker BH+, *J Clin Epidemiol* 45, 1177
(1992): Vial T+, *Ann Pharmacother* 26, 910
(1991): Hebert AA+, *J Am Acad Dermatol* 25, 805
(1990): Heckbert SB+, *Am J Epidemiol* 132, 336
(1988): Platt R+, *J Infect Dis* 158, 474
(1987): Norrby SR, *Drugs* 34 (Suppl 2), 105 (1–5%)
(1985): Callahan CW+, *J Am Osteopath Assoc* 85, 450
(1985): Levine LR, *Ped Infect Dis* 4, 358 (0.5%)
(1985): Murray DL+, *Pediatr Inf Dis* 4, 706
(1983): Johnson T+, *J Ark Med Soc* 80, 110
(1982): Lovell SJ+, *Can Med Assoc J* 126, 1032
(1980): Murray DL+, *N Engl J Med* 303, 1003

CEFADROXIL

Trade names: Baxan; Bidocef; Cedrox; Cefamox; Duracef; Duricef (Warner Chilcott); Moxacef; Oracefal; Sumacef
Indications: Various infections caused by susceptible organisms
Category: Cephalosporin, 1st generation
Half-life: 1.2–1.5 hours

Note: Penicillin and cephalosporins share a common beta-lactam structure. People who are allergic to penicillin are approximately 4 times more likely to develop an allergic reaction to a cephalosporin than those people who have no penicillin allergy. (From 5 to 16% of patients allergic to penicillin develop allergic reactions to cephalosporins)

Reactions

Skin
Angioedema (<1%)
Erythema
  (1986): Tanrisever B+, *Drugs* 32(Suppl 3), 1
Erythema multiforme (<1%)
Exanthems (<1%)
  (1986): Tanrisever B+, *Drugs* 32(Suppl 3), 1 (0.3%)
Pemphigus
  (1986): Wilson JP+, *Drug Intell Clin Pharm* 20, 219
Pruritus (<1%)
  (1986): Tanrisever B+, *Drugs* 32(Suppl 3), 1 (0.3%)
Rash (sic) (<1%)
Stevens–Johnson syndrome (<1%)
Toxic epidermal necrolysis
Urticaria (<1%)
  (1993): Shelley WB+, *Cutis* 52, 262 (observation)
  (1986): Tanrisever B+, *Drugs* 32(Suppl 3), 1 (0.1%)

Mucosal/ENT
Glossitis
  (1986): Tanrisever B+, *Drugs* 32 (Suppl 3), 1, 21, 43
Oral candidiasis
Oral mucosal eruption
  (1986): Tanrisever B+, *Drugs* 32(Suppl 3), 1 (0.1%)
Oral ulceration
  (1986): Wilson JP+, *Drug Intell Clin Pharm* 20, 219
Vaginitis (<1%)
  (1986): Tanrisever B+, *Drugs* 32(Suppl 3), 1

Other
Anaphylactoid reactions/Anaphylaxis (<1%)
Candidiasis
Hypersensitivity
Serum sickness (<1%)

CEFAMANDOLE

Trade names: Cedol; Cefadol; Kefadol; Kefdole; Mancef; Mandokef
Indications: Various infections caused by susceptible organisms
Category: Cephalosporin, 2nd generation
Half-life: 0.5–1.0 hours

Note: Penicillin and cephalosporins share a common beta-lactam structure. People who are allergic to penicillin are approximately 4 times more likely to develop an allergic reaction to a cephalosporin than those people who have no penicillin allergy. (From 5 to 16% of patients allergic to penicillin develop allergic reactions to cephalosporins)

Reactions

Skin
Acne
Diaper rash
Diaphoresis
Edema
Erythema multiforme
  (1987): Argenyi ZB+, *Cleve Clin J Med* 54, 445
Exanthems
  (1985): Richards DM+, *Drugs* 29, 281 (1.7%)
  (1985): Sanders CV+, *Ann Intern Med* 103, 70 (2%)
Linear IgA dermatosis
  (2003): Avci O+, *J Am Acad Dermatol* 48(2), 299 (passim)
  (1987): Argenyi ZB+, *Cleve Clin J Med* 54, 445
Pruritus (<1%)
Purpura
Rash (sic) (<1%)
Stevens–Johnson syndrome (<1%)
Toxic epidermal necrolysis
  (1985): Sanders CV+, *Ann Intern Med* 103, 70 (2%)
  (1982): Seifter EJ+, *Johns Hopkins Med J* 151, 326
Toxic erythema
  (1995): Rademaker M, *N Z Med J* 108, 165
Urticaria (<1%)

Mucosal/ENT
Dysgeusia
Glossitis
Oral candidiasis (<1%)
Vaginitis
Vulvovaginal candidiasis

Other
Anaphylactoid reactions/Anaphylaxis (<1%)
  (1992): Lin RY, *Arch Intern Med* 152, 930
Hypersensitivity
Injection-site burning
Injection-site cellulitis
Injection-site edema
Injection-site inflammation
Injection-site pain (<1%)
  (1985): Sanders CV+, *Ann Intern Med* 103, 70 (7%)
Injection-site thrombophlebitis (1–10%)
  (1985): Sanders CV+, *Ann Intern Med* 103, 70 (15%)
Paresthesias
Serum sickness (<1%)

CEFAZOLIN

Trade names: Ancef; Basocef; Cefacidal; Cefamezin; Elzogram; Gramaxin; Kefarin; Totacef; Zolin
Indications: Various infections caused by susceptible organisms
Category: Cephalosporin, 1st generation
Half-life: 1.4–1.8 hours

Note: Penicillin and cephalosporins share a common beta-lactam structure. People who are allergic to penicillin are approximately 4 times more likely to develop an allergic reaction to a cephalosporin than those people who have no penicillin allergy. (From 5 to 16% of patients allergic to penicillin develop allergic reactions to cephalosporins)

Reactions

Skin
Acute generalized exanthematous pustulosis (AGEP)
  (1995): Moreau A+, *Int J Dermatol* 34, 263 (passim)
  (1994): Manders SM+, *Cutis* 54, 194 (with metronidazole)
Allergic reactions (sic)
  (1994): Pleasants RA+, *Chest* 106, 1124 (in patients with cystic fibrosis)
  (1993): Faulk D+, *Nurse Anesth* 4, 188 (3–5%)
Dermatitis
  (2000): Straube MD+, *Contact Dermatitis* 42, 44
Erythema multiforme
Exanthems
  (1990): Flax SH+, *Cutis* 46, 59
  (1988): Fayol J+, *J Am Acad Dermatol* 19, 571
  (1986): Szylit JA+, *Cutis* 37, 390
Fixed eruption (linear)
  (1988): Sigal-Nahum M+, *Br J Dermatol* 118, 849
Pemphigus
  (1997): Brenner S+, *J Am Acad Dermatol* 36, 919
Photo-recall
  (2004): Garza LA+, *Cutis* 73(1), 79
  (1990): Flax SH+, *Cutis* 46, 59
Photosensitivity
  (1990): Flax SH+, *Cutis* 46, 59
Pruritus (<1%)
  (1987): Stough D+, *J Am Acad Dermatol* 16, 1051
Pruritus ani et vulvae
Pustules
  (1990): Rustin MHA+, *Br J Dermatol* 123, 119
  (1988): Fayol J+, *J Am Acad Dermatol* 19, 571
  (1987): Stough D+, *J Am Acad Dermatol* 16, 1051
Rash (sic) (<1%)
Stevens–Johnson syndrome (<1%)
Toxic epidermal necrolysis
  (1999): Egan CA+, *J Am Acad Dermatol* 40, 458 (6 cases)
  (1994): Julsrud ME, *J Foot Ankle Surg* 33, 255
Urticaria (<1%)

Mucosal/ENT
Oral candidiasis (<1%)
Vaginitis (<1%)

Other
Anaphylactoid reactions/Anaphylaxis (<1%)
  (2004): Lee CW+, *Allergy Asthma Proc* 25(1), 23
  (2003): Gibbs MW+, *Acta Anaesthesiol Scand* 47(2), 230
  (1996): Warrington RJ+, *J Allergy Clin Immunol* 98, 460
  (1995): Konno R+, *J Obstet Gynaecol* 21, 577
  (1992): Lin RY, *Arch Intern Med* 152, 930
Hypersensitivity
  (2001): Romano AG+, *Allergy Clin Immunol* 107, 134 (delayed)

Injection-site induration
Injection-site pain (<1%)
Injection-site phlebitis (<1%)
Phlebitis
Seizures
  (2006): Arkaravichien W+, *J Med Assoc Thai* 89(11), 1981
Serum sickness (<1%)
  (2006): Brucculeri M+, *BMC Clin Pharmacol* 6, 3

CEFDINIR

Synonym: CFDN
Trade name: Omnicef (Medicis)
Indications: Community-acquired pneumonia and various infections caused by susceptible organisms
Category: Cephalosporin, 3rd generation
Half-life: 1–2 hours

Note: Penicillin and cephalosporins share a common beta-lactam structure. People who are allergic to penicillin are approximately 4 times more likely to develop an allergic reaction to a cephalosporin than those people who have no penicillin allergy. (From 5 to 16% of patients allergic to penicillin develop allergic reactions to cephalosporins)

Reactions

Skin
Erythema multiforme
Erythema nodosum
Exanthems (0.2%)
Exfoliative dermatitis
Facial edema
Pruritus (0.2%)
Purpura
Rash (sic) (3%)
Stevens–Johnson syndrome (<1%)
Toxic epidermal necrolysis
Urticaria (<1%)
Vasculitis

Mucosal/ENT
Stomatitis
Vaginitis (1%)
Vulvovaginal candidiasis (5%)

Other
Anaphylactoid reactions/Anaphylaxis
Candidiasis (1%)
Headache
Serum sickness (<1%)

CEFDITOREN

Trade name: Spectracef (Meiji)
Indications: Various infections caused by susceptible organisms
Category: Cephalosporin, 3rd generation
Half-life: ~1.6 hours
Clinically important, potentially hazardous interactions with: famotidine

Note: Penicillin and cephalosporins share a common beta-lactam structure. People who are allergic to penicillin are approximately 4 times more likely to develop an allergic reaction to a cephalosporin than those people who have no penicillin allergy. (From 5 to 16% of patients allergic to penicillin develop allergic reactions to cephalosporins)

Reactions

Skin
Allergic reactions (sic) (<1%)
Diaphoresis (<1%)
Erythema multiforme
Fungal dermatitis (<1%)
Peripheral edema (<1%)
Pruritus (<1%)
Rash (sic) (<1%)
Stevens–Johnson syndrome
Toxic epidermal necrolysis
Urticaria (<1%)

Mucosal/ENT
Dysgeusia (<1%)
Oral candidiasis (<1%)
Oral ulceration (<1%)
Stomatitis (<1%)
Vaginitis (<1%)
Vulvovaginal candidiasis (3–6%)
Xerostomia (<1%)

Other
Abdominal pain
 (2002): Darkes MJ+, Drugs 62(2), 319
Anaphylactoid reactions/Anaphylaxis
Candidiasis
 (2002): Darkes MJ+, Drugs 62(2), 319
Headache
 (2002): Balbisi EA, Pharmacotherapy 22(10), 1278
 (2002): Darkes MJ+, Drugs 62(2), 319
Myalgia/Myositis/Myopathy/Myotoxicity (<1%)
Pain (<1%)
Serum sickness

CEFEPIME

Trade names: Maxcef; Maxipime (Elan)
Indications: Various infections caused by susceptible organisms
Category: Cephalosporin, 4th generation
Half-life: 2–2.3 hours

Note: Penicillin and cephalosporins share a common beta-lactam structure. People who are allergic to penicillin are approximately 4 times more likely to develop an allergic reaction to a cephalosporin than those people who have no penicillin allergy. (From 5 to 16% of patients allergic to penicillin develop allergic reactions to cephalosporins)

Reactions

Skin
Angioedema
Erythema multiforme
Exanthems (1.8%)
Pruritus (1–10%)
 (1993): Giamarellou H, J Antimicrob Chemother 32 Suppl B, 123 (2%)
 (1993): Jauregui L+, J Antimicrob Chemother 32 Suppl B, 141
 (1993): Mouton Y+, J Antimicrob Chemother 32 Suppl B, 133 (4%)
Rash (sic) (51%)
 (2001): Mustafa MM+, Pediatr Infect Dis J 20(3), 362
 (2000): Sheng WH+, J Microbiol Immunol Infect 33, 109
 (1996): Holloway WJ+, Am J Med 100, 52S
 (1995): Schrank JH+, Clin Infect Dis 20(1), 56
 (1994): Okamoto MP+, Am J Hosp Pharm 51, 463
 (1993): Barckow D+, J Antimicrob Chemother 32 Suppl B, 187
 (1993): Giamarellou H, J Antimicrob Chemother 32 Suppl B, 123 (2%)
 (1993): Mouton Y+, J Antimicrob Chemother 32 Suppl B, 133 (4%)
 (1993): Newton ER+, J Antimicrob Chemother 32 Suppl B, 195
Stevens–Johnson syndrome
Toxic epidermal necrolysis
Urticaria (1.8%)
 (1993): Mouton Y+, J Antimicrob Chemother 32 Suppl B, 133 (4%)

Mucosal/ENT
Oral candidiasis
Vaginitis (<1%)

Other
Anaphylactoid reactions/Anaphylaxis
Candidiasis (<1%)
Death
Fever
 (2000): Sheng WH+, J Microbiol Immunol Infect 33(2), 109
Headache
 (1995): Schrank JH Jr+, Clin Infect Dis 20(1), 56
 (1993): Giamarellou H, J Antimicrob Chemother 32 Suppl B, 123 (2%)
 (1993): Newton ER+, J Antimicrob Chemother 32 Suppl B, 195
Hypersensitivity
 (2004): Orhan F+, Allergy 59(2), 239
Injection-site inflammation (0.6%)
Injection-site pain (0.6%)
Injection-site phlebitis (1.3%)
Injection-site reactions
 (1993): Hoepelman AI+, J Antimicrob Chemother 32 Suppl B, 175
 (1993): Mouton Y+, J Antimicrob Chemother 32 Suppl B, 133 (9%)
Myoclonus
 (2006): Lam S+, Pharmacotherapy 26(8), 1169
Neurotoxicity
 (2006): Fernandez-Torre JL, Neurology 67(2), 367
 (2006): Lam S+, Pharmacotherapy 26(8), 1169
 (2006): Lin CM+, Acta Neurol Taiwan 15(4), 269
 (2001): Barbey F+, Ann Intern Med 135(11), 1011
Pseudoporphyria
 (2004): Phung TL+, J Am Acad Dermatol 51(2), S80 (with ampicillin)
Seizures
 (2006): Maganti R+, Epilepsy Behav 8(1), 312
 (2005): Bragatti JA+, Arq Neuropsiquiatr 63(1), 87
 (2004): Abanades S+, Ann Pharmacother 38(4), 606
 (2004): Alpay H+, Pediatr Nephrol 19(4), 445
 (2004): Plensa E+, Bone Marrow Transplant 33(1), 119
 (2004): Primavera A+, Neuropsychobiology 49(4), 218
 (2003): Chow KM+, Pharmacotherapy 23(3), 369 (42 cases)
 (2003): Ferrara N+, Clin Nephrol 59(5), 388
 (2002): Chatellier D+, Intensive Care Med 28(2), 214 (5 cases)
 (2001): Martinez-Rodriguez JE+, Am J Med 111, 115
 (2000): Dixit S+, Neurology 54(11), 2153
 (2000): Saurina A+, Nefrologia 20(6), 554

CEFIXIME

Trade names: Cefspan; Cephoral; Fixime; Oroken; Supran; Suprax (Lupin); Uro-cephoral
Indications: Various infections caused by susceptible organisms
Category: Cephalosporin, 3rd generation
Half-life: 3–4 hours

Note: Penicillin and cephalosporins share a common beta-lactam structure. People who are allergic to penicillin are approximately 4 times more likely to develop an allergic reaction to a cephalosporin than those people who have no penicillin allergy. (From 5 to 16% of patients allergic to penicillin develop allergic reactions to cephalosporins)

Reactions

Skin
Angioedema
Erythema multiforme (<2%)
Facial edema
Pruritus (<2%)
  (1987): Tally FP+, *Pediatr Infect Dis J* 6, 976
Pruritus ani et vulvae
Rash (sic) (<2%)
  (2001): Ho MW+, *J Microbiol Immunol Infect* 34(3), 185 (3.2%)
  (1987): Tally FP+, *Pediatr Infect Dis J* 6, 976
Stevens–Johnson syndrome (<2%)
Toxic epidermal necrolysis
Urticaria (<2%)
  (1987): Tally FP+, *Pediatr Infect Dis J* 6, 976

Mucosal/ENT
Vaginitis (<2%)
Vulvovaginal candidiasis
Xerostomia
  (1987): Tally FP+, *Pediatr Infect Dis J* 6, 976

Other
Anaphylactoid reactions/Anaphylaxis
  (1996): Vilas Martinez F+, *Med Clin* (Barc) (Spanish) 106, 439
Candidiasis
Hypersensitivity
  (1999): Gaig P+, *Allergy* 54(8), 901
Pseudolymphoma
  (1998): Jabbar A+, *Br J Haematol* 101, 209
Serum sickness (<2%)
  (1987): Tally FP+, *Pediatr Infect Dis J* 6, 976

CEFMETAZOLE

Trade names: Cefmetazon; Cefotazol; Cemetol; Cetazone; Gomcefa; Metalin; Zefazone
Indications: Various infections caused by susceptible organisms
Category: Cephalosporin, 2nd generation
Half-life: 72 minutes

Note: Penicillin and cephalosporins share a common beta-lactam structure. People who are allergic to penicillin are approximately 4 times more likely to develop an allergic reaction to a cephalosporin than those people who have no penicillin allergy. (From 5 to 16% of patients allergic to penicillin develop allergic reactions to cephalosporins)

Note: The disulfiram-like reaction consists of facial flushing, diaphoresis, tachycardia, and pounding headache

Reactions

Skin
Allergic reactions (sic)
  (1989): Saito A, *J Antimicrob Chemother* 23, 131
Pruritus (<1%)
Purpura
Rash (sic) (1–10%)
Stevens–Johnson syndrome (<1%)
Toxic epidermal necrolysis
Urticaria (<1%)

Mucosal/ENT
Dysgeusia
Oral candidiasis
  (1989): Yangco BG+, *J Antimicrob Chemother* 23 Suppl D, 39
Vaginitis (<1%)

Eyes
Periorbital edema

Other
Anaphylactoid reactions/Anaphylaxis
  (1989): Saito A, *J Antimicrob Chemother* 23, 131
Candidiasis (<1%)
Disulfiram-like reaction
  (1989): Saito A, *J Antimicrob Chemother* 23, 131
Headache
Hot flashes (<1%)
Hypersensitivity
Injection-site edema
Injection-site induration
Injection-site pain
Injection-site thrombophlebitis (<1%)
Neurotoxicity
  (1988): Uchihara T+, *Clin Neurol Neurosurg* 90(4), 369
Phlebitis (<1%)
Serum sickness (<1%)

CEFONICID

Trade names: Dinacid; Monocef; Monocid; Monocidur
Indications: Various infections caused by susceptible organisms
Category: Cephalosporin, 2nd generation
Half-life: 3–6 hours

Note: Penicillin and cephalosporins share a common beta-lactam structure. People who are allergic to penicillin are approximately 4 times more likely to develop an allergic reaction to a cephalosporin than those people who have no penicillin allergy. (From 5 to 16% of patients allergic to penicillin develop allergic reactions to cephalosporins)

Note: The disulfiram-like reaction consists of facial flushing, diaphoresis, tachycardia, and pounding headache

Reactions

Skin
Allergic reactions (sic)
  (1994): Martin JA+, *Ann Allergy* 72, 341
Erythema (<1%)
Erythema multiforme
Pruritus (<1%)
Purpura
Rash (sic) (<1%)

Stevens–Johnson syndrome (<1%)
Toxic epidermal necrolysis
Urticaria (<1%)

Mucosal/ENT

Vaginitis

Other

Anaphylactoid reactions/Anaphylaxis (<1%)
Candidiasis (<1%)
Disulfiram-like reaction
  (1990): Marcon G+, *Recenti Prog Med* (Italian) 81, 47
Hypersensitivity
  (2007): Testi S+, *J Investig Allergol Clin Immunol* 17(4), 281
Injection-site edema (>1%)
Injection-site induration (>1%)
Injection-site pain (5.7%)
Injection-site phlebitis (>1%)
Myalgia/Myositis/Myopathy/Myotoxicity
Serum sickness (<1%)
  (1995): Ortega Calvo M+, *An Med Interna* (Spanish) 12, 289

CEFOPERAZONE

Trade names: Cefobid (Pfizer); Cefobis; Cefogram; Cefozone; CPZ; Mediper; Tomabef; Zoncef
Indications: Various infections caused by susceptible organisms
Category: Cephalosporin, 3rd generation
Half-life: 1.6–2.6 hours

Note: Penicillin and cephalosporins share a common beta-lactam structure. People who are allergic to penicillin are approximately 4 times more likely to develop an allergic reaction to a cephalosporin than those people who have no penicillin allergy. (From 5 to 16% of patients allergic to penicillin develop allergic reactions to cephalosporins)

Note: The disulfiram-like reaction consists of facial flushing, diaphoresis, tachycardia, and pounding headache

Reactions

Skin

Erythema multiforme
Exanthems (<1%)
Pruritus (<1%)
Rash (sic) (2%)
  (1983): Lyon JA, *Drug Intell Clin Pharm* 17, 7
Stevens–Johnson syndrome (<1%)
Toxic epidermal necrolysis
Urticaria (<1%)
  (1983): Lyon JA, *Drug Intell Clin Pharm* 17, 7

Other

Anaphylactoid reactions/Anaphylaxis
  (2005): Kunitake A+, *Masui* 54(10), 1156
Candidiasis (<1%)
Disulfiram-like reaction
  (1981): Vonhogen LH+, *Ned Tijdschr Geneeskd* (Dutch) 125, 1610
  (1980): Foster TS+, *Am J Hosp Pharm* 37, 858
Hypersensitivity (>2%)
Injection-site induration (<1%)
Injection-site pain (<1%)
  (1983): Lyon JA, *Drug Intell Clin Pharm* 17, 7
Phlebitis (<1%)

  (1983): Lyon JA, *Drug Intell Clin Pharm* 17, 7
Serum sickness (<1%)
Thrombophlebitis

CEFOTAXIME

Trade names: Alfotax; Benaxima; Biosint; Cefaxim; Cefotax; Claforan (Sanofi-Aventis); Molelant; Oritaxim; Primafen; Spirosine; Zariviz
Indications: Various infections caused by susceptible organisms
Category: Cephalosporin, 3rd generation
Half-life: adults: 60 minutes

Note: Penicillin and cephalosporins share a common beta-lactam structure. People who are allergic to penicillin are approximately 4 times more likely to develop an allergic reaction to a cephalosporin than those people who have no penicillin allergy. (From 5 to 16% of patients allergic to penicillin develop allergic reactions to cephalosporins)

Reactions

Skin

Erythema multiforme
  (1990): Todd PA+, *Drugs* 40, 608
  (1986): Green ST+, *Postgrad Med J* 62, 415
Exanthems
  (1990): Todd PA+, *Drugs* 40, 608
  (1984): Smith CR+, *Ann Intern Med* 101, 469 (3.4%)
  (1983): Carmine AA+, *Drugs* 25, 223 (2%)
Pruritus (2.4%)
  (1993): Newton ER+, *J Antimicrob Chemother* 32 Suppl B, 195
  (1990): Todd PA+, *Drugs* 40, 608
  (1983): Carmine AA+, *Drugs* 25, 223 (2%)
Rash (sic) (2.4%)
  (2005): Mazzeo F+, *Pharmacol Res* 51(3), 269
  (1993): Newton ER+, *J Antimicrob Chemother* 32 Suppl B, 195
  (1982): LeFrock JL+, *Clin Ther* 5, 19
Stevens–Johnson syndrome
  (2003): Liberopoulos EN+, *Ann Pharmacother* 37(6), 812
Toxic epidermal necrolysis
  (2002): Paquet P+, *Crit Care Med* 30(11), 2580
Urticaria (2.4%)

Mucosal/ENT

Vaginitis (<1%)

Other

Anaphylactoid reactions/Anaphylaxis (2.4%)
Aseptic meningitis
  (2007): Nakajima W+, *J Child Neurol* 22(6), 780
Candidiasis
Headache
Hypersensitivity
  (1993): Papakonstantinou G+, *Clin Investig* 71, 165
Injection-site inflammation (4.3%)
  (1983): Carmine AA+, *Drugs* 25, 223 (5%)
Injection-site pain (1–10%)
  (1983): Carmine AA+, *Drugs* 25, 223 (32%)
Injection-site thrombophlebitis
Nephrotoxicity
  (2005): Mazzeo F+, *Pharmacol Res* 51(3), 269
Paresthesias
Phlebitis (<1%)
Serum sickness

CEFOTETAN

Trade names: Apacef; Apatef; Cefotan (AstraZeneca); Ceftenon; Cepan; Yamatetan
Indications: Various infections caused by susceptible organisms
Category: Cephalosporin, 2nd generation
Half-life: 3–5 hours

Note: Penicillin and cephalosporins share a common beta-lactam structure. People who are allergic to penicillin are approximately 4 times more likely to develop an allergic reaction to a cephalosporin than those people who have no penicillin allergy. (From 5 to 16% of patients allergic to penicillin develop allergic reactions to cephalosporins)

Reactions

Skin
Erythema multiforme
Exanthems
Photo-recall
   (2006): Ayoola A+, *Oncologist* 11(10), 1118
Pruritus (<1%)
Rash (sic) (<1%)
   (1994): Lapointe RW+, *Can J Surg* 37(4), 313
   (1990): Nguyen VD+, *Am J Kidney Dis* 16(3), 259
Stevens–Johnson syndrome (<1%)
Toxic epidermal necrolysis
Urticaria (<1%)

Other
Abdominal pain
   (1989): Gesualdo L+, *Drugs Exp Clin Res* 15(6–7), 309
Anaphylactoid reactions/Anaphylaxis (<1%)
   (1990): Faro S+, *Am J Obstet Gynecol* 162, 296
   (1988): Bloomberg RJ, *Am J Obstet Gynecol* 159, 125
Candidiasis (<1%)
Chills
   (1989): Gesualdo L+, *Drugs Exp Clin Res* 15(6–7), 309
Death
   (2000): Moes GS+, *Arch Pathol Lab Med* 124(9), 1344
   (1994): Peano GM+, *Vox Sang* 66(1), 84
   (1992): Garratty G+, *Transfusion* 32(3), 269
Fever
   (1990): Nguyen VD+, *Am J Kidney Dis* 16(3), 259
Headache
   (1989): Gesualdo L+, *Drugs Exp Clin Res* 15(6–7), 309
Hypersensitivity (1.2%)
   (2001): Romano A+, *Allergy* 56, 260
Injection-site erythema
   (1989): Gesualdo L+, *Drugs Exp Clin Res* 15(6–7), 309
Injection-site pain (<1%)
   (1989): Gesualdo L+, *Drugs Exp Clin Res* 15(6–7), 309
Phlebitis (<1%)
Serum sickness (<1%)
Thrombophlebitis

CEFOXITIN

Trade names: Cefmore; Cefoxin; Lephocin; Mefoxil; Mefoxin (Merck); Mefoxitin
Indications: Various infections caused by susceptible organisms
Category: Cephalosporin, 2nd generation
Half-life: 40–60 minutes

Note: Penicillin and cephalosporins share a common beta-lactam structure. People who are allergic to penicillin are approximately 4 times more likely to develop an allergic reaction to a cephalosporin than those people who have no penicillin allergy. (From 5 to 16% of patients allergic to penicillin develop allergic reactions to cephalosporins)

Reactions

Skin
Angioedema (<1%)
Exanthems
Exfoliative dermatitis (<1%)
   (1987): Norrby SR, *Drugs* 34 (Suppl 2), 105
   (1985): Sanders CV+, *Ann Intern Med* 103, 70 (2%)
   (1983): Tietze KJ+, *Clin Pharmacy* 2, 582
   (1982): Kannangara DW+, *Arch Intern Med* 142, 1031
Pruritus (<1%)
   (1983): Tietze KJ+, *Clin Pharmacy* 2, 582
Purpura
   (1990): Burstein M+, *Drug Intell Clin Pharm* 24, 206
Pustules
   (1994): Spencer JM+, *Br J Dermatol* 130, 514
Rash (sic) (<1%)
Stevens–Johnson syndrome (<1%)
Toxic epidermal necrolysis (<1%)
Urticaria

Other
Anaphylactoid reactions/Anaphylaxis (<1%)
   (1992): Lin RY, *Arch Intern Med* 152, 930 (11 cases)
Candidiasis (<1%)
Injection-site induration
Injection-site pain
   (1985): Sanders CV+, *Ann Intern Med* 103, 70 (10%)
Serum sickness (<1%)
   (1986): Panwalker AP+, *Drug Intell Clin Pharm* 20, 953
Thrombophlebitis

CEFPODOXIME

Trade names: Cefodox; Orelox; Podomexef; Vantin (Pfizer)
Indications: Various infections caused by susceptible organisms
Category: Cephalosporin, 3rd generation
Half-life: 2.1–2.8 hours

Note: Penicillin and cephalosporins share a common beta-lactam structure. People who are allergic to penicillin are approximately 4 times more likely to develop an allergic reaction to a cephalosporin than those people who have no penicillin allergy. (From 5 to 16% of patients allergic to penicillin develop allergic reactions to cephalosporins)

Reactions

Skin
Acne
Diaper rash (12.1%)

Diaphoresis
Edema
Erythema multiforme
Exfoliative dermatitis (<1%)
Pruritus (<1%)
Rash (sic) (1.4%)
   (2001): Fulton B+, *Paediatr Drugs* 3(2), 137
   (1994): Asmar BI+, *Pediatrics* 94(6 Pt 1), 847
   (1989): Fujii R+, *Jpn J Antibiot* 42(7), 1439
Stevens–Johnson syndrome (<1%)
Toxic epidermal necrolysis
Urticaria (<1%)

Mucosal/ENT
Dysgeusia (<1%)
Glossitis
Oral candidiasis
Sialopenia (<1%)
Tinnitus
Vaginitis
   (1991): Tack KJ+, *Drugs* 42, 51
Vulvovaginal candidiasis (<1%)

Other
Anaphylactoid reactions/Anaphylaxis (<1%)
Candidiasis (<1%)
   (1989): Fujii R+, *Jpn J Antibiot* 42(7), 1439
Hypersensitivity
Injection-site burning
Injection-site cellulitis
Injection-site edema
Injection-site inflammation
Injection-site thrombophlebitis
Paresthesias
Serum sickness (<1%)

CEFPROZIL

Trade name: Cefzil (Bristol-Myers Squibb)
Indications: Various infections caused by susceptible organisms
Category: Cephalosporin, 2nd generaton
Half-life: 1.3 hours

Note: Penicillin and cephalosporins share a common beta-lactam structure. People who are allergic to penicillin are approximately 4 times more likely to develop an allergic reaction to a cephalosporin than those people who have no penicillin allergy. (From 5 to 16% of patients allergic to penicillin develop allergic reactions to cephalosporins)

Reactions

Skin
Angioedema (<1%)
Diaper rash (1.5%)
Erythema multiforme (<1%)
Exanthems
Genital pruritus (1.6%)
Pallor
   (1992): Woo M+, *Jpn J Antibiot* 45(12), 1635
Pruritus
Rash (sic) (<1%)
Stevens–Johnson syndrome (<1%)
Toxic epidermal necrolysis
Urticaria (<1%)

Mucosal/ENT
Glossitis
Oral candidiasis
Vaginitis (1.6%)

Other
Anaphylactoid reactions/Anaphylaxis (<1%)
Candidiasis
   (1991): Christenson JC+, *J Antimicrob Chemother* 28(4), 581
Headache
Hypersensitivity
Paresthesias
Serum sickness (<1%)
   (1994): Lowery N+, *J Pediatr* 125, 325

CEFTAZIDIME

Trade names: Ceftazim; Ceptaz (GSK); Fortaz (GSK); Fortum; Tagal; Taloken; Tazicef (Hospira); Waytrax
Indications: Various infections caused by susceptible organisms
Category: Cephalosporin, 3rd generation
Half-life: 1–2 hours

Note: Penicillin and cephalosporins share a common beta-lactam structure. People who are allergic to penicillin are approximately 4 times more likely to develop an allergic reaction to a cephalosporin than those people who have no penicillin allergy. (From 5 to 16% of patients allergic to penicillin develop allergic reactions to cephalosporins)

Reactions

Skin
Acne
Acute generalized exanthematous pustulosis (AGEP)
   (2003): Mysore V+, *J Dermatolog Treat* 14(1), 54
Allergic reactions (sic)
   (1994): Pleasants RA+, *Chest* 106, 1124 (in patients with cystic fibrosis)
Angioedema (2%)
Diaper rash
Diaphoresis
Edema
Erythema multiforme (2%)
   (1983): Pierce TH+, *J Antimicrob Chemother* 12 (Suppl A), 21
Exanthems
   (1985): Richards DM+, *Drugs* 29, 105 (1.6%)
Pemphigus erythematodes
   (1993): Iannantuono M+, *Int J Dermatol* 32, 675
   (1993): Pellicano R+, *Int J Dermatol* 32, 675
Photosensitivity
   (1993): Vinks SA+, *Lancet* 341, 1221
Pruritus (2%)
   (1996): Holloway WJ+, *Am J Med* 100, 52S
   (1985): Richards DM+, *Drugs* 29, 105
Rash (sic) (2%)
   (2001): Mustafa MM+, *Pediatr Infect Dis J* 20(3), 362
   (2000): Fang CT+, *Chemotherapy* 46(5), 371
   (2000): Feld R+, *J Clin Oncol* 18(21), 3690
   (1996): Holloway WJ+, *Am J Med* 100, 52S
Stevens–Johnson syndrome (2%)
Toxic epidermal necrolysis (2%)
   (2000): Thestrup-Pedersen K+, *Acta Derm Venereol* 80(4), 316 (with vancomycin)
Toxic erythema
   (1995): Rademaker M, *N Z Med J* 108, 165

Toxic pustuloderma
  (1990): Rustin MHA+, *Br J Dermatol* 123, 119
Urticaria (<1%)

Mucosal/ENT
Dysgeusia
Glossitis
Oral candidiasis
Vaginitis (1%)
Vulvovaginal candidiasis

Other
Anaphylactoid reactions/Anaphylaxis (2%)
  (2005): Punchihewa GL+, *Ceylon Med J* 50(1), 34
  (1985): Richards DM+, *Drugs* 29, 105
Candidiasis (<1%)
Death
  (1998): Basto E+, *Therapie* 53(6), 608
Hypersensitivity (2%)
  (2001): Romano A+, *Allergy* 56, 84
Injection-site burning
Injection-site cellulitis
Injection-site edema
Injection-site inflammation (2%)
Injection-site pain (1.4%)
  (1989): Gaut PL+, *Am J Med* 87 (Suppl 5A), 169S
Injection-site reactions
  (1993): Hoepelman AI+, *J Antimicrob Chemother* 32 Suppl B, 175
Injection-site thrombophlebitis (2%)
Paresthesias (<1%)
Phlebitis (<1%)
Seizures
  (2003): Chow KM+, *Pharmacotherapy* 23(3), 369 (12 cases)
  (2001): Martinez-Rodriguez JE+, *Am J Med* 111(2), 115
Serum sickness

CEFTIBUTEN

Trade names: Cedax (Shionogi); Ceten; Cilecef; Keimax; Seftem
Indications: Various infections caused by susceptible organisms
Category: Cephalosporin, 3rd generation
Half-life: 2 hours

Note: Penicillin and cephalosporins share a common beta-lactam structure. People who are allergic to penicillin are approximately 4 times more likely to develop an allergic reaction to a cephalosporin than those people who have no penicillin allergy. (From 5 to 16% of patients allergic to penicillin develop allergic reactions to cephalosporins)

Reactions

Skin
Diaper rash (<1%)
Pruritus (0.3%)
Pustules
  (2000): Novalbos A+, *J Investig Allergol Clin Immunol* 10(3), 178
Rash (sic) (0.3%)
Stevens–Johnson syndrome (<1%)
Toxic epidermal necrolysis
Urticaria (<1%)

Mucosal/ENT
Dysgeusia (<1%)
Oral candidiasis
Vaginitis (<1%)

Xerostomia (<1%)

Other
Candidiasis (<1%)
Hypersensitivity
  (2005): Atanaskovic-Markovic M+, *Allergy* 60(11), 1454
Paresthesias (<1%)
Serum sickness (<1%)

CEFTIZOXIME

Trade names: Cefizox (Astellas); Ceftix; Ceftrax; Epocelin; Lyceft; Tefidox; Ultracef
Indications: Various infections caused by susceptible organisms
Category: Cephalosporin, 3rd generation
Half-life: 1.6 hours

Note: Penicillin and cephalosporins share a common beta-lactam structure. People who are allergic to penicillin are approximately 4 times more likely to develop an allergic reaction to a cephalosporin than those people who have no penicillin allergy. (From 5 to 16% of patients allergic to penicillin develop allergic reactions to cephalosporins)

Reactions

Skin
Pruritus (1–5%)
Rash (sic) (1–5%)
Stevens–Johnson syndrome (<1%)
Toxic epidermal necrolysis
Urticaria (<1%)

Mucosal/ENT
Oral candidiasis
Vaginitis (<1%)

Other
Anaphylactoid reactions/Anaphylaxis (<1%)
Candidiasis (<1%)
Injection-site edema
Injection-site induration
Injection-site pain (1–5%)
Injection-site phlebitis (1–5%)
Paresthesias (1–5%)
Phlebitis (<1%)
Serum sickness (<1%)

CEFTOBIPROLE

Trade name: BAL5788 (Basilea) (Cilag AG)
Indications: Bacterial infections, MRSA
Category: Cephalosporin antibiotic
Half-life: 3 hours
Clinically important, potentially hazardous interactions with: alcohol, anticoagulants, carbenicillin, dipyridamole, heparin, pentoxifylline, plicamycin, sulfinpyrazone, ticarcillin, valproic acid

Reactions

Skin
Erythema (9%)
Pruritus (9%)

Rash (sic)

Mucosal/ENT

Dysgeusia (8%)
   (2004): Schmitt-Hoffmann A+, *Antimicrob Agents Chemother*
      48(7), 2570

Other

Fever
Headache
Injection-site pain
Vertigo

CEFTRIAXONE

Trade names: Benaxona; Cefaxona; Cefaxone; Rocefin;
Rocephalin; Rocephin (Roche); Tacex; Triaken; Zefone
Indications: Various infections caused by susceptible organisms
Category: Cephalosporin, 3rd generation
Half-life: 5–9 hours

Note: Penicillin and cephalosporins share a common beta-lactam
structure. People who are allergic to penicillin are approximately 4
times more likely to develop an allergic reaction to a cephalosporin
than those people who have no penicillin allergy. (From 5 to 16% of
patients allergic to penicillin develop allergic reactions to
cephalosporins)

Reactions

Skin

Acute generalized exanthematous pustulosis (AGEP)
   (2005): Belda Junior W+, *Rev Inst Med Trop Sao Paulo* 47(3), 171
Angioedema
   (1984): Richards DM+, *Drugs* 27, 469
Dermatitis
   (1989): Baba S+, *Jap J Antibiotics* 42, 212 (4%)
   (1984): Richards DM+, *Drugs* 27, 469 (0.4%)
Diaphoresis (0.2%)
   (1984): Moskowitz BL, *Am J Med* 77 (Suppl 4C), 84
Erythema multiforme
   (1984): Richards DM+, *Drugs* 27, 469
Exanthems
   (2003): Zhang YM+, *Zhonghua Er Ke Za Zhi* 41(2), 135 (2 cases)
   (1990): Schaad UB+, *N Engl J Med* 322, 141 (4%)
   (1988): Richards DM+, *Drugs* 35, 604
   (1985): Judson FN+, *JAMA* 253, 1417 (1.2%)
   (1984): Moskowitz BL, *Am J Med* 77 (Suppl 4C), 84 (1.74%)
   (1984): Richards DM+, *Drugs* 27, 469 (1.4%)
   (1983): Eron LJ+, *J Antimicrob Chemother* 12, 65 (6%)
Jarisch–Herxheimer reaction
   (1994): Strominger MB+, *J Neuroophthalmol* 14, 77
Linear IgA dermatosis
   (1999): Yawalker N+, *Dermatology* 199, 25
Pemphigus
   (1992): Ruocco V+, *Acta Derm Venereol* (Stockh) 72, 48
Pigmentation
   (2003): Zhang YM+, *Zhonghua Er Ke Za Zhi* 41(2), 135 (2 cases)
Pruritus (<1%)
   (1984): Moskowitz BL, *Am J Med* 77 (Suppl 4C), 84 (0.34%)
   (1984): Richards DM+, *Drugs* 27, 469 (0.3%)
Purpura
Rash (sic) (1.7%)
   (2003): Zhang YM+, *Zhonghua Er Ke Za Zhi* 41(2), 135
   (2002): Lamb HM+, *Drugs* 62(7), 1041
   (2000): San Miguel MM+, *Allergy* 55(10), 977

   (1992): Francioli P+, *JAMA* 267, 264
   (1983): Eron LJ+, *J Antimicrob Chemother* 12, 65
Side effects (sic) (3%)
   (1984): Richards DM+, *Drugs* 27, 469
Stevens–Johnson syndrome
   (2003): Narayanan VS+, *Indian J Dent Res* 14(4), 220
Toxic epidermal necrolysis
Urticaria (0.1%)
   (2003): Zhang YM+, *Zhonghua Er Ke Za Zhi* 41(2), 135 (2 cases)
   (2002): Litt JZ, Beachwood, OH (personal case) (observation)
   (1984): Richards DM+, *Drugs* 27, 469

Mucosal/ENT

Dysgeusia (<1%)
   (1992): Francioli P+, *JAMA* 267, 264
Glossitis
   (1984): Moskowitz BL, *Am J Med* 77 (Suppl 4C), 84
   (1984): Richards DM+, *Drugs* 27, 469
Oral mucosal eruption
   (1984): Richards DM+, *Drugs* 27, 469
Tongue black
   (2007): Naimushin A+, *Harefuah* 146(7), 564
Vaginitis (<1%)

Other

Anaphylactoid reactions/Anaphylaxis
   (2007): Belliard CR+, *Arch Pediatr* 14(2), 199
   (2006): Polimeni G+, *Drug Saf* 29(5), 449
   (2002): Baumgartner-Bonnevay C+, *Arch Pediatr* 9(10), 1050
   (2002): Ernst MR+, *Acta Paediatr* 91(3), 355
   (1999): Romano A+, *J Allergy Clin Immunol* 104, 1113
   (1992): Lin RY, *Arch Intern Med* 152, 930 (17 cases)
   (1984): Richards DM+, *Drugs* 27, 469
Anticonvulsant hypersensitivity syndrome
   (2006): Gaig P+, *J Investig Allergol Clin Immunol* 16(5), 321
Aseptic meningitis
   (2007): Nakajima W+, *J Child Neurol* 22(6), 780
Candidiasis (5%)
   (2002): Lamb HM+, *Drugs* 62(7), 1041
   (1983): Bittner MJ+, *Antimicrob Agents Chemother* 23, 261
      (superficial) (sic)
   (1983): Harrison CJ+, *Am J Dis Child* 137, 1048 (superficial) (sic)
      (5%)
Chills (<1%)
DRESS syndrome
   (2006): Akcam FZ+, *J Infect* 53(2), e51
Hepatotoxicity
   (2005): Rivkin AM+, *Am J Health Syst Pharm* 62(19), 2006
Hypersensitivity
   (2002): Hausermann P+, *Contact Dermatitis* 47(5), 311
   (2000): Demoly P+, *Allergy* 55, 418 (immediate)
   (2000): Romano A+, *Allergy* 55, 415 (immediate)
Injection-site induration
Injection-site pain (1–10%)
   (1992): Francioli P+, *JAMA* 267, 264
   (1984): Moskowitz BL, *Am J Med* 77 (Suppl 4C), 84 (1%)
   (1984): Richards DM+, *Drugs* 27, 469 (1–15%)
Injection-site phlebitis (<1%)
   (1984): Moskowitz BL, *Am J Med* 77 (Suppl 4C), 84 (0.95%)
   (1984): Richards DM+, *Drugs* 27, 469
Nephrotoxicity
   (2006): Demirkaya E+, *Pediatr Nephrol* 21(5), 733
   (2005): Bickford CL+, *Pharmacotherapy* 25(10), 1389
   (2005): Costa DL+, *Rev Soc Bras Med Trop* 38(6), 521
Seizures
   (2001): Martinez-Rodriguez JE+, *Am J Med* 111
Serum sickness
   (1984): Moskowitz BL, *Am J Med* 77 (Suppl 4C), 84 (0.04%)

CEFUROXIME

Trade names: Ceftin (GSK); Cefuril; Cepazine; Elobact; Froxal; Zinacef (GSK); Zinacet; Zinat; Zinnat; Zoref
Indications: Various infections caused by susceptible organisms
Category: Cephalosporin, 2nd generation
Half-life: 1–2 hours

Note: Penicillin and cephalosporins share a common beta-lactam structure. People who are allergic to penicillin are approximately 4 times more likely to develop an allergic reaction to a cephalosporin than those people who have no penicillin allergy. (From 5 to 16% of patients allergic to penicillin develop allergic reactions to cephalosporins)

Reactions

Skin
Acute generalized exanthematous pustulosis (AGEP)
  (2001): Cohen AD+, *Int J Dermatol* 40(7), 458
  (1995): Moreau A+, *Int J Dermatol* 34, 263 (passim)
Angioedema (<1%)
Baboon syndrome
  (2003): Wolf R+, *Dermatol Online J* 9(3), 2
Erythema multiforme (<1%)
Exanthems
  (1997): Litt JZ, Beachwood, OH (personal case) (observation)
  (1990): Schaad UB+, *N Engl J Med* 332, 141 (6%)
Jarisch–Herxheimer reaction
  (1992): Nadelman RB+, *Ann Intern Med* 117, 273
Lupus erythematosus
  (2007): Uz E+, *J Natl Med Assoc* 99(9), 1066
Pemphigus
  (1997): Brenner S+, *J Am Acad Dermatol* 36, 919
Pruritus (<1%)
Purpura
Pustules
  (1990): Rustin MHA+, *Br J Dermatol* 123, 119
Rash (sic) (<1%)
  (1988): *Med Lett* 30, 57
Stevens–Johnson syndrome (<1%)
Toxic epidermal necrolysis (<1%)
  (1997): Yossepowitch O+, *Eur J Med Res* 2, 182
  (1993): Correia O+, *Dermatology* 186, 32
Urticaria (<1%)
  (2002): Namyslowski G+, *J Chemother* 14(5), 508
  (1995): Litt JZ, Beachwood, OH (personal case) (observation)
  (1987): Parish LC+, *Int J Dermatol* 26, 389

Mucosal/ENT
Oral candidiasis
  (1985): Cooper TJ+, *J Antimicrobial Chemother* 16, 373
Perianal candidiasis
  (1987): Carson JWK+, *J Antimicrob Chemother* 19, 109
Vaginitis (<1%)
  (1988): *Med Lett* 30, 57

Other
Anaphylactoid reactions/Anaphylaxis (<1%)
  (2007): Hasdenteufel F+, *Ann Pharmacother* 41(6), 1069
  (2005): Villada JR+, *J Cataract Refract Surg* 31(3), 620
  (2002): Prosser DP+, *Paediatr Anaesth* 12(1), 73
Hypersensitivity
  (2000): Saeed SA+, *Postgrad Med J* 76(899), 577 (lymphomatoid)
  (1998): Romano A+, *J Allergy Clin Immunol* 101, 564
  (1992): Romano A+, *Contact Dermatitis* 27, 270
  (1991): Powell DA+, *Drug Intell Clin Pharm* 25, 1236
Injection-site pain (<1%)

Serum sickness (<1%)
Thrombophlebitis (1–10%)

CELECOXIB

Trade name: Celebrex (Pfizer)
Indications: Osteoarthritis, rheumatoid arthritis
Category: COX-2 inhibitor; Non-steroidal anti-inflammatory
Half-life: 11 hours
Clinically important, potentially hazardous interactions with: aliskiren, dexibuprofen

Note: Celecoxib is a sulfonamide and can be absorbed systemically. Sulfonamides can produce severe, possibly fatal, reactions such as toxic epidermal necrolysis and Stevens–Johnson syndrome

Reactions

Skin
Acute febrile neutrophilic dermatosis (Sweet's syndrome)
  (2001): Fye KH+, *J Am Acad Dermatol* 45, 300
Acute generalized exanthematous pustulosis (AGEP)
  (2004): Goeschke B+, *Dermatology* 209(1), 53
  (2004): Yang CC+, *J Formos Med Assoc* 103(7), 555
  (2003): Marques S+, *Ann Dermatol Venereol* 130(11), 1051
Allergic reactions (sic) (<2%)
Angioedema
  (2006): Downing A+, *Br J Clin Pharmacol* 62(4), 496
  (2002): Schneider F+, *Lancet* 359, 852
  (2001): Kelkar PS+, *J Rheumatol* 28(11), 2553
Bacterial infections (<2%)
Bullous dermatitis
  (2003): Marques S+, *Ann Dermatol Venereol* 130(11), 1051
Dermatitis (<2%)
Diaphoresis (<2%)
Edema (<2%)
Erythema
  (2002): Friedman B+, *South Med J* 95(10), 1213
Erythema multiforme
  (1999): Puritz E, Smithtown, NY (from Internet) (observation)
Exanthems (<2%)
  (2003): Marques S+, *Ann Dermatol Venereol* 130(11), 1051
  (2002): Schneider F+, *Lancet* 359, 852
  (2002): Verbeiren S+, *Ann Dermatol Venereol* 129(2), 203
  (2000): Grob M+, *Dermatology* 201, 383
  (2000): Valentine MC, Everett, WA (from internet) (observation) (patient was allergic to sulfa)
  (1999): Fisher BJ, Toronto, Ontario (from Internet) (observation)
  (1999): Graedon J+, *People's Pharmacy* (anecdote from a reader)
  (1999): Jaffe PG, Columbia, SC (from Internet) (observation)
  (1999): Litt JZ, Beachwood, OH (personal case) (observation)
  (1999): Rudolph RI, Wyomissing, PA (from Internet) (observation)
Exfoliative dermatitis
  (2002): Friedman B+, *South Med J* 95(10), 1213
Facial edema (<2%)
Fixed eruption
  (2003): Bandyopadhyay D, *Clin Exp Dermatol* 28(4), 452
Herpes simplex (<2%)
Herpes zoster (<2%)
Keratoderma
  (2005): Vildosola S+, *Actas Dermosifiliogr* 96(8), 537
Lupus erythematosus
  (2003): Poza-Guedes P+, *Rheumatology* (Oxford) 42(7), 916
Nodular eruption (<2%)
Peripheral edema (2.1%)

(2002): Chan FK+, *N Engl J Med* 347(26), 2104
(2000): Fetterman MR, Miami, FL (from Internet) (observation) (leg)
(2000): Panagotacos PJ, San Francisco, CA (pedal) (from Internet) (observation)
(1999): Simon LS+, *JAMA* 282, 1921
Photoallergic reaction
  (2004): Yazici AC+, *Int J Dermatol* 43(6), 459
Photosensitivity (<2%)
  (1999): Zabawski E, Dallas, TX (from Internet) (observation)
Pruritus (<2%)
  (2006): Forrester MB, *Hum Exp Toxicol* 25(5), 261 (2%)
  (1999): Rudolph RI, Wyomissing, PA (from Internet) (observation)
Psoriasis (palmoplantar)
  (2000): Catalano PM, Bradenton, FL (from Internet) (observation)
Purpura
  (2003): Marques S+, *Ann Dermatol Venereol* 130(11), 1051
Pustules
  (2003): Marques S+, *Ann Dermatol Venereol* 130(11), 1051
Rash (sic) (2.2%)
  (2006): Forrester MB, *Hum Exp Toxicol* 25(5), 261 (3%)
Stevens–Johnson syndrome
  (2005): La Grenade L+, *Drug Saf* 28(10), 917 (43 cases)
  (1999): Puritz E, Smithtown, NY (from Internet) (observation)
Toxic epidermal necrolysis
  (2005): La Grenade L+, *Drug Saf* 28(10), 917 (43 cases)
  (2003): Giglio P, *South Med J* 96(3), 320
  (2003): Perna AG+, *Dermatol Online J* 9(5), 25
  (2002): Berger P+, *Pharmacotherapy* 22(9), 1193
  (2002): Friedman B+, *South Med J* 95(10), 1213
  (2000): Mitchell D, Thomasville, GA (from Internet) (observation)
Urticaria (<2%)
  (2004): Senna G+, *Allerg Immunol* (Paris) 36(6), 215
  (2002): Schneider F+, *Lancet* 359, 852
  (2001): Kelkar PS+, *J Rheumatol* 28(11), 2553
Vasculitis
  (2002): Gscheidel D+, *Hautarzt* 53(7), 488
  (2002): Jordan KM+, *Rheumatology* (Oxford) 41(12), 1453
  (2002): Schneider F+, *Lancet* 359, 852
  (2002): Skowron F+, *Dermatology* 204(4), 305
Xerosis (<2%)

Mucosal/ENT
Dysgeusia (<2%)
Stomatitis (<2%)
Vaginitis (<2%)
Vulvovaginal candidiasis (<2%)
Xerostomia (<2%)

Hair
Hair – alopecia (<2%)

Nails
Nails – changes (sic) (<2%)

Eyes
Visual disturbances
  (2003): Coulter DM+, *BMJ* 327(7425), 1214 (2 cases)
  (2001): Lund BC+, *Pharmacotherapy* 21(1), 114

Other
Anaphylactoid reactions/Anaphylaxis
  (2003): Gagnon R+, *J Allergy Clin Immunol* 111(6), 1404
  (2003): Schuster C+, *Allergy* 58(10), 1072 (with sulfamethoxazole)
  (2001): Habki R+, *Ann Med Interne* (Paris) 152(5), 355
  (2001): Levy MB+, *Ann Allergy Asthma Immunol* 87, 72

Application-site cellulitis (<2%)
Application-site reactions (<2%)
Aseptic meningitis
  (2004): Papaioannides DH+, *Ann Pharmacother* 38(1), 172
Asthenia
  (2006): Forrester MB, *Hum Exp Toxicol* 25(5), 261 (3%)
Candidiasis (<2%)
  (1999): McClain SA, Bronx, NY (from Internet) (observation)
Death
  (2005): Solomon SD+, *N Engl J Med* 352(11), 1071
  (2002): Schneider F+, *Lancet* 359, 852
  (2001): Weaver J+, *Am J Gastroenterol* 96(12), 3449
Hot flashes (<2%)
Hypersensitivity
  (2003): Fradet G+, *Ann Med Interne* (Paris) 154(3), 181
  (2003): Marques S+, *Ann Dermatol Venereol* 130(11), 1051
Infections (<2%)
Myalgia/Myositis/Myopathy/Myotoxicity (<2%)
Nephrotoxicity
  (2005): Clifford TM+, *Pharmacotherapy* 25(5), 773
  (2002): Galli G+, *G Ital Nefrol* 19(2), 199
Paresthesias (<2%)
Pseudoporphyria
  (2000): Cummins R+, *J Rheumatol* 27, 2938
Stroke
  (2005): Solomon SD+, *N Engl J Med* 352(11), 1071
Tendinopathy/Tendon rupture (<2%)
Thrombophlebitis (<0.1%)

CELIPROLOL

Trade names: Cardem; Celectol; Celipres; Celipro; Celol (Pacific); Cordiax; Dilanorm; Selectol (Sanofi-Aventis)
Indications: Hypertension, Angina Pectoris
Category: Beta blocker
Half-life: 5–6 hours
Clinically important, potentially hazardous interactions with: amiodarone, bepridil, diltiazem, disopyramide, floctafenine, quinidine, verapamil

Reactions

Skin
Cold extremities
Lupus erythematosus
  (2006): Charniot JC+, *Acta Cardiol* 61(6), 661
Raynaud's phenomenon

Eyes
Vision impaired

Other
Abdominal pain
Asthenia
  (1991): Roman O+, *Rev Med Chil* 119(1), 50
  (1986): Capone P+, *J Cardiovasc Pharmacol* 8(Suppl 4), S119
Bronchospasm
Cardiac failure
Depression
Headache
  (1991): Roman O+, *Rev Med Chil* 119(1), 50 (4 patients)
  (1986): Capone P+, *J Cardiovasc Pharmacol* 8(Suppl 4), S119
Paresthesias
Tremor
  (1985): Belovezhdov N+, *Vutr Boles* 24(5), 74

Vertigo
(1986): Capone P+, *J Cardiovasc Pharmacol* 8(Suppl 4), S119
(1985): Belovezhdov N+, *Vutr Boles* 24(5), 74

CEPHALEXIN

Trade names: Apo-Cephalex; Biocet; Ceforal; Ceporex; Ceporexine; Kefarol; Keflex (Advancis); Keftab (Biovail); Novo-Lexin; Ospexin
Indications: Various infections caused by susceptible organisms
Category: Cephalosporin, 1st generation
Half-life: 0.9–1.2 hours
Clinically important, potentially hazardous interactions with: amikacin, gentamicin

Note: Penicillin and cephalosporins share a common beta-lactam structure. People who are allergic to penicillin are approximately 4 times more likely to develop an allergic reaction to a cephalosporin than those people who have no penicillin allergy. (From 5 to 16% of patients allergic to penicillin develop allergic reactions to cephalosporins)

Reactions

Skin
Acute generalized exanthematous pustulosis (AGEP)
(2002): Arroyo MP+, *J Drugs Dermatol* 1(1), 63
(1995): Moreau A+, *Int J Dermatol* 34, 263 (passim)
Allergic reactions
Angioedema (<1%)
Baboon syndrome
(2003): Wolf R+, *Dermatol Online J* 9(3), 2 (2 cases)
Bullous pemphigoid
(2004): Paul J, *Conn Med* 68(10), 611
(2001): Czechowicz RT, *Australas J Dermatol* 42(2), 132
Dermatitis
(1986): Milligan A+, *Contact Dermatitis* 15, 91
Erythema multiforme (<1%)
(1998): Blumenthal HL, Beachwood, OH (personal case) (observation)
(1992): Murray KM+, *Ann Pharmacotherapy* 26, 1230
(1988): Platt R+, *J Infect Dis* 158, 474
(1987): Norrby SR, *Drugs* 34 (Suppl 2), 105
Exanthems
(1999): Litt JZ, Beachwood, OH (personal case) (observation)
(1997): McCloskey GL+, *Cutis* 59, 251
(1995): Litt JZ, Beachwood, OH (personal case) (observation)
Fixed eruption
(1991): Baran R+, *Br J Dermatol* 125, 592
Pemphigus
(1992): Vaillant L+, *Int J Dermatol* 31, 67
(1991): Wolf R+, *Int J Dermatol* 30, 213
Pruritus
(1999): Litt JZ, Beachwood, OH (personal case) (observation)
(1988): Kumar A+, *Antimicrob Agents Chemother* 32, 882
Pruritus ani et vulvae
Purpura
Pustules
(1994): Spencer JM+, *Br J Dermatol* 130, 514
(1988): Jackson H+, *Dermatologica* 177, 292
Rash (sic) (<1%)
Side effects (sic) (2%)
Stevens–Johnson syndrome (<1%)
(1992): Murray KM+, *Ann Pharmacother* 26, 1230
(1988): Platt R+, *J Infect Dis* 158, 474
Toxic epidermal necrolysis (<1%)

(1995): Jick H+, *Pharmacotherapy* 15, 428
(1991): Dave J+, *J Antimicrob Chemotherapy* 28, 477
(1987): Harnar TJ+, *J Burn Care Rehabil* 8, 554
(1987): Hogan DJ+, *J Am Acad Dermatol* 17, 852
Urticaria (<1%)
(1993): Litt JZ, Beachwood, OH (personal case) (observation)

Mucosal/ENT
Oral candidiasis
Vaginitis

Hair
Hair – hypertrichosis
(2006): Kerob D+, *Arch Dermatol* 142(12), 1656

Nails
Nails – paronychia
(1991): Baran R+, *Br J Dermatol* 125, 592

Other
Anaphylactoid reactions/Anaphylaxis (<1%)
(1999): Nordt SP+, *Am J Emerg Med* 17, 492
(1992): Lin RY, *Arch Intern Med* 152, 930 (17 cases)
(1989): Hoffman DR+, *Ann Allergy* 62, 91 (fatal)
Hypersensitivity
Serum sickness (<1%)
(1988): Platt R+, *J Infect Dis* 158, 474

CEPHALOTHIN

Trade names: Ceftina; Ceporacin; Cepovenin; Keflin Neutral; Keflin Neutro; Keflin-N; Practogen
Indications: Various infections caused by susceptible organisms
Category: Cephalosporin, 1st generation
Half-life: 30–50 minutes
Clinically important, potentially hazardous interactions with: amphotericin B, colistin, gentamicin

Note: Penicillin and cephalosporins share a common beta-lactam structure. People who are allergic to penicillin are approximately 4 times more likely to develop an allergic reaction to a cephalosporin than those people who have no penicillin allergy. (From 5 to 16% of patients allergic to penicillin develop allergic reactions to cephalosporins)

Reactions

Skin
Allergic reactions (sic)
Erythema multiforme
(1996): Munoz-D+, *Contact Dermatitis* 34, 227
Exanthems (1–5%)
Pruritus (<1%)
Purpura
(1980): Miescher PA+, *Clin Haematol* 9, 505
Rash (sic)
Stevens–Johnson syndrome (<1%)
Toxic epidermal necrolysis
(1988): Dreyfuss DA+, *Ann Plast Surg* 20, 146
Urticaria

Other
Anaphylactoid reactions/Anaphylaxis
(1987): Norrby SR, *Drugs* 34 (Suppl 2), 105
Candidiasis (<1%)
Injection-site induration (<1%)
Injection-site pain (<1%)
Phlebitis

(1980): Meguro S+, *Jpn J Antibiot* 33, 1163
Serum sickness (<1%)

CEPHAPIRIN

Trade names: Brisfirina; Cefadyl; Cefaloject; Cefatrex;
Cefatrexyl; Lopitrex; Unipirin
Indications: Various infections caused by susceptible organisms
Category: Cephalosporin, 1st generation
Half-life: 36–60 minutes

Note: Penicillin and cephalosporins share a common beta-lactam structure. People who are allergic to penicillin are approximately 4 times more likely to develop an allergic reaction to a cephalosporin than those people who have no penicillin allergy. (From 5 to 16% of patients allergic to penicillin develop allergic reactions to cephalosporins)

Reactions

Skin
Erythema multiforme
Exanthems
  (1983): Watanabe A+, *Jpn J Antibiot* 36(12), 3395
Pruritus (1–5%)
Rash (sic) (1–5%)
  (1989): Vidal Pan C+, *Chemotherapy* 35(6), 449
Stevens–Johnson syndrome (<1%)
Toxic epidermal necrolysis
Urticaria (<1%)

Other
Anaphylactoid reactions/Anaphylaxis
Candidiasis (<1%)
Fever
  (1989): Vidal Pan C+, *Chemotherapy* 35(6), 449
  (1983): Watanabe A+, *Jpn J Antibiot* 36(12), 3395
Hypersensitivity
Injection-site pain (1–5%)
Injection-site phlebitis (1–5%)
Paresthesias (1–5%)
Phlebitis
  (1983): Watanabe A+, *Jpn J Antibiot* 36(12), 3395
  (1980): Meguro S+, *Jpn J Antibiot* 33, 1163
Serum sickness (<1%)

CEPHRADINE

Trade names: Anspor; Cefro; Celex; Doncef; Eskacef;
Maxisporin; Opebrin; Sefril; Velosef (Bristol-Myers Squibb);
Veracef
Indications: Various infections caused by susceptible organisms
Category: Cephalosporin, 1st generation
Half-life: 1–2 hours

Note: Penicillin and cephalosporins share a common beta-lactam structure. People who are allergic to penicillin are approximately 4 times more likely to develop an allergic reaction to a cephalosporin than those people who have no penicillin allergy. (From 5 to 16% of patients allergic to penicillin develop allergic reactions to cephalosporins)

Reactions

Skin
Acute generalized exanthematous pustulosis (AGEP)
  (1995): Moreau A+, *Int J Dermatol* 34, 263 (passim)
Erythema multiforme
Exanthems
Pruritus (<1%)
Purpura
Pustules
  (1986): Kalb RE+, *Cutis* 38, 58
Rash (sic) (<1%)
Stevens–Johnson syndrome (<1%)
Toxic epidermal necrolysis
  (1990): Balcar-Boron A+, *Wiad Lek* (Polish) 43, 988
Toxic pustuloderma
  (1990): Rustin MHA+, *Br J Dermatol* 123, 119
Urticaria (<1%)

Mucosal/ENT
Vaginitis

Other
Anaphylactoid reactions/Anaphylaxis
Hypersensitivity
Injection-site pain (<1%)
Injection-site phlebitis (<1%)
Serum sickness

CERTOLIZUMAB PEGOL

Trade name: Cimzia (Celltech) (UCB)
Indications: Crohn's disease, rheumatoid arthritis
Category: TNF inhibitor
Half-life: 14 days
Clinically important, potentially hazardous interactions with: abatacept, anakinra, **live and dead vaccines**

Reactions

Skin
Allergic reactions (sic)
Angioedema (<1%)
Dermatitis (<1%)
Erythema nodosum (<1%)
Lupus syndrome (<1%)
Lymphoma
Rash (sic) (<1%)
Urticaria (<1%)
Vasculitis (<1%)

Mucosal/ENT
Aphthous stomatitis (<1%)
Nasopharyngitis (4–13%)

Hair
Hair – alopecia (<1%)

Eyes
Ocular hemorrhage (<1%)
Optic neuritis (<1%)
Uveitis (<1%)
Vision blurred (<1%)

Other

Abdominal pain
Anxiety (<1%)
Asthenia (<1%)
Cardiac failure
Fever (5%)
Headache (7–18%)
Hepatotoxicity (<1%)
Hypersensitivity (<1%)
Hypotension (<1%)
Infections (sic) (14–38%)
  (2007): Schreiber S+, *N Engl J Med* 357(3), 239
Injection-site reactions (~7%)
Nephrotoxicity
Seizures (<1%)
Serum sickness (<1%)
Suicidal ideation (<1%)
Upper respiratory infection (20%)
Vertigo (~6%)

CETIRIZINE

Synonyms: P-071; UCB-P071
Trade names: Alercet; Alerid; Cetrine; Cezin; Reactine; Triz; Virlix; Zirtin; Zyrtec (Pfizer)
Indications: Allergic rhinitis, urticaria
Category: Histamine H1 receptor antagonist
Half-life: 8–11 hours
Clinically important, potentially hazardous interactions with: alcohol, CNS depressants, pilsicainide

Reactions

Skin

Acne (<2%)
Angioedema (<2%)
Bullous dermatitis (<2%)
Dermatitis (<2%)
Diaphoresis (<2%)
Edema (ankle) (generalized)
Exanthems (<2%)
  (1998): Rehbein H, Jacksonville, FL (generalized) (from Internet) (observation)
  (1997): Stingeni L+, *Contact Dermatitis* 37, 249
Facial edema
  (2002): Schroer S+, *Clin Exp Dermatol* 27, 185
Fixed eruption
  (2007): Cravo M+, *Int J Dermatol* 46(7), 760
  (2005): Guptha SD+, *Indian J Dermatol Venereol Leprol* 71(5), 361
  (2002): Assouere MN+, *Ann Dermatol Venereol* 129(11), 1295
  (2002): Inamadar AC+, *Br J Dermatol* 147(5), 1025
  (2000): Kranke B+, *J Allergy Clin Immunol* 106(5), 988 (multilocalized and bullous)
Furunculosis (<2%)
Hyperkeratosis (<2%)
Peripheral edema
Photosensitivity (<2%)
Phototoxicity (<2%)
Pruritus (<2%)
  (2002): Schroer S+, *Clin Exp Dermatol* 27, 185
Purpura (<2%)
Rash (sic) (<2%)
Seborrhea (<2%)

Urticaria (<2%)
  (2002): Schroer S+, *Clin Exp Dermatol* 27, 185
  (2001): Calista D+, *Br J Dermatol* 144, 196
  (1999): Karamfilov T+, *Br J Dermatol* 140, 979
  (1997): Stingeni L+, *Contact Dermatitis* 37, 249
Xerosis (<2%)

Mucosal/ENT

Ageusia (<2%)
Dysgeusia (<2%)
Parosmia (<2%)
Sialorrhea (<2%)
Stomatitis (<2%)
Tongue edema (<2%)
Tongue pigmentation (<2%)
Vaginitis (<2%)
Xerostomia (5.7%)
  (2001): Wellington K+, *Drugs* 61(15), 2231 (with pseudoephedrine)
  (1995): Breneman D+, *J Am Acad Dermatol* 33, 192

Hair

Hair – alopecia (<2%)
  (1998): Reed BR, Denver, CO (from Internet) (observation)
Hair – hypertrichosis (<2%)

Eyes

Periorbital edema

Other

Anaphylactoid reactions/Anaphylaxis (<2%)
Asthenia
  (2001): Wellington K+, *Drugs* 61(15), 2231 (with pseudoephedrine)
Headache
  (2001): Wellington K+, *Drugs* 61(15), 2231 (with pseudoephedrine)
Myalgia/Myositis/Myopathy/Myotoxicity (<2%)
Paresthesias (<2%)

CETRORELIX

Trade name: Cetrotide (Merck)
Indications: Inhibition of premature luteinizing hormone surges in women undergoing controlled ovarian stimulation
Category: Gonadotropin-releasing hormone antagonist
Half-life: 5 hours

Reactions

Skin

Edema
Erythema
Peripheral edema
Pruritus
Purpura

Other

Anaphylactoid reactions/Anaphylaxis
  (2003): Verschraegen CF+, *Gynecol Oncol* 90(3), 552
Headache
  (2003): Verschraegen CF+, *Gynecol Oncol* 90(3), 552
Hot flashes
  (2003): Verschraegen CF+, *Gynecol Oncol* 90(3), 552
Injection-site edema
Injection-site erythema
  (1994): Leroy I+, *Fertil Steril* 62, 461

Injection-site pruritus
(1994): Leroy I+, *Fertil Steril* 62, 461
Injection-site purpura
Injection-site reactions
(2003): Verschraegen CF+, *Gynecol Oncol* 90(3), 552

CETUXIMAB

Trade name: Erbitux (Bristol-Myers Squibb)
Indications: Metastatic colorectal cancer
Category: Antineoplastic; Monoclonal antibody
Half-life: 75–188 hours
Clinically important, potentially hazardous interactions with: None

Reactions

Skin
Acne (88%)
(2007): Alexandrescu DT+, *Clin Exp Dermatol* 32(1), 71
(2007): Cotena C+, *Acta Dermatovenerol Croat* 15(4), 246
(2007): Gencoglan G+, *Skin Pharmacol Physiol* 20(5), 260 (2 cases)
(2007): Labianca R+, *Int J Biol Markers* 22(1 Suppl 4), S40
(2007): Saif MW+, *Expert Opin Drug Saf* 6(2), 175
(2006): Gebbia V+, *Clin Colorectal Cancer* 5(6), 422 (13%)
(2006): Gutzmer R+, *Hautarzt* 57(6), 509
(2006): Hanna N+, *J Clin Oncol* 24(33), 5253 (6%)
(2006): Hannoud S+, *Ann Dermatol Venereol* 133(3), 239
(2006): Lenz HJ, *Oncology (Williston Park)* 20(5 Suppl 2), 5
(2006): Roe E+, *J Am Acad Dermatol* 55(3), 429
(2006): Tscharner GG+, *Dermatology* 213(1), 37
(2005): *Prescrire Int* 14(80), 215
(2005): Ely EH, Grass Valley, CA (from Internet) (observation)
(2005): Grafton LH, Thiboudaux, LA (from Internet) (observation)
(2005): Herrera-Acosta E+, *Actas Dermosifiliogr* 96(4), 252
(2005): Martinez de Lagran Z+, *Actas Dermosifiliogr* 96(7), 450
(2005): Micantonio T+, *Arch Dermatol* 141(9), 1173
(2005): Molinari E+, *Dermatology* 211(4), 330
(2005): Moss JE+, *N Engl J Med* 353(19), e17
(2004): Saltz LB+, *J Clin Oncol* 22(7), 1201
(2003): Walon L+, *Ann Dermatol Venereol* 130(4), 443 (2 cases)
(2000): Baselga J+, *J Clin Oncol* 18, 904
Allergic reactions (sic)
(2001): Herbst RS+, *Expert Opin Biol Ther* 1(4), 719
(2001): Robert F+, *J Clin Oncol* 19(13), 3234
Burning
(2006): Roe E+, *J Am Acad Dermatol* 55(3), 429
Erythema
(2006): Hannoud S+, *Ann Dermatol Venereol* 133(3), 239
Exanthems (with irinotecan)
Fissures
(2006): Roe E+, *J Am Acad Dermatol* 55(3), 429
Folliculitis
(2006): Adams DH+, *Am J Clin Dermatol* 7(5), 333
(2006): Hannoud S+, *Ann Dermatol Venereol* 133(3), 239
(2006): Roe E+, *J Am Acad* 55(3), 429
(2005): Egana JI+, *Neuroscience* 134(3), 1069
(2005): Ely EH, Grass Valley. CA (from Internet) (observation)
(2002): Kimyai-Asadi A, *Arch Dermatol* 138, 129
(1999): Ezekiel MP+, *Am Soc Clin Oncol meeting* Abstract 1501
(1999): Mendelsohn J+, *Am Soc Clin Oncol meeting* Abstract 1502
Papulopustular eruption
(2007): Bragg J+, *Dermatol Online J* 13(1), 1
Peripheral edema (10%)

Pruritus (10%)
(2006): Porzio G+, *J Pain Symptom Manage* 32(5), 397
(2003): Walon L+, *Ann Dermatol Venereol* 130(4), 443 (2 cases)
Rash (sic)
(2007): Saif MW+, *Expert Opin Drug Saf* 6(2), 175
(2005): Rhee J+, *Clin Colorectal Cancer* 5 Suppl 2, S101
(2004): Yamamoto DS+, *Clin J Oncol Nurs* 8(6), 654
(2001): Herbst RS+, *Expert Opin Biol Ther* 1(4), 719
Toxicity (sic)
(2006): Modi S+, *Clin Breast Cancer* 7(3), 270 (with paclitaxel)
(2003): Monti M+, *J Clin Oncol* 21(24), 4651
(2001): Robert F+, *J Clin Oncol* 19(13), 3234
Transient acantholytic dermatosis (Grover's disease)
(2006): Tscharner GG+, *Dermatology* 213(1), 37
Xerosis
(2006): Gutzmer R+, *Hautarzt* 57(6), 509
(2006): Roe E+, *J Am Acad Dermatol* 55(3), 429

Mucosal/ENT
Aphthous stomatitis
(2006): Roe E+, *J Am Acad Dermatol* 55(3), 429
Stomatitis (11%)

Hair
Hair – alopecia (5%)

Nails
Nails – changes (sic) (16%)
Nails – paronychia
(2006): Gutzmer R+, *Hautarzt* 57(6), 509
(2006): Roe E+, *J Am Acad Dermatol* 55(3), 429
(2006): Shu KY+, *Br J Dermatol* 154(1), 191
(2002): Boucher KW+, *J Am Acad Dermatol* 47(4), 632 (14%)
(2001): Williamson K, *Dermatol Online J* 7(1), 24D

Eyes
Blepharitis
(2006): Dranko S+, *Clin Colorectal Cancer* 6(3), 224
Conjunctivitis (7%)
Ectropion
(2007): Garibaldi DC+, *Ophthal Plast Reconstr Surg* 23(1), 62
Eyelashes – hypertrichosis
(2006): Roe E+, *J Am Acad Dermatol* 55(3), 429
Ocular pruritus
(2006): Roe E+, *J Am Acad Dermatol* 55(3), 429
Trichomegaly
(2005): Bouche O+, *Ann Oncol* 16(10), 1711

Other
Abdominal pain (25%)
Anaphylactoid reactions/Anaphylaxis
(2006): Hanna N+, *J Clin Oncol* 24(33), 5253 (1%)
(2006): Lenz HJ, *Oncology (Williston Park)* 20(5 Suppl 2), 5
Application-site reactions (sic) (~3%)
(2006): Hannoud S+, *Ann Dermatol Venereol* 133(3), 239
(2006): Patel DD+, *Oncology (Williston Park)* 20(11), 1373
Asthenia
(2006): Gebbia V+, *Clin Colorectal Cancer* 5(6), 422 (13%)
(2001): Robert F+, *J Clin Oncol* 19(13), 3234 (49%)
Chills (with irinotecan)
Cough (9%)
Depression (9%)
Fever
(2007): Saif MW+, *Expert Opin Drug Saf* 6(2), 175
(2001): Robert F+, *J Clin Oncol* 19(13), 3234 (33%)
Headache (25%)
(2007): Saif MW+, *Expert Opin Drug Saf* 6(2), 175
Hypersensitivity
(2008): Chung CH+, *N Engl J Med* 358(11), 1109
(2007): Saif MW+, *Expert Opin Drug Saf* 6(2), 175

(2005): *Prescrire Int* 14(80), 215
Pain (19%)

CEVIMELINE

Trade name: Exovac
Indications: Sicca syndrome in patients with Sjøgren's syndrome
Category: Muscarinic cholinergic agonist
Half-life: 3–4 hours

Reactions

Skin
Allergic reactions (sic) (1–10%)
Bullous dermatitis (<1%)
Dermatitis (<1%)
Diaphoresis (20%)
Eczema (<1%)
Edema (1–10%)
Exanthems (1–10%)
Fungal dermatitis (1–10%)
Genital pruritus (<1%)
Hyperhidrosis
   (2002): Petrone D+, *Arthritis Rheum* 46(3), 748
Peripheral edema (1–10%)
Photosensitivity (<1%)
Pruritus (1–10%)
Rash (sic) (4%)
Ulcerations (<1%)
Vasculitis (<1%)
Xerosis (<1%)

Mucosal/ENT
Dysgeusia (<1%)
Gingival hyperplasia/hypertrophy (<1%)
Parosmia (<1%)
Sialorrhea (2%)
Stomatitis (<1%)
Tongue pigmentation (<1%)
Tongue ulceration (<1%)
Ulcerative stomatitis (1–10%)
Vaginitis (1–10%)
Xerostomia (1–10%)

Hair
Hair – alopecia (<1%)

Other
Abdominal pain
   (2002): Petrone D+, *Arthritis Rheum* 46(3), 748
Headache
   (2002): Petrone D+, *Arthritis Rheum* 46(3), 748
Hot flashes (2%)
Myalgia/Myositis/Myopathy/Myotoxicity (1–10%)
Paresthesias (<1%)
Tendinopathy/Tendon rupture (<1%)
Thrombophlebitis (<1%)
Tremor (1–10%)

CHAMOMILE

Scientific names: *Chamomilla recutita; Matricaria chamomilla; Matricaria recutita*
Family: Asteraceae; Compositae
Trade and other common names: Camomille; German Chamomile; Manzanilla; Pin Heads
Category: Sedative
Purported indications and other uses: Flatulence, travel sickness, nervous diarrhea, restlessness, menstrual cramps, hemorrhoids, mastitis, leg ulcers, inflammation of the respiratory tract. Used in flavoring, cosmetics, soaps and mouthwashes
Half-life: N/A
Clinically important, potentially hazardous interactions with: warfarin

Reactions

Skin
Allergic reactions (sic) (to those allergic to ragweed, marigolds, daisies)
Dermatitis
   (2002): Schempp CM+, *Hautarzt* 53(2), 93
   (2000): Foti C+, *Contact Dermatitis* 42(6), 360
   (2000): Giordano-Labadie F+, *Contact Dermatitis* 42(4), 247
Irritation
Sensitization
   (2002): Paulsen E, *Contact Dermatitis* 47(4), 189

Eyes
Ocular adverse effects
   (2004): Fraunfelder FW, *Am J Ophthalmol* 138(4), 639

Other
Anaphylactoid reactions/Anaphylaxis
   (2001): Thien FC, *Med J Aust* 175(1), 54 (from enema)
   (1989): Subiza J+, *J Allergy Clin Immunol* 84, 353
Hypersensitivity

CHARCOAL

Synonyms: Activated carbon; activated charcoal; liquid antidote
Trade names: Actidose-Aqua (Cambridge); Carbomix (Meadow); Char-Caps; Charcadole; Charcoal Plus; Charcocaps; EZ-Char; Kerr Insta-Char
Indications: Emergency treatment in poisoning
Category: Antidote; Antimotility
Half-life: N/A
Clinically important, potentially hazardous interactions with: carbamazepine

Reactions

Other
Abdominal pain
   (2003): Eroglu A+, *J Toxicol Clin Toxical* 41(1), 71
Asthenia
   (2002): Sato RL+, *Hawaii Med J* 61(11), 251
Headache
   (2002): Sato RL+, *Hawaii Med J* 61(11), 251
Seizures
   (2003): Pellitero Rodriguez S+, *Rev Clin Esp* 203(7), 358

CHASTEBERRY

Scientific name: *Vitex agnus-castus*
Family: Verbenaceae
Trade and other common names: Abraham's Balm; Agno Casto; Agnocasto; Agnolyt (Madaus); Bish Barmagh Aghaji; Chaste Lamb-Tree; Chaste tree; Daribrahim; Gatilier; Hayit; Hemp Tree; Kaff Maryam; Keuschlamm; Lygos; Monks Pepper; Panjangusht; Ranukabija; Safe Tree; Sauzgatillo; Seiyo-Ninzin-Boku; Shajerat Ebrahim; Strotan; Vitex; Ze 440
Category: Hormone modulator
Half-life: N/A
Clinically important, potentially hazardous interactions with: dopamine-receptor antagonists

Reactions

Skin
Abscess
  (2001): Schellenberg R, *BMJ* 322(7279), 134 (mild)
Acne
  (2001): Schellenberg R, *BMJ* 322(7279), 134 (mild)
Adverse effects (sic)
  (2001): Schellenberg R, *BMJ* 322(7279), 134 (mild)
  (2000): Loch EG+, *J Womens Health Gend Based Med* 9(3), 315 (1.2%)
Formication
Pruritus
Rash (sic)
Urticaria
  (2001): Schellenberg R, *BMJ* 322(7279), 134 (mild)

Other
Asthenia
  (2000): Berger D+, *Arch Gynecol Obstet* 264(3), 150
Headache
  (2000): Berger D+, *Arch Gynecol Obstet* 264(3), 150

CHICORY

Scientific name: *Cichorium intybus*
Family: Compositae
Trade and other common names: Barbe de Capucin; Belgian endive; Hendibeh; Succory; Wild Succory
Category: Diuretic
Purported indications and other uses: coffee substitute, jaundice, liver enlargement, gout, rheumatism, skin eruptions connected with gout, inflammation. **Topical:** leaves used for swelling and inflammation. Culinary spice, flavoring
Half-life: N/A

Reactions

Skin
Allergic reactions (sic)
  (2003): Cadot P+, *Int Arch Allergy Immunol* 131(1), 19
  (1997): Helbling A+, *J Allergy Clin Immunol* 99(6), 854
  (1996): Cadot P+, *Clin Exp Allergy* 26(8), 940
Dermatitis
  (1983): Malten KE, *Contact Dermatitis* 9(3), 232

CHLORAL HYDRATE

Synonyms: chloral; hydrated chloral
Trade names: Aquachloral; Chloraldurat; Medianox; Noctec; Novochlorhydrate; Somnox; Welldorm
Indications: Insomnia, sedation
Category: Anesthetic, general; Hypnotic
Half-life: 8–11 hours
Clinically important, potentially hazardous interactions with: antihistamines, azatadine, brompheniramine, buclizine, chlorpheniramine, clemastine, dexchlorpheniramine, diphenhydramine, meclizine, tripelennamine

Reactions

Skin
Acne
Angioedema
Bullous dermatitis
Dermatitis
  (1987): de Groot AC+, *Contact Dermatitis* 16, 229
Eczema
Erythema
Erythema multiforme
  (1991): Porteous DM+, *Arch Dermatol* 127, 740 (in AIDS)
Exanthems
  (1990): Lindner K+, *Dermatol Monatsschr* (German) 176, 483
Fixed eruption
Lichenoid eruption
Perioral dermatitis
  (2001): Caksen H+, *Pediatr Dermatol* 18(5), 454
Pruritus
  (1990): Lindner K+, *Dermatol Monatsschr* (German) 176, 483
Purpura
Rash (sic) (1–10%)
Ulcerations
Urticaria (1–10%)

Mucosal/ENT
Dysgeusia
Oral lesions
  (2001): Caksen H+, *Pediatr Dermatol* 18(5), 454
Oral ulceration
Stomatitis

Other
Death
  (2003): Thurau K+, *Arch Kriminol* 211(3), 90
  (2001): Gaulier JM+, *J Forensic Sci* 46(6), 1507 (2 cases)
Headache
Hypersensitivity
Hypertension
  (2006): Heistein LC+, *Pediatrics* 117(3), e434 (6%)

CHLORAMBUCIL

Trade names: Chloraminophene; Leukeran (GSK); Linfolysin
Indications: Chronic lymphocytic leukemia, lymphomas, carcinomas
Category: Alkylating agent
Half-life: 1.5 hours
Clinically important, potentially hazardous interactions with: aldesleukin, antineoplastics, azathioprine, bone marrow suppressants, prednisone, **vaccines**

Reactions

Skin
Angioedema
Dermatitis
 (2002): Goon AT+, *Contact Dermatitis* 47(5), 309 (with
   melphalan)
Edema
Erythema multiforme
 (1987): Hitchens RN+, *Aust N Z J Med* 17, 600
Exanthems
 (1992): Breathnach SM+, *Adverse Drug Reactions and the Skin*
   Blackwell, Oxford, 289 (passim)
 (1987): Hitchens RN+, *Aust N Z J Med* 17, 600
 (1986): Peterman A+, *Arch Dermatol* 122, 1358
Exfoliative dermatitis
 (2006): Kilickap S+, *Am J Hematol* 81(11), 891
 (1987): Hitchens RN+, *Aust N Z J Med* 17, 600
Facial erythema
 (1986): Peterman A+, *Arch Dermatol* 122, 1358
Herpes simplex
 (1984): Sahgal SM+, *J R Soc Med* 77, 144
Herpes zoster
 (2003): Martinelli G+, *Br J Haematol* 123(2), 271 (2 cases) (with
   rituximab)
 (2002): Goldstein DA+, *Ophthalmology* 109(2), 370
Kaposi's sarcoma
Lupus erythematosus
 (1986): Peterman A+, *Arch Dermatol* 122, 1358
Necrosis
Perianal irritation
 (2003): Martinelli G+, *Br J Haematol* 123(2), 271 (with
   rituximab)
Peripheral edema
 (1987): Schmutz JL+, *Ann Dermatol Venereol* (French) 114, 569
Photosensitivity
 (1987): Schmutz JL+, *Ann Dermatol Venereol* (French) 114, 569
Pruritus
Psoriasis (exacerbation)
Purpura
 (1990): Pietrantonio F+, *Cancer Lett* 54, 109
Rash (sic) (1–10%)
Sezary syndrome
 (1981): Ferme F+, *Leuk Res* 5, 169
Side effects (sic)
Stevens–Johnson syndrome
Toxic epidermal necrolysis
 (1997): Aydogdu I+, *Anticancer Drugs* 8, 468
 (1990): Barone C+, *Eur J Cancer* 26, 1262
 (1990): Pietrantonio F+, *Cancer Lett* 54, 109
Urticaria
 (1992): Breathnach SM+, *Adverse Drug Reactions and the Skin*
   Blackwell, Oxford, 289 (passim)

Mucosal/ENT
Oral lesions
Oral ulceration (<1%)
 (1987): Hitchens RN+, *Aust N Z J Med* 17, 600
Stomatitis
Tinnitus
 (1984): Snavely SR+, *Ann Intern Med* 101(1), 92

Hair
Hair – alopecia
 (1992): Breathnach SM+, *Adverse Drug Reactions and the Skin*
   Blackwell, Oxford, 289 (passim)

Eyes
Periorbital edema
 (1992): Breathnach SM+, *Adverse Drug Reactions and the Skin*
   Blackwell, Oxford, 289 (passim)
 (1986): Peterman A+, *Arch Dermatol* 122, 1358
Visual hallucinations
 (1984): Walsh KP+, *Ir Med J* 77(9), 288

Other
Hypersensitivity (<1%)
Inappropriate secretion of antidiuretic hormone (SIADH)
 (1999): Wagner AM+, *Ann Hematol* 78(1), 37
Seizures
 (2006): Lau CP+, *Intern Med J* 36(10), 683

CHLORAMPHENICOL

Trade names: AK-Chlor; Aquamycetin; Cebenicol; Chloroptic;
Diochloram; Kloramfenicol; Oleomycetin; Ophthochlor;
Pentamycetin; Sopamycetin; Tifomycine
Indications: Various infections caused by susceptible organisms
Category: Antibiotic
Half-life: 1.5–3.5 hours
**Clinically important, potentially hazardous interactions
with:** amoxicillin, ampicillin, ethotoin, fosphenytoin,
mephenytoin, phenytoin

Note: Gray syndrome: toxic reactions in premature infants and
newborns. Signs and symptoms include: abdominal distension, blue-
gray skin color, low body temperature, and uneven breathing

Reactions

Skin
Acute generalized exanthematous pustulosis (AGEP)
 (1999): Lee AY+, *Acta Derm Venereol* 79, 412
 (1995): Moreau A+, *Int J Dermatol* 34, 263 (passim)
Angioedema (<1%)
 (1985): Schewach-Millet M+, *Arch Dermatol* 121, 587
Bullous dermatitis
Dermatitis
 (2001): Sachs B+, *Allergy* 56(1), 69
 (1998): Le Coz CJ+, *Contact Dermatitis* 38, 108 (face)
 (1996): Moyano JC+, *Allergy* 51, 67
 (1992): Urrutia I+, *Contact Dermatitis* 26, 66
 (1991): Vincenzi C+, *Contact Dermatitis* 25, 64
 (1987): Kubo Y+, *Contact Dermatitis* 17, 245
 (1987): Raulin C+, *Derm Beruf Umwelt* 35, 64
 (1986): Rebandel P+, *Contact Dermatitis* 15, 92
 (1986): van Joost T+, *Contact Dermatitis* 14, 176
 (1985): Linss G+, *Dermatol Monatsschr* (German) 171, 250
Eczema
Erythema (sheet-like)
Erythema multiforme (<1%)
 (1996): Lazarov A+, *Cutis* 58, 263 (from eyedrops)
 (1986): Fisher AA, *Cutis* 37, 158 (topical application)
Exanthems (1–5%)
 (1992): Breathnach SM+, *Adverse Drug Reactions and the Skin*
   Blackwell, Oxford, 157 (passim)
Fixed eruption
 (1985): Pandhi RK+, *Australasian J Dermatol* 26, 88
Gray syndrome
Jarisch–Herxheimer reaction
 (1983): Perine PL+, *Am J Trop Med Hyg* 32(5), 1096
Leukoderma
 (1980): Chalfin J+, *Ophthalmic Surg* 11, 194 (eyelid)

Peripheral edema
Pruritus (<1%)
(1992): Breathnach SM+, *Adverse Drug Reactions and the Skin*
Blackwell, Oxford, 157 (passim)
Purpura
Pustules
Rash (sic) (<1%)
Sensitization
(1992): Urrutia I+, *Contact Dermatitis* 26, 66
(1986): van Joost T+, *Contact Dermatitis* 14, 176
Stevens–Johnson syndrome
Toxic epidermal necrolysis (<1%)
Urticaria
(1992): Breathnach SM+, *Adverse Drug Reactions and the Skin*
Blackwell, Oxford, 157 (passim)
(1987): Perkins JB+, *Drug Intell Clin Pharm* 21, 343
(1985): Schewach-Millet M+, *Arch Dermatol* 121, 587
Vasculitis

Mucosal/ENT
Glossitis
Oral mucosal eruption
Oral ulceration
Stomatitis (<1%)
Tinnitus
(1984): Snavely SR+, *Ann Intern Med* 101(1), 92
Tongue black
Xerostomia

Hair
Hair – alopecia

Nails
Nails – photo-onycholysis
(1985): Kechijian P, *J Am Acad Dermatol* 12, 552
(1984): Daniel CR+, *J Am Acad Dermatol* 10, 250

Other
Anaphylactoid reactions/Anaphylaxis
Headache
Hypersensitivity
Paresthesias
(1988): Ramilo O+, *Pediatr Infect Dis* 7, 358
Porphyria

CHLORDIAZEPOXIDE

Trade names: Corax; Huberplex; Libritabs (Valeant); Librium (Valeant); Limbitrol (Valeant); Medilium; Mitran; Multum; Novopoxide; Psicofar; Reposans-10; Solium; Tropium
Indications: Anxiety
Category: Benzodiazepine
Half-life: 6–25 hours
Clinically important, potentially hazardous interactions with: chlorpheniramine, clarithromycin, efavirenz, esomeprazole, imatinib, indinavir, ketoconazole, nelfinavir, nilutamide, ritonavir

Note: Limbitrol is amitriptyline and chlordiazepoxide

Reactions

Skin
Angioedema (<1%)
Dermatitis (1–10%)
Diaphoresis (>10%)
Edema (1–10%)

Erythema multiforme (<1%)
(1992): Breathnach SM+, *Adverse Drug Reactions and the Skin*
Blackwell, Oxford, 200 (passim)
(1985): Kauppinen K+, *Br J Dermatol* 112, 575
(1981): Edwards JG, *Drugs* 22, 495 (passim)
Erythema nodosum (<1%)
(1981): Edwards JG, *Drugs* 22, 495 (passim)
Exanthems
(2005): Sakai H+, *Int J Dermatol* 44(3), 260
Fixed eruption (<1%)
(2005): Sakai H+, *Int J Dermatol* 44(3), 260
(1990): Gaffoor PMA+, *Cutis* 45, 242 (passim)
(1981): Edwards JG, *Drugs* 22, 495 (passim)
Lupus erythematosus
Photosensitivity
(1986): Morliere P, *Biochemie* 68, 849
(1981): Edwards JG, *Drugs* 22, 495 (passim)
(1980): Bjellerup M+, *J Invest Dermatol* 75, 228
Pigmented purpuric eruption
(1989): Nishioka K+, *J Dermatol* (Tokio) 16, 220
Pruritus
Purpura
(2001): Alexopoulou A+, *Arch Intern Med* 161(14), 1778 (with clidinium)
(1981): Edwards JG, *Drugs* 22, 495 (passim)
Rash (sic) (>10%)
Stevens–Johnson syndrome
(2005): Huang PH+, *J Chin Med Assoc* 68(6), 276
Urticaria
(1981): Edwards JG, *Drugs* 22, 495 (passim)
Vasculitis
(1989): Nishioka K+, *J Dermatol* 16, 220

Mucosal/ENT
Sialopenia (>10%)
Sialorrhea (1–10%)
Xerostomia (>10%)

Hair
Hair – alopecia

Other
Gynecomastia
Headache
Injection-site phlebitis
Paresthesias
Porphyria
(1983): Eubanks SW+, *Int J Dermatol* 22, 337

CHLORHEXIDINE

Trade names: Alcloxidine; Bactoscrub; BactoShield; Betasept; Chlorhexamed; Corsodyl; Dyna-Hex; Exidine Scrub; Hexol; Hibiclens (SSL); Hibident; Hibidil; Hibiscrub; Hibistat; Hibitane; Peridex; PerioChip; Periogard; Savlon; Spectro Gram
Indications: Skin antisepsis, gingivitis
Category: Antiseptic
Half-life: N/A

Reactions

Skin
Allergic reactions (sic)
(2003): Jayathillake A+, *Urology* 61(4), 837
(2001): Garvey LH+, *Acta Anaesthesiol Scand* 45(10), 1290 (4 cases)

(1995): Yong D+, *Med J Aust* 162, 257
(1992): Ramselaar CG+, *Br J Urol* 70, 451
(1985): Cheung J+, *Anaesth Intensive Care* 13, 429
(1982): Staab W+, *Stomatol DDR* (German) 32, 700

Dermatitis
(2007): Kaminska R+, *Contact Dermatitis* 56(6), 358 (contact)
(2001): Barnett L+, *Ostomy Wound Manage* 47(9), 47
(2001): Barrazza V, *Contact Dermatitis* 45(1), 42
(1998): Ebo DG+, *J Allergy Clin Immunol* 101, 128
(1998): Thune P, *Tidsskr Nor Laegeforen* (Norwegian) 18, 3295
(1995): Stingeni L+, *Contact Dermatitis* 33, 172
(1990): Reynolds NJ+, *Contact Dermatitis* 22, 103
(1988): Bergqvist-Karlsson A, *Contact Dermatitis* 18, 84
(1987): Osmundsen PE+, *Ugeskr Laeger* (Danish) 149, 3048
(1985): Lasthein Andersen B+, *Contact Dermatitis* 13, 307
    (5.4%)
(1983): Shoji A, *Contact Dermatitis* 9, 156
(1982): Osmundsen PE, *Contact Dermatitis* 8, 81
(1981): Roberts DL+, *Contact Dermatitis* 7, 326

Facial edema (<1%)

Fixed eruption
(1991): Moghadam BK+, *Oral Surg Oral Med Oral Pathol* 71, 431

Photosensitivity

Rash (sic)
(2001): Garvey LH+, *Acta Anaesthesiol Scand* 45(10), 1290 (4
    cases)

Urticaria
(1998): Stables GI+, *Br J Urol* 82, 756
(1990): Wong WK+, *Contact Dermatitis* 22, 52 (contact)
(1989): Fisher AA, *Cutis* 43, 17
(1988): Bergqvist-Karlsson A, *Contact Dermatitis* 18, 84

Mucosal/ENT

Ageusia

Dysgeusia (>10%)
(2006): Gurgan CA+, *J Periodontol* 77(3), 370
(2001): Quirynen M+, *J Clin Periodontol* 28(12), 1127

Gingival pigmentation
(2006): Gurgan CA+, *J Periodontol* 77(3), 370
(2005): Ernst CP+, *Quintessence Int* 36(8), 641

Gingivitis
(1984): Asikainen S+, *J Clin Periodontol* 11, 87
(1982): Ainamo J+, *J Clin Periodontol* 9, 337

Glossitis (1–10%)

Oral mucosal irritation
(2006): Gurgan CA+, *J Periodontol* 77(3), 370

Oral mucositis
(1982): Skoglund LA+, *Int J Oral Surg* 11, 380 (3 cases)

Stomatitis (1–10%)

Tongue irritation (1–10%)

Tongue pigmentation (>10%)

Vaginal pruritus
(2004): Wilson CM+, *J Acquir Immune Defic Syndr* 35(2), 138

Other

Anaphylactoid reactions/Anaphylaxis
(2004): Beaudouin E+, *Allerg Immunol* (Paris) 36(4), 123
(2004): Krautheim AB+, *Contact Dermatitis* 50(3), 113
(2001): Garvey LH+, *Acta Anaesthesiol Scand* 45(10), 1204 (4
    cases)
(2001): Knight BA+, *Intern Med J* 31(7), 436
(2001): Lockhart AS+, *Br J Anaesth* 87(6), 940
(2001): Stephens R+, *Br J Anaesth* 87(2), 306 (with sulfadiazine)
(2000): Pham NH+, *Clin Exp Allergy* 30, 1001
(1999): Autegarden JE+, *Contact Dermatitis* 40, 215
(1999): Snellman E+, *J Am Acad Dermatol* 40, 771
(1998): Ebo DG+, *J Allergy Clin Immunol* 101, 128
(1998): Nikaido S+, *Masui* (Japanese) 47, 330
(1998): Olivieri J+, *Schweiz Med Wochenschr* 128, 1508

(1998): Terazawa E+, *Anesthesiology* 89, 1296
(1998): Thune P, *Tidsskr Nor Laegeforen* (Norwegian) 118, 3295
(1997): Chisholm DG+, *BMJ* 315, 785
(1997): Fujita S+, *Masui* (Japanese) 46, 1118 (2 cases)
(1996): Torricelli R, *Clin Exp Allergy* 26, 112
(1995): Parker F+, *Anaesth Intensive Care* 23, 126
(1994): de Groot AC+, *Ned Tijdschr Geneeskd* (Dutch)
    138, 1342
(1994): Okuda T+, *Masui* (Japanese) 43, 1352
(1994): Russ BR+, *Anaesth Intensive Care* 22, 611
(1994): Visser LE+, *Ned Tijdschr Geneeskd* (Dutch) 138, 778
(1992): Evans RJ, *BMJ* 304, 686
(1992): Harukuni I+, *Masui* (Japanese) 41, 455
(1992): Peutrell JM, *Anaesthesia* 47, 1013
(1990): Wong WK+, *Contact Dermatitis* 22, 52

Hypersensitivity
(2001): Lauerma AL, *Contact Dermatitis* 44(1), 59
(1998): Burlington B, *Ostomy Wound Manage* 44, 84
(1994): Aalto-Korte K+, *Duodecim* (Finnish) 110, 2013
(1989): Okano M+, *Arch Dermatol* 125, 50 (6 cases)
(1988): Bergqvist-Karlsson A, *Contact Dermatitis* 18, 84
(1986): Ohtoshi T+, *Clin Allergy* 16, 155
(1986): Yaacob H+, *J Oral Med* 41, 145

CHLORMEZANONE

Trade name: Trancopal
Indications: Anxiety
Category: Anxiolytic; Central muscle relaxant
Half-life: 24 hours

Reactions

Skin

Edema

Erythema multiforme

Exanthems
(1989): Alanko K+, *Acta Derm Venereol* (Stockh) 69, 223

Fixed eruption
(1998): Leal G, Fortaleza, Brazil (from Internet) (observation)
(1998): Lee AY, *Contact Dermatitis* 38(5), 258
(1998): Mahboob A+, *Int J Dermatol* 37, 833
(1995): Rademacher D+, *Contact Dermatitis* 32, 117
(1992): el-Sayed F+, *Ann Dermatol Venereol* (French) 119, 671
(1991): Lee AY+, *Drug Intell Clin Pharm* 25, 604
(1989): Alanko K+, *Acta Derm Venereol* (Stockh) 69, 223
(1988): McFadden N, *Dermatologica* 176, 106
(1985): Kauppinen K+, *Br J Dermatol* 112, 575
(1985): Verbov J, *Dermatologica* 171, 60 (with acetaminophen)
(1983): Mohamed KN+, *Int J Dermatol* 22, 548

Peripheral edema

Pruritus

Rash (sic)
(1991): Lee AY+, *Drug Intell Clin Pharm* 25, 604 (passim)

Stevens–Johnson syndrome
(1995): Roujeau JC+, *N Engl J Med* 333(24), 1600
(1995): Wolkenstein P+, *Drug Saf* 13, 56

Toxic epidermal necrolysis
(1998): von Boxberg C+, *Dtsch Med Wochenschr* (German)
    123, 866 (fatal)
(1996): Blum L+, *J Am Acad Dermatol* 34, 1088
(1995): Roujeau JC+, *N Engl J Med* 333(24), 1600
(1993): Correia O+, *Dermatology* 186, 32
(1992): Saiag P+, *J Am Acad Dermatol* 26, 567
(1991): Rosenthal E+, *Presse Med* (French) 20, 1459
(1987): Guillaume JC+, *Arch Dermatol* 123, 1166
(1983): Tagami H+, *Arch Dermatol* 119, 910

Urticaria
Mucosal/ENT
Dysgeusia
Xerostomia
Other
Death

CHLOROQUINE

Trade names: Aralen (Sanofi-Aventis); Avloclor; Chlorquin; Emquin; Heliopar; Lagaquin; Malarivon
Indications: Malaria, rheumatoid arthritis, lupus erythematosus
Category: Antimalarial; Antiprotozoal; Disease-modifying antirheumatic
Half-life: 3–5 days
Clinically important, potentially hazardous interactions with: acitretin, antacids, cholestyramine, dapsone, furazolidone, hydroxychloroquine, methotrexate, methoxsalen, penicillamine, sulfonamides

Reactions

Skin
Acute generalized exanthematous pustulosis (AGEP)
    (1998): Janier M+, *Dermatology* 196, 271
Angioedema (<1%)
    (1993): *Lakartidningen* (Swedish) 90, 54
Bullous pemphigoid
    (1999): Millard TP+, *Clin Exp Dermatol* 24, 263
Dermatitis
    (1984): Kellett JK+, *Contact Dermatitis* 11, 17
Desquamation
    (2002): Pages F+, *Trop Med Int Health* 7(11), 919 (with proguanil)
Ephelides
    (1985): Dupre A+, *Arch Dermatol* 121, 1164
Erythema annulare centrifugum
    (1982): Koralewski F, *Dermatosen* (German) 30, 125
Erythema multiforme (<1%)
Erythroderma
    (1990): Simoneaux PW, *Curr Concept Skin Dis* Winter, 15
    (1986): Langtry JA+, *Br Med J Clin Res Ed* 292, 1107
    (1985): Slagel GA+, *J Am Acad Dermatol* 12, 857
Exanthems (1–5%)
    (1991): Ochsendorf FR+, *Hautarzt* (German) 42, 140
    (1990): Simoneaux PW, *Curr Concept Skin Dis* Winter, 15
Exfoliative dermatitis
    (1986): Lavrijsen APM+, *Acta Derm Venereol* (Stockh) 66, 536
    (1985): Slagel GA+, *J Am Acad Dermatol* 12, 857
    (1980): Koranda FC, *J Am Acad Dermatol* 4, 650 (passim)
Fixed eruption (<1%)
Lichenoid eruption
    (1990): Simoneaux PW, *Curr Concept Skin Dis* Winter, 15
    (1981): Koranda FC, *J Am Acad Dermatol* 4, 650 (passim)
Necrotizing vasculitis
    (2003): Luong MS+, *Acta Derm Venereol* 83(2), 141
Photosensitivity
    (2002): Pages F+, *Trop Med Int Health* 7(11), 919 (with proguanil)
    (1993): *Lakartidningen* (Swedish) 90, 54
    (1992): Seideman P+, *Scand J Rheumatol* 21, 101
    (1991): Ochsendorf FR+, *Hautarzt* (German) 42, 140
    (1989): Ortel B+, *Dermatologica* 178, 39
    (1982): van Weelden H, *Arch Dermatol* 118, 290

Pigmentation
    (2006): Anders HJ+, *Med Klin* (Munich) 101(5), 421
    (2006): Reynaert S+, *J Eur Acad Dermatol Venereol* 20(4), 487
    (1998): Guedira N+, *Rev Rhum Engl Ed* 65, 58
    (1991): Ochsendorf FR+, *Hautarzt* (German) 42, 140
    (1987): Krebs A, *Schweiz Rundsch Med Prax* (German) 76, 1069
    (1982): Levy H, *S Afr Med J* 62, 735
    (1981): Koranda FC, *J Am Acad Dermatol* 4, 650 (passim)
    (1980): Bentsi-Enchill KO, *Trop Geogr Med* 32, 216
Pruritus
    (2004): Ajayi AA+, *Int J Dermatol* 43(12), 972
    (2000): Ademowo OG+, *Clin Pharm Ther* 67, 237
    (1999): Millard TP+, *Clin Exp Dermatol* 24, 263
    (1997): Adebayo RA+, *Br J Clin Pharmacol* 44, 157
    (1997): Sowunmi A+, *Trans R Trop Med Hyg* 91, 63
    (1996): George AO, *Int J Dermatol* 35, 323
    (1995): Osifo NG, *Afr J Med Sci* 24, 67
    (1992): Ogunranti JO+, *Eur J Clin Pharmacol* 43, 323
    (1991): Ajayi AA+, *Eur J Clin Pharmacol* 41, 383
    (1991): Ezeamuzie IC+, *J Trop Med Hyg* 94, 184
    (1991): Mnyika KS, *East Afr Med J* 68, 139
    (1991): Mnyika KS+, *J Trop Med Hyg* 94, 27 (47%)
    (1991): Okor RS, *J Clin Pharm Ther* 16, 463
    (1990): Abdulkadir SA+, *Trans Roy Soc Trop Med Hyg* 84, 898
    (1990): Okor RS, *J Clin Pharm Ther* 15, 147
    (1990): Simoneaux PW, *Curr Concept Skin Dis* Winter, 15
    (1989): Abila B+, *J Trop Med Hyg* 92, 356
    (1989): Burnham G+, *Trans R Soc Trop Med Hyg* 83, 527
    (1989): Hallwood PM+, *Lancet* 2, 397
    (1989): Osifo NG, *Afr J Med Sci* 18, 121
    (1989): Soro B+, *Bull Soc Pathol Exot Filiales* (French) 82, 88
    (1989): Sowunmi A+, *Lancet* 2, 213
    (1987): Spencer HC+, *Ann Trop Med Parasitol* 81, 124
    (1986): Harries AD+, *Ann Trop Med Parasitol* 80, 479
    (1984): Bhasin V+, *J Indian Med Assoc* 82, 447
    (1984): Caussade P, *Arch Fr Pediatr* (French) 41, 727
    (1984): Osifo NG, *Arch Dermatol* 120, 80
    (1982): Spencer HC+, *BMJ* 285, 1703
Psoriasis
    (1999): Capper N, Mobile, AL (from Internet) (observation)
    (1998): Wilairatana P+, *Int J Dermatol* 37, 713
    (1997): Wilairatana P+, *Int J Dermatol* 36, 634
    (1993): Schopt RE+, *Dermatology* 187, 100
    (1992): Vestey JP+, *J Infect* 24, 211
    (1991): Damstra RJ+, *Ned Tijdschr Geneeskd* (Dutch) 135, 671
    (1990): Abdulkadir SA+, *Trans R Soc Trop Med Hyg* 84, 898
    (1990): Katugampola G+, *Int J Dermatol* 29, 153
    (1990): Okor RS, *J Clin Pharm Ther* 15, 147
    (1989): Mallett R+, *BMJ* 299, 1400
    (1988): Nicolas J-F+, *Ann Dermatol Venereol* (French) 115, 289
    (1987): Friedman SJ, *J Am Acad Dermatol* 16, 1256
    (1985): Stone OJ, *Int J Dermatol* 24, 539
    (1982): Abel EA+, *J Am Acad Dermatol* 15, 2007
    (1982): Luzar MJ, *J Rheumatol* 9, 462
    (1981): Olsen TG, *Ann Intern Med* 94, 546
    (1980): Kuflik EG, *Cutis* 26, 153
Pustules
    (1990): Lotem M+, *Acta Derm Venereol* (Stockh) 70, 250
Stevens–Johnson syndrome
    (2000): Madnani N, Mumbai, India (from Internet) (observation)
    (1989): Ortel B+, *Dermatologica* 178, 39
    (1987): Lenox-Smith I, *J Infect* 14, 90 (fatal)
    (1986): Bamber MG+, *J Infect* 13, 31 (fatal)
Toxic epidermal necrolysis (<1%)
    (1994): Boffa MJ+, *Br J Dermatol* 131, 444
    (1988): Phillips-Howard PA+, *Br Med J Clin Res Ed* 296, 1605
Urticaria
    (2002): Pages F+, *Trop Med Int Health* 7(11), 919 (with proguanil)
    (1990): Simoneaux PW, *Curr Concept Skin Dis* Winter, 15

(1980): Koranda FC, *J Am Acad Dermatol* 4, 650 (passim)
Vasculitis
Vitiligo
  (2003): Martin-Garcia RF+, *J Am Acad Dermatol* 48(6), 981
  (2002): Martin R+, *World Congress Dermatol* Poster, 0114
  (1997): Selvaag E, *Ann Trop Pediatr* 17, 45
  (1996): Selvaag E, *Acta Derm Venereol* 76, 166
  (1996): Selvaag E, *Trans R Trop Med Hyg* 90, 683
  (1995): Selvaag E+, American Academy of Dermatology
    Meeting, New Orleans (observation)
  (1992): Gonggryp LA+, *Br J Rheumatol* 31, 790
  (1980): Bentsi-Enchill KO, *Trop Geogr Med* 32, 216

Mucosal/ENT

Gingival pigmentation
  (1992): Veraldi S+, *Cutis* 49, 281
Mucosal membrane pigmentation
  (2005): Fardet L+, *Ann Dermatol Venereol* 132(8-9 Pt 1), 665
Oral pigmentation
  (1992): Veraldi S+, *Cutis* 49, 281
  (1991): Zic JA+, *Arch Dermatol* 127, 1037
  (1990): Wollina U+, *Dtsch Z Mund Kiefer Gesichtschir* (German)
    14, 104
  (1981): Koranda FC, *J Am Acad Dermatol* 4, 650 (passim)
  (1980): Bentsi-Enchill KO, *Trop Geogr Med* 32, 216
Oral ulceration
  (2002): Pages F+, *Trop Med Int Health* 7(11), 919 (with
    proguanil)
Stomatitis (<1%)
Stomatopyrosis
Tinnitus
  (2007): Bortoli R+, *Clin Rheumatol* 26(11), 1809

Hair

Hair – alopecia
Hair – pigmentation (<1%)
  (1997): Asch PH+, *Ann Dermatol Venereol* (French) 124, 552
  (1992): Bublin JG+, *J Clin Pharm Ther* 17, 297
  (1991): Ochsendorf FR+, *Hautarzt* (German) 42, 140
  (1981): Koranda FC, *J Am Acad Dermatol* 4, 650 (passim)
Hair – poliosis
  (1985): Dupre A+, *Arch Dermatol* 121, 1164

Nails

Nails – discoloration
  (1991): Zic JA+, *Arch Dermatol* 127, 1037
Nails – pigmentation
  (1981): Koranda FC, *J Am Acad Dermatol* 4, 650 (passim)
Nails – shoreline
  (1993): Pavithran K, *Indian J Lepr* 65, 225

Eyes

Maculopathy
  (1985): Taylor F, *Aust Fam Physician* 14(8), 744
Ocular toxicity
  (2002): Grana Gil+, *An Med Interna* 19(4), 189
Retinopathy
  (2007): Ferreras A+, *Arch Soc Esp Oftalmol* 82(2), 103
  (2006): Ingster-Moati I+, *J Fr Ophtalmol* 29(6), 642
  (2006): Kellner U+, *Invest Ophthalmol Vis Sci* 47(8), 3531
  (2005): Fardet L+, *Ann Dermatol Venereol* 132(8-9 Pt 1), 665
  (2004): Araiza-Casillas R+, *Lupus* 13(2), 119
Vision impaired
  (2005): Tzekov R, *Doc Ophthalmol* 110(1), 111

Other

Cardiac failure
  (1999): Baguet JP+, *Heart* 81(2), 221
Congestive heart failure
  (2005): Naqvi TZ+, *J Am Soc Echocardiogr* 18(4), 383

(1993): Iglesias Cubero G+, *Br Heart J* 69(5), 451
Death
Headache
Myalgia/Myositis/Myopathy/Myotoxicity
  (2005): Haberl A+, *Z Rheumatol* 64(4), 274
  (1998): Guedira N+, *Rev Rhum Engl Ed* 65, 58
Porphyria
  (1980): Gerwel M, *Pol Tyg Lek* (Polish) 35, 1351
Porphyria cutanea tarda
  (1985): Handa F+, *Indian J Dermatol* 30, 49
Seizures
  (2004): Tristano AG+, *Rheumatol Int* 24(5), 315
  (2003): Reuther LO+, *Ugeskr Laeger* 165(14), 1447

CHLOROTHIAZIDE

Trade names: Aldoclor (Merck); Azide; Chlothin; Chlotride;
Diurazide; Diuret; Diuril (Merck); Saluretil; Saluric
Indications: Hypertension, edema
Category: Diuretic, thiazide
Half-life: 1–2 hours
**Clinically important, potentially hazardous interactions
with:** cisplatin, digoxin, lithium, zinc

Note: Chlorothiazide is a sulfonamide and can be absorbed
systemically. Sulfonamides can produce severe, possibly fatal,
reactions such as toxic epidermal necrolysis and Stevens–Johnson
syndrome

Reactions

Skin

Bullous dermatitis
Erythema multiforme
Exanthems
Exfoliative dermatitis
Fixed eruption
  (1984): Chan HL, *Int J Dermatol* 23, 607
Lichenoid eruption
  (1986): Gonzalez JG+, *J Am Acad Dermatol* 15, 87
Lupus erythematosus
Photosensitivity (<1%)
  (1994): Enta T, *Can Fam Physicians* 40, 1269
  (1993): Iwamoto Y, *Nippon Saikingaku Zasshi* (Japanese) 48, 523
  (1984): Horio T, *Int J Dermatol* 23, 376
  (1980): Stern RS+, *Arch Dermatol* 116, 1269
Pruritus
Purpura
  (1992): Breathnach SM+, *Adverse Drug Reactions and the Skin*
    Blackwell, Oxford, 46
  (1980): Miescher PA+, *Clin Haematol* 9, 505
Rash (sic) (<1%)
Stevens–Johnson syndrome
Toxic epidermal necrolysis
Urticaria
Vasculitis

Mucosal/ENT

Dysgeusia
Oral lesions

Hair

Hair – alopecia

Eyes

Dyschromatopsia

Other
 Anaphylactoid reactions/Anaphylaxis
 Paresthesias (<1%)

CHLOROTRIANISENE

Trade names: Estregur; Merbentul; Tace
Indications: Inoperable prostate cancer, atrophic vaginitis
Category: Selective estrogen receptor modulator (SERM)
Half-life: N/A
Clinically important, potentially hazardous interactions with: hydrocortisone

Reactions

Skin
 Acne
 Chloasma (<1%)
 Dermatitis
 Edema (>1%)
 Erythema
 Erythema multiforme
 Erythema nodosum
 Melasma (<1%)
 Peripheral edema (>10%)
 Photosensitivity
 Rash (sic) (<1%)
 Urticaria

Mucosal/ENT
 Vaginitis
 Vulvovaginal candidiasis

Hair
 Hair – alopecia
 Hair – hirsutism

Other
 Candidiasis
 Gynecomastia (>10%)
 Porphyria cutanea tarda

CHLORPHENIRAMINE

Trade names: AL-R; Aller-Chlor; Chlo-Amine; Chlor-Pro; Chlor-Trimeton (Schering); Chlor-Tripolon; Chlorate; Ornade; Phenetron; Telachlor; Teldrin; Triaminic (Novartis)
Indications: Allergic rhinitis, urticaria
Category: Histamine H1 receptor antagonist; Muscarinic antagonist
Half-life: 20–40 hours
Clinically important, potentially hazardous interactions with: alcohol, anticholinergics, barbiturates, benzodiazepines, butabarbital, chloral hydrate, chlordiazepoxide, chlorpromazine, clonazepam, clorazepate, diazepam, ethchlorvynol, fluphenazine, flurazepam, hypnotics, lorazepam, MAO inhibitors, mephobarbital, mesoridazine, midazolam, narcotics, oxazepam, pentobarbital, phenobarbital, phenothiazines, phenylbutazone, primidone, prochlorperazine, promethazine, quazepam, secobarbital, sedatives, temazepam, thioridazine, tranquilizers, trifluoperazine, zolpidem

Reactions

Skin
 Angioedema (1–10%)
 Dermatitis (1–10%)
  (2005): Brown VL+, *Contact Dermatitis* 52(1), 49
  (2002): Kuroda K+, *Dermatology* 205(3), 281
  (2001): Hayashi K+, *Contact Dermatitis* 44(1), 38
  (1990): Tosti A+, *Contact Dermatitis* 22, 55 (eye-drops)
 Diaphoresis
 Photosensitivity (1–10%)
 Pruritus
  (1997): Sowunmi A+, *Trans R Soc Trop Med Hyg* 91(1), 63

Mucosal/ENT
 Tinnitus
 Xerostomia (1–10%)

Other
 Hypersensitivity
 Myalgia/Myositis/Myopathy/Myotoxicity (<1%)
 Paresthesias (<1%)

CHLORPROMAZINE

Trade names: Chloractil; Chlorazin; Chlorpromanyl; Esmino; Largactil; Novo-Chlorpromazine; Ormazine; Propaphenin; Prozin; Thorazine (GSK)
Indications: Psychosis, manic-depressive disorders
Category: Antipsychotic, phenothiazine; Muscarinic antagonist
Half-life: initial: 2 hours; terminal: 30 hours
Clinically important, potentially hazardous interactions with: alcohol, antihistamines, arsenic, chlorpheniramine, dofetilide, epinephrine, **evening primrose**, guanethidine, quinolones, sparfloxacin

Note: The prolonged use of chlorpromazine can produce a gray-blue or purplish pigmentation over light-exposed areas. This is a result of either dermal deposits of melanin, a chlorpromazine metabolite, or to a combination of both. Chlorpromazine melanosis is seen more often in women

Reactions

Skin
 Angioedema (<1%)
 Bullous dermatitis (<1%)
 Dermatitis
 Erythema multiforme (<1%)
 Exanthems (>5%)
 Exfoliative dermatitis
 Facial edema
  (2006): McCulley TJ+, *Ophthal Plast Reconstr Surg* 22(4), 283
 Fixed eruption (<1%)
 Lichenoid eruption
 Lupus erythematosus
  (1996): Matsukawa Y+, *J Int Med Res* 24, 147
  (1995): Price EJ+, *Drug Saf* 12(4), 283
  (1994): Yung RL+, *Rheum Dis Clin North Am* 20, 61
  (1990): Roche-Bayard P, *Chest* 98, 1545
  (1985): Pavlidakey GP+, *J Am Acad Dermatol* 13, 109
  (1981): Grossman J+, *Arthritis Rheum* 24, 927
  (1980): Condemi JJ, *Geriatrics* 35(3), 81
  (1980): Goldman LS+, *Am J Psychiatry* 137, 1613
 Miliaria

Peripheral edema
Photosensitivity (1–10%)
  (1995): Kim TH+, *Photodermatol Photoimmunol Photomed* 11, 170
  (1993): Jeanmougin M+, *Ann Dermatol Venereol* (French) 120, 840
  (1993): Wolf ME+, *Int J Clin Pharmacol* 31, 365
  (1989): Hoshino T+, *Arch Dermatol Res* 281, 60
  (1989): Rosen C, *Semin Dermatol* 8, 149
  (1986): Lovell CR+, *Contact Dermatitis* 14, 290
  (1982): Amblard P+, *Ann Dermatol Venereol* (French) 109, 225
Phototoxicity
  (1997): Eberlein-Konig B+, *Dermatology* 194, 131
Pigmentation (<1%)
  (2001): Kass J+, *Cutis* 68(4), 260
  (2000): Lal+, *J Psychiatry Neurosci* 25, 281
  (1993): Bloom D+, *Acta Psychiatr Scand* 87, 223
  (1993): Lal S+, *J Psychiatry Neurosci* 18, 173
  (1993): Wolf ME+, *Int J Clin Pharmacol* 31, 365 (blue-gray)
  (1988): Benning TL+, *Arch Dermatol* 124, 1541
  (1988): Thompson TR+, *Acta Psychiatr Scand* 78, 763
Pruritus (1–10%)
Purpura
  (1987): Aram H, *J Am Acad Dermatol* 17, 139
Pustules
  (1994): Burrows NP+, *BMJ* 309, 97
Rash (sic) (1–10%)
Seborrheic dermatitis
  (1983): Binder RL+, *Arch Dermatol* 119, 473 (1–5%)
  (1981): Kanwar AJ+, *Arch Dermatol* 117, 65 (passim)
Toxic epidermal necrolysis (<1%)
  (1996): Purcell P+, *Postgrad Med J* 72, 186
  (1990): Ward DJ+, *Burns* 16, 97
Urticaria
  (1992): Loesche C+, *Contact Dermatitis* 26, 278
  (1986): Lovell CR+, *Contact Dermatitis* 14, 290
Vasculitis
  (1987): Aram H, *J Am Acad Dermatol* 17, 139
Xerosis

Mucosal/ENT

Oral mucosal eruption
Oral pigmentation
Oral ulceration
Xerostomia (1–10%)

Nails

Nails – photo-onycholysis
  (1985): Kechijian P, *J Am Acad Dermatol* 12, 552
Nails – pigmentation

Eyes

Cataract
  (2002): Shahzad S+, *Psychosomatics* 43(5), 354
Corneal opacity
  (2001): Webber SK+, *Cornea* 20(2), 217
Eyelid edema
  (2006): McCulley TJ+, *Ophthal Plast Reconstr Surg* 22(4), 283
  (2005): Cesaro S+, *J Clin Virol* 34(2), 129
Retinopathy
  (1985): Taylor F, *Aust Fam Physician* 14(8), 744

Other

Anaphylactoid reactions/Anaphylaxis (<1%)
  (2001): Nikolic S+, *Srp Arh Celok Lek* 129(7), 203
Death
  (2001): Nikolic S+, *Srp Arh Celok Lek* 129(7), 203
Gynecomastia (1–10%)
Headache

Hypotension
  (2004): Strachan EM+, *Eur J Clin Pharmacol* 60(8), 541
Inappropriate secretion of antidiuretic hormone (SIADH)
  (1983): Tildesley HD+, *Can J Psychiatry* 28(6), 487
Injection-site necrosis
Polyarteritis nodosa
Pseudolymphoma
  (1995): Magro CM+, *J Am Acad Dermatol* 32, 419
Rhabdomyolysis
  (1984): Hashimoto F+, *Arch Intern Med* 144(3), 629 (with haloperidol)
Somnambulism
  (1986): Glassman JN+, *J Clin Psychiatry* 47(10), 523 (along with lithium, benztropine, and triazolam)
Tremor
  (2001): Chetty M+, *Ther Drug Monit* 23(5), 556 (with oral contraceptives)

CHLORPROPAMIDE

Trade names: Apo-Chlorpropamide; Arodoc C; Chlormide; Diabemide; Diabenese; Diabinese (Pfizer); Insogen; Melormin; Tesmel
Indications: Diabetes
Category: Sulfonylurea
Half-life: 30–42 hours
Clinically important, potentially hazardous interactions with: alcohol, garlic, phenylbutazones

Note: Chlorpropamide is a sulfonamide and can be absorbed systemically. Sulfonamides can produce severe, possibly fatal, reactions such as toxic epidermal necrolysis and Stevens–Johnson syndrome

Reactions

Skin

Allergic granulomatous angiitis (Churg–Strauss syndrome)
Angioedema
  (1991): Chinchmanian RM+, *Therapie* (French) 46, 163
Bullous dermatitis (<1%)
Dermatitis
  (1982): Fisher AA, *Cutis* 29, 551
Edema (<1%)
Erythema multiforme (<1%)
  (1980): Kanefsky TM+, *Arch Intern Med* 140, 1543
Erythema nodosum (<1%)
Exanthems (1–5%)
Exfoliative dermatitis
Fixed eruption
Lichenoid eruption
  (1990): Franz CB+, *J Am Acad Dermatol* 22, 128
  (1984): Barnett JH+, *Cutis* 34, 542
Lupus erythematosus
Photosensitivity (1–10%)
Pruritus (<3%)
Purpura
Rash (sic) (1–10%)
  (1985): Baciewicz AM+, *Diabetes Care* 8, 200
Side effects (sic)
Stevens–Johnson syndrome
  (1980): Kanefsky TM+, *Arch Intern Med* 140, 1543
Toxic epidermal necrolysis
  (1989): Stern RS+, *J Am Acad Dermatol* 21, 317
Urticaria (1–10%)

(1991): Chinchmanian RM+, *Therapie* (French) 46, 163
Vasculitis
   (1983): Batko B, *Wiad Lek* (Polish) 36, 761

Mucosal/ENT
Oral lichenoid eruption
   (1988): Zain RB+, *Dent J Malays* 10, 15
   (1984): Barnett J+, *Cutis* 34, 542
Tongue ulceration
   (1984): Barnett J+, *Cutis* 34, 542

Hair
Hair – alopecia

Other
Death
Inappropriate secretion of antidiuretic hormone (SIADH)
   (1991): Ravat HK+, *J Assoc Physicians india* 39(8), 645
   (1980): Fonseca VA+, *J Postgrad Med* 26(2), 127
Paresthesias
Porphyria
Porphyria cutanea tarda

CHLORTETRACYCLINE

Trade names: Aureomicina; Aureomycin
Indications: Various infections due to susceptible organisms
Category: Antibiotic, tetracycline
Half-life: N/A

Reactions

Skin
Edema (topical)
Erythema (topical)
Irritation (topical)
Photosensitivity
Pruritus (topical)
Rash (sic) (topical)
Xerosis (topical)

Mucosal/ENT
Xerostomia (ophthalmic)

Eyes
Corneal edema
Ocular burning (topical)
Ocular stinging (topical)

CHLORTHALIDONE

Trade names: Combipres; Higroton; Hydro-Long; Hygroton; Hypertol; Igroton; Tenoretic (AstraZeneca); Thalidone; Thalitone (Monarch); Uridon
Indications: Hypertension
Category: Diuretic, thiazide
Half-life: 35–50 hours
Clinically important, potentially hazardous interactions with: digoxin, lithium, zinc

Note: Combipres is chlorthalidone and clonidine

Note: Chlorthalidone is a sulfonamide and can be absorbed systemically. Sulfonamides can produce severe, possibly fatal, reactions such as toxic epidermal necrolysis and Stevens–Johnson syndrome

Reactions

Skin
Angioedema
   (2006): Piller LB+, *J Clin Hypertens* 8(9), 649 (Greenwich) (15%)
Erythema multiforme
Exanthems
Exfoliative dermatitis
Lupus erythematosus
Necrotizing vasculitis
Photosensitivity (1–10%)
   (1989): Baker EJ+, *J Am Acad Dermatol* 21, 1026
   (1988): Lehmann P+, *Hautarzt* (German) 39, 38
Psoriasis
   (1987): Wolf R+, *Cutis* 40, 162
Purpura (<1%)
Rash (sic) (<1%)
Stevens–Johnson syndrome
Toxic epidermal necrolysis
   (1999): Egan CA+, *J Am Acad Dermatol* 40(3), 458
Urticaria (<1%)
   (1993): Neaton JD+, *JAMA* 279, 713 (passim)
Vasculitis (<1%)

Hair
Hair – alopecia

Eyes
Dyschromatopsia
Myopia
   (1996): Krieg PH+, *Eye* 10 (Pt 1), 121

Other
Fever
Headache
Inappropriate secretion of antidiuretic hormone (SIADH)
Paresthesias (<1%)
Pseudoporphyria
   (1989): Baker EJ+, *J Am Acad Dermatol* 21, 1026

CHLORZOXAZONE

Trade names: Escoflex; Flexaphen; Klorzoxazon; Muscol; Paraflex (Ortho-McNeil); Parafon Forte DSC (Ortho-McNeil); Prolax; Remular-S; Solaxin
Indications: Painful musculoskeletal conditions
Category: Central muscle relaxant
Half-life: 1–2 hours

Reactions

Skin
Acute generalized exanthematous pustulosis (AGEP)
   (2004): Padial MA+, *Br J Dermatol* A(1), 139
Angioedema (1–10%)
Erythema multiforme (<1%)
Exanthems
Petechiae
Pruritus
Rash (sic) (<1%)
Urticaria (<1%)
Vasculitis
   (2004): Chiu CS+, *Br J Dermatol* A(1), 153

Other
  Anaphylactoid reactions/Anaphylaxis
  Hypersensitivity

CHOLESTYRAMINE

Trade names: Chol-Less; Colestrol; Lismol; PMS-
Cholestyramine; Prevalite; Quantalan; Questran (Par); Questran
Lite
Indications: Pruritus associated with biliary obstruction, primary
hypercholesterolemia
Category: Bile acid sequestrant
Half-life: N/A
**Clinically important, potentially hazardous interactions
with:** acetaminophen, acitretin, aspirin, chloroquine, digoxin,
doxepin, fat-soluble vitamins A, D, E, K, hydroxychloroquine,
isotretinoin, lovastatin, mycophenolate, raloxifene, sulfasalazine,
sulfonylureas, tetracycline, tricyclic antidepressants, valproic acid

Reactions

Skin
  Edema
  Exanthems
  Hemorrhage
    (1986): Shojania AM+, *CMAJ* 134(6), 609
  Palmar erythema
    (2007): Serrao R+, *Am J Clin Dermatol* 8(6), 347
  Pruritus
    (2003): Vroonhof K+, *Neth J Med* 61(1), 19
  Rash (sic) (<1%)
  Urticaria

Mucosal/ENT
  Dysgeusia
    (1993): Liacouras CA+, *J Pediatr* 122(3), 477 (73%)
  Tinnitus
  Tongue irritation (<1%)

Eyes
  Amblyopia

Other
  Myalgia/Myositis/Myopathy/Myotoxicity
    (1992): Stugaard M+, *Tidsskr Nor Laegeforen* 112(20), 2642
  Paresthesias
  Rhabdomyolysis
    (1992): Chrysanthopoulos C+, *BMJ* 304(6836), 1225 (with
      lovastatin)

CHONDROITIN

Scientific names: *Chondroitin 4- and 6-sulfate; Chondroitin 4-
sulfate; Condrosulf; Structum*
Family: None
Trade and other common names: CDS; Chondroitin Sulfate
C; CSA; CSC; GAG
Category: Amino sugar; Food supplement
Purported indications and other uses: Osteoarthritis (often
with glucosamine), ischemic heart disease, osteoporosis,
hyperlipidemia, keratoconjunctivitis, agent in cataract surgery
Half-life: N/A
**Clinically important, potentially hazardous interactions
with:** warfarin with chondroitin

Reactions

Skin
  Allergic reactions (sic)
  Peripheral edema

Hair
  Hair – alopecia

Eyes
  Corneal opacity
    (1986): Coffman MR+, *Am J Ophthalmol* 102(2), 279
  Eyelid edema
    (2000): Leeb BF+, *J Rheumatology* 27, 205
  Keratopathy
    (1987): Binder PS+, *Arch Ophthalmol* 105(9), 1243

CICLESONIDE

Trade names: Alvesco (Oral inhalation) (Altana); Omnaris
(Intranasal) (Altana)
Indications: Allergic rhinitis, asthma
Category: Corticosteroid
Half-life: 5–7 hours
**Clinically important, potentially hazardous interactions
with:** itraconazole, ketoconazole, nelfinavir, ritonavir

Reactions

Skin
  Angioedema
  Eczema
  Rash (sic)

Mucosal/ENT
  Dysgeusia
  Dysphonia (1%)
  Ear pain
  Epistaxis
  Nasopharyngitis
  Oropharyngeal candidiasis
  Pharyngitis
  Xerostomia

Eyes
  Cataract
  Intraocular pressure increased
  Vision blurred

Other
  Application-site reactions
  Bronchospasm
  Cough
  Headache
  Weight gain

CIDOFOVIR

Trade names: Forvade; Vistide (Gilead)
Indications: Cytomegalovirus (CMV) retinitis in patients with AIDS
Category: Antiviral, nucleotide analog
Half-life: ~2.6 hours
Clinically important, potentially hazardous interactions with: amphotericin B, tenofovir

Reactions

Skin
Acne (>10%)
Allergic reactions (sic) (1–10%)
Burning
  (2000): Calista D, *J Eur Acad Dermatol Venereol* 14(6), 484
Dermatitis
  (2001): Holdiness MR, *Contact Dermatitis* 44(5), 265
Diaphoresis (1–10%)
Edema
Erosions
  (2000): Calista D, *J Eur Acad Dermatol Venereol* 14(6), 484
Erythema
  (2001): Martinelli C+, *J Eur Acad Dermatol Venereol* 15(6), 568
Facial edema
Herpes simplex
Inflammation
  (2000): Calista D, *J Eur Acad Dermatol Venereol* 14(6), 484
Irritation (sic)
  (1998): Zabawski EJ+, *J Am Acad Dermatol* 39, 741
Pallor (1–10%)
Photosensitivity
Pigmentation (>10%)
  (2000): Calista D, *J Eur Acad Dermatol Venereol* 14(6), 484
Pruritus (1–10%)
Rash (sic) (27%)
  (2005): Kuypers DR+, *Am J Transplant* 5(8), 1997
  (2005): Shehab N+, *Pharmacotherapy* 25(7), 977
Toxicity (sic)
  (2003): Ljungman P+, *Bone Marrow Transplant* 31(6), 481
Urticaria (1–10%)
Xerosis

Mucosal/ENT
Aphthous stomatitis
Dysgeusia (1–10%)
Oral candidiasis
Oral ulceration
Stomatitis (1–10%)
Tongue pigmentation
Xerostomia

Hair
Hair – alopecia (22%)
  (2000): Calista D, *J Eur Acad Dermatol Venereol* 14(6), 484 (transient)
  (2000): Seijas M+, *Rev Clin Esp* 200(10), 584

Eyes
Iritis
  (2006): Kottke MD+, *J Am Acad Dermatol* 55(3), 533
  (1999): Neau D+, *Clin Infect Dis* 28(1), 156
  (1999): Tseng AL+, *Ann Pharmacother* 33(2), 167
  (1997): Davis JL+, *Arch Ophthalmol* 115(6), 733
  (1997): Palau LA+, *Clin Infect Dis* 25(2), 337
  (1997): Taskintuna I+, *Ophthalmology* 104(11), 1827 (32%)

Ocular hypotension
  (2003): Hackethal U+, *Klin Monatsbl Augenheilkd* 220(6), 391
Retinal detachment
  (2003): Hackethal U+, *Klin Monatsbl Augenheilkd* 220(6), 391
  (1998): Akler ME+, *Ophthalmology* 105(4), 651 (44%)
  (1997): Taskintuna I+, *Ophthalmology* 104(11), 1827 (6%)
Uveitis
  (2006): Kottke MD+, *J Am Acad Dermatol* 55(3), 533
  (2005): Cano Parra J+, *Arch Soc Esp Oftalmol* 80(3), 137
  (2003): Hackethal U+, *Klin Monatsbl Augenheilkd* 220(6), 391
  (2003): Tacconelli E+, *Eur J Clin Microbiol Infect Dis* 22(2), 114
  (2001): Accorinti M+, *Ocul Immunol Inflamm* 9(3), 211
  (2001): Chakrabarti S+, *Bone Marrow Transplant* 28(9), 879
  (2001): Martinez de la Casa JM+, *Arch Soc Esp Oftalmol* 76(4), 213
  (2001): Rougier MB+, *J Fr Ophtalmol* 24(5), 491
  (2001): Soltau JB, *Ocul Immunol Inflamm* 9(3), 137
  (2000): *AIDS* 14(11), 1571
  (2000): Scott RA+, *Am J Ophthalmol* 130(1), 126
  (1999): Ambati J+, *Br J Ophthalmol* 83(10), 1153
  (1999): Cochereau I+, *Ocul Immunol Inflamm* 7(3–4), 223
  (1999): Plosker GL+, *Drugs* 58(2), 325
  (1997): Chavez-de la Paz E+, *Ophthalmology* 104(3), 539
Vision impaired
  (2003): Rapp P+, *J Fr Ophtalmol* 26(7), 717
  (1999): Bainbridge JW+, *Eye* 13 (Pt 3a), 353
  (1998): *Prescrire Int* 7(37), 135
Vision loss
  (2003): Hackethal U+, *Klin Monatsbl Augenheilkd* 220(6), 391
  (1997): Friedberg DN, *Arch Ophthalmol* 115(6), 801
  (1997): Taskintuna I+, *Ophthalmology* 104(11), 1827

Other
Application-site reactions (sic) (39%)
  (1998): Sacks SL+, *Antimicrob Agents Chemother* 42(11), 2996
  (1998): Zabawski EJ+, *J Am Acad Dermatol* 39, 741
Chills (24%)
Headache
  (2005): Shehab N+, *Pharmacotherapy* 25(7), 977
Myalgia/Myositis/Myopathy/Myotoxicity
Nephrotoxicity
  (2005): Izzedine H+, *Am J Kidney Dis* 45(5), 804
  (2005): Ortiz A+, *Antivir Ther* 10(1), 185
  (2002): Verhelst D+, *Am J Kidney Dis* 40(6), 1331
Paresthesias (>10%)

CILAZAPRIL

Trade names: Inhibase (Roche); Vascace (Roche)
Indications: Hypertension
Category: Angiotensin-converting enzyme inhibitor
Half-life: 9 Hours
Clinically important, potentially hazardous interactions with: alcohol, diuretics

Reactions

Skin
Angioedema
  (1997): Schiller PI+, *Allergy* 52(4), 432
  (1992): Szucs T+, *Cardiology* 80(1), 34
Edema
  (1992): Szucs T+, *Cardiology* 80(1), 34 (facial)
Lupus erythematosus
  (1995): Fernandez-Diaz ML+, *Lancet* 345(8946), 398
Pemphigus foliaceus

(1998): Buzon E+, *Acta Derm Venereol* 78(3), 227
Pemphigus vulgaris
  (2005): Goldberg I+, *Acta Dermatovenerol Croat* 13(3), 153
  (2000): Orion E+, *Acta Derm Venereol* 80(3), 220
Rash (sic)
  (1996): Abraham G+, *Orv Hetil* 137(29), 1583

Mucosal/ENT
Dysgeusia

Other
Asthenia
  (1994): Dossegger L+, *J Cardiovasc Pharmacol* 24(Suppl 3), S38
  (1993): Coulter DM, *N Z Med J* 106(968), 497 (1.1%)
  (1992): Szucs T+, *Cardiology* 80(1), 34
  (1988): Goldszer RC+, *Am J Hypertens* 1(3 Pt 3), 300S
Chest pain
  (1992): Szucs T+, *Cardiology* 80(1), 34
Cough
  (2007): Tumanan-Mendoza BA+, *J Clin Epidemiol* 60(6), 547
  (2003): Buranakitjaroen P+, *J Med Assoc Thai* 86(7), 647
  (1996): Rosenthal JR+, *Cardiology* 87(1), 54
  (1994): Dossegger L+, *J Cardiovasc Pharmacol* 24(Suppl 3), S38
  (1994): Karpov YA+, *J Cardiovasc Pharmacol* 24(Suppl 3), S86
  (1993): Coulter DM, *N Z Med J* 106(968), 497 (2.9%)
  (1993): Reisin L, *Cardiology* 82(Suppl 2), 47
  (1992): Szucs T+, *Cardiology* 80(1), 34
Headache
  (1994): Dossegger L+, *J Cardiovasc Pharmacol* 24(Suppl 3), S38
  (1993): Coulter DM, *N Z Med J* 106(968), 497
  (1992): Szucs T+, *Cardiology* 80(1), 34
Hypotension
  (1992): Szucs T+, *Cardiology* 80(1), 34
Inappropriate secretion of antidiuretic hormone (SIADH)
  (2001): Arinzon ZH+, *J Am Geriatr Soc* 49(12), 1735
Somnolence
Vertigo
  (1994): Dossegger L+, *J Cardiovasc Pharmacol* 24(Suppl 3), S38
  (1992): Szucs T+, *Cardiology* 80(1), 34

CILOSTAZOL

Synonym: OPC13013
Trade name: Pletal (Pfizer)
Indications: Peripheral vascular disease, intermittent claudication
Category: Antiplatelet; Phosphodiesterase inhibitor; Vasodilator, peripheral
Half-life: 11–13 hours
Clinically important, potentially hazardous interactions with: clarithromycin, erythromycin, fondaparinux

Reactions

Skin
Edema (<2%)
Facial edema (<2%)
Furunculosis (<2%)
Hypertrophy
Peripheral edema (7–9%)
Pruritus
Purpura (<2%)
Rash (sic) (2%)
  (1998): Yoshitomi Y+, *Heart* 80(4), 393
Stevens–Johnson syndrome
Urticaria (<2%)
Xerosis (<2%)

Mucosal/ENT
Tongue edema (<2%)
Vaginitis (<2%)

Other
Chills (<2%)
Headache
  (2006): Birk S+, *Cephalalgia* 26(11), 1304
  (2002): Thompson PD+, *Am J Cardiol* 90(12), 1314
  (2001): Doggrell SA, *Expert Opin Pharmacother* 2(11), 1725
  (2001): Liu Y+, *Cardiovasc Drug Rev* 19(4), 369
  (2001): Pratt CM, *Am J Cardiol* 87(12A), 28D
  (2000): Dawson DL+, *Am J Med* 109(7), 523
  (1998): Torigoe R+, *No To Shinkei* 50(9), 829
  (1995): Fujimura M+, *Am J Respir Crit Care Med* 151(1), 222
  (1985): Niki T+, *Arzneimittelforschung* 35(7A), 1173
Infections
Myalgia/Myositis/Myopathy/Myotoxicity (2–3%)
Paresthesias (2%)
Thrombosis
  (2006): Patel TN+, *J Invasive Cardiol* 18(7), E211
Upper respiratory infection
  (1995): Suzuki K+, *Nihon Kyobu Shikkan Gakkai Zasshi* 33(2), 156
Vertigo
  (2001): Liu Y+, *Cardiovasc Drug Rev* 19(4), 369

CIMETIDINE

Trade names: Apo-Cimetidine; Azucimet; Blocan; Cimedine; Cimehexal; Ciuk; Dyspamet; Novocimetine; Nu-Cimet; Peptol; Stomedine; Tagamet (GSK); Ulcedine; Zymerol
Indications: Duodenal ulcer
Category: Histamine H2 receptor antagonist
Half-life: 2 hours
Clinically important, potentially hazardous interactions with: acenocoumarol, alfuzosin, aminophylline, anisindione, anticoagulants, buprenorphine, butorphanol, **caffeine**, carmustine, clobazam, **cocoa**, dicumarol, dofetilide, duloxetine, epirubicin, eszopiclone, fentanyl, floxuridine, fluorouracil, galantamine, hydromorphone, itraconazole, ketoconazole, lidocaine, midazolam, moclobemide, morphine, narcotic analgesics, oxycodone, pentazocine, phenytoin, posaconazole, prednisone, propranolol, sufentanil, theophylline, tolazoline, warfarin, xanthines, zaleplon, zolmitriptan, zolpidem

Reactions

Skin
Acne
Angioedema (<1%)
  (1985): Whelan JP, *J Clin Pharmacol* 25, 610
  (1982): Sandhu BS+, *Ann Intern Med* 97, 138
Baboon syndrome
  (1998): Helmbold P+, *Dermatology* 197, 402
Erythema annulare centrifugum
  (1982): Merrett AC+, *N Z J Med* 12, 107
  (1981): Merrett AC+, *BMJ* 283, 698
Erythema multiforme (<1%)
  (1987): Talvard O+, *Presse Med* (French) 16, 825
  (1983): Guan R+, *Aust N Z J Med* 13, 182
  (1982): Wallach D+, *Dermatologica* 165, 197
  (1981): Bjaeldager PA, *Ugeskr Laeger* (Danish) 143, 1406
Erythroderma
Erythrosis

Exanthems
  (1986): Peters K, *Contact Dermatitis* 15, 190
  (1982): Freston JW, *Ann Intern Med* 97, 728
Exfoliative dermatitis
  (1983): Mitchell GG, *Am J Med* 75, 875
  (1980): Yantis PL+, *Dig Dis Sci* 25, 73
Fixed eruption
  (1998): Helmbold P+, *Dermatology* 197, 402 (baboon syndrome)
  (1995): Inoue A+, *Acta Derm Venereol* 75, 250
Ichthyosis
  (1984): Aram H, *Int J Dermatol* 23, 458
Id reaction
  (1987): Sander-Jensen K+, *Dermatologica* 174, 103
Lupus erythematosus
  (1982): Davidson BL+, *Arch Intern Med* 142, 166 (exacerbation)
Pruritus (<1%)
  (1994): Warner DMc+, *J Am Acad Dermatol* 31, 677 (passim)
  (1982): Freston JW, *Ann Intern Med* 97, 728
  (1982): Sandhu BS+, *Ann Intern Med* 97, 138
  (1982): Wallach D+, *Dermatologica* 165, 197
  (1981): Taillandier J+, *Nouv Presse Med* (French) 10, 258
Psoriasis
  (1991): Andersen M, *Ugeskr Laeger* (Danish) 153, 132
  (1986): Peters K, *Contact Dermatitis* 15, 190
  (1983): Mitchell GG, *Am J Med* 75, 875
  (1982): Wallach D+, *Dermatologica* 165, 197
  (1980): Yates VM+, *BMJ* 280, 1453
Purpura
Rash (sic) (<2%)
  (1991): Marshall J+, *Chest* 99, 1016
Seborrheic dermatitis
  (1981): Kanwar AJ, *Arch Dermatol* 117, 65
Side effects (sic) (0.4%)
  (1982): Freston JW, *Ann Intern Med* 97, 728
Stevens–Johnson syndrome
  (1987): Talvard O+, *Presse Med* (French) 16, 825
  (1983): Guan R+, *Aust N Z J Med* 13, 182
Toxic dermatitis (sic)
  (1981): Pasquier P+, *Nouv Presse Med* (French) 10, 2994
Toxic epidermal necrolysis (<1%)
  (1998): Tidwell BH+, *Am J Health Syst Pharm* 55, 163
  (1983): Dabadie H+, *Gastroenterol Clin Biol* (French) 7, 425
Urticaria
  (1985): Goolamali SK, *Postgrad Med J* 61, 925
  (1983): Mitchell GG, *Am J Med* 75, 875
  (1982): Freston JW, *Ann Intern Med* 97, 728
  (1982): Sandhu BS+, *Ann Intern Med* 97, 138
  (1981): Brandrup E, *Ugeskr Laeger* (Danish) 143, 1715
Vasculitis
  (1983): Mitchell GG, *Am J Med* 75, 875
  (1982): Wallach D+, *Dermatologica* 165, 197
  (1981): Dernbach WK+, *JAMA* 246, 331
Xerosis
  (1982): Greist MC+, *Arch Dermatol* 118, 253

Mucosal/ENT
  Xerostomia

Hair
  Hair – alopecia
  (1985): Tullio CJ+, *Clin Pharm* 4, 145
  (1983): Khalsa JH+, *Int J Dermatol* 22, 202
  (1981): Vircburger MI+, *Lancet* 1, 1160

Other
  Anaphylactoid reactions/Anaphylaxis
  (1982): Knapp AB+, *Ann Intern Med* 97, 374
  Gynecomastia (<1%)
  (2004): Stratakis CA+, *Clin Endocrinol* (Oxf) 61(6), 779

  (2000): Hugues FC+, *Ann Med Interne* (Paris) (French) 151, 10
    (passim)
  (1994): Garcia-Rodriguez LA+, *BMJ* 308, 503
  (1991): Barth JA, *Zentralbl Gynakol* (German) 113, 667
  (1983): Jensen RT+, *N Engl J Med* 308, 883
  (1982): Peden NR+, *Br J Clin Pharmacol* 14, 565
Headache
Hypersensitivity
  (2000): Evans RD+, *Clin Podiatr Med Surg* 17, 371
  (1986): Peters K, *Contact Dermatitis* 15, 190
  (1985): Whalen JP, *J Clin Pharmacol* 25, 610
Injection-site pain
Myalgia/Myositis/Myopathy/Myotoxicity
  (1982): Kaplinsky N+, *J Rheumatol* 9, 156
  (1980): Feest TG+, *BMJ* 281, 1284
Nephrotoxicity
  (2005): Ueda H+, *Clin Exp Nephrol* 9(4), 332
  (2001): Fisher AA+, *Drug Saf* 24(1), 39
Porphyria
  (1985): Singh R+, *J Assoc Physicians India* 33, 187
Pseudolymphoma
  (1995): Magro CM+, *J Am Acad Dermatol* 32, 419
  (1988): Kardaun SH+, *Br J Dermatol* 118(4), 545

CINACALCET

Trade name: Sensipar (Amgen)
Indications: Secondary hyperparathyroidism, parathyroid carcinoma
Category: Calcimimetic
Half-life: 30–40 hours
Clinically important, potentially hazardous interactions with: ketoconazole

Reactions

Other
  Asthenia (7%)
  Chest pain (6%)
  Myalgia/Myositis/Myopathy/Myotoxicity (15%)
  Seizures (1.4%)
  (2006): *Prescrire Int* 15(83), 90
  Vertigo (10%)

CINNARIZINE

Trade names: Arlevert; Cerepar; Cinarizins; Cinazyn; Cinnabene; Cinnacet; Cinnageron; Cinnarisine; Cinnipirine; Clinadil; Derozin; Diclamina; Ederal; Libotacin; Medozine; Pericephal; Pervasum; Sepan; Stugeron (Janssen); Surepil; Sureptil; Touristil; Vertizin (Ram)
Indications: Dizziness, tinnitus, nystagmus, nausea and vomiting, motion sickness
Category: Histamine H1 receptor antagonist; Muscarinic antagonist; Peripheral vasodilator
Half-life: 4 hours
Clinically important, potentially hazardous interactions with: alcohol, barbiturates, hypnotics, narcotic analgesics, sedatives, tranquilizers, tricyclic antidepressants

Reactions

Skin
Diaphoresis
Lichen planus
  (1990): Suys E+, *Dermatologica* 181(1), 71
  (1985): Miyagawa S+, *Br J Dermatol* 112(5), 607
Lichenoid eruption
  (2002): Ramallal M+, *Pharm World Sci* 24(6), 215
Lupus erythematosus
  (1998): Toll A+, *Lupus* 7(5), 364 (with sunbathing)

Mucosal/ENT
Xerostomia

Eyes
Blepharospasm
  (2006): Alonso-Navarro H+, *Clin Neuropharmacol* 29(4), 187
Vision blurred

Other
Abdominal pain
  (1989): Hausler R+, *Acta Otorhinolaryngol Belg* 43(2), 177
Adverse effects (sic)
  (1989): Bhatia RS, *J Assoc Physicians India* 37(11), 733
Depression
  (2005): Kuzuhara S, *Nippon Ronen Igakkai Zasshi* 42(1), 21
  (1999): Stucchi-Portocarrero S+, *Rev Neurol* 28(9), 876
  (1989): Micheli FE+, *Mov Disord* 4(2), 139
  (1988): Capella D+, *BMJ* 297(6650), 722
  (1987): Micheli F+, *Neurology* 37(5), 881
  (1986): Chouza C+, *Lancet* 1(8493), 1303
  (1986): Meyboom RH+, *Lancet* 2(8501), 292
Headache
  (2002): Pianese CP+, *Otol Neurotol* 23(3), 357
  (1989): Hausler R+, *Acta Otorhinolaryngol Belg* 43(2), 177
Myalgia/Myositis/Myopathy/Myotoxicity
Tremor
  (1988): Capella D+, *BMJ* 297(6650), 722
Vertigo
  (2003): Tosoni C+, *Eur J Dermatol* 13(1), 54

CINOXACIN

Trade names: Cerexin; Cinobac (Lilly); Cinobact; Cinobactin; Gugecin; Nossacin; Noxigram; Uronorm
Indications: Various urinary tract infections caused by susceptible organisms
Category: Antibiotic, quinolone
Half-life: 1.5 hours

Reactions

Skin
Allergic reactions (sic)
Angioedema (<3%)
Edema (<3%)
Erythema multiforme
Photosensitivity
Pruritus (<3%)
Rash (sic)
Stevens–Johnson syndrome
Toxic epidermal necrolysis
Urticaria (<3%)

Mucosal/ENT
Dysgeusia (<1%)
Tinnitus
Vaginitis
  (1987): Goldstein EJ+, *Am J Med* 82(4A), 284

Other
Anaphylactoid reactions/Anaphylaxis
  (2003): Quercia O+, *Allerg Immunol* (Paris) 35(2), 61
  (1988): Stricker BH+, *BMJ* 297, 1434
Headache
  (1987): Goldstein EJ+, *Am J Med* 82(4A), 284
Hypersensitivity
  (1984): Burt RA, *Urology* 23(1), 101 (2%)
  (1982): Scavone JM+, *Pharmacotherapy* 2, 266
Paresthesias (<1%)

CIPROFIBRATE

Trade names: Lipanor; Modalim (Sanofi-Aventis)
Indications: Hyperlipidemia
Category: Fibrate; Lipid regulator
Half-life: 1.5 hours
Clinically important, potentially hazardous interactions with: atorvastatin, fluvastatin, ibuprofen, norfloxacin, pravastatin, rosuvastatin, simvastatin

Reactions

Skin
Pruritus
Radiodermatitis
  (1998): Gironet N+, *Ann Dermatol Venereol* 125(9), 598
Urticaria

Hair
Hair – alopecia

Other
Abdominal pain
Asthenia
Headache
Hepatotoxicity
  (2003): Pflumio F+, *Ann Endocrinol* (Paris) 64(3), 232
  (1999): Dumortier J+, *Gastroenterol Clin Biol* 23(12), 1399
  (1992): Perault MC+, *Gastroenterol Clin Biol* 16(6–7), 609
Myalgia/Myositis/Myopathy/Myotoxicity
Nephrotoxicity
  (2000): Broeders N+, *Nephrol Dial Transplant* 15(12), 1993
  (2000): Sharobeem KM+, *J Cardiovasc Pharmacol Ther* 5(1), 33
Rhabdomyolysis
  (1997): Ramachandran S+, *BMJ* 314(7094), 1593 (with ibuprofen)
  (1996): Blain H+, *Rev Med Interne* 17(10), 859 (with norfloxacin)
  (1990): Delangre T+, *Presse Med* 19(39), 1811
  (1987): Baglin A+, *Therapie* 42(2), 247
Vertigo

CIPROFLOXACIN

Trade names: Ciflox; Ciloxan Ophthalmic (Alcon); Cimogal; Ciplox; Cipro (Alcon); Ciprobay Uro; Cipromycin; Ciproxin; Italnik; Kenzoflex; Uniflox
Indications: Various infections caused by susceptible organisms
Category: Antibiotic, quinolone
Half-life: 4 hours
Clinically important, potentially hazardous interactions with: amiodarone, antacids, antineoplastics, arsenic, bepridil, bismuth, bismuth subsalicylate, bretylium, calcium salts, **cocoa**, didanosine, disopyramide, duloxetine, erythromycin, iron, magnesium salts, methylxanthines, NSAIDs, phenothiazines, procainamide, quinidine, rasagiline, sotalol, sucralfate, theophylline, tizanidine, tricyclic antidepressants, zinc

Note: Ciprofloxacin is chemically related to nalidixic acid

Reactions

Skin
Acne
  (1989): Rahm V+, *Scand J Infect Dis* 60, 120
  (1988): Campoli-Richards DM+, *Drugs* 35, 373
  (1988): Schacht P+, *Infection* 16, S29
Acute generalized exanthematous pustulosis
  (2005): Hausermann P+, *Dermatology* 211(3), 277
Allergic reactions (sic)
  (2000): Burke P+, *BMJ* 320, 679
Angioedema (<1%)
  (1995): Vidal C+, *Postgrad Med J* 71, 318
  (1989): Davis H+, *Ann Intern Med* 111, 1041
  (1989): Rahm V+, *Scand J Infect Dis* 60, 120
  (1989): Schacht P1, *Am J Med* 87, 90S
  (1988): Campoli-Richards DM+, *Drugs* 35, 373
  (1988): Schacht P+, *Infection* 16, S29
Bullous dermatitis
  (1988): Kaufmann I+, *Z Hautkr* (German) 63, 679
Bullous pemphigoid
  (2000): Kimyadi-Asadi A+, *J Am Acad Dermatol* 42, 847
Diaphoresis
  (1990): Karimi K, *Indiana Med* 83, 266
  (1989): Rahm V+, *Scand J Infect Dis* 60, 120
  (1988): Campoli-Richards DM+, *Drugs* 35, 373 (0.05%)
  (1988): Schacht P+, *Infection* 16, S29
Edema (<1%)
  (1995): Shelley ED, Toledo, OH (personal case) (observation)
Elastolysis
  (1993): Lien YH+, *Am J Kidney Dis* 22, 598
Erythema multiforme
  (1994): Win A+, *Int J Dermatol* 33, 512
  (1993): Imrie K+, *Am J Hematol* 43, 159
Erythema nodosum (<1%)
  (2007): Bhalla M+, *Clin Exp Dermatol* 32(1), 115
Erythroderma (<1%)
  (1989): Wurtz RM+, *Lancet* 1, 955
Exanthems
  (2002): Litt JZ, Beachwood, OH (personal case) (observation)
  (2000): Litt JZ, Beachwood, OH (personal case) (observation)
  (1999): Litt JZ, Beachwood, OH (anecdote from lay person on the Internet)
  (1999): Litt JZ, Beachwood, OH (personal case) (observation)
  (1997): Bircher AJ+, *Allergy* 52, 1246
  (1996): McCarty JR, Fort Worth, TX (from Internet) (observation)
  (1989): Gaut PL+, *Am J Med* 87 (Suppl 5A), 169S
  (1988): Campoli-Richards DM+, *Drugs* 35, 373 (0.7%)

Exfoliative dermatitis (<1%)
Fixed eruption
  (2001): Hamamoto Y+, *Clin Exp Dermatol* 26(1), 48
  (2001): Rodriguez-Morales A+, *Contact Dermatitis* 44(4), 255
  (2001): Sharma R, Aligarh, India (from Internet) (observation) (recurrence after fixed eruption from sparfloxacin)
  (1998): Litt JZ, Beachwood, OH (personal case) (observation)
  (1998): Maquirriain Gorriz MT+, *Aten Primaria* (Spanish) 21, 585
  (1996): Dhar S+, *Br J Dermatol* 134, 156
  (1995): Lozano-Ayllon M+, *Allergy* 50, 598
  (1994): Kawada A+, *Contact Dermatitis* 31, 182
  (1993): Alonso MD+, *Allergy* 48, 296
  (1992): Alonso MD+, *Allergy* 47, 194
Jarisch–Herxheimer reaction
  (2002): Webster G+, *Pediatr Infect Dis J* 21(6), 571
Linear IgA dermatosis
  (2001): Wiadrowski TP+, *Austral J Dermatol* 42, 196 (with vancomycin)
Livedo reticularis
  (1999): Verros CD, Tripolis, Greece (from Internet) (observation) (occurred on rechallenge)
Petechiae
Photo-recall
  (2001): Krishnan RS+, *J Am Acad Dermatol* 44, 1045 (with piperacillin & tobramycin)
Photosensitivity (<1%)
  (2006): Urbina F+, *Photodermatol Photoimmunol Photomed* 22(2), 111
  (2000): Ferguson J+, *J Antimicrob Chemother* 45, 503
  (1999): Jaffe A+, *Pediatr Pulmonol* 28(6), 449
  (1998): Kimura M+, *Contact Dermatitis* 38, 180
  (1997): Ferguson J+, *J Antimicrob Chemother* 40, 93
  (1995): Burdge DR+, *Antimicrob Agents Chemother* 39, 793
  (1993): Jick SS+, *Pharmacotherapy* 13(5), 461
  (1993): Shelley WB+, *Cutis* 51, 154 (observation)
  (1993): Shelley WB+, *Cutis* 52, 27 (observation)
  (1990): Ferguson J+, *Br J Dermatol* 123, 9
  (1989): Granowitz EV, *J Infect Dis* 160, 910
  (1989): Nedorost ST+, *Arch Dermatol* 125, 433
  (1989): Rahm V+, *Scand J Infect Dis* 60, 120
  (1988): Campoli-Richards DM+, *Drugs* 35, 373
  (1988): Kaufmann I+, *Z Hautkr* (German) 63, 679
  (1988): Schacht P+, *Infection* 16, S29
  (1987): Jensen T+, *J Antimicrob Chemother* 20, 585
  (1986): Ball P, *J Antimicrob Chemother* 18 (Suppl D), 187
Phototoxicity
  (2000): Traynor NJ+, *Toxicol Vitr* 14, 275
  (1998): Martinez LJ+, *Photochem Photobiol* 67, 399
  (1993): Ferguson J+, *Br J Dermatol* 128, 285
Pigmentation (<1%)
Pruritus (<1%)
  (2006): Urbina F+, *Photodermatol Photoimmunol Photomed* 22(2), 111
  (2002): Litt JZ, Beachwood, OH (personal case) (observation)
  (1999): Litt JZ, Beachwood, OH (2 personal cases) (observation)
  (1989): Davis H+, *Ann Intern Med* 111, 1041
  (1989): Gaut PL+, *Am J Med* 87 (Suppl 5A), 169S
  (1989): Rahm V+, *Scand J Infect Dis* 60, 120
  (1989): Schacht P+, *Am J Med* 87, 98S
  (1989): Yangco BG+, *Clin Ther* 11, 503
  (1988): Campoli-Richards DM+, *Drugs* 35, 373 (0.3%)
  (1988): Sanders WE, *Rev Infect Dis* 10, 528
  (1988): Schacht P+, *Infection* 16, S29
  (1988): Thorsteinsson SB+, *Chemotherapy* 34, 256
Purpura
  (2006): Urbina F+, *Photodermatol Photoimmunol Photomed* 22(2), 111
  (2002): Mouraux A+, *Rev Neurol* (Paris) 158(11), 1115
  (1999): Goldberg EI+, *J Clin Dermatol* 2, 25

(1997): Sapadin A+, New York, American Academy of
Dermatology Meeting (SF), Poster #110
(1994): Gamboa F+, *Ann Pharmacol* 29, 84

Rash (sic) (1–10%)
(2006): Matsuoka H+, *Leuk Lymphoma* 47(8), 1618
(2000): Johansson A+, *Pediatr Infect Dis J* 19, 449
(2000): Talan DA+, *JAMA* 283, 1583 (4%)
(1995): Chaisson RE, *Infections in Medicine* 12, 48
(1989): Fass RJ+, *Am J Med* 87, 164S
(1989): Modai J, *Am J Med* 87, 243S
(1989): Rahm V+, *Scand J Infect Dis* 60, 120
(1989): Schacht P+, *Am J Med* 87, 98S
(1988): Sanders WE, *Rev Infect Dis* 10, 528
(1988): Schacht P+, *Infection* 16, S29

Stevens–Johnson syndrome (<1%)
(2003): Hallgren J+, *J Am Acad Dermatol* 49(5 Suppl), S267
(2003): Leone R+, *Drug Saf* 26(2), 109
(1994): Bhatia RS, *J Assoc Physicians India* 42(4), 344
(1994): Gohel DR+, *J Assoc Physicians India* 42, 665
(1994): Kamili MA+, *J Assoc Physicians India* 42, 755
(1994): Win A+, *Int J Dermatol* 33, 512

Toxic epidermal necrolysis (<1%)
(2004): Mandal B+, *Age Ageing* 33(4), 405
(2003): Jongen-Lavrencic M+, *Infection* 31(6), 428
(2003): Leone R+, *Drug Saf* 26(2), 109
(1997): Livasy CA+, *Dermatology* 195, 173 (fatal)
(1997): Yerasi AB+, *Ann Pharmacother* 30, 297
(1993): Moshfeghi M+, *Ann Pharmacother* 27, 1467
(1991): Sakellariou G+, *Int J Artif Organs* 14, 634
(1991): Tham TC+, *Lancet* 338, 522

Urticaria (<1%)
(1999): Litt JZ, Beachwood, OH (personal case) (observation)
(1994): Guharoy SR, *Vet Hum Toxicol* 36, 540
(1993): Litt JZ, Beachwood, OH (personal case) (observation)
(1989): Davis H+, *Ann Intern Med* 111, 1041
(1989): Rahm V+, *Scand J Infect Dis* 60, 120
(1989): Schacht P+, *Am J Med* 87, 98S
(1988): Campoli-Richards DM+, *Drugs* 35, 373 (0.05%)
(1988): Schacht P+, *Infection* 16, S29
(1986): Ball P, *J Antimicrob Chemother* 18 (Suppl D), 187

Vasculitis (<1%)
(2007): Storsley L+, *Nephrol Dial Transplant* 22(2), 660
(2000): Perez Vazquez A+, *An Med Interna* (Spanish) 17, 225
(1999): Goldberg EI+, *J Clin Dermatol* 2, 25
(1997): Lieu PK+, *Allergy* 52, 593
(1997): Reano M+, *Allergy* 52, 599
(1994): Beuselinck B+, *Acta Clin Belg* 49, 173
(1993): Wagh SS+, *Indian J Pediatr* 60, 610
(1992): Stubbings J+, *BMJ* 305, 29
(1991): Kanuga J+, *Ann Allergy* 66, 76
(1989): Choe U+, *N Engl J Med* 320, 257

Mucosal/ENT
Anosmia
Dysgeusia (<1%)
(1988): Schacht P+, *Infection* 16, S29
Oral candidiasis
(1988): Esposito S+, *Infection* 16, S57
Oral lesions
(1988): Campoli-Richards DM+, *Drugs* 35, 373
Stomatitis
(1989): Rahm V+, *Scand J Infect Dis* 60, 120
(1989): Schacht P+, *Am J Med* 87, 98S
(1988): Schacht P+, *Infection* 16, S29
Tinnitus
Vaginitis (<1%)
(1990): Karimi K, *Indiana Med* 83, 266
(1987): Arcieri G+, *Am J Med* 82, 381
Xerostomia

(1989): Rahm V+, *Scand J Infect Dis* 60, 120
(1988): Campoli-Richards DM+, *Drugs* 35, 373
(1988): Schacht P+, *Infection* 16, S29

Eyes
Optic neuropathy
(2007): Samarakoon N+, *Clin Experiment Ophthalmol* 35(1), 102
Visual hallucinations
(2007): Asensio-Sanchez VM+, *Arch Soc Esp Oftalmol* 82(5), 299
(2001): Prakken H, *Ned Tijdschr Geneeskd* 145(51), 2497
(1993): Jick SS+, *Pharmacotherapy* 13(5), 461
(1987): Davies BI+, *Pharm Weekbl Sci* 9, S53
(1986): Davies BI+, *Eur J Clin Microbiol* 5(2), 226
(1986): Davies BI+, *Pharm Weekbl Sci* 8(1), 53

Other
Anaphylactoid reactions/Anaphylaxis (<1%)
(2006): Sachs B+, *Drug Saf* 29(11), 1087
(2003): Ho DY+, *Ann Pharmacother* 37(7), 1018
(1999): Corcoy M+, *Rev Esp Anestesiol Reanim* (Spanish) 46, 419
(1999): Erdem G+, *Pediatr Infect Dis J* 18, 563
(1997): Clutterbuck DJ+, *Int J STD AIDS* 8, 707
(1997): Salon EJ+, *Ann Pharmacother* 31, 119
(1995): Assouad M+, *Ann Intern Med* 122, 396
(1994): Beuselinck B+, *Acta Clin Belg* (Dutch; French) 49, 173
(1993): Soetikno RM+, *Ann Pharmacother* 27, 1404 (in AIDS)
(1992): Berger TG+, *J Am Acad Dermatol* 26, 256
(1992): Deamer RL+, *Ann Pharmacother* 26, 1081
(1989): Davis H+, *Ann Intern Med* 111, 1041
(1989): Wurtz RM+, *Lancet* 1, 955
Asthenia
(2006): Mannaerts L+, *Ned Tijdschr Geneeskd* 150(14), 804
Candidiasis (<1%)
(1997): Litt JZ, Beachwood, OH (penile) (personal case)
(observation)
(1989): Yangco BG+, *Clin Ther* 11, 503
(1988): Schacht P+, *Infection* 16, S29
Death
(2004): Mandal B+, *Age Ageing* 33(4), 405
Delusions of parasitosis
(2006): Steinert T+, *Pharmacopsychiatry* 39(4), 159
Gynecomastia (<1%)
(1991): MacGowan AP+, *J Infect* 22, 100
Headache
(1993): Jick SS+, *Pharmacotherapy* 13(5), 461
Hepatotoxicity
(2006): Matsuoka H+, *Leuk Lymphoma* 47(8), 1618
(2004): Zimpfer A+, *Virchows Arch* 444(1), 87
Hypersensitivity
(2001): Scala E+, *Int J Dermatol* 40(9), 603
(1992): Deamer RL+, *Ann Pharmacother* 26, 1081
(1991): Bhatia RS, *J Assoc Physicians India* 39, 972
Injection-site pain
(1988): Thorsteinsson SB+, *Chemotherapy* 34, 256
(1987): Thorsteinsson SB+, *Chemotherapy* 33, 448 (with itching
and burning)
Lobular panniculitis (erythematous tender nodules of
extremities)
(1990): Rodriguez E+, *BMJ* 300, 1468
Mania
(2006): Bhalerao S+, *Psychosomatics* 47(6), 539
Myoclonus
(2004): Post B+, *Mov Disord* 19(5), 595
Nephrotoxicity
(2007): Storsley L+, *Nephrol Dial Transplant* 22(2), 660
(2007): Stratta P+, *Am J Kidney Dis* 50(2), 330
(2006): Mannaerts L+, *Ned Tijdschr Geneeskd* 150(14), 804
(2006): Sedlacek M+, *Nephrol Dial Transplant* 21(8), 2339
(2005): Montagnac R+, *Nephrol Ther* 1(1), 44

(2005): Paszkowska M+, *Wiad Lek* 58(1-2), 131
(2003): Moffett BS+, *J Cyst Fibros* 2(3), 152
Paresthesias
  (1989): Rahm V+, *Scand J Infect Dis* 60, 120
Pseudoporphyria
  (2007): Degiovanni CV+, *Clin Exp Dermatol*
Seizures
  (2005): Kisa C+, *J ECT* 21(1), 43
  (2003): Orr CF+, *Med J Aust* 178(7), 343
  (2001): Kushner JM+, *Ann Pharmacother* 35(10), 1194
Serum sickness
  (1994): Guharoy SR, *Vet Hum Toxicol* 36, 540
  (1990): Slama TG, *Antimicrob Agents Chemother* 34, 904
Tendinopathy/Tendon rupture
  (2006): Palin SL+, *Diabet Med* 23(12), 1386
  (2006): Shortt P+, *Emerg Med J* 23(12), e63 (2 cases)
  (2005): Mouzopoulos G+, *Acta Orthop Belg* 71(6), 743
  (2003): Khaliq Y+, *Clin Infect Dis* 36(11), 1404
  (2003): Ozaras R+, *Clin Rheumatol* 22(6), 500
  (2003): van der Linden PD+, *Arch Intern Med* 163(15), 1801
  (2002): Chhajed PN+, *Eur Respir J* 19(3), 469 (15 cases)
  (2002): Chhajed PN+, *Eur Respir J* 19(3), 469 (5 cases)
  (2002): Corps AN+, *Arthritis Rheum* 46(11), 3034
  (2001): Malaguti M+, *J Nephrol* 14(5), 431
  (2001): van der Linden PD+, *Arthritis Rheum* 45(3), 235
  (2000): Casparian JM+, *South Med J* 93, 488 (2 cases)
  (2000): Saint F+, *Rev Chir Orthop Reparatrice Appar Mot* 86(5), 495
  (1999): Harrell RM, *South Med J* 92, 622 (passim)
  (1998): Blanco Andres C+, *Aten Primaria* (Spanish) 21, 184 (bilateral)
  (1998): Petersen W+, *Umfallchirurg* (German) 101, 731 (bilateral)
  (1998): West MB+, *N Z Med J* 111, 18
  (1998): West MB+, *N Z Med J* 111, 18 (bilateral)
  (1997): Carrasco JM+, *Ann Pharmacother* 31, 120
  (1997): Movin T+, *Foot Ankle Int* 18, 297 (2 cases)
  (1997): Peyrade F+, *Presse Med* (French) 26, 1489
  (1997): Poon CC+, *Med J Aust* 166, 665
  (1997): Shinohara YT+, *J Rheumatol* 24, 238
  (1996): Hugo-Persson M, *Lakartidningen* (Swedish) 93, 1520
  (1996): Jagose JT+, *N Z Med J* 109, 471
  (1996): McGarvey WC+, *Foot Ankle Int* 17, 496
  (1993): Boulay I+, *Ann Med Interne* (Paris) (French) 144, 493
  (1992): Lee TW+, *Aust N Z J Med*, 22, 500
Tremor
  (2007): Cheung YF+, *Mov Disord* 22(7), 1038 (palatal)

CISATRACURIUM

Trade name: Nimbex (Abbott)
Indications: Adjunct to general anesthesia, relaxes skeletal muscle
Category: Non-depolarizing neuromuscular blocker
Half-life: 22 minutes
Clinically important, potentially hazardous interactions with: aminoglycosides, clindamycin, cyclopropane, enflurane, halothane, isoflurane, methoxyflurane, piperacillin, rocuronium

Reactions

Skin
Pruritus
Rash (sic) (0.1%)

Other
Anaphylactoid reactions/Anaphylaxis

(2005): Dewachter P+, *Ann Fr Anesth Reanim* 24(5), 543
(2005): Fraser BA+, *Anaesth Intensive Care* 33(6), 816
(2004): Sanchez Palacios A+, *Allergol Immunopathol (Madr)* 32(6), 352
(2003): Rieder J+, *Anesth Analg* 96(1), 301
(2002): Iannuzzi E+, *Eur J Anaesthesiol* 19(9), 691
(2001): Krombach J+, *Anesth Analg* 93(5), 1257
(2001): Legros CB+, *Anesth Analg* 92(3), 648
(2000): Briassoulis G+, *Paediatr Anaesth* 10(4), 429
(1999): Toh KW+, *Anesth Analg* 88(2), 462
(1997): Clendenen SR+, *Anesthesiology* 87(3), 690
Hypersensitivity
Myalgia/Myositis/Myopathy/Myotoxicity
  (1998): Davis NA+, *Crit Care Med* 26(7), 1290

CISPLATIN

Synonym: CDDP
Trade names: Cisplatyl; Plasticin; Platiblastin; Platinex; Platinol (Bristol-Myers Squibb); Platinol-AQ; Platistil
Indications: Carcinomas, lymphomas
Category: Alkylating agent; Antineoplastic
Half-life: α phase: 25–49 minutes; β phase: 58–73 hours
Clinically important, potentially hazardous interactions with: aldesleukin, atenolol, chlorothiazide, methotrexate, selenium, zinc

Reactions

Skin
Acral erythema
  (1998): Vakalis D+, *Br J Dermatol* 139, 750
Actinic keratoses
  (1987): Johnson TM+, *J Am Acad Dermatol* 17(2 Pt 1), 192
Allergic reactions (sic)
  (2002): Cantu MG+, *J Clin Oncol* 20(5), 1232 (2%) (with cyclophosphamide and doxorubicin)
Angioedema
  (1984): Loehrer PJ+, *Ann Intern Med* 100, 704
  (1983): Bronner AK+, *J Am Acad Dermatol* 9, 645 (1–5%)
  (1981): Weiss RB+, *Ann Intern Med* 94, 66 (1–5%)
Dermatitis
  (1996): Schena D+, *Contact Dermatitis* 34, 220
Diaphoresis
  (1983): Bronner AK+, *J Am Acad Dermatol* 9, 645
Erythema
  (2001): Robinson JB+, *Gynecol Oncol* 82(3), 550
  (1983): Bronner AK+, *J Am Acad Dermatol* 9, 645
  (1980): Vogl SE+, *Cancer* 45, 11
Exanthems
  (2003): Lin XG+, *Ai Zheng* 22(4), 411 (with paclitaxel)
  (1984): Loehrer PJ+, *Ann Intern Med* 100, 704
  (1981): Weiss RB+, *Ann Intern Med* 94, 66 (1–5%)
  (1980): Vogl SE+, *Cancer* 45, 11
Exfoliative dermatitis
  (1994): Lee TC+, *Mayo Clin Proc* 69, 80
Facial edema
  (1994): Lee TC+, *Mayo Clin Proc* 69, 80
Necrosis
  (2006): Stijelja B+, *Srp Arh Celok Lek* 134(5-6), 244 (penis)
  (1983): Leyden M+, *Cancer Treat Rep* 67, 199
Pigmentation
  (2006): Yanagi T+, *J Am Acad Dermatol* 54(2), 362
  (2002): Kim KJ+, *Clin Exp Dermatol* 27(2), 118
  (1996): Al-Lamki Z+, *Cancer* 77, 1578
Pruritus

Extravasation

Hypersensitivity
(2002): Koren C+, *Am J Clin Oncol* 25(6), 625
(2001): Robinson JB+, *Gynecol Oncol* 82(3), 550

Inappropriate secretion of antidiuretic hormone (SIADH)
(2006): Saegusa T+, *Gan To Kagaku Ryoho* 33(13), 2053
(2005): Yamamoto Y+, *Gan To Kagaku Ryoho* 32(1), 107
(2004): Kusuki M+, *Acta Otolaryngol Suppl* 554, 74
(2002): Ishii K+, *Gynecol Oncol* 87(1), 150
(2001): Kagawa K+, *Intern Med* 40(10), 1020
(1996): Otsuka F+, *Intern Med* 35(4), 290
(1987): Vassal G+, *Pediatr Hematol Oncol* 4(4), 337 (3 cases)
(1986): Hayes DF+, *J Surg Oncol* 32(3), 150
(1984): Littlewood TJ+, *Thorax* 39(8), 636
(1982): Levin L+, *Cancer* 50(11), 2279

Injection-site cellulitis
(1994): Lee TC+, *Mayo Clin Proc* 69, 80 (passim)
(1990): Fields S+J, *Natl Cancer Inst* 82, 1649
(1989): Kerker BJ+, *Semin Dermatol* 8, 173
(1980): Lewis KP+, *Cancer Treat Rep* 64, 1162

Injection-site pain
(1998): Kempf W+, *Arch Dermatol* 134, 1343

Injection-site thrombophlebitis

Lymphedema
(2005): Bellati F+, *Gynecol Oncol* 96(1), 227 (3 cases)

Myalgia/Myositis/Myopathy/Myotoxicity
(2006): Panichpisal K+, *BMC Nephrol* 7, 10
(2002): Cantu MG+, *J Clin Oncol* 20(5), 1232 (4%) (with cyclophosphamide and doxorubicin)

Nephrotoxicity
(2007): Stohr W+, *Pediatr Blood Cancer* 48(2), 140 (mild)
(2006): Ali BH+, *Food Chem Toxicol* 44(8), 1173
(2006): Panichpisal K+, *BMC Nephrol* 7, 10
(2006): Shord SS+, *Anticancer Drugs* 17(2), 207
(2005): Taguchi T+, *Contrib Nephrol* 148, 107
(2004): Fisher MJ+, *Pediatr Blood Cancer* 43(7), 780
(2003): Arany I+, *Semin Nephrol* 23(5), 460
(2003): Chaudhary UB+, *Drugs* 63(15), 1565
(2003): Goren MP, *Med Pediatr Oncol* 41(3), 186
(2003): Hayek M+, *Pediatr Hematol Oncol* 20(3), 253
(2003): Kuhnt T+, *Strahlenther Onkol* 179(10), 673
(2003): Miyazaki J+, *Nippon Rinsho* 61(6), 973
(2003): Perazella MA+, *Am J Med Sci* 325(6), 349
(2003): Santoso JT+, *Cancer Chemother Pharmacol* 52(1), 13
(2002): Caglar K+, *Nephrol Dial Transplant* 17(11), 1931 (23%)
(2002): Kern W+, *Anticancer Res* 22(5), 3099
(2002): Nisar S+, *Ren Fail* 24(4), 529
(2001): Erdlenbruch B+, *Eur J Clin Pharmacol* 57(5), 393
(2001): Kintzel PE, *Drug Saf* 24(1), 19
(2001): Rojanasthien N+, *Int J Clin Pharmacol Ther* 39(3), 121
(2001): Waszkiewicz K, *Postepy Hig Med Dosw* 55(3), 387
(2000): Lyubimova NV+, *Bull Exp Biol Med* 130(9), 886
(1999): Alberts DS, *Semin Oncol* 26(2 Suppl 7), 125
(1999): Capizzi RL, *Semin Oncol* 26(2 Suppl 7), 72
(1999): Kollmannsberger C+, *Semin Surg Oncol* 17(4), 275
(1999): Takayama K+, *Gan To Kagaku Ryoho* 26(4), 503
(1998): Koch Nogueira PC+, *Pediatr Nephrol* 12(7), 572
(1998): Nishikawa H+, *Gan To Kagaku Ryoho* 25(1), 89
(1998): Nishikawa H+, *Gan To Kagaku Ryoho* 25(1), 97
(1997): Hayashi M+, *Acta Obstet Gynecol Scand* 76(6), 590
(1997): Hu YJ+, *Biol Trace Elem Res* 56(3), 331
(1997): Ramnath N+, *Am J Clin Oncol* 20(4), 368
(1997): Tesar V+, *Cas Lek Cesk* 136(7), 205
(1996): Bokemeyer C+, *Br J Cancer* 74(12), 2036
(1992): Hansen SW, *Dan Med Bull* 39(5), 391 (with vinblastine & bleomycin)

Neurotoxicity
(2005): Winton T+, *N Engl J Med* 352(25), 2589 (48%) (with vinorelbine)

(2001): Waszkiewicz K, *Postepy Hig Med Dosw* 55(3), 387
(1999): Alberts DS, *Semin Oncol* 26(2 Suppl 7), 125
(1999): Kollmannsberger C+, *Semin Surg Oncol* 17(4), 275
(1997): Ramnath N+, *Am J Clin Oncol* 20(4), 368
(1996): Bokemeyer C+, *Br J Cancer* 74(12), 2036
(1992): Hansen SW, *Dan Med Bull* 39(5), 391 (with vinblastine & bleomycin)

Pain
(2005): Lena MD+, *Lung Cancer* 48(1), 129 (with vinorelbine)

Phlebitis

Porphyria
(1986): Aramburo-Gonzalez P+, *Med Clin* (Barc) (Spanish) 87, 738

Rhabdomyolysis
(1995): Anderlini P+, *Cancer* 76(4), 678

Seizures
(2006): Panichpisal K+, *BMC Nephrol* 7, 10

CITALOPRAM

Synonym: nitalapram
Trade name: Celexa (Forest)
Indications: Depression, obsessive-compulsive disorder, panic disorder
Category: Antidepressant; Selective serotonin reuptake inhibitor
Half-life: 33 hours
Clinically important, potentially hazardous interactions with: dexibuprofen, isocarboxazid, MAO inhibitors, phenelzine, selegiline, **St John's wort**, sumatriptan, tramadol, tranylcypromine, trazodone

Reactions

Skin

Acute febrile neutrophilic dermatosis (Sweet's syndrome)
(2004): Mecca P+, *J Cutan Pathol* 31(2), 189 (with perphenazine and amoxapine) (photodistributed)

Angioedema

Cellulitis

Dermatitis

Diaphoresis (11%)
(2005): Tseng WP+, *Kaohsiung J Med Sci* 21(7), 326
(2001): Bostic JQ+, *J Child Adole Pyschopharmacol* 11(2), 159 (33%)
(1999): Feighner JP+, *J Clin Psychiatry* 60(12), 824

Eczema

Erythema multiforme

Exanthems
(2001): Richard MA+, *Ann Dermatol Venereol* 128(6), 759

Facial edema

Photosensitivity

Pigmentation
(2001): Inaloz HS+, *J Dermatol* 28(12), 742

Pruritus (<10%)
(2001): Richard MA+, *Ann Dermatol Venereol* 128(6), 759

Pruritus ani et vulvae

Psoriasis
(2000): Elliott P, Logan Central, Australia (from Internet) (observation)

Purpura
(2001): Robinson MJ, *Can Psychiatry* 46, 286

Rash (sic) (<10%)

Urticaria

Vasculitis
(2001): Richard MA+, *Ann Dermatol Venereol* 128(6), 759

Xerosis

Mucosal/ENT

Dysgeusia

Gingivitis

Sialorrhea

(2003): Lavretsky H+, *J Clin Psychiatry* 64(12), 1410 (with methylphenidate)

Stomatitis

Xerostomia (20%)

(2003): Lavretsky H+, *J Clin Psychiatry* 64(12), 1410 (with methylphenidate)

(1999): Feighner JP+, *J Clin Psychiatry* 60(12), 824

Hair

Hair – alopecia

(2006): Hedenmalm K+, *Pharmacoepidemiol Drug Saf* 15(10), 719

Hair – hypertrichosis

Eyes

Diplopia

(2005): Mowla A+, *J Clin Psychopharmacol* 25(6), 623

Glaucoma

(2005): Croos R+, *BMC Ophthalmol* 5, 23

Ocular allergy (sic)

(2004): Campo JV+, *J Am Acad Child Adolesc Psychiatry* 43(10), 1234 (4 cases)

Visual hallucinations

(2007): Bez Y+, *J Psychopharmacol* 21(6), 665

Other

Asthenia

(2007): Bez Y+, *J Psychopharmacol* 21(6), 665

Death

(2002): Jonasson B+, *Forensic Sci Int* 126(1), 1 (5 cases)

(2001): Dams R+, *J Anal Toxicol* 25(2), 147 (with moclobemide)

(2001): Isbister GK+, *J Anal Toxicol* 25(8), 716 (with moclobemide)

(1999): Musshoff F+, *Forensic Sci Int* 106(2), 125

Gynecomastia

Headache

(2006): von Knorring AL+, *J Clin Psychopharmacol* 26(3), 311

(2003): Barak Y+, *Prog Neuropsychopharmacol Biol Psychiatry* 27(3), 545

Hot flashes

Hypotension

(2001): Isbister GK+, *Ann Pharmacother* 35(12), 1552

Inappropriate secretion of antidiuretic hormone (SIADH)

(2007): Bez Y+, *J Psychopharmacol* 21(6), 665

(2006): Bavbek N+, *Am J Kidney Dis* 48(4), e61

(2005): Miehle K+, *Pharmacopsychiatry* 38(4), 181

(2004): Flores G+, *BMC Nephrol* 5, 2

(2004): Iraqi A+, *J Am Med Dir Assoc* 5(1), 64

(2002): Bourgeois JA+, *Psychosomatics* 43(3), 241

(2002): Fisher A+, *Adverse Drug React Toxicol Rev* 21(4), 179

(2001): Odeh M+, *Am J Med Sci* 321(2), 159

(2000): Zullino D+, *Therapie* 55(5), 651

(1998): Pradalier A+, *Therapie* 53(6), 600

(1996): Christensen O+, *Ugeskr Laeger* 158(48), 6920

Myalgia/Myositis/Myopathy/Myotoxicity (>2%)

Neurotoxicity

(2006): Thwaites JH+, *N Z Med J* 119(1235), U2019

Paresthesias

(2007): Bez Y+, *J Psychopharmacol* 21(6), 665

Rhabdomyolysis

(2000): Zullino D+, *Therapie* 55(5), 651

Suicidal ideation

(2006): von Knorring AL+, *J Clin Psychopharmacol* 26(3), 311

Tremor (jaw)

(2004): Tarlaci S, *Clin Neurol Neurosurg* 107(1), 73

Vertigo

(2001): Bostic JQ+, *J Child Adolesc Psychopharmacol* 11(2), 159

CLADRIBINE

Synonyms: 2-CdA; 2-chlorodeoxyadenosine
Trade name: Leustatin (Ortho)
Indications: Leukemias
Category: Antimetabolite; Antineoplastic
Half-life: α phase: 25 minutes; β phase: 6.7 hours

Reactions

Skin

Allergic reactions (sic)

(1997): Robak T+, *J Med* 28, 199

Diaphoresis (1–10%)

Edema (6%)

Eosinophilic cellulitis

(2004): Rossini MS+, *J Eur Acad Dermatol Venereol* 18(5), 538

Erythema (6%)

Erythroderma

(2006): Kokunai A+, *Arerugi* 55(6), 662

Exanthems (27–50%)

(2004): Rossini MS+, *J Eur Acad Dermatol Venereol* 18, 538

(1996): Meunier P+, *Acta Derm Venereol* 76, 385 (21%)

Halogenoderma

(1996): Zevin S+, *Am J Hematol* 53, 209

Herpes

(2002): Robak T+, *Eur J Haematol* 69(1), 27 (10 cases)

Petechiae (8%)

Pruritus (6%)

Purpura (10%)

Rash (sic) (27%)

(2000): Grey MR+, *Clin Lab Haematol* 22, 111

Stevens–Johnson syndrome

Toxic epidermal necrolysis

(1996): Meunier P+, *Acta Derm Venereol* 76, 385

Transient acantholytic dermatosis (Grover's Disease)

(1997): Cohen PR+, *Acta Derm Venereol* 77, 412

Urticaria

Vasculitis

(2002): Tousi B+, *Clin Lab Haematol* 24(4), 259 (1 case)

Other

Death

(2004): Ogura M+, *Int J Hematol* 80(3), 267 (2 cases)

Gynecomastia

(2001): Abhyankar D+, *Leuk Lymphoma* 42(1), 243

Headache

Infections

(2003): Byrd JC+, *Leukemia* 17(2), 323 (43%)

Injection-site edema (9%)

Injection-site erythema (9%)

Injection-site pain (9%)

Injection-site phlebitis (2%)

Injection-site thrombosis (2%)

Myalgia/Myositis/Myopathy/Myotoxicity (7%)

CLARITHROMYCIN

Trade names: Biaxin (Abbott); Biaxin HP; Clacine; Clarith; Klacid; Klaricid; Macladin; Veclam
Indications: Various infections caused by susceptible organisms
Category: Antibiotic, macrolide
Half-life: 5–7 hours
Clinically important, potentially hazardous interactions with: alprazolam, aprepitant, astemizole, atorvastatin, benzodiazepines, carbamazepine, chlordiazepoxide, cilostazol, clonazepam, clorazepate, colchicine, conivaptan, cyclosporine, dasatinib, diazepam, digoxin, dihydroergotamine, disopyramide, ergot alkaloids, fluoxetine, flurazepam, fluvastatin, HMG-CoA reductase inhibitors, imatinib, ixabepilone, lapatinib, lorazepam, lovastatin, methylprednisolone, methysergide, midazolam, oxazepam, paroxetine, pimozide, pravastatin, prednisone, quazepam, repaglinide, rimonabant, sertraline, simvastatin, solifenacin, temazepam, temsirolimus, triazolam, warfarin, zidovudine

Reactions

Skin
Baboon syndrome
    (2003): Wolf R+, *Dermatol Online J* 9(3), 2 (with amoxicillin and omeprazole)
Exanthems
Fixed eruption
    (2001): Hamamoto Y+, *Clin Exp Dermatol* 26(1), 48
    (1988): Rosina P+, *Contact Dermatitis* 38, 105
Henoch–Schönlein purpura
    (2003): Borras-Blasco J+, *Int J Clin Pharmacol Ther* 41(5), 213
Phototoxicity
    (2002): Parkash P+, *J Assoc Physicians India* 50, 1192
Pruritus
    (1991): Poirier R, *J Antimicrob Chemother* 27 (Suppl A), 109
Psoriasis
    (1994): Ellerin P, *The Schoch Letter* 44, 47 (#185) (observation)
Purpura
    (2006): Zink A+, *Dtsch Med Wochenschr* 131(40), 2217
    (2003): Borras-Blasco J+, *Int J Clin Pharmacol Ther* 41(5), 213
    (2002): Alexopoulou A+, *Eur J Haematol* 69(3), 191
Pustules
Rash (sic) (3%)
Stevens–Johnson syndrome (<1%)
Toxic epidermal necrolysis
    (2007): Clayton TH+, *Clin Exp Dermatol* 32(6), 755
    (2005): Khaldi N+, *Can J Clin Pharmacol* 12(3), e264
    (2002): Masia M+, *Arch Intern Med* 162(4), 474 (with disulfiram)
Urticaria
Vasculitis
    (2006): Zink A+, *Dtsch Med Wochenschr* 131(40), 2217
    (1998): Gavura SR+, *Ann Pharmacol* 32, 543
    (1993): de Vega T+, *Eur J Clin Microbiol Infect Dis* 12, 563

Mucosal/ENT
Dysgeusia (3%)
    (2006): Dean NC+, *Antimicrob Agents Chemother* 50(4), 1164
    (2001): Litt JZ, Beachwood, OH (personal case)
    (2001): McCarty JM+, *Ann Allergy Asthma Immunol* 87(4), 327
    (1997): Saluja A+, *Derm Surg* 23, 539
Glossitis
    (1997): Greco S+, *Ann Pharmacother* 31, 1548
Oral candidiasis
Parosmia
Stomatitis

    (1997): Greco S+, *Ann Pharmacother* 31, 1548
Tinnitus
    (2003): Uzun C, *J Laryngol Otol* 117(12), 1006
Tongue black
    (1997): Greco S+, *Ann Pharmacother* 31, 1548
Xerostomia
    (2001): McCarty JM+, *Ann Allergy Asthma Immunol* 87(4), 327

Hair
Hair – alopecia
    (2004): Rollot F+, *Ann Pharmacother* 38(12), 2074 (with colchicine)

Other
Abdominal pain
    (2004): Rollot F+, *Ann Pharmacother* 38(12), 2074 (with colchicine)
Anaphylactoid reactions/Anaphylaxis (<1%)
Death
    (2002): Masia M+, *Arch Intern Med* 162(4), 474
Fever
    (2004): Rollot F+, *Ann Pharmacother* 38(12), 2074 (with colchicine)
Headache
Hepatotoxicity
    (2006): Giannattasio A+, *Ann Pharmacother* 40(6), 1196
    (2005): Peters TS, *Toxicol Pathol* 33(1), 146
Hypersensitivity
    (1998): Igea JM+, *Allergy* 53, 107
    (1998): Kruppa A+, *Dermatology* 196(3), 335
Injection-site extravasation
    (2001): Zimmerman T+, *Clin Drug Invest* 21, 527 (8%)
Injection-site pain
    (2001): Zimmerman T+, *Clin Drug Invest* 21, 527 (100%)
    (1996): Peck KD+, *Pharm Res* 13, PT6028 (9 Suppl)
Nephrotoxicity
    (2006): Audimoolam VK+, *Nephrol Dial Transplant* 21(9), 2654
Phlebitis
    (2001): De Dios Garcia-Diaz J+, *Med Clin* (Barc) 116(4), 133 (from intravenous administration)
Pseudolymphoma
    (1995): Magro CM+, *J Am Acad Dermatol* 32, 419
Rhabdomyolysis
    (2007): Molden E+, *Pharmacotherapy* 27(4), 603 (with simvastatin)
    (2004): Kahri AJ+, *Ann Pharmacother* 38(4), 719 (with simvastatin)
    (2004): Trieu J+, *Clin Nucl Med* 29(12), 803 (with simvastatin)
    (2003): Mah Ming+, *AIDS Patient Care STDS* 17(5), 207 (with atorvastatin and lopinavir/ritonavir)
    (2003): Sipe BE+, *Ann Pharmacother* 37(6), 808 (with atorvastatin and esomeprazole)
    (2001): Lee AJ, *Ann Pharmacother* 35(1), 26 (with simvastatin)
    (1999): Shimada N+, *Nippon Jinzo Gakkai Shi* 41(4), 460 (with theophylline)
Tremor (<1%)

CLEMASTINE

Trade names: Aller-Eze; Antihist-1; Clema; Darvine; Tavegil; Tavegyl; Tavist (Novartis)
Indications: Allergic rhinitis, urticaria
Category: Histamine H1 receptor antagonist
Half-life: 4–6 hours
Clinically important, potentially hazardous interactions with: barbiturates, chloral hydrate, ethchlorvynol, phenothiazines, zolpidem

Reactions

Skin
Angioedema (<1%)
Diaphoresis
Edema (<1%)
Exanthems
Photosensitivity (<1%)
Purpura
Rash (sic) (<1%)
Toxic pustuloderma
(1996): Feind-Koopmans A+, *Clin Exp Dermatol* 21, 293
Urticaria
(1984): Savchak VI, *Vestn Dermatol Venerol* (Russian) 1, 47

Mucosal/ENT
Tinnitus
Xerostomia (1–10%)
(1996): Gwaltney JM+, *Clin Infect Dis* 22(4), 656 (6%)
(1990): Frolund L+, *Allergy* 45, 254

Other
Anaphylactoid reactions/Anaphylaxis
Hypersensitivity
Myalgia/Myositis/Myopathy/Myotoxicity (<1%)
Paresthesias (<1%)

CLEVIDIPINE

Trade name: Cleviprex (The Medicines Company)
Indications: Reduction of blood pressure
Category: Calcium channel blocker
Half-life: Initial: Minute; Terminal: 15 Minutes

Reactions

Other
Cardiac arrest (<1%)
Headache (6.3%)
(1999): Ericsson H+, *Br J Clin Pharmacol* 47(5), 531
Hypotension
Renal failure (9%)
Vertigo (<1%)

CLIDINIUM

Trade names: Bralix; Diporax; Epirax; Librax (Valeant); Libraxin; Librocol; Nirvaxal; Quarzan; Spasmoten
Indications: Duodenal and gastric ulcers
Category: Muscarinic antagonist
Half-life: N/A
Clinically important, potentially hazardous interactions with: anticholinergics, arbutamine

Note: Librax is clidinium and chlordiazepoxide (see chlordiazepoxide)

Reactions

Skin
Purpura
(2001): Alexopoulou A+, *Arch Intern Med* 161(14), 1778 (with chlordiazepoxide)

Urticaria
Mucosal/ENT
Ageusia
Dysgeusia
Xerostomia
Other
Anaphylactoid reactions/Anaphylaxis

CLINDAMYCIN

Trade names: Aclinda; BB; Benzaclin (cream) (Dermik); Cleocin (Pfizer); Cleocin-T (Pfizer); Clindacin; Clindagel (Galderma); Clindets (Stiefel); Dalacin; Dalacin C; Dalacine; Galecin; Sobelin
Indications: Various serious infections caused by susceptible organisms
Category: Antibiotic, lincosamide
Half-life: 2–3 hours
Clinically important, potentially hazardous interactions with: cisatracurium, erythromycin, kaolin, rocuronium, saquinavir

Reactions

Skin
Acute febrile neutrophilic dermatosis (Sweet's syndrome)
(2007): Clark BM+, *Pharmacotherapy* 27(9), 1343
Acute generalized exanthematous pustulosis (AGEP)
(2006): Kapoor R+, *Arch Dermatol* 142(8), 1080
(2003): Valois M+, *Contact Dermatitis* 48(3), 169
(2000): Schwab RA+, *Cutis* 65, 391
Allergic reactions (sic)
(1996): Garcia R+, *Contact Dermatitis* 35, 116
Dermatitis (from topical preparations)
(1995): Vejlstrup E+, *Contact Dermatitis* 32, 110
(1994): Rietschel RL, *Infect Dis Clin North Am* 8, 607
(1992): de Groot AC, *Contact Dermatitis* 8, 428
(1991): Yokayama R+, *Contact Dermatitis* 25, 125
(1983): Conde-Salazar L, *Contact Dermatitis* 9, 225
Eczema
(1991): Yokoyama R+, *Contact Dermatitis* 25, 125
Edema of lip
(1993): Segars LW+, *Ann Pharmacother* 27, 885
Erythema multiforme (<1%)
(1996): Munoz D+, *Contact Dermatitis* 34, 227
Erythroderma
(2006): Gonzalo-Garijo MA+, *J Investig Allergol Clin Immunol* 16(3), 210
(2002): Horiuchi Y+, *J Dermatol* 29(2), 115
Exanthems
(2002): Lammintausta K+, *Br J Dermatol* 146, 643 (6 cases)
(1999): Mazur N+, *Ann Allergy Asthma Immunol* 82, 443
(1984): Brenner S+, *Harefuah* (Hebrew) 106, 570
Facial edema
(1999): Mazur N+, *Ann Allergy Asthma Immunol* 82, 443
Fixed eruption
(1998): Mahboob A+, *Int J Dermatol* 37, 833
Pruritus (<1%)
Pruritus ani et vulvae
Purpura
Rash (sic) (1–10%)
(2002): Maraqa NF+, *Clin Infect Dis* 34(1), 50 (1.4%)
Rosacea
(1989): de Kort WJ+, *Contact Dermatitis* 20, 72
Stevens–Johnson syndrome (<1%)
Toxic epidermal necrolysis

(1995): Paquet P+, *Br J Dermatol* 132, 665
(1993): Correia O+, *Dermatology* 186, 32
(1992): Saiag P+, *J Am Acad Dermatol* 26, 567
Urticaria (<1%)
Vasculitis
(1982): Lambert WC+, *Cutis* 30, 615
Xerosis (from topical preparations)

Mucosal/ENT
Dysgeusia
Tinnitus
(2006): Scissors B+, *J Am Acad Dermatol* 54(5 Suppl), S243
Vulvovaginal pruritus
(2001): Sobel J+, *Infect Dis Obstet Gynecol* 9(1), 9

Other
Anaphylactoid reactions/Anaphylaxis
(2006): Chiou CS+, *J Chin Med Assoc* 69(11), 549
Hypersensitivity
(2002): Kim P+, *Clin Experiment Ophthalmol* 30(2), 147
(2002): Lammintausta K+, *Br J Dermatol* 146(4), 643
Injection-site phlebitis (<1%)
Thrombophlebitis

CLIOQUINOL

Synonyms: Iodochlorhydroxyquin; chloroiodoquin
Trade names: Iodo Plain; Vioform (Novartis)
Indications: Athlete's foot, eczema, fungal infections, parkinsonism
Category: Antibacterial; Antifungal; Chelator
Half-life: N/A
Clinically important, potentially hazardous interactions with: bacitracin

Reactions

Skin
Contact dermatitis
(2006): Kiec-Swierczynska M+, *Med Pr* 57(3), 245
(1994): Beck MH+, *Contact Dermatitis* 31(1), 54
(1991): Rivara G+, *Photodermatol Photoimmunol Photomed* 8(5), 225
Dermatitis
Edema
Erythema
Fixed eruption
(1995): Janier M+, *Br J Dermatol* 133(6), 1013
Pruritus
Urticaria
(1991): Palungwachira P, *J Med Assoc Thai* 74(1), 43 (with bacitracin)
Xerosis

Eyes
Optic atrophy
Optic neuritis
Vision loss

Other
Amnesia
(1984): Kaeser HE, *Acta Neurol Scand Suppl* 100, 175 (global)
Anaphylactoid reactions/Anaphylaxis
(1991): Palungwachira P, *J Med Assoc Thai* 74(1), 43
Hypersensitivity
(2002): Morris SD+, *Br J Dermatol* 146(6), 1047

Neurotoxicity
(1984): Clifford Rose F+, *Acta Neurol Scand Suppl* 100, 137
(1984): Gilland O, *Acta Neurol Scand Suppl* 100, 165
(1984): Wadia NH, *Acta Neurol Scand Suppl* 100, 159
(1983): Devoize JL+, *Presse Med* 12(40), 2532
(1983): Herxheimer A+, *J R Coll Gen Pract* 33(253), 535
(1980): *Lancet* 1(8173), 857
(1980): Mackiewicz J+, *Neurol Neurochir Pol* 14(1), 121

CLOBAZAM

Trade names: Castillium; Frisium (Sanofi-Aventis); Mystan; Odipam; Urbanil; Urbanyl
Indications: Epilepsy adjunct therapy, psychosis
Category: Benzodiazepine
Half-life: 18 hours
Clinically important, potentially hazardous interactions with: alcohol, carbamazepine, cimetidine, phenytoin, valproic acid

Reactions

Skin
Bullae
(2000): Setterfield JF+, *Clin Exp Dermatol* 25(3), 215
Lupus erythematosus
(1995): Caramaschi P+, *Clin Rheumatol* 14(1), 116
Pruritus
Rash (sic)
(2007): Arif H+, *Neurology* 68(20), 1701
(1992): Machet L+, *Contact Dermatitis* 26(5), 347 (from patch testing) (relapse)
Toxic epidermal necrolysis
(2005): Mansur AT+, *Photodermatol Photoimmunol Photomed* 21(2), 100
(1996): Redondo P+, *Br J Dermatol* 135(6), 999 (photo-induced)
Urticaria

Mucosal/ENT
Xerostomia

Eyes
Vision blurred

Other
Adverse effects (47%)
(2004): Sugai K, *Epilepsia* 45 Suppl 8, 20
Death
(2004): Proenca P+, *Forensic Sci Int* 143(2–3), 205
Depression
(1995): Sheth RD+, *J Child Neurol* 10(3), 205
Headache
Side effects (35%)
(1995): Sheth RD+, *J Child Neurol* 10(3), 205
(1990): Davila-Gutierrez G+, *Bol Med Hosp Infant Mex* 47(10), 694
Suicidal ideation
(1995): Sheth RD+, *J Child Neurol* 10(3), 205
Sweat gland necrosis
(2000): Setterfield JF+, *Clin Exp Dermatol* 25(3), 215
Toxicity (sic)
(1991): Zifkin B+, *Neurology* 41(2 (Pt 1)), 313 (with phenytoin)
Tremor
Vertigo
(1987): Koeppen D+, *Epilepsia* 28(5), 495

CLOBETASOL

Trade names: Clobex (Galderma); Embeline (Healthpoint);
Olux (Connetics); Temovate (GSK)
Indications: Dermatoses
Category: Corticosteroid, topical
Half-life: N/A
**Clinically important, potentially hazardous interactions
with:** live vaccines

Reactions

Skin

Acne
 (1990): Prawer SE+, *Am Fam Physician* 41(5), 1531
Allergic reactions (sic)
 (2002): Brazzini B+, *Am J Clin Dermatol* 3(1), 47
 (1988): Cox NH, *Arch Dermatol* 124(6), 911
 (1983): Bachmann-Buffle, *Dermatologica* 167(2), 104
 (1981): van Ketel WG+, *Contact Dermatitis* 7(5), 278
Atrophy
 (2003): Lepe V+, *Arch Dermatol* 139(5), 581 (3 cases)
 (1999): Zimmermann R+, *Ann Dermatol Venereol* 126(1), 13
 (1995): Lubach D+, *Dermatology* 190(1), 51
 (1992): Lubach D+, *Dermatology* 185(1), 44
 (1990): Prawer SE+, *Am Fam Physician* 41(5), 1531
 (1988): Harris DW+, *Dermatol Clin* 6(4), 643
 (1985): Serup J+, *Dermatologica* 170(4), 189
 (1981): Black MM+, *Curr Med Res Opin* 7(7), 463 (3 cases)
Burning
 (1991): Olsen EA+, *J Am Acad Dermatol* 24(3), 443 (11%)
Dermatitis
 (2000): Murata T+, *Contact Dermatitis* 42(5), 305
 (1991): Dunkel FG+, *Contact Dermatitis* 25(2), 97 (2 cases)
 (1988): Camarasa JG+, *Med Cutan Ibero Lat Am* 16(4), 328
 (1987): Tosti A+, *Contact Dermatitis* 17(4), 256
 (1986): Spiro JG+, *Contact Dermatitis* 14(2), 116
 (1985): Corbett JR, *Contact Dermatitis* 13(4), 281
 (1984): Boyle J+, *Contact Dermatitis* 11(1), 50
 (1983): Dooms-Goossens A+, *Contact Dermatitis* 9(6), 470 (2
   cases)
Erythema
 (2001): Smith YR+, *Obstet Gynecol* 98(4), 588
 (1993): Dalziel KL+, *J Reprod Med* 38(1), 25
Milia
 (1989): Iacobelli D+, *J Am Acad Dermatol* 21(2), 215
Perioral dermatitis
 (1990): Prawer SE+, *Am Fam Physician* 41(5), 1531
Pigmentation
 (1990): Prawer SE+, *Am Fam Physician* 41(5), 1531
Porokeratosis
 (2006): Yazkan F+, *J Cutan Pathol* 33(7), 516
Stinging
 (1991): Olsen EA+, *J Am Acad Dermatol* 24(3), 443
Striae
 (1988): Harris DW+, *Dermatol Clin* 6(4), 643
Telangiectasia
 (2004): Vazquez-Lopez F+, *J Am Acad Dermatol* 51(5), 811
 (2003): Lepe V+, *Arch Dermatol* 139(5), 581 (2 cases)
 (1985): Serup J+, *Dermatologica* 170(4), 189

Hair

Hair – hypertrichosis
 (1990): Prawer SE+, *Am Fam Physician* 41(5), 1531

Eyes

Glaucoma
 (1993): Aggarwal RK+, *Eye* 7, 664

Other

Hypersensitivity
 (2002): Sommer S+, *Br J Dermatol* 147(2), 266
 (1983): Chalmers RJ+, *Contact Dermatitis* 9(4), 317
 (1983): Kuhlwein A+, *Z Hautkr* 58(11), 794
Infections
 (1999): Zimmermann R+, *Ann Dermatol Venereol* 126(1), 13
 (1990): Prawer SE+, *Am Fam Physician* 41(5), 1531

CLOFARABINE

Trade name: Clolar (Genzyme)
Indications: Acute lymphoblastic leukemia
Category: Antimetabolite
Half-life: 5.2 hours
**Clinically important, potentially hazardous interactions
with:** hepatotoxic & nephrotoxic drugs

Reactions

Skin

Acral erythema
 (2003): Chiao N+, *Leuk Lymphoma* 44(8), 1405 (2 cases)
Cellulitis (11%)
Dermatitis (sic) (41%)
Edema (20%)
Erythema (18%)
Hand–foot syndrome
 (2005): Faderl S+, *Blood* 105(3), 940
 (2005): Kline JP+, *Expert Opin Pharmacother* 6(15), 2711
 (2003): Chiao N+, *Leuk Lymphoma* 44(8), 1405 (13%)
Herpes simplex (11%)
Petechiae (29%)
Pruritus (47%)
Rash (sic)
 (2005): Faderl S+, *Blood* 105(3), 940
Xerosis (10%)

Mucosal/ENT

Gingival bleeding (15%)
Mucosal inflammation (18%)
Mucositis
 (2005): Faderl S+, *Blood* 105(3), 940
Oral candidiasis (13%)
Stomatitis
 (2005): Kline JP+, *Expert Opin Pharmacother* 6(15), 2711

Other

Abdominal pain (36%)
Asthenia (36%)
Cough (19%)
Depression (11%)
Headache (46%)
 (2005): Kline JP+, *Expert Opin Pharmacother* 6(15), 2711
Hypertension (11%)
Hypotension (29%)
 (2006): Jeha S+, *J Clin Oncol* 24(12), 1917
Injection-site pain (14%)
Myalgia/Myositis/Myopathy/Myotoxicity (14%)
 (2005): Kline JP+, *Expert Opin Pharmacother* 6(15), 2711
Pain (19%)
Tremor (10%)
Vertigo (11%)

CLOFAZIMINE

Trade names: Clofozine; Hansepran; Lampren; Lamprene (Novartis); Lapren
Indications: Leprosy
Category: Anti-inflammatory; Antimycobacterial
Half-life: 10 days after a single dose
Clinically important, potentially hazardous interactions with: fludarabine, pentostatin

Reactions

Skin

Acne (<1%)
  (1992): Breathnach SM+, *Adverse Drug Reactions and the Skin* Blackwell, Oxford, 161 (passim)
Acute febrile neutrophilic dermatosis (Sweet's syndrome)
  (1994): Tacke J+, *Hautarzt* (German) 45, 184
Chromhidrosis (red sweat) (1–10%)
  (1987): Kumar B+, *Indian J Lepr* 59, 63
Erythroderma (<1%)
Exanthems
Exfoliative dermatitis
  (1985): Pavithran K, *Int J Lepr* 53, 645
Ichthyosis (8–28%)
  (1989): Patki AH+, *Indian J Lepr* 61, 92
  (1987): Kumar B+, *Indian J Lepr* 59, 63
  (1984): Aram H, *Int J Dermatol* 23, 458
  (1982): Caver CV, *Cutis* 29, 341
Nodular eruption
  (1993): Iyagi PY+, *Int J Lepr Other Mycobact Dis* 61, 636
Peripheral edema (<1%)
  (1990): Oommen T, *Leprosy Review* 61, 289
Photosensitivity (<1%)
  (1992): Breathnach SM+, *Adverse Drug Reactions and the Skin* Blackwell, Oxford, 161 (passim)
Pigmentation (pink to brownish-black) (75–100%)
  (1993): Krop LC+, *N Engl J Med* 329, 1582
  (1992): Fitzpatrick JE, *Derm Clinics* 10, 19
  (1992): Gallais V+, *Ann Dermatol Venereol* (French) 119, 471
  (1991): Garrelts JC, *Ann Pharmacother* 25, 525 (orange-pink)
  (1990): Job CK+, *J Am Acad Dermatol* 23, 236
  (1989): Langford A+, *Oral Surg Oral Med Oral Pathol* 67, 301 (oral)
  (1989): Patki AH+, *Indian J Lepr* 61, 92 (oral)
  (1989): Zhang X+, *J Oral Pathol Med* 18, 471
  (1988): Mensing H, *Dermatologica* 177, 232
  (1987): Kossard S+, *J Am Acad Dermatol* 17, 867 (reddish-blue)
  (1987): Kumar B+, *Indian J Lepr* 59, 63
  (1983): Burte NP+, *Lepr India* 55, 265
  (1983): Moore VJ, *Lepr Rev* 54, 327
  (1981): Granstein RD+, *J Am Acad Dermatol* 5, 1 (red)
Pruritus (1–5%)
  (1992): Breathnach SM+, *Adverse Drug Reactions and the Skin* Blackwell, Oxford, 161 (passim)
Rash (sic) (1–5%)
  (1995): Chaisson RE, *Infections in Medicine* 12, 48
  (1992): Breathnach SM+, *Adverse Drug Reactions and the Skin* Blackwell, Oxford, 161 (passim)
Urticaria
Vitiligo
  (1996): Brown-Harrell V+, *Clin Infect Dis* 22, 581
Xerosis (8–28%)
  (1992): Breathnach SM+, *Adverse Drug Reactions and the Skin* Blackwell, Oxford, 161 (passim)

Mucosal/ENT

Cheilitis (candidal) (<1%)
Dysgeusia (<1%)

Nails

Nails – discoloration
  (1989): Dixit VB+, *Indian J Lepr* 61, 476
  (1982): Caver CV, *Cutis* 29, 341
Nails – subungual hyperkeratosis
  (1989): Dixit VB+, *Indian J Lepr* 61, 476

Other

Abdominal pain
  (2004): Jadhav MV+, *Indian J Pathol Microbiol* 47(2), 281
Death
  (2004): Jadhav MV+, *Indian J Pathol Microbiol* 47(2), 281

CLOFIBRATE

Trade names: Abitrate; Atromid-S; Claripex; Col; Lipavlon; Novo-Fibrate; Regelan N; Skleromexe
Indications: Type III hyperlipidemia
Category: Fibrate
Half-life: 6–25 hours after a single dose
Clinically important, potentially hazardous interactions with: anisindione, anticoagulants, dicumarol, warfarin

Reactions

Skin

Dermatitis
  (1988): Murata Y+, *J Am Acad Dermatol* 18, 381
Diaphoresis
Erythema multiforme
  (1988): Murata Y+, *J Am Acad Dermatol* 18, 381
Exanthems
  (1988): Murata Y+, *J Am Acad Dermatol* 18, 381
  (1980): Cumming A, *BMJ* 281, 1529
Exfoliative dermatitis
Facial rash
Lupus erythematosus
Photosensitivity
  (1990): Leroy D+, *Photodermatology* 7, 136
  (1988): Murata Y+, *J Am Acad Dermatol* 18, 381
Pruritus (<1%)
Purpura
Rash (sic) (<1%)
Sarcoidosis
  (1986): Yamada S+, *J Dermatol* (Tokio) 13, 217
Stevens–Johnson syndrome
  (1994): Wong SS, *Acta Derm Venereol* 74, 475
Toxic epidermal necrolysis
Urticaria (<1%)
Vesiculobullous eruption
Xerosis

Mucosal/ENT

Dysgeusia
Hypogeusia
Oral ulceration
Stomatitis

Hair

Hair – alopecia (<1%)
Hair – dry (<1%)

Other

Gynecomastia
Myalgia/Myositis/Myopathy/Myotoxicity (<1%)
Rhabdomyolysis
  (1992): Schneider S+, *Rev Med Interne* 13(5), 398

CLOMIPHENE

Trade names: Clom 50; Clomid (Sanofi-Aventis); Clomifen; Dyneric; Milophene; Omifin; Pergotime; Phenate; Serophene (Merck)
Indications: Ovulatory failure
Category: Selective estrogen receptor modulator (SERM)
Half-life: 5–7 days

Reactions

Skin

Acne
  (2001): Guzick ND, Houston, TX (from Internet) (several observations)
Allergic reactions (sic)
Dermatitis (<1%)
Diaphoresis
Edema
Erythema
Erythema multiforme
Erythema nodosum
  (1980): Salvatore MA+, *Arch Dermatol* 116, 557
Exanthems
  (1996): Coots NV+, *Cutis* 57, 91
Melanoma
  (2001): Young P+, *Melanoma Res* 11(5), 535
  (1999): Fuller PN, *Am J Obstet Gynecol* 180, 1499
  (1995): Rossing MA+, *Melanoma Res* 5, 123
  (1992): Kuppens E+, *Melanoma Res* 2, 71
Pruritus
Purpura (palpable)
  (1996): Coots NV+, *Cutis* 57, 91
Rash (sic) (<1%)
Urticaria

Hair

Hair – alopecia (<1%)
Hair – hypertrichosis
  (2001): Smith KC, Niagara Falls, ON, Canada (from Internet) (several observations)

Other

Gynecomastia (1–10%)
Headache
Hot flashes (>10%)
Myalgia/Myositis/Myopathy/Myotoxicity

CLOMIPRAMINE

Trade names: Anafranil (Mallinckrodt); Anafranil Retard; Apo-Clomipramine; Clofranil; Clopress; Placil
Indications: Obsessive-compulsive disorder
Category: Antidepressant, tricyclic; Muscarinic antagonist
Half-life: 21–31 hours
Clinically important, potentially hazardous interactions with: amprenavir, arbutamine, clonidine, epinephrine, formoterol, guanethidine, isocarboxazid, linezolid, MAO inhibitors, moclobemide, phenelzine, quinolones, sparfloxacin, tranylcypromine

Reactions

Skin

Acne (2%)
Allergic reactions (sic) (<3%)
Cellulitis (2%)
Chloasma
Dermatitis (2%)
  (1991): Ljunggren B+, *Contact Dermatitis* 24, 259
Diaphoresis (29%)
  (1992): Guelfi JD+, *Br J Psychiatry* 160, 519
  (1990): McTavish D+, *Drugs* 38, 19 (43%)
Edema (2%)
Erythema
Exanthems
Folliculitis
Photosensitivity (<1%)
  (1991): Ljunggren B+, *Contact Dermatitis* 24, 259
  (1989): Tunca Z+, *Am J Psychiatry* 146, 552
Pigmentation (pseudocyanotic)
  (1989): Tunca Z+, *Am J Psychiatry* 146, 552
Pruritus (6%)
Psoriasis
Purpura (3%)
Pustules
Rash (sic) (8%)
Seborrhea
Urticaria (1%)
  (2006): Gallelli L+, *Pharmacopsychiatry* 39(4), 154
Vasculitis
Xerosis (2%)

Mucosal/ENT

Ageusia
Cheilitis
Dysgeusia (8%)
Gingivitis
Glossitis
Sialorrhea
Stomatitis
Tinnitus
  (1996): Ackerman DL+, *J Clin Psychopharmacol* 16(4), 324
Tongue black
Tongue ulceration
Vaginitis (2%)
Xerostomia (84%)
  (1992): Cohen DJ+, *Psychiatr Clin North Am* 15, 109
  (1992): DeVeaugh-Geiss J+, *J Am Acad Child Adolesc Psychiatry* 31, 45
  (1992): Guelfi JD+, *Br J Psychiatry* 160, 519
  (1990): McTavish D+, *Drugs* 38, 19
  (1981): Rafaelsen OJ+, *Acta Psychiatr Scand Suppl* 290, 364

Hair

Hair – alopecia (<1%)
Hair – alopecia areata
  (1993): Kubota T+, *Acta Neurol Napoli* (Italian) 15, 200
Hair – hypertrichosis

Other

Gynecomastia (2%)
Headache
Hypersensitivity
  (2006): Kano Y+, *J Am Acad Dermatol.* 55(4), 727
  (2005): Nishimura Y+, *J Am Acad Dermatol* 53(5 Suppl 1), S231
Hypertension
  (2005): Stage KB+, *Nord J Psychiatry* 59(4), 298
Inappropriate secretion of antidiuretic hormone (SIADH)
  (1997): Sommer BR, *Am J Geriatr Psychiatry* 5(3), 268
  (1994): Assal F+, *Encephale* 20(5), 527
  (1989): Pledger DR+, *Br J Psychiatry* 154, 263
Myalgia/Myositis/Myopathy/Myotoxicity (13%)
Paresthesias

CLONAZEPAM

Trade names: Clonex; Iktorivil; Klonopin (Roche); Landsen;
Lonazep; Rivotril
Indications: Petit mal and myoclonic seizures
Category: Benzodiazepine
Half-life: 18–50 hours
**Clinically important, potentially hazardous interactions
with:** amprenavir, chlorpheniramine, clarithromycin, efavirenz,
esomeprazole, imatinib, indinavir, nelfinavir, oxycodone

Reactions

Skin

Allergic reactions (sic) (1–10%)
Angioedema
Dermatitis (1–10%)
Diaphoresis (>10%)
Erythema multiforme
  (1998): Amichai B+, *Clin Exp Dermatology* 23, 206
Exanthems
Facial edema
Hypermelanosis
Mycosis fungoides
  (1996): Gordon KB+, *J Am Acad Dermatol* 34, 304
Peripheral edema
Pruritus
Purpura
Rash (sic) (>10%)
Urticaria

Mucosal/ENT

Burning mouth syndrome
  (2001): Culhane NS+, *Ann Pharmacother* 35(7), 874
Dysgeusia
  (2000): Heymann WR, *Cutis* 66, 25
Gingivitis
Oral mucosal eruption
  (1986): Bernard K, *Lijec Vjesn* (Serbo-Croatian-Roman) 108, 235
Oral ulceration
Sialopenia (>10%)
Sialorrhea (1–10%)
Tongue black
  (2000): Heymann WR, *Cutis* 66, 25

Xerostomia (>10%)
  (2000): Heymann WR, *Cutis* 66, 25

Hair

Hair – alopecia
  (2000): Mercke Y+, *Ann Clin Psychiatry* 12, 35
Hair – hirsutism

Other

Death
  (2003): Burrows DL+, *J Forensic Sci* 48(3), 683 (with
    oxycodone)
Depression
  (2006): Grabowska-Grzyb A+, *Epilepsy Behav* 8(2), 411
Headache
Injection-site phlebitis
Injection-site thrombosis
Paresthesias
Pseudolymphoma
  (1995): Magro CM+, *J Am Acad Dermatol* 32, 419
  (1988): Kardaun SH+, *Br J Dermatol* 118(4), 545

CLONIDINE

Trade names: Barclyd; Catapres (Boehringer Ingelheim);
Catapresan; Combivent (Boehringer Ingelheim); Daipres; Dixarit;
Duraclon; Haemiton; Nu-Clonidine; Sulmidine
Indications: Hypertension
Category: Adrenergic alpha-receptor agonist
Half-life: 6–24 hours
**Clinically important, potentially hazardous interactions
with:** acebutolol, amitriptyline, amoxapine, atenolol, betaxolol,
carteolol, clomipramine, desipramine, dexmethylphenidate,
doxepin, esmolol, imipramine, insulin detemir, insulin glulisine,
metoprolol, nadolol, nortriptyline, penbutolol, pindolol,
propranolol, protriptyline, timolol, tricyclic antidepressants,
trimipramine, verapamil

Note: Combipres is clonidine and chlorthalidone

Reactions

Skin

Angioedema (<1%)
  (1995): Waldfahrer F+, *HNO* (German) 43, 35
Burning
Depigmentation
  (2002): Prisant LM, *J Clin Hypertens* (Greenwich) 4(2), 136
  (1995): Doe N+, *Arch Intern Med* 155, 2129 (from patch)
Dermatitis (from patch) (20%)
  (2002): Prisant LM, *J Clin Hypertens* (Greenwich) 4(2), 136
  (1999): Polster AM+, *Cutis* 63, 154
  (1997): Shelley ED+, *J Geriatr Dermatol* 4, 192
  (1995): Corazza M+, *Contact Dermatitis* 32, 246
  (1994): Tom GR+, *Ann Pharmacother* 28, 889
  (1992): Breathnach SM+, *Adverse Drug Reactions and the Skin*
    Blackwell, Oxford, 226 (passim)
  (1991): Ito MK+, *Am J Med* 91, 42S
  (1991): McChesney JA, *West J Med* 154, 736
  (1990): Hogan DJ+, *J Am Acad Dermatol* 22, 811
  (1990): Scheper RJ+, *Contact Dermatitis* 23, 81
  (1989): Fillingim JM+, *Clin Ther* 11, 398
  (1989): Holdiness MR, *Contact Dermatitis* 20, 3
  (1988): Horning JR+, *Chest* 93, 941
  (1987): Bigby M+, *JAMA* 258, 1819 (letter)
  (1987): Maibach HI, *Contact Dermatitis* 16, 1
  (1986): Hollifield J, *Am Heart J* 112, 900

(1986): Weber MA, *Am Heart J* 112, 906
(1986): White TM+, *West J Med* 145, 104
(1985): Grattan CEH+, *Contact Dermatitis* 2, 225
(1985): Maibach H, *Contact Dermatitis* 12, 192
(1984): van Ketel WG, *Ned Tijdschr Geneeskd* (Dutch) 128, 34
(1983): Boekhorst JC, *Lancet* 2, 1031
(1983): Groth H+, *Lancet* 2, 850

Diaphoresis
(1990): Leeman CP, *J Clin Psychiatry* 51, 258

Eczema
(1987): Dick JBC+, *Lancet* 1, 516
(1985): Grattan CEH+, *Contact Dermatitis* 12, 225

Edema

Erythema
(2002): Prisant LM, *J Clin Hypertens* (Greenwich) 4(2), 136
(1987): Dick JBC+, *Lancet* 1, 516

Exanthems

Excoriations
(2002): Prisant LM, *J Clin Hypertens* (Greenwich) 4(2), 136

Herpes simplex
(1987): Wiser TH+, *J Am Acad Dermatol* 17, 143

Induration
(2002): Prisant LM, *J Clin Hypertens* (Greenwich) 4(2), 136

Irritation (from patch)
(1999): Dias VC+, *Am J Ther* 6, 19

Lupus erythematosus
(1994): Heilmann G+, *Dtsch Med Wochenschr* (German) 119, 858
(1994): Yung RL+, *Rheum Dis Clin North Am* 20, 61
(1992): Breathnach SM+, *Adverse Drug Reactions and the Skin* Blackwell, Oxford, 226 (passim)
(1981): Witman G+, *R I Med J* 64, 147

Pemphigus (anogenital and cicatricial)
(1980): van Joost T+, *Br J Dermatol* 102, 715

Peripheral edema

Pigmentation
(2002): Prisant LM, *J Clin Hypertens* (Greenwich) 4(2), 136
(1987): Wiser TH+, *J Am Acad Dermatol* 17, 143 (from patch)

Pityriasis rosea
(1998): Reed BR, Denver, CO (2 cases – in siblings) (from Internet) (observation)
(1992): Breathnach SM+, *Adverse Drug Reactions and the Skin* Blackwell, Oxford, 226 (passim)

Pruritus (>5%)
(1999): Dias VC+, *Am J Ther* 6, 19
(1987): Dick JBC+, *Lancet* 1, 516
(1984): Weber MA+, *Arch Intern Med* 144, 1211
(1984): Weber MA+, *Lancet* 1, 9
(1983): Boekhorst JC, *Lancet* 2, 1031

Psoriasis
(1981): Wilkin J, *Arch Dermatol* 117, 4

Rash (sic) (1–10%)
(1988): Glassman AH, *JAMA* 259, 2863

Raynaud's phenomenon (<1%)

Scaling
(2002): Prisant LM, *J Clin Hypertens* (Greenwich) 4(2), 136

Ulcerations (1–10%)

Urticaria (<1%)

Vesiculation
(2002): Prisant LM, *J Clin Hypertens* (Greenwich) 4(2), 136

Mucosal/ENT
Dysgeusia (from patch)
Xerostomia (40%)
(2000): Geyer O+, *Graefes Arch Clin Exp Ophthalmol* 238, 149
(2000): Litt JZ, Beachwood, OH (personal case) (observation)
(1999): Dias VC+, *Am J Ther* 6, 19
(1995): Johnson MA+, *Br J Clin Pharmacol* 39(5), 477

(1991): Warren JB+, *Clin Pharmacol Ther* 50(1), 71
(1989): Warren JB+, *Clin Pharmacol Ther* 46(1), 103
(1988): Glassman AH, *JAMA* 259, 2863
(1984): Weber MA+, *Arch Intern Med* 144, 1211
(1984): Weber MA+, *Lancet* 1, 9
(1983): Boekhorst JC, *Lancet* 2, 1031
(1980): Jaattela A, *Br J Clin Pharmacol* 10 Suppl, 67S

Hair
Hair – alopecia (<1%)

Other
Application-site vesicles
(1987): Dick JBC+, *Lancet* 1, 516

Gynecomastia (<1%)
(2005): Mendhekar DN, *J Clin Psychiatry* 66(12), 1616

Headache
(1995): Johnson MA+, *Br J Clin Pharmacol* 39(5), 477

Hypotension
(2006): Roelants F, *Curr Opin Anaesthesiol* 19(3), 233
(2005): Marui S+, *Arq Bras Endocrinol Metabol* 49(4), 510 (5%)
(1996): Chan CK+, *J Hypertens* 14(7), 855
(1995): Klimscha W+, *Anesth Analg* 80(2), 322
(1994): Singh H+, *Anesth Analg* 79(6), 1113
(1991): Park KH+, *J Pharmacol Exp Ther* 259(3), 1221
(1987): Orko R+, *Acta Anaesthesiol Scand* 31(4), 325

Pseudolymphoma
(1997): Shelley WB+, *Lancet* 350, 1223 (at site of patch)

Seizures
(2004): Ahmed SU+, *Anesth Analg* 99(2), 593 (with lidocaine)

CLOPIDOGREL

Trade name: Plavix (Bristol-Myers Squibb) (Sanofi-Aventis)
Indications: Atherosclerotic events
Category: Antiplatelet, thienopyridine
Half-life: ~8 hours
Clinically important, potentially hazardous interactions with: anisindione, anticoagulants, atorvastatin, dicumarol, fondaparinux, simvastatin, warfarin

Reactions

Skin
Allergic reactions (sic) (1–2.5%)

Angioedema
(2003): Fischer TC+, *Am J Med* 114(1), 77

Bullous dermatitis (1–2.5%)

Cellulitis
(2003): Wolf I+, *Mayo Clin Proc* 78(5), 618

Eczema (1–2.5%)

Edema (3–5%)

Erythema multiforme

Exanthems (1–2.5%)
(2001): Blumenthal HL, Beachwood, OH (personal communication)
(1999): Smith JG, Mobile, AL (generalized) (from Internet) (observation)

Lichenoid eruption (photosensitive)
(2003): Dogra S+, *Br J Dermatol* 148(3), 609

Photosensitivity (lichenoid)
(2003): Dogra S+, *Br J Dermatol* 148(3), 609

Pruritus (3.3%)
(2006): Makkar K+, *Ann Pharmacother* 40(6), 1204
(1999): Smith JG, Mobile, AL (from Internet) (observation)

Psoriasis

(2006): Meissner M+, *Br J Dermatol* 155(3), 630
Purpura
  (2006): Oo TH, *Am J Hematol* 81(11), 890
  (2006): Patel TN+, *J Invasive Cardiol* 18(7), E211
  (2005): Szuldrzynski K+, *Kardiol Pol* 63(4), 411
  (2004): Andersohn F+, *Heart* 90(9), e57
  (2002): Paradiso-Hardy FL+, *Can J Cardiol* 18(7), 771 (5 cases)
  (2001): Briguori C+, *Ital Heart J* 2(12), 935
  (2001): Medina PJ+, *Curr Opin Hematol* 8(5), 286
  (2001): Nara W+, *Am J Med Sci* 322(3), 170
  (2000): Bennett CL+, *N Engl J Med* 342, 1773 (11 patients)
  (2000): Brooker JZ, *N Engl J Med* 343(16), 1192
  (2000): Cheung RT, *N Engl J Med* 343(16), 1192
  (2000): Chinnakotla S+, *Transplantation* 70, 550
  (2000): Goldstein MR, *N Engl J Med* 343(16), 1192
  (2000): Salliere D+, *N Engl J Med* 343(16), 1191
  (2000): SoRelle R, *Circulation* 101, E9036
  (2000): Trontell AE+, *N Engl J Med* 343(16), 1191
  (1999): Carwile JM+, *Blood* 94, 1:78
  (1999): Connors JM+, *Transfusion* 39, 56S
Rash (sic) (4.2%)
  (2006): Makkar K+, *Ann Pharmacother* 40(6), 1204 (with
    ticlopidine)
Stevens–Johnson syndrome
Toxic dermatitis (sic)
  (2001): El-Majjaoui S+, *J Mal Vasc* 26(3), 207
Toxic epidermal necrolysis
Ulcerations (1–2.5%)
Urticaria (1–2.5%)
  (1997): Coukell AJ+, *Drugs* 54, 745
Vasculitis

Mucosal/ENT
Ageusia
  (2006): Koc F+, *Neurol India* 54(2), 218
  (2000): Golka K+, *Lancet* 355, 465
Oral ulceration
  (2005): Adelola OA+, *Ir Med J* 98(9), 282

Eyes
Ocular hemorrhage
  (2004): Davies BR, *Br J Ophthalmol* 88(9), 1226 (with aspirin)

Other
Fever
  (2006): Ng JA+, *Pharmacotherapy* 26(7), 1023
  (2003): Wolf I+, *Mayo Clin Proc* 78(5), 618
Headache
  (2006): Soman T+, *Stroke* 37(4), 1120
Hepatotoxicity
  (2006): Ng JA+, *Pharmacotherapy* 26(7), 1023
  (2005): Chau TN+, *Hong Kong Med J* 11(5), 414
Hypersensitivity
  (2006): Nebeker JR+, *J Am Coll Cardiol* 47(1), 175
  (2006): Walker NE+, *J Invasive Cardiol* 18(7), 341
  (2005): Comert A+, *Int J Dermatol* 44(10), 882
  (2005): Doogue MP+, *Mayo Clin Proc* 80(10), 1368
  (2001): Sarrot-Reynauld F+, *Ann Intern Med* 135(4), 305
Paresthesias (1–2.5%)
Rhabdomyolysis
  (2007): Burton JR+, *Ann Pharmacother* 41(1), 133
  (2003): Uber PA+, *J Heart Lung Transplant* 22(1), 107

CLORAZEPATE

Trade names: Gen-XENE; Novoclopate; Transene; Tranxal; Tranxen; Tranxene (Ovation) (Abbott); Tranxilen; Tranxilium
Indications: Anxiety and panic disorders
Category: Benzodiazepine
Half-life: 48–96 hours
Clinically important, potentially hazardous interactions with: amprenavir, antacids, carbamazepine, carmustine, chlorpheniramine, clarithromycin, efavirenz, esomeprazole, imatinib, indinavir, itraconazole, ketoconazole, MAO inhibitors, midazolam, moclobemide, nelfinavir, phenytoin, sucralfate, theophylline, warfarin

Reactions

Skin
Dermatitis (1–10%)
Diaphoresis (>10%)
Exanthems
  (2001): Sachs B+, *Br J Dermatol* 144(2), 316 (generalized)
Photosensitivity
  (1989): Torras H+, *J Am Acad Dermatol* 21, 1304
Pruritus
Purpura
Rash (sic) (>10%)
Urticaria
  (1981): Bonnetblanc JM+, *Ann Dermatol Venereol* (French)
    108, 177
Vasculitis
  (1985): Sanchez NP+, *Arch Dermatol* 121, 220
Vesiculation

Mucosal/ENT
Oral ulceration
Sialopenia (>10%)
Sialorrhea (1–10%)
Xerostomia (>10%)

Nails
Nails – photo-onycholysis
  (1989): Torras H+, *J Am Acad Dermatol* 21, 1304

Other
Headache
Paresthesias
Porphyria
  (2001): Rassiat E+, *Gastroenterol Clin Biol* 25(8), 832
Tremor

CLOTRIMAZOLE

Trade names: Agisten; Candid; Canestene; Gyne-Lotrimin (Schering); Imazol; Lotrimin (Schering); Lotrisone (Schering); Mycelex (Bayer); Taon
Indications: Candidiasis, dermatophyte infections of the skin
Category: Antibiotic, imidazole
Half-life: N/A
Clinically important, potentially hazardous interactions with: betamethasone

Reactions

Skin
Burning
    (1994): Binet O+, *Mycoses* 37, 455
    (1983): Higashide K+, *J Int Med Res* 11, 21 (from vaginal tablets)
Dermatitis
    (1999): Cooper SM+, *Contact Dermatitis* 41, 168
    (1999): Erdmann S+, *Contact Dermatitis* 40, 47
    (1997): Dharmagunawardena B+, *Contact Dermatitis* 32, 187
    (1995): Baes H, *Contact Dermatitis* 32, 187
    (1994): Valsecchi R+, *Contact Dermatitis* 30, 248
    (1987): Raulin C+, *Derm Beruf Umwelt* (German) 35, 64
    (1985): Balato N+, *Contact Dermatitis* 12, 110
    (1985): Kalb RE+, *Cutis* 36, 240
Edema
Erythema
Exfoliative dermatitis
Irritation (sic)
    (1994): Binet O+, *Mycoses* 37, 455
Pruritus
Stinging
Urticaria
Vesiculation

Mucosal/ENT
Dysgeusia

CLOXACILLIN

Trade names: Alclox; Apo-Cloxi; Cloxapen (GSK); Ekvacillin; Loxavit; Nu-Cloxi; Orbenin; Orbenine; Tegopen
Indications: Various infections caused by susceptible organisms
Category: Antibiotic, penicillin
Half-life: 0.5–1.1 hours
Clinically important, potentially hazardous interactions with: anticoagulants, cyclosporine, demeclocycline, doxycycline, imipenem/cilastatin, methotrexate, minocycline, oxytetracycline, proguanil, tetracycline

Reactions

Skin
Angioedema
    (2006): Dominguez-Ortega J+, *Allergol Immunopathol (Madr)* 34(1), 37
    (1996): Torres MJ+, *Clin Exp Allergy* 26(1), 108 (facial)
Dermatitis
    (1996): Gamboa P+, *Contact Dermatitis* 34, 75
Erythema
    (1996): Torres MJ+, *Clin Exp Allergy* 26(1), 108
Erythema multiforme
Exanthems
    (2006): Dominguez-Ortega J+, *Allergol Immunopathol (Madr)* 34(1), 37
Exfoliative dermatitis
Facial edema
    (2006): Dominguez-Ortega J+, *Allergol Immunopathol (Madr)* 34(1), 37
Hematomas
Jarisch–Herxheimer reaction
Pruritus
    (1996): Torres MJ+, *Clin Exp Allergy* 26(1), 108
Rash (sic) (<1%)

Stevens–Johnson syndrome
Urticaria
    (2006): Dominguez-Ortega J+, *Allergol Immunopathol (Madr)* 34(1), 37

Mucosal/ENT
Glossitis
Glossodynia
Oral candidiasis
Stomatitis
Tongue black
Vaginitis

Nails
Nails – loss
    (1984): Daniel CR, *J Am Acad Dermatol* 10, 250

Other
Anaphylactoid reactions/Anaphylaxis
    (2006): Rodriguez Trabado A+, *Allergy Asthma Proc* 27(3), 269
Hypersensitivity
    (2003): Moreno-Ancillo A+, *Contact Dermatitis* 49(1), 44
Injection-site pain
Phlebitis
    (1980): Svedhem A+, *Antimicrob Agents Chemother* 18(2), 349 (13%)
Serum sickness (<1%)

CLOZAPINE

Trade names: Clozaril (Novartis); Entumin; Entumine; Leponex; Lozapin; Sizopin
Indications: Schizophrenia
Category: Antipsychotic, tricyclic
Half-life: 8–12 hours
Clinically important, potentially hazardous interactions with: caffeine, carbamazepine, **cocoa**, fluoxetine, **guarana**, insulin glulisine, risperidone, ritonavir, selenium, uracil/tegafur

Reactions

Skin
Acute febrile neutrophilic dermatosis (Sweet's syndrome)
    (2002): Schonfeldt-Lecuona C+, *Am J Psychiatry* 159(11), 1947
Acute generalized exanthematous pustulosis (AGEP)
    (1997): Bosonnet S+, *Ann Dermatol Venereol* (French) 124, 547
Allergic reactions (sic)
    (1992): Stoppe G+, *Br J Psychiatry* 161, 259
Angioedema
    (2007): Mishra B+, *Gen Hosp Psychiatry* 29(1), 78 (2 cases)
Dermatitis (<1%)
Diaphoresis (6%)
    (2001): Kane JM+, *Arch Gen Psychiatry* 58(10), 965
    (2001): Richardson C+, *Am J Psychiatry* 158(8), 1329
    (1991): Safferman A+, *Schizophr Bull* 17, 247 (31%)
    (1990): Fitton A+, *Drugs* 40, 722
Eczema (<1%)
    (1994): Shelley WB+, *Cutis* 53, 33 (observation)
Edema (<1%)
Erythema (<1%)
Erythema multiforme (<1%)
Exanthems
    (1999): Stanislav SW+, *Ann Pharmacother* 33(9), 1008
Facial erosions
    (1994): Shelley WB+, *Cutis* 53, 33 (observation)
Lupus erythematosus

(2006): Rami AF+, *Ann Pharmacother* 40(5), 983
(2004): Wolf J+, *J Clin Psychopharmacol* 24(2), 236
(1994): Wickert WA+, *Postgrad Med J* 70, 940
Nodular eruption
(2000): Durst R+, *Isr Med Assoc* 2, 485
Petechiae (<1%)
(1994): Shelley WB+, *Cutis* 53, 33 (observation)
Photosensitivity
(1995): Howanitz E+, *J Clin Psychiatry* 56, 589
Pruritus (<1%)
Purpura (<1%)
Rash (sic) (2%)
(2005): Bhatti MA+, *J Clin Psychiatry* 66(11), 1490
(1999): Hauben M, *Ann Pharmacother* 33(12), 1374
Stevens–Johnson syndrome (<1%)
Urticaria (<1%)
Vasculitis (<1%)

Mucosal/ENT

Dysgeusia (<1%)
Glossodynia (1%)
Parotitis
(1995): Robinson D+, *Am J Psychiatry* 152(2), 297
Sialorrhea (31%)
(2008): Robb AS+, *J Child Adolesc Psychopharmacol* 18(1), 99
(2007): Duggal HS, *Prog Neuropsychopharmacol Biol Psychiatry* 31(7), 1546
(2007): Praharaj SK+, *Br J Clin Pharmacol* 63(1), 128
(2007): Sockalingam S+, *Can J Psychiatry* 52(6), 377
(2006): Fleischhaker C+, *J Child Adolesc Psychopharmacol* 16(3), 308
(2006): Kontaxakis VP+, *Eur Arch Psychiatry Clin Neurosci* 256(6), 350 (with risperidone)
(2006): Kreinin A+, *Int Clin Psychopharmacol* 21(2), 99
(2006): Praharaj SK+, *Psychopharmacology (Berl)* 185(3), 265
(2005): Boyce HW+, *J Clin Gastroenterol* 39(2), 89 (passim)
(2005): Croissant B+, *Pharmacopsychiatry* 38(1), 38
(2005): Freudenreich O, *Drugs Today (Barc)* 41(6), 411
(2005): Kahl KG+, *Nervenarzt* 76(2), 205
(2005): Kreinin A+, *Isr J Psychiatry Relat Sci* 42(1), 61
(2005): Praharaj SK+, *J Psychopharmacol* 19(4), 426
(2004): Freudenreich O+, *J Clin Psychopharmacol* 24(1), 98
(2004): Gaftanyuk O+, *Psychiatr Serv* 55(3), 318
(2004): Kahl KG+, *Psychopharmacology (Berl)* 173(1-2), 229
(2004): Schneider B+, *Pharmacopsychiatry* 37(2), 43
(2004): Sharma A+, *Ann Pharmacother* 38(9), 1538
(2004): Webber MA+, *J Clin Psychopharmacol* 24(6), 675
(2003): Fernandez HH+, *Drug Saf* 26(9), 643
(2002): Tuunainen A+, *Schizophr Res* 56(1-2), 1
(2001): Bai YM+, *J Clin Psychopharmacol* 21(6), 608
(2001): Kane JM+, *Arch Gen Psychiatry* 58(10), 965
(2001): Tessier P+, *J Psychiatry Neurosci* 26(3), 253
(2000): Calderon J+, *Int Clin Psychopharmacol* 15(1), 49
(2000): Davydov L+, *Ann Pharmacother* 34(5), 662
(2000): Littrell KH+, *J Clin Psychiatry* 61(12), 912
(2000): Miller DD, *J Clin Psychiatry* 61, 14
(2000): Wahlbeck K+, *Cochran Database Syst Rev* (2):CD000059
(1999): Antonello C+, *J Psychiatry Neurosci* 24, 250
(1999): Campbell M+, *Br J Clin Pharmacol* 47, 13
(1998): Young CR+, *Schizophr Bull* 24, 381
(1997): Spivak B+, *Int Clin Psychopharmacol* 12, 213
(1995): Fritze J+, *Lancet* 346, 1034
(1991): Bourgeois JA+, *Hosp Community Psychiatry* 42, 1174
(1991): Calabrese JR+, *J Clin Psychopharmacol* 11, 396
(1991): Copp PJ+, *Br J Psychiatry* 159, 166
(1991): Goumeniouk AD+, *Can J Psychiatry* 36, 234
(1991): Kahn N+, *Neurology* 41, 1699
(1991): Ogle MR+, *Indiana Med* 84, 606
(1991): Safferman A+, *Schizophr Bull* 17, 247

(1990): Fitton A+, *Drugs* 40, 722
Xerostomia (6%)
(2001): Kane JM+, *Arch Gen Psychiatry* 58(10), 965
(1991): Safferman A+, *Schizophr Bull* 17, 247 (6%)
(1990): Fitton A+, *Drugs* 40, 722

Eyes

Blepharospasm
(2007): Duggal HS+, *J Neuropsychiatry Clin Neurosci* 19(1), 86
Periorbital edema (<1%)

Other

Congestive heart failure
(2003): Ansari A+, *Tex Heart Inst J* 30(1), 76
Death
(2006): Gambassi G+, *Aging Clin Exp Res* 18(3), 266 (with paroxetine)
(2006): Townsend G+, *BMC Psychiatry* 6, 43
(2004): Farah RE+, *Ann Pharmacother* 38(9), 1435 (with paroxetine)
(2002): Levin TT+, *Psychosomatics* 43(1), 71
(2001): Gillespie JA, *Ann Pharmacother* 35(12), 1671
(2001): Hoehns JD+, *Ann Pharmacother* 35(7), 862 (with sertraline)
(2001): Tie H+, *J Clin Psychopharmacol* 21(6), 630
Fever
(2002): Jeong SH+, *Schizophr Res* 56(1), 191
(2000): Miller DD, *J Clin Psychiatry* 61 (Suppl 8), 14
Headache
Hepatotoxicity
(2007): Luo D+, *Intern Med J* 37(3), 204
Hypertension
(2005): Henderson DC+, *J Clin Psychiatry* 66(9), 1116
(2000): Miller DD, *J Clin Psychiatry* 61 (Suppl 8), 14
Hypotension
(2000): Miller DD, *J Clin Psychiatry* 61 (Suppl 8), 14
Rhabdomyolysis
(2006): Tenyi T+, *Pharmacopsychiatry* 39(4), 157
(2002): Jung HH+, *Muscle Nerve* 26(3), 424
(1998): Koren W+, *Clin Neuropharmacol* 21(4), 262
(1998): Wicki J+, *Ann Pharmacother* 32(9), 892
(1996): Meltzer HY+, *Neuropsychopharmacology* 15(4), 395
Seizures
(2006): Shaw P+, *Arch Gen Psychiatry* 63(7), 721
(2004): Gazdag G+, *Ideggyogy Sz* 57(11-12), 385 (50%)
(2003): Reuther LO+, *Ugeskr Laeger* 165(14), 1447
(2002): Duggal HS+, *Am J Psychiatry* 159(2), 315
(2001): Landry P, *Am J Psychiatry* 158(11), 1930
(2001): Navarro V+, *Am J Psychiatry* 158(6), 968
(1997): Popli AP+, *J Clin Psychiatry* 58(3), 108
(1992): Lieberman JA+, *Psychiatr Q* 63(1), 51
Somnolence
(2006): Kontaxakis VP+, *Eur Arch Psychiatry Clin Neurosci* 256(6), 350 (with risperidone)
(2004): Levoyer D+, *Encephale* 30(3), 285
(2000): Miller DD, *J Clin Psychiatry* 61 (Suppl 8), 14
(1997): Popli AP+, *J Clin Psychiatry* 58(3), 108
(1992): Lieberman JA+, *Psychiatr Q* 63(1), 51
Thrombosis
(2006): Gallien S+, *Dermatol Online J* 12(2), 13
Tremor (1–10%)
(2002): Zesiewicz TA+, *Mov Disord* 17(6), 1365 (withdrawal)
Vertigo
(1992): Lieberman JA+, *Psychiatr Q* 63(1), 51
Weight gain
(2006): Fleischhaker C+, *J Child Adolesc Psychopharmacol* 16(3), 308
(2005): Ness-Abramof R+, *Drugs Today (Barc)* 41(8), 547
(2004): Levoyer D+, *Encephale* 30(3), 285

(2000): Miller DD, *J Clin Psychiatry* 61 (Suppl 8), 14
(2000): Remschmidt H+, *Paediatr Drugs* 2(4), 253
(1997): Popli AP+, *J Clin Psychiatry* 58(3), 108

CO-TRIMOXAZOLE

Synonyms: sulfamethoxazole-trimethoprim; SMX-TMP; SMZ-TMP; TMP-SMX; TMP-SMZ
Trade names: Anitrim; Apo-Sulfatrim; Bactelan; Bactrim (GSK); Batrizol; Cotrim; Ectaprim; Esteprim; Isobac; Pro-Trin; Roubac; Septra (Monarch); Sulfatrim; Trimzol; Trisulfa
Indications: Various infections caused by susceptible organisms
Category: Antibiotic, sulfonamide
Half-life: 6–10 hours
Clinically important, potentially hazardous interactions with: anticoagulants, cyclosporine, dofetilide, isotretinoin, methotrexate, warfarin

Note: Co-trimoxazole is sulfamethoxazole and trimethoprim

Note: Co-trimoxazole is a sulfonamide and can be absorbed systemically. Sulfonamides can produce severe, possibly fatal, reactions such as toxic epidermal necrolysis and Stevens–Johnson syndrome

Reactions

Skin

Acute febrile neutrophilic dermatosis (Sweet's syndrome)
(1996): Walker DC+, *J Am Acad Dermatol* 34, 918
(1989): Cobb MW, *J Am Acad Dermatol* 21, 339 (passim)
(1986): Su WPD+, *Cutis* 37, 167
Acute generalized exanthematous pustulosis (AGEP)
(2003): Anliker MD+, *J Investig Allergol Clin Immunol* 13(1), 66 (with sulfamethoxazole)
(2003): Saissi EH+, *Ann Dermatol Venereol* 130(6-7), 612
(1995): Moreau A+, *Int J Dermatol* 34, 263 (passim)
Allergic reactions (sic)
(2002): Choquet-Kastylevsky G+, *Curr Allergy Asthma Rep* 2(1), 16
(1999): ter Hofstede HJ+, *Br Clin Pharmacol* 47, 571
Angioedema
(2006): Ruscin JM+, *Am J Geriatr Pharmacother* 4(4), 325
(1988): Fihn SD+, *Ann Intern Med* 108, 350 (1–5%)
Bullous dermatitis
(1995): Roholt NS+, *J Am Acad Dermatol* 32(2 Pt 2), 367
(1989): Caumes E+, *Presse Med* (French) 18, 1708
Dermatitis
(1989): Atahan IL+, *Br J Radiol* 62, 1107 (at previously irradiated area)
(1987): Vukelja SJ+, *Cancer Treat Rep* 71, 668 (at previously irradiated area)
(1984): Shelley WB+, *J Am Acad Dermatol* 11, 53 (at site of previous sunburn)
Erythema multiforme
(1999): Lehman DF+, *J Clin Pharmacol* 39, 533
(1998): Siegfried EC+, *J Am Acad Dermatol* 39, 797 (passim)
(1997): Rieder MJ+, *Pediatr Infect Dis J* 16, 1028 (70% in children with HIV)
(1995): Jick H+, *Pharmacotherapy* 15, 428
(1991): Tilden ME+, *Arch Ophthalmol* 109, 67
(1990): Chan HL+, *Arch Dermatol* 126, 43
(1989): Alanko K+, *Acta Derm Venereol* (Stockh) 69, 223
(1988): Hira SK+, *J Am Acad Dermatol* 19, 451
(1988): Platt R+, *J Infect Dis* 158, 474
(1987): Penmetcha M, *BMJ* 295, 556
(1987): Schöpf E, *Infection* 15 (Suppl 5P), S254

(1985): Heer M+, *Gastroenterology* 88, 1954
(1982): Brettle RP+, *J Infect* 4, 149
Erythema nodosum
Erythroderma
Exanthems
(2006): Eastern JS, NJ (from Internet) (observation)
(2005): Beer AM+, *Forsch Komplementarmed Klass Naturheilkd* 12(1), 32
(1999): Iborra C+, *Arch Dermatol* 135, 350
(1998): Blumenthal HL, Beachwood, OH (personal case) (observation)
(1998): Hattori N+, *J Dermatol* 25, 269
(1998): Litt JZ, Beachwood, OH (personal case) (observation)
(1997): Blumenthal HL, Beachwood, OH (personal case) (observation)
(1997): Palau LA+, *Infect Med* 14, 846
(1996): Caumes E, *Rev Mal Respir* (French) 13, 101 (passim)
(1995): Hertl M+, *Br J Dermatol* 132, 215
(1995): Wolkenstein P+, *Arch Dermatol* 131, 544
(1994): Litt JZ, Beachwood, OH (personal case) (observation)
(1993): Agarwal BR+, *Indian Pediatr* 30, 1026
(1993): Litt JZ, Beachwood, OH (personal case) (observation)
(1993): Malnick SDH+, *Ann Pharmacotherapy* 27, 1139
(1990): Medina I+, *N Engl J Med* 323, 776 (47% in AIDS)
(1988): DeRaeve L+, *Br J Dermatol* 119, 521
(1988): Fihn SD+, *Ann Intern Med* 108, 350 (1–5%)
(1988): Sattler FR+, *Ann Intern Med* 109, 280 (44% in AIDS)
(1988): Weinke T+, *Dtsch Med Wochenschr* (German) 113, 1129 (25% in AIDS)
(1987): Goa KL+, *Drugs* 33, 242 (65% in AIDS)
(1987): Schöpf E, *Infection* 15 (Suppl 5P), S254
(1986): Sonntag MR+, *Schweiz Med Wochenschr* (German) 116, 142
(1985): DeHovitz JA+, *Ann Intern Med* 103, 479
(1985): Maayan S+, *Arch Intern Med* 145, 1607
(1984): Gordon FM+, *Ann Intern Med* 100, 495 (51% in AIDS)
(1984): Kovacs JA+, *Ann Intern Med* 100, 663 (29% in AIDS)
(1983): Mitsuyasu R+, *N Engl J Med* 308, 1535 (69% in AIDS)
(1982): Goetz MB+, *JAMA* 247, 3118
(1980): Fennell RS+, *Clin Pediatr* 19, 124
Exfoliative dermatitis
(1990): Ponte CD+, *Drug Intell Clin Pharm* 24, 140 (feet)
Fixed eruption
(2006): Nnoruka EN+, *Int J Dermatol* 45(9), 1062
(2006): Ozkaya E, *Eur J Dermatol* 16(5), 591
(2006): Rasi A+, *Dermatol Online J* 12(6), 12 (non-pigmenting)
(2006): Ruscin JM+, *Am J Geriatr Pharmacother* 4(4), 325
(2004): Ozkaya-Bayazit E, *J Am Acad Dermatol* 51(2 Suppl), S102
(2004): Zawar V+, *Int J STD AIDS* 15(8), 560 (3 cases)
(2002): Litt JZ, Beachwood, OH (glans penis) (recurrent) (personal case)
(2001): Bayazit-Ozkaya E+, *J Am Acad Dermatol* 45(5), 712
(2000): Ozkaya-Bayazit E+, *Eur J Dermatol* 10, 288
(1999): Mohamed KB, *J Pediatr* 135, 396
(1999): Morelli JG+, *J Pediatr* 134, 365
(1999): Ozkaya-Bayazit E+, *Contact Dermatitis* 41(4), 185 (27 cases)
(1998): Lee AY, *Contact Dermatitis* 38(5), 258
(1998): Mahboob A+, *Int J Dermatol* 37, 833
(1998): Ozkaya-Bayazit E+, *Contact Dermatitis* 39, 87 (trimethoprim)
(1997): Gruber F+, *Clin Exp Dermatol* 22, 144
(1997): Ozkaya-Bayazit E+, *Br J Dermatol* 137, 1028 (linear) (trimethoprim)
(1996): Sharma VK+, *J Dermatol* 23, 530
(1995): Wolkenstein P+, *Arch Dermatol* 131, 544
(1993): Oleaga JM+, *Contact Dermatitis* 29, 155
(1993): Ramam M+, *Indian Pediatr* 30, 110 (in an infant)
(1992): Arifhodzic F+, *Vojnosanit Pregl* 49(1), 30
(1992): Lim JT+, *Ann Acad Med Singapore* 21, 408

(1991): Jain VK+, *Ann Dent* 50, 9 (oral mucous membrane)
(1991): Smoller BR+, *J Cutan Pathol* 18, 13
(1991): Thankappen TP+, *Int J Dermatol* 30, 867 (36.3%)
(1990): Gaffoor PMA+, *Cutis* 45, 242 (genitalia)
(1989): Basomba A+, *J Allergy Clin Immunol* 84, 409
(1989): Bharija SC+, *Australas J Dermatol* 30, 43
(1989): Gupta R, *Indian J Dermatol* 55, 181 (in an infant)
(1989): Varsano I+, *Dermatologica* 178, 232
(1988): Baird BJ+, *Int J Dermatol* 27, 170 (bullous and generalized)
(1988): Bharija SC+, *Dermatologica* 176, 108 (in an infant)
(1987): Amir J+, *Drug Intell Clin Pharm* 21, 41
(1987): Hughes BR+, *Br J Dermatol* 116, 241
(1987): Van Voorhees A+, *Am J Dermatopathol* 9, 528
(1986): Kanwar AJ+, *Dermatologica* 172, 230
(1985): Gomez B+, *Allergol Immunopathol Madr* (Spanish) 13, 87
(1984): Pandhi RK+, *Sex Transm Dis* 11, 164
(1982): Gibson JR, *BMJ* 284, 1529
(1980): Talbot MD, *Practitioner* 224, 823

Hand–foot syndrome
(1999): van Rooijen MM+, *Hautarzt* 50(4), 280

Jarisch–Herxheimer reaction
(2001): Peschard S+, *Presse Med* 30(31), 1549
(1992): Playford RJ+, *Gut* 33(1), 132 (with streptomycin)

Lichenoid eruption
(1994): Berger TG+, *Arch Dermatol* 130, 609

Linear IgA dermatosis
(2002): Cohen LM+, *J Am Acad Dermatol* 46, S32 (passim)
(1997): Paul C+, *Br J Dermatol* 136, 406
(1994): Kuechle MK+, *J Am Acad Dermatol* 30, 187

Lupus erythematosus
(1985): Stratton MA, *Clin Pharm* 4, 657

Photo-recall
(1990): Leslie MD+, *Br J Radiol* 63, 661
(1987): Vukelja SJ+, *Cancer Treat Rep* 71, 668 (at previously irradiated area)
(1984): Shelley WB+, *J Am Acad Dermatol* 11, 53 (at site of previous sunburn)

Photosensitivity
(1994): Berger TG+, *Arch Dermatol* 130, 609 (in HIV-infected) (4 cases)
(1994): Shelley WB+, *Cutis* 53, 162 (observation)
(1987): Schöpf E, *Infection* 15 (Suppl 5P), S254
(1986): Chandler MJ, *J Infect Dis* 153, 1001

Pruritus
(1997): Caumes E+, *Arch Dermatol* 133, 465
(1997): Thaler D, Monona, WI (from Internet) (observation)
(1996): Litt JZ, Beachwood, OH (from Internet) (observation)
(1990): Medina I+, *N Engl J Med* 323, 776 (1–5%)
(1987): Colebunders R+, *Ann Intern Med* 107, 599 (4% in AIDS)
(1986): Sher MR, *J Allergy Clin Immunol* 77, 133
(1984): Kramer BS+, *Cancer* 53, 329

Pruritus ani et vulvae
(1981): *Modern Medicine* 49, 111

Psoriasis

Purple gloves and socks syndrome
(1999): van Rooijen MM+, *Hautarzt* (German) 50, 280

Purpura
(1993): Kaufman DW+, *Blood* 82, 2714
(1989): Saxena SK, *J Assoc Physicians India* 37, 479

Pustules
(1994): Spencer JM+, *Br J Dermatol* 130, 514
(1990): Guy C+, *Nouv Dermatol* (French) 9, 540
(1989): Grattan CEH, *Dermatologica* 179, 57 (passim)
(1986): Macdonald KJS+, *BMJ* 293, 1279

Rash (sic) (>10%)
(2001): Meyers B+, *Liver Transpl* 7(8), 750
(2000): Talan DA+, *JAMA* 283, 1583 (14%)
(1995): Williams JW+, *JAMA* 273, 1015

(1993): Malnick SD+, *Ann Pharmacother* 27, 1139
(1984): Gordin FM+, *Ann Intern Med* 100, 495

Side effects (sic)
(1994): Roudier C+, *Arch Dermatol* 130, 1383 (48% in AIDS patients)

Stevens–Johnson syndrome (1–10%)
(2006): Gimnig JE+, *Am J Trop Med Hyg* 74(5), 738
(2006): Panagotacos P, San Francisco, CA (personal communication)
(2001): Brett AS+, *South Med J* 94, 342
(1998): Arola O+, *Lancet* 351, 1102 (trimethoprim)
(1998): Siegfried EC+, *J Am Acad Dermatol* 39, 797 (passim)
(1997): Douglas R+, *Clin Infect Dis* 25, 1480 (2 cases)
(1997): Rieder MJ+, *Pediatr Infect Dis J* 16, 1028 (10% in children with HIV)
(1996): Caumes E, *Rev Mal Respir* (French) 13, 101
(1996): Eastham JH+, *Ann Pharmacother* 30, 606
(1996): McCarty J, Fort Worth, TX (from Internet) (observation)
(1995): Jick H+, *Pharmacotherapy* 15(4), 428
(1995): Kuper K+, *Ophthalmologe* (German) 92, 823
(1995): Lewis RJ, *Br J Rheumatol* 34, 84
(1995): Sharma VK+, *Pediatr Dermatol* 12, 178
(1995): Wolkenstein P+, *Arch Dermatol* 131, 544
(1994): Shelley WB+, *Cutis* 53, 159 (observation)
(1993): Gompels M+, *Int J STD AIDS* 4(5), 293
(1993): Litt JZ, Beachwood, OH (personal case) (observation)
(1990): Chan HL+, *Arch Dermatol* 126, 43
(1988): Platt R+, *J Infect Dis* 158, 474
(1987): Schopf E, *Infection* 15 Suppl 5, S254 (1%)
(1985): Heer M+, *Gastroenterology* 88, 1954
(1982): Brettle RP+, *J Infect* 4, 149

Toxic epidermal necrolysis (1–10%)
(2006): Gimnig JE+, *Am J Trop Med Hyg* 74(5), 738
(2002): Correia O+, *Arch Dermatol* 138, 29 (3 cases)
(2002): John T+, *Ophthalmology* 109(2), 351
(2002): Nassif A+, *J Invest Dermatol* 118(4), 728
(2001): Paquet P+, *Burns* 27(6), 652
(2001): See S+, *Ann Pharmacother* 35(6), 694
(2001): Spies M+, *Pediatrics* 108, 1162
(2000): Moussala M+, *J Fr Ophtalmol* (French) 23, 229
(2000): Yang CH+, *Int J Dermatol* 39, 621 (with methotrexate)
(1999): Egan CA+, *J Am Acad Dermatol* 40, 458 (6 cases)
(1998): Arora VK+, *Indian J Chest Dis Allied Sci* 40, 125
(1998): Rademaker M+, *New Zealand Adverse Drug Reactions Committee*, April, 1998 (from Internet)
(1998): Siegfried EC+, *J Am Acad Dermatol* 39, 797 (passim)
(1996): Caumes E, *Rev Mal Respir* (French) 13, 101
(1996): Rehbein H, Jacksonville, FL (from Internet) (observation)
(1996): Wagner FF+, *N Engl J Med* 334, 922
(1995): Jick H+, *Pharmacotherapy* 15, 428
(1995): Sharma VK+, *Pediatr Dermatol* 12, 178
(1995): Wolkenstein P+, *Arch Dermatol* 131, 544 (7 cases)
(1993): Correia O+, *Dermatology* 186, 32
(1990): Chan HL+, *Arch Dermatol* 126, 43
(1990): Kobza Black A+, *Br J Dermatol* 123, 277
(1990): Roujeau JC+, *Arch Dermatol* 126, 37
(1990): Ward DJ+, *Burns* 16, 97
(1989): Carmichael AJ+, *Lancet* 2, 808
(1989): Whittington RM, *Lancet* 2, 574
(1988): De Raeve L+, *Br J Dermatol* 119, 521 (passim)
(1987): Guillaume JC+, *Arch Dermatol* 123, 1166
(1987): Schöpf E, *Infection* 15 (Suppl 5P), S254
(1986): Miller KD+, *Am J Trop Med Hyg* 33, 451
(1986): Revuz J, *J Dermatol Paris* 153 (abstract)
(1986): Roman O+, *Rev Pediatr Obstet Ginecol Pediatr* (Romanian) 35, 261
(1984): Fong PH+, *Singapore Med J* 25, 184
(1984): Westly ED+, *Arch Dermatol* 120, 721
(1983): Petersen P+, *Ugeskr Laeger* (Danish) 145, 3345
(1982): Ortiz JE+, *Ann Plast Surg* 9, 249

Urticaria
(2006): Padilla Serrato MT+, *Rev Alerg Mex* 53(5), 179
(2005): Feiza BA+, *Tunis Med* 83(11), 714
(1994): Blumenthal HL, Beachwood, OH (personal case)
(observation)
(1993): Litt JZ, Beachwood, OH (personal case) (observation)
(1991): Greenberger PA, *JAMA* 265, 458
(1987): Schöpf E, *Infection* 15 (Suppl 5P), S254
(1985): Goolamali SK, *Postgrad Med J* 61, 925
(1985): Maayan S+, *Arch Intern Med* 145, 1607
(1984): Kramer BS+, *Cancer* 53, 329
(1981): Abi-Mansur P+, *Am J Gastroenterol* 76, 356
Vasculitis
(2005): Feiza BA+, *Tunis Med* 83(11), 714
(1998): Tonev S+, *J Eur Acad Dermatol Venereol* 11, 165
(1995): Lewis RJ, *Br J Rheumatol* 34, 84
(1989): Verne-Pignatelli J+, *Postgrad Med J* 65, 51
(1987): Schöpf E, *Infection* 15 (Suppl 5P), S254

Mucosal/ENT
Aphthous stomatitis
(1981): *J Antimicrob Chemother* 7, 179
Dysgeusia
(1988): Fischl MA+, *JAMA* 259, 1185
Genital ulceration
(2001): Cherian G, *Int J Clin Pract* 55(2), 151
Gingival hyperplasia/hypertrophy
(1997): Caron F+, *Therapie* (French) 52, 73
Glossitis
Mucocutaneous syndrome
(1982): Brettle RP+, *J Infect* 4, 149
Oral mucosal eruption
(1991): Tilden ME+, *Arch Ophthalmol* 109, 67
(1988): Fihn SD+, *Ann Intern Med* 108, 350 (1–5%)
Oral ulceration
(1987): Hughes WT+, *N Engl J Med* 316, 1627
(1981): Orenstein WA+, *Am J Med Sci* 282, 27
Stomatitis (<1%)
(1999): Iborra C+, *Arch Dermatol* 135, 350
Tinnitus
Tongue black
(1993): Blumenthal HL, Beachwood, OH (personal case)
(observation)
Tongue ulceration
(1981): *J Antimicrob Chemother* 7, 179
Vaginitis
(1985): Wong ES+, *Ann Intern Med* 102, 302

Hair
Hair – straight
(1999): Oakley A, Hamilton, New Zealand (from Internet)
(observation)

Nails
Nails – loss
(2000): Canning DA, *J Urol* 163, 1386

Other
Anaphylactoid reactions/Anaphylaxis
(1998): Bijl AM+, *Clin Exp Allergy* 28, 510 (trimethoprim)
(1998): Siegfried EC+, *J Am Acad Dermatol* 39, 797 (passim)
(1988): Arnold PA+, *Drug Intell Clin Pharm* 22, 43
(1985): Gossius G+, *Scand J Infect Dis* 16, 373
Aseptic meningitis
(2005): Wambulwa C+, *J Natl Med Assoc* 97(12), 1725
(2004): Therrien R, *Ann Pharmacother* 38(11), 1863
Death
(1995): Lewis RJ, *Br J Rheumatol* 34(1), 84
Hypersensitivity
(2006): Mohammedi I+, *Rev Med Interne* 27(6), 499

(2006): Morimoto T+, *Intern Med* 45(2), 101
(2001): Moran KA+, *South Med J* 94(3), 350 ('sepsis-like')
(2000): Pirmohamed M+, *Pharmacogenetics* 10(8), 705
(1999): Lehman DF+, *J Clin Pharmacol* 39, 533
(1999): Pakianathan MR+, *AIDS* 13, 1787
(1998): Mohanasundaram J+, *J Indian Med Assoc* 96, 21
(1998): Ryan C+, *WMJ* 97, 23
(1997): Hicks ME+, *Ann Pharmacother* 31, 1259
(1994): Carr A+, *AIDS* 8, 333
(1993): Marinac JS+, *Clin Infect Dis* 16, 178
(1993): Martin GJ+, *Clin Infect Dis* 16, 175
(1993): Mathelier-Fusade P+, *Presse Med* (French) 22, 1363
(1993): Mehta J+, *J Assoc Physicians India* 41, 235
Myalgia/Myositis/Myopathy/Myotoxicity
Pseudolymphoma
Rhabdomyolysis
(2006): Walker S+, *Am J Med Sci* 331(6), 339
(1998): Singer SJ+, *Clin Infect Dis* 26(1), 233
(1997): Anders HJ+, *Eur J Med Res* 2(5), 198
(1988): Arnold PA+, *Drug Intell Clin Pharm* 22, 43
Serum sickness (<1%)
(1988): Platt R+, *J Infect Dis* 158, 474
Tremor
(2005): Bua J+, *Pediatr Infect Dis J* 24(10), 934
(1999): Patterson RG+, *Pharmacotherapy* 19, 1456

COCAINE

Trade name: Cocaine
Indications: Topical anesthesia
Category: Anesthetic, local; CNS stimulant
Half-life: 75 minutes
Clinically important, potentially hazardous interactions with: epinephrine

Note: Cocaine is a benzoylmethylecogonine alkaloid derived from the leaves of the *Erythroxylon coca* tree. Street names for cocaine include: coke; flake; snow; toot, etc. Crack cocaine is a highly potent smokable form of cocaine

Reactions

Skin
Allergic granulomatous angiitis (Churg–Strauss syndrome)
(foreign body)
(1985): Posner DI+, *J Am Acad Dermatol* 13, 869
Angioedema
(2003): Kestler A+, *N Engl J Med* 349(9), 867
(1999): Castro-Villamor MA+, *Ann Emerg Med* 34, 296
Bullous dermatitis
(1985): Tomecki KJ+, *J Am Acad Dermatol* 12, 585
Diaphoresis
(1998): Winbery S+, *Am J Emerg Med* 16(5), 529
(1994): Hollander JE+, *Acad Emerg Med* 1(4), 330
(1983): Jonsson S+, *Am J Med* 75(6), 1061
Formication
Hyperkeratosis (fingers and palms)
(1992): Feeney CM+, *Cutis* 50, 193 (from crack cocaine)
Necrosis
(2003): Jouary T+, *Ann Dermatol Venereol* 130(5), 537
(2000): Carter EL+, *Cutis* 65, 73 (mid-facial)
(1988): Zamora-Quezada JC+, *Ann Intern Med* 108, 564
Nodular eruption
(1989): Heng MCY+, *J Am Acad Dermatol* 21, 570
Pruritus
Raynaud's phenomenon

(2001): Balbir-Gurman A+, *Clin Rheumatol* 20(5), 376
(1987): Lohr KM, *Semin Arthritis Rheum* 17(2), 90
Scleroderma (reversible)
(1992): Lam M+, *N Engl J Med* 326, 1435
(1991): Bourgeois P+, *Baillieres Clin Rheumatol* 5, 13
(1989): Kerr HD, *South Med J* 82, 1275
Stevens–Johnson syndrome
(2000): Hofbauer GF+, *Dermatology* 201(3), 258
Urticaria
(1999): Castro-Villamor MA+, *Ann Emerg Med* 34, 296
Vasculitis
(1999): Hofbauer GF+, *Br J Dermatol* 141, 600
Verrucae (snorters' warts)
(1987): Schuster DS, *Arch Dermatol* 123, 571

Mucosal/ENT
Ageusia (>10%)
Anosmia (>10%)
Gingival ulceration
(1999): Fazzi M+, *Minerva Stomatol* (Italian) 48, 485
Nasal septal perforation
(2001): Millard DR+, *Plast Reconstr Surg* 107(2), 419
(2000): Patel R+, *J Natl Med Assoc* 92, 39
(1986): Schwartz RH+, *Am Fam Physician* 43, 187
Palatal perforation
(2007): Lypka MA+, *N Engl J Med* 357(19), 1956
(2005): Jewers WM+, *Oral Surg Oral Med Oral Pathol Oral Radiol Endod* 99(5), 594
(2002): Smith JC+, *Ear Nose Throat J* 81(3), 172
(1998): Gendeh BS+, *Med J Malaysia* 53(4), 435
(1991): Mattson-Gates G+, *Ann Plast Surg* 26(5), 466
Tongue black
(1999): Burnett LB+, *Online Textbook of Emergency Medicine* (from crack cocaine)

Eyes
Visual hallucinations
(2006): Tapp AM+, *J Clin Psychiatry* 67(11), 1819
(1993): Barroso Moguel R+, *Gac Med Mex* 129(1), 13

Other
Cardiac arrest
(1992): Menon D, *CMAJ* 146(2), 113
Chest pain
(2006): Jones JH+, *Clin Lab Med* 26(1), 127
(2003): Honderick T+, *Am J Emerg Med* 21(1), 39
(1999): Schar B+, *Schweiz Rundsch Med Prax* 88(4), 129
(1994): Hollander JE+, *Acad Emerg Med* 1(4), 330
Death
(2006): Williams J+, *J Emerg Med* 31(2), 181
(1994): Hollander JE+, *Acad Emerg Med* 1(4), 330
Depression
(1993): Barroso Moguel R+, *Gac Med Mex* 129(1), 13
Injection-site scarring
Nephrotoxicity
(2006): Rivero M+, *J Nephrol* 19(1), 108
Porphyria
(1987): Dick AD+, *Lancet* 2, 1150
Rhabdomyolysis
(2003): Doctora JS+, *J Oral Maxillofac Surg* 61(8), 964
(2000): Richards JR, *J Emerg Med* 19(1), 51
(1999): Hedetoft C+, *Ugeskr Laeger* 161(50), 6907
(1996): Bakir AA+, *Curr Opin Nephrol Hypertens* 5(2), 122
(1996): Lampley EC+, *Obstet Gynecol* 87(5), 804
(1994): Villalba Garcia MV+, *An Med Interna* 11(3), 119
(1992): Garcia Castano J+, *An Med Interna* 9(7), 340 (13 cases)
(1992): Zele I+, *Minerva Med* 83(12), 847 (24%)
(1991): Horst E+, *South Med J* 84(2), 269
(1991): Welch RD+, *Ann Emerg Med* 20(2), 154 (24%)

(1990): Kanel GC+, *Hepatology* 11(4), 646
(1989): Fox AW, *N Engl J Med* 321(18), 1271
(1989): Loper KA, *Med Toxicol Adverse Drug Exp* 4(3), 174
(1989): VanDette JM+, *Clin Pharm* 8(6), 401
(1988): Leung AK, *West J Med* 149(1), 93
Seizures
(1998): Winbery S+, *Am J Emerg Med* 16(5), 529
(1993): Barroso Moguel R+, *Gac Med Mex* 129(1), 13
(1983): Jonsson S+, *Am J Med* 75(6), 1061
Suicidal ideation
(2003): Garlow SJ+, *Drug Alcohol Depend* 70(1), 101
(1993): Barroso Moguel R+, *Gac Med Mex* 129(1), 13
Thrombophlebitis
(1987): Heng MC+, *J Am Acad Dermatol* 16, 462
Tremor (1–10%)

COCOA

Scientific names: *Theobroma cacao; Theobroma sativum*
Family: Sterculiaceae
Trade and other common names: Cacao; Chocola; Cocoa Oleum; Theobromine
Category: Food supplement
Purported indications and other uses: Oral: asthma, bronchitis, cardiovascular disease, diarrhea. **Topical:** cosmetics, pharmaceutical preparations, foods. Chocolate is produced from cocoa powder
Half-life: 5 hours
Clinically important, potentially hazardous interactions with: caffeine, cimetidine, ciprofloxacin, clozapine, **ephedra**, lithium, phenylpropanolamine, theophylline

Reactions

Skin
Allergic granulomatous angiitis (Churg–Strauss syndrome)
(2004): Taibjee SM+, *Br J Dermatol* 150(3), 595
Allergic reactions
Henoch–Schönlein purpura
Prurigo
(2004): Cederberg J+, *BMC Psychiatry* 4, 36 (with fluoxetine or sertraline)
(1998): Rudzki E+, *Przegl Lek* 55(5), 239
Pruritus ani et vulvae
Rash
(2004): Cederberg J+, *BMC Psychiatry* 4, 36 (with fluoxetine or sertraline)

Other
Headache
(2003): Jansen SC+, *Ann Allergy Asthma Immunol* 91(3), 233
(2002): Savi L+, *Panminerva Med* 44(1), 27
(1995): Peatfield RC, *Headache* 35(6), 355
(1991): Gibb CM+, *Cephalalgia* 11(2), 93
(1984): Peatfield RC+, *Cephalalgia* 4(3), 179
(1982): Seltzer S+, *Cephalalgia* 2(2), 111
Tremor

CODEINE

Synonym: methylmorphine
Trade names: Actacode; Calcidrine; Cheracol; Codicept; Codiforton; Guaituss AC; Halotussin (Watson); Novahistine DH; Nucofed (Monarch); Paveral; Robitussin AC (Wyeth); Solcodein; Tricodein; Tussar-2; Tussi-Organidin (MedPointe)
Indications: Pain, cough suppressant
Category: Opiate agonist
Half-life: 2.5–4 hours
Clinically important, potentially hazardous interactions with: alcohol, CNS depressants, MAO inhibitors, mianserin, **raspberry leaf**

Reactions

Skin
Acute generalized exanthematous pustulosis (AGEP)
    (1995): Lee S+, *Australas J Dermatol* 36, 25
Angioedema
    (1992): Breathnach SM+, *Adverse Drug Reactions and the Skin*
        Blackwell, Oxford, 211 (passim)
Bullous dermatitis
    (1992): Breathnach SM+, *Adverse Drug Reactions and the Skin*
        Blackwell, Oxford, 211 (passim)
Dermatitis
    (2005): Rodriguez A+, *Contact Dermatitis* 53(4), 240
    (1995): Waclawski ER+, *Contact Dermatitis* 33, 51
    (1983): Romaguera C+, *Contact Dermatitis* 9, 170
Diaphoresis
Edema
    (2001): Estrada JL+, *Contact Dermatitis* 44(3), 185 (generalized)
Erythema multiforme (<1%)
    (1992): Breathnach SM+, *Adverse Drug Reactions and the Skin*
        Blackwell, Oxford, 211 (passim)
    (1983): Ponte CD, *Drug Intell Clin Pharm* 17, 128
Erythema nodosum (<1%)
    (1992): Breathnach SM+, *Adverse Drug Reactions and the Skin*
        Blackwell, Oxford, 211 (passim)
Exanthems
    (1985): Hunskaar S+, *Ann Allergy* 54, 240
    (1980): Voorhorst R+, *Ann Allergy* 44, 116
Exfoliative dermatitis
    (1995): Rodriguez F+, *Contact Dermatitis* 32, 120
Facial edema
Fixed eruption (<1%)
    (1996): Gonzalo-Garijo MA+, *Br J Dermatol* 135, 498
    (1992): Breathnach SM+, *Adverse Drug Reactions and the Skin*
        Blackwell, Oxford, 211 (passim)
    (1990): Gaffoor PMA+, *Cutis* 45, 242 (passim)
Photo-recall (sunlight and electronic beam)
    (1984): Shelley WB+, *J Am Acad Dermatol* 11, 53
Pityriasis rosea
    (1993): Yosipovitch G+, *Harefuah* (Hebrew) 124, 198; 247
Pruritus (<1%)
    (1986): de Groot AC+, *Contact Dermatitis* 14, 209
Purpura
    (2006): Santoro D+, *Clin Nephrol* 66(2), 131 (with acetaminophen)
Rash (sic) (1–10%)
Toxic epidermal necrolysis (<1%)
Urticaria (1–10%)
    (2006): Santoro D+, *Clin Nephrol* 66(2), 131 (with acetaminophen)
    (2000): Vidal C+, *Allergy* 55, 416
    (1986): de Groot AC+, *Contact Dermatitis* 4, 209

    (1986): Rosenstreich DL, *J Allergy Clin Immunol* 78, 1099
    (1985): Hunskaar S+, *Ann Allergy* 54, 240

Mucosal/ENT
Dysgeusia
Oral ulceration
Xerostomia (1–10%)

Nails
Nails – shoreline
    (1985): Shelley WB+, *Cutis* 35, 220

Other
Anaphylactoid reactions/Anaphylaxis
Death
    (2005): Reith D+, *N Z Med J* 118(1209), U1293 (12 cases)
Headache
Injection-site pain (1–10%)
Paresthesias
Seizures
    (2001): Zolezzi M+, *Ann Pharmacother* 35(10), 1211

COENZYME Q-10

Scientific names: *Mitoquinone; Ubidecarenone; Ubiquinone*
Family: None
Trade and other common names: Co Q10; Co-Q10; CoQ; CoQ-10; Q10
Category: Food supplement
Purported indications and other uses: Congestive heart failure, angina, diabetes, hypertension, breast cancer, increasing exercise tolerance, muscular dystrophy, chronic fatigue
Half-life: N/A
Clinically important, potentially hazardous interactions with: warfarin

Reactions

None

COLCHICINE

Trade names: Cochiquim; ColBenemid; Colchineos; Colgout; Goutnil; Kolkicin; Konicine
Indications: Gouty arthritis
Category: Alkaloid; Anti-inflammatory
Half-life: 20 minutes
Clinically important, potentially hazardous interactions with: clarithromycin, erythromycin, troleandomycin

Note: ColBenemid is colchicine and probenecid

Note: Colchicine, by itself, is generic

Reactions

Skin
Allergic reactions (sic)
    (2001): Vittori F+, *Therapie* 56(1), 63
Angioedema
Behçet's disease
    (2003): Fujii Y+, *Ryumachi* Feb 43(1), 44
Bullous dermatitis (<1%)
Erythema nodosum
    (2002): Guven AG+, *Pediatrics* 109(5), 971

Erythroderma
Exanthems
  (2006): Mason SE+, *J Cutan Pathol* 33(4), 309 (violaceous)
Fixed eruption
  (1996): Mochida K+, *Dermatology* 192, 61
Lichenoid eruption
Necrosis
Photosensitivity
  (1992): Foti C+, *Contact Dermatitis* 27, 201
Pruritus (<1%)
Purpura
Pyoderma
Rash (sic) (<1%)
Side effects (sic) (14%)
Staphylococcal scalded skin syndrome
  (1993): Khuong MA+, *Dermatology* 186, 153
Toxic epidermal necrolysis
  (2004): Arroyo MP+, *Br J Dermatol* 150(3), 581
  (1994): Alfandari S+, *Infection* 22, 365
  (1990): Roujeau JC+, *Arch Dermatol* 126, 37
Urticaria
  (1991): Anderson MH+, *Ann Allergy* 66, 207
Vasculitis
  (1993): Barash J+, *Isr J Med Sci* 29, 310
Vesiculation (palms)

Hair
Hair – alopecia (1–10%)
  (2004): Rollot F+, *Ann Pharmacother* 38(12), 2074 (with
    erythromycin, clarithromycin)
  (2002): Guven AG+, *Pediatrics* 109(5), 971
  (1980): Harms M, *Hautarzt* (German) 31, 161 (20–50%)

Other
Abdominal pain
  (2004): Rollot F+, *Ann Pharmacother* 38(12), 2074 (with
    erythromycin, clarithromycin)
Anaphylactoid reactions/Anaphylaxis
Death
  (2006): Huynh-Do U, *Ther Umsch* 63(12), 783
  (2002): Maxwell MJ+, *Emerg Med J* 19(3), 265 (overdose)
  (2002): Sannohe S+, *J Forensic Sci* 47(6), 1391 (overdose)
Fever
  (2004): Rollot F+, *Ann Pharmacother* 38(12), 2074 (with
    erythromycin, clarithromycin)
Hypersensitivity
Injection-site thrombophlebitis
Myalgia/Myositis/Myopathy/Myotoxicity
  (2005): Alayli G+, *Ann Pharmacother* 39(7-8), 1358 (with
    pravastatin)
  (2005): Sugie M+, *No To Shinkei* 57(9), 785 (with bezafibrate)
  (2002): Atmaca H+, *Ann Pharmacother* 36(11), 1719 (with
    gemfibrozil)
  (2002): Ayllon-Munoz JA+, *Rev Neurol* 35(2), 195
  (2002): Caglar K+, *Nephron* 92(4), 922
  (2002): Fernandez C+, *Acta Neuropathol* (Berlin) 103(2), 100
  (2002): Guven AG+, *Pediatrics* 109(5), 971
  (2002): Hsu WC+, *Clin Neuropharmacol* 25(5), 266 (with
    simvastatin)
  (1999): Gruberg L+, *Transplant Proc* 31, 2157
  (1998): Duarte J+, *Muscle Nerve* 21, 550
  (1997): Ducloux D+, *Nephrol Dial Transplant* 12, 2389
  (1997): Sinsawaiwong S+, *J Med Assoc Thai* 80, 667
  (1992): Himmelmann F+, *Acta Neuropathologica* 83, 440
Nephrotoxicity
  (2005): Krysiak R+, *Pol Arch Med Wewn* 114(3), 882
Porphyria cutanea tarda
Rhabdomyolysis

  (2006): Tufan A+, *Ann Pharmacother* 40(7-8), 1466 (with
    atorvastatin)
  (2006): Varughese GI+, *Nephrology* (Carlton) 11(5), 481
  (2005): Atasoyu EM+, *Ann Pharmacother* 39(7–8), 1368 (with
    fluvastatin)
  (2004): Baker SK+, *Muscle Nerve* 30(6), 799 (with simvastatin)
  (2003): Phanish MK+, *Am J Med* 114(2), 166
  (2003): Vasudevan AR+, *Am J Med* 115(3), 249
  (2002): Atmaca H+, *Ann Pharmacother* 36(11), 1719 (with
    gemfibrozil)
  (2002): Boomershine KH, *Ann Pharmacother* 36(5), 824
  (2001): Chattopadhyay I+, *Postgrad Med J* 77(905), 191
  (1998): Rosset L+, *Schweiz Med Wochenschr* 128(49), 1953
  (1997): Dawson TM+, *J Rheumatol* 24(10), 2045
  (1992): Stefanidis I+, *Dtsch Med Wochenschr* 117(33), 1237

COLESEVELAM

Trade name: Welchol (Sankyo)
Indications: Hypercholesterolemia
Category: Bile acid sequestrant
Half-life: N/A

Reactions

Mucosal/ENT
Oral ulceration

Other
Myalgia/Myositis/Myopathy/Myotoxicity (2%)

COLESTIPOL

Trade names: Cholestabyl; Colestid (Pfizer); Lestid
Indications: Primary hypercholesterolemia
Category: Anion exchange resin; Lipid regulator
Half-life: N/A

Reactions

Skin
Dermatitis (<1%)
Edema
Exanthems (<1%)
Urticaria (<1%)

COLISTIN

Synonyms: Colomycin; Polymixin E
Trade names: Colomycin (Forest); Promixin
Indications: Gram-negative bacterial infections, cystic fibrosis
Category: Antibiotic, polymixin
Half-life: 8 hours
**Clinically important, potentially hazardous interactions
with:** aminoglycosides, cephalothin

Reactions

Skin
Dermatitis
  (2005): Sowa J+, *Contact Dermatitis* 53(3), 175
  (1998): Sasaki S+, *J Dermatol* 25(6), 415

(1995): Inoue A+, *Contact Dermatitis* 33(3), 200
Pruritus
Rash (sic)
(1998): Ledson MJ+, *Eur Respir J* 12(3), 592

Mucosal/ENT
Tinnitus
(1984): Snavely SR+, *Ann Intern Med* 101(1), 92

Other
Asthenia
(2001): Reed MD+, *J Clin Pharmacol* 41(6), 645
Headache
(2001): Reed MD+, *J Clin Pharmacol* 41(6), 645
Hypotension
(2006): Hakeam HA+, *Ann Pharmacother* 40(9), 1677
Myalgia/Myositis/Myopathy/Myotoxicity
(1998): Ledson MJ+, *Eur Respir J* 12(3), 592
Nephrotoxicity
(2006): Falagas ME+, *Eur J Clin Microbiol Infect Dis* 25(9), 596
(2005): Falagas ME+, *Int J Antimicrob Agents* 26(6), 504 (14%)
(2005): Kallel H+, *J Nephrol* 18(3), 323
(2005): Michalopoulos AS+, *Clin Microbiol Infect* 11(2), 115
(2001): Reed MD+, *J Clin Pharmacol* 41(6), 645
(1999): Levin AS+, *Clin Infect Dis* 28(5), 1008 (27%)
(1991): Bosso JA+, *DICP* 25(11), 1168
Neurotoxicity
(2001): Reed MD+, *J Clin Pharmacol* 41(6), 645
(1984): Snavely SR+, *Ann Intern Med* 101(1), 92
Paresthesias
(2001): Reed MD+, *J Clin Pharmacol* 41(6), 645
(1991): Bosso JA+, *DICP* 25(11), 1168
(1984): Snavely SR+, *Ann Intern Med* 101(1), 92
Vertigo

COLLAGEN

Synonym: gluteraldehyde cross-linked (GAX) collagen
Trade names: Artecoll (contains polymethyl-methacrylate microspheres); Autologen; Avitene; Contigen; Dermalogen; Fibrel; Zyderm-I (Inamed); Zyplast
Indications: Cataract surgery (collagen shields), depressed cutaneous scars, facial lines, wrinkles, glottic insufficiency, phonosurgey, urinary incontinence
Category: Protein
Half-life: Several months to years
Clinically important, potentially hazardous interactions with: avitene

Note: A reaction to the anesthetic, lidocaine, in liquid collagen injections may occur

Reactions

Skin
Abscess
(1999): Sweat SD+, *J Urol* 161(1), 93
(1998): McLennan MT+, *Obstet Gynecol* 92(4 Pt 2), 650
Adverse effects (sic)
(2001): Klein AW, *Facial Plast Surg Clin North Am* 9(2), 205
(2000): Moody BR+, *Dermatol Surg* 26(10), 936
(1999): Constantinides M+, *Otolaryngol Head Neck Surg* 120(4), 557
(1998): Stothers L+, *J Urol* 159(3), 806 (0.9%)
(1995): Gold MH, *Dermatol Clin* 13(2), 353
(1994): Moscona R+, *Plast Reconstr Surg* 93(7), 1525
(1989): Clark DP+, *J Am Acad Dermatol* 21(5 Pt 1), 992

(1989): Elson ML, *J Am Acad Dermatol* 20(5 Pt 1), 861
(1986): Vanderveen EE+, *Arch Dermatol* 122(6), 650
(1985): Cooperman LS+, *Aesthetic Plast Surg* 9(2), 145 (1.3%)
(1985): Klein AW+, *J Dermatol Surg Oncol* 11(3), 337
Allergic granulomatous angiitis (Churg–Strauss syndrome)
(2006): O'Shaughnessy BA+, *J Neurosurg* 104(1 Suppl), 33
(2006): Poveda R+, *Med Oral Patol Oral Cir Bucal* 11(1), E1
(2006): Sidwell RU+, *Clin Exp Dermatol* 31(2), 208
(2001): Heise H+, *J Craniomaxillofac Surg* 29(4), 238
(2000): Garcia-Domingo MI+, *J Investig Allergol Clin Immunol* 10(2), 107
(1986): Schurig V+, *Hautarzt* 37(1), 42
(1982): Barr RJ+, *J Am Acad Dermatol* 6(5), 867
Allergic reactions (sic)
(2002): Echols KT+, *Int Urogynecol J Pelvic Floor Dysfunct* 13(1), 52
(1999): Gorton E+, *BJU Int* 84(9), 966
(1999): Su TH+, *Int Urogynecol J Pelvic Floor Dysfunct* 10(3), 200
(1998): Stothers L+, *J Urol* 159(5), 1507
(1985): Pieyre JM, *Aesthetic Plast Surg* 9(2), 153 (4 cases)
(1985): Robinson JK+, *J Dermatol Surg Oncol* 11(2), 124
(1984): Webster RC+, *Arch Otolaryngol* 110(10), 652
Bruising
Dermatomyositis
(1993): Cukier J+, *Ann Intern Med* 118(12), 920
(1993): Elson ML, *J Dermatol Surg Oncol* 19(2), 165
Edema
(1985): Cooperman L+, *J Int Med Res* 13(2), 109 (localized)
(1985): Cooperman LS+, *Aesthetic Plast Surg* 9(2), 145 (localized)
Erythema
(1987): DeLustro F+, *Plast Reconstr Surg* 79(4), 581
(1985): Cooperman L+, *J Int Med Res* 13(2), 109
(1985): Cooperman LS+, *Aesthetic Plast Surg* 9(2), 145
Erythema multiforme
(1993): Moscona RR+, *Plast Reconstr Surg* 92(2), 331
Granuloma annulare
(1984): Rapaport MJ, *Arch Dermatol* 120(7), 837
Herpes simplex
Induration
(1987): DeLustro F+, *Plast Reconstr Surg* 79(4), 581
(1985): Cooperman L+, *J Int Med Res* 13(2), 109
Inflammation
(1995): Gold MH, *Dermatol Clin* 13(2), 353
Nodular eruption
(2005): Thaler MP+, *Dermatol Surg* 31(11 Pt 2), 1566
Pigmentation
(1999): Davis PK, *Br J Plast Surg* 52(1), 81
Pruritus
Rash (sic)
Scar
(1995): Lemperle G+, *Plast Reconstr Surg* 1995 Sep; 96(3), 627
Urticaria

Other
Asthenia
Death
(2003): McCarthy DM+, *Arch Pathol Lab Med* 127(2), E67
Hypersensitivity
(2002): Echols KT+, *Int Urogynecol J Pelvic Floor Dysfunct* 13(1), 52
(2000): Garcia-Domingo MI+, *J Investig Allergol Clin Immunol* 10(2), 107
(1993): Cukier J+, *Ann Intern Med* 118(12), 920
(1991): Frank DH+, *Plast Reconstr Surg* 87(6), 1080
(1991): Schnitzler L, *Rev Fr Gynecol Obstet* 86(6), 469
(1989): Elson ML, *J Dermatol Surg Oncol* 15(3), 301 (2.5%)
(1988): Elson ML, *J Am Acad Dermatol* 18(4), 707 (3%)
(1987): DeLustro F+, *Plast Reconstr Surg* 79(4), 581

(1984): Kamer FM+, *Arch Otolaryngol* 110(2), 93
Infections
  (1998): Faerber GJ+, *Tech Urol* 4(3), 124
Myalgia/Myositis/Myopathy/Myotoxicity
Panniculitis
  (2000): Garcia-Domingo MI+, *J Investig Allergol Clin Immunol* 10(2), 107
  (1999): Biasi D+, *Clin Rheumatol* 18(4), 328
Polymyositis
  (1993): Cukier J+, *Ann Intern Med* 118(12), 920
  (1993): Elson ML, *J Dermatol Surg* 19(2), 165

COMFREY

Scientific names: *Symphytum asperum; Symphytum officinale; Symphytum peregrinum; Symphytum x uplandicum*
Family: Boraginaceae
Trade and other common names: Ass ear; Blackwort; Boneset; Bruisewort; consolida; consormol; consound; gum plant; knitback; Knitbone; nipbone; Russian comfrey; Slippery Root; Wallwort
Category: Carminative
Purported indications and other uses: Leaf: Gastric and duodenal ulcer, rheumatic pain, gout, arthritis. **Topical:** poultice for bruises, sprains, athlete's foot, crural ulcers, mastitis, varicose ulcers. **Root:** Gastric and duodenal ulcers, hematemesis, colitis, diarrhea. **Topical:** ulcers, wounds, fractures, hernia
Half-life: N/A
Clinically important, potentially hazardous interactions with: eucalyptus

Reactions

Other
Death
  (2003): Dasgupta A, *Am J Clin Pathol* 120(1), 127
  (1990): Yeong ML+, *J Gastroenterol Hepatol* 5(2), 211
Toxicity (sic)
  (2002): Rode D, *Trends Pharmacol Sci* 23(11), 497
Tumors
  (1988): Abbott PJ, *Med J Aust* 149(11–12), 678

CONIVAPTAN

Trade name: Vaprisol (Astellas)
Indications: Hyponatremia, SIADH
Category: Vasopressin receptor antagonist
Half-life: 5 hours
Clinically important, potentially hazardous interactions with: clarithromycin, digoxin, indinavir, itraconazole, ketoconazole, ritonavir

Note: Conivaptan is a potent inhibitor of CYP3A4

Reactions

Skin
Erythema (3%)
Peripheral edema (5%)

Mucosal/ENT
Oral candidiasis (2%)
Xerostomia (4%)

Other
Application-site edema (3%)
Application-site erythema (5%)
Application-site pain (8%)
Application-site reactions (52%)
Confusion
Fever (4%)
Headache (12%)
  (2006): Ghali JK+, *J Clin Endocrinol Metab* 91(6), 2145
Hypertension (5%)
Hypotension (3%)
  (2006): Ghali JK+, *J Clin Endocrinol metab* 91(6), 2145
Injection-site reactions
Insomnia
Phlebitis (5%)

CORDYCEPS

Scientific name: *Cordyceps sinensis*
Family: Ascomycetes; Clavicipitaceae
Trade and other common names: Caterpillar Fungus; CordyMax Cs-4 (Pharmanex); Dong Chong Xia Cao; Dong Chong Zia Cao; Hsia Ts'Ao Tung Ch'Ung; Jinshuibaom; Tochukaso; Vegetable Caterpillar
Category: Immunomodulator
Purported indications and other uses: Anemia, arrhythmia, anti-aging, atherosclerosis, bronchitis, cough, dizziness, hyperlipidemia, athletic performance, lethargy, liver disorders, male sexual dysfunction, nocturia, tinnitus
Half-life: N/A
Clinically important, potentially hazardous interactions with: N/A

Reactions

None

CORTISONE

Trade name: Cortone (Merck)
Indications: Arthralgia, dermatoses, ophthalmia, (many others)
Category: Corticosteroid
Half-life: N/A
Clinically important, potentially hazardous interactions with: chlorpropamide, diuretics, ethambutol, **live vaccines,** pancuronium, rifampicin, rifampin

Reactions

Skin
Atrophy
  (1981): Kikuchi I+, *J Dermatol* 8(5), 419
Edema
Leukoderma
Scleroderma

Eyes
Cataract
  (1993): Pirga H, *Oftalmologia* 37(2), 154
  (1991): No Authors, *Am J Epidemiol* 133(6), 541
  (1989): Ndiaye PA+, *Dakar Med* 34(1-4), 161
Glaucoma

(1993): Pirga H, *Oftalmologia* 37(2), 154
(1989): Ndiaye PA+, *Dakar Med* 34(1-4), 161
(1986): Peyresblanques J+, *Bull Soc Ophtalmol Fr* 86(8-9), 1053
(1983): Calixto N+, *Bull Mem Soc Fr Ophtalmol* 95, 525
(1981): Espildora J+, *J Fr Ophtalmol* 4(6-7), 503 (22 cases)
(1980): Stocker S+, *J Fr Ophtalmol* 3(6-7), 415

Other
Adverse effects (sic)
(1990): Gerster JC, *Rev Med Suisse Romande* 110(10), 847
Lipomatosis
(1988): Bischoff C, *Dtsch Med Wochenschr* 113(50), 1964
Myalgia/Myositis/Myopathy/Myotoxicity
Neurotoxicity
Osteoporosis
(2004): Trombetti A+, *Schweiz Rundsch Med Prax* 93(11), 407
(2003): Kaiser H, *Wien Klin Wochenschr* 115(1-2), 6
(2000): Andress HJ+, *Arch Orthop Trauma Surg* 120(7-8), 484
(1996): Mora S+, *Bone* 18(4), 337
(1994): Meunier PJ, *Rev Rhum Ed Fr* 61(11), 797
(1991): Stazi C+, *Clin Ter* 137(1), 9
(1990): Terreaux F+, *Rev Prat* 40(6), 549
(1987): Charbon SA, *Rev Prat* 37(27), 1619
(1987): Oesterreich FU+, *Rofo* 147(5), 572
Tendinopathy/Tendon rupture

CRANBERRY

Scientific name: *Vaccinium oxycoccus*
Family: Ericaceae
Trade and other common names: Kranbeere; Ronce d'Amerique; Tsuru-kokemomo
Category: Diuretic; Proanthocyanadin
Purported indications and other uses: Erythema, hyperplasia, thrush, cystitis, prevention of urinary tract infections, tumor inhibition, influenza, common cold, scurvy, pleurisy
Half-life: N/A

Reactions

Other
Toxicity (sic)
(2002): Garcia-Calatayud S+, *An Esp Pediatr* 56(1), 72

CREATINE

Scientific names: *N-(aminoiminomethyl)-N methyl glycine; N-amidinosarcosine*
Family: None
Trade and other common names: Cr; Creatine monohydrate
Category: Food supplement
Purported indications and other uses: Improve exercise performance, increase muscle mass, heart failure, neuromuscular disease, cholesterol-lowering, amyotrophic lateral sclerosis (ALS), rheumatoid arthritis, cardiac surgery (IV)
Half-life: N/A

Reactions

Skin
Acne
(1998): Gregg LJ, Tulsa, OK (from Internet) (2 observations)
Facial rash (sic)
(1998): US Food & Drug Administration

Pigmented purpuric eruption
(2006): Chorny JA+, *Arch Dermatol* 142(12), 1662
Purpura
(2006): Chorny JA+, *Arch Dermatol* 142(12), 1662 (pigmented)

Eyes
Periorbital edema
(1998): US Food & Drug Administration

Other
Anaphylactoid reactions/Anaphylaxis
(1998): US Food & Drug Administration
Myalgia/Myositis/Myopathy/Myotoxicity
(1998): US Food & Drug Administration
Nephrotoxicity
(2006): Sheth NP+, *Clin Nephrol* 65(2), 134
(2006): Thorsteinsdottir B+, *J Ren Nutr* 16(4), 341
Polymyositis
(1998): US Food & Drug Administration
Rhabdomyolysis
(2007): Do KD+, *Clin J Sport Med* 17(1), 78
(2006): Sheth NP+, *Clin Nephrol* 65(2), 134
(2001): Ray TR+, *South Med J* 94(6), 608
(2000): Robinson SJ, *J Am Board Fam Pract* 13(2), 134
(1998): US Food & Drug Administration
Side effects (sic)
(2002): Lawrence ME+, *J Clin Gastroenterol* 35(4), 299

CROMOLYN

Synonyms: cromolyn sodium; disodium cromoglycate
Trade names: Colimune; Crolom; Cromlom; Cromoptic; Fivent; Gastrocrom (Celltech); Intal (Monarch); Nalcrom; Nasalcrom (Pfizer); Opticrom (Allergan); Rynacrom
Indications: Allergic rhinitis, asthma, mastocytosis
Category: Mast cell stabilizer
Half-life: 80 minutes

Reactions

Skin
Angioedema (1–10%)
(1992): Breathnach SM+, *Adverse Drug Reactions and the Skin* Blackwell, Oxford, 235 (passim)
Dermatitis (generalized)
(1997): Camarasa JG+, *Contact Dermatitis* 36, 160 (from eye drops)
(1993): Lewis FM+, *Contact Dermatitis* 28, 246
(1988): Kudo H+, *Contact Dermatitis* 19, 312
Eczema
Edema
Erythema
Exanthems
Exfoliative dermatitis
Facial rash (sic)
Photosensitivity
Pruritus
Purpura
Rash (sic) (<1%)
Rosacea
Urticaria (<1%)
(1992): Breathnach SM+, *Adverse Drug Reactions and the Skin,* Blackwell, Oxford, 235 (passim)
Vasculitis

Mucosal/ENT
Anosmia
(1998): Graedon J+Newspaper anecdote from, *People's Pharmacy* column
Dysgeusia (>10%)
Xerostomia (1–10%)

Eyes
Conjunctivitis
(1998): Valdivieso R+, *J Investig Allergol Clin Immunol* 8(1), 58

Other
Anaphylactoid reactions/Anaphylaxis (<1%)
(1996): Ibanez MD+, *Ann Allergy Asthma Immunol* 77, 185
(1996): Shearer WT, *Ann Allergy Asthma Immunol* 77, 165
(1992): Breathnach SM+, *Adverse Drug Reactions and the Skin* Blackwell, Oxford, 235 (passim)
(1983): Ahmad S, *Ann Intern Med* 99, 882
Hypersensitivity (immediate type)
(1987): Skarpass IJK, *Allergy* 42, 318
Myalgia/Myositis/Myopathy/Myotoxicity
Paresthesias
Serum sickness

CYANOCOBALAMIN

Synonym: vitamin B_{12}
Trade names: Anacobin; Berubigen; Betolvex; Cobex; Crystamine; Crysti-12; Cyanoject; Cyomin; Cytamen; Dobetin; Ener-B; Lifaton B_{12}; Nascobal (Nastech); Redisol; Rubesol-1000; Rubramin; Sytobex; Vicapan N; Vitamin B_{12}
Indications: Vitamin B_{12} deficiency, pernicious anemia
Category: Vitamin
Half-life: 6 days

Reactions

Skin
Acne
(1991): Sherertz EF, *Cutis* 48, 119
Allergic reactions (sic)
(1986): Bigby M+, *JAMA* 256, 3358 (1.79%)
Angioedema
Bullous dermatitis (<1%)
Dermatitis
(1994): Rodriguez A+, *Contact Dermatitis* 31, 271
Eczema
Exanthems
(1986): Woodliff HJ, *Med J Aust* 144, 223
Folliculitis
(1989): Gallastegui C+, *Drug Intell Clin Pharm* 23, 1033
Pruritus (1–10%)
Rosacea fulminans
(2001): Jansen T+, *J Eur Acad Dermatol Venereol* 15(5), 484
Scleroderma
(2004): Ho J+, *Dermatol Surg* 30(9), 1252
Urticaria (<1%)
(1996): Denis R+, *Clin Lab Haematol* 18, 129
(1986): Woodliff HJ, *Med J Aust* 144, 223

Mucosal/ENT
Cheilitis
(1981): Price ML+, *Contact Dermatitis* 7, 352

Other
Anaphylactoid reactions/Anaphylaxis (<1%)
(1998): Tordjman R+, *Eur J Haematol* 60, 269

(1984): Sobolevskii AI+, *Vestn Dermatol Venerol* (Russian) April, 66
Embolia cutis medicamentosa (Nicolau syndrome)
(2006): Luton K+, *Int J Dermatol* 45(11), 1326
(2002): Poletti E+, *World Congress Dermatol* Poster, 0124
(1995): Kunzi T+, *Schweiz Rundsch Med Prax* (German) 84, 640
Headache
Hypersensitivity
Injection-site necrosis
(1995): Kunzi T+, *Schweiz Rundsch Med Prax* (German) 84, 640
Injection-site pain
Injection-site scleroderma
(2004): Ho J+, *Dermatol Surg* 30(9), 1252
Paresthesias
Porphyria cutanea tarda
Seizures
(2007): Benbir G+, *Seizure* 16(1), 69 (in infants)

CYCLAMATE

Trade name: Sucaryl (Abbott)
Indications: Sweetening
Category: Sweetening agent
Half-life: N/A

Note: Cyclamate is a sulfonamide and can be absorbed systemically. Sulfonamides can produce severe, possibly fatal, reactions such as toxic epidermal necrolysis and Stevens–Johnson syndrome

Reactions

Skin
Angioedema
Bullous dermatitis
Exanthems
Photosensitivity
(1981): Fujita M+, *Arch Dermatol* 117, 246 (passim)
Pruritus
Urticaria
(1981): Fujita M+, *Arch Dermatol* 117, 246

Other
Hypersensitivity (nonallergic)
(1998): Ehlers I+, *Allergy* 53, 1074
Paresthesias
(1992): Shelley WB+, *Advanced Dermatologic Diagnosis* WB Saunders, 1039

CYCLESONIDE

Synonyms: BY 9010; EL 876
Trade name: Omnaris (Altana)
Indications: Allergic rhinitis, asthma
Category: Corticosteroid, inhaled
Half-life: N/A
Clinically important, potentially hazardous interactions with: ketoconazole

Reactions

Mucosal/ENT
Epistaxis (5%)

Other
Headache (6%)

CYCLOBENZAPRINE

Trade names: Benzamin; Cloben; Cyben; Flexeril (McNeil) (Merck); Flexiban; Novo-Cycloprine; Yurelax
Indications: Muscle spasms
Category: Central muscle relaxant
Half-life: 1–3 days
Clinically important, potentially hazardous interactions with: cisapride, droperidol, phendimetrazine

Reactions

Skin
Allergic reactions (sic)
Angioedema (<1%)
Dermatitis (<1%)
Diaphoresis
  (1984): Heckerling PS+, *Ann Intern Med* 101, 881
Facial edema (<1%)
Photosensitivity
Pruritus (<1%)
Purpura
Rash (sic) (<1%)
Urticaria (<1%)

Mucosal/ENT
Ageusia (<1%)
Dysgeusia (3%)
Stomatitis
Tinnitus
Tongue edema (<1%)
Tongue pigmentation
Xerostomia (27%)
  (1988): Bennett RM+, *Arthritis Rheum* 31, 1535
  (1988): Katz WA+, *Clin Ther* 10, 216

Hair
Hair – alopecia

Other
Anaphylactoid reactions/Anaphylaxis (<1%)
Asthenia
  (2005): Childers MK+, *Curr Med Res Opin* 21(9), 1485
  (2004): Toth PP+, *Clin Ther* 26(9), 1355
  (1995): Spiller HA+, *J Emerg Med* 13(6), 781
Gynecomastia
Headache
Paresthesias (<1%)
Vertigo
  (2005): Childers MK+, *Curr Med Res Opin* 21(9), 1485
  (2004): Toth PP+, *Clin Ther* 26(9), 1355

CYCLOPHOSPHAMIDE

Synonyms: CPM; CTX; CYT
Trade names: Cycloblastin; Cyclostin; Cytoxan (Mead Johnson); Endoxan; Endoxana; Genoxal; Ledoxina; Neosar (Gensia); Procytox; Sendoxan
Indications: Lymphomas
Category: Alkylating agent
Half-life: 4–7 hours
Clinically important, potentially hazardous interactions with: aldesleukin, **astragalus root**, azathioprine, cyclosporine, dexamethasone, etanercept, mycophenolate, prednisone, **vaccines**

Reactions

Skin
Acral erythema
  (1995): Komamura H+, *J Dermatol* 22(2), 116 (with vincristine, doxorubicin and GCSF)
  (1993): Vukelja SJ+, *Cutis* 52, 89
  (1986): Crider MK+, *Arch Dermatol* 122, 1023
Allergic reactions (sic)
  (2002): Cantu MG+, *J Clin Oncol* 20(5), 1232 (2%) (with doxorubicin and cisplatin)
  (2001): Stratton J+, *Nephrol Dial Transplant* 16(8), 1724
Angioedema
Carcinoma
  (2003): Cummins DL+, *J Am Acad Dermatol* 49, 276 (8%)
Condylomata acuminata
  (1996): D'Hondt L+, *Acta Gastroenterol Belg* (French) 59, 254
Dermatitis
Dermatitis herpetiformis
  (1986): Gottlieb D+, *Med J Aust* 145, 241
Dermatofibromas
  (1986): Bargman HB+, *J Am Acad Dermatol* 14, 351
Diaphoresis
Eccrine squamous syringometaplasia
  (1997): Valks R+, *Arch Dermatol* 133, 873
Edema
  (2007): Tashiro H+, *Gan To Kagaku Ryoho* 34(3), 393 (with docetaxel) (25%)
Eosinophilic pustular folliculitis
  (2007): Laing ME+, *Photodermatol Photoimmunol Photomed* 23(2-3), 62
Erythema multiforme (<1%)
Exanthems
  (1992): Breathnach SM+, *Adverse Drug Reactions and the Skin* Blackwell, Oxford, 289 (passim)
  (1992): Hann SK+, *J Dermatol* 20, 94
  (1982): Bailin PL+, *Clin Rheum Dis* 8, 493 (passim)
Facial burning
  (1994): Kosirog-Glowacki JL+, *Ann Pharmacother* 28, 197
Graft-versus-host reaction
  (2001): Valks R+, *Arch Dermatol* 137, 61 (3 cases)
Hand–foot syndrome
  (2003): Leighl NB+, *Clin Lung Cancer* 5(2), 107 (with doxorubicin and vincristine)
  (1989): Matsuyama JR+, *Drug Intell Clin Pharm* 23, 776
Herpes zoster
  (2004): Riley P+, *Rheumatology* (Oxford) 43(4), 491
  (2003): Cummins DL+, *J Am Acad Dermatol* 49, 276
Keratoacanthoma
Lupus erythematosus
  (2001): McClain S, New York, NY (from Internet) (observation)
Lymphoma
  (1992): Pandya AG+, *Arch Dermatol* 128, 1626 (passim)
  (1983): Goslen JB+, *Arch Dermatol* 119, 326
Myxedema
Neutrophilic eccrine hidradenitis
  (2003): Lienesch DW+, *Lupus* 12(9), 707
Palmar–plantar erythema
  (1990): Pagliuca A+, *Postgrad Med J* 66, 242
Paraneoplastic pemphigus
  (2004): Preisz K+, *Br J Dermatol* 150(5), 1018
Pemphigus
  (2004): Preisz K+, *Br J Dermatol* 150(5), 1018
Photo-recall (UV)
  (2004): Borroni G+, *Am J Dermatopathol* 26(3), 213
  (1993): Williams BJ+, *Clin Exp Dermatol* 18, 452
  (1984): Andersen KE+, *Photodermatol* 1, 129

Pigmentation (<1%)
 (2001): Viana G, Belo Horizonte, Brazil (from Internet)
  (observation)
 (1993): Pai BH, *J Assoc Physicians India* 41, 124
 (1992): Babu KG, *J Assoc Physicians India* 40, 211
 (1992): Pandya AG+, *Arch Dermatol* 128, 1626 (passim)
 (1991): Dutta TK+, *J Assoc Physicians India* 39, 230
 (1991): Singal R+, *Pediatr Dermatol* 8, 231
 (1981): Nixon DW+, *Cutis* 27, 181
Pruritus
Purpura
Rash (sic) (1–10%)
Scleroderma
 (2005): Alexandrescu DT+, *Clin Exp Dermatol* 30(2), 141 (with
  doxorubicin)
Squamous cell carcinoma
 (1992): Pandya AG+, *Arch Dermatol* 128, 1626 (passim)
Stevens–Johnson syndrome
 (1996): Assier-Bonnet H+, *Br J Dermatol* 135, 864
 (1985): Leititis JU+, *Klin Padiatr* (German) 197, 441
Toxic epidermal necrolysis (<1%)
Toxicity (sic)
 (2007): Tashiro H+, *Gan To Kagaku Ryoho* 34(3), 393 (with
  docetaxel) (13%)
Urticaria
 (1992): Breathnach SM+, *Adverse Drug Reactions and the Skin*
  Blackwell, Oxford, 289 (passim)
 (1987): Grosbois B+, *Rev Med Interne* (French) 8, 208
 (1982): Anku V, *Cancer Treat Rep* 66, 2106
 (1980): Diaz-Rubio E+, *Rev Clin Esp* (Spanish) 156, 461
Vasculitis
 (1989): Green RM+, *Aust N Z J Med* 19, 55

Mucosal/ENT

Gingival pigmentation
Oral mucositis
 (2000): Wardley AM+, *Br J Haematol* 110, 292
Oral ulceration
 (1992): Pandya AG+, *Arch Dermatol* 128, 1626 (passim)
 (1982): Bailin PL+, *Clin Rheum Dis* 8, 493 (passim)
Stomatitis (10%)
 (2007): Tashiro H+, *Gan To Kagaku Ryoho* 34(3), 393 (with
  docetaxel) (25%)
 (1982): Bailin PL+, *Clin Rheum Dis* 8, 493 (passim)

Hair

Hair – alopecia (universal and severe in one-third)
 (2007): Perini P+, *Expert Opin Drug Saf* 6(2), 183
 (2007): Tashiro H+, *Gan To Kagaku Ryoho* 34(3), 393 (with
  docetaxel)
 (2004): Riley P+, *Rheumatology* (Oxford) 43(4), 491
 (2002): de Jonge ME+, *Bone Marrow Transplantation* 30(9), 593
  (permanent) (with carboplatin and thiotepa)
 (2002): Klasa RJ+, *J Clin Oncol* 20(24), 4649 (with vincristine and
  prednisone)
 (2001): Viana G, Belo Horizonte, Brazil (from Internet)
  (observation)
 (2000): Tran D+, *Australas J Dermatol* 41(2), 106 (with
  busulphan)
 (1996): Infanti L+, *Haematologica* 81, 521
 (1992): Pandya AG+, *Arch Dermatol* 128, 1626 (passim)
 (1987): David J+, *Nurs Times* 83, 36
 (1987): Parker R, *Oncol Nurs Forum* 14, 49
 (1985): Middleton J+, *Cancer Treat Rep* 69, 373
 (1984): Ahmed AR+, *J Am Acad Dermatol* 11, 1115
 (1984): Cline BW, *Cancer Nurs* 7, 221
 (1982): Bailin PL+, *Clin Rheum Dis* 8, 493 (passim)
 (1980): Maxwell MB, *Am J Nursing* 80, 900

Nails

Nails – Beau's lines (transverse nail bands)
 (1994): Ben-Dyan D+, *Acta Haematol* 91, 89
Nails – dystrophy
 (1992): Breathnach SM+, *Adverse Drug Reactions and the Skin*
  Blackwell, Oxford, 289 (passim)
Nails – leukonychia (Muehrcke's lines)
 (1992): Bianchi L+, *Dermatology* 185, 216 (longitudinal)
 (1990): Bader-Meunier B+, *Ann Pediatr Paris* (French) 37, 337
 (1983): James WD+, *Arch Dermatol* 119, 334
Nails – onychodermal band
 (1993): Kowal-Vern A+, *Cutis* 52, 43
Nails – pigmentation (<1%)
 (2003): Dave S+, *Dermatol Online J* 9(3), 14
 (2002): Srikant M+, *Br J Haematol* 117(1), 2
 (2001): Viana G, Belo Horizonte, Brazil (from Internet)
  (observation)
 (1992): Bianchi L+, *Dermatology* 185, 216 (longitudinal)
 (1989): Baran R+, *J Am Acad Dermatol* T(6), 1165 (longitudinal)
 (1983): Manigand G+, *Sem Hop* (French) 59, 1840
 (1982): Bailin PL+, *Clin Rheum Dis* 8, 493 (passim)
 (1981): Adam BA, *Singapore Med J* 22, 35
 (1980): Daniel CR+, *Cutis* 25, 595
 (1980): Sulis E+, *Eur J Cancer* 16, 1517

Other

Abdominal pain
 (2003): Cummins DL+, *J Am Acad Dermatol* 49, 276
Anaphylactoid reactions/Anaphylaxis (<1%)
 (1992): Breathnach SM+, *Adverse Drug Reactions and the Skin*
  Blackwell, Oxford, 289 (passim)
Cardiotoxicity
 (2005): de Jonge ME+, *Clin Pharmacokinet* 44(11), 1135
Congestive heart failure
 (2004): Libersa C I, *Therapie* 59(1), 127
Hepatotoxicity
 (2006): Akay H+, *South Med J* 99(12), 1399
 (2006): de Jonge ME+, *Br J Cancer* 94(9), 1226
 (2005): Muratori L+, *Dig Dis Sci* 50(12), 2364
Hypersensitivity
 (1996): Popescu NA+, *J Allergy Clin Immunol* 97, 26
 (1992): Weiss RB, *Semin Oncol* 19, 458
Inappropriate secretion of antidiuretic hormone (SIADH)
 (1996): Juan O+, *Sangre* (Barc) 41(1), 69
Infections
 (2003): Cummins DL+, *J Am Acad Dermatol* 49, 276 (26%)
Injection-site pain
Myalgia/Myositis/Myopathy/Myotoxicity
 (2004): Borroni G+, *Am J Dermatopathol* 26(3), 213
 (2002): Cantu MG+, *J Clin Oncol* 20(5), 1232 (4%) (with
  doxorubicin and cisplatin)
Panniculitis
 (2004): Borroni G+, *Am J Dermatopathol* 26(3), 213
Polyarteritis nodosa
 (1983): Goslen JB+, *Arch Dermatol* 119, 326
Porphyria cutanea tarda
 (1988): Manzione NC+, *Gastroenterology* 95, 1119
Rhabdomyolysis
Scalp burning
 (1994): Kosirog-Glowacki JL+, *Ann Pharmacother* 28, 197

CYCLOSERINE

Trade names: Closerin; Closerina; Cyclomycin; Cyclorine; Cycosin; Orientomycin; Seromycin (Lilly)
Indications: Tuberculosis
Category: Antibiotic
Half-life: 10 hours

Reactions

Skin

Allergic reactions (sic)
Dermatitis
Exanthems
  (1985): Holdiness R, *Int J Dermatol* 24, 280
Lichenoid eruption
  (1995): Shim JH+, *Dermatology* 191, 142
Peripheral edema
  (2006): Zver S+, *Int J Hematol* 83(3), 238
Pruritus
Purpura
  (2005): Zakarija A+, *Semin Thromb Hemost* 31(6), 681
Rash (sic) (<1%)
  (2006): Doan S+, *Am J Ophthalmol* 141(1), 62
Stevens–Johnson syndrome
  (1997): Akula SK+, *Int J Tuberc Lung Dis* 1, 187 (in AIDS)
Urticaria

Mucosal/ENT

Gingival hyperplasia/hypertrophy
  (2006): Argani H+, *Exp Clin Transplant* 4(1), 420
  (2006): de Oliveira Costa F+, *J Periodontol* 77(6), 969 (29%)
  (2006): Grassi FR+, *Minerva Stomatol* 55(1-2), 59
Oral lesions

Other

Cardiotoxicity
  (2006): Rezzani R, *Histol Histopathol* 21(3), 301
Headache
Hepatotoxicity
  (2006): Rezzani R, *Histol Histopathol* 21(3), 301
Nephrotoxicity
  (2006): Kim CD+, *Transplant Proc* 38(5), 1314
  (2006): Rezzani R, *Histol Histopathol* 21(3), 301
Paresthesias
Seizures
  (2006): Munoz R+, *Transplant Proc* 38(3), 921

CYCLOSPORINE

Synonyms: CsA; CyA; cyclosporin A
Trade names: Ciclosporin; Consupren; Implanta; Neoral (Novartis); Sandimmun; Sandimmune (Novartis)
Indications: Prophylaxis of organ rejection in transplants
Category: Calcineurin inhibitor; Disease-modifying antirheumatic; Immunosuppressant
Half-life: 10–27 hours (adults)
Clinically important, potentially hazardous interactions with: amiloride, aminoglycosides, amphotericin B, ampicillin, anisindione, anticoagulants, armodafinil, atorvastatin, azathioprine, azithromycin, bacampicillin, basiliximab, bosentan, bupropion, carbenicillin, caspofungin, cholestyramine, clarithromycin, cloxacillin, co-trimoxazole, corticosteroids, cyclophosphamide, daclizumab, danazol, dicloxacillin, dicumarol, digoxin, diltiazem, disulfiram, **echinacea**, erythromycin, ethotoin, etoposide, ezetimibe, flunisolide, fluoxymesterone, fluvastatin, foscarnet, fosphenytoin, gemfibrozil, **hemophilus B vaccine**, HMG-CoA reductase inhibitors, imatinib, imipenem/cilastatin, **influenza vaccines**, ketoconazole, lanreotide, lovastatin, mephenytoin, methicillin, methoxsalen, methylphenidate, methylprednisolone, methyltestosterone, mezlocillin, mycophenolate, nafcillin, nisoldipine, NSAIDs, orlistat, oxacillin, penicillins, **phellodendron**, phenytoin, pravastatin, prednisolone, prednisone, ranolazine, **red rice yeast**, rifabutin, rifampin, rifapentine, ritonavir, rosuvastatin, simvastatin, sirolimus, spironolactone, **St John's wort**, sulfacetamide, sulfadiazine, sulfamethoxazole, sulfisoxazole, sulfonamides, tacrolimus, telithromycin, testosterone, ticarcillin, triamterene, troleandomycin, **vaccines**, vecuronium, warfarin

Note: A good discussion of cyclosporine in dermatology can be found in (1989): Gupta AK+, *J Am Acad Dermatol* 21, 1245

Reactions

Skin

Acne
  (2001): Reitamo S+, *Br J Dermatol* 145(3), 438 (13%) (with sirolimus)
  (2001): Werth V, *Dermatology Times* 15
Acne keloid
  (2001): Carnero L+, *Br J Dermatol* 144(2), 429 (nuchal scalp)
Allergic granulomatous angiitis (Churg–Strauss syndrome)
  (2002): Kim SS+, *J Korean Med Sci* 17(5), 704
Angioedema
  (1980): Isenberg DA+, *N Engl J Med* 303, 754
Angiomas
  (1998): De Felipe I+, *Arch Dermatol* 134, 1487
Basal cell carcinoma
  (2004): Lain EL+, *J Drugs Dermatol* 3(6), 680 (Nodular)
  (2001): Otley CC+, *Arch Dermatol* 137, 459
  (1992): Pakula A+, *J Am Acad Dermatol* 26, 139
  (1987): Penn I, *Transplantation* 43, 32
Bullous dermatitis (1%)
  (1990): Petit D+, *J Am Acad Dermatol* 22, 851
Burning
  (2002): Pucci N+, *Ann Allergy Asthma Immunol* 89(3), 298 (topical)
Buschke–Lowenstein penile carcinoma
  (1993): Piepkorn M+, *J Am Acad Dermatol* 29, 321
Cellulitis
Cyst
  (1993): Richter A+, *Hautarzt* (German) 44, 521
  (1993): Valicenti JMK+, *Arch Dermatol* 129, 794 (passim)

(1992): Schoendorff C+, *Cutis* 50, 36 (epidermoid)
(1986): Bencini PL+, *Dermatologica* 172, 24

Dermatitis

Dyshidrosis
(2002): Sharma AK+, *Transpl Int* 15(9), 519

Eccrine squamous syringometaplasia
(1997): Valks R+, *Arch Dermatol* 133, 873

Eczema

Edema
(1997): Shapiro J+, *J Am Acad Dermatol* 36, 114

Erythema
(2001): Takamatsu Y+, *Bone Marrow Transplant* 28(4), 421

Exanthems
(1985): Chapius B+, *N Engl J Med* 312, 1259

Facial edema
(1986): Schmitz-Schumann M, *Prog Allergy* 38, 436

Fixed eruption
(2002): Verma SB, Baroda, India (from Internet) (observation)

Folliculitis
(2003): Harman KE+, *Clin Exp Dermatol* 28(3), 341
(2001): Werth V, *Dermatology Times* 15
(1995): Ojeda-Vargas M+, *Enferm Infecc Microbiol Clin* (Spanish) 13, 637
(1993): Richter A+, *Hautarzt* (German) 44, 521
(1993): Sepp N+, *Br J Dermatol* 128, 213
(1993): Valicenti JMK+, *Arch Dermatol* 129, 794 (passim)
(1986): Bencini PL+, *Dermatologica* 172, 24

Herpes simplex
(2006): Spolidorio LC+, *Oral Dis* 12(3), 309
(1993): Sepp N+, *Br J Dermatol* 128, 213
(1993): Valicenti JMK+, *Arch Dermatol* 129, 794 (passim)
(1986): Bencini PL I, *Dermatologica* 172, 24

Herpes zoster
(1986): Bencini PL+, *Dermatologica* 172, 24

Hidradenitis
(1984): Palestine AG+, *Am J Med* 4:77, 652

Hyperkeratosis (follicular spiny)
(1995): Izakovic J+, *Hautarzt* (German) 46, 841

Hypertrophy (Lip)
(2006): Bhattacharyya I+, *Oral Surg Oral Med Oral Pathol Oral Radiol Endod* 102(4), 469

Ichthyosis
(1986): Bencini PL+, *Dermatologica* 172, 24

Kaposi's sarcoma
(1997): Vella JP+, *N Engl J Med* 336, 1761
(1996): Ozen S+, *Nephrol Dial Transplant* 11, 1162
(1988): Bencini PL+, *Br J Dermatol* 118, 709
(1987): Penn I, *Transplantation* 43, 32

Keloid
(2007): Shivaswamy KN+, *J Eur Acad Dermatol Venereol* 21(1), 111

Keratoacanthoma
(2004): Lain EL+, *J Drugs Dermatol* 3(6), 680 (Multiple)

Keratoses
(1995): Yamamoto T+, *J Dermatol* 22, 298
(1993): Piepkorn M+, *J Am Acad Dermatol* 29, 321
(1992): Ross M+, *J Am Acad Dermatol* 26, 128

Keratosis pilaris
(1993): Valicenti JMK+, *Arch Dermatol* 129, 794 (passim)
(1986): Bencini PL+, *Dermatologica* 172, 24

Lichenoid eruption
(1995): Shim JH+, *Dermatology* 191, 142

Linear IgA dermatosis
(2003): Avci O+, *J Am Acad Dermatol* 48(2), 299 (passim)
(1990): Petit D+, *J Am Acad Dermatol* 22, 851

Lupus erythematosus
(1990): Cooper KD, *Dermatology* 1(2), 3

Lymphocytic infiltration

(1992): Bagot M+, *J Am Acad Dermatol* 26, 283
(1991): Sabourin JC, *Ann Pathol* 11, 208
(1990): Gupta AK+, *J Am Acad Dermatol* 22, 242
(1990): Gupta AK+, *J Am Acad Dermatol* 23, 1137
(1988): Brown MD+, *Arch Dermatol* 124, 1097

Lymphoma
(2007): Madan V+, *Dermatol Ther* 20(4), 239 (passim)
(2002): Kirby B+, *J Am Acad Dermatol* 47(2 Suppl), S165
(1999): Cliff S+, *Br J Dermatol* 140(4), 763
(1999): Zackheim HS, *J Am Acad Dermatol* 40(6 Pt 1), 1015
(1993): Masouye I+, *Arch Dermatol* 129, 914
(1992): Koo JY+, *J Am Acad Dermatol* 26, 836
(1992): Zijlmans JM+, *N Engl J Med* 326, 1363
(1991): Tomson CR+, *Nephrol Dial Transplant* 6, 896
(1989): Walker RJ+, *Aust N Z J Med* 19, 154
(1987): Penn I, *Transplantation* 43, 32
(1984): Beveridge T+, *Lancet* 1, 788
(1983): Inglehart JK, *N Engl J Med* 309, 123

Lymphomatoid papulosis
(2005): Laube S+, *Br J Dermatol* 152(6), 1346

Melanoma
(1990): Merot Y+, *Br J Dermatol* 123, 237

Mycosis fungoides
(2002): Zackheim HS+, *J Am Acad Dermatol* 47(1), 155
(1990): Fradin MS+, *J Am Acad Dermatol* 23, 1265

Neoplasms
(1995): Kohler LD+, *Hautarzt* (German) 46, 638

Papillomas (facial)
(1993): Valicenti JMK+, *Arch Dermatol* 129, 794

Papulovesicular eruption
(1988): Frosch PJ+, *Hautarzt* (German) 39, 611

Peripheral edema
(1997): Berthe-Jones J+, *Br J Dermatol* 136, 76

Pigmentation
(1997): Oakley A, Hamilton, New Zealand (from Internet) (observation)

Poikiloderma
(1986): Bencini PL+, *Dermatologica* 172, 24

Porokeratosis (superficial actinic)
(1997): Matsushita S+, *J Dermatol* 24, 110

Pruritus (<2%)
(1992): Goodman MM+, *J Am Acad Dermatol* 27, 594

Psoriasis
(1998): Mahendran R+, *Br J Dermatol* 139, 934
(1997): Drugge R, Stamford, CT (from Internet) (observation)
(1986): Bencini PL+, *Dermatologica* 172, 24

Purpura (3%)
(2005): Orion E+, *Clin Dermatol* 23(2), 182
(2001): Medina PJ+, *Curr Opin Hematol* 8(5), 286
(1998): Roberts P+, *Transplant Proc* 30, 1512
(1986): Bencini PL+, *Dermatologica* 172, 24

Pyogenic granuloma
(2001): al-Zayer M+, *Spec Care Dentist* 21(5), 187

Rash (sic) (10%)
(1992): Goodman MM+, *J Am Acad Dermatol* 27, 594

Raynaud's phenomenon
(2002): Sharma AK+, *Transpl Int* 15(9), 517
(1986): Deray G+, *Lancet* 2, 1092

Sebaceous hyperplasia
(2005): Engel F+, *Ann Dermatol Venereol* 132(4), 342
(2005): Pang SM+, *Ann Acad Med Singapore* 34(5), 391
(2003): Boschnakow A+, *Br J Dermatol* 149(1), 198
(1998): Walther T+, *Dtsch Med Wochenschr* 123, 798
(1993): Valicenti JMK+, *Arch Dermatol* 129, 794 (passim)
(1992): Pakula A+, *J Am Acad Dermatol* 26, 139
(1986): Bencini PL+, *Dermatologica* 172, 24

Shivering
(2000): Lepine EM, Rock Hill, SC (from Internet) (observation)

Squamous cell carcinoma
(2003): Paul CF+, *J Invest Dermatol* 120(2), 211
(2001): Marcil I+, *Lancet* 358(9287), 1042
(2001): Otley CC+, *Arch Dermatol* 137, 459
(1997): van de Kerkhof PC+, *Br J Dermatol* 136, 275
(1996): Cox NH, *Clin Exp Dermatol* 21, 323
(1993): Piepkorn M+, *J Am Acad Dermatol* 29, 321 (penis)
(1990): Fradin MS+, *J Am Acad Dermatol* 23, 1265 (passim)
(1989): Bos JD+, *J Am Acad Dermatol* 21, 1305
(1985): Bencini PL+, *Br J Dermatol* 113, 373
(1985): Price ML+, *N Engl J Med* 313, 1420
(1985): Thompson JF+, *Lancet* 1, 158
(1983): Mortimer PS+, *J R Soc Med* 76, 786
Striae
(1986): Bencini PL+, *Dermatologica* 172, 24
Toxic epidermal necrolysis
(1997): Jarrett P+, *Clin Exp Dermatol* 22, 254
Ulcerations (1%)
Urticaria
(2001): Takamatsu Y+, *Bone Marrow Transplant* 28(4), 421 (with tacrolimus)
(1985): Ptachcinski RJ+, *Lancet* 1, 636
Vasculitis
(2000): Gupta MN+, *Ann Rheum Dis* 59, 319
(1994): Henckes M+, *Transpl Int* 7, 292
Verruca vulgaris
(1998): Irimajiri J+, *J Dermatol* 25, 688
Vitiligo
(1986): Bencini PL+, *Dermatologica* 172, 24
Xerosis

Mucosal/ENT

Aphthous stomatitis
(2001): Reitamo S+, *Br J Dermatol* 145(3), 438 (9%) (with sirolimus)
(1986): Bencini PL+, *Dermatologica* 172, 24
Gingival hyperplasia/hypertrophy (>10%)
(2007): Buduneli N+, *J Periodontol* 78(2), 282
(2007): Ciavarella D+, *Med Oral Patol Oral Cir Bucal* 12(1), E19
(2007): de Oliveira Costa F+, *J Periodontol* 78(2), 254
(2007): Madan V+, *Dermatol Ther* 20(4), 239 (passim)
(2007): Tamilselvan S+, *J Periodontol* 78(2), 290
(2006): Argani H+, *Exp Clin Transplant* 4(1), 420
(2006): Bhattacharyya I+, *Oral Surg Oral Med Oral Pathol Oral Radiol Endod* 102(4), 469
(2006): Dannewitz B+, *Cell Tissue Res* 325(3), 513
(2006): de Oliveira Costa F+, *J Periodontol* 77(6), 969
(2006): Smith JM+, *Pediatr Nephrol* 21(11), 1753
(2006): Spolidorio LC+, *Oral Dis* 12(3), 309
(2006): Stefanidou V+, *Transplant Proc* 38(9), 2905
(2005): Bulut S+, *J Periodontol* 76(5), 691
(2005): Keglevich T+, *Fogorv Sz* 98(5), 199
(2005): Lucas VS+, *Pediatr Nephrol* 20(10), 1388
(2005): Mahmoud I+, *Nephrol Dial Transplant* 20(4), 735
(2005): Torrezan PR+, *Rev Assoc Med Bras* 51(4), 200 (with nifedipine)
(2005): V'lckova-Laskoska MT, *Acta Dermatovenerol Croat* 13(2), 108
(2004): Tokgoz B+, *Transplant Proc* 36(9), 2699
(2003): Afonso M+, *J Periodontol* 74(1), 51
(2003): Bunetel L+, *J Periodontol* 74(4), 552
(2003): Gnoatto N+, *J Periodontol* 74(12), 1747
(2003): Guelmann M+, *J Clin Pediatr Dent* 27(2), 123
(2003): Hernandez G+, *J Periodontol* 74(12), 1816
(2003): Hyland PL+, *J Periodontol* 74(4), 437
(2003): Jaiarj N, *J Mass Dent Soc* 52(3), 16
(2003): Perez-Espana L+, *Nefrologia* 23(2), 179
(2003): Strachan D+, *J Clin Pharm Ther* 28(4), 329
(2002): Bulut S+, *J Periodontol* 73(8), 892
(2002): Das SJ+, *J Dent Res* 81(10), 683

(2002): Hood KA, *Prog Transplant* 12(1), 17
(2002): Hosey MT+, *Int J Paediatr Dent* 12(4), 236
(2002): Keglevich T+, *Fogorv Sz* 95(1), 15
(2002): McKaig SJ+, *Int J Paediatr Dent* 12(6), 398
(2002): Voulgari PV+, *J Rheumatol* 29(11), 2466
(2001): Brennan MT+, *Oral Surg Oral Med Oral Pathol Oral Radiol Endod* 92(5), 503
(2001): Buduneli N+, *Acta Odontol Scand* 59(6), 367
(2001): Bustos DA+, *J Periodontol* 72(6), 741
(2001): Derici U+, *Acta Neurol Belg* 101(2), 124
(2001): Irshied J+, *J Clin Pediatr Dent* 26(1), 93
(2001): Oettinger-Barak O+, *J Periodontol* 72(9), 1236
(2001): Thomas DW+, *J Clin Periodontol* 28(7), 706
(2001): Uzel MI+, *J Periodontol* 72(7), 921
(2001): Vallejo C+, *Haematologica* 86(1), 110
(2001): Werth V, *Dermatology Times* 15
(2001): Wondimu B+, *Int J Paediatr Dent* 11(6), 424
(2000): Czech W+, *J Am Acad Dermatol* 42, 653
(2000): Hernandez G+, *J Periodontol* 71(10), 1630
(2000): Kirby B+, *Clin Exp Dermatol* 25, 97
(2000): Oettinger-Barak O+, *J Periodontol* 71, 650
(2000): Thomas DW+, *Transplantation* 69, 522
(2000): Thorp M+, *Transplantation* 69(6), 1218
(1999): Busque S+, *Ann Chir* 53(8), 687
(1999): Spratt H+, *Oral Dis* 5, 27
(1999): Wirnsberger GH+, *Transplantation* 67, 1289
(1998): Cebeci I+, *J Periodontol* 69, 1435
(1998): Desai P+, *J Can Dent Assoc* 64, 263
(1998): Garzino-Demo P+, *Minerva Stomatol* 47(9), 387
(1998): Jucgla A+, *Br J Dermatol* 138, 198
(1998): Kohnle M+, *Transplant Proc* 30, 2122
(1998): Mattson JS+, *J Am Dent Assoc* 129, 78
(1998): Nash MM+, *Transplantation* 65, 1611
(1998): Nohl F+, *Ther Umsch* (German) 55, 573
(1998): Nowicki M+, *Ann Transplant* 3, 25
(1998): Pilloni A+, *J Periodontol* 69, 791
(1998): Santi E+, *Int J Periodontics Restorative Dent* 18(1), 80
(1998): Varga E+, *J Clin Periodontol* 25, 225
(1998): Wirnsberger GH+, *Transplant Proc* 30, 2117
(1997): Aufricht C+, *Pediatr Nephrol* 11(5), 552
(1997): Avci O+, *J Am Acad Dermatol* 36, 796
(1997): Brehler R+, *J Am Acad Dermatol* 36, 983 (passim)
(1997): Cecchin E+, *Ann Intern Med* 126, 409
(1997): Dodd DA, *J Heart Lung Transplant* 16, 579
(1997): Ellis CN, *Int J Dermatol* 36 (Supplement), 7 (passim)
(1997): Gómez E+, *Nephrol Dial Transplant* 12, 2694
(1997): Hall EE, *Curr Opin Peridontology* 4, 59 (passim)
(1997): Iacopino AM+, *J Periodontol* 68, 73
(1997): Jackson C+, *N Y State Dent J* 63, 46
(1997): Puig JM+, *Transplant Proc* 29, 2379
(1997): Silverstein LH+, *Gen Dent* 45, 371
(1997): Vescovi P+, *Minerva Stomatol* 46(4), 155
(1996): Ashrafi SH+, *Scanning Microsc* 10, 219
(1996): Boran M+, *Transplant Proc* 28, 2316
(1996): Cebeci I+, *J Periodontol* 67, 1201
(1996): Darbar UR+, *J Clin Periodontol* 23, 941
(1996): Montebugnoli L+, *J Clin Periodontol* 23, 868
(1996): Seymour RA+, *J Clin Periodontol* 23(3 Pt 1), 165
(1996): Somacarrera ML+, *Spec Care Dent* 16, 18
(1996): Thomason JM+, *J Clin Periodontol* 23(4), 367
(1996): Vescovi P+, *Minerva Stomatol* 45(11), 523
(1995): Moghadam BKH+, *Cutis* 56, 46 (passim)
(1995): O'Valle F+, *J Clin Periodontol* 22(8), 591
(1995): Thomason JM+, *J Periodontol* 66(8), 742
(1995): Wahlstrom E+, *N Engl J Med* 332, 753
(1994): Bokenkamp A+, *Pediatr Nephrol* 8(2), 181
(1994): Hefti AF+, *J Periodontol* 65(8), 744
(1994): O'Valle F+, *J Periodontol* 65(7), 724
(1994): Roehrich N+, *Schweiz Monatsschr Zahnmed* 104(12), 1471

(1994): Schincaglia GP+, *Minerva Stomatol* 43(9), 429
(1994): Somacarrera ML+, *J Periodontol* 65(7), 671
(1994): Wong W+, *Lancet* 343, 986
(1993): Arda O+, *J Marmara Univ Dent Fac* 1(4), 290
(1993): Belazi M+, *J Submicrosc Cytol Pathol* 25(4), 591
(1993): King GN+, *J Clin Periodontol* 20, 286
(1993): Seymour RA, *Adverse Drug React Toxicol Rev* 12, 215
(1993): Seymour RA+, *J R Coll Surg Edinb* 38, 328
(1993): Thomason JM+, *J Clin Periodontol* 20, 37
(1993): Valicenti JMK+, *Arch Dermatol* 129, 794 (passim)
(1992): Humphreys TR+, *J Am Acad Dermatol* 29, 490 (passim)
(1992): Mastrolonardo M+, *Dermatol Clin* (Italian) 4, 246
(1992): Seymour RA+, *J Clin Periodontol* 19, 1
(1991): Gonzalez-Jaranay Ruiz M+, *Rev Eur Odontoestomatol* 3(4), 265
(1991): Nassouti A+, *Parodontol* 2(4), 309
(1991): Puelacher W+, *Z Stomatol* (German) 88, 7
(1990): Cooper KD, *Dermatology* 1(2), 3
(1990): Gotze G+, *Stomatol DDR* 40(1), 15
(1990): Krupp P+, *Br J Dermatol* 122 Suppl 36, 47
(1990): Niimi A+, *J Oral Pathol Med* 19(9), 397
(1989): Ross PJ+, *J Dent Child* 56, 56
(1988): Frosch PJ+, *Hautarzt* (German) 39, 611
(1988): Veraldi S+, *Int J Dermatol* 27, 730
(1987): Keown PA+, *Hospital Practice* 22, 207
(1987): Reznik VM, *Lancet* 1, 1405
(1986): Kahan BD+, *World J Surg* 10, 348
Gingivitis
(2003): Leichter C, Oceanside, NY (from Internet) (observation)
Glossitis (atrophic)
(1986): Bencini PL+, *Dermatologica* 172, 24
Oral ulceration
(1986): Bencini PL+, *Dermatologica* 172, 24
Stomatitis (7%)
Tinnitus
(2002): Ozkaya O+, *Pediatr Nephrol* 17(7), 544
Tongue fungiform papillae hypertrophy
(1996): Silverberg NB+, *Lancet* 348, 967

Hair

Hair – alopecia (3%)
(1998): Hunt M, *Cosmetic Dermatology* 23
(1987): Keown PA+, *Hospital Practice* 22, 207
Hair – alopecia areata
(2005): Phillips MA+, *J Am Acad Dermatol* 53(5 Suppl 1), S252
(1999): Cerottini JP+, *Dermatology* 198, 415
(1996): Misciali C+, *Arch Dermatol* 132, 843 (universalis)
(1996): Parodi A+, *Br J Dermatol* 135, 657 (universalis)
(1995): Davies MG+, *Br J Dermatol* 132, 835
(1994): Roger D+, *Acta Derm Venereol* 74, 154
Hair – brittle
Hair – hirsutism
(2004): Willetts IE+, *Transplant Proc* 36(2 Suppl), 211S
Hair – hypertrichosis (19%)
(2007): Madan V+, *Dermatol Ther* 20(4), 239 (passim)
(2006): Tanaka H+, *Tohoku J Exp Med* 209(3), 191
(2005): Mahmoud I+, *Nephrol Dial Transplant* 20(4), 735
(2001): Werth V, *Dermatology Times* 15
(2000): Ionnides D+, *Arch Dermatol* 136, 868
(2000): Thorp M+, *Transplantation* 69(6), 1218
(1999): Busque S+, *Ann Chir* 53(8), 687
(1997): Avci O+, *J Am Acad Dermatol* 36, 796
(1997): Brehler R+, *J Am Acad Dermatol* 36, 983 (passim)
(1997): Ellis CN, *Int J Dermatol* 36 (Supplement), 7 (passim)
(1997): Shapiro J+, *J Am Acad Dermatol* 36, 114
(1997): Shupack J+, *J Am Acad Dermatol* 36, 423
(1996): el Shahawy MA+, *Nephron* 72, 679
(1996): Jayamanne DG+, *Nephrol Dial Transplant* 11, 1159 (eyelashes)
(1996): Vescovi P+, *Minerva Stomatol* 45(11), 523

(1995): Honeyman JF+, *Int J Dermatol* 34, 583
(1995): Mannes GP+, *Transpl Int* 8(3), 247
(1994): Yamamoto S+, *J Dermatol Sci* 7, s47
(1993): Sepp N+, *Br J Dermatol* 128, 213
(1993): Valicenti JMK+, *Arch Dermatol* 129, 794 (passim)
(1992): Humphreys TR+, *J Am Acad Dermatol* 29, 490 (passim)
(1990): Fradin MS+, *J Am Acad Dermatol* 23, 1265
(1988): Frosch PJ+, *Hautarzt* (German) 39, 611
(1988): Penmetcha M+, *Int J Dermatol* 27, 53
(1987): Keown PA+, *Hospital Practice* 22, 207
(1987): Wysocki GP+, *Clin Exp Dermatol* 12, 191
(1986): Bencini PL+, *Br J Dermatol* 114, 396
(1986): Kahan BD+, *World J Surg* 10, 348
(1984): Harper JL+, *Br J Dermatol* 110, 469
Hair – perifolliculitis barbae
(2002): Moderer M+, *World Congress Dermatol* Poster, 0117
Hair – pseudofolliculitis barbae
(1997): Lear J+, *Br J Dermatol* 136, 132

Nails

Nails – abnormal growth
(1986): Gratwohl A+, *Prog Allergy* 38, 404
Nails – brittle (<2%)
Nails – changes (sic)
(1994): Wakelin SH+, *Br J Dermatol* 131, 147
Nails – leukonychia
(1986): Bencini PL+, *Dermatologica* 172, 24
Nails – onychocryptosis
(1993): Olujohungbe A+, *Lancet* 342, 1111
Nails – periungual granuloma
(1995): Higgins EM+, *Br J Dermatol* 132, 829

Eyes

Trichomegaly
(1990): Weaver DT+, *Am J Ophthalmol* 109(2), 239

Other

Acromegaloid features
(1987): Reznik VM, *Lancet* 1, 1405
Anaphylactoid reactions/Anaphylaxis (<1%)
(2001): Ebo DG+, *Ann Allergy Asthma Immunol* 87(3), 243
(2001): Riegert-Johnson DL+, *Bone Marrow Transplant* 28(12), 1176
(2001): Takamatsu Y+, *Bone Marrow Transplant* 28(4), 421
(1989): Gupta AK+, *J Am Acad Dermatol* 21, 1245
(1985): Chapuis B+, *N Engl J Med* 312, 1259
(1985): Leunissen KML+, *Lancet* 1, 636
(1985): Ptachcinski RJ+, *Lancet* 1, 636
Asthenia
(2007): Madan V+, *Dermatol Ther* 20(4), 239 (passim)
(1993): Yamanishi Y+, *Ryumachi* 33(1), 63
Death
(2002): Zackheim HS+, *J Am Acad Dermatol* 47(1), 155
Erythromelalgia
(2003): Thami GP+, *BMJ* 326(7395), 910
Facial numbness
(2002): Ozkaya O+, *Pediatr Nephrol* 17(7), 544
Fibroadenoma
(2001): Muttarak M+, *Australas Radiol* 45(4), 517
(2001): Weinstein SP+, *Radiology* 220(2), 465
Gynecomastia (>3%)
(1998): Kollias J+, *Aust N Z J Surg* 68, 679
(1994): Jacobs U+, *Transplant Proc* 26, 3122
(1987): Beris P+, *Schweiz Med Wochenschr* (German) 117, 1751
Headache
(2007): Madan V+, *Dermatol Ther* 20(4), 239 (passim)
Hepatotoxicity
(2001): Derici U+, *Acta Neurol Belg* 101(2), 124
(1996): Vescovi P+, *Minerva Stomatol* 45(11), 523

Hot flashes
(2001): Reitamo S+, *Br J Dermatol* 145(3), 438 (12%) (with sirolimus)

Hypersensitivity
(2003): Harman KE+, *Clin Exp Dermatol* 28, 364
(2001): Sumpton JE+, *Transplant Proc* 33(6), 3015

Hypertension
(2007): Madan V+, *Dermatol Ther* 20(4), 239 (passim)
(2005): Mahmoud I+, *Nephrol Dial Transplant* 20(4), 735
(2004): Willetts IE+, *Transplant Proc* 36(2 Suppl), 211S
(2003): Suwelack B+, *Transpl Int* 16(5), 313
(2002): Isnard Bagnis+, *J Am Soc* 13(12), 2962
(2001): Campistol JM+, *Transplantation* 71(11 Suppl), SS42
(2001): Derici U+, *Acta Neurol Belg* 101(2), 124
(1998): Bagnis C+, *Arch Mal Coeur Vaiss* 91(4), 411
(1998): Branten AJ+, *Nephrol Dial Transplant* 13(2), 423
(1997): Charnick SB+, *Ther Drug Monit* 19(1), 17
(1997): Pratschke J+, *Transplantation* 64(6), 938
(1996): Vescovi P+, *Minerva Stomatol* 45(11), 523

Infections (sic)
(2007): Madan V+, *Dermatol Ther* 20(4), 239 (passim)

Lymphoproliferative disease
(1989): Walker RJ+, *Aust N Z J Med* 19, 154
(1988): Brown MD+, *Arch Dermatol* 124, 1097

Myalgia/Myositis/Myopathy/Myotoxicity
(2007): Madan V+, *Dermatol Ther* 20(4), 239 (passim)
(2005): Wahie S+, *Br J Dermatol* 153(6), 1238
(2003): Spencer L, Crawfordsville, IN (from Internet) (observation)
(2001): Kappers-Klunne MC+, *Br J Haematol* 114(1), 121
(1993): Yamanishi Y+, *Ryumachi* 33(1), 63
(1990): Fernandez-Sola J+, *Lancet* 335, 362
(1989): Chassagne P+, *Lancet* 2(8671), 1104
(1988): Brown MD+, *Arch Dermatol* 124, 1097 (passim)

Nephrotoxicity
(2007): Lim AK+, *Intern Med J* 37(1), 55
(2007): Madan V+, *Dermatol Ther* 20(4), 239 (passim)
(2007): Tejedor A+, *Curr Med Res Opin* 23(3), 505
(2007): Tostivint I+, *Nephrol Dial Transplant* 22(3), 880
(2006): Anglicheau D+, *Kidney Int* 70(6), 1019
(2006): Chapman JR+, *Nephrol Dial Transplant* 21(8), 2060
(2006): Dziewanowski K+, *Kardiol Pol* 64(5), 522
(2005): Cantarovich D+, *Transplantation* 79(1), 72
(2005): Dubus I+, *Life Sci* 77(26), 3366
(2005): Kuypers DR, *Drug Saf* 28(2), 153
(2005): Mahmoud I+, *Nephrol Dial Transplant* 20(4), 735
(2005): Mention K+, *Pediatr Transplant* 9(2), 201
(2005): Orion E+, *Clin Dermatol* 23(2), 182
(2005): Ulinski T+, *Pediatr Nephrol* 20(4), 482
(2004): Baran DA+, *Am J Cardiovasc Drugs* 4(1), 21
(2004): Busauschina A+, *Transplant Proc* 36(2 Suppl), 229S
(2004): Cattaneo D+, *Transplant Proc* 36(2 Suppl), 234S
(2004): Hesselink DA+, *Transplant Proc* 36(2 Suppl), 372S
(2004): Kuypers DR+, *Transplantation* 78(8), 1204
(2004): Parekh K+, *Transplant Proc* 36(2 Suppl), 318S
(2004): Paul LC+, *Transplant Proc* 36(2 Suppl), 224S
(2004): Raafat RH+, *Am J Kidney Dis* 44(1), 50
(2004): Willetts IE+, *Transplant Proc* 36(2 Suppl), 211S
(2003): Burdmann EA+, *Semin Nephrol* 23(5), 465
(2003): Cattran DC, *Semin Nephrol* 23(2), 234
(2003): Dudley J+, *Nephrol Dial Transplant* 18(2), 403
(2003): Flechner SM, *Transplant Proc* 35(3 Suppl), 118S
(2003): Parra Cid T+, *Toxicology* 189(1–2), 99
(2003): Suwelack B+, *Transpl Int* 16(5), 313
(2003): Ziolkowski J+, *Transplant Proc* 35(6), 2307
(2002): Assan R+, *Diabetes Metab Res Rev* 18(6), 464
(2002): Furrer K+, *Swiss Med Wkly* 132(23–24), 316
(2002): Ganesan V+, *Pediatr Nephrol* 17(3), 225
(2002): Iijima K+, *Kidney Int* 61(5), 1801
(2002): Isnard Bagnis C+, *J Am Soc Nephrol* 13(12), 2962

(2002): Israni A+, *Am J Kidney Dis* 39(3), E16
(2002): Khanna A+, *Kidney Int* 62(6), 2257
(2002): Lytton SD+, *Clin Exp Immunol* 127(2), 293
(2002): Markham T+, *Clin Exp Dermatol* 27(2), 111
(2002): McClure SL+, *Drug Saf* 25(13), 913
(2001): Campistol JM+, *Transplantation* 71(11 Suppl), SS42
(2001): Derici U+, *Acta Neurol Belg* 101(2), 124
(2001): Gossmann J+, *Kidney Blood Press Res* 24(2), 111
(2001): Jankauskiene A+, *Clin Nephrol* 56(6), S27
(2001): Morales JM+, *Nephrol Dial Transplant* 16 Suppl 1, 121
(2001): Pescovitz MD+, *Am J Kidney Dis* 38(4 Suppl 2), S16
(2001): Sijpkens YW+, *Clin Nephrol* 55(2), 149
(2001): Takeda A+, *Clin Transplant* 15 Suppl 5, 22
(2001): Wondimu B+, *Int J Paediatr Dent* 11(6), 424
(2000): Davison SC+, *Br J Dermatol* 143(2), 405
(2000): de Mattos AM+, *Am J Kidney Dis* 35(2), 333
(2000): Seikaly MG+, *Pediatr Nephrol* 14(3), 214
(1999): Ponticelli C+, *Kidney Int* 55(5), 2075
(1999): Soccal PM+, *Transplantation* 68(1), 164
(1998): Andoh TF+, *Curr Opin Nephrol Hypertens* 7(3), 265
(1998): Bagnis C+, *Arch Mal Coeur Vaiss* 91(4), 411
(1998): Branten AJ+, *Nephrol Dial Transplant* 13(2), 423
(1998): Fisher NC+, *Transplantation* 66(1), 59
(1998): Madsen JK+, *Nephrol Dial Transplant* 13(9), 2327
(1998): Min DI+, *Pharmacotherapy* 18(2), 282
(1998): Powles AV+, *Br J Dermatol* 138(3), 443
(1998): Solez K+, *Transplantation* 66(12), 1736
(1998): Vercauteren SB+, *Kidney Int* 54(2), 536
(1997): Andoh TF+, *Semin Nephrol* 17(1), 34
(1997): Bennett WM, *Int J Dermatol* 36 Suppl 1, 11
(1997): Carmellini M+, *Transplantation* 64(1), 164
(1997): Chan C+, *Transplantation* 63(10), 1435
(1997): Charnick SB+, *Ther Drug Monit* 19(1), 17
(1997): Filler G+, *Nephrol Dial Transplant* 12(8), 1668
(1997): Goldstein DJ+, *Transplantation* 63(5), 664
(1997): Goral S+, *J Heart Lung Transplant* 16(11), 1106
(1997): Pratschke J+, *Transplantation* 64(6), 938
(1997): Simon N+, *Int J Clin Pharmacol Res* 17(4), 133
(1997): Simon N+, *Therapie* 52(2), 151
(1997): Woolfson RG+, *Nephrol Dial Transplant* 12(10), 2054
(1996): Bennett WM, *Int J Clin Pharmacol Ther* 34(11), 515
(1996): Vescovi P+, *Minerva Stomatol* 45(11), 523
(1996): Wissmann C+, *J Am Soc Nephrol* 7(12), 2677

Neurotoxicity
(2001): Derici U+, *Acta Neurol Belg* 101(2), 124
(2001): Wondimu B+, *Int J Paediatr Dent* 11(6), 424
(1997): Pratschke J+, *Transplantation* 64(6), 938

Paresthesias (>8%)
(2007): Madan V+, *Dermatol Ther* 20(4), 239 (passim)
(2001): Capper RN, Mobile, AL (tingling lips & fingers) (from Internet) (observation)
(2001): Laws RA, Providence, RI (hands & feet) (from Internet) (observation)
(2001): Thaler D, Monona, WI (numb lips) (from Internet) (observation)
(2000): Baumgaertnet J, LaCrosse, WI (from Internet) (3 observations)
(2000): Lepine EM, Rock Hill, SC (from Internet) (observation)
(2000): Thaler D, Monona, WI (from internet) (observation)
(1997): Berthe-Jones J+, *Br J Dermatol* 136, 76
(1997): Ellis CN, *Int J Dermatol* 36 (Supplement), 7 (passim)
(1997): Shupack J+, *J Am Acad Dermatol* 36, 423
(1992): Goodman MM+, *J Am Acad Dermatol* 27, 594
(1990): Cooper KD, *Dermatology* 1(2), 3
(1988): Bennett WM+, *Ann Rev Med* 37, 215 (passim)
(1987): Dougados M+, *Arthritis Rheum* 30, 83

Pseudolymphoma
(2003): Hivnor C+, *Arch Dermatol* 139(10), 1373
(1993): Kerl H+, *Dermatology in General Medicine* McGraw-Hill New York

(1990): Gupta AK+, *J Am Acad Dermatol* 23(6), 1137
(1988): Brown MD+, *Arch Dermatol* 124(7), 1097
(1988): Thestrup-Pedersen K+, *Dermatologica* 177, 376
Pseudoporphyria
(2003): Hivnor C+, *Arch Dermatol* 139(10), 1373
Rhabdomyolysis
(2007): Burton JR+, *Ann Pharmacother* 41(1), 133
(2005): Tong J+, *Bone Marrow Transplant* 36(8), 739 (with simvastatin)
(2003): Chiffoleau A+, *Therapie* 58(2), 168 (with verapamil and simvastatin)
(2003): Gumprecht J+, *Med Sci Monit* 9(9), CS89 (with simvastatin)
(2002): Cassidy JV+, *Paediatr Anaesth* 12(8), 729
(1999): Maltz HC+, *Ann Pharmacother* 33(11), 1176 (with atorvastatin)
(1995): Meier C+, *Schweiz Med Wochenschr* 125(27), 1342 (with simvastatin)
(1994): Alejandro DS+, *J Am Soc Nephrol* 5(2), 153 (with lovastatin)
(1992): Blaison G+, *Rev Med Interne* 13(1), 61 (with simvastatin)
(1988): Corpier CL+, *JAMA* 260(2), 239 (lovastatin)
(1988): Tobert JA, *Am J Cardiol* 62, 28J (with lovastatin)
Seizures
(2006): Gaggero R+, *J Child Neurol* 21(10), 861
(2003): Reuther LO+, *Ugeskr Laeger* 165(14), 1447
Thrombosis
(1996): Vescovi P+, *Minerva Stomatol* 45(11), 523
Tremor (>10%)
(2007): Madan V+, *Dermatol Ther* 20(4), 239 (passim)
Tumors
(2001): Werth V, *Dermatology Times* 15

CYCLOTHIAZIDE

Trade names: Anhydron; Doburil; Valmiran
Indications: Edema, hypertension
Category: Diuretic, thiazide
Half-life: N/A
Clinically important, potentially hazardous interactions with: digoxin

Note: Cyclothiazide is a sulfonamide and can be absorbed systemically. Sulfonamides can produce severe, possibly fatal, reactions such as toxic epidermal necrolysis and Stevens–Johnson syndrome

Reactions

Skin
Exanthems (<1%)
Photosensitivity
Purpura
Rash (sic)
Urticaria
Vasculitis

Other
Inappropriate secretion of antidiuretic hormone (SIADH)
Paresthesias

CYPROHEPTADINE

Trade names: Ciplactin; Ciproral; Nuran; Periactin; Periactine; Periactinol; Peritol; Sigloton
Indications: Allergic rhinitis, urticaria
Category: Histamine H1 receptor antagonist
Half-life: 1–4 hours
Clinically important, potentially hazardous interactions with: anticholinergics, MAO inhibitors, phenelzine, tranylcypromine

Reactions

Skin
Allergic reactions (sic) (<1%)
Angioedema (<1%)
Dermatitis
  (1995): Li LF+, *Contact Dermatitis* 33, 50
Diaphoresis
Edema (<1%)
Erythema
Exanthems
Lichenoid eruption
Lupus erythematosus
Peripheral edema
Photosensitivity
Purpura
Rash (sic) (<1%)
Urticaria
Vasculitis
  (1984): Ekenstam E+, *Arch Dermatol* 120, 484

Mucosal/ENT
Dysgeusia
  (1997): Neufeld-Kaiser W+, *Arch Dermatol* 133, 251
Tinnitus
Xerostomia (1–10%)
  (1990): Kardinal CG+, *Cancer* 65, 2657
  (1990): Pontius EB, *J Clin Psychopharmacol* 8, 230

Other
Anaphylactoid reactions/Anaphylaxis
Myalgia/Myositis/Myopathy/Myotoxicity (<1%)
Paresthesias (<1%)

CYTARABINE

Synonyms: arabinosylcytosine; ara-C
Trade names: Alexan; Arabitin; Arace; Aracytine; Cytarbel; Cytosar; Cytosar-U (Sicor); Uducil
Indications: Leukemias
Category: Antimetabolite; Antineoplastic; Antiviral
Half-life: initial: 10–15 minutes
Clinically important, potentially hazardous interactions with: aldesleukin

Note: Vasculitis, a part of the cytarabine syndrome, consists of fever, malaise, myalgia, conjunctivitis, arthralgia and a diffuse erythematous maculopapular eruption that occurs from 6 to 12 hours following the administration of the drug

Reactions

Skin

Acral erythema
(2002): Cetkovska P+, *J Eur Acad Dermatol Venereol* 16(5), 481
(2001): Takeuchi M+, *Rinsho Ketsueki* 42(3), 216
(1999): Azurdia RM+, *Clin Exp Dermatol* 24, 64
(1998): Calista D+, *J Eur Acad Dermatol Venereol* 10, 274
(1997): Arranz FR+, *Arch Dermatol* 133, 499
(1997): Demircay Z+, *Int J Dermatol* 36, 593
(1997): Whitlock JA+, *Leukemia* 11(2), 185 (4 cases) (with etopside)
(1995): Dechaufour F+, *Ann Dermatol Venereol* (French) 120, 219
(1992): Doll DC+, *Semin Oncol* 19(5), 580
(1992): Rongioletti F+, *J Am Acad Dermatol* 26, 284
(1991): Brown J+, *J Am Acad Dermatol* 24, 1023
(1991): Rongioletti F+, *J Cutan Pathol* 18, 453
(1989): Alexander J, *Oncol Nurs Forum* 16, 829
(1989): Kroll SS+, *Ann Plast Surg* 23, 263
(1989): Oksenhendler E+, *Eur J Cancer Clin Oncol* 25, 1181
Actinic keratoses (with pruritus and erythema)
(1989): Kerker BJ+, *Semin Dermatol* 8, 173
Acute febrile neutrophilic dermatosis (Sweet's syndrome)
(1993): Torri O+, *Ann Dermatol Venereol* (French) 120, 884
Acute generalized exanthematous pustulosis (AGEP)
(2002): Chiu A+, *J Am Acad Dermatol* 47(4), 633
Bullous dermatitis
(1992): Richards C+, *Oncol Nurs Forum* 19, 1191
Desquamation
(1992): Richards C+, *Oncol Nurs Forum* 19, 1191
Edema
Ephelides (1–10%)
Erythema
(2002): Tay J, *CMAJ* 167(6), 672
(1998): Taverna C+, *Schweiz Med Wochenschr* (German) 128, 1117
(1992): Richards C+, *Oncol Nurs Forum* 19, 1191
(1990): Krulder JWM+, *Eur J Cancer* 26, 649
Erythroderma (generalized)
(1988): Benson PM+, *J Assoc Military Derm* XIV, 28 (passim)
Exanthems
(2002): Cetkovska P+, *J Eur Acad Dermatol Venereol* 16(5), 481 (44.4%)
(2002): Chiu A+, *J Am Acad Dermatol* 47(4), 633
(1988): Benson PM+, *J Assoc Military Derm* XIV, 28
(1986): Morant R+, *Schweiz Med Wochenschr* (German) 116, 1415 (60%)
(1983): Herzig RH+, *Blood* 62, 361 (1–5%)
(1983): Shah SS+, *Cancer Treat Rep* 67, 405
Exfoliative dermatitis
(1989): Williams SF+, *Br J Haematol* 73, 274
Hand–foot syndrome
(2002): Crawford JH+, *Eur J Haematol* 69(5), 315
(1997): Whitlock JA+, *Leukemia* 11(2), 185 (with etoposide)
(1993): Cohen PR, *Cutis* 51(3), 175
(1993): Waltzer JF+, *Arch Dermatol* 129, 43 (bullous variety)
(1991): Baack BR+, *J Am Acad Dermatol* 24, 457
(1989): Kampmann KK+, *Cancer* 63, 2482 (bullous variety)
(1988): Shall L+, *Br J Dermatol* 119, 249
(1986): Crider MK+, *Arch Dermatol* 122, 1023 (>5%)
(1985): Baer MR+, *Ann Intern Med* 102, 556 (bullous variety)
(1985): Cardonnier C+, *Ann Intern Med* 97, 783
(1985): Levine LE+, *Arch Dermatol* 121, 102
(1985): Peters WG+, *Ann Intern Med* 103, 805 (bullous variety)
(1985): Walker IR+, *Arch Dermatol* 121(10), 1240 (10–67%) (dose-related)
(1983): Herzig RH+, *Blood* 62, 361 (1–5%)

(1982): Burgdorf WHC+, *Ann Intern Med* 97, 61
Herpes zoster
Neutrophilic dermatosis
(2008): Uhara H+, *J Am Acad Dermatol* 59(2), S10 (with idarubicin)
Neutrophilic eccrine hidradenitis
(2007): Srivastava M+, *J Am Acad Dermatol* 56(4), 693
(1997): Jegasothy SM+, Pittsburgh, American Academy of Dermatology Meeting (SF) (gross and microscopic)
(1995): Kanzaki H+, *J Dermatol* 22, 137
(1993): Nikkels AF+, *Acta Clin Belg* 48(6), 397
(1993): Thorisdottir K+, *J Am Acad Dermatol* 28, 775
(1992): Bernstein EF+, *Br J Dermatol* 127, 529 (recurrent)
(1991): Vion B+, *Dermatologica* 183, 70
(1990): Hurt MA+, *Arch Dermatol* 126, 73
(1989): Bailey DL+, *Pediatr Dermatol* 6, 33
(1989): Kerker BJ+, *Semin Dermatol* 8, 173
(1987): Katsanis E+, *Am J Pediatr Hematol Oncol* 9, 204
(1984): Flynn TC+, *J Am Acad Dermatol* 11, 584
Petechiae
(1998): Taverna C+, *Schweiz Med Wochenschr* (German) 128, 1117
Photo-recall
(2006): Kaya TI+, *J Eur Acad Dermatol Venereol* 20(3), 353 (with methotrexate)
Pruritus (1–10%)
Rash (sic) (>10%)
(2002): Cetkovska P+, *J Eur Acad Dermatol Venereol* 16(5), 481 (40–73%)
Seborrheic keratoses (inflammation of) (Leser–Trélat syndrome)
(1999): Williams JV+, *J Am Acad Dermatol* 40, 643
Squamous syringometaplasia
(1990): Bhawan J+, *Am J Dermatopathol* 12, 1
Toxic epidermal necrolysis
(2001): Özkan A+, *Pediatr Dermatol* 18(1), 38
(1998): Figueiredo MS+, *Rev Assoc Med Bras* (Portuguese) 44, 53
Ulcerations
Urticaria
(2002): Cetkovska P+, *J Eur Acad Dermatol Venereol* 16(5), 481
Vasculitis
(1998): Ahmed I+, *Mayo Clin Proc* 73, 239
(1989): Kerker BJ+, *Semin Dermatol* 8, 173
(1989): Williams SF+, *Br J Haematol* 73, 274

Mucosal/ENT

Oral lesions
(1986): Morant R+, *Schweiz Med Wochenschr* (German) 116, 1415 (1–5%)
Oral ulceration (>10%)
Perianal ulcerations (>10%)
Stomatitis
(1988): Benson PM+, *J Assoc Military Derm* XIV, 28 (passim)

Hair

Hair – alopecia (1–10%)
(1988): Benson PM+, *J Assoc Military Derm* XIV, 28 (passim)
(1986): Morant R+, *Schweiz Med Wochenschr* (German) 116, 1415 (100%)

Nails

Nails – leukonychia
(1990): Bader-Meunier B+, *Ann Pediatr Paris* (French) 37, 337
Nails – Mees' lines
(1982): Jeanmougin M+, *Ann Dermatol Venereol* (French) 109, 169

Eyes

Conjunctivitis
(2006): Matteucci P+, *Haematologica* 91(2), 255

Other

Anaphylactoid reactions/Anaphylaxis
 (1997): Blanca M+, *Allergy* 52, 1009
 (1989): Williams SF+, *Br J Haematol* 73, 274
 (1980): Rassiga AL+, *Arch Intern Med* 104, 425
Cardiotoxicity
 (2006): Hengel CL+, *Heart Lung Circ* 15(1), 59
Headache
 (2006): *Prescrire Int* 15(81), 11
Hypersensitivity
 (1992): Weiss RB, *Semin Oncol* 19, 458
Infections
 (1997): Whitlock JA+, *Leukemia* 11(2), 185 (39%) (with
  etopside)
Injection-site cellulitis (1–10%)
Myalgia/Myositis/Myopathy/Myotoxicity (1–10%)
Neurotoxicity
 (2006): Nakajima D+, *No To Hattatsu* 38(3), 195
 (2006): Saito T+, *J Infect Chemother* 12(3), 148
Rhabdomyolysis
 (2002): Truica CI+, *Am J Hematol* 70(4), 320
 (1997): Morales-Polanco M+, *Arch Med Res* 28(3), 377 (5 cases)
 (1987): Margolis D+, *Cancer Treat Rep* 71(12), 1325
Thrombophlebitis (>10%)

DACARBAZINE

Synonym: DIC
Trade names: D.T.I.C; Dacatic; Deticene; Detimedac; DTIC-Dome (Bayer)
Indications: Malignant melanoma, carcinomas
Category: Alkylating agent; Antineoplastic
Half-life: Initial: 20–40 minutes
Clinically important, potentially hazardous interactions with: aldesleukin

Reactions

Skin

Actinic keratoses
 (1987): Johnson TM+, *J Am Acad Dermatol* 17(2 Pt 1), 192
Angioedema
 (1981): Wassilew SW+, *Hautarzt* (German) 32 (Suppl 5), 453
Erythema
Exanthems
 (1981): Wassilew SW+, *Hautarzt* (German) 32 (Suppl 5), 453
Fixed eruption
 (1982): Koehn GG+, *Arch Dermatol* 118, 1018
Photo-recall
 (2001): Kennedy RD+, *Clin Oncol (R Coll Radiol)* 13(6), 470
Photosensitivity (<1%)
 (2004): Treudler R+, *J Am Acad Dermatol* 50(5), 783
 (1989): Serrano G+, *Photodermatol* 6, 140
 (1982): Koehn GG+, *Arch Dermatol* 118, 1018
 (1981): Bonifazi E+, *Contact Dermatitis* 7, 161
 (1981): Wassilew SW+, *Hautarzt* (German) 32 (Suppl 5), 453
 (1981): Yung CW+, *J Am Acad Dermatol* 4, 541
 (1980): Beck TM+, *Cancer Treat Rep* 64, 725
 (1980): Bolling R+, *Hautarzt* (German) 31, 602
 (1980): Ippen H, *Dtsch Med Wochenschr* (German) 105, 531
 (1980): Kunze J+, *Z Hautkr* (German) 55, 100
Phototoxicity
 (2006): Schmutz JL+, *Ann Dermatol Venereol* 133(5 Pt 1), 500
Rash (sic) (1–10%)
 (2004): Buesa JM+, *Cancer* 101(10), 2261 (with gemcitabine)

Urticaria
 (1995): Bourry C+, *Therapie* (French) 50, 588
 (1981): Wassilew SW+, *Hautarzt* (German) 32 (Suppl 5), 453
Vasculitis

Mucosal/ENT

Dysgeusia (1–10%) (metallic taste)
Stomatitis (48%)
 (2004): Buesa JM+, *Cancer* 101(10), 2261 (with gemcitabine)

Hair

Hair – alopecia (1–10%)
 (2004): Buesa JM+, *Cancer* 101(10), 2261 (with gemcitabine)

Nails

Nails – pigmentation
 (1984): Daniel CR+, *J Am Acad Dermatol* 10, 250

Other

Anaphylactoid reactions/Anaphylaxis (1–10%)
Asthenia (75%)
 (2004): Buesa JM+, *Cancer* 101(10), 2261 (with gemcitabine)
Death
 (2001): Ramanathan RK+, *Ann Oncol* 12(8), 1139
Depression
 (2001): Ramanathan RK+, *Ann Oncol* 12(8), 1139
Fever
 (2004): Buesa JM+, *Cancer* 101(10), 2261 (with gemcitabine)
Headache
Hypersensitivity
 (2006): Levy A+, *Ann Dermatol Venereol* 133(2), 157 (20%)
 (1992): Weiss RB, *Semin Oncol* 19, 458
Injection-site burning (>10%)
Injection-site cellulitis
 (1989): Kerker BJ+, *Semin Dermatol* 8, 173
Injection-site dermatitis
 (1987): Dufresne RG, *Cutis* 39, 197
Injection-site necrosis (>10%)
 (1987): Dufresne RG, *Cutis* 39, 197
Injection-site pain (>10%)
Injection-site phlebitis
 (1989): Kerker BJ+, *Semin Dermatol* 8, 173
Myalgia/Myositis/Myopathy/Myotoxicity (1–10%)
Paresthesias (facial)
Rhabdomyolysis
 (1995): Anderlini P+, *Cancer* 76(4), 678

DACLIZUMAB

Trade name: Zenapax (Roche)
Indications: Transplant rejection
Category: Immunosupressant; Monoclonal antibody
Half-life: N/A
Clinically important, potentially hazardous interactions with: corticosteroids, cyclosporine, **hemophilus B vaccine**, methylprednisolone, mycophenolate, prednisolone

Reactions

Skin

Acne
Cellulitis
Pruritus
Rash (sic)
Urticaria

Other
  Application-site reactions
  Hypersensitivity
  Infections
    (2004): Huang XS+, *Di Yi Jun Yi Da Xue Xue Bao* 24(2), 126

DACTINOMYCIN

Synonyms: ACT; actinomycin D
Trade names: Ac-De; Cosmegen (Merck); Cosmegen Lyovac; Lyovac
Indications: Melanomas, sarcomas
Category: Antibiotic, anthracycline
Half-life: 36 hours
Clinically important, potentially hazardous interactions with: aldesleukin

Reactions

Skin
  Acne (>10%)
    (1993): Blatt J+, *Med Pediatr Oncol* 21, 373
    (1983): Bronner AK+, *J Am Acad Dermatol* 9, 645
    (1982): Dunagin WG, *Semin Oncol* 9, 14
  Actinic keratoses
    (1987): Johnson TM+, *J Am Acad Dermatol* 17(2 Pt 1), 192
  Bullous pemphigoid
    (1982): Amer MH+, *Int J Dermatol* 21, 32
  Cellulitis
    (1989): Kerker BJ+, *Semin Dermatol* 8, 173
  Dermatitis
  Erythema
    (1997): Coppes MJ+, *Med Pediatr Oncol* 29, 226
  Erythema multiforme
  Exanthems
  Folliculitis
    (1981): Henkes J+, *Actas Dermosifiliogr* (Spanish) 72, 469
  Keratoses (reactivation of)
    (1989): Kerker BJ+, *Semin Dermatol* 8, 173
  Lichenoid eruption
    (2006): Ridola V+, *Pediatr Dermatol* 23(5), 503
  Photo-recall (>10%)
    (1997): Coppes MJ+, *Med Pediatr Oncol* 29, 226
  Pigmentation
    (2000): Marcoux D+, *J Am Acad Dermatol* 43, 540 (with vincristine)
    (1995): Kanwar VS+, *Med Pediatr Oncol* 24, 329
  Pruritus
    (2006): Ridola V+, *Pediatr Dermatol* 23(5), 503
    (1989): Kerker BJ+, *Semin Dermatol* 8, 173
  Pustules
    (1983): Bronner AK+, *J Am Acad Dermatol* 9, 645
  Toxic epidermal necrolysis
  Urticaria

Mucosal/ENT
  Cheilitis
  Oral lesions
    (1983): Bronner AK+, *J Am Acad Dermatol* 9, 645 (>5%)
  Stomatitis (ulcerative) (>5%)

Hair
  Hair – alopecia (>10%)

Other
  Anaphylactoid reactions/Anaphylaxis (<1%)

Injection-site extravasation (>10%)
  (1997): Coppes MJ+, *Med Pediatr Oncol* 29, 226
Injection-site necrosis (>10%)
  (1987): Dufresne RG, *Cutis* 39, 197
Injection-site phlebitis (>10%)
Myalgia/Myositis/Myopathy/Myotoxicity
Phlebitis
  (1989): Kerker BJ+, *Semin Dermatol* 8, 173

DALTEPARIN

Trade names: Fragmin (Pfizer); Fragmine
Indications: Prophylaxis of deep vein thrombosis
Category: Heparin, low molecular weight
Half-life: 4–8 hours
Clinically important, potentially hazardous interactions with: butabarbital, danaparoid

Reactions

Skin
  Allergic reactions (sic) (1–10%)
    (2003): Myers B+, *Blood Coagul Fibrinolysis* 14(5), 485
    (1999): Ensom MH+, *Pharmacotherapy* 19(9), 1013
    (1993): Phillips JK+, *Br J Haematol* 84(2), 349
  Bullous dermatitis (1–10%)
    (1999): Tong, M, Kota Kinabalu, Malaysia (from Internet) (observation)
  Exanthems (<1%)
  Necrosis
  Pruritus (1–10%)
  Rash (sic) (1–10%)

Hair
  Hair – alopecia
    (2001): Apsner R+, *Blood* 97(9), 2914–5
    (2000): Barnes C, *Blood* 96, 1618

Other
  Anaphylactoid reactions/Anaphylaxis (1–10%)
    (2001): Ueda A+, *Nephron* 87(1), 93
  Injection-site edema
    (2000): Szolar-Platzer C+, *J Am Acad Dermatol* 43, 920
  Injection-site hematoma (1–10%)
  Injection-site pain (1–10%)
  Injection-site pruritus
    (2000): Szolar-Platzer C+, *J Am Acad Dermatol* 43, 920

DAN-SHEN

Scientific name: *Salvia miltiorrhiza*
Family: Labiatae; Lamiaceae
Trade and other common names: Huang Ken; Red Rooted Sage; Red Sage; Salvia Root; Tzu Tan-Ken
Category: Food supplement; Platelet aggregation inhibitor
Purported indications and other uses: Circulation problems, ischemic stroke, angina pectoris, menstrual problems, chronic hepatitis, abdominal masses, insomnia, acne, psoriasis, eczema, bruising, hearing loss
Half-life: N/A
Clinically important, potentially hazardous interactions with: digoxin, warfarin

Reactions

Skin
Pruritus

DANAPAROID

Trade name: Orgaran (Organon)
Indications: Prevention of postoperative deep thrombosis
Category: Anticoagulant; Heparinoid
Half-life: ~24 hours
**Clinically important, potentially hazardous interactions
with:** butabarbital, dalteparin, enoxaparin, heparin

Reactions

Skin
Allergic reactions (sic) (<1%)
  (2000): de Saint-Blanquat L+, *Ann Fr Anesth Reanim* 19, 751
Edema (2.6%)
Peripheral edema (3.3%)
Pruritus (3.9%)
Purpura
Rash (sic) (2.1–4.8%)
  (1999): Wutschert R+, *Drug Saf* 20, 515

Other
Infections (2.1%)
Injection-site hematoma (5%)
Injection-site pain (7.6–13.7%)
Injection-site plaques
  (2000): Koch P+, *J Am Acad Dermatol* 42, 612
  (2000): Martin L+, *Contact Dermatitis* 42, 295
  (2000): Szolar-Platzer C+, *J Am Acad Dermatol* 43, 920
Injection-site reactions
  (2001): Figarella I+, *Ann Dermatol Venereol* 128, 35
Paresthesias

DANAZOL

Trade names: Azol; Bonzol; Cyclomen; D-Zol; Danocrine;
Danol; Ladogal; Winobanin; Zoldan-A
Indications: Endometriosis, fibrocystic breast disease
Category: Pituitary hormone inhibitor
Half-life: ~4.5 hours
**Clinically important, potentially hazardous interactions
with:** acenocoumarol, acitretin, cyclosporine, insulin detemir,
oral contraceptives, tacrolimus, warfarin

Reactions

Skin
Acne (>10%)
  (1982): Madanes AE+, *Ann Intern Med* 96, 625 (20%)
  (1980): Hosea SW+, *Ann Intern Med* 93, 809 (8%)
Angioedema
  (1993): Litt JZ, Beachwood, OH (personal case) (observation)
  (1988): Guillet G+, *Dermatologica* 177, 370
Diaphoresis (3%)
Edema (>10%)
Erythema multiforme
  (1992): Reynolds NJ+, *Clin Exp Dermatol* 17, 140

  (1988): Gately LE+, *Ann Intern Med* 109, 85
Exanthems
  (1993): Litt JZ, Beachwood, OH (personal case) (observation)
  (1989): Ahn YS+, *Ann Intern Med* 111, 723 (6%)
  (1982): Madanes AE+, *Ann Intern Med* 96, 625
Lupus erythematosus
  (1994): Yung RL+, *Rheum Dis Clin North Am* 20, 61
  (1991): Sassolas B+, *Br J Dermatol* 125, 190
  (1988): Guillet G+, *Dermatologica* 177, 370
  (1982): Fretwell MD, *Allergy Clin Immunol* 69, 306
Lymphomatoid papulosis
  (1985): Wise C+, *Fertil Steril* 44, 702
Petechiae
Photosensitivity (<1%)
Pruritus
  (1989): Ahn YS+, *Ann Intern Med* 111, 723 (3.5%)
Purpura
  (1990): Taillan B+, *Presse Med* (French) 19, 721
Rash (sic) (3%)
Seborrhea
  (1989): Ahn YS+, *Ann Intern Med* 111, 723
  (1982): Madanes AE+, *Ann Intern Med* 96, 625 (30%)
  (1981): Duff P+, *Am J Obstet Gynecol* 141, 349 (passim)
Stevens–Johnson syndrome
Urticaria
Vesiculation

Mucosal/ENT
Candidal vaginitis (<1%)
Gingivitis
Vaginal dryness

Hair
Hair – alopecia
  (1989): Ahn YS+, *Ann Intern Med* 111, 723 (3.5%)
  (1981): Duff P+, *Am J Obstet Gynecol* 141, 349
  (1980): Hosea SW+, *Ann Intern Med* 93, 809 (17%)
Hair – hirsutism (<10%)
  (2004): Zawar V+, *Cutis* 74(5), 301
  (1991): Bates GW+, *Clin Obstet Gynecol* 34, 848
  (1989): Ahn YS+, *Ann Intern Med* 111, 723 (3.5%)
  (1982): Madanes AE+, *Ann Intern Med* 96, 625 (7%)
  (1980): Hosea SW+, *Ann Intern Med* 93, 809 (8%)

Other
Death
  (2001): Hayashi T+, *J Gastroenterol* 36(11), 783
Paresthesias
Rhabdomyolysis
  (2003): Andreou ER+, *Can J Clin Pharmacol* 10(4), 172 (with
   simvastatin)
  (1994): Dallaire M+, *CMAJ* 150(12), 1991 (with lovastatin)

DANTROLENE

Trade names: Dantamacrin; Dantrium (Procter & Gamble);
Dantrolen
Indications: Spasticity, malignant hyperthermia
Category: Skeletal muscle relaxant, hydantoin
Half-life: 8.7 hours
**Clinically important, potentially hazardous interactions
with:** verapamil

Reactions

Skin

Acne
(1981): Pembroke AC+, *Br J Dermatol* 104, 465
(1980): Dykes MHM, *JAMA* 231, 862
Dermatitis
Diaphoresis
Erythema
Exanthems
(1980): Dykes MHM, *JAMA* 231, 862
Jaundice
(1990): Chan CH, *Neurology* 40(9), 1427
Photosensitivity
Pruritus
Rash (sic) (>10%)
Urticaria

Mucosal/ENT

Dysgeusia

Hair

Hair – hypertrichosis

Other

Anaphylactoid reactions/Anaphylaxis
Asthenia
(1995): Wedel DJ+, *Mayo Clin Proc* 70(3), 241
Chills (1–10%)
Death
(1990): Chan CH, *Neurology* 40(9), 1427
(1980): Cornette M+, *Acta Neurol Belg* 80(6), 336
Headache
Myalgia/Myositis/Myopathy/Myotoxicity
(1995): Wedel DJ+, *Mayo Clin Proc* 70(3), 241
Thrombophlebitis
Tremor
Vertigo
(1995): Wedel DJ+, *Mayo Clin Proc* 70(3), 241

DAPSONE

Trade names: Avlosulfon; Dapson; Dapson-Fatol; Maloprim (Combination); Protogen; Sulfona
Indications: Leprosy, dermatitis herpetiformis
Category: Antibiotic; Antimycobacterial
Half-life: 10–50 hours
Clinically important, potentially hazardous interactions with: chloroquine, didanosine, furazolidone, ganciclovir, hydroxychloroquine, methotrexate, pyrimethamine, rifabutin, rifampin, sulfonamides

Note: A hypersensitivity reaction – termed the "sulfone syndrome" or "dapsone syndrome" – may infrequently develop during the first six weeks of treatment. This syndrome consists of exfoliative dermatitis, fever, malaise, nausea, anorexia, hepatitis, jaundice, lymphadenopathy and hemolytic anemia. See (1982): Kromann NP+, *Arch Dermatol* 118, 531

Reactions

Skin

Bullous dermatitis (<1%)
(1984): Alarcon GS+, *Arthritis Rheum* 27, 1071
Cyanosis
(1981): Editorial, *Lancet* 2, 184

Dapsone syndrome
(2006): Sener O+, *J Investig Allergol Clin Immunol* 16(4), 268
(2005): Agrawal S+, *J Dermatol* 32(11), 883
(2005): Alves-Rodrigues EN+, *Am J Kidney Dis* 46(4), e51
(2004): Bucaretchi F+, *Rev Inst Med Trop Sao Paulo* 46(6), 331
(2003): Itha S+, *BMC Gastroenterol* 3, 21
(1998): Kumar RH+, *Indian J Lepr* 70, 271 (17 cases)
(1997): McKenna KE+, *Br J Dermatol* 137, 657
(1994): Barnard GF+, *Am J Gastroenterol* 89, 2057
(1994): Hiran S+, *J Assoc Physicians India* 42, 497
(1994): Risse L+, *Ann Dermatol Venereol* (French) 121, 242
(1994): Saito S+, *Clin Exp Dermatol* 19, 152
(1994): Stephen G+, *J Assoc Physicians India* 42, 72
(1992): Kraus A+, *J Rheumatol* 19, 178
(1991): Ramanan C+, *Indian J Lepr* 63, 226
(1988): Grayson ML+, *Lancet* 1, 531
(1987): Khare AK+, *Indian J Lepr* 59, 106
(1985): Sharma VK+, *Indian J Lepr* 57, 807
(1982): Kromann NP+, *Arch Dermatol* 118, 531
(1981): Tomecki KJ+, *Arch Dermatol* 117, 38
Epidermolysis bullosa
(1992): Kong LN, *Chung Hua Li Tsa Chih* (Chinese) 27, 495
Erythema multiforme (<1%)
(2001): Werth V, *Dermatology Times* 15
(1994): Pertel P+, *Clin Infect Dis* 18, 630
(1993): Stern RS, *Arch Dermatol* 129, 301 (passim)
(1981): Frey HM+, *Ann Intern Med* 94, 777
(1980): Dutta RK, *Lepr India* 52, 306
Erythema nodosum
(1993): Stern RS, *Arch Dermatol* 129, 301 (passim)
(1981): Editorial, *Lancet* 2, 184
Erythroderma
(1989): Patki AH+, *Lepr Rev* 60, 274
Exanthems (1–5%)
(2002): Thong BY+, *Ann Allergy Asthma Immunol* 88(5), 527 (with pyrimethamine)
(2001): Werth V, *Dermatology Times* 15
(1993): Stern RS, *Arch Dermatol* 129, 301 (passim)
(1986): Lindskov R+, *Dermatologica* 172, 214 (6%)
(1981): Frey HM+, *Ann Intern Med* 94, 777
(1981): Tomecki KJ+, *Arch Dermatol* 117, 38
Exfoliative dermatitis (<1%)
(1993): Stern RS, *Arch Dermatol* 129, 301 (passim)
(1981): Frey HM+, *Ann Intern Med* 94, 777
(1981): Tomecki KJ+, *Arch Dermatol* 117, 38
(1980): Lal S+, *Lepr India* 52, 302
Fixed eruption
(1988): Tham SN+, *Singapore Med J* 29, 300
(1982): Sinha MR, *Lepr India* 54, 152
Lichenoid eruption
Lupus erythematosus (<1%)
(1992): Kraus A+, *J Rheumatol* 19, 178
(1984): Alarcon GS+, *Arthritis Rheum* 27, 1071 (bullous)
Photosensitivity (<1%)
(2001): Stockel S+, *Eur J Dermatol* 11(1), 50
(1994): Berger TG+, *Arch Dermatol* 130, 609 (in HIV-infected) (4 cases)
(1989): Dhanapaul S, *Lepr Rev* 60, 147
(1988): Fumey SM+, *Z Hautkr* (German) 63, 53
(1987): Joseph MS, *Lepr Rev* 58, 425
Pigmentation
(1997): David KP+, *Trans R Soc Trop Med Hyg* 91, 204 (hyperpigmented dermal macules)
Pruritus
Purpura
Rash (sic)
(2000): Chogle A+, *Indian J Gastroenterol* 19, 85
(1996): Beumont MG+, *Am J Med* 100, 611
Scleroderma

(1990): May DG+, *Clin Pharm Ther* 48, 286
Stevens–Johnson syndrome
  (1994): Pertel P+, *Clin Infect Dis* 18, 630
Subcorneal pustular dermatosis (Sneddon-Wilkinson)
  (2001): Kishimoto K+, *Eur J Dermatol* 11(1), 41
Toxic epidermal necrolysis (<1%)
  (1993): Fitzpatrick TB+, *Dermatologic Capsule and Comment*
    15, 10 (observation)
  (1993): Stern RS, *Arch Dermatol* 129, 301 (passim)
  (1988): Phillips-Howard PA+, *Br Med J Clin Res Ed* 296, 1605
  (1983): Katoch K+, *Lepr India* 55, 133
  (1981): Editorial, *Lancet* 2, 184
Toxic erythema
  (1993): Stern RS, *Arch Dermatol* 129, 301 (passim)
Urticaria

Mucosal/ENT
Oral mucosal eruption
  (1981): Frey HM+, *Ann Intern Med* 94, 777
Oral pigmentation
Tinnitus

Nails
Nails – Beau's lines (transverse nail bands)
  (1989): Patki AH+, *Lepr Rev* 60, 274
  (1988): Grayson ML+, *Lancet* 1, 531
  (1984): Daniel CR+, *J Am Acad Dermatol* 10, 250

Eyes
Myopia
  (2006): Gopalani VV+, *Indian J Dermatol Venereol Leprol*
    72(6), 455

Other
DRESS syndrome
  (2003): Itha S+, *BMC Gastroenterol* 3(1), 21
Headache
Hypersensitivity
  (2006): Takahashi H+, *Clin Exp Dermatol* 31(1), 33
  (2006): Teo RY+, *Ann Acad Med Singapore* 35(11), 833 (with
    pyrimethamine)
  (2005): Agrawal S+, *J Dermatol* 32(11), 883
  (2003): Leslie KS+, *Clin Exp Dermatol* 28(5), 496
  (2002): Thong BY+, *Ann Allergy Asthma Immunol* 88(5), 527
    (with pyrimethamine)
  (2001): Rao PN+, *Lepr Rev* 72(1), 57
  (2001): Werth V, *Dermatology Times* 15
  (2000): Chogle A+, *Indian J Gastroenterol* 19, 85
  (1998): Holtzer CD+, *Pharmacotherapy* 18(4), 831
  (1998): Pei-Lin Ng P+, *J Am Acad Dermatol* 39, 646
  (1998): Schlienger RG+, *Epilepsia* 39, S3 (passim)
  (1998): Siegfried EC+, *J Am Acad Dermatol* 39, 797 (passim)
  (1996): Prussick R+, *J Am Acad Dermatol* 35, 346
  (1995): Bocquet H+, *Ann Dermatol Venereol* (French) 122, 514
  (1984): Mohamed KN, *Lepr Rev* 55, 385
Nephrotoxicity
  (2005): Alves-Rodrigues EN+, *Am J Kidney Dis* 46(4), e51
Nodular panniculitis
  (1986): Uplekar MW+, *Indian J Lepr* 58, 286
Porphyria cutanea tarda
  (1992): Shelley WB+, *Advanced Dermatologic Diagnosis* WB
    Saunders, 414 (passim)
Pseudolymphoma
  (1993): Kerl H+, *Dermatology In General Medicine* McGraw-Hill
    New York

DAPTOMYCIN

Trade name: Cubicin (Cubist)
Indications: Complicated skin & skin structure infections
Category: Antibiotic, glycopeptide
Half-life: ~8 hours
**Clinically important, potentially hazardous interactions
with:** HMG-CoA reductase inhibitors, warfarin

Reactions

Skin
Cellulitis (1–2%)
Eczema (<1%)
Edema (1–2%)
Erythema
Fungal dermatitis (2.6%)
Pruritus (2.8%)
  (2004): Spencer L, Crawfordsville, IN (with vancomycin) (from
    Internet) (observation)
Rash (sic) (4.3%)

Mucosal/ENT
Dysgeusia (<1%)
Stomatitis (<1%)

Other
Abdominal pain (1–2%)
Asthenia (<1%)
Cough (1–2%)
Fever (1.9%)
Headache (5.4%)
  (2004): Jeu L+, *Clin Ther* 26(11), 1728
Hypersensitivity (<1%)
Injection-site reactions (5.8%)
  (2004): Jeu L+, *Clin Ther* 26(11), 1728
Myalgia/Myositis/Myopathy/Myotoxicity (<1%)
  (2005): Echevarria K+, *J Antimicrob Chemother* 55(4), 599
  (2004): Veligandla SR+, *Ann Pharmacother* 38(11), 1860
Paresthesias (<1%)
Rhabdomyolysis
  (2006): Kazory A+, *J Antimicrob Chemother* 57(3), 578
  (2006): Papadopoulos S+, *Clin Infect Dis* 42(12), e108
Vertigo (2.2%)

DARBEPOETIN ALFA

Synonym: Erythropoiesis stimulating protein
Trade name: Aranesp (Amgen)
Indications: Anemia associated with renal failure and
chemotherapy
Category: Colony stimulating factor; Erythropoietin
Half-life: Terminal: I.V. = 21 hours

Reactions

Skin
Edema (21%)
  (2003): Cvetkovic RS+, *Drugs* 63(11), 1067
Peripheral edema (11%)
Pruritus (8%)
Rash (sic) (7%)
  (2003): Cvetkovic RS+, *Drugs* 63(11), 1067
Urticaria

Other
Abdominal pain (12%)
Asthenia (9–33%)
Cough (10%)
Death (7%)
Fever (9–19%)
Headache
Infections
Injection-site pain (7%)
Myalgia/Myositis/Myopathy/Myotoxicity (21%)
Seizures (<1%)
Thrombosis
  (2006): Bohlius J+, *J Natl Cancer Inst* 98(10), 708
  (2005): *Prescrire Int* 14(79), 174 (6%)
Upper respiratory infection (14%)
Vertigo (8–14%)

DARIFENACIN

Trade name: Enablex (Novartis)
Indications: Overactive bladder
Category: Muscarinic antagonist
Half-life: 13–19 hours
Clinically important, potentially hazardous interactions with: flecainide, imipramine, potent CYP3A4 inhibitors, thioridazine, tricyclic antidepressants

Reactions

Skin
Peripheral edema (~1%)
Pruritus (~1%)
Rash (sic) (~1%)
Xerosis (~1%)

Mucosal/ENT
Vaginitis (~1%)
Xerostomia (20%)
  (2006): Haab F+, *BJU Int* 98(5), 1025
  (2006): Hill S+, *Int Urogynecol J Pelvic Floor Dysfunct* 17(3), 239
  (2006): Zinner N+, *Int J Clin Pract* 60(1), 119
  (2005): *Med Lett Drugs Ther* 14;47(1204), 23
  (2005): Chapple C+, *BJU Int* 95(7), 993
  (2005): Steers W+, *BJU Int* 95(4), 580
  (2004): Sand PK, *J Am Acad Nurse Pract* 16(10 Suppl), 8

Eyes
Vision blurred
Visual disturbances (~1%)
Xerophthalmia

Other
Abdominal pain (2.4%)
Asthenia
Chills
Cough
Headache
Paresthesias
Vertigo

DARUNAVIR

Synonym: TMC-114
Trade name: Prezista (Tibotec)
Indications: HIV infection
Category: Antiretroviral; Protease inhibitor
Half-life: 15 hours
Clinically important, potentially hazardous interactions with: astemizole, carbamazepine, cisapride, dihydroergotamine, ergotamine, lovastatin, midazolam, phenobarbital, phenytoin, pimozide, pravastatin, rifampin, saquinavir, simvastatin, **St John's wort**, terfenadine, triazolam

Note: Darunavir is a sulfonamide and can be absorbed systemically. Sulfonamides can produce severe, possibly fatal, reactions such as toxic epidermal necrolysis and Stevens–Johnson syndrome

Reactions

Skin
Dermatitis (with ritonavir)
Eczema (with ritonavir)
Erythema multiforme (with ritonavir)
Exanthems (with ritonavir)
Folliculitis (with ritonavir)
Hyperhidrosis (with ritonavir)
Peripheral edema (with ritonavir)
Rash (sic) (with ritonavir) (7%)
Stevens–Johnson syndrome (with ritonavir)

Mucosal/ENT
Xerostomia (with ritonavir)

Hair
Hair – alopecia (with ritonavir)

Other
Abdominal pain (with ritonavir) (2%)
Asthenia (with ritonavir)
Cough (with ritonavir)
Fever (with ritonavir)
Gynecomastia (with ritonavir)
Headache (with ritonavir) (4%)
Hypertension (with ritonavir)
Lipoatrophy (with ritonavir)
Myalgia/Myositis/Myopathy/Myotoxicity (with ritonavir)
Neurotoxicity (with ritonavir)
Paresthesias (with ritonavir)
Vertigo (with ritonavir)

DASATINIB

Synonym: BMS354825
Trade name: SPRYCEL (Bristol-Myers Squibb)
Indications: Leukemia (chronic myeloid), acute lymphoblastic leukemia
Category: Antineoplastic; Tyrosine kinase inhibitor
Half-life: 4–6 hours
Clinically important, potentially hazardous interactions with: atazanavir, carbamazepine, clarithromycin, dexamethasone, erythromycin, indinavir, itraconazole, ketoconazole, nefazodone, nelfinavir, phenobarbital, phenytoin, rifampicin, ritonavir, saquinavir, **St John's wort**

Reactions

Skin
Acne
Dermatitis
Hyperhidrosis
Photosensitivity
Pigmentation
Pruritus (11%)
Rash (sic) (39%)
Urticaria
Xerosis

Mucosal/ENT
Dysgeusia
Mucositis (16%)
Tinnitus

Hair
Hair – alopecia

Eyes
Conjunctivitis

Other
Abdominal pain (25%)
Anxiety
Asthenia (19%)
Cardiac failure (3%)
Chest pain (13%)
Chills (11%)
Confusion
Cough (28%)
Depression
Fever (39%)
Gynecomastia
Headache (40%)
Hypertension
Hypotension
Infections (sic)
Insomnia
Myalgia/Myositis/Myopathy/Myotoxicity (12%)
Neurotoxicity (13%)
Pain (26%)
Panniculitis
    (2006): Assouline S+, N Engl J Med 354(24), 2623
Seizures
Somnolence
Tremor
Vertigo (14%)

DAUNORUBICIN

Synonyms: daunomycin; DNR; rubidomycin
Trade names: Cerubidine; Daunoxome
Indications: Acute leukemias
Category: Antibiotic, anthracycline
Half-life: 14–20 hours
Clinically important, potentially hazardous interactions with: aldesleukin

Reactions

Skin
Angioedema
    (1983): Bronner AK+, J Am Acad Dermatol 9, 645
    (1981): Weiss RB+, Ann Intern Med 94, 66 (1–5%)
Dermatitis
    (1986): Eddy JL+, Oncol Nurs Forum 13, 9
Erythema
Exanthems
Exfoliative dermatitis
    (2004): Huang JY+, Anticancer Drugs 15(3), 239
Folliculitis
    (1997): Fournier S+, Arch Dermatol 133, 918 (disseminated)
Hand–foot syndrome
    (2000): Hui YF+, Pharmacotherapy 20(10), 1221
Hypomelanosis
Neutrophilic eccrine hidradenitis
    (1993): Nikkels AF+, Acta Clin Belg 48(6), 397
    (1993): Thorisdottir K+, J Am Acad Dermatol 28, 775
Pigmentation
    (2002): Kroumpouzos G+, J Am Acad Dermatol 46(2), S1
        (generalized)
    (1992): Anderson LL+, J Am Acad Dermatol 26, 255
    (1984): Kelly TM+, Arch Dermatol 120, 262
Pruritus
Rash (sic) (<1%)
    (2004): Huang JY+, Anticancer Drugs 15(3), 239
Urticaria (<1%)
    (1983): Bronner AK+, J Am Acad Dermatol 9, 645
    (1981): Weiss RB+, Ann Intern Med 94, 66 (1–5%)

Mucosal/ENT
Mucositis
    (2002): Fassas A+, Br J Haematol 116(2), 308
Oral lesions
    (1983): Bronner AK+, J Am Acad Dermatol 9, 645 (>5%)
Stomatitis (>10%)

Hair
Hair – alopecia (>10%)
    (1997): Fournier S+, Arch Dermatol 133, 918

Nails
Nails – pigmentation (<1%)
    (1983): James WD+, Arch Dermatol 119, 334
    (1982): Daniel CR+, Cutis 30, 348

Other
Anaphylactoid reactions/Anaphylaxis
Chills (<1%)
Congestive heart failure
    (1981): Von Hoff DD+, Cancer Treat Rep 65 Suppl 4, 19
Death
    (2002): Fassas A+, Br J Haematol 116(2), 308
Fever
    (2004): Huang JY+, Anticancer Drugs 15(3), 239
Headache
Injection-site cellulitis
    (1989): Kerker BJ+, Semin Dermatol 8, 173
Injection-site extravasation
    (2000): Kassner E, J Pediatr Oncon Nurs 17, 135
Injection-site necrosis (1–10%)
    (1987): Dufresne RG, Cutis 39, 197
Injection-site phlebitis
    (1989): Kerker BJ+, Semin Dermatol 8, 173
Injection-site ulceration (1–10%)
    (1984): Cox RF, Am J Hosp Pharm 41, 2410

DECITABINE

Synonyms: 5AZA-CdR; DAC; Aza-dC
Trade name: Dacogen (MGI Pharma)
Indications: Myelodysplastic syndromes, leukemia
Category: Antineoplastic
Half-life: ~30 minutes
Clinically important, potentially hazardous interactions with: None

Reactions

Skin
Bacterial infections (5%)
Cellulitis (12%)
Edema (18%)
Erythema (14%)
Facial edema (6%)
Hematomas (5%)
Pallor (23%)
Peripheral edema (25%)
Petechiae (39%)
Pruritus (11%)
Purpura
Rash (sic) (19%)
  (2000): Schwartsmann G+, *Invest New Drugs* 18(1), 83 (with cisplatin)
Urticaria (6%)

Mucosal/ENT
Dysphagia (6%)
Gingival bleeding (8%)
Glossodynia (5%)
Lip ulceration (5%)
Mucositis
  (2000): Schwartsmann G+, *Invest New Drugs* 18(1), 83 (with cisplatin)
  (1997): Schwartsmann G+, *Leukemia* Suppl 1, S28 (with daunorubicin)
Oral candidiasis (6%)
Sinusitis (5%)
Stomatitis (12%)
Tongue ulceration (7%)

Hair
Hair – alopecia
  (1997): Schwartsmann G+, *Leukemia* Suppl 1, S28 (with daunorubicin)

Eyes
Vision blurred (6%)

Other
Abdominal pain (14%)
Anaphylactoid reactions/Anaphylaxis
Asthenia
Chest pain
Confusion
Congestive heart failure
Cough (40%)
Depression
Fever (53%)
Headache (28%)
Hypersensitivity
Hypotension (6%)
Infections

  (2000): Wijermans P+, *J Clin Oncol* 18(5), 956
Injection-site edema (5%)
Injection-site irritation
Insomnia
Myalgia/Myositis/Myopathy/Myotoxicity (5%)
Pain (13%)
Upper respiratory infection
Vertigo (18%)

DEFERASIROX

Trade name: Exjade (Novartis)
Indications: Chronic iron overload due to blood transfusions
Category: Chelator, iron
Half-life: 8–16 hours
Clinically important, potentially hazardous interactions with: N/A

Reactions

Skin
Purpura
Rash (sic) (8%)
  (2007): Vichinsky E+, *Br J Haematol* 136(3), 501
  (2006): Cappellini MD+, *Blood* 107(9), 3455
  (2006): Vanorden HE+, *Ann Pharmacother* 40(6), 1110
Urticaria (4%)

Mucosal/ENT
Hearing loss

Eyes
Cataract
Ocular pressure
Visual disturbances

Other
Abdominal pain (14%)
  (2007): Vichinsky E+, *Br J Haematol* 136(3), 501
Asthenia (6%)
Cough (14%)
Fever
Headache (16%)
Hepatotoxicity
Upper respiratory infection (9%)

DEFEROXAMINE

Trade names: Desferal (Novartis); Desferin
Indications: Hemochromatosis, acute iron overload
Category: Chelator, iron
Half-life: 6.1 hours
Clinically important, potentially hazardous interactions with: ascorbic acid, zinc

Reactions

Skin
Acne
Angioedema
  (1984): Romeo MA+, *J Inherited Metab Dis* 7, 121
Depigmentation
  (2001): Lopez L+, *Dermatol Surg* 27(9), 795

Dermatitis
  (1988): Venencie PY+, *Ann Dermatol Venereol* (French)
    115, 1174
Edema (<1%)
Erythema (<1%)
Erythema multiforme
Exanthems
Pigmentation
Pruritus (<1%)
  (1984): Romeo MA+, *J Inherited Metab Dis* 7, 121
Purpura
Rash (sic) (<1%)
Toxic epidermal necrolysis
Urticaria (<1%)

Mucosal/ENT
Oral lesions
Ototoxicity
  (2005): Chen SH+, *J Pediatr Hematol Oncol* 27(12), 651
  (2002): Karimi M+, *Acta Haematol* 108(2), 79
  (1997): Chiodo AA+, *J Otolaryngol* 26(2), 116
  (1996): Styles LA+, *J Pediatr Hematol Oncol* 18(1), 42
  (1995): Kanno H+, *Am J Otolaryngol* 16(3), 148
  (1994): Sacco M+, *Minerva Pediatr* 46(5), 225
  (1992): de Espana R+, *An Otorrinolaringol Ibero Am* 19(4), 341
Tinnitus
  (1981): Marsh MN+, *Postgrad Med J* 57(671), 582

Eyes
Cataract
  (2004): Arora A+, *Am J Hematol* 76(4), 386
Dyschromatopsia
  (1990): Charton N+, *Bull Soc Ophtalmol Fr* 90(6-7), 599
Night blindness
  (2004): Arora A+, *Am J Hematol* 76(4), 386
  (1995): Dennerlein JA+, *Ophthalmologe* 92(1), 38
Optic neuropathy
  (2004): Arora A+, *Am J Hematol* 76(4), 386
Retinopathy
  (2006): Lai TY+, *Br J Ophthalmol* 90(2), 243
  (2004): Arora A+, *Am J Hematol* 76(4), 386
  (2004): Hidajat RR+, *Doc Ophthalmol* 109(3), 273
  (2004): Kertes PJ+, *Can J Ophthalmol* 39(6), 656
  (2002): Haimovici R+, *Ophthalmology* 109(1), 164
  (2002): Szwarcberg J+, *J Fr Ophtalmol* 25(6), 609
  (1996): Albalate M+, *Nephron* 73(4), 726
  (1996): Sanchez Dalmau BF+, *Med Clin (Barc)* 107(16), 636
  (1996): Spraul CW+, *Klin Monatsbl Augenheilkd* 209(1), 31
  (1995): Dennerlein JA+, *Ophthalmologe* 92(1), 38
  (1994): Mehta AM+, *Am J Ophthalmol* 118(2), 260
  (1991): Marciani MG+, *Haematologica* 76(2), 131

Other
Anaphylactoid reactions/Anaphylaxis (<1%)
  (1996): La Rosa M+, *J Allergy Clin Immunol* 97(1 Pt 1), 127
  (1995): Donikyan R+, *Arch Pediatr* 2(7), 703
  (1994): Di Marco JN+, *Arch Pediatr* 1(10), 959
Cardiotoxicity
  (2006): Borgna-Pignatti C+, *Blood* 107(9), 3733
Death
  (2006): Wu VC+, *Kidney Int* 70(11), 1888
  (1992): Tenenbein M+, *Lancet* 339(8795), 699
Hypersensitivity
  (2006): Gulen F+, *Minerva Pediatr* 58(6), 571
  (1995): Patriarca G+, *J Investig Allergol Clin Immunol* 5(5), 294
Hypotension
  (1991): Bentur Y+, *Drug Saf* 6(1), 37
Infections
  (1991): Bentur Y+, *Drug Saf* 6(1), 37

Injection-site erythema
Injection-site inflammation (1–10%)
Injection-site pain (1–10%)
Injection-site reactions
  (2006): Pennell DJ+, *Blood* 107(9), 3738
Neurotoxicity
  (1997): Levine JE+, *J Pediatr Hematol Oncol* 19(2), 139
  (1991): Bentur Y+, *Drug Saf* 6(1), 37

DELAVIRDINE

Synonym: U-90152S
Trade name: Rescriptor (Agouron)
Indications: HIV-1 infection
Category: Antiretroviral; Non-nucleoside reverse transcriptase inhibitor
Half-life: 5.8 hours
Clinically important, potentially hazardous interactions with: adefovir, alprazolam, amprenavir, anisindione, anticoagulants, buprenorphine, carbamazepine, dicumarol, dihydroergotamine, ergot, fosamprenavir, indinavir, ixabepilone, lovastatin, methadone, methysergide, midazolam, phenobarbital, phenytoin, quinidine, rifabutin, rifampin, sildenafil, simvastatin, triazolam, warfarin

Reactions

Skin
Allergic reactions (sic) (<2%)
Angioedema (<2%)
Cyst (<2%)
Dermatitis (<2%)
Desquamation (<2%)
Diaphoresis (<2%)
Edema of lip (<2%)
Erythema (<2%)
Erythema multiforme (<2%)
Exanthems (6.6%)
Folliculitis (<2%)
Fungal dermatitis (<2%)
Nodular eruption (<2%)
Peripheral edema (<2%)
Petechiae (<2%)
Pruritus (<2%)
Purpura (<2%)
Rash (sic) (9.8%)
  (2003): Justesen US+, *Br J Clin Pharmacol* 55(1), 100 (with amprenavir)
  (2000): Gangar M+, *Ann Pharmacother* 34(7–8), 839
  (2000): Scott LJ+, *Drugs* 60(6), 1411
  (1999): Para MF+, *Antimicrob Agents Chemother* 43(6), 1373
  (1997): James JS, *AIDS Treat News* 269, 1
Seborrhea (<2%)
Stevens–Johnson syndrome (<2%)
  (2000): Scott LJ+, *Drugs* 60(6), 1411
Urticaria (<2%)
Vasculitis (<2%)
Vesiculobullous eruption (<2%)
Xerosis (<2%)

Mucosal/ENT
Aphthous stomatitis (<2%)
Dysgeusia (<2%)
Gingivitis (<2%)

Oral ulceration (<2%)
Sialorrhea (<2%)
Stomatitis (<2%)
Tongue edema (<2%)
Vulvovaginal candidiasis (<2%)
Xerostomia (<2%)

Hair
Hair – alopecia (<2%)

Nails
Nails – changes (sic) (<2%)

Other
Gynecomastia (<2%)
Headache
Hypersensitivity
  (1999): Mills G+, *Antivir Ther* 4(1), 51
Myalgia/Myositis/Myopathy/Myotoxicity (<2%)
Paresthesias (<2%)
Rhabdomyolysis
  (2002): Castro JG+, *Am J Med* 112(6), 505 (with atorvastatin)

DEMECLOCYCLINE

Trade names: Declomycin (ESP Pharma); Ledermicina;
Ledermycin; Rynabron
Indications: Various infections caused by susceptible organisms
Category: Antibiotic, tetracycline
Half-life: 10–17 hours
**Clinically important, potentially hazardous interactions
with:** amoxicillin, ampicillin, antacids, bacampicillin, calcium
carbonate, carbenicillin, cloxacillin, digoxin, methotrexate,
methoxyflurane, mezlocillin, nafcillin, oxacillin, penicillins,
piperacillin, ticarcillin, zinc

Reactions

Skin
Acne
Angioedema
Bullous dermatitis
Erythema multiforme
Exanthems
Exfoliative dermatitis (<1%)
Fixed eruption
Lichenoid eruption
Lupus erythematosus
Perianal rash
Photosensitivity (1–10%)
  (1984): Kromann N+, *Ugeskr Laeger* (Danish) 146, 515
  (1980): Stern RS+, *Arch Dermatol* 116, 1269
Phototoxicity
Pigmentation
Pruritus (<1%)
Pruritus ani et vulvae
Purpura
Stevens–Johnson syndrome
Toxic epidermal necrolysis
  (1988): Massullo RE+, *J Am Acad Dermatol* 19, 358
Urticaria

Mucosal/ENT
Glossitis
Mucosal membrane pigmentation

Oral mucosal eruption
Tongue pigmentation

Nails
Nails – photo-onycholysis
Nails – pigmentation (<1%)

Other
Anaphylactoid reactions/Anaphylaxis (<1%)
Candidiasis
Nephrotoxicity
  (2002): Curtis NJ+, *Age Ageing* 31(2), 151
Paresthesias (<1%)
Porphyria

DENILEUKIN

Trade name: Ontak (Ligand)
Indications: Cutaneous T-cell lymphoma
Category: Antineoplastic
Half-life: distribution: 2–5 minutes; terminal: 70–80 minutes

Reactions

Skin
Allergic reactions (sic) (1%)
Bullous dermatitis
Diaphoresis (10%)
Edema (47%)
  (1998): Duvic M+, *Am J Hematol* 58(1), 87
Erythroderma
  (2008): Kazin R+, *J Am Acad Dermatol* 58(2 Suppl), S31
Exanthems
Petechiae
Pruritus (20%)
Purpura
Rash (sic) (34%)
  (2001): Foss FM+, *Clin Lymphoma* 1(4), 298
Toxic epidermal necrolysis
  (2005): Polder K+, *Leuk Lymphoma* 46(12), 1807
Urticaria
Vesiculation

Other
Anaphylactoid reactions/Anaphylaxis (1%)
Application-site reactions
  (2001): Foss FM+, *Clin Lymphoma* 1(4), 298
Asthenia
  (2001): Foss FM+, *Clin Lymphoma* 1(4), 298
Chills (81%)
  (1998): Saleh MN+, *J Am Acad Dermatol* 39(1), 63
Fever
  (1998): Saleh MN+, *J Am Acad Dermatol* 39(1), 63
Headache
Hypersensitivity (69%)
  (2001): Foss FM+, *Clin Lymphoma* 1(4), 298
Hypotension
  (1998): Saleh MN+, *J Am Acad Dermatol* 39(1), 63
Infections (48%)
Injection-site reactions (sic) (8%)
Myalgia/Myositis/Myopathy/Myotoxicity (18%)
  (1998): Duvic M+, *Am J Hematol* 58(1), 87
Paresthesias (13%)
Phlebitis
Thrombophlebitis

Tremor
(2006): Ghori F+, *J Clin Endocrinol Metab* 91(6), 2205

DESFLURANE

Trade names: Sulorane; Suprane (Baxter)
Indications: Induction or maintenance of anesthesia
Category: Anesthetic, inhalation
Half-life: Onset of action: 1–2 minutes
Clinically important, potentially hazardous interactions with: tramadol

Reactions

Skin
Pruritus
Shivering
(1998): Horn EP+, *Anesthesiology* 89(4), 878

Other
Cardiac failure
(2005): Smelt WL, *Acta Anaesthesiol Scand* 49(2), 267
Cough (34%)
(2005): Arain SR+, *Anesthesiology* 103(3), 495
(2003): Valley RD+, *Anesth Analg* 96(5), 1320
Death
(1998): Murray JM+, *Can J Anaesth* 45(12), 1200 (4 cases)
Hypertension
(2002): Marret E+, *Anesth Analg* 95(2), 319
Myalgia/Myositis/Myopathy/Myotoxicity

DESIPRAMINE

Trade names: Deprexan; Nebril; Nortimil; Pertofran; Pertofrane; Petylyl; PMS-Desipramine
Indications: Depression
Category: Antidepressant, tricyclic; Norepinephrine reuptake inhibitor
Half-life: 7–60 hours
Clinically important, potentially hazardous interactions with: amprenavir, arbutamine, clonidine, epinephrine, formoterol, guanethidine, isocarboxazid, linezolid, MAO inhibitors, phenelzine, quinolones, sparfloxacin, tranylcypromine

Reactions

Skin
Acne
Allergic reactions (sic) (<1%)
(1987): Joffe RT+, *Can J Psychiatry* 32, 695
(1987): Richter MA+, *Am J Psychiatry* 144, 526
Angioedema
Diaphoresis (1–10%)
Edema
Erythema
Exanthems
(1988): Biederman J+, *J Clin Psychiatry* 49, 178 (5.8%)
(1988): McLean JD, *Can J Psychiatry* 33, 331
(1987): Ellsworth A+, *Drug Intell Clin Pharm* 21, 510
(1987): Joffe RT+, *Can J Psychiatry* 32, 695 (6.2%)
Exfoliative dermatitis
Petechiae
Photosensitivity (1.4%)

Pigmentation (blue-gray) (photosensitive)
(1993): Narurkar V+, *Arch Dermatol* 129, 474
(1993): Steele TE+, *J Clin Psychopharmacol* 13, 76
Pruritus
(1988): Biederman J+, *J Clin Psychiatry* 49, 178
(1987): Ellsworth A+, *Drug Intell Clin Pharm* 21, 510
(1987): Pohl R+, *Am J Psychiatry* 144, 237
Purpura
(1980): Miescher PA+, *Clin Haematol* 9, 505
Rash (sic)
Side effects (sic)
(2002): Galanter CA+, *J Child Adolesc Psychopharmacol* 12(2), 137
Urticaria
(1991): Bajwa WK+, *J Nerv Ment Dis* 179, 108
(1988): Biederman J+, *J Clin Psychiatry* 49, 178
(1987): Pohl R+, *Am J Psychiatry* 144, 237
Vasculitis
Xerosis

Mucosal/ENT
Bromhidrosis
Dysgeusia (>10%)
Mucosal membrane desquamation
Stomatitis
Tinnitus
Tongue black
Xerostomia (>10%)
(2006): Choi SY+, *J Dent Res* 85(9), 839
(2002): Galanter CA+, *J Child Adolesc Psychopharmacol* 12(2), 137
(1993): Pataki CS+, *J Am Acad Child Adolesc Psychiatry* 32, 1065

Hair
Hair – alopecia (<1%)
(1991): Warnock JK+, *J Nerv Ment Dis* 179, 441

Other
Death
(2004): Amitai Y+, *Ther Drug Monit* 26(5), 468
Gynecomastia (<1%)
Hypersensitivity
Inappropriate secretion of antidiuretic hormone (SIADH)
(1983): Lydiard RB, *J Clin Psychiatry* 44(4), 153
Paresthesias
Pseudolymphoma
(1995): Magro CM+, *J Am Acad Dermatol* 32, 419
(1988): Kardaun SH+, *Br J Dermatol* 118(4), 545
Rhabdomyolysis
(1992): Petit P+, *Can Assoc Radiol J* 43(6), 443

DESLORATADINE

Trade name: Clarinex (Schering)
Indications: Allergic rhinitis, urticaria
Category: Histamine H1 receptor antagonist
Half-life: 27 hours

Reactions

Skin
Edema
Pruritus
Urticaria

Mucosal/ENT
Xerostomia

(2007): Scharf M+, *Curr Med Res Opin* 23(2), 313

Other
Anaphylactoid reactions/Anaphylaxis
Asthenia
   (2007): Scharf M+, *Curr Med Res Opin* 23(2), 313
Hypersensitivity
Myalgia/Myositis/Myopathy/Myotoxicity

DESMOPRESSIN

Trade names: DDAVP (Sanofi-Aventis); Defirin; Desmospray; Minirin; Minurin; Octostim; Stimate (ZLB Behring)
Indications: Primary nocturnal enuresis
Category: Antidiuretic hormone analog
Half-life: 75 minutes

Reactions

Skin
Allergic reactions (sic)
   (1982): Yokota M+, *Endocrinol Jpn* 29, 475
Diaphoresis
   (1985): Richardson DW+, *Ann Intern Med* 103, 228
Edema
Rash (sic)

Other
Death
   (2003): Lose G+, *Am J Obstet Gynecol* 189(4), 1106
Headache
   (2006): Dehoorne JL+, *J Urol* 176(2), 754
   (2003): Lose G+, *Am J Obstet Gynecol* 189(4), 1106 (22%)
Inappropriate secretion of antidiuretic hormone (SIADH)
   (2006): Rembratt A+, *Neurourol Urodyn* 25(2), 105
   (2005): van den Born BJ+, *Ned Tijdschr Geneeskd* 149(29), 1612
Injection-site edema
Injection-site erythema
Injection-site pain (1–10%)
Seizures
   (2006): Dehoorne JL+, *J Urol* 176(2), 754
   (2006): Larney V+, *Eur J Anaesthesiol* 23(10), 895
   (2002): Pruthi RS+, *J Urol* 168(1), 187

DESONIDE

Trade names: Desonide (Taro); DesOwen (Galderma); Tridesilon
Indications: Dermatoses
Category: Corticosteroid, topical
Half-life: N/A
Clinically important, potentially hazardous interactions with: live vaccines

Reactions

Skin
Allergic reactions (sic)
   (2004): Wong VK+, *J Drugs Dermatol* 3(4), 393
Dermatitis
   (1999): Garner LA+, *Am J Contact Dermat* 10(2), 81
   (1997): Hernandez N+, *Contact Dermatitis* 36(2), 111
   (1989): Rivara G+, *Contact Dermatitis* 21(2), 83
   (1983): Sturtz RP+, *Arch Dermatol* 119(12), 1023

Pruritus
   (2002): Freeman S+, *Australas J Dermatol* 43(3), 186
Rash (sic)
   (2002): Freeman S+, *Australas J Dermatol* 43(3), 186

DESOXIMETASONE

Trade name: Topicort (Taro)
Indications: Dermatoses
Category: Corticosteroid, topical
Half-life: N/A
Clinically important, potentially hazardous interactions with: live vaccines

Reactions

Skin
Adverse effects (sic)
   (1989): Brambilla L+, *Contact Dermatitis* 21(4), 272
   (1986): Garden JM+, *Arch Dermatol* 122(9), 1007
Erythema multiforme
   (1996): Stingeni L+, *Contact Dermatitis* 35(6), 363
Photosensitivity
   (1988): Stierstorfer MB+, *Arch Dermatol* 124(12), 1870

Eyes
Glaucoma
   (1993): Aggarwal RK+, *Eye* 7, 664 (3 cases)
Ocular hypertension
   (1993): Aggarwal RK+, *Eye* 7, 664 (2 cases)

DESVENLAFAXINE

Trade name: Pristiq (Wyeth)
Indications: Major depressive disorder
Category: Serotonin-norepinephrine reuptake inhibitor
Half-life: 12 hours
Clinically important, potentially hazardous interactions with: alcohol, antidepressants, aspirin, heparin, linezolid, lithium, NSAIDs, sibutramine, tramadol, warfarin

Reactions

Skin
Hyperhidrosis
   (2007): DeMartinis NA+, *J Clin Psychiatry* 68(5), 677 (10–14%)
Rash (sic) (1%)

Mucosal/ENT
Xerostomia (11–17%)
   (2007): DeMartinis NA+, *J Clin Psychiatry* 68(5), 677
   (2007): Liebowitz MR+, *J Clin Psychiatry* 68(11), 1663

Eyes
Mydriasis (2%)
Vision blurred (3–4%)
Visual hallucinations

Other
Abdominal pain
Agitation
Anxiety (3–5%)
Asthenia (7%)
   (2007): DeMartinis NA+, *J Clin Psychiatry* 68(5), 677

Headache
Hypersensitivity (2%)
Hypertension
Hypotension (~2%)
Insomnia (9–12%)
  (2007): DeMartinis NA+, J Clin Psychiatry 68(5), 677
Paresthesias (~2%)
Seizures (~2%)
Somnolence (~9%)
  (2007): DeMartinis NA+, J Clin Psychiatry 68(5), 677
  (2007): Liebowitz MR+, J Clin Psychiatry 68(11), 1663
Suicidal ideation
Tremor (~3%)
Vertigo (10–13%)
  (2007): DeMartinis NA+, J Clin Psychiatry 68(5), 677
Weight loss (~2%)

DEVIL'S CLAW

Scientific names: *Harpagophytum procumbens; Harpagophytum zeyheri*
Family: Pedaliaceae
Trade and other common names: Doloteffin; Grapple plant; Griffe du diable; Harpadol; wood spider
Category: Analgesic; Anti-inflammatory
Purported indications and other uses: Oral: anorexia, arteriosclerosis, rheumatoid arthritis, GI disorders, fibromyalgia, loss of appetite, headache, fever, high cholesterol, menstrual complaints, liver and gallbladder problems. **Topical:** rash, ulcers
Half-life: 3–6 hours
Clinically important, potentially hazardous interactions with: anesthetics, antacids, antiarrhythmic drugs, anticoagulants, aspirin, beta-blockers, digoxin, famotidine, histamine 2 blockers (e.g. ranitidine), hypoglycemics, NSAIDs, ranitidine, sympathomimetics, terfenadine, warfarin

Reactions

Skin
Adverse effects (sic)
  (2003): Chrubasik S+, Rheumatology (Oxford) 42(1), 141
  (2002): Chrubasik S+, Phytomedicine 9(3), 181
  (2001): Gobel H+, Schmerz 15(1), 10
  (2000): Chantre P+, Phytomedicine 7(3), 177

Mucosal/ENT
Dysgeusia
  (1981): Grahame R+, Ann Rheum Dis 40, 632
Tinnitus
  (1981): Grahame R+, Ann Rheum Dis 40, 632

DEXAMETHASONE

Trade names: Cortastat; Decadron (Merck); Dexone (Solvay); Hexadrol
Indications: Antiemetic, Arthralgias, Dermatoses, Diagnostic aid (many more)
Category: Corticosteroid, systemic; Corticosteroid, topical
Half-life: N/A
Clinically important, potentially hazardous interactions with: albendazole, aminoglutethimide, aspirin, bexarotene, carbamazepine, cyclophosphamide, dasatinib, diuretics, ephedrine, imatinib, itraconazole, lapatinib, **live vaccines**, methotrexate, phenobarbital, phenytoin, praziquantel, primidone, rifampicin, rifampin, temsirolimus, warfarin

Reactions

Skin
Acne
  (2006): Mentink LF+, Arch Dermatol 142(5), 570
  (2006): Vardy J+, Br J Cancer 94(7), 1011 (15%)
  (1997): Borgna-Pignatti+, J Pediatr 130(1), 13
Acute generalized exanthematous pustulosis
  (1995): Demitsu T+, Dermatology 193, 56
Allergic reactions (sic)
  (1989): Brambilla L+, Contact Dermatitis 21(4), 272
Dermatitis
  (2003): Hall VC+, J Am Acad Dermatol 48(4), 548 (with thalidomide)
  (2002): Nucera E+, Dermatology 204(3), 248
  (2000): Chew AL+, Cutis 65, 307
  (1994): Whitmore SE, Br J Dermatol 131, 296 (generalized)
  (1989): Rivara G+, Contact Dermatitis 21(2), 83
Edema
  (1998): Berinstein TH+, Ear Nose Throat J 77(1), 40
Erythema multiforme
  (2003): Hall VC+, J Am Acad Dermatol 48(4), 548 (with thalidomide)
  (1999): Alexiou C+, Laryngorhinootologie 78(10), 573
Exanthems
  (1987): Maucher OM+, Hautarzt (German) 38, 577
Exfoliative erythroderma
  (2003): Hall VC+, J Am Acad Dermatol 48(4), 548 (with thalidomide)
Peripheral edema
  (2002): Hempen C+, Support Care Cancer 10(4), 322
  (1991): Weissman DE+, J Neurooncol 11(3), 235
Photosensitivity
  (1988): Stierstorfer MB+, Arch Dermatol 124(12), 1870
Pruritus
  (2004): Crandell JT, Can J Anaesth 51(4), 398
  (2004): Kuczkowski KM, Anaesthesia 59(3), 308
  (2003): Perron G+, Can J Anaesth 50(7), 749
  (2001): Dong Y+, Chin Med J (Engl) 114(7), 764 (with methotrexate)
  (1999): Alexiou C+, Laryngorhinootologie 78(10), 573
  (1988): Taleb N+, Eur J Cancer Clin Oncol 24(3), 495
Rash (sic)
  (2003): Jain R+, J Dermatol 30(10), 713 (3 cases) (with cyclophosphamide)
Seborrheic dermatitis
  (2003): Hall VC+, J Am Acad Dermatol 48(4), 548 (with thalidomide)
Striae
  (1997): Borgna-Pignatti C+, J Pediatr 130(1), 13
  (1992): Pang S+, J Clin Endocrinol 75(1), 249
  (1985): Job JC+, Arch Fr Pediatr 42(9), 765

(1983): Guest G+, *Arch Fr Pediatr* 40(6), 453

Toxic epidermal necrolysis
(2003): Hall VC+, *J Am Acad Dermatol* 48(4), 548 (with thalidomide)

Mucosal/ENT
Dysgeusia
(2005): Herr BD+, *Otolaryngol Head Neck Surg* 132(4), 527
(2003): Jain R+, *J Dermatol* 30(10), 713 (13%) (with cyclophosphamide)
(1993): Pasricha JS+, *Int J Dermatol* 32(10), 753

Oral candidiasis
(2001): Hardy JR+, *Palliat Med* 15(1), 3
(1983): Hanks GW+, *Postgrad Med J* 59(697), 702

Ototoxicity
(1998): Abello P+, *Acta Otorrinolaringol Esp* 49(5), 353
(1998): Arditi M+, *Pediatrics* 102(5), 1087
(1994): Syrogiannopoulos GA+, *J Infect Dis* 169(4), 853

Hair
Hair – alopecia
(2003): Jain R+, *J Dermatol* 30(10), 713 (9%) (with cyclophosphamide)

Hair – hirsutism
(1997): Borgna-Pignatti+, *J Pediatr* 130(1), 13

Hair – hypertrichosis
(2006): Mentink LF+, *Arch Dermatol* 142(5), 570

Eyes
Cataract
(2003): Jain R+, *J Dermatol* 30(10), 713 (with cyclophosphamide)
(1994): Zheng Y+, *Yan Ke Xue Bao* 10(2), 102
(1989): Mohan R+, *Indian J Ophthalmol* 37(1), 13
(1986): Bluming AZ+, *J Clin Oncol* 4(2), 221

Glaucoma
(2006): Mentink LF+, *Arch Dermatol* 142(5), 570
(2003): Jain R+, *J Dermatol* 30(10), 713 (3 cases) (with cyclophosphamide)
(1999): Tan DT+, *Ophthalmology* 106(2), 223
(1995): Kong L+, *Yan Ke Xue Bao* 11(1), 53
(1993): Aggarwal RK+, *Eye* 7, 664
(1993): Kong LX, *Zhonghua Yan Ke Za Zhi* 29(3), 151
(1989): Mohan R+, *Indian J Ophthalmol* 37(1), 13

Ocular hypertension
(2001): Dinning WJ+, *Ophthalmology* 108(10), 1715
(2000): Ng JS+, *Ophthalmology* 107(11), 2097
(1999): Deng Y+, *Hua Xi Yi Ke Da Xue Xue Bao* 30(2), 205

Ocular keratitis
(2003): Davidson RS+, *J Glaucoma* 12(1), 23

Ocular pain
(1999): Deng Y+, *Hua Xi Yi Ke Da Xue Xue Bao* 30(2), 205
(1997): Kwok AK+, *Ophthalmology* 104(12), 2112
(1995): Clark AF+, *Invest Ophthalmol Vis Sci* 36(2), 478
(1986): Kass M+, *Am J Ophthalmol* 102(2), 159
(1984): Stewart RH+, *Curr Eye Res* 3(6), 835

Retinopathy
(1995): Ramanathan R+, *J Perinatol* 15(3), 178 (12 cases)

Vision blurred
(2003): Jain R+, *J Dermatol* 30(10), 713 (9%) (with cyclophosphamide)

Visual halos
(1999): Deng Y+, *Hua Xi Yi Ke Da Xue Xue Bao* 30(2), 205

Other
Abdominal pain (sic)
(1997): Borgna-Pignatti C+, *J Pediatr* 130(1), 13

Adverse effects
(2005): Richardson PG+, *N Engl J Med* 352(24), 2487 (60%)
(2004): Borst F+, *Ann Hematol* 83(12), 764
(2004): May C+, *Monaldi Arch Chest Dis* 61(3), 162

(2004): Odd DE+, *J Paediatr Child Health* 40(5-6), 282
(2004): Palladini G+, *Blood* 103(8), 2936 (11%) (with melphalan)
(1998): Yeh TF+, *Pediatrics* 101(5), E7
(1986): Garden JM+, *Arch Dermatol* 122(9), 1007

Anaphylactoid reactions/Anaphylaxis
(1997): Figueredo E+, *Allergy* 52(8), 877

Asthenia
(2005): Richardson PG+, *N Engl J Med* 352(24), 2487
(2003): Jain R+, *J Dermatol* 30(10), 713 (54%) (with cyclophosphamide)
(1997): Borgna-Pignatti C+, *J Pediatr* 130(1), 13
(1993): Pasricha JS+, *Int J Dermatol* 32(10), 753

Candidiasis
(2002): Pera A+, *J Perinatol* 22(3), 204

Death
(1994): Malik IA+, *South Med J* 87(3), 409
(1992): Heimdal K+, *J Neurooncol* 12(2), 141
(1992): O'Neil EA+, *Arch Dis Child* 67(1), 10
(1991): Friedenberg WR+, *Am J Hematol* 36(3), 171
(1990): Ferrara TB+, *J Perinatol* 10(2), 137

Embolia cutis medicamentosa (Nicolau syndrome)
(1997): Kohler LD+, *Int J Dermatol* 36(3), 197 (with diclofenac)

Fever
(1997): McIntyre PB+, *JAMA* 278(11), 925
(1994): Pichard E+, *Isr J Med Sci* 30(5-6), 408

Headache
(2003): Jain R+, *J Dermatol* 30(10), 713 (16%) (with cyclophosphamide)
(2001): Dong Y+, *Chin Med J* (Engl) 114(7), 764 (with methotrexate)
(1998): Goedhals L+, *Ann Oncol* 9(6), 661 (with granisetron)
(1998): Martoni A+, *Anticancer Res* 18(4B), 2799 (with granisetron)
(1993): Pasricha JS+, *Int J Dermatol* 32(10), 753

Hypersensitivity
(1993): Chan AT, *BMJ* 306, 109
(1993): Williams WR, *BMJ* 306(6877), 585
(1986): Baldinger J+, *Ann Ophthalmol* eact(3), 95 (with polymyxin B/neomycin)

Hypertension
(2006): Mentink LF+, *Arch Dermatol* 142(5), 570
(2006): Wallenborn J+, *BMJ* 333(7563), 324 (with metoclopramide)
(2003): Halliday HL+, *Cochrane Database Syst* (1), CD001146
(2003): Jain R+, *J Dermatol* 30(10), 713 (3%) (with cyclophosphamide)
(2001): Halliday HL+, *Pediatrics* 107(2), 232
(1999): Fuchs M+, *HNO* 47(7), 647
(1998): Hari P+, *Indian J Pediatr* 65(4), 557
(1996): Smets K+, *Eur J Pediatr* 155(7), 573
(1995): Caulier MT+, *Br J Haematol* 91(2), 477
(1992): Greenough A+, *Eur J Pediatr* 151(2), 134
(1992): Pang S+, *J Clin Endocrinol Metab* 75(1), 249
(1990): Ferrara TB+, *J Perinatol* 10(2), 137
(1989): Merz U+, *Klin Padiatr* 201(1), 11

Infections
(2004): Mantadakis E+, *Pediatr Hematol Oncol* 21(1), 27
(2003): Belgaumi AF+, *Cancer* 97(11), 2898 (36%)
(1999): Stoll BJ+, *Pediatrics* 104(5), e63
(1998): Hari P+, *Indian J Pediatr* 65(4), 557
(1998): Papile LA+, *N Engl J Med* 338(16), 1112
(1998): Thomas MC+, *Int J Clin Pract* 52(7), 520
(1995): Koehler PJ, *Anticancer Drugs* 6(1), 19
(1994): Keogh P+, *Neurosurgery* 34(2), 364
(1994): Sharada B+, *Rheumatol Int* 14(3), 91
(1991): Friedenberg WR+, *Am J Hematol* 36(3), 171
(1990): Ferrara TB+, *J Perinatol* 10(2), 137
(1990): Karnik R+, *Wien Klin Wochenschr* 102(1), 1
(1990): Ng PC+, *Arch Dis Child* 65(1 Spec No), 54

(1985): Moskopp D, *Neurochirurgia* (Stuttg) 28(3), 147
(1983): Hanks GW+, *Postgrad Med J* 59(697), 702
(1980): West BC+, *Am J Ophthalmol* 89(6), 854
Myalgia/Myositis/Myopathy/Myotoxicity
(2006): Mentink LF+, *Arch Dermatol* 142(5), 570
(2005): Richardson PG+, *N Engl J Med* 352(24), 2487
(2001): Hardy JR+, *Palliat Med* 15(1), 3
(1995): Koehler PJ, *Anticancer Drugs* 6(1), 19
(1991): Dropcho EJ+, *Neurology* 41(8), 1235
Osteoporosis
(2004): Raff H, *Trends Endocrinol Metab* 15(8), 351
(1999): Fuchs M+, *HNO* 47(7), 647
(1988): Kruse K+, *Monatsschr Kinderheilkd* 136(5), 237
Paresthesias
(1986): Rasche H+, *Dtsch Med Wochenschr* 111(37), 1406
Seizures
(2003): Jain R+, *J Dermatol* 30(10), 713 (with cyclophosphamide)
Side effects (sic)
(2001): Hamon I+, *J Gynecol Obstet Biol Reprod* (Paris) 30(6), S50
(1997): Kuhne T+, *J Pediatr* 130(1), 17
(1996): Ralls JE, *Aust Fam Physician* 25(5), 713
Toxicity (sic)
(2003): Belgaumi AF+, *Cancer* 97(11), 2898 (with daunomycin)

DEXCHLORPHENIRAMINE

Trade names: Delamin; Poladex; Polaramin; Polaramine; Polaronil; Polazit; Tanafed (First Horizon); Trenolone
Indications: Allergic rhinitis, urticaria
Category: Histamine H1 receptor antagonist
Half-life: 20–24 hours
Clinically important, potentially hazardous interactions with: barbiturates, chloral hydrate, ethchlorvynol, glutethimide, phenothiazines, zolpidem

Reactions

Skin
Angioedema (<1%)
Dermatitis
  (1989): Cusano F+, *Contact Dermatitis* 21, 340
Diaphoresis
Edema (<1%)
Photosensitivity (<1%)
Rash (sic) (<1%)
Urticaria

Mucosal/ENT
Xerostomia (1–10%)

Other
Anaphylactoid reactions/Anaphylaxis
  (2007): Thurot-Guillou C+, *Eur J Dermatol* A(2), 170
Aseptic meningitis
  (2003): Lafaurie M+, *Ann Med Interne* (Paris) 154(3), 179
Asthenia
  (1987): Johansen LV+, *Rhinology* 25(1), 35
Chills
Headache
Infections
  (2003): Lafaurie M+, *Ann Med Interne* (Paris) 154(3), 179
Myalgia/Myositis/Myopathy/Myotoxicity (<1%)
Paresthesias (<1%)

DEXIBUPROFEN

Trade names: Actifen (Gebro); Deltaran (Strathmann); Dexoptifen (Spirig); Seractil (Genus)
Indications: Dental pain, dysmenorrhea, muscular pain and osteoarthritis
Category: Non-steroidal anti-inflammatory
Half-life: 2 hours
Clinically important, potentially hazardous interactions with: aspirin, celecoxib, citalopram, etoricoxib, fluoxetine, NSAIDs, paroxetine, venlafaxine, warfarin

Reactions

Skin
Allergic reactions (sic)
Angioedema
Erythema multiforme
Lupus erythematosus
Peripheral edema
Photosensitivity
Pruritus
Purpura
Rash (sic)
Stevens–Johnson syndrome
Toxic epidermal necrolysis
Urticaria
Vasculitis

Mucosal/ENT
Rhinitis
Tinnitus

Hair
Hair – alopecia

Eyes
Visual disturbances

Other
Abdominal pain
Anaphylactoid reactions/Anaphylaxis
Anxiety
Asthenia
Bronchospasm
Confusion
Depression
Headache
Somnolence
Vertigo

DEXKETOPROFEN

Trade names: Enangel (Topical); Keral (Menarini); Ketesse (Pharmaforte)
Indications: Pain
Half-life: N/A

Reactions

Skin
Photocontact dermatitis
  (2006): Goday-Bujan JJ+, *Contact Dermatitis* 55(1), 59

(2004): Lopez-Abad R+, *J Investig Allergol Clin Immunol*
    14(3), 247
(2003): Cuerda Galindo E+, *Contact Dermatitis* 48(5), 283
(2002): Valenzuela N+, *Contact Dermatitis* 47(4), 237

Other
Asthenia
    (1999): Krappweis J+, *Dtsch Med Wochenschr* 124(41), 1206

DEXMEDETOMIDINE

Trade name: Precedex (Abbott)
Indications: Sedation for intensive care unit intubation
Category: Adrenergic alpha-receptor agonist
Half-life: 2 hours
**Clinically important, potentially hazardous interactions
with:** digoxin, opioids

Reactions

Skin
Diaphoresis (<1%)
Xerosis

Mucosal/ENT
Sialopenia
    (1990): Aantaa RE+, *Anesth Analg* 70, 407

Eyes
Photopsia (<1%)

Other
Hypotension
    (2006): Aryan HE+, *Brain Inj* 20(8), 791
    (2006): Chrysostomou C+, *Pediatr Crit Care Med* 7(2), 126
        (15%)
    (2004): Dasta JF+, *Ann Pharmacother* 38(7–8), 1130
Infections (2%)
Pain (3%)

DEXMETHYLPHENIDATE

Trade name: Focalin (Novartis)
Indications: Attention deficit disorder
Category: CNS stimulant
Half-life: 2.0–4.5 hours
**Clinically important, potentially hazardous interactions
with:** clonidine, MAO inhibitors

Reactions

Skin
Erythema multiforme
Exfoliative dermatitis
Purpura
Rash (sic)
Urticaria

Hair
Hair – alopecia

Other
Abdominal pain (15%)
Fever (5%)
Headache

Hypertension
Hypotension
Vertigo

DEXRAZOXANE

Trade names: Cardioxane (Novartis); Totect; Zinecard (Pfizer)
Indications: Protective agent against cardiomyopathy,
anthracycline-induced extravasation
Category: Cardioprotective agent
Half-life: 2–4 hours
**Clinically important, potentially hazardous interactions
with:** None

Reactions

Skin
Erythema (streaking)
Rash (sic)
Urticaria

Mucosal/ENT
Stomatitis

Hair
Hair – alopecia

Other
Abdominal pain
Anaphylactoid reactions/Anaphylaxis
    (2004): Leoni V+, *Allergy* 59(2), 241
Asthenia
Cough
Depression
Fever
Headache
Infections (sic)
Injection-site burning
Injection-site pain (12–16%)
    (2007): Mouridsen HT+, *Ann Oncol* 18(3), 546
Insomnia
Neurotoxicity
Phlebitis
Vertigo

DEXTROAMPHETAMINE

Trade names: Adderall (Shire); Dexamphetamine;
Dexamphetamini; Dexedrine (Alliant); Dextrostat; Ferndex;
Oxydess
Indications: Narcolepsy, attention deficit disorder (ADD)
Category: Amphetamine
Half-life: 10–12 hours
**Clinically important, potentially hazardous interactions
with:** fluoxetine, fluvoxamine, MAO inhibitors, paroxetine,
phenelzine, sertraline, tranylcypromine

Reactions

Skin
Diaphoresis (1–10%)
Rash (sic) (<1%)
Toxic epidermal necrolysis

Urticaria (<1%)

Mucosal/ENT
Dysgeusia
Xerostomia (1–10%)

Other
Chills
Headache
Rhabdomyolysis
(2000): Richards JR, *J Emerg Med* 19(1), 51
(1999): Hedetoft C+, *Ugeskr Laeger* 161(50), 6907
(1998): Robertsen A+, *Tidsskr Nor Laegeforen* 118(28), 4340
(1996): Hofland E+, *Ned Tijdschr Geneeskd* 140(12), 681
(1996): Roebroek RM+, *Ned Tijdschr Geneeskd* 140(29), 1519
(1996): Roebroek RM+, *Ned Tijdschr Geneeskd* 140(4), 205
(1996): Sultana SR+, *J R Coll Surg Edinb* 41(6), 419
(1992): Kao CH+, *Clin Nucl Med* 17(2), 101
(1990): Yamazaki F+, *Nippon Naika Gakkai* 79(1), 100

DEXTROMETHORPHAN

Trade names: Balminil; Benylin; Cheracol-D; Delsym; Koffex; Pertussin; Robitussin (Wyeth); Sucrets; Suppress; Triaminic DM; Trocal; Vicks Formula 44 (Procter & Gamble)
Indications: Nonproductive cough
Category: Analgesic, narcotic; NMDA receptor antagonist
Half-life: N/A
Clinically important, potentially hazardous interactions with: linezolid, memantine, moclobemide, phenelzine, rasagiline, sibutramine, tranylcypromine, valdecoxib

Reactions

Skin
Bullous dermatitis
(1999): Sahn EE, *Dermatology Times* April, 5 (infant with urticaria pigmentosa)
(1996): Cook J+, *Pediatr Dermatol* 13, 410 (infant with urticaria pigmentosa)
Fixed eruption
(1991): Smoller BR+, *J Cutan Pathol* 18, 13
(1990): Stubb S+, *Arch Dermatol* 126, 970

Other
Anaphylactoid reactions/Anaphylaxis
(1998): Knowles SR+, *J Allergy Clin Immunol* 102, 316
Headache
Neurotoxicity
(2006): Cherkes JK+, *Neurology* 66(12), 1952
Vertigo
(2006): Panitch HS+, *Ann Neurol* 59(5), 780 (with quinidine)

DIACETYLMORPHINE

(See HEROIN)

DIATRIZOATE

Trade name: Gastrografin (Schering)
Indications: Imaging (gastrointestinal tract)
Category: Iodine-containing radiocontrast medium
Half-life: N/A
Clinically important, potentially hazardous interactions with: N/A

Reactions

Skin
Dermatitis
Pruritus
(1992): Choyke PL+, *Radiology* 183(1), 111
Rash (sic)
(1992): Choyke PL+, *Radiology* 183(1), 111
Toxic epidermal necrolysis
(1998): Schmidt BJ+, *Am J Roentgenol* 171(5), 1215
Urticaria

Other
Anaphylactoid reactions/Anaphylaxis (rare)
(2004): Seymour CW+, *J Trauma* 57(5), 1105 (rare)
(1997): Miller SH, *Am J Roentgenol* 168(4), 959 (rare)
(1992): Ishiyama T+, *Masui* 41(8), 1314 (rare)
(1982): Boden WE, *Chest* 81(6), 759 (rare)
Death
(1983): Schneiderman H+, *JAMA* 250(17), 2340
Rhabdomyolysis
(1991): Carena J+, *Medicina (B Aires)* 51(4), 348
Seizures
(1996): Muruve DA+, *Clin Nephrol* 45(6), 406
Vertigo
(1992): Choyke PL+, *Radiology* 183(1), 111

DIAZEPAM

Trade names: Assival; Dialar; Diapax; Diastat (Xcel); Diazemuls; Dizac; Ducene; E-Pam; Meval; Novazam; Solis; Valium (Roche); Vivol
Indications: Anxiety
Category: Benzodiazepine; Skeletal muscle relaxant
Half-life: 20–70 hours
Clinically important, potentially hazardous interactions with: alcohol, amprenavir, barbiturates, buprenorphine, chlorpheniramine, clarithromycin, CNS depressants, efavirenz, esomeprazole, **eucalyptus**, fluoroquinolones, imatinib, indinavir, ivermectin, macrolide antibiotics, MAO inhibitors, methadone, mianserin, nalbuphine, narcotics, nelfinavir, nilutamide, phenothiazines, ritonavir, SSRIs

Reactions

Skin
Acne
Acute febrile neutrophilic dermatosis (Sweet's syndrome)
(2000): Guimera FJ+, *Int J Dermatol* 39(10), 795
Allergic reactions (sic)
(1982): Allin DM, *Curr Med Res Opin* 8, 33
Angioedema
Bullous dermatitis
Dermatitis (1–10%)
(1995): Fisher AA, *Cutis* 55, 327 (systemic)

(1995): Kampgen E+, *Contact Dermatitis* 33, 356
(1994): Garcia-Bravo B+, *Contact Dermatitis* 30, 40
Diaphoresis (>10%)
Eczema
Exanthems
  (1986): Bigby M+, *JAMA* 256, 3358 (0.04%)
  (1981): Adverse Drug Reaction List, *Jpn Med Gaz* (Japanese)
    18:6–7, 16
Exfoliative dermatitis
Fixed eruption (<1%)
Melanoma
  (1981): Adam S+, *Lancet* 2, 1344
Peripheral edema
  (1982): Stadler R+, *Hautarzt* (German) 33, 276
Pigmentation
  (2002): Viale PH+, *Clin J Oncol Nurs* 6(5), 310
  (1980): Ferreira JA, *Aesthetic Plast Surg* 4, 343
Pruritus
  (1995): Kampgen E+, *Contact Dermatitis* 33, 356
Purpura
  (1985): Ambriz-Fernandez R+, *Rev Invest Clin* (Spanish) 37, 347
  (1980): Miescher PA+, *Clin Haematol* 9, 505
Rash (sic) (>10%)
  (1983): O'Brien JE+, *Curr Ther Res* 34, 825
Urticaria
  (1987): Deardon DJ+, *Br J Anaesth* 59, 391
Vasculitis
  (1999): Olcina GM+, *Am J Psychiatry* 156, 972

Mucosal/ENT
Sialorrhea
Tongue furry
Xerostomia (>10%)

Nails
Nails – parrot-beak

Other
Anaphylactoid reactions/Anaphylaxis
  (1987): Deardon DJ+, *Br J Anaesth* 59, 391
Gynecomastia
  (2005): Jelenkovic AV+, *Ann Pharmacother* 39(1), 201
  (2000): Hugues FC+, *Ann Med Interne* (Paris) (French) 151, 10
    (passim)
  (1994): Llop R+, *Ann Pharmacother* 28, 671
Headache
Hypersensitivity
  (2002): Asero R, *Allergy* 57(12), 1209
Hypotension
  (1990): Ruff R+, *J Cardiothorac Anesth* 4(3), 314
Injection-site pain
  (2002): Majedi H+, *Anesth Analg* 95(5), 1297
Injection-site phlebitis (>10%)
  (1981): Clarke RSJ, *Drugs* 22, 26 (39%)
  (1980): Schou-Olesen A+, *Br J Anaesth* 52, 609
Paresthesias
Porphyria
Porphyria variegata
Rhabdomyolysis
  (1982): Bogaerts Y+, *Clin Nephrol* 17(4), 206
Vertigo
  (2002): Cereghino JJ+, *Arch Neurol* 59(12), 1915

DIAZOXIDE

Trade names: Eudimine; Hyperstat (Schering); Proglicem; Proglycem; Sefulken
Indications: Hypoglycemia, hypertension
Category: Vasodilator
Half-life: 20–36 hours
Clinically important, potentially hazardous interactions with: phenytoin

Reactions

Skin
Cellulitis (<1%)
Diaphoresis
Edema
Exanthems
Herpes
Leukomelanosis
Lichenoid eruption
Photosensitivity
Pruritus
Purpura
Rash (sic) (<1%)
Urticaria
Xerosis

Mucosal/ENT
Ageusia
Dysgeusia
Sialorrhea
Tinnitus
Xerostomia

Hair
Hair – alopecia
Hair – hypertrichosis (<1%)
  (1989): Rousseau C+, *Dermatologica* 179, 221
  (1988): Prigent F+, *Ann Dermatol Venereol* (French) 115, 191
  (1987): Turpin G+, *Presse Med* (French) 16, 398
  (1983): Schiazza L+, *G Ital Dermatol Venereol* (Italian) 118, 113
  (1981): Perez-Mijares R+, *Rev Clin Esp* (Spanish) 162, 225

Other
Candidiasis
Headache
Hypersensitivity
Injection-site pain (<1%)
Injection-site phlebitis (<1%)
Paresthesias

DICLOFENAC

Trade names: Allvoran; Apo-Diclo; Arthrotec (Pfizer); Fenac; Galedol; Liroken; Monoflam; Nu-Diclo; Remethan; Solaraze Gel (Doak); Taks; Voltaren (Novartis); Voltarene; Voltarol
Indications: Rheumatoid and osteoarthritis
Category: Non-steroidal anti-inflammatory
Half-life: 1–2 hours
Clinically important, potentially hazardous interactions with: methotrexate

Note: Arthrotec is diclofenac and misoprostol

Reactions

Skin

Adverse effects (sic)
  (1986): Catalano MA, *Am J Med* 80, 81
Allergic reactions (sic)
  (1992): Schiavino D+, *Contact Dermatitis* 26, 357
Angioedema (1–3%)
  (2000): Hadar A+, *Harefuah* (Hebrew) 138, 211 (from suppository)
Bullous dermatitis (1–3%)
  (1982): Valsecchi R+, *G Ital Derm Venereol* (Italian) 117, 221
  (1981): Gabrielsen TO+, *Acta Derm Venereol* (Stockh) 61, 439
Dermatitis (1–3%)
  (2004): Bohannon JS, Midlothian, VA (topical) (2 cases) (from Internet) (observation)
  (2004): Foti C+, *Clin Exp Dermatol* 29(1), 91
  (2004): Marmelzat JA, Los Angeles, CA (topical) (2 cases) (from Internet) (observation)
  (2004): Smith JG, Mobile, AL (topical) (from Internet) (observation)
  (2002): Bohannon JS, Midlothian, VA (from Internet) (observation)
  (2002): Kerr OA+, *Contact Dermatitis* 47(3), 175
  (2002): Sorkin M, Denver, CO (from Internet) (observation)
  (1998): Ueda K+, *Contact Dermatitis* 39, 323
  (1996): Gonzalo MA+, *Dermatology* 193, 59
  (1996): Valsecchi R+, *Contact Dermatitis* 34, 150
  (1994): Gebhardt M+, *Contact Dermatitis* 30, 183
  (1994): Romano A+, *Allergy* 49, 57
Dermatitis herpetiformis
  (1989): Grob JJ+, *Dermatologica* 178, 58
  (1981): Gabrielsen TO+, *Acta Derm Venereol* (Stockh) 61, 439
Dermatomyositis
  (1989): Grob JJ+, *Dermatologica* 178, 58
Diaphoresis (<1%)
Eczema (1–3%)
Edema
Erythema
  (1998): Schaad HJ+, *Ther Umsch* (German) 55, 586 (generalized)
  (1992): Barrett PJ+, *Anaesthesia* 47, 83
Erythema multiforme (<1%)
  (1999): Emmett SD, Solana Beach, CA (from internet) (observation)
  (1996): Delrio FG+, *Am J Med Sci* 312(2), 95
  (1995): Dhar S+, *Dermatology* 191, 76
  (1993): Khalil H+, *Arch Intern Med* 153, 1649
  (1988): Todd PA+, *Drugs* 35, 244
  (1985): Morris BAP+, *Can Med Assoc J* 133, 665
  (1982): Seigneuric C+, *Ann Dermatol Venereol* (French) 109, 287
Erythema nodosum (<1%)
Exanthems (1–5%)
  (1994): Romano A+, *Allergy* 49, 57
  (1992): Breathnach SM+, *Adverse Drug Reactions and the Skin* Blackwell, Oxford, 188 (passim)
  (1988): Todd PA+, *Drugs* 35, 244
  (1986): Halevy S+, *Harefuah* (Hebrew) 110, 30
  (1985): Morris BAP+, *Can Med Assoc J* 133, 665
Exfoliative dermatitis (<1%)
Fixed eruption
  (1998): Mahboob A+, *Int J Dermatol* 37, 833
Lichenoid eruption
  (1999): Fetterman M, Miami, FL (from Internet) (observation)
Linear IgA dermatosis
  (2003): Avci O+, *J Am Acad Dermatol* 48(2), 299 (passim)
  (2002): Cohen LM+, *J Am Acad Dermatol* 46, S32 (passim)
  (1997): Paul C+, *Br J Dermatol* 136, 406
  (1982): Valsecchi R+, *G Ital Derm Venereol* (Italian) 117, 221
  (1981): Gabrielsen TO+, *Acta Derm Venereol* (Stockh) 61, 439
Lupus erythematosus
Necrosis
  (2003): Mayrink M+, *Plast Reconstr Surg* 112(7), 1970
Necrotizing fasciitis
  (2002): Verfaillie G+, *Eur J Emerg Med* 9(3), 270
Pemphigus
  (1997): Matz H+, *Dermatology* 195, 48
Peripheral edema
  (2002): Chan FK+, *N Engl J Med* 347(26), 2104 (with omeprazole)
Photoallergic reaction
  (2003): Montoro J+, *Contact Dermatitis* 48(2), 115
Photosensitivity (1–3%)
  (1998): Encinas S+, *Chem Res Toxicol* 11, 946
  (1997): O'Reilly FM+, American Academy of Dermatology Meeting, Poster #14
  (1996): Becker L+, *Acta Derm Venereol* (Stockh) 76, 337
  (1992): Le Corre Y+, *Ann Dermatol Venereol* (French) 119, 923 (granuloma annulare type)
  (1988): Todd PA+, *Drugs* 35, 244
Pruritus (1–10%)
  (1995): Litt JZ, Beachwood, OH (personal case) (observation)
  (1994): Litt JZ, Beachwood, OH (personal case) (observation)
  (1992): Breathnach SM+, *Adverse Drug Reactions and the Skin* Blackwell, Oxford, 188 (passim)
  (1988): Todd PA+, *Drugs* 35, 244
  (1981): Gabrielsen TO+, *Acta Derm Venereol* (Stockh) 61, 439
Psoriasis
  (1999): Dintiman B, Fairfax, VA (from Internet) (observation)
  (1999): Fetterman M, Miami, FL (from Internet) (observation)
  (1987): Sendagorta E+, *Dermatologica* 175, 300
Purpura (1–3%)
  (1988): Todd PA+, *Drugs* 35, 244
Purpura fulminans
  (2002): Hengge UR+, *Hautarzt* 53(7), 483
Rash (sic) (>10%)
Stevens–Johnson syndrome (1–3%) (1 fatal case)
  (1988): Todd PA+, *Drugs* 35, 244
Toxic epidermal necrolysis
  (1998): Choi KL, Toronto, Canada (from Internet) (observation)
  (1993): Correia O+, *Dermatology* 186, 32
  (1985): Kamanabroo D+, *Arch Dermatol* 121, 1548
Urticaria (1–3%)
  (1998): Gala G+, *Allergy* 53, 623
  (1995): Litt JZ, Beachwood, OH (personal case) (observation)
  (1995): Rademaker M, *N Z Med J* 108, 165
  (1992): Breathnach SM+, *Adverse Drug Reactions and the Skin* Blackwell, Oxford, 188 (passim)
  (1988): Todd PA+, *Drugs* 35, 244
Vasculitis
  (1999): Emmet S, Solana Beach, CA (from ophthalmic solution) (from Internet) (observation)
  (1997): Morros R+, *Br J Rheumatol* 36, 503
  (1992): Breathnach SM+, *Adverse Drug Reactions and the Skin* Blackwell, Oxford, 188 (passim)
  (1982): Bonafe JL+, *Ann Dermatol Venereol* (French) 109, 283

Mucosal/ENT

Aphthous stomatitis
  (1988): Todd PA+, *Drugs* 35, 244
Dysgeusia (1–3%)
Oral ulceration
  (2000): Madinier I+, *Ann Med Interne* (Paris) (French) 151, 248
Stomatitis (<1%)
Tinnitus
Tongue edema (1–3%)
Xerostomia (1–3%)

(1988): Todd PA+, *Drugs* 35, 244

Hair

Hair – alopecia (1–3%)

Other

Anaphylactoid reactions/Anaphylaxis (1–3%)
  (2003): Jonker MJ+, *Contact Dermatitis* 49, 114
  (2002): Meuleman C+, *Arch Mal Coeur Vaiss* 95(12), 1230 (with misoprostol)
  (2000): Hadar A+, *Harefuah* (Hebrew) 138, 211 (from suppository)
  (2000): Ray M+, *Indian Pediatr* 36, 1067 (fatal)
  (1999): Enrique E+, *Allergy* 54, 529
  (1996): Levy JH+, *N Engl J Med* 335, 1925
  (1993): Alkhawajah AM+, *Forensic Sci Int* 60, 107
  (1993): van der Klauw MM+, *Br J Clin Pharmacol* 35, 400
  (1992): *Australian Adverse Drug Reactions Bulletin* 11, 7
Aseptic meningitis
  (2003): Chazan B+, *J Neurol* 250(12), 1503
Death
  (2006): Gislason GH+, *Circulation* 113(25), 2906
  (2002): Hengge UR+, *Hautarzt* 53(7), 483
  (2002): Verfaillie G+, *Eur J Emerg Med* 9(3), 270
Embolia cutis medicamentosa (Nicolau syndrome)
  (2008): Seiel E+, *J Dermatol* 35(1), 18
  (2007): Sarifakioglu E, *J Eur Acad Dermatol Venereol* 21(2), 266
  (2006): Lie C+, *J Orthop Surg* 14(1), 104
  (2006): Luton K+, *Int J Dermatol* 45(11), 1326
  (2006): Mutalik S+, *J Drug Dermatol* 5(4), 377
  (2005): *Reactions* 1, 1001, 7
  (2005): Bajaj DR+, *J Coll Physicians Surg Pak* 15(3), 187
  (2004): Ezzedine K+, *Br J Dermatol* 150(2), 385
  (2003): Reding EL+, *J Am Acad Dermatol* 48(3), 472 (passim)
  (2002): McGee AM+, *Br J Anaesth* 88(1), 139
  (2002): Poletti E+, *World Congress Dermatol* Poster, 0124
  (2001): Corazza M+, *J Eur Acad Dermatol Venereol* 15(6), 585
  (1999): Forsbach Sanchez G+, *Rev Invest Clin* (Spanish) 51, 71
  (1995): Rygnestad T+, *Acta Anaesthesiol Scand* 39(8), 1128
  (1992): Stricker BH+, *Ann Intern Med* 117(12), 1058
Headache
Hypersensitivity
  (2003): Klingenberg RD+, *Allergy* 58(10), 1076
  (2000): del Pozo MD+, *Allergy* 55, 412
  (1998): Romano A+, *Ann Allergy Asthma Immunol* 81, 373
Injection-site necrosis
  (1989): Tweedie DG, *Anaesthesia* 44, 932
Injection-site pain
  (1998): Schaad HJ+, *Ther Umsch* (German) 55, 586
Nephrotoxicity
  (2001): Hickey EJ+, *Free Radic Biol Med* 31(2), 139
Paresthesias (<1%)
Pseudolymphoma
  (2001): Werth V, *Dermatology Times* 18
Rhabdomyolysis
  (2002): Hengge UR+, *Hautarzt* 53(7), 483
  (1996): Delrio FG+, *Am J Med Sci* 312(2), 95
Serum sickness
Systemic reactions
  (2004): Macchia L+, *Allergy* 59(3), 367

DICLOXACILLIN

Trade names: Brispen; Dichlor-Stapenor; Diclo; Diclocil; Diclocillin; Diclox; Dycill (GSK); Dynapen; Novapen; Pathocil; Posipen
Indications: Infections due to penicillinase-producing staphylococci
Category: Antibiotic, penicillin
Half-life: 0.5–1.0 hours
Clinically important, potentially hazardous interactions with: anticoagulants, cyclosporine, imipenem/cilastatin, methotrexate, tetracycline, warfarin

Reactions

Skin

Angioedema
Bullous dermatitis
Dermatitis
Erythema multiforme
  (1991): Porteous DM+, *Arch Dermatol* 127, 740
Erythema nodosum
Erythroderma
  (1985): Shelley WB+, *Cutis* 220, 224
Exanthems (<1%)
Exfoliative dermatitis (<1%)
Hematomas
Jarisch–Herxheimer reaction
Jaundice
  (1993): Siegmund JB+, *Am J Gastroenterol* 88(8), 1299
Pruritus
  (1998): Siegfried EC+, *J Am Acad Dermatol* 39, 797 (passim)
Purpura
Rash (sic) (<1%)
Stevens–Johnson syndrome
  (1991): Porteous DM+, *Arch Dermatol* 127, 740
Toxic epidermal necrolysis
Urticaria
  (1998): Siegfried EC+, *J Am Acad Dermatol* 39, 797 (passim)
  (1985): Green RL+, *JAMA* 254, 531 (postcoital)
Vasculitis
Vesiculation

Mucosal/ENT

Dysgeusia
Glossitis
Glossodynia
Oral candidiasis
Stomatitis
Stomatodynia
Tongue black
Vaginitis (<1%)
Xerostomia

Nails

Nails – shoreline
  (1985): Shelley WB+, *Cutis* 220, 224

Other

Anaphylactoid reactions/Anaphylaxis
  (1998): Siegfried EC+, *J Am Acad Dermatol* 39, 797 (passim)
Hypersensitivity (<1%)
Injection-site pain
Myalgia/Myositis/Myopathy/Myotoxicity
Phlebitis
  (2004): Lanbeck P+, *J Antimicrob Chemother* 53(2), 174

(2003): Lanbeck P+, *Scand J Infect Dis* 35(6–7), 397
Serum sickness (<1%)
Thrombophlebitis
  (1982): Bergman BR, *Acta Orthop Scand* 53(1), 57 (16%)

DICUMAROL

Synonym: bishydroxycoumarin
Trade names: Apekumarol; Dicumarol; Dicumol; Embolin
Indications: Atrial fibrillation, pulmonary embolism, venous thrombosis
Category: Coumarin
Half-life: 1–4 days
Clinically important, potentially hazardous interactions with: allopurinol, amiodarone, amobarbital, anabolic steroids, anti-thyroid agents, aprobarbital, aspirin, barbiturates, bivalirudin, butabarbital, butalbital, cimetidine, clofibrate, clopidogrel, cyclosporine, delavirdine, disulfiram, fenofibrate, fluconazole, gemfibrozil, glutethimide, imatinib, itraconazole, ketoconazole, levothyroxine, liothyronine, mephobarbital, methimazole, metronidazole, miconazole, penicillins, pentobarbital, phenobarbital, phenylbutazones, piperacillin, prednisone, primidone, propylthiouracil, quinidine, quinine, rifabutin, rifampin, rifapentine, rofecoxib, salicylates, secobarbital, sulfinpyrazone, sulfonamides, testosterone, thyroid, zileuton

Reactions

Skin
Acral purpura
  (1986): Stone MS+, *J Am Acad Dermatol* 14, 796
Angioedema (<1%)
Bullous dermatitis
  (1986): Stone MS+, *J Am Acad Dermatol* 14, 796 (passim)
Dermatitis
  (1992): Breathnach SM+, *Adverse Drug Reactions and the Skin* Blackwell, Oxford, 248 (passim)
  (1991): Quintavalla R+, *Int Angiol* 10, 103
Exanthems
  (1989): Kruis-de Vries MH+, *Dermatologica* 178, 109
  (1988): Cole MS+, *Surgery* 103, 271 (passim)
Hemorrhage
  (1989): Geoghegan+, *BMJ* 298, 902
  (1988): Cole MS, *Surgery* 103, 271
  (1980): Schleicher SM+, *Arch Dermatol* 116, 444
Necrosis
  (2002): Cirafici P+, *Dermatology* 204(2), 157
  (1992): Sharafuddin MA+, *Arch Dermatol* 128, 105
  (1989): Grimaudo V+, *BMJ* 289, 233
  (1988): Cole MS+, *Surgery* 103, 271
  (1987): Gladson CL+, *Arch Dermatol* 123, 1701a
  (1984): Slutzki S+, *Int J Dermatol* 23, 117
  (1982): Faraci PA, *Int J Dermatol* 21, 329
  (1981): Horn JR+, *Am J Hosp Pharm* 38, 1763
Pigmentation
Pruritus (<1%)
Purplish erythema (feet and toes)
Purpura
  (1988): Cole MS+, *Surgery* 103, 271 (passim)
Rash (sic)
Urticaria
  (1988): Cole MS+, *Surgery* 103, 271 (passim)
  (1986): Stone MS+, *J Am Acad Dermatol* 14, 796 (passim)
Vesiculation
  (1986): Stone MS+, *J Am Acad Dermatol* 14, 796 (passim)

Mucosal/ENT
Oral ulceration

Hair
Hair – alopecia (1–10%)
  (1989): Kruis-de Vries MH+, *Dermatologica* 178, 109 (passim)
  (1988): Umlas J+, *Cutis* 42, 63
  (1986): Stone MS+, *J Am Acad Dermatol* 14, 796 (passim)

Other
Hypersensitivity

DICYCLOMINE

Trade names: Antispaz; Bemote; Bentyl (Axcan); Bentylol; Byclomine; Di-Spaz; Dibent; Formulex; Lomine; Merbentyl; Neoquess; Notensyl; OrTyl; Panakiron; Spasmoban; Spasmoject; Swityl
Indications: Irritable bowel syndrome
Category: Anticholinergic; Muscarinic antagonist
Half-life: initial: 1.8 hours; terminal: 9–10 hours
Clinically important, potentially hazardous interactions with: anticholinergics, arbutamine

Reactions

Skin
Exanthems
  (1987): Castleden CM+, *J Clin Exp Gerontol* 9, 265
Pruritus
Rash (sic) (<1%)
Urticaria
Xerosis (>10%)

Mucosal/ENT
Ageusia
Dysgeusia
Xerostomia (>10%)

Other
Anaphylactoid reactions/Anaphylaxis
Headache
Injection-site reactions (sic) (>10%)
Tremor

DIDANOSINE

Trade name: Videx (Bristol-Myers Squibb)
Indications: Advanced HIV infection
Category: Antiretroviral; Nucleoside analog reverse transcriptase inhibitor
Half-life: 1.5 hours
Clinically important, potentially hazardous interactions with: acetaminophen, ciprofloxacin, corticosteroids, dapsone, itraconazole, ketoconazole, lomefloxacin, sulfones, tenofovir, tetracycline

Reactions

Skin
Acral erythema
  (1993): Pedailles S+, *Ann Dermatol Venereol* (French) 120, 837
Diaphoresis
Erythema multiforme

(2001): Scully C+, *Oral Dis* 7(4), 205 (passim)
(1992): Parneix-Spake A+, *Lancet* 340, 847
Exanthems
Pruritus (9%)
Purpura
Rash (sic) (9%)
Stevens–Johnson syndrome
   (2003): Rotunda A+, *Acta Derm Venereol* 83(1), 1
   (1992): Parneix-Spake A+, *Lancet* 340, 847
Urticaria
Vasculitis
   (1994): Herranz P+, *Lancet* 344, 680

Mucosal/ENT
Xerostomia
   (2001): Scully C+, *Oral Dis* 7(4), 205 (up to 33%) (passim)
   (1993): Allan JD+, *Clin Infect Dis* 16 Suppl 1, S46
   (1992): Dodd CL+, *Lancet* 340(8822), 790
   (1992): Valentine C+, *Lancet* 340(8834–8835), 1542

Hair
Hair – alopecia (<1%)

Eyes
Retinopathy
   (2006): Fernando AI+, *Eye* 20(12), 1435

Other
Anaphylactoid reactions/Anaphylaxis (<1%)
Chills
Death
   (2001): Hwang SW+, *Singapore Med J* 42(6), 247 (2 cases) (with stavudine)
Gynecomastia
   (2001): Aquilina C+, *Int J STD AIDS* 12(7), 481 (with stavudine)
   (2001): Manfredi R+, *Ann Pharmacother* 35(4), 438 (with stavudine)
Headache
Hepatotoxicity
   (2006): Maida I+, *J Acquir Immune Defic Syndr* 42(2), 177
Hypersensitivity (<1%)
Lipodystrophy
   (2001): Aquilina C+, *Int J STD AIDS* 12(7), 481 (with didanosine)
Myalgia/Myositis/Myopathy/Myotoxicity
Neurotoxicity
   (2006): Young B+, *AIDS Patient Care STDS* 20(4), 238
   (1993): Allan JD+, *Clin Infect Dis* 16 Suppl 1, S46
Paresthesias
Rhabdomyolysis
   (1994): Chariot P+, *Neurology* 44(9), 1692

DIDEOXYCYTIDINE (ddC)

(See ZALCITABINE)

DIETHYLPROPION

Synonym: amfepramone
Trade names: Anorex; Linea; Nobesine; Prefamone; Regenon; Tenuate (Sanofi-Aventis); Tenuate Retard; Tepanil
Indications: Weight reduction
Category: Amphetamine
Half-life: 4–6 hours
Clinically important, potentially hazardous interactions with: fluoxetine, fluvoxamine, MAO inhibitors, paroxetine, phenelzine, sertraline, tranylcypromine

Reactions

Skin
Diaphoresis (<1%)
Erythema (<1%)
Erythema multiforme
   (1997): Thaler D, Monona, WI (from Internet) (observation)
Exanthems (<1%)
Pruritus (<1%)
Purpura (<1%)
Rash (sic)
Scleroderma
   (1991): Bourgeois P+, *Baillieres Clin Rheumatol* 5, 13
   (1990): Aeschlimann A+, *Scand J Rheumatol* 19, 87
Systemic sclerosis
   (1984): Tomlinson JW+, *J Rheumatol* 11, 254
Urticaria

Mucosal/ENT
Dysgeusia
Xerostomia

Hair
Hair – alopecia (<1%)

Other
Gynecomastia
Headache
Myalgia/Myositis/Myopathy/Myotoxicity (<1%)
Tremor

DIETHYLSTILBESTROL

Synonyms: DES; stilbestrol
Trade names: Diethyl Stilbestrol; Diethylstilbestrol; Distilbene; Honvol; Stilboestrol; Stilphostrol
Indications: Metastatic prostate carcinoma, progressive breast cancer
Category: Estrogen
Half-life: 2–3 days

Reactions

Skin
Acanthosis nigricans
Acne
Angioedema
Bullous dermatitis
Chloasma (<1%)
Edema
Erythema multiforme
Erythema nodosum
Exanthems
   (1984): Lee M+, *J Urol* 131, 767
Exfoliative dermatitis
Hyperkeratosis
   (1980): Mold DE+, *Cutis* 26, 95
Lupus erythematosus
   (1989): Collins D, *J Rheumatol* 16, 408
Melasma (<1%)
Peripheral edema (>10%)
Pruritus
Purpura
   (1984): Lee M+, *J Urol* 131, 767

Rash (sic) (<1%)
Urticaria
(1989): Collins D, *J Rheumatol* 16, 408
(1984): Lee M+, *J Urol* 131, 767

Mucosal/ENT
Vulvovaginal candidiasis

Hair
Hair – alopecia
Hair – hirsutism
(1982): Peress MR+, *Am J Obstet Gynecol* 144, 135

Other
Gynecomastia (>10%)
Polyarteritis nodosa
Porphyria cutanea tarda
(1989): Coulson IH+, *Br J Urol* 63, 648

DIFLUNISAL

Trade names: Ansal; Apo-Diflunisal; Diflonid; Diflusal; Dolobid (Merck); Dolobis; Donobid; Fluniget; Flustar; Nu-Diflunisal
Indications: Rheumatoid and osteoarthritis
Category: Non-steroidal anti-inflammatory
Half-life: 8–12 hours
Clinically important, potentially hazardous interactions with: indomethacin

Reactions

Skin
Adverse effects (sic)
(1985): Lee P+, *J Rheumatol* 12, 544
(1983): McQueen EG, *N Z Med J* 96, 95
Angioedema (<1%)
Bullous dermatitis
(1989): Street ML+, *J Am Acad Dermatol* 20, 850
Diaphoresis (<1%)
(1986): Muncie HL+, *J Fam Pract* 23, 125
Edema (<1%)
Erythema multiforme (<1%)
(1986): Grom JA+, *Hosp Formul Manage* 21, 353
(1985): Bigby M+, *J Am Acad Dermatol* 12, 866 (5%)
(1985): O'Brien WM+, *J Rheumatol* 12, 13
(1982): Dubois A+, *Presse Med* (French) 11, 606
Erythroderma
(1989): Street ML+, *J Am Acad Dermatol* 20, 850
(1980): Chan LK+, *BMJ* 280, 84
Exanthems
(1992): Breathnach SM+, *Adverse Drug Reactions and the Skin*
Blackwell, Oxford, 180 (passim)
(1988): Cook DJ+, *Can Med Assoc J* 138, 1029
(1985): Bigby M+, *J Am Acad Dermatol* 12, 866 (5%)
(1985): Bocanegra TS+, *Curr Res Med Opin* 9, 568 (1.7%)
Exfoliative dermatitis (<1%)
(1985): Bigby M+, *J Am Acad Dermatol* 12, 866
Fixed eruption
(1998): Mahboob A+, *Int J Dermatol* 37, 833
(1991): Roetzheim RG+, *J Am Acad Dermatol* 24, 1021 (non-pigmenting)
Lichenoid eruption
(1989): Street ML+, *J Am Acad Dermatol* 20, 850
Peripheral edema
Photosensitivity (<1%)
(1989): Street ML+, *J Am Acad Dermatol* 20, 850

Pruritus (1–10%)
(1992): Breathnach SM+, *Adverse Drug Reactions and the Skin*
Blackwell, Oxford, 180 (passim)
(1986): Hurme M+, *Int J Clin Pharmacol Res* 6, 53
(1985): Bigby M+, *J Am Acad Dermatol* 12, 866 (5%)
Purpura
Rash (sic) (3–9%)
(1987): Masden JJ+, *Curr Ther Res* 42, 319
(1986): Bennett RM, *Clin Ther* 9, 27
(1986): Turner RA+, *Clin Ther* 9, 37
Stevens–Johnson syndrome (<1%)
(1999): Yusin JS+, *Ann Allergy Asthma Immunol* 83(5), 353
(1992): Breathnach SM+, *Adverse Drug Reactions and the Skin*
Blackwell, Oxford, 180 (passim)
(1986): Grom JA+, *Hosp Formul Manage* 21, 353
(1986): Szczeklik A, *Drugs* 32 (Suppl 4), 148
(1985): Bigby M+, *J Am Acad Dermatol* 12, 866
(1982): Dubois A+, *Presse Med* (French) 11, 606
Toxic epidermal necrolysis (<1%)
(1990): Roujeau JC+, *Arch Dermatol* 126, 37
Urticaria (>1%)
(1995): Arias J+, *Ann Allergy Asthma Immunol* 74, 160
(1992): Breathnach SM+, *Adverse Drug Reactions and the Skin*
Blackwell, Oxford, 180 (passim)
(1987): Morse DR+, *Clin Ther* 9, 500
(1985): Bigby M+, *J Am Acad Dermatol* 12, 866 (5%)
(1983): Griffin JP, *Practitioner* 227, 1283 (passim)
(1980): Chan LK+, *BMJ* 280, 84
Vasculitis (<1%)

Mucosal/ENT
Aphthous stomatitis
Oral lichen planus
(1983): Hamburger J+, *BMJ* 287, 1258
Oral ulceration
Stomatitis (<1%)
Tinnitus
Xerostomia
(1982): Ankri J+, *Clin Ther* 5, 85

Hair
Hair – alopecia

Other
Anaphylactoid reactions/Anaphylaxis (<1%)
Headache
Hypersensitivity (<1%)
Paresthesias (<1%)
Pseudolymphoma
(2001): Werth V, *Dermatology Times* 18
Pseudoporphyria
(1987): Taylor BJ+, *N Z Med J* 100, 322

DIFLUPREDNATE

Trade names: Durezol; Epitopic; Myser (Sirion)
Indications: Corticosteroid responsive dermatoses, inflammation and pain associated with ocular surgery
Category: Corticosteroid, topical

Reactions

Eyes
Blepharitis
Cataract
Conjunctival edema

Conjunctival hyperemia
Corneal edema
Eyelid pain
Intraocular pressure increased
Photophobia
Posterior capsule opacification

DIGOXIN

Trade names: Cardigox; Digacin; Digoxine; Eudigox; Lanicor; Lanoxin (GSK); Lenoxin; Novo-Digoxin
Indications: Congestive heart failure, atrial fibrillation
Category: Antiarrhythmic class IV; Cardiac glycoside; Inotrope
Half-life: 36–48 hours
Clinically important, potentially hazardous interactions with: alprazolam, amiodarone, amphotericin B, arbutamine, bendroflumethiazide, benzthiazide, bisacodyl, bumetanide, carbimazole, chlorothiazide, chlorthalidone, cholestyramine, clarithromycin, conivaptan, cyclosporine, cyclothiazide, **danshen**, demeclocycline, **devil's claw**, dexmedetomidine, doxycycline, erythromycin, esomeprazole, ethacrynic acid, flunisolide, furosemide, **ginseng, hawthorn (fruit, leaf, flower extract), horsetail**, hydrochlorothiazide, hydroflumethiazide, indapamide, **licorice**, mepenzolate, methyclothiazide, metolazone, minocycline, **mistletoe**, oxytetracycline, paroxetine, phenylbutazone, polythiazide, propafenone, propantheline, quinethazone, quinidine, rabeprazole, rifampin, roxithromycin, **sarsaparilla, senna, siberian ginseng, squill, St John's wort**, telithromycin, teriparatide, tetracycline, thiazide diuretics, trichlormethiazide, verapamil

Note: This is the pure form of Digitalis

Reactions

Skin
Angioedema
Bullous dermatitis
   (1992): Breathnach SM+, *Adverse Drug Reactions and the Skin* Blackwell, Oxford, 216 (passim)
Diaphoresis
   (1980): Lofgren RP, *N Engl J Med* 302, 919
Exanthems (1.6%)
   (1994): Martin SJ+, *JAMA* 271, 1905 (generalized)
   (1994): Shelley WB+, *Cutis* 54, 76 (observation)
   (1992): Breathnach SM+, *Adverse Drug Reactions and the Skin* Blackwell, Oxford, 216 (passim)
Pruritus
   (1994): Martin SJ+, *JAMA* 271, 1905 (generalized)
Psoriasis
   (1981): David M+, *J Am Acad Dermatol* 5, 702
Purpura
   (1992): Breathnach SM+, *Adverse Drug Reactions and the Skin* Blackwell, Oxford, 216 (passim)
Rash (sic)
Urticaria
   (1994): Shelley WB+, *Cutis* 54, 76 (observation)
   (1992): Breathnach SM+, *Adverse Drug Reactions and the Skin* Blackwell, Oxford, 216 (passim)
Vasculitis

Hair
Hair – alopecia

Nails
Nails – loss (finger- and toenails)

Eyes
Dyschromatopsia (green)
   (2002): Lawrenson JG+, *Br J Ophthalmol* 86(11), 1259
   (2001): Nagai N+, *Nippon Ganka Gakkai Zasshi* 105(1), 24
   (1993): Piltz JR+, *J Clin Neuroophthalmol* 13(4), 275 (3 cases)
   (1991): Arnold WN+, *Eye* 5(Pt 5), 503
   (1989): Lanthony P, *Bull Soc Ophtalmol Fr* 89(10), 1133
   (1981): Lee TC, *JAMA* 245(7), 727
Photopsia
   (2006): Oishi A+, *Can J Ophthalmol* 41(5), 603

Other
Dementia
   (2007): *Prescrire Int* 16(87), 15
Gynecomastia
   (2000): Hugues FC+, *Ann Med Interne* (Paris) (French) 151, 10 (passim)
Headache

DIHYDROERGOTAMINE

Trade names: D.H.E. 45 (Xcel); Dergiflux; Dihydergot; Ergont; Ergovasan; Ikaran; Migranal (Xcel); Orstanorm; Seglor; Verladyn; Verteblan
Indications: Prevention of vascular headaches
Category: Ergot alkaloid
Half-life: 1.3–3.9 hours
Clinically important, potentially hazardous interactions with: almotriptan, amprenavir, clarithromycin, darunavir, delavirdine, efavirenz, erythromycin, fosamprenavir, indinavir, naratriptan, nelfinavir, ritonavir, rizatriptan, saquinavir, sibutramine, sumatriptan, telithromycin, tipranavir, troleandomycin, zolmitriptan

Reactions

Skin
Edema (>10%)
Necrosis
   (1998): Hahne T+, *Hautarzt* 49(9), 722
   (1991): Bongard O+, *Vasa* 20(2), 153
   (1983): Jehn U+, *Dtsch Med Wochenschr* 108(30), 1148 (with heparin)
Pruritus

Mucosal/ENT
Dysgeusia
   (1995): Beubler E, *Wien Med Wochenschr* 145(14), 326
Xerostomia (>10%)

Other
Abdominal pain
   (1991): Iaquinto G+, *Ital J Gastroenterol* 23(4), 219
Gangrene
   (1996): Gupta VL+, *Acta Anaesthesiol Scand* 40(3), 389
Headache
   (1996): Evans MS+, *Clin Neuropharmacol* 19(2), 177
   (1996): Queiroz LP+, *Headache* 36(5), 291
   (1993): Walker J+, *South Med J* 86(11), 1202
   (1992): Saadah HA, *Headache* 32(1), 18
Hypertension
   (1993): Hopson JR+, *Herz* 18(3), 164
Injection-site burning
   (1992): Robbins L+, *Headache* 32(9), 455

Injection-site reactions (sic)
Myalgia/Myositis/Myopathy/Myotoxicity
Paresthesias (>10%)
Thrombosis
(1991): Iaquinto G+, *Ital J Gastroenterol* 23(4), 219
Vertigo
(1996): Queiroz LP+, *Headache* 36(5), 291
(1990): Jenzer G+, *Schweiz Rundsch Med Prax* 79(31–32), 914

DIHYDROTACHYSTEROL

Trade names: AT 10; DHT (Roxane); Dihydral; Dygratyl;
Hytakerol (Sanofi-Aventis)
Indications: Hypocalcemia associated with hypoparathyroidism
Category: Vitamin D receptor agonist
Half-life: N/A

Reactions

Skin
Calcification
(1985): Michel B+, *Schweiz Med Wochenschr* (German) 115, 418
Exanthems
Livedo reticularis
(1985): Michel B+, *Schweiz Med Wochenschr* (German) 115, 418
Pruritus (1–10%)
Ulcerative necrosis
(1985): Michel B+, *Schweiz Med Wochenschr* (German) 115, 418

Mucosal/ENT
Dysgeusia (metallic taste)
Xerostomia

Other
Myalgia/Myositis/Myopathy/Myotoxicity

DILTIAZEM

Trade names: Alti-Diltiazem; Britiazem; Calcicard; Cardizem
(Biovail); Cartia-XT; Deltazen; Dilacor XR (Watson); Dilrene;
Diltahexal; Diltia-XT; Nu-Diltiaz; Presoken; Teczem (Sanofi-
Aventis); Tiamate; Tiazac (Forest); Tilazem; Tildiem
Indications: Angina, essential hypertension
Category: Antiarrhythmic class IV; Calcium channel blocker
Half-life: 5–8 hours (for extended-release capsules)
**Clinically important, potentially hazardous interactions
with:** alfuzosin, amiodarone, aprepitant, carbamazepine,
celiprolol, corticosteroids, cyclosporine, epirubicin, erythromycin,
mistletoe, moricizine, ranolazine, simvastatin

Note: Teczem is diltiazem and enalapril

Reactions

Skin
Acne
(1989): Stern R+, *Arch Intern Med* 149, 829
Acute generalized exanthematous pustulosis (AGEP)
(2003): Saissi EH+, *Ann Dermatol Venereol* 130(6-7), 612
(2002): Arroyo MP+, *J Drugs Dermatol* 1(1), 63
(1998): Jan V+, *Dermatology* 197, 274
(1998): Knowles S+, *J Am Acad Dermatol* 38, 201 (passim)
(1997): Blodgett TP+, *Cutis* 60, 45
(1997): Vincente-Calleja JM+, *Br J Dermatol* 137, 837

(1996): Wolkenstein P+, *Contact Dermatitis* 35, 234
(1995): Krasovec M+, *Schweiz Rundsch Med Prax* (German)
84, 814
(1995): Moreau A+, *Int J Dermatol* 34, 263 (passim)
(1995): Wakelin SH+, *Clin Exp Dermatol* 20, 341
(1993): Janier M+, *Br J Dermatol* 129, 354
(1992): Wittal RA+, *Australas J Dermatol* 33, 11
(1988): Lambert DG+, *Br J Dermatol* 118, 308
Adverse effects (sic)
(1993): Barbaud A+, *Therapie* (French) 48, 499
Angioedema
(1998): Knowles S+, *J Am Acad Dermatol* 38, 201 (passim)
(1989): Sadick NS+, *J Am Acad Dermatol* 21, 132
Capillaritis (Schamberg's)
(1999): Eastern JS, Belleville, NJ (from Internet) (observation)
Dermatitis
Diaphoresis
(1988): Lambert DG+, *Br J Dermatol* 118, 308 (passim)
(1985): Scolnick B+, *Ann Intern Med* 102, 558
Edema (1–10%)
(2001): Chugh SK+, *J Cardiovasc Pharmacol* 38(3), 356
(1998): Knowles S+, *J Am Acad Dermatol* 38, 201 (passim)
(1982): Hossack KF, *Am J Cardiol* 49, 567
(1982): McGraw BF, *Drug Intell Clin Pharm* 16, 366
Erythema
(1998): Knowles S+, *J Am Acad Dermatol* 38, 201 (passim)
(1982): McGraw BF, *Drug Intell Clin Pharm* 16, 366
Erythema multiforme (1–31%)
(2001): Swale VJ+, *Br J Dermatol* 144(4), 920
(1998): Knowles S+, *J Am Acad Dermatol* 38, 201 (passim)
(1995): Avila JR+, *Ann Pharmacother* 29, 317
(1993): Kitamura K+, *J Dermatol* 20, 279 (psoriasiform) (31%)
(1993): Sanders CJ+, *Lancet* 341, 967
(1993): Sousa-Basto A+, *Contact Dermatitis* 29, 44
(1992): Wittal RA+, *Australas J Dermatol* 33, 11
(1989): Berbis P+, *Dermatologica* 179, 90
(1989): Brown FH+, *Ann Dent* 48, 39
(1989): Stern R+, *Arch Intern Med* 149, 829
Exanthems
(2000): Heymann WR, *Cutis* 66, 129
(1998): Knowles S+, *J Am Acad Dermatol* 38, 201 (passim)
(1994): Baker BA+, *Ann Pharmacother* 28, 118
(1993): Kitamura K+, *J Dermatol* 20, 279 (psoriasiform) (31%)
(1993): Sousa-Basto A+, *Contact Dermatitis* 29, 44
(1992): Romano A+, *Ann Allergy* 69, 31
(1992): Wittal RA+, *Australas J Dermatol* 33, 11 (erythroderma)
(1990): Wirebaugh SR+, *Drug Intell Clin Pharm* 24, 1046
(1989): Jones SK+, *Clin Exp Dermatol* 14, 457
(1989): Stern R+, *Arch Intern Med* 149, 829
(1988): Hammentgen R+, *Dtsch Med Wochenschr* (German)
113, 1283
(1988): Lambert DG+, *Br J Dermatol* 118, 308 (passim)
(1988): Wakeel RA+, *BMJ* 296, 1071 (passim)
(1986): Gibson RS+, *N Engl J Med* 315, 423 (0.7%)
(1985): Chaffman M+, *Drugs* 29, 387 (1.3%)
(1985): Scolnick B+, *Ann Intern Med* 102, 558
Exfoliative dermatitis (<1%)
(1998): Knowles S+, *J Am Acad Dermatol* 38, 201 (passim)
(1997): Odeh M, *J Toxicol Clin Toxicol* 35, 101
(1993): Sousa-Basto A+, *Contact Dermatitis* 29, 44
(1989): Stern R+, *Arch Intern Med* 149, 829
(1988): Wakeel RA+, *BMJ* 296, 1071 (passim)
(1986): Lavrijsen APM+, *Acta Derm Venereol* 66, 536 (in a
patient with psoriasis)
Hyperkeratosis (feet)
(1992): Ilia R+, *Int J Cardiol* 35, 115
Leg ulceration
(1989): Jones SK+, *Clin Exp Dermatol* 14, 457
(1988): Carmichael AJ+, *BMJ* 297, 562 (vasculitic)

Lichenoid eruption (photosensitive)
  (2001): Gladstone GC, *Dermatology Times* Worcester, MA
    (personal communication)
  (1988): Lambert DG+, *Br J Dermatol* 118, 308
Lupus erythematosus
  (1998): Callen JP, Academy '98 Meeting (4 patients)
  (1998): Knowles S+, *J Am Acad Dermatol* 38, 201 (passim)
  (1997): Crowson AN+, *Hum Pathol* 28(1), 67
  (1995): Crowson AN+, *N Engl J Med* 333, 1429
  (1989): Stern R+, *Arch Intern Med* 149, 829
Palmar–plantar desquamation
  (1985): Scolnick B+, *Ann Intern Med* 102, 558
Peripheral edema (5–8%)
  (2002): No Author, *Medscape Primary Care* 4
  (1994): Litt JZ, Beachwood, OH (personal case) (observation)
Petechiae (<1%)
Photoallergic reaction
  (2007): Ramirez A+, *Contact Dermatitis* 56(2), 118
Photosensitivity (<1%)
  (2007): Ramirez A+, *Contact Dermatitis* 56(2), 118
  (1998): Knowles S+, *J Am Acad Dermatol* 38, 201 (passim)
  (1997): O'Reilly FM+, American Academy of Dermatology
    Meeting, Poster #14
  (1996): Seggev JS+, *J Allergy Clin Immunol* 97, 852
  (1994): Shelley WB+, *Cutis* 53, 161 (observation)
  (1992): Wittal RA+, *Australas J Dermatol* 33, 11 (erythroderma)
  (1990): Young L+, *Clin Exp Dermatol* 15, 467
  (1989): Berbis P+, *Dermatologica* 179, 90
  (1988): Lambert DG+, *Br J Dermatol* 118, 308
  (1986): Lavrijsen APM+, *Acta Derm Venereol* 66, 536
Pigmentation
  (2006): Berendzen SM+, *Int J Dermatol* 45(12), 1450
    (photodistributed)
  (2006): Saladi RN+, *Arch Dermatol* 142(2), 206
    (photodistributed)
  (2004): Kuykendall-Ivy T+, *Cutis* 73(4), 239
  (2004): Mendelsohn D, Phoenix, AZ (personal communication)
    (gray)
  (2003): Boyer M+, *Dermatol Online J* 9(5), 10 (photodistributed)
  (2002): Chawla A+, *J Am Acad Dermatol* 46(3), 468
  (2002): Schmutz JL+, *Ann Dermatol Venereol* 129(11), 1332
  (2001): Scherschun L+, *Arch Dermatol* 137(2), 179 (4 cases)
    (photodistributed)
Pruritus (<1%)
  (2001): Gladstone GC, *Dermatology Times* (personal
    communication)
  (2000): Heymann WR, *Cutis* 66, 129
  (1998): Knowles S+, *J Am Acad Dermatol* 38, 201 (passim)
  (1994): Baker BA+, *Ann Pharmacother* 28, 118
  (1989): Stern R+, *Arch Intern Med* 149, 829
  (1986): Gibson RS+, *N Engl J Med* 315, 423 (0.7%)
  (1982): McGraw BF, *Drug Intell Clin Pharm* 16, 366
Psoriasis
  (2001): Smith KC, Niagara Falls, Ontario (from Internet)
    (observation)
  (1998): Knowles S+, *J Am Acad Dermatol* 38, 201 (passim)
  (1993): Kitamura K+, *J Dermatol* 20, 279 (psoriasiform) (31%)
  (1989): Stern R+, *Arch Intern Med* 149, 829
Purpura (<1%)
  (2001): Inui S+, *J Dermatol* 28(2), 100 (lichenoid)
  (1998): Knowles S+, *J Am Acad Dermatol* 38, 201 (passim)
  (1992): Kuo M+, *Ann Pharmacother* 26, 1089
Pustules
  (1993): Janier M+, *Br J Dermatol* 129, 354
  (1988): Lambert DG+, *Br J Dermatol* 118, 308
Rash (sic) (1.3%)
  (2006): Glasser SP, *Adv Ther* 23(2), 284 (%)
  (1998): Knowles S+, *J Am Acad Dermatol* 38, 201 (passim)
  (1989): Stern R+, *Arch Intern Med* 149, 829

  (1982): McGraw BF, *Drug Intell Clin Pharm* 16, 366
Side effects (sic)
  (1993): Kitamura K+, *J Dermatol* 20, 279 (psoriasiform) (31%)
  (1993): Sousa-Basto A+, *Contact Dermatitis* 29, 44
Stevens–Johnson syndrome
  (1998): Knowles S+, *J Am Acad Dermatol* 38, 201 (passim)
  (1993): Sanders CJ+, *Lancet* 341, 967
  (1990): Taylor J+, *Clin Pharmacy* 9, 948
  (1989): Stern R+, *Arch Intern Med* 149, 829
Subcorneal pustular dermatosis (Sneddon-Wilkinson)
  (2001): Reed B, Denver, CO (from internet) (observation)
  (1992): Wittal RA+, *Australas J Dermatol* 33(1), 11
Thickening
  (1998): Knowles S+, *J Am Acad Dermatol* 38, 201 (passim)
  (1992): Ilia R+, *Int J Cardiol* 35, 115
Toxic dermatitis (sic)
  (1988): Wakeel RA+, *BMJ* 296, 1071
Toxic epidermal necrolysis
  (1998): Knowles S+, *J Am Acad Dermatol* 38, 201 (passim)
  (1991): No Author, *Lakartidningen* (Swedish) 88, 3489
  (1989): Stern R+, *Arch Intern Med* 149, 829
  (1988): Wakeel RA+, *BMJ* 296, 1071 (passim)
Toxic erythema
  (1998): Knowles S+, *J Am Acad Dermatol* 38, 201 (passim)
  (1988): Wakeel RA+, *BMJ* 296, 1071
Urticaria (<1%)
  (1998): Knowles S+, *J Am Acad Dermatol* 38, 201 (passim)
  (1989): Jones SK+, *Clin Exp Dermatol* 14, 457
  (1989): Sadick NS+, *J Am Acad Dermatol* 21, 132
  (1989): Stern R+, *Arch Intern Med* 149, 829
Vasculitis (<1%)
  (1998): Knowles S+, *J Am Acad Dermatol* 38, 201 (passim)
  (1992): Kuo M+, *Ann Pharmacother* 26, 1089
  (1992): Wittal RA+, *Australas J Dermatol* 33, 11
  (1989): Stern R+, *Arch Intern Med* 149, 829
  (1988): Sheehan-Dare RA+, *Br J Dermatol* 119, 134
  (1988): Sheehan-Dare RA+, *Postgrad Med J* 64, 467

Mucosal/ENT
Dysgeusia (<1%)
  (2000): Zervakis J+, *Physiol Behav* 68, 405
  (1985): Berman JL, *Ann Intern Med* 102(5), 717
Gingival hyperplasia/hypertrophy (21%)
  (2005): Miranda J+, *J Clin Periodontol* 32(3), 294 (50%)
  (1999): Ellis JS+, *J Periodontol* 70, 63 (74%)
  (1998): Knowles S+, *J Am Acad Dermatol* 38, 201 (passim)
  (1998): Young PC+, *Cutis* 62(indu), 41
  (1995): Bullon P+, *Oral Surg Oral Med Oral Pathol Oral Radiol
    Endod* 79(3), 300
  (1995): Moghadam BKH+, *Cutis* 56, 46 (passim)
  (1993): King GN+, *J Clin Periodontol* 20, 286
  (1990): Brown RS+, *Oral Surg* 70, 593
  (1987): Giustiniani S+, *Int J Cardiol* 15, 247
Oral ulceration
  (1999): Cohen DM+, *J Am Dent Assoc* 130(11), 1611
Tinnitus
Xerostomia (<1%)
  (1983): Lewis JG, *Drugs* 25, 196
  (1981): Pepine CJ+, *Am Heart J* 101, 719

Hair
Hair – alopecia (<1%)
  (1998): Knowles S+, *J Am Acad Dermatol* 38, 201 (passim)
  (1989): Stern R+, *Arch Intern Med* 149, 829
Hair – hirsutism
  (1989): Stern R+, *Arch Intern Med* 149, 829

Nails
Nails – dystrophy
  (1989): Stern R+, *Arch Intern Med* 149, 829

Eyes

Periorbital edema
  (1993): Friedland S+, *Arch Ophthalmol* 111, 1027

Other

Erythromelalgia
  (1989): Stern R+, *Arch Intern Med* 149, 829
Fever
  (2003): Jover-Saenz A+, *Med Clin* (Barc) 120(13), 517
Gynecomastia
  (1994): Otto C+, *Arch Intern Med* 154, 351
Headache
  (2006): Glasser SP, *Adv Ther* 23(2), 284 (%)
Hypersensitivity
  (1998): Knowles S+, *J Am Acad Dermatol* 38, 201 (passim)
  (1986): Lavrijsen AP+, *Acta Derm Venereol* 66(6), 536
Hypertension
  (1985): Schroeder JS+, *Acta Pharmacol Toxicol* (Copenh) 57
    Suppl 2, 55
Paresthesias (<1%)
  (1982): McGraw BF, *Drug Intell Clin Pharm* 16, 366
Pseudolymphoma
  (1995): Magro CM+, *J Am Acad Dermatol* 32, 419
Rhabdomyolysis
  (2002): Lewin JJ 3rd+, *Ann Pharmacother* 36(10), 1546 (with
    atorvastatin)
  (2001): Kanathur N+, *Tenn Med* 94(9), 339 (with simvastatin)
  (2001): Peces R+, *Nephron* 89(1), 117 (with simvastatin)
Tremor (<1%)
Vertigo
  (2006): Glasser SP, *Adv Ther* 23(2), 284 (%)

DIMENHYDRINATE

Trade names: Andrumin; Calm-X; Dimetabs; Dramamine
(Pfizer); Lomarin; Marmine; Nauseatol; Nausicalm; Nico-Vert;
Tega-Cert; Tega-Vert; Travel Tabs; Triptone; Vertab; Vomacur;
Vomex A; Vomisen; Wehamine
Indications: Motion sickness, dizziness, nausea, vomiting
Category: Cholinesterase absorption inhibitor
Half-life: N/A

Reactions

Skin

Angioedema (<1%)
Dermatitis (systemic)
Diaphoresis
Eczema
Edema (<1%)
Exanthems
Fixed eruption (<1%)
  (2000): Ozkaya-Bayazit E+, *Eur J Dermatol* 10, 288
  (2000): Saenz de San Pedro B+, *Allergy* 55, 297
  (2000): Smith KC, Niagara Falls, Ontario (recurrent) (from
    Internet) (observation)
  (1999): Gallagher W, *The Schoch Letter*, 49, #1, 2
  (1998): Smola H+, *Br J Dermatol* 138, 920
  (1997): Gonzalo-Garijo MA+, *Br J Dermatol* 135, 661
  (1992): Hatzis J+, *Cutis* 50, 50
  (1989): Hogan DJ+, *J Am Acad Dermatol* 20, 503
  (1982): Schnyder UW+, *Dermatologica* 165, 292
Photosensitivity (<1%)
Rash (sic) (<1%)
Urticaria

Mucosal/ENT

Xerostomia (1–10%)

Other

Anaphylactoid reactions/Anaphylaxis
Headache
Injection-site pain (<1%)
Myalgia/Myositis/Myopathy/Myotoxicity (<1%)
Paresthesias (<1%)

DIMERCAPROL

Synonyms: Dicaptol; Dithioglycerol; British Anti-Lewisite
Trade names: BAL (Taylor); Sulfactin
Indications: Heavy metal poisoning (Arsenic, Gold, Mercury,
Lead)
Category: Antidote; Chelator
Half-life: N/A
**Clinically important, potentially hazardous interactions
with:** insulin, iron, selenium

Reactions

Skin

Burning
Diaphoresis

Mucosal/ENT

Rhinorrhea
Sialorrhea

Eyes

Blepharospasm
Conjunctivitis
Epiphora

Other

Abdominal pain
Fever
Headache
Hypertension
Injection-site abscess
Injection-site pain
Paresthesias
Seizures

DINOPROSTONE

Trade names: Cervidel (Forest); Cerviprime; Cerviprost; KP-E;
Miniprostin E(2); Prandin E2; Prepidil (Pfizer); Primiprost;
Propess; Prostarmon; Prostin; Prostin E2; Prostin VR; Prostine
Indications: Pregnancy termination, uterine content evacuation,
cervical ripening
Category: Prostaglandin
Half-life: 2.5–5.0 minutes

Note: Dinoprostone is the naturally occurring form of Prostaglandin
E2 (PGE2)

Reactions

Skin

Diaphoresis
Pigmentation

Rash (sic)
Shivering

Mucosal/ENT
Vaginitis

Eyes
Ocular pain

Other
Anaphylactoid reactions/Anaphylaxis
  (2005): Cusick W+, *J Reprod Med* 50(3), 225
Chills
Cough
Fever
Headache
Hot flashes
Myalgia/Myositis/Myopathy/Myotoxicity
Paresthesias
Tremor
Vertigo

DIPHENHYDRAMINE

Trade names: Allerdryl; Allermax; Allermin; Banophen; Benadryl (Pfizer); Benahist; Benylin; Compoz; Dibrondrin; Dolestan; Genahist; Insomnal; Nytol; Resmin; Sediat; Sominex 2; Valdrene
Indications: Allergic rhinitis, urticaria
Category: Histamine H1 receptor antagonist; Muscarinic antagonist
Half-life: 2–8 hours
Clinically important, potentially hazardous interactions with: alcohol, anticholinergics, chloral hydrate, CNS depressants, glutethimide, MAO inhibitors

Reactions

Skin
Allergic reactions (sic)
Angioedema (<1%)
  (1988): Self F+, *J R Soc Med* 81, 544
Dermatitis
  (1998): Yamada S+, *Contact Dermatitis* 38, 282
  (1983): Coskey RJ, *J Am Acad Dermatol* 8, 204
Diaphoresis
Eczema
  (1981): Lawrence CM+, *Contact Dermatitis* 7, 276
Edema (<1%)
Exanthems
Fixed eruption
  (1993): Dwyer CM+, *J Am Acad Dermatol* 29, 496
Livedo reticularis
  (1996): Morell A+, *Dermatology* 193, 50
Photosensitivity (<1%)
  (2000): Danby FW, Manchester, NH (from Internet)
    (observation)
Pruritus
  (1998): Litt JZ, Beachwood, OH (following varicella) (personal
    case) (observation)
Purpura
  (1996): Morell A+, *Dermatology* 193, 50
Rash (sic) (<1%)
Toxic epidermal necrolysis
  (1991): Epishin AV+, *Klin Med Mosk* (Russian) 69, 92
Urticaria

Vasculitis
Mucosal/ENT
Tinnitus
Xerostomia (1–10%)

Eyes
Visual hallucinations

Other
Anaphylactoid reactions/Anaphylaxis
  (1998): Barranco P+, *Allergy* 53, 814
  (1995): Manhart AR+J, *Toxicol Clin Toxicol* 33, 189
  (1994): Watanabe T+, *J Toxicol Clin Toxicol* 32, 593
  (1980): Sandler BB, *Sov Med* (Russian) 9, 119
Death
  (2003): Baker AM+, *J Forensic Sci* 48(2), 425
Hypersensitivity
Injection-site gangrene
  (1989): Ramsdell WM, *J Am Acad Dermatol* 21, 1318
Injection-site necrosis
  (1989): Ramsdell WM, *J Am Acad Dermatol* 21, 1318
Myalgia/Myositis/Myopathy/Myotoxicity (<1%)
Paresthesias (<1%)
Rhabdomyolysis
  (2004): Coco TJ+, *Curr Opin Pediatr* 16(2), 206
  (2003): Haas CE+, *Ann Pharmacother* 37(4), 538
  (2003): Stucka KR+, *Pediatr Emerg Care* 19(1), 25
  (1996): Emadian SM+, *Am J Emerg Med* 14(6), 574
Tremor

DIPHENOXYLATE

Trade names: Lamocot; Lofene; Logen; Lomanate; Lomotil (Pfizer); Lonox; Low-Quel
Indications: Diarrhea
Category: Antimotility; Opioid agonist
Half-life: 2.5 hours

Note: Diphenoxylate is almost always prescribed with atropine sulfate

Reactions

Skin
Angioedema
Diaphoresis (<1%)
Pruritus (<1%)
Urticaria (<1%)

Mucosal/ENT
Gingivitis
Xerostomia (3%)

Eyes
Keratoconjunctivitis
  (1991): Mader TH+, *Am J Ophthalmol* 111(3), 377

Other
Anaphylactoid reactions/Anaphylaxis
Headache
Paresthesias

DIPHENYLHYDANTOIN

(See PHENYTOIN)

DIPHTHERIA ANTITOXIN

Indications: Diphtheria immunization
Category: Vaccine
Half-life: N/A
**Clinically important, potentially hazardous interactions
with:** N/A

Reactions

Skin
Erythema
Facial edema
Pruritus
Rash (sic)

Other
Allergic reactions
Asthenia
Chills
Fever
Myalgia/Myositis/Myopathy/Myotoxicity

DIPYRIDAMOLE

Trade names: Aggrenox (Boehringer Ingelheim); Cardoxin;
Cleridium; Coronarine; Coroxin; Curantyl N; Dipridacot;
Lodimol; Novo-Dipiradol; Persantin; Persantine (Boehringer
Ingelheim)
Indications: Thromboembolic complications following cardiac
valve replacement
Category: Adensosine reuptake inhibitor; Antiplatelet
Half-life: 10–12 hours
**Clinically important, potentially hazardous interactions
with:** adenosine, ceftobiprole, **dong quai**, fondaparinux,
reteplase

Note: Aggrenox is dipyridamole and aspirin

Reactions

Skin
Allergic reactions (sic) (<1%)
Angioedema
Diaphoresis (0.4%)
Edema (0.3%)
Erythema multiforme
Exanthems
Pruritus
Psoriasis
Purpura (1.4%)
  (1993): Kaufman DW+, *Blood* 82, 2714
Rash (sic) (2.3%)
Stevens–Johnson syndrome
Toxic epidermal necrolysis
  (1993): Seoane-Leston JM+, *Rev Stomatol Chir Maxillofac*
    (French) 94, 281
Ulcerations (<1%)
Urticaria
Xanthoderma
  (2007): Haught JM+, *J Am Acad Dermatol* 57(6), 1051

Mucosal/ENT
Auditory hallucinations

  (2007): Tomar A+, *Int Psychogeriatr* 19(6), 1169
Dysgeusia (0.1%)
  (1985): Goy JJ+, *Arzneimittelforschung* 35(5), 854
Gingivitis (<1%)

Eyes
Photophobia
  (2006): Kruuse C+, *Cephalalgia* 26(8), 925

Other
Anaphylactoid reactions/Anaphylaxis
  (1994): Weinmann P+, *Am J Med* 97, 488
Headache
  (2006): Kruuse C+, *Cephalalgia* 26(8), 925
Injection-site pain (0.1%)
Injection-site reactions (sic) (0.4%)
Migraine
  (2006): Kruuse C+, *Cephalalgia* 26(8), 925
Myalgia/Myositis/Myopathy/Myotoxicity (0.9%)
Paresthesias (1.3%)
Pseudopolymyalgia
  (1990): Chassagne P+, *BMJ* 301, 875
Tremor (<1%)

DIRITHROMYCIN

Trade name: Dynabac (Muro)
Indications: Various infections caused by susceptible organisms
Category: Antibiotic, macrolide
Half-life: 8 hours
**Clinically important, potentially hazardous interactions
with:** pimozide, warfarin

Reactions

Skin
Allergic reactions (sic) (<1%)
Bullous dermatitis
Diaphoresis (<1%)
Edema (<1%)
Peripheral edema (<1%)
Pruritus (1.2%)
Rash (sic) (1.4%)
Urticaria (1.2%)

Mucosal/ENT
Dysgeusia (<1%)
Oral ulceration (<1%)
Vaginitis (<1%)
Vulvovaginal candidiasis (<1%)
Xerostomia (<1%)

Other
Abdominal pain
  (1993): Jacobson K, *J Antimicrob Chemother* 31 Suppl C, 121
Anaphylactoid reactions/Anaphylaxis
Headache
  (1999): Wasilewski MM+, *J Antimicrob Chemother* 43(4), 541
    (8%)
Myalgia/Myositis/Myopathy/Myotoxicity (<1%)
Paresthesias (<1%)
Tremor (<1%)

DISOPYRAMIDE

Trade names: Dimodan; Dirythmin SA; Disonorm; Durbis; Isorythm; Norpace (Pfizer)
Indications: Ventricular arrhythmias
Category: Antiarrhythmic class Ia; Muscarinic antagonist
Half-life: 4–10 hours
Clinically important, potentially hazardous interactions with: amisulpride, arsenic, astemizole, celiprolol, ciprofloxacin, clarithromycin, enoxacin, erythromycin, gatifloxacin, lomefloxacin, moxifloxacin, norfloxacin, ofloxacin, quinolones, roxithromycin, sparfloxacin

Reactions

Skin
Angioedema
Dermatitis
Edema (1–3%)
Erythema nodosum
  (1985): Niv Y+, *Harefuah* (Hebrew) 108, 490
Exanthems (1–5%)
  (1987): Brogden RN+, *Drugs* 34, 151 (1–2%)
Lupus erythematosus (<1%)
  (1985): Epstein A+, *Arthritis Rheum* 28, 158
  (1981): Wanner WR+, *Am Heart J* 101, 687
Photosensitivity
  (1987): Brogden RN+, *Drugs* 34, 151
Pruritus (1–3%)
Purpura
  (1987): Brogden RN+, *Drugs* 34, 151
Rash (sic) (generalized) (1–3%)
Urticaria
Xerosis

Mucosal/ENT
Oral lesions (40%)
  (1987): Brogden RN+, *Drugs* 34, 151
Xerostomia (32%)
  (1987): Brogden RN+, *Drugs* 34, 151 (40%)

Hair
Hair – alopecia

Other
Gynecomastia (<1%)
Headache
Paresthesias (<1%)

DISULFIRAM

Trade names: Antabus; Antabuse (Odyssey); Busetal; Esperal; Nocbin; Refusal; Tetradin
Indications: Alcoholism
Category: Antialcoholism; Antioxidant
Half-life: N/A
Clinically important, potentially hazardous interactions with: acenocoumarol, **alcohol**, anisindione, anticoagulants, **capsicum**, cyclosporine, dicumarol, ethanolamine, ethotoin, fosphenytoin, mephenytoin, metronidazole, phenytoin, warfarin

Reactions

Skin
Acne
Adverse effects (sic) (from beer-containing shampoo)
  (1980): Stoll D+, *JAMA* 244, 2045
Allergic reactions (sic)
Bullous dermatitis
  (1990): Larbre B+, *Ann Dermatol Venereol* (French) 117, 721
Dermatitis
  (1996): Rebandel P+, *Contact Dermatitis* 35, 48
  (1995): Fisher AA, *Cutis* 56, 131
  (1994): Mathelier-Fusade P+, *Contact Dermatitis* 31, 121
  (1992): Baptista A+, *Contact Dermatitis* 26, 140
  (1989): Minet A+, *Ann Dermatol Venereol* (French) 116, 543
  (1988): Olfson M, *Am J Psychiatry* 145, 651
  (1984): van Hecke E+, *Contact Dermatitis* 10, 254
  (1982): Fisher AA, *Cutis* 30, 461 (passim)
Diaphoresis (<1%) (with alcohol)
Eczema
  (1994): Mathelier-Fusade P+, *Contact Dermatitis* 31, 121
  (1981): Goitre M+, *Contact Dermatitis* 7, 272
Exanthems
  (1992): Breathnach SM+, *Adverse Drug Reactions and the Skin*
    Blackwell, Oxford, 204 (passim)
  (1989): Minet A+, *Ann Dermatol Venereol* (French) 116, 543
Fixed eruption (<1%)
  (2000): Sorkin M, Denver, CO (from Internet) (observation)
Purpura
  (1982): Thompson CC+, *J Am Dent Assoc* 105, 465
Pustules
  (1990): Larbre R+, *Ann Dermatol Venereol* (French) 117, 721
Rash (sic) (1–10%)
Recall reaction (nickel)
  (1993): Gamboa P+, *Contact Dermatitis* 28, 255
  (1992): Klein LR+, *J Am Acad Dermatol* 26, 645
  (1987): Grondahl-Hansen V+, *Ugeskr Laeger* (Danish) 149, 2401
  (1987): Kaaber K+, *Derm Beruf Umwelt* (German) 35, 209
Toxic epidermal necrolysis
  (1989): Stern RS+, *J Am Acad Dermatol* 21, 317
Urticaria
  (1992): Breathnach SM+, *Adverse Drug Reactions and the Skin*
    Blackwell, Oxford, 204 (passim)
  (1989): Minet A+, *Ann Dermatol Venereol* (French) 116, 543
  (1982): Fisher AA, *Cutis* 30, 461 (passim)
Vasculitis
  (1985): Sanchez NP+, *Arch Dermatol* 121, 220
Yellow palms
  (1997): Santonastaso M+, *Lancet* 350, 266

Mucosal/ENT
Dysgeusia (metallic or garlic aftertaste) (1–10%)
Hypogeusia

Eyes
Optic neuropathy
  (2006): Bessero AC+, *J Fr Ophtalmol* 29(8), 924

Other
Asthenia
Headache
Hepatotoxicity
Paresthesias
Polyarteritis nodosa
Somnolence

DIVALPROEX

(See VALPROIC ACID)

DOBUTAMINE

Trade names: Cardiject; Dobril; Dobuject; Dobutamin; Dobutrex (Lilly); Inotrex; Oxiken; Tobrex
Indications: Cardiac surgery, heart failure
Category: Adrenergic beta-receptor agonist; Catecholamine; Inotropic sympathomimetic
Half-life: 2 minutes
Clinically important, potentially hazardous interactions with: furazolidone

Reactions

Skin
Cellulitis
  (1994): Cernek PK, *Ann Pharmacother* 28, 964
Erythema
  (1991): Wu CC+, *Chest* 99, 1547
Necrosis
Pruritus
  (1991): Wu CC+, *Chest* 99, 1547
  (1986): McCauley CS+, *Ann Intern Med* 105, 966 (scalp)

Other
Cardiotoxicity
  (2006): Bonvini RF+, *Heart* 92(8), 1054
Headache
Hypersensitivity
  (1991): Wu CC+, *Chest* 99, 1547
Hypotension
  (2006): Siddiqui TS+, *J Am Soc Echocardiogr* 19(9), 1144
  (2004): Kuijpers D+, *Eur Radiol* 14(10), 1823 (1.5%)
Injection-site pain
Injection-site phlebitis
Myoclonus
  (2007): Boord A+, *Am J Health Syst Pharm* 64(21), 2241
  (2005): Hauben M+, *Nephrol Dial Transplant* 20(2), 471
Paresthesias (1–10%)
Phlebitis

DOCETAXEL

Trade name: Taxotere (Sanofi-Aventis)
Indications: Metastatic breast cancer
Category: Taxane
Half-life: 11–18 hours
Clinically important, potentially hazardous interactions with: aldesleukin, aprepitant, prednisone

Reactions

Skin
Allergic reactions (sic)
  (2001): Talla M+, *Therapie* 56(5), 632
Angioedema
Edema (1–20%)
  (2007): Tashiro H+, *Gan To Kagaku Ryoho* 34(3), 393 (with cyclophosphamide) (25%)
  (2007): Tashiro H+, *Gan To Kagaku Ryoho* 34(3), 453 (100%)

  (2004): Furugen Y+, *Gan To Kagaku Ryoho* 31(8), 1205 (30%) (with carboplatin)
  (2003): Qin YK+, *Ai Zheng* 22(4), 415
  (2002): Eich D+, *Am J Clin Oncol* 25(6), 599 (passim)
  (1996): Edmonson JH+, *Am J Clin Oncon* 19, 574
  (1993): Schrijvers D+, *Ann Oncol* 4, 610 (20%)
Erythema (0.9%)
  (2002): Hirai K+, *Gynecol Obstet Invest* 53(2), 118
  (1995): Cortes JE+, *J Clin Oncol* 13, 2643
Exanthems
  (1995): Cortes JE+, *J Clin Oncol* 13, 2643
  (1995): Zimmerman GC+, *Arch Dermatol* 131, 202
Facial erythema
  (2004): Katoh M+, *J Dermatol* 31(5), 403
Fixed eruption (erythematous plaque)
  (2000): Chu CY+, *Br J Dermatol* 142, 808
Hand–foot syndrome
  (2007): Kanaji N+, *Nihon Kokyuki Gakkai Zasshi* 45(6), 474 (with uracil/tegafur)
  (2006): Kara IO+, *Breast* 15(3), 414 (with capecitabine)
  (2005): Levy C+, *Cancer Treat Rev* 31 Suppl 4, S17 (with capecitabine)
  (2005): Ramanathan RK+, *Cancer Chemother Pharmacol* 55(4), 354 (with capecitabine)
  (2004): Katoh M+, *J Dermatol* 31(5), 403
  (2004): Lebowitz PF+, *Clin Cancer Res* 10(20), 6764 (with capecitabine)
  (2004): Mackey JR+, *Clin Breast Cancer* 5(4), 287 (30%) (with capecitabine)
  (2004): Park YH+, *Br J Cancer* 90(7), 1329 (with capecitabine)
  (2004): Pavlick AC+, *Anticancer Drugs* 15(2), 119 (with doxorubicin)
  (2003): Han JY+, *Cancer* 98(9), 1918 (33%) (with capecitabine)
  (2002): Eich D+, *Am J Clin Oncol* 25(6), 599 (2 cases)
  (2002): O'Shaughnessy J+, *J Clin Oncol* 20(12), 2812 (with capecitabine)
  (2000): Chu CY+, *Br J Dermatol* 142(4), 808
  (1995): Zimmerman GC+, *Arch Dermatol* 131, 202
  (1994): Zimmerman GC+, *J Natl Cancer Inst* 86, 557
  (1993): Vukelja SJ+, *J Natl Cancer Inst* 85, 1432
Lupus erythematosus
  (2004): Chen M+, *J Rheumatol* 31(4), 818 (4 cases) (subacute)
Peripheral edema
  (2002): Koukourakis MI+, *Anticancer Res* 22(4), 2491
  (1998): Hainsworth JD+, *J Clin Oncol* 16(6), 2164
  (1995): Zimmerman GC+, *Arch Dermatol* 131, 202
Photo-recall
  (2006): Mizumoto M+, *Int J Radiat Oncol Biol Phys* 66(4), 1187
  (2005): Borgia F+, *Br J Dermatol* 153(3), 674
  (2005): Chu CY+, *Br J Dermatol* 153(2), 441
  (2005): Kandemir EG+, *Swiss Med Wkly* 135(1-2), 34
  (2002): Magne N+, *Cancer Radiother* 6(5), 281 (2 cases) (with radiation therapy)
  (2002): Morkas M+, *J Clin Oncol* 20(3), 867
  (2002): Piroth MD+, *Onkologie* 25(5), 438
  (2001): Giesel BU+, *Strahlenther Onkol* 177(9), 487
  (1995): Zimmerman GC+, *Arch Dermatol* 101, 202
Photosensitivity
  (2002): Eich D+, *Am J Clin Oncol* 25(6), 599 (passim)
  (1995): Zimmerman GC+, *Arch Dermatol* 131, 202
Pigmentation
  (2005): Aydogan I+, *J Eur Acad Dermatol Venereol* 19(3), 345 (supravenous)
Pruritus
  (1995): Cortes JE+, *J Clin Oncol* 13, 2643
Radiodermatitis
  (2005): Borgia F+, *Br J Dermatol* 153(3), 674
Rash (sic) (0.9%)
  (1996): Edmonson JH+, *Am J Clin Oncon* 19, 574

Recall reaction
(2005): Chu CY+, *Br J Dermatol* 153(2), 441
Scleroderma
(2002): Eich D+, *Am J Clin Oncol* 25(6), 599 (passim)
(2001): Hassett G+, *Clin Exp Rheumatol* 19(2), 197
(2000): Cleveland MG+, *Cancer* 88(5), 1078
(1995): Battafarano DF+, *Cancer* 76, 110
Seborrheic keratoses
(2001): Chu CY+, *Acta Derm Venereol* 81(4), 316
Squamous syringometaplasia
(2002): Karam A+, *Br J Dermatol* 146(3), 524
Stevens–Johnson syndrome
(2007): Ohlmann CH+, *Urologe A* 46(10), 1425
Toxic epidermal necrolysis
(2002): Dourakis SP+, *J Clin Oncol* 20(13), 3030
Toxicity (sic)
(2007): Tashiro H+, *Gan To Kagaku Ryoho* 34(3), 393 (with cyclophosphamide) (13%)
(2007): Tinker AV+, *Gynecol Oncol* 104(3), 647 (3%)
(2003): Fracasso PM+, *Cancer* 98(3), 610
Urticaria
(2005): Feldweg AM+, *Gynecol Oncol* 96(3), 824
Xerosis
(1995): Cortes JE+, *J Clin Oncol* 13, 2643

Mucosal/ENT
Dysgeusia
(2003): Maisano R+, *Anticancer Res* 23(2C), 1923
Dysphagia
(2002): Koukourakis MI+, *Anticancer Res* 22(4), 2491
Mucositis
(2004): Culp LR+, *Head Neck* 26(2), 197 (photo-recall)
(2003): Suzuki M+, *Jpn J Clin Oncol* 33(6), 297
(2002): Marx G+, *Br J Cancer* 87(8), 846 (with ifosfamide)
(2002): Rein DT+, *Gynecol Oncol* 87(1), 98 (with carboplatin)
Nasal septal perforation
(2006): Tan TH+, *Intern Med J* 36(7), 471
Stomatitis (5–42%)
(2007): Tashiro H+, *Gan To Kagaku Ryoho* 34(3), 393 (with cyclophosphamide) (25%)
(2006): Izquierdo MA+, *Eur J Cancer* 42(12), 1789 (with paclitaxel)
(2005): G Oumlker E+, *Neth J Med* 63(9), 364
(2003): Han JY+, *Cancer* 98(9), 1918 (33%) (with capecitabine)
(2003): Qin YK+, *Ai Zheng* 22(4), 415
(2002): Bonneterre J+, *Br J Cancer* 87(11), 1210 (5%)
(2002): Eich D+, *Am J Clin Oncol* 25(6), 599 (passim)
(1998): Amodio A+, *Clin Ter* 149(2), 121
(1996): Edmonson JH+, *Am J Clin Oncon* 19, 574

Hair
Hair – alopecia (80%)
(2007): Tashiro H+, *Gan To Kagaku Ryoho* 34(3), 393 (with cyclophosphamide) (100%)
(2007): Tashiro H+, *Gan To Kagaku Ryoho* 34(3), 453 (100%)
(2004): Gridelli C+, *Br J Cancer* 91(12), 1996
(2003): Qin YK+, *Ai Zheng* 22(4), 415
(2003): Yoshida K+, *Gan To Kagaku Ryoho.* 30(12), 1927
(2002): Eich D+, *Am J Clin Oncol* 25(6), 599 (passim)
(2002): Koukourakis MI+, *Anticancer Res* 22(4), 2491
(2002): Rein DT+, *Gynecol Oncol* 87(1), 98 (with carboplatin)
(1998): Amodio A+, *Clin Ter* 149(2), 121
(1995): Lemenager M+, *Lancet* 346, 371

Nails
Nails – Beau's lines (transverse nail bands)
(2001): Camidge DR+, *Lancet Oncol* 2(6), 342
(1999): Correia O+, *Dermatology* 198, 288
Nails – changes (sic)
(2003): Kuroi K+, *Breast Cancer* 10(1), 10

(2003): Rafi L+, *Eur J Dermatol* 13(6), 610 (severe)
(2003): Yoshida K+, *Gan To Kagaku Ryoho.* 30(12), 1927
(2002): Pavithran K+, *Br J Dermatol* 146(4), 709
(2001): Kuroi K+, *Gan To Kagaku Ryoho* (Japanese) 28(6), 797
(2001): Wasner G+, *Lancet* 357(9260), 910
Nails – discoloration
(2003): Mourad YA+, *Dermatol Online J* 9(3), 15
(2002): Nicolopoulos J+, *Australas J Dermatol* 43(4), 293
Nails – dystrophy
(2006): Alexandrescu DT+, *Int J Dermatol* 45(11), 1334 (with Trastuzumab)
Nails – hyponychial dermatitis
(2003): Chen GY+, *Br J Dermatol* 148, 1071 (with capecitabine)
Nails – loss
(2004): Mackey JR+, *Clin Breast Cancer* 5(4), 287 (45%) (with capecitabine)
(2003): Maisano R+, *Anticancer Res* 23(2C), 1923
(2003): Mourad YA+, *Dermatol Online J* 9(3), 15
Nails – paronychia
(2002): Nicolopoulos J+, *Australas J Dermatol* 43(4), 293
(1999): Correia O+, *Dermatology* 198, 288 (painful)
Nails – pigmentation
(2002): Eich D+, *Am J Clin Oncol* 25(6), 599 (passim)
(1999): Correia O+, *Dermatology* 198, 288 (orange discoloration)
(1998): Jacob CI+, *Arch Dermatol* 134, 1167 (nail bed dyschromia)
Nails – subungual abscess
(2002): Nicolopoulos J+, *Australas J Dermatol* 43(4), 293
(2000): Vanhooteghem O+, *Br J Dermatol* 143, 462
Nails – subungual hemorrhages
(2002): Nicolopoulos J+, *Australas J Dermatol* 43(4), 293
(1999): Correia O+, *Dermatology* 198, 288
Nails – subungual hyperkeratosis
(1999): Correia O+, *Dermatology* 198, 288
Nails – transverse superficial loss of nail plate
(1999): Correia O+, *Dermatology* 198, 288
(1997): Llombart-Cussac A+, *Arch Dermatol* 133, 1466

Eyes
Epiphora
(2007): Tinker AV+, *Gynecol Oncol* 104(3), 647 (8%)
(2006): Esmaeli B+, *J Clin Oncol* 24(22), 3619 (64%)
(2006): Kintzel PE+, *Pharmacotherapy* 26(6), 853
(2006): Tsalic M+, *Med Oncol* 23(1), 57 (33%)
(2005): Esmaeli B, *Clin Breast Cancer* 5(6), 455
(2003): Kuroi K+, *Breast Cancer* 10(1), 10
(2003): Maisano R+, *Anticancer Res* 23(2C), 1923

Other
Abdominal pain
(2003): Viret F+, *Pancreas* 27(3), 214
Anaphylactoid reactions/Anaphylaxis
(2007): Gunthert AR+, *Gynecol Oncol* 104(1), 86
Application-site fixed eruption
(1995): Zimmerman GC+, *Arch Dermatol* 131, 202
Asthenia
(2007): Tinker AV+, *Gynecol Oncol* 104(3), 647 (14%)
(2006): Feliu J+, *Cancer Chemother Pharmacol* 58(4), 527 (11%) (with mitomycin)
(2006): Izquierdo MA+, *Eur J Cancer* 42(12), 1789 (with paclitaxel)
(2004): Mackey JR+, *Clin Breast Cancer* 5(4), 287 (30%) (with capecitabine)
(2004): Morales S+, *Cancer Chemother Pharmacol* 53(1), 75 (6%)
(2003): Han JY+, *Cancer* 98(9), 1918 (51%) (with capecitabine)
(2003): Kuroi K+, *Breast Cancer* 10(1), 10
(2003): Qin YK+, *Ai Zheng* 22(4), 415
(2003): Viret F+, *Pancreas* 27(3), 214
(2002): Paciucci PA+, *Anticancer Drugs* 13(8), 791

(1998): Hainsworth JD+, *J Clin Oncol* 16(6), 2164
Cough
  (2004): Gridelli C+, *Br J Cancer* 91(12), 1996
Death
  (2006): Laber DA+, *Am J Clin Oncol* 29(4), 389 (4%)
  (2003): Han JY+, *Cancer* 98(9), 1918 (2 cases) (with capecitabine)
  (2002): Morris MJ+, *Urology* 60(6), 1111
Extravasation
  (2005): Barcelo R+, *Arch Dermatol* 141(10), 1326
Fever
  (2006): Yip AY+, *Breast Cancer* 13(2), 192 (19%)
Fibrosis
  (2000): Cleveland MG+, *Cancer* 88, 1078 (generalized)
Hypersensitivity (1–28%)
  (2005): Feldweg AM+, *Gynecol Oncol* 96(3), 824
  (2004): Furugen Y+, *Gan To Kagaku Ryoho* 31(8), 1205 (25%) (with carboplatin)
  (2002): Denman JP+, *J Clin Oncol* 20(11), 2760 (previous hypersensitivity to paclitaxel)
  (2002): Eich D+, *Am J Clin Oncol* 25(6), 599 (passim)
  (1996): Hudis CA+, *J Clin Oncol* 14, 58
  (1995): Bedikian AY+, *J Clin Oncol* 13, 2895
  (1993): Schrijvers D+, *Ann Oncol* 4, 610 (28%)
Inappropriate secretion of antidiuretic hormone (SIADH)
  (2000): Langer-Nitsche C+, *Acta Oncol* 39(8), 1001
Infections
  (2002): Bonneterre J+, *Br J Cancer* 87(11), 1210 (2%)
  (2002): Koukourakis MI+, *Anticancer Res* 22(4), 2491
  (2002): Souglakos J+, *Cancer* 95(6), 1326 (11.7%)
Injection-site dermatitis
  (2002): Hirai K+, *Gynecol Obstet Invest* 53(2), 118
Injection-site erythema
  (2002): Hirai K+, *Gynecol Obstet Invest* 53(2), 118
  (1995): Zimmerman GC+, *Arch Dermatol* 131, 202
Injection-site exanthems
  (2002): Hirai K+, *Gynecol Obstet Invest* 53(2), 118
Injection-site extravasation
  (2000): Raley J+, *Gynecol Oncol* 78, 259
  (1995): Zimmerman GC+, *Arch Dermatol* 131, 202
Injection-site pigmentation
  (2005): Aydogan I+, *J Eur Acad Derm Ven* 19, 345 (supravenous, serpentine)
  (2000): Schrijvers D+, *Br J Dermatol* 142, 1069
  (1995): Zimmerman GC+, *Arch Dermatol* 131, 202
Injection-site reactions
  (2002): Eich D+, *Am J Clin Oncol* 25(6), 599 (passim)
Myalgia/Myositis/Myopathy/Myotoxicity (>10%)
  (2006): Izquierdo MA+, *Eur J Cancer* 42(12), 1789 (with paclitaxel)
  (2005): Hughes BG+, *Intern Med J* 35(6), 369
  (2003): Qin YK+, *Ai Zheng* 22(4), 415
Neurotoxicity
  (2006): Izquierdo MA+, *Eur J Cancer* 42(12), 1789 (with paclitaxel)
  (2006): Lee JJ+, *J Clin Oncol* 24(10), 1633
  (2005): Wampler MA+, *Clin J Oncol Nurs* 9(2), 189
  (2004): Furugen Y+, *Gan To Kagaku Ryoho* 31(8), 1205 (6%) (with carboplatin)
  (1998): Hainsworth JD+, *J Clin Oncol* 16(6), 2164
Pain
  (2004): Gridelli C+, *Br J Cancer* 91(12), 1996
  (2002): Paciucci PA+, *Anticancer Drugs* 13(8), 791
Paresthesias (3.9%)
  (2002): Eich D+, *Am J Clin Oncol* 25(6), 599 (passim)
Thrombosis
  (2006): Laber DA+, *Am J Clin Oncol* 29(4), 389 (8%)

DOCOSANOL

Synonyms: Behenyl Alcohol; n-Docosanol
Trade name: Abreva (GSK)
Indications: Herpes simplex (labialis)
Category: Antiviral, topical
Half-life: N/A
Clinically important, potentially hazardous interactions with: None

Reactions

Skin
  Irritation (sic) (local)

DOCUSATE

Trade names: Colase (Purdue); Coloxyl; Dialose; Diocto; Disonate; DOK; Doxate-S; Doxinate; Hisof; Jamylene; Lambanol; Mollax; Peri-Colase (Purdue); Regulex; Regutol; Selax; SoFlax; Softon; Sulfalax; Surfak (Pfizer)
Indications: Constipation
Category: Stimulant laxative
Half-life: N/A
Onset of action: 12–72 hours

Reactions

Skin
  Dermatitis
    (1998): Lee AY+, *Contact Dermatitis* 38, 355
  Diaphoresis
  Exanthems (1%)
  Rash (sic)

Mucosal/ENT
  Dysgeusia

DOFETILIDE

Trade name: Tikosyn (Pfizer)
Indications: Conversion of atrial fibrillation and atrial flutter to normal sinus rhythm
Category: Antiarrhythmic class III
Half-life: 10 hours
Clinically important, potentially hazardous interactions with: atazanavir, chlorpromazine, cimetidine, co-trimoxazole, fluphenazine, ketoconazole, medroxyprogesterone, megestrol, mesoridazine, phenothiazines, prochlorperazine, progestins, promethazine, ranolazine, thioridazine, trifluoperazine, trimethoprim, verapamil

Reactions

Skin
  Angioedema (<2%)
  Diaphoresis (>2%)
  Edema
  Peripheral edema (>2%)
  Rash (sic) (3%)

Other

Headache
Paresthesias (<2%)

DOLASETRON

Trade name: Anzemet (Sanofi-Aventis)
Indications: Prevention of nausea and vomiting
Category: 5-HT3 antagonist; Serotonin type 3 receptor antagonist
Half-life: 7.3 hours

Reactions

Skin

Diaphoresis
Edema
Facial edema
Peripheral edema
Pruritus
Purpura
Rash (sic)
Urticaria

Mucosal/ENT

Dysgeusia
   (1995): Hunt TL+, J Clin Pharmacol 35(7), 705

Eyes

Ocular pigmentation

Other

Anaphylactoid reactions/Anaphylaxis
Chills (>2%)
   (2007): Bock M+, Anaesthesist 56(1), 63
Headache
   (2003): Kovac AL, Drug Saf 26(4), 227
   (1998): Diemunsch P+, J Clin Anesth 10(2), 145
   (1997): Balfour JA+, Drugs 54(2), 273
   (1997): Kasimis BS+, Cancer Invest 15(4), 304
   (1997): Keung AC+, Biopharm Drug Dispos 18(4), 361
   (1997): Rubenstein EB+, Cancer 79(6), 1216
   (1996): Audhuy B+, Eur J Cancer 32A(5), 807
   (1996): Dixon RM+, Pharmacotherapy 16(2), 245
   (1996): Hunt TL+, Pharmacotherapy 16(2), 253
   (1995): Hunt TL+, J Clin Pharmacol 35(7), 705
   (1994): Conroy T+, Am J Clin Oncol 17(2), 97 (11%)
Hot flashes
   (1997): Keung AC+, Biopharm Drug Dispos 18(4), 361
Myalgia/Myositis/Myopathy/Myotoxicity
Paresthesias
Thrombophlebitis
Vertigo
   (2003): Kovac AL, Drug Saf 26(4), 227
   (1997): Balfour JA+, Drugs 54(2), 273
   (1997): Keung AC+, Biopharm Drug Dispos 18(4), 361
   (1996): Dixon RM+, Pharmacotherapy 16(2), 245
   (1996): Hunt TL+, Pharmacotherapy 16(2), 253
   (1995): Hunt TL+, J Clin Pharmacol 35(7), 705

DOMPERIDONE

Trade names: Evoxin; Motilium (Johnson & Johnson)
Indications: Investigational antiemetic, gastroesophageal reflux disease (GERD), nausea and vomiting
Category: Dopamine receptor antagonist
Half-life: 7–8 hours
Clinically important, potentially hazardous interactions with: ketoconazole

Note: Domperamol is domperidone & acetaminophen

Reactions

Skin

Diaphoresis
Edema
Edema of lip
Facial edema
Facial erythema
Lupus erythematosus
   (1986): Yasue T+, J Dermatol 13(4), 292
Pruritus
Rash (sic)
   (1981): Nagler J+, Am J Gastroenterol 76(6), 495
Urticaria

Mucosal/ENT

Dry mucous membranes

Other

Anaphylactoid reactions/Anaphylaxis
Death
   (1984): Giaccone G+, Lancet 2(8415):1336 (2 cases)
   (1982): Joss RA+, Lancet 1(8279):1019
Depression
   (1999): Patterson D+, Am J Gastroenterol 95(5), 1230
Gynecomastia
   (1991): Keating JP+, Postgrad Med J 67(786), 401
   (1982): van der Steen M+, Lancet 2(8303), 884 (in a male infant)
Hypersensitivity
Rhabdomyolysis
   (2002): Bourlon S+, Therapie 57(6), 597 (with rabeprazole)
Tremor

DONEPEZIL

Synonym: E2020
Trade name: Aricept (Eisai) (Endo)
Indications: Mild dementia of the Alzheimer's type
Category: Cholinesterase inhibitor
Half-life: 50–70 hours
Clinically important, potentially hazardous interactions with: galantamine

Reactions

Skin

Dermatitis (<1%)
Diaphoresis (>1%)
Erythema (<1%)
Facial edema (<1%)
Hyperkeratosis (<1%)
Neurodermatitis (<1%)

Pigmentation (<1%)
Pruritus (>1%)
Purpura (1–10%)
  (1998): Bryant CA+, *BMJ* 317, 787
Rash (sic)
Striae (<1%)
Ulcerations (<1%)
Urticaria (>1%)

Mucosal/ENT

Dysgeusia (<1%)
Gingivitis (<1%)
Rhinitis
  (2002): Pratt RD+, *Int J Clin Pract* 56(9), 710
Tongue edema (<1%)
Vaginitis (<1%)
Xerostomia (<1%)

Hair

Hair – alopecia (<1%)
Hair – hirsutism (<1%)

Eyes

Periorbital edema (<1%)

Other

Asthenia
  (2002): Pratt RD+, *Int J Clin Pract* 56(9), 710
Depression
  (2002): Gauthier S+, *Int Psychogeriatr* 14(4), 389 (52%)
Headache
  (2004): Reyes JF+, *Br J Clin Pharmacol* 58 Suppl 1:, 9
  (2002): Pratt RD+, *Int J Clin Pract* 56(9), 710
Pain (leg)
  (2006): Kuloor CB+, *Age Ageing* 35(6), 639
Paresthesias (<1%)
Vertigo
  (2002): Pratt RD+, *Int J Clin Pract* 56(9), 710

DONG QUAI

Scientific name: *Angelica sinensis (Angelica polymorpha sinensis)*
Family: Umbelliferae; Apioideae
Trade and other common names: Dang Gui; Dang Kwai; Danggui; Dong qua; Tan Kue; Tang Quai; Tank Kuei
Category: Immunomodulator; Phytoestrogen
Purported indications and other uses: Menopausal symptoms, PMS, menstrual disorders, anemia, constipation, insomnia, rheumatism, neuralgia, hypertension, hypopigmentation, psoriasis
Half-life: N/A
Clinically important, potentially hazardous interactions with: acetaminophen, dipyridamole, heparin, tamoxifen, ticlopidine, warfarin

Reactions

Skin

Photosensitivity
Phototoxicity

Other

Gynecomastia
  (2001): Goh SY+, *Singapore Med J* 42(3), 115
  (2001): Kiong HN, *Singapore Med J* 42(6), 286

DOPAMINE

Trade names: Cardiosteril; Dopamin; Dopamin AWD; Dopastat; Dynatra; Intropin; Revimine
Indications: Hemodynamic imbalances present in shock
Category: Adrenergic alpha-receptor agonist; Catecholamine; Inotropic sympathomimetic
Half-life: 2 minutes
Clinically important, potentially hazardous interactions with: ethotoin, fosphenytoin, furazolidone, MAO inhibitors, mephenytoin, phenelzine, phenytoin, tranylcypromine

Reactions

Skin

Exanthems
Necrosis
  (2001): Subhani M+, *J Perinatol* 21(5), 324
Pruritus
Raynaud's phenomenon (<1%)
Urticaria

Hair

Hair – alopecia
Hair – piloerection

Other

Gangrene
  (1997): Weinberg JM+, *Arch Dermatol* 133, 249
Headache
Injection-site extravasation
  (1998): Chen JL+, *Ann Pharmacother* 32, 545
  (1989): Denkler KA+, *Plast Reconstr Surg* 84, 811
Injection-site gangrene
Injection-site necrosis (<1%)
  (1992): Breathnach SM+, *Adverse Drug Reactions and the Skin*
    Blackwell, Oxford, 233 (passim)
  (1982): Pillgram-Larsen J+, *Tidsskr Nor Laegeforen* (Norwegian)
    102, 1583
Injection-site piloerection and vasoconstriction
  (1991): Ross M, *Arch Dermatol* 127, 586

DORIPENEM

Trade name: Doribax (Ortho-McNeil)
Indications: Complicated Infections
Category: Carbapenem antibiotic
Half-life: 1 hour
Clinically important, potentially hazardous interactions with: probenecid, valproic acid

Reactions

Skin

Rash (sic) (0.1%)
Stevens–Johnson syndrome
Toxic epidermal necrolysis

Mucosal/ENT

Oral candidiasis (1%)
Vulvomycotic infection (sic) (2%)

Other

Headache (16%)
Hepatotoxicity

Phlebitis
Seizures

DORNASE ALFA

Trade name: Pulmozyme (Genentech)
Indications: Cystic fibrosis
Category: Recombinant DNase
Half-life: N/A
Clinically important, potentially hazardous interactions with: None

Reactions

Skin
Rash (sic) (3%)
  (1995): Hodson ME, *Am J Respir Crit Care Med* 151(3), S70
Urticaria

Mucosal/ENT
Rhinitis (30%)
Sinusitis

Eyes
Conjunctivitis (4%)
  (1995): Hodson ME, *Am J Respir Crit Care Med* 151(3), S70

Other
Abdominal pain
Asthenia
Chest pain (25%)
  (1995): Hodson ME, *Am J Respir Crit Care Med* 151(3), S70
Cough
Fever (32%)

DORZOLAMIDE

Trade names: Cosopt (Merck); Trusopt (Banyu)
Indications: Glaucoma, ocular hypertension
Category: Carbonic anhydrase inhibitor; Diuretic
Half-life: about 4 months

Note: Cosopt is dorzolamide and timolol

Note: Dorzolamide is a sulfonamide and can be absorbed systemically. Sulfonamides can produce severe, possibly fatal, reactions such as toxic epidermal necrolysis and Stevens–Johnson syndrome

Reactions

Skin
Dermatitis
  (2008): Kluger N+, *Contact Dermatitis* 58(3), 167 (contact)
  (2006): Kalavala M+, *Contact Dermatitis* 54(6), 345 (contact)
  (2005): Linares Mata T+, *Contact Dermatitis* 52(2), 111
  (2001): Shimada M+, *Contact Dermatitis* 45(1), 52
  (1998): Aalto-Korte K, *Contact Dermatitis* 39, 206
Erythema multiforme
  (2008): Munshi V+, *J Ocul Pharmacol Ther* 24(1), 91
Lichenoid eruption
  (2004): Mullins RJ+, *Australas J Dermatol* 45(2), 151 (with timolol)
Rash (sic) (<1%)
Toxic epidermal necrolysis

  (2005): Florez A+, *J Am Acad Dermatol* 53(5), 909 (with timolol & latanoprost)

Mucosal/ENT
Anosmia
  (2007): Bell MA+, *Dev Neuropsychol* 31(1), 21
Dysgeusia (25%)
  (2005): Konstas AG+, *Ophthalmology* 112(4), 603
  (2000): Sall K, *Surv Ophthalmol* 44, S155
  (2000): Sugrue MF, *Prog Retin Eye Res* 19(1), 87

Eyes
Blepharoconjunctivitis
  (2001): Mancuso G+, *Contact Dermatitis* 45(4), 243
Ectropion
  (2007): Hegde V+, *Ophthalmology* 114(2), 362 (53%)
Eyelid edema
  (1998): Adamsons IA+, *J Glaucoma* 7, 395
Ocular burning (33%)
  (2003): Hommer A+, *Br J Ophthalmol* 87(5), 592
Ocular lichenoid eruption
  (2004): Mullins RJ+, *Australas J Dermatol* 45(2), 151
Ocular stinging
  (2004): Fechtner RD+, *Acta Ophthalmol Scand* 82(1), 42 (with timolol)
  (2003): Hommer A+, *Br J Ophthalmol* 87(5), 592 (with timolol)
  (2001): Seong GJ+, *Ophthalmologica* 215(3), 188
  (2000): Stewart WC+, *Am J Ophthalmol* 129(6), 723
  (1998): Adamsons IA+, *J Glaucoma* 7(6), 395
Periorbital dermatitis
  (2002): Delaney YM+, *Br J Ophthalmol* 86(4), 378

Other
Headache

DOXACURIUM

Trade name: Nuromax (GSK)
Indications: Neuromuscular blockade
Category: Non-depolarizing neuromuscular blocker
Half-life: 100–200 minutes
Clinically important, potentially hazardous interactions with: amikacin, aminoglycosides, carbamazepine, cyclopropane, enflurane, gentamicin, halothane, isoflurane, kanamycin, methoxyflurane, neomycin, piperacillin, streptomycin, tobramycin

Reactions

Skin
Rash (sic)
Urticaria (<1%)

Other
Asthenia
  (1997): Brandom BW+, *Anesth Analg* 84(2), 307
Hypotension
  (1989): Reich DL, *Anesthesiology* 71(5), 783

DOXAPRAM

Trade name: Dopram (Baxter)
Indications: Chronic obstructive pulmonary disease, drug-induced CNS depression
Category: Analeptic
Half-life: N/A
Duration of action: 3.4 hours

Reactions

Skin
Diaphoresis (<1%)
Pruritus

Mucosal/ENT
Oral lesions

Other
Injection-site erythema
Injection-site pain
Injection-site phlebitis (<1%)
Paresthesias

DOXAZOSIN

Trade names: Alfadil; Cardoxan; Cardular; Cardura (Pfizer); Dedralen; Diblocin; Supressin
Indications: Hypertension
Category: Adrenergic alpha-receptor antagonist
Half-life: 19–22 hours
Clinically important, potentially hazardous interactions with: tadalafil, vardenafil

Reactions

Skin
Angioedema
 (2006): Piller LB+, *J Clin Hypertens* 8(9), 649 (Greenwich) (9%)
Bruising
 (1991): Anon, *Arch Intern Med* 151, 1413
Diaphoresis (1.4%)
 (1988): Young JL+, *Drugs* 35, 525
Eczema (<0.5%)
Edema (4%)
Exanthems (1.7%)
 (1988): Young JL+, *Drugs* 35, 525
Facial edema (1%)
Lichen planus
 (2001): Madnani N, Mumbai, India (from Internet) (observation)
Lichenoid eruption
 (2002): Mittal A, Udaipur, India (from Internet) (observation)
Lupus erythematosus
 (1992): Feurle GE, *Dtsch Med Wochenschr* (German) 117, 157
Pallor (<1%)
Peripheral edema
Pruritus (1%)
Purpura (<0.5%)
Rash (sic) (1%)
 (1991): Anon, *Arch Intern Med* 151, 1413
Urticaria
 (1991): Anon, *Arch Intern Med* 151, 1413
Xerosis (<0.5%)

Mucosal/ENT
Dysgeusia (<0.5%)
 (1991): Anon, *Arch Intern Med* 151, 1413
Parosmia (<0.05%)
Tinnitus
Xerostomia (2%)
 (2006): Chung BH+, *BJU Int* 97(1), 90 (1%)
 (1991): Anon, *Arch Intern Med* 151, 1413

Hair
Hair – alopecia (<0.5%)
 (1991): Anon, *Arch Intern Med* 151, 1413
Hair – hypertrichosis
 (1991): Anon, *Arch Intern Med* 151, 1413

Other
Asthenia
 (2004): MacDonald R+, *BJU Int* 94(9), 1263
Headache
Hot flashes (<1%)
Hypotension
 (2006): Chung BH+, *BJU Int* 97(1), 90 (%)
Myalgia/Myositis/Myopathy/Myotoxicity (1%)
Paresthesias
Vertigo
 (2006): Chung BH+, *BJU Int* 97(1), 90 (3%)
 (2006): Rahardjo D+, *Int J Urol* 13(11), 1405 (22%)
 (2004): MacDonald R+, *BJU Int* 94(9), 1263

DOXEPIN

Trade names: Adapin; Alti-Doxepin; Anten; Aponal; Doneurin; Gilex; Mareen; Novo-Doxepin; Sinequan (Pfizer); Sinquan; Triadapin; Zonalon (topical) (Bioglan)
Indications: Mental depression, anxiety
Category: Antidepressant, tricyclic; Muscarinic antagonist
Half-life: 6–8 hours
Clinically important, potentially hazardous interactions with: alcohol, amprenavir, arbutamine, cholestyramine, clonidine, CNS depressants, epinephrine, formoterol, guanethidine, isocarboxazid, linezolid, MAO inhibitors, phenelzine, QT interval prolonging agents, quinolones, **selegiline,** sparfloxacin, sympathomimetics, tranylcypromine

Reactions

Skin
Allergic reactions (sic)
Dermatitis (from topical)
 (2004): Drayton G, Los Angeles, CA (from Internet) (observation)
 (2003): Bonnel RA+, *J Am Acad Dermatol* 48(2), 294
 (2003): Brancaccio RR+, *J Drugs Dermatol* 2(4), 409
 (1999): Wakelin SH+, *Contact Dermatitis* 40, 214
 (1997): Koehn G, *The Schoch Letter* 47, 20 (observation)
 (1996): Bilbao I+, *Contact Dermatitis* 35, 254
 (1996): Rapaport MJ, *Arch Dermatol* 132, 1516
 (1996): Shama S, *The Schoch Letter* 46, 36 (observation)
 (1996): Shelley WB+, *J Am Acad Dermatol* 34, 143
 (1996): Smith KC, Niagara Falls, Ontario (from Internet) (observation)
 (1996): Taylor JS+, *Arch Dermatol* 132, 515
 (1995): Goldblum O, *The Schoch Letter* 45, 26 (observation)
 (1995): Greenberg JH, *Contact Dermatitis* 33, 281
 (1995): Porres J, *The Schoch Letter* 45, 39 (observation)
Diaphoresis (1–10%)
Edema
Erythema
Erythroderma
 (1991): Kastrup O+, *Dtsch Med Wochenschr* (German) 116, 1748
Exanthems
Peripheral edema
 (1991): Dalack GW+, *Am J Psychiatry* 148, 1601

Photosensitivity (<1%)
  (1985): Walter-Ryan WG+, *JAMA* 254, 357
  (1982): *Patient Care* June 15, 208 (list)
Pruritus
Purpura
Rash (sic)
  (1991): Roose SP+, *J Clin Psychiatry* 52, 338
Toxic dermatitis (sic)
  (1995): Vo MY, *Arch Dermatol* 131, 1468
Urticaria
Vasculitis

Mucosal/ENT

Aphthous stomatitis
  (1980): Ives TJ+, *Am J Hosp Pharm* 37, 1551 (passim)
Dysgeusia (>10%)
Glossitis
  (1980): Ives TJ+, *Am J Hosp Pharm* 37, 1551
Glossodynia
  (1980): Ives TJ+, *Am J Hosp Pharm* 37, 1551 (passim)
Stomatitis
  (1981): Salem RB+, *Drug Intell Clin Pharm* 15, 992
Tinnitus
  (1983): Golden RN+, *South Med J* 76(9), 1204
Xerostomia (>10%)
  (1998): Foster M+, *J Clin Dermatol* Winter, 7 (5%)
  (1989): Assalian P+, *Drugs* 38(Suppl 1), 32
  (1989): Lose G+, *J Urol* 142, 1024
  (1985): Feighner JP+, *J Clin Psychiatry* 46(3 Pt 2), 20

Hair

Hair – alopecia (<1%)

Other

Application-site burning
Application-site edema
Gynecomastia (<1%)
Headache
Paresthesias
Pseudolymphoma
  (1995): Magro CM+, *J Am Acad Dermatol* 32, 419
  (1988): Kardaun SH+, *Br J Dermatol* 118(4), 545
Rhabdomyolysis
  (1988): Hojgaard AD+, *Acta Med Scand* 223, 79 (with
    nitrazepam)
Tremor

DOXERCALCIFEROL

Trade name: Hectorol (Bone Care)
Indications: Secondary hyperparathyroidism
Category: Vitamin D receptor agonist wakefulness promoting
agent
Half-life: 32–37 hours

Reactions

Skin

Edema (34.4%)
Pruritus (8.2%)

DOXORUBICIN

Trade names: Adiblastine; Adriablastine; Adriacin; Adriamycin
(Bedford); Adriblatina; Doxil (Tibotec); Farmablastina; Rubex
(Mead Johnson)
Indications: Carcinomas, leukemias, sarcomas
Category: Antibiotic, anthracycline
Half-life: α phase: 0.6 hours; β phase: 16.7 hours
**Clinically important, potentially hazardous interactions
with:** aldesleukin, sorafenib

Reactions

Skin

Acral erythema
  (1995): Komamura H+, *J Dermatol* 22(2), 116 (with vincristine,
    cyclophosphamide and GCSF)
Actinic keratoses
  (2001): Eisner J, Mt. Vernon, WA (from Internet) (observation)
  (1987): Johnson TM+, *J Am Acad Dermatol* 17(2 pT 1), 192
Adverse effects (sic)
  (2001): Verschraegen CF+, *Cancer* 92(9), 2327
Allergic reactions (sic) (<1%)
  (2002): Cantu MG+, *J Clin Oncol* 20(5), 1232 (2%) (with
    cyclophosphamide and cisplatin)
  (2002): McMenemin R+, *Invest New Drugs* 20(3), 331
Angioedema
  (1984): Collins JA, *Drug Intell Clin Pharm* 18, 402
  (1983): Bronner AK+, *J Am Acad Dermatol* 9, 645
  (1981): von Eyben FE+, *Cancer* 48, 1535 (passim)
  (1981): Weiss RB+, *Ann Intern Med* 94, 66
Cellulitis
Dermatitis
Dermatitis herpetiformis
  (1986): Gottlieb D+, *Med J Aust* 145, 241
Diaphoresis
  (1987): Lee M+, *J Urol* eact(1), 143
Exanthems
  (1987): Lee M+, *J Urol* 138, 143
  (1984): Collins JA, *Drug Intell Clin Pharm* 18, 402
Exfoliative dermatitis
  (2004): Huang JY+, *Anticancer Drugs* 15(3), 239
Fixed eruption
  (2006): Cady FM+, *Am J Dermatopathol* 28(2), 168
Hand–foot syndrome
  (2006): Cady FM+, *Am J Dermatopathol* 28(2), 168
  (2006): Campanelli A+, *J Eur Acad Dermatol Venereol* 20(8), 1022
  (2006): Chou HH+, *Gynecol Oncol* 101(3), 423
  (2006): Gordinier ME+, *Gynecol Oncol* 103(1), 72
  (2006): Palaia I+, *Am J Obstet Gynecol* 195(4), e1
  (2006): Sehouli J+, *Ann Oncol* 17(6), 957
  (2005): Rose PG, *Oncologist* 10(3), 205
  (2005): Schmook T+, *Dermatology* 210(3), 237
  (2005): Wilkes GM+, *Clin J Oncol Nurs* 9(1), 103
  (2004): Arcuri C+, *Tumori* 90(6), 556 (10%)
  (2004): Martin M+, *Clin Breast Cancer* 5(5), 353 (6%) (with
    vinorelbine)
  (2004): Pavlick AC+, *Anticancer Drugs* 15(2), 119
  (2003): Campos SM+, *Gynecol Oncol* 90(3), 610
  (2003): Chao TC+, *Cancer Invest* 21(6), 837
  (2003): Escobar PF+, *J Cancer Res Clin Oncol* 129(11), 651
  (2003): Leighl NB+, *Clin Lung Cancer* 5(2), 107 (with
    cyclophosphamide and vincristine)
  (2003): Risum S+, *Ugeskr Laeger* 165(33), 3161
  (2003): Skubitz KM, *Cancer Invest* 21(2), 167
  (2003): Tomb R+, *Ann Dermatol Venereol* 130(11), 1057
  (2003): Travitzky M+, *Anticancer Drugs* 14(3), 247

(2002): Fracasso PM+, *Cancer* 95(10), 2223 (with gemcitabine)
(2002): Hussein MA+, *Cancer* 95(10), 2160 (with vincristine and dexamethasone)
(2002): Numico G+, *Lung Cancer* 35(1), 59
(2002): Skubitz KM, *Cancer Invest* 20(5–6), 693
(2002): Skubitz KM, *Invest New Drugs* 20(1), 101
(2001): Goram AL+, *Pharmacotherapy* 21(6), 751
(2001): Verschraegen CF+, *Cancer* 92(9), 2327
(2000): Hubert A+, *Anticancer Drugs* 11(2), 123
(2000): Lotem M+, *Arch Dermatol* 136(12), 1475
(2000): Markman M+, *Gynecol Oncol* 78(3 Pt 1), 369 (8%)
(1999): Lopez AM+, *Cancer Chemother Pharmacol* 44(4), 303
(1997): Muggia FM+, *J Clin Oncol* 15(3), 987
(1995): Gordon KB+, *Cancer* 75, 2169
(1995): Uziely B+, *J Clin Oncol* 13(7), 1777
(1994): Sella A+, *J Clin Oncol* 12(4), 683 (with ketoconazole)
(1991): Baack BR+, *J Am Acad Dermatol* 24, 457
(1989): Jones AP+, *Br J Cancer* 59, 814
(1985): Levine LE+, *Arch Dermatol* 121, 102
(1985): Vogelzang NJ+, *Ann Intern Med* 103, 303
(1985): Walker IR+, *Arch Dermatol* 121, 1240
(1984): Lokich JJ+, *Ann Intern Med* 101, 798
(1982): Cordonnier C+, *Ann Intern Med* 97, 783

Inflammation
(2005): Ilyas EN+, *Cutis* 75, 167

Intertrigo
(2006): Campanelli A+, *J Eur Acad Dermatol Venereol* 20(8), 1022
(2006): Korver GE+, *J Drugs Dermatol* 5(9), 901
(2000): Lotem M+, *Arch Dermatol* 136, 1475

Keratoderma

Melanosis
(2000): Lotem M+, *Arch Dermatol* 136, 1475

Necrosis (local)
(2006): Palaia I+, *Am J Obstet Gynecol* 195(4), e1 (distal phalange)
(1998): Bekerecioglu M+, *J Surg Res* 75, 61
(1982): Riegels-Nielsen P+, *Ugeskr-Laeger* (Danish) 144, 1313
(1981): von Eyben FE+, *Cancer* 48, 1535 (passim)

Palmar–plantar erythema (painful)
(1990): Pagliuca A+, *Postgrad Med J* 66, 242
(1989): Jones AP+, *Br J Cancer* 59, 814
(1989): Oksenhendler E+, *Eur J Cancer Clin Oncol* 25, 1181
(1988): Shall L+, *Br J Dermatol* 119, 249

Palmar–plantar toxicity
(2004): Chua SL+, *Neuro-oncol* 6(1), 38 (4%)

Photo-recall (<1%)
(2004): Muggia FM, *Anticancer Drugs* 15(1), 35
(2003): Jimeno A+, *Anticancer Drugs* 14(7), 575
(2002): Stratman EJ, *J Am Acad Dermatol* 46(5), 797 (passim)
(2000): Lotem M+, *Arch Dermatol* 136, 1475

Pigmentation
(2006): Chou HH+, *Gynecol Oncol* 101(3), 423
(1996): Schulte-Huermann P+, *Dermatology* 191, 65
(1992): Konohana A, *J Dermatol* 19, 250
(1990): Curran CF, *N Z Med J* 103, 517
(1990): Kumar L+, *N Z Med J* 103, 165
(1987): Loureiro C+, *J Clin Oncol* 5, 1705
(1983): Bronner AK+, *J Am Acad Dermatol* 9, 645 (palms and soles)
(1982): Alagaratnam TT+, *Aust N Z J Surg* 52, 531
(1981): Granstein RD+, *J Am Acad Dermatol* 5, 1 (brown-black)
(1980): Orr LE+, *Arch Dermatol* 116, 273

Postirradiation erythema

Pruritus
(1987): Lee M+, *J Urol* 138, 143
(1984): Solimando DA+, *Drug Intell Clin Pharm* 18, 808

Psoriasis
(2001): Kreuter A+, *Acta Derm Venereol* 81(3), 224

Purpura

(1987): Lee M+, *J Urol* 138, 143

Rash (sic)
(2004): Chua SL+, *Neuro-oncol* 6(1), 38 (14%) (with temozolomide)
(2004): Huang JY+, *Anticancer Drugs* 15(3), 239
(2004): Zervas K+, *Ann Oncol* 15(1), 134 (5%)
(2002): Fracasso PM+, *Cancer* 95(10), 2223 (with gemcitabine)
(2000): Israel VP+, *Gynecol Oncol* 78, 143
(1981): Karlin DA+, *Lancet* 2, 534

Raynaud's phenomenon
(1993): von Gunten CF+, *Cancer* 72, 2004

Scleroderma
(2005): Alexandrescu DT+, *Clin Exp Dermatol* 30(2), 141 (with cyclophosphamide)

Toxic erythema
(2008): Ziemer M+, *J Am Acad Dermatol* 58(2 Suppl), S44

Toxicity (sic)
(2003): Chao TC+, *Cancer Invest* 21(6), 837
(2003): Fiets WE+, *Eur J Cancer* 39(8), 1081
(2003): Fracasso PM+, *Cancer* 98(3), 610
(2003): Gabizon A+, *Clin Pharmacokinet* 42(5), 419
(2003): Skubitz KM, *Cancer Invest* 21(2), 167
(1981): von Eyben FE+, *Cancer* 48, 1535

Urticaria (<1%)
(1986): Wandt H, *Dtsch Med Wochenschr* (German) 111, 356
(1984): Collins JA, *Drug Intell Clin Pharm* 18, 402
(1984): Solimando DA+, *Drug Intell Clin Pharm* 18, 808
(1983): Bronner AK+, *J Am Acad Dermatol* 9, 645
(1981): Hatfield AK+, *Cancer Treat Rep* 65, 353
(1981): von Eyben FE+, *Cancer* 48, 1535 (passim)
(1981): Weiss RB+, *Ann Intern Med* 94, 66

Mucosal/ENT

Ageusia
(2004): Kiewe P+, *Ann Pharmacother* 38(7-8), 1212

Mucositis
(2006): Al-Batran SE+, *Oncology* 70(2), 141 (4%)
(2004): Arcuri C+, *Tumori* 90(6), 556 (10%)
(2004): Martin M+, *Clin Breast Cancer* 5(5), 353 (15%) (with vinorelbine)
(2003): Skubitz KM, *Cancer Invest* 21(2), 167
(2002): McMenemin R+, *Invest New Drugs* 20(3), 331
(2001): Verschraegen CF+, *Cancer* 92(9), 2327
(2000): Lotem M+, *Arch Dermatol* 136, 1475

Oral lesions

Oral pigmentation
(1989): Kerker BJ+, *Semin Dermatol* 8, 173

Oral ulceration

Stomatitis (>10%)
(2005): Rose PG, *Oncologist* 10(3), 205
(2003): Chao TC+, *Cancer Invest* 21(6), 837
(2002): Fracasso PM+, *Cancer* 95(10), 2223 (with gemcitabine)
(2002): Numico G+, *Lung Cancer* 35(1), 59
(2001): Goram AL+, *Pharmacotherapy* 21(6), 751
(2001): Verschraegen CF+, *Cancer* 92(9), 2327
(2000): Israel VP+, *Gynecol Oncol* 78, 143
(2000): Lotem M+, *Arch Dermatol* 136, 1475
(1994): Bogner JR+, *J Acquir Immune Defic Syndr* 7, 463
(1994): Sella A+, *J Clin Oncol* 12(4), 683 (with ketoconazole)
(1989): Henderson IC+, *J Clin Oncol* 7, 560 (8.4%)
(1981): von Eyben FE+, *Cancer* 48, 1535 (passim)

Tongue pigmentation
(1989): Kerker BJ+, *Semin Dermatol* 8, 173

Hair

Hair – alopecia (>10%)
(2006): Selleri S+, *J Invest Dermatol*
(2004): Martin M+, *Clin Breast Cancer* 5(5), 353 (53%) (with vinorelbine)
(2000): Lotem M+, *Arch Dermatol* 136, 1475 (passim)

(1995): Bonadonna G+, *JAMA* 273, 542 (96%)
(1994): Bogner JR+, *J Acquir Immune Defic Syndr* 7, 463
(1994): Rodrigeuz R+, *Ann Oncol* 5, 769
(1989): Henderson IC+, *J Clin Oncol* 7, 560 (>5%)
(1988): Giaccone G+, *Cancer Nurs* 11, 170
(1986): Martin-Jiminez M+, *N Engl J Med* 315, 894
(1986): Perez JE+, *Cancer Treat Rep* 70, 1213
(1984): Satterwhite B+, *Cancer* 54, 34
(1984): Wheelock JB+, *Cancer Treat Rep* 68, 1387
(1983): Howard N+, *Br J Radiol* 56, 963
(1983): Tigges FJ, *MMW Munch Med Wochenschr* (German) 125, 19
(1982): Gregory RP+, *Br Med J Clin Res Ed* 284, 1674
(1982): Hunt JM+, *Cancer Nurs* 5, 25
(1981): Anderson JE+, *Br Med J Clin Res* 282, 423
(1981): Cooke T+, *Br Med J Clin Res Ed* 282, 734
(1981): Hallett N, *Nurs Mirror* 152, 32
(1981): Tigges FJ, *MMW Munch Med Wochenschr* (German) 123, 737
(1980): Presser SE, *N Engl J Med* 302, 921
(1980): Timothy AR+, *Lancet* 1, 663

Nails

Nails – Beau's lines (transverse nail bands)
(2006): Dasanu CA+, *Dermatol Online J* 12(6), 10 (with vincristine and dexamethasone)
(1994): Ben-Dayan D+, *Acta Haematol* 91, 89
Nails – melanonychia
(2003): Khairkar PH, *Indian Pediatr* 40(11), 1094
Nails – muehrcke's lines
(2006): Dasanu CA+, *Dermatol Online J* 12(6), 10 (with vincristine and dexamethasone)
Nails – pigmentation
(2006): Dasanu CA+, *Dermatol Online J* 12(6), 10 (with vincristine and dexamethasone)
(1999): Ghoshal UC+, *J Diarrhoeal Dis Res* 17, 43
(1983): Bronner AK+, *J Am Acad Dermatol* 9, 645
(1983): James WD+, *Arch Dermatol* 119, 334 (white lines)
(1983): Manigand G+, *Sem Hop* (French) 59, 1840
(1982): Sans-Ortiz J+, *Med Clin* (Barc) (Spanish) 79, 49
(1981): Giacobetti R+, *Am J Dis Child* 135, 317
(1980): Runne U+, *Z Haut* (German) 55, 1590
(1980): Sulis E+, *Eur J Cancer* 16, 1517

Other

Anaphylactoid reactions/Anaphylaxis (<1%)
(1984): Collins JA, *Drug Intell Clin Pharm* 18, 402
(1982): Dunagin WG, *Semin Oncol* 9, 14
Asthenia
(2007): Cooley T+, *Oncologist* 12(1), 114 (16.7%)
Cardiotoxicity
(2006): Elbl L+, *Vnitr Lek* 52(4), 328 (4%)
(2006): Katamadze NA+, *Georgian Med News* (130), 61
(2006): Lipshultz SE+, *Leuk Lymphoma* 47(8), 1454
(2006): Lowis S+, *Br J Cancer* 95(5), 571
(2006): Tokarska-Schlattner M+, *J Mol Cell Cardiol* 41(3), 389
Chest pain
(2003): Saisho S+, *Gan To Kagaku Ryoho* 30(13), 2063
Congestive heart failure
(1985): Speyer JL+, *Am J Med* 78(4), 555
(1983): Lenzhofer R+, *Z Kardiol* 72(5), 297
Death
(2002): Escudier B+, *J Urol* 168(3), 959 (with ifosfamide)
(2002): McMenemin R+, *Invest New Drugs* 20(3), 331
(1994): Sella A+, *J Clin Oncol* 12(4), 683 (with ketoconazole)
Fever
(2004): Huang JY+, *Anticancer Drugs* 15(3), 239
(2003): Saisho S+, *Gan To Kagaku Ryoho* 30(13), 2063
Headache
Hypersensitivity

(2004): Chua SL+, *Neuro-oncol* 6(1), 38 (14%)
Injection-site erythema
(1984): Collins JA, *Drug Intell Clin Pharm* 18, 402
(1983): Bronner AK+, *J Am Acad Dermatol* 9, 645
(1982): Dunagin WG, *Semin Oncol* 9, 14
(1981): von Eyben FE+, *Cancer* 48, 1535 (passim)
(1981): Weiss RB+, *Ann Intern Med* 94, 66 (>5%)
Injection-site extravasation (>10%)
(2000): Kassner E, *J Pediatr Oncon Nurs* 17, 135
(2000): Lotem M+, *Arch Dermatol* 136, 1475
(1999): Fleming A+, *J Hand Surg [Br]* 24, 390
(1998): Emiroglu M+, *Ann Plast Surg* 41, 103
(1989): Harwood KV+, *Oncol Nurs Forum* 16, 10
(1984): Hankin FM+, *J Pediatr Orthop* 4, 96
(1984): Sonneveld P+, *Cancer Treat Rep* 68, 895
(1983): Cohen FJ+, *J Hand Surg Am* 8, 43
(1983): Olver IN+, *Cancer Treat Rep* 67, 407
(1983): Pitkanen J+, *J Surg Oncol* 23, 259
(1980): Barden GA, *South Med J* 73, 1543
Injection-site necrosis (>10%)
(1998): Bekerecioglu M+, *J Surg Res* 75, 61
(1987): Dufresne RG, *Cutis* 39, 197
(1983): Bronner AK+, *J Am Acad Dermatol* 9, 645
Injection-site reactions
(2001): Verschraegen CF+, *Cancer* 92(9), 2327
Injection-site ulceration (>10%)
Myalgia/Myositis/Myopathy/Myotoxicity
(2002): Cantu MG+, *J Clin Oncol* 20(5), 1232 (4%) (with cyclophosphamide and cisplatin)

DOXYCYCLINE

Trade names: Adoxa (Bioglan); Apo-Dox; Apo-Doxy; Atridox; Azudoxat; Bactidox; Doryx (Warner Chilcott); Doximed; Doxy-100; Doxylin; Doxytec; Monodox; Vibra-Tabs (Pfizer); Vibramycin (Pfizer); Vibramycine; Vibravenos
Indications: Various infections caused by susceptible organisms
Category: Antibiotic, tetracycline
Half-life: 12–22 hours
Clinically important, potentially hazardous interactions with: amoxicillin, ampicillin, antacids, bacampicillin, bismuth, calcium, carbenicillin, cloxacillin, corticosteroids, digoxin, iron, methoxyflurane, mezlocillin, nafcillin, oxacillin, penicillins, piperacillin, retinoids, ticarcillin, zinc

Reactions

Skin

Actinic granuloma
(2003): Lim DS+, *Australas J Dermatol* 44(1), 67
Acute generalized exanthematous pustulosis (AGEP)
(1993): Trueb RM+, *Dermatology* 186, 75
Allergic reactions (sic) (0.47%)
(1986): Bigby M+, *JAMA* 256, 3358
Angioedema
(1997): Shapiro LE+, *Arch Dermatol* 133, 1224
Erythema multiforme
(1988): Lewis-Jones MS+, *Clin Exp Dermatol* 13, 245
(1987): Curley RK+, *Clin Exp Dermatol* 12, 124
(1985): Albengres E+, *Therapie* (French) 38, 577
Erythroderma
(2003): Batinac T+, *Tumori* 89(1), 91
Exanthems
(2003): Batinac T+, *Tumori* 89(1), 91
(1987): Bryant SG+, *Pharmacotherapy* 7, 125 (4.4%)
Exfoliative dermatitis

Fixed eruption (<1%)
  (2003): Drayton GE, Los Angeles, CA (from Internet) (observation)
  (2003): Gregg LJ, Tulsa, OK (3 cases – all on glans penis) (from Internet) (observation)
  (2002): Walfish AE+, *Cutis* 69, 207 (metronidazole, in the same patient, also produced a fixed eruption)
  (1999): Correia O+, *Clin Exp Dermatol* 24, 137 (genital) (with minocycline)
  (1996): Marmelzat J, Los Angeles, CA (from Internet) (observation)
  (1989): Alanko K+, *Acta Derm Venereol* (Stockh) 69, 223
  (1988): Budde J+, *Aktuel Dermatol* (German) 14, 304
  (1987): Jolly HW+, *Arch Dermatol* 114, 1484
  (1984): Bargman H, *J Am Acad Dermatol* 11, 900
Jarisch–Herxheimer reaction
  (1983): Perine PL+, *Am J Trop Med Hyg* 32(5), 1096
Lupus erythematosus
Painful eruption of hands
  (1995): Levine N, *Geriatrics* 50, 23
Perforating Dermatosis
  (2006): Gonul M+, *Int J Dermatol* 45(12), 1461
Photosensitivity (<1%)
  (2004): Donta ST+, *Ann Intern Med* 141(2), 85
  (2002): Baxter BT+, *J Vasc Surg* 36(1), 1
  (2002): Litt JZ, Beachwood, OH (personal observation)
  (2002): Maffei K, Athens, GA (from Internet) (observation)
  (2002): Pages F+, *Trop Med Int Health* 7(11), 919
  (1997): O'Reilly FM+, American Academy of Dermatology Meeting, Poster #14
  (1997): Shapiro LE+, *Arch Dermatol* 133, 1224
  (1997): Tanaka N+, *Contact Dermatitis* 37, 93
  (1995). Nowakowski J+, *J Am Acad Dermatol* 32, 223
  (1992): Bennett MJ, *J R Army Med Corps* 138, 56
  (1987): Bryant SG+, *Pharmacotherapy* 7(4), 125
  (1987): Edwards R, *N Z Med J* 100, 640
  (1980): Möller H+, *Acta Derm Venereol* (Stockh) 60, 495
Phototoxicity
  (2006): Habif TP, *N Engl J Med* 355(2), 182
  (2002): Bohannon JS, Midlothian, VA (from Internet) (observation)
  (2002): Fishman CB, San Luis Obispo, CA (from Internet) (observation)
  (2002): Litt JZ, Beachwood, OH (personal case) (observation)
  (2002): Sorkin M, Denver, CO (from Internet) (observation)
  (2002): Thaler D, Monona, WI (from Internet) (observation)
  (1999): Litt JZ, Beachwood, OH (personal case) (observation)
  (1996): McCarty JR, Fort Worth, TX (from Internet) (observation)
  (1995): Smith EL+, *Br J Dermatol* 132, 316
  (1994): Bjellerup AM+, *Br J Dermatol* 130, 356
  (1993): Layton A+, *Clin Exp Dermatol* 18, 425
  (1993): Shea CR+, *J Invest Dermatol* 101, 329
  (1982): Rosen K+, *Acta Derm Venereol* 62, 246
Pigmentation
  (2006): Adisen E+, *Int J Dermatol* 45(10), 1245
  (2006): Pichardo RO+, *Am J Dermatopathol* A(3), 235
  (2002): Bohm M+, *Am J Dermatopathol* 24(4), 345
  (1999): Westermann GW+, *J Intern Med* 246, 591
  (1980): Möller H+, *Acta Derm Venereol* (Stockh) 60, 495
Pruritus ani et vulvae
Psoriasis
  (1988): Tsankov NK+, *Australas J Dermatol* 29, 111
Purpura
Rash (sic) (<1%)
  (1997): Shapiro LE+, *Arch Dermatol* 133, 1224
Seborrhea
  (1997): Rademaker M, New Zealand (from Internet) (observation)

Stevens–Johnson syndrome
  (2007): Cac NN+, *Cutis* 79(2), 119
  (1997): Gallais V+, *Presse Med* 26(18), 855
  (1987): Curley RK+, *Clin Exp Dermatol* 12, 124
Toxic epidermal necrolysis
  (1999): Egan CA+, *J Am Acad Dermatol* 40, 458
Urticaria
  (2002): Pages F+, *Trop Med Int Health* 7(11), 919
  (1997): Shapiro LE+, *Arch Dermatol* 133, 1224
  (1992): Deluze C+, *Allergol Immunopathol Madr* (Spanish) 20, 215
  (1989): Alanko K+, *Acta Derm Venereol* (Stockh) 69, 223
Vasculitis
  (1981): Rockl H, *Hautarzt* (German) 32, 467

Mucosal/ENT
Anosmia
  (1990): Bleasel AF+, *Med J Aust* 152, 440
Dysgeusia
  (2001): Bunker C, United Kingdom (personal communication)
Glossitis
Oral ulceration
  (2002): Pages F+, *Trop Med Int Health* 7(11), 919
Tongue black
  (2007): Ramsakal A+, *N Engl J Med* 357(23), 2388
  (2006): Tamam L+, *Mt Sinai J Med* 73(6), 891
Vaginitis
  (1995): Nowakowski J+, *J Am Acad Dermatol* 32, 223

Nails
Nails – discoloration (painful)
  (1993): Coffin SE+, *Pediatr Infect Dis J* 12, 702
Nails – photo-onycholysis
  (2005): Fitch MH, Aiken, SC (from Internet) (observation)
  (2004): Passier A+, *BMJ* 329(7460), 265
  (2004): Rabar D+, *J Travel Med* 11(6), 386
  (2003): Carroll LA+, *J Drugs Dermatol* 2(6), 662
  (2000): Yong CK+, *Pediatrics* 106, E13
  (1995): Shapero H, *The Schoch Letter* 45 #6, 21 (observation)
  (1988): Quirce-Gancedo S+, *Med Clin* (Barc) (Spanish) 90, 636
  (1987): Baran R+, *J Am Acad Dermatol* 17, 1012
  (1985): Gventer M+, *J Am Podiatr Med Assoc* 75, 658
  (1982): Jeanmougin M+, *Ann Dermatol Venereol* (French) 109, 165
  (1981): Cavens TR, *Cutis* 27, 53
Nails – pigmentation
  (2005): Akcam M+, *Pediatr Infect Dis J* 24(9), 845

Other
Anaphylactoid reactions/Anaphylaxis
Candidiasis
  (2002): Baxter BT+, *J Vasc Surg* 36(1), 1
Fever
  (2003): Batinac T+, *Tumori* 89(1), 91
Headache
Hypersensitivity
  (2008): Robles DT+, *Dermatology* 217(1), 23
Injection-site phlebitis (<1%)
Paresthesias
  (1995): Shapero H, *The Schoch Letter* 45, 21 (observation)
  (1994): Blanchard L, *The Schoch Letter* 44, 6 (observation)
  (1994): Liss W, *The Schoch Letter* 44, 16 (observation)
  (1993): Held J, *The Schoch Letter* 43, 27 (observation)
Phlebitis (<1%)
Serum sickness
  (1997): Shapiro LE+, *Arch Dermatol* 133, 1224

DRONABINOL

Synonyms: tetrahydrocannabinol; THC
Trade name: Marinol (Unimed)
Indications: Chemotherapy-induced nausea
Category: Cannabinoid
Half-life: 19–24 hours

Reactions

Skin
Diaphoresis (<1%)

Mucosal/ENT
Tinnitus
Xerostomia (1–10%)

Other
Myalgia/Myositis/Myopathy/Myotoxicity (<1%)
Paresthesias
Vertigo
  (2004): Svendsen KB+, *BMJ* 329(7460), 253

DROPERIDOL

Trade names: Dehydrobenzperidol; Droleptan; Droperidol;
Inapsin; Inapsine (Akorn); Sintodian
Indications: Tranquilizer and antiemetic in surgical procedures
Category: Antipsychotic; Butyrophenone
Half-life: 2.3 hours
**Clinically important, potentially hazardous interactions
with:** amisulpride, cyclobenzaprine, fluoxetine

Note: In 2001, droperidol was removed from the European market
and the US FDA issued a 'black box' warning, citing cases of QT
prolongation and/or torsades de pointes.

Reactions

Skin
Angioedema
  (1996): Palombaro JF+, *Ann Emerg Med* 27(3), 379
  (1993): Corke PJ+, *Anaesth Intensive Care* 21(3), 375
Diaphoresis
Pruritus
  (2003): Culebras X+, *Anesth Analg* 97(3), 816 (6.1%)
Shivering

Other
Anaphylactoid reactions/Anaphylaxis
  (1984): Aguilera Celorrio L+, *Rev Esp Anestesiol Reanim*
    31(6), 249
  (1984): Aren Frontera JJ+, *Rev Esp Anestesiol Reanim* 31(2), 75
  (1984): Occelli G+, *Ann Fr Anesth Reanim* 3(6), 440
Chills
Death
  (2004): Cox RD+, *Vet Hum Toxicol* 46(1), 21 (2 cases)
  (2004): Mullins M+, *Am J Emerg Med* 22(1), 27 (99 cases)
  (2001): Glassman AH+, *Am J Psychiatry* 158(11), 1774
Hypertension
  (1982): Takino Y+, *Masui* 31(5), 522
Rhabdomyolysis
  (1983): Reis J+, *Rev Neurol (Paris)* 139(10), 595
Seizures
  (2002): Chase PB+, *Acad Emerg Med* 9(12), 1402 (3 cases)

DROTRECOGIN ALFA

Trade name: Xigris (Lilly)
Indications: Severe sepsis
Category: Recombinant protein C
Half-life: 1.6 hours
**Clinically important, potentially hazardous interactions
with:** None

Reactions

Skin
Purpura (>10%)

DULOXETINE

Trade name: Cymbalta (Lilly)
Indications: Depression
Category: Antidepressant; Noradrenaline reuptake inhibitor;
Serotonin reuptake inhibitor
Half-life: 8–17 hours
**Clinically important, potentially hazardous interactions
with:** cimetidine, ciprofloxacin, enoxacin, fluoxetine,
fluvoxamine, MAO inhibitors, paroxetine, quinidine, thioridazine

Reactions

Skin
Acne (<1%)
Diaphoresis (6%)
  (2007): Gahimer J+, *Curr Med Res Opin* 23(1), 175
  (2004): Detke MJ+, *Eur Neuropsychopharmacol* 14(6), 457
Eczema (<1%)
Erythema (<1%)
Facial edema (<1%)
Hyperhidrosis
  (2005): Wernicke JF+, *Expert Opin Drug Saf* 4(6), 987
Peripheral edema (<1%)
Photosensitivity (<1%)
Pruritus (<1%)
Purpura (<1%)
Rash (sic) (<1%)

Mucosal/ENT
Dysphagia (<1%)
Gingivitis (<1%)
Xerostomia (15%)
  (2007): Gahimer J+, *Curr Med Res Opin* 23(1), 175
  (2007): Nierenberg AA+, *Curr Med Res Opin* 23(2), 401
  (2006): Stewart DE+, *J Affect Disord* 94(1-3), 183
  (2006): Weinstein DL+, *Curr Med Res Opin* 22(11), 2121
  (2005): Brannan SK+, *J Psychiatr Res* 39(1), 43
  (2005): Wernicke JF+, *Expert Opin Drug Saf* 4(6), 987
  (2005): Wohlreich MM+, *J Clin Psychopharmacol* 25(6), 552
  (2002): Detke MJ+, *J Psychiatr Res* 36(6), 383
  (2000): Sharma A+, *J Clin Pharmacol* 40(2), 161

Hair
Hair – alopecia (<1%)

Eyes
Vision blurred
  (2005): Wernicke JF+, *Expert Opin Drug Saf* 4(6), 987

Other

Abdominal pain (>2%)

Asthenia
  (2007): Gahimer J+, *Curr Med Res Opin* 23(1), 175
  (2006): Weinstein DL+, *Curr Med Res Opin* 22(11), 2121
  (2005): Brannan SK+, *J Psychiatr Res* 39(1), 43
  (2005): Wernicke JF+, *Expert Opin Drug Saf* 4(6), 987
  (2003): Mallinckrodt CH+, *Prim Care Companion J Clinical Psychiatry* 5(1), 19 (8%)
  (2002): Goldstein DJ+, *J Clin Psychiatry* 63(3), 225

Cough (>2%)

Headache (>2%)
  (2007): Gahimer J+, *Curr Med Res Opin* 23(1), 175
  (2006): Bailey RK+, *J Natl Med Assoc* 98(3), 437
  (2006): Stewart DE+, *J Affect Disord* 94(1-3), 183
  (2005): Wernicke JF+, *Expert Opin Drug Saf* 4(6), 987
  (2005): Wohlreich MM+, *J Clin Psychopharmacol* 25(6), 552

Hepatotoxicity (rare)
  (2006): Hanje AJ+, *Clin Gastroenterol Hepatol* 4(7), 912 (fatal)
  (2005): *Prescrire Int* 14(80), 218
  (2005): Wernicke JF+, *Expert Opin Drug Saf* 4(6), 987

Hot flashes (2%)

Inappropriate secretion of antidiuretic hormone (SIADH)
  (2007): Kruger S+, *J Clin Psychopharmacol* 27(1), 101 (5 cases)
  (2006): Maramattom BV, *Neurology* 66(5), 773
  (2006): Safdieh JE+, *J Clin Psychopharmacol* 26(6), 675

Insomnia
  (2007): Gahimer J+, *Curr Med Res Opin* 23(1), 175

Phlebitis (<1%)

Porphyria
  (2007): Loper T+, *Psychosomatics* 48(2), 179

Seizures
  (2006): Maramattom BV, *Neurology* 66(5), 773

Suicidal ideation
  (2005): *Prescrire Int* 14(80), 218

Tremor (3%)

Upper respiratory infection (>2%)

Vertigo (9%)
  (2007): Gahimer J+, *Curr Med Res Opin* 23(1), 175
  (2006): Bailey RK+, *J Natl Med Assoc* 98(3), 437
  (2005): Wernicke JF+, *Expert Opin Drug Saf* 4(6), 987
  (2003): Mallinckrodt CH+, *Prim Care Companion J Clinical Psychiatry* 5(1), 19
  (2003): Raskin J+, *J Clin Psychiatry* 64(10), 1237
  (2002): Detke MJ+, *J Psychiatr Res* 36(6), 383

DUTASTERIDE

Trade name: Avodart (GSK)
Indications: Benign prostatic hyperplasia, male pattern baldness (anecdotal)
Category: 5-alpha reductase inhibitor; Androgen antagonist
Half-life: 3–5 weeks
Clinically important, potentially hazardous interactions with: None

Reactions

Other

Asthenia
  (2006): Dolder CR+, *Ann Pharmacother* 40(4), 658
Gynecomastia (1%)
  (2006): Schulman C+, *BJU Int* 97(1), 73
Headache
  (2006): Dolder CR+, *Ann Pharmacother* 40(4), 658

Infections
  (2006): Dolder CR+, *Ann Pharmacother* 40(4), 658
Myalgia/Myositis/Myopathy/Myotoxicity
  (2006): Dolder CR+, *Ann Pharmacother* 40(4), 658
Vertigo
  (2006): Dolder CR+, *Ann Pharmacother* 40(4), 658

ECHINACEA

Scientific names: *Echinacea angustifola; Echinacea pallida; Echinacea purpurea*
Family: Asteraceae; Compositae
Trade and other common names: Black Sampson; Black Susans; Comb Flower; Indian Head; Purple-Cone Flower; Snakeroot
Category: Immunomodulator
Purported indications and other uses: Colds, upper respiratory infections, peripheral vasodilator, urinary tract infections, yeast infections, ulcers, psoriasis, herpes simplex, septicemia, boils, abscesses, rheumatism, migraine, dyspepsia, eczema, bee stings and hemorrhoids
Half-life: N/A
Clinically important, potentially hazardous interactions with: corticosteroids, cyclosporine

Reactions

Skin

Adverse effects (sic)
  (2002): Bielory L, *Ann Allergy Asthma Immunol* 88(1), 7
  (2002): Ernst E, *Ann Intern Med* 136(1), 42
  (2002): Haller CA+, *Adverse Drug React Toxicol Rev* 21(3), 143
  (2002): Mattsson K+, *Lakartidningen* 99(50), 5095
Allergic reactions (sic)
  (2005): Huntley AL+, *Drug Saf* 28(5), 387
Angioedema
  (2000): www.aaaai.org/media/pressreleases/2000/03/000307.html
Bullae
  (2004): Lee AN+, *Arch Dermatol* 140(6), 723 (flare)
Erythema nodosum
  (2001): Crawford R, *J Am Acad Dermatol* 44, 298 (recurrent)
Rash (sic)
  (2005): Huntley AL+, *Drug Saf* 28(5), 387
  (2002): Mullins RJ+, *Ann Allergy Asthma Immunol* 88(1), 42
Sensitization
  (2002): Paulsen E, *Contact Dermatitis* 47(4), 189
Urticaria
  (2002): Mullins RJ+, *Ann Allergy Asthma Immunol* 88(1), 42
  (2000): www.aaaai.org/media/pressreleases/2000/03/000307.html

Mucosal/ENT

Oral lesions
  (2004): Lee AN+, *Arch Dermatol* 140(6), 723 (flare)
Sialorrhea
Tongue numb
  (2003): Abebe W, *J Dent Hyg* 77(1), 37

Eyes

Ocular adverse effects
  (2004): Fraunfelder FW, *Am J Ophthalmol* 138(4), 639

Other

Anaphylactoid reactions/Anaphylaxis
  (2004): Bielory L, *Ann Allergy Asthma Immunol* 93(2 Suppl), S45

(2002): Mullins RJ+, *Ann Allergy Asthma Immunol* 88(1), 42
(2000):
  www.aaaai.org/media/pressreleases/2000/03/000307.html
(1998): Mullins RJ, *Med J Aust* 168, 170
Hypersensitivity
(2002): Mullins RJ+, *Ann Allergy Asthma Immunol* 88(1), 42
(2000):
  www.aaaai.org/media/pressreleases/2000/03/000307.html (23
  cases)
Paresthesias
Vertigo
(2003): Kligler B, *Am Fam Physician* 2003 Jan 67(1), 77

ECULIZUMAB

Trade name: Soliris (Alexion)
Indications: Paroxysmal nocturnal hemoglobinuria (PNH)
Category: Monoclonal antibody
Half-life: 272 Hours
**Clinically important, potentially hazardous interactions
with:** N/A

Reactions

Skin
Edema
Herpes simplex
Rash (sic)

Mucosal/ENT
Nasopharyngitis (23%)
Sinusitis

Other
Abdominal pain
Asthenia (12%)
Cough (12%)
Fever
Headache (44%)
Hypersensitivity
Injection-site reactions
Meningococcal infection
Myalgia/Myositis/Myopathy/Myotoxicity
Upper respiratory infection
Vertigo

EDROPHONIUM

Trade names: Enlon (Baxter); Tensilon (Valeant)
Indications: Myasthenia gravis diagnosis
Category: Anesthetic; Cholinesterase inhibitor
Half-life: 1.8 hours
**Clinically important, potentially hazardous interactions
with:** corticosteroids, digitalis, galantamine

Reactions

Skin
Allergic reactions
Diaphoresis (>10%)
Rash (sic)
Urticaria

Mucosal/ENT
Sialorrhea (>10%)

Other
Abdominal pain
Anaphylactoid reactions/Anaphylaxis
Cardiac failure
Chest pain
  (1990): Dalton CB+, *Dig Dis Sci* 35(12), 1445
Headache
Hypersensitivity (<1%)
Myalgia/Myositis/Myopathy/Myotoxicity
  (1984): Macchi G+, *Ital J Neurol Sci* 5(2), 225
Seizures
  (2000): Ing EB+, *Can J Ophthalmol* 35(3), 141
Thrombophlebitis (<1%)
Vertigo

EFALIZUMAB

Trade name: Raptiva (Genentech)
Indications: Psoriasis
Category: Immunomodulator; Monoclonal antibody
Half-life: 12–35 days
**Clinically important, potentially hazardous interactions
with:** immunosuppressives, **live vaccines**

Reactions

Skin
Abscess
Acne (4%)
Allergic reactions (sic)
Angioedema
Basal cell carcinoma
Cellulitis
Dermatitis
  (2005): de Groot M+, *Br J Dermatol* 153(4), 843
Erythema multiforme
Erythroderma
  (2004): Gaylor M-L G+, *J Drugs Dermatol* 3(1), 77 (following
    withdrawal)
Exanthems
Inflammatory papules (sic)
  (2007): Lowes MA+, *BMC Dermatol* 7, 2 (15 cases)
Lupus erythematosus
  (2007): Heffernan MP+, *J Drugs Dermatol* 6(3), 310
  (2006): Bentley DD+, *J Am Acad Dermatol* 54(5 suppl), S242
Lymphoma
  (2006): Berthelot C+, *Clin Lymphoma Myeloma* 6(4), 329
Peripheral edema
  (2006): Scheinfeld N, *Expert Opin Drug Saf* 5(2), 197
Psoriasis (0.7%)
  (2007): Chacko M+, *Dermatol Ther* 20(4), 265 (passim)
  (2006): Descamps V, *Ann Dermatol Venereol* 133(8-9 Pt 1), 666
  (2006): Golda N+, *J Drugs Dermatol* 5(1), 63
  (2005): Gregg LJ, Tulsa, OK (2 cases) (from Internet)
    (observation)
  (2005): Howard B, Santa Maria, CA (from Internet)
    (observation)
  (2004): Gaylor M-L G+, *J Drugs Dermatol* 3(1), 77 (recurrence)
    (following withdrawal)
Skin cancer
  (2006): *Prescrire Int* 15(81), 8
Squamous cell carcinoma

Urticaria
(2007): Heffernan MP+, *J Drugs Dermatol* 6(3), 310
Vitiligo
(2008): Wakkee M+, *J Am Acad Dermatol* 59(2), S57

Mucosal/ENT
Ototoxicity
(2006): Scheinfeld N, *Expert Opin Drug Saf* 5(2), 197
Sialadenitis
(2006): Scheinfeld N, *Expert Opin Drug Saf* 5(2), 197
Sinusitis

Other
Aseptic meningitis
(2007): Kluger N+, *Br J Dermatol* 156(1), 189
(2007): Rivas-Rodriguez R+, *Farm Hosp* 31(1), 70
Asthenia
(2006): Scheinfeld N, *Expert Opin Drug Saf* 5(2), 197
Chills (13%)
(2007): Chacko M+, *Dermatol Ther* 20(4), 265 (passim)
(2006): Scheinfeld N, *Expert Opin Drug* 5(2), 197
(2004): Gaylor M-L G+, *J Drugs Dermatol* 3(1), 77 (13%)
DRESS syndrome
(2007): White JM+, *Clin Exp Dermatol* 33(1), 50
Fever
(2007): Chacko M+, *Dermatol Ther* 20(4), 265 (passim)
(2006): Scheinfeld N, *Expert Opin Drug Saf* 5(2), 197
(2004): Gaylor M-L G+, *J Drugs Dermatol* 3(1), 77
Headache
(2007): Chacko M+, *Dermatol Ther* 20(4), 265 (passim)
(2006): Scheinfeld N, *Expert Opin Drug Saf* 5(2), 197
(2003): Gauvreau GM+, *J Allergy Clin Immunol* 112(2), 331 (40%)
Hepatotoxicity
(2006): Scheinfeld N, *Expert Opin Drug Saf* 5(2), 197
Hypersensitivity
(2006): *Prescrire Int* 15(81), 8
(2006): Descamps V, *Ann Dermatol Venereol* 133(8-9 Pt 1), 666
(2006): Scheinfeld N, *Expert Opin Drug Saf* 5(2), 197
Infections (29%)
(2007): Chacko M+, *Dermatol Ther* 20(4), 265 (passim)
(2007): Heffernan MP+, *J Drugs Dermatol* 6(3), 310 (staphylococcal abscess)
(2006): *Prescrire Int* 15(81), 8
(2004): Gaylor M-L G+, *J Drugs Dermatol* 3(1), 77 (29%)
Myalgia/Myositis/Myopathy/Myotoxicity (8%)
(2007): Chacko M+, *Dermatol Ther* 20(4), 265 (passim)
(2006): Scheinfeld N, *Expert Opin Drug Saf* 5(2), 197
Pain (10%)
(2004): Gaylor M-L G+, *J Drugs Dermatol* 3(1), 77 (10%)
Serum sickness

EFAVIRENZ

Trade name: Sustiva (Bristol-Myers Squibb)
Indications: HIV infection
Category: Antiretroviral; Non-nucleoside reverse transcriptase inhibitor
Half-life: 52–76 hours
Clinically important, potentially hazardous interactions with: alprazolam, benzodiazepines, chlordiazepoxide, clonazepam, clorazepate, diazepam, dihydroergotamine, ergot, flurazepam, lorazepam, methysergide, midazolam, oral contraceptives, oxazepam, quazepam, temazepam, triazolam

Reactions

Skin
Diaphoresis
Eczema (<2%)
Erythema
(2003): Foti JL+, *AIDS Patient Care STDS* 17(1), 1
Exanthems (27%)
(2002): Phillips EJ+, *Ann Pharmacother* 36(3), 430
(2001): Hartmann M+, *HIV Clin Trials* 2(5), 421
(1998): Adkins JC+, *Drugs* 56, 1055
Exfoliative dermatitis (<2%)
Folliculitis (<2%)
Peripheral edema (<2%)
Photosensitivity
(2004): Furue M, *Intern Med* 43(7), 533
(2004): Yoshimoto E+, *Intern Med* 43(7), 630
(2000): Newell A+, *Sex Transm Infect* 76, 221
Pruritus (<2%)
Rash (sic) (5–20%)
(2003): Arribas JR, *Int J STD AIDS* 14 Suppl 1, 6
(2002): Perez-Molina JA, *HIV Clin Trials* 3(4), 279 (5.8%)
Stevens–Johnson syndrome
(2004): Colebunders R+, *Infection* 32(5), 306
Urticaria (<2%)
Vasculitis
(2002): Domingo P+, *Arch Intern Med* 162(3), 355

Mucosal/ENT
Burning mouth syndrome
(2006): Borras-Blasco J+, *Ann Pharmacother* 40(7-8), 1471
Dysgeusia (<2%)
Parosmia (<2%)
Xerostomia (<2%)

Hair
Hair – alopecia (<2%)

Other
Aseptic meningitis
(2007): Kluger N+, *Br J Dermatol* 156(1), 189
Asthenia
(2006): Ward DJ+, *AIDS Patient Care* 20(8), 542
Depression
(2006): Ward DJ+, *AIDS Patient Care STDS* 20(8), 542
(2005): Gutierrez F+, *Clin Infect Dis* 41(11), 1648
(2005): Hawkins T+, *HIV Clin Trials* 6(4), 187
(2002): Puzantian T, *Pharmacotherapy* 22(7), 930
Fever
(2003): Foti JL+, *AIDS Patient Care STDS* 17(1), 1
Gynecomastia
(2004): Braunstein GD, *AIDS Read* 14(1), 38
(2004): Rahim S+, *AIDS Read* 14(1), 23
(2002): Qazi NA+, *AIDS* 16(3), 506
(2001): Arranz Caso JA+, *AIDS* 15(11), 1447
(2001): Caso JA+, *AIDS* 15(11), 1447
(2001): Mercie P+, *AIDS* 15(1), 126
Headache
Hot flashes (<2%)
Hypersensitivity
(2003): Foti JL+, *AIDS Patient Care STDS* 17(1), 1
(2002): Phillips EJ+, *Ann Pharmacother* 36(3), 430
(2000): Bossi P+, *Clin Infect Dis* 30, 227
Myalgia/Myositis/Myopathy/Myotoxicity (<2%)
Paresthesias (<2%)
Suicidal ideation
(2005): Gutierrez F+, *Clin Infect Dis* 41(11), 1648
(2003): Lochet P+, *HIV Med* 4(1), 62 (9.2%)

Thrombophlebitis (<2%)
Tremor (<2%)
Vertigo
(2005): Fumaz CR+, *J Acquir Immune Defic Syndr* 38(5), 560

EFLORNITHINE

Synonym: DFMO
Trade names: Ornidyl; Vaniqa (Women First)
Indications: Sleeping sickness, hypertrichosis
Category: Ornithine decarboxylase inhibitor
Half-life: IV: 3–3.5 hours; topical: 8 hours

Reactions

Skin
Acne (24.3%)
(2001): Thaler D, Monona, WS (perioral) (from Internet)
(observation))
Burning (4.3%)
Dermatitis (<1%)
Edema of lip (<1%)
Erythema (1.3%)
(2001): Hickman JG+, *Curr Med Res Opin* 16, 235
Facial edema (0.3–3%)
Folliculitis (0.5%)
Herpes simplex (<1%)
Irritation (1%)
Pruritus (3.8%)
(2001): Hickman JG+, *Curr Med Res Opin* 16, 235
Rash (sic) (2.8%)
Rosacea (<1%)
Stinging (7.9%)
Xerosis (1.8%)
(2001): Hickman JG+, *Curr Med Res Opin* 16, 235

Mucosal/ENT
Cheilitis (<1%)

Hair
Hair – alopecia (5–10%)
(2003): Burri C+, *Parasitol Res* 90(Suppl 1), S49 (5–10%)
Hair – ingrown (0.3–2%)
Hair – pseudofolliculitis barbae (5–15%)

Other
Paresthesias (3.6%)
Seizures (7%)
(2003): Burri C+, *Parasitol Res* 90(Suppl 1), S49 (7%)

ELETRIPTAN

Trade name: Relpax (Pfizer)
Indications: Migraine headaches
Category: 5-HT1 agonist; Serotonin receptor agonist; Triptan
Half-life: 4–5 hours

Reactions

Skin
Abscess (<1%)
Allergic reactions (sic) (<1%)
Diaphoresis (<1%)

Edema (<1%)
Exanthems (<1%)
Exfoliative dermatitis (<1%)
Facial edema (<1%)
Peripheral edema (<1%)
Pigmentation (<1%)
Pruritus (<1%)
Psoriasis (<1%)
Rash (sic) (<1%)
Urticaria (<1%)
Xerosis (<1%)

Mucosal/ENT
Dysgeusia (<1%)
Gingivitis (<1%)
Parosmia (<1%)
Sialorrhea (<1%)
Stomatitis (<1%)
Tinnitus (<1%)
Tongue disorder (<1%)
Vaginitis (<1%)

Hair
Hair – alopecia

Other
Asthenia
(2003): Farkkila M+, *Cephalalgia* 23(6), 463
Candidiasis (<1%)
Chest pain
(2003): Farkkila M+, *Cephalalgia* 23(6), 463
Chills (<1%)
Depression (<1%)
Headache
Myalgia/Myositis/Myopathy/Myotoxicity (<1%)
Paresthesias (<1%)
Tremor (<1%)

EMTRICITABINE

Synonyms: 524W91; BW 524W91
Trade name: Emtriva (Gilead)
Indications: HIV-1 infection in adults
Category: Antiretroviral; Nucleoside analog reverse
transcriptase inhibitor
Half-life: ~10 hours

Note: Emtricitabine is a fluorinated derivative of lamivudine

Reactions

Skin
Allergic reactions (sic) (17%)
Exanthems (17%)
Pigmentation (palms & soles)
(2004): *AIDS Patient Care STDS* 18(10), 616
Pruritus (17%)
Pustules (17%)
Rash (sic)
(2000): Molina JM+, *J Infect Dis* 182(2), 599
Urticaria (17%)
Vesiculobullous eruption

Mucosal/ENT
Rhinitis (12%)

Other

Abdominal pain (14%)
  (2005): *Prescrire Int* 14(76), 54
Asthenia
  (2005): *Prescrire Int* 14(76), 54
Cough (14%)
Depression (10%)
Fever
  (2005): *Prescrire Int* 14(76), 54
Headache (16%)
  (2005): *Prescrire Int* 14(76), 54
Myalgia/Myositis/Myopathy/Myotoxicity (6%)
Pain
  (2005): *Prescrire Int* 14(76), 54
Paresthesias (6%)
Vertigo (25%)

ENALAPRIL

Trade names: Amprace; Apo-Enalapril; Enaladil; Enapren;
Glioten; Innovace; Lexxel (AstraZeneca); Pres; Renitec; Reniten;
Teczem (Sanofi-Aventis); Vasotec (Biovail); Xanef
Indications: Hypertension
Category: Angiotensin-converting enzyme inhibitor
Half-life: 11 hours
**Clinically important, potentially hazardous interactions
with:** amiloride, **licorice**, spironolactone, triamterene

Note: Lexxel is enalapril and felodipine; Teczem is enalapril and
diltiazem; Vaseretic is enalapril and hydrochlorothiazide

Reactions

Skin

Acantholysis
  (1999): Lo Schiavo A+, *Dermatology* 198, 391
Angioedema (<1%)
  (2007): Cupido C+, *S Afr Med J* 97(4), 244 (fatal)
  (2007): Garcia-Pavia P+, *Can J Cardiol* 23(4), 315
  (2007): Llinares Tello F+, *Farm Hosp* 31(3), 193
  (2004): Stevenson HA+, *Prim Dent Care* 11(1), 17 (2 cases)
  (2003): Mlynarek A+, *Otolaryngol Head Neck Surg* 129(5), 593
  (2003): Olesen AL+, *Ugeskr Laeger* 165(10), 1041
  (2003): Panaszek B+, *Pol Arch Med Wewn* 110(5), 1339
  (2003): Regner KR+, *Mayo Clin Proc* 78(5), 655
  (2002): Abdi R+, *Pharmacotherapy* 22(9), 1173
  (2002): Kaur S+, *J Dermatol* 29(6), 336
  (2001): Cohen EG+, *Ann Otol Rhinol Laryngol* 110(8), 701 (64
    cases)
  (2000): Babadzhan VD+, *Lik Sprava* (Russian) Apr–Jun, (3–4), 54
  (1998): *Prescrire Int* 7, 92
  (1998): Leuwer A+, *HNO* (German) 46, 56 (9 cases)
  (1997): Brown NJ+, *JAMA* 278, 232
  (1996): Kind B+, *Schweiz Rundsch Med Prax* (German) 85, 567
  (1996): Langauer-Messmer S+, *Postgrad Med J* 72, 383
  (1996): Mullins RJ+, *Med J Aust* 165, 319 (visceral)
  (1996): Pillans PI+, *Eur J Clin Pharmacol* 51, 123
  (1995): Forslund T+, *J Intern Med* 238, 179
  (1995): Juarez-Giminez JC+, *Ann Pharmacother* 29, 317
  (1995): Kozel MM+, *Clin Exp Dermatol* 20, 60
  (1995): Waldfahrer F+, *HNO* (German) 43, 35
  (1994): Dupasquier E, *Arch Mal Coeur Vaiss* (French) 87, 1371
  (1994): Dyer PD, *J Allergy Clin Immunol* 93, 947
  (1994): Farraye FA+, *Am J Gastroenterol* 89, 1117
  (1994): Lehmke J, *Med Klin* (German) 89, 508

  (1994): Nielsen EW+, *Tidsskr Nor Laegeforen* (Norwegian)
    114, 804
  (1994): Varma JR+, *J Am Board Fam Pract* 7, 433
  (1993): Oike Y+, *Intern Med* 32, 308 (fatal)
  (1993): Thompson T+, *Laryngoscope* 103, 10
  (1992): Bielory L+, *Allergy Proc* 13, 85
  (1992): Diehl KL+, *Dtsch Med Wochenschr* (German) 117, 727
  (1992): Dobroschke R+, *Anasthesiol Intensivmed Notfallmed
    Schmerzther* (German) 27, 510
  (1992): Finley CJ+, *Am J Emerg Med* 10, 550
  (1992): Hedner T+, *BMJ* 304, 941
  (1992): Jain M+, *Chest* 102, 871
  (1992): Venable RJ, *J Fam Pract* 34, 201
  (1991): Abidin MR+, *Arch Otolaryngol Head Neck Surg* 117, 1059
  (1991): Candelaria LM+, *J Oral Maxillofac Surg* 49, 1237
  (1991): Lanting PJ+, *Ned Tijdschr Geneeskd* (Dutch) 135, 335
  (1991): Roberts JR+, *Ann Emerg Med* 20, 555
  (1990): Chin HL+, *Ann Intern Med* 112, 312
  (1990): DiNardo LJ+, *Trans Pa Acad Ophthalmol Otolaryngol*
    42, 998
  (1990): Gannon TH+, *Laryngoscope* 100, 1156
  (1990): Gianos ME+, *Am J Emerg Med* 8, 124
  (1990): Gonnering RS+, *Am J Ophthalmol* 110, 566
  (1990): McAreavey D+, *Drugs* 40, 326 (0.2%)
  (1990): Orfan N+, *JAMA* 264, 1287
  (1990): Seidman MD+, *Otolaryngol Head Neck Surg* 102, 727
  (1990): Zech J+, *HNO* (German) 38, 143
  (1989): Barna JS+, *Va Med* 116, 147
  (1989): Giannoccaro PJ+, *Can J Cardiol* 5, 335 (fatal)
  (1989): Huwyler T+, *Schweiz Med Wochenschr* (German)
    119, 1253
  (1989): Smith ME+, *Otolaryngol Head Neck Surg* 101, 93
  (1989): Todd PA+, *Drugs* 37, 141 (<0.1%)
  (1989): Werber JL+, *Otolaryngol Head Neck Surg* 101, 96
  (1988): Inman WH+, *BMJ* 297, 826
  (1988): Schilling H+, *Z Kardiol* 77 (German) (Suppl 3), 47
  (1988): Slater EE+, *JAMA* 260, 967 (0.1%)
  (1988): Wernze H, *Z Kardiol* (German) 77, 61
  (1987): Ferner RE+, *BMJ* 294, 1119
  (1987): Inman WHW, *BMJ* 294, 578
  (1987): Vaillant L+, *Therapie* (French) 42, 411
  (1987): Wood SM+, *BMJ* 294, 91
  (1986): Marichal JF+, *Therapie* (French) 41, 517
Bullous pemphigoid
  (1994): Mullins PD+, *BMJ* 309, 1411
  (1993): Smith EP+, *J Am Acad Dermatol* 29, 879
Diaphoresis (<1%)
  (1994): Nachbar F+, *Dtsch Med Wochenschr* (German) 119, 321
Erythema
  (1993): Carrington PR+, *Cutis* 51, 121
Erythema multiforme (<1%)
Erythroderma
  (2006): Antonov D+, *Skinmed* 5(2), 90
Exanthems (1%)
  (1993): Carrington PR+, *Cutis* 51, 121
  (1990): McAreavey D+, *Drugs* 40, 326 (1.4%)
  (1990): Ruiz AM+, *Drugs* 39 (Suppl 2), 77 (0.9%)
  (1989): Todd PA+, *Drugs* 37, 141
  (1988): Warner NJ+, *Drugs* 35 (Suppl 5), 89 (1.4%)
  (1986): Gavras H, *Clin Ther* 9, 24
  (1986): Todd PA+, *Drugs* 31, 198 (0.5%)
  (1984): Kubo SH+, *Ann Intern Med* 100, 616
  (1983): Barnes JN+, *Lancet* 2, 41
Exfoliative dermatitis (<1%)
Herpes zoster (<1%)
Lichen planus
  (2003): Ruiz Villaverde R+, *J Eur Acad Dermatol Venereol*
    17(5), 612
Lichenoid eruption

(1995): Roten SV+, *J Am Acad Dermatol* 32, 293
(1993): Kanwar AJ+, *Dermatology* 187, 80 (photosensitive)

Lupus erythematosus
(1990): Schwarz D+, *Lancet* 336, 187

Mycosis fungoides
(1986): Furness PN+, *J Clin Pathol* 39, 902

Pemphigus
(2003): Stavropoulos PG+, *Dermatology* 207(3), 336
(2001): Thami GP+, *Dermatology* 202(4), 341
(1997): Brenner S+, *J Am Acad Dermatol* 36, 919
(1996): Mitchell DF, Charleston, SC (from Internet)
(observation)
(1995): Frangogiannis NG+, *Ann Intern Med* 122, 803 (larynx and esophagus)
(1994): Kuechle MK+, *Mayo Clin Proc* 69, 1166
(1994): Wolf R+, *Dermatology* 189, 1
(1993): Brenner S+, *Clin Dermatol* 11, 501
(1992): de Angelis E+, *Int J Dermatol* 31(10), 722
(1992): Ruocco V+, *Int J Dermatol* 31, 33

Pemphigus foliaceus
(2000): Ong CS+, *Australas J Dermatol* 41(4), 242
(1991): Shelton RM, *J Am Acad Dermatol* 24, 503

Pemphigus vegetans
(1994): Bastiaens MT+, *Int J Dermatol* 33, 168 (3 cases)

Photosensitivity (<1%)
(1997): O'Reilly FM+, *American Academy of Dermatology Meeting* Poster #14
(1993): Kanwar AJ+, *Dermatology* 187, 80
(1993): Shelley WB+, *Cutis* 52, 81 (observation)

Pruritus (<1%)
(1993): Litt JZ, Beachwood, OH (personal case) (observation)
(1990): Heckerling PS, *Ann Intern Med* 112, 879 (vulvovaginal)
(1987): Nugent LW+, *J Clin Pharmacol* 27, 461
(1986): Gavras H, *Clin Ther* 9, 24 (0.75%)

Psoriasis
(2003): Stavropoulos PG+, *Dermatology* 207(3), 336
(1993): Coulter DM+, *N Z Med J* 106, 392
(1990): Wolf R+, *Dermatologica* 181, 51

Purpura
(1989): Grosbois B+, *BMJ* 298, 189 (with quinidine)

Rash (sic) (1.4%)
(2000): Babadzhan VD+, *Lik Sprava* (Russian) Apr–Jun, (3–4), 54
(1986): DiBianco R, *Med Toxicol* 1, 122 (passim)
(1986): Irvin JD+, *Am J Med* 81, 46
(1984): Davies RO+, *Am J Med* 77, 23
(1984): McFate Smith W+, *J Hypertens* Suppl 2, S113

Stevens–Johnson syndrome (<1%)

Toxic epidermal necrolysis (<1%)

Toxic pustuloderma
(1996): Ferguson JE+, *Clin Exp Dermatol* 21, 54

Urticaria (<1%)
(1996): Pillans PI+, *Eur J Clin Pharmacol* 51, 123
(1993): Carrington PR+, *Cutis* 51, 121
(1988): Inman WH+, *BMJ* 297, 826
(1988): Slater EE+, *JAMA* 260, 967
(1987): Wood SM+, *BMJ* 294, 91

Vasculitis (<1%)
(1993): Carrington PR+, *Cutis* 51, 121
(1991): Ayani I+, *Med Clin* (Barc) (Spanish) 95, 596

Mucosal/ENT

Ageusia
(1988): Rumboldt Z+, *Int J Clin Pharmacol Res* 8(3), 181
(1984): Davies RO+, *Am J Med* 77, 23
(1984): Gutierrez Fuentes JA+, *Rev Clin Esp* 172(3), 149
(1984): McFate Smith W+, *J Hypertens* Suppl 2, S113

Anosmia (<1%)

Burning mouth syndrome
(1992): Savino LB+, *Ann Pharmacother* 26(11), 1381

Dysgeusia (1–10%)
(2004): Unnikrishnan D+, *J Am Med Dir Assoc* 5(2), 107
(2000): Zervakis J+, *Physiol Behav* 68, 405
(1989): Perronne C+, *Therapie* 44(1), 67
(1988): Schilling H+, *Z Kardiol* (German) 77 (Suppl 3), 47
(1986): DiBianco R, *Med Toxicol* 1, 122
(1986): Irvin JD+, *Am J Med* 81, 46
(1984): Davies RO+, *Am J Med* 77, 23

Glossitis (<1%)

Glossopyrosis
(1989): Drucker CR+, *Arch Dermatol* 125, 1437

Oral bleeding
(1984): Kubo SH+, *Ann Intern Med* 100, 616

Oral burn
(1982): Vlasses PH+, *BMJ* 284, 1672

Oral lesions (<0.5%)
(1986): Gavras H, *Clin Ther* 9, 24 (0.37%)
(1986): Todd PA+, *Drugs* 31, 198 (0.5%)
(1985): Gomez HJ+, *Drugs* 30 (Suppl 1), 13
(1984): Kubo SH+, *Ann Intern Med* 100, 616

Oral mucosal lichenoid eruption
(1989): Firth NA+, *Oral Surg Oral Med Oral Pathol* 67, 41

Oral ulceration
(2000): Madinier I+, *Ann Med Interne* (Paris) 151, 248
(1982): Viraben R+, *Arch Dermatol* 118, 959

Stomatitis (<1%)

Tinnitus

Tongue edema
(1996): Litt JZ, Beachwood, OH (personal case) (observation)
(1990): Zech J+, *HNO* (German) 38, 143
(1986): Marichal JF+, *Therapie* (French) 41, 517

Xerostomia (<1%)

Hair

Hair – alopecia (<1%)
(1991): Ahmad S, *Arch Intern Med* 151, 404

Nails

Nails – dystrophy
(1986): Gupta S+, *BMJ* 293, 140

Nails – subungual hyperkeratosis
(2006): Antonov D+, *Skinmed* 5(2), 90

Other

Anaphylactoid reactions/Anaphylaxis (<1%)
(1989): Todd PA+, *Drugs* 37, 141

Cough (8–23%)
(2007): Tumanan-Mendoza BA+, *J Clin Epidemiol* 60(6), 547
(2006): Cicolin A+, *Mayo Clin Proc* 81(1), 53
(2005): Ko GT+, *Adv Ther* 22(2), 155 (35%)
(2004): Chen JH+, *Int J Clin Pract Suppl* 156(145), 29 (18%)
(2004): Tomlinson B+, *Clin Ther* 26(8), 1292 (32%)
(2002): Amerena J+, *J Int Med Res* 30(6), 543 (8.9%) (with telmisartan)
(2002): Chowta KN+, *J Assoc Physicians India* 50, 1236 (30%)
(2002): Coca A+, *Clin Ther* 24(1), 126
(2002): Cuspidi C+, *J Hypertens* 20(11), 2293
(2001): Adigun AQ+, *West Afr J Med* 20(1), 46
(2001): Breeze E+, *J Hum Hypertens* 15(12), 857
(2001): Dunselman PH+, *Int J Cardiol* 77(2–3), 131
(2001): Gryglas P, *Pol Arch Med Wewn* 105(2), 109
(2001): Lee SC+, *Hypertension* 38(2), 166
(2001): Rake EC+, *J Hum Hypertens* 15(12), 863 (23%)
(2001): Ruilope L+, *Blood Press* 10(4), 223
(2000): Babadzhan VD+, *Lik Sprava* (Russian) Apr–Jun, (3–4), 54
(2000): Chiou KR+, *Zhonghua Yi Xue Za Zhi* (Taipei) 63(5), 368
(2000): Lacourciere Y+, *Kidney Int* 58(2), 762
(2000): Taseva T, *Vutr Boles* 32(2), 27
(1998): Sabir M+, *J Assoc Physicians India* 46(4), 355
(1998): Singh NP+, *J Assoc Physicians India* 46(5), 448

(1992): Aggarwal P+, *J Emerg Med* 10(6), 689
(1992): Kaufman J+, *Chest* 101(4), 922
(1992): Reisin L+, *Am J Cardiol* 70(3), 398
(1991): Kaku T+, *Nippon Ronen Igakkai Zasshi* 28(3), 365
(1991): Katsumata U+, *Tohoku J Exp Med* 164(2), 103
(1991): Yeo WW+, *Q J Med* 80(293), 763
(1990): Nuss DW+, *Ear Nose Throat J* 69(9), 649
(1988): Rumboldt Z+, *Int J Clin Pharmacol Res* 8(3), 181
Death
  (2007): Cupido C+, *S Afr Med J* 97(4), 244
  (2001): Gonzalez de la Puente MA+, *Ann Pharmacother* 35(11), 1492
Gynecomastia
  (1994): Llop R+, *Ann Pharmacother* 28, 671
Headache
Inappropriate secretion of antidiuretic hormone (SIADH)
  (2002): Izzedine H+, *Clin Pharmacol Ther* 71(6), 503
  (1993): Castrillon JL+, *J Intern Med* 233(1), 89
Myalgia/Myositis/Myopathy/Myotoxicity (<1%)
Paresthesias (<1%)
Pseudopolymyalgia
  (1989): Leloët X+, *BMJ* 298, 325
  (1986): Furness PN+, *J Clin Pathol* 39, 902
Stroke
  (2006): Sandstrom H, *Lakartidningen* 103(8), 564

ENFLURANE

Trade names: Alyrane; Efrane; Ethrane (Baxter); Etrane
Indications: Maintenance of general anesthesia
Category: Anesthetic, inhalation
Half-life: N/A
Clinically important, potentially hazardous interactions with: cisatracurium, doxacurium, pancuronium, rapacuronium

Reactions

Skin
Jaundice
Shivering
  (1981): Lindgren L, *Br J Anaesth* 53(5), 537

Other
Anaphylactoid reactions/Anaphylaxis
  (1988): Ganzuka A+, *Masui* 37(11), 1382
Death
  (1998): Asai K+, *Eur J Pediatr* 157(2), 169
  (1995): Schneider M, *Anaesth Intensive Care* 23(2), 225
  (1987): Paull JD+, *Anaesthesia* 42(11), 1191
Headache
  (1998): van den Berg AA+, *Acta Anaesthesiol Scand* 42(6), 658
  (1980): Ng AT, *Can Anaesth Soc* 27(5), 502
Hypotension
  (1986): Sorensen O+, *Acta Anaesthesiol Scand* 30(8), 630
Myalgia/Myositis/Myopathy/Myotoxicity
Rhabdomyolysis
  (1987): Lee SC+, *J Oral Maxillofac Surg* 45(9), 789 (with succinylcholine)
  (1987): Lee SC+, *Ma Zui Xue Za Zhi* 25(2), 97
Seizures
  (2003): Reuther LO+, *Ugeskr Laeger* 165(14), 1447
  (1994): Vohra SB, *Can J Anaesth* 41(5 Pt 1), 420
  (1992): Khan AA+, *J Pak Med Assoc* 42(2), 46
  (1992): Parke TJ+, *Anaesthesia* 47(1), 79
  (1989): Christys AR+, *Br J Anaesth* 62(6), 624
  (1988): Helmy ES+, *J Oral Maxillofac Surg* 46(1), 52

(1987): Fahy LT, *Anaesthesia* 42(12), 1327
(1986): Grant IS, *Anaesthesia* 41(10), 1024
(1986): Nicoll JM, *Anaesthesia* 41(9), 927
(1984): *Anaesthesia* 39(6), 605
(1984): DeWolf AM+, *Anesth Prog* 31(3), 136
(1984): Jenkins J+, *Anaesthesia* 39(1), 44
(1984): Yazji NS+, *Anaesthesia* 39(12), 1249
(1982): Sprague DH+, *Anesth Analg* 61(1), 67 (with amitriptyline)
(1981): Wolf S, *Can Anaesth Soc J* 28(2), 185

ENFUVIRTIDE

Trade names: Fuzeon (Roche); T-20
Indications: HIV-1 Infection (in combination with other antiretroviral agents)
Category: Antiretroviral; HIV cell fusion inhibitor
Half-life: 3.8 hours
Clinically important, potentially hazardous interactions with: None

Reactions

Skin
Allergic reactions (sic)
  (2005): Hayashi T, *Nippon Rinsho* 63(1), 173
Edema
  (2004): Church JA+, *Pediatr Infect Dis J* 23(8), 713
Exanthems
Folliculitis (2%)
Herpes simplex (5%)
Papillomas (4.2%)
Pruritus (62%)
Rash (sic)

Mucosal/ENT
Dysgeusia (2.4%)
Sinusitis (6.2%)

Eyes
Conjunctivitis (2.4%)

Other
Abdominal pain (3%)
Asthenia (16.1%)
  (2005): Trottier B+, *J Acquir Immune Defic Syndr* 40(4), 413
Chills
Cough (7.4%)
Depression (8.65)
Fever
Hypersensitivity (<1%)
  (2005): Shahar E+, *AIDS* 19(4), 451
  (2004): Beilke MA, *Scand J Infect Dis* 36(10), 778
  (2004): DeSimone JA+, *Clin Infect Dis* 39(10), e110
Infections
  (2005): Trottier B+, *J Acquir Immune Defic Syndr* 40(4), 413
  (2004): Jamjian MC+, *Am J Health Syst Pharm* 61(12), 1242
  (2003): Dando TM+, *Drugs* 63(24), 2755
Injection-site erythema (89%)
Injection-site granuloma
  (2003): Ball RA+, *J Am Acad Dermatol* 49(5), 826
Injection-site induration (89%)
Injection-site nodules (76%)
  (2004): Church JA+, *Pediatr Infect Dis J* 23(8), 713
  (2004): Maggi P+, *J Antimicrob Chemother* 53(4), 678
Injection-site pain (95%)

Injection-site pruritus
Injection-site reactions (sic) (98%)
  (2007): Agampodi SB+, *Indian J Med Sci* 61(4), 192
  (2007): Loutfy MR+, *HIV Clin Trials* 8(1), 36
  (2007): Luther J+, *Am J Clin Dermatol* 8(4), 221
  (2005): Espona M+, *Farm Hosp* 29(6), 375
  (2005): Hayashi T, *Nippon Rinsho* 63(1), 173
  (2005): Kapic E+, *Med Arh* 59(5), 313
  (2005): Trottier B+, *J Acquir Immune Defic Syndr* 40(4), 413
    (98%)
  (2004): Church JA+, *Pediatr Infect Dis J* 23(8), 713
  (2004): Foy K+, *J Assoc Nurses AIDS Care* 15(6), 65
  (2004): Jamjian MC+, *Am J Health Syst Pharm* 61(12), 1242
    (98%)
  (2004): Raffi F, *Med Mal Infect* 34 Spec No 1, 8
  (2003): Ball RA+, *J Am Acad Dermatol* 49(5), 826
  (2003): Dando TM+, *Drugs* 63(24), 2755
  (2003): Duffalo ML+, *Ann Pharmacother* 37(10), 1448
  (2003): Koopmans PP, *Ned Tijdschr Geneeskd* 147(36), 1726
  (2003): Lalezari JP+, *AIDS* 17(5), 691
  (2003): Lalezari JP+, *Antivir Ther* 8(4), 279 (68.5%)
  (2003): Lalezari JP+, *N Engl J Med* 348(22), 2175 (98%)
  (2002): Chen RY+, *Expert Opin Investig Drugs* 11(12), 1837
  (2002): Kilby JM+, *AIDS Res Hum Retroviruses* 18(10), 685
Injection-site scleroderma
  (2004): Maggi P+, *J Antimicrob Chemother* 53(4), 678
Injection-site urticaria
  (2004): Maggi P+, *J Antimicrob Chemother* 53(4), 678
Injection-site vasculitis
  (2004): Maggi P+, *J Antimicrob Chemother* 53(4), 678
Myalgia/Myositis/Myopathy/Myotoxicity (5%)
Paresthesias
Vertigo

ENOXACIN

Trade names: Bactidan; Comprecin; Enoxacine; Enoxen; Enoxor; Gyramid; Penetrex (Sanofi-Aventis)
Indications: Urinary tract infections
Category: Antibiotic, quinolone
Half-life: 3–6 hours
Clinically important, potentially hazardous interactions with: amiodarone, arsenic, bepridil, bretylium, disopyramide, duloxetine, erythromycin, fenbufen, phenothiazines, procainamide, quinidine, sotalol, tricyclic antidepressants

Reactions

Skin
Diaphoresis (<1%)
Edema (<1%)
Erythema multiforme (<1%)
Erythema nodosum
Exanthems (0.5%)
  (1988): Henwood JM+, *Drugs* 32, 32 (0.57%)
Exfoliative dermatitis (<1%)
Photosensitivity (<1%)
  (1993): Kang JS+, *Photodermatol Photoimmunol Photomed* 9, 159
  (1992): Izu R+, *Photodermatol Photoimmunol Photomed* 9, 86
  (1990): Schauder S, *Z Hautkr* (German) 65, 253
  (1989): Kawabe Y+, *Photodermatology* 6, 57
  (1988): Henwood JM+, *Drugs* 32, 32 (0.57%)
Phototoxicity
  (2003): Dawe RS+, *Br J Dermatol* 149(6), 1232
  (1998): Martinez LJ+, *Photochem Photobiol* 67, 399

  (1994): Fujita H+, *Photodermatol Photoimmunol Photomed* 10, 202
  (1990): Przybilla B+, *Dermatologica* 181, 98
  (1990): Schauder S, *Z Hautkr* (German) 65, 253
Pigmentation
  (2003): Dawe RS+, *Br J Dermatol* 149(6), 1232
Pruritus (<1%)
Purpura (<1%)
Rash (sic) (<1%)
Stevens–Johnson syndrome (<1%)
Toxic epidermal necrolysis (<1%)
Urticaria (<1%)
  (1988): Henwood JM+, *Drugs* 32, 32 (0.57%)

Mucosal/ENT
Dysgeusia
Stomatitis (<1%)
Tinnitus
Vaginitis (<1%)
Vulvovaginal candidiasis (<1%)
Xerostomia (<1%)

Eyes
Visual hallucinations
  (1986): Davies BI+, *Pharm Weekbl Sci* 8(1), 53

Other
Chills (<1%)
Hypersensitivity
Injection-site phlebitis
Insomnia
  (2006): Rafalsky V+, *Cochrane Database Syst Rev* 3
Myalgia/Myositis/Myopathy/Myotoxicity (<1%)
Paresthesias (<1%)
Rhabdomyolysis
  (1988): Morita H+, *Nippon Naika Gakkai Zasshi* 77(5), 744 (with fenbufen)
Tendinopathy/Tendon rupture (<1%)
Tremor (<1%)

ENOXAPARIN

Trade names: Clexan; Clexane 40; Klexane; Lovenox (Sanofi-Aventis)
Indications: Prevention of deep vein thrombosis
Category: Heparin, low molecular weight
Half-life: 4.5 hours
Clinically important, potentially hazardous interactions with: butabarbital, danaparoid

Reactions

Skin
Allergic reactions (sic)
  (2004): Tiu A+, *N Z Med J* 117(1204), U1126
Angioedema
  (1992): Odeh M+, *Lancet* 340, 972
Bullous pemphigoid
  (2004): Dyson SW+, *J Am Acad Dermatol* 51(1), 141
Eczema
  (2006): White JM+, *Contact Dermatitis* 54(1), 18 (3 cases)
Edema (3%)
Erythema (1–10%)
  (1993): Phillips JK+, *Br J Haematol* 85, 837
Erythema multiforme
  (2002): MacLaughlin EJ+, *Pharmacotherapy* 22(11), 1511

Exanthems
(2003): Kim KH+, *Cutis* 72(1), 57
(2002): MacLaughlin EJ+, *Pharmacotherapy* 22, 1511
(2001): Kim K & Lynfield Y, New York, NY (personal
communication)
Hematomas
(2005): Khan FY+, *Saudi Med J* 26(2), 336 (with rofecoxib)
(2004): Anton E+, *Age Ageing* 33(6), 641
(2000): Antonelli D+, *Am Surg* 66(8), 797 (2 cases)
Necrosis (<1%)
(2006): Nadir Y+, *Eur J Haematol* 77(2), 166
(2003): Scharf Y+, *Harefuah* 142(11), 742
(2002): Toll A+, *World Congress Dermatol* Poster, 0130
Peripheral edema (3%)
Pruritus
(2002): MacLaughlin EJ+, *Pharmacotherapy* 22, 1511
(2001): Kim K & Lynfield Y, New York, NY (personal
communication)
Purpura (1–10%)
Side effects (sic) (0.2%)
(2000): Enrique E+, *Contact Dermatitis* 42, 43
Urticaria
(1997): Downham TF, Taylor, MI (from Internet) (observation)
(1992): Odeh M+, *Lancet* 340, 972
Vesiculation (<1%)

Hair
Hair – alopecia
(2006): Wang YY+, *J Clin Pharm Ther* 31(5), 513

Other
Anaphylactoid reactions/Anaphylaxis (<1%)
(2002): MacLaughlin EJ 1, *Pharmacotherapy* 22(11), 1511
Cough
(2002): MacLaughlin EJ+, *Pharmacotherapy* 22(11), 1511
Death
(2006): Nadir Y+, *Eur J Haematol* 77(2), 166
Hypersensitivity
(2000): Romero Ortega MR+, *Aten Primaria* (Spanish) 25, 521
(1998): Cabanas R+, *J Investig Allergol Clin Immunol* 8, 383
(1998): Mendez J+, *Allergy* 53, 999
(1996): Koch P+, *Contact Dermatitis* 34, 156
(1996): Mendez J+, *Allergy* 51, 853
Injection-site erythema
(2001): Kim K & Lynfield Y, New York, NY (personal
communication)
Injection-site exanthems
(2000): Szolar-Platzer C+, *J Am Acad Dermatol* 43, 920
Injection-site hematoma
(2002): Robb DM+, *Pharmacotherapy* 22(9), 1105
Injection-site necrosis
(1997): Lefebvre I+, *Ann Dermatol Venereol* (French) 124, 397
(1997): Tonn ME+, *Ann Pharmacother* 31, 323
(1996): Fried M+, *Ann Intern Med* 125, 521
Injection-site pain
(2002): Robb DM+, *Pharmacotherapy* 22(9), 1105
Injection-site plaques
(1998): Mendez J+, *Allergy* 53, 999
(1998): Valdes F+, *Allergy* 53, 625
Injection-site pruritus
(2000): Szolar-Platzer C+, *J Am Acad Dermatol* 43, 920

ENTACAPONE

Trade names: Comtan (Novartis); Comtess
Indications: Parkinsonism
Category: Catechol-O-methyl transferase inhibitor
Half-life: 2.4 hours
**Clinically important, potentially hazardous interactions
with:** MAO inhibitors, phenelzine, rasagiline, tranylcypromine

Reactions

Skin
Bacterial infections (1%)
Bullous dermatitis
(2004): Foti C+, *Int J Dermatol* 43, 471
Diaphoresis (2%)
Purpura (2%)

Mucosal/ENT
Dysgeusia (1%)
Xerostomia (3%)

Eyes
Nystagmus
(2005): *Prescrire Int* 14(76), 51

Other
Abdominal pain
(2004): Gordin A+, *J Neural Transm* 111(10-11), 1343
Headache
Vertigo (20%)
(2003): Larsen JP+, *Eur J Neurol* 10(2), 137 (20%)

ENTECAVIR

Trade name: Baraclude (Bristol-Myers Squibb)
Indications: Chronic hepatitis B virus infection
Category: Antiviral; Guanosine nucleoside analog
Half-life: ~24 hours
**Clinically important, potentially hazardous interactions
with:** None

Reactions

Other
Asthenia (1%)
Headache (2%)
Vertigo (<1%)

EPHEDRA

Scientific names: *Ephedra equisetina; Ephedra intermedia; Ephedra sinica; Ephedra vulgaris*
Family: Gnetaceae
Trade and other common names: Joint Fir; Ma Huang; Popotillo; Sea Grape; Teamster's Tea; Yellow Astringent; Yellow Horse
Category: Ephedrine alkaloid; Stimulant
Purported indications and other uses: Bronchospasm, asthma, bronchitis, allergy, appetite suppressant, colds, flu, fever, chills, edema, headache, anhidrosis, diuretic, joint and bone pain
Half-life: N/A
Clinically important, potentially hazardous interactions with: acetazolamide, amitriptyline, **caffeine**, **cocoa**, corticosteroids, ephedrine, epinephrine, guanethidine, **guarana**, MAO inhibitors, olmesartan, phenelzine, phenylpropanolamine, selegiline, sibutramine, sodium bicarbonate

Reactions

Skin
Adverse effects (sic)
(2003): Bent S+, *Ann Intern Med* 138(6), 468
(2002): Arditti J+, *Acta Clin Belg* Suppl (1), 34 (slimming pills)
(2002): Haller CA+, *Adverse Drug React Toxicol Rev* 21(3), 143

Mucosal/ENT
Xerostomia
(2002): Boozer CN+, *Int J Obes Relat Metab Disord* 26(5), 593

Eyes
Vision impaired
(2006): Moawad FJ+, *South Med J* 99(5), 511 (transient)
Visual hallucinations
(2005): Maglione M+, *Am J Psychiatry* 162(1), 189

Other
Agitation
(2005): Maglione M+, *Am J Psychiatry* 162(1), 189
Death
(2005): Woolf AD+, *Clin Toxicol (Phila)* 43(5), 347
(2003): Charatan F, *BMJ* 326(7387), 464
(2003): Schulman S, *Public Health Rep* 118(6), 487
(2002): Arditti J+, *Acta Clin Belg* Suppl (1), 34 (slimming pills)
(2000): Haller CA+, *N Engl J Med* 343(25), 1833 (10 cases)
Depression
(2005): Maglione M+, *Am J Psychiatry* 162(1), 189
Hypersensitivity
Hypertension
(2000): Haller CA+, *N Engl J Med* 343(25), 1833 (17 cases)
Mania
(2005): Maglione M+, *Am J Psychiatry* 162(1), 189
Seizures
(2005): Haller CA+, *Clin Toxicol* (Phila) 43(1), 23
(2003): Schulman S, *Public Health Rep* 118(6), 487
(2002): Arditti J+, *Acta Clin Belg* Suppl (1), 34
(2002): van der Hooft CS+, *Ned Tijdschr Geneeskd* 146(28), 1335
(2001): Kockler DR+, *Pharmacotherapy* 21(5), 647 (with caffeine)
(2000): Haller CA+, *N Engl J Med* 343(25), 1833 (7 cases)
Side effects (sic)
(2002): Lawrence ME+, *J Clin Gastroenterol* 35(4), 299
Stroke
(2000): Haller CA+, *N Engl J Med* 343(25), 1833 (10 cases)
Suicidal ideation
(2005): Maglione M+, *Am J Psychiatry* 162(1), 189
Tremor

EPHEDRINE

Trade names: Ectasule; Efedron; Ephedsol; Marax; Pretz-D; Rynatuss (MedPointe); Vicks Vatronol (Procter & Gamble)
Indications: Nasal congestion, acute hypotensive states, asthma
Category: Adrenergic alpha-receptor agonist; Sympathomimetic
Half-life: 3–6 hours
Clinically important, potentially hazardous interactions with: antihypertensives, dexamethasone, **ephedra**, furazolidone, guanethidine, **guarana**, MAO inhibitors, methyldopa, phenelzine, phenylpropanolamine, selegiline, tranylcypromine, tricyclic antidepressants

Reactions

Skin
Bullous dermatitis
Dermatitis
(1993): Villas-Martinez F+, *Contact Dermatitis* 29, 215
(1991): Audicana M+, *Contact Dermatitis* 24, 223
Diaphoresis (1–10%)
Edema
Exanthems
Exfoliative dermatitis
(1981): Serup J, *Ugeskr Laeger* (Danish) 143, 1660
Fixed eruption
(2003): Matsumoto K+, *J Am Acad Dermatol* 48(4), 628
(2000): Tanimoto K+, *Masui* 49(12), 1374
(1997): Garcia Ortiz JC+, *Allergy* 52, 229
(1994): Krivda SJ+, *J Am Acad Dermatol* 31, 291 (non-pigmenting)
Pallor (1–10%)
Purpura
Toxic epidermal necrolysis
(2002): Yung A+, *Australas J Dermatol* 43(1), 35
Urticaria
Vasculitis

Mucosal/ENT
Xerostomia (1–10%)

Other
Death
(2003): Kanstrup MH+, *Ugeskr Laeger* 165(3), 239 (with caffeine)
Headache
Hypertension
(1993): Hopson JR+, *Herz* 18(3), 164
Myalgia/Myositis/Myopathy/Myotoxicity
(2002): Gonzalez Rodriguez JL+, *Rev Esp Anestesiol Reanim* 49(9), 501
Seizures
(2002): van der Hooft CS+, *Ned Tijdschr Geneeskd* 146(28), 1335
Tremor (1–10%)
(2002): Gonzalez Rodriguez JL+, *Rev Esp Anestesiol Reanim* 49(9), 501

EPINASTINE

Synonyms: Relastat; WAL-801-CL
Trade name: Elestat (Allergan)
Indications: Allergic conjunctivitis
Category: Histamine H1 receptor antagonist
Half-life: 12 hours
Clinically important, potentially hazardous interactions with: None

Reactions

Mucosal/ENT
Rhinitis (~10%)
Sinusitis (~10%)

Eyes
Ocular burning (1–10)
Ocular hemorrhage (1–10%)
Ocular pruritus (1–10%)

Other
Cough (1–3%)
Headache (~10%)
Upper respiratory infection (~10%)
  (2004): Abelson MB+, *Clin Ther* 26(1), 35

EPINEPHRINE

Synonym: adrenaline
Trade names: Adrenalin (Monarch); Adrenaline; Ana-Guard; AsthmaHaler; Bronitin; Bronkaid; Epi E-Z Pen; Epifrin; Epipen (DEY); Eppy; Eppystabil; Isopto-Epinal; MedihalerEpi; Primatene; Primatene Mist; S-2; Simplene
Indications: Cardiac arrest, hay fever, asthma, anaphylaxis
Category: Catecholamine; Sympathomimetic
Half-life: N/A
Duration of action: 1–4 hours
Clinically important, potentially hazardous interactions with: albuterol, alpha-blockers, amitriptyline, amoxapine, atenolol, beta-blockers, carteolol, chlorpromazine, clomipramine, cocaine, desipramine, doxepin, **ephedra**, ergotamine, furazolidone, halothane, imipramine, insulin detemir, MAO inhibitors, metoprolol, nadolol, nortriptyline, penbutolol, phenelzine, phenoxybenzamine, phenylephrine, pindolol, prazosin, propranolol, protriptyline, sympathomimetics, terbutaline, thioridazine, timolol, tranylcypromine, tricyclic antidepressants, trimipramine, vasopressors

Reactions

Skin
Dermatitis
  (1993): Gaspari AA, *Contact Dermatitis* 28, 35
  (1980): Romaguera C+, *Contact Dermatitis* 6, 364
Diaphoresis (1–10%)
Exanthems
Fixed eruption
Necrosis
  (1984): Antrum RM+, *Br J Clin Pract* 38, 191
Pallor (<1%)
Pemphigus (cicatricial)
  (1981): Vadot E+, *Bull Soc Ophtalmol Fr* (French) 81, 693
Urticaria

Mucosal/ENT
Xerostomia (<1%)

Hair
Hair – alopecia

Other
Chest pain
  (2006): Putland M+, *Ann Emerg Med* 47(6), 559
Headache
Hypotension
  (2006): Putland M+, *Ann Emerg Med* 47(6), 559
  (2006): Yang JJ+, *J Pharm Pharm Sci* 9(2), 190
Injection-site necrosis
Injection-site pain
Injection-site urticaria

EPIRUBICIN

Trade name: Ellence (Pfizer)
Indications: Adjuvant therapy in primary breast cancer
Category: Antibiotic, anthracycline
Half-life: 33 hours
Clinically important, potentially hazardous interactions with: amlodipine, bepridil, cimetidine, diltiazem, felodipine, isradipine, nicardipine, nifedipine, nimodipine, nisoldipine, verapamil

Reactions

Skin
Allergic reactions (sic)
  (1999). Ormrod D+, *Drugs Aging* 15, 389
Erythema
Erythroderma (0.7–5%)
Exfoliative dermatitis
Facial flushing
Photo-recall
  (1999): Wilson J+, *Clin Oncol (R Coll Radiol)* 11, 424
Photosensitivity
Pigmentation
Pruritus (9%)
Rash (sic) (1–9%)
Ulcerations
Urticaria
Vasculitis
  (2005): Nakazawa Y+, *Gan To Kagaku Ryoho* 32 suppl 1, 24

Mucosal/ENT
Mucositis
  (1999): Ormrod D+, *Drugs Aging* 15, 389
Oral ulceration
Stomatitis
  (2006): Pacilio C+, *Br J Cancer* 94(9), 1233
  (2005): Serin D+, *Br J Cancer* 92(11), 1989 (with vinorelbine)
  (1995): Fountzilas G+, *Med Pediatr Oncol* 24, 23
  (1991): Carmo-Pereira J+, *Cancer Chemother Pharmacol* 27, 394
    (35%)
  (1991): Fountzilas G+, *Tumori* 77, 232 (24%)
  (1986): Kimura K+, *Gan To Kagaku Ruoho* (Japanese) 13, 2440
    (12.5%)
  (1986): Sakata Y+, *Gan To Kagaku Ryoho* (Japanese) 13, 1887
  (1980): Bonfante V+, *Recent Results Cancer Res* 74, 192

Hair
Hair – alopecia (69–95%) (reversible)

(2005): Berruti A+, *Anticancer Res* 25(6C), 4475
(2002): Colozza M+, *Eur J Cancer* 38(17), 2279
(1999): Ormrod D+, *Drugs Aging* 15, 389
(1991): Carmo-Pereira J+, *Cancer Chemother Pharmacol* 27, 394 (95%)
(1991): Fountzilas G+, *Tumori* 77, 232 (81%)
(1986): Kimura K+, *Gan To Kagaku Ryoho* (Japanese) 13, 2440 (71.4%)
(1986): Sakata Y+, *Gan To Kagaku Ryoho* (Japanese) 13, 1887
(1986): Tominaga T+, *Gan To Kagaku Ryoho* (Japanese) 13, 2187 (66.7%)
(1985): Holdener EE+, *Invest New Drugs* 3, 63 (54%)
(1984): Lopez M+, *Invest New Drugs* 2, 315
(1984): Schutte J+, *J Cancer Res Clin Oncol* 107, 38 (88%)
(1980): Bonfante V+, *Recent Results Cancer Res* 74, 192

Nails
Nails – pigmentation

Other
Anaphylactoid reactions/Anaphylaxis
Asthenia (6%)
  (2004): Morales S+, *Cancer Chemother Pharmacol* 53(1), 75 (6%)
Hot flashes (5–39%)
Hypersensitivity
Injection-site extravasation
  (1999): Fleming A+, *J Hand Surg [Br]* 24, 390
Injection-site inflammation
Injection-site necrosis
Injection-site reactions (sic) (3–20%)
Injection-site ulceration
Myalgia/Myositis/Myopathy/Myotoxicity (55%)
  (1995): Fountzilas G+, *Med Pediatr Oncol* 24, 23 (55%)
Phlebitis
Sjøgren's (Sicca) syndrome
  (1986): Oxholm A+, *Lancet* 2(8507), 629

EPLERENONE

Trade name: Inspra (Pfizer)
Indications: Hypertension
Category: Aldosterone antagonist; Diuretic
Half-life: 4–6 hours
Clinically important, potentially hazardous interactions with: ACE inhibitors, angiotensin ii receptor antagonists, erythromycin, fluconazole, **grapefruit juice**, itraconazole, ketoconazole, saquinavir, **St John's wort**, verapamil

Reactions

Other
Asthenia (2%)
Cough (2%)
Gynecomastia (males <1%)
Headache
Vertigo (3%)

EPOETIN ALFA

Synonyms: erythropoietin; EPO
Trade names: Epogen (Amgen); Epoxitin; Eprex; Erypo; Procrit (Ortho)
Indications: Anemia
Category: Erythropoietin
Half-life: 4–13 hours (in patients with chronic renal failure)

Reactions

Skin
Acne
  (1989): Faulds D+, *Drugs* 38, 863
Angioedema (1–5%)
Dermatitis
  (1993): Hardwick N+, *Contact Dermatitis* 28, 123
Edema (17%)
Erythroderma
  (2005): Wolf IH+, *J Cutan Pathol* 32(5), 371
Exanthems
  (1990): Schröder-Kolb B, *Derm Beruf Umwelt* (German) 38, 12 (papular)
Lichenoid eruption
  (1997): Puritz E, Smithtown, NY (from Internet) (observation)
Photosensitivity
  (1992): Harvey E+, *J Pediatr* 121, 749
Pruritus
  (1990): Schröder-Kolb B, *Derm Beruf Umwelt* (German) 38, 12 (papular)
  (1989): Faulds D+, *Drugs* 38, 863
Rash (sic) (1–10%)
  (2005): Norgard N+, *Am J Health Syst Pharm* 62(23), 2524
Urticaria

Hair
Hair – alopecia
  (2001): Reddy V+, *Nephrol Dial Transplant* 16(7), 1525
Hair – alopecia totalis
  (2001): Reddy V+, *Nephrol Dial Transplant* 16(7), 1525
Hair – hypertrichosis
  (1991): Kleiner MJ+, *Am J Kidney Dis* 18, 689

Other
Anaphylactoid reactions/Anaphylaxis
Headache
Hypersensitivity (<1%)
Injection-site pain
  (1998): Veys N+, *Clin Nephrol* 49, 41
Injection-site reactions (sic) (7%)
Injection-site thrombophlebitis
Injection-site ulceration
  (1997): Siegel DM, New York, NY (from Internet) (observation)
Myalgia/Myositis/Myopathy/Myotoxicity
Paresthesias (11%)
Porphyria cutanea tarda
  (1992): Harvey E+, *J Pediatr* 121, 749

EPOPROSTENOL

Trade name: Flolan (GSK) (Gilead)
Indications: Pulmonary Arterial Hypertension
Category: Peripheral vasodilator
Half-life: 6 minutes
**Clinically important, potentially hazardous interactions
with:** anticoagulants, antihypertensives, diuretics, vasodilators

Reactions

Skin
 Diaphoresis (41%)
 Eczema (sic)
 Edema
 Pruritus (4%)
 Rash (sic) (10%)
  (2004): Myers SA+, *J Am Acad Dermatol* 51(1), 98
 Urticaria

Other
 Abdominal pain (14%)
  (1982): Pickles H+, *Br J Clin Pharmacol* 14(2), 177
 Agitation (11%)
 Anxiety (21%)
  (1981): Data JL+, *Circulation* 64(1), 4
 Cardiac failure (31%)
 Chest pain (11%)
  (1982): Pickles H+, *Br J Clin Pharmacol* 14(2), 177
 Chills (25%)
 Fever (25%)
 Headache (83%)
  (2008): Wienecke T+, *Pain*
  (2004): Myers SA+, *J Am Acad Dermatol* 51(1), 98
  (1982): Hassan S+, *Br J Clin Pharmacol* 14(3), 369
  (1982): Pickles H+, *Br J Clin Pharmacol* 14(2), 177
  (1981): Data JL+, *Circulation* 64(1), 4
 Hypotension (16%)
  (1982): Pickles H+, *Br J Clin Pharmacol* 14(2), 177
 Injection-site erythema
  (1982): Pickles H+, *Br J Clin Pharmacol* 14(2), 177
 Injection-site infection (21%)
 Injection-site pain (13%)
 Insomnia (9%)
 Myalgia/Myositis/Myopathy/Myotoxicity (44%)
  (2004): Myers SA+, *J Am Acad Dermatol* 51(1), 98
 Paresthesias (12%)
 Seizures (4%)
 Sepsis (25%)
  (2000): Badesch DB+, *Ann Intern Med* 132(6), 425
 Somnolence (4%)
  (1982): Pickles H+, *Br J Clin Pharmacol* 14(2), 177
 Thrombosis
 Tremor (21%)
 Vertigo
 Weight loss (27%)

EPROSARTAN

Trade name: Teveten (Biovail)
Indications: Hypertension
Category: Angiotensin II receptor antagonist
Half-life: 5–9 hours

Reactions

Skin
 Angioedema
 Diaphoresis (<1%)
 Eczema (<1%)
 Exanthems (<1%)
 Facial edema (<1%)
 Furunculosis (<1%)
 Herpes simplex (<1%)
 Peripheral edema (<1%)
 Pruritus (<1%)
 Purpura (<1%)
 Rash (sic) (<1%)

Mucosal/ENT
 Burning mouth syndrome
  (2002): Castells X+, *BMJ* 325(7375), 1277
 Dysgeusia
  (2004): Chen C+, *Nephrologie* 25(3), 97
  (2002): Castells X+, *BMJ* 325(7375), 1277
 Gingivitis (<1%)
 Xerostomia (<1%)

Other
 Cough (5%)
  (2001): Breeze E+, *J Hum Hypertens* 15(12), 857
  (2001): Rake EC+, *J Hum Hypertens* 15(12), 863 (5%)
 Headache
  (2002): Bohm M+, *Drug Saf* 25(8), 599 (with
   hydrochlorothiazide)
 Hot flashes (<1%)
 Myalgia/Myositis/Myopathy/Myotoxicity
  (2002): Bohm M+, *Drug Saf* 25(8), 599 (with
   hydrochlorothiazide)
 Paresthesias (<1%)
 Tendinopathy/Tendon rupture (<1%)
 Tremor (<1%)
 Upper respiratory infection
  (2002): Bohm M+, *Drug Saf* 25(8), 599 (with
   hydrochlorothiazide)
  (2001): Levine B, *Curr Med Res Opin* 17(1), 8
 Vertigo
  (2002): Bohm M+, *Drug Saf* 25(8), 599 (with
   hydrochlorothiazide)

EPTIFIBATIDE

Trade name: Integrilin (Millennium) (Schering)
Indications: Acute coronary syndrome, unstable angina
Category: Antiplatelet; Glycoprotein IIb / IIIa inhibitor
Half-life: 2.5 hours
**Clinically important, potentially hazardous interactions
with:** fondaparinux

Reactions

Other
 Anaphylactoid reactions/Anaphylaxis (<1%)
 Hypotension
  (2003): Rezkalla SH+, *Catheter Cardiovasc Interv* 58(1), 76
 Injection-site reactions (sic)

ERDOSTEINE

Trade name: Erdotin (Galen Ltd)
Indications: Chronic obstructive pulmonary disease (COPD)
Category: Mucolytic
Half-life: N/A
Clinically important, potentially hazardous interactions with: N/A

Reactions

Skin
Eczema
Erythema
Facial flushing
Urticaria

Mucosal/ENT
Dysgeusia
(1995): Marchioni CF+, *Int J Clin Pharmacol Ther* 33(11), 612

Other
Abdominal pain
Headache

ERGOCALCIFEROL

Synonyms: viosterol; vitamin D_2
Trade names: Drisdol (Sanofi-Aventis); Kalciferol; Ostoforte; Radiostol Forte; Sterogyl-15; Vigantol; Vitaminol
Indications: Rickets, hypoparathyroidism
Category: Vitamin
Half-life: 19–48 hours

Reactions

Skin
Allergic granulomatous angiitis (Churg–Strauss syndrome) (perforating)
(1982): Aliaga A+, *Dermatologica* 164, 62
Pruritus (1–10%)

Mucosal/ENT
Dysgeusia (1–10%) (metallic taste)
Xerostomia

Other
Myalgia/Myositis/Myopathy/Myotoxicity

ERLOTINIB

Trade name: Tarceva (Genentech) (Roche)
Indications: Non-small cell lung cancer
Category: Tyrosine kinase inhibitor
Half-life: ~36 hours
Clinically important, potentially hazardous interactions with: atazanavir, carbamazepine, clarithromycin, itraconazole, ketoconazole, nefazodone, nelfinavir, phenobarbital, phenytoin, rifabutin, rifampin, rifapentine, ritonavir, saquinavir, **St John's wort**, troleandomycin, voriconazole, warfarin

Reactions

Skin
Acne
(2008): Kardaun SH+, *Clin Exp Dermatol* 33(1), 46
(2007): Alexandrescu DT+, *Clin Exp Dermatol* 32(1), 71
(2007): Jackman DM+, *J Clin Oncol* 25(7), 760 (79%)
(2006): Journagan S+, *J Am Acad Dermatol* 54(2), 358
(2006): Roe E+, *J Am Acad Dermatol* 55(3), 429
(2005): Martinez de Lagran Z+, *Actas Dermosifiliogr* 96(7), 450
Acute generalized exanthematous pustulosis
(2006): Mitchell D+ (Thomasville, GA) (observation) (from Internet)
(2006): Román Peréz-Soler, L, *Department of Oncology, Montefiore Medical Center* (Bronx, NY)
Erythema (18%)
Fissures
(2006): Roe E+, *J Am Acad Dermatol* 55(3), 429
Follicular pustular eruption
(2006): Roe E+, *J Am Acad Dermatol* 55(3), 429
Folliculitis
(2006): Cuetara MS+, *Br J Dermatol* 155(2), 477
(2006): Gerdes S+, *J Dtsch Dermatol* 4(10), 855
(2006): Roe E+, *J Am Acad Dermatol* 55(3), 429
Papulopustular eruption
(2008): Lubbe J+, *Dermatology* 216(3), 247
(2007): Bragg J+, *Dermatol Online J* 13(1), 1
Photosensitivity
(2007): Luu M+, *Photodermatol Photoimmunol Photomed* 23(1), 42
Pruritus (13%)
(2006): Roe E+, *J Am Acad Dermatol* 55(3), 429
Rash (sic) (75%)
(2008): Tan AR+, *Ann Oncol* 19(1), 185
(2007): Dragovich T+, *Cancer Chemother Pharmacol* 60(2), 295 (with gemcitabine)
(2007): Gatzemeier U+, *J Clin Oncol* 25(12), 1545
(2007): Lacouture ME+, *J Clin Oncol* 25(15), 2140
(2006): *Prescrire Int* 15(83), 86
(2006): Lu JF+, *Clin Pharmacol Ther* 80(2), 136
(2006): Mitra SS+, *J Clin Oncol* 24(16), e28
(2006): Philip PA+, *J Clin Oncol* 24(19), 3069
(2006): Roe E+, *J Am Acad Dermatol* 55(3), 429
(2006): Tang PA+, *Expert Opin Pharmacother* 7(2), 177
(2006): Townsley CA+, *Br J Cancer* 94(8), 1136
(2005): *Med Lett Drugs* 47(1205), 25
(2005): Herbst RS+, *J Clin Oncol* 23(11), 2544 (with bevacizumab)
(2005): Iannitti D+, *Am J Clin Oncol* 28(6), 570
(2005): Rhee J+, *Clin Colorectal Cancer* 5 suppl 2, S101
(2004): Messersmith WA+, *Clin Cancer Res* 10(19), 6522
(2004): Perez-Soler+, *J Clin Oncol* 22(16), 3238
(2004): Soulieres D+, *J Clin Oncol* 22(1), 77
(2003): Bonomi P, *Expert Opin Investig Drugs* 12(8), 1395
(2003): Bonomi P, *Lung Cancer* 41 Suppl 1, S43
(2003): Perez-Soler R, *Oncology (Williston Park)* 17(11 Suppl 12), 23
(2003): Soulieres D, *Oncology (Williston Park)* 17(11 Suppl 12), 29
Skin reactions (sic)
(2006): Zoller A+, *Br J Dermatol* 155(6), 1293
Telangiectasia
(2006): Roe E+, *J Am Acad Dermatol* 55(3), 429
Xerosis (12%)
(2008): Lubbe J+, *Dermatology* 216(3), 247 (generalized)
(2006): Roe E+, *J Am Acad Dermatol* 55(3), 429

Mucosal/ENT
Aphthous stomatitis
(2006): Roe E+, *J Am Acad Dermatol* 55(3), 429

Oral ulceration
(2006): Roe E+, J Am Acad Dermatol 55(3), 429
Stomatitis (17%)

Hair

Hair – alopecia
(2007): Costa DB+, J Thorac Oncol 2(12), 1136
(2006): Roe E+, J Am Acad Dermatol 55(3), 429
Hair – changes (sic)
(2008): Gerber PA+, N Engl J Med 358(11), 1175

Nails

Nails – paronychia
(2006): Roe E+, J Am Acad Dermatol 55(3), 429
Nails – pyogenic granulomas (passim)
(2008): Lubbe J+, Dermatology 216(3), 247

Eyes

Conjunctivitis (12%)
(2007): Methvin AB+, Ophthal Plast Reconstr Surg 23(1), 63
(2006): Prescrire Int 15(83), 86 (12%)
Ectropion
(2007): Methvin AB+, Ophthal Plast Reconstr Surg 23(1), 63
Epiphora
(2007): Methvin AB+, Ophthal Plast Reconstr Surg 23(1), 63
Eyelashes – hypertrichosis
(2006): Roe E+, J Am Acad Dermatol 55(3), 429
Keratoconjunctivitis
Periorbital rash
(2007): Methvin AB+, Ophthal Plast Reconstr Surg 23(1), 63
Trichomegaly
(2007): Lane K+, Ophthal Plast Reconstr Surg 23(1), 65
(2006): Carser JF+, J Thorac Oncol 1(9), 1040

Other

Abdominal pain (11%)
Asthenia (52%)
Cough (33%)
Death
Hepatotoxicity
(2007): Ramanarayanan J+, JOP 8(1), 39
Infections (24%)

ERTAPENEM

Synonyms: L-749,345; MK-0826
Trade name: Invanz (Merck)
Indications: Severe resistant bacterial infections caused by susceptible organisms
Category: Antibiotic, beta-lactam
Half-life: 4 hours
Clinically important, potentially hazardous interactions with: probenecid

Reactions

Skin

Dermatitis (>1%)
Desquamation (>1%)
Diaphoresis (>1%)
Edema (3%)
Erythema (1–2%)
Facial edema (>1%)
Facial flushing
Hematomas (<1%)
Necrosis (<1%)

Pruritus (1–2%)
Rash (sic) (2–3%)
Urticaria (>1%)

Mucosal/ENT

Dysgeusia (>1%)
Oral candidiasis (0.1%)
Oral ulceration (>1%)
Stomatitis (>1%)
Vaginal pruritus (>1%)
Vaginitis (1–3%)
Vulvovaginal candidiasis (>1%)

Other

Anaphylactoid reactions/Anaphylaxis (some fatal)
Candidiasis (>1%)
Chills (>1%)
Cough (1–2%)
Death (2.5%)
Depression (>1%)
Headache
Hypersensitivity
Injection-site extravasation (0.7–2%)
Injection-site induration (>1%)
Injection-site pain (>1%)
(2002): Legua P+, Clin Ther 24(3), 434
Pain (>1%)
Paresthesias (>1%)
Phlebitis (1.5–2%)
Seizures (0.5%)
(2005): Seto AH+, Ann Pharmacother 39(2), 352
Thrombophlebitis (1.5–2%)
Tremor (>1%)

ERYTHROMYCIN

Trade names: E-Mycin; E.E.S; Eramycin; Ery-Ped; Ery-Tab; Eryc (Warner Chilcott); Erypar; Erythrocin; Eryzole; Ilosone; Ilotycin; PCE (Abbott); Pediazole (Abbott); Robimycin; Wintrocin; Wyamicin S
Indications: Various infections caused by susceptible organisms
Category: Antibiotic, macrolide
Half-life: 1.4–2 hours
Clinically important, potentially hazardous interactions with: alfentanil, aminophylline, amisulpride, amoxicillin, ampicillin, anticonvulsants, astemizole, atorvastatin, benzodiazepines, bromocriptine, buprenorphine, bupropion, carbamazepine, cilostazol, ciprofloxacin, cisapride, clindamycin, colchicine, cyclosporine, dasatinib, digoxin, dihydroergotamine, diltiazem, disopyramide, enoxacin, eplerenone, ergotamine, eszopiclone, everolimus, fluconazole, fluoxetine, fluvastatin, gatifloxacin, HMG-CoA reductase inhibitors, imatinib, itraconazole, ketoconazole, lomefloxacin, lorazepam, lovastatin, methadone, methylprednisolone, methysergide, midazolam, moxifloxacin, nitrazepam, norfloxacin, ofloxacin, paroxetine, pimozide, pravastatin, quinolones, ranolazine, repaglinide, sertraline, sildenafil, simvastatin, sparfloxacin, tacrolimus, terfenadine, theophylline, triazolam, troleandomycin, vardenafil, verapamil, vinblastine, warfarin, zaleplon, zolpidem

Note: Eryzole and Pediazole are combinations of erythromycin and sulfisoxazole

Reactions

Skin

Acne

Acute generalized exanthematous pustulosis (AGEP)
  (1995): Moreau A+, *Int J Dermatol* 34, 263 (passim)
  (1991): Roujeau J-C+, *Arch Dermatol* 127, 1333

Allergic reactions (sic) (<2%)
  (1986): Bigby M+, *JAMA* 256, 3358 (2.04%)

Baboon syndrome
  (1997): Goossens C+, *Dermatology* 194, 421

Dermatitis (systemic)
  (1996): Valsecchi R+, *Contact Dermatitis* 34, 428
  (1995): Martins C+, *Contact Dermatitis* 33, 360
  (1994): Fernandez Redondo V+, *Contact Dermatitis* 30, 311
  (1994): Fernandez Redondo V+, *Contact Dermatitis* 30, 43

Eczema

Erythema multiforme
  (1985): Ting HC+, *Int J Dermatol* 24, 587

Exanthems (1–5%)
  (1995): Litt JZ, Beachwood, OH (personal case) (observation)
  (1991): Igea JM+, *Ann Allergy* 66, 216
  (1989): Pendleton N+, *Br J Clin Prac* 43, 464

Fixed eruption
  (1998): Mahboob A+, *Int J Dermatol* 37, 833
  (1991): Florido-Lopez JF+, *Allergy* 46, 77
  (1991): Mutalik S, *Int J Dermatol* 30, 751
  (1986): Kanwar AJ+, *Dermatologica* 172, 315
  (1984): Pigatto PD, *Acta Derm Venereol (Stockh)* 64, 272

Jarisch–Herxheimer reaction
  (1983): Perine PL+, *Am J Trop Med Hyg* 32(5), 1096

Pruritus

Pustules
  (1993): Manu Shah R+, *Eur J Dermatol* 3, 576

Rash (sic) (<1%)
  (1992): Shirin H+, *Ann Pharmacother* 26, 1522
  (1989): Pendleton N+, *Br J Clin Pract* 43, 464
  (1983): Furniss LD, *Drug Intell Clin Pharm* 17, 631

Red neck syndrome
  (1992): Estrada V+, *Rev Clin Esp* (Spanish) 190, 100

Stevens–Johnson syndrome
  (2000): Williams DA, *Mil Med* 165(8), 636
  (1999): Sullivan S+, *Ann Pharmacother* 33(12), 1369
  (1998): N Z Medicines Adverse Reactions Committee (from Internet) (observation)
  (1995): Kuper K+, *Ophthalmologe* 92(6), 823
  (1995): Lestico MR+, *Am J Health Syst Pharm* 52, 1805
  (1995): Pandha HS+, *N Z Med J* 108, 13
  (1993): Leenutaphong V+, *Int J Dermatol* 32, 428
  (1983): Fischer PR+, *Am J Dis Child* 137, 914

Toxic epidermal necrolysis
  (1995): Kuper K+, *Ophthalmologe* (German) 92, 823
  (1995): Raymond F+, *Arch Pediatr* (French) 2, 494
  (1993): Leenutaphong V+, *Int J Dermatol* 32, 428
  (1991): Porteous DM+, *Arch Dermatol* 127, 740 (in AIDS)
  (1987): Guillaume JC+, *Arch Dermatol* 123, 1166
  (1985): Lund-Kofoed ML+, *Contact Dermatitis* 13, 273

Urticaria
  (1998): Siegfried EC+, *J Am Acad Dermatol* 39, 797 (passim)
  (1993): Lopez-Serrano C+, *Allergol Immunopathol Madr* (Spanish) 21, 225

Vasculitis
  (1985): Sanchez NP+, *Arch Dermatol* 121, 220

Mucosal/ENT

Gingival hyperplasia/hypertrophy
  (1992): Valsecchi R+, *Acta Derm Venereol (Stockh)* 72, 157

Glossodynia

Oral candidiasis (1–10%)

Oral ulceration
  (1980): Evens RP+, *Drug Intell Clin Pharm* 14, 217

Stomatodynia

Tinnitus
  (1993): Vasquez EM+, *Arch Intern Med* 153(7), 879
  (1992): Swanson DJ+, *Am J Med* 92(1), 61
  (1984): Snavely SR+, *Ann Intern Med* 101(1), 92

Hair

Hair – alopecia
  (2004): Rollot F+, *Ann Pharmacother* 38(12), 2074 (with colchicine)

Other

Abdominal pain
  (2004): Rollot F+, *Ann Pharmacother* 38(12), 2074 (with colchicine)

Anaphylactoid reactions/Anaphylaxis
  (1998): Siegfried EC+, *J Am Acad Dermatol* 39, 797 (passim)
  (1996): Jorro G+, *Ann Allergy Asthma Immunol* 77, 456

Death
  (2005): Amory JK+, *N Engl J Med* 352(3), 301
  (2005): Harris JD+, *N Engl J Med* 352(3), 301
  (2005): Kaplan EL, *N Engl J Med* 352(3), 301
  (2005): Schoenholtz JC, *N Engl J* 352(3), 301
  (2005): Winston AP, *N Engl J Med* 352(3), 301
  (2004): Ray WA+, *N Engl J Med* 351(11), 1089

Fever
  (2004): Rollot F+, *Ann Pharmacother* 38(12), 2074 (with colchicine)

Headache

Hypersensitivity (1–10%)
  (1999): Gallardo MA+, *Cutis* 64, 129
  (1998): Kruppa A+, *Dermatology* 196(3), 335
  (1982): Lombardi P+, *Contact Dermatitis* 8, 416

Inappropriate secretion of antidiuretic hormone (SIADH)
  (1985): Carranco E+, *Arch Neurol* 42(2), 187 (with carbamazepine)

Injection-site extravasation (58%)
  (2001): Zimmerman T+, *Clin Drug Invest* 21, 527 (58%)

Injection-site irritation
  (1983): Marlin GE+, *Hum Toxicol* 3, 593

Injection-site pain (25%)
  (2001): Zimmerman T+, *Clin Drug Invest* 21, 527 (25%)

Injection-site phlebitis (1–10%)
  (1987): David LM, *Am J Hosp Pharm* 44, 732
  (1986): Holt RJ+, *Clin Pharm* 5, 787

Phlebitis
  (2001): de Dios Garcia-Diaz J+, *Med Clin* (Barc) 116(4), 133 (from intravenous administration)

Rhabdomyolysis
  (2007): Molden E+, *Pharmacotherapy* 27(4), 603 (with simvastatin)
  (1991): Spach DH+, *West J Med* 154(2), 213 (with lovastatin)
  (1988): Tobert JA, *Am J Cardiol* 62, 28J (with cyclosporine)

Thrombophlebitis

ESCITALOPRAM

Synonyms: Lu-26-054; S-Citalopram
Trade name: Lexapro (Forest)
Indications: Major depressive disorders, anxiety
Category: Antidepressant; Selective serotonin reuptake inhibitor
Half-life: 27–32 hours
Clinically important, potentially hazardous interactions with: alcohol, bupropion, **kava**, MAO inhibitors, methylphenidate, selegiline, **St John's wort**, sumatriptan, **valerian**

Reactions

Skin
Acne (<1%)
Allergic reactions (sic) (1–10%)
Dermatitis
Diaphoresis (5%)
  (2005): Buecking A+, *Eur J Clin Pharmacol* 61(7), 543
Eczema (<1%)
Edema (<1%)
Facial edema
Folliculitis (<1%)
Furunculosis (<1%)
Peripheral edema
Pruritus (<1%)
Purpura (<1%)
Rash (sic) (1–10%)
Shivering
Xerosis (<1%)

Mucosal/ENT
Dysgeusia (<1%)
Oral vesiculation (1–19%)
Tinnitus (1–10%)
Xerostomia (6%)

Hair
Hair – alopecia (<1%)

Eyes
Conjunctivitis (<1%)
Glaucoma
  (2006): Zelefsky JR+, *Am J Ophthalmol* 141(6), 1144

Other
Anaphylactoid reactions/Anaphylaxis
Chills (<1%)
Cough (1–10%)
Depression (<1%)
Headache
Hot flashes (1–10%)
Inappropriate secretion of antidiuretic hormone (SIADH)
  (2006): Adiga GU+, *Clin Drug Investig* 26(10), 607
  (2006): Nirmalani A+, *CNS Spectr* 11(6), 429
  (2004): Nahshoni E+, *J Clin Psychiatry* 65(12), 1722
Lipomatosis
Myalgia/Myositis/Myopathy/Myotoxicity (1–10%)
Paresthesias (1–10%)
Thrombosis
  (2004): Kurne A+, *Gen Hosp Psychiatry* 26(6), 481
Tremor (1–10%)
Upper respiratory infection
  (2005): Bielski RJ+, *Ann Clin Psychiatry* 17(2), 65

Vertigo (5%)
  (2006): Mohamed S+, *Am J Geriatr Pharmacother* 4(3), 201

ESMOLOL

Trade name: Brevibloc (Baxter)
Indications: Tachyarrhythmias, tachycardia
Category: Adrenergic beta-receptor antagonist; Antiarrhythmic class II
Half-life: 9 minutes
Clinically important, potentially hazardous interactions with: clonidine, verapamil

Reactions

Skin
Acne (<1%)
Cold extremities
Diaphoresis (>10%)
Eczema (<1%)
Edema (<1%)
Erythema (<1%)
Exfoliative dermatitis (<1%)
Facial edema
Facial flushing
Necrosis (<1%)
Pallor (<1%)
Pigmentation (<1%)
Psoriasis (<1%)
Purpura
Rash (sic)
Urticaria

Mucosal/ENT
Dysgeusia
Xerostomia (<1%)

Hair
Hair – alopecia

Other
Asthenia
  (1988): Schwartz M+, *Chest* 93(4), 705 (transient)
Death
  (1995): Barone JE, *Crit Care Med* 23(1), 212
  (1993): Herschman Z+, *Crit Care Med* 21(12), 1975
Hypotension
  (1991): Wolman RL+, *AANA J* 59(6), 541
  (1988): Schwartz M+, *Chest* 93(4), 705 (transient)
  (1987): Askenazi J+, *J Clin Pharmacol* 27(8), 567
  (1986): *Am Heart J* 112(3), 498
  (1986): Anderson S+, *Am Heart J* 111(1), 42 (12%)
  (1986): Angaran DM+, *Clin Pharm* 5(4), 288
  (1985): Abrams J+, *Am Heart J* 110(5), 913
  (1985): Gray RJ+, *J Am Coll Cardiol* 5(6), 1451 (transient)
Injection-site inflammation
  (1987): Benfield P+, *Drugs* 33, 392
Injection-site pain (8%)
Injection-site reactions (sic) (1–10%)
Paresthesias (<1%)
Phlebitis
  (1986): Angaran DM+, *Clin Pharm* 5(4), 288
Seizures
  (1988): Das G+, *Drug Intell Clin Pharm* 22(6), 484
Thrombophlebitis (<1%)

ESOMEPRAZOLE

Synonyms: Perprazole; H 19918
Trade name: Nexium (AstraZeneca)
Indications: Gastroesophageal Reflux Disease (GERD)
Category: Proton pump inhibitor
Half-life: 1.5 hours
**Clinically important, potentially hazardous interactions
with:** benzodiazepines, chlordiazepoxide, clonazepam,
clorazepate, diazepam, digoxin, flurazepam, lorazepam,
midazolam, oxazepam, quazepam, temazepam

Reactions

Skin
Acne (<1%)
Allergic reactions (sic) (<1%)
Angioedema (<1%)
Dermatitis (<1%)
Diaphoresis (<1%)
Edema (<1%)
Erythema multiforme
Exanthems (<1%)
Facial flushing (<1%)
Fungal dermatitis (<1%)
Hyperhidrosis
Peripheral edema (<1%)
Photosensitivity
  (2003): Zabawski E, Longwood, TX (from Internet)
    (observation)
Pruritus (<1%)
Pruritus ani et vulvae (<1%)
Stevens–Johnson syndrome
Toxic epidermal necrolysis
Urticaria (<1%)
Xerosis
  (2005): Chen CY+, *World J Gastroenterol* 11(20), 3112

Mucosal/ENT
Dysgeusia (<1%)
Parosmia (<1%)
Tinnitus (<1%)
Tongue edema (<1%)
Ulcerative stomatitis (<1%)
Vaginitis (<1%)
Xerostomia

Other
Candidiasis (<1%)
Depression (<1%)
Fever
  (2005): Grattagliano I+, *Ann Pharmacother* 39(4), 757
Headache
  (2005): Grattagliano I+, *Ann Pharmacother* 39(4), 757
  (2002): Johnson TJ+, *Am J Health Syst Pharm* 59(14), 1333
Hepatotoxicity
  (2005): Capitain O+, *Presse Med* 34(17), 1235
Myalgia/Myositis/Myopathy/Myotoxicity
  (2005): Grattagliano I+, *Ann Pharmacother* 39(4), 757
Nephrotoxicity
  (2006): Geevasinga N+, *Clin Gastroenterol Hepatol* 4(5), 597
Paresthesias (<1%)
Polymyositis (<1%)
Rhabdomyolysis
  (2003): Sipe BE+, *Ann Pharmacother* 37(6), 808 (with
    atorvastatin and clarithromycin)

ESTAZOLAM

Trade names: Domnamid; Esilgan; Eurodin; Kainever; Nuctalon;
ProSom; Tasedan
Indications: Insomnia
Category: Benzodiazepine
Half-life: 10–24 hours
**Clinically important, potentially hazardous interactions
with:** indinavir, ritonavir

Reactions

Skin
Acne (<1%)
Allergic reactions (sic) (<1%)
Dermatitis (<1%)
Diaphoresis (1–10%)
Edema (<1%)
Facial flushing
Photosensitivity
Pruritus (1–10%)
Purpura (<1%)
Rash (sic) (>10%)
Urticaria (1–10%)
Xerosis (<1%)

Mucosal/ENT
Dysgeusia (1–10%)
Glossitis
Oral ulceration (<1%)
Sialopenia (>10%)
Sialorrhea (<1%)
Vaginal pruritus (1–10%)
Xerostomia (>10%)

Eyes
Eyelid edema (<1%)

Other
Chills (<1%)
Gynecomastia (<1%)
Myalgia/Myositis/Myopathy/Myotoxicity (1–10%)
Paresthesias (1–10%)

ESTRAMUSTINE

Trade names: Cellmusin; Emcyt (Pfizer)
Indications: Prostate carcinoma
Category: Alkylating agent; Nitrosourea
Half-life: 20 hours
**Clinically important, potentially hazardous interactions
with:** aldesleukin

Reactions

Skin
Acne
  (1984): Halpern J+, *J Med* 15(1), 35
Allergic reactions (sic)
  (2001): Zelek L+, *Ann Oncol* 12(9), 1265
Angioedema
  (2006): Kamata Y+, *J Investig Allergol Clin Immunol* 16(6), 388
    (with an ACE-inhibitor)
  (2003): Haas NB+, *Cancer* 98(9), 1837 (with vinblastine)

Edema (>10%)
 (1990): Asakawa M+, *Hinyokika Kiyo* 36(11), 1361
 (1986): de Voogt HJ+, *J Urol* 135(2), 303
 (1984): Halpern J+, *J Med* 15(1), 35
Exanthems
Facial flushing
Pigmentation (<1%)
Pruritus (2%)
 (1984): Halpern J+, *J Med* 15(1), 35
Purpura (3%)
Rash (sic) (1%)
Urticaria
Xerosis (2%)

Mucosal/ENT
Tinnitus

Hair
Hair – alopecia (<1%)

Other
Asthenia
 (2002): Hudes G+, *J Clin Oncol* 20(4), 1115
Chest pain
 (1986): Nishio S+, *Hinyokika Kiyo* 32(11), 1763
Death
 (2001): Zelek L+, *Ann Oncol* 12(9), 1265
Gynecomastia (>10%)
 (1990): Asakawa M+, *Hinyokika Kiyo* 36(11), 1361
 (1986): Nishio S+, *Hinyokika Kiyo* 32(11), 1763
 (1982): Veronesi A+, *Prostate* 3(2), 159
 (1980): Kuss R+, *Br J Urol* 52(1), 29
Hot flashes (<1%)
Hypotension
 (2002): Hudes G+, *J Clin Oncol* 20(4), 1115
Injection-site thrombophlebitis (1–10%)
 (1981): Rambausek M+, *Urologe A* 20(4), 223
Thrombophlebitis (3%)

ESTROGENS

Generic:
 Chlorotrianisene
  Trade name: Tace
 Diethylstilbestrol
  Trade names: Cyren A; Destrol; Stilphostrol
 Estradiol
  Trade names: Estrace (Warner Chilcott); Estraderm (Novartis)
 Estrogens, conjugated
  Trade name: Premarin (Wyeth)
 Estrogens, esterified
  Trade names: Estratab (Solvay); Menest (Monarch)
 Estrone
  Trade names: Estroject; Estronol; Gynogen; Theelin, etc.
 Estropipate
  Trade name: Ogen (Pfizer)
 Ethinyl estradiol
  Trade name: Estinyl
 Quinestrol
  Trade name: Estrovis
Category: Estrogen
Half-life: N/A
Clinically important, potentially hazardous interactions with: beclomethasone, **black cohosh**, flunisolide, hydrocortisone, insulin detemir, penicillin g, penicillin V, prednisone, triamcinolone

Reactions

Skin
Acanthosis nigricans
Acne (5%)
 (2003): Phillips EH+, *Clin Ther* 25(12), 3027 (5.6%)
Allergic granulomatous angiitis (Churg–Strauss syndrome)
 (1998): Somogyi A+, *Adverse Drug React Toxicol Rev* 17(2–3), 63
Angioedema
 (2002): van der Klooster JM+, *Ned Tijdschr Geneeskd* 146(34), 1599
 (2000): McGlinchey PG+, *Am J Med Sci* 320, 212
Bullous dermatitis
Chloasma (<1%)
Dermatitis
 (1995): Shelley WB+, *J Am Acad Dermatol* 32, 25
 (1981): Ljunggren B, *Contact Dermatitis* 7(3), 141
Eczema
 (1995): Shelley WB+, *J Am Acad Dermatol* 32, 25
Edema (<1%)
Erythema multiforme
 (1998): Moghadam BK+, *Oral Surg Oral Med Oral Pathol Oral Radiol Endod* 85, 537
Erythema nodosum
 (1990): Bartelsmeyer JA+, *Clin Obstet Gynecol* 33, 777
 (1980): Salvatore MA+, *Arch Dermatol* 116, 557
Exanthems
 (2003): Murano K+, *J Dermatol* 30(10), 719
 (1999): Coustou D+, *Ann Dermatol Venereol* 125, 484
 (1999): Kumar A+, *Australas J Dermatol* 40, 96
 (1997): Litt JZ, Beachwood, OH (personal case) (observation)
 (1984): Lee M+, *J Urol* 131, 767
Exfoliative dermatitis
Fixed eruption (<1%)
Hyperkeratosis
 (1980): Mold DE+, *Cutis* 26, 95
Irritation (sic) (from transdermal system)
Livedo reticularis
Lupus erythematosus
 (2007): Carroll DG+, *Ann Pharmacother* 41(4), 702
 (2005): Vanini G+, *Rev Med Suisse* 1(15), 991
 (1989): Colins D, *J Rheumatol* 16, 408
 (1986): Barrett C+, *Br J Rheumatol* 25, 300
Melasma (<1%)
 (1992): Breathnach SM+, *Adverse Drug Reactions and the Skin* Blackwell, Oxford, 274 (passim)
Mucha–Habermann disease
Osteoma cutis
 (2002): Stockel S+, *Hautarzt* 53(1), 37
Papulovesicular eruption
 (1999): Coustou D+, *Ann Dermatol* 125, 484
 (1998): Coustou D+, *Ann Dermatol Venereol* (French) 125, 505
Peripheral edema
Photosensitivity
Pigmentation
 (1999): Oakley A, Auckland, New Zealand (from topical, over vulva) (from Internet) (observation)
Pruritus
 (2003): Murano K+, *J Dermatol* 30(10), 719
 (2000): Siepmann M+, *Dtsch Med Wochenschr* (German) 125, 557
 (1999): Coustou D+, *Ann Dermatol Venereol* 125, 484
 (1999): Kumar A+, *Australas J Dermatol* 40, 96
 (1998): Coustou D+, *Ann Dermatol Venereol* (French) 125, 505
 (1995): Shelley WB+, *J Am Acad Dermatol* 32, 25
Purpura
 (1984): Lee M+, *J Urol* 131, 767

Rash (sic) (<1%)
Raynaud's phenomenon
  (1998): Fraenkel L+, Ann Intern Med 129, 208
Scleroderma
  (2000): D'Cruz D, Toxicol Lett 112 and 421
Spider nevi
  (1992): Breathnach SM+, Adverse Drug Reactions and the Skin
    Blackwell, Oxford, 274 (passim)
Striae
Telangiectasia
Urticaria
  (1998): Moghadam BK+, Oral Surg Oral Med Oral Pathol Oral
    Radiol Endod 85, 537
  (1995): Shelley WB+, J Am Acad Dermatol 32, 25
  (1984): Lee M+, J Urol 131, 767
Vasculitis (cutaneous polyarteritis nodosa)
  (1998): Cvancara JL+, J Am Acad Dermatol 39, 643
Vesiculation
  (1999): Kumar A+, Australas J Dermatol 40, 96

Mucosal/ENT
Gingival hyperplasia/hypertrophy
Oral mucosal eruption
  (1998): Moghadam BK+, Oral Surg Oral Med Oral Pathol Oral
    Radiol Endod 85, 537
Oral pigmentation
  (1991): Perusse R+, Cutis 48, 61
Vulvovaginal candidiasis

Hair
Hair – alopecia (9%)
  (2003): Phillips EH+, Clin Ther 25(12), 3027 (8.8%)
  (1992): Breathnach SM+, Adverse Drug Reactions and the Skin
    Blackwell, Oxford, 233 (passim)
Hair – hirsutism (<5%)
  (2003): Phillips EH+, Clin Ther 25(12), 3027 (4.5%)
Hair – straight
  (1994): Litt JZ, Beachwood, OH (personal case) (observation)

Eyes
Xerophthalmia
  (2001): Schaumberg DA+, JAMA 286(17), 2114

Other
Gynecomastia (>10%)
  (2000): Felner EI+, Pediatrics 105, E55 (3 prepubertal boys from
    an estrogen cream)
  (1987): Schmidt KU+, Dtsch Med Wochenschr (German)
    112, 926
  (1984): Gottswinter JM+, Haarwasser Med Klin (German)
    79, 181
Headache
Hot flashes
  (2001): Spetz AC+, J Urol 166(2), 517
Injection-site pain (1–10%)
Porphyria
  (1994): Siersema PD+, Eur J Gastroenterol Hepatol 6, 371
  (1989): CoulsonDH+, Br J Urol 63, 648
Porphyria cutanea tarda
  (1995): Nonaka S+, Nippon Rinsho (Japanese) 53, 1427
  (1990): Roger D+, Ann Dermatol Venereol (French) 117, 127
  (1982): Enriquez de Salamanca R+, Arch Dermatol Res 274, 179
Pseudolymphoma
  (1996): Magro CM+, Hum Pathol 27(2), 125

ESZOPICLONE

Synonyms: Esopiclone; Estorra; S-zopiclone; S(+)-zopiclone
Trade names: Imovane; Lunesta (Sepracor); Zimovane (Aventis)
Indications: Insomnia
Category: Hypnotic, non-benzodiazepine
Half-life: 6 hours
**Clinically important, potentially hazardous interactions
with:** alcohol, cimetidine, CNS depressant, erythromycin,
ethanol, ketoconazole, nefazodone, nelfinavir, olanzapine,
rifampin, ritonavir, tricyclic antidepressants

Reactions

Skin
Acne
Allergic reactions (sic)
Angioedema
Cellulitis
Dermatitis
Diaphoresis
Eczema
Erythema multiforme
  (2005): White RE, Rock Hill, SC (from Internet) (observation)
Exanthems
Facial edema
Furunculosis
Herpes zoster
Hyperhidrosis
Peripheral edema (>1%)
Photosensitivity
Pigmentation
Pruritus (4%)
Rash (<5%)
Urticaria
Vesiculobullous eruption
Xerosis

Mucosal/ENT
Dysgeusia (34%)
  (2006): Brielmaier BD, Proc (Bayl Univ Med Cent) 19(1), 54
  (2006): Halas CJ, Am J Health Syst Pharm 63(1), 41
  (2006): Najib J, Clin Ther 28(4), 491
  (2005): Rosenberg R+, Sleep Med 6(1), 15
  (2005): Roth T+, Sleep Med 6(6), 487
  (2005): Scharf M+, Sleep 28(6), 720
  (2004): Zammit GK+, Curr Med Res Opin 20(12), 1979
  (2003): Krystal AD+, Sleep 26(7), 793
  (2001): Tsutsui S+, J Int Med Res 29(3), 163 (5.8%)
  (1999): Hajak G, Drug Saf 21(6), 457 (%)
  (1998): Disayavanish C+, J Med Assoc Thai 81(6), 393
Dysphagia
Tinnitus
Xerostomia
  (2006): Halas CJ, Am J Health Syst Pharm 63(1), 41
  (2006): Najib J, Clin Ther 28(4), 491 (5–7%)
  (2001): Georgiev V, Curr Opin Invest Drugs 2(2), 271

Hair
Hair – alopecia
Hair – hirsutism

Eyes
Conjunctivitis
Iritis
Mydriasis

Photophobia
Ptosis

Other
Abdominal pain
Agitation
  (2007): Moloney I+, *Ir Med J* 100(6), 511
Amnesia
  (2005): *Med Lett Drugs* 47(1203), 17
  (2004): Goulle JP+, *Ther Drug Monit* 26(2), 206
Anxiety
Asthenia
Chest pain (>1%)
Chills
Depression (4%)
  (2007): Kripke DF, *BMC Psychiatry* 7, 42
Gynecomastia (3%)
Headache
  (2006): Brielmaier BD, *Proc (Bayl Univ Med Cent)* 19(1), 54
  (2006): Halas CJ, *Am J Health Syst Pharm* 63(1), 41
  (2003): Krystal AD+, *Sleep* 26(7), 793
  (1998): Disayavanish C+, *J Med Assoc Thai* 81(6), 393
Infections (sic)
Pain (5%)
Paresthesias
Seizures
Somnolence
Suicidal ideation
Tremor (<1%)
Vertigo (7%)
  (2006): Brielmaier BD, *Proc (Bayl Univ Med Cent)* 19(1), 54
  (2006): Najib J, *Clin Ther* 28(4), 491 (5–7%)
Weight loss

ETANERCEPT

Trade name: Enbrel (Amgen) (Wyeth)
Indications: Rheumatoid arthritis
Category: Cytokine inhibitor; TNF inhibitor
Half-life: 98–300 hours
Clinically important, potentially hazardous interactions with: anakinra, cyclophosphamide

Reactions

Skin
Abscess
  (2007): Borras-Blasco J+, *Ann Pharmacother* 41(2), 341 (parapharyngeal)
  (2006): D'Amore M+, *Panminerva Med* 48(3), 199
Adverse effects (sic)
  (2002): Brocq O+, *Presse Med* 31(39), 1836
  (2001): Sandborn WJ+, *Gastroenterology* 121(5), 1088
Allergic reactions (sic) (<3%)
Angioedema
Carcinoma
  (2006): *Prescrire Int* 15(81), 8
  (2006): Stone JH+, *Arthritis Rheum* 54(5), 1608 (with cyclophosphamide)
Cellulitis
  (2002): Gorman JD+, *N Engl J Med* 346, 1349
Dermatomyositis
  (2006): Hall HA+, *Arthritis Rheum* 55(6), 982
Erythema
Exanthems

(2003): Hashkes PJ+, *Clin Exp Rheumatol* 21(5), 645
(2002): Conaghan P+, *Skin & Allergy News* June, 40
Facial flushing
Folliculitis (perforating)
  (2007): Gilaberte Y+, *Br J Dermatol* 156(2), 368
Granuloma annulare
  (2006): Deng A+, *Arch Dermatol* 142(2), 198
Granulomatous tattoo reaction (sic)
  (2007): Bachmeyer C+, *J Eur Acad Dermatol Venereol* 21(4), 550
Henoch–Schönlein purpura
  (2006): Duffy TN+, *Clin Exp Rheumatol* 24(2 suppl 41), S106
  (2006): Lee A+, *J Clin Rheumatol* 12(5), 249
Herpes zoster
  (2001): Hogarty T (generalized) (from Internet) (observation)
Lichen planus
  (2007): Battistella M+, *Br J Dermatol* 158(1), 188
Lupus erythematosus
  (2007): Ramos-Casals M+, *Medicine (Baltimore)* 86(4), 242 (37 cases)
  (2006): Kang MJ+, *J Korean Med Sci* 21(5), 946
  (2005): Richez C+, *Clin Exp Rheumatol* 23(2), 273
  (2004): Scheinfeld N, *J Drugs Dermatol* 3(6), 653
  (2003): Carlson E+, *Arthritis Rheum* 48(4), 1165
  (2003): Debandt M+, *Clin Rheumatol* 22(1), 56
  (2003): Lepore L+, *Clin Exp Rheumatol* 21(2), 276
  (2003): Swale VJ+, *Clin Exp Dermatol* 28(6), 604 (systemic)
  (2002): Cairns AP+, *Ann Rheum Dis* 61(11), 1031
  (2002): Ferraccioli GF+, *Lancet* 360(9333), 645
  (2002): Mohan AK+, *Lancet* 360(9333), 646
  (2002): Shakoor N+, *Lancet* 359 (4 cases)
  (2002): Takeuchi T+, *Nippon Rinsho* 60(12), 2390
  (2001): Bleumink GS+, *Rheumatology (Oxford)* 40, 1317
  (2001): Werth V, *Dermatology Times* 18
  (1999): Brion PH+, *Ann Intern Med* 131, 634 (discoid)
Lymphoma
  (2005): Geborek P+, *Ann Rheum Dis* 64(5), 699
  (2002): Brown SL+, *Arthritis Rheum* 46(12), 3151 (18 cases)
Malignancies (sic) (<3%)
Nevi
  (2006): Bovenschen HJ+, *Br J Dermatol* 154(5), 880 (Eruptive)
Nodular eruption
  (2003): Goffe B+, *J Am Acad Dermatol* 49(2), S105
  (2002): Cunnane G+, *Arthritis Rheum* 47(4), 445
Peripheral edema
  (2003): Goffe B+, *J Am Acad Dermatol* 49(2), S105
Pruritus
  (2003): Goffe B+, *J Am Acad Dermatol* 49(2), S105
Psoriasis
  (2008): Boms S+, *Hautarzt* (generalized)
  (2007): Cohen JD+, *J Rheumatol* 34(2), 380
  (2007): Ubriani R+, *Arch Dermatol* 143(2), 270
  (2006): Kary S+, *Ann Rheum Dis* 65(3), 405
  (2006): Peek R+, *Ann Rheum Dis* 65(9), 1259
  (2006): Sari I+, *J Rheumatol* 33(7), 1411
  (2005): Sfikakis PP+, *Arthritis Rheum* 52(8), 2513
  (2004): Hess K, Marion, IN (from Internet) (observation) (recurrence, 2 cases)
  (2004): Mitchell D, Thomasville, GA (from Internet) (observation) (recurrence)
Purpura
  (2006): Lee A+, *J Clin Rheumatol* 12(5), 249
  (2002): Mitchell DF, Thomasville, MD (from Internet) (observation)
Rash (sic) (5%)
  (2006): Klareskog L+, *Ann Rheum Dis* 65(12), 1578
  (2003): Goffe B+, *J Am Acad Dermatol* 49(2), S105
  (2000): *Nurses' Drug Alert* 24, 4
  (1999): Brion PH+, *Ann Int Med* 131, 634
Sarcoidosis

(2007): Kudrin A+, *J Rheumatol* 34(3), 648
(2006): Gonzalez-Lopez MA+, *Arthritis Rheum* 55(5), 817
(2006): Grunewald J+, *Lakartidningen* 103(26-27), 2045

Squamous cell carcinoma (penis)
(2004): Fryrear RS 2nd+, *J Am Acad Dermatol* 51(6), 1026
(2001): Smith KJ+, *J Am Acad Dermatol* 45(6), 953 (7 cases)
(2000): Smith KJ+, Academy of Dermatology Meeting San Francisco Poster Exhibit

Ulcerations

Urticaria
(2003): Goffe B+, *J Am Acad Dermatol* 49(2), S105
(2000): Skytta E+, *Clin Exp Rheumatol* 18, 533

Vasculitis
(2007): Ramos-Casals M+, *Medicine* (Baltimore) 86(4), 242 (59 cases)
(2006): Lee A+, *J Clin Rheumatol* 12(5), 249 (passim)
(2006): Saint Marcoux B+, *Joint Bone Spine* 73(6), 710
(2005): Mor A+, *J Rheumatol* 32(4), 740
(2005): Srivastava MD+, *Scand J Immunol* 61(4), 329
(2004): Mohan N+, *J Rheumatol* 31(10), 1955 (20 cases)
(2004): Olsen C, Minneapolis, MN (from Internet) (observation)
(2004): Scheinfeld N, *J Drugs Dermatol* 3(6), 653
(2003): Goffe B+, *J Am Acad Dermatol* 49(2), S105
(2002): Conaghan P+, *Skin & Allergy News* June, 40
(2002): Cunnane G+, *Arthritis Rheum* 47(4), 445
(2002): Livermore PA+, *Rheumatology* (Oxford) 41(12), 1450
(2001): Werth V, *Dermatology Times* 18
(2000): Galaria NA+, *J Rheumatol* 27, 2041 (leukocytoclastic)
(1999): Brion PH+, *Ann Intern Med* 131, 634 (necrotizing)

Mucosal/ENT

Oral ulceration
(2003): Goffe B+, *J Am Acad Dermatol* 49(2), S105

Rhinitis
(2003): Fleischmann RM+, *J Rheumatol* 30(4), 691
(2003): Goffe B+, *J Am Acad Dermatol* 49(2), S105

Sinusitis
(2003): Goffe B+, *J Am Acad Dermatol* 49(2), S105

Tinnitus
(2002): Gorman JD+, *N Engl J Med* 346, 1349

Hair

Hair – alopecia
(2005): Posten W+, *Arch Dermatol* 141(6), 759
(2003): Goffe B+, *J Am Acad Dermatol* 49(2), S105

Eyes

Optic neuritis
(2005): Tauber T+, *Rheumatology* (Oxford) 44(3), 405

Uveitis
(2006): Saurenmann RK+, *J Pediatr* 149(6), 833
(2006): Taban M+, *Ocul Immunol Inflamm* 14(3), 145
(2003): Hashkes PJ+, *Clin Exp Rheumatol* 21(5), 645

Other

Abdominal pain
(2003): Goffe B+, *J Am Acad Dermatol* 49(2), S105

Anaphylactoid reactions/Anaphylaxis
(2006): Houtman PM+, *J Clin Rheumatol* 12(6), 321 (with methotrexate)

Asthenia
(2006): de Groot M+, *Br J Dermatol* 155(4), 808
(2004): Madhusudan S+, *Clin Cancer Res* 10(19), 6528 (5 cases)
(2003): Goffe B+, *J Am Acad Dermatol* 49(2), S105

Congestive heart failure
(2004): Scheinfeld N, *J Drugs Dermatol* 3(6), 653

Cough
(2003): Goffe B+, *J Am Acad Dermatol* 49(2), S105

Death
(2006): Thomas JE+, *Hawaii Med J* 65(1), 12

(2002): Phillips K+, *Arthritis Rheum* 47(1), 17
(2001): Baghai M+, *Mayo Clin Proc* 76(6), 653

Depression
(2003): Goffe B+, *J Am Acad Dermatol* 49(2), S105

Headache
(2004): Madhusudan S+, *Clin Cancer Res* 10(19), 6528 (1 case)
(2003): Fleischmann RM+, *J Rheumatol* 30(4), 691
(2003): Goffe B+, *J Am Acad Dermatol* 49(2), S105

Hypersensitivity
(2006): *Prescrire Int* 15(81), 8

Infections (<3%)
(2007): Salliot C+, *Rheumatology* (Oxford) 46(2), 327 (34%)
(2006): *Prescrire Int* 15(81), 8
(2006): Combe B+, *Ann Rheum Dis* 65(10), 1357
(2006): Klareskog L+, *Ann Rheum Dis* 65(12), 1578 (respiratory)
(2006): Strady C+, *Presse Med* 35(11 Pt 2), 1765 (tuberculosis)
(2006): Thomas JE+, *Hawaii Med J* 65(1), 12
(2006): Winthrop KL, *Nat Clin Pract Rheumatol* 2(11), 602 (tuberculosis)
(2005): Ehlers S, *J Rheumatol Suppl* 74, 35
(2005): Feltelius N+, *Ann Rheum Dis* 64(2), 246 (22%)
(2004): Dunlop H, *CMAJ* 171(8), 992
(2004): Giles JT+, *J Intensive Care Med* 19(6), 320
(2004): Hyrich KL+, *Ann Rheum Dis* 63(12), 1538
(2004): Scheinfeld N, *J Drugs Dermatol* 3(6), 653
(2003): Goffe B+, *J Am Acad Dermatol* 49(2), S105
(2003): Kroesen S+, *Rheumatology* (Oxford) 42(5), 617
(2002): Gorman JD+, *N Engl J Med* 346, 1349
(2002): Phillips K+, *Arthritis Rheum* 47(1), 17
(2002): Steensma DP+, *Blood* 99(6), 2252
(2001): Baghai M+, *Mayo Clin Proc* 76(6), 653

Injection-site cellulitis
(2006): Winfield H+, *Arch Dermatol* 142(2), 218

Injection-site reactions (sic) (20–40%)
(2007): Dore RK+, *Clin Exp Rheumatol* 25(1), 40
(2007): Gonzalez-Lopez MA+, *Clin Exp Dermatol* 32(6), 672 (recall) (2 cases)
(2006): Combe B+, *Ann Rheum Dis* 65(10), 1357
(2006): Klareskog L+, *Ann Rheum Dis* 65(12), 1578
(2005): Clelland S+, *Dermatol Nurs* 17(5), 375
(2004): Calin A+, *Ann Rheum Dis* 63(12), 1594
(2004): Madhusudan S+, *Clin Cancer Res* 10(19), 6528 (6 cases)
(2004): Papp KA, *Expert Opin Pharmacother* 5(10), 2139
(2004): Rajakulendran S+, *Rheumatology* (Oxford) 43(12), 1588
(2004): Scheinfeld N, *J Drugs Dermatol* 3(6), 653
(2003): *Prescrire Int* 12(66), 127
(2003): Arnold EL+, *Arthritis Rheum* 48(7), 2078
(2003): Edwards KR+, *J Drugs Dermatol* 2(2), 184
(2003): Fleischmann RM+, *J Rheumatol* 30(4), 691
(2002): Gorman JD+, *N Engl J Med* 346, 1349
(2002): Steensma DP+, *Blood* 99(6), 2252
(2001): Alldred A, *Expert Opin Pharmacother* 2(7), 1137
(2001): Girolomoni G+, *Arch Dermatol* 137, 784
(2001): Sandborn WJ+, *Gastroenterology* 121(5), 1088
(2001): Werth V, *Dermatology Times* 18
(2001): Werth VP+, *Arch Dermatol* 137(7), 953
(2001): Zeltser R+, *Arch Dermatol* 137, 893 (20%)
(2000): Bathon JM+, *N Engl J Med* 343, 1586
(2000): Lovell DJ+, *N Engl J Med* 342, 763
(2000): Mease PJ, *Lancet* 356, 385
(2000): Murphy FT+, *Arch Dermatol* 136, 556
(1999): Jarvis B+, *Drugs* 57, 945
(1999): Moreland LW+, *Ann Intern Med* 130, 478
(1999): Moreland LW+, *Arthritis Rheum* 41, S364 (Suppl)
(1999): Weinblatt ME+, *N Engl J Med* 340, 253

Lymphoproliferative disease
(2002): Brown SL+, *Arthritis Rheum* 46(12), 3151 (18 cases)

Mania
(2005): Kaufman KR, *Int Clin Psychopharmacol* 20(4), 239

Multiple sclerosis-like syndrome

(2008): Mitchell D, Thomasville, GA (from internet) (observation)
Nephrotoxicity
(2005): Mor A+, *J Rheumatol* 32(4), 740
(2003): Icardi A+, *Reumatismo* 55(2), 76 (rare)
Polymyositis
(2003): Goffe B+, *J Am Acad Dermatol* 49(2), S105
Thrombophlebitis
(2003): Goffe B+, *J Am Acad Dermatol* 49(2), S105
Upper respiratory infection
(2006): Johnsen AK+, *J Rheumatol* 33(4), 659
(2001): Alldred A, *Expert Opin Pharmacother* 2(7), 1137
Vertigo
(2004): Madhusudan S+, *Clin Cancer Res* 10(19), 6528 (1 case)
(2003): Goffe B+, *J Am Acad Dermatol* 49(2), S105

ETHACRYNIC ACID

Trade names: Edecril; Edecrin (Merck); Edecrina; Hydromedin; Reomax
Indications: Edema
Category: Diuretic, loop
Half-life: 2–4 hours
Clinically important, potentially hazardous interactions with: amikacin, aminoglycosides, digoxin, gentamicin, kanamycin, neomycin, streptomycin, tobramycin

Reactions

Skin
Allergic reactions (sic)
Exanthems
Photosensitivity
Purpura (<1%)
Rash (sic) (<1%)
Urticaria
Vasculitis
(1992): Breathnach SM+, *Adverse Drug Reactions and the Skin* Blackwell, Oxford, 229 (passim)

Mucosal/ENT
Ototoxicity
(1999): Humes HD, *Ann N Y Acad Sci* 884, 15
(1988): Rybak LP, *J Laryngol Otol* 102(6), 518
(1980): Gomolin IH+, *N Engl J Med* 303(12), 702
Tinnitus
Xerostomia

Eyes
Nystagmus
(1980): Gomolin IH+, *N Engl J Med* 303(12), 702

Other
Chills (<1%)
Injection-site pain
Thrombophlebitis (<1%)

ETHAMBUTOL

Trade names: Apo-Ethambutol; Dexambutol; EMB; Etapiam; Etibi; Myambutol (Stat Trade); Stambutol
Indications: Tuberculosis
Category: Antimycobacterial
Half-life: 3–4 hours
Clinically important, potentially hazardous interactions with: cortisone, zinc

Reactions

Skin
Acne
Angioedema
(1985): Holdiness MR, *Int J Dermatol* 24, 280
Bullous dermatitis
(1985): Holdiness MR, *Int J Dermatol* 24, 280
(1981): Frentz G+, *Acta Derm Venereol* (Stockh) 61, 89
Dermatitis
(1986): Holdiness MR, *Contact Dermatitis* 15, 282
(1986): Holdiness MR, *Contact Dermatitis* 15, 96
Diaphoresis
(1985): Holdiness MR, *Int J Dermatol* 24, 280
Erythema multiforme
(1985): Holdiness MR, *Int J Dermatol* 24, 280
(1981): Frentz G+, *Acta Derm Venereol* (Stockh) 61, 89
Erythroderma
(1999): Morar N+, *Int J Dermatol* 38(12), 895
Exanthems (<5%)
(1985): Holdiness MR, *Int J Dermatol* 24, 280
(1981): Frentz G+, *Acta Derm Venereol* (Stockh) 61, 89 (1–5%)
Exfoliative dermatitis
(1985): Holdiness MR, *Int J Dermatol* 24, 280
Lichenoid eruption
(1995): Grossman ME+, *J Am Acad Dermatol* 33, 675
(1981): Frentz G+, *Acta Derm Venereol* (Stockh) 61, 89
Lupus erythematosus
(1986): Layer P+, *Dtsch Med Wochenschr* (German) 111, 1603
Photosensitivity
(1994): Berger TG+, *Arch Dermatol* 130, 609 (in HIV-infected)
Pruritus (<1%)
(1985): Holdiness MR, *Int J Dermatol* 24, 280
(1981): Frentz G+, *Acta Derm Venereol* (Stockh) 61, 89
Purpura
Rash (sic) (<1%)
(1995): Chaisson RE, *Infections in Medicine* 12, 48
(1995): Wong PC+, *Eur Respir J* 8, 866
Stevens–Johnson syndrome
Toxic epidermal necrolysis
(1985): Heng MCY, *Br J Dermatol* 106, 107
(1981): Pegram PS+, *Arch Intern Med* 141, 1677
Urticaria
(1985): Holdiness MR, *Int J Dermatol* 24, 280
(1981): Frentz G+, *Acta Derm Venereol* (Stockh) 61, 89

Mucosal/ENT
Tinnitus
(1984): Snavely SR+, *Ann Intern Med* 101(1), 92

Hair
Hair – alopecia
(1985): Holdiness MR, *Int J Dermatol* 24, 280

Eyes
Dyschromatopsia
Ocular toxicity (sic)

(2006): Chan RY+, *Hong Kong Med J* 12(1), 56
(2006): Hernandez Prats C+, *Farm Hosp* 30(4), 262
Optic neuritis
  (2005): Balal M+, *Mt Sinai J Med* 72(2), 124
Optic neuropathy
  (2006): Fraunfelder FW+, *Expert Opin Drug Saf* 5(5), 615
  (2006): Ikeda A+, *Jpn J Ophthalmol* 50(3), 280
Vision impaired
  (2006): Sobota I+, *Acta Med Croatica* 60(2), 181
Vision loss
  (2006): Kardon RH+, *Semin Ophthalmol* 21(4), 215

Other
Anaphylactoid reactions/Anaphylaxis (<1%)
Chills
Headache
Hypersensitivity
  (1995): Dhamgaye T+, *Tuber Lung Dis* 76, 181
Paresthesias

ETHANOLAMINE

Trade names: Ethamolin (GSK); Ethanolamine oleate
Indications: Bleeding esophageal varices
Category: Sclerosant, local
Half-life: N/A
**Clinically important, potentially hazardous interactions
with:** acitretin, amobarbital, aprobarbital, butabarbital, disulfiram,
insulin, mephobarbital, pentobarbital, phenobarbital, primidone,
secobarbital, thiopental

Reactions

Skin
Dermatitis
  (2002): Bowling JC+, *Contact Dermatitis* 47(2), 116
  (1995): Kock P, *Contact Dermatitis* 33, 273
  (1994): Aranzabal A+, *Contact Dermatitis* 31, 121
  (1994): Ortiz-Frutos FJ+, *Contact Dermatitis* 31, 193
  (1994): Schnuch A, *Contact Dermatitis* 30, 243

Other
Anaphylactoid reactions/Anaphylaxis (<1%)
Injection-site necrosis

ETHCHLORVYNOL

Trade names: Arvynol; Nostel
Indications: Insomnia
Category: Sedative
Half-life: 10–20 hours
**Clinically important, potentially hazardous interactions
with:** antihistamines, brompheniramine, buclizine,
chlorpheniramine, clemastine, dexchlorpheniramine, meclizine,
tripelennamine

Reactions

Skin
Allergic reactions (sic)
Bullous dermatitis (from overdose)
  (1990): Yell RP, *Am J Emerg Med* 8, 246
  (1980): Brodin MD+, *J Cutan Pathol* 7, 326
Diaphoresis

Fixed eruption
Pressure necrosis
  (1990): Chamberlain JM+, *Am J Emerg Med* 8, 467
Pruritus
Purpura
Rash (sic) (1–10%)
Urticaria

Mucosal/ENT
Dysgeusia (>10%)

Other
Death
Facial numbness
Hypersensitivity
Paresthesias

ETHIONAMIDE

Trade names: Ethatyl; Etiocidan; Myobid-250; Trecator-SC
(Wyeth); Tubermin
Indications: Tuberculosis
Category: Antibiotic
Half-life: 2–3 hours

Reactions

Skin
Acne
  (1992): Breathnach SM+, *Adverse Drug Reactions and the Skin*
    Blackwell, Oxford (passim)
Allergic reactions (sic) (1%)
Butterfly eruption on the face
  (1992): Breathnach SM+, *Adverse Drug Reactions and the Skin*
    Blackwell, Oxford (passim)
Eczema (chiefly involving the forehead)
  (1992): Breathnach SM+, *Adverse Drug Reactions and the Skin*
    Blackwell, Oxford, 159 (passim)
Exanthems
Ichthyosis
Lupus erythematosus
Peripheral edema
  (1987): Schmutz JL+, *Ann Dermatol Venereol* (French) 114, 569
Photosensitivity
Purpura
  (1992): Breathnach SM+, *Adverse Drug Reactions and the Skin*
    Blackwell, Oxford (passim)
Rash (sic) (<1%)
Seborrheic dermatitis
Urticaria (1–5%)

Mucosal/ENT
Dysgeusia (1–10%) (metallic taste)
Oral ulceration
Sialorrhea
Stomatitis (<1%)
  (1992): Breathnach SM+, *Adverse Drug Reactions and the Skin*
    Blackwell, Oxford (passim)
Stomatodynia
Xerostomia

Hair
Hair – alopecia (<1%)
  (1992): Breathnach SM+, *Adverse Drug Reactions and the Skin*
    Blackwell, Oxford, 159 (passim)

Other

Gynecomastia (<1%)

Headache

Inappropriate secretion of antidiuretic hormone (SIADH)
(2006): Nakashita T+, *Kekkaku* 81(12), 731

ETHOSUXIMIDE

Trade names: Emeside; Ethymal; Petnidan; Pyknolepsinum;
Simatin; Zarondan; Zarontin (Pfizer)
Indications: Absence (petit mal) seizures
Category: Antiepileptic, succinimide
Half-life: 50–60 hours

Reactions

Skin

Erythema multiforme (<1%)

Exanthems (1–5%)
(1991): Pelekanos J+, *Epilepsia* 32, 554

Exfoliative dermatitis (<1%)

Lupus erythematosus (>10%)
(1996): Miyasaka N, *Intern Med* 35, 527
(1996): Takeda S+, *Intern Med* 35, 587
(1996): Wallace SJ, *Drug Saf* 15, 378
(1994): Riviello JJ+, *J Epilepsy* 7, 23
(1994): Yung RL+, *Rheum Dis Clin North Am* 20, 61
(1993): Ansell BM, *Lupus* 2, 193
(1993): Drory VE+, *Clin Neuropharmacol* 16, 19 (passim)
(1985): Lovisetto P+, *Recenti Prog Med* (Italian) 76, 84
(1984): Koike K+, *Rinsho Ketsueki* 25, 1635
(1981): Grossman J+, *Arthritis Rheum* 24, 927
(1980): Condemi JJ, *Geriatrics* 35(3), 81

Pruritus

Purpura

Rash (sic) (<1%)

Raynaud's phenomenon
(1990): Rose CD+, *Arthritis Rheum* 33 (Suppl) R23

Side effects (sic) (3.4%)

Stevens–Johnson syndrome (>10%)

Urticaria (1–5%)

Mucosal/ENT

Gingival hyperplasia/hypertrophy

Oral ulceration

Tongue edema

Hair

Hair – alopecia

Hair – hirsutism

Eyes

Periorbital edema

Other

Anticonvulsant hypersensitivity syndrome
(2004): Papp Z+, *Orv Hetil* 145(32), 1665

Headache

Hypersensitivity
(1999): Conilleau V+, *Contact Dermatitis* 41(3), 141

Pseudolymphoma
(2005): Masruha MR+, *J Neurol Neurosurg Psychiatry*
76(11), 1610

ETHOTOIN

Trade names: Accenon; Peganone (Ovation)
Indications: Tonic–clonic (grand mal) seizures
Category: Antiepileptic, hydantoin
Half-life: 3–9 hours
**Clinically important, potentially hazardous interactions
with:** chloramphenicol, cyclosporine, disulfiram, dopamine,
imatinib, itraconazole

Reactions

Skin

Bullous dermatitis

Fixed eruption

Lupus erythematosus

Purpura

Rash (sic)

Stevens–Johnson syndrome

Mucosal/ENT

Gingival hyperplasia/hypertrophy

Other

Pseudolymphoma

ETIDRONATE

Trade names: Didronate; Didronel (Procter & Gamble);
Difosfen; Dinol; Diphos; Osteum
Indications: Paget's disease, osteoporosis
Category: Bisphosphonate
Half-life: 6 hours

Reactions

Skin

Angioedema (<1%)

Exanthems

Pruritus
(1985): Holzmann H+, *Hautarzt* (German) 36, 326

Rash (sic) (<1%)

Stevens–Johnson syndrome

Toxic epidermal necrolysis
(1995): Coakley G+, *Br J Rheumatol* 34, 798

Urticaria

Mucosal/ENT

Ageusia
(1987): Jones PB+, *Lancet* 2(8559), 637

Dysgeusia (<1%)

Glossitis

Stomatitis

Hair

Hair – alopecia

Eyes

Conjunctivitis
(2003): Frauenfelder FW+, *N Engl J Med* 348, 1187

Visual disturbances
(2004): Coleman CI+, *Pharmacotherapy* 24(6), 799 (rare)

Other

Hypersensitivity (<1%)

Paresthesias

ETODOLAC

Trade names: Antilak; Ecridoxan; Edolan; Elderin; Lodine
(Wyeth); Lonine; Tedolan; Utradol; Zedolac
Indications: Pain
Category: COX-2 inhibitor; Non-steroidal anti-inflammatory
Half-life: 7 hours
**Clinically important, potentially hazardous interactions
with:** aspirin, methotrexate

Reactions

Skin

Allergic reactions
Angioedema (<1%)
 (1991): Astorga-Paulsen G+, *Curr Med Res Opin* 12, 401
Bullous dermatitis
Dermatitis
Diaphoresis
Edema
Erythema multiforme (<1%)
Exanthems
 (1998): Litt JZ, Beachwood, OH (personal case) (observation)
 (1997): Litt JZ, Beachwood, OH (personal case) (observation)
 (1990): Schattenkirchner M, *Eur J Rheumatol Inflamm* 10, 56
 (1986): Lynch S+, *Drugs* 31, 288 (3%)
Exfoliative dermatitis
Facial edema
 (1991): Astorga-Paulsen G+, *Curr Res Med Opin* 12, 401
 (1990): Freitas GG, *Curr Med Res Opin* 12, 255
Fixed eruption
 (2007): Ozkaya E+, *Clin Exp Dermatol* 32(3), 332
 (1997): Blumenthal HL, Beachwood, OH (personal case)
  (observation)
Furunculosis
 (1987): Waltham-Weeks CD, *Curr Med Res Opin* 10, 540
Peripheral edema
 (1990): Freitas GG, *Curr Med Res Opin* 12, 255
Photosensitivity
 (1987): Waltham-Weeks CD, *Curr Med Res Opin* 10, 540
Pigmentation
Pruritus (1–10%)
 (1998): Litt JZ, Beachwood, OH (personal case) (observation)
 (1991): *Med Lett Drug Ther* 33, 79
 (1991): Astorga-Paulsen G+, *Curr Res Med Opin* 12, 401
 (1991): Balfour JA+, *Drugs* 42, 274
 (1991): Bianchi-Porro G+, *J Intern Med* 229, 5
 (1991): Karbowski A, *Curr Med Res Opin* 12, 309
 (1990): Schattenkirchner M, *Eur J Rheumatol Inflamm* 10, 56
 (1989): Ciocci A, *Curr Med Res Opin* 11, 471
Purpura
Rash (sic) (>10%)
 (1991): Anon, *Med Lett Drug Ther* 33, 79
 (1991): Astorga-Paulsen G+, *Curr Med Res Opin* 12, 401
 (1991): Balfour JA+, *Drugs* 42, 274
 (1989): Ciocci A, *Curr Med Res Opin* 11, 471
 (1989): Williams PI+, *Curr Med Res Opin*
Stevens–Johnson syndrome (<1%)
Toxic epidermal necrolysis (<1%)
Urticaria (<1%)
 (2000): Mitchell D, Thomasville, GA (from Internet)
  (observation)
 (1996): Thaler D, Monona, WI (pressure) (personal case)
  (observation)
Vasculitis
 (1996): Lie JT+, *J Rheumatol* 23, 183 (hypersensitivity)

 (1989): Willemin B+, *Ann Méd Int* (French) 140, 529
Vesiculobullous eruption

Mucosal/ENT

Dysgeusia
Gingival ulceration
Glossitis
Sialorrhea
Stomatitis
Tinnitus
Ulcerative stomatitis
Xerostomia

Hair

Hair – alopecia

Other

Gynecomastia
Paresthesias

ETOPOSIDE

Synonyms: epipodophyllotoxin; VP-16; VP-16–213
Trade names: Aside; Etopos; Etosid; Lastet; Serozide; VePesid
(Bristol-Myers Squibb); Vepeside; VP-TEC
Indications: Lymphomas, carcinomas
Category: Topoisomerase 2 inhibitor
Half-life: terminal: 4–15 hours
**Clinically important, potentially hazardous interactions
with:** aldesleukin, cyclosporine, prednisolone, **St John's wort**

Reactions

Skin

Acral erythema
 (1997): Whitlock JA+, *Leukemia* 11(2), 185 (4 cases) (with
  cytarabine)
Allergic reactions (sic) (1–2%)
Diaphoresis
Eccrine squamous syringometaplasia
 (1997): Valks R+, *Arch Dermatol* 133, 873
Erythema
 (1994): Portal I+, *Cancer Chemother Pharmacol* 34, 181 (acral)
 (1993): Dechaufour F+, *Ann Dermatol Venereol* (French)
  120, 219 (acral)
 (1993): Vukelja SJ+, *Cutis* 52, 89 (acral)
Erythema multiforme
 (1987): Yokel BK+, *J Cutan Pathol* 14, 326
Exanthems
 (1992): Beyer J+, *Bone Marrow Transplant* 10, 491
 (1992): Breathnach SM+, *Adverse Drug Reactions and the Skin*
  Blackwell, Oxford, 301 (passim)
 (1987): Yokel BK+, *J Cutan Pathol* 14, 326
 (1981): Weiss RB+, *Ann Intern Med* 94, 66
Facial edema
Hand–foot syndrome
 (2005): Marigny K+, *Cancer Chemother Pharmacol* 55(3), 244
 (1997): Whitlock JA+, *Leukemia* 11(2), 185 (with cytarabine)
 (1994): Portal I+, *Cancer Chemother Pharmacol* 34(2), 181
Neutrophilic eccrine hidradenitis
 (1993): Nikkels AF+, *Acta Clin Belg* 48(6), 397
Photo-recall
 (1993): Williams BJ+, *Clin Exp Dermatol* 18, 452 (ultraviolet)
 (1992): Breathnach SM+, *Adverse Drug Reactions and the Skin*
  Blackwell, Oxford, 301 (passim)
 (1987): Yokel BK+, *J Cutan Pathol* 14, 326

Pigmentation
   (2001): Mutafoglu-Uysal K+, *Turk J Pediatr* 43(2), 172
   (1991): Singal R+, *Pediatr Dermatol* 8, 231
Pruritus
Purpura
Rash (sic)
Stevens–Johnson syndrome
   (1992): Breathnach SM+, *Adverse Drug Reactions and the Skin*
      Blackwell, Oxford, 301 (passim)
   (1987): Yokel BK+, *J Cutan Pathol* 14, 326
   (1983): Jameson CH+, *Cancer Treat Rep* 67, 1050
Urticaria

Mucosal/ENT
Dysgeusia
Mucositis (>10%)
Oral lesions (<5%)
   (1990): Henwood JM+, *Drugs* 39, 438 (1–5%)
Stomatitis (1–10%)
Tinnitus
   (1988): Evans WK+, *Br J Cancer* 58(4), 464
Tongue edema

Hair
Hair – alopecia (8–66%)
   (1990): Henwood JM+, *Drugs* 39, 438 (100%, dose-dependent)
   (1989): Smit EF+, *Thorax* 44, 631
   (1989): Wander HE+, *Cancer Chemother Pharmacol* 24, 261
   (1989): Yoshino M+, *Jpn J Clin Oncol* 19, 120 (57%)

Nails
Nails – Beau's lines (transverse nail bands)
   (1994): Ben-Dayan D+, *Acta Haematol* 91, 89
Nails – onychopathy
   (2005): Marigny K+, *Cancer Chemother Pharmacol* 55(3), 244

Other
Anaphylactoid reactions/Anaphylaxis (<2%)
   (2003): Taguchi A+, *Gan To Kagaku Ryoho* 30(8), 1187
   (1989): Siddall SJ+, *Lancet* 1, 394
   (1989): Wander HE+, *Cancer Chemother Pharmacol* 24, 261
Hypersensitivity (<1%)
   (2002): Siderov J+, *Br J Cancer* 86(1), 12
   (2001): Mutafoglu-Uysal K+, *Turk J Pediatr* 43(2), 172
   (1993): Hudson MM+, *J Clin Oncol* 11, 1080
   (1992): Weiss RB, *Semin Oncol* 19, 458
   (1991): Kellie SJ+, *Cancer* 67, 1070
   (1988): Ogle KM+, *Am J Clin Oncol* 11, 663
   (1985): Tucci E+, *Chemioterapia* 4, 460
   (1984): O'Dwyer PJ+, *Cancer Treat Rep* 68, 959
Infections
   (2002): Evans SR+, *J Clin Oncol* 20(15), 3236
   (1997): Whitlock JA+, *Leukemia* 11(2), 185 (39%) (with
      cytarabine)
Injection-site pain
Nephrotoxicity
   (2000): Gerke P+, *J Cancer Res Clin Oncol* 126(3), 173
   (1997): Beyer J+, *Bone Marrow Transplant* 20(10), 813
Paresthesias
Thrombophlebitis (<1%)

ETORICOXIB

Trade names: Algix; Arcoxia (Merck); Tauxib
Indications: Rheumatoid arthritis, osteoarthritis, ankylosing
spondylitis, chronic low back pain, dysmenorrhea, acute gouty
arthritis
Category: COX-2 inhibitor; Non-steroidal anti-inflammatory
Half-life: 22 Hours
**Clinically important, potentially hazardous interactions
with:** ACE inhibitors, cyclosporin, dexibuprofen, lithium,
methotrexate, rifampicin, tacrolimus, warfarin. and other oral
anticoagulants

Reactions

Skin
Angioedema
   (2005): Sanchez-Borges M+, *Ann Allergy Asthma Immunol*
      95(2), 154
Erythema
   (2006): Augustine M+, *Indian J Dermatol Venereol Leprol*
      72(4), 307 (generalized)
Erythema multiforme
   (2008): Thirion L+, *Dermatology* 216(3), 227
Exanthems
   (2006): Atzori L+, *J Cutan Med Surg* 10(1), 31
Fixed eruption
   (2006): Augustine M+, *Indian J Dermatol Venereol Leprol*
      72(4), 307
Stevens–Johnson syndrome
   (2006): Layton D+, *Drug Saf* 29(8), 687
Urticaria
   (2007): Muratore L+, *Ann Allergy Asthma Immunol* 98(2), 168
   (2005): Nettis E+, *Ann Allergy Asthma Immunol* 95(5), 438
   (2005): Sanchez-Borges M+, *Ann Allergy Asthma Immunol*
      95(2), 154

Other
Abdominal pain
Cardiotoxicity
   (2006): Cannon CP+, *Lancet* 368(9549), 1771
   (2006): Curtis SP+, *Curr Med Res Opin* 22(12), 2365
   (2006): Hilario MO+, *J Pediatr* (Rio J) 82(5 Suppl), S206
   (2006): Niederberger E+, *Biochem Biophys Res Commun*
      342(3), 940
   (2006): Nielsen OH+, *Aliment Pharmacol Ther* 23(1), 27
   (2005): Aldington S+, *N Z Med J* 118(1223), U168
Headache
   (2006): Tsoukas C+, *Blood* 107(5), 1785
Hypertension
   (2007): Baraf HS+, *J Rheumatol* 34(2), 408
   (2005): Capone ML+, *Expert Opin Drug Metab Toxicol* 1(2), 269
Stroke
   (2007): Wong EH+, *J Neuroimaging* 17(1), 87
   (2006): Andersohn F+, *Stroke* 37(7), 1725
Upper respiratory infection
   (2006): Tsoukas C+, *Blood* 107(5), 1785

ETRAVIRINE

Trade name: Intelence (Tibotec)
Indications: HIV infection
Category: Non-nucleoside reverse transcriptase inhibitor
Half-life: 41 hours
**Clinically important, potentially hazardous interactions
with:** atazanavir, fosamprenavir, nnrtis, ritonavir, tipranavir

Reactions

Skin
Erythema multiforme
Rash (sic) (9%)
  (2008): Knoll BM+, *Drugs Today (Barc)* 44(1), 23
  (2007): Madruga JV+, *Lancet* 370(9581), 29
  (2007): Nadler JP+, *AIDS* 21(6), F1
Stevens–Johnson syndrome

Mucosal/ENT
Stomatitis (>2%)
Xerostomia (>2%)

Eyes
Vision blurred (>2%)

Other
Abdominal pain (3%)
Amnesia (>2%)
Anxiety (>2%)
Asthenia (3.3%)
Bronchospasm (>2%)
Gynecomastia (>2%)
Headache (2.7%)
  (2003): Gazzard BG+, *AIDS* 17(18), F49
Hepatotoxicity
  (2007): Nadler JP+, *AIDS* 21(6), F1
Hypersensitivity
Hypertension (2.8%)
Insomnia (>2%)
Paresthesias (>2%)
Somnolence (>2%)
Tremor (>2%)
Vertigo (>2%)

EUCALYPTUS

Scientific names: *Eucalyptus bicostata; Eucalyptus fruticetorum; Eucalyptus globulus; Eucalyptus odorata; Eucalyptus pauciflora; Eucalyptus polybractea; Eucalyptus smithii*
Family: Myrtacceae
Trade and other common names: Blue gum; Blue mallee oil; Dristan Nasal Decongestant Spray; Fever tree; Gully gum oil; Listerine; Red gum; Stringy bark; Vicks VapoRub. Mentho-Lyptus (Hall) in mouthwash; toothpaste, cough drops, lozenges
Category: Anti-inflammatory; Diuretic
Purported indications and other uses: Asthma, bronchitis, cough, croup, fever, joint and muscle pains, nasal congestion, sore throats, rheumatism.
Flavoring, fragrance, toothpaste, substances used in root canal fillings
Half-life: N/A
**Clinically important, potentially hazardous interactions
with:** amitriptyline, borage, carisoprodol, coltsfoot, **comfrey**, diazepam, haloperidol, insulin, lansoprazole, nelfinavir, omeprazole, ondansetron, pantoprazole, propranolol, theophylline, verapamil

Reactions

Skin
Cyanosis
Dermatitis
  (1995): Schaller M+, *Clin Exp Dermatol* 20(2), 143
Rash
  (2000): Ernst E, *Br J Dermatol* 143(5), 923

Eyes
Miosis

Other
Death [O]
Seizures
  (1999): Burkhard PR+, *J Neurol* 246(8), 667
Toxicity (sic)
Vertigo

EVENING PRIMROSE

Scientific names: *Oenothera biennis; Oenothera muricata; Oenothera purpurata; Oenothera rubricaulis; Oenothera suaveolens*
Family: Onagraceae
Trade and other common names: EPO; Fever Plant; Gamma Linolenic Acid; GLA; Night Willow-Herb; Scabish; Sun Drop
Category: Anti-inflammatory; Gamma linoleic acid
Purported indications and other uses: Mastalgia, osteoporosis, atopic dermatitis, rheumatoid arthritis, hypercholesterolemia, chronic fatigue syndrome, neurodermatitis, ulcerative colitis, irritable bowel syndrome.
Used in soaps and cosmetics
Half-life: N/A
**Clinically important, potentially hazardous interactions
with:** aspirin, chlorpromazine, fluphenazine, phenothiazine, thioridazine, warfarin

Reactions

Skin
Adverse effects (sic)
(2004): Werneke U+, *Br J Cancer* 90(2), 408

Other
Seizures

EVEROLIMUS

Trade name: Certican (Novartis)
Indications: Immunosuppressant
Category: mTOR inhibitor
Half-life: 24–35 hours
Clinically important, potentially hazardous interactions with: erythromycin, verapamil

Reactions

Skin
Acne
Edema
(2007): Moro J+, *Transplant Proc* 39(7), 2365
Rash (sic)
(2008): Awada A+, *Eur J Cancer* 44(1), 84 (with letrozole)

Mucosal/ENT
Stomatitis
(2008): Awada A+, *Eur J Cancer* 44(1), 84 (with letrozole)

Other
Abdominal pain
Asthenia
(2008): Awada A+, *Eur J Cancer* 44(1), 84 (with letrozole)
Fever
(2004): Dorschner L+, *Transplantation* 78(2), 303
Headache
(2008): Awada A+, *Eur J Cancer* 44(1), 84 (with letrozole)
Hepatotoxicity
Hypertension
Infections (sic)
(2007): Moro J+, *Transplant Proc* 39(7), 2365
Myalgia/Myositis/Myopathy/Myotoxicity
Pain
Pancreatitis

EXEMESTANE

Trade name: Aromasin (Pfizer)
Indications: advanced breast cancer
Category: Aromatase inhibitor
Half-life: 24 hours

Reactions

Skin
Diaphoresis (6–12%)
(2000): Clemett D+, *Drugs* 59, 1279
(1997): Thurlimann B+, *Eur J Cancer* 33, 1767 (12%)
Edema (7%)
Hyperhidrosis
Peripheral edema (9%)

(1997): Thurlimann B+, *Eur J Cancer* 33, 1767 (9%)
Pruritus (2–5%)
Rash (sic) (2–5%)

Hair
Hair – alopecia (2–5%)

Other
Headache
(2002): Tabei T+, *Gan To Kagaku Ryocho* 29(7), 1199
Hot flashes (30%)
(2002): Tabei T+, *Gan To Kagaku Ryoho* 29(7), 1199
(2000): Clemett D+, *Drugs* 59, 1279
(1999): Jones S+, *J Clin Oncol* 17, 3418
(1998): Paridaens R+, *Anticancer Drugs* 9, 675 (30%)
(1997): Thurlimann B+, *Eur J Cancer* 33, 1767 (21%)
Infections
Lymphedema (2–5%)
Paresthesias (2–5%)
Tumor pain (30%)
(1998): Paridaens R+, *Anticancer Drugs* 9, 675 (30%)

EZETIMIBE

Trade names: Vytorin; Zetia
Indications: Hypercholesterolemia
Category: Cholesterol inhibitor
Half-life: 22 hours
Clinically important, potentially hazardous interactions with: cyclosporine, fenofibrate, gemfibrozil, HMG-CoA inhibitors (statins), ritonavir

Note: Vytorin is a combination of ezetimibe and simvastatin

Reactions

Skin
Angioedema
Rash (sic)
Urticaria

Hair
Hair – alopecia
(2004): Smith JG, Mobile, AL (from Internet) (observation)

Other
Abdominal pain (2.2%)
Cough (2.3%)
Hepatotoxicity
(2006): Stolk MF+, *Clin Gastroenterol Hepatol* 4(7), 908
Myalgia/Myositis/Myopathy/Myotoxicity (5%)
(2007): Patel AR+, *J Heart Lung* 26(3), 281
(2007): Weffald LA+, *Pharmacotherapy* 27(2), 309
(2006): Davidson MH+, *Am J Cardiol* 97(2), 223
(2006): Havranek JM+, *Am J Med* 119(3), 285
(2006): Kohnle M+, *Am J Transplant* 6(1), 205
(2006): Simard C+, *Can J Cardiol* 22(2), 141
(2005): Perez-Calvo J+, *QJM* 98(6), 461
(2004): Litt JZ, Beachwood, OH (personal case) (observation)

FAMCICLOVIR

Trade name: Famvir (Novartis)
Indications: Acute herpes zoster, recurrent genital herpes
Category: Antiviral; Guanine nucleoside analog
Half-life: 2–3 hours

Reactions

Skin
Dermatitis
  (1996): Sacks SL+, *JAMA* 276, 44
Pruritus (3.7%)
Vasculitis
  (2005): Ali SO+, *J Drugs Dermatol* 4(4), 486

Other
Abdominal pain
  (2004): Sra KK+, *Skin Therapy Lett* 9(8), 1
Headache
  (1994): Saltzman R+, *Antimicrob Agents Chemother* 38(10), 2454
Hypersensitivity
  (2001): Kawsar M+, *Sex Transm Infect* 77(3), 204
Paresthesias (2.6%)

FAMOTIDINE

Trade names: Amfamox; Apo-Famotidine; Durater; Famodil; Famoxal; Ganor; Gastro; Motiax; Mylanta AR; Nu-Famotidine; Pepcid (Merck); Pepcidine; Pepdul; Sigafam
Indications: Duodenal ulcer, Gastroesophageal Reflux Disease (GERD)
Category: Histamine H2 receptor antagonist
Half-life: 2.5–3.5 hours
Clinically important, potentially hazardous interactions with: cefditoren, **devil's claw**

Reactions

Skin
Acne (<1%)
Acute generalized exanthematous pustulosis (AGEP)
  (2003): Scheinfeld N+, *Acta Derm Venereol* 83(1), 76
Allergic reactions (sic) (<1%)
Angioedema (<1%)
  (1986): Campoli-Richards DM+, *Drugs* 32, 197 (0.05%)
Dermatitis
  (1994): Guimaraens D+, *Contact Dermatitis* 31, 259
  (1990): Monteseirin J+, *Contact Dermatitis* 22, 290
Dermographism
  (1994): Warner DMc+, *J Am Acad Dermatol* 31, 677
Erythema multiforme
  (1999): Horiuchi Y+, *Ann Intern Med* 131, 795
Exanthems
Facial edema
Pruritus (<1%)
  (1994): Warner DMc+, *J Am Acad Dermatol* 31, 677
  (1990): Edge DP, *N Z Med J* 103, 150
Purpura
  (1996): Kallal SM+, *West J Med* 164, 446
Rash (sic)
  (1989): McCullough AJ+, *Gastroenterology* 97, 860
  (1989): Schunack W, *J Int Med Res* 17 (Suppl 1), 9A
Side effects (sic)

  (1986): Campoli-Richards DM+, *Drugs* 32, 197 (0.4%)
Toxic epidermal necrolysis
  (1995): Brunner M+, *Br J Dermatol* 133, 814
Urticaria (<1%)
  (1994): Warner DMc+, *J Am Acad Dermatol* 31, 677
  (1986): Campoli-Richards DM+, *Drugs* 32, 197 (0.1%)
Vasculitis
  (1993): Torralba M+, *An Med Interna* (Spanish) 10, 621
  (1990): Andreo JA+, *Med Clin* (Barc) (Spanish) 95, 234
Xerosis (<1%)

Mucosal/ENT
Dysgeusia
Oral lesions
  (1986): Campoli-Richards DM+, *Drugs* 32, 197 (0.15%)
Tinnitus
Xerostomia
  (1986): Campoli-Richards DM+, *Drugs* 32, 197 (0.15%)

Hair
Hair – alopecia

Eyes
Periorbital edema

Other
Candidiasis
  (2003): Orenstein SR+, *Aliment Pharmacol Ther* 17(9), 1097 (1 case)
Gynecomastia
Headache
  (2003): Orenstein SR+, *Aliment Pharmacol Ther* 17(9), 1097 (2 cases)
Injection-site pain
Myalgia/Myositis/Myopathy/Myotoxicity
Paresthesias (<1%)
  (1997): Litt JZ, Beachwood, OH (personal case) (observation)
  (1997): Litt JZ, Beachwood, OH (prickly sensation) (personal case) (observation)
Seizures
  (2002): von Einsiedel RW+, *Pharmacopsychiatry* 35(4), 152

FELBAMATE

Trade names: Felbamyl; Felbatol (MedPointe); Taloxa
Indications: Partial seizures
Category: Anticonvulsant
Half-life: 13–23 hours

Reactions

Skin
Acne (3.4%)
Bullous dermatitis (<1%)
Diaphoresis
Edema
Facial edema (3.4%)
Idiosyncratic drug reactions
  (2002): Dieckhaus CM+, *Chem Biol Interact* 142(1), 99
Lichen planus
Livedo reticularis
Lupus erythematosus
Photosensitivity (<0.01%)
Pruritus (>1%)
Purpura
Pustules

(1994): Shelley WB+, *Cutis* 53, 282 (observation)
Rash (sic) (3.5%)
(2007): Arif H+, *Neurology* 68(20), 1701
Stevens–Johnson syndrome
(1994): Jackel RA, *Epilepsia* 35, 98
Toxic epidermal necrolysis
(1995): Travaglini MT+, *Pharmacotherapy* 15, 260
Urticaria (<1%)

Mucosal/ENT
Dysgeusia (6.1%)
Gingivitis
Glossitis
Oral edema (>1%)
Xerostomia (2.6%)

Hair
Hair – alopecia

Other
Anaphylactoid reactions/Anaphylaxis (<0.01%)
Anticonvulsant hypersensitivity syndrome
(2002): Galindo PA+, *J Investig Allergol Clin Immunol* 12(4), 299
Depression
(2007): Mula M+, *Drug Saf* 30(7), 555 (4%)
Headache
Myalgia/Myositis/Myopathy/Myotoxicity (2.6%)
Paresthesias (3.5%)
Thrombophlebitis
Weight loss
(2007): Ben-Menachem, *Epilepsia* 48, 42

FELODIPINE

Trade names: AGON SR; Hydac; Lexxel (AstraZeneca); Modip; Munobal; Penedil; Plendil (AstraZeneca); Renedil; Splendil
Indications: Hypertension
Category: Calcium channel blocker
Half-life: 11–16 hours
Clinically important, potentially hazardous interactions with: carbamazepine, epirubicin, **grapefruit juice**, imatinib

Note: Lexxel is enalapril and felodipine

Reactions

Skin
Diaphoresis
(1988): Saltiel E+, *Drugs* 36, 387
Edema
(1991): *Med Lett Drugs Ther* 33, 115
Erythema (1.5%)
Exanthems
(1993): Litt JZ, Beachwood, OH (personal case) (observation)
(1985): Lorimer AR+, *Drugs* 29 (Suppl 2), 154
Facial edema (1.5%)
Peripheral edema (22%)
(1992): Morgan TO+, *Am J Hypertens* 5, 238
(1992): Morgan TO+, *Kidney Int* Suppl 36, S78
(1991): Dimenas E+, *Eur J Clin Pharmacol* 40, 141
(1991): Frewin DB+, *Eur J Clin Pharmacol* 41, 393 (22%)
(1991): Liedholm H+, *Drug Intell Clin Pharm* 25, 1007
Pruritus (<1%)
Purpura
(1991): Capewell S+, *Eur J Clin Pharmacol* 41, 95
Rash (sic) (1.5%)

Telangiectasia
(2001): Silvestre JF+, *J Am Acad Dermatol* 45, 323 (facial; photodistributed)
(1998): Karonen T+, *Dermatology* 196, 272 (truncal)
Urticaria (1.5%)

Mucosal/ENT
Gingival hyperplasia/hypertrophy (2–10%)
(2005): Fay AA+, *J Periodontol* 76(7), 1217
(2004): Hansen KW+, *Ugeskr Laeger* 166(43), 3828
(1998): Young PC+, *Cutis* 62, 41
(1991): Lombardi T+, *J Oral Pathol Med* 20(2), 89
Tinnitus
Xerostomia (<1%)
(1991): Dimenas E+, *Eur J Clin Pharmacol* 40, 141

Nails
Nails – brittle (44%)
(1985): Aberg H+, *Drugs* 29 (Suppl 2), 117 (44%)

Other
Gynecomastia (<1%)
Headache
Myalgia/Myositis/Myopathy/Myotoxicity (1.5%)
Paresthesias (2.5%)

FENBUFEN

Trade name: Lederfen (Goldshield)
Indications: Rheumatism
Category: Non-steroidal anti-inflammatory
Half-life: 8 hours
Clinically important, potentially hazardous interactions with: enoxacin

Reactions

Skin
Dermatitis
(1983): Crossley RJ, *Am J Med* 75(4B), 84
(1983): Nicolas C+, *Ann Dermatol Venereol* 110(5), 419
Erythema multiforme
(1984): Chagnon A+, *Presse Med* 13(38), 2326
(1981): Peacock A+, *Br Med J (Clin Res Ed)* 283(6291), 582
Rash (sic)
(1994): Crosse BA+, *Br J Clin Pract* 48(5), 277
(1990): Burton GH, *BMJ* 300(6717), 82
(1988): Edwards IR, *N Z Med J* 101(852), 550
(1981): Solomon L+, *S Afr Med J* 60(10), 384
Stevens–Johnson syndrome
(1993): Leenutaphong V+, *Int J Dermatol* 32(6), 428
Toxic dermatitis (sic)
(1984): Martin T+, *Presse Med* 13(1), 43
Toxic epidermal necrolysis
(1997): Krivoy N+, *Clin Rheumatol* 16(5), 489
(1993): Leenutaphong V+, *Int J Dermatol* 32(6), 428
(1990): Roujeau JC+, *Arch Dermatol* 126(1), 37
Vasculitis
(1984): Jean-Pastor MJ+, *Therapie* 39(3), 305
(1983): Teillac D+, *Presse Med* 12(20), 1297

Other
Hypersensitivity
(1988): Muthiah MM, *BMJ* 297(6663), 1614
Nephrotoxicity
(1997): Krivoy N+, *Clin Rheumatol* 16(5), 489

(1988): Morita H+, *Nippon Naika Gakkai Zasshi* 77(5), 744 (with enoxacin)
(1987): Levy M+, *Clin Nephrol* 28(2), 103
Rhabdomyolysis
(1988): Morita H+, *Nippon Naika Gakkai Zasshi* 77(5), 744 (with enoxacin)
Seizures
(1988): Morita H+, *Nippon Naika Gakkai Zasshi* 77(5), 744 (with enoxacin)

FENOFIBRATE

Synonyms: procetofene; proctofene
Trade names: Apo-Fenofibrate; Tricor (Abbott)
Indications: Hyperlipidemia
Category: Fibrate; Lipid regulator
Half-life: 20 hours
Clinically important, potentially hazardous interactions with: dicumarol, ezetimibe, lovastatin, nicotinic acid, statins, warfarin

Reactions

Skin
Adverse effects (sic) (1–10%)
  (1989): Goldberg AC+, *Clin Ther* 11, 69
Exanthems
  (1990): Balfour JA+, *Drugs* 40, 260
Photosensitivity
  (1997): Leroy D+, *Photodermatol Photoimmunol Photomed* 13, 93
  (1997): Machet L+, *J Am Acad Dermatol* 37, 808
  (1996): Diemer S+, *J Dermatol Sci* 13, 172
  (1996): Leenutaphong V+, *J Am Acad Dermatol* 35, 775
  (1994): Miranda MA+, *Photochem Photobiol* 59, 171
  (1993): Gardeazabal J+, *Photodermatol Photoimmunol Photomed* 9, 156
  (1993): Jeanmougin M+, *Ann Dermatol Venereol* (French) 120, 549
  (1992): Serrano G+, *J Am Acad Dermatol* 27, 204
  (1990): Leroy D+, *Photodermatol Photoimmunol Photomed* 7, 136
  (1989): Merino MV+, *Actas Dermo-Sif* (Spanish) 80, 703
Phototoxicity
  (1993): Vargas F+, *Photochem Photobiol* 58, 471
  (1990): Merino V+, *Contact Dermatitis* 23, 284
Pruritus (4%)
Rash (sic) (2–8%)
  (2002): Najib J, *Clin Ther* 24(12), 2022
  (1989): *Am J Med* 83, 26 (2%)
  (1989): Blane GF, *Cardiology* 76, 1
Toxic epidermal necrolysis
  (2002): Correia O+, *Arch Dermatol* 138, 29 (2 cases)
Urticaria

Mucosal/ENT
Vaginitis

Hair
Hair – alopecia
  (1990): Gollnick H+, *Z Hautkr* (German) 65, 1128

Other
Gynecomastia
  (2007): Gardette V+, *Ann Pharmacother* 41(3), 508 (unilateral)
Headache
Hepatotoxicity
  (2007): Alexander MS+, *Carbohydr Res* 342(1), 31

(2005): Dohmen K+, *World J Gastroenterol* 11(48), 7702
(2004): Ho CY+, *J Chin Med Assoc* 67(5), 245
(2003): Pichon N+, *Gastroenterol Clin Biol* 27(10), 947
(2001): Fartoux-Heymann L+, *Ann Med Interne* (Paris) 152(5), 353
(1998): Ganne-Carrie N+, *Gastroenterol Clin Biol* 22(5), 525
(1996): Rouhier ML+, *Gastroenterol Clin Biol* 20(12), 1137
(1994): Bernard PH+, *Gastroenterol Clin Biol* 18(11), 1048
(1993): Chatrenet P+, *Gastroenterol Clin Biol* 17(8-9), 612
(1992): Bravo ML+, *Aten Primaria* 10(3), 697
(1992): Lelouch S+, *Gastroenterol Clin Biol* 16(6-7), 597
(1989): Rigal J+, *Rev Med Interne* 10(1), 65
(1986): Massen H+, *Cah Anesthesiol* 34(3), 249
(1980): Couzigou P+, *Therapie* 35(3), 403
Myalgia/Myositis/Myopathy/Myotoxicity
  (2007): Dedhia V+, *J Assoc Physicians India* (India) 55, 152 (with rosuvastatin)
  (2006): Lukjanowicz M+, *Pol Arch Med Wewn* 115(1), 45
  (2005): Litt JZ, Beachwood, OH (personal case) (observation)
  (2004): Ghosh B+, *Neurol India* 52(2), 268
  (2002): Najib J, *Clin Ther* 24(12), 2022
  (2001): Rabasa-Lhoret R+, *Diabetes Metab* 27(1), 66
  (1993): Berger O+, *Nervenarzt* 64(8), 539
  (1991): Solsona L+, *Med Clin* (Barc) (Spanish) 97, 677
  (1989): *Am J Med* 83, 26 (1%)
  (1989): Muller JP+, *Presse Med* 18(20), 1033
  (1982): Giraud P+, *Rev Rhum Mal* 49(2), 162
Paresthesias
Polymyositis
  (1991): Sauvaget F+, *Rev Med Interne* (French) 12, 52
Rhabdomyolysis
  (2006): Archambeaud-Mouveroux F+, *Rev Med Interne* 27(7), 573
  (2005): Ireland JH+, *Ann Intern Med* 142(11), 949 (with rosuvastatin)
  (2005): Jones PH+, *Am J Cardiol* 95(1), 120 (with statins)
  (2005): Kursat S+, *Clin Nephrol* 64(5), 391 (with statins)
  (2003): Barker BJ+, *Diabetes Care* 26(8), 2482
  (2000): Duda-Krol W+, *Wiad Lek* 53(7), 454
  (1999): Clouatre Y+, *Nephrol Dial Transplant* 14(4), 1047
  (1993): Berger O+, *Nervenarzt* 64(8), 539
  (1992): Raimondeau J+, *Presse Med* 21(14), 663 (with pravastatin)
Septic–toxic shock
  (2000): Duda-Krol W+, *Wiad Lek* 53(7), 454

FENOLDOPAM

Trade name: Corlopam (Abbott) (Neurex)
Indications: Hypertension (severe), hypertensive emergency
Category: Dopamine receptor agonist
Half-life: ~5 minutes
Clinically important, potentially hazardous interactions with: None

Reactions

Skin
Diaphoresis

Other
Chest pain
Headache
Injection-site reactions
Vertigo

FENOPROFEN

Trade names: Fenoprex; Fenopron; Fepron; Feprona; Nalfon (Ranbaxy); Nalgesic; Progesic
Indications: Arthritis
Category: Non-steroidal anti-inflammatory
Half-life: 2.5–3 hours
Clinically important, potentially hazardous interactions with: methotrexate

Reactions

Skin
Acne
Angioedema (<1%)
Bruising (<1%)
Bullous dermatitis
Diaphoresis (<0.5%)
Erythema multiforme (<1%)
  (1988): Stotts JS+, *J Am Acad Dermatol* 18, 755
Exanthems
  (1985): Bigby M+, *J Am Acad Dermatol* 12, 866
Exfoliative dermatitis (<1%)
Peripheral edema (<1%)
Pruritus (3–9%)
  (1992): Breathnach SM+, *Adverse Drug Reactions and the Skin*
    Blackwell, Oxford, 186 (passim)
  (1985): Bigby M+, *J Am Acad Dermatol* 12, 866
Purpura (<1%)
  (1992): Breathnach SM+, *Adverse Drug Reactions and the Skin*
    Blackwell, Oxford, 186 (passim)
Rash (sic) (>10%)
Stevens Johnson syndrome (<1%)
Toxic epidermal necrolysis (<1%)
  (1988): Stotts JS+, *J Am Acad Dermatol* 18, 755
Urticaria (1–3%)
  (1992): Breathnach SM+, *Adverse Drug Reactions and the Skin*
    Blackwell, Oxford, 186 (passim)
  (1985): Bigby M+, *J Am Acad Dermatol* 12, 866
Vesiculobullous eruption
  (1992): Breathnach SM+, *Adverse Drug Reactions and the Skin*
    Blackwell, Oxford, 186 (passim)

Mucosal/ENT
Aphthous stomatitis (<1%)
Dysgeusia (<1%) (metallic taste)
Glossopyrosis (<1%)
Oral ulceration
Stomatitis
Tinnitus
Xerostomia (>1%)

Hair
Hair – alopecia (<1%)

Other
Anaphylactoid reactions/Anaphylaxis
Headache
Hot flashes (<1%)

FENTANYL

Trade names: Actiq (Cephalon); Beatryl; Durogesic; Fentanest; Leptanal; Sublimaze
Indications: Chronic pain
Category: Analgesic, opioid; Anesthetic
Half-life: 1.5–6 hours
Clinically important, potentially hazardous interactions with: amiodarone, amprenavir, atazanavir, cimetidine, indinavir, itraconazole, ketoconazole, nelfinavir, ranitidine, ritonavir, saquinavir

Reactions

Skin
Clammy skin (<1%)
Diaphoresis (>10%)
  (2001): Litt JZ, Beachwood, OH (personal case) (observation)
  (1992): Calis KA+, *Clin Pharm* 11, 22
  (1992): Friesen RH+, *Anesthesiology* 76, 46
Edema
  (1990): Ducker P+, *Z Hautkr* (German) 65, 734
Erythema (at application site) (<1%)
  (2006): Schmid-Grendelmeier P+, *Curr Med Res Opin* 22(3), 501
  (1992): Mosser KH, *Am Fam Physician* 45, 2289
  (1990): Ducker P+, *Z Hautkr* (German) 65, 734
Exanthems
Exfoliative dermatitis
Fixed eruption
  (2001): Vaughan K, Lakewood, WA (from patch) (from Internet)
    (observation)
Papulo-nodular lesions (>1%)
Pruritus (3–44%)
  (2006): Sarvela PJ+, *Acta Anaesthesiol Scand* 50(2), 239
  (2002): Gurkan Y+, *Anesth Analg* 95(6), 1763
  (2002): Henry A+, *Reg Anesth Pain Med* 27(5), 538 (intrathecal)
  (2002): Nelson KE+, *Anesthesiology* 96(5), 1070
  (1999): Herman NL+, *Anesth Analg* 89, 378
  (1996): Larijani GE+, *Pharmacotherapy* 16, 958
  (1994): Gerwels JW+, *J Dermatol Surg Oncol* 20, 823
  (1992): Badner NH+, *Can J Anaesth* 39, 330
  (1992): Belzarena SD, *Anesth Analg* 74, 653
  (1992): Calis KA+, *Clin Pharm* 11, 22
  (1992): Friesen RH+, *Anesthesiology* 76, 46 (facial)
  (1992): Mosser KH, *Am Fam Physician* 45, 2289
  (1992): Mourisse J+, *Acta Anaesthesiol Scand* 36, 70
  (1992): Paech MJ, *Anaesth Intensive Care* 20, 15
  (1992): Sandler ES+, *Pediatrics* 89, 631
  (1992): Varrassi G+, *Anaesthesia* 47, 558
  (1992): White MJ+, *Can J Anaesth* 39, 594
  (1989): Ackerman WE+, *Can J Anaesth* 36, 388
  (1989): Jorrot JC+, *Ann Fr Anesth Réanim* (French) 8, 321 (22%)
  (1988): Davies GG+, *Anesthesiology* 69, 763
  (1988): Monk JP+, *Drugs* 36, 286 (40%)
  (1986): Shipton EA+, *S Afr Med J* 70, 325 (13%)
Purpura
  (2001): Tweed WA+, *Anesth Analg* 92, 1442
Pustules (<1%)
Rash (sic) (>1%)
  (1992): Sandler ES+, *Pediatrics* 89, 631
  (1992): Stoukides CA+, *Clin Pharm* 11, 222
Urticaria (<1%)

Mucosal/ENT
Dysgeusia (<1%)
Stomatitis
  (2004): Hanks GW+, *Palliat Med* 18(8), 698

Xerostomia (>10%)
  (2001): Litt JZ, Beachwood, OH (personal case) (observation)
  (1992): Calis KA+, *Clin Pharm* 11, 22

Other

Abdominal pain
Anaphylactoid reactions/Anaphylaxis
  (2007): Cummings KC 3rd+, *Can J Anaesth* 54(4), 301
  (2001): Girgis Y, *Anaesthesia* 56(10), 1016
  (2001): Konarzewski W+, *Anaesthesia* 56(5), 497 (with
    propofol) (fatal)
  (2001): Lewis S+, *Anaesthesia* 56(11), 1128
  (1990): Ducker P+, *Z Hautkr* (German) 65, 734
Application-site reactions
Asthenia
Confusion
Cough
  (2007): Yeh CC+, *J Clin Anesth* 19(1), 53
  (2006): Oshima T+, *Can J Anaesth* 53(8), 753
  (2005): Schlimp CJ+, *Can J Anaesth* 52(2), 207
  (2004): Pandey CK+, *Anesth Analg* 99(6), 1696
  (2002): Tsou CH+, *Acta Anaesthesiol Sin* 40(4), 165
  (2001): Tweed WA+, *Anesth Analg* 92(6), 1442
Death
  (2005): Ekedahl A+, *Lakartidningen* 102(39), 2788
  (2002): Mertes PM+, *Anaesthesia* 57(8), 821 (with propofol)
  (2002): Reeves MD+, *Med J Aust* 177(10), 552
  (2001): Girgis Y, *Anaesthesia* 56(10), 1016
Depression
Headache
Hypertension
  (2006): Sato Y+, *Masui* 55(10), 1260
Hypotension
  (1990): Ruff R+, *J Cardiothorac Anesth* 4(3), 314
Inappropriate secretion of antidiuretic hormone (SIADH)
  (2002): Kokko H+, *Pharmacotherapy* 22(9), 1188
Insomnia
Paresthesias (<1%)
Somnolence
Vertigo
  (2004): Hanks GW+, *Palliat Med* 18(8), 698
  (2002): *Prescrire Int* 11(60), 106

FEVERFEW

Scientific names: *Chrysanthemum parthenium; Pyrethrum
parthenium; Tanacetum parthenium*
Family: Asteraceae; Compositae
Trade and other common names: Atamisa; Featerfoiul;
Featherfew; Featherfoil; MIG-99; Santa Maria
Category: Antipyretic
Purported indications and other uses: Fever, headache,
migraine, menstrual irregularities, arthritis, psoriasis, allergy,
asthma, tinnitus, vertigo, nausea, cold, earache, orthopedic
disorders, swollen feet, diarrhea, dyspepsia
Half-life: N/A
**Clinically important, potentially hazardous interactions
with:** anticoagulants, NSAIDs, warfarin

Reactions

Skin

Adverse effects (sic) (mild)
  (2000): Ernst E+, *Public Health Nutr* 3(4A), 509
Allergic reactions (sic)

(1983): Hausen BM+, *Acta Derm Venereol* 63(4), 308
Angioedema (lips)
  (1998): Awang DVC, *Int Med* 1, 11
  (1985): Johnson ES+, *BMJ (Clin Res Ed)* 291, 569
Dermatitis
  (2006): Verma KK+, *Indian J Dermatol Venereol Leprol* 72(1), 24
  (2002): Paulsen E+, *Contact Dermatitis* 47(1), 14
  (1996): Lamminpaa A+, *Contact Dermatitis* 34, 330
Prurigo nodularis
  (2000): Sharma VK+, *Contact Dermatitis* 42(4), 235

Mucosal/ENT

Ageusia
  (1998): Awang DVC, *Int Med* 1, 11
  (1985): Johnson ES+, *BMJ (Clin Res Ed)* 291, 569
Oral ulceration
  (1998): Awang DVC, *Int Med* 1, 11
  (1985): Johnson ES+, *BMJ (Clin Res Ed)* 291, 569

FEXOFENADINE

Trade name: Allegra (Sanofi-Aventis)
Indications: Allergic rhinitis, pruritus, urticaria
Category: Histamine H1 receptor antagonist
Half-life: 14.4 hours
**Clinically important, potentially hazardous interactions
with: St John's wort**

Reactions

Skin

Acne
  (1998): Litt JZ, Beachwood, OH (personal case) (observation)
Psoriasis
  (2006): Saraswat A+, *Clin Exp Dermatol* 31(3), 477 (pustular)
Pustules
  (2006): Saraswat A+, *Clin Exp Dermatol* 31(3), 477

Other

Headache
  (2004): Meltzer EO+, *Pediatr Allergy Immunol* 15(3), 253
  (2001): Kulthanan K+, *J Med Assoc Thai* 84(2), 153

FILGRASTIM

(See GRANULOCYTE COLONY-STIMULATING FACTOR
(GCSF))

FINASTERIDE

Trade names: Pro-Cure; Propecia (Merck); Proscar (Merck);
Proscar 5
Indications: Benign prostatic hypertrophy, male-pattern
baldness
Category: 5-alpha reductase inhibitor; Androgen antagonist
Half-life: 4.8–6 hours

Reactions

Skin

Edema of lip
Erythema annulare centrifugum
  (2007): Al Hammadi A+, *J Drugs Dermatol* 6(4), 460

Folliculitis
  (2000): Price VH+, *J Am Acad Dermatol* 43, 768
Rash (sic)
  (1999): Cather JC+, *Cutis* 64, 167
Urticaria

Hair

Hair – hypotrichosis
  (1998): Panagotacos PJ (reversal of graying hair) (from Internet)
    (observation)
Hair – patchy hair, loss of beard
  (1999): Mitchell D, Thomasville, GA (from Internet)
    (observation)
  (1998): Drayton GE, Los Angeles, CA (from Internet)
    (observation)

Nails

Nails – onychomycosis
  (1999): Mitchell D, Thomasville, GA (from Internet)
    (observation)

Other

Depression
  (2006): Rahimi-Ardabili B+, *BMC Clin Pharmacol* 6, 7
  (2002): Altomare G+, *J Dermatol* 29(10), 665 (19 cases)
Gynecomastia
  (2002): Ferrando J+, *Arch Dermatol* 138, 543
  (2000): Wade MS+, *Australas J Dermatol* 41, 55 (painful and
    reversible)
  (2000): Zimmerman RL+, *Arch Pathol Lab Med* 124, 625
  (1999): Cather JC+, *Cutis* 64, 167 (passim)
  (1999): Miller JA+, *South Med J* 92, 615
  (1997): Carlin BI+, *J Urol* 158, 547
  (1997): Staiman VR+, *Urology* 50, 929
  (1996): Green L+, *New Engl J Med* 335, 823
  (1996): Wilton L+, *Br J Urol* 78, 379
  (1995): Volpi R+, *Am J Med Sci* 309, 322
Hepatotoxicity
  (2006): Martinez de Guzman M+, *Farm Hosp* 30(6), 385
Myalgia/Myositis/Myopathy/Myotoxicity (severe)
  (1999): Cather JC+, *Cutis* 64, 167

FISH OILS

Scientific names: *docosahexaenoic acid (DHA); eicosapentaenoic
acid (EPA); Omega-3 fatty acids*
Trade and other common names: Cod liver oil; n-3 fatty
acids; polyunsaturated fatty acids (PUFA)
Category: Anti-inflammatory; Lipid regulator
Purported indications and other uses: Albuminuria, anorexia
nervosa, cardiovascular disease, hypertension, lupus
erythematosus, macular degeneration, osteoarthritis, otitis media,
psoriasis
Half-life: N/A

Note: More than 25 mL or 3 g per day can decrease blood
coagulation and increase the risk of bleeding. Fish oils contain a
significant amount of vitamins A and D and high doses may be toxic

Reactions

Skin

Malignant melanoma
  (1997): Veierod MB+, *Int J Cancer* 71(4), 600

Mucosal/ENT

Dysgeusia
  (2002): Carroll DN+, *Ann Pharmacother* 36(12), 1950

  (1992): Zakaria B+, *Fortschr Med* 110(10), 178

Eyes

Glaucoma
  (2004): Kang JH+, *Am J Clin Nutr* 79(5), 755

Other

Lymphoid hyperplasia
  (1988): Ogden P+, *Ann Intern Med* 109(10), 843

FLAVOXATE

Trade names: Bladderon; Genurin; Harnin; Patricin; Spasuret;
Urispadol; Urispas (Ortho-McNeil); Uronid
Indications: Dysuria, urgency, nocturia
Category: Anticholinergic; Muscarinic antagonist
Half-life: Onset of action: 55–60 minutes
**Clinically important, potentially hazardous interactions
with:** anticholinergics, arbutamine

Reactions

Skin

Exanthems
Fixed eruption
  (1999): Enomoto U+, *Contact Dermatitis* 40(6), 337
Jaundice
  (1999): Sevenoaks M+, *J R Soc Med* 92(11), 589
Rash (sic) (<1%)
  (1999): Enomoto U+, *Contact Dermatitis* 40, 337
Urticaria

Mucosal/ENT

Oral ulceration
Xerostomia (>10%)

Other

Headache
Hypersensitivity
  (1986): Hirohata S+, *Arch Intern Med* 146, 2409

FLECAINIDE

Trade names: Almarytm; Apocard; Corflene; Flecaine; Tabco;
Tambocor (3M)
Indications: Atrial fibrillation
Category: Antiarrhythmic class 1c
Half-life: 7–22 hours
**Clinically important, potentially hazardous interactions
with:** amisulpride, darifenacin, fosamprenavir, ritonavir, tipranavir

Reactions

Skin

Diaphoresis (<3%)
Edema (3.5%)
Exanthems (>1%)
  (2003): Litt JZ, Beachwood, OH (personal case) (observation)
  (1985): Holmes B+, *Drugs* 27, 301 (1.4%)
Exfoliative dermatitis (<1%)
Pruritus (<1%)
  (2003): Litt JZ, Beachwood, OH (personal case) (observation)
Psoriasis
  (1988): Mancuso G+, *G Ital Dermatol Venerol* (Italian) 123, 171

(1985): Holmes B+, *Drugs* 27, 301
Rash (sic) (<3%)
Urticaria (<1%)

Mucosal/ENT
Dysgeusia (<1%) (metallic taste)
Oral edema
Tinnitus
Tongue edema (<1%)
Xerostomia (<1%)

Hair
Hair – alopecia (<1%)

Other
Cardiotoxicity
   (2007): Khavandi A+, *Emerg Med J* 24(5), e26
Congestive heart failure
   (1985): Platia EV+, *Am J Cardiol* 55(8), 956
Depression
   (1988): Drerup U, *Dtsch Med Wochenschr* 113(10), 386
Headache
Myalgia/Myositis/Myopathy/Myotoxicity (<1%)
Paresthesias (<1%)
Tremor (5%)

FLOXURIDINE

Trade name: FUDR (Roche)
Indications: Gastrointestinal carcinoma, metastatic to the liver
Category: Antimetabolite; Antineoplastic
Half-life: N/A
Clinically important, potentially hazardous interactions with: cimetidine, phenytoin

Reactions

Skin
Abscess
Acne
Allergic reactions (sic)
Bullous dermatitis
Dermatitis
   (1986): Hohn DC+, *Cancer* 57(3), 465
Erythema
Exanthems
Fissures
Palmar–plantar erythema
   (1993): Conroy T+, *Cancer* 72(7), 2190
   (1987): Neuss MN+, *J Natl Med Assoc* 79(6), 669
Petechiae
Photosensitivity
Pigmentation
Pruritus
Purpura
Rash (sic)
Xerosis

Mucosal/ENT
Gingivitis
Glossitis
Mucositis
   (1999): Soori GS+, *Cancer Invest* 17(6), 379 (11%) (with interferon alfa)
   (1996): Baiocchi C+, *Tumori* 82(3), 225
   (1993): Falcone A+, *Cancer* 72(2), 564

Oral ulceration
Stomatitis
   (1986): Hohn DC+, *Cancer* 57(3), 465
Stomatodynia
Tongue edema

Hair
Hair – alopecia
Hair – brittle

Nails
Nails – loss

Eyes
Epiphora
Vision blurred

Other
Anaphylactoid reactions/Anaphylaxis
Asthenia
   (1999): Soori GS+, *Cancer Invest* 17(6), 379 (50%) (with interferon alfa)
   (1993): Falcone A+, *Cancer* 72(2), 564
Chills
Cough
Depression
Fever
   (1999): Soori GS+, *Cancer Invest* 17(6), 379 (22%) (with interferon alfa)
   (1993): Falcone A+, *Cancer* 72(2), 564
Paresthesias
Seizures
Thrombophlebitis
Vertigo

FLUCONAZOLE

Trade names: Biozolene; Diflucan (Pfizer); Flucazol; Flukezol; Fluzone; Fungata; Triflucan
Indications: Candidiasis
Category: Antibiotic, triazole
Half-life: 25–30 hours
Clinically important, potentially hazardous interactions with: alprazolam, amphotericin B, anisindione, anticoagulants, dicumarol, eplerenone, erythromycin, methadone, midazolam, phenobarbital, phenytoin, ramelteon, sulfonylureas, vinblastine, vincristine, warfarin

Reactions

Skin
Acne
   (1998): Drake L, *J Am Acad Dermatol* 38, S87
Acute generalized exanthematous pustulosis (AGEP)
   (2002): Alsadhan A+, *J Cutan Med Surg* 6(2), 122
   (2002): Di Lernia V, Italy (from Internet) (observation)
   (2002): Fabre B+, *Ann Dermatol Venereol* 129(3), 294
Angioedema
   (1999): Errico MR, Buenos Aires, Argentina (from Internet) (observation)
   (1991): Abbott M+, *Lancet* 2, 633
Bullous dermatitis
   (1994): Gupta AK+, *J Am Acad Dermatol* 30, 911
Erythema multiforme
   (1994): Gupta AK+, *J Am Acad Dermatol* 30, 911
   (1991): Gussenhoven MJE+, *Lancet* 338, 120

Exanthems (>1%)
 (2001): Altman EM, West Orange, NJ (from Internet)
  (observation)
 (1990): Grant SM+, *Drugs* 39, 877 (1.8%) (in AIDS patients)
Exfoliative dermatitis
 (1994): Gupta AK+, *J Am Acad Dermatol* 30, 911 (passim)
 (1990): Grant SM+, *Drugs* 39, 877
Fixed eruption
 (2006): Mahendra A+, *Indian J Dermatol Venereol Leprol*
  72(5), 391 (oral)
 (2004): Goel A+, *J Dermatol* 31(4), 345
 (2003): Lane JE+, *Oral Surg Oral Med Oral Pathol Oral Radiol*
  Endod 95(2), 129
 (2002): Ghislain P-D, *J Am Acad Dermatol* 46, 47 (recurrence)
 (2001): Hudson TF, Conway, AR (from Internet) (observation)
 (2000): Heikkilä H+, *J Am Acad Dermatol* 42, 883
 (1997): Danby B, Kingston, Ontario (from Internet)
  (observation)
 (1997): Jaffe P, Columbia, SC (from Internet) (observation)
 (1994): Morgan JM+, *BMJ* 308, 454
Hypertrophy
 (1998): Drake L+, *J Am Acad Dermatol* 38, S87
Pallor (<1%)
Petechiae
 (1995): Mercurio MG+, *J Am Acad Dermatol* 32, 525
Pruritus
 (1999): Errico MR, Buenos Aires, Argentina (from Internet)
  (observation)
 (1991): Neuhaus G+, *BMJ* 302, 1341
Purpura
 (1990): Agarwal A+, *Ann Intern Med* 113, 899
Rash (sic) (1.8%)
 (1998): Scher RK+, *J Am Acad Dermatol* 38, S77
 (1995): Powderly WG, *Infections in Medicine* 257 (passim)
 (1994): Gupta AK+, *J Am Acad Dermatol* 30, 911 (1.8%)
Stevens–Johnson syndrome
 (1995): Powderly WG, *Infections in Medicine* 257 (passim)
 (1991): Gussenhoven MJE+, *Lancet* 1, 120
 (1990): Sugar AM+, *Rev Infect Dis* 12, S338
Toxic epidermal necrolysis
 (1993): Azon-Masoliver A+, *Dermatology* 187, 268
 (1990): Grant SM+, *Drugs* 39, 877
Urticaria

Mucosal/ENT

Dysgeusia
 (1998): Quart AM+, *Infect Med* 15, 379
 (1991): Neuhaus G+, *BMJ* 302, 1341
Oral ulceration
 (1998): Ling MR+, *J Am Acad Dermatol* 38, S95
 (1991): Abbott M+, *Lancet* 2, 633
Xerostomia
 (1998): Quart AM+, *Infect Med* 15, 379

Hair

Hair – alopecia
 (2001): Ondo A, Las Cruces, NM (from Internet) (observation)
 (1996): Goldsmith LA, *Ann Intern Med* 125, 153
 (1995): Pappas PG+, *Ann Intern Med* 123, 354
 (1993): Weinroth SE+, *Ann Intern Med* 119, 637

Nails

Nails – changes (sic)
 (1998): Drake L+, *J Am Acad Dermatol* 38, S87
 (1998): Ling MR+, *J Am Acad Dermatol* 38, S95
Nails – melanonychia (longitudinal)
 (1998): Kar HK, *Int J Dermatol* 37, 719

Eyes

Ocular hemorrhage

 (2002): Mootha VV+, *Arch Ophthalmol* 120(1), 94 (with
  warfarin)

Other

Anaphylactoid reactions/Anaphylaxis (in AIDS patients)
Headache
Hypersensitivity (1–4%)
 (1997): Craig TJ, *J Am Osteopath Assoc* 97, 584
Nephrotoxicity
 (2007): Shin GT+, *Am J Kidney* 49(2), 318
Paresthesias
 (1991): Neuhaus G+, *BMJ* 302, 1341
Rhabdomyolysis
 (2004): Moro H+, *AIDS Patient Care STDS* 18(12), 687 (with
  simvastatin)
 (2003): Shaukat A+, *Ann Pharmacother* 37(7), 1032 (with
  simvastatin)

FLUCYTOSINE

Trade names: 5-FC; Alcobon; Ancobon; Ancotil
Indications: Candidal and cryptococcal infections
Category: Antimycobacterial
Half-life: 3–8 hours
**Clinically important, potentially hazardous interactions
with:** amphotericin B

Reactions

Skin

Exanthems
 (1987): Thyss A+, *Ann Dermatol Venereol* (French) 114, 1131
Photosensitivity (<1%)
 (1987): Thyss A+, *Ann Dermatol Venereol* (French) 114, 1131
 (1983): Shelley WB+, *J Am Acad Dermatol* 8, 229
Pruritus
Purpura
Rash (sic) (1–10%)
Urticaria

Mucosal/ENT

Xerostomia

Other

Anaphylactoid reactions/Anaphylaxis (<1%)
 (1988): Kotani S+, *JAMA* 260(22), 3275
Headache
Paresthesias (<1%)
Thrombophlebitis
 (2005): Natarajan G+, *J Perinatol* 25(12), 770

FLUDARABINE

Trade name: Fludara (Schering)
Indications: Chronic lymphocytic leukemia (B-cell)
Category: Antimetabolite; Antineoplastic
Half-life: 9 hours
**Clinically important, potentially hazardous interactions
with:** aldesleukin, clofazimine

Reactions

Skin

Edema (>10%)

Exanthems
  (2004): Huang HQ+, *Ai Zheng* 23(4), 448
Herpes simplex
  (2007): Satzger I+, *Eur J Dermatol* 17(2), 165
Paraneoplastic pemphigus
  (2007): Yildiz O+, *Med Oncol* 24(1), 115
  (2004): Powell AM+, *J Eur Acad Dermatol Venereol* 18(3), 360
  (2001): Gooptu C+, *Br J Dermatol* 144(6), 1255 (3 cases)
  (1995): Bazarbachi A+, *Ann Oncol* 6, 730
Petechiae
  (2001): Churn M+, *Clin Oncol* 13, 273
Rash (sic) (>10%)
  (2003): Leitman SF+, *Transfusion* 43(12), 1667
Squamous cell carcinoma
  (1997): Davidovitz Y+, *Acta Haematol* 98, 44 (flare-up)

Mucosal/ENT
Dysgeusia (<1%) (metallic taste)
Stomatitis (>10%)

Hair
Hair – alopecia (1–10%)

Other
Application-site reactions
  (2002): Rai KR+, *J Clin Oncol* 20(18), 3891 (with alemtuzumab)
Chills (>10%)
Death
  (2002): Klasa RJ+, *J Clin Oncol* 20(24), 4649 (3 patients)
Fever
  (2003): Leitman SF+, *Transfusion* 43(12), 1667
Infections
  (2002): Rai KR+, *J Clin Oncol* 20(18), 3891 (with alemtuzumab)
Myalgia/Myositis/Myopathy/Myotoxicity (>10%)
Paresthesias (>10%)

FLUMAZENIL

Trade names: Anexate; Lanexat; Romazicon (Roche)
Indications: Benzodiazepine overdose
Category: Benzodiazepine antagonist
Half-life: terminal: 41–79 minutes
Clinically important, potentially hazardous interactions with: alcohol, neuromuscular blockers

Reactions

Skin
Diaphoresis (3–9%)
Rash (sic)
Urticaria (<1%)

Mucosal/ENT
Tinnitus
Tongue disorder (sic) (<1%)
Xerostomia (1–10%)

Other
Asthenia
  (1993): Spivey WH+, *Ann Emerg Med* 22(12), 1813 (3%)
Headache
  (1993): Spivey WH+, *Ann Emerg Med* 22(12), 1813 (3%)
Hot flashes (1–10%)
Injection-site pain (3–9%)
  (1993): Spivey WH+, *Ann Emerg Med* 22(12), 1813 (10%)
Injection-site reactions (sic)
Paresthesias (1–10%)

Seizures
  (1996): Davis CO+, *J Emerg Med* 14(3), 331
  (1996): Taki H+, *Masui* 45(10), 1247
  (1995): McDuffee AT+, *Pediatr Emerg Care* 11(3), 186
  (1995): Proudfoot AT, *Toxicol Lett* 82–83, 779
  (1994): Ng KO+, *Zhonghua Yi Xue Za Zhi* (Taipei) 53(6), 383
  (1993): Hoffman EJ+, *Clin Pharm* 12(9), 641
  (1993): Longmire AW+, *Am J Med Sci* 306(1), 49
  (1993): Spivey WH+, *Ann Emerg Med* 22(12), 1813
  (1991): O'Connor HJ, *Endoscopy* 23(1), 53
  (1991): Pietila K+, *Duodecim* 107(23–24), 1985
  (1990): Nielsen J+, *Ugeskr Laeger* 152(38), 2737
  (1989): Marchant B+, *BMJ* 299(6703), 860
Thrombophlebitis
Tremor (1–10%)
Vertigo
  (2006): Ondo WG+, *Mov Disord* 21(10), 1614

FLUMETASONE

Trade names: Locacorten (Bioglan); Locasalen (Bioglan)
Indications: Dermatoses
Category: Corticosteroid, topical
Half-life: N/A
Clinically important, potentially hazardous interactions with: live vaccines

Reactions

Skin
Atrophy
Bruising
Burning
Dermatitis
Erythema
Folliculitis
Irritation
Pruritus
Rash (sic)
Rosacea
Scaling
Sensitivity
Thinning

Other
Infections
Paresthesias

FLUNISOLIDE

Trade names: Aerobid (Roche); Nasalide (Ivax); Nasarel (Ivax)
Indications: Asthma, rhinitis
Category: Corticosteroid, inhaled
Half-life: N/A
Clinically important, potentially hazardous interactions with: aspirin, cyclosporine, digoxin, diuretics, estrogens, ketoconazole, **live vaccines**, oral contraceptives, phenobarbital, phenytoin, rifampin, warfarin

Reactions

Skin
Edema

Rash (sic)
Rosacea
Xerosis

Mucosal/ENT
Dysgeusia
  (1994): Conley SF, *Ann Allergy* 72(6), 529
  (1988): Greenbaum J+, *Ann Allergy* 61(4), 305
  (1985): Dry J+, *J Int Med Res* 13(5), 289
Oral candidiasis
  (1999): Jackson LD+, *Can J Clin* 6(1), 26

Eyes
Cataract
Epiphora
Glaucoma
Visual disturbances

Other
Adverse effects (sic)
  (2001): Terzano C+, *Adv Ther* 18(6), 253
Cough
Headache
  (2002): Trangsrud AJ+, *Pharmacotherapy* 22(11), 1458
  (1992): Bryson HM+, *Drugs* 43(5), 760
  (1988): Greenbaum J+, *Ann Allergy* 61(4), 305
  (1980): Sahay JN+, *Clin Allergy* 10(1), 65
Infections
Myalgia/Myositis/Myopathy/Myotoxicity
Paresthesias

FLUOCINOLONE

Trade names: Capex (Galderma); Synalar (Medicis)
Indications: Dermatoses, Asthma, Ophthalmology
Category: Corticosteroid, topical
Half-life: N/A
Clinically important, potentially hazardous interactions with: live vaccines

Reactions

Skin
Adverse effects (sic)
Atrophy
Burning
Facial erythema
  (1981): Tirlapur VG+, *Br J Clin Pract* 35(7-8), 275
Pigmentation
Pruritus
Rash (sic)
  (1993): Hisa T+, *Contact Dermatitis* 28(3), 174
Rosacea
Sensitivity
  (1983): Pasricha JS+, *Contact Dermatitis* 9(4), 330
Telangiectasia
  (1981): Tirlapur VG+, *Br J Clin Pract* 35(7-8), 275
Thinning
  (1984): Somerma S+, *Acta Derm Venereol* 64(1), 41
Ulcerative necrosis

Eyes
Cataract
  (2006): Jaffe GJ+, *Ophthalmology* 113(6), 1020
  (2005): Holekamp NM+, *Am J Ophthalmol* 139(3), 421
Glaucoma

  (1995): Katsushima H, *Nippon Ganka Gakkai Zasshi* 99(2), 238
Intraocular pressure increased
  (2006): Jaffe GJ+, *Ophthalmology* 113(6), 1020
Ocular pressure
  (2005): Holekamp NM+, *Am J Ophthalmol* 139(3), 421
  (2005): Jaffe GJ+, *Ophthalmology* 112(7), 1192
  (2000): Jaffe GJ+, *Ophthalmology* 107(11), 2024
Retinitis
  (2007): Ufret-Vincenty RL+, *Am J Ophthalmol* 143(2), 334

Other
Infections
Side effects (sic)
  (1985): Jegasothy B+, *Int J Dermatol* 24(7), 461

FLUOCINONIDE

Trade names: Fluonex; Lidex (Medicis); Lonide; Topsyn
Indications: Dermatoses
Category: Corticosteroid, topical
Half-life: N/A
Clinically important, potentially hazardous interactions with: live vaccines

Reactions

Skin
Acne
Adverse effects (sic)
  (1994): Bruce S+, *J Am Acad Dermatol* 31(5), 755
  (1985): Jegasothy B+, *Int J Dermatol* 24(7), 461 (12%)
Burning
Dermatitis
  (1999): Miura Y+, *Contact Dermatitis* 41(2), 118
  (1993): Hisa T+, *Contact Dermatitis* 28, 174
Erythema
Pigmentation
Pruritus
  (1996): Carbone M+, *Minerva Stomatol* 45(3), 61
Rash (sic)
Rosacea
Xerosis

Mucosal/ENT
Mucosal bleeding
  (1996): Carbone M+, *Minerva Stomatol* 45(3), 61

Eyes
Keratopathy
  (2005): Savage HI+, *Cornea* 24(3), 342 (with ketoconazole)

Other
Infections

FLUORIDES

Trade names: Acidulated phosphate fluoride; F;
Fluorophosphate; Hydrogen fluoride [HF]; Monofluorophosphate
[MFP]; Silicofluoride; Sodium fluoride [NaF]; Sodium
monofluorophosphate; Stannous fluoride [SF]; Sulfur hexafluoride
[SF6]
Indications: Caries prevention (topical), osteoporosis prevention
(oral)
Category: Chemical
Half-life: N/A
**Clinically important, potentially hazardous interactions
with: caffeine**

Reactions

Skin

Acne
Atopic dermatitis
Burning
  (2002): Fujimoto K+, *J Nippon Med Sch* 69(2), 180 (HF)
  (1995): Saada V+, *Ann Dermatol Venereol* 122(8), 512 (HF)
  (1993): Bordelon BM+, *J Trauma* 34(3), 437 (HF)
  (1992): Mistry DG+, *Am Fam Physician* 45(4), 1748 (HF)
  (1988): MacKinnon MA, *Dermatol Clin* 6(1), 67 (HF)
  (1987): Modly CE+, *Cutis* 40(2), 89
  (1987): Mullett T+, *J Burn Care Rehabil* 8(3), 216 (HF) (fatal)
  (1986): Edelman P, *Occup Med* 1(1), 89 (HF)
  (1986): Vance MV+, *Ann Emerg Med* 15(8), 890 (HF)
  (1985): Mayer TG+, *Ann Emerg Med* 14(2), 149 (HF)
  (1980): Tepperman PB, *J Occup Med* 22(10), 691 (HF)
Calcification
Carcinoma
  (1996): Tohyama E, *J Epidemiol* 6(4), 184 (uterine)
Dermatitis
  (2003): McCaffery K, *J Am Dent Assoc* 134(9), 1166
  (1997): Ganter G+, *Contact Dermatitis* 37(5), 248
  (1993): Isaksson M+, *Scand J Dent Res* 101(1), 49 (Duraphat)
Dermatitis herpetiformis
  (1985): Bovenmyer DA, *J Am Acad Dermatol* 12(4), 719
    (aggravataion)
Edema
  (1995): Saada V+, *Ann Dermatol Venereol* 122(8), 512 (HF)
Erythema
  (2002): Fujimoto K+, *J Nippon Med Sch* 69(2), 180 (HF)
  (1995): Saada V+, *Ann Dermatol Venereol* 122(8), 512 (HF)
Folliculitis
  (1982): Andersen KE+, *Contact Dermatitis* 8(3), 173 (Triphenyl
    tin fluoride in paint)
Inflammation
  (2002): Lund K+, *Inhal Toxicol* 14(2), 119 (HF)
Necrosis
  (1999): Sjostrom S+, *J Clin Periodontol* 26(4), 257 (SF gel)
  (1995): Saada V+, *Ann Dermatol Venereol* 122(8), 512 (HF)
Papulo-nodular lesions
Perioral dermatitis
  (1992): Ferlito TA, *J Clin Orthod* 26(1), 43
Pruritus
Pustules
  (1985): Dooms-Goossens A+, *Contact Dermatitis* 12(1), 42
    (NaF)
Side effects (sic)
  (1987): Rubenstein LK+, *ASDC J Dent Child* 54(4), 245 (topical F)
Urticaria
  (1993): Camarasa JG+, *Contact Dermatitis* 28(5), 294 (NaF)
Vesiculation

  (2002): Fujimoto K+, *J Nippon Med Sch* 69(2), 180 (HF)

Mucosal/ENT

Aphthous stomatitis
Gingival lesions
  (2000): Banks PA+, *Eur J Orthod* 22(4), 401 (50% [SF])
Mucosal irritation
Oral ulceration
Rhinitis
Stomatitis
  (1997): Ganter G+, *Contact Dermatitis* 37(5), 248
  (1993): Isaksson M+, *Scand J Dent Res* 101(1), 49 (Duraphat)
Xerostomia
  (1985): Grad H+, *J Can Dent Assoc* 51(4), 296

Eyes

Cataract
  (1985): Thienpont P+, *Bull Soc Ophtalmol Fr* 85(2), 253 (SF6)
  (1983): Werry H+, *Klin Monatsbl Augenheilkd* 182(4), 331 (SF6)
Conjunctivitis
Ocular allergy
Ocular stinging
  (1997): Lund K+, *Occup Environ Med* 54(1), 32 (HF)

Other

Abdominal pain
  (1994): Das TK+, *J Clin Gastroenterol* 18(3), 194
Adverse effects (sic)
  (2003): Marinho VC+, *J Dent Educ* 67(4), 448
  (2002): Ringe JD+, *Rheumatol Int* 22(1), 27 (mild)
  (1997): Gotjamanos T+, *Aust Dent J* 42(1), 52
  (1993): Spittle B, *Fluoride* 26(4), 267
  (1992): Garcia-Sanchez MJ+, *Rev Esp Anestesiol Reanim*
    39(5), 285 (isoflurane)
  (1992): Muller P+, *Z Gastroenterol* 30(4), 252 (NaF) (4 cases)
  (1987): Hasling C+, *Miner Electrolyte Metab* 13(2), 96 (51%)
    (NaF + Ca + vitamin D)
  (1985): Dubovsky J+, *Ala Med* 54(12), 47
Chest pain
  (1993): Uyama T+, *Surg Today* 23(9), 807 (SF6)
Death
  (1998): Klasner AE+, *Ann Emerg Med* 31(4), 525
  (1998): Mullins ME+, *Ann Emerg Med* 31(4), 524 (HF)
  (1996): Tohyama E, *J Epidemiol* 6(4), 184
  (1994): Arnow PM+, *Ann Intern Med* 121(5), 339 (hemodialysis)
  (1987): Mullett T+, *J Burn Care Rehabil* 8(3), 216 (HF)
  (1985): Mayer TG+, *Ann Emerg Med* 14(2), 149 (HF)
  (1980): Tepperman PB, *J Occup Med* 22(10), 691 (HF)
Headache
Hypersensitivity
  (1996): Lopez-Serrano MC+, *J Investig Allergol Clin Immunol*
    6(5), 324 (F-containing corticosteroids)
  (1996): Soyseth V+, *Allergy* 51(10), 719 (environmental
    exposure)
  (1993): Isaksson M+, *Scand J Dent Res* 101(1), 49 (Duraphat)
  (1993): Spittle B, *Fluoride* 26(4), 267
  (1990): Kaminsky LS+, *Crit Rev Oral Biol Med* 1(4), 261
  (1988): Razak IA+, *Ann Dent* 47(2), 37 (SF)
Toxicity (sic)
  (2001): Chang YC+, *Oral Surg Oral Med Oral Pathol Oral Radiol
    Endod* 91(2), 230
  (2001): Gupta SK+, *Indian Pediatr* 38(2), 139
  (2001): Kleinsasser NH+, *Laryngorhinootologie* 80(4), 187
  (2001): Lubben B+, *Laryngorhinootologie* 80(4), 214
  (2000): Masters RD+, *Neurotoxicology* 21(6), 1091
  (1999): Sjostrom S+, *J Clin Periodontol* 26(4), 257 (SF gel)
  (1997): Gotjamanos T+, *Aust Dent J* 42(1), 52
  (1997): Lochhead KM+, *Am J Pathol* 150(6), 2209 (F anesthetics)
  (1997): Shulman JD+, *J Public Health Dent* 57(3), 150
  (1996): Cittanova ML+, *Anesthesiology* 84(2), 428 (F anesthetics)

(1996): Klasaer AE+, *Ann Emerg Med* 28(6), 713 (HF)
(1994): Das TK+, *J Clin Gastroenterol* 18(3), 194
(1993): Bordelon BM+, *J Trauma* 34(3), 437 (HF)
(1992): Whitford GM, *J Dent Res* 71(5), 1249
(1990): Spak CJ+, *J Dent Res* 69(2), 426
(1988): Caravati EM, *Am J Emerg Med* 6(2), 143 (HF)
(1988): Greco RJ+, *J Trauma* 28(11), 1593 (HF) (3 cases)
(1987): Lantz O+, *Am J Kidney Dis* 10(2), 136 (Vichy water)
(1987): Whitford GM, *J Dent Res* 66(5), 1056 (5.0 mg F/kg)
(1987): Whitford GM+, *J Dent Res* 66(5), 1072 (APF gel)
(1987): Zaborra G+, *Stomatol Mediterr* 7(3), 387
(1985): Bayless JM+, *J Am Dent Assoc* 110(2), 209
(1984): Mazze RI, *Can Anaesth Soc J* 31(3 Pt 2), S16 (methoxyflurane)

FLUOROURACIL

Trade names: Carac (Dermik); Efudex (Valeant); Efudix; Efurix; Fluoroplex (Allergan)
Category: Antimetabolite; Antineoplastic
Half-life: 8–20 minutes
Clinically important, potentially hazardous interactions with: aldesleukin, **bromelain**, cimetidine, granulocyte colony-stimulating factor (GCSF)), metronidazole

Reactions

Skin
Acral erythema
(2007): Adachi A+, *Dermatology* 214(1), 85
(1995): Esteve E+, *Ann Med Interne Paris* (French) 146, 192
(1992): Doll DC+, *Semin Oncol* 19(5), 580
(1989): Vukelja SJ+, *Ann Intern Med* 111, 688
Actinic keratoses
(1999): Nabai H+, *Cutis* 64, 43
(1987): Johnson TM+, *J Am Acad Dermatol* 17(2 Pt 1), 192
Angioedema
Bullous dermatitis
Dermatitis (>10%)
(1999): Sanchez-Perez J+, *Contact Dermatitis* 41, 106
(1997): Anderson LL+, *J Am Acad Dermatol* 36, 478
(1996): Nadal C+, *Contact Dermatitis* 35, 124 (systemic)
Diaphoresis
(1994): Anand AJ, *Ann Pharmacother* 28(3), 374
Eczema
(2003): Salim A+, *Br J Dermatol* 148(3), 539
Eosinophilic pustular folliculitis
(2007): Laing ME+, *Photodermatol Photoimmunol Photomed* 23(2-3), 62
Erosion of psoriatic plaques
(2002): Wetzig T+, *Br J Dermatol* 147(4), 824
Erosions
(2003): Salim A+, *Br J Dermatol* 148(3), 539
Erythema
(1987): Dudley K+, *Cutis* 39(1), 64
(1980): Hrushesky WJ, *Cutis* 26, 181
Erythema gyratum
(1998): Pujol RM+, *J Am Acad Dermatol* 39, 839
Erythema multiforme
(1980): Ueki H+, *Hautarzt* (German) 31, 207
Exanthems (1–10%)
(1994): Leo S+, *J Chemother* 6, 423
(1994): Sollitto RB+, *Arch Dermatol* 130, 1194 (sun-exposed areas)
Fissures
Folliculitis (forehead)

(2001): Schmid-Wendtner M-H+, *Lancet* 358, 1575 (passim)
Hand–foot syndrome (<38%)
(2006): Janusch M+, *Eur J Dermatol* 16(5), 494
(2004): Feng JF+, *Ai Zheng* 23(12), 1704 (with paclitaxel)
(2004): Kuhfahl J+, *Onkologie* 27(5), 449 (12%)
(2004): Lienemann AO+, *Cutis* 73(5), 303
(2003): Moehler M+, *Chemotherapy* 49(1–2), 85
(2003): Risum S+, *Ugeskr Laeger* 165(33), 3161
(2002): Cure H+, *J Clin Oncol* 20(5), 1175 (38%)
(2002): Emens LA+, *Breast Cancer Res Treat 2002 Nov* 76(2), 145
(2002): Hofheinz RD+, *Onkologie* 25(3), 255
(2001): Elasmar SA+, *Jpn J Clin Oncol* 31(4), 172 (passim)
(2001): Hartung G+, *Onkologie 2001 Oct* 24(5), 457 (12%)
(1999): Bertolini A+, *Minerva Cardioangiol* 47(7–8), 269
(1999): Lim WT+, *Ann Acad Med Singapore* 28(2), 256 (24%)
(1998): *J Clin Oncol* 16(11), 3537 (13–34%)
(1998): Chiara S+, *Cancer Chemother Pharmacol* 42(4), 336 (13%)
(1998): Rustum YM+, *Cancer J Sci Am* 4(1), 12
(1997): Chiara S+, *Eur J Cancer* 33, 967
(1997): Iurio A+, *Acta Oncol* 36, 653
(1997): Thaler D, Monona, WI (from internet) (observation)
(1996): Aranda E+, *J Infus Chemother* 6(3), 118 (4%)
(1995): Banfield GK+, *J R Soc Med* 88, 356
(1995): Tralongo P+, *Anticancer Res* 15(2), 635
(1995): Yamao T+, *Jpn J Clin Oncol* 25(2), 46 (40%)
(1994): Leo S+, *J Chemother* 6, 423
(1993): Beard JS+, *J Am Acad Dermatol* 29, 325
(1993): Comandone A+, *Anticancer Res* 13(5C), 1781 (7%)
(1993): John WJ+, *Cancer* 72(11), 3191
(1991): Ardalan B+, *Cancer 1991 Sep 15* 68(6), 1242
(1991): Jorda E+, *Int J Dermatol* 30, 653
(1990): Fabian CJ+, *Invest New Drugs* 8(1), 57
(1989): Curran CF+, *Ann Intern Med* 111, 858
(1989): Jabboury K+, *Cancer* 64(4), 793
(1989): Lokich J+, *Cancer* 64(5), 1021 (10%)
(1989): Vukelja SJ+, *Ann Intern Med* 111, 688
(1988): Bellmunt J+, *Tumori* 74(3), 329
(1988): Guillaume J-C+, *Ann Dermatol Venereol* (French) 115, 1167
(1987): Molina R+, *Proc Am Soc Clin Oncol* 4, 92
(1985): Atkins JN, *Ann Intern Med* 102, 419
(1985): Caballero GA+, *Cancer Treat Rep* 69(1), 13
(1985): Feldman LD+, *JAMA* 254, 3479
(1984): Lokich JJ+, *Ann Intern Med* 101, 798
Irritation
(2002): Jorizzo J+, *Cutis* 70(6), 335
Keratoderma (palms)
(2001): Schmid-Wendtner M-H+, *Lancet* 358, 1575 (passim)
Keratoses
(2001): Kurzman MA, Staten Island, NY (from Internet) (observation)
(2001): Lamberts RJ, Grand Rapids, MI (inflammation) (from Internet) (observation)
Lupus erythematosus (systemic)
(2008): Weger W+, *J Am Acad Dermatol* 59(2), S4 (with capecitabine)
(2007): Adachi A+, *Dermatology* 214(1), 85
(2006): Kluger N+, *J Dermatolog Treat* 17(1), 51 (Cutaneous)
(2002): Moazzam N+, *J Clin Oncol* 20(13), 3032
Necrosis
(1980): Yaffee HS+, *Cutis* 25, 649 (ecdysis)
Palmar–plantar pigmentation
(2001): Schmid-Wendtner M-H+, *Lancet* 358, 1575 (passim)
Peripheral edema
(1992): Breathnach SM+, *Adverse Drug Reactions and the Skin* Blackwell, Oxford, 193 (passim)
Photo-recall
(1993): Prussick R+, *Arch Dermatol* 129, 644

(1992): Breathnach SM+, *Adverse Drug Reactions and the Skin*
Blackwell, Oxford, 193 (passim)

Photoallergic reaction
(2006): Tsoussis S+, *Clin Oncol (R Coll Radiol)* 18(2), 158
Photosensitivity (<1%)
(1999): von Moos R+, *Schweiz Med Wochenschr* (German)
129, 52
(1992): Breathnach SM+, *Adverse Drug Reactions and the Skin*
Blackwell, Oxford, 193 (passim)
Phototoxicity
Pigmentation (<1%)
(2005): Jain V+, *J Am Acad Dermatol* 53(3), 529 (serpentine)
(1997): Miller BH+, *J Am Acad Dermatol* 36, 72
(1995): Allen BJ+, *Int J Dermatol* 34, 219 (reticulate)
(1994): Leo S+, *J Chemother* 6, 423
(1991): Vukelja SJ+, *J Am Acad Dermatol* 25, 905 (serpentine)
(1980): Hrushesky WJ, *Cutis* 26, 181 (sun-exposed areas)
Pruritus
Psoriasis
(2002): Wetzig T+, *Br J Dermatol* 147(4), 824
Pyogenic granuloma
(2006): Curr N+, *Australas J Dermatol* 47(2), 130
Recall reaction
(2003): Kirkup ME+, *Dermatology* 206(2), 175
(1997): Anderson LL+, *J Am Acad Dermatol* 36, 478
(1993): Prussick R+, *Arch Dermatol* 129, 644
Seborrheic dermatitis
Side effects (sic)
(2002): Moazzam N+, *J Clin Oncol* 20(13), 3032
Ulcerations
(2006): Lambert T+, *J Drugs Dermatol* 5(3), 282
(2003): Salim A+, *Br J Dermatol* 148(3), 539
Urticaria
Xerosis (1–10%)

Mucosal/ENT
Dysgeusia
Mucositis (1–79%)
(2005): Chansky K+, *Cancer* 103(6), 1165
(2003): Chen JY+, *Ai Zheng* 22(4), 418
(2003): Nottage M+, *Support Care Cancer* 11(1), 41 (79%)
(2003): Tsalic M+, *Am J Clin Oncol* 26(1), 103 (10%) (with
leucovorin)
(2002): Cure H+, *J Clin Oncol* 20(5), 1175 (26%)
(2001): Hejna M+, *Eur J Cancer* 37(16), 1994
Oral mucositis
(2006): Alter P+, *Cardiovasc Hematol Agents Med Chem* 4(1), 1
(2006): Baek JH+, *Korean J Intern Med* 21(1), 43
(2006): Cerchietti LC+, *Int J Radiat Oncol Biol Phys* 65(5), 1330
(2006): Jones JA+, *Support Care Cancer* 14(6), 505
Oral ulceration
(2002): Xu D+, *Zhonghua Zhong Liu Za Zhi* 24(1), 93 (with
leucovorin)
Rectal mucosal ulceration
(2006): Navarro M+, *Int J Radiat Oncol Biol Phys* 66(1), 201 (8%)
Stomatitis (>10%)
(2007): Papadeas E+, *Eur J Oncol* 11(1), 60
(2005): D'Andre S+, *Clin Colorectal Cancer* 4(5), 325 (17%)
(2003): Rossi A+, *Oncology* 64(4), 353
(2003): Saini A+, *Br J Cancer* 88(12), 1859
(2003): Tebbutt NC+, *Br J Cancer* 88(10), 1510
(2002): Bonneterre J+, *Br J Cancer* 87(11), 1210 (40%) (with
vinorelbine)
(2002): Ito A+, *Gan To Kagaku Ryoho* 29(4), 563
(2002): McCollum AD+, *J Natl Cancer Inst* 94(15), 1160
(2002): Sloan JA+, *J Clin Oncol* 20(6), 1491
(2002): Ueno H+, *Cancer Chemother Pharmacol* 49(2), 155
Tongue pigmentation
(2001): Schmid-Wendtner M-H+, *Lancet* 358, 1575 (passim)

Hair
Hair – alopecia (>10%)
(2003): Saini A+, *Br J Cancer* 88(12), 1859
(2002): Sloan JA+, *J Clin Oncol* 20(6), 1491
(2001): Madnani N, Mumbai, India (from Internet) (observation)
(1992): Breathnach SM+, *Adverse Drug Reactions and the Skin*
Blackwell, Oxford, 193 (passim)

Nails
Nails – periungual granuloma
(2006): Curr N+, *Australas J Dermatol* 47(2), 130
Nails – pigmentation (<1%)
(2001): Schmid-Wendtner M-H+, *Lancet* 358, 1575 (passim)

Eyes
Ectropion
(1997): Lewis JE, *Int J Dermatol* 36, 79
(1994): Hecker D+, *Cutis* 53, 137

Other
Abdominal pain
(2006): Navarro M+, *Int J Radiat Oncol Biol Phys* 66(1), 201 (8%)
Anaphylactoid reactions/Anaphylaxis
(1992): Breathnach SM+, *Adverse Drug Reactions and the Skin*
Blackwell, Oxford, 193 (passim)
Asthenia
(2006): Navarro M+, *Int J Radiat Oncol Biol Phys* 66(1), 201 (9%)
Cardiotoxicity
(2007): Georgieva S+, *J BUON* 12(1), 113
(2006): Gundling F+, *Z Gastroenterol* 44(9), 975
(2006): Lu JI+, *J Clin Oncol* 24(18), 2959
(2006): Tsibiribi P+, *Bull Cancer* 93(3), E27
(2002): Tsavaris N+, *Med Sci Monit* 8(6), PI51
(1997): Meyer CC+, *Pharmacotherapy* 17(4), 729
(1993): Akhtar SS+, *Oncology* 50(6), 441
Coma
(2006): Heluwaert F+, *Gastroenterol Clin Biol* 30(2), 325
Death
(2004): Teixeira L+, *Bull Cancer* 91 Suppl 3, 154 (2.2–13%)
(2003): Tsalic M+, *Am J Clin Oncol* 26(1), 103 (2%) (with
leucovorin)
(2003): van Kuilenburg AB+, *Ann Oncol* 14(2), 341
Hepatotoxicity
(2007): Brooks AJ+, *Intern Med J* 37(5), 344
(2006): Alazmi WM+, *J Clin Gastroenterol* 40(4), 353
Infections
(2005): D'Andre S+, *Clin Colorectal Cancer* 4(5), 325 (4%)
(2002): Bonneterre J+, *Br J Cancer* 87(11), 1210 (7%) (with
vinorelbine)
Injection-site burning
(1998): Kraus S+, *J Am Acad Dermatol* 38, 438
(1997): Miller BH+, *J Am Acad Dermatol* 36, 72
Injection-site desquamation
(1998): Kraus S+, *J Am Acad Dermatol* 38, 438
(1997): Miller BH+, *J Am Acad Dermatol* 36, 72
(1997): Swinehart JM+, *Arch Dermatol* 133, 67
(1992): Breathnach SM+, *Adverse Drug Reactions and the Skin*
Blackwell, Oxford, 193 (passim)
Injection-site edema
(1997): Miller BH+, *J Am Acad Dermatol* 36, 72
(1997): Swinehart JM+, *Arch Dermatol* 133, 67
(1992): Breathnach SM+, *Adverse Drug Reactions and the Skin*
Blackwell, Oxford, 193 (passim)
Injection-site erythema
(1998): Kraus S+, *J Am Acad Dermatol* 38, 438
(1997): Miller BH+, *J Am Acad Dermatol* 36, 72
(1997): Swinehart JM+, *Arch Dermatol* 133, 67
(1992): Breathnach SM+, *Adverse Drug Reactions and the Skin*
Blackwell, Oxford, 193 (passim)
Injection-site necrosis

(1998): Kraus S+, *J Am Acad Dermatol* 38, 438
(1997): Swinehart JM+, *Arch Dermatol* 133, 67
Injection-site pain
(1998): Kraus S+, *J Am Acad Dermatol* 38, 438
(1997): Swinehart JM+, *Arch Dermatol* 133, 67
Injection-site pigmentation
(2001): Schmid-Wendtner M-H+, *Lancet* 358, 1575 (passim)
Injection-site ulceration
(1997): Miller BH+, *J Am Acad Dermatol* 36, 72
(1997): Swinehart JM+, *Arch Dermatol* 133, 67
Neurotoxicity
(2006): Lucato LT+, *Australas Radiol* 50(4), 364
(2006): Saif MW+, *Anticancer Drugs* 17(9), 1095
Paresthesias (<1%)
Phlebitis
(2002): Xu D+, *Zhonghua Zhong Liu Za Zhi* 24(1), 93 (with leucovorin)
Pseudoporphyria
(1992): Laidman PJ+, *Aust N Z J Med* 22(4), 385
Rhabdomyolysis
(1986): Schmied E+, *Dermatologica* 173(5), 257 (topical)

FLUOXETINE

Trade names: Adofen; Apo-Fluoxetine; Dom-Fluoxetine; Fluctin; Fluctine; Fludac; Fluoxac; Fluoxeren; Fluxil; Fontex; Prozac (Lilly); Sarafem (Warner Chilcott)
Indications: Depression, obsessive-compulsive disorder
Category: Antidepressant; Selective serotonin reuptake inhibitor
Half-life: 2–3 days
Clinically important, potentially hazardous interactions with: alprazolam, amphetamines, astemizole, clarithromycin, clozapine, desipramine, dexibuprofen, dextroamphetamine, diethylpropion, droperidol, duloxetine, erythromycin, haloperidol, imipramine, isocarboxazid, linezolid, lithium, MAO inhibitors, mazindol, meperidine, methamphetamine, midazolam, moclobemide, nortriptyline, phendimetrazine, phenelzine, phentermine, phenylpropanolamine, phenytoin, pimozide, pseudoephedrine, selegiline, serotonin agonists, sibutramine, **St John's wort**, sumatriptan, sympathomimetics, tramadol, tranylcypromine, trazodone, tricyclic antidepressants, troleandomycin, **tryptophan**, zolmitriptan

Reactions

Skin

Acne (<1%)
Allergic reactions (sic)
(1998): Beauquier B+, *Encephale* (French) 24, 62
Angioedema
(1991): Olfson M+, *J Nerv Mental Dis* 179, 504
Bruising
(1996): Pai VB+, *Ann Pharmacother* 30, 786
Bullous dermatitis (<1%)
Bullous pemphigoid
(1999): Rault S+, *Br J Dermatol* 141(4), 755
Cellulitis
Dermatitis (<1%)
Diaphoresis (8.4%)
(1997): Amir I+, *Isr J Psychiatry Relat Sci* 34(2), 119
(1985): Wernicke JF, *J Clin Psychiatry* 46, 59
Eczema (<1%)
Erythema multiforme
(1985): Wernicke JF, *J Clin Psychiatry* 46, 59

Erythema nodosum (<1%)
Exanthems (4%)
(2002): Sannicandro TJ+, *Pharmacotherapy* 22(4), 516
(1993): Gupta MA+, *Cutis* 51, 386 (3%) (passim)
(1993): Gupta RK+, *Med J Aust* 158, 722
(1993): Litt JZ, Beachwood, OH (personal case) (observation)
(1991): Olfson M+, *J Nerv Mental Dis* 159, 504
(1989): Miller LG+, *Am J Psychiatry* 146, 1616
(1988): Cooper GL, *Br J Psychiatry* 153, 77
(1985): Wernicke JF, *J Clin Psychiatry* 46, 59
Exfoliative dermatitis
Facial edema (<1%)
Furunculosis (<1%)
Herpes simplex (reactivation)
(1991): Reed SM+, *Am J Psychiatry* 148, 949
Herpes zoster
Lichenoid eruption
Lupus erythematosus (discoid)
Lymphocytoma cutis
(2006): Breza TS Jr+, *J Cutan Pathol* 33(7), 522
Mycosis fungoides
(1996): Gordon KB+, *J Am Acad Dermatol* 34, 304
(1996): Vermeer MH+, *J Am Acad Dermatol* 35, 635
Nodular eruption
Peripheral edema (<1%)
Petechiae (<1%)
Photosensitivity
(1998): Pazzagli L+, *Pharm World Sci* 20, 136 (with alprazolam)
Phototoxicity (<1%)
(1995): Gaufberg E+, *J Clin Psychiatry* 56, 486
(1995): O'Brien T, *Australas J Dermatology* 36, 103
Pigmentation (<1%)
Pruritus (2.4%)
(2002): Sannicandro TJ+, *Pharmacotherapy* 22(4), 516
(1993): Gupta RK+, *Med J Aust* 158, 722
(1991): Olfson M+, *J Nerv Mental Dis* 159, 504
(1985): Wernicke JF, *J Clin Psychiatry* 46, 59
Psoriasis (<1%)
(1992): Hemlock C+, *Ann Pharmacother* 26, 211
Purpura (<1%)
Pustules (<1%)
Rash (sic) (6%)
(1989): Miller LG+, *Am J Psychiatry* 146, 1616
(1987): Zerbe RL, *Int J Obes* 11 (Suppl 3), 191
(1985): Wernicke JF, *J Clin Psychiatry* 46, 59
Raynaud's phenomenon
(2000): De Broucker +, *Ann Med Interne* (Paris) 151(5), 424
(1997): Rudnick A+, *Biol Psychiatry* 41(12), 1218
Seborrhea (<1%)
Stevens–Johnson syndrome
(1998): N Z Medicines Adverse Reactions Committee (from Internet) (observation)
(1992): Bodokh I+, *Therapie* (French) 47, 441
Toxic epidermal necrolysis
(1992): Bodokh I+, *Therapie* (French) 47, 441
(1991): Rosenthal E+, *Presse Med* (French) 20, 1459
Ulcerations (<1%)
Urticaria (4%)
(1994): Blumenthal HL, Beachwood, OH (personal case) (observation)
(1993): Gupta RK+, *Med J Aust* 158, 722
(1992): Leznoff A+, *J Clin Psychopharmacol* 12, 355
(1991): Olfson M+, *J Nerv Mental Dis* 159, 504
(1989): Miller LG+, *Am J Psychiatry* 146, 1616
Vasculitis
(1999): Fisher A+, *Aust N Z J Med* 29, 375 (focal necrotizing)
(1995): Roger D+, *Dermatology* 191, 164

Xerosis

Mucosal/ENT

Ageusia (<1%)
Aphthous stomatitis (<1%)
Dysgeusia (1.8%)
  (2000): Heymann WR, *Cutis* 66, 25
Gingivitis (<1%)
Glossitis (<1%)
Glossodynia
  (1994): Shelley WB+, *Cutis* 53, 242 (observation)
Oral ulceration (<1%)
  (2000): Madinier I+, *Ann Med Interne (Paris)* (French) 151, 248
Parosmia (<1%)
Sialorrhea (<1%)
Stomatitis (<1%)
Tinnitus
Tongue black
  (2004): Hommes M+, *Ned Tijdschr Geneeskd* 148(20), 984
  (2000): Heymann WR, *Cutis* 66, 25
Tongue edema (<1%)
Xerostomia (12%)
  (2003): Corya SA+, *J Clin Psychiatry* 64(11), 1349 (with
    olanzapine)
  (2002): Krymchantowski AV+, *Headache* 42(6), 510 (with
    amitriptyline)
  (2000): Heymann WR, *Cutis* 66, 25
  (1997): Boyd LD+, *Nutr Rev* 55(10), 362
  (1993): Beasley CM+, *Ann Clin Psychiatry* 5, 199
  (1985): Wernicke JF, *J Clin Psychiatry* 46, 59

Hair

Hair – alopecia (<1%)
  (2000): Murlidhar MD, Madras, India (from Internet)
    (observation)
  (1996): Bhatara VS+, *J Clin Psychiatry* 57, 227
  (1995): Seifritz E+, *Can J Psychiatry* 40, 362
  (1995): Shelley WB+, *Cutis* 55, 144 (observation)
  (1994): Mareth TR, *J Clin Psychiatry* 55, 163
  (1994): Shelley WB+, *Cutis* 53, 282 (observation)
  (1993): Ogilvie AD, *Lancet* 342, 1423
  (1991): Ananth J+, *J Psychiatry* 36, 621
  (1991): Gupta S+, *Br J Psychiatry* 159, 737
  (1991): Jenike MA, *Am J Psychiatry* 148, 392
Hair – hirsutism (<1%)

Other

Anaphylactoid reactions/Anaphylaxis (<1%)
Candidiasis
Delirium
  (2006): Chan CH+, *J Clin Psychopharmacol* 26(6), 677 (with
    bupropion)
Depression
  (2007): Cusin C+, *J Clin Psychiatry* 68(1), 52
  (2004): Jick H+, *JAMA* 292(3), 338
Gynecomastia (<1%)
  (2003): Boulenger A+, *J Eur Acad Dermatol Venereol* 17(1), 109
Headache (<27%)
  (2003): Calabrese JR+, *J Clin Psychiatry* 64(5), 562 (27%)
  (2003): Corya SA+, *J Clin Psychiatry* 64(11), 1349 (with
    olanzapine)
Hot flashes
Hypersensitivity
  (1994): Beer K+, *Arch Dermatol* 130, 803
Inappropriate secretion of antidiuretic hormone (SIADH)
  (2006): Twardowshy CA+, *Arq Neuropsiquiatr* 64(1), 142
  (2005): Bogdanovic Z+, *Ann Pharmacother* 39(10), 1755
  (2000): Romerio SC+, *Schweiz Rundsch Med Prax* 89(10), 404
  (1996): Burke D+, *Aust N Z J Psychiatry* 30(2), 295

(1996): Burke D+, *Aust N Z J Psychiatry* 30(2), 299
(1996): Christensen O+, *Ugeskr Laeger* 158(48), 6920
(1996): Flint AJ+, *Am J Psychiatry* 153(1), 134
(1996): Schattner A+, *J Am Geriatr Soc* 44(11), 1413 (75%)
(1995): Jackson C+, *Am J Psychiatry* 152(5), 809
(1994): Druckenbrod R+, *J Geriatr Psychiatry Neurol* 7(4), 254
(1994): ten Holt WL+, *Ned Tijdschr Geneeskd* 138(23), 1181
(1993): Kazal LA Jr+, *J Fam Pract* 36(3), 341
(1991): Vishwanath BM+, *Am J Psychiatry* 148(4), 542
(1990): Cohen BJ+, *Am J Psychiatry* 147(7), 948
(1990): Staab JP+, *Am J Psychiatry* 147(11), 1569
(1989): Hwang AS+, *Am J Psychiatry* 146(3), 399
Myalgia/Myositis/Myopathy/Myotoxicity (<1%)
Paresthesias
  (2001): Ribeiro L+, *Braz J Med Biol Res* 34(10), 1303
  (1996): Bhatara VS+, *J Clin Psychiatry* 57, 227
Pseudolymphoma
  (1995): Crowson AN+, *Arch Dermatol* 131, 925
  (1995): Magro CM+, *J Am Acad Dermatol* 32, 419
  (1988): Kardaun SH+, *Br J Dermatol* 118(4), 545
Rhabdomyolysis
  (1990): Lazarus A, *J Clin Psychopharmacol* 10 (overdose)
Serum sickness
  (1991): Vincent A+, *Am J Psychiatry* 148, 1602
  (1989): Miller LG+, *Am J Psychiatry* 146, 1616
Suicidal ideation
  (2007): Perlis RH+, *Psychother Psychosom* 76(1), 40
  (2005): Giner L+, *Int J Adolesc Med Health* 17(3), 211
  (2003): Hansen L, *J Psychopharmacol* 17(4), 451
  (2002): Falsetti AE, *Food Drug Law J* 57(2), 247
  (1997): Lancon C+, *Encephale* 23(3), 218
  (1992): Hamilton MS+, *J Clin Psychiatry* 53(11), 401
  (1992): Hawthorne ME+, *J Affect Disord* 26(3), 205
  (1991): Rothschild AJ+, *J Clin Psychiatry* 52(12), 491 (3 cases)
  (1990): *Am J Psychiatry* 147(11), 1570
Thrombophlebitis (<1%)
Tremor (2–10%)

FLUOXYMESTERONE

Trade names: Android-F; Halotestin (Pfizer); Stenox; Vewon
Indications: Breast carcinoma, hypogonadism, anemia
Category: Anabolic steroid
Half-life: 9.2 hours
**Clinically important, potentially hazardous interactions
with:** anticoagulants, cyclosporine, warfarin

Reactions

Skin

Acne (>10%)
  (1992): Fryand O+, *Acta Derm Venereol* 72, 148
  (1990): Fuchs E+, *J Am Acad Dermatol* 23, 125
  (1989): Fryand O+, *Tidsskr Nor Laegeforen* (Norwegian)
    109, 239
  (1989): Hartmann AA+, *Monatsschr Kinderheilkd* (German)
    137, 466
  (1989): Heydenreich G, *Arch Dermatol* 125, 571 (fulminans)
  (1989): Scott MJ+, *Cutis* 44, 30
  (1989): von Muhlendahl KE+, *Dtsch Med Wochenschr* (German)
    114, 712
  (1988): Traupe H+, *Arch Dermatol* 124, 414 (fulminans)
  (1987): Kiraly CL+, *Am J Dermatopathol* 9, 515
  (1984): Lamb DR, *Am J Sports Med* 12, 31
Dermatitis
  (1989): Holdiness MR, *Contact Dermatitis* 20, 3 (from patch)
Edema (>10%)

Exanthems
Furunculosis
  (1989): Scott MJ+, *Cutis* 44, 30
Lichenoid eruption
  (1989): Aihara M+, *J Dermatol* (Tokio) 16, 330
Lupus erythematosus
Pruritus
Psoriasis
  (1990): O'Driscoll JB+, *Clin Exp Dermatol* 15, 68
Purpura
Seborrhea
Seborrheic dermatitis
  (1989): Scott MJ+, *Cutis* 44, 30
Striae
  (1989): Scott MJ+, *Cutis* 44, 30
Urticaria

Mucosal/ENT
Stomatitis

Hair
Hair – alopecia
  (1989): Scott MJ+, *Cutis* 44, 30
Hair – hirsutism (1–10%)
  (1994): Castillo-Ceballos A+, *Med Clin* (Barc) (Spanish) 102, 78
  (1991): Bates GW+, *Clin Obstet Gynecol* 34, 848
  (1991): No Author, *Obstet Gynecol* 78, 474
  (1991): Parker LU+, *Cleve Clin J Med* 58, 43
  (1991): Urman B+, *Obstet Gynecol* 77, 595
  (1989): Scott MJ+, *Cutis* 44, 30

Other
Anaphylactoid reactions/Anaphylaxis
Gynecomastia (<1%)
Hypersensitivity (<1%)
Injection-site pain
Paresthesias

FLUPHENAZINE

Trade names: Anatensol; Apo-Fluphenazine; Dapatum D25; Dapotum D; Fludecate; Modecate; Moditen; Prolixin
Indications: Psychoses
Category: Antipsychotic, phenothiazine
Half-life: 84–96 hours
Clinically important, potentially hazardous interactions with: antihistamines, arsenic, chlorpheniramine, dofetilide, **evening primrose**, quinolones, sparfloxacin

Reactions

Skin
Angioedema (<1%)
Dermatitis
Diaphoresis
Eczema
Edema
Erythema
Exanthems
Exfoliative dermatitis
Lupus erythematosus
Peripheral edema
Photosensitivity
Pigmentation (<1%) (blue-gray)
  (1987): Krebs A, *Schweiz Rundsch Med Prax* (German) 76, 1069

Pruritus (<1%)
Purpura
Rash (sic) (1–10%)
Seborrhea
Toxic epidermal necrolysis
Urticaria
Vitiligo
  (1987): Krebs A, *Schweiz Rundsch Med Prax* (German) 76, 1069
  (1985): Rampertaap MP, *Mo Med* 82, 24
Xerosis

Mucosal/ENT
Sialorrhea
Xerostomia (<1%)

Eyes
Maculopathy
  (2004): Lee MS+, *Ophthalmic Res* 36(4), 237
  (1992): Neki AS, *Br J Ophthalmol* 76(4), 255
  (1991): Power WJ+, *Br J Ophthalmol* 75(7), 433
Ocular pigmentation
  (2001): Panzitt M+, *Klin Monatsbl Augenheilkd* 218(4), 273
Retinopathy
  (2005): Toler SM, *J Ocul Pharmacol Ther* 21(4), 259

Other
Anaphylactoid reactions/Anaphylaxis
Gynecomastia (1–10%)
Headache
Injection-site reactions
Rhabdomyolysis

FLURAZEPAM

Trade names: Apo-Flurazepam; Benozil; Dalmadorm; Dalmane (Valeant); Flunox; Flurazepam (Watson); Nergart; Novoflupam; Som Pam; Somnol; Valdorm
Indications: Insomnia
Category: Benzodiazepine
Half-life: 40–114 hours
Clinically important, potentially hazardous interactions with: amprenavir, chlorpheniramine, clarithromycin, efavirenz, esomeprazole, imatinib, indinavir, nelfinavir, ritonavir

Reactions

Skin
Dermatitis (1–10%)
Diaphoresis (>10%)
Exanthems
Pruritus
Purpura
Rash (sic) (>10%)
Toxic epidermal necrolysis
  (2005): Loncar C+, *Psychiatr Danub* 17(3-4), 236
Urticaria

Mucosal/ENT
Dysgeusia (3.4%) (metallic taste)
  (1984): Greenblatt DJ+, *J Clin Psychiatry* 45, 192 (3%)
Oral lesions
  (1984): Greenblatt DJ+, *J Clin Psychiatry* 45, 192 (3%)
Sialopenia (>10%)
Sialorrhea (1–10%)
Xerostomia (>10%)

Other
Headache
Paresthesias

FLURBIPROFEN

Trade names: Ansaid (Pfizer); Apo-Flurbiprofen; Cebutid; Flurofen; Flurozin; Froben; Lapole; Nu-Flurprofen
Indications: Arthritis
Category: Non-steroidal anti-inflammatory
Half-life: 3–4 hours
Clinically important, potentially hazardous interactions with: methotrexate

Reactions

Skin
Angioedema (<1%)
   (1997): Romano A+, J Intern Med 241, 81
Dermatitis
   (2000): Kawada A+, Contact Dermatitis 42, 167
Dermatitis herpetiformis
   (1994): Tousignant J+, Int J Dermatol 33, 199
Diaphoresis
Eczema (3–9%)
Edema (3–9%)
Erythema multiforme (<1%)
Exanthems
   (1997): Romano A+, J Intern Med 241, 81
Exfoliative dermatitis (<1%)
Fixed eruption
   (1993): Dermatology 186, 164
Furunculosis
Herpes simplex
Herpes zoster
Peripheral edema
Photosensitivity (<1%)
Pigmentation
Pruritus (1–5%)
Purpura
Rash (sic) (1–3%)
Seborrhea
Side effects (sic) (6%)
   (1986): Buson M, J Int Med Res 14, 1
Stevens–Johnson syndrome (<1%)
Toxic epidermal necrolysis (<1%)
   (1987): Gillaume JC+, Arch Dermatol 123, 1166
Ulcerations
Urticaria (<1%)
Vasculitis
   (1990): Wei M, Ann Intern Med 112, 550
Xerosis

Mucosal/ENT
Aphthous stomatitis
Dysgeusia (<1%)
Oral lichenoid eruption
   (2000): Madinier I+, Ann Med Interne (Paris) (French) 151, 248
   (1983): Hamburger J+, BMJ 287, 1258
Parosmia (<1%)
Stomatitis
Tinnitus
Vaginitis
Xerostomia (<1%)

Hair
Hair – alopecia (<1%)

Nails
Nails – changes (sic) (<1%)
Nails – pigmentation

Eyes
Ocular burning
Ocular stinging

Other
Anaphylactoid reactions/Anaphylaxis (<1%)
Headache
Hot flashes (<1%)
Hypersensitivity
   (1997): Romano A+, J Intern Med 241, 81
Paresthesias (<1%)

FLUTAMIDE

Trade names: Drogenil; Euflex; Eulexin (Schering); Eulexine; Flucinom; Fluken; Flulem; Fugerel; Novo-Flutamide
Indications: Metastatic prostate carcinoma
Category: Androgen antagonist
Half-life: 6 hours

Reactions

Skin
Bullous dermatitis
Diaphoresis
   (1992): Schmeller N, Internist Berl (German) 33, 284
Edema (4%)
Erythema
Exanthems
   (1999): Fisher BJ, Toronto, Ontario (generalized) (from Internet) (observation)
   (1989): Brogden RN+, Drugs 38, 185
Lupus erythematosus
   (1998): Reid MB+, J Urol 159, 2098
Photosensitivity
   (2003): Kaur C+, Br J Dermatol 148(3), 603
   (1999): Tsien C+, J Urol 162, 494
   (1998): Vilaplana J+, Contact Dermatitis 38, 68
   (1998): Yokote R+, Eur J Dermatol 8, 427
   (1996): Fujimoto M+, Br J Dermatol 135, 496
   (1996): Leroy D+, Photodermatol Photoimmunol Photomed 12(5), 216
   (1991): Moraillon I+, Photodermatol Photoimmunol Photomed 8, 264
Rash (sic) (3%)
Toxic epidermal necrolysis
Urticaria

Other
Gynecomastia (9%)
   (1997): Staiman VR+, Urology 50, 929
   (1993): Aso Y+, Hinyokika Kiyo (Japanese) 39, 391
Hepatotoxicity
   (2005): Papaioannides D+, Int Urol Nephrol 37(3), 515
Hot flashes (61%)
Injection-site irritation (3%)
Paresthesias (1–10%)
Pseudoporphyria
   (1999): Mantoux F+, Ann Dermatol Venereol (French) 126, 150

(1999): Schmutz JL+, *Ann Dermatol Venereol* (French) 126, 374
(1998): Borroni G+, *Br J Dermatol* 138, 711

FLUTICASONE

Trade names: Cutivate (GSK); Flonase (GSK); Flovent (GSK)
Indications: Dermatoses, rhinitis
Category: Corticosteroid, inhaled; Corticosteroid, topical
Half-life: N/A
**Clinically important, potentially hazardous interactions
with:** ketoconazole, **live vaccines**, oral contraceptives, ritonavir

Reactions

Skin
Acne
Atrophy
  (1996): Johnson M, *Cutis* 57(2), 10
Bruising
  (2005): Man SF+, *Drugs* 65(5), 579
Burning
  (1996): Johnson M, *Cutis* 57(2), 10
  (1996): Lebwohl M, *Cutis* 57(2), 62
Edema
Pruritus
  (1996): Johnson M, *Cutis* 57(2), 10
  (1996): Lebwohl M, *Cutis* 57(2), 62
Rash (sic)
Vasculitis
  (2003): English J 3rd+, *J Drugs Dermatol* 2(3), 326
  (2002): Koya T+, *Arerugi* 51(11), 1127
  (2001): Termeer C+, *Arch Dermatol* 137(11), 1527

Mucosal/ENT
Dysphonia
  (2005): Man SF+, *Drugs* 65(5), 579
  (2003): Randell TL+, *Paediatr Drugs* 5(7), 481 (rare)
  (2002): DelGaudio JM, *Arch Otolaryngol Head Neck Surg* 128(6), 677
  (2002): Lyseng-Williamson KA+, *Am J Respir Med* 1(4), 273
  (1999): Spencer CM+, *Drugs* 57(6), 933
Oral candidiasis
  (2005): Adams NP+, *Cochrane Database Syst Rev* (4), CD003135
  (2005): Lipworth BJ+, *Ann Allergy Asthma* 94(4), 465 (22%)
  (2005): Man SF+, *Drugs* 65(5), 579
  (2004): Donohue JF+, *Treat Respir Med* 3(3), 173
  (2003): Fukushima C+, *Ann Allergy Asthma Immunol* 90(6), 646
  (2003): Hanania NA+, *Chest* 124(3), 834
  (2003): Powell H+, *Med J Aust* 178(5), 223
  (2003): Randell TL+, *Paediatr Drugs* 5(7), 481 (rare)
  (2002): Lyseng-Williamson KA+, *Am J Respir Med* 1(4), 273
  (1999): Spencer CM+, *Drugs* 57(6), 933

Eyes
Cataract
  (2004): Bisgaard H+, *Pediatrics* 113(2), e87
Ocular pressure
  (2004): Sihota R+, *Indian J Ophthalmol* 52(2), 170

Other
Adverse effects (sic)
  (2003): Coghlan D+, *Paediatr Drugs* 5(10), 685 (rare)
  (2000): Kokot M, *Pol Merkuriusz Lek* 8(47), 330 (%)
  (1999): Todd GR, *Eur Respir J* 13(3), 707
  (1996): Lebwohl M, *Cutis* 57(2), 62
Chills
Cough

(2004): Bisgaard H+, *Pediatrics* 113(2), e87
(2003): Dubus JC+, *Fundam Clin Pharmacol* 17(5), 627
Death
  (2006): Li AM, *J Pediatr* 148(3), 294 (with ritonavir)
Depression
Fever
Headache
  (2002): Bratton RL+, *Mayo Clin Proc* 77(12), 1353
  (1999): Spencer CM+, *Drugs* 57(6), 933
Infections
  (2002): Bratton RL+, *Mayo Clin Proc* 77(12), 1353
  (2002): Peter E+, *Clin Infect Dis* 35(5), e54
  (2000): Leav BA+, *N Engl J Med* 343(8), 586
  (1999): Fairfax AJ+, *Thorax* 54(9), 860
Myalgia/Myositis/Myopathy/Myotoxicity
  (2004): De Swert+, *N Engl J Med* 350(11), 1157
Osteoporosis
  (2005): Licata AA, *Endocr Pract* 11(3), 194
Paresthesias
Tremor
  (1999): Spencer CM+, *Drugs* 57(6), 933
Vertigo
  (1999): Spencer CM+, *Drugs* 57(6), 933

FLUVASTATIN

Trade names: Cranoc; Lescol (Novartis); Locol
Indications: Hypercholesterolemia
Category: HMG-CoA reductase inhibitor; Statin
Half-life: 1.2 hours
**Clinically important, potentially hazardous interactions
with:** azithromycin, bosentan, ciprofibrate, clarithromycin,
cyclosporine, erythromycin, gemfibrozil, imatinib, **red rice yeast**

Reactions

Skin
Allergic reactions (sic) (2.6%)
Angioedema
Dermatomyositis
  (2005): Thual N+, *Ann Dermatol Venereol* 132(12), 996
Erythema multiforme
Lichenoid eruption
  (2004): Sebok B+, *Acta Derm Venereol* 84(3), 229
Lupus erythematosus
  (1998): Sridhar MK+, *Lancet* 352, 114 (fatal)
Photosensitivity
Pigmentation
Pruritus
Purpura
Rash (sic) (2.7%)
  (1998): N Z Medicines Adverse Reactions Committee (2 patients) (from Internet) (observation)
Stevens–Johnson syndrome
Toxic epidermal necrolysis
Urticaria
Vasculitis
Xerosis

Mucosal/ENT
Dysgeusia

Hair
Hair – alopecia
  (2002): Litt JZ, Beachwood, OH (personal case) (observation)

Hair – changes (sic)

Nails

Nails – changes (sic)

Other

Anaphylactoid reactions/Anaphylaxis
Death
Gynecomastia
Headache
Myalgia/Myositis/Myopathy/Myotoxicity
   (2002): Lawrence JM+, *Expert Opin Pharmacother* 3(11), 1631
   (1997): 16(1), February
   (1997): 61(1), February
   (1995): Garnett WR, *Am J Health Syst Pharm* 52(15), 1639
Paresthesias
Rhabdomyolysis
   (2005): Andrejak M+, *Therapie* 60(3), 299
   (2005): Atasoyu EM+, *Ann Pharmacother* 39(7–8), 1368 (with colchicine)
   (2005): Deak G+, *J Nephrol* 18(6), 773
   (2002): Lawrence JM+, *Expert Opin Pharmacother* 3(11), 1631
   (2002): Modi JR+, *Ann Pharmacother* 36(12), 1870
   (2002): Sica DA+, *Am J Geriatr Cardiol* 11(1), 48
   (2002): Sica DA+, *Curr Opin Nephrol Hypertens* 11(2), 123
   (1999): Bottorff M, *Atherosclerosis* 147(Suppl 1), S23
   (1995): Farmer JA+, *Baillieres Clin Endocrinol Metab* 9(4), 825
   (1995): Garnett WR, *Am J Health Syst Pharm* 52(15), 1639
Upper respiratory infection (16%)

FLUVOXAMINE

Trade names: Apo-Fluvoxamine; Dumirox; Dumyrox; Faverin; Favoxil; Fevarin; Luvox (Solvay); Maveral
Indications: Obsessive-compulsive disorder, depression
Category: Antidepressant; Selective serotonin reuptake inhibitor
Half-life: 15 hours
Clinically important, potentially hazardous interactions with: alprazolam, amphetamines, astemizole, dextroamphetamine, diethylpropion, duloxetine, isocarboxazid, linezolid, MAO inhibitors, mazindol, methadone, methamphetamine, phendimetrazine, phenelzine, phentermine, phenylpropanolamine, pseudoephedrine, ramelteon, ropivacaine, selegiline, sibutramine, **St John's wort**, sumatriptan, sympathomimetics, tacrine, theophyllines, tizanidine, tramadol, tranylcypromine, trazodone, troleandomycin, **tryptophan**, zolmitriptan

Reactions

Skin

Acne (<1%)
Allergic reactions (sic) (<1%)
   (1998): Beauquier B+, *Encephale* (French) 24, 62
Angioedema
   (1993): No Author, *Lakartidningen* (Swedish) 90, 54
Bullae
   (2006): Ke CL+, *J Am Acad Dermatol* 55(2), 355
Bullous dermatitis
   (2006): Ke CL+, *J Am Acad Dermatol* 55(2), 355
Dermatitis (<1%)
Diaphoresis (<7%)
   (1986): Benfield P+, *Drugs* 32, 313 (5%)
Edema (<1%)
Exanthems

Exfoliative dermatitis (<1%)
Furunculosis (<1%)
Intertrigo
   (2006): Ke CL+, *J Am Acad Dermatol* 55(2), 355
Photosensitivity (<1%)
   (1996): Gillet-Terver MN+, *Australas J Dermatol* 37, 62
   (1993): *Lakartidningen* (Swedish) 90, 54
Pigmentation (<1%)
Pruritus
Purpura (<1%)
Rash (sic)
Seborrhea (<1%)
Stevens–Johnson syndrome
Toxic epidermal necrolysis (<1%)
   (1993): Wolkenstein P+, *Lancet* 342, 304
Urticaria (<1%)
Xerosis (<1%)

Mucosal/ENT

Ageusia (<1%)
Dysgeusia (3%)
Gingivitis (<1%)
Glossitis (<1%)
Oral lesions (10%)
   (1986): Benfield P+, *Drugs* 32, 313 (10%)
Parosmia (<1%)
Sialorrhea
   (2006): Hori T+, *Prog Neuropsychopharmacol Biol Psychiatry* 30(4), 758 (with olanzapine)
Stomatitis (<1%)
Vaginitis (<1%)
   (2003): Versea L+, *Clin J Oncol Nurs* 7(3), 307
Xerostomia (<14%)
   (1997): Kiev A+, *J Clin Psychiatry* 58(4), 146
   (1986): Benfield P+, *Drugs* 32, 313 (10%)

Hair

Hair – alopecia (<1%)
Hair – alopecia areata
   (1996): Parameshwar E, *Am J Psychiatry* 153, 581

Eyes

Visual hallucinations
   (2006): Kito S+, *Int Psychogeriatr* 18(4), 749 (with zolpidem)

Other

Anaphylactoid reactions/Anaphylaxis
Asthenia
   (2003): Sugie Y+, *No To Hattatsu* 35(3), 233
   (1997): Kiev A+, *J Clin Psychiatry* 58(4), 146
Headache
   (1997): Kiev A+, *J Clin Psychiatry* 58(4), 146
Inappropriate secretion of antidiuretic hormone (SIADH)
   (2002): Arinzon ZH+, *Ann Pharmacother* 36(7-8), 1175
   (1996): Liu BA+, *CMAJ* 155(5), 519
Myalgia/Myositis/Myopathy/Myotoxicity (<1%)
Paresthesias

FOLIC ACID

Synonyms: folacin; folate; vitamin B$_9$
Trade names: Acfol; Apo-Folic; Dalisol; Flodine; Folacin; Folina; Folinsyre; Folitab; Folsan; Lexpec
Indications: Anemias
Category: Vitamin
Half-life: N/A

Reactions

Skin
Acne
Allergic reactions (sic) (<1%)
Dermatitis
Erythema
Exanthems
   (1985): Sparling R+, *Clin Lab Haematol* 7, 184
Pruritus (<1%)
Rash (sic) (<1%)
Urticaria
   (1985): Sparling R+, *Clin Lab Haematol* 7, 184

Other
Anaphylactoid reactions/Anaphylaxis
   (2007): Pfab F+, *Allergy* 62(7), 823
   (2000): Dykewicz MS+, *J Allergy Clin Immunol* 106, 386

FOMEPIZOLE

Synonyms: 4-Methylpyrazole; 4-MP
Trade name: Antizol (Orphan Medical)
Indications: Toxicity to methanol and ethylene glycol
Category: Antidote
Half-life: N/A (varies with dose)
Clinically important, potentially hazardous interactions with: alcohol

Reactions

Skin
Facial flushing (~3%)
Rash (sic) (~3%)
   (2002): Dean P+, *Pharmacotherapy* 22(3), 365 (passim)
   (1986): Baud FJ+, *J Toxicol Clin Toxicol* 24(6), 463

Mucosal/ENT
Dysgeusia (6%)
Oral vesiculation (~3%)
   (1988): Jacobsen D+, *Alcohol Clin Exp Res* 12(4), 516
Parosmia (1–10%)

Other
Application-site reactions (1–10%)
Injection-site inflammation (1–10%)
Injection-site pain (1–10%)
Phlebitis (1–10%)
Seizures (~3%)
Vertigo (6%)
   (2002): Dean P+, *Pharmacotherapy* 22(3), 365
   (1988): Jacobsen D+, *Alcohol Clin Exp Res* 12(4), 516

FOMIVIRSEN

Synonym: ISIS 2922
Trade name: Vitravene (CIBA Vision)
Indications: Cytomegalovirus retinitis
Category: Oligonucleotide
Half-life: ~7–10 days (in animals)
Clinically important, potentially hazardous interactions with: N/A

Reactions

Skin
Allergic reactions (sic) (2–5%)
Diaphoresis (2–5%)
Rash (sic) (5–20%)

Mucosal/ENT
Sinusitis (5–20%)

Eyes
Cataract (5–20%)
Intraocular inflammation
   (1999): Perry CM+, *Drugs* 57(3), 375
Intraocular pressure increased
   (2002): *Am J Ophthalmol* 133(4), 484
   (1999): Perry CM+, *Drugs* 57(3), 375
Maculopathy
   (2000): Stone TW+, *Am J Ophthalmol* 130(2), 242
Ocular pain (5–20%)
Photophobia (5–20%)
Retinal detachment (5–20%)
Retinopathy
   (2002): Uwaydat SH+, *Arch Ophthalmol* 120(6), 854
      (pigmentary)
Uveitis (5–10%)
Vision blurred (5–20%)

Other
Abdominal pain (5–20%)
Asthenia (5–20%)
Chest pain (2–5%)
Cough (2–5%)
Depression (2–5%)
Fever (5–10%)
Headache (5–20%)
Infections (>5%)
Neurotoxicity (2–5%)
Pain (2–5%)
Vertigo (2–5%)

FONDAPARINUX

Trade name: Arixtra (GSK) (Organon)
Indications: Prophylaxis of deep vein thrombosis
Category: Anticoagulant; Heparinoid
Half-life: 17–21 hours
Clinically important, potentially hazardous interactions with: abciximab, anagrelide, anticoagulants, cilostazol, clopidogrel, dipyridamole, eptifibatide, salicylates, ticlopidine, tirofiban. Many **herbals** that possess anticoagulant or antiplatelet activity

Reactions

Skin
Bullous dermatitis (3%)
Edema (9%)
Purpura (4%)
Rash (sic) (8%)

Other
Hypersensitivity
  (2005): Maetzke J+, *Allergy* 60(3), 413
  (2005): Utikal J+, *Thromb Haemost* 94(4), 895
  (2004): Hohenstein E+, *Contact Dermatitis* 51(3), 149
  (2004): Jappe U+, *Contact Dermatitis* 51(2), 67
Injection-site bleeding (1–10%)
Injection-site pruritus (1–10%)
Pain (2%)

FORMOTEROL

Synonym: Formoterol fumarate
Trade name: Oxeze
Indications: Asthma, bronchospasm
Category: Adrenergic beta2-receptor agonist
Half-life: 10–14 hours
Clinically important, potentially hazardous interactions with: clomipramine, desipramine, doxepin, imipramine, nortriptyline, protriptyline, trimipramine

Reactions

Skin
Angioedema
Erythema
Pruritus
Rash (sic) (1.1%)
Urticaria

Mucosal/ENT
Xerostomia (1%)
  (1990): Schultze-Werninghaus G, *Lung* 168 (Suppl 83–9) (1%)

Other
Anaphylactoid reactions/Anaphylaxis (1%)
Cough
  (1990): Schultze-Werninghaus G, *Lung* 168 (Suppl 83-9)
Death
  (2006): Aaronson DW, *J Allergy Clin Immunol* 117(1), 40
Headache
  (2005): Randell J+, *Respir Med* 99(12), 1485
Infections (3%)
Myalgia/Myositis/Myopathy/Myotoxicity
Tremor (1–6%)
  (2005): Randell J+, *Respir Med* 99(12), 1485
  (1998): Bartow RA+, *Drugs* 55(2), 303
  (1995): van den Berg BT+, *Fundam Clin Pharmacol* 9(6), 593
  (1992): Lipworth BJ, *Drug Saf* 7(1), 54
  (1991): Faulds D+, *Drugs* 42(1), 115
  (1990): Schultze-Werninghaus G, *Lung* 168 (Suppl 83–9) (6%)

FOSAMPRENAVIR

Trade name: Lexiva (GSK)
Indications: HIV infections (in combination with other antiretrovirals)
Category: Antiretroviral; Protease inhibitor, HIV
Half-life: 7.7 hours
Clinically important, potentially hazardous interactions with: amiodarone, atorvastatin, bepridil, carbamazepine, delavirdine, dihydroergotamine, etravirine, flecainide, itraconazole, ketoconazole, lidocaine, lovastatin, midazolam, phenobarbital, phenytoin, pimozide, propafenone, quinidine, rifabutin, rifampin, sildenafil, simvastatin, **St John's wort**, triazolam, vardenafil, warfarin

Note: Fosamprenavir is a prodrug of amprenavir

Note: Fosamprenavir is a sulfonamide and can be absorbed systemically. Sulfonamides can produce severe, possibly fatal, reactions such as toxic epidermal necrolysis and Stevens–Johnson syndrome

Reactions

Skin
Exanthems
Pruritus (7%)
Rash (sic) (~19%)
  (2004): Chapman TM+, *Drugs* 64(18), 2101
Stevens–Johnson syndrome

Other
Abdominal pain (5%)
  (2004): Chapman TM+, *Drugs* 64(18), 2101
Asthenia (10%)
Depression (8%)
Headache (19%)
Hypersensitivity
  (2006): Gathe JC Jr+, *Clin Ther* 28(5), 745 (7%) (with ritonavir)
  (2004): Chapman TM+, *Drugs* 64(18), 2101
Infections
Paresthesias (2%) (oral)

FOSCARNET

Trade names: Foscavir (AstraZeneca); Foscovir
Indications: Cytomegalovirus retinitis in patients with AIDS
Category: Antiviral; DNA & RNA polymerase inhibitor
Half-life: ~3 hours
Clinically important, potentially hazardous interactions with: adefovir, cyclosporine

Reactions

Skin
Acne
Dermatitis (<1%)
Diaphoresis (>5%)
Edema (<1%)
Eosinophilic pustular folliculitis
  (2001): Roos TC+, *J Am Acad Dermatol* 44, 546
Exanthems (>5%)
  (2001): Roos TC+, *J Am Acad Dermatol* 44, 546
  (1990): Green ST, *J Infection* 21, 227
Facial edema (>5%)

Fixed eruption
  (1990): Connolly GM+, *Genitourin Med* 66, 97
Herpes simplex (<1%)
Penile ulcers (4–30%)
  (1997): English JC+, *J Am Acad Dermatol* 37, 1
  (1996): Agcaoili DJ+, *Infect Med* 13, 35
  (1996): Papini M+, *Ann Dermatol Venereol* (French) 123, 679
  (1995): Fitzgerald E+, *Arch Dermatol* 131, 1447
  (1993): Bodian AB, *Int J Dermatol* 32, 526
  (1993): Brockmeyer NH+, *Int J Clin Pharmacol Ther Toxicol* 31, 204
  (1993): Gross AS+, *Clin Infect Dis* 17, 1076
  (1993): Moyle G+, *AIDS* 7, 140
  (1993): Schiff TA+, *Int J Dermatol* 32, 526
  (1992): Evans LM+, *J Am Acad Dermatol* 27, 124
  (1992): Katlama C+, *J Acquir Immune Defic Syndr* 5 (Suppl 1), S18
  (1991): Chrisp P+, *Drugs* 41, 104
  (1990): Fégueux S+, *Lancet* 335, 547
  (1990): Gilquin J+, *Lancet* 335, 287
  (1990): Lernestedt J-O+, *Lancet* 335, 548
  (1990): Moyle G+, *Lancet* 335, 547 (4.7%)
  (1990): Van Der Pijl JW+, *Lancet* 335, 286 (30%)
Peripheral edema (<1%)
Pigmentation (>5%)
Pruritus (>5%)
  (2001): Roos TC+, *J Am Acad Dermatol* 44, 546
Pruritus ani et vulvae (<1%)
Psoriasis (<1%)
Rash (sic) (generalized) (>5%)
  (1991): Blanshard C, *J Infect* 23, 336
  (1990): Green ST+, *J Infect* 21, 227
Seborrhea (>5%)
Toxic epidermal necrolysis
  (1999): Wharton JR+, *Cutis* 63, 333
  (1997): Lauglin CL, Little Rock, Arkansas, American Academy of Dermatology Meeting, (SF) (gross and microscopic)
Ulcerations (>5%)
Urticaria (<1%)
  (2001): Roos TC+, *J Am Acad Dermatol* 44, 546
Verrucae (<1%)
Xerosis (<1%)

Mucosal/ENT
Dysgeusia (>5%)
Oral leukoplakia
Oral ulceration
  (2000): Madinier I+, *Ann Med Interne* (Paris) (French) 151, 248
  (1997): Schiodt M, *Oral Dis* 3 Suppl 1, S208
  (1990): Fégueux S+, *Lancet* 335, 547
  (1990): Gilquin J+, *Lancet* 335, 287
  (1990): Moyle G+, *Lancet* 335, 547
Stomatitis (<1%)
Tinnitus
Tongue ulceration (<1%)
Ulcerative stomatitis (>5%)
Vulvar ulceration
  (1993): Caumes E+, *J Am Acad Dermatol* 28, 799 (erosion)
  (1992): Lacey HB+, *Genitourin Med* 68, 182
Xerostomia

Hair
Hair – alopecia (<1%)

Eyes
Periorbital edema

Other
Gynecomastia (<1%)
Headache

Injection-site pain (1–10%)
Injection-site thrombophlebitis
  (1991): Chrisp P+, *Drugs* 41, 104
Myalgia/Myositis/Myopathy/Myotoxicity (>5%)
Nephrotoxicity
  (1997): Jayaweera DT, *Drug Saf* 16(4), 258
Paresthesias (1–10%)
  (1990): Safrin S+, *J Infect Dis* 161, 1078
Thrombophlebitis (<1%)

FOSFOMYCIN

Trade name: Monurol (Forest)
Indications: Urinary tract infections
Category: Antibiotic
Half-life: 3–9 hours

Reactions

Skin
Angioedema
Exanthems (<1%)
Necrosis
Pruritus (<1%)
Rash (sic) (1.4%)
  (2005): Rudenko N+, *Arzneimittelforschung* 55(7), 420
  (1993): Mayama T+, *Int J Clin Pharmacol Ther Toxicol* 31(2), 77

Mucosal/ENT
Vaginitis (7.6%)
Xerostomia (<1%)

Other
Abdominal pain
  (1993): Mayama T+, *Int J Clin Pharmacol Ther Toxicol* 31(2), 77
  (1989): Takahashi H+, *Jpn J Antibiot* 42(1), 179
Anaphylactoid reactions/Anaphylaxis
  (1998): Rosales MJ+, *Allergy* 53, 905
Injection-site pain
Myalgia/Myositis/Myopathy/Myotoxicity (<1%)
Paresthesias (<1%)

FOSINOPRIL

Trade names: Acenor-M; Dynacil; Fosinorm; Fozitec; Monopril (Bristol-Myers Squibb); Staril; Vasopril
Indications: Hypertension
Category: Angiotensin-converting enzyme inhibitor
Half-life: 11.5 hours
Clinically important, potentially hazardous interactions with: amiloride, spironolactone, triamterene

Reactions

Skin
Angioedema (<1%)
  (2006): Kahegeshe NL+, *Acta Gastroenterol Belg* 69(4), 381 (bowel)
  (2001): Cohen EG+, *Ann Otol Rhinol Laryngol* 110(8), 701 (64 cases)
  (1997): Graumuller S+, *HNO* (German) 45, 1016
Bullous pemphigoid
Dermatitis

(2004): Pfutzner W+, *Acta Derm Venereol* 84(1), 91 (with
captopril)
Diaphoresis (<1%)
Edema (<1%)
Eosinophilic fasciitis
(1997): Biasi D+, *J Rheumatol* 24(6), 1242
Eosinophilic vasculitis
Exfoliative dermatitis
Pemphigus
(2002): Parodi A+, *Dermatology* 204, 139
Pemphigus foliaceus
(2000): Ong CS+, *Australas J Dermatol* 41(4), 242
Photosensitivity (<1%)
Pruritus (<1%)
(2001): Nunes AC+, *Eur J Gastroenterol Hepatol* 13, 279
Rash (sic) (<1%)
(1990): Pool JL, *Clin Ther* 12, 520 (0.9%)
Scleroderma
(1997): Biasi D+, *J Rheumatol* 24(6), 1242
Urticaria (<1%)
Vasculitis

Mucosal/ENT
Ageusia (<1%)
Dysgeusia (<1%)
(1992): Murdoch D+, *Drugs* 43, 123
Tinnitus
Xerostomia (<1%)

Other
Anaphylactoid reactions/Anaphylaxis
Cough
(2001): Adigun AQ+, *West Afr J Med* 20(1), 46–7
(2001): Lee SC+, *Hypertension* 38(2), 166
(2001): Rosolova H+, *Vnitr Lek* 47(12), 834
Gynecomastia
Headache
Myalgia/Myositis/Myopathy/Myotoxicity (<1%)
Paresthesias (<1%)
Tremor (<1%)

FOSPHENYTOIN

Trade name: Cerebyx (Eisai)
Indications: Seizure prophylaxis, status epilepticus
Category: Antiepileptic, hydantoin
Half-life: 15 minutes
**Clinically important, potentially hazardous interactions
with:** chloramphenicol, cyclosporine, disulfiram, dopamine,
imatinib, itraconazole

Note: Fosphenytoin is a prodrug of phenytoin

Reactions

Skin
Acne (<1%)
Bullous dermatitis
(2001): Hebert AA+, *J Clin Psychiatry* 62(suppl 14), 22
Erythema multiforme (<1%)
(2001): Hebert AA+, *J Clin Psychiatry* 62(suppl 14), 22
Exanthems
Exfoliative dermatitis (<1%)
(2001): Hebert AA+, *J Clin Psychiatry* 62(suppl 14), 22
Facial edema
Lupus erythematosus

(2001): Hebert AA+, *J Clin Psychiatry* 62(suppl 14), 22
Pruritus (48.9%)
(2002): Coplin WM+, *Neurol Res* 24(8), 842
(2001): Hebert AA+, *J Clin Psychiatry* 62(suppl 14), 22
(1998): Knapp LE+, *J Child Neurol* 13, S15
(1998): Luer MS, *Neurol Res* 20, 178
Rash (sic) (<1%)
Stevens–Johnson syndrome
Toxic epidermal necrolysis

Mucosal/ENT
Dysgeusia (3.3%)
Gingival hyperplasia/hypertrophy
(2001): Hebert AA+, *J Clin Psychiatry* 62(suppl 14), 22
Tongue disorder (sic)
Xerostomia (4.4%)

Other
Application-site pain
(2002): Coplin WM+, *Neurol Res* 24(8), 842
Cardiotoxicity
Chills
Headache
Paresthesias (4.4%)
(2002): Coplin WM+, *Neurol Res* 24(8), 842
(1998): Luer MS, *Neurol Res* 20, 178

FROVATRIPTAN

Trade name: Frova (Vernalis)
Indications: Migraine headaches
Category: 5-HT1 agonist; Serotonin receptor agonist; Triptan
Half-life: 26 hours

Reactions

Skin
Bullous dermatitis (<1%)
Diaphoresis (1%)
Pruritus (<1%)
Purpura (<1%)
Rash (sic)

Mucosal/ENT
Cheilitis (<1%)
Dysgeusia (<1%)
Sialopenia (3%)
Sialorrhea (<1%)
Stomatitis (<1%)
Tinnitus (1%)
Xerostomia
(2004): Balbisi EA+, *Int J Clin Pract* 58(7), 695

Eyes
Conjunctivitis (<1%)

Other
Asthenia
(2004): Balbisi EA+, *Int J Clin Pract* 58(7), 695
(2001): Easthope SE+, *CNS Drugs* 15(12), 969
Depression (<1%)
Headache
Hot flashes (<1%)
Myalgia/Myositis/Myopathy/Myotoxicity (<1%)
Pain (1%)
Paresthesias (4%)

(2004): Balbisi EA+, *Int J Clin Pract* 58(7), 695
(2001): Easthope SE+, *CNS Drugs* 15(12), 969
Tremor (<1%)
Vertigo
(2004): Balbisi EA+, *Int J Clin Pract* 58(7), 695

FULVESTRANT

Synonyms: ICI 182; 780
Trade name: Faslodex (AstraZeneca)
Indications: Metastatic breast cancer
Category: Estrogen receptor antagonist
Half-life: ~40 days

Reactions

Skin
Diaphoresis (5%)
Edema (9%)
Peripheral edema
Rash (sic) (7%)

Mucosal/ENT
Vaginitis
(2003): Versea L+, *Clin J Oncol Nurs* 7(3), 307

Other
Cough (10%)
Depression (6%)
Headache
(2004): Watanabe T+, *Anticancer Res* 24(2C), 1275 (23%)
Hot flashes
(2003): Bross PF+, *Clin Cancer Res* 9(12), 4309
(2002): Lynn J, *Cancer Nurs* 25, 12S
Injection-site reactions (11%)
(2003): Bross PF+, *Clin Cancer Res* 9(12), 4309
(2002): Lynn J, *Cancer Nurs* 25, 12S
Myalgia/Myositis/Myopathy/Myotoxicity (<1%)
Pain (19%)
Paresthesias (6%)

FURAZOLIDONE

Trade names: Furion; Furoxona; Fuxol
Indications: Various infections caused by susceptible organisms
Category: Antibiotic, nitrofuran
Half-life: N/A
**Clinically important, potentially hazardous interactions
with:** amphetamines, benzphetamine, chloroquine, dapsone,
dobutamine, dopamine, ephedrine, epinephrine, meperidine,
morphine, phenylephrine, phenylpropanolamine,
pseudoephedrine, sympathomimetics

Note: The disulfiram-like reaction consists of facial flushing,
diaphoresis, tachycardia, and pounding headache

Reactions

Skin
Dermatitis
(1990): de Groot AC+, *Contact Dermatitis* 22, 202
(1980): Goette DK+, *Cutis* 26, 406
Erythema multiforme
(1986): Fisher AA, *Cutis* 37, 158

(1980): Goette DK+, *Cutis* 26, 406
Exanthems (<1%)
Palmar–plantar fixed eruption
(2005): Tan C+, *Allergy* 60(7), 972
Photosensitivity
(1980): Goette DK+, *Cutis* 26, 406
Pruritus
Pruritus ani et vulvae
Rash (sic) (<1%)
Urticaria (<1%)

Other
Disulfiram-like reaction (with alcohol) (<1%)
Serum sickness

FUROSEMIDE

Trade names: Apo-Furosemide; Discoid; Dryptal; Edenol;
Frusid; Furorese; Furoside; Fusid; Henexal; Lasilix; Lasix (Sanofi-
Aventis); Novo-Semide; Urex; Uritol
Indications: Edema
Category: Diuretic, loop
Half-life: 0.5–1 hour
**Clinically important, potentially hazardous interactions
with:** aliskiren, amikacin, amyl nitrite, digoxin, gentamicin,
hydrocortisone, kanamycin, neomycin, probenecid, streptomycin,
tobramycin

Note: Furosemide is a sulfonamide and can be absorbed systemically.
Sulfonamides can produce severe, possibly fatal, reactions such as
toxic epidermal necrolysis and Stevens–Johnson syndrome

Note: Grinspan's syndrome is the triad of oral lichen planus, diabetes
mellitus, and hypertension

Reactions

Skin
Acute febrile neutrophilic dermatosis (Sweet's syndrome)
(2005): Govindarajan G+, *South Med J* 98(5), 570
(1989): Cobb MW, *J Am Acad Dermatol* 21, 339
Acute generalized exanthematous pustulosis (AGEP)
(2006): Davidovici BB+, *Harefuah* 145(7), 477 (with
vancomycin)
(1995): Moreau A+, *Int J Dermatol* 34, 263 (passim)
Bullous dermatitis (<1%)
(1995): Tamimi NA+, *Nephrol Dial Transplant* 10, 1943
(1993): Landor M+, *Ann Allergy* 70, 196
(1992): Van Olden RW+, *Am J Nephrol* 12, 351 (photosensitive)
(1989): Sfar Z+, *Tunis Med* (French) 67, 805
(1985): Anderson CD+, *Photodermatol* 2, 111
(1982): Hallan H+, *Tidsskr Nor Laegeforen* (Norwegian) 102, 630
(1980): Guin JD, *Cutis* 25, 534
(1980): Rees RB+, *J Am Acad Dermatol* 2, 244
Bullous pemphigoid
(2006): Lee JJ+, *J Drugs Dermatol* 5(6), 562
(2003): Ng C, Jackson Beach, FL (from Internet) (observation)
(2002): Thaler D, Monona, WI (from Internet) (observation)
(1997): Panayiotou BN+, *Br J Clin Pract* 51, 49 (2 patients)
(1996): Koch CA+, *Cutis* 58, 340
(1995): Siddiqui MA+, *J Am Geriatr Soc* 43, 1183
(1991): Shelley WB+, *Cutis* 48, 367 (passim)
(1986): Ingber A+, *Z Hautarzt* (German)
(1984): Halevy S+, *Harefuah* (Hebrew) 106, 125
(1981): Castel T, *Clin Exp Dermatol* 6, 635
(1980): Neufeld R+, *Cutis* 26, 290
Diaphoresis

Epidermolysis bullosa
Erythema multiforme (<1%)
　(1980): Zugerman C, *Arch Dermatol* 116, 518
Erythema nodosum
Exanthems (0.2–12%)
　(1999): Litt JZ, Beachwood, OH (personal case) (observation)
　(1988): Lin RY, *N Y State J Med* 88, 439
Exfoliative dermatitis
　(1992): Breathnach SM+, *Adverse Drug Reactions and the Skin*
　　　Blackwell, Oxford, 230 (passim)
Fixed eruption
　(2004): Tornero P+, *Contact Dermatitis* 51(2), 57
Grinspan's syndrome
　(1990): Lamey PJ+, *Oral Surg Oral Med Oral Path* 70, 184
Lichenoid eruption
　(1990): West AJ+, *J Am Acad Dermatol* 23, 689
　(1981): Ota J+, *Skin Res* (Japanese) 23, 639
Linear IgA dermatosis
　(2003): Avci O+, *J Am Acad Dermatol* 48(2), 299 (passim)
　(1999): Cerottini J-P+, *J Am Acad Dermatol* 41, 103
Lupus erythematosus
　(1988): Lin RY, *N Y State J Med* 88, 439
Papuloerythroderma of Ofuji
　(2008): Sugita K+, *J Am Acad Dermatol* 58(2 Suppl), S54
Photosensitivity (1–10%)
　(1989): Cobb MW, *J Am Acad Dermatol* 21, 339
Phototoxicity
　(1998): Vargas F+, *J Photochem Photobiol B* 42, 219
Porokeratosis (disseminated superficial)
　(2000): Kroiss MM+, *Acta Derm Venereol* 80, 52
Pruritus (<1%)
　(1993): Litt JZ, Beachwood, OH (personal case) (observation)
　(1987): Hansbrough JR+, *J Allergy Clin Immunol* 80, 538
Purpura
　(1989): Nishioka K+, *J Dermatol* 16, 220 (pigmented)
　(1983): Michel M+, *Rev Geriat* (French) 8/10, 505
Pustules
　(1990): Mothiron C+, *Presse Med* (French) 19, 1504
　(1989): Cobb MW, *J Am Acad Dermatol* 21, 339
Rash (sic) (<1%)
Side effects (sic)
　(1986): Bigby M+, *JAMA* 256, 3358 (0.05%)
Stevens–Johnson syndrome
　(1991): Chan JC+, *Drug Saf* 6, 230
Toxic epidermal necrolysis
　(2004): Marmelzat J, Los Angeles, CA (from Internet)
　　　(observation)
　(1999): Egan CA+, *J Am Acad Dermatol* 40, 458
Urticaria
　(1987): Hansbrough JR+, *J Allergy Clin Immunol* 80, 538
Vasculitis
　(1990): Bourgain C+, *Presse Med* (French) 19, 1504
　(1989): Cobb MW, *J Am Acad Dermatol* 21, 339
　(1988): Lin RY, *N Y State J Med* 88, 439
　(1982): de la Chapelle C+, *LARC Med* (French) 2, 760

Mucosal/ENT
Ototoxicity
　(2005): Shine NP+, *East Afr Med J* 82(10), 536
　(1999): Humes HD, *Ann N Y Acad Sci* 884, 15
Tinnitus
Ulcerative stomatitis
　(1988): Lin RY, *N Y State J Med* 88, 439
Xerostomia
　(2004): Nederfors T+, *Arch Oral Biol* 49(7), 507
　(1989): Atkinson JC+, *Gerodontology* 8(1), 23

Eyes
Dyschromatopsia
Periorbital edema
　(1987): Hansbrough JR+, *J Allergy Clin Immunol* 80, 538

Other
Anaphylactoid reactions/Anaphylaxis
　(2003): Dominguez-Ortega J+, *Allergol Immunopathol* (Madr)
　　　31(6), 345
　(1987): Hansbrough JR+, *J Allergy Clin Immunol* 80, 538
Headache
Injection-site erythema (<1%)
Injection-site pain
Paresthesias
Porphyria
　(1984): Harber LC+, *J Invest Dermatol* 82, 207
Porphyria cutanea tarda
　(1992): Shelley WB+, *Advanced Dermatologic Diagnosis* WB
　　　Saunders, 414 (passim)
　(1983): Goldsman CI+, *Cleve Clin Q* 50, 151
Pseudolymphoma
　(1995): Magro CM+, *J Am Acad Dermatol* 32, 419
Pseudoporphyria cutanea tarda
　(1998): Breier F+, *Dermatology* 197, 271
Thrombophlebitis

FUSIDIC ACID

Trade names: Fucidin (Leo); Fucithalmic (Leo)
Indications: Angular cheilitis, Bacterial infections, Ocular
infections
Category: Antibacterial
Half-life: N/A
**Clinically important, potentially hazardous interactions
with:** atorvastatin, simvastatin

Reactions

Skin
Acanthosis nigricans
　(1993): Teknetzis A+, *J Am Acad Dermatol* 28(3), 501
Dermatitis
　(2000): Lee AY+, *Contact Dermatitis* 42(1), 53
　(1999): Christiansen K, *Int J Antimicrob Agents* 12 Suppl 2, S3
　(1996): Giordano-Labadie F+, *Contact Dermatitis* 34(2), 159
　(1990): Baptista A+, *Contact Dermatitis* 23(3), 186
　(1988): Hogan DJ, *CMAJ* 138(4), 336 (widespread)
　(1985): Romaguera C+, *Contact Dermatitis* 12(3), 176
　(1982): de Groot AC+, *Contact Dermatitis* 8(6), 429
Jaundice
　(1993): Haddad M+, *Eur J Clin Microbiol Infect Dis* 12(9), 725
　(1983): McAreavey D+, *Scott Med J* 28(2), 179
　(1980): Humble MW+, *Br Med J* 280(6230), 1495 (34%)
Rash (sic)
　(1990): Stonelake PS, *BMJ* 301(6763), 1281
　(1989): Youle MS+, *J Acquir Immune Defic Syndr* 2(1), 59

Eyes
Ocular burning
　(1996): Malminiemi K+, *Acta Ophthalmol Scand* 74(3), 280
Ocular edema
　(1996): Adenis JP+, *Eur J Ophthalmol* 6(4), 368

Other
Abdominal pain
　(1989): Youle MS+, *J Acquir Immune Defic Syndr* 2(1), 59

Asthenia
Headache
(1999): Christiansen K, *Int J Antimicrob Agents* 12 Suppl 2, S3
Hepatotoxicity
(1999): Christiansen K, *Int J Antimicrob Agents* 12 Suppl 2, S3
Hypersensitivity
(1990): Riess CE+, *Lancet* 335(8704), 1525
Nephrotoxicity
(1997): Davies JP+, *Int J Clin Pract* 51(4), 264
(1993): Phillips AO+, *Nephrol Dial Transplant* 8(6), 572
Rhabdomyolysis
(2003): Yuen SL+, *Med J Aust* 179(3), 172 (with simvastatin)
(2000): Wenisch C+, *Am J Med* 109(1), 78 (with atorvastatin)
Thrombophlebitis
(1981): Iwarson S+, *Scand J Infect Dis* 13(1), 65

GABAPENTIN

Trade name: Neurontin (Pfizer)
Indications: Seizures
Category: Anticonvulsant
Half-life: 5–6 hours

Reactions

Skin
Acne (>1%)
Acute febrile neutrophilic dermatosis (Sweet's syndrome)
(2001): Popescu C, Bucharest, Romania (from Internet)
(observation)
(1999): Smith W (from Internet) (observation)
Bullous pemphigoid
(2002): Zachariae CO, *Acta Derm Venereol* 82(5), 396
Edema
(2006): Kanbay M+, *Clin Neuropharmacol* 29(3), 186
(2003): Huber B+, *Seizure* 12(8), 602 (2 cases)
(2002): *Prescrire Int* 11(60), 111
(2002): Gueguen A+, *Presse Med* 31(33), 1559
Exanthems
(2003): Warnock JK+, *Am J Clin Dermatol* 4(1), 21
(1999): DeToledo JC+, *Ther Drug Monit* 21(1), 137
Facial edema (<1%)
Peripheral edema (1.7%)
(2002): *Prescrire Int* 11(60), 111
(1998): Rowbotham M+, *JAMA* 280, 1837
Pruritus (1.3%)
(2006): Ho KY+, *Pain* 126(1-3), 91
Purpura (<1%)
(2003): Poon DY+, *Singapore Med J* 44(1), 42
Rash (sic) (>1%)
(2007): Arif H+, *Neurology* 68(20), 1701
Stevens–Johnson syndrome
(1998): Gonzalez-Sicilia L+, *Am J Med* 105, 455
Urticaria
Vasculitis

Mucosal/ENT
Gingivitis (<1%)
Glossitis
Sialorrhea
Stomatitis
Tinnitus
Xerostomia (1.7%)

Hair
Hair – alopecia

(1997): Picard C+, *Ann Pharmacother* 31, 1260

Eyes
Nystagmus
(2005): Lipson J+, *Am J Kidney Dis* 45(6), e100

Other
Anticonvulsant hypersensitivity syndrome
(2004): Papp Z+, *Orv Hetil* 145(32), 1665
(2001): Ragucci MV+, *Clin Neuropharmacol* 24(2), 103
Asthenia
(2007): Tiippana EM+, *Anesth Analg* 104(6), 1545
(2006): Ho KY+, *Pain* 126(1-3), 91
(2006): Yamauchi T+, *Psychiatry Clin Neurosci* 60(4), 507
(2005): Lipson J+, *Am J Kidney Dis* 45(6), e100
Coma
(2006): Dogukan A+, *Hemodial Int* 10(2), 168
Gynecomastia
(2000): Zylicz Z, *J Pain Symptom Manage* 20, 2
Headache
(2006): Reddy SY+, *Obstet Gynecol* 108(1), 41
Myalgia/Myositis/Myopathy/Myotoxicity
(2005): Lipson J+, *Am J Kidney Dis* 45(6), e100
Neurotoxicity
(2005): Bookwalter T+, *Pharmacotherapy* 25(12), 1817
Paresthesias (<1%)
Somnolence
(2008): Zaccara G+, *Seizure* nd, 182
(2005): Lipson J+, *Am J Kidney Dis* 45(6), e100
Tremor (1–10%)
(2005): Lipson J+, *Am J Kidney Dis* 45(6), e100
(2002): Viteri C, *Rev Neurol* 34(3), 292
Vertigo
(2008): Zaccara G+, *Seizure* nd, 182
(2007): Tiippana EM+, *Anesth Analg* 104(6), 1545
(2006): Reddy SY+, *Obstet Gynecol* 108(1), 41
(2006): Yamauchi T+, *Psychiatry Clin Neurosci* 60(4), 507
(2002): *Prescrire Int* 11(60), 111
(2002): Serpell MG, *Pain* 99(3), 557
(2002): Wilton LV+, *Epilepsia* 43(9), 983
Weight gain
(2007): Ben-Menachem, *Epilepsia* 48, 42
(2005): Ness-Abramof R+, *Drugs Today* (Barc) 41(8), 547

GADOBUTROL

Trade name: Gadovist (Bayer Schering pharma)
Indications: Magnetic resonance imaging
Category: Contrast agent
Half-life: 90 minutes
Clinically important, potentially hazardous interactions with: N/A

Reactions

Skin
Erythema
Hyperhidrosis
Pruritus
Rash (sic) (0.3%)
Urticaria

Mucosal/ENT
Dysgeusia
Xerostomia

Other

Abdominal pain
Anaphylactoid reactions/Anaphylaxis
Bronchospasm
Chills
Headache (0.9%)
Hypersensitivity
Hypotension
Injection-site pain (0.4%)
Injection-site reactions
Insomnia
Nephrotoxicity
  (2006): Briguori C+, *Catheter Cardiovasc Interv* 67(2), 175
Paresthesias (2.5%)
Seizures
Vertigo

GADODIAMIDE

Trade name: Omniscan (Mallinckrodt)
Indications: Magnetic resonance imaging (MRI)
Category: Diagnostic aid; Magnetic resonance imaging contrast medium
Half-life: N/A
Clinically important, potentially hazardous interactions with: N/A

Note: Nephrogenic systemic fibrosis has been reported in patients with end-stage renal failure who were treated with gadodiamide. However, this serious side effect has not been reported in patients with normal renal function

Reactions

Skin

Allergic reactions (sic)
  (1999): Murphy KP+, *Acad Radiol* 6(11), 656
Diaphoresis
Exanthems
Facial edema
Pigmentation
Pruritus
  (1996): Ekholm S+, *Acta Radiol* 37(2), 223
Purpura
Rash (sic)
Urticaria
  (1996): Ekholm S+, *Acta Radiol* 37(2), 223

Mucosal/ENT

Dysgeusia
  (1996): Ekholm S+, *Acta Radiol* 37(2), 223
Rhinitis
Sialorrhea
Tinnitus
Xerostomia

Eyes

Visual disturbances

Other

Abdominal pain
Anaphylactoid reactions/Anaphylaxis
Asthenia
Chest pain
Cough

Fever
Headache
  (1996): Aslanian V+, *Neuroradiology* 38(6), 537
  (1996): Ekholm S+, *Acta Radiol* 37(2), 223
  (1995): Aslanian V+, *J Radiol* 76(7), 431
Hot flashes
Injection-site reactions
  (1996): Aslanian V+, *Neuroradiology* 38(6), 537
  (1996): Hogstrom B+, *J Magn Reson* 6(1), 255
  (1995): Aslanian V+, *J Radiol* 76(7), 431
Myalgia/Myositis/Myopathy/Myotoxicity
Nephrotoxicity
  (2007): Broome DR+, *AJR Am J Roentgenol* 188(2), 586
  (2007): High WA+, *J Am Acad Dermatol* 56(4), 710
  (2007): Karlik SJ, *AJR Am J Roentgenol* 188(6), W584
  (2007): Khurana A+, *Invest Radiol* 42(2), 139
  (2006): Briguori C+, *Catheter Cardiovasc Interv* 67(2), 175
  (2006): Grobner T, *Nephrol Dial Transplant* 21(4), 1104
  (2006): Marckmann P+, *J Am Soc Nephrol* 17(9), 2359
  (2006): Thomsen HS, *Eur Radiol* 16(12), 2619
  (2006): Thomsen HS+, *Clin Radiol* 61(11), 905
  (2004): Thomsen HS, *Eur Radiol* 14(9), 1654
Pain
Paresthesias
Seizures
Thrombophlebitis
Tremor
Vertigo
  (1996): Ekholm S+, *Acta Radiol* 37(2), 223

GADOFOSVESET

Trade name: Vasovist (Schering)
Indications: Radiological contrast agent
Category: Gadolinium-containing intravascular contrast agent
Half-life: ~16 hours
Clinically important, potentially hazardous interactions with: electrolyte-altering agents, qt-prolonging agents

Reactions

Skin

Burning (2%)
Diaphoresis
Erythema
Pruritus (4%)
Urticaria

Mucosal/ENT

Ageusia
Dysgeusia (2%)
Xerostomia

Eyes

Visual hallucinations

Other

Anaphylactoid reactions/Anaphylaxis
Headache (2%)
Hypersensitivity
Hypertension
Hypotension
Injection-site pain
Myalgia/Myositis/Myopathy/Myotoxicity
Paresthesias (3%)
Phlebitis

Tremor
Vertigo

GALANTAMINE

Trade name: Reminyl (Janssen)
Indications: Alzheimer's disease
Category: Cholinesterase inhibitor
Half-life: 6–8 hours
**Clinically important, potentially hazardous interactions
with:** bethanechol, cimetidine, donepezil, edrophonium,
physostigmine, pilocarpine, rivastigmine, succinylcholine, tacrine

Note: Derived from snowdrop (*Galanthus* sp) bulbs

Reactions

Skin
Acute generalized exanthematous pustulosis (AGEP)
  (2002): Gantcheva M+, *World Congress Dermatol* Poster, 1588
Edema
Peripheral edema (>2%)
Purpura (>2%)

Mucosal/ENT
Sialorrhea
Xerostomia

Other
Death
  (2006): *Prescrire Int* 15(83), 103
Delirium
  (2008): Fisher AA+, *Ann Pharmacother*
Depression (5%)
  (2003): Kurz AF+, *Eur J Neurol* 10(6), 633
Headache
  (2002): Zhao Q+, *J Clin Pharmacol* 42(4), 428
Paresthesias
  (2002): Zhao Q+, *J Clin Pharmacol* 42(4), 428
Tremor (1–10%)
Upper respiratory infection (>2%)
Vertigo
  (2005): Levin OS, *Zh Nevrol Psikhiatr Im S S Korsakova*
    105(10), 15

GALSULFASE

Trade name: Naglazyme (BioMarin)
Indications: Mucopolysaccharidosis
Category: Enzyme
Half-life: 9–26 minutes
**Clinically important, potentially hazardous interactions
with:** N/A

Reactions

Skin
Angioedema
Facial edema (11%)
Rash (sic)
Urticaria

Mucosal/ENT
Ear pain

Eyes
Conjunctivitis
Corneal opacity (11%)

Other
Abdominal pain (53%)
Application-site reactions (>50%)
Asthenia (11%)
Chest pain (21%)
Chills
Cough
Fever
Headache
Hypertension (11%)
Pain (26%)

GANCICLOVIR

Trade names: Cymevan; Cymeven; Cymevene; Cytovene
(Roche); Vitrasert
Indications: Cytomegalovirus retinitis in immunocompromised
patients
Category: Antiviral; Guanine nucleoside analog
Half-life: 2.5–3.6 hours
**Clinically important, potentially hazardous interactions
with:** amphotericin B, dapsone, imipenem/cilastatin, zidovudine

Reactions

Skin
Acne (<1%)
Bullous dermatitis (<1%)
Diaphoresis
Edema (<1%)
Exanthems (2–5%)
  (1987): Chachoua A+, *Ann Intern Med* 107, 133 (4.9%)
Exfoliative dermatitis
Facial edema (<1%)
Fixed eruption (<1%)
Photosensitivity (<1%)
Pigmentation (<1%)
Pruritus (5%)
Psoriasis
Purpura
Rash (sic) (>10%)
  (2003): Lorenzi S+, *J Dermatolog Treat* 14(3), 177
Stevens–Johnson syndrome
Urticaria (<1%)
Vitiligo
  (2000): Aubin F+, *Lancet* 355(9204), 626

Mucosal/ENT
Anosmia
Dysgeusia (<1%)
Gingival hyperplasia/hypertrophy
Oral ulceration (<1%)
Tongue disorder (sic) (<1%)
Xerostomia (<1%)

Hair
Hair – alopecia (<1%)
  (1990): Faulds D+, *Drugs* 39, 597

Other
Anaphylactoid reactions/Anaphylaxis

Chills (<1%)
Headache
Injection-site edema (<1%)
Injection-site inflammation (2%)
Injection-site pain (4%)
  (1990): Faulds D+, *Drugs* 39, 597 (4%)
Myalgia/Myositis/Myopathy/Myotoxicity (<1%)
Paresthesias (6–10%)
Phlebitis (2%)
Seizures
  (2003): Reuther LO+, *Ugeskr Laeger* 165(14), 1447
Tremor (<1%)

GANIRELIX

Trade name: Antagon (Organon)
Indications: Infertility
Category: Gonadotropin-releasing hormone antagonist
Half-life: 16.2 hours

Reactions

Skin
Pruritus

Other
Asthenia
  (2000): Gillies PS+, *Drugs* 59(1), 107
Headache
  (2000): Gillies PS+, *Drugs* 59(1), 107
Hot flashes (4–5%)
Injection-site reactions (11%)
  (2001): Fluker M+, *Fertil Steril* 75(1), 38 (11.9%)
  (2000): Gillies PS+, *Drugs* 59, 107
  (2000): Oberye J+, *Hum Reprod* 15, 245

GARLIC

Scientific name: *Allium sativum*
Family: Liliaceae
Trade and other common names: Ail; Ajo; Camphor of the Poor; Nectar of the Gods; Poor Man's Treacle; Rust Treacle; Stinking Rose
Category: Immunomodulator
Purported indications and other uses: Hypertension, hypercholesterolemia, atherosclerosis, earache, menstrual disorders, allergy, flu, arthritis, diarrhea, bacterial and fungal infections, tinea corporis, tinea pedis, onychomycosis, vaginitis
Half-life: N/A
Clinically important, potentially hazardous interactions with: atazanavir, chlorpropamide, HIV medications, lisinopril, olmesartan, saquinavir, ticlopidine, warfarin

Reactions

Skin
Allergic reactions (sic)
  (2002): Moneret-Vautrin DA+, *Allerg Immunol* (Paris) 34(4), 135
  (2002): Pires G+, *Allergy* 57(10), 957
  (2000): Sanchez-Hernandez MC+, *Allergy* 55(3), 297
Bullous dermatitis
  (1993): Garty BZ, *Pediatrics* 91, 658
Burning

(2006): Friedman T+, *Int J Dermatol* 45(10), 1161 (self-inflicted)
(2003): Lachter J+, *Mil Med* 168(6), 499
(2002): Groppo FC+, *Int Dent J* 52(6), 433
(2001): Baruchin AM+, *Burns* 27(7), 781
(2000): Hviid K+, *Ugeskr Laeger* 162(50), 6853
(2000): Rafaat M+, *Peditar Dermatol* 17(6), 475
(1997): Roberge RJ+, *Am J Emerg Med* 15(5), 548
(1987): Parish RA+, *Pediatr Emerg Care* 3(4), 258
Dermatitis
  (2002): Hughes TM+, *Contact Dermatitis* 47(1), 48
  (2001): McGovern TW+, *Cutis* 67, 193
  (2000): Fernandez-Vozmediano JM+, *Contact Dermatitis* 42(2), 108
  (1999): Eming SA+, *Br J Dermatol* 141(2), 391 (toxic)
  (1999): Jappe U+, *Am J Contact Dermat* 10, 37
  (1997): Bruynzeel DP, *Contact Dermatitis* 37, 70
  (1996): Delaney TA+, *Australas J Dermatol* 37, 109
  (1996): Kanerva L+, *Contact Dermatitis* 35(3), 157
  (1994): Burden AD+, *Contact Dermatitis* 30(5), 299 (systemic)
  (1993): Acciai MC+, *Contact Dermatitis* 29, 48
  (1992): McFadden JP+, *Contact Dermatitis* 27(5), 333
  (1991): Lee TY+, *Contact Dermatits* 24(3), 193
  (1991): Lembo G+, *Contact Dermatitis* 25(5), 330
  (1987): Cronin E, *Contact Dermatitis* 17, 265
  (1985): Fernandez de Corres L+, *Allergol Immunopathol* (Madr) 13(4), 291
  (1983): Papegeorgiou C+, *Arch Dermatol Res* 275(4), 229
  (1981): Martinescu E, *Rev Med Chir Soc Med Nat Iasi* 85(3), 541
  (1980): Mitchell JC, *Contact Dermatitis* 6(5), 356
Hemorrhage
  (2002): Carden SM+, *Clin Experiment Ophthalmol* 30(4), 303
Pemphigus
  (1996): Ruocco V+, *Dermatology* 192(4), 373
Sensitization
  (2002): Moneret-Vautrin DA+, *Allerg Immunol* (Paris) 34(4), 135
Urticaria
  (2001): McGovern TW+, *Cutis* 67, 193 (passim)

Mucosal/ENT
Cheilitis
  (2007): Ekeowa-Anderson AL+, *Contact Dermatitis* 56(3), 174
Stomatodynia

Eyes
Rhinoconjunctivitis
  (2002): Jimenez-Timon A+, *Allergol Immunopathol* (Madr) 30(5), 295

Other
Anaphylactoid reactions/Anaphylaxis
  (1999): Perez-Pimiento AJ+ 54(6), 626
Hypersensitivity
  (2001): McGovern TW+, *Cutis* 67, 193 (passim)
  (1982): Campolmi P+, *Contact Dermatitis* 8(5), 352

GATIFLOXACIN

Trade name: Tequin (Bristol-Myers Squibb)
Indications: Various infections caused by susceptible organisms
Category: Antibiotic, quinolone
Half-life: 7–14 hours
Clinically important, potentially hazardous interactions with: amiodarone, arsenic, bepridil, bretylium, disopyramide, erythromycin, phenothiazines, procainamide, quinidine, sotalol, tricyclic antidepressants, zinc

Reactions

Skin

Allergic reactions (sic) (0.1–3%)
  (2002): Medeiros EA, *Braz J Infect Dis* 6(4), 149 (0.18%)
Angioedema
Burning
Diaphoresis (0.1–3%)
Edema (<0.1%)
Erythema
Exanthems (<0.1%)
Facial edema (<0.1%)
Fixed eruption
  (2000): Zabawski E, Longwood, TX (from Internet)
    (observation)
Peripheral edema (0.1–3%)
Photosensitivity
  (2006): Chawla S+, *J Assoc Physicians India* 54, 827
  (2000): Stein GE+, *Inf Med* 17, 564
Phototoxicity
  (2006): Chawla S+, *J Assoc Physicians india* 54, 827
Pruritus (<0.1%)
Rash (sic) (0.1–3%)
Stevens–Johnson syndrome
Toxic epidermal necrolysis
Urticaria
Vasculitis
Vesiculobullous eruption (<0.1%)

Mucosal/ENT

Cheilitis (<0.1%)
Dysgeusia (0.1–3%)
  (2002): Medeiros EA, *Braz J Infect Dis* 6(4), 149 (0.46%)
  (2000): Stein GE+, *Inf Med* 17, 564
Gingivitis (<0.1%)
Glossitis (0.1–3%)
Oral candidiasis (0.1–3%)
Oral ulceration (0.1–3%)
Parosmia (<0.1%)
Stomatitis (0.1–3%)
Tongue edema (<0.1%)
Vaginitis (6%)
  (2000): Stein GE+, *Inf Med* 17, 564

Eyes

Corneal abnormalities
  (2004): Awwad ST+, *Eye Contact Lens* 30(3), 169
Visual hallucinations
  (2006): Adams M+, *Psychosomatics* 47(4), 360

Other

Anaphylactoid reactions/Anaphylaxis
Candidiasis
Chills (0.1–3%)
  (2002): Nicholson SC+, *Diagn Microbiol Infect Dis* 44(1), 117
Delirium
  (2006): Satyanarayana S+, *J Am Geriatr Soc* 54(5), 871
  (2003): Sumner CL+, *Psychosomatics* 44(1), 85
Headache
  (2002): Medeiros EA, *Braz J Infect Dis* 6(4), 149 (0.42%)
Hepatotoxicity
  (2005): Tunuguntla A+, *Tenn Med* 98(3), 133
  (2004): Cheung O+, *Ann Intern Med* 140(1), 73
  (2002): Artymowicz RJ, *Ann Pharmacother* 36(11), 1810
  (2001): Henann NE+, *Pharmacotherapy* 21(12), 1579
Hypersensitivity
Injection-site reactions (sic) (5%)

(2002): Perry CM+, *Drugs* 62(1), 169
(2000): Gajjar DA+, *Pharmacotherapy* 20, 49S
Myalgia/Myositis/Myopathy/Myotoxicity (<0.1%)
Paresthesias (0.1–3%)
Seizures
  (2007): Koussa S+, *Rev Neurol* (Paris) 163(1), 99
  (2006): Koussa SF+, *Eur J Neurol* 13(6), 671
  (2004): Quigley CA+, *Ann Pharmacother* 38(2), 235
Serum sickness
Tendinopathy/Tendon rupture
Tremor (0.1–3%)
Vertigo (<2%)
  (2002): Medeiros EA, *Braz J Infect Dis* 6(4), 149
  (2002): Sher LD+, *Otolaryngol Head Neck Surg* 127(3), 182
    (1.8%)

GEFITINIB

Trade names: Iressa (AstraZeneca); ZD1839
Indications: Advanced non-small cell lung cancer
Category: Tyrosine kinase inhibitor
Half-life: 12–51 hours
**Clinically important, potentially hazardous interactions
with:** None

Reactions

Skin

Acne (39–52%)
  (2007): Ijin-A-Ion ML+, *Ned Tijdschr Geneeskd* 151(17), 945 (2
    cases)
  (2006): Fernandez-Guarino M+, *Actas Dermosifiliogr* 97(8), 503
  (2006): Graves JE+, *J Am Acad Dermatol* 55(2), 349
  (2006): Niho S+, *J Clin Oncol* 24(1), 64
  (2005): Martinez de Lagran Z+, *Actas Dermosifiliogr* 96(7), 450
  (2004): Cappuzzo F+, *Br J Cancer* 90(1), 82 (52.6%)
  (2004): Fernandez-Galar M+, *Clin Exp Dermatol* 29(2), 138
  (2004): Forsythe B+, *Drug Saf* 27(14), 1081
  (2004): Jacot W+, *Br J Dermatol* 151(1), 238
  (2004): Lee MW+, *Acta Derm Venereol* 84(1), 23 (39%)
  (2004): Mittal A, Udipur, India (from Internet) (observation)
  (2004): Mu XL+, *BMC Cancer* 4, 51
  (2004): Purdom M, *Clin J Oncol Nurs* 8(3), 316
  (2004): Tong M, Maylasia (pustular) (from Internet) (observation)
  (2004): Warthan MM+, *J Drugs Dermatol* 3(5), 569
  (2003): Ieki R+, *Eur Respir J* 22(1), 179
  (2003): Johnson DH, *Lung Cancer* 41, S23
  (2003): Kris MG+, *JAMA* 290(16), 2149
  (2003): Nakagawa K+, *Ann Oncol* 14(6), 922
  (2002): Baselga J+, *J Clin Oncol* 20(21), 4292
  (2002): Herbst RS+, *J Clin Oncol* 20(18), 3815 (46%) (follicular)
  (2002): Van Doorn R+, *Br J Dermatol* 147(3), 598
  (1995): Salomon DS+, *Crit Rev Oncol Hematol* 19(3), 183
Acute generalized exanthematous pustulosis (AGEP)
  (2006): Shih HC+, *Br J Dermatol* 155(5), 1101 (2 cases)
Adverse effects (sic)
  (2004): Perras C, *Issues Emerg Health Technol* 150(55), 1
  (2004): Ranson M+, *J Clin Pharm Ther* 29(2), 95
  (2004): Rich JN+, *J Clin Oncol* 22(1), 133
Desquamation (39%)
  (2006): Graves JE+, *J Am Acad* 55(2), 349
  (2004): Lee MW+, *Acta Derm Venereol* 84(1), 23 (39%)
Erosive pustular dermatosis
  (2008): Wu CY+, *Clin Exp Dermatol* 33(1), 106 (scalp)
Exanthems
  (2005): Kurokawa I+, *Int J Dermatol* 44(2), 167

(2004): Schlessinger J, Omaha, NE (from Internet) (observation)

Exfoliative dermatitis
(2006): Cersosimo RJ, *Expert Opin Drug Saf* 5(3), 469

Folliculitis
(2006): Kirby AM+, *Br J Cancer* 94(5), 631
(2006): Matheis P+, *J Am Acad Dermatol* 55(4), 710 (3 cases)
(2005): Treudler R+, *Dermatology* 211(4), 375
(2002): Van Doorn R+, *Br J Dermatol* 147(3), 598

Glucagonoma syndrome
(2003): Trojan A+, *Swiss Med Wkly* 133(1), 22

Hand–foot syndrome
(2006): Razis E+, *Cancer Invest* 24(5), 514 (recall) (3 cases)

Pigmentation
(2004): Chang GC+, *J Clin Oncol* 22(22), 4646

Pruritus (52%)
(2004): Cappuzzo F+, *Br J Cancer* 90(1), 82 (52.6%)
(2004): Forsythe B+, *Drug Saf* 27(14), 1081

Pyoderma gangrenosum
(2006): Sagara R+, *Int J Dermatol* 45(8), 1002

Rash (sic) (52%)
(2007): Fury MG+, *Cancer Chemother Pharmacol* 59(4), 467
(2007): Gadgeel SM+, *J Thorac Oncol* 2(4), 299
(2006): Chang A+, *J Thorac Oncol* 1(8), 847
(2006): Chou LS+, *Clin Lung Cancer* 8 Suppl 1, S15
(2006): Dudek AZ+, *Lung Cancer* 51(1), 89
(2006): Jubelirer SJ+, *W V Med J* 102(6), 14
(2006): Maurel J+, *Int J Radiat Oncol Biol Phys* 66(5), 1391 (with gemcitabine)
(2006): Perez-Soler R, *Clin Lung Cancer* 8 Suppl 1, S7
(2006): Seiverling EV+, *J Drugs Dermatol* 5(4), 368
(2005): Canil CM+, *J Clin Oncol* 23(3), 455
(2005): Mohamed MK+, *Ann Oncol* 16(5), 780
(2005): Pascual JC+, *Br J Dermatol* 153(6), 1222
(2005): Perez-Soler R+, *J Clin Oncol* 23(22), 5235
(2005): Razis E+, *Anticancer Drugs* 16(2), 191
(2004): Argiris A+, *Lung Cancer* 43(3), 317
(2004): Cappuzzo F+, *Br J Cancer* 90(1), 82 (52.6%)
(2004): Cersosimo RJ, *Am J Health Syst Pharm* 61(9), 889
(2004): Forsythe B+, *Drug Saf* 27(14), 1081
(2004): Janne PA+, *Lung Cancer* 44(2), 221
(2004): Mu XL+, *BMC Cancer* 4, 51
(2003): Perez-Soler R, *Oncology (Huntingt)* 17(11 Suppl 12), 23
(2002): Culy CR+, *Drugs* 62(15), 2237
(2000): Meric JB+, *Bull Cancer* 87(12), 873

Rosacea
(2004): Aylesworth R, Rhinelander, WI (from Internet) (observation)

Scaling
(2002): Van Doorn R+, *Br J Dermatol* 147(3), 598

Seborrhea
(2006): Cersosimo RJ, *Expert Opin Drug Saf* 5(3), 469
(2005): Graves JE+, *J Am Acad* 55(2), 349

Toxicity (sic)
(2007): Yoshida K+, *J Thorac Oncol* 2(1), 22
(2006): Cusatis G+, *J Natl Cancer Inst* 98(23), 1739
(2006): Lin WC+, *Lung Cancer* 54(2), 193
(2004): Herbst RS+, *J Clin Oncol* 22(5), 785

Ulcerations
(2004): Lee MW+, *Acta Derm Venereol* 84(1), 23 (nasal)

Urticaria
(2004): Lee MW+, *Acta Derm Venereol* 84(1), 23

Xerosis (39–52%)
(2006): Cersosimo RJ, *Expert Opin Drug Saf* 5(3), 469
(2006): Graves JE+, *J Am Acad Dermatol* 55(2), 349
(2004): Cappuzzo F+, *Br J Cancer* 90(1), 82 (52.6%)
(2004): Forsythe B+, *Drug Saf* 27(14), 1081
(2004): Lee MW+, *Acta Derm Venereol* 84(1), 23 (39%)

Mucosal/ENT

Epistaxis
(2006): Cersosimo RJ, *Expert Opin Drug Saf* 5(3), 469

Oral ulceration
(2004): Lee MW+, *Acta Derm Venereol* 84(1), 23

Stomatitis
(2006): Cersosimo RJ, *Expert Opin Drug Saf* 5(3), 469

Hair

Hair – abnormal texture
(2006): Graves JE+, *J Am Acad Dermatol* 55(2), 349

Hair – alopecia
(2006): Graves JE+, *J Am Acad Dermatol* 55(2), 349

Hair – hypertrichosis
(2002): Van Doorn R+, *Br J Dermatol* 147(3), 598

Nails

Nails – changes (sic) (17%)
(2006): Lin WC+, *Lung Cancer* 54(2), 193

Nails – paronychia (6%)
(2007): Tjin-A-Ton ML+, *Ned Tijdschr Geneeskd* 151(17), 945 (2 cases)
(2006): Graves JE+, *J Am Acad Dermatol* 55(2), 349
(2004): Chang GC+, *J Clin Oncol* 22(22), 4646
(2004): Davidson D, Groton, CT (all fingers) (from Internet) (observation)
(2004): Lee MW+, *Acta Derm Venereol* 84(1), 23 (6%)
(2004): Thaler D, Monona, WI (from Internet) (observation)
(2003): Dainichi T+, *Dermatology* 207(3), 324
(2003): Nakano J+, *J Dermatol* 30(3), 261
(2002): Di Lernia V Reggio Emilia, Italy (from Internet) (observation)

Nails – pyogenic granulomas
(2006): High WA, *Arch Dermatol* 142(7), 939

Eyes

Blepharitis
(2006): Cersosimo RJ, *Expert Opin Drug Saf* 5(3), 469

Conjunctivitis
(2006): Cersosimo RJ, *Expert Opin Drug Saf* 5(3), 469

Eyelashes – hypertrichosis
(2004): Pascual JC+, *Br J Dermatol* 151(5), 1111

Other

Abdominal pain
(2006): Cersosimo RJ, *Expert Opin Drug Saf* 5(3), 469

Anaphylactoid reactions/Anaphylaxis
(2004): Perras C, *Issues Emerg Health Technol* 55, 1

Asthenia
(2007): Fury MG+, *Cancer Chemother Pharmacol* 59(4), 467
(2006): Hofheinz RD+, *Onkologie* 29(12), 563
(2006): Maurel J+, *Int J Radiat Oncol Biol Phys* 66(5), 1391
(2005): Canil CM+, *J Clin Oncol* 23(3), 455
(2004): Forsythe B+, *Drug Saf* 27(14), 1081

Death
(2005): Aoe K+, *Anticancer Res* 25(1B), 415
(2003): Rabinowits G+, *Anticancer Drugs* 14(8), 665

Hepatotoxicity
(2006): Carlini P+, *J Clin Oncol* 24(35), e60
(2005): Ho C+, *J Clin Oncol* 23(33), 8531

Nephrotoxicity
(2004): Kumasaka R+, *J Clin Oncol* 22(12), 2504

Pain
(2006): Cersosimo RJ, *Expert Opin Drug Saf* 5(3), 469

Thrombophlebitis
(2004): Perras C, *Issues Emerg Health Technol* 55, 1

GEMCITABINE

Trade name: Gemzar (Lilly)
Indications: Pancreatic carcinoma
Category: Antimetabolite; Antineoplastic
Half-life: 42–94 minutes
Clinically important, potentially hazardous interactions with: aldesleukin

Reactions

Skin

Acral necrosis
  (2003): D'Alessandro V+, *Clin Ter* 154(3), 207
Allergic reactions (sic) (4%)
Cellulitis
  (2003): Schwartz BM+, *Gynecol Oncol* 91(2), 421
Dermatitis
  (2001): Fogarty G+, *Lung Cancer* 33(2), 299
Diaphoresis
Edema (13%)
  (2003): Schwartz BM+, *Gynecol Oncol* 91(2), 421
  (2000): Geffen DB+, *Isr Med Assoc J* 2, 552
  (1995): Tonato M+, *Anticancer Drugs* 6, 27
Erysipelas
  (2000): Brandes A+, *Anticancer Drugs* 11, 15 (confined to areas of lymphedema)
Exanthems
  (2001): Chu CY+, *Acta Derm Venereol* 81(6), 426
  (1996): Chen YM+, *J Clin Oncol* 14, 1743
Hand–foot syndrome
  (2005): Rini BI+, *Cancer* 103(3), 553 (with capecitabine)
  (2003): Michaelson MD+, *Cancer* 97(1), 148
  (2003): Scheithauer W+, *Ann Oncol* 14(1), 97
  (2002): Dalbagni G+, *J Clin Oncol* 20(15), 3193
  (2002): Fracasso PM+, *Cancer* 95(10), 2223 (with doxorubicin)
  (2001): Laack E+, *Ann Oncol* 12(12), 1761 (with vinorelbine)
Linear IgA dermatosis
  (2001): del Pozo J+, *Ann Pharmacother* 35(7–8), 891
Lipodermatosclerosis
  (2001): Chia-Yu C+, *Acta Dermato-Venereol* 81(6), 426
Livedo reticularis
  (2005): Gibbs MB+, *J Am Acad Dermatol* 52(6), 1009
Necrotizing vasculitis
  (2003): Venat-Bouvet L+, *Anticancer Drugs* 14(10), 829
Petechiae (16%)
Photo-recall (<74%)
  (2006): Fakih MG, *JOP* 7(3), 306
  (2006): Pinson PJ+, *Ned Tijdschr Geneeskd* 150(34), 1891 (myositis) (with carboplatin)
  (2006): Saif MW+, *Anticancer Drugs* 17(1), 107
  (2006): Squire S+, *Am J Clin Oncol* 29(6), 636
  (2005): Badger J+, *J Clin Oncol* 23(28), 7224
  (2005): Marisavljevic D+, *Am J Hematol* 80(1), 91
  (2004): Aguilar-Ponce J+, *Ann Oncol* 15(2), 301 (74%)
  (2004): Friedlander PA+, *Cancer* 100(9), 1793
  (2003): Miura G+, *Nippon Igaku Hoshasen Gakkai Zasshi* 63(8), 420
  (2003): Schwartz BM+, *Gynecol Oncol* 91(2), 421
  (2002): Jeter MD+, *Int J Radiat Oncol Biol Phys* 53(2), 394
  (2001): Bar-Sela G+, *Tumori* 87(6), 428
  (2001): Fogarty G+, *Lung Cancer* 33(2–3), 299
  (2000): Burstein HJ, *J Clin Oncol* 18, 693
Pruritus (13%)
Pruritus ani et vulvae
  (1999): Hejna M+, *N Engl J Med* 340, 655
Rash (sic) (30%)

  (2007): Dragovich T+, *Cancer Chemother Pharmacol* 60(2), 295 (with erlotinib)
  (2006): Maurel J+, *Int J Radiat Oncol Biol Phys* 66(5), 1391 (with gefitinib)
  (2004): Buesa JM+, *Cancer* 101(10), 2261 (with dacarbazine)
  (2003): Sumii T+, *Gan To Kagaku Ryoho* 30(7), 971
  (2002): Fracasso PM+, *Cancer* 95(10), 2223 (with doxorubicin)
Raynaud's phenomenon
  (2003): Clowse ME+, *J Rheumatol* 30(6), 1341 (with carboplatin)
  (2003): D'Alessandro V+, *Clin Ter* 154(3), 207
Scleroderma
  (2004): Bessis D+, *J Am Acad Dermatol* 51(2 Suppl), S73
Stevens–Johnson syndrome
  (2003): Sommers KR+, *Anticancer Drugs* 14(8), 659
Toxic epidermal necrolysis
  (2003): Mermershtain W+, *J Chemother* 15(5), 510
  (2003): Sommers KR+, *Anticancer Drugs* 14(8), 659
Toxicity (sic)
  (2005): Tendo M+, *Gan To Kagaku Ryoho* 32(6), 795
Vasculitis
  (2004): Geisler JP+, *Gynecol Oncol* 92(2), 705
  (2002): Voorburg AM+, *Lung Cancer* 36(2), 203
  (2000): Banach MJ+, *Arch Ophthalmol* 118, 726 (necrotizing)

Mucosal/ENT

Dysgeusia
  (2001): Johnson FM, *Cancer Nurs* 24(2), 149
Mucositis
  (2002): Eckel F+, *Cancer Invest* 20(2), 180
Stomatitis (11%)
  (2006): Ochi T+, *Nippon Hinyokika Gakkai Zasshi* 97(6), 777 (with cisplatin)
  (2006): von der Masse H+, *Ann Oncol* 17(10), 1533 (with pemetrexed)
  (2005): Schmid P+, *Invest New Drugs* 23(2), 139
  (2004): Buesa JM+, *Cancer* 101(10), 2261 (with dacarbazine)
  (2003): Michaelson MD+, *Cancer* 97(1), 148
  (2002): Bass AJ+, *J Clin Oncol* 20(13), 2995
  (2002): Brugnatelli S+, *Oncology* 62(1), 33
  (2002): Fracasso PM+, *Cancer* 95(10), 2223 (with doxorubicin)

Hair

Hair – alopecia (15%)
  (2006): Ochi T+, *Nippon Hinyokika Gakkai Zasshi* 97(6), 777 (with cisplatin)
  (2004): Buesa JM+, *Cancer* 101(10), 2261 (with dacarbazine)
  (2003): Belpomme D+, *Gynecol Oncol* 91(1), 32 (with cisplatin)
  (2002): Brugnatelli S+, *Oncology* 62(1), 33
  (2001): Chu CY+, *Acta Derm Venereol* 81(6), 426 (passim)
  (1999): Akrivakis K+, *Anticancer Drugs* 10, 525
  (1995): Tonato M+, *Anticancer Drugs* 6, 27
  (1994): Abratt RP+, *J Clin Oncol* 12, 1535

Other

Anaphylactoid reactions/Anaphylaxis
Asthenia (18%)
  (2005): Schmid P+, *Invest New Drugs* 23(2), 139
  (2004): Buesa JM+, *Cancer* 101(10), 2261 (with dacarbazine)
  (2004): Nobutani K+, *Gan To Kagaku Ryoho* 31(2), 199 (18.8%)
  (2003): Markman M+, *Gynecol Oncol* 90(3), 593
  (2002): Poggi MM+, *Int J Radiat Oncol Biol Phys* 54(3), 670
Chills
  (2003): Markman M+, *Gynecol Oncol* 90(3), 593
Death
  (2004): Geisler JP+, *Gynecol Oncol* 92(2), 705
  (2003): Belpomme D+, *Gynecol Oncol* 91(1), 32 (with cisplatin)
  (2003): Maniwa K+, *Intern Med* 42(10), 1022
Fever
  (2004): Buesa JM+, *Cancer* 101(10), 2261 (with dacarbazine)
  (2003): D'Alessandro V+, *Clin Ter* 154(3), 207

(2003): Markman M+, *Gynecol Oncol* 90(3), 593
Gangrene (digital)
(2003): D'Alessandro V+, *Clin Ter* 154(3), 207
Headache
Infections (16%)
(2002): Poggi MM+, *Int J Radiat Oncol Biol Phys* 54(3), 670
Injection-site reactions (4%)
Lymphedema
(2000): Brandes A+, *Anticancer Drugs* 11, 15 (confined to areas of erysipeloid rash)
Myalgia/Myositis/Myopathy/Myotoxicity (>10%)
(2007): Huang YJ+, *Chin Med J* (Engl) 120(6), 458
(2002): Voorburg AM+, *Lung Cancer* 36(2), 203 (with cisplatin)
(2001): Fogarty G+, *Lung Cancer* 33(2), 299
Nephrotoxicity
(2007): Yamamoto A+, *Pancreas* 34(3), 378
(2001): Kintzel PE, *Drug Saf* 24(1), 19
Neurotoxicity
(2007): Huang YJ+, *Chin Med J* (Engl) 120(6), 458
Paresthesias (10%)
(2003): D'Alessandro V+, *Clin Ter* 154(3), 207
Pseudolymphoma
(2001): Marucci G+, *Br J Dermatol* 145(4), 650
Seizures
(2007): Huang YJ+, *Chin Med J* (Engl) 120(6), 458

GEMFIBROZIL

Trade names: Bolutol; Decrelip; Fibrocit; Gemlipid; Gen-Fibro; Gevilon Uno; Jezil; Lipur; Lopid (Pfizer); Nu-Gemfibrozil
Indications: Hyperlipidemia
Category: Fibrate; Lipid regulator
Half-life: 1.5 hours
Clinically important, potentially hazardous interactions with: atorvastatin, bexarotene, cyclosporine, dicumarol, ezetimibe, fluvastatin, interferon alfa, lovastatin, nicotinic acid, pioglitazone, pravastatin, repaglinide, rosuvastatin, roxithromycin, simvastatin, statins, warfarin

Reactions

Skin
Abscess
Acanthosis nigricans
Angioedema
Basal cell carcinoma
Dermatitis (0.4%)
(1988): Todd PA+, *Drugs* 36, 314
Dermatomyositis (<1%)
Eczema (1.9%)
Erythema multiforme
Exanthems (3%)
(1990): Fusella J+, *J Rheumatol* 17, 572
(1988): Todd PA+, *Drugs* 36, 314 (2.1%)
Exfoliative dermatitis (<1%)
Ichthyosis
Lichen planus
Lupus erythematosus
Melanoma
Palmar erythema
(2007): Serrao R+, *Am J Clin Dermatol* 8(6), 347
Petechiae
Pruritus (0.8%)
(1988): Todd PA+, *Drugs* 36, 314

Psoriasis
(1989): Frick MH, *Arch Dermatol* 125, 132
(1988): Fisher DA+, *Arch Dermatol* 124, 854
Rash (sic) (1.7%)
Raynaud's phenomenon (<1%)
(1993): Smith GW+, *Br J Rheumatol* 32, 84
Seborrhea
Thickening
Urticaria (0.1%)
(1988): Todd PA+, *Drugs* 36, 314
Vasculitis (<1%)
(1993): Smith GW+, *Br J Rheumatol* 32, 84
Xerosis

Mucosal/ENT
Dysgeusia (<1%)

Hair
Hair – alopecia
Hair – hirsutism

Nails
Nails – discoloration
(1990): Klein ME, *The Schoch Letter* 40 (#7), 29 (#120) (observation)
Nails – growth

Other
Anaphylactoid reactions/Anaphylaxis
Death
(2001): Federman DG+, *South Med J* 94(10), 1023
(2000): Ozdemir O+, *Angiology* 51(8), 695 (with cerivastatin)
Headache
Hepatotoxicity
(2006): Grubisic-Cabo F+, *Med Oncol* 23(1), 121 (with interferon alfa)
Myalgia/Myositis/Myopathy/Myotoxicity (<1%)
(2002): Atmaca H+, *Ann Pharmacother* 36(11), 1719 (with colchicine)
(2001): Litt JZ (personal case) (observation)
Paresthesias (<1%)
Polymyositis
(1990): Fusella J+, *J Rheumatol* 17, 572
Pseudolymphoma
(1995): Magro CM+, *J Am Acad Dermatol* 32, 419
Rhabdomyolysis
(2006): Barquero-Romero J+, *An Med Interna* 23(10), 504
(2005): Jones PH+, *Am J Cardiol* 95(1), 120 (with statins)
(2004): Alsheikh-Ali AA+, *Am J Cardiol* 94(7), 935 (with cerivastatin)
(2004): Layne RD+, *Ann Pharmacother* 38(2), 232
(2003): Yen TH+, *Ren Fail* 25(1), 139
(2002): Atmaca H+, *Ann Pharmacother* 36(11), 1719 (with colchicine)
(2002): Backman JT+, *Clin Pharmacol Ther* 72(6), 685 (with cerivastatin)
(2002): Carretero MM+, *Br J Gen Pract* 52(476), 235 (with cerivastatin)
(2002): Kind AH+, *WMJ* 101(7), 53 (with cerivastatin)
(2002): Roca B+, *Ann Pharmacother* 36(4), 730 (with cerivastatin)
(2002): SantaCruz PL+, *Nefrologia* 22(3), 301 (with cerivastatin)
(2002): Su M+, *Am J Forensic Med Pathol* 23(3), 305 (with cerivastatin)
(2001): Bosch Rovira T+, *Rev Clin Esp* 201(12), 731 (with cerivastatin)
(2001): Bruno-Joyce J+, *Ann Pharmacother* 35(9), 1016 (with cerivastatin)
(2001): de Arriba Mendez JJ+, *Med Clin* (Barc) 117(7), 278 (with cerivastatin)

(2001): Federman DG+, *South Med J* 94(10), 1023 (with simvastatin)
(2001): Hendriks F+, *Nephrol Dial Transplant* 16(12), 2418 (with cerivastatin)
(2001): Sirvent AE+, *Nefrologia* 21(5), 497 (with cerivastatin)
(2001): Tomlinson B+, *Am J Med* 110(8), 669 (with cerivastatin)
(2000): Oldemeyer JB+, *Cardiology* 94(2), 127 (with simvastatin)
(2000): Ozdemir O+, *Angiology* 51(8), 695 (with cerivastatin)
(1998): Duell PB+, *Am J Cardiol* 81(3), 368 (with atorvastatin)
(1998): Torbet JA, *Am J Cardiol* 62, 28J (with cyclosporine)
(1997): Tal A+, *South Med J* 1997 May; 90(5), 546 (with simvastatin)
(1996): Gorriz JL+, *Nephron* 74(2), 437
(1996): van Puijenbroek EP+, *J Intern Med* 240(6), 403 (with simvastatin)
(1995): Abdul-Ghaffar NU+, *J Clin Gastroenterol* 21(4), 340 (with lovastatin)
(1993): Knoll RW+, *Conn Med* 57(9), 593 (with lovastatin)
(1991): Magarian GJ+, *Arch Intern Med* 151(9), 1873
(1990): *JAMA* 264(23), 2991 (with lovastatin)
(1990): Marais GE+, *Ann Intern Med* 112(3), 228 (with lovastatin)
(1990): Pierce LR+, *JAMA* 264(1), 71 (with lovastatin)

GEMIFLOXACIN

Synonyms: DW286; LA 20304a; SB-265805
Trade name: Factive
Indications: Infections due to various microorganisms
Category: Antibiotic, quinolone
Half-life: 4–12 hours
Clinically important, potentially hazardous interactions with: None

Note: The incidence of rash increases significantly when duration of therapy exceeds seven days, reaching 7.4% at 14 days

Reactions

Skin
Angioedema
Dermatitis (<1%)
Eczema (<1%)
Exanthems
  (2004): File TM Jr+, *Expert Rev Anti Infect Ther* 2(6), 831 (2.8%)
Fungal dermatitis (<1%)
Photosensitivity (<1%)
  (2002): Lode H+, *Clin Ther* 24(11), 1915
  (2000): Lowe MN+, *Drugs* 59(5), 1137
Rash (sic)
  (2006): Iannini P+, *J Chemother* 18(1), 3
  (2004): Ball P+, *Int J Antimicrob Agents* 23(5), 421
  (2004): File TM+, *Expert Rev Anti Infect Ther* 2(6), 831
  (2004): Leophonte P+, *Respir Med* 98(8), 708
Urticaria (<1%)

Mucosal/ENT
Dysgeusia (<1%)
Vaginitis (<1%)
  (2003): Wilson R+, *Respir Med* 97, 242
  (2002): Lode H+, *Clin Ther* 24, 1915
  (2001): Ball P+, *Int J Antimicrob Agents* 18, 19
  (2001): Hammerschlag MR+, *Antimicrob Chemother* 48, 735
Xerostomia (<1%)

Other
Abdominal pain (1%)
  (2000): Lowe MN+, *Drugs* 59(5), 1137

Anaphylactoid reactions/Anaphylaxis
Asthenia (<1%)
Candidiasis (genital) (<1%)
Headache
Hot flashes (<0.1%)
Hypersensitivity
Myalgia/Myositis/Myopathy/Myotoxicity (<1%)
Pseudoporphyria
  (2005): Valentine MC, Everett, WA (from Internet) (observation)
Seizures
Tremor (<1%)
Vertigo (1%)

GEMTUZUMAB

Trade name: Mylotarg (Wyeth)
Indications: Acute myeloid leukemia
Category: Antineoplastic; Monoclonal antibody
Half-life: 45 hours (initial dose)

Reactions

Skin
Herpes simplex (22%)
Peripheral edema (21%)
Petechiae (21%)
Rash (sic) (23%)

Mucosal/ENT
Mucositis (<4–25%)
  (2001): Larson RA, *Semin Hematol* 38(Suppl 6), 24 (4%)
  (2001): Sievers EL+, *Curr Opin Oncol* 13(6), 522
  (2001): Sievers EL+, *J Clin Oncol* 19(13), 3244 (4%)
Stomatitis (32%)

Other
Chills (66%)
  (2001): Larson RA, *Semin Hematol* 38(Suppl 6), 24
Headache
Hepatotoxicity
  (2005): Kurt M+, *Am J Hematol* 80(3), 213
Hypersensitivity
  (2007): Hanbali A+, *Am J Health* 64(13), 1401
Infections (<28%)
  (2001): Larson RA, *Semin Hematol* 38(Suppl 6), 24 (23%)
  (2001): Sievers EL+, *Curr Opin Oncol* 13(6), 522
  (2001): Sievers EL+, *J Clin Oncol* 19(13), 3244 (28%)
Infusion-related syndrome
  (2001): Larson RA, *Semin Hematol* 38(Suppl 6), 24
Injection-site reactions (sic) (<3–25%)
  (2003): Giles FJ+, *Ann Pharmacother* 37(9), 1182 (3%)
Pain
  (2001): Larson RA, *Semin Hematol* 38(SUppl 6), 24

GENTAMICIN

Trade names: Alcomicinx; Cidomycin; Diogent; Garamycin (Schering); Garatec; Genoptic (Allergan); Gentacidin; Gentalline; Gentalol; I-Gent; Jenamicin; Ocumycin; Pred-G; Refobacin; Sedanazin
Indications: Various infections caused by susceptible organisms
Category: Antibiotic, aminoglycoside
Half-life: 2–4 hours
Clinically important, potentially hazardous interactions with: adefovir, aldesleukin, aminoglycosides, atracurium, bumetanide, carbenicillin, cephalexin, cephalothin, doxacurium, ethacrynic acid, furosemide, methoxyflurane, non-polarizing muscle relaxants, pancuronium, pipecuronium, polypeptide antibiotics, rocuronium, succinylcholine, torsemide, tubocurarine, vecuronium

Reactions

Skin
Dermatitis
    (2002): Paniagua MJ+, *Allergy* 57(11), 1086
    (2001): Sanchez-Perez J+, *Contact Dermatitis* 44(1), 54 (with kanamycin)
    (1996): Merlob P+, *Cutis* 57, 429 (neonatal orbital)
    (1996): Munoz-Bellido FJ+, *Allergy* 51, 758
    (1989): van Ketel WG+, *Contact Dermatitis* 20, 303
    (1988): Robinson PM, *J Laryngol Otol* 102, 577
Eczema
    (1988): Ghadially R+, *J Am Acad Dermatol* 19, 428
Edema (1–10%)
Erythema (1–10%)
Exanthems (<1%)
    (2002): Spigarelli MG+, *Pediatr Pulmonol* 33(4), 311
    (1990): Flax SH+, *Cutis* 46, 59
Exfoliative dermatitis
    (1989): Guin JD+, *Cutis* 43, 564
Photosensitivity (<1%)
    (1990): Flax SH+, *Cutis* 46, 59 (photo recall)
Pruritus (1–10%)
Purpura
Rash (sic)
    (2002): Spigarelli MG+, *Pediatr Pulmonol* 33(4), 311
Toxic epidermal necrolysis
    (1984): Sluchenkova LD+, *Pediatriia* (Russian) July, 57
Urticaria
Vasculitis
    (1980): Bonnetblanc JM+, *Ann Dermatol Vénéréol* (French) 107, 1089

Mucosal/ENT
Ototoxicity
    (2006): Dobie RA+, *Arch Otolaryngol Head Neck Surgngol Head* 132(3), 253
    (2006): Ishiyama G+, *Acta Otolaryngol* 126(10), 1057
    (2006): Sha SH+, *N Engl J Med* 354(17), 1856
    (2004): Nagai J+, *Drug Metab Pharmacokinet* 19(3), 159
    (1998): El Bakri F+, *Lancet* 351(9113), 1407
Sialorrhea (<1%)
Stomatitis
Tinnitus
    (2004): Black FO+, *Otol Neurotol* 25(4), 559
    (2004): Pino Rivero+, *An Otorrinolaringol Ibero Am* 31(6), 531
    (1991): Magnusson M+, *Acta Otolaryngol* 111(4), 671
    (1986): Esterhai JL+, *Clin Orthop Relat Res* 348(209), 185

Hair
Hair – alopecia

Other
Anaphylactoid reactions/Anaphylaxis
    (2003): Schulze S+, *Allergy* 58(1), 88
    (1983): Fisher AA, *Cutis* 32, 510
Headache
Hypersensitivity
    (2002): Spigarelli MG+, *Pediatr Pulmonol* 33(4), 311
Injection-site erythema
    (1990): Shen K, *Lancet* 336, 689
Injection-site induration
Injection-site necrosis
    (1990): Grob JJ+, *Dermatologica* 180, 258
    (1985): Doutre MS+, *Therapie* (French) 40, 266
    (1985): Duterque M+, *Ann Dermatol Venereol* (French) 112, 707
    (1984): Penso D+, *Presse Méd* (French) 13, 1575
    (1984): Taillandier J+, *Presse Méd* (French) 13, 1574
Injection-site pain (<1%)
Nephrotoxicity
    (2006): Hung CC+, *Nephrol Dial Transplant* 21(2), 547
    (2004): Nagai J+, *Drug Metab Pharmacokinet* 19(3), 159
    (2003): Ali BH, *Food Chem Toxicol* 41(11), 1447
    (2003): Bartal C+, *Am J Med* 114(3), 194
    (2000): Shetty AK+, *Clin Pediatr (Phila)* 39(9), 529
    (1997): Landau D+, *Pediatr Nephrol* 11(6), 737
    (1996): Prins JM+, *Antimicrob Agents Chemother* 40(11), 2494
Paresthesias
    (2005): Chou CL+, *Am J Med Sci* 329(3), 144
Phlebitis
Thrombophlebitis
Tremor (<1%)
Vertigo
    (2005): Dallan I+, *Acta Otorhinolaryngol Ital* 25(6), 370

GINGER

Scientific name: *Zingiber officinale*
Family: Zingiberaceae
Trade and other common names: African Ginger; Cochin Ginger; Gingembre; Jamaica Ginger; Race Ginger
Category: Carminative; Oleoresin
Purported indications and other uses: Colic, dyspepsia, flatulence, rheumatoid arthritis, loss of appetite, nausea, vomiting, upper respiratory infections, cough, bronchitis, burns, tinnitus, flavoring agent, fragrance component
Half-life: N/A
Clinically important, potentially hazardous interactions with: heparin, **squill**, ticlopidine, warfarin

Reactions

Skin
Dermatitis
    (1996): Kanerva L+, *Contact Dermatitis* 35(3), 157

Other
Abdominal pain
    (2006): Chaiyakunapruk N+, *Am J Obstet Gynecol* 194(1), 95

GINKGO BILOBA

Scientific name: *Ginkgo biloba (Mericon)*
Family: Ginkgoaceae
Trade and other common names: Fossil Tree; Japanese Silver Apricot; Maidenhair Tree; Salisburia; Tanakan; Tebonin
Category: Food supplement; Vascular stimulant
Purported indications and other uses: Dementia, memory loss, headache, tinnitus, dizziness, mood disturbances, hearing disorders, intermittent claudication, attention deficit hyperactivity disorder, premenstrual syndrome, heart disease
Half-life: N/A
Clinically important, potentially hazardous interactions with: anticoagulants, aspirin, diuretics, NSAIDs, phenytoin, platelet inhibitors, SSRIs, **St John's wort**, thiazide diuretics, trazodone, valproic acid, warfarin

Reactions

Skin
Acute generalized exanthematous pustulosis
   (2006): Pennisi RS, *Med J Aust* 184(11), 583
Adverse effects (sic)
   (2002): Ernst E, *Ann Intern Med* 136(1), 42
   (2002): Haller CA+, *Adverse Drug React Toxicol Rev* 21(3), 143
   (2002): Mattsson K+, *Lakartidningen* 99(50), 5095
Allergic reactions (sic)
Dermatitis
   (1989): Lepoittevin JP+, *Arch Dermatol* 281, 227
   (1988): Tomb RR+, *Contact Dermatitis* 19, 281
Erythema
Exanthems
   (2002): Chiu AE+, *J Am Acad Dermatol* 46(1), 145
Pruritus
Rash (sic)
Vasculitis
Vesiculation

Mucosal/ENT
Rectal burning
Stomatitis

Eyes
Hyphema
   (2002): Schneider C+, *J Fr Ophtalmol* 25(7), 731
Ocular adverse effects
   (2004): Fraunfelder FW, *Am J Ophthalmol* 138(4), 639

Other
Death
   (2005): Kupiec T+, *J Anal Toxicol* 29(7), 755 (with valproic acid)
Phlebitis
Seizures
   (2006): Hasegawa S+, *Pediatr Neurol* 35(4), 275
   (2002): Kajiyama Y+, *Pediatrics* 109(2), 325 (overdose)
   (2001): Granger AS, *Age Ageing* 30(6), 523
   (2001): Gregory PJ, *Ann Intern Med* 134(4), 344
   (2001): Miwa H+, *Epilepsia* Feb 42(2), 280

GINSENG

Scientific name: *Panax ginseng*
Family: Araliaceae
Trade and other common names: Asian Ginseng; Asiatic Ginseng; Chinese Ginseng; Japanese Ginseng; Jintsam; Korean Ginseng; Korean Red; Ninjin; Red Ginseng; Ren She; Sang; Seng
Category: Immunomodulator
Purported indications and other uses: General tonic, improving stamina, cognitive function, concentration, diuretic, antidepressant, gastritis, neurasthenia, impotence, fever, hangover, cancer, cardiovascular diseases
Half-life: N/A
Clinically important, potentially hazardous interactions with: **alcohol**, aspirin, **caffeine**, digoxin, olmesartan, phenelzine, **squill**, tamoxifen, ticlopidine, warfarin

Reactions

Skin
Adverse effects (sic)
   (2002): Ellis JM+, *Ann Pharmacother* 36(3), 375
   (2002): Ernst E, *Ann Intern Med* 136(1), 42
   (2002): Haller CA+, *Adverse Drug React Toxicol Rev* 21(3), 143
Allergic reactions (sic)
Burning (sensation)
   (1999): Choi HK+, *Int J Impot Res* 11(5), 261
Edema
Pruritus
Stevens-Johnson syndrome
   (2001): Boniel T+, *Harefuah* 140(8), 780
   (1996): Dega H+, *Lancet* 313, 756

Other
Gynecomastia
   (1999): Palop V+, *Med Clin* (Barc) 112(19), 758
Side effects (sic)
   (2002): Tesch BJ, *Dis Mon* Oct 48(10), 671

GLATIRAMER

Trade name: Copaxone (Teva)
Indications: Multiple sclerosis
Category: Immunomodulator
Half-life: N/A
Clinically important, potentially hazardous interactions with: hemophilus B vaccine. None

Note: Also known as Copolymer-1

Reactions

Skin
Acne (>2%)
Allergic reactions (sic)
Angioedema
Atrophy
Cellulitis
Cyst (2%)
Dermatitis
Diaphoresis (15%)
   (2004): Munari L+, *Cochrane Database Syst Rev* (1), CD004678
Eczema
Edema (3%)

Erythema (4%)
Erythema nodosum
Exanthems
Facial edema (6%)
Fungal dermatitis
Furunculosis
Herpes simplex (4%)
Herpes zoster
Lupus erythematosus
Lymphocytic infiltration
   (2005): Nolden S+, *Mult Scler* 11(2), 245
Nodular eruption (2%)
Peripheral edema (7%)
Photosensitivity
Pigmentation
Pruritus (185)
Psoriasis
Purpura
Pustules
Rash (sic) (18%)
Striae
Urticaria
Vesiculobullous eruption
Xanthomas
Xerosis

Mucosal/ENT
Ageusia
Dysgeusia (>2%)
Gingival bleeding
Glossodynia
Oral candidiasis
Oral ulceration
Oral vesiculation (6%)
Sinusitis (>2%)
Stomatitis
Tinnitus (>2%)
Tongue edema
Tongue pigmentation
Ulcerative stomatitis
Vaginitis
Xerostomia (>2%)

Hair
Hair – alopecia (>2%)

Nails
Nails – changes (>2%)

Eyes
Xerophthalmia

Other
Anaphylactoid reactions/Anaphylaxis
   (2005): Rauschka H+, *Neurology* 64(8), 1481
Chills (4%)
Cough (>2%)
Depression (>2%)
Embolia cutis medicamentosa (Nicolau syndrome)
   (2003): Gaudez C+, *Rev Neurol* (Paris) 159(5), 571
Facial numbness
Gynecomastia
Headache
Infections (50%)
Injection-site abscess
Injection-site atrophy
Injection-site bleeding (5%)

Injection-site ecchymoses (>2%)
Injection-site edema
Injection-site erythema (66%)
   (2005): Nolden S+, *Mult Scler* 11(2), 245
   (2001): Ziemssen T+, *Drug Saf* 24(13), 979
Injection-site fibrosis
Injection-site hematoma
Injection-site hypersensitivity
Injection-site induration (13%)
   (2005): Nolden S+, *Mult Scler* 11(2), 245
   (2004): Soos N+, *Am J Clin Dermatol* 5(5), 357
   (2001): Ziemssen T+, *Drug Saf* 24(13), 979
Injection-site inflammation (49%)
   (2001): Ziemssen T+, *Drug Saf* 24(13), 979
Injection-site lipoatrophy
   (2004): Edgar CM+, *Can J Neurol Sci* 31(1), 58 (45%)
   (2004): Soos N+, *Am J Clin Dermatol* 5(5), 357
Injection-site necrosis
   (2007): *Prescrire Int* 16(92), 251
Injection-site pain (73%)
   (2005): Nolden S+, *Mult Scler* 11(2), 245
Injection-site panniculitis
   (2004): Soos N+, *Am J Clin Dermatol* 5(5), 357
Injection-site pigmentation
Injection-site pruritus (40%)
   (2005): Nolden S+, *Mult Scler* 11(2), 245
Injection-site reactions (6–67%)
   (2006): Gordon PH+, *Neurology* 66(7), 1117
   (2005): Fiore AP+, *Arq Neuropsiquiatr* 63(3B), 738
   (2004): *Prescrire Int* 13(69), 10
   (2002): Flechter S+, *J Neurol Sci* 197(1), 51 (67%)
   (2002): Ziemssen T+, *Nervenarzt* 73(4), 321
Injection-site urticaria (5%)
Lipoatrophy
   (2001): Hwang L+, *Cutis* 68(4), 287
   (1999): Drago F+, *Arch Dermatol* 135(10), 1277 (localized)
Lipomatosis
Lymphedema
Moon face
Myalgia/Myositis/Myopathy/Myotoxicity (>2%)
Pain (28%)
Panniculitis
   (2006): Soares Almeida LM+, *J Am Acad Dermatol* 55(6), 968
Paresthesias (>2%)
Serum sickness
Tremor (7%)
Tumors
Vertigo (>2%)

GLIMEPIRIDE

Trade name: Amaryl (Sanofi-Aventis)
Indications: Non-insulin dependent diabetes type II
Category: Sulfonylurea
Half-life: 5–9 hours

Note: Glimepiride is a sulfonamide and can be absorbed systemically. Sulfonamides can produce severe, possibly fatal, reactions such as toxic epidermal necrolysis and Stevens–Johnson syndrome

Reactions

Skin
Allergic reactions (sic) (<1%)
Diaphoresis

Edema (<1%)
Erythema (<1%)
Exanthems (<1%)
Exfoliative dermatitis
Lichenoid eruption
  (2003): Noakes R, *Australas J Dermatol* 44(4), 302
Photosensitivity (<1%)
Pruritus (<1%)
Psoriasis
  (1997): Leal G, Fortaleza, Brazil (from Internet) (observation)
Rash (sic) (<1%)
  (2001): Deerochanawong C+, *J Med Assoc Thai* 84(9), 1221
Urticaria (<1%)

Other
Headache
  (1998): Campbell RK+, *Ann Pharmacother* 32(10), 1044
  (1997): Sonnenberg GE+, *Ann Pharmacother* 31(6), 671
Porphyria cutanea tarda
Vertigo
  (1998): Campbell RK+, *Ann Pharmacother* 32(10), 1044

GLIPIZIDE

Trade names: Glibenese; Glipid; Glucotrol (Pfizer); Glyde; Melizide; Metaglip (Bristol-Myers Squibb); Mindiab; Minidiab; Minodiab
Indications: Non-insulin dependent diabetes type II
Category: Sulfonylurea
Half-life: 2–4 hours

Note: Glipizide is a sulfonamide and can be absorbed systemically. Sulfonamides can produce severe, possibly fatal, reactions such as toxic epidermal necrolysis and Stevens–Johnson syndrome

Note: Grinspan's syndrome: the triad of oral lichen planus, diabetes mellitus, and hypertension

Reactions

Skin
Eczema
Edema (<1%)
Erythema (<1%)
Exanthems (<1%)
Exfoliative dermatitis
Fixed eruption
  (2004): Tornero P+, *Contact Dermatitis* 51(2), 57
Grinspan's syndrome
  (1990): Lamey PJ+, *Oral Surg Oral Med Oral Path* 70, 184
Lichenoid eruption
Photosensitivity (1–10%)
Phototoxicity
  (2000): Vargas F+, *In Vitr Mol Toxicol* 13, 17
Pigmented purpuric eruption
  (1999): Adams BB+, *J Am Acad Dermatol* 41, 827
Pruritus (<3%)
Psoriasis (induced)
  (1994): Litt JZ, Beachwood, OH (2 personal cases) (observation)
Purpura
Rash (sic) (1–10%)
Stevens–Johnson syndrome
  (2006): Cheng JB+, *Dermatitis* 17(1), 36
Urticaria (1–10%)

Mucosal/ENT
Oral lichen planus
  (1990): Lamey PJ+, *Oral Surg Oral Med Oral Path* 70, 184
Other
Headache
Myalgia/Myositis/Myopathy/Myotoxicity (<3%)
Paresthesias (<3%)
Porphyria (coproporphyria-like)
  (1991): Moder KG+, *Mayo Clin Proc* 66, 312
Porphyria cutanea tarda

GLUCAGON

Trade name: Glucagon Emergency Kit (Lilly)
Indications: Hypoglycemic reactions
Category: Hormone, polypeptide
Half-life: 3–10 minutes
Clinically important, potentially hazardous interactions with: warfarin

Reactions

Skin
Acute febrile neutrophilic dermatosis (Sweet's syndrome)
  (1996): Glass LF+, *J Am Acad Dermatol* 34, 455 (passim)
  (1994): Fukutoku M+, *Br J Haematol* 86, 645
  (1994): Johnson ML+, *Arch Dermatol* 130, 77
  (1993): Paydas S+, *Br J Haematol* 85, 191
  (1992): Karp DL, *Ann Intern Med* 117, 875
  (1992): Park JW+, *Ann Intern Med* 116, 996
  (1991): Cohen PR+, *J Am Acad Dermatol* 25, 734
Angioedema
  (1985): Gelfand DW+, *Am J Roentgenol* 144, 405
Epidermolysis bullosa acquisita
  (1992): Ward JC+, *Br J Haematol* 81, 27
Erythema multiforme
  (1980): Edell SL, *Am J Roentgenol* 134, 385
Erythema necrolyticum migrans
  (2003): Case CC+, *Endocr Pract* 9(1), 22
  (2002): Wald M+, *Eur J Pediatr* 161(11), 600
Erythema nodosum
  (1994): Nomiyama J+, *Am J Hematol* 47, 333
Exanthems
  (1996): Glass LF+, *J Am Acad Dermatol* 34, 455
  (1995): Scott GA, *Am J Dermatopathol* 17, 107
  (1994): Sasaki O+, *Intern Med* 33, 641
  (1993): Peters MS+, *J Cutan Pathol* 20, 465
  (1993): Yamashita N+, *J Dermatol* 20, 473
  (1992): Mehregan DR+, *Arch Dermatol* 128, 1055
Folliculitis
  (1996): Glass LF+, *J Am Acad Dermatol* 34, 455 (passim)
  (1992): Ostlere LS+, *Br J Dermatol* 127, 193
Glucagonoma syndrome (necrolytic migratory erythema)
  (1988): Benhamou PY+, *Ann Dermatol Venereol* (French) 115, 717
Pyoderma gangrenosum
  (1996): Glass LF+, *J Am Acad Dermatol* 34, 455 (passim)
  (1994): Johnson ML+, *Arch Dermatol* 130, 77
  (1991): Ross HJ+, *Cancer* 68, 441 (bullous)
Rash (sic)
Urticaria (1–10%)
  (1985): Gelfand DW+, *Am J Roentgenol* 144, 405
Vasculitis
  (1996): Glass LF+, *J Am Acad Dermatol* 34, 455 (passim)
  (1995): Couderc LJ+, *Respir Med* 89, 237

(1995): Vidarsson B+, *Am J Med* 98, 589
(1994): Jain KK, *J Am Acad Dermatol* 31, 213
(1994): Johnson ML+, *Arch Dermatol* 130, 77
(1994): van Kamp H+, *Br J Haematol* 86, 415
(1991): Wodzinski MA+, *Br J Haematol* 77, 249
(1990): Welte Z+, *Blood* 75, 1056
(1989): Dreicer R+, *Ann Intern Med* 111, 91

Mucosal/ENT
Cheilitis
(2003): Case CC+, *Endocr Pract* 9(1), 22

Other
Headache
Injection-site reactions (sic)
(1996): Glass LF+, *J Am Acad Dermatol* 34, 455 (passim)
(1993): Samlaska CP+, *Arch Dermatol* 129, 645
(1992): Mehregan DR+, *Arch Dermatol* 128, 1055

GLUCOSAMINE

Trade names: 2-amino-2-deoxyglucose hydrochloride; 2-amino-deoxyglucose sulfate; Arthro-Aid (NutraSense); Chitosamine; Glucosamine sulfate (Rottapharm); N-acetyl-glucosamine (NAG)
Indications: Arthritis, osteoarthritis, cartilage repair and maintenance, strained joints, improving joint function and range of motion, alleviating joint pain
Category: Amino sugar; Food supplement
Half-life: N/A
Clinically important, potentially hazardous interactions with: None

Reactions

Skin
Adverse effects (sic) (6%)
(1998): Barclay TS+, *Ann Pharmacother* 32(5), 574
(1998): Qiu GX+, *Arzneimittelforschung* 48(5), 469 (6%)
(1994): Muller-Fassbender H+, *Osteoarthritis Cartilage* 2(1), 61 (6%)
Allergic reactions (sic) (4%)
(2006): *Prescrire Int* 15(84), 139
(2001): Reginster JY+, *Lancet* 357(9252), (4%)
Eczema
(2003): Maffei KR, Athens, GA (from Internet) (observations)
Pruritus
(2003): Matheson AJ+, *Drugs Aging* 20(14), 1041

Mucosal/ENT
Oral vesiculation (7%)
(2001): Reginster JY+, *Lancet* 357(9252), (7%)

Other
Asthenia (9%)
(2003): Matheson AJ+, *Drugs Aging* 20(14), 1041
(2001): Reginster JY+, *Lancet* 357(9252), (9%)
Depression (6%)
(2001): Reginster JY+, *Lancet* 357(9252), (6%)
Hepatotoxicity
(2007): Ossendza RA+, *Gastroenterol Clin Biol* 31(4), 449
Hypersensitivity
(1999): Matheu V+, *Allergy* 54(6), 643

GLYBURIDE

Synonyms: glibenclamide; glybenclamide
Trade names: Albert (Glyburide); Daonil; Diabeta (Sanofi-Aventis); Euglucan; Euglucon; Glimel; Glucal; Glucovance (Bristol-Myers Squibb); Glynase (Pfizer); Hemi-Daonil; Med-Glibe; Micronase (Pfizer); Miglucan; Norboral
Indications: Non-insulin dependent diabetes type II
Category: Sulfonylurea
Half-life: 5–16 hours
Clinically important, potentially hazardous interactions with: bosentan

Note: Glucovance is glyburide and metformin

Note: Glyburide is a sulfonamide and can be absorbed systemically. Sulfonamides can produce severe, possibly fatal, reactions such as toxic epidermal necrolysis and Stevens–Johnson syndrome

Reactions

Skin
Allergic reactions (sic) (0.21%)
(1986): Bigby M+, *JAMA* 256, 3358
Angioedema
Bullous dermatitis
(1981): Wongpaitoon V+, *Postgrad Med J* 57, 244
Eczema
Erythema (1–5%)
(1988): Chee Ching S, *Photodermatol* 5, 42
Exanthems (1–5%)
Exfoliative dermatitis
Lichenoid eruption
(2005): Fox GN+, *Cutis* 76(1), 41
Linear IgA dermatosis
(2003): Avci O+, *J Am Acad Dermatol* 48(2), 299 (passim)
(1983): Väätäinen N+, *Acta Derm Venereol* (Stockh) 63, 169
Pemphigus
(2005): Goldberg I+, *Acta Dermatovenerol Croat* 13(3), 153
(1993): Paterson AJ+, *J Oral Pathol Med* 22, 92
Peripheral edema
(1988): Berova N+, *Dermatol Monatsschr* (German) 174, 50
Photosensitivity (1–10%)
(1995): Fujii S+, *Am J Hematol* 50, 223
(1994): Shelley WB+, *Cutis* 53, 287 (observation)
(1994): Shelley WB+, *Cutis* 53, 77 (observation)
(1988): Chee-Ching S, *Photodermatology* 5, 42
(1988): Sun CC, *Photodermatol* 5, 42
(1987): Henrietta G, *Nursing* 17, 56
Pruritus (1–10%)
(1988): Chee Ching S, *Photodermatol* 5, 42
(1987): *Physicians Drug Alert* 7, 71
Psoriasis
(1988): Milner JE, *The Schoch Letter* 38(5), Item 64 (obervation)
(1987): Goh CL, *Australas J Dermatol* 28, 30
Purpura
(1986): Dickey W+, *BMJ* 293, 823
(1983): Väätäinen N+, *Acta Derm Venereol* (Stockh) 63, 169
Rash (sic) (1–10%)
Urticaria (1–5%)
(1994): Shelley WB+, *Cutis* 53, 77 (observation)
(1991): Chichmanian RM+, *Therapie* (French) 46, 163
(1986): Jordan NS+, *Hosp Pharm* 21, 462
(1986): Kure J, *NC Med J* 47, 149
Vasculitis
(2003): Bukhalo M+, *Cutis* 71(3), 235
(1986): Dickey W+, *BMJ* 293, 823

(1980): Ingelmo M+, *Med Clin* (Barc) (Spanish) 75, 306
Vesiculobullous eruption
(1993): Landor M+, *Ann Allergy* 70, 196

Mucosal/ENT
Dysgeusia

Eyes
Eyelid edema
(1985): Yitalo P+, *Arzneimittelforsch* (German) 35, 1596

Other
Headache
Hypersensitivity (generalized)
Myalgia/Myositis/Myopathy/Myotoxicity
Paresthesias (<1%)
Porphyria cutanea tarda

GLYCOPYRROLATE

Trade names: Gastrodyn; Robinul (First Horizon); Sroton;
Strodin
Indications: Duodenal ulcer, irritable bowel syndrome
Category: Anticholinergic; Muscarinic antagonist; Non-
depolarizing muscle relaxant
Half-life: N/A
**Clinically important, potentially hazardous interactions
with:** anticholinergics, arbutamine

Reactions

Skin
Allergic reactions (sic)
Photosensitivity (1–10%)
Rash (sic) (<1%)
Urticaria
Xerosis (>10%)

Mucosal/ENT
Dysgeusia
(1999): Wolff MS+, *Arch Oral Biol* 44(2), 97
Sialorrhea
(1999): Evans JS+, *Curr Opin Pediatr* 11(5), 396
Xerostomia (>10%)
(2001): Patel PS+, *Spec Care Dentist* 21(5), 176
(1999): Marples IL+, *Br J Anaesth* 83(3), 537
(1999): Wolff MS+, *Arch Oral Biol* 44(2), 97
(1993): Gorcsan J+, *J Am Soc Echocardiogr* 6(2), 200

Eyes
Mydriasis
(2006): Izadi S+, *J Neuroophthalmol* 26(3), 232

Other
Anhidrosis
Headache
Injection-site irritation (>10%)

GOLD and GOLD COMPOUNDS

Generic names:
    Auranofin
        Trade name: Ridaura (GSK)
    Aurothioglucose
        Trade name: Solganal (Schering)
    Gold sodium thiomalate (sodium aurothiomalate)
        Trade name: Myochrysine (Merck)
Indications: Rheumatoid arthritis
Category: Disease-modifying antirheumatic
Half-life: 5 days

Note: Adverse reactions can occur months after therapy has been
discontinued

Reactions

Skin
Acne
(1982): Bailin PL+, *Clin Rheum Dis* 8, 493 (passim)
Angioedema (<1%)
(1989): Herbst WM+, *Hautarzt* (German) 40, 568
Angiofibromatosis
(1989): Herbst WM+, *Hautarzt* (German) 40, 568
Bullous dermatitis
Bullous pemphigoid
(1983): Wozel G+, *Dermatol Monatsschr* (German) 169, 125
Chrysiasis (blue-green pigmentation)
(2001): Werth V, *Dermatology Times* 18
Dermatitis
(2007): Conde-Taboada A+, *Contact Dermatitis* 56(3), 179
(Contact) (lymphomatoid)
(2002): Ahlgren C+, *Acta Derm Venereol* 82(1), 41 (dental gold
alloy)
(2001): Lee AY+, *Contact Dermatitis* 45(4), 214
(2000): ter Borg EJ+, *Arthritis Rheum* 43, 1420
(2000): Trattner A+, *Contact Dermatitis* 42, 301
(2000): Vamnes JS+, *Contact Dermatitis* 42, 128
(1999): Bruze M+, *Contact Dermatitis* 40, 295
(1999): Fowler JF, *Skin and Allergy News* September, 34 (9.5%)
(1999): Räsänen L+, *Br J Dermatol* 141, 683
(1998): Estlander T+, *Contact Dermatitis* 38, 40
(1998): Moller H+, *Am J Contact Dermat* 9, 15
(1998): Wiesner M+, *Contact Dermatitis* 38, 52
(1997): Armstrong DK+, *Br J Dermatol* 136, 776
(1997): Choy EH+, *Br J Rheumatol* 36, 1054
(1997): Fleming C+, *Contact Dermatitis* 37, 298 (lymphomatoid)
(1997): Hostynek JJ, *Food Chem Toxicol* 35, 839
(1997): Kilpikari I, *Contact Dermatitis* 37, 130
(1997): Moller H+, *Acta Derm Venereol* 77, 370
(1997): Silva R+, *Contact Dermatitis* 37, 78
(1996): Bonnetblanc JM, *Presse Med* (French) 25, 1555
(1996): Sabroe RA+, *Contact Dermatitis* 34, 345
(1996): Tan E+, *Australas J Dermatol* 37, 218
(1994): Björkner B+, *Contact Dermatitis* 30, 144
(1994): Bruze M+, *J Am Acad Dermatol* 31, 579
(1994): Collet E+, *Ann Dermatol Venereol* (French) 121, 21
(1994): Osawa J+, *Contact Dermatitis* 31, 89
(1994): Webster CG+, *Cutis* 54, 25
(1993): Aro T+, *Contact Dermatitis* 28, 276
(1993): Hisa T+, *Contact Dermatitis* 28, 174
(1993): Koga T+, *Br J Dermatol* 128, 227
(1993): Koga T+, *Contact Dermatitis* 28, 303
(1990): Miller RA+, *J Am Acad Dermatol* 23, 360
(1990): Wijnands MJ+, *Lancet* 335, 867
(1989): Camarasa JG+, *Med Cutan Ibero Lat Am* (Spanish)
17, 187
(1988): Fowler JF, *Arch Dermatol* 124, 181

(1988): Goh CL, *Contact Dermatitis* 18, 122
(1988): Wicks IP+, *Ann Rheum Dis* 47, 421
(1987): Fisher AA, *Cutis* 39, 473
(1987): Fisher AA, *J Am Acad Dermatol* 17, 853
(1986): Minghetti G+, *G Ital Dermatol Venereol* (Italian) 121, 425
(1985): Kalamkarian AA+, *Vestn Dermatol Venerol* (8), 4
(1985): Rapson WS, *Contact Dermatitis* 13, 56
(1985): Silvennoinen-Kassinen S+, *Contact Dermatitis* 11, 156
(1985): Tosi S+, *Int J Clin Pharmacol Res* 5, 265
(1983): Monti M+, *Contact Dermatitis* 9, 150
(1983): Sigler JW, *Am J Med* 75, 59
(1982): Iwatsuki K+, *Arch Dermatol* 118, 608
(1980): Raith L+, *Dermatol Monatsschr* (German) 166, 382

Eczema
(1994): Lizeaux-Parneix V+, *Ann Dermatol Venereol* (French) 121, 793
(1986): Hofmann C+, *Z Rheumatol* (German) 45, 100

Erythema annulare centrifugum
(1992): Tsuji T+, *J Am Acad Dermatol* 27, 284

Erythema multiforme
(1982): Bailin PL+, *Clin Rheum Dis* 8, 493 (passim)

Erythema nodosum
(1998): Pandya AG+, *Arch Dermatol* 134, 1104 (passim)
(1982): Bailin PL+, *Clin Rheum Dis* 8, 493 (passim)

Exanthems (>5%)
(2003): Sperber BR+, *Contact Dermatitis* 48(4), 204
(1999): Räsänen L+, *Br J Dermatol* 141, 683
(1998): Pandya AG+, *Arch Dermatol* 134, 1104 (passim)
(1996): Bonnetblanc JM, *Presse Med* (French) 25, 1555
(1994): Shelley WB+, *Cutis* 52, 87 (observation)

Exfoliative dermatitis
(2000): Lancucki J+, *Wiad Lek* (Polish) 21, 1347 (erythroderma)
(1998): Pandya AG+, *Arch Dermatol* 134, 1104 (passim)
(1996): Sigurdsson V+, *J Am Acad Dermatol* 35, 53
(1991): Wilson CL+, *Int J Dermatol* 30, 148
(1989): Ranki A+, *Am J Dermatopathol* 11, 22
(1984): Adachi JD+, *J Rheumatol* 11, 355
(1982): Bailin PL+, *Clin Rheum Dis* 8, 493 (passim)

Fixed eruption

Graft-versus-host reaction
(1998): Jappe U+, *Hautarzt* (German) 49, 126 (passim)

Granuloma annulare
(1990): Martin N+, *Arch Dermatol* 126, 1370
(1980): Rothwell RS+, *Arch Dermatol* 116, 863

Herpes zoster
(1987): Murav'ev Iu V+, *Ter Arkh* 59(4), 136
(1981): Fam AG+, *Ann Intern Med* 94, 712

Lichen planus (<32%)
(2005): Yokozeki H+, *Br J Dermatol* 152(5), 1087
(1996): Russell MA+, *N Engl J Med* 334, 603
(1990): Torrelo A+, *Actas Dermo-Sif* (Spanish) 81, 743
(1986): Hofmann C+, *Z Rheumatol* (German) 45, 100
(1986): Ingber A+, *Z Hautkr* (German) 61, 315
(1982): Bailin PL+, *Clin Rheum Dis* 8, 493 (passim)

Lichen spinulosus

Lichenoid eruption
(2001): Werth V, *Dermatology Times* 18
(1999): Räsänen L+, *Br J Dermatol* 141, 683
(1998): Pandya AG+, *Arch Dermatol* 134, 1104 (passim)
(1997): Choy EH+, *Br J Rheumatol* 36, 1054
(1996): Bonnetblanc JM, *Presse Med* (French) 25, 1555
(1994): Alzieu PH+, *Ann Dermatol Venereol* (French) 121, 798
(1994): Lizeaux-Parneix V+, *Ann Dermatol Venereol* (French) 121, 793

Lupus erythematosus
(1988): Balsa A+, *Rev Clin Esp* (Spanish) 182, 505

Lymphocytoma cutis
(1992): Kobayashi Y+, *J Am Acad Dermatol* 27, 457

Pemphigus

(1995): Ciompi ML+, *Rheumatol Int* 15(3), 95

Photosensitivity

Pigmentation
(1998): Pandya AG+, *Arch Dermatol* 134, 1104 (passim)
(1997): Miller ML+, *Cutis* 59, 256
(1996): Fleming CJ+, *J Am Acad Dermatol* 34, 349
(1992): Cremer B+, *Dtsch Med Wochenschr* (German) 117, 558
(1990): Bonet M+, *Clin Rheumatol* 9, 254
(1984): Fam AG+, *Arthritis Rheum* 27, 119
(1984): Larsen FS+, *Clin Exp Dermatol* 9, 174
(1984): Pelachyk IM+, *J Cutan Pathol* 11, 491
(1982): Bailin PL+, *Clin Rheum Dis* 8, 493 (passim)
(1982): Beckett VL+, *Mayo Clin Proc* 57, 773
(1981): Granstein RD+, *J Am Acad Dermatol* 5, 1 (blue-gray)

Pityriasis rosea
(1999): Räsänen L+, *Br J Dermatol* 141, 683
(1998): Pandya AG+, *Arch Dermatol* 134, 1104 (passim)
(1994): Lizeaux-Parneix V+, *Ann Dermatol Venereol* (French) 121, 793
(1992): Tsuji T+, *J Am Acad Dermatol* 27, 284
(1986): Hofmann C+, *Z Rheumatol* (German) 45, 100
(1982): Bailin PL+, *Clin Rheum Dis* 8, 493 (passim)

Pruritus (<84%)
(2003): Sperber BR+, *Contact Dermatitis* 48(4), 204
(1998): Pandya AG+, *Arch Dermatol* 134, 1104
(1996): Bonnetblanc JM, *Presse Med* (French) 25, 1555
(1982): Bailin PL+, *Clin Rheum Dis* 8, 493 (passim)

Psoriasis
(1991): Smith DL+, *Arch Dermatol* 127, 268

Purpura
(1984): Adachi JD+, *J Rheumatol* 11, 355
(1982): Bailin PL+, *Clin Rheum Dis* 8, 493 (passim)

Pyoderma gangrenosum

Radiation keratosis
(1996): Helm KF+, *Cutis* 57, 435

Rash (sic) (>10%)
(1990): Fremont-Smith P+, *Ann Rheum Dis* 49, 271
(1989): Caspi D+, *Ann Rheum Dis* 48, 730
(1984): Grindulis KA+, *Ann Rheum Dis* 43, 398
(1982): Smith PJ+, *Br Med J* (Clin Res Ed) 285, 595

Seborrheic dermatitis
(1982): Bailin PL+, *Clin Rheum Dis* 8, 493 (passim)
(1981): Kanwar AJ+, *Arch Dermatol* 117, 65 (passim)

Squamous cell carcinoma
(1990): Miller RA+, *J Am Acad Dermatol* 23, 360 (from radioactive gold)

Toxic dermatitis (sic)

Toxic epidermal necrolysis
(1998): Pandya AG+, *Arch Dermatol* 134, 1104 (passim)
(1982): Braun-Falco O+, *MMM Munch Med Wochenschr* (German) 124, 757 (with benoxaprofen)
(1982): Feldman C+, *Rheumatol Rehabil* 21, 222 (with benoxaprofen)

Toxicoderma
(1985): Kalamkarian AA+, *Vestn Dermatol Venerol* (8), 4

Urticaria (1–10%)
(1998): Pandya AG+, *Arch Dermatol* 134, 1104 (passim)
(1994): Lizeaux-Parneix V+, *Ann Dermatol Venereol* (French) 121, 793
(1982): Bailin PL+, *Clin Rheum Dis* 8, 493 (passim)

Vasculitis
(1984): Hauteville D+, *Rev Rhum Mal Osteoartic* (French) 51, 56
(1982): Bailin PL+, *Clin Rheum Dis* 8, 493 (passim)

Vitiligo

Xerosis
(1984): Grindulis KA+, *Ann Rheum Dis* 43, 398

Mucosal/ENT

Aphthous stomatitis

(1989): Caspi D+, *Ann Rheum Dis* 48, 730
(1988): Tishler M+, *Ann Rheum Dis* 47(3), 215
Burning mouth syndrome
  (1994): Laeijendecker R+, *J Am Acad Dermatol* 30, 205
Cheilitis
  (1982): Bailin PL+, *Clin Rheum Dis* 8, 493 (passim)
Dysgeusia
  (1996): Bonnetblanc JM, *Presse Med* (French) 25, 1555
Gingivitis (>10%)
Gingivostomatitis
  (1982): Izumi AK, *Arch Dermatol Res* 272, 387 (allergic contact)
Glossitis (>10%)
Mucocutaneous reactions
  (1996): Cheatum DE, *J Rheumatol* 23, 944
  (1995): Klinkhoff AV+, *J Rheumatol* 22, 1657
Oral lichen planus
  (1994): Laeijendecker R+, *J Am Acad Dermatol* 30, 205
  (1994): Lizeaux-Parneix V+, *Ann Dermatol Venereol* (French) 121, 793
  (1993): Brown RS+, *Cutis* 51, 183
Oral lichenoid eruption
  (1990): Vallejo-Irastorza G+, *Av Odontoestomatol* (Spanish) 6, 131
Oral mucosal eruption
Oral pigmentation
  (1990): Torrelo A+, *Actas Dermo-Sif* (Spanish) 81, 743
  (1984): Sutak J+, *Prakt Zubn Lek* (Czech) 32, 166
Oral ulceration
  (2000): Madinier I+, *Ann Med Interne* (Paris) (French) 151, 248
  (1999): Räsänen L+, *Br J Dermatol* 141, 683
  (1984): Glenert U, *Oral Surg* 58, 52
  (1982): Bailin PL+, *Clin Rheum Dis* 8, 493 (passim)
Stomatitis (>10%)
  (2001): Werth V, *Dermatology Times* 18
  (1997): Tosti A+, *Semin Cutan Med Surg* 16, 314
  (1996): Bonnetblanc JM, *Presse Med* (French) 25, 1555
  (1994): Laeijendecker R+, *J Am Acad Dermatol* 30, 205
  (1992): Svensson A+, *Ann Rheum Dis* 51, 326
  (1989): Caspi D+, *Ann Rheum Dis* 48, 730
  (1987): Tumiati B+, *J Rheumatol* 14, 177
  (1984): Glenert U, *Oral Surg* 58, 52
  (1983): Sigler JW, *Am J Med* 75, 59
  (1982): Bailin PL+, *Clin Rheum Dis* 8, 493 (passim)
Vaginitis

Hair

Hair – alopecia (1–10%)
  (1998): Pandya AG+, *Arch Dermatol* 134, 1104 (passim)
  (1984): Grindulis KA+, *Ann Rheum Dis* 43, 398
  (1982): Bailin PL+, *Clin Rheum Dis* 8, 493 (passim)
Hair – pigmentation

Nails

Nails – dystrophy
  (2005): Yokozeki H+, *Br J Dermatol* 152(5), 1087
Nails – exfoliation
Nails – lichen planus
  (1990): Torrelo A+, *Actas Dermo-Sif* (Spanish) 81, 743
Nails – loss
  (2000): ter Borg EJ+, *Arthritis Rheum* 43, 1420
Nails – pigmentation
  (2001): Roest MA+, *Br J Dermatol* 145, 186
  (1984): Fam AG+, *Arthritis Rheum* 27, 119 (gold nails)

Other

Anaphylactoid reactions/Anaphylaxis
Death
  (1991): Van Linthoudt D+, *Schweiz Med Wochenschr* 121(30), 1099

Headache
Hypersensitivity
Injection-site pain
  (1984): Grindulis KA+, *Ann Rheum Dis* 43, 398
Nephrotoxicity
  (2004): Ohno I+, *Nippon Rinsho* 62(10), 1919
Pseudolymphoma
  (2002): Kim KJ+, *Br J Dermatol* 146, 882 (gold acupuncture)
  (1996): Kalimo K+, *J Cutan Pathol* 23, 328
  (1993): Kerl H+, *Dermatology in General Medicine* McGraw-Hill New York

GOLDENSEAL

Scientific name: *Hydrastis canadensis*
Family: Ranunculaceae
Trade and other common names: Eye balm; Goldenroot; Ground raspberry; Huanglian; Indian dye; Jaundice root; Orange root; Warnera; Yellow puccoon; Yellow root
Category: Immunomodulator; Isoquinolone alkaloid
Purported indications and other uses: Oral: Anorexia, fever, hemorrhoids, hemorrhage, liver disorders, menstrual disorders, rhinitis, upper respiratory tract infections, urinary tract infections. **Topical:** Acne, conjunctivitis, dandruff, earache, eczema, eye inflammation, herpes, itching, mouthwash, rash, ringworm, tinnitus, wounds
Half-life: N/A

Reactions

Skin

Photosensitivity
  (2003): Palanisamy A+, *J Toxicol Clin Toxicol* 41(6), 865 (with ginseng, bee pollen)
Phototoxicity
  (2001): Inbaraj JJ+, *Chem Res Toxicol* 14(11), 1529

Mucosal/ENT

Mucosal irritation

Other

Death (overdose)
Depression (overdose)
Seizures (overdose)

GOSERELIN

Trade names: Prozoladex; Zoladex (AstraZeneca)
Indications: Breast and prostate carcinoma, endometriosis
Category: Gonadotropin-releasing hormone agonist
Half-life: 5 hours

Reactions

Skin

Diaphoresis (1–10%)
  (2006): Nikolov A+, *Akush Ginekol* (Sofiia) 45(4), 13
Edema (1–10%)
Rash (sic) (1–10%)
Urticaria

Mucosal/ENT

Vaginal dryness
  (2006): Nikolov A+, *Akush Ginekol* (Sofiia) 45(4), 13

Hair

Hair – alopecia
   (2002): Jonat W+, *J Clin Oncol* 20(24), 4628

Eyes

Cataract
   (2007): Al-Enezi A+, *Med Princ Pract* 16(2), 161

Other

Anaphylactoid reactions/Anaphylaxis
   (2006): Lam C+, *Pharmacotherapy* 26(12), 1811
   (2006): Lam C+, *Pharmacotherapy* 26(12), 1811 (recurrent)
   (1996): Raj SG+, *Am J Med Sci* 312, 187
Chills
Depression
   (2006): Kohen I+, *Psychosomatics* 47(4), 360
Gynecomastia (>10%)
Hot flashes (>10%)
   (2006): Nikolov A+, *Akush Ginekol (Sofiia)* 45(4), 13
   (2005): Franco S+, *Acta Med Port* 18(2), 123
   (2002): Gommersall LM+, *Expert Opin Pharmacother* 3(12), 1685
   (1993): Bressler LR+, *Ann Pharmacother* 27, 182
Hypersensitivity
   (1996): Raj SG+, *Am J Med Sci* 312, 187
Injection-site pain (1–10%)
Injection-site papules & nodules
   (2002): Cunha AP+, *World Congress Dermatol* Poster, 0095

GRANISETRON

Trade names: Kevatril; Kytril (Roche)
Indications: Chemotherapy-related emesis
Category: 5-HT3 antagonist; Serotonin type 3 receptor antagonist
Half-life: 3–4 hours; cancer patients: 10–12 hours

Reactions

Skin

Allergic reactions (sic)
   (2001): Kanny G+, *J Allergy Clin Immunol* 108(6), 1059
Exanthems
Rash (sic)
Urticaria

Mucosal/ENT

Dysgeusia (2%)
Xerostomia
   (2005): Moreno J+, *Support Care Cancer* 13(10), 850 (11%)

Hair

Hair – alopecia (3%)

Other

Anaphylactoid reactions/Anaphylaxis
Asthenia
   (2001): Lanciano R+, *Cancer Invest* 19(8), 763
   (1998): Perez EA+, *J Clin Oncol* 16(2), 754
Headache
   (2005): Moreno J+, *Support Care Cancer* 13(10), 850 (35%)
   (1998): Carmichael J+, *Anticancer Drugs* 9(5), 381
   (1998): Perez EA+, *J Clin Oncol* 16(2), 754
   (1997): Sismondi P+, *Anticancer Drugs* 8(3), 225 (7%)
   (1995): Gebbia V+, *Cancer* 76(10), 1821 (8%)
   (1995): Golaszewski T+, *Wien Klin Wochenschr* 107(20), 613 (8%)
   (1994): Soukop M, *Support Care Cancer* 2(3), 177 (14%)

Hot flashes (<1%)
Hypersensitivity

GRANULOCYTE COLONY-STIMULATING FACTOR (GCSF)

Generic name:
   Filgrastim (rG-CSF)
      Trade name: Neupogen (Amgen)
   Pegfilgrastim (rG-CSF)
      Trade name: Neulasta (Amgen)
   Sargramostin (rGM-CSF)
      Trade names: Leukine (Berlex); Prokine
Indications: Bone marrow allograft and autograft
Category: Colony stimulating factor; Hematopoietic
Half-life: filgrastim: 3.5 hours; sargramostin: 2–3 hours; pegfilgrastim: 15–80 hours
Clinically important, potentially hazardous interactions with: fluorouracil

Note: rGM-CSF is granulocyte-macrophage colony-stimulating factor; rG-CSF is granulocyte colony-stimulating factor

Reactions

Skin

Abscess
   (2000): Hilbe W+, *Bone Marrow Transplant* 26(7), 811
Acne
   (1996): Lee PK+, *J Am Acad Dermatol* 34, 855
Acral erythema
   (1995): Komamura H+, *J Dermatol* 22(2), 116
Acute febrile neutrophilic dermatosis (Sweet's syndrome)
   (2007): Cohen PR, *Orphanet J Rare Dis* 2, 34
   (2007): Thompson DF+, *Ann Pharmacother* 41(5), 802
   (2006): Hara I+, *Int J Urol* 13(4), 481
   (2006): Oiso N+, *Br J Haematol* 135(2), 148
   (2006): Thompson MA+, *Am J Hematol* 81(9), 703
   (2006): White JM+, *Clin Exp Dermatol* 31(2), 206 (3 cases)
   (2004): Kumar G+, *Am J Hematol* 76(3), 283
   (2002): Brazzelli V+, *World Congress Dermatol* Poster, 0089
   (2001): Magro CM+, *J Cutan Pathol* 28(2), 90
   (2001): Matsumura T+, *Br J Haematol* 113(1), 1
   (2001): Prendiville J+, *Pediatr Dermatol* 18(5), 417 (2 cases)
   (2000): Malone JC+, *Arch Dermatol* 345 (passim)
   (1999): Arbetter KR+, *Am J Hematol* 61, 126
   (1999): Veres K+, *Orv Hetil* (Hungarian) 140, 1059
   (1998): Chao SC+, *J Formos Med Assoc* 96, 276
   (1998): Hasegawa M+, *Eur J Dermatol* 8, 503 (2 patients)
   (1998): Merkel PA, *Curr Opin Rheumatol* 10, 45
   (1996): Garty BZ+, *Pediatrics* 97, 401
   (1996): Jain KK, *Cutis* 57, 107
   (1996): Petit T+, *Lancet* 347, 690
   (1996): Prevost-Blank PL+, *J Am Acad Dermatol* 35, 995
   (1996): Richard MA+, *J Am Acad Dermatol* 35, 629
   (1996): Shimizu T+, *J Pediatr Hematol Oncol* 18, 282
   (1995): Shiga Y+, *Rinsho Ketsueki* (Japanese) 36, 353
   (1995): Suzuki Y+, *Br J Dermatol* 133, 483
   (1994): Fukutoku M+, *Br J Haematol* 86, 645
   (1994): Johnson ML+, *Arch Dermatol* 130, 77
   (1994): Reuss-Borst MA+, *Leuk Lymphoma* 15, 261
   (1994): van Kamp H+, *Br J Haematol* 86, 415
   (1993): Paydas S+, *Br J Haematol* 85, 191
   (1992): Karp DL, *Ann Intern Med* 117, 875
   (1992): Park JW+, *Ann Intern Med* 116, 996
   (1991): Ross HJ+, *Cancer* 68, 441
   (1990): Morioka N+, *J Am Acad Dermatol* 23, 247

(1989): Groopman JE+, *N Engl J Med* 321, 1449
(1989): Kluin-Nelemans JC+, *Br J Haematol* 73, 419

Adverse effects (sic) (19%)
(2002): De la Rubia J+, *J Hematother Stem Cell Res* 11(4), 705
(2002): Heuft HG+, *Transfusion* 42(7), 928
(2001): Kashiwagi H+, *Gan To Kagaku Ryoho* 28(8), 1105
(1998): Caballero MD+, *Haematologica* 83(6), 514 (19%)
(1997): Hanauske AR+, *Oncology* 54(5), 363
(1997): Yano T+, *Int J Hematol* 66(2), 169

Allergic granulomatous angiitis (Churg–Strauss syndrome)
(2006): Ferran M+, *Dermatology. 2006* 212(2), 188

Allergic reactions (sic) (19%)
(2003): van der Kolk LE+, *Leukemia* 17(8), 1658 (19%)

Diaphoresis
(2000): Khoury H+, *Bone Marrow Transplant* 25, 1197

Edema
(2000): Milkovich G+, *Pharmacotherapy* 20(12), 1432

Erythema
(2003): Lenczowski JM+, *J Am Acad Dermatol* 49(1), 105
(2001): Prendiville J+, *Pediatr Dermatol* 18(5), 417
(2001): Tomita Y+, *Acta Derm Venereol* 81(6), 436
(1990): Farmer KL+, *Arch Dermatol* 126, 1243
(1989): Groopman JE+, *N Engl J Med* 321, 1449

Erythema nodosum
(2005): George S+, *Biol Blood Marrow Transplant* 11(10), 816
(1994): Nomiyama J+, *Am J Hematol* 47, 333

Exanthems (5–63%)
(1996): Glass LF+, *J Am Acad Dermatol* 34, 455
(1995): McMullin MF+, *Clin Rheumatol* 14, 204
(1995): Scott GA, *Am J Dermatopathol* 17, 107
(1994): Sasaki O+, *Intern Med* 33, 641
(1993): Samlaska CP+, *Arch Dermatol* 129, 645
(1993): Yamashita N+, *J Dermatol* 20, 473
(1991): Cohen PR+, *J Am Acad Dermatol* 25, 734
(1991): Horn TD+, *Arch Dermatol* 127, 49 (>5%)
(1990): Farmer KL+, *Arch Dermatol* 126, 1243
(1990): Lazarus H+, *Proc Am Soc Clin Oncol* 9, 15
(1988): Brandt SJ+, *N Engl J Med* 318, 869 (63%)

Exfoliative dermatitis (10%)
(1988): Brandt SJ+, *N Engl J Med* 318, 869 (10%)

Folliculitis
(1992): Ostlere LS+, *Br J Dermatol* 127, 193

Graft-versus-host reaction
(2005): Mohty M+, *Leukemia* 19(4), 500
(2002): Law L+, *Int J Hematol* 76(4), 360
(2001): Deeg HJ, *Int J Hematol* 74(1), 26
(2001): Ji S+, *Chin Med J* (Engl) 114(2), 191

Lichenoid eruption
(2002): Brazzelli V+, *World Congress Dermatol* Poster, 0089

Linear IgA dermatosis
(1999): Kano Y+, *Eur J Dermatol* 9, 122

Lupus erythematosus
(2006): Vasiliu IM+, *J Rheumatol* 33(9), 1878

Neutrophilic eccrine hidradenitis
(1998): Bachmeyer C+, *Br J Dermatol* 139, 354

Palmar–plantar pustulosis
(2005): Kurokawa I+, *Int J Dermatol* 44(6), 529

Peripheral edema (1–10%)

Pruritus (1–5%)
(1990): Farmer KL+, *Arch Dermatol* 126, 1243
(1990): Steward WP+, *Int J Cell Cloning* 8, 335
(1989): Steward WP+, *Br J Cancer* 59, 142 (1–5%)

Psoriasis
(2004): Mossner R+, *Exp Dermatol* 13(6), 340
(2001): Yonei T+, *Nihon Kokyuki Gakkai Zasshi* 39(6), 438
(1998): Cho SG+, *J Korean Med Sci* 13, 685
(1997): Feliu J+, *J Natl Cancer Inst* 89(17), 1315
(1996): Kavanaugh A, *Am J Med* 101, 567

Pyoderma gangrenosum
(2006): Miall FM+, *Br J Haematol* 132(1), 115
(2006): White LE+, *Skinmed* 5(2), 96
(1998): Merkel PA, *Curr Opin Rheumatol* 10, 45
(1991): Ross HJ+, *Cancer* 68, 441

Rash (sic) (<40%)
(2003): Brumit MC+, *Transfusion* 43(10), 1343
(2003): Prosper F+, *Leukemia* 17(2), 437
(1996): Johnson RJ+, *Br J Haematol* 93(4), 863 (40%)
(1993): Dale DC+, *Blood* 81(10), 2496

Side effects (sic)
(1999): Will R+, *Urologe A* 38(3), 258 (G-CSF: 38.5%, GM-CSF: 69.3%)

Urticaria

Vasculitis
(1999): Andavolu MV+, *Ann Hematol* 78, 79
(1998): Merkel PA, *Curr Opin Rheumatol* 10, 45
(1995): Couderc LJ+, *Respir Med* 89, 237
(1995): Farhey YD+, *J Rheumatol* 22, 1179
(1995): Vidarsson B+, *Am J Med* 98, 589
(1994): Jain KK, *J Am Acad Dermatol* 31, 213
(1994): Johnson ML+, *Arch Dermatol* 130, 77
(1990): Farmer KL+, *Arch Dermatol* 126, 1243
(1989): Kluin-Nelemans JC+, *Br J Haematol* 73, 419

Mucosal/ENT
Dysgeusia
Mucositis (40%)
(1999): Crawford J+, *Cytokines Cell Mol Ther* 5, 187
(1996): Johnson RJ+, *Br J Haematol* 93(4), 863 (40%)

Oral lesions
(1990): Lazarus H+, *Proc Am Soc Clin Oncol* 9, 15

Stomatitis (>10%)

Hair
Hair – alopecia (>10%)
(1990): Lazarus H+, *Proc Am Soc Clin Oncol* 9, 15

Eyes
Keratitis
(2007): Fraunfelder FW+, *Cornea* 26(3), 368

Other
Abdominal pain
(2002): Otaibi AA+, *J Pediatr Surg* 37(5), 770

Anaphylactoid reactions/Anaphylaxis (<1%)
(2000): Khoury H+, *Bone Marrow Transplant* 25, 1197
(1999): Dupre D+, *Ann Dermatol Venereol* (French) 126, 161
(1999): Keung YK+, *Bone Marrow Transplant* 23, 200

Asthenia
(2002): Cesaro S+, *Haematologica* 87(8), 35 (31%)
(2002): Kroger N+, *Bone Marrow Transplant* 29(9), 727
(2000): Milkovich G+, *Pharmacotherapy* 20(12), 1432
(1999): Martinez C+, *Bone Marrow Transplant* 24(12), 1273

Death
(2003): O'Malley DP+, *Am J Hematol* 73(4), 294
(2002): Kikuchi M+, *Nippon Ronen Igakkai Zasshi* 39(4), 433
(2001): Adler BK+, *Blood* 97(10), 3313

Depression
(1996): Cousins JP+, *Cancer Lett* 110(1), 163 (with paclitaxel)

Fever (5–50%)
(2003): Aoyama Y+, *Gan To Kagaku Ryoho* 30(6), 829
(2003): van der Kolk LE+, *Leukemia* 17(8), 1658 (29%)
(2002): Cesaro S+, *Haematologica* 87(8), 35 (5%)
(2002): Takatsuka H+, *Chest* 121(5), 1716
(2001): Mayer J+, *Vnitr Lek* 47, 15
(2001): Weaver CH+, *Bone Marrow Transplant* 27, S23 (G-CSF 18%, GM-CSF 52%)
(2000): Hilbe W+, *Bone Marrow Transplant* 26(7), 811

(2000): Milkovich G+, *Pharmacotherapy* 20(12), 1432
  (sargramostim 7% filgrastim 1%)
(1999): Alvarado Ibarra+, *Rev Invest Clin* 51(2), 77
(1999): Anderlini P+, *Transfusion* 39(6), 555 (34%)
(1997): Hanauske AR+, *Oncology* 54(5), 363
(1996): Anderlini P+, *Transfusion* 36(7), 590 (20%)
(1996): Johnson RJ+, *Br J Haematol* 93(4), 863 (50%)
(1996): Rackoff WR+, *Blood* 88(5), 1588
(1996): Stroncek DF+, *Transfusion* 36(7), 601 (14%)
Headache (39–80%)
  (2007): Andre N+, *Anticancer Drugs* 18(3), 277
  (2003): Aoyama Y+, *Gan To Kagaku Ryoho* 30(6), 829
  (2002): Beelen DW+, *Ann Hematol* 81(12), 701 (80%)
  (2002): Cesaro S+, *Haematologica* 87(8), 35 (54%)
  (2002): Kroger N+, *Bone Marrow Transplant* 29(9), 727
  (1999): Anderlini P+, *Transfusion* 39(6), 555 (54%)
  (1999): Martinez C+, *Bone Marrow Transplant* 24(12), 1273
  (1996): Anderlini P+, *Transfusion* 36(7), 590 (70%)
  (1996): Stroncek DF+, *Transfusion* 36(7), 601 (39%)
  (1993): Dale DC+, *Blood* 81(10), 2496
Injection-site bullous eruption
  (1990): Farmer KL+, *Arch Dermatol* 126, 1243
Injection-site erythema
  (1995): Scott GA, *Am J Dermatopathol* 17, 107
Injection-site lichenoid reaction
  (1999): Viallard AM+, *Dermatology* 198, 301
Injection-site nodules
  (1990): Farmer KL+, *Arch Dermatol* 126, 1243
Injection-site pain (1–10%)
Injection-site pruritus
  (1990): Farmer KL+, *Arch Dermatol* 126, 1243
Injection-site reactions (>5%)
  (2002): Cesaro S+, *Haematologica* 87(8), 35 (5%)
  (2000): Milkovich G+, *Pharmacotherapy* 20(12), 1432
  (1999): Facon T+, *Blood* 94(4), 1218
  (1997): Moskowitz CH+, *Blood* 89(9), 3136
Injection-site urticaria
  (1995): Scott GA, *Am J Dermatopathol* 17, 107
Lymphoproliferative disease
  (1994): De la Rubia J+, *Bone Marrow Transplantation* 14, 475
  (1994): Kawach Y+, *Leukemia and Lymphoma* 13, 509
Myalgia/Myositis/Myopathy/Myotoxicity (>10%)
  (2002): Sevilla J+, *Bone Marrow Transplant* 30(7), 417
Panniculitis (necrotizing)
  (2000): Dereure O+, *Br J Dermatol* 142, 834
Systemic reactions
  (1999): Alvarado Ibarra ML+, *Rev Invest Clin* 51(2), 77
Vertigo (>5%)
  (2002): Cesaro S+, *Haematologica* 87(8), 35 (5%)

GRAPEFRUIT JUICE

Scientific names: *Citrus decumana; Citrus maxima; Citrus paradisi*
Family: Rutaceae
Trade and other common names: Paradisapfel; Pomelo; Toronja
Category: Food supplement
Purported indications and other uses: atherosclerosis, anti-cancer agent, cholesterol reduction, psoriasis, weight reduction. Source of potassium, vitamin C, and fiber
Half-life: N/A
Clinically important, potentially hazardous interactions with: alprazolam, amiodarone, astemizole, buspirone, corticosteroids, eplerenone, felodipine, itraconazole, lapatinib, lercanidipine, lovastatin, midazolam, nifedipine, nisoldipine, pimozide, prednisolone, prednisone, propafenone, **red rice yeast**, repaglinide, simvastatin, tacrolimus, terfenadine, warfarin

Reactions

Skin
Urticaria
  (2006): Kumar A+, *Clin Rev Allergy Immunol* 30(1), 61

Other
Adverse effects (sic)
  (2003): Bailey DG+, *Clin Pharmacol Ther* 73(6), 529 (with felodipine) (1 case)
Headache
  (2000): Takanaga H+, *Clin Pharmacol Ther* 67(3), 201 (with nisoldipine)
  (1995): Lundahl J+, *Eur J Clin Pharmacol* 49(1-2), 61 (with felodipine)
Rhabdomyolysis
  (2002): Sardi A+, *Ann Ital Med Int* 17(2), 126 (with licorice) (1 case)

GREEN TEA

Scientific names: *Camellia sinensis; Camellia thea; Camellia theifera; Thea bohea; Thea sinensis; Thea viridis*
Family: Theaceae
Trade and other common names: Chinese tea
Category: Food supplement; TNF inhibitor; Xanthine alkaloid NSAID
Purported indications and other uses: Improving cognitive performance, stomach disorders, nausea, vomiting, diarrhea, anticancer, headaches, Crohn's disease. **Topical:** soothe sunburn, bleeding gums, reduce sweating
Half-life: N/A
Clinically important, potentially hazardous interactions with: warfarin

Reactions

Skin
Rosacea
  (2007): Lleonart R+, *Allergy* 62(1), 89

Other
Hepatotoxicity
  (2006): Bonkovsky HL, *Ann Intern Med* 144(1), 68
  (2006): Jimenez-Saenz M+, *J Hepatol* 44(3), 616

GREPAFLOXACIN

Trade name: Raxar
Indications: Various infections caused by susceptible organisms
Category: Antibiotic, quinolone
Half-life: 5–12 hours

Note: Grepafloxacin has been withdrawn

Reactions

Skin
Acne (<1%)
Diaphoresis (<1%)
Edema (<1%)
Exanthems (<1%)
Exfoliative dermatitis (<1%)
Facial edema (<1%)
Fungal dermatitis (<1%)
Herpes simplex (<1%)
Peripheral edema (<1%)
Photosensitivity
 (1997): Ferguson J+, *J Antimicrob Chemother* 40, 93
 (1997): Stahlmann R+, *J Antimicrob Chemother* 40, 83
Phototoxicity (2%)
 (2000): Traynor NJ+, *Toxicol Vitr* 14, 275
 (1998): Lode H, *Infect Med* 15 (Suppl 1), 28
Pruritus (<1%)
Rash (sic) (1.9%)
 (1998): Lode H, *Infect Med* 15 (Suppl 1), 28
 (1997): Stahlmann R+, *J Antimicrob Chemother* 40, 83
Toxic epidermal necrolysis (<1%)
Urticaria (<1%)
Vesiculobullous eruption (<1%)
Xerosis (<1%)

Mucosal/ENT
Ageusia (<1%)
Balanitis (<1%)
Bromhidrosis (<1%)
Cheilitis (<1%)
Dysgeusia (17%) (metallic taste)
 (1998): Chodosh S+, *Antimicrob Agents Chemother* 42, 114
 (1998): Lode H, *Infect Med* 15 (Suppl 1), 28
 (1997): Stahlmann R+, *J Antimicrob Chemother* 40, 83
Gingivitis (<1%)
Glossitis (<1%)
Oral candidiasis (<1%)
Oral ulceration (<1%)
Parosmia (<1%)
Stomatitis (<1%)
Tongue disorder (sic) (<1%)
Tongue edema (<1%)
Tongue pigmentation (<1%)
Vaginitis (3.3%)
Xerostomia (1.1%)

Hair
Hair – alopecia (<1%)

Other
Hypersensitivity
Myalgia/Myositis/Myopathy/Myotoxicity (<1%)
Paresthesias (<1%)
Tendinopathy/Tendon rupture

GRISEOFULVIN

Trade names: Fulcin; Fulvina P/G; Grifulvin V (Ortho); Gris-PEG (Pedinol); Grisefuline; Griseostatin; Grisovin; Likudin M; Polygris
Indications: Fungal infections of the skin, hair and nails
Category: Antimycobacterial
Half-life: 9–24 hours
Clinically important, potentially hazardous interactions with: alcohol, midazolam

Reactions

Skin
Allergic reactions (sic) (1–5%)
Angioedema (<1%)
 (1994): Gupta AK+, *J Am Acad Dermatol* 30, 677 (passim)
 (1989): Rustin MHA+, *Br J Dermatol* 120, 455
Bullous dermatitis (<1%)
 (1995): Meffert JJ+, *Cutis* 56, 279
Cold urticaria
 (1989): Rustin MHA+, *Br J Dermatol* 120, 455
Erythema multiforme (<1%)
 (2001): Thami GP+, *Dermatology* 203(1), 84
 (1994): Gupta AK+, *J Am Acad Dermatol* 30, 677 (passim)
 (1990): Almeida L+, *J Am Acad Dermatol* 23, 855
 (1989): Rustin MHA+, *Br J Dermatol* 120, 455
 (1981): Walinga H+, *Ned Tijdschr Geneeskd* (Dutch) 125, 729
Exanthems
 (2001): Develoux M, *Ann Dermatol Venereol* 128(12), 1317
 (1997): Litt JZ, Beachwood, OH (personal case) (observation in a 10–year-old boy)
 (1994): Gupta AK+, *J Am Acad Dermatol* 30, 677 (passim)
 (1993): Gaudin JL+, *Gastroenterol Clin Biol* 17, 145
 (1992): Breathnach SM+, *Adverse Drug Reactions and the Skin* Blackwell, Oxford, 169 (passim)
 (1989): Miyagawa S+, *Am J Med* 87, 100
Exfoliative dermatitis
 (1989): Rustin MHA+, *Br J Dermatol* 120, 455
Fixed eruption (<1%)
 (1998): Mahboob A+, *Int J Dermatol* 37, 833
 (1994): Gupta AK+, *J Am Acad Dermatol* 30, 677 (passim)
 (1989): Boudghene-Stambouli O+, *Dermatologica* 179, 92
 (1989): Rustin MHA+, *Br J Dermatol* 120, 455
 (1984): Feinstein A+, *J Am Acad Dermatol* 10, 915
 (1981): Thyagarajan K+, *Mykosen* (German) 24, 482
Hemorrhage
 (1992): Breathnach SM+, *Adverse Drug Reactions and the Skin* Blackwell, Oxford, 169 (passim)
Herpes zoster
Jarisch–Herxheimer reaction
 (1993): Amita DB+, *Clin Exp Dermatol* 18, 389
Lichenoid eruption
 (1994): Gupta AK+, *J Am Acad Dermatol* 30, 677 (passim)
Lupus erythematosus
 (1995): Bonilla-Felix M+, *Pediatr Nephrol* 9, 478
 (1994): Gupta AK+, *J Am Acad Dermatol* 30, 677 (passim)
 (1994): Yung RL+, *Rheum Dis Clin North Am* 20, 61
 (1990): Okazaki H+, *Ryumachi* (Japanese) 30, 418
 (1989): Miyagawa S+, *Am J Med* 87, 100
 (1989): Miyagawa S+, *J Am Acad Dermatol* 21, 343
 (1985): Madhok R+, *BMJ* 291, 249 (fatal)
 (1980): Condemi JJ, *Geriatrics* 35(3), 81
Petechiae
 (1994): Gupta AK+, *J Am Acad Dermatol* 30, 677 (passim)
Photosensitivity (1–10%)
 (1994): Gupta AK+, *J Am Acad Dermatol* 30, 677 (passim)
 (1989): Kojima K+, *J Dermatol* (Tokio) 15, 76

(1989): Miyagawa S+, *Am J Med* 87, 100
(1989): Rustin MHA+, *Br J Dermatol* 120, 455
(1988): Kawabe Y+, *Photodermatol* 5, 272
(1988): Kojima T+, *J Dermatol* 15, 76
(1986): Ljunggren B+, *Photodermatol* 3, 26
(1983): Hawk JLM, *Clin Exp Dermatol* 9, 300
Pigmentation
Pityriasis rosea
Pruritus (<1%)
(1994): Gupta AK+, *J Am Acad Dermatol* 30, 677 (passim)
(1989): Rustin MHA+, *Br J Dermatol* 120, 455
Purpura
Rash (sic) (>10%)
Seborrheic dermatitis
Stevens–Johnson syndrome
(1989): Rustin MHA+, *Br J Dermatol* 120, 455
(1981): Walinga H+, *Ned Tijdschr Geneeskd* (Dutch) 125, 729
Toxic epidermal necrolysis
(1991): Correia O+, *Ann Fr Anesth Reanim* (French) 10, 493
(1990): Mion G+, *Ann Fr Anesth Reanim* (French) 9, 305 (fatal)
(1989): Mion G+, *Lancet* 2, 1331 (fatal)
(1988): Taylor B+, *J Am Acad Dermatol* 19, 565
Urticaria (>10%)
(1989): Rustin MHA+, *Br J Dermatol* 120, 455
(1984): Feinstein A+, *J Am Acad Dermatol* 10, 915
Vasculitis
(1994): Gupta AK+, *J Am Acad Dermatol* 30, 677 (passim)

Mucosal/ENT
Angular stomatitis
(1994): Gupta AK+, *J Am Acad Dermatol* 30, 677 (passim)
Dysgeusia
(1995): Hofmann H+, *Arch Dermatol* 131, 919
(1994): Gupta AK+, *J Am Acad Dermatol* 30, 677 (passim)
Glossodynia
(1994): Gupta AK+, *J Am Acad Dermatol* 30, 677 (passim)
Hypogeusia
Mucocutaneous lymph node syndrome (Kawasaki syndrome)
Oral candidiasis (1–10%)
(1994): Gupta AK+, *J Am Acad Dermatol* 30, 677 (passim)
Stomatodynia
Tongue black
(1994): Gupta AK+, *J Am Acad Dermatol* 30, 677 (passim)
Xerostomia
(1994): Gupta AK+, *J Am Acad Dermatol* 30, 677 (passim)

Nails
Nails – pigmentation
(1986): Duvanel T, *Ann Dermatol Venereol* (French) 113, 471
Nails – subungual hemorrhages

Other
Anaphylactoid reactions/Anaphylaxis
Candidiasis
Death
Gynecomastia
(1994): Gupta AK+, *J Am Acad Dermatol* 30, 677 (passim)
Headache
(2001): Develoux M, *Ann Dermatol Venereol* 128(12), 1317
Paresthesias
(1994): Gupta AK+, *J Am Acad Dermatol* 30, 677 (passim)
Porphyria
(1990): Gederaas OA+, *Photodermatol Photoimmunol Photomed* 7, 82
(1983): Poh-Fitzpatrick MB+, *J Clin Invest* 72, 1449
(1980): Smith AG+, *Clin Haematol* 9, 399
Porphyria cutanea tarda

Serum sickness
(2004): Colton RL+, *Ann Pharmacother* 38(4), 609
(1994): Gupta AK+, *J Am Acad Dermatol* 30, 677 (passim)
(1989): Rustin MHA+, *Br J Dermatol* 120, 455

GUANABENZ

Trade names: Rexitene; Wytens
Indications: Hypertension
Category: Adrenergic alpha-receptor agonist
Half-life: 7–10 hours

Reactions

Skin
Edema (<3%)
Hyperhidrosis
Pruritus (<3%)
Rash (sic) (<3%)

Mucosal/ENT
Dysgeusia (<3%)
Sialorrhea
Xerostomia (28%)
(1988): Bork K, *Cutaneous Side Effects of Drugs* WB Saunders, 307
(1984): Walson PD+, *Pediatr Pharmacol (New York)* 4(1), 1
(1983): Holmes B+, *Drugs* 26(3), 212
(1981): Walker BR+, *Clin Ther* 4(3), 217

Other
Asthenia
Gynecomastia (<3%)
Headache
(1984): Walson PD+, *Pediatr Pharmacol (New York)* 4(1), 1
Vertigo
(1981): Walker BR+, *Clin Ther* 4(3), 217

GUANADREL

Trade name: Hylorel
Indications: Hypertension
Category: Adrenergic alpha-receptor agonist
Half-life: 5–45 hours (terminal)

Reactions

Skin
Peripheral edema (28.6%)

Mucosal/ENT
Glossitis (8.4%)
Xerostomia (1.7%)

Other
Asthenia
(1988): Owens SD+, *Arch Intern Med* 148(7), 1515
Headache
Paresthesias (25.1%)
Vertigo
(1988): Owens SD+, *Arch Intern Med* 148(7), 1515

GUANETHIDINE

Trade names: Apo-Guanethidine; Ismelin (Novartis); Ismeline
Indications: Hypertension
Category: Adrenergic alpha-receptor agonist
Half-life: 5–10 days
Clinically important, potentially hazardous interactions
with: amitriptyline, amoxapine, benzphetamine, chlorpromazine, clomipramine, desipramine, doxepin, **ephedra**, ephedrine, imipramine, insulin, insulin glargine, minoxidil, nortriptyline, protriptyline, tricyclic antidepressants, trimipramine, zuclopentixol acetate, zuclopentixol decanoate, zuclopentixol dihydrochloride

Reactions

Skin
Dermatitis
Exanthems
Fixed eruption
Lupus erythematosus
Peripheral edema (>10%)
Purpura
Urticaria
Vasculitis

Mucosal/ENT
Glossitis (5%)
Sialorrhea
Xerostomia (1 10%)

Hair
Hair – alopecia

Other
Headache
Hypotension
  (1991): Park KH+, *J Pharmacol Exp Ther* 259(3), 1221
Myalgia/Myositis/Myopathy/Myotoxicity
Paresthesias (16%)
Vertigo
  (1996): Kaplan R+, *Acta Anaesthesiol Scand* 40(10), 1216

GUANFACINE

Trade names: Entulic; Estulic; Tenex (ESP)
Indications: Hypertension
Category: Adrenergic alpha-receptor agonist
Half-life: 10–30 hours

Reactions

Skin
Dermatitis (<3%)
Diaphoresis (<3%)
  (1991): Wilson MF+, *J Clin Pharmacol* 31, 318
  (1990): Mosqueda-Garcia R, *Am J Med Sci* 299, 73
  (1986): Sorkin EM+, *Drugs* 31, 301 (3%)
Edema
Exanthems
Exfoliative dermatitis
Peripheral edema
  (1991): Oster JR+, *Arch Intern Med* 151, 1638
Pruritus (<3%)

  (1991): Wilson MF+, *J Clin Pharmacol* 31, 318
Purpura (<3%)
Rash (sic)
  (1990): Lewin A+, *J Clin Pharmacol* 30, 1081
Urticaria

Mucosal/ENT
Dysgeusia (<3%)
  (1988): Cornish LA, *Clin Pharm* 7, 187
Sialorrhea
Tinnitus
Xerostomia (47%)
  (1991): Wilson MF+, *J Clin Pharmacol* 31, 318
  (1990): Lewin A+, *J Clin Pharmacol* 30, 1081
  (1990): Mosqueda-Garcia R, *Am J Med Sci* 299, 73
  (1988): Board AW+, *Clin Ther* 10, 761
  (1988): Cornish LA, *Clin Pharm* 7, 187
  (1988): Van Zweiten PA, *Am J Cardiol* 61, 6D
  (1980): Jaattela A, *Br J Clin Pharmacol* 10 Suppl 1, 67S

Hair
Hair – alopecia

Eyes
Visual hallucinations

Other
Headache
Paresthesias (<3%)

GUARANA

Scientific names: *Paullinia cupana; Paullinia sorbilis*
Family: Sapindaceae
Trade and other common names: Brazilian Cocoa; Cupana; Uabano; Uaranzeiro; Zoom
Category: Stimulant, mild
Purported indications and other uses: Aphrodisiac, diarrhea, fatigue, fever, heart problems, headache, mental alertness, neuralgia, weight loss. Cosmetic products, anti-cellulite creams, shampoo for hair loss. Flavoring
Half-life: N/A
Clinically important, potentially hazardous interactions
with: **caffeine**, clozapine, **ephedra**, ephedrine, lithium, MAO inhibitors, phenylpropanolamine, warfarin

Note: The main constituent of Guarana is caffeine. It contains more than twice as much caffeine as coffee or tea. Excessive consumption of caffeine is contraindicated for persons with high blood pressure, cardiac disorders, diabetes, ulcers, and epilepsy

Reactions

Mucosal/ENT
Tinnitus

Other
Abdominal pain
Adverse effects (sic)
  (2002): Arditti J+, *Acta Clin Belg* 1(Suppl), 34 (with ephedra)
  (2002): Haller CA+, *Adverse Drug React Toxicol Rev* 21(3), 143
  (2001): Cannon ME+, *Med J Aust* 174(10), 520
  (2001): du Boisgueheneuc F+, *Presse Med* 30(4), 166 (with ephedra)
  (2000): Donadio V+, *Neurol Sci* 21(2), 124
Death
  (2002): Arditti J+, *Acta Clin Belg* 1(Suppl), 34 (with ephedra)
Nephrotoxicity

(2007): Vagasi K+, *Orv Hetil* 148(9), 421
Seizures
  (2002): Arditti J+, *Acta Clin Belg* 1(Suppl), 34 (with ephedra)
  (2001): Kockler DR+, *Pharmacotherapy* 21(5), 647 (with ephedra)
Vertigo

HALCINONIDE

Trade name: Halog (Bristol-Myers Squibb)
Indications: Dermatoses
Category: Corticosteroid, topical
Half-life: N/A
Clinically important, potentially hazardous interactions with: live vaccines

Reactions

Skin
Acne
Burning
  (1981): Guenther L+, *Cutis* 28(4), 461
  (1980): Akers WA, *Arch Dermatol* 116(7), 786
Irritation
  (1981): Guenther L+, *Cutis* 28(4), 461
  (1980): Akers WA, *Arch Dermatol* 116(7), 786
Pigmentation
Pruritus
  (1981): Guenther L+, *Cutis* 28(4), 461
  (1980): Akers WA, *Arch Dermatol* 116(7), 786
Rash (sic)
Xerosis
  (1980): Akers WA, *Arch Dermatol* 116(7), 786

Other
Hypersensitivity
  (1986): Reitamo S+, *J Am Acad Dermatol* 14(4), 582
Infections

HALOBETASOL

Trade name: Ultravate (Ranbaxy)
Indications: Dermatoses
Category: Corticosteroid, topical
Half-life: N/A
Clinically important, potentially hazardous interactions with: live vaccines

Reactions

Skin
Adverse effects (sic)
  (1991): Blum G+, *J Am Acad Dermatol* 25(6), 1153
  (1991): Brunner N+, *J Am Acad Dermatol* 25(6), 1160 (rare)
  (1991): Datz B+, *J Am Acad Dermatol* 25(6), 1157 (5%)
  (1991): Goldberg B+, *J Am Acad Dermatol* 25(6), 1145 (7%)
  (1991): Herz G+, *J Am Acad Dermatol* 25(6), 1166 (2%)
Atrophy
  (1991): Herz G+, *J Am Acad Dermatol* 25(6), 1166 (1 case)
Burning
Erythema
Pruritus
  (1991): Yawalkar SJ+, *J Am Acad Dermatol* 25(6), 1163
  (1990): Watson WA+, *Pharmacotherapy* 10(2), 107 (2 cases)

Stinging
Xerosis
  (1991): Yawalkar SJ+, *J Am Acad Dermatol* 25(6), 1163 (1 case)

HALOMETASONE

Trade name: Sicorten
Indications: Dermatoses
Category: Corticosteroid, topical
Half-life: N/A
Clinically important, potentially hazardous interactions with: live vaccines

Reactions

Skin
Adverse effects (sic)
  (1983): Maeder E+, *J Int Med Res* 11, 48 (mild)
Pruritus
  (1983): Weitgasser H+, *J Int Med Res* 11, 34 (4%)
Pustules
  (1983): Galbiati G+, *J Int Med Res* 11, 31 (1 case)

HALOPERIDOL

Trade names: Dozic; Duraperidol; Haldol (Ortho-McNeil); Haloper; Peridol; Seranace; Serenace
Indications: Psychoses, Tourette's disorder
Category: Antipsychotic, butyrophenone
Half-life: 20 hours
Clinically important, potentially hazardous interactions with: benztropine, **eucalyptus**, fluoxetine, lithium, methotrexate, propranolol

Reactions

Skin
Acne
Cellulitis
  (1982): Sacks HS, *Hosp Pract Off Ed* 17, 179
Dermatitis (<1%)
Diaphoresis
  (2001): Kane JM+, *Arch Gen Psychiatry* 58(10), 965
  (1999): Wilkinson R+, *Brain Inj* 13(12), 1025
Exanthems
Exfoliative dermatitis
Pemphigus foliaceus
  (2003): Perez Espana+, *Med Clin* (Barc) 120(3), 117
Photo-recall
  (2002): Thami GP+, *Postgrad Med J* 78(916), 116
Photosensitivity (<1%)
  (2002): Thami GP+, *Postgrad Med* 78(916), 116 (pellagra-like)
Pigmentation (<1%)
Pruritus (<1%)
Purpura
Rash (sic) (<1%)
Seborrheic dermatitis
  (1984): Binder RL+, *J Clin Psychiatry* 45, 125
  (1983): Binder RL+, *Arch Dermatol* 119, 473
Urticaria

Mucosal/ENT
Dysphagia

(2007): Dziewas R+, *Dysphagia* 22(1), 63
Sialorrhea
  (2001): Kane JM+, *Arch Gen Psychiatry* 58(10), 965
Xerostomia (<1%)
  (2003): Tohen M+, *Am J Psychiatry* 160(7), 1263
  (2001): Kane JM+, *Arch Gen Psychiatry* 58(10), 965

Hair
Hair – alopecia (<1%)
  (2000): Mercke Y+, *Ann Clin Psychiatry* 12, 35
Hair – alopecia areata
  (1994): Kubota T+, *Jpn J Psychiatry Neurol* 48, 579
  (1993): Kubota T+, *Acta Neurol Napoli* 15, 200 (3 cases)
Hair – poliosis

Other
Death
  (2006): Hollis J+, *Aust N Z J Psychiatry* 40(11-12), 981
  (2002): Remijnse PL+, *Ned Tijdschr Geneeskd* 146(16), 768
  (2002): Veltkamp R, *Ned Tijdschr Geneeskd* 146(27), 1301
  (2002): Vorel-Havelkova E+, *Ned Tijdschr Geneeskd* 146(27), 1301
  (2001): Glassman AH+, *Am J Psychiatry* 158(11), 1774
  (1995): Guadagnucci A+, *Minerva Med* 86(7–8), 327
Gynecomastia (<1%)
Headache
Inappropriate secretion of antidiuretic hormone (SIADH)
  (2006): van den Heuvel OA+, *Ned Tijdschr Geneeskd* 150(35), 1944
  (1981): Husband C+, *Can J Psychiatry* 26(3), 196
Injection-site hypersensitivity
  (1992): Hay J, *J Clin Psychiatry* 53, 256
Injection-site pain
  (1990): Hamann GL+, *J Clin Psychiatry* 51, 502
Injection-site reactions (sic)
  (1995): Maharaj K+, *J Clin Psychiatry* 56, 172
  (1992): Reinke M+, *J Clin Psychiatry* 53, 415
  (1990): Hamann GL+, *J Clin Psychiatry* 51, 502
Rhabdomyolysis
  (2000): Yoshikawa H+, *Brain Dev* 22(4), 256
  (1996): Meltzer HY+, *Neuropsychopharmacology* 15(4), 395
  (1995): Marsh SJ+, *Ren Fail* 17(4), 475
  (1984): Cavanaugh JJ+, *J Clin Psychiatry* 45, 356
  (1984): Hashimoto F+, *Arch Intern Med* 144(3), 629 (with chlorpromazine)
  (1982): Eiser AR+, *Arch Intern Med* 142(3), 601
Somnolence
  (2006): Tariot PN+, *Am J Geriatr Psychiatry* 14(9), 767
Tremor
  (2001): Russell CS+, *Obstet Gynecol* 98(5), 906

HALOTHANE

Trade names: Fluothane; Halothan; Trothane
Indications: Induction and maintenance of general anesthesia
Category: Anesthetic, inhalation
Half-life: N/A
Clinically important, potentially hazardous interactions with: aminophylline, atracurium, cisatracurium, doxacurium, epinephrine, non-depolarizing muscle relaxants, pancuronium, rapacuronium, rifampin, theophylline, vecuronium, xanthines

Reactions

Skin
Acne
  (1987): Guldager H, *Lancet* 1, 1211

Angioedema
  (1988): Slegers-Karsmakers S+, *Anesthesia* 43, 506
Exanthems
  (1988): Slegers-Karsmakers S+, *Anesthesia* 43, 506
Sensitivity (sic)
Urticaria

Hair
Hair – alopecia
  (1990): Gollnick H+, *Z Haut* (German) 65, 1128

Other
Rhabdomyolysis
  (1993): Blank JW+, *J Clin Anesth* 5(1), 69
  (1987): Rubiano R+, *Anesthesiology* 67(5), 856
  (1985): Sodano R+, *Minerva Anestesiol* 51(3), 109

HAWTHORN (FRUIT, LEAF, FLOWER EXTRACT)

Scientific names: *Crataegus laevigata; Crataegus monogyna; Crataegus oxyacantha; Crataegus pentagyna*
Family: Rosaceae
Trade and other common names: Arterio-K; Aubepine; Basticrat; Born; Cardiplant; Cordapur; Coronal; Cratamed; Harthorne; Haw; HeartCare (Nature's Way); Hedgethorne; Maythorn; Nan Shanzha; Naranocor; Regulacor; Shanzha; Thorn Plum; Whitethorn
Category: Cardio-stimulant
Purported indications and other uses: Amenorrhea, arrhythmias, atherosclerosis, diuretic, hyperlipidemia, hypertension, hypotension, sedative, appetite stimulant, arthritis, enteritis, indigestion, sore throats. **Topical:** boils, sores and ulcers
Half-life: N/A
Clinically important, potentially hazardous interactions with: digoxin, vasodilators

Note: The American Herbal Products Association (AHPA) gives hawthorn a class 1 safety rating, indicating that it is very safe. However, hawthorn should be used with caution in patients with heart disease

Reactions

Skin
Allergic reactions (sic)
Diaphoresis
  (2002): Rigelsky JM+, *Am J Health Syst Pharm* 59(5), 417
Rash (sic) (hands)
  (2002): Rigelsky JM+, *Am J Health Syst Pharm* 59(5), 417
  (1996): Newall CA+, *A Guide For Healthcare Professionals* London UK, Pharmaceutical Press
Toxicoderma
  (1984): Rogov VD, *Vestn Dermatol Venerol* 7, 46

Other
Hypersensitivity
  (1984): Steinman HK+, *Contact Dermatitis* 11(5), 321
Vertigo
  (2003): Pittler MH+, *Am J Med* 114(8), 665
  (2002): Rigelsky JM+, *Am J Health Syst Pharm* 59(5), 417

HEMOPHILUS B VACCINE

Trade names: ActHIB (Sanofi-Aventis); Comvax (Merck);
HibTITER (Lederle); OmniHIB (GSK); PedivaxHIB (Merck);
ProHIBIT (Connaught)
Indications: Haemophilus b immunization
Category: Vaccine
Half-life: N/A
**Clinically important, potentially hazardous interactions
with:** azathioprine, basiliximab, corticosteroids, cyclosporine,
daclizumab, glatiramer, mycophenolate, sirolimus, tacrolimus

Reactions

Skin
Angioedema
Erythema
  (1993): de Montalembert M+, *Arch Fr Pediatr* 50(10), 863
  (1991): *MMWR Recomm Rep* 40(RR), 1
Erythema multiforme
Facial edema
Pigmentation
Pruritus
Rash (sic)
Urticaria

Other
Anaphylactoid reactions/Anaphylaxis
Asthenia
Fever
  (1991): *MMWR Recomm Rep* 40(RR), 1
Hypersensitivity
Injection-site edema
  (1991): *MMWR Recomm Rep* 40(RR), 1
Injection-site induration
Injection-site pain
  (1993): de Montalembert M+, *Arch Fr Pediatr* 50(10), 863
Seizures

HENNA

Scientific names: *Lawsonia alba; Lawsonia inermis*
Family: Lythraceae
Trade and other common names: Alcanna; Egyptian Privet;
Hinai; Hinna; Inai; Jamaica Kina; Lawsone (2-hydroxy-
1:4naphthaquione); Mehandi; Mehndi
Category: Anti-inflammatory
Purported indications and other uses: Analgesic, antipyretic,
seborrheic dermatitis, fungal infections, gastrointestinal ulcers,
sunscreen, dandruff, scabies, headache, jaundice, decorative
tattoos, Used in cosmetics, body paint, hair dyes, hair care
products
Half-life: N/A

Note: Black Henna is Henna plus paraphenylenediamine (PPD). PPD
is added to henna to make it stain black. PPD is a transdermal toxin
and may be used alone as hair dye or to stain skin black. Other
products called 'black henna' may have indigo or food dyes added,
and are generally not harmful to the skin

Reactions

Skin
Adverse effects (sic)

  (2003): De Souza B+, *Plast Reconstr Surg* 111(7), 2487
  (2003): Wolf R+, *Dermatol Online J* 9(1), 3
Allergic reactions (sic)
  (2000): US Food and Drug Administration, Office of Cosmetics
    and Colors Fact Sheet
Angioedema
  (2006): Gulen F+, *Minerva Pediatr* 58(6), 583
Bullous dermatitis
Burning
Dermatitis
  (2007): Reyes Balaguer J+, *Med Clin* (Barc) 128(8), 318
  (2003): Leggiadro RJ+, *J Pediatr* 142(5), 586
  (2003): Wolf R+, *Dermatol Online J* 9(1), 3
  (2002): Marcoux D+, *Pediatr Dermatol* 19(6), 498
  (2002): Neri I+, *Pediatr Dermatol* 19(6), 503
  (2002): Pegas JR+, *J Investig Allergol Clin Immunol* 12(1), 62
  (2002): Temesvari E+, *Contact Dermatitis* 47(4), 240
  (2002): van Zuuren+, *Ned Tijdschr Geneeskd* 146(28), 1332
  (2001): Di Lando A+, *Am J Contact Dermat* 12(3), 186
  (2001): Kulkarni PD+, *Cutis* 68(3):187, 229 (+PPD)
  (2001): Lauchl S+, *Swiss Med Wkly* 131, 199 (+PPD)
  (2001): Onder M+, *Int J Dermatol* 40(9), 577 (+PPD)
  (2001): Oztass MO+, *J Eur Acad Dermatol Venereol* 15(1), 91
  (2001): Thami GP+, *Allergy* 56(10), 1013
  (2000): Le Coz CJ+, *Arch Dermatol* 136(12), 1515 (+PPD)
  (2000): Lyon MJ+, *Arch Dermatol* 136(1), 124
  (2000): Nikkels AF+, *J Eur Acad Dermatol Venereol* 15(2), 140
    (+PPD)
  (2000): Raison-Peyron N+, *Ann Dermatol Venereol* 127(12), 1083
    (+PPD)
  (2000): Sidbury R+, *Am J Contact Dermat* 11(3), 182 (+PPD)
  (2000): Tosti A+, *Contact Dermatitis* 42(6), 356
  (1999): Gallo R+, *Contact Dermatitis* 40(1), 57
  (1999): Lestringant GG+, *Br J Dermatol* 141(3), 598
  (1999): Lewin PK, *CMAJ* 160(3), 310
  (1998): Nigam PK+, *Contact Dermatitis* 18(1), 55
  (1998): Wakelin SH+, *Contact Dermatitis* 39(2), 92 (+PPD)
  (1997): Downs AMR+, *Br Med J* 315, 1772 (+PPD)
  (1997): Etienne A+, *Contact Dermatitis* 37(4), 183
  (1997): Garcia Ortiz JC+, *Int Arch Allergy Immunol* 114(3), 298
  (1996): al-Sheik OA+, *Int J Dermatol* 35(7), 493
  (1992): Wantke F+, *Contact Dermatitis* 27(5), 346 (from Azo
    dyes)
  (1986): Gupta BN+, *Contact Dermatitis* 15(5), 303
  (1980): Pasricha JS+, *Contact Dermatitis* 6(4), 288
Eczema
  (2002): Suarez Fernandez R+, *Allergol Immunopathol* (Madr)
    30(5), 292
Edema
  (2002): Marcoux D+, *Pediatr Dermatol* 19(6), 498
  (2001): Lauchl S+, *Swiss Med Wkly* 131, 199 (+PPD)
  (2001): Wohrl S+, *Eur Acad Dermatol Venereol* 15(5), 470
    (+PPD)
Erythema
  (2002): Marcoux D+, *Pediatr Dermatol* 19(6), 498
  (2002): Schultz E+, *Int J Dermatol* 41(5), 301
  (2001): Lauchl S+, *Swiss Med Wkly* 131, 199 (+PPD)
Erythema multiforme
  (2001): Jappe U+, *Contact Dermatitis* 45(4), 249 (+PPD)
Keloid
  (1999): Lewkin PK, *CMAJ* 160(3), 310
Leukoderma
  (2007): Valsecchi R+, *Contact Dermatitis* 56(2), 108
Lichenoid eruption
  (2002): Chung WH+, *Arch Dermatol* 138(1), 88 (+PPD)
  (2002): Ferrer P+, *Cosmetic Dermatology* 15, 11
  (2002): Schultz E+, *Int J Dermatol* 41(5), 301
  (2000): Rubegni P+, *Contact Dermatitis* 42(2), 117
Photosensitivity

Pigmentation
(2002): Marcoux D+, *Pediatr Dermatol* 19(6), 498
(2002): van Zuuren+, *Ned Tijdschr Geneeskd* 146(28), 1332
(2001): Wohrl S+, *J Eur Acad Dermatol Venereol* 15(5), 470
(+PPD)
Pruritus
(2002): Suarez Fernandez+, *Allergol Immunopathol* (Madr)
30(5), 292
(2001): Lauchl S+, *Swiss Med Wkly* 131, 199 (+PPD)
(2000): Sidbury R+, *Am J Contact Dermat* 11(3), 182 (+PPD)
Psoriasis
(1991): El-Gammal SY, *Bull Indian Inst Hist Med Hyderabad*
121(2), 125
Rash (sic)
Sensitivity
(2004): Lim SP+, *Br J Dermatol* 151(6), 1271 (+PPD)
Urticaria
(2006): Gulen F+, *Minerva Pediatr* 58(6), 583
(1997): Downs AMR+, *Br Med J* 315, 1722
(1996): Majoie IM+, *Am J Contact Dermat* 7(1), 38

Other
Death
(2001): Devecioglu C+, *Turk J Pediatr* 43(1), 65
(2001): Raupp P+, *Arch Dis Child* 85(5), 411
(1992): Sir Hashim M+, *Ann Trop Paediatr* 12(1), 3 (+PDD)
Hypersensitivity
(2001): Bolhaar ST+, *Allergy* 56(3), 248
(2001): Kulkarni PD+, *Cutis* 68(3), 187 (+PPD)
(2000): Lyon MJ+, *Arch Dermatol* 136(1), 124
(2000): Nikkels AF+, *J Eur Acad Dermatol Venereol* 15(2), 140
(+PPD)
(1996): Abdulla KA+, *Lancet* 348(9028), 658 (+PPD)
(1996): Majoie IM+, *Am J Contact Dermat* 7(1), 38
(1996): Ozsoylu S, *Lancet* 348(9035), 1173
(1982): Starr JC+, *Ann Allergy* 48(2), 98
Side effects (sic)
(2000): Ernst E, *Br J Dermatol* 143(5), 923

HEPARIN

Trade names: Calcilean; Calciparin; Caprin; Hep-Flush (Wyeth);
Hepalean; Heparin-Leo; Heparine; Liquemin; Uniparin
Indications: Venous thrombosis, pulmonary embolism
Category: Anticoagulant; Heparinoid
Half-life: 1.5 hours
**Clinically important, potentially hazardous interactions
with:** acenocoumarol, aspirin, bivalirudin, butabarbital,
capsicum, ceftobiprole, danaparoid, desvenlafaxine, **dong quai**,
ginger, **horse chestnut (bark, flower, leaf, seed)**, palifermin,
red clover, salicylates, tirofiban

Reactions

Skin
Allergic reactions (sic) (1–10%)
(2004): Tiu A+, *N Z Med J* 117(1204), U1126
(1997): Hermes B+, *Acta Derm Venereol* 77, 35
Angioedema (<1%)
Baboon syndrome
(1993): Herfs H+, *Hautarzt* (German) 44, 466
Burning (soles)
(1992): Breathnach SM+, *Adverse Drug Reactions and the Skin*
Blackwell,Oxford, 249 (passim)
Dermatitis
(1996): Boehncke WH+, *Contact Dermatitis* 35, 73

(1996): Koch P+, *Contact Dermatitis* 34, 1256
(1995): Krasovec M+, *Contact Dermatitis* 32, 135
(1992): Valsecchi R+, *Contact Dermatitis* 26, 129
(1988): Young E, *Contact Dermatitis* 19, 152
Erythema
(2005): Warkentin TE+, *Chest* 127(5), 1857 (4 cases)
Erythema nodosum
Exanthems
(1996): Warkentin TE, *Br J Haematol* 92, 494
(1994): Greiner D+, *Hautarzt* (German) 45, 569
Fixed eruption
(1995): Mohammed KN, *Dermatology* 190, 91
Hemorrhage
(1992): Breathnach SM+, *Adverse Drug Reactions and the Skin*
Blackwell, Oxford, 249 (passim)
(1986): Levine M+, *Semin Thromb Hemost* 12, 39
Livedo reticularis
(2005): Gibbs MB+, *J Am Acad Dermatol* 52(6), 1009
(1993): Gross AS+, *Int J Dermatol* 32, 276
Necrosis
(2005): Warkentin TE+, *Chest* 127(5), 1857 (4 cases)
(2004): Housholder-Hughes SD, *Am J Nurs* 104(10), 16
(2003): Takwale A+, *Br J Dermatol* 148(6), 1292
(2002): Denoel C+, *Rev Med Liege* 57(8), 502
(2002): Wong G+, *World Congress Dermatol* Poster, 0133
(2001): Andolfatto S+, *Ann Biol Clin* (Paris) 59(5), 651 (2 cases)
(2001): Denton MD+, *Am J Nephrol* 21(4), 289
(1997): Carter RL, *N Engl J Med* 336, 589
(1997): Kumar PD, *N Engl J Med* 336, 588
(1997): Libow LF+, *Cutis* 59, 242
(1997): McCloskey RV, *N Engl J Med* 336, 588
(1997): Schechter FG, *N Engl J Med* 336, 589
(1996): Christiaens GC+, *N Engl J Med* 335, 715
(1996): Whitmore SE+, *Arch Dermatol* 132, 341
(1995): Balestra B, *Schweiz Med Wochenschr* (German) 125, 361
(1994): Griffin JP, *Adverse Drug React Toxicol Rev* 13, 157
(1994): Leblanc M+, *Nephron* 68, 133
(1994): Peluso AM+, *Eur J Dermatol* 4, 127
(1994): Yoon TY+, *Ann Dermatol* 6, 74
(1993): Humphries JE, *Acta Haematol* 90, 52
(1993): Warkentin TE+, *Am J Med* 95, 662
(1993): Yates P+, *Clin Exp Dermatol* 18, 138
(1992): Calzavara-Pinton PG+, *EJD* 2, 171
(1992): Soundararajan R+, *Am J Med* 93, 467
(1992): Thomas D+, *Chest* 102, 1578
(1991): Humphries JE+, *Am J Kidney Dis* 17, 233
(1991): Ritchie AJ+, *Ulster Med J* 60, 248
(1990): Adcock DM+, *Semin Thromb Hemost* 16, 283
(1990): Bircher AJ+, *Br J Dermatol* 123, 507 (passim)
(1990): Fowlie J+, *Postgrad Med J* 66, 573
(1989): Armengol R+, *Med Clin* (Barc) (Spanish) 93, 699
(1989): Diem E, *Hautarzt* (German) 40, 239
(1989): Rongioletti F+, *Dermatologica* 178, 47
(1989): Vinti H+, *Presse Med* (French) 18, 128
(1988): Cohen GR+, *Obstet Gynecol* 73, 498
(1988): Hartman AR+, *J Vasc Surg* 7, 781
(1987): Alegre A+, *Med Clin* (Barc) (Spanish) 88, 170
(1987): Jones BF+, *Australas J Dermatol* 28, 117
(1986): Lim KB+, *Singapore Med J* 27, 356
(1985): Barthelemy H+, *Ann Dermatol Venereol* (French)
112, 245
(1985): Tuneu A+, *J Am Acad Dermatol* 12, 1072
(1984): Hasegawa GR, *Drug Intell Clin Pharm* 18, 313
(1984): Mathieu A+, *Ann Dermatol Venereol* (French) 111, 733
(1984): Monreal M+, *Lancet* 2, 820
(1984): Nodel'son SE+, *Ter Arkh* (Russian) 56, 118
(1984): Ulrick PJ+, *Med J Aust* 140, 287
(1983): Jehn U+, *Dtsch Med Wochenschr* (German) 108, 1148
(1983): Levine LE+, *Arch Dermatol* 119, 400
(1982): Isaacs P+, *Br Med J Clin Res Ed* 284, 201

(1982): No Author, *Am J Hosp Pharm* 39, 412
(1982): Shelley WB+, *J Am Acad Dermatol* 7, 674
(1981): Berkessy S+, *Orv Hetil* (Hungarian) 122, 3075
(1981): Jackson AM+, *Br Med J Clin Res Ed* 283, 1087
(1981): Kelly RA+, *JAMA* 246, 1582
(1980): Hall JC+, *JAMA* 244, 1831

Peripheral edema
(1993): Phillips JK+, *Br J Haematol* 84, 349

Petechiae
(2006): Perrinaud A+, *J Am Acad Dermatol* 54(2 Suppl), S5

Pruritus (<1%)

Purpura (>10%)

Rash (sic)

Scleroderma
(1985): Barthelemy H+, *Ann Dermatol Venereol* (French)
112, 245

Toxic dermatitis (sic)
(1996): Gallais V+, *Presse Med* (French) 25, 1040

Toxic epidermal necrolysis
(1991): Lemziakov TG+, *Vrach Delo* (Ukrainian) November, 113
(1985): Leung A, *JAMA* 253, 201

Ulcerations
(2001): Denton MD+, *Am J Nephrol* 21(4), 289

Urticaria (<1%)
(1992): Breathnach SM+, *Adverse Drug Reactions and the Skin*
Blackwell, Oxford, 249 (passim)
(1990): Bircher AJ+, *Br J Dermatol* 123, 507 (passim)

Vasculitis
(1989): Guillet G+, *J Am Acad Dermatol* 20, 1130
(1989): Korstanje MJ+, *Contact Dermatitis* 20, 283
(1982): Kearsley JH+, *Aust N Z J Med* 12, 288

Mucosal/ENT

Gingivitis (>10%)

Hair

Hair – alopecia
(1980): Jaques LB, *Pharmacol Rev* 31, 99

Nails

Nails – discoloration

Other

Anaphylactoid reactions/Anaphylaxis
(2005): Warkentin TE+, *Chest* 127(5), 1857
(2004): Berkun Y+, *Clin Exp Allergy* 2004 Dec;34(12), 1916
(1992): Breathnach SM+, *Adverse Drug Reactions and the Skin*
Blackwell, Oxford, 249 (passim)
(1990): Bircher AJ+, *Br J Dermatol* 123, 507 (passim)

Chills

Headache

Hypersensitivity
(2005): Gaigl Z+, *Br J Haematol* 128(3), 389 (28 cases)
(2004): Liew G+, *ANZ J Surg* 74(11), 1020
(2002): Mora A+, *Contact Dermatitis* 47(3), 177
(2002): Nicolie B+, *Allerg Immunol* (Paris) 34(2), 47
(2000): Koch P+, *J Am Acad Dermatol* 42, 612
(1995): Sanders MN+, *Int J Dermatol* 34, 443
(1994): Patriarca G+, *Allergy* 49, 292
(1993): Dupin N+, *Ann Dermatol Venereol* (French) 120, 845
(1993): O'Donnell BF+, *Br J Dermatol* 129, 634
(1992): de Kort WJ+, *Ned Tijdschr Geneeskd* (Dutch) 136, 2379
(1992): Manoharan A, *Eur J Haematol* 48, 234
(1991): Rivers JK+, *Aust N Z J Surg* 61, 865
(1989): Korstanje MJ+, *Contact Dermatitis* 20, 383
(1989): Patrizi A+, *Contact Dermatitis* 20, 309

Injection-site eczematous eruption (<1%)
(2000): Koch P+, *J Am Acad Dermatol* 42, 612
(1995): Mathelier-Fusade P+, *Presse Med* (French) 24, 323
(1993): Phillips JK+, *Br J Haematol* 84, 349 (erythema)

(1990): Bircher AJ+, *Br J Dermatol* 123, 507

Injection-site hematoma

Injection-site induration
(1993): Phillips JK+, *Br J Haematol* 84, 349
(1989): Guillet G+, *J Am Acad Dermatol* 20, 1130
(1989): Klein GF+, *J Am Acad Dermatol* 21, 703
(1987): Mayou SC+, *Br J Dermatol* 117, 664

Injection-site necrosis (<1%)
(1995): Mar AW+, *Australas J Dermatol* 36, 201
(1988): Cohen GR+, *Obstet and Gyn* 72, 498
(1984): Hasegawa GR, *Drug Intell Clin Pharm* 18, 313
(1980): Hall JC+, *JAMA* 244, 1831

Injection-site nodules
(2002): Funt SA+, *J Comput Assist Tomogr* 26(4), 520

Injection-site pain
(2001): Chan H, *J Adv Nurs* 35(6), 882

Injection-site plaques
(2000): Koch P+, *J Am Acad Dermatol* 42, 612
(1990): Bircher AJ+, *Br J Dermatol* 123, 507

Injection-site purpura
(2001): Chan H, *J Adv Nurs* 35(6), 882

Injection-site urticaria
(1995): Mathelier-Fusade P+, *Presse Med* (French) 24, 323

HEPATITIS A VACCINE

Trade names: Avaxim (Sanofi-Aventis); Epaxal; Havrix (GSK);
Vaqta (Merck)
Indications: Hepatitis A immunization
Category: Vaccine
Half-life: 2 years
**Clinically important, potentially hazardous interactions
with:** none

Reactions

Skin

Pruritus

Rash (sic)

Vitiligo
(2005): Maubec E+, *J Am Acad Dermatol* 52(4), 623 (1 case)

Other

Abdominal pain

Asthenia

Fever
(2006): Bhave S+, *Indian Pediatr* 43(11), 983
(2001): Lopez EL+, *Pediatr Infect Dis J* 20(1), 48

Headache

Injection-site erythema
(2000): Lee CY+, *Southeast Asian J Trop Med Public Health*
31(1), 29

Injection-site pain
(2005): Bovier PA+, *Vaccine* 23(19), 2424
(2001): Abarca K+, *Arch Med Res* 32(5), 468
(2000): Bryan JP+, *Vaccine* 19(7-8), 743
(2000): Lee CY+, *Southeast Asian J Trop Med Public Health*
31(1), 29

Injection-site reactions
(2003): Ferreira CT+, *J Pediatr Gastroenterol Nutr* 37(3), 258
(2001): Clarke P+, *Vaccine* 19(31), 4429
(2001): Connor BA+, *Clin Infect Dis* 32(3), 396
(2001): Lopez EL+, *Pediatr Infect Dis J* 20(1), 48

Myalgia/Myositis/Myopathy/Myotoxicity
(2005): Maubec E+, *J Am Acad* 52(4), 623 (2 cases)

Neurotoxicity

(2003): George DL+, *Am J Med Dermatol* 115(7), 587
Pseudolymphoma
  (2005): Maubec E+, *J Am Acad Dermatol* 52(4), 623

HEPATITIS B VACCINE

Trade names: Comvax (Merck); Engerix B (GSK); Pediatrix (GSK); Recombivax HB (Merck); Twinrix (GSK)
Other common trade name: *Heptavax-B*
Indications: For immunization of infection caused by all known subtypes of hepatitis B virus
Category: Vaccine
Half-life: N/A

Reactions

Skin
Allergic granulomatous angiitis (Churg–Strauss syndrome)
  (1998): Ajithkumar K+, *Clin Exp Dermatol* 23(5), 222 (necrobiotic)
  (1998): Vanoli M+, *Ann Rheum Dis* 57(4), 256
Anetoderma
  (1997): Daoud MS+, *J Am Acad Dermatol* 36 (5 Pt 1), 779
Angioedema
  (1998): Barbaud A+, *Br J Dermatol* 139(5), 925
Bullous lichen planus
  (2005): Miteva L, *Int J Dermatol* 44(2), 142
Bullous pemphigoid
  (2002): Erbagci Z, *J Dermatol* 29(12), 781
  (2002): Erbagci Z, *World Congress Dermatol* Poster 0315
Dermatomyositis
  (1998): Fernandez-Funez A+, *Med Clin* (Barc) 111(17), 675
Diaphoresis
Eczema
  (1999): Mc Kenna KE, *Contact Dermatitis* 40(3), 158
Erythema
Erythema multiforme
  (2000): Loche F+, *Clin Exp Dermatol* 25(2), 167
  (1994): Di Lernia+, *Pediatr Dermatol* 11(4), 363
Erythema nodosum
  (1993): Castresana-Isla CJ+, *J Rheumatol* 20(8), 1417
  (1990): Rogerson SJ+, *BMJ* 301, 345
  (1989): Goolsby PL, *N Engl J Med* 321, 1198
Gianotti–Crosti syndrome
  (2007): Karakas M+, *J Dermatol* 34(2), 117
  (2001): Tay YK, *Pediatr Dermatol* 18(3), 262
Granuloma annulare
  (2004): Criado PR+, *J Eur Acad Dermatol Venereol* 18(5), 603
  (1998): Wolf F+, *Eur J Dermatol* 8(6), 435 (generalized)
Herpes zoster
Lichen nitidus
  (2004): Fetil E+, *Int J Dermatol* 43(12), 956
Lichen planus
  (2004): Calista D+, *Int J Dermatol* 43(8), 562
  (2004): Criado PR+, *J Eur Acad Dermatol Venereol* 18(5), 603
  (2002): Calista D+, *World Congress Dermatol* Poster, 0090
  (2002): Schuh T+, *Hautarzt* 53(10), 650
  (2001): Al-Khenaizan S, *J Am Acad Dermatol* 45(4), 614
  (2001): Aron-Moar A+, *Lupus* 10(3), 237
  (2000): Agrawal S+, *J Dermatol* 27(9), 618
  (1999): Rebora A+, *Dermatology* 198(1), 1
  (1999): Schupp P+, *Int J Dermatol* 38(10), 799
  (1998): Ferrando MN+, *Br J Dermatol* 139(2), 350
  (1998): Merigou D+, *Ann Dermatol Venereol* 125(6-7), 399
  (1997): Gisserot O+, *Presse Med* 26(16), 760
  (1995): Lefort A+, *Ann Dermatol Venereol* 122(10), 701

  (1994): Aubin F+, *Arch Dermatol* 130(10), 1329
  (1993): Trevisan G+, *Acta Derm Venereol* 73(1), 73
  (1990): Ciaccio M+, *Br J Dermatol* 122, 424
Lichenoid eruption
  (2004): Fetil E+, *Int J Dermatol* 43(12), 956
  (2001): Usman A+, *Pediatr Dermatol* 18(2), 123
  (1997): Saywell CA+, *Australas J Dermatol* 38(3), 152
Lupus erythematosus
  (2005): Geier DA+, *Autoimmunity* 38(4), 295
  (2000): Maillefert JF+, *Arthritis Rheum* 43(2), 468
  (1999): Senecal JL+, *Arthritis Rheum* 42(6), 1307
  (1998): Grotto I+, *Vaccine* 16(4), 329
  (1996): Grezard P+, *Ann Dermatol Venereol* 123(10), 657
  (1996): Guiserix J, *Nephron* 74(2), 441
  (1994): Mamoux V+, *Arch Pediatr* 1(3), 307
  (1992): Tudela P+, *Nephron* 62(2), 236
Morphea
  (2000): Schmutz JL+, *Presse Med* 29(19), 1046
Petechiae
Purpura
  (2004): Nuevo H+, *Pediatr Infect Dis J* 23(2), 183
  (2002): Chave TA+, *World Congress Dermatol* Poster, 0093
  (2001): Conesa V+, *Haematologica* 86(3), E09
  (1999): Lliminana C+, *Med Clin* (Barc) 113(1), 39
  (1999): Muller A+, *Eur J Pediatr* 158 Suppl 3, S209
  (1998): Ronchi F+, *Arch Dis Child* 78(3), 273 (3 cases)
  (1994): Poullin P+, *Lancet* 344(8932), 1293
Rash (sic)
Raynaud's phenomenon
  (1990): Cockwell P+, *BMJ* 301, 1281
Sclerotic plaques
  (1998): Gout O+, *Rev Neurol* (Paris) 154(3), 205
Stevens–Johnson syndrome
Urticaria
  (2000): Barbaud A+, *Ann Dermatol Venereol* 127(6-7), 662
  (1998): Barbaud A+, *Br J Dermatol* 139(5), 925
  (1998): Grotto I+, *Vaccine* 16(4), 329
Vasculitis
  (2005): Geier DA+, *Autoimmunity* 38(4), 295
  (2001): Saadoun D+, *Rev Med Interne* 22(2), 172
  (1999): Le Hello C, *Pathol Biol* (Paris) 47(3), 252
  (1999): Le Hello+, *J Rheumatol* 26(1), 191 (3 cases)
  (1998): Bui-Quang D+, *Presse Med* 27(26), 1321
  (1998): Grotto I+, *Vaccine* 16(4), 329
  (1998): Masse I+, *Presse Med* 27(20), 965
  (1997): Kerleau JM+, *Rev Interne Med* 18(6), 491 (necrotizing)
  (1993): Allen MB+, *Thorax* 48(5), 580
  (1990): Cockwell P+, *BMJ* 301, 1281

Mucosal/ENT
Aphthous stomatitis
  (1996): Grezard P+, *Ann Dermatol Venereol* 123(10), 657
Oral lichenoid eruption
  (2000): Pemberton MN+, *Oral Surg Oral Med Oral Pathol Oral Radiol Endod* 89(6), 717
Tinnitus
  (2001): DeJonckere PH+, *Int Tinnitus J* 7(1), 59

Hair
Hair – alopecia
  (2005): Geier DA+, *Autoimmunity* 38(4), 295
  (1997): Wise RP+, *JAMA* 278(14), 1176 (46 cases)

Nails
Nails – lichen planus
  (2005): Miteva L, *Int J Dermatol* 44(2), 142

Eyes
Optic neuropathy
  (2005): Geier DA+, *Autoimmunity* 38(4), 295

(2004): Geier MR+, *Clin Exp Rheumatol* 22(6), 749

White dot syndrome
  (1996): Baglivo E+, *Am J Ophthalmol* 122(3), 431

Other

Anaphylactoid reactions/Anaphylaxis
  (2004): *Prescrire Int* 13(74), 218 (rare)
  (2000): *Prescrire Int* 9(46), 59
  (1998): Grotto I+, *Vaccine* 16(4), 329
  (1996): *MMWR Morb Mortal Wkly Rep* 45(RR-12), 1
  (1994): Stratton KR+, *JAMA* 271(20), 1602
Chills
Death
  (1999): Niu MT+, *Pediatr Adolesc Med* 153(12), 1279
Erythromelalgia
  (1999): Rabaud C+, *J Rheumatol* 26(1), 233
Headache
Hypersensitivity
Injection-site ecchymoses
Injection-site edema
  (2005): Chowdhury A+, *World J Gastroenterol* 11(7), 1037
Injection-site erythema
  (2005): Chowdhury A+, *World J Gastroenterol* 11(7), 1037
Injection-site induration
Injection-site nodules
Injection-site pain (22%)
  (2005): Chowdhury A+, *World J Gastroenterol* 11(7), 1037
Injection-site pruritus
Injection-site reactions
  (2005): Saenger R+, *Vaccine* 23(9), 1135 (2.3%)
Myalgia/Myositis/Myopathy/Myotoxicity
  (2004): Geier MR+, *Clin Exp Rheumatol* 22(6), 749
Nephrotoxicity
  (2007): Santoro D+, *Clin Nephrol* 67(1), 61
Pain
  (2003): Jastaniah WA+, *J Pediatr* 143(6), 802
Paresthesias
Polyarteritis nodosa
  (2004): Begier EM+, *J Rheumatol* 31(11), 2181 (9 cases)
  (2003): Bourgeais AM+, *Ann Dermatol Venereol* 130(2), 205
  (2001): Saadoun D+, *Rev Med Interne* 22(2), 172
  (1988): Le Goff P+, *Presse Med* 17, 1763
Polymyositis
  (2001): Saadoun D+, *Rev Med Interne* 22(2), 172
Pseudolymphoma
  (2005): Maubec E+, *J Am Acad Dermatol* 52(4), 623
Serum sickness
  (2002): Arkachaisri T, *J Med Assoc Thai* 85, S607
Sjøgren's (Sicca) syndrome
  (2000): Toussirot E+, *Arthritis Rheum* 43(9), 2139

HEROIN

Trade name: Heroin
Indications: Recreational drug
Category: Opiate agonist
Half-life: N/A

Reactions

Skin

Abscess
  (1990): Rasokat H, *Z Haut* (German) 65, 351
  (1987): Muller F+, *Infection* 15, 201
  (1987): Podzamczer D+, *J Am Acad Dermatol* 16, 386
  (1984): O'Sullivan M+, *Ir Med J* 77, 68

(1980): Espiritu MB+, *Laryngoscope* 90, 1111 (neck)
Acanthosis nigricans
Acne
Angioedema
Bullous impetigo
Burning (24%)
  (2002): Warner-Smith M+, *Addiction* 97(8), 963 (24%)
Cellulitis
  (1988): O'Rourke MG+, *Med J Aust* 148, 54
  (1984): Alguire PC, *Cutis* 34, 93 (necrotizing of the scrotum)
Dermatitis
Ecthyma
  (1990): Rasokat H, *Z Haut* (German) 65, 351
Ecthyma gangrenosum
Edema
  (1990): Rasokat H, *Z Haut* (German) 65, 351
Exanthems
Excoriations
  (1990): Rasokat H, *Z Haut* (German) 65, 351
Fixed eruption
  (1983): Westerhof W+, *Br J Dermatol* 109, 605 (tongue)
Folliculitis (candidal)
  (1987): Cristobal-Rodriguez P+, *Med Cutan Ibero Lat Am* (Spanish) 15, 411
  (1986): Darcis JM+, *Am J Dermatopathol* 8, 501 (with septicemia)
  (1986): Leclerc G+, *Int J Dermatol* 25, 100
  (1985): Calandra T+, *Eur J Clin Microbiol* 4, 340
Glucagonoma syndrome (necrolytic migratory erythema)
  (1994): Bencini PL+, *Dermatology* 189, 72
Kaposi's sarcoma
  (1986): Schofer H+, *Hautarzt* (German) 37, 159
Necrosis
  (2002): Oehler U+, *Pathologe* 23(4), 318
  (1990): Rasokat H, *Z Haut* (German) 65, 351
Necrotizing fasciitis
  (1990): Rasokat H, *Z Haut* (German) 65, 351
Necrotizing vasculitis (tongue)
  (1995): Jurgensen O+, *Schweiz Monatsschr Zahnmed* (German, French) 105, 54
Pemphigus
  (1989): Civatte J, *Dermatol Monatsschr* (German) 175, 1
Pemphigus erythematodes
Pemphigus vegetans
  (1998): Downie JB+, *J Am Acad Dermatol* 39, 872
Perforating collagenosis
  (1989): Bank DE+, *J Am Acad Dermatol* 21, 371
Photosensitivity
Pigmentation
  (1990): Rasokat H, *Z Haut* (German) 65, 351
Pruritus
  (1990): Rasokat H, *Z Haut* (German) 65, 351
Purpura
Pustules
  (1993): Badillet G+, *Ann Dermatol Venereol* (French) 110, 691 (candidal)
  (1992): Gallais V+, *Presse Med* (French) 21, 677 (candidal)
  (1990): Altes J+, *Enferm Infecc Microbiol Clin* (Spanish) 8, 464
  (1985): Cabre L+, *Med Clin* (Barc) (Spanish) 84, 542 (candidal)
  (1984): Pinilla-Moraza J+, *Med Clin* (Barc) (Spanish) 83, 557
Side effects (sic) (85%)
Toxic epidermal necrolysis
  (1990): Llibre LM+, *Med Clin* (Barc) (Spanish) 94, 799
Ulcerations
  (1990): Abidin MR+, *Ann Plast Surg* 24, 268
  (1990): Rasokat H, *Z Haut* (German) 65, 351
Urticaria
  (1990): Shaikh WA, *Allergy* 45, 555

Vasculitis
(1984): Rosman JB+, *Neth J Med* 27, 50
Vesiculation (arms)
(1995): Mielke-Ibrahim R+, *Dtsch Med Wochenschr* (German) 120, 55

Mucosal/ENT
Oral ulceration (tongue)
(1983): Westerhof W+, *Br J Dermatol* 109, 605
Tongue pigmentation (fixed eruption)
(1983): Westerhof W+, *Br J Dermatol* 109, 605

Eyes
Diplopia
(2005): Firth AY, *Addiction* 100(1), 46
Eyelid edema

Other
Anaphylactoid reactions/Anaphylaxis
(2006): Gooch I+, *Resuscitation* 70(3), 470
Candidiasis
(1987): Bielsa I+, *Int J Dermatol* 26, 314 (systemic)
(1987): Puig L+, *Int J Dermatol* 26, 257
(1985): Calandra T+, *Eur J Clin Microbiol* 4, 340 (disseminated)
Death
(2003): Sheedy DL+, *Am J Addict* 12(1), 52
(2002): Darke S+, *Addiction* 97(8), 977
(2002): Davidson PJ+, *Addiction* 97(12), 1511
(1996): Amoiridis G+, *Nervenarzt* 67(12), 1023
Hypersensitivity
(1990): Rasokat H, *Z Haut* (German) 65, 351
Infections (13%)
(2002): Warner-Smith M+, *Addiction* 97(8), 963 (13%)
Injection-site scarring
(1990): Rasokat H, *Z Haut* (German) 65, 351
Injection-site ulceration
(1995): Hatton MQ+, *Clin Oncol R Coll Radiol* 7, 268
(1982): White WB+, *Cutis* 29, 63 (penis)
Myalgia/Myositis/Myopathy/Myotoxicity
(1990): Shoji S, *Nippon* (Rinsho) (Japanese) 48, 1517
Neurotoxicity
(2006): Dabby R+, *J Peripher Nerv Syst* 11(4), 304
Polyarteritis nodosa
(1982): Ojeda E+, *Rev Clin Esp* (Spanish) 167, 275
Rhabdomyolysis
(2006): Gomez M+, *An Sist Sanit Navar* 29(1), 131
(2002): Oehler U+, *Pathologe* 23(4), 318
(2001): Lee BF+, *Clin Nucl Med* 26(4), 289
(2000): Richards JR, *J Emerg Med* 19(1), 51
(1996): Amoiridis G+, *Nervenarzt* 67(12), 1023 (fatal)
(1994): Rasmussen FO+, *Tidsskr Nor Laegeforen* 114(4), 432
(1992): Zele I+, *Minerva Med* 83(12), 847 (30%)
(1991): Nolte KB+, *Am J Forensic Med Pathol* 12(3), 273
(1991): Vitris M+, *Dakar Med* 36(1), 15
(1990): Larpin R+, *Presse Med* 19(30), 1403
(1988): Hecker E+, *Schweiz Med Wochenschr* 118(52), 1982 (5 cases)
(1988): Uzan M+, *Nephrologie* 9(5), 217 (13 cases)
(1981): Palmucci L+, *Ital J Neurol Sci* 2(3), 275
Seizures (2%)
(2002): Warner-Smith M+, *Addiction* 97(8), 963 (2%)
Serum sickness
Sweat gland necrosis
(1986): Rocamora A+, *J Dermatol* 13, 49

HISTRELIN

Trade names: Supprelin (Shire); Vantas (Valera)
Indications: Advanced prostate cancer (palliative treatment), Control of precocious puberty
Category: Gonadotropin-releasing hormone agonist
Half-life: 4 hours
Clinically important, potentially hazardous interactions with: N/A

Reactions

Skin
Acne (3–10%)
Angioedema (1–3%)
Diaphoresis (3–10%)
Edema (2%)
Erythema (1%)
Keratoderma (1–3%)
Pallor (1%)
Pruritus (1–3%)
Purpura (2%)
Rash (sic) (7%)
Urticaria (4%)

Eyes
Photophobia (1–3%)
Visual disturbances (2%)

Other
Abdominal pain (>1%)
Asthenia (>1%)
Chills (>1%)
Cough (3–10%)
Depression (>1%)
Gynecomastia
Headache (>1%)
Hot flashes (2%)
Hypersensitivity
Infections (>1%)
Injection-site edema (45%)
Injection-site erythema (45%)
Injection-site pruritus (45%)
Myalgia/Myositis/Myopathy/Myotoxicity (2–3%)
Pain (>1%)
Paresthesias (2–3%)
Seizures (2%)
Tremor (>1%)
Upper respiratory infection (3–10%)
Vertigo

HOPS

Scientific name: *Humulus lupulus*
Family: Cannabaceae
Trade and other common names: Hop Strobile;
Hopfenzapfen; Houblon
Category: Cannabinoid; Phytoestrogen; Sedative
Purported indications and other uses: Insomnia, anxiety,
diuretic, appetite stimulant. Flavoring in foods and beverages
Half-life: N/A

Reactions

Skin
    Urticaria
      (2002): Estrada JL+, *Contact Dermatitis* 46(2), 127
      (2002): Pradalier A+, *Allerg Immunol (Paris)* 34(9), 330

Other
    Fever
      (2002): Pradalier A+, *Allerg Immunol (Paris)* 34(9), 330

HORSE CHESTNUT (BARK, FLOWER, LEAF, SEED)

Scientific name: *Aesculus hippocastanum*
Family: Hippocastanaceae
Trade and other common names: Buckeye; Hippocastani;
Marron Europeen; Venostat; Venostatin Retard
Category: Diuretic
Purported indications and other uses: Oral: malaria,
dysentery, tinnitus, pancreatitis, cough, arthritis, rheumatism,
chronic venous insufficiency. **Topical:** lupus, skin ulcers eczema,
phlebitis, varicose veins, hemorrhoids, rectal problems
Half-life: N/A
**Clinically important, potentially hazardous interactions
with:** heparin, NSAIDs, ticlopidine, warfarin

Reactions

Skin
    Adverse effects (sic) (mild)
      (2002): Pittler MH+, *Cochrane Database Syst Rev* (1), CD003230
    Dermatitis (flower)
      (1980): Comaish JS+, *Contact Dermatitis* 6(2), 150
    Purpura
      (1998): Brinker F, *Herb Contraindications & Interactions* Eclectic
        Medical Publications (2nd Ed)

Other
    Anaphylactoid reactions/Anaphylaxis (seed)
      (1998): Gruenwald J+, *PDR for Herbal Medicines. 1st ed*
        Montvale, NJ: Medical Economics Company, Inc
    Depression (seed)

HORSETAIL

Scientific names: *Equisetum arvense; Equisetum myriochaetum;
Equisetum ramosissimum; Equisetum telmateia*
Family: Equisetaceae
Trade and other common names: Bottle Brush; Cavalinha;
Dutch Rush; Horse Herb; Mepentol; Paddock-Pipes;
Pewterwort; Prele; Scouring Rush; Shave Grass; Toadpipe
Category: Anti-inflammatory; Antioxidant; Diuretic
Purported indications and other uses: Oral: Alopecia,
diabetes, hepatitis, bacterial infections, osteoarthritis, pressure
ulcers, urinary tract infections. **Topical:** burns
Half-life: N/A
**Clinically important, potentially hazardous interactions
with:** digoxin, diuretics, nicotine

Reactions

Skin
    Rash (sic)
    Seborrheic dermatitis
      (1985): Sudan BJ, *Contact Dermatitis* 13(3), 201

Other
    Anaphylactoid reactions/Anaphylaxis
      (2004): Agustin-Ubide MP+, *Allergy* 59(7), 786

HUMAN PAPILLOMAVIRUS VACCINE

Trade name: Gardasil (Merck)
Indications: For prevention of HPV genital warts, cervical
cancers and vulvar dysplasias
Category: Vaccine
Half-life: N/A
**Clinically important, potentially hazardous interactions
with:** N/A

Note: Against Types 6, 11, 16 and 18 Human Papillomavirus

Reactions

Other
    Fever (10.3%)
    Injection-site edema (25.4%)
    Injection-site erythema (24.6%)
    Injection-site pain (83.9%)
    Injection-site pruritus (3.1%)
    Injection-site reactions
      (2004): Fife KH+, *Vaccine* 22(21–2), 2943

HYALURONIC ACID

Synonyms: Hyaluronidase; Hyaluronan; Hyaluran; Hyaluronate sodium

Trade names: Adant; Aquamid; ARTZ; BioHy; DermaDeep; DermaLive; Hyalgan; Hylaform; Hylan G-F 20 (Synvisc); Juvederm; Orthovisc; Perlane (Q-Med AB); Restylane Fine Lines (Medicis); Supartz

Indications: Oral: joint disorders. **Injection:** adjunct in eye surgery, viscosupplementation in orthopedics, cosmetic surgery. **Topical:** wounds, burns, skin ulcers, stomatitis

Category: Food supplement; Glycoaminoglycan

Half-life: 2.5–5.5 minutes

Clinically important, potentially hazardous interactions with: NSAIDs, oral anticoagulants

Note: Most reported reactions relate to orthopedic use

Reactions

Skin

Acne (0.1–29%)
(2002): Friedman PM+, *Dermatol Surg* 28(6), 491 (0.15%)

Adverse effects (sic)
(2003): Tomas Gil+, *Arthritis Rheum* 48(3), 866
(2002): Leopold SS+, *J Bone Joint Surg Am* 84-A(9), 1619 (2–21%)
(2001): Evanich JD+, *Clin Orthop* 390, 173 (15%)
(2000): Allen E+, *J Rheumatol* 27(6), 1572
(2000): Kroesen S+, *Clin Rheumatol* 19(2), 147 (2 cases)
(2000): Shafir R+, *Plast Reconstr Surg* 106(5), 1215
(2000): Wen DY, *Am Fam Physician* 62(3), 565–70, 572 (rare)
(1997): Kirwan JR+, *Baillieres Clin Rheumatol* 11(4), 769 (%)
(1997): McEwan LE+, *Australas J Dermatol* 38(4), 187 (29%) (with diclofenac)

Allergic granulomatous angiitis (Churg–Strauss syndrome)
(2007): Bardazzi F+, *J Dermatolog Treat* 18(1), 59
(2006): Ghislanzoni M+, *Br J Dermatol* 154(4), 755
(2006): Vargas-Machuca I+, *Am J Dermatopathol* 28(2), 173
(2004): Lombardi T+, *J Oral Pathol Med* 33(2), 115
(2003): Fernandez-Acenero MJ+, *Dermatol Surg* 29(12), 1225
(2003): Honig JF+, *J Craniofac Surg* 14(2), 197
(2003): Marino AA+, *J Bone Joint Surg Am* 85-A(10), 2051
(2003): Rongioletti F+, *Arch Dermatol* 139(6), 815
(2003): Zardawi IM, *J Bone Joint Surg Am* 85-A(12), 2484
(2002): Friedman PM+, *Dermatol Surg* 28(6), 491 (rare)
(2001): Zardawi IM+, *Pathology* 33(4), 519
(2000): Raulin C+, *Contact Dermatitis* 43(3), 178

Angioedema
(2005): Leonhardt JM+, *Dermatol Surg* 31(5), 577

Dermatitis (24%)
(1997): Rivers JK+, *Arch Dermatol* 133(10), 1239 (24%) (with diclofenac)

Erythema multiforme
(2007): Calvo M+, *J Investig Allergol Clin Immunol* 17(2), 127
(2003): Young J, *J Dermatolog Treat* 14(3), 189

Herpes simplex

Inflammation
(2007): Bisaccia E+, *Cutis* 79(5), 388
(2005): Christensen L+, *Aesthetic Plast Surg* 29(1), 34
(2005): Soparkar CN+, *Ophthal Plast Reconstr Surg* 21(2), 151
(2003): Hamburger MI+, *Semin Arthritis Rheum* 32(5), 296
(2001): Filion MC+, *J Pharm Pharmacol* 53(4), 555
(2001): Martens PB, *Arthritis Rheum* 44(4), 978

Irritation
(1999): Peters DC+, *Drugs Aging* 14(4), 313 (with diclofenac)

Necrosis

(2007): Hirsch RJ+, *J Drugs Dermatol* 6(3), 325

Sarcoidosis
(2005): Dal Sacco D+, *Int J Dermatol* 44(5), 411

Mucosal/ENT

Sinusitis

Other

Anaphylactoid reactions/Anaphylaxis
(2003): Hamburger MI+, *Semin Arthritis Rheum* 32(5), 296 (rare)

Depression

Headache

Hypersensitivity
(2006): Matarasso SL+, *J Am Acad Dermatol* 55(1), 128
(2006): Patel VJ+, *Plast Reconstr Surg* 117(6), 92e
(2002): Friedman PM+, *Dermatol Surg* 28(6), 491 (rare)

Infections
(2002): Friedman PM+, *Dermatol Surg* 28(6), 491 (rare)
(2000): Adams ME+, *Drug Saf* 23(2), 115 (rare)

Injection-site bruising

Injection-site edema (0.1–20%)
(2003): Hamburger MI+, *Semin Arthritis Rheum* 32(5), 296
(2003): Waddell DD, *Curr Med Res Opin* 19(7), 575
(2002): Chen AL+, *J Bone Joint Surg Am* 84-A(7), 1142 (20%)
(2002): Friedman PM+, *Dermatol Surg* 28(6), 491 (0.15%)
(2000): Adams ME+, *Drug Saf* 23(2), 115 (2–4%)
(1996): Lussier A+, *J Rheumatol* 23(9), 1579 (8.3%)
(1995): Puttick MP+, *J Rheumatol* 22(7), 1311 (11%)

Injection-site erythema (0.1–47%)
(2002): Friedman PM+, *Dermatol Surg* 28(6), 491 (0.15%)
(2000): Lupton JR+, *Dermatol Surg* 26(2), 135
(1994): Henderson EB+, *Ann Rheum Dis* 53(8), 529 (47%)

Injection-site granuloma
(2004): Sidwell RU+, *Clin Exp Dermatol* 29(6), 630

Injection-site infection
(2005): Christensen L+, *Aesthetic Plast Surg* 29(1), 34

Injection-site nodules
(2001): Bergeret-Galley C+, *Aesthetic Plast Surg* 25(4), 249 (0.12%)
(2000): Lupton JR+, *Dermatol Surg* 26(2), 135

Injection-site pain (8–47%)
(2003): Hamburger MI+, *Semin Arthritis Rheum* 32(5), 296
(2003): Waddell DD, *Curr Med Res Opin* 19(7), 575
(2002): Brocq O+, *Joint Bone Spine* 69(4), 388 (3 cases)
(2002): Chen AL+, *J Bone Joint Surg Am* 84(-A7), 1142 (20%)
(2002): Pavelka K+, *Acta Chir Orthop Traumatol Cech* 69(5), 302 (6.8%)
(2000): Altman RD, *Semin Arthritis Rheum* 30(2), 11
(2000): Roman JA+, *Clin Rheumatol* 19(3), 204 (8–16%)
(1998): Altman RD+, *J Rheumatol* 25(11), 2203 (23%)
(1996): Lussier A+, *J Rheumatol* 23(9), 1579 (8.3%)
(1995): Puttick MP+, *J Rheumatol* 22(7), 1311 (11%)
(1994): Henderson EB+, *Ann Rheum Dis* 53(8), 529 (47%)

Injection-site pruritus

Injection-site reactions (sic) (<11%)
(2003): Magilavy D+, *J Bone Joint Surg Am* 85-A(8), 1618
(2003): Morton AH+, *J Bone Joint Surg Am* 85-A(10), 2050
(2003): Waddell DD, *J Bone Joint Surg Am* 85-A(8), 1620
(2001): Micheels P, *Dermatol Surg* 27(2), 185 (8 cases)
(2000): Oswald A+, *Schweiz Rundsch Med Prax* 89(46), 1929
(2000): Rosier RN+, *Instr Course Lect* 49, 495
(1996): Adams ME, *J Rheumatol* 23(5), 944
(1996): O'Hanlon D, *J Rheumatol* 23(5), 945
(1995): Puttick MP+, *J Rheumatol* 22(7), 1311 (11%)

Systemic reactions
(2001): Rees JD+, *Rheumatology* (Oxford) 40(12), 1425

Upper respiratory infection

HYDRALAZINE

Trade names: Alphapress; Apdormin; Apresazide (Novartis); Apresolin; Apresoline (Novartis); Novo-Hylazin; Nu-Hydral; Ser-Ap-Es (Novartis); Solesorin; Stable
Indications: Hypertension
Category: Vasodilator
Half-life: 3–7 hours

Note: Apresazide is hydralazine and hydrochlorothiazide; Ser-Ap-Es is hydralazine, reserpine and hydrochlorothiazide

Reactions

Skin
Acute febrile neutrophilic dermatosis (Sweet's syndrome)
  (1995): Gilmour E+, *Br J Dermatol* 133, 490
  (1991): Juanola X+, *J Rheumatol* 18, 948
  (1990): Ramsay-Goldman R+, *J Rheumatol* 17, 682
  (1987): Servitje O+, *Arch Dermatol* 123, 1436
  (1986): Sequeira W+, *Am J Med* 81, 558
Allergic reactions (sic)
  (1986): Bigby M+, *JAMA* 236, 3358
Angioedema (<1%)
Bullous dermatitis
  (1988): Dodd HJ+, *Br J Dermatol* 119 (Suppl 33), 27
Dermatitis (systemic)
Diaphoresis
Edema (<1%)
Erythema nodosum
  (1984): Peterson LL, *J Am Acad Dermatol* 10, 379
Exanthems
  (1984): Peterson LL, *J Am Acad Dermatol* 10, 379
  (1984): Schapel GJ, *Med J Aust* 141, 765
  (1981): Finlay AY+, *BMJ* 282, 1703
Fixed eruption (<1%)
  (1986): Sehgal VN+, *Int J Dermatol* 25, 394
Lupus erythematosus (6.7%)
  (2006): Birnbaum B+, *Arthritis Rheum* 55(3), 501
  (2006): Finks SW+, *South Med J* 99(1), 18
  (2006): Singh S, *South Med J* 99(1), 6
  (2003): Deng C+, *Arthritis Rheum* 48(3), 746
  (2002): Pape L+, *Pediatr Transplant* 6(4), 337
  (2002): Siddiqui MA+, *Am J Ther* 9(2), 163 (passim)
  (1998): Hari CK+, *J Laryngol Otol* 112, 875
  (1997): Yung R+, *Arthritis Rheum* 40, 1436
  (1996): Miyasaka N, *Intern Med* 35, 587
  (1996): Pirmohamed M, *Hum Exp Toxicol* 15, 361
  (1995): Price EJ+, *Drug Saf* 12(4), 283
  (1994): Cohen MG, *J Rheumatol* 21, 578
  (1994): Hofstra AH, *Drug Metab Rev* 26, 485
  (1994): Nassberger L+, *Scand J Rheumatol* 23, 206
  (1994): Yung RL+, *Rheum Dis Clin North Am* 20, 61
  (1992): Rubin RL, *Clin Biochem* 25, 223
  (1992): Skaer TL, *Clin Ther* 14, 496
  (1992): Yonga GO, *East Afr Med J* 69, 649
  (1991): Alarcon-Segovia D+, *Baillieres Clin Rheumatol* 5, 1
  (1991): Hess EV, *Curr Opin Rheumatol* 3, 809
  (1991): Juanola X+, *J Rheumatol* 18, 948
  (1990): Mulder H, *Eur J Clin Pharmacol* 38, 303
  (1990): Nassberger L+, *Clin Exp Immunol* 81, 380
  (1990): Ramsay-Goldman R+, *J Rheumatol* 17, 682
  (1990): Richards FM+, *Am J Med* 88, 56N
  (1989): Fleming MG+, *Int J Dermatol* 28, 321 (bullous)
  (1989): Mitchell JA+, *Clin Exp Immunol* 78, 354
  (1989): Palsson L+, *Clin Pharmacol Ther* 46, 177
  (1989): Sim E, *Complement Inflamm* 6, 119
  (1989): Speirs C+, *Lancet* 1, 922

  (1989): Yemini M+, *Eur J Obstet Gynecol Reprod Biol* 30, 193
  (1988): Chong WK+, *BMJ* 297, 660
  (1988): Dodd HJ+, *Br J Dermatol* 119 (Suppl 33), 27
  (1988): Jiang M, *Chung Kuo I Hsueh Yuan Hsueh Pao* (Chinese) 10, 379
  (1988): Sturman SG+, *Lancet* 2, 1304 (fatal)
  (1988): Uetrecht JP, *Chem Res Toxicol* 1, 133
  (1987): Andersson OK, *Eur J Clin Pharmacol* 31, 741
  (1987): Craft JE+, *Arthritis Rheum* 30, 689
  (1987): Hobbs RN+, *Ann Rheum Dis* 46, 408
  (1987): Martinez-Vea A+, *Am J Nephrol* 7, 71
  (1987): Servitje O+, *Arch Dermatol* 123, 1436
  (1986): Asherson RA+, *Ann Rheum Dis* 45, 771
  (1986): Innes A+, *Br J Rheumatol* 25, 225
  (1986): Sequeira W+, *Am J Med* 81, 558
  (1985): Cush JJ+, *Am J Med Sci* 290, 36
  (1985): Doherty M+, *Br Med J Clin Res Ed* 290, 675
  (1985): Epstein A+, *Arthritis Rheum* 28, 158
  (1985): Kale SA, *Postgrad Med* 77, 231
  (1985): Lovisetto P+, *Recenti Prog Med* (Italian) 76, 110
  (1985): Stratton MA, *Clin Pharm* 4, 657
  (1985): Totoritis MC+, *Postgrad Med* 78, 149
  (1984): Brand C+, *Lancet* 1, 462
  (1984): Cameron HA+, *BMJ* 289, 410 (6.7%)
  (1984): Christophidis N, *Lancet* 2, 868
  (1984): French WJ, *Ala J Med Sci* 21, 427
  (1984): Naparstek Y+, *Arthritis Rheum* 27, 822
  (1984): No Author, *Lancet* 2, 441
  (1984): Peterson LL, *J Am Acad Dermatol* 10, 379
  (1984): Ramsay LE+, *Br Med J Clin Res Ed* 289, 1310
  (1984): Shapiro KS+, *Am J Kidney Dis* 3, 270
  (1984): Sim E+, *Lancet* 2, 422
  (1984): Timbrell JA+, *Eur J Clin Pharmacol* 27, 555
  (1984): Weiser GA+, *Arch Intern Med* 144, 2271
  (1984): Wollina U, *Z Gesamte Inn Med* (German) 39, 69
  (1983): Macleod WN, *Scott Med J* 28, 181
  (1983): Shoenfeld Y+, *Br Med J Clin Res Ed* 286, 224
  (1982): Aylward PE+, *Aust N Z J Med* 12, 546
  (1982): Freestone S+, *Br Med J Clin Res Ed* 285, 1536
  (1982): Harmon CE+, *Clin Rheum Dis* 8, 121
  (1982): Hess EV, *Arthritis Rheum* 25, 857
  (1982): Mansilla-Tinoco R+, *BMJ* 284, 936
  (1982): Ohe A+, *Osaka City Med J* 28, 149
  (1982): Portanova JP+, *Clin Immunol Immunopathol* 25(1), 67
  (1982): Ramsay LE+, *Br Med J Clin Res Ed* 284, 1711
  (1981): Chisholm JC, *J Natl Med Assoc* 73, 278
  (1981): Dubroff LM+, *Arthritis Rheum* 24, 1082
  (1981): Grossman J+, *Arthritis Rheum* 24, 927
  (1981): Neville E+, *Postgrad Med* 57, 378
  (1981): Perry HM, *Arthritis Rheum* 24, 1093
  (1981): Reidenberg MM, *Arthritis Rheum* 24, 1004
  (1981): Sinclair AJ+, *Hum Toxicol* 1, 65
  (1980): Batchelor JR+, *Lancet* 1, 1107
  (1980): Condemi JJ, *Geriatrics* 35(3), 81
  (1980): Harland SJ+, *BMJ* 281, 273
  (1980): Weinstein A, *Prog Clin Immunol* 4, 1
Photosensitivity
Pruritus
  (1984): Peterson LL, *J Am Acad Dermatol* 10, 379
Purpura
  (1984): Peterson LL, *J Am Acad Dermatol* 10, 379
  (1980): Petty R+, *BMJ* 280, 482
Pyoderma gangrenosum
  (1984): Peterson LL, *J Am Acad Dermatol* 10, 379
Rash (sic) (<1%)
Ulcerations
  (1980): Brooks AP+, *BMJ* 280, 482
  (1980): Petty R+, *BMJ* 280, 482
Urticaria
Vasculitis

(2003): Norris JH+, *Ren Fail* 25(2), 311
(1998): Merkel PA, *Curr Opin Rheumatol* 10, 45
(1995): Short AK+, *QJ Med* 88, 775
(1993): Reynolds NJ+, *Br J Dermatol* 129, 82
(1982): Kincaid-Smith P+, *Lancet* 2, 348
(1981): Finlay AY+, *Br Med J Clin Res Ed* 282, 1703
(1981): Peacock A+, *BMJ* 282, 1121
(1980): Bernstein RM+, *BMJ* 280, 156
(1980): Brooks AP+, *BMJ* 280, 482

Mucosal/ENT
Oral ulceration
(1984): Peterson LL, *J Am Acad Dermatol* 10, 379
(1980): Brooks AP+, *BMJ* 280, 482
Orogenital ulceration
(1984): Peterson LL, *J Am Acad Dermatol* 10, 379
(1981): Neville E+, *Postgrad Med* 57, 378

Other
Chills
Death
Headache
Hypersensitivity
Myalgia/Myositis/Myopathy/Myotoxicity
(2002): Pape L+, *Pediatr Transplant* 6(4), 337
Paresthesias
Sjøgren's (Sicca) syndrome
(1988): Darwaza A+, *Int J Oral Maxillopfac* 17, 92
Somnolence
Tremor
Vertigo

HYDROCHLOROTHIAZIDE

Trade names: Accuretic (Pfizer); Aldactazide (Pfizer); Aldoril (Merck); Apo-Hydro; Atacand HCT (AstraZeneca); Avalide (Bristol-Myers Squibb); Capozide (Par); Clothia; Dichlotride; Diovan (Novartis); Diu-Melsin; Diuchlor H; Dyazide (GSK); Esidrex; Hydrosaluric; Hyzaar (Merck); Inderide (Wyeth); Lopressor (Novartis); Lotensin (Novartis); Maxzide; Micardis (Boehringer Ingelheim); Microzide (Watson); Moduretic (Merck); Prinzide (Merck); Teveten HCT (Biovail); Uniretic (Schwarz); Urozide; Vaseretic (Biovail); Zestoretic (AstraZeneca); Ziac (Barr)
Indications: Edema
Category: Diuretic, thiazide
Half-life: 5.6–14.8 hours
Clinically important, potentially hazardous interactions with: digoxin, lithium, zinc

Note: Aldactazide is spironolactone and hydrochlorothiazide; Aldoril is methyldopa and hydrochlorothiazide; Avalide is irbesartan and hydrochlorothiazide; Capozide is captopril and hydrochlorothiazide; Dyazide is triamterene and hydrochlorothiazide; Maxzide is triamterene and hydrochlorothiazide; Moduretic is amiloride and hydrochlorothiazide; Prinizide is lisinopril and hydrochlorothiazide

Note: Hydrochlorothiazide is a sulfonamide and can be absorbed systemically. Sulfonamides can produce severe, possibly fatal, reactions such as toxic epidermal necrolysis and Stevens–Johnson syndrome

Reactions

Skin
Acute generalized exanthematous pustulosis (AGEP)
(2001): Petavy-Catala C+, *Acta Derm Venereol* 81(3), 209

Angioedema
(2006): Ruscin JM+, *Am J Geriatr Pharmacother* 4(4), 325
Bullous dermatitis (<1%)
Dermatitis
(1984): Fisher RS+, *J Am Acad Dermatol* 11, 146
Diaphoresis
(1984): Levay ID, *Drug Intell Clin Pharm* 18(3), 238
Erythema annulare centrifugum
(1988): Goette DK+, *Int J Dermatol* 27, 129
Erythema multiforme (<1%)
(1985): Ting HC+, *Int J Dermatol* 24, 587
Exanthems
Exfoliative dermatitis
Fixed eruption
(1985): Kauppinen K+, *Br J Dermatol* 112, 575
Lichenoid eruption
(2006): Pfab F+, *Allergy* 61(6), 786 (with irbesartan)
(1986): Halevy S+, *Ann Allergy* 56, 402
Lupus erythematosus
(2002): Boye T+, *World Congress Dermatol* Poster, 0088
(1998): Callen JP, *Academy '98 Meeting* (5 patients)
(1996): Litt JZ, Beachwood, OH (personal case) (observation)
(1995): Brown CW+, *Clin Toxicol* 33, 729
(1995): Rich MW+, *J Rheumatol* 22, 1001
(1993): Goodrich AL+, *J Am Acad Dermatol* 28, 1001
(1991): Wollenberg A+, *Hautarzt* (German) 42, 709
(1989): Alanko K+, *Acta Derm Venereol* (Stockh) 69, 223
(1989): Fine RM, *Int J Dermatol* 28, 375 (Comment)
(1989): Parodi A+, *Photodermatology* 6, 100
(1988): Darken M+, *J Am Acad Dermatol* 18, 38
(1986): Berbis Ph, *Ann Dermatol Venereol* 113, 1245 (thiazides)
(1985): Reed BR+, *Ann Intern Med* 103, 49
Photosensitivity (<1%)
(2002): Johnston GA, *Clin Exp Dermatol* 27(8), 670 (lichenoid)
(2000): Wagner SN+, *Contact Dermatitis* 43, 245 (with ramipril)
(1994): Bielan B, *Dermatol Nurs* 6, 30
(1994): Shelley WB+, *Cutis* 53, 77 (observation)
(1987): Addo HA+, *Br J Dermatol* 116, 749
(1985): Reed BR+, *Ann Intern Med* 103, 49
(1985): Robinson HN+, *Arch Dermatol* 121, 522
(1984): Ophir O+, *Harefuah* (Hebrew) 107, 14
(1983): White IR, *Contact Dermatitis* 9, 237
(1982): No Author, *Ugeskr Laeger* (Danish) 144, 1101
(1981): Journet M, *Union Med Can* 110, 356
(1980): Okrasinski H, *Lakartidningen* (Swedish) 77, 2718
(1980): Torinuki W, *J Dermatol* (Tokio) 7, 293
Phototoxicity
(1989): Diffey BL, *Arch Dermatol* 125, 1355
(1987): Addo HA+, *Br J Dermatol* 116, 749
(1982): Rosen K+, *Acta Derm Venereol* (Stockh) 62, 246
Pityriasis rosea
(2006): Atzori L+, *Dermatology Online Journal* 12(1), 1
Porokeratosis (Mibelli)
(1984): Inamoto N+, *J Am Acad Dermatol* 11, 359
Pruritus (<1%)
(1992): Shelley WB+, *Cutis* 49, 391 (observation)
Purpura
(1980): Miescher PA+, *Clin Haematol* 9, 505
Rash (sic)
(2006): Ruscin JM+, *Am J Geriatr Pharmacother* 4(4), 325
Stevens–Johnson syndrome
Toxic epidermal necrolysis
Urticaria
Vasculitis
(1989): Grunwald MH+, *Isr J Med Sci* 25, 572

Mucosal/ENT
Dysgeusia

(2000): Zervakis J+, *Physiol Behav* 68, 405
Dysphagia
(2006): Ruscin JM+, *Am J Geriatr Pharmacother* 4(4), 325
Oral lichenoid eruption (erosive)
(1990): Espana A+, *Med Clin* (Barc) (Spanish) 94, 559
Xerostomia

Eyes
Dyschromatopsia
Glaucoma
(2007): Lee GC+, *Clin Experiment Ophthalmol* 35(1), 55

Other
Depression
(2003): Ullrich H+, *Dtsch Med Wochenschr* 128(48), 2534 (with valsartan)
Headache
Inappropriate secretion of antidiuretic hormone (SIADH)
(1999): van Assen S+, *Neth J Med* 54(3), 108
(1990): Emsley RA+, *S Afr Med J* 77(6), 307
Paresthesias
Pseudoporphyria
(1990): Motley RJ, *BMJ* 300, 1468

HYDROCODONE

Trade names: Bacomine; Ban-Tuss HC; Codamine; Duratuss (UCB); Entex HC (Andrx); Hycotuss (Endo); Lortab (UCB); Maxidone (Watson); Morcomine; Norco (Watson); Prolex-DH; Propachem; Ru-Tuss; Tussgen; Tussionex (Celltech); Tussogest; Vicodin (Abbott); Vicoprofen (Abbott); Zydone (Endo)
Indications: Acute pain, coughing
Category: Opiate agonist
Half-life: 3.8 hours

Note: Hydrocodone is included in many combination drugs. Other medications that can be included in these preparations include: phenylpropanolamine, phenylephrine, pyrilamine, pseudoephedrine, acetaminophen, ibuprofen, and others

Reactions

Skin
Diaphoresis
Edema
Erythema multiforme
Exanthems
(2000): Litt JZ, Beachwood, OH (personal case) (observation)
Pruritus (1–10%)
(2000): Litt JZ, Beachwood, OH (personal case) (observation)
(1999): Litt JZ, Beachwood, OH (personal case) (observation)
(1999): Sorkin MJ, Denver, CO (from Internet) (observation)
Rash (sic) (>10%)
Stevens–Johnson syndrome
Toxic epidermal necrolysis
Urticaria (>10%)

Mucosal/ENT
Ototoxicity
(2007): Ho T+, *Pain Physician* 10(3), 467
Xerostomia

Other
Headache
Hot flashes
Myoclonus
(1999): Lauterbach EC, *Clin Neuropharmacol* 22(2), 87

HYDROCORTISONE

Trade names: Ala-Cort (Del-Ray); Cortef (Pharmacia); Cortenema (Solvay); Hydrocortone (Merck); Hytone (Dermik); Solu-Cortef (Pharmacia)
Indications: Arthralgias, Ophthalmology, Asthma, Rhinitis (many more)
Category: Corticosteroid, topical
Half-life: N/A
Clinically important, potentially hazardous interactions with: amphotericin B, chlorotrianisene, colestyramine, diuretics, estrogens, furosemide, insulin, **live vaccines**, methotrexate, oral contraceptives, pancuronium, phenobarbital, rifampicin

Reactions

Skin
Acne
Allergic reactions (sic)
(2004): Keegel T+, *Contact Dermatitis* 50(1), 6
(1999): Kamm GL+, *Ann Pharmacother* 33(4), 451
(1995): Lepoittevin JP+, *Arch Dermatol* 131(1), 31
(1992): Schoenmakers A+, *Contact Dermatitis* 26(3), 159
(1991): Lauerma AI+, *J Am Acad Dermatol* 24(2), 182
(1989): Reitamo S+, *J Am Acad Dermatol* 21(3), 506
(1986): Dooms-Goossens A+, *Contact Dermatitis* 14(2), 94
(1980): Brown R, *Contact Dermatitis* 6(7), 504
Angioedema
(1980): Ashford RF+, *Postgrad Med J* 56(656), 437
Atrophy
(1985): Serup J+, *Dermatologica* 170(4), 189
Bruising
Burning
(1997): Sears HW+, *Clin Ther* 19(4), 710
Dermatitis
(1998): Isaksson M+, *Am J Contact Dermat* 9(2), 136
(1997): Vestergaard L+, *Ugeskr Laeger* (Danish) 159, 5662
(1995): Wilkinson SM+, *Br J Dermatol* 132(5), 766
(1993): Hisa T+, *Contact Dermatitis* 28, 174
(1993): Torres V+, *Contact Dermatitis* 29(2), 106
(1992): Wilkinson SM+, *Contact Dermatitis* 27(3), 197
(1991): Dunkel FG+, *Contact Dermatitis* 25(2), 97
(1991): Marston S, *Contact Dermatitis* 24(5), 372
(1985): Yoshikawa K+, *Contact Dermatitis* 12, 55
Eczema
(1996): Juhlin L, *Cutis* 57(2), 51 (exacerbation)
(1993): Torres V+, *Contact Dermatitis* 29, 106
(1992): Lauerma AI+, *Arch Dermatol* 128, 275
(1991): Wilkinson SM+, *Lancet* 337(8744), 761 (4.8%)
Molluscum contagiosum
(1990): Ratka P+, *Dermatol Monatsschr* 176(12), 735
Photoallergic reaction
(1996): Stitt WZ+, *Am J Contact Dermat* 7(3), 166
Pruritus
(2004): El Mekki+, *Presse Med* 33(9 Pt 1), 604
Purpura
(2004): El Mekki+, *Presse Med* 33(9 Pt 1), 604
Rash (sic)
(1999): Vaghjimal A+, *Int J Clin Pract* 53(7), 567
(1993): Hisa T+, *Contact Dermatitis* 28(3), 174
Sensitivity
(2000): Bircher AJ+, *Dermatology* 200(4), 349
Telangiectasia
(1985): Serup J+, *Dermatologica* 170(4), 189
Urticaria
(2001): Borja JM+, *Allergy* 56(8), 802

(2001): Nettis E+, *Allergy* 56(8), 791
(2001): Rasanen L+, *Allergy* 56, 352
(1987): Kuokkanen K+, *Clin Ther* 9(2), 223 (1 case)
(1980): Ashford RF+, *Postgrad Med J* 56(656), 437

Hair
Hair – hypertrichosis

Eyes
Cataract
    (1996): Phillips CI+, *Acta Derm Venereol* 76(4), 314
Visual disturbances

Other
Anaphylactoid reactions/Anaphylaxis
    (2004): Calogiuri GF+, *Br J Dermatol* 151(3), 707
    (2002): Holz W+, *Anaesthesist* 51(3), 187
    (1993): Yoshikawa T+, *Nihon Kyobu Shikkan Gakkai Zasshi*
        31(8), 1024
    (1992): Corominas N+, *Pharm Weekbl Sci* 14(3), 93
    (1991): Fulcher DA+, *Med J Aust* 154(3), 210
    (1991): Kawane H, *Med J Aust* 154(11), 783
    (1991): Murrieta-Aguttes M+, *J Asthma* 28(5), 329
    (1990): Suenaga N+, *Nihon Kyobu Shikkan Gakkai Zasshi*
        28(6), 900
    (1986): Mansfield LE+, *J Asthma* 23(2), 81
    (1985): Goldstein DA+, *Ann Allergy* 55(4), 599
    (1985): Murata Y+, *Nihon Kyobu Shikkan Gakkai Zasshi*
        23(3), 375
    (1985): Peller JS+, *Ann Allergy* 54, 302
    (1984): Chan CS+, *Med J Aust* 141(7), 444
    (1984): Rogov VD, *Vestn Otorinolaringol* 647(4), 66
    (1982): Tada T+, *Kokyu To Junkan* 30(11), 1173
    (1981): Dajani BM+, *J Allergy Clin* 68, 201
Depression
    (2004): Sher L, *Gen Hosp Psychiatry* 26(3), 241
Fever
    (1999): Vaghjimal A+, *Int J Clin Pract* 53(7), 567
Headache
Hypersensitivity
    (2002): Le Coz, *Ann Dermatol Venereol* 129(6-7), 931
    (1994): Wilkinson SM+, *Br J Dermatol* 131(4), 495
    (1993): Lauerma AI+, *Contact Dermatitis* 28(1), 10
    (1993): Wilkinson SM+, *Contact Dermatitis* 28(5), 295
    (1992): Burden AD+, *Br J Dermatol* 127(5), 497 (2.5%)
Hypertension
    (1989): Hasaerts D+, *Arch Fr Pediatr* 46(9), 635
    (1989): Sudhir K+, *Hypertension* 13(5), 416
Infections
    (2003): Lionakis MS+, *Lancet* 362(9398), 1828
Myalgia/Myositis/Myopathy/Myotoxicity
    (2004): Tsai WS+, *Am J Med Sci* 327(3), 152
    (1990): Shee CD, *Respir Med* 84(3), 229
    (1990): Shee CD, *Respiratory Medicine* 84, 229
    (1988): Sury MR+, *Lancet* 2(8609), 515
    (1986): Knox AJ+, *Thorax* 41, 411
    (1986): Knox AJ+, *Thorax* 41(5), 411
    (1980): Van Marle W+, *BMJ* 281, 271
    (1980): Van Marle W+, *Br Med J* 281(6235), 271
Seizures
    (2003): Odeh M+, *J Toxicol Clin Toxicol* 41(7), 995
Vertigo

HYDROFLUMETHIAZIDE

Trade names: Diademil; Hydravern; Hydrenox; Leodrine; Rivosil; Rontyl
Indications: Hypertension, edema
Category: Diuretic, thiazide
Half-life: 12–24 hours
Clinically important, potentially hazardous interactions with: digoxin, lithium

Note: Hydroflumethiazide is a sulfonamide and can be absorbed systemically. Sulfonamides can produce severe, possibly fatal, reactions such as toxic epidermal necrolysis and Stevens–Johnson syndrome

Reactions

Skin
Photosensitivity (<1%)
Purpura
Rash (sic) (<1%)
Urticaria
Vasculitis

Mucosal/ENT
Dysgeusia

Eyes
Dyschromatopsia

Other
Paresthesias (<1%)

HYDROMORPHONE

Trade names: Dilaudid (Abbott); Dilaudid HP; HydroStat IR; Palladone
Indications: Pain
Category: Opiate agonist
Half-life: 1–3 hours
Clinically important, potentially hazardous interactions with: cimetidine

Note: This drug has been withdrawn

Reactions

Skin
Diaphoresis
Exanthems
    (1992): de Cuyper C+, *Contact Dermatitis* 27, 220 (generalized)
Pruritus (1–11%)
    (1996): Halpern SH+, *Can J Anaesth* 43(6), 595
    (1992): Chaplan SR+, *Anesthesiology* 77, 1090 (11.5%)
    (1989): Dougherty TB+, *Anesth Analg* 68(3), 318
    (1986): Chestnut DH+, *Obstet Gynecol* 68(1), 65
Rash (sic) (<1%)
Urticaria (<1%)

Mucosal/ENT
Dysgeusia
    (2004): Rudy AC+, *Anesth Analg* 99(5), 1379
    (2003): Coda BA+, *Anesth Analg* 97(1), 117
Xerostomia (1–10%)

Hair
Hair – alopecia

Other

Anaphylactoid reactions/Anaphylaxis
  (2007): Mushlin N+, *South Med J* 100(6), 611
Injection-site reactions (sic)
Myoclonus
  (2006): Hofmann A+, *J Neurol Neurosurg Psychiatry* 77(8), 994
  (2004): Thwaites D+, *J Palliat Med* 7(4), 545
Paresthesias
Seizures
  (2004): Thwaites D+, *J Palliat Med* 7(4), 545
Vertigo
  (2004): Rudy AC+, *Anesth Analg* 99(5), 1379
  (2003): Coda BA+, *Anesth Analg* 97(1), 117

HYDROXYCHLOROQUINE

Trade names: Ercoquin; Oxiklorin; Plaquenil (Sanofi-Aventis); Plaquinol; Quensyl; Toremonil; Yuma
Indications: Malaria, lupus erythematosus, rheumatoid arthritis
Category: Antimalarial; Antiprotozoal; Disease-modifying antirheumatic
Half-life: elimination in blood: 50 days
Clinically important, potentially hazardous interactions with: chloroquine, cholestyramine, dapsone, penicillamine

Reactions

Skin

Acute generalized exanthematous pustulosis (AGEP)
  (2004): Evans CC+, *J Am Acad Dermatol* 50(4), 650
  (2003): Saissi EH+, *Ann Dermatol Venereol* 130(6-7), 612
  (1996): Assier-Bonnet H+, *Dermatology* 193, 70
  (1995): Bonnetblanc JM+, *Ann Dermatol Venereol* (French) 122, 604
  (1995): Moreau A+, *Int J Dermatol* 34, 263 (passim)
  (1993): Assier H+, *Ann Dermatol Venereol* (French) 120, 848
Angioedema (<1%)
Atrophy
  (2001): Vassallo C+, *Clin Exp Dermatol* 26(2), 141
Bullous dermatitis
  (2008): Mitchell D, Thomasville, GA (from internet) (observation)
  (2001): Klein AD, Statesboro, GA (from Internet) (observation)
  (1995): Kutz DC+, *Arthritis Rheum* 38, 440
Dermatitis
  (1999): Meier H+, *Hautarzt* (German) 50, 665
Dermatomyositis
  (1994): Bloom BJ+, *J Rheumatology* 21, 2171
Erythema annulare centrifugum
  (1985): Hudson LD, *J Am Acad Dermatol* 36, 129
  (1982): Koralewski F, *Dermatosen* (German) 30, 125
Erythema multiforme (<1%)
  (1997): Rudolph R, Wyomissing, PA (from Internet) (observation)
Erythema nodosum
  (1996): Jarrett P+, *Br J Dermatol* 134, 373 (chronic)
Erythroderma
  (1990): Simoneaux PW, *Curr Concept Skin Dis* Winter, 15
  (1985): Slagel GA+, *J Am Acad Dermatol* 12, 857
Exanthems (1–5%)
  (2001): Werth V, *Dermatology Times* 18
  (1995): Blumenthal HL, Beachwood, OH (personal case) (observation)
  (1991): Ochsendorf FR+, *Hautarzt* (German) 42, 140
  (1990): Simoneaux PW, *Curr Concept Skin Dis* Winter, 15
Exfoliative dermatitis

  (1995): Blumenthal HL, Beachwood, OH (personal case) (observation)
  (1986): Lavrijsen APM+, *Acta Derm Venereol* (Stockh) 66, 536
  (1985): Slagel GA+, *J Am Acad Dermatol* 12, 857
  (1980): Koranda FC, *J Am Acad Dermatol* 4, 650 (passim)
Fixed eruption (<1%)
Lichenoid eruption
  (1990): Simoneaux PW, *Curr Concept Skin Dis* Winter, 15
  (1980): Koranda FC, *J Am Acad Dermatol* 4, 650 (passim)
Photoallergic reaction
  (2004): Lisi P+, *Contact Dermatitis* 50(4), 255
Photosensitivity
  (2002): Litt JZ, Beachwood, OH (personal observation)
  (2001): Metayer I+, *Ann Dermatol Venereol* 128(6), 729 (4 cases)
  (2000): Ainsworth GE, Salina, KS (from Internet) (observation)
  (1991): Ochsendorf FR+, *Hautarzt* (German) 42, 140
  (1982): van Weelden H, *Arch Dermatol* 118, 290
  (1981): Journet M, *Union Med Can* (French) 110, 356
Phototoxicity
  (2004): Lisi P+, *Contact Dermatitis* 50(4), 255
  (2001): Metayer I+, *Ann Dermatol Venereol* 128(6), 729 (4 cases)
Pigmentation (1–10%)
  (2006): Reynaert S+, *J Eur Acad Dermatol Venereol* 20(4), 487
  (2005): Fardet L+, *Ann Dermatol Venereol* 132(8-9 Pt 1), 665
  (2004): Millard TP+, *Clin Exp Dermatol* 29(1), 92
  (1991): Ochsendorf FR+, *Hautarzt* (German) 42, 140
  (1982): Levy H, *S Afr Med J* 2, 735
  (1980): Koranda FC, *J Am Acad Dermatol* 4, 650 (passim)
Pruritus (>10%)
  (2006): Gul U+, *Eur J Dermatol* 16(5), 586
  (2004): Jimenez-Alonso J+, *Rev Clin Esp* 204(11), 588 (1.5%)
  (2002): Litt JZ, Beachwood, OH (personal observation)
  (2001): Silver B, Deerfield, IL (from Internet) (observation)
  (1999): Holme SA+, *Acta Derm Venereol* (Stockh) 79, 333
  (1995): Blumenthal HL, Beachwood, OH (personal case) (observation)
  (1994): Fain O+, *Rev Med Interne* (French) 15, 433
  (1991): Mnyika KS+, *J Trop Med Hyg* 94, 27 (47%)
  (1990): Abdulkadir SA+, *Trans Roy Soc Trop Med Hyg* 84, 898
  (1990): Simoneaux PW, *Curr Concept Skin Dis* Winter, 15
  (1984): Osifo NG, *Arch Dermatol* 120, 80
  (1982): Spencer HC+, *BMJ* 285, 1703
Psoriasis (exacerbation)
  (2003): Welsch MJ, *J Drugs Dermatol* 2, 193
  (2001): Spencer L, Crawfordsville, IN (from Internet) (2 observations)
  (2001): Thaler D, Monona, WI (exacerbation) (from Internet) (observation)
  (1996): Vine JE+, *J Dermatol* 23, 357
  (1993): Potter B, *Cutis* 52, 229 (passim)
  (1988): Nicolas J-F+, *Ann Dermatol Venereol* (French) 115, 289
  (1987): Friedman SJ, *J Am Acad Dermatol* 16, 1256
  (1985): Gray RG, *J Rheumatol* 12, 391
  (1982): Abel EA+, *J Am Acad Dermatol* 15, 2007
  (1982): Luzar MJ, *J Rheumatol* 9, 462
  (1981): Olsen TG, *Ann Intern Med* 94, 546
Purpura
Pustules
  (1990): Lotem M+, *Acta Derm Venereol* (Stockh) 70, 250
Rash (sic) (1–10%)
  (2006): Mates M+, *J Rheumatol* 33(4), 814
  (2001): Levy RA+, *Lupus* 10(6), 401
Stevens–Johnson syndrome
  (2002): Leckie MJ+, *Rheumatology* (Oxford) 41(4), 473
Telangiectasia
  (2001): Vassallo C+, *Clin Exp Dermatol* 26(2), 141
Toxic epidermal necrolysis
  (2002): Chavez JS, Santiago, Chile, March AAD Poster
  (2001): Murphy M+, *Clin Exp Dermatol* 26(5), 457 (fatal)

Urticaria
  (2002): Litt JZ, Beachwood, OH (personal case) (observation)
  (1990): Simoneaux PW, *Curr Concept Skin Dis* Winter, 15
  (1980): Koranda FC, *J Am Acad Dermatol* 4, 650 (passim)
Vasculitis
  (2003): Welsch MJ, *J Drugs Dermatol* 2(2), 193

Mucosal/ENT
Dysgeusia
  (2004): Jimenez-Alonso J+, *Rev Clin Esp* 204(11), 588 (64%)
  (1996): Weber JC+, *Presse Med* (French) 25, 213
Gingival pigmentation
  (1992): Veraldi S+, *Cutis* 49, 281
Mucosal atrophy
  (2001): Vassallo C+, *Clin Exp Dermatol* 26(2), 141
Oral pigmentation
  (2005): Fardet L+, *Ann Dermatol Venereol* 132(8-9 Pt 1), 665
  (2001): Vassallo C+, *Clin Exp Dermatol* 26(2), 141
  (1992): Veraldi S+, *Cutis* 49, 281
  (1991): Zic JA+, *Arch Dermatol* 127, 1037
  (1980): Koranda FC, *J Am Acad Dermatol* 4, 650 (passim)
Oral ulceration
Stomatitis
  (2001): Vassallo C+, *Clin Exp Dermatol* 26(2), 141
Stomatopyrosis
Tinnitus

Hair
Hair – alopecia
Hair – pigmentation (bleaching) (1–10%)
  (1999): Lecocq P+, *Presse Med* (French) 28, 741
  (1991): Ochsendorf FR+, *Hautarzt* (German) 42, 140
  (1985): Dupré A+, *Arch Dermatol* 121, 1164
  (1980): Koranda FC, *J Am Acad Dermatol* 4, 650 (passim)

Nails
Nails – discoloration
  (1991): Zic JA+, *Arch Dermatol* 127, 1037
Nails – pigmentation
  (2001): Vassallo C+, *Clin Exp Dermatol* 26(2), 141
  (1980): Koranda FC, *J Am Acad Dermatol* 4, 650 (passim)

Eyes
Maculopathy
  (2001): Warner AE, *Arthritis Rheum* 44(8), 1959
  (1985): Taylor F, *Aust Fam Physician* 14(8), 744
Ocular toxicity
  (2002): Grana Gil+, *An Med Interna* 19(4), 189
Retinopathy
  (2007): Ferreras A+, *Arch Soc Esp Oftalmol* 82(2), 103
  (2006): Tripp JM+, *Am J Clin Dermatol* 7(3), 171
  (2005): Fardet L+, *Ann Dermatol Venereol* 132(8-9 Pt 1), 665
  (2005): Lai TY+, *Am J Ophthalmol* 140(5), 794
  (2005): Tzekov R, *Doc Ophthalmol* 110(1), 111
  (2004): Constable S+, *Expert Opin Drug Saf* 3(3), 249

Other
Cardiotoxicity
  (2005): Keating RJ+, *J Am Soc Echocardiogr* 18(9), 981
Death
  (2001): Murphy M+, *Clin Exp Dermatol* 26(5), 457
Headache
Lymphoproliferative disease
  (1980): Schechter SL+, *Arthritis Rheum* 23, 256
Myalgia/Myositis/Myopathy/Myotoxicity
  (1998): Richards AJ, *J Rheumatol* 25, 1642
Porphyria
  (1993): Potter B, *Cutis* 52, 229 (passim)
Rhabdomyolysis
  (2005): Creel N+, *J Drugs Dermatol* 4(2), 225 (with quinacrine)

Seizures
  (2000): Malcangi G+, *Rheumatol Int* 20(1), 31

HYDROXYUREA

Trade names: Droxia (Bristol-Myers Squibb); Hydrea (Bristol-Myers Squibb); Litalir; Mylocel; Onco-Carbide
Indications: Leukemia, malignant tumors
Category: Antineoplastic; Antiretroviral
Half-life: 3–4 hours
Clinically important, potentially hazardous interactions with: adefovir, aldesleukin

Reactions

Skin
Acral erythema
  (1993): Brincker H+, *Cancer Chemother Pharmacol* 32, 496 (edema and soreness)
  (1992): Parodi A+, *G Ital Dermatol Venereol* (Italian) 127, 361 (fingers and toes)
  (1991): Baack BR+, *J Am Acad Dermatol* 24, 457
  (1989): Kampmann KK+, *Cancer* 63, 2482 (passim)
  (1984): Sigal M+, *Ann Dermatol Venereol* (French) 111, 895 (band-like)
  (1983): Silver FS+, *Ann Intern Med* 98, 675
Acute febrile neutrophilic dermatosis (Sweet's syndrome)
  (2002): Guennoc B+, *World Congress Dermatol* Poster 0102
Atrophy
  (1997): Ena P+, *J Geriatr Dermatol* 5, 310
Baboon syndrome
  (1999): Chowdhury MM+, *Clin Exp Dermatol* 24, 336
Café-au-lait macules
  (2004): Zargari O+, *Pediatr Dermatol* 21(6), 633
Collodion-like skin
  (1996): Gauthier O+, *Ann Dermatol Venereol* (French) 123, 727
Dermatitis
  (2001): Eming SA+, *J Am Acad Dermatol* 45, 321
  (1984): Sigal M+, *Ann Dermatol Venereol* (French) 111, 895
Dermatomyositis
  (2006): Elliott R+, *J Dermatolog Treat* 17(1), 59
  (2006): Haniffa MA+, *Clin Exp Dermatol* 31(5), 733
  (2006): Slobodin G+, *Rheumatol Int* 26(8), 768 (Gottron's papules)
  (2006): Zaccaria E+, *J Dermatolog Treat* 17(3), 176
  (2005): Bouldouyre MA+, *Eur J Dermatol* 15(4), 268
  (2005): Yoshida K+, *Clin Exp Dermatol* 30(2), 191
  (2003): Oh ST+, *J Am Acad Dermatol* 49, 339 (2 cases)
  (2002): Dacey MJ+, Louisville, KY, March AAD Poster
  (2002): Oskay T+, *Eur J Dermatol* 12(6), 586
  (2001): Vassallo C+, *Clin Exp Dermatol* 26(2), 141
  (2000): Kirby B+, *Clin Exp Dermatol* 25, 256
  (2000): Rocamora V+, *J Eur Acad Dermatol Venereol* 14(3), 227
  (1999): Varma S+, *Clin Exp Dermatol* 24(3), 164
  (1998): Suehiro M+, *Br J Dermatol* 139, 748
  (1998): Velez A+, *Clin Exp Dermatol* 23, 94
  (1997): Ena P+, *J Geriatr Dermatol* 5, 310
  (1996): Bahadoran P+, *Br J Dermatol* 134, 1161
  (1995): Senet P+, *Br J Dermatol* 133, 455
  (1995): Weber L+, *Hautarzt* 46, 717
  (1994): Kelly RI+, *Australas J Dermatol* 35, 61
  (1994): Perrot JL+, *Ann Dermatol Venereol* (French) 121, 499
  (1989): Richard M+, *J Am Acad Dermatol* 21, 797
  (1984): Sigal M+, *Ann Dermatol Venereol* (French) 111, 895
Erythema gyratum
  (1984): Sigal M+, *Ann Dermatol Venereol* (French) 111, 895 (fingers and toes)

(1995): Weber L+, *Hautarzt* (German) 46, 717
(1989): Richard M+, *J Am Acad Dermatol* 21, 797 (passim)
(1984): Sigal M+, *Ann Dermatol Venereol* (French) 111, 895

Mucosal/ENT

Glossitis
  (2001): Vassallo C+, *Clin Exp Dermatol* 26(2), 141
Mucocutaneous eruption
  (2002): Kumar B+, *Clin Exp Dermatol* 27(1), 8
Oral lesions
Oral pigmentation (<29%)
  (2002): Kumar B+, *Clin Exp Dermatol* 27(1), 8
  (2001): Chaine B+, *Arch Dermatol* 137, 467 (29%)
Oral squamous cell carcinoma
  (2004): De Benedittis M+, *Clin Exp Dermatol* 29(6), 605
  (2001): Esteve E+, *Ann Dermatol Venereol* 128(8), 919
Oral ulceration
  (2006): Saravu K+, *J Korean Med Sci* 21(1), 177
  (2006): Steels E+, *Rev Med Brux* 27(1), 39
  (2002): Kumar B+, *Clin Exp Dermatol* 27(1), 8
  (2001): Vassallo C+, *Clin Exp Dermatol* 26(2), 141
  (1997): Norhaya MR+, *Singapore Med J* 38, 283
  (1989): Richard M+, *J Am Acad Dermatol* 21, 797 (passim)
Stomatitis (>10%)
  (1993): Brincker H+, *Cancer Chemother Pharmacol* 32, 496
  (1992): Breathnach SM+, *Adverse Drug Reactions and the Skin* Blackwell, Oxford, 303 (passim)
  (1989): Richard M+, *J Am Acad Dermatol* 21, 797 (passim)
Tongue pigmentation (<29%)
  (2001): Chaine B+, *Arch Dermatol* 137, 467 (29%)
  (1997): Ena P+, *J Geriatr Dermatol* 5, 310
  (1993): Gropper CA+, *Int J Dermatol* 32, 731

Hair

Hair – alopecia (1–10%)
  (2002): Kumar B+, *Clin Exp Dermatol* 27(1), 8 (diffuse)
  (1992): Breathnach SM+, *Adverse Drug Reactions and the Skin* Blackwell, Oxford, 303 (passim)
  (1989): Layton AM+, *Br J Dermatol* 121, 647
  (1989): Richard M+, *J Am Acad Dermatol* 21, 797 (passim)

Nails

Nails – atrophic
  (1984): Daniel CR+, *J Am Acad Dermatol* 10, 250
  (1984): Sigal M+, *Ann Dermatol Venereol* (French) 111, 895
Nails – blue lunulae
  (2003): Jeevankumar B+, *J Dermatol* 30(8), 628
Nails – dystrophy
  (1992): Breathnach SM+, *Adverse Drug Reactions and the Skin* Blackwell, Oxford, 303 (passim)
  (1989): Richard M+, *J Am Acad Dermatol* 21, 797 (passim)
Nails – leukonychia
  (2004): Zargari O+, *Pediatr Dermatol* 21(6), 633
Nails – melanonychia
  (2006): Teo RY+, *Int J Dermatol* 45(11), 1329
  (2004): Zargari O+, *Pediatr Dermatol* 21(6), 633 (longitudinal)
  (2003): Oh ST+, *J Am Acad Dermatol* 49, 339 (7 cases)
Nails – pigmentation (9%)
  (2004): Liss W, Pleasanton, CA (gray) (from Internet) (observation)
  (2003): Jeevankumar B+, *J Dermatol* 30(8), 628
  (2002): Aste N+, *J Am Acad Dermatol* 47(1), 146 (9 cases)
  (2002): Kumar B+, *Clin Exp Dermatol* 27(1), 8
  (2001): Chaine B+, *Arch Dermatol* 137, 467 (9%)
  (2001): O'Branski EE+, *J Am Acad Dermatol* 44, 859 (longitudinal bands) (patient had sickle cell anemia)
  (1999): Hernández-Martin A+, *J Am Acad Dermatol* 40, 333
  (1997): Cakir B+, *Int J Dermatol* 36, 234
  (1997): Ena P+, *J Geriatr Dermatol* 5, 310
  (1996): Kwong YL, *J Am Acad Dermatol* 35, 275

(1995): Delmas-Marsalet B+, *Nouv Rev Fr Hematol* (French) 37, 205
(1994): Pirard C+, *Ann Dermatol Venereol* (French) 121, 106 (longitudinal)
(1993): Gropper CA+, *Int J Dermatol* 32, 731
(1992): Kelsey PR, *Clin Lab Haematol* 14, 337
(1991): Vomvouras S+, *J Am Acad Dermatol* 24, 1016
(1989): Baran R+, *J Am Acad Dermatol* 21, 1165
(1984): Sigal M+, *Ann Dermatol Venereol* (French) 111, 895
(1982): Jeanmougin M+, *Ann Dermatol Venereol* 109, 169
Nails – ridging
  (2004): Zargari O+, *Pediatr Dermatol* 21(6), 633

Eyes

Scleral pigmentation
  (2002): Kumar B+, *Clin Exp Dermatol* 27(1), 8

Other

Death
  (2001): Young HS+, *Clin Exp Dermatol* 26(8), 664
Gangrene (toes)
  (2002): Leo E+, *Ann Hematol* 81(8), 467
Inappropriate secretion of antidiuretic hormone (SIADH)
  (2004): Watanabe N+, *Rinsho Ketsueki* 45(3), 243
Infections
  (2002): Venigalla P+, *Blood* 100(1), 363
Myalgia/Myositis/Myopathy/Myotoxicity
  (1998): Ikeda K+, *Rinsho Ketsueki* (Japanese) 39, 676
Porphyria cutanea tarda
  (2002): Zweegman S+, *Ned Tijdschr Geneeskd* 146(49), 2353
Tumors
  (1998): Best PJ+, *Mayo Clin Proc* 73, 961 (multiple malignant)
  (1998): De Simone C+, *Eur J Dermatol* 8, 114 (multiple squamous cell)
  (1998): Salmon-Her V+, *Dermatology* 196, 274
  (1993): Papi M+, *J Am Acad Dermatol* 28, 485 (on light-exposed areas)
  (1992): Stasi R+, *Eur J Haematol* 48, 121

HYDROXYZINE

Trade names: AH3 N; Anaxanil; Atarax (Pfizer); Bobsule; Iremofar; Marax; Masmoran; Multipax; Otarex; Paxistil; Quiess; Rezine; Vamate; Vistaril (Pfizer)
Indications: Anxiety and tension, pruritus
Category: Histamine H1 receptor antagonist; Muscarinic antagonist
Half-life: 3–7 hours
Clinically important, potentially hazardous interactions with: alcohol, barbiturates, CNS depressants, narcotics, non-narcotic analgesics

Reactions

Skin

Acute generalized exanthematous pustulosis (AGEP)
  (2007): Tsai YS+, *Br J Dermatol* 157(6), 1296
Angioedema (<1%)
Dermatitis
  (1997): Menne T, *Am J Contact Dermat* 8, 1
Diaphoresis
Edema (<1%)
Erythema multiforme (<1%)
  (2006): Tamagawa R+, *Arerugi* 55(1), 34
Exanthems
Fixed eruption

(2002): Assouere MN+, *Ann Dermatol Venereol* 129(11), 1295
(1997): Cohen HA+, *Ann Pharmacother* 31, 327 (penis)
(1996): Cohen HA+, *Cutis* 57, 431 (scrotum)
Photosensitivity (<1%)
Purpura
(2006): Tamagawa R+, *Arerugi* 55(1), 34
Rash (sic) (<1%)
Urticaria

Mucosal/ENT
Xerostomia (12%)
(1998): Foster M+, *J Clin Dermatol* Winter, 7 (12.5%)
(1990): Kalivas J+, *J Allergy Clin Immunol* 86, 1014

Other
Hypersensitivity
Injection-site necrosis
(1995): Tokodi G+, *J Am Osteopath Assoc* 95, 609
Myalgia/Myositis/Myopathy/Myotoxicity (<1%)

HYOSCYAMINE

Synonyms: Hyoscyamine sulfate; hyoscyamine sulfate
Trade names: Anaspaz; Cytospaz; Donnamar; Duboisine; ED-SPAZ; Egacene Durettes; Egazil; Gastrosed; Hyco; Hycosol Sl; Hyospaz; IB-Stat (InKline); Levbid (Schwarz); Levsin (Schwarz); Levsin/SL (Schwarz); Levsinex (Schwarz); Medispaz; Nulev (Schwarz); Pasmex; Peptard; Setamine; Urised
Indications: Treatment of gastrointestinal tract disorders caused by spasm, Adjunctive therapy for peptic ulcers, cystitis, parkinsonism, biliary & renal colic
Category: Anticholinergic; Muscarinic antagonist
Half-life: N/A
Duration of action: 13–38 min
Clinically important, potentially hazardous interactions with: anticholinergics, arbutamine

Reactions

Skin
Allergic reactions (sic)
Photosensitivity (1–10%)
Rash (sic) (<1%)
Urticaria
Xerosis (>10%)

Mucosal/ENT
Ageusia
Dysgeusia
Mucositis
(2004): Borghaei H+, *Semin Nucl Med* 34(1 Suppl 1), 4
Xerostomia (>10%)

Hair
Hair – alopecia
(2004): Borghaei H+, *Semin Nucl Med* 34(1 Suppl 1), 4

Eyes
Ocular pain
Vision blurred

Other
Anaphylactoid reactions/Anaphylaxis
Asthenia
Headache
Infections
(2004): Borghaei H+, *Semin Nucl Med* 34(1 Suppl 1), 4

Injection-site inflammation (>10%)
Vertigo

IBANDRONATE

Synonyms: Ibandroic acid; Ibandrosaeure; CAS 114084-78-5; BM 21.0955
Trade name: Boniva (Roche)
Indications: Postmenopausal osteoporosis
Category: Bisphosphonate
Half-life: 10–60 hours
Clinically important, potentially hazardous interactions with: None

Reactions

Skin
Allergic reactions (sic) (2.5%)
Diaphoresis
Rash (sic)

Eyes
Scleritis
Uveitis

Other
Fever (~9%)
(2007): Body JJ+, *Ann Oncol* 18(7), 1165
(1996): Pecherstorfer M+, *J Clin Oncol* 14(1), 268
Headache (6.5%)
Hot flashes
Infections
Myalgia/Myositis/Myopathy/Myotoxicity (5.7%)
Upper respiratory infection (33.7%)
Vertigo (3.7%)

IBRITUMOMAB

Synonyms: In-111 Zevalin; Y-90 Zevalin
Trade name: Zevalin (Biogen)
Indications: Non-Hodgkin's lymphoma
Category: Antineoplastic; Monoclonal antibody
Half-life: 30 hours

Reactions

Skin
Allergic reactions (sic) (2%)
Angioedema (5%)
Bullous dermatitis
Diaphoresis (4%)
Erythema multiforme
Exfoliative dermatitis
Peripheral edema (8%)
Petechiae (3%)
Pruritus (9%)
Purpura (7%)
Rash (sic) (8%)
Stevens–Johnson syndrome
Toxic epidermal necrolysis
Urticaria (4%)

Mucosal/ENT

Mucositis
   (2004): Borghaei H+, *Semin Nucl Med* 34(1 Suppl 1), 4

Hair

Hair – alopecia
   (2004): Borghaei H+, *Semin Nucl Med* 34(1 Suppl 1), 4

Other

Anaphylactoid reactions/Anaphylaxis
Chills (24%)
Cough (10%)
Death
Extravasation
   (2006): Williams G+, *Cancer Biother Radiopharm* 21(2), 101
Hypersensitivity
Infections (29%)
   (2004): Borghaei H+, *Semin Nucl Med* 34(1 Suppl 1), 4
   (2003): Hagenbeek A, *Leuk Lymphoma* 44 Suppl 4, S37 (7%)
   (2003): Witzig TE+, *J Clin Oncol* 21(7), 1263 (3%)
Injection-site reactions (sic) (fatal)
Myalgia/Myositis/Myopathy/Myotoxicity (7%)
Pain (13%)

IBUPROFEN

Trade names: Act-3; Actiprofen; Advil (Wyeth); Anco; Apsifen;
Brufen; Ebufac; Genpril; Haltran; Lidifen; Medipren; Midol 220;
Motrin (McNeil); Nuprin; Pamprin; Profen; Proflex; Rufen;
Tabalom; Trendar; Urem; Vicoprofen (Abbott)
Indications: Arthritis, pain
Category: Non-steroidal anti-inflammatory
Half-life: 2–4 hours
**Clinically important, potentially hazardous interactions
with:** aspirin, **boswellia**, ciprofibrate, diuretics, methotrexate,
NSAIDs, oxycodone hydrochloride, salicylates, tacrine,
tacrolimus, urokinase

Reactions

Skin

Acute generalized exanthematous pustulosis (AGEP)
   (2004): Yesudian PD+, *Int J Dermatol* 43(3), 208
Angioedema (<1%)
   (1994): Halpern SM, *Arch Dermatol* 130, 259 (passim)
   (1987): Shelley ED+, *J Am Acad Dermatol* 17, 1057
   (1985): Bigby M+, *J Am Acad Dermatol* 12, 866
   (1984): Stern RS+, *JAMA* 252, 1433
   (1982): Bailin PL+, *Clinics in Rheumatic Diseases* WB Saunders 8,
      493 (passim)
Bullous dermatitis (<1%)
   (1994): Halpern SM, *Arch Dermatol* 130, 259 (passim)
   (1988): Laing VB+, *J Am Acad Dermatol* 19, 91
   (1984): Stern R+, *JAMA* 252, 1433
Bullous pemphigoid
   (1993): Fellner MJ, *Clin Dermatol* 11, 515
   (1981): Pompeova L, *Cesk Dermatol* (Czech) 56, 256
Dermatitis (<1%)
   (1993): Ophaswongse S+, *Contact Dermatitis* 29, 57
   (1986): Veronesi S+, *Contact Dermatitis* 15, 103
   (1985): Valsecchi R+, *Contact Dermatitis* 12, 286
Dermatitis herpetiformis
   (1994): Tousignant J+, *Int J Dermatol* 33, 199
Diaphoresis
Eczema
   (1986): Veronesi S+, *Contact Dermatitis* 15, 103

Edema (<1%)
Erythema multiforme (<1%)
   (2007): Dore J+, *J Burn Care Res* 28(6), 865
   (1995): Lesko SM+, *JAMA* 273, 929
   (1994): Halpern SM, *Arch Dermatol* 130, 259 (passim)
   (1992): Breathnach SM+, *Adverse Drug Reactions and the Skin*
      Blackwell, Oxford, 186 (passim)
   (1985): Bigby M+, *J Am Acad Dermatol* 12, 866
   (1985): O'Brien WM+, *J Rheumatol* 12, 13
   (1984): Stern R+, *JAMA* 252, 1433
Erythema nodosum (1–5%)
   (1994): Halpern SM, *Arch Dermatol* 130, 259 (passim)
Exanthems
   (1994): Halpern SM, *Arch Dermatol* 130, 259 (passim)
   (1994): Litt JZ, Beachwood, OH (personal case) (observation)
   (1985): Bigby M+, *J Am Acad Dermatol* 12, 866
   (1980): Shoenfeld Y+, *JAMA* 244, 547
Fixed eruption (<1%)
   (2007): Fischer G, *J Reprod Med* 52(2), 81 (vulva) (2 cases)
   (2003): Al Aboud K+, *J Drugs Dermatol* 2(6), 658
   (2003): Litt JZ, Beachwood, OH (glans penis) (observation)
   (2003): Litt JZ, Beachwood, OH (personal case) (observation)
   (2001): Diaz Jara M+, *Pediatr Dermatol* 18, 66
   (2000): Zabawski E, Longview, TX (from Internet) (observation)
   (1998): Mahboob A+, *Int J Dermatol* 37, 833
   (1996): Eichwald M, Redding, CA (from Internet) (observation)
   (1994): Shelley WB+, *Cutis* 53, 282 (observation)
   (1992): Breathnach SM+, *Adverse Drug Reactions and the Skin*
      Blackwell, Oxford, 186 (passim)
   (1991): Kuligowski ME+, *Contact Dermatitis* 25, 259
   (1990): Bharija SC+, *Dermatologica* 181, 237
   (1985): Bigby M+, *J Am Acad Dermatol* 12, 866
   (1981): Kanwar AJ 1, *J Dermatol* 11, 383
   (1984): Stern R+, *JAMA* 252, 1433
Lichenoid eruption
   (2004): Danby W, Manchester, NH (from Internet) (observation)
Linear IgA dermatosis
   (2002): Au S+, Vancouver, Canada, March AAD Poster
Livedo reticularis
Lupus erythematosus
   (1996): Vigouroux C+, *Rev Med Interne* (French) 14, 856
   (1985): O'Brien WM+, *J Rheumatol* 12, 13
   (1980): Bar-Sela S+, *J Rheumatol* 7, 379
Pemphigus
   (1988): Laing VB+, *J Am Acad Dermatol* 19, 91
Photosensitivity
   (1994): Berger TG+, *Arch Dermatol* 130, 609 (in HIV-infected) (5
      cases)
   (1994): Halpern SM, *Arch Dermatol* 130, 259 (passim)
   (1992): Bergner T+, *J Am Acad Dermatol* 26, 114
   (1990): Bergner T+, *J Allergy Clin Immunol* 85, 177
   (1985): Bigby M+, *J Am Acad Dermatol* 12, 866
   (1982): Bailin PL+, *Clinics in Rheumatic Diseases* WB Saunders 8,
      493
Pruritus (1–5%)
   (1994): Halpern SM, *Arch Dermatol* 130, 259 (passim)
   (1992): Breathnach SM+, *Adverse Drug Reactions and the Skin*
      Blackwell, Oxford, 186 (passim)
   (1985): Bigby M+, *J Am Acad Dermatol* 12, 866 (1–5%)
Psoriasis (palms)
   (1986): Ben-Chetrit E+, *Cutis* 38, 45 (exacerbation)
   (1985): Bigby M+, *J Am Acad Dermatol* 12, 866
Purpura
Rash (sic) (>10%)
Stevens–Johnson syndrome (<1%)
   (2007): Dore J+, *J Burn Care Res* 28(6), 865
   (2007): Neuman M+, *Transl Res* 149(5), 254
   (1994): Halpern SM, *Arch Dermatol* 130, 259 (passim)
Toxic epidermal necrolysis (<1%)

(2007): Dore J+, *J Burn Care Res* 28(6), 865
(1994): Halpern SM, *Arch Dermatol* 130, 259 (passim)
(1980): Sternlieb P+, *Ann Intern Med* 92, 570
Urticaria (>10%)
(2004): Litt JZ, Beachwood, OH (observation)
(2001): Diaz Jara M+, *Pediatr Dermatol* 18, 66
(1994): Halpern SM, *Arch Dermatol* 130, 259 (passim)
(1993): Litt JZ, Beachwood, OH (personal case) (observation)
(1987): Shelley ED+, *J Am Acad Dermatol* 17, 1057
(1985): Bigby M+, *J Am Acad Dermatol* 12, 866
(1984): Stern RS+, *JAMA* 252, 1433
(1982): Bailin PL+, *Clinics in Rheumatic Diseases* WB Saunders 8, 493 (passim)
Vasculitis
(2001): Davidson KA+, *Cutis* 67, 303 (bullous leukocytoclastic)
(1996): Peters F+, *J Rheumatol* 23, 2008
(1994): Halpern SM, *Arch Dermatol* 130, 259 (passim)
(1992): Breathnach SM+, *Adverse Drug Reactions and the Skin* Blackwell, Oxford, 186 (passim)
(1985): Bigby M+, *J Am Acad Dermatol* 12, 866
(1984): Stern R+, *JAMA* 252, 1433
(1982): Labbe A+, *Ann Dermatol Venereol* (French) 109, 995
Vesiculobullous eruption
(1992): Breathnach SM+, *Adverse Drug Reactions and the Skin* Blackwell, Oxford, 186 (passim)
(1988): Laing VB+, *J Am Acad Dermatol* 19, 91 (passim)
Wound complications
(1988): Proper SA+, *J Am Acad Dermatol* 18, 1173

Mucosal/ENT

Aphthous stomatitis
Gingival ulceration (<1%)
Oral lesions
Oral lichenoid eruption
(1983): Hamburger J+, *BMJ* 287, 1258
Oral ulceration
Stomatitis
Tinnitus
(1998): Davison SP+, *Ear Nose Throat J* 77(10), 820
Xerostomia (<1%)

Hair

Hair – alopecia (<1%)
(1985): O'Brien WM+, *J Rheumatol* 12, 13
Hair – disorders
(1994): Halpern SM, *Arch Dermatol* 130, 259 (passim)

Nails

Nails – changes (sic)
(1994): Halpern SM, *Arch Dermatol* 130, 259 (passim)

Eyes

Eyelid edema
(2005): Bock G, Stockton, CA (from Internet) (observation) (unilateral)
Optic neuritis
(2006): Gamulescu MA+, *Ann Pharmacother* 40(3), 571
Periorbital edema
(2005): Palungwachira P+, *J Dermatol* 32(12), 969
Visual disturbances
(1989): Nicastro NJ, *Ann Ophthalmol* 21(12), 447
(1981): Tullio CJ, *Am J Hosp Pharm* 38(9), 1362

Other

Anaphylactoid reactions/Anaphylaxis (<1%)
(2001): Verma S, Baroda, India (with acetaminophen) (from Internet) (observation)
(2000): Takahama H+, *J Dermatol* 27, 337
(1998): Menendez R+, *Ann Allergy Asthma Immunol* 80, 225
(1985): O'Brien WM+, *J Rheumatol* 12, 13

Aseptic meningitis
(2006): Cano Vargas-Machuca E+, *Rev Neurol* 42(4), 217
(2006): Rodriguez SC+, *Medicine* (Baltimore) 85(4), 214 (2 cases)
(2004): Hidalgo Natera A+, *Med Clin* (Barc) 122(17), 678
(2004): Nguyen HT+, *Ann Pharmacother* 38(3), 408
(2002): Lee RZ+, *Rheumatology* (Oxford) 41(3), 353
(1999): Pisani E+, *Ital J Neurol Sci* 20(1), 59
(1993): Colamarino R+, *Therapie* 48(5), 516
(1989): Gilbert GJ+, *South Med J* 82(4), 514
(1987): Jensen S+, *Acta Med Scand* 221(5), 509
(1983): Treves R+, *Rev Rhum Mal Osteoartic* 50(1), 75
(1980): Giansiracusa DF+, *Arch Intern Med* 140(11), 1553
Death
(2001): Stevenson R+, *Scott Med J* 46(3), 84
DRESS syndrome
(2001): Descamps V+, *Arch Dermatol* 137, 301
Embolia cutis medicamentosa (Nicolau syndrome)
(2003): Reding EL+, *J Am Acad Dermatol* 48(3), 472 (passim)
(2001): Corazza M+, *J Eur Acad Dermatol Venereol* 15(6), 585
Fever
(2006): Gonzalo-Garijo MA+, *J Investig Allergol Clin Immunol* 16(4), 266
Gynecomastia (<1%)
Headache
Hot flashes (<1%)
Hypersensitivity
(2006): Mou SS+, *J Rheumatol* 33(1), 171
(2001): McMahon AD+, *J Clin Epidemiol* 54(12), 1271
(1981): Ruppert GB+, *South Med J* 74, 241
Myalgia/Myositis/Myopathy/Myotoxicity
(1987): Ross NS+, *JAMA* 257, 62
Paresthesias
Pseudolymphoma
(2001): Werth V, *Dermatology Times* 18
Pseudoporphyria
(2000): De Silva B+, *Pediatr Dermatol* 17, 480
(1992): Petersen CS+, *Ugeskr Laeger* (Danish) 154, 1713
Rhabdomyolysis
(2007): Nelson H+, *Pharmacotherapy* 27(4), 608 (overdose)
(1997): Ramachandran S+, *BMJ* 1997 May 31; 314(7094), 1593 (with ciprofibrate)
(1989): Menzies DG+, *Med Toxicol Adverse* 4(6), 468
Serum sickness
(1995): Lesko SM+, *JAMA* 273, 929

IBUTILIDE

Trade name: Corvert (Pfizer)
Indications: Atrial fibrillation and flutter
Category: Antiarrhythmic class III
Half-life: 2–12 hours

Reactions

Skin

Bullous dermatitis
(1998): Dodds ES+, *Pharmacotherapy* 18, 880

Other

Headache

ICODEXTRIN

Trade name: Extraneal (Baxter)
Indications: Peritoneal dialysis (continuous, ambulatory)
Category: Dialysis solution
Half-life: N/A
Clinically important, potentially hazardous interactions with: None

Reactions

Skin

Acute generalized exanthematous pustulosis (AGEP)
 (2001): Al-Hoqail IA+, *Br J Dermatol* 145(6), 1026
 (2001): Valance A+, *Arch Dermatol* 137(3), 309
Allergic reactions (sic) (>5%)
Eczema (<5%)
Edema (6%)
Erythema multiforme (<5%)
Exanthems
 (2002): Ekart R+, *Acta Med Croatica* 56(4-5), 185
 (2001): Valance A+, *Arch Dermatol* 137(3), 309
Exfoliative dermatitis (<5%)
 (2002): Ekart R+, *Acta Med Croatica* 56(4-5), 185
Facial edema (<5%)
Peripheral edema (>5%)
Pruritus (>5%)
Rash (sic)
 (2003): Frampton JE+, *Drugs* 63(19), 2079 (5%)
Vesiculobullous eruption (<5%)

Other

Abdominal pain (8%)
Asthenia (>5%)
Chest pain (5%)
Cough (7%)
Headache (9%)
Hypotension (>5%)
Infections (>5%)
Pain (>5%)
Upper respiratory infection (15%)
Vertigo (>5%)

IDARUBICIN

Synonyms: 4-demethoxydaunorubicin; 4-DMDR
Trade names: Idamycin (Pfizer); Zavedos
Indications: Acute myeloid leukemia
Category: Antibiotic, anthracycline
Half-life: 14–35 hours (oral)
Clinically important, potentially hazardous interactions with: aldesleukin

Reactions

Skin

Acral erythema
 (1993): Cohen PR, *Cutis* 51, 175
Bullous dermatitis (palms and soles)
Exanthems (<1%)
Neutrophilic dermatosis
 (2008): Uhara H+, *J Am Acad Dermatol* 59(2), S10 (with cytarabine)

Photo-recall
 (1995): Gabel C+, *Gynecol Oncol* 57, 266
Rash (sic) (>10%)
 (1998): Stuart NS+, *Cancer Chemother Pharmacol* 21, 351
 (1997): Maloney DG+, *J Clin Oncol* 15, 3266
Urticaria (>10%)
 (1997): Maloney DG+, *J Clin Oncol* 15, 3266

Mucosal/ENT

Mucositis (50%)
 (2000): Creutzig U+, *Klin Padiatr* 212, 163
 (1986): Dodion P+, *Invest New Drugs* 4, 31
Stomatitis (>10%)

Hair

Hair – alopecia (77%)
 (2000): No author, *Prescrire Int* 9, 103
 (1993): Ogawa M+, *Gan To Kaguku Ryoho* (Japanese) 20, 897
 (1993): Ogawa M+, *Gan To Kaguku Ryoho* (Japanese) 20, 907
 (1991): Hollingshead LM+, *Drugs* 42, 690
 (1988): Gillies H+, *Cancer Chemother Pharmacol* 21, 261
 (1986): Dodion P+, *Invest New Drugs* 4, 31
 (1986): Lopez M+, *Invest New Drugs* 4, 39

Nails

Nails – pigmentation
 (1997): Borecky Derrick J+, *Cutis* 59, 203

Other

Injection-site urticaria

IDEBENONE

Synonym: 6-(10-hydroxydecyl)-2,3-dimethoxy-5-methyl-1,4-benzoquinone
Trade names: Avan; Mnesis
Indications: Alzheimer's dementia, cardiovascular disease, cerebrovascular disease, demyelination, depression, Friedreich's ataxia, improving memory, Leber's hereditary optic neuropathy
Category: Coenzyme Q10 analog
Half-life: N/A
Clinically important, potentially hazardous interactions with: None

Reactions

None

IDURSULFASE

Trade name: Elaprase (Shire)
Indications: Hunter syndrome, Mucopolysaccharidosis II
Category: Enzyme
Half-life: 46 minutes
Clinically important, potentially hazardous interactions with: N/A

Reactions

Skin

Pruritus (28%)
Rash (sic) (13%)
Urticaria (16%)

Eyes
Visual disturbances (22%)

Other
Anaphylactoid reactions/Anaphylaxis
Application-site edema (13%)
Asthenia (22%)
Chest pain (16%)
Fever (63%)
Headache (59%)
Hypersensitivity
Hypertension (25%)

IFOSFAMIDE

Trade names: Holoxan; Ifex (Bristol-Myers Squibb); Ifoxan;
Mitoxana; Tronoxal
Indications: Cancers, sarcomas, leukemias, lymphomas
Category: Alkylating agent
Half-life: 4–15 hours
**Clinically important, potentially hazardous interactions
with:** aldesleukin, aprepitant

Reactions

Skin
Allergic reactions (sic) (1–10%)
Dermatitis (1–10%)
Pigmentation (1–10%)
  (1994): Yule SM+, *Cancer* 73, 240
  (1993): Teresi ME+, *Cancer* 71, 2873

Mucosal/ENT
Oral lesions
Sialorrhea (<1%)
Stomatitis (<1%)

Hair
Hair – alopecia (50–100%)
  (1988): Negretti E+, *Tumori* (Italian) 74, 163 (100%)

Nails
Nails – ridging (1–10%)
  (1994): Ben Dayan D+, *Acta Haematol* 91, 89

Other
Anaphylactoid reactions/Anaphylaxis
Death
  (2002): Escudier B+, *J Urol* 168(3), 959 (with doxorubicin)
Inappropriate secretion of antidiuretic hormone (SIADH)
  (1997): Kirch C+, *Eur J Cancer* 33(14), 2438
Nephrotoxicity
  (2005): Aleksa K+, *Pediatr Nephrol* 20(7), 872
  (2005): Benesic A+, *Kidney Int* 68(5), 2029
  (2005): Berrak SG+, *Pediatr Blood Cancer* 44(3), 215
  (2005): Ferrari S+, *J Clin Oncol* 23(34), 8845 (10%)
  (2005): Zielinska E+, *J Pediatr Hematol Oncol* 27(11), 582
  (2004): McCune JS+, *Pediatr Blood Cancer* 42(5), 427
  (2004): Rogowska E+, *Med Wieku Rozwoj* 8(2 Pt 1), 289
  (2003): Miyazaki J+, *Nippon Rinsho* 61(6), 973
  (2003): Skinner R, *Med Pediatr Oncol* 41(3), 190
  (2001): Aleksa K+, *Pediatr Nephrol* 16(12), 1153
  (2001): Caglar M+, *Nucl Med Commun* 22(12), 1325
  (2001): Kerbusch T+, *Clin Pharmacokinet* 40(1), 41
  (2001): Kintzel PE, *Drug Saf* 24(1), 19
  (2001): Lee BS+, *Pediatr Nephrol* 16(10), 796

  (2000): Gerke P+, *J Cancer Res Clin Oncol* 126(3), 173
  (1999): Ferrari S+, *Anticancer Drugs* 10(1), 25 (mild)
  (1999): Loebstein R+, *J Clin Pharmacol* 39(5), 454 (9%)
  (1999): Rossi R+, *Med Pediatr Oncol* 32(3), 177
  (1998): Koch Nogueira PC+, *Pediatr Nephrol* 12(7), 572
  (1998): Loebstein R+, *Pediatrics* 101(6), E8
  (1998): MacLean FR+, *Cancer Chemother Pharmacol* 41(5), 413
  (1997): Ashraf MS+, *Med Pediatr Oncol* 28(1), 62
  (1997): Beyer J+, *Bone Marrow Transplant* 20(10), 813
  (1997): Foxall PJ+, *Clin Cancer Res* 3(9), 1507
  (1997): Rossi R, *Nephrol Dial Transplant* 12(6), 1091
  (1997): Tesar V+, *Cas Lek Cesk* 136(7), 205
  (1997): Tokuc G+, *J Exp Clin Cancer Res* 16(2), 227
Neurotoxicity
  (2006): Dufour C+, *Arch Pediatr* 13(2), 140
  (2006): Kerdudo C+, *Pediatr Blood Cancer* 47(1), 100
  (2005): Zielinska E+, *J Pediatr Hematol Oncol* 27(11), 582
  (2001): Kerbusch T+, *Clin Pharmacokinet* 40(1), 41
  (1997): Foxall PJ+, *Clin Cancer Res* 3(9), 1507
Phlebitis (2%)
Seizures
  (2006): Kerdudo C+, *Pediatr Blood Cancer* 47(1), 100
  (2006): Kilickap S+, *Ann Pharmacother* 40(2), 332

ILOPROST

Trade name: Ventavis (Schering) (Cotherix)
Indications: Pulmonary arterial hypertension, peripheral
neuropathy
Category: Prostaglandin; Vasodilator
Half-life: 20–30 minutes
**Clinically important, potentially hazardous interactions
with:** anticoagulants

Reactions

Skin
Peripheral edema

Other
Chest pain
  (1992): Wigley FM+, *J Rheumatol* 19(9), 1407
Cough (39%)
  (2004): Goldsmith DR+, *Drugs* 64(7), 763
  (2000): Hoeper MM+, *N Engl J Med* 342(25), 1866
Headache (30%)
  (2004): Goldsmith DR+, *Drugs* 64(7), 763
  (2004): Zulian F+, *Rheumatology (Oxford)* 43(2), 229
  (2000): Hoeper MM+, *N Engl J Med* 342(25), 1866
  (1998): Arosio E+, *Eur Rev Med Pharmacol Sci* 2(2), 53
  (1996): Staben P+, *Prostaglandins Leukot Essent Fatty Acids*
    54(5), 327
  (1996): Zachariae H+, *Acta Derm Venereol* 76(3), 236
  (1993): Kecsker A+, *Arzneimittelforschung* 43(4), 450
  (1993): Poggesi L+, *Ann Ital Med Int 1993 Oct* 8 Suppl, 71S
  (1992): Wigley FM+, *J Rheumatol* 19(9), 1407
  (1991): Shindo H+, *Prostaglandins* 41(1), 85
  (1990): Brock FE+, *Schweiz Med Wochenschr* 120(40), 1477
  (1990): Norgren L+, *Eur J Vasc Surg* 4(5), 463
Hypotension (11%)
  (2004): Zulian F+, *Rheumatology (Oxford)* 43(2), 229
  (1993): Poggesi L+, *Ann Ital Med Int 1993 Oct* 8 Suppl, 71S
Injection-site reactions
  (2004): Zulian F+, *Rheumatology (Oxford)* 43(2), 229
Myalgia/Myositis/Myopathy/Myotoxicity (6%)
Vertigo (8%)

IMATINIB

Synonyms: CGP57148; ST1571; STi571
Trade names: Gleevec (Novartis); Glivec
Indications: Chronic myeloid leukemia
Category: Tyrosine kinase inhibitor
Half-life: 18 hours
**Clinically important, potentially hazardous interactions
with:** amlodipine, anisindione, anticoagulants, aprepitant,
atorvastatin, barbiturates, benzodiazepines, butabarbital,
carbamazepine, chlordiazepoxide, clarithromycin, clonazepam,
clorazepate, corticosteroids, cyclosporine, dexamethasone,
diazepam, dicumarol, erythromycin, ethotoin, felodipine,
flurazepam, fluvastatin, fosphenytoin, isradipine, itraconazole,
ketoconazole, lorazepam, lovastatin, mephenytoin,
mephobarbital, midazolam, nicardipine, nifedipine, nimodipine,
nisoldipine, oxazepam, pentobarbital, phenobarbital, pimozide,
pravastatin, primidone, quazepam, rifampin, secobarbital,
simvastatin, **St John's wort**, temazepam, warfarin

Reactions

Skin

Acne
   (2006): Martin JM+, *J Eur Acad Dermatol Venereol* 20(10), 1368
   (2005): Emmet S, San Diego, CA (from Internet) (observation)
Acute febrile neutrophilic dermatosis (Sweet's syndrome)
   (2005): Ayirookuzhi SJ+, *Arch Dermatol* 141(3), 368
Acute generalized exanthematous pustulosis (AGEP)
   (2006): Nelson RP Jr+, *Ann Allergy Asthma Immunol* 97(2), 216
   (2006): Scheinfeld N, *J Drugs Dermatol* 5(3), 228
   (2002): Schwarz M+, *Eur J Haematol* 69(4), 254 (2 cases)
   (2001): Brouard MC+, *Dermatology* 203(1), 57
Carcinoma
   (2005): Breccia M+, *Eur J Haematol* 74(2), 121
Dermatomyositis
   (2006): Kuwano Y+, *Int J Dermatol* 45(10), 1249
Eccrine squamous syringometaplasia
   (2006): Van de Voorde K+, *J Am Acad Dermatol* 55(2), S58
Edema (1–5%)
   (2006): Scheinfeld N, *J Drugs Dermatol* 5(3), 228
   (2005): Modi S+, *Breast Cancer Res* 90(2), 157 (38%)
   (2005): Severino G+, *Ann Pharmacother* 39(1), 162
   (2004): Curran MP+, *BioDrugs* 18(3), 207
   (2003): *Prescrire Int* 12(64), 49 (2%)
   (2003): Shimazaki C+, *Leukemia* 17(4), 804
   (2003): Valeyrie L+, *J Am Acad Dermatol* 48(2), 201 (35 cases)
   (2002): Dagher R+, *Clin Cancer Res* 8(10), 3034
   (2002): Demetri GD+, *N Engl J Med* 347(7), 472
   (2002): Pindolia VK+, *Pharmacotherapy* 22(10), 1249
   (2002): Tefferi A+, *Blood* 99(10), 3854
   (2001): van Oosterom AT+, *Lancet* 358(9291), 1421
Erythema
   (2006): Scheinfeld N, *J Drugs Dermatol* 5(3), 228
   (2005): Sugito M+, *Rinsho Ketsueki* 46(11), 1226
   (2003): Duncan E+, *Br J Haematol* 122(1), 1
   (2003): Pasmatzi E+, *Acta Derm Venereol* 83(5), 391
Erythroderma
   (2007): Vano-Galvan S+, *Eur J Dermatol* 17(6), 538
   (2006): Oztas P+, *Acta Derm Venereol* 86(2), 174
Exanthems
   (2006): Nelson RP Jr+, *Ann Allergy Asthma Immunol* 97(2), 216
   (2006): Scheinfeld N, *J Drugs Dermatol* 5(3), 228
   (2004): Park MA+, *Allergy Asthma Proc* 25(5), 345
   (2003): Dogra S+, *Natl Med J India* 16(5), 285
   (2002): Dagher R+, *Clin Cancer Res* 8(10), 3034

Exfoliative dermatitis
   (2006): Nelson RP Jr+, *Ann Allergy Asthma Immunol* 97(2), 216
   (2003): Tanvetyanon T+, *Ann Pharmacother* 37(12), 1818
Hypomelanosis
   (2006): Brazzelli V+, *Pediatr Dermatol* 23(2), 175
   (2005): McPartlin S+, *Br J Haematol* 129(4), 448
   (2004): Grossman WJ+, *J Pediatr Hematol Oncol* 26(3), 214
   (2003): Tsao AS+, *Cancer* 98(11), 2483
Lichen planus
   (2004): Roux C+, *Ann Dermatol Venereol* 131(6-7 Pt 1), 571
Lichenoid eruption
   (2007): Chan CY+, *Dermatol Online J* 13(2), 29
   (2006): Dalmau J+, *Br J Dermatol* 154(6), 1213
   (2006): Scheinfeld N, *J Drugs Dermatol* 5(3), 228
   (2005): Prabhash K+, *Indian J Derm, Venereol Leprol* 71(4), 287
Mycosis fungoides
   (2006): Scheinfeld N, *J Drugs Dermatol* 5(3), 228
Necrolysis
   (2003): Schaich M+, *Ann Hematol* 82(5), 303
Neutrophilic eccrine hidradenitis
   (2006): Scheinfeld N, *J Drugs Dermatol* 5(3), 228
   (2005): Dib EG+, *Leuk Res* 29(2), 233
Palmar–plantar hyperkeratosis
   (2006): Deguchi N+, *Br J Dermatol* 154(6), 1216
Peripheral edema
Petechiae (1–10%)
Photosensitivity
   (2003): Rousselot P+, *Br J Haematol* 120(6), 1091
Pigmentation
   (2006): Scheinfeld N, *J Drugs Dermatol* 5(3), 228
   (2004): Arora B+, *Ann Oncol* 15(2), 358
Pityriasis rosea
   (2006): Scheinfeld N, *J Drugs Dermatol* 5(3), 228
   (2005): Brazzelli V+, *J Am Acad Dermatol* 53(5 Suppl 1), S240
   (2003): Pasmatzi E+, *Acta Derm Venereol* 83(5), 391
   (2002): Konstantopoulos K+, *Dermatology* 205(2), 172
Pruritus (6–10%)
   (2003): Valeyrie L+, *J Am Acad Dermatol* 48(2), 201 (22 cases)
Psoriasis
   (2005): Shimizu K+, *Rinsho Ketsueki* 46(10), 1152
Rash (sic) (32–39%)
   (2005): Breccia M+, *Eur J Haematol* 74(2), 121
   (2005): Modi S+, *Breast Cancer Res Treat* 90(2), 157 (25%)
   (2005): Severino G+, *Ann Pharmacother* 39(1), 162
   (2004): Curran MP+, *BioDrugs* 18(3), 207
   (2003): Valeyrie L+, *J Am Acad Dermatol* 48(2), 201 (36 cases)
   (2003): Verweij J+, *Eur J Cancer* 39(14), 2006 (69%)
   (2001): van Oosterom+, *Lancet* 358(9291), 1421
Squamous cell carcinoma
   (2003): Baskaynak G+, *Eur J Haematol* 70(4), 231
Stevens–Johnson syndrome
   (2006): Nelson RP Jr+, *Ann Allergy Asthma Immunol* 97(2), 216
   (2006): Scheinfeld N, *J Drugs Dermatol* 5(3), 228
   (2005): Pavithran K+, *Indian J Dermatol Venereol Leprol* 71(4), 288
   (2005): Severino G+, *Ann Pharmacother* 39(1), 162 (with lansoprazole)
   (2002): Hsiao LT+, *Br J Haematol* 117(3), 620
   (2002): Vidal D+, *Br J Haematol* 119(1), 274
Toxic epidermal necrolysis
   (2006): Scheinfeld N, *J Drugs Dermatol* 5(3), 228
Toxicity (sic)
   (2003): Ugurel S+, *Br J Cancer* 88(8), 1157
Urticaria
   (2006): Nelson RP Jr+, *Ann Allergy Asthma Immunol* 97(2), 216
Vasculitis
   (2006): Scheinfeld N, *J Drugs Dermatol* 5(3), 228

Mucosal/ENT

Oral lichenoid eruption
  (2004): Ena P+, J Dermatol Treatment 15(4), 253
  (2002): Lim DS+, Dermatology 205(2), 169

Hair

Hair – follicular mucinosis
  (2006): Scheinfeld N, J Drugs Dermatol 5(3), 228
  (2004): Yanagi T+, Br J Dermatol 151(6), 1276

Nails

Nails – dystrophy
  (2006): Deguchi N+, Br J Dermatol 154(6), 1216
Nails – pigmentation
  (2006): Prabhash K+, Indian J Dermatol Venereol Leprol 72(1), 63

Eyes

Epiphora
  (2003): Fraunfelder FW+, J Ocul Pharmacol Ther 19(4), 371
    (18%)
Eyelid edema
  (2004): Maalouf T+, J Fr Ophtalmol 27(1), 107
Macular edema
  (2005): Masood I+, J Cataract Refract Surg 31(12), 2427
Periorbital edema
  (2006): Scheinfeld N, J Drugs Dermatol 5(3), 228
  (2003): Fraunfelder FW+, J Ocul Pharmacol Ther 19(4), 371
    (70%)
  (2003): Ramar K+, J Clin Oncol 21(1), 172
  (2003): Verweij J+, Eur J Cancer 39(14), 2006 (84%)
  (2002): Esmaeli B+, Cancer 95(4), 881

Other

Asthenia
  (2005): Modi S+, Breast Cancer Res Treat 90(2), 157 (56%)
  (2003): Prescrire Int 12(68), 216
  (2003): Verweij J+, Eur J Cancer 39(14), 2006 (76%)
  (2002): Demetri GD+, N Engl J Med 347(7), 472
Cardiotoxicity
  (2006): Kerkela R+, Nat Med 12(8), 908
Depression
  (2003): Prescrire Int 12(68), 216
DRESS syndrome
  (2006): Le Nouail P+, Ann Dermatol Venereol 133(8-9 Pt 1), 686
Gynecomastia (male)
  (2003): Gambacorti-Passerini C+, Lancet 361(9373), 1954
Headache
Hematotoxicity
Hepatotoxicity
  (2006): Cross TJ+, Am J Hematol 81(3), 189
  (2006): Ikeda K+, Leuk Lymphoma 47(1), 155
Myalgia/Myositis/Myopathy/Myotoxicity
  (2004): Curran MP+, BioDrugs 18(3), 207
  (2003): Prescrire Int 12(64), 49
  (2002): Dagher R+, Clin Cancer Res 8(10), 3034
  (2002): Tefferi A+, Blood 99(10), 3854
Panniculitis
  (2003): Ugurel S+, Br J Dermatol 149, 678
Porphyria cutanea tarda
  (2004): Breccia M+, Leukemia 18(1), 182
  (2003): Ho AY+, Br J Haematol 121(2), 375
Pseudolymphoma
  (2006): Scheinfeld N, J Drugs Dermatol 5(3), 228

IMIDAPRIL

Trade names: Cardipril; Novarok; Tanatril (Trinity Pharmaceuticals Ltd)
Indications: Hypertension
Category: Angiotensin-converting enzyme inhibitor
Half-life: 2 hours
Clinically important, potentially hazardous interactions with: allopurinol, azathioprine, procainamide

Reactions

Skin

Angioedema
Pruritus
  (2002): Zweiker R+, Acta Med Austriaca 29(2), 72
Rash (sic)

Mucosal/ENT

Dysgeusia

Eyes

Vision blurred

Other

Abdominal pain
Asthenia
Cough
  (2007): Robinson DM+, Drugs 67(9), 1359
  (2007): Tumanan-Mendoza BA+, J Clin Epidemiol 60(6), 547
  (2002): Zweiker R+, Acta Med Austriaca 29(2), 72
  (2001): Huang PJ+, Cardiology 95(3), 146
  (1998): Shionoiri H+, J Clin Pharmacol 38(5), 442
  (1995): Saruta T+, J Hypertens Suppl 13(3), 523
Headache
  (2002): Zweiker R+, Acta Med Austriaca 29(2), 72
Hypotension
Somnolence
Vertigo
  (2002): Zweiker R+, Acta Med Austriaca 29(2), 72

IMIGLUCERASE

Trade name: Cerezyme (Genzyme)
Indications: Gaucher's disease
Category: Enzyme
Half-life: 3.6–10.4 hours
Clinically important, potentially hazardous interactions with: None

Reactions

Skin

Angioedema (<1.5%)
Diaphoresis
  (1999): Aviner S+, Blood Cells Mol Dis 25(5), 90
Peripheral edema
Pruritus (<1.5%)
Rash (sic) (6.5%)
Urticaria (<1.5%)

Other

Abdominal pain
Anaphylactoid reactions/Anaphylaxis (<1%) (2 cases)
  (1999): Aviner S+, Blood Cells Mol Dis 25(2), 92

Asthenia (6.5%)
Chest pain
  (1999): Aviner S+, *Blood Cells Mol Dis* 25(5), 90
Chills (6.5%)
Cough
  (1999): Aviner S+, *Blood Cells Mol Dis* 25(5), 90
Headache (6.5%)
Hypersensitivity (6.6%)
Injection-site burning (<1.5%)
Injection-site edema (<1.5%)
Injection-site pruritus (<1.5%)
Vertigo (6.5%)

IMIPENEM/CILASTATIN

Synonym: imipemide
Trade names: Primaxin (Merck); Tenacid; Tienam; Tienam 500; Zienam
Indications: Various infections caused by susceptible organisms
Category: Antibiotic, beta-lactam; Thienamycin
Half-life: 1 hour
Clinically important, potentially hazardous interactions with: amoxicillin, ampicilin, azlocillin, bacampicillin, carbenicillin, cloxacillin, cyclosporine, dicloxacillin, ganciclovir, methicillin, mezlocillin, nafcillin, oxacillin, penicillin g, penicillin V, piperacillin, ticaracillin

Reactions

Skin
Acute generalized exanthematous pustulosis (AGEP)
  (1989): Escallier F I, *Ann Dermatol Venereol* (French) 116, 407
Allergic reactions (sic) (1–3%)
  (1994): Pleasants RA+, *Chest* 106, 1124 (in patients with cystic fibrosis)
Angioedema (0.2%)
  (1987): Clissold SP+, *Drugs* 33, 183
Diaphoresis (0.2%)
Erythema multiforme (0.2%)
  (1987): Clissold SP+, *Drugs* 33, 183
Exanthems (1–5%)
  (1989): Escallier F+, *Ann Dermatol Venereol* (French) 116, 407
  (1987): Clissold SP+, *Drugs* 33, 183
  (1985): Calandra GB+, *Am J Med* 78, 73 (1–5%)
Pruritus (0.3%)
  (1991): Machado ARL+, *J Allergy Clin Immunol* 87, 754
  (1989): Escallier F+, *Ann Dermatol Venereol* (French) 116, 407
  (1987): Clissold SP+, *Drugs* 33, 183
Pruritus ani et vulvae (0.2%)
Pustules
  (1994): Spencer JM+, *Br J Dermatol* 130, 514
Rash (sic) (4%)
  (1994): Grayson ML+, *Clin Infect Dis* 18, 683
Stevens–Johnson syndrome
  (2005): Ely EH, Grass Valley, CA (from Internet) (observation)
Toxic epidermal necrolysis (0.2%)
Urticaria (0.2%)
  (1991): Hantson P+, *BMJ* 302, 294
  (1989): Escallier F+, *Ann Dermatol Venereol* (French) 116, 407
  (1987): Clissold SP+, *Drugs* 33, 183
Vasculitis
  (1997): Reiner MR+, *J Am Podiatr Med Assoc* 87, 245

Mucosal/ENT
Dysgeusia (0.2%)
Glossitis (0.2%)
Oral lesions
Sialorrhea (0.2%)
Tinnitus

Other
Candidiasis (0.2%)
Hypersensitivity
  (1988): Donowitz GR+, *N Engl J Med* 318, 490
Injection-site erythema (0.4%)
Injection-site pain (<1%)
  (1991): *Drug Ther Bull* 29, 43
  (1985): Calandra GB+, *Am J Med* 78, 73 (0.7%)
Injection-site phlebitis (<4%)
  (1991): *Drug Ther Bull* 29, 43
  (1988): Gould IM+, *Drugs Exp Clin Res* 14, 555
  (1987): Clissold SP+, *Drugs* 33, 183 (2%)
  (1985): Calandra GB+, *Am J Med* 78, 73 (3.8%)
Paresthesias (0.2%)
Phlebitis (3%)
Seizures
  (2003): Reuther LO+, *Ugeskr Laeger* 165(14), 1447
Thrombophlebitis (3.1%)

IMIPRAMINE

Trade names: Apo-Imipramine; Imidol; Imipramin; Impril; Novo-Pramine; Primonil; Pryleugan; Tofranil (Mallinckrodt) (Novartis)
Indications: Depression
Category: Antidepressant, tricyclic; Muscarinic antagonist
Half-life: 6–18 hours
Clinically important, potentially hazardous interactions with: amprenavir, arbutamine, clonidine, darifenacin, epinephrine, fluoxetine, formoterol, guanethidine, isocarboxazid, linezolid, MAO inhibitors, phenelzine, quinolones, sparfloxacin, tranylcypromine, zaleplon

Reactions

Skin
Acne
Allergic reactions (sic)
Angioedema (<1%)
Bullous dermatitis
Diaphoresis (1–25%)
  (2002): Mavissakalian M+, *J Clin Psychopharmacol* 22(2), 155
  (1990): Leeman CP, *J Clin Psychiatry* 51, 258
  (1989): Butt MM, *J Clin Psychiatry* 50, 146
Edema
Erythema
Exanthems (1–6%)
  (1992): Breathnach SM+, *Adverse Drug Reactions and the Skin* Blackwell, Oxford, 197 (passim)
  (1988): Warnock JK+, *Am J Psychiatry* 145, 425 (6%)
  (1985): Walter-Ryan WG+, *JAMA* 254, 357
Exfoliative dermatitis
  (1992): Breathnach SM+, *Adverse Drug Reactions and the Skin* Blackwell, Oxford, 197 (passim)
Fixed eruption (<1%)
Lichen planus
Lupus erythematosus
Peripheral edema
Petechiae
Photosensitivity (<1%)

(1985): Walter-Ryan WG+, *JAMA* 354, 357

Pigmentation
(2005): Mendhekar DN, *Indian J Med Sci* 59(9), 405
(2005): Metelitsa AI+, *J Cutan Med Surg* 9(6), 341
(2003): Dean CE+, *Ann Pharmacother* 37(6), 825
(2002): Angel TA+, *Int J Dermatol* 41(6), 327 (slate gray)
(photodistributed)
(2000): Atkin DH+, *J Am Acad Dermatol* 43(1 Pt 1), 77
(1999): Ming ME+, *J Am Acad Dermatol* 40, 159 (4 cases)
(1999): Sicari MC+, *J Am Acad Dermatol* 40(2), 290 (slate gray)
(2 cases)
(1991): Hashimoto K+, *J Am Acad Dermatol* 25, 357 (slate-gray)
(1990): Goldberg NC, *Dermatology Perspectives* 6, 8
(1989): Hashimoto K+, *Am Soc Dermatopath* San Francisco, CA
(abstract)
(1988): Warnock JK+, *Am J Psychiatry* 145, 425

Pruritus (3%)
(1988): Warnock JK+, *Am J Psychiatry* 145, 425 (3%)
(1987): Pohl R+, *Am J Psychiatry* 144, 237

Purpura
(1988): Warnock JK+, *Am J Psychiatry* 145, 425

Rash (sic)
Urticaria
(1992): Breathnach SM+, *Adverse Drug Reactions and the Skin*
Blackwell, Oxford, 197 (passim)
(1987): Pohl R+, *Am J Psychiatry* 144, 237
(1985): Burnett GB+, *South Med J* 78, 71

Vasculitis
(1992): Breathnach SM+, *Adverse Drug Reactions and the Skin*
Blackwell, Oxford, 197 (passim)

Xerosis

Mucosal/ENT

Dysgeusia (>10%) (metallic taste)
Glossitis
(1992): Breathnach SM+, *Adverse Drug Reactions and the Skin*
Blackwell, Oxford, 197 (passim)
Glossodynia
Hypogeusia
Mucosal membrane desquamation
Oral lesions
Oral ulceration
Stomatitis
(1992): Breathnach SM+, *Adverse Drug Reactions and the Skin*
Blackwell, Oxford, 197 (passim)
Tinnitus
(1989): Laird LK+, *J Clin Psychiatry* 50(4), 146
(1987): *J Clin Psychiatry* 48(12), 496
(1987): Tandon R+, *J Clin Psychiatry* 48(3), 109
(1987): Tandon R+, *J Clin Psychiatry* 48(3), 109 (5 cases)
(1980): Racy J+, *Am J Psychiatry* 137(7), 854
Tongue black
Vaginitis
Xerostomia (>10%)
(2004): Akhondzadeh S+, *BMC Complement Altern Med* 4, 12
(2002): Mavissakalian M+, *J Clin Psychopharmacol* 22(2), 155
(1997): Berzewski H+, *Eur Neuropsychopharmacol* 7 Suppl 1, S37
(1985): Cohn JB+, *J Clin Psychiatry* 46(3 Pt 2), 26
(1984): Bremner JD+, *J Clin Psychiatry* 45(4 Pt 2), 56
(1984): Garvey MJ+, *Am J Psychiatry* 141(7), 853
(1981): Rafaelsen OJ+, *Acta Psychiatr Scand Suppl* 290, 364

Hair

Hair – alopecia (<1%)
(1994): Friedman M, *J Fam Pract* 39, 114
(1991): Warnock JK+, *J Nerv Ment Dis* 179, 441
Hair – alopecia areata
(1987): Baral J+, *Int J Dermatol* 26, 198

Nails

Nails – parrot-beak

Other

Gynecomastia (<1%)
Inappropriate secretion of antidiuretic hormone (SIADH)
(1993): Colgate R, *Br J Psychiatry* 163, 819
(1992): Bozzolo M+, *Schweiz Rundsch Med Prax* 81(47), 1435
(1986): Mitsch RA+, *Drug Intell Clin Pharm* 20(10), 787
(1984): Liskin B+, *J Clin Psychopharmacol* 4(3), 146
Paresthesias
Tremor

IMIQUIMOD

Trade name: Aldara (3M)
Indications: External genital and perianal warts
Category: Antiviral; Immunomodulator
Half-life: N/A

Reactions

Skin

Angioedema
(2004): Barton JC, *J Am Acad Dermatol* 2004 Sep 51(3), 477
Bullous dermatitis
(2002): Chen TM+, *Dermatol Surg* 28, 344 (for BCCs)
Burning (9–31%)
(2006): *Prescrire Int* 15(84), 130
(2003): Bayerl C+, *Br J Dermatol* 149 Suppl 66, 25 (23%)
(2001): Gollnick H+, *Int J STD AIDS* 12(1), 22
(1999): Perry CM+, *Drugs* 58(2), 375
(1998): Beutner KR+, *J Am Acad Dermatol* 38(2), 230 (31.3%)
Crusting
(2006): Hadley G+, *J Invest Dermatol* 126(6), 1251 (21%)
(2005): Nikkels AF+, *Acta Clin Belg* 60(5), 227
Eczema
(2006): Taylor CL+, *Sex Transm Infect* 82(3), 227 (from topical)
Edema (12–17%)
(2006): Hadley G+, *J Invest Dermatol* 126(6), 1251 (4%)
(2004): Marchitelli C+, *J Reprod Med* 49(11), 876 (12.5%)
Erosions (10–32%)
(2006): Hadley G+, *J Invest Dermatol* 126(6), 1251 (6%)
(2004): Marchitelli C+, *J Reprod Med* 49(11), 876 (12.5%)
(1999): Perry CM+, *Drugs* 58(2), 375
(1998): Beutner KR+, *J Am Acad Dermatol* 38(2), 230 (10.4%)
Erythema (33–85%)
(2006): Garland SM+, *Int J STD AIDS* 17(7), 448
(2006): Hadley G+, *J Invest Dermatol* 126(6), 1251 (27%)
(2005): Nikkels AF+, *Acta Clin Belg* 60(5), 227
(2004): Haidopoulos D+, *Arch Gynecol Obstet* 270(4), 240
(2004): Marchitelli C+, *J Reprod Med* 49(11), 876 (100%)
(2003): Bayerl C+, *Br J Dermatol* 149 Suppl 66, 25 (85%)
(2002): Chen TM+, *Dermatol Surg* 28, 344 (for BCCs)
(2001): Fife KH+, *Sex Transm Dis* 28(4), 226
(2001): Garland SM+, *Int J STD AIDS* 12(11), 722 (67%)
(2001): Gollnick H+, *Int J STD AIDS* 12(1), 22
(1999): Gilson RJ+, *AIDS* 13(17), 2397 (41.9%)
(1999): Perry CM+, *Drugs* 58(2), 375 (67%)
(1998): Beutner KR+, *J Am Acad Dermatol* 38(2), 230 (33.3%)
(1998): Edwards L+, *Arch Dermatol* 134(1), 25
Excoriations (18–25%)
(2001): Fife KH+, *Sex Transm Dis* 28(4), 226
(1999): Perry CM+, *Drugs* 58(2), 375
Flaking (18–67%)
(2006): Hadley G+, *J Invest Dermatol* 126(6), 1251 (9%)

(1999): Perry CM+, *Drugs* 58(2), 375 (67%)
Fungal dermatitis (2–11%)
Hypomelanosis
(2006): Mendonca CO+, *Clin Exp Dermatol* 31(5), 721
Induration (5%)
Irritation (sic) (16%)
(1998): Beutner KR+, *J Am Acad Dermatol* 38(2), 230 (16.7%)
Pemphigus
(2004): Ruocco E+, *Eur J Obstet Gynecol Reprod Biol* 115(2), 242
(2003): Campagne G+, *Eur J Obstet Gynecol Reprod Biol* 109(2), 224
Pemphigus foliaceus
(2005): Mashiah J+, *Arch Dermatol* 141(7), 908
(2004): Lin R+, *Arch Dermatol* 140(7), 889
Pigmentation
(2005): Brown T+, *J Am Acad Dermatol* 52(4), 715
(2000): Geisse JK, *Dermatol Surg* 26, 579
Pruritus (22–75%)
(2006): *Prescrire Int* 15(84), 130
(2004): Barton JC, *J Am Acad Dermatol* 2004 Sep 51(3), 477
(2003): Bayerl C+, *Br J Dermatol* 149 Suppl 66, 25 (75%)
(2001): Gollnick H+, *Int J STD AIDS* 12(1), 22
(1999): Perry CM+, *Drugs* 58(2), 375 (67%)
(1998): Beutner KR+, *J Am Acad Dermatol* 38(2), 230 (54.2%)
Psoriasis
(2006): Fanti PA+, *Int J Dermatol* 45(12), 1464
(2006): Rajan N+, *Clin Exp Dermatol* 31(1), 140
Scabbing (4%)
Tenderness (local) (12%)
(2002): Schroeder TL+, *J Am Acad Dermatol* 46(4), 545
(1998): Beutner KR+, *J Am Acad Dermatol* 38(2), 230 (12.5%)
Ulcerations (5–10%)
(2005): Nikkels AF+, *Acta Clin Belg* 60(5), 227
(2002): Chen TM+, *Dermatol Surg* 28, 344 (for BCCs) (focal)
(2002): Emmet S, Solana Beach, CA (topical on lips) (from Internet) (observation)
(2001): Fife KH+, *Sex Transm Dis* 28(4), 226
(1998): Beutner KR+, *J Am Acad Dermatol* 38(2), 230 (10.4%)
Vesiculation (2–3%)
(2001): Fife KH+, *Sex Transm Dis* 28(4), 226
Vitiligo
(2007): Al-Dujaili+, *Dermatol Online J* 13(2), 10
(2007): Senel E+, *Indian J Dermatol Venereol Leprol* 73(6), 423

Mucosal/ENT
Aphthous stomatitis
(2005): Chakrabarty AK+, *J Am Acad Dermatol* 52(2 Suppl 1), 35
(2004): Emmet S, San Diego, CA (from Internet) (observation)
(2004): Emmet S, Solana Beach, CA (3 cases) (from Internet) (observation)
(2004): Panagotacos P, San Francisco, CA (from Internet) (observation)
(2002): Goldblum O, Pittsburgh, PA (topical on face and lips) (from Internet) (observation)
(2002): Kaufmann MD, New York, NY (topical on face) (from Internet) (observation)
Dysgeusia
(2004): Capper N, Mobile, AL (from Internet) (observation)
Stomatitis
(2005): Chakrabarty AK+, *J Am Acad Dermatol* 52(2 Suppl 1), 35
Tongue edema
(2004): Barton JC, *J Am Acad Dermatol* 2004 Sep 51(3), 477

Hair
Hair – pigmentation (of white hair)
(2002): Kirschenbaum MB, Chicago, IL (from Internet) (observation)

Eyes
Ocular pigmentation
(2004): Emmet S, Solana Beach, CA (from Internet) (observation)

Other
Application-site reactions (sic)
(2001): Barba AR+, *Dermatol Online J* 7(1), 20
(2001): Gollnick H+, *Int J STD AIDS* 12, 22
(2000): Kagy MK+, *Dermatol Surg* 26(6), 577 (for BCCs)
Asthenia
(2004): Emmet S, Solana Beach, CA (from Internet) (observation)
Cough
(2004): Emmet S, Solana Beach, CA (from Internet) (observation)
Depression
(1998): Goldstein D+, *J Infect Dis* 178(3), 858 (oral intake)
Headache
(2004): Emmet S, Solana Beach, CA (from Internet) (observation)
Injection-site Varicella-like eruption
(2006): Holcomb K+, *J Drugs Dermatol* 5(9), 863
Myalgia/Myositis/Myopathy/Myotoxicity (1%)
(2002): Sorkin MJ, Denver, CO (topical) (from Internet) (observation)
Pain (2–11%)
(2006): *Prescrire Int* 15(84), 130
(2003): Bayerl C+, *Br J Dermatol* 149 Suppl 66, 25 (11%)
(2001): Gollnick H+, *Int J STD AIDS* 12(1), 22
(1998): Beutner KR+, *J Am Acad Dermatol* 38(2), 230
Vertigo
(2005): Huether M, Tuscon, AR (from Internet) (observation)
(2005): Teller C, Bellaire, TX (from Internet) (observation)

IMMUNE GLOBULIN I.V.

Synonyms: IGIV; IVIG
Trade names: Allerglobuline; Baygam; Beriglobulin; Citax; Endobulin; Gamafine; Gamastan; Gamimune (Bayer); Gamma 16; Gammabulin; Gammagard (Baxter); Gammar P.I.V (ZLB Behring); Gammer-IV; Gammonayiv; Gamunex (Bayer); IG Gamma; IGIM; Interglobin; IV Globulin-S; Iveegam (Baxter); Octagam; Panglobulin (American Red Cross); Pentaglobin; Polygam S/D (American Red Cross); Sandoglobulin; Sandoglobulina; Sandoglobuline; Venoglobulin (Alpha Therapeutics)
Category: Immunomodulator
Half-life: N/A
Clinically important, potentially hazardous interactions with: live vaccines

Reactions

Skin
Baboon syndrome
(1999): Barbaud A+, *Dermatology* 199(3), 258
Cyanosis
Diaphoresis
Dyshidrosis
(2003): Uyttendaele H+, *J Drugs Dermatol* 2(3), 337
Eczema
(2003): Eastern J, N Caldwell, NJ (generalized) (from Internet) (observation)
Lichenoid eruption
(2007): Fernandez AP+, *Dermatol Ther* 20(4), 288 (passim)

(1998): Smith KJ+, *J Cutan Med Surg* 3(2), 96
Lymphocytic vasculitis
  (2006): Bodemer AA+, *J Am Acad Dermatol* A(5), S112
Pallor
Petechiae
  (2007): Fernandez AP+, *Dermatol Ther* 20(4), 288 (passim)
Pompholyx
  (1999): Iannaccone S+, *Neurology* 53(5), 1154
Pruritus
  (2007): Fernandez AP+, *Dermatol Ther* 20(4), 288 (palms)
    (passim)
Rash (sic)
  (2003): Wittstock M+, *Eur Neurol* 50(3), 172
Stevens–Johnson syndrome
  (2007): Fernandez AP+, *Dermatol Ther* 20(4), 288 (passim)
Toxic epidermal necrolysis
  (2006): Trent J+, *Seminars Cutan Med Surg* 25(2), 91
Urticaria
Vasculitis
  (2001): Odum J+, *Nephrol Dial Transplant* 16(2), 403
  (1998): Howse M+, *BMJ* 317(7168), 1291
  (1996): Hashkes PJ+, *Clin Exp Rheumatol* 14(6), 673

Mucosal/ENT

Rhinitis
  (2007): Fernandez AP+, *Dermatol Ther* 20(4), 288 (passim)

Hair

Hair – alopecia
  (2007): Fernandez AP+, *Dermatol Ther* 20(4), 288 (passim)

Other

Abdominal pain
  (2007): Fernandez AP+, *Dermatol Ther* 20(4), 288 (passim)
Anaphylactoid reactions/Anaphylaxis
  (2007): Fernandez AP+, *Dermatol Ther* 20(4), 288 (passim)
Application-site pain (16%)
Aseptic meningitis
  (2007): Fernandez AP+, *Dermatol Ther* 20(4), 288 (passim)
Asthenia
  (1997): Benincasa P+, *Ann Allergy Asthma Immunol* 79(3), 189
Chills
  (2007): Fernandez AP+, *Dermatol Ther* 20(4), 288 (passim)
Cough
  (1997): Benincasa P+, *Ann Allergy Asthma Immunol* 79(3), 189
Death
Fever
  (2007): Fernandez AP+, *Dermatol Ther* 20(4), 288 (passim)
  (1997): Benincasa P+, *Ann Allergy Asthma Immunol* 79(3), 189
Headache
  (2007): Fernandez AP+, *Dermatol Ther* 20(4), 288 (passim)
  (2003): Wittstock M+, *Eur Neurol* 50(3), 172 (mild)
Hypersensitivity
Myalgia/Myositis/Myopathy/Myotoxicity
  (2007): Fernandez AP+, *Dermatol Ther* 20(4), 288 (passim)
Nephrotoxicity
  (2007): Fernandez AP+, *Dermatol Ther* 20(4), 288 (passim)
  (2004): Orbach H+, *Semin Arthritis Rheum* 34(3), 593 (from
    sucrose)
  (2000): Dilhuydy MS+, *Presse Med* 29(17), 942
  (2000): Levy JB+, *QJM* 93(11), 751 (7%)
Seizures
  (2007): Fernandez AP+, *Dermatol Ther* 20(4), 288 (passim)
Serum sickness
  (2007): Fernandez AP+, *Dermatol Ther* 20(4), 288 (passim)
Stroke
  (2007): Fernandez AP+, *Dermatol Ther* 20(4), 288 (passim)
Vertigo

INAMRINONE

Trade names: Amcoral; Cartonic; Vestistol
Indications: Congestive heart failure
Category: Phosphodiesterase inhibitor
Half-life: 4.6 hours

Reactions

Other

Hypersensitivity
Injection-site burning (0.2%)

INDAPAMIDE

Trade names: Dapa-tabs; Fludex; Ipamix; Lozide; Lozol (Sanofi-Aventis); Naplin; Natrilix; Pamid
Indications: Edema
Category: Diuretic, thiazide
Half-life: 14–18 hours
Clinically important, potentially hazardous interactions with: digoxin, lithium, zinc

Note: Indapamide is a sulfonamide and can be absorbed systemically. Sulfonamides can produce severe, possibly fatal, reactions such as toxic epidermal necrolysis and Stevens–Johnson syndrome

Reactions

Skin

Angioedema
  (1994): Gales BJ+, *Am J Hosp Pharm* 51, 118
  (1992): Spinler SA+, *Cutis* 50, 200
  (1987): Stricker BHC+, *Br Med J Clin Res Ed* 295, 1313
Bullous dermatitis
Diaphoresis
Erythema multiforme
  (1994): Gales BJ+, *Am J Hosp Pharm* 51, 118
  (1987): Stricker BHC+, *Br Med J Clin Res Ed* 295, 1313
Exanthems
  (1987): Stricker BHC+, *Br Med J Clin Res Ed* 295, 1313
Fixed eruption
  (1998): De Barrio M+, *J Investig Allergol Clin Immunol* 8, 253
Necrotizing vasculitis
Pemphigus foliaceus
  (2002): Schmutz JL+, *Ann Dermatol Venereol* 129(8-9), 1085
  (2001): Bayramgurler D+, *J Dermatolog Treat* 12(3), 175
Peripheral edema (<5%)
Photosensitivity (<1%)
Pigmentation
  (2002): Roy-Peaud F+, *Rev Med Interne* 23(7), 674
Pruritus (<5%)
  (1985): Kirsten R+, *Z Kardiol* (German) 74, 66
  (1982): Brennan L+, *Clin Ther* 5, 121
Purpura
Rash (sic) (<5%)
  (1988): Kandela D+, *BMJ* 296, 573
  (1985): Kirsten R+, *Z Kardiol* (German) 74, 66
  (1983): Slotkoff L, *Am Heart J* 106, 233
  (1982): Brennan L+, *Clin Ther* 5, 121
Stevens–Johnson syndrome
  (1992): Spinler SA+, *Cutis* 50, 200
Toxic epidermal necrolysis
  (1993): Partanen J+, *Arch Dermatol* 129, 793
  (1990): Black RJ+, *Br Med J Clin Res Ed* 301, 1280

(1987): Stricker BHC+, *Br Med J Clin Res Ed* 295, 1313
Urticaria (<5%)
  (1987): Stricker BHC+, *Br Med J Clin Res Ed* 295, 1313
Vasculitis (<5%)

Mucosal/ENT
Xerostomia (<5%)
  (1985): Kirsten R+, *Z Kardiol* (German) 74, 66
  (1982): Brennan L+, *Clin Ther* 5, 121

Nails
Nails – photo-onycholysis
  (2007): Rutherford T+, *Australas J Dermatol* 48(1), 35

Eyes
Dyschromatopsia

Other
Anaphylactoid reactions/Anaphylaxis
Headache
Paresthesias (<5%)

INDINAVIR

Trade name: Crixivan (Merck)
Indications: HIV infection
Category: Antiretroviral; Protease inhibitor, HIV
Half-life: ~1.8 hours
**Clinically important, potentially hazardous interactions
with:** alprazolam, astemizole, atazanavir, chlordiazepoxide,
clonazepam, clorazepate, conivaptan, dasatinib, delavirdine,
diazepam, dihydroergotamine, ergot alkaloids, estazolam,
fentanyl, flurazepam, halazepam, ixabepilone, lapatinib,
methysergide, midazolam, pimozide, quazepam, rifapentine,
sildenafil, solifenacin, **St John's wort**, temsirolimus, triazolam,
vardenafil

Note: Protease inhibitors cause dyslipidemia which includes elevated
triglycerides and cholesterol and redistribution of body fat centrally to
produce the so-called 'protease paunch,' breast enlargement, facial
atrophy, and 'buffalo hump'

Reactions

Skin
Allergic reactions (sic)
  (1998): Rijnders B+, *Clin Infect Dis* 26, 523
Dermatitis (<2%)
Diaphoresis (<2%)
Erythema multiforme
Exanthems
  (1999): Fung HB+, *Pharmacotherapy* 19, 1328
Folliculitis (<2%)
Herpes simplex (<2%)
Herpes zoster (<2%)
Pigmentation
Pruritus (11–86%)
  (2000): Calista D+, *Eur J Dermatol* 10, 292 (11.9%)
  (1999): Gajewski LK+, *Ann Pharmacother* 33, 17 (86%)
Pyogenic granuloma
  (1998): Bouscarat F+, *N Engl J Med* 338, 1776 (great toes)
Rash (sic) (<67%)
  (2002): Albrecht D+, *AIDS* 16(15), 2098
  (1999): Gajewski LK+, *Ann Pharmacother* 33, 17 (67%)
Seborrhea (<2%)
Stevens–Johnson syndrome
  (2003): Rotunda A+, *Acta Derm Venereol* 83(1), 1

(1998): Teira R+, *Scand J Infect Dis* 30, 634
Striae
  (1999): Darvay A+, *J Am Acad Dermatol* 41, 467
Urticaria (<2%)
Vasculitis
  (2001): Rachline A+, *Br J Dermatol* 143, 1112
Xerosis (11%)
  (2000): Bonfanti P+, *J Acquir Immune Defic Syndr* 23(3), 236
  (2000): Calista D+, *Eur J Dermatol* 10, 292 (11.9%)

Mucosal/ENT
Aphthous stomatitis (<2%)
Bromhidrosis (<2%)
Cheilitis (<51%)
  (2001): Scully C+, *Oral Dis* 7, 205 (passim)
  (2000): Bonfanti P+, *J Acquir Immune Defic Syndr* 23(3), 236
  (2000): Calista D+, *Eur J Dermatol* 10, 292 (51.7%)
  (2000): Fox PA+, *Sex Transm Infect* 76, 323
Dysgeusia (2.6%)
Gingivitis (<2%)
Xerostomia (0.5%)

Hair
Hair – alopecia (11%)
  (2002): Ginarte M+, *AIDS* 16(12), 1695 (with ritonavir)
  (2000): Bonfanti P+, *J Acquir Immune Defic Syndr* 23(3), 236
  (2000): Calista D+, *Eur J Dermatol* 10, 292 (11.9%)
  (1999): Bouscarat F+, *N Engl J Med* 341, 618
  (1998): d'Arminio Monforte A+, *AIDS* 12, 328

Nails
Nails – onychocryptosis
  (2001): James CW+, *Ann Pharmacother* 35(7), 881 (with
    ritonavir)
  (2000): Heim M+, *Haemophilia* 6, 191
  (2000): Miot HA, Sao Paulo, Brazil (from Internet) (observation)
Nails – paronychia
  (2001): Colson AE+, *Clin Infect Dis* 32, 140
  (2001): Garcia Garcia+, *Rev Clin Esp* 201(8), 455
  (2000): Dauden E+, *Br J Dermatol* 142, 1063 (toes and finger)
  (2000): Sass JO+, *Dermatology* 200(1), 40
  (1998): Bouscarat F+, *N Engl J Med* 338, 1776 (great toes)
Nails – pyogenic granulomas (<6%)
  (2000): Calista D+, *Eur J Dermatol* 10, 292 (5.9%)
  (2000): Sass JO+, *Dermatology* 200(1), 40

Eyes
Eyelid edema (<2%)
Ocular pigmentation
  (2003): Huitema AD+, *Ther Drug Monit* 25(6), 735

Other
Abdominal pain (14%)
  (2007): McMahon DK+, *HIV Clin Trials* 8(5), 269 (28%) (with
    zidovudine & lamivudine)
  (2003): Hirsch MS+, *Clin Infect Dis* 37(8), 1119 (14%)
Asthenia
  (2007): McMahon DK+, *HIV Clin Trials* 8(5), 269 (49%) (with
    zidovudine & lamivudine)
Gynecomastia
  (2001): Manfredi R+, *Ann Pharmacother* 35, 438
  (1998): Caeiro JP+, *Clin Infect Dis* 27, 1539
  (1998): Lui A+, *Clin Infect Dis* 26, 1482
  (1998): Toma E+, *AIDS* 12, 681
Headache
  (2007): McMahon DK+, *HIV Clin Trials* 8(5), 269 (28%) (with
    zidovudine & lamivudine)
Lipoatrophy
  (2001): Lichtenstein KA+, *AIDS* 15(11), 1389
Lipodystrophy (<14%)

(2002): Reid S, *Can Adv Drug Reaction Newsletter* 12, 5
(2000): Calista D+, *Eur J Dermatol* 10, 292 (14.3%)
(2000): Hartmann M+, *Hautarzt* (German) 51, 159
(1999): Hermieu JF+, *Prog Urol* (French) 9, 537
(1999): Krautheim A, *Schweiz Rundsch Med Prax* (German)
    88, 285
(1998): Miller KD+, *Lancet* 351, 871
(1998): Viraben R+, *AIDS* 12, F37
(1997): Herry I+, *Clin Infect Dis* 25, 937 (breast hypertrophy)
Lipomatosis
(2000): Calista D+, *Eur J Dermatol* 10, 292
(1997): Hengel RL+, *Lancet* 350, 1596 (benign symmetric)
Myalgia/Myositis/Myopathy/Myotoxicity (<2%)
Nephrotoxicity
(2006): Boyd MA+, *J Antimicrob Chemother* 57(6), 1161
(2006): Servais A+, *Ann Urol (Paris)* 40(2), 57
(2005): Izzedine H+, *Am J Kidney Dis* 45(5), 804
(2003): Aarnoutse RE+, *Antivir Ther* 8(4), 309
(2003): Burger D+, *J Antimicrob Chemother* 51(5), 1231
(2003): Dieleman JP+, *J Acquir Immune Defic Syndr* 32(2), 135
(2002): van Rossum AM+, *Pediatrics* 110(2 Pt 1), e19
(2001): Dieleman JP+, *Infection* 29(4), 232
(1998): Trainor LD+, *Arch Pathol Lab Med* 122(3), 256
Paresthesias (<2%)
(2001): McMahon D+, *Antivir Ther* 6(2), 105
Porphyria (acute)
(2001): Schmutz JL+, *Ann Dermatol Venereol* 128(2), 184
(1999): Fox PA+, *AIDS* 16, 322
Tendinopathy/Tendon rupture
(2002): Florence E+, *Ann Rheum Dis* 61(1), 82

INDOMETHACIN

Synonym: indometacin
Trade names: Amuno; Apo-Indomethacin; Durametacin;
Imbrilon; Indochron; Indocin; Indolar SR; Indotec; Nu-Indo;
Rhodacine; Vonum
Indications: Arthritis
Category: Non-steroidal anti-inflammatory
Half-life: 4.5 hours
**Clinically important, potentially hazardous interactions
with:** aldesleukin, aspirin, diflunisal, diuretics, methotrexate,
NSAIDs, prednisolone, prednisone, sermorelin, tiludronate,
triamterene, urokinase

Reactions

Skin
Allergic granulomatous angiitis (Churg–Strauss syndrome)
    (plasma cell)
Angioedema (<1%)
(1981): Juhlin L, *Br J Dermatol* 104, 369
Bullous dermatitis (<1%)
(1986): Harrington CI+, *Br J Dermatol* 114, 265
Dermatitis
(1999): Pulido Z+, *Contact Dermatitis* 41, 112
(1998): Ueda K+, *Contact Dermatitis* 39, 323
(1993): Goday-Bujan JJ+, *Contact Dermatitis* 28, 111
(1993): Ophaswongse S+, *Contact Dermatitis* 29, 57
(1987): Beller U+, *Contact Dermatitis* 17, 121
Dermatitis herpetiformis (exacerbation)
(1986): Harrington CI+, *Br J Dermatol* 114, 265
(1985): Griffiths CEM+, *Br J Dermatol* 112, 443
Diaphoresis (<1%)
Eczema
(1987): Beller U+, *Contact Dermatitis* 17, 121

Edema (3–9%)
Erythema multiforme (<1%)
(1985): Ting HC+, *Int J Dermatol* 24, 58
Erythema nodosum (<1%)
(1982): Elizaga FV, *Ann Intern Med* 96, 383
Exanthems (1–5%)
Exfoliative dermatitis (<1%)
(1983): O'Sullivan M+, *Br J Rheumatol* 22, 47
Fixed eruption
(1998): Mahboob A+, *Int J Dermatol* 37, 833
Generalized eruption (sic)
Lichen planus
(1983): Hamburger J+, *BMJ* 287, 1258
Pemphigus
Peripheral edema
Petechiae (>1%)
Photosensitivity
(1984): Stern RS+, *JAMA* 252, 1433
Pruritus (1–10%)
Psoriasis
(1993): Shelley WB+, *Cutis* 51, 415 (observation)
(1989): Lazarova AZ+, *Clin Exp Dermatol* 14, 260 (from topical
    application)
(1987): Powles AV+, *Br J Dermatol* 117, 799
(1987): Sendagorta E+, *Dermatologica* 175, 300
(1986): Abel EA+, *J Am Acad Dermatol* 15, 1007
(1981): Katayama H+, *J Dermatol* (Tokio) 8, 323
(1980): Katayama H+, *Nippon Hifuka Gakkai Zasshi* (Japanese)
    90, 1027
Purpura (<1%)
(1984): Camba L+, *Acta Hematol* 71, 350
Rash (sic) (>10%)
Side effects (sic)
(1986): Bigby M+, *JAMA* 256, 3358 (0.21%)
Stevens–Johnson syndrome (<1%)
Toxic epidermal necrolysis (<1%)
(1996): Lear JT+, *Postgrad Med J* 72, 186
(1990): Roujeau JC+, *Arch Dermatol* 126, 37
(1989): Roth DE+, *Med Clin North Am* 73, 1275
(1986): Johnson VB+, *La Pharm* 45, 4
(1985): Heng MCY, *Br J Dermatol* 113, 597
(1983): O'Sullivan M+, *Br J Rheumatol* 22, 47
Urticaria
(1995): Gebhardt M+, *Z Rheumatol* (German) 54, 405
(1992): Shelley WB+, *Cutis* 50, 87 (observation)
(1985): O'Brien WM+, *J Rheumatol* 12, 13
(1981): Juhlin L, *Br J Dermatol* 104, 369
Urticaria pigmentosa
Vasculitis (<1%)
(1988): Gamboa PM+, *Allergol Immunopathol Madr* (Spanish)
    16, 53
(1985): Bigby M, *J Am Acad Dermatol* 12, 866
(1985): O'Brien WM+, *J Rheumatol* 12, 13

Mucosal/ENT
Ageusia
Aphthous stomatitis
Oral lesions (<7%)
Oral lichenoid eruption
(1983): Hamburger J+, *BMJ* 287, 1258
Oral ulceration
(2000): Madinier I+, *Ann Med Interne* (Paris) (French) 151, 248
(1983): Hamburger J+, *BMJ* 287, 1258
Tinnitus
(1981): Ekstrand R+, *Scand J Rheumatol* 10(2), 69 (with aspirin)
Tongue edema
Ulcerative stomatitis (<1%)
(1982): Bailin PL+, *Clin Rheum Dis* 8, 493 (passim)

Xerostomia

Hair

Hair – alopecia (<1%)

Eyes

Periorbital edema

Other

Anaphylactoid reactions/Anaphylaxis (<1%)
Gynecomastia (<1%)
Headache
Hot flashes (<1%)
Hypersensitivity (<1%)
Paresthesias (<1%)
Pseudolymphoma
  (2000): Werth V, *Dermatology Times* 18
Pseudoporphyria
  (2000): De Silva B+, *Pediatr Dermatol* 17, 480
Serum sickness
  (1985): Ferraccioli G+, *Acta Haematol* 73, 45

INFLIXIMAB

Trade name: Remicade (Centocor)
Indications: Crohn's disease, psoriasis and rheumatoid arthritis
Category: Cytokine inhibitor; TNF inhibitor
Half-life: 9.5 days

Reactions

Skin

Acne
  (2008): Sladden MJ+, *Br J Dermatol* 158(1), 172
  (2008): Sun G+, *J Drugs Dermatol* 7(1), 69
  (2007): Bassi E+, *Br J Dermatol* 156(2), 402 (2 cases)
  (2006): Krathen RA+, *J Drugs Dermatol* 5(3), 251
Acute febrile neutrophilic dermatosis (Sweet's syndrome)
  (2003): Matzkies FG+, *Ann Rheum Dis* 62(1), 81
Acute generalized exanthematous pustulosis (AGEP)
  (2007): Meiss F+, *J Eur Acad Dermatol Venereol* 21(5), 717
Adverse effects (sic)
  (2001): Serrano MS+, *Ann Pharmacother* 35(7), 823
Allergic reactions (sic)
  (2002): Brocq O+, *Presse Med* 31(39), 1836
Bullous dermatitis
  (2002): Kent PD+, *Arthritis Rheum* 46(8), 2257
Cellulitis
  (2004): Colombel JF+, *Gastroenterology* 126(1), 19 (1 case)
Dermatitis
  (2006): Huang F+, *Zhonghua Nei Ke Za Zhi* 45(2), 122
  (2004): Chan JL+, *J Drugs Dermatol* 3(3), 315 (Atopic)
Eczema
  (2004): Dumont-Berset M+, *Br J Dermatol* 151(6), 1272
Edema
  (2004): Krishnan RS+, *J Drugs Dermatol* 3(3), 305
  (1999): Lichenstein GR+, *Biologics in Clinical Practice Symposium,* Orlando, FL, May 19 (from Internet) (observation)
Exanthems
  (2005): Jaffe P, Columbia, SC (from Internet) (observation)
  (2004): Dumont-Berset M+, *Br J Dermatol* 151(6), 1272
  (2004): Scheinfeld N, *J Drugs Dermatol* 3(3), 273 (passim)
  (2003): Gottlieb AB, *J Am Acad Dermatol* 49(2), S112
Facial edema
  (2004): Scheinfeld N, *J Drugs Dermatol* 3(3), 273 (passim)
Folliculitis

(2007): Gilaberte Y+, *Br J Dermatol* 156(2), 368 (perforating)
  (2003): Devos SA+, *Dermatology* 206(4), 388
Granuloma annulare
  (2003): Devos SA+, *Dermatology* 206(4), 388
Herpes simplex
  (2001): Voigtländer C+, *Arch Dermatol* 137, 1571
Herpes zoster
  (2004): Kinder A+, *Postgrad Med J* 80(939), 26
  (2002): Baumgart DC+, *Ann Rheum Dis* 61(7), 661
Impetigo
  (2007): Wegscheider BJ+, *Eye* 21(4), 547
Keratoacanthoma
  (2004): Esser AC+, *J Am Acad Dermatol* 50(5 Suppl), S75
Lichenoid eruption
  (2003): Devos SA+, *Dermatology* 206(4), 388
Lupus erythematosus
  (2007): de Langen–Wouterse, JJ+, *Ned Tijdschr Geneeskd* 151(6), 367
  (2007): Ramos-Casals M+, *Medicine* (Baltimore) 86(4), 242 (40 cases)
  (2006): Bratcher JM+, *Expert Opin Drug Saf* 5(1), 9 (passim)
  (2006): Chadha T+, *Arthritis Rheum* 55(1), 163
  (2006): Pallotta P+, *Rheumatology* (Oxford) 45(1), 116
  (2006): Perez-Garcia C+, *Rheumatology* (Oxford) 45(1), 114
  (2006): Schneider SW+, *Arch Dermatol* 142(1), 115
  (2005): Benucci M+, *J Clin Rheumatol* 11(1), 47
  (2005): High WA+, *J Am Acad Dermatol* 52(4), E5
  (2005): Richez C+, *J Rheumatol* 32(4), 760
  (2005): Vabre-Latre CM+, *Ann Dermatol Venereol* 132(4), 349
  (2004): Elkayam O+, *Clin Exp Rheumatol* 22(4), 502
  (2004): Novak S+, *Clin Exp Rheumatol* 22(2), 268
  (2004): Stratigos AJ+, *Clin Exp Dermatol* 29(2), 150
  (2003): Debandt M+, *Clin Rheumatol* 22(1), 56
  (2003): Jarrett SJ+, *J Rheumatol* 30(10), 2287 (8 cases)
  (2003): Klapman JB+, *Inflamm Bowel Dis* 9(3), 176
  (2003): Mikuls TR+, *Drug Saf* 26(1), 23
  (2002): Ali Y+, *Ann Intern Med* 137(7), 625
  (2000): Charles PJ+, *Arthritis Rheum* 43(11), 2383
Lupus syndrome
  (2006): Pallotta P+, *Rheumatology* (Oxford) 45(1), 116
  (2005): Atzeni F+, *Aliment Pharmacol Ther* 22(5), 453 (1 case)
  (2004): Colombel JF+, *Gastroenterology* 126(1), 19 (3 cases)
  (2003): Christopher-Stine L+, *J Rheumatol* 30(12), 2725
  (2003): Sarzi-Puttini P+, *Dig Liver Dis* 35(11), 814
Lymphoma
  (2006): Bratcher JM+, *Expert Opin Drug Saf* 5(1), 9 (passim)
  (2005): Doty JD+, *Chest* 127(3), 1064
  (2002): Brown SL+, *Arthritis Rheum* 46(12), 3151 (8 cases)
  (2001): Aithal GP+, *Aliment Pharmacol Ther* 15(8), 1101
  (1992): Greenstein AJ+, *Cancer* 69, 1119
Molluscum contagiosum (eyelids)
  (2002): Cursiefen C+, *Am J Ophthalmol* 134(2), 270
Necrotizing fasciitis
  (2002): Chan AT+, *Postgrad Med J* 78(915), 47
Nevi
  (2008): Fabre C+, *Dermatology* 216(2), 185 (Halo) (multiple)
  (2006): Bovenschen HJ+, *Br J Dermatol* 154(5), 880 (Eruptive)
Palmar–plantar pustulosis
  (2007): Roux CH+, *J Rheumatol* 34(2), 434
  (2007): Sladden MJ+, *Arch Dermatol* 143(11), 1449
  (2005): Michaelsson G+, *Br J Dermatol* 153(6), 1243
Peripheral edema
  (2003): Gottlieb AB, *J Am Acad Dermatol* 49(2), S112
Pernio
  (2003): Devos SA+, *Dermatology* 206(4), 388
Photosensitivity
  (2002): Smith JG, Mobile, AL (2 cases) (from Internet) (observation)
Pruritus (5%)

(2004): Scheinfeld N, *J Drugs Dermatol* 3(3), 273 (passim)
(2003): Gottlieb AB, *J Am Acad Dermatol* 49(2), S112
(2001): Finkelstein RP, Stratford, NJ (from Internet)
(observation)
(1999): Lichenstein GR+, *Biologics in Clinical Practice Symposium*,
Orlando, FL, May 19

Psoriasis
(2007): Cavailhes A+, *Ann Dermatol Venereol* 134(4 Pt 1), 363
(2007): Cohen JD+, *J Rheumatol* 34(2), 380
(2007): Roux CH+, *J Rheumatol* 34(2), 434 (pustular) (2 cases)
(2007): Ubriani R+, *Arch Dermatol* 143(2), 270
(2007): Wegscheider BJ+, *Eye* 21(4), 547 (pustular)
(2006): Adams DR+, *J Drugs Dermatol* 5(2), 178
(2006): Gonzalez-Lopez MA+, *Med Clin* (Barc) 127(8), 316
(2005): Grinblat B+, *Arthritis Rheum* 52(4), 1333
(2005): Michaelsson G+, *Br J Dermatol* 153(6), 1243 (pustular)
(2005): Peramiquel L+, *Clin Exp Dermatol* 30(6), 713 (flexural)
(2005): Sfikakis PP+, *Arthritis Rheum* 52(8), 2513
(2004): Thurber M+, *J Drugs Dermatol* 3(4), 439 (pustular)
(2004): Verea MM+, *Ann Pharmacother* 38(1), 54
(2002): Smith SZ, Louisville, KY (from Internet) (observation)
(2001): Finkelstein RP, Stratford, NJ (from Internet)
(observation)

Pustules
(2005): Starmans-Kool MJ+, *Rheumatol Int* 25(7), 550 (2 cases)
(2002): Chan AT+, *Postgrad Med J* 78(915), 47
(2001): Finkelstein RP, Stratford, NJ (from Internet)
(observation)

Rash (sic) (6%)
(2006): Krathen RA+, *J Drugs Dermatol* 5(3), 251
(2004): Scheinfeld N, *J Drugs Dermatol* 3(3), 273 (passim)
(2003): Gottlieb AB, *J Am Acad Dermatol* 49(2), S112
(2002): Ljung T+, *Scand J Gastroenterol* 37(9), 1108
(2001): Serrano MS+, *Ann Pharmacother* 35(7), 823
(2000): Hyams JS+, *J Pediatr* 137(2), 192
(1999): Baert S+, *Int J Colorectal Dis* 14, 47
(1999): Lichenstein GR+, *Biologics in Clinical Practice Symposium*
Orlando, FL, May 19

Red man syndrome
(2003): Lobel EZ+, *J Clin Gastroenterol* 36(2), 186

Sarcoidosis
(2006): O'Shea FD+, *Arthritis Rheum* 55(6), 978

Scleredema
(2005): Ranganathan P, *J Clin Rheumatol* 11(6), 319

Squamous cell carcinoma
(2004): Esser AC+, *J Am Acad Dermatol* 50(5 Suppl), S75

Stevens–Johnson syndrome
(2002): Kiely PD+, *Rheumatology (Oxford)* 41(6), 631

Toxic epidermal necrolysis
(2007): Meiss F+, *J Eur Acad Dermatol Venereol* 21(5), 717

Ulcerations (foot)
(2002): Conaghan P+, *Skin & Allergy News* June, 40

Urticaria
(2004): Scheinfeld N, *J Drugs Dermatol* 3(3), 273 (passim)
(2003): Gottlieb AB, *J Am Acad Dermatol* 49(2), S112
(2001): Schaible TF, *Presse Med* 30(12), 610 (17%)
(1999): Lichenstein GR+, *Biologics in Clinical Practice Symposium*,
Orlando, FL, May 19
(1997): Van Deventer SJH, *Clin Nutr* 16, 271

Vasculitis
(2007): Ramos-Casals M+, *Medicine* (Baltimore) 86(4), 242 (47
cases)
(2006): Saint Marcoux B+, *Joint Bone Spine* 73(6), 710
(2005): Srivastava MD+, *Scand J Immunol* 61(4), 329
(2004): Mohan N+, *J Rheumatol* 31(10), 1955 (15 cases)
(2003): Devos SA+, *Dermatology* 206(4), 388
(2003): Jarrett SJ+, *J Rheumatol* 30(10), 2287 (8 cases)
(2003): McIlwain L+, *J Clin Gastroenterol* 36(5), 411

Vitiligo

(2005): Ramirez-Hernandez M+, *Dermatology* 210(1), 79

Mucosal/ENT
Oral candidiasis
(2005): Doty JD+, *Chest* 127(3), 1064
Oral mucositis
(2002): Kugathasan S+, *Am J Gastroenterol* 97(6), 1408
Rhinitis
(2003): Gottlieb AB, *J Am Acad Dermatol* 49(2), S112
Sinusitis
(2003): Gottlieb AB, *J Am Acad Dermatol* 49(2), S112
Ulcerative stomatitis
(2003): Gottlieb AB, *J Am Acad Dermatol* 49(2), S112

Hair
Hair – alopecia areata
(2008): Fabre C+, *Dermatology* 216(2), 185 (worsening)
(2004): Ettefagh L+, *Arch Dermatol* 140(8), 1012

Eyes
Orbital cellulitis
(2006): Roos JC+, *Am J Ophthalmol* 141(4), 767

Other
Abdominal pain
(2003): Gottlieb AB, *J Am Acad Dermatol* 49(2), S112
Anaphylactoid reactions/Anaphylaxis
(2005): Chavez-Lopez MA+, *Allergol Immunopathol* (Madr)
33(5), 291
(2004): Scheinfeld N, *J Drugs Dermatol* 3(3), 273 (passim)
(2004): Stallmach A+, *Eur J Gastroenterol Hepatol* 16(6), 627
(2002): Diamanti A+, *J Pediatr* 140(5), 636
(2002): O'Connor M+, *Dig Dis Sci* 47(6), 1323
(2002): Sample C+, *Can J Gastroenterol* 16(3), 165
(2000): Soykan I+, *Am J Gastroenterol* 95(9), 2395
Application-site reactions (<4%) (mild)
(2004): Colombel JF+, *Gastroenterology* 126(1), 19 (3.8%)
(2004): McNamara DA+, *Surgeon* 2(5), 258
(2004): Scheinfeld N, *J Drugs Dermatol* 3(3), 273 (10%) (passim)
(2003): Mikuls TR+, *Drug Saf* 26(1), 23
(2003): Stone WJ, *J Infus Nurs* 26(6), 380
(2002): Sandborn WJ+, *Am J Gastroenterol* 97(12), 2962
Aseptic meningitis
(2005): Hegde N+, *South Med J* 98(5), 564
(2001): Marotte H+, *Lancet* 358(9295), 1784
Asthenia
(2003): Gottlieb AB, *J Am Acad Dermatol* 49(2), S112
Candidiasis (5%)
(2003): Gottlieb AB, *J Am Acad Dermatol* 49(2), S112
Chest pain
(2003): Gottlieb AB, *J Am Acad Dermatol* 49(2), S112
(2001): Schaible TF, *Presse Med* 30(12), 610 (17%)
Chills (5–9%)
(2004): Scheinfeld N, *J Drugs Dermatol* 3(3), 273 (passim)
(2001): Schaible TF, *Presse Med* 30(12), 610 (17%)
Congestive heart failure
(2003): Mikuls TR+, *Drug Saf* 26(1), 23
Cough
(2003): Gottlieb AB, *J Am Acad Dermaol* 49(2), S112
Death
(2004): Colombel JF+, *Gastroenterology* 126(1), 19 (10 cases)
(2002): de' Clari F+, *Circulation* 105(21), E183
(2002): Su C+, *Am J Gastroenterol* 97(10), 2577
(2001): Lankarani KB, *J Clin Gastroenterol* 33(3), 255
(2001): Srinivasan R, *Am J Gastroenterol* 96, 2274 (neonatal)
Depression
(2003): Gottlieb AB, *J Am Acad Dermatol* 49(2), S112
Fever
(2006): Krathen RA+, *J Drugs Dermatol* 5(3), 251
(2005): Hegde N+, *South Med J* 98(5), 564

(2004): Krishnan RS+, *J Drugs Dermatol* 3(3), 305
(2004): Scheinfeld N, *J Drugs Dermatol* 3(3), 273 (passim)
(2003): Gottlieb AB, *J Am Acad Dermatol* 49(2), S112
(2001): Schaible TF, *Presse Med* 30(12), 610 (17%)
Headache
   (2005): Hegde N+, *South Med J* 98(5), 564
   (2004): Scheinfeld N, *J Drugs Dermatol* 3(3), 273 (passim)
   (2003): Gottlieb AB, *J Am Acad Dermatol* 49(2), S112
   (2001): Schaible TF, *Presse Med* 30(12), 610 (17%)
Hepatotoxicity
   (2006): Bratcher JM+, *Expert Opin Drug Saf* 5(1), 9 (passim)
   (2006): Soto-Fernandez S+, *Gastroenterol Hepatol* 29(5), 321
   (2006): Wahie S+, *Clin Exp Dermatol* 31(3), 460
Hypersensitivity
   (2005): Voulgari PV+, *Am J Med* 118(5), 515 (11%)
   (2002): Riegert-Johnson DL+, *Inflamm Bowel Dis* 8(3), 186
   (2002): Sandborn WJ+, *Am J Gastroenterol* 97(12), 2962
   (1999): Lichenstein GR+, *Biologics in Clinical Practice Symposium* Orlando, FL, May 19
   (1997): Van Deventer SJH, *Clin Nutr* 16, 271
Hypertension
   (2003): Gottlieb AB, *J Am Acad Dermatol* 49(2), S112
Infections (21%)
   (2006): Imaizumi K+, *Intern Med* 45(10), 685
   (2006): Krathen RA+, *J Drugs Dermatol* 5(3), 251
   (2006): Scollard DM+, *Clin Infect Dis* 43(2), e19
   (2005): Mufti AH+, *Diagn Microbiol Infect Dis* 53(3), 233
   (2005): Voulgari PV+, *Am J Med* 118(5), 515 (7%)
   (2004): Broholm B+, *Ugeskr Laeger* 166(43), 3827
   (2004): Colombel JF+, *Gastroenterology* 126(1), 19 (8.2%)
   (2004): Dunlop H, *CMAJ* 171(8), 992
   (2003): Kroesen S+, *Rheumatology* (Oxford) 42(5), 617
   (2003): Mikuls TR+, *Drug Saf* 26(1), 23
   (2002): Brocq O+, *Presse Med* 31(39), 1836
   (2001): Ouraghi A+, *Gastroenterol Clin Biol* 25(11), 949
   (2001): Schaible TF, *Presse Med* 30(12), 610 (26%)
   (2001): Serrano MS+, *Ann Pharmacother* 35(7), 823
Injection-site reactions (sic) (6%)
   (2004): Lamireau T+, *Inflamm Bowel Dis* 10(6), 745 (15%)
   (2003): Cheifetz A+, *Am J Gastroenterol* 98(6), 1315 (6.1%)
   (2003): Crandall WV+, *Aliment Pharmacol Ther* 17(1), 75 (35 cases)
   (2002): Kugathasan S+, *Am J Gastroenterol* 97(6), 1408
   (2002): Steinfeld SD+, *Arthritis Rheum* 46(12), 3301
   (1989): Morrison SL, *Hosp Prac* 24, 65
Lymphoproliferative disease
   (2002): Brown SL+, *Arthritis Rheum* 46(12), 3151 (8 cases)
Myalgia/Myositis/Myopathy/Myotoxicity (5%)
   (2005): Hegde N+, *South Med J* 98(5), 564
   (2004): Scheinfeld N, *J Drugs Dermatol* 3(3), 273 (passim)
   (2002): Kugathasan S+, *Am J Gastroenterol* 97(6), 1408
   (2002): Riegert-Johnson DL+, *Inflamm Bowel Dis* 8(3), 186
   (1999): Baert S+, *Int J Colorectal Dis* 14, 47
   (1999): Lichenstein GR+, *Biologics in Clinical Practice Symposium* Orlando, FL, May 19
Nephrotoxicity
   (2005): Chin G+, *Nephrol Dial Transplant* 20(12), 2824
Neurotoxicity
   (2007): Tektonidou MG+, *Clin Rheumatol* 26(2), 258 (2 cases)
   (2005): Chin G+, *Nephrol Dial Transplant* 20(12), 2824
Pain
   (2006): Pontikaki I+, *Reumatismo* 58(1), 31
   (2003): Gottlieb AB, *J Am Acad Dermatol* 49(2), S112
Paresthesias (1–4%)
   (2002): Conaghan P+, *Skin & Allergy News* June, 40
Polymyositis
   (2003): Kane D+, *Rheumatology* (Oxford) 42(12), 1564
   (2003): Musial J+, *Rheumatology* (Oxford) 42(12), 1566
Seizures

(2004): Scheinfeld N, *J Drugs Dermatol* 3(3), 273 (passim)
Serum sickness (<3%)
   (2004): Colombel JF+, *Gastroenterology* 126(1), 19 (2.8%)
   (2004): Krishnan RS+, *J Drugs Dermatol* 3(3), 305
Upper respiratory infection
   (2006): Huang F+, *Zhonghua Nei Ke Za Zhi* 45(2), 122
   (2003): Gottlieb AB, *J Am Acad Dermatol* 49(2), S112
Vertigo
   (2003): Gottlieb AB, *J Am Acad Dermatol* 49(2), S112

INFLUENZA VACCINES

Trade names: Agrippal (Chiron); Begrivac; Comvax (Merck); Fluad (Chiron); Fluarix (GSK); FluMist (MedImmune) (Wyeth); Flurix (GSK); Fluviral (Shire); Fluzone; Imovax; Inflexal V (Berna Biotech); Influsome; Invivac (Solvay); Vaxigrip (Sanofi-Aventis)
Indications: Influenza prevention
Category: Vaccine
Half-life: N/A
Clinically important, potentially hazardous interactions with: carbamazepine, cyclosporine, mercaptopurine, methotrexate, phenobarbital, prednisone, theophylline, vincristine, warfarin

Note: Inactivated influenza vaccine should not be given to persons with anaphylactic hypersensitivity to eggs or other components of the vaccine. For current data on influenza consult http://www.cdc.gov/flu

Note: Oculorespiratory syndrome (ORS) is defined as the presence of bilateral conjunctivitis, facial edema, or respiratory symptoms occurring between 2 and 24h following immunization

Reactions

Skin
Acute febrile neutrophilic dermatosis (Sweet's syndrome)
   (2005): Jovanovic M+, *J Am Acad Dermatol* 52(2), 367
Adverse effects (sic)
   (2004): Kenney RT+, *N Engl J Med* 351(22), 2295 (mild & transient)
   (2004): Lawrence G+, *Commun Dis Intell* 28(3), 324
   (2003): Ben-Yehuda A+, *Vaccine* 21(23), 3169
   (2002): Galaj A+, *Wiad Lek* 55(7-8), 366
   (2001): Holdiness MR, *Int J Dermatol* 40(7), 427
   (2000): Poole PJ+, *Cochrane Database Syst Rev* (4), CD002733
Angioedema
Bullous dermatitis
   (2003): Augey F+, *Ann Dermatol Venereol* 130(11), 1058
Bullous pemphigoid
   (2006): Garcia-Doval I+, *Br J Dermatol* 155(4), 820 (%)
Fixed eruption
   (2001): Garcia-Doval I+, *Acta Derm Venereol* 81(6), 450
Gianotti–Crosti syndrome
   (2002): Haug S+, *Hautarzt* 53(10), 683 (4 cases)
Henoch–Schönlein purpura
   (2001): Watanabe T+, *Pediatr Nephrol* 16(5), 458
Impetigo
   (2004): France EK+, *Arch Pediatr Adolesc Med* 158(11), 1031 (9 cases)
Linear IgA dermatosis
   (2000): Boyce TG+, *Vaccine* 19(2-3), 217 (26–35%)
Pemphigus
   (2000): Mignogna MD+, *Int J Dermatol* 39(10), 800
Purpura
   (2006): Tishler M+, *Isr Med Assoc J* 8(5), 322
   (2002): Yanai-Berar N+, *Clin Nephrol* 58(3), 220 (1 case)

Rash (sic)
(2004): *Prescrire Int* 13(74), 206 (with squalene adjuvant)
(2004): Hesley TM+, *Pediatr Infect Dis J* 23(3), 240 (with hepatitis B, measles-mumps-rubella, and varicella vaccine)
(2000): Lohiya GS, *Am J Infect Control* 28(5), 386

Shivering
(2004): Kanra G+, *Pediatr Infect Dis J* 23(4), 300 (%)

Side effects (sic)
(2004): de Bruijn IA+, *Virus Res* 103(1-2), 139 (transient)
(2003): Allsup S+, *Health Technol Assess* 7(24), iii
(2003): Bodkin C+, *Int J Nurs Pract* 9(6), 382
(2002): Williams JP+, *Am J Manag Care* 8(5 Suppl), S143 (mild)

Toxicoderma
(2000): Manzano E+, *Aten Primaria* 26(6), 429

Vasculitis
(2006): Famularo G+, *J Clin Rheumatol* 12(1), 48
(2004): Hull JH+, *J Neurol Neurosurg Psychiatry* 75(10), 1507
(2004): Walker SL+, *Clin Exp Dermatol* 29(1), 95
(2003): Iyngkaran P+, *Rheumatology* (Oxford) 42(7), 907
(2003): Ritter O+, *Z Kardiol* 92(11), 962
(2003): Tavadia S+, *Clin Exp Dermatol* 28(2), 154 (4 cases)
(2002): Yanai-Berar N+, *Clin Nephrol* 58(3), 220 (1 case)

Mucosal/ENT

Rhinitis
(2002): Piedra PA+, *Pediatrics* 110(4), 662

Eyes

Oculorespiratory syndrome
(2005): *Can Commun Dis Rep* 31(21), 217
(2004): De Serres G+, *Arch Intern Med* 164(20), 2266 (15–34%)
(2004): Grenier JL+, *Can Commun Dis Rep* 30(2), 9
(2003): De Serres G+, *Vaccine* 21(19-20), 2346 (4–5%)
(2003): Fredette MJ+, *Clin Infect Dis* 37(8), 1136 (6 cases)
(2003): Scheifele DW+, *Clin Infect Dis* 36(7), 850 (3%)
(2003): Skowronski DM+, *Clin Infect Dis* 36(6), 705 (13–27%)
(2003): Skowronski DM+, *Clin Infect Dis* 37(8), 1059
(2003): Skowronski DM+, *J Infect Dis* 187(3), 495
(2002): Orr P, *Can Commun Dis Rep* 28, 1
(2002): Skowronski DM+, *CMAJ* 167(8), 853 (5%)
(2002): Skowronski DM+, *Vaccine* 20(21-22), 2713
(2001): Boulianne N+, *Can Commun Dis Rep* 27(10), 85
(2000): *Can Commun Dis Rep* 26(23), 201
(2000): Vilain S+, *Bull Soc Belge Ophtalmol* (277), 71

Other

Abdominal pain
(2002): Piedra PA, *Semin Pediatr Infect Dis* 13(2), 90 (2%)
(2002): Piedra PA+, *Pediatrics* 110(4), 662

Anaphylactoid reactions/Anaphylaxis (rare)
(2005): Izurieta HS+, *JAMA* 294(21), 2720

Asthenia
(2004): *Prescrire Int* 13(74), 206 (with squalene adjuvant)
(2004): D'Alessandro D+, *Indian J Med Res* 119 Suppl, 108
(2004): Kanra G+, *Pediatr Infect Dis J* 23(4), 300 (12%)
(2004): Socan M+, *Vaccine* 22(23-24), 3087
(2000): Banzhoff A+, *Immunol Lett* 71(2), 91 (53%)
(2000): Schaad UB+, *Antimicrob Agents Chemother* 44(5), 1163

Chills
(2003): Frey S+, *Vaccine* 21(27-30), 4234 (mild)

Cough
(2000): Schaad UB+, *Antimicrob Agents Chemother* 44(5), 1163

Fever
(2006): Skowronski DM+, *Pediatrics* 117(6), 1963
(2004): D'Alessandro D+, *Indian J Med Res* 119 Suppl, 108
(2004): Hesley TM+, *Pediatr Infect Dis J* 23(3), 240 (with hepatitis B, measles-mumps-rubella, and varicella vaccine)
(2004): Kanra G+, *Pediatr Infect Dis J* 23(4), 300 (6–8%)
(2004): Socan M+, *Vaccine* 22(23-24), 3087

(2003): Dong PM+, *Zhonghua Liu Xing Bing Xue Za Zhi* 24(7), 570 (2–6%)
(2003): Squarcione S+, *Vaccine* 21(11-12), 1268 (%)
(2002): Galaj A+, *Pol Merkuriusz Lek* 12(72), 496 (1%)
(2002): Piedra PA+, *Pediatrics* 110(4), 662
(2001): Zangwill KM+, *Pediatr Infect Dis J* 20(8), 740

Headache
(2004): *Prescrire Int* 13(74), 206 (with squalene adjuvant)
(2004): Cooper CL+, *Vaccine* 22(23-24), 3136
(2004): Socan M+, *Vaccine* 22(23-24), 3087
(2002): Galaj A+, *Pol Merkuriusz Lek* 12(72), 496 (1%)
(2000): Banzhoff A+, *Immunol Lett* 71(2), 91 (53%)
(2000): Schaad UB+, *Antimicrob Agents Chemother* 44(5), 1163

Hypersensitivity
(2003): Skowronski DM+, *J Infect Dis* 187(3), 495

Injection-site edema
(2004): Socan M+, *Vaccine* 22(23-24), 3087
(2002): Galaj A+, *Pol Merkuriusz Lek* 12(72), 496 (7%)
(2002): Kawahara H+, *Arerugi* 51(7), 559 (1 case)
(2001): Schmitt-Grohe S+, *Klin Padiatr* 213(6), 338

Injection-site erythema
(2004): Kanra G+, *Pediatr Infect Dis J* 23(4), 300 (9–11%)
(2004): Socan M+, *Vaccine* 22(23-24), 3087
(2002): Gaeta GB+, *Vaccine* 20 Suppl 5, B33
(2002): Galaj A+, *Pol Merkuriusz Lek* 12(72), 496 (1%)
(2001): Schmitt-Grohe S+, *Klin Padiatr* 213(6), 338
(2000): Banzhoff A+, *Immunol Lett* 71(2), 91 (53%)
(2000): Murayama N+, *Kansenshogaku Zasshi* 74(1), 30

Injection-site induration
(2004): *Prescrire Int* 13(74), 206 (with squalene adjuvant)
(2004): D'Alessandro D+, *Indian J Med Res* 119 Suppl, 108
(2004): Kanra G+, *Pediatr Infect Dis J* 23(4), 300 (9%)
(2001): Schmitt-Grohe+, *Klin Padiatr* 213(6), 338
(2000): Banzhoff A+, *Immunol Lett* 71(2), 91 (53%)

Injection-site inflammation
(2004): Belshe RB+, *N Engl J Med* 351(22), 2286
(2003): Frey S+, *Vaccine* 21(27-30), 4234 (mild)
(2003): Squarcione S+, *Vaccine* 21(11-12), 1268

Injection-site pain (20–28%)
(2004): *Prescrire Int* 13(74), 206 (with squalene adjuvant)
(2004): Belshe RB+, *N Engl J Med* 351(22), 2286
(2004): Cooper CL+, *Vaccine* 22(23-24), 3136
(2004): Kanra G+, *Pediatr Infect Dis J* 23(4), 300 (24–25%)
(2003): Ben-Yehuda A+, *J Med Virol* 69(4), 560
(2003): Donalisio MR+, *Rev Soc Bras Med Trop* 36(4), 467 (12%)
(2003): Frey S+, *Vaccine* 21(27-30), 4234 (mild)
(2002): Galaj A+, *Pol Merkuriusz Lek* 12(72), 496 (1%)
(2001): Gasparini R+, *Eur J Epidemiol* 17(2), 135 (mild)
(2001): Jackson LA+, *Vaccine* 19(32), 4703
(2001): Schmitt-Grohe S+, *Klin Padiatr* 213(6), 338
(2000): Banzhoff A+, *Immunol Lett* 2000 Feb 1;71(2), 91 (53%)
(2000): Schaad UB+, *Antimicrob Agents Chemother* 44(5), 1163 (42–57%)

Injection-site papules & nodules
(2000): Gonzalez M+, *Arch Dis Child* 2000 Dec; 83(6), 488 (mild)

Injection-site reactions (sic)
(2002): Redding G+, *Pediatr Infect Dis J* 21(1), 44
(2001): Allsup SJ+, *Gerontology* 47(6), 311 (11%)

Myalgia/Myositis/Myopathy/Myotoxicity
(2004): *Prescrire Int* 13(74), 206 (with squalene adjuvant)
(2004): D'Alessandro D+, *Indian J Med Res* 119 Suppl, 108
(2004): Iyoda K+, *No To Hattatsu* 36(5), 401
(2004): Socan M+, *Vaccine* 22(23-24), 3087
(2003): Frey S+, *Vaccine* 21(27-30), 4234 (mild)
(2002): Piedra PA+, *Pediatrics* 110(4), 662
(2002): Yanai-Berar N+, *Clin Nephrol* 58(3), 220 (1 case)
(2001): *N Engl J Med* 345(21), 1529
(2000): Larner AJ+, *Eur J Neurol* 7(6), 731

Neurotoxicity
 (2003): Shoji H+, *Intern Med* 42(2), 139
Polymyositis
 (2004): Marti J+, *J Am Geriatr Soc* 52(8), 1412
 (2001): Saadoun D+, *Rev Med Interne* 22(2), 172
 (2000): Liozon E+, *J Am Geriatr Soc* 48(11), 1533
 (2000): Perez C+, *Muscle Nerve* 23(5), 824
Rhabdomyolysis
 (2000): Plotkin E+, *Nephrol Dial Transplant* 15(5), 740 (with cerivastatin and bezafibrate)
Seizures
 (2003): Nakamura N+, *Intern Med* 42(2), 191 (1 case)
Systemic reactions (injection site)
 (2002): Halperin SA+, *Vaccine* 20(7-8), 1240 (10–12%)
 (2001): Allsup SJ+, *Gerontology* 47(6), 311 (5%)
 (2001): Pregliasco F+, *Aging* (Milano) 13(1), 38
 (2001): Zangwill KM+, *Pediatr Infect Dis J* 20(8), 740
 (2000): Gonzalez M+, *Arch Dis Child* 2000 Dec; 83(6), 488 (mild)
Vertigo
 (2004): Chen YH+, *Vaccine* 22(21-22), 2806 (2–3%)

INH

(See ISONIAZID)

INSULIN

Trade names: Humalog; Huminsulin; Humulin (Lilly); Iletin Lente (Lilly); Insuman; Monotard; Novolin R (Novo Nordisk); Velosulin (Novo Nordisk); Velosuline Humaine
Indications: Diabetes
Category: Hormone, polypeptide
Half-life: N/A
Duration of action: 5–28 hours
Clinically important, potentially hazardous interactions with: alcohol, dimercaprol, ethanolamine, **eucalyptus,** guanethidine, hydrocortisone, lanreotide, pegvisomant, propranolol, sermorelin, vidarabine

Note: About 25% of patients with insulin allergy have a concomitant history of penicillin allergy

Reactions

Skin

Allergic granulomatous angiitis (Churg–Strauss syndrome) (zinc)
 (1989): Jordaan HF+, *Clin Exp Dermatol* 14, 227
Allergic reactions (sic) (local)
 (2002): Lee AY+, *Acta Derm Venereol* 82(2), 114
 (1989): Zinman B, *N Engl J Med* 321, 363
 (1988): Plantin P+, *Ann Dermatol Venereol* (French) 115, 813 (>5%)
 (1985): Bruni B+, *Diabetes Care* 8, 201
 (1984): Grammer LC+, *JAMA* 251, 1459
 (1982): Carveth-Johnson AO+, *Lancet* 2, 1287
 (1982): Patterson R+, *JAMA* 248, 2637 (passim)
 (1981): Hasche H+, *Dtsch Med Wochenschr* (German) 106, 1451
 (1981): Kahn CB, *Handbook of Diabetes Mellitus* Garland STPM, 75
 (1980): Jegasothy BV, *Int J Dermatol* 19, 139 (immediate and delayed) (10–56%)
Angioedema
 (1983): Grammer LC+, *J Allergy Clin Immunol* 71, 250

 (1981): Kahn CB, *Handbook of Diabetes Mellitus* Garland STPM, 75
Atrophy
Bullous dermatitis
Dermatitis
 (1994): Goldfine AB+, *Curr Ther Endocrinol Metab* 5, 461
 (1989): Geldof BA+, *Contact Dermatitis* 20, 384
Diaphoresis (1–10%)
Edema (1–10%)
 (2004): Kalambokis G+, *J Endocrinol Invest* 27(10), 957
 (2004): Kalambokis GN+, *Am J Kidney Dis* 44(4), 575
 (1981): Galloway JA+, *Diabetes Mellitus* Bowie 5, 117
Erythema
 (2005): Wonders J+, *Ned Tijdschr Geneeskd* 149(50), 2783
Exanthems
Hematomas
 (2003): Camata DG, *Rev Lat Am Enfermagem* 11(1), 119
Hyperkeratosis
 (1989): Jordaan HF+, *Clin Exp Dermatol* 14, 277
 (1986): Fleming MG+, *Arch Dermatol* 122, 1054 (resembling acanthosis nigricans)
Keloid
Necrosis
Pallor (1–10%)
Pigmentation
Pigskin appearance
Pruritus (1–10%)
 (2005): Wonders J+, *Ned Tijdschr Geneeskd* 149(50), 2783
 (2002): Lee AY+, *Acta Derm Venereol* 82(2), 114
 (1981): Knick B, *Munch Med Wochenschr* (German) 123, 1197
Purpura
Urticaria (1–10%)
 (1996): Rowland-Payne CM+, *Br J Dermatol* 134, 184
 (1995): Chng HH+, *Allergy* 50, 984
 (1988): Plantin P+, *Ann Dermatol Venereol* (French) 115, 813
 (1983): Grammer LC+, *J Allergy Clin Immunol* 71, 250
 (1982): Mirouze J+, *Nouv Presse Med* (French) 11, 3121
 (1982): Patterson R+, *JAMA* 248, 2637 (passim)
 (1981): Kahn CB, *Handbook of Diabetes Mellitus* Garland STPM, 75
Vasculitis
 (2002): Mandrup-Poulsen T+, *Diabetes Care* 25(1), 242
 (1983): Grammer LC+, *J Allergy Clin Immunol* 71, 250
Xanthomas

Mucosal/ENT
Xerostomia

Other
Anaphylactoid reactions/Anaphylaxis (1–10%)
 (2007): Kaya A+, *J Diabetes Complications* 21(2), 124 (fatal)
 (2005): Wonders J+, *Ned Tijdschr Geneeskd* 149(50), 2783
 (1983): Grammer LC+, *J Allergy Clin Immunol* 71, 250
 (1982): Patterson R+, *JAMA* 248, 2637 (passim)
 (1981): Kahn CB, *Handbook of Diabetes Mellitus* Garland STPM, 75
Cough
Headache
Hypersensitivity
 (2003): Wittrup M+, *Ugeskr Laeger* 165(21), 2207
 (1983): Berman BA+, *Cutis* 32, 320
 (1982): deShazo RD+, *J Allergy Clin Immunol* 69, 229
Hypertension
 (2006): Tseng CH, *Arch Intern Med* 166(11), 1184
Hypertrophic lipodystrophy
 (1983): Johnson DA+, *Cutis* 32, 273
Injection-site calcification
 (1995): Ullman HR+, *J Comput Assist Tomogr* 19, 657

Injection-site cancer
Injection-site erythema
  (2006): Moyes V+, *Diabet Med* 23(2), 204
Injection-site induration
  (1983): White WB+, *Am J Med* 74, 909
  (1981): Galloway JA+, *Diabetes Mellitus* Bowie 5, 117
Injection-site pain
  (2006): Moyes V+, *Diabet Med* 23(2), 204
Injection-site pruritus
  (1988): Plantin P+, *Ann Dermatol Venereol* (French) 115, 813
Injection-site reactions (sic)
  (2003): HOE 901/2004, *Diabet Med* 20(7), 545 (1 case)
Lipoatrophy (1–10%)
  (2006): Beltrand J+, *Horm Res* 65(5), 253
  (2003): Ampudia-Blasco FJ+, *Diabetes Care* 26(3), 953
  (2003): Chowdhury TA+, *BMJ* 327(7411), 383
  (2003): Felner EI, *J Pediatr* 142(4), 448
  (1998): Murao S+, *Intern Med* 37, 1031
  (1996): Logwin S+, *Diabetes Care* 19, 255
  (1993): Chantelau E+, *Exp Clin Endocrinol* 101, 194
  (1992): Igea JM+, *Allergol Immunopathol Madr* (Spanish) 20, 173
  (1989): Gyimesi A+, *Orv Hetil* (Hungarian) 130, 2751
  (1989): Zinman B, *N Engl J Med* 321, 363
  (1988): McNally PG+, *Postgrad Med J* 64, 850
  (1988): Perrot H, *Ann Dermatol Venereol* (French) 115, 523
  (1983): Blickle JF+, *Presse Med* (French) 12, 2534
  (1982): Levandoski LA+, *Diabetes Care* 5, 6
  (1981): Jones GR+, *BMJ* 282, 190
  (1981): Kahn CB, *Handbook of Diabetes Mellitus* Garland STPM, 75
  (1980): Reeves WG+, *BMJ* 280, 1500
Lipodystrophy
  (2006): Olsovsky J, *Vnitr Lek* 52(5), 474
  (1990): Kohli V+, *Indian Pediatr* 27, 1120
  (1988): Field LM, *J Am Acad Dermatol* 19, 570
  (1988): Verbenko EV+, *Sov Med* (Russian) 3, 104
  (1987): Goldman JM+, *Am J Med* 83, 195
  (1985): Valenta LJ+, *Ann Intern Med* 102, 790
  (1984): Campbell IW+, *Postgrad Med J* 60, 439
  (1984): De Mattia G+, *Clin Ter* (Italian) 111, 169
  (1984): Tebuev AM, *Pediatriia* (Russian) December, 59
  (1982): Levandoski LA+, *Diabetes Care* 5, 6
  (1981): Libman E+, *Med Pregl* (Serbo-Croatian-Roman) 34, 49
  (1981): Pisarskaia IV+, *Med Sestra* (Russian) 40, 54
Lipohypertrophy (1–10%)
  (1996): Hauner H+, *Exp Clin Endocrinol Diabetes* 104, 106
  (1990): Schiazza L+, *J Am Acad Dermatol* 22, 148
  (1989): Zinman B, *N Engl J Med* 321, 363
  (1988): McNally PG+, *Postgrad Med J* 64, 850
  (1987): Samadaei A+, *J Am Acad Dermatol* 17, 506
  (1984): Young RJ+, *Diabetes Care* 7, 479
  (1983): Johnson DA+, *Cutis* 32, 273
  (1982): Mier A+, *BMJ* 285, 1539
Panniculitis
  (1988): Verbenko EV+, *Vestn Dermatol Venerol* (Russian) 1, 63
Paresthesias (1–10%)
Tremor (1–10%)
Tumors (nodules)
  (1981): Galloway JA+, *Diabetes Mellitus* Bowie 5, 117

INSULIN DETEMIR

Synonym: NN304
Trade name: Levemir (Novo Nordisk)
Indications: Diabetes (Type 1 or 2)
Category: Human Insulin analog, long-acting
Half-life: 5–7 hours
Clinically important, potentially hazardous interactions with: albuterol, **alcohol**, clonidine, corticosteroids, danazol, diuretics, epinephrine, estrogens, isoniazid, lithium, oral contraceptives, pentamidine, phenothiazines, propranolol, somatropin, terbutaline, thyroid

Reactions

Skin
Allergic reactions (sic)
  (2007): Sola-Gazagnes A+, *Lancet* 369(9562), 637 (type I and IV)
  (2006): Stechemesser L+, *Diabetes Care* 29(12), 2758 (type III)
  (2005): Darmon P+, *Diabetes Care* 28(12), 2980
Pruritus
Rash (sic)

Other
Headache
  (2004): Jhee SS+, *J Clin Pharmacol* 44(3), 258
Injection-site edema
Injection-site erythema
Injection-site inflammation
Injection-site pruritus
Injection-site reactions (3–4%)
  (2006): Blumer IR, *Diabetes Care* 29(4), 946
  (2006): No authors listed, *Prescrire Int* 15(85), 163
  (2004): Jhee SS+, *J Clin Pharmacol* 44(3), 258
Injection-site urticaria
Vertigo
  (2004): Jhee SS+, *J Clin Pharmacol* 44(3), 258

INSULIN GLARGINE

Trade name: Lantus (Sanofi-Aventis)
Indications: Type 1 & type 2 diabetes
Category: Hormone analog, polypeptide
Half-life: N/A
Clinically important, potentially hazardous interactions with: alcohol, guanethidine, propranolol

Reactions

Skin
Allergic reactions (sic)
Edema
Pruritus
Rash (sic)

Other
Injection-site pain (2.7%)
Lipoatrophy
  (2005): Ampudia-Blasco FJ+, *Diabetes Care* 28(12), 2983
Lipodystrophy
Seizures
  (2004): Tan CY+, *Pediatr Diabetes* 5(2), 80

INSULIN GLULISINE

Trade name: Apidra (Sanofi-Aventis)
Indications: Diabetes
Category: Insulin analog
Half-life: 1.5 hours
**Clinically important, potentially hazardous interactions
with:** albuterol, **alcohol**, clonidine, clozapine, lithium,
pentamidine, propranolol, somatropin

Reactions

Skin
Diaphoresis
Pruritus (<1%)
Rash (sic)
Urticaria (<1%)

Other
Anaphylactoid reactions/Anaphylaxis (<1%)
Hypersensitivity (<1%)
Hypotension
Injection-site edema
Injection-site erythema
Injection-site pruritus
Injection-site reactions (10.3%)
  (2007): Kamal AD+, *Expert Opin Drug Saf* 6(1), 5
  (2006): Hoogma RP+, *Horm Metab Res* 38(6), 429
Lipodystrophy (<0.1%   )

INTERFERON ALFA

Synonyms: IFLrA; IFN; rLFN-A; INF; INF-alpha-2
Trade names: Alferon N; Green-Alpha; Infergen (Intermune);
Intron A (Schering); Introna; Introne; Laroferon; Rebetron
(Schering); Roceron-A; Roferon-A (Roche)
Indications: Chronic hepatitis C virus infection
Category: Immunomodulator; Interferon
Half-life: 2 hours
**Clinically important, potentially hazardous interactions
with:** gemfibrozil

Note: Many of the adverse reactions depend on the nature of the
disease being treated. Either hairy cell leukemia [L] or AIDS-related
Kaposi's sarcoma [K]

Reactions

Skin
Acne (1%)
Acral sclerosis
  (2002): Saydam G+, *Acta Haematol* 107(1), 43
Allergic reactions (sic)
  (1996): Azagury M+, *Eur J Cancer* 32A, 1821 (severe)
Angioedema
  (2004): Guillot B+, *Dermatology* 208(1), 49
  (2001): Ohmoto K, *Am J Gastroenterol* 96, 1311
Atrophie blanche
  (2002): Bugatti L+, *Dermatology* 204(2), 154
Behçet's disease
  (1995): Segawa F+, *J Rheumatol* 22, 1183
Bullous dermatitis
  (2002): Pouthier D+, *Nephrol Dial Transplant* 17(1), 174
  (1995): Chang LW+, *Cutis* 56, 144

  (1993): Andry P+, *Ann Dermatol Venereol* (French) 120, 843
  (1993): Parodi A+, *Dermatology* 186, 155
Dermatitis
  (1995): Chang LW+, *Cutis* 56, 144
Dermatitis herpetiformis
  (1995): Dmochowski M+, *Postepy Dermatol* 12, 7
Dermatomyositis
  (2000): Dietrich LL+, *Med Oncol* 17(1), 64
Diaphoresis (22%) [L]; (7%) [K]
  (1999): Angulo MP+, *Pediatr Cardiol* 20, 293 [L]
Eczema (sic)
  (2004): Guillot B+, *Dermatology* 208(1), 49 (39%)
  (2004): Vazquez-Lopez F+, *Br J Dermatol* 150(5), 1046 (with
    ribavirin)
  (2002): Dereure O+, *Br J Dermatol* 147(6), 1142 (with ribavirin)
  (2000): Berger L+, *Ann Dermatol Venereol* 127(1), 51
  (1999): Sookoian S+, *Arch Dermatol* 135, 999 [K] (with ribavirin)
  (1989): Detmar U+, *Contact Dermatitis* 20, 149
Edema (11%) [L]
  (2002): Goldberg JS+, *Cancer* 95(6), 1220 (1 case)
Erythema
  (1999): Sookoian S+, *Arch Dermatol* 135, 999 [K] (with ribavirin)
    (malar)
Erythema nodosum
  (2001): Leveque L+, *Rev Med Interne* 22(12), 1248 (with
    ribavirin)
Exanthems
  (2002): Farady KK, Austin, TX (with ribavirin) (from Internet)
    (observation)
  (1994): Sollitto RB+, *Arch Dermatol* 130, 1194
  (1994): Toyofuku K+, *J Dermatol* 21, 732
  (1986): Quesada JR+, *Lancet* 1, 1466
Fungal dermatitis (<1%)
Halo dermatitis
  (1999): Krischer J 1, *J Am Acad Dermatol* 40, 105
Herpes simplex (1%)
  (1995): Chang LW+, *Cutis* 56, 144
  (1992): Breathnach SM+, *Adverse Drug Reactions and the Skin*
    Blackwell, Oxford, 322 (passim)
Kaposi's sarcoma
  (2002): Giuliani M+, *Arch Dermatol* 138(4), 535
  (1993): Ariad S+, *South Afr Med J* 83, 430
Keratoses
  (1994): Sollitto RB+, *Arch Dermatol* 130, 1194
Lichen myxedematosus
  (1998): Rongioletti F+, *J Am Acad Dermatol* 38, 760
Lichen planus
  (1999): Herstoff JK, Newport, RI (from Internet) (observation)
  (1999): Sookoian S+, *Arch Dermatol* 135, 999 [K] (with ribavirin)
  (1998): Dalekos GN+, *Eur J Gastroenterol Hepatol* 10, 933
  (1995): Chang LW+, *Cutis* 56, 144
  (1995): Fornaciari G+, *J Clin Gastroenterol* 20, 346
  (1995): Hyrailles V+, *Gastroenterol Clin Biol* (French) 19, 833
  (1993): Boccia S+, *Gastroenterology* 105, 1921
  (1993): Heintges T+, *J Hepatol* 18, 129
  (1993): Protzer U+, *Gastroenterology* 104, 903
Lichenoid eruption
  (2002): Bohannon JS, Midlothian, VA (from Internet)
    (observation)
Linear IgA dermatosis
  (1993): Parodi A+, *Dermatology* 187, 155
  (1990): Guillaume JC+, *Ann Dermatol Venereol* (French) 117, 899
Livedo reticularis
  (2004): Guillot B+, *Dermatology* 208(1), 49 (10 cases)
Lupus erythematosus
  (2005): Goldman KE+, *Oral Surg Oral Med Oral Pathol Oral Radiol
    Endod* 100(3), 285
  (2005): Niewold TB+, *Clin Rheumatol* 24(2), 178

(2004): Martinez Alfaro E+, *Med Clin* (Barc) 123(15), 597
(2002): Tothova E+, *Neoplasma* 49(2), 91
(2001): Werth V, *Dermatology Times* 18
(1998): Garcia-Porrua C+, *Clin Exp Rheumatol* 16, 107
(1994): Flores A+, *Br J Rheumatol* 33, 787
(1994): Fritzler MJ, *Lupus* 3, 455
(1994): Sanchez Roman J+, *Med Clin* (Barc) (Spanish) 102, 198
(1992): Mehta ND+, *Am J Hematol* 41, 141
(1992): Tolaymat A+, *J Pediatr* 120, 429
(1991): Hess EV, *Curr Opin Rheumatol* 3, 809
(1991): Schilling JP+, *Cancer* 68, 1536

Lupus syndrome
(2005): Fritz M+, *J Perinatol* 25(8), 552 (neonatal)
(2002): Pouthier D+, *Nephrol Dial Transplant* 17(1), 174

Malignancies (sic)
(1991): Wagner RF+, *Arch Dermatol* 127, 272

Melanoma
(1988): Bork K+, *Dermatologica* 177, 249 (exacerbation)

Necrosis
(1998): Sickler JB+, *Am J Gastroenterol* 93, 463
(1997): de Ledinghen V+, *Gastroenterol Clin Biol* 21, 523
(1995): Chang LW+, *Cutis* 56, 144
(1995): Trautinger F+, *N Engl J Med* 333, 1222
(1991): Cnudde F+, *Int J Dermatol* 30, 147
(1989): Rasokat H+, *Dtsch Med Wochenschr* (German) 114, 458

Nodular eruption (painful)
(1995): Chang LW+, *Cutis* 56, 144

Pemphigus
(1995): Kirsner RS+, *Br J Dermatol* 132, 474
(1994): Niizeki H+, *Dermatology* 189 (Suppl), 129

Photo-recall
(2002): Thomas R+, *J Clin Oncol* 20(1), 355

Photosensitivity (<1%)
(2002): Dereure O+, *Br J Dermatol* 147(6), 1142 (with ribavirin)
(1994): Sollitto RB+, *Arch Dermatol* 130, 1194

Pigmentation (<1%)
(2003): Willems M+, *Br J Dermatol* 149(2), 390

Pigmented purpuric eruption (capillaritis)
(2000): Gupta G+, *J Am Acad Dermatol* 43, 937

Pityriasis versicolor
(2004): Guillot B+, *Dermatology* 208(1), 49

Pruritus (13%) [L]; (5%) [K]
(2004): Guillot B+, *Dermatology* 208(1), 49 (30%)
(2002): Bohannon JS, Midlothian VA (from Internet) (observation)
(2001): Beaudet LD (from Internet) (observation)
(1994): Czarnetzki BM+, *J Am Acad Dermatol* 30, 500
(1992): Breathnach SM+, *Adverse Drug Reactions and the Skin* Blackwell, Oxford, 322 (passim)

Psoriasis
(2004): Seckin D+, *Pediatr Dermatol* 21(5), 577
(2002): Oliveira-Soares+, *World Congress Dermatol* Poster, 0123 (aggravation in 3 cases)
(2001): Werth V, *Dermatology Times* 18
(2000): Downs AM+, *Clin Exp Dermatol* 25(4), 351
(2000): Taylor C+, *Postgrad Med J* 76, 365
(1997): Brenard R, *Acta Gastroenterol Belg* 60(3), 211
(1996): Wolfer LU+, *Hautarzt* (German) 47, 124
(1995): Chang LW+, *Cutis* 56, 144
(1995): Wolfe JT+, *J Am Acad Dermatol* 32, 887
(1994): Matsuoka H+, *Rinsho Ketsueki* (Japanese) 35, 309
(1993): Cleveland MG+, *J Am Acad Dermatol* 29, 788
(1993): Garcia-Lora E+, *Dermatology* 187, 280
(1993): Georgetson MJ+, *Am J Gastroenterol* 88, 756
(1993): Pauluzzi P+, *Acta Derm Venereol* 73, 395
(1991): Funk J+, *Br J Dermatol* 125, 463
(1990): Fierlbeck G+, *Arch Dermatol* 126, 351 (at injection site)
(1990): Jucgla A+, *Arch Dermatol* 127, 910 (exacerbation)

(1990): Kowalzick L+, *Arch Dermatol* 126, 1515 (at injection site)
(1990): Kusec R+, *Dermatologica* 181, 170
(1989): Harrison P, *J Invest Dermatol* 93, 555
(1989): Hartmann F+, *Dtsch Med Wochenschr* (German) 114, 96 (exacerbation)
(1986): Quesada JR+, *Lancet* 1, 1466 (exacerbation)

Purpura
(2003): Al-Zahrani H+, *Leuk Lymphoma* 44(3), 471
(2001): Toubai T+, *Nippon Naika Gakkai Zasshi* 90(7), 1330

Rash (sic) (44%) [L]; (11%) [K]
(2000): Stafford-Fox V+, *Clin J Oncol Nurs* 4(4), 164
(1999): Sookoian S+, *Arch Dermatol* 135, 999 [K] (with ribavirin)

Raynaud's phenomenon
(2004): Guillot B+, *Dermatology* 208(1), 49 (10 cases)
(2003): Al-Zahrani H+, *Leuk Lymphoma* 44(3), 471
(2003): Iorio R+, *Pediatr Infect Dis J* 22(2), 195
(2002): Schapira D+, *Semin Arthritis Rheum* 32(3), 157
(2002): Tothova E+, *Neoplasma* 49(2), 91
(2000): Kruit WH+, *Ann Oncol* 11(11), 1501
(1998): Campo-Voegeli A+, *Dermatology* 196(3), 361
(1997): Liozon E+, *Rev Med Interne* 18(4), 316
(1996): Bachmeyer C+, *Br J Dermatol* 1996 Sep 135(3), 481
(1996): Creutzig A+, *Ann Intern Med* 125, 423
(1994): Arslan M+, *J Intern Med* 235, 503

Sarcoidosis
(2006): Akay BN+, *J Eur Acad Dermatol Venereol* 20(4), 442
(2006): Alazemi S+, *Int J Clin Pract* 60(2), 201
(2006): Alonso-Perez A+, *J Eur Acad Dermatol Venereol* 20(10), 1328
(2006): Goldberg HJ+, *Respir Med* 100(11), 2063
(2006): Pellova A+, *Klin Mikrobiol Infekc Lek* 12(5), 200
(2006): Perera GK+, *Clin Exp Dermatol* 31(3), 387 (with ribavirin)
(2005): Bolukbas C+, *Acta Gastroenterol Belg* 68(4), 432 (with ribavirin)
(2005): Butnor KJ, *Am J Surg Pathol* 29(7), 976
(2005): Celik G+, *Respirology* 10(4), 535
(2005): Farah R+, *Int J Clin Pharmacol Ther* 43(9), 441
(2005): Hirano A+, *Respirology* 10(4), 529
(2005): Rosen Y, *Am J Surg Pathol* 29(11), 1544
(2004): Kreutzer K+, *J Dtsch Dermatol Ges* 2(8), 689
(2004): Massaguer S+, *Eur Radiol* 14(9), 1716
(2004): Menon Y+, *Am J Med Sci* 328(3), 173
(2004): Papaioannides D+, *Med Sci Monit* 10(1), CS5
(2004): Rogers CJ+, *J Am Acad Dermatol* 50(4), 649 (with ribavirin)
(2004): Salvio A+, *Ann Ital Med Int* 19(1), 58 (with ribavirin)
(2004): Tortorella C+, *J Interferon Cytokine Res* 24(11), 655
(2004): Toulemonde A+, *Ann Dermatol Venereol* 131(1 Pt 1), 49
(2003): Luchi S+, *Scand J Infect Dis* 35(10), 775 (2 cases)
(2003): Rubinowitz AN+, *J Comput Assist Tomogr* 27(2), 279
(2003): Tahan V+, *Dig Dis Sci* 48(1), 169 (with ribavirin)
(2002): Cogrel O+, *Br J Dermatol* 146(2), 320 (with ribavirin)
(2002): Gitlin N, *Eur J Gastroenterol Hepatol* 14(8), 883 (with ribavirin)
(2002): Li SD+, *J Gastroenterol* 37(1), 50
(2002): Misery L, *J Interferon Cytokine Res* 22(8), 881 (with ribavirin)
(2002): Nawras A+, *Dig Dis Sci* 47(7), 1627
(2002): Noguchi K+, *J Clin Gastroenterol* 35(3), 282
(2002): Perez-Alvarez R+, *J Viral Hepat* 9(1), 75 (with ribavirin)
(2002): Wendling J+, *Arch Dermatol* 138, 546 (2 cases) (with ribavirin)
(2001): Krehmeier H+, *Dtsch Med Wochenschr* 126(16), 460
(2001): Leveque L+, *Rev Med Interne* 22(12), 1248 (with ribavirin)
(2001): Miwa H+, *Eur Neurol* 45(4), 288
(2001): Neglia V+, *J Cutan Med Surg* 5(5), 406
(2001): Ravenel JG+, *Am J Roentgenol* 177(1), 199

(2000): Cacoub P+, *Gastroenterol Clin Biol* 24(3), 364
(2000): Fiorani C+, *Haematologica* 85(9), 1006
(2000): Pohl J+, *Z Gastroenterol* 38(12), 951
(2000): Savoye G+, *Gastroenterol Clin Biol* 24(6-7), 679 (with ribavirin)
(2000): Vallina E+, *An Med Interna* 17(10), 538
(1999): Pietropaoli A+, *Chest* 116, 569
(1998): Kikawada M+, *Respirology* 3(1), 41
(1996): Teragawa H+, *Intern Med* 35(1), 19
(1993): Blum L+, *Rev Med Interne* (Paris) (French) 14, 1161

Scleroderma
(2004): Solans R+, *Clin Exp Rheumatol* 22(5), 625

Seborrheic dermatitis
(2004): Guillot B+, *Dermatology* 208(1), 49 (3 cases)
(1986): Quesada JR+, *Lancet* 1, 1466

Systemic sclerosis
(2002): Beretta L+, *Br J Dermatol* 147(2), 385

Telangiectasia
(1989): Dreno B+, *Ann Intern Med* 111, 95

Toxicity (sic)
(1993): Miglino M+, *Haematologica* 78(6), 411
(1989): Dreno B+, *Ann Intern Med* 111, 95

Ulcerations
(1992): Orlow SJ+, *Arch Dermatol* 128, 566

Urticaria (<3%) [K]
(2004): Guillot B+, *Dermatology* 208(1), 49
(1994): Czarnetzki BM+, *J Am Acad Dermatol* 30, 500
(1992): Breathnach SM+, *Adverse Drug Reactions and the Skin* Blackwell, Oxford, 322 (passim)

Vasculitis
(2001): Toubai T+, *Nippon Naika Gakkai Zasshi* 90(7), 1330
(2001): Werth V, *Dermatology Times* 18
(1998): Gordon AC+, *J Infect* 36, 229
(1996): Pateron D+, *Clin Exp Rheumatol* 14, 79
(1995): Chang LW+, *Cutis* 56, 144
(1992): Liet JM+, *Rev Med Interne* (French) 13, 169
(1983): Sangster G+, *Eur J Cancer Clin Oncol* 19, 1647

Vitiligo
(2006): Tinio P+, *Skinmed* 5(1), 50 (with ribavirin)
(2004): Guillot B+, *Dermatology* 208(1), 49
(2004): Seckin D+, *Pediatr Dermatol* 21(5), 577
(1997): Nouri K+, *Cutis* 60, 289
(1996): Le Gal F-A+, *J Am Acad Dermatol* 35, 650
(1996): Simsek H+, *Dermatology* 193, 65
(1995): Bernstein D+, *Am J Gastroenterol* 90, 1176
(1994): Scheibenbogen C+, *Eur J Cancer* 30A, 1209

Xerosis (17%) [L]; (22%) [K]

Mucosal/ENT

Ageusia
(2003): Irigoien Aleixandre S+, *Rev Esp Enferm Dig* 95(5), 364
(2001): Manzano Alonso ML+, *Gastroenterol Hepatol* 24(8), 412

Anosmia
(2001): Manzano Alonso ML+, *Gastroenterol Hepatol* 24(8), 412
(2000): Fernandez Fernandez FJ+, *Gastroenterol Hepatol* 23(10), 499
(2000): Kraus I+, *Int J Clin Pharmacol Ther* 38(7), 360
(1998): Maruyama S+, *Am J Gastroenterol* 93, 122

Aphthous stomatitis
(2004): Guillot B+, *Dermatology* 208(1), 49
(1998): Dalekos GN+, *Eur J Gastroenterol Hepatol* 10, 933

Dysgeusia (25%) (metallic taste) [K]
(1995): Chang LW+, *Cutis* 56, 144

Oral lichen planus
(2005): Nagao Y+, *Int J Mol Med* 15(2), 237 (with ribavirin)
(1997): Kutting B+, *Br J Dermatol* 137, 836
(1997): Schlesinger TE+, *J Am Acad Dermatol* 36, 1023 (erosive)
(1995): Chang LW+, *Cutis* 56, 144
(1994): Papini M+, *Int J Dermatol* 33, 221

(1994): Perreard M+, *Gastroenterol Clin Biol* (French) 18, 1051
(1993): Sassigneux P+, *Gastroenterol Clin Biol* (French) 17, 764

Oral pemphigus
(2001): Marinho RT+, *Eur J Gastroenterol Hepatol* 13(7), 869

Ototoxicity
(1995): Kanda Y+, *Audiology* 34(2), 98

Sialopenia

Stomatitis (1–10%)

Tinnitus
(2004): Tunca A+, *Turk J Gastroenterol* 15(2), 97
(2001): Tsushima K+, *Nihon Kokyuki Gakkai Zasshi* 39(11), 893
(2000): Zhang H+, *Zhonghua Shi Yan He Lin Chuang Bing Du Xue Za Zhi* 14(4), 376
(1995): Kanda Y+, *Audiology* 34(2), 98

Xerostomia (>10%)
(2004): Guillot B+, *Dermatology* 208(1), 49 (10 cases)

Hair

Hair – alopecia (1–10%)
(2004): Guillot B+, *Dermatology* 208(1), 49 (48%)
(2002): Alpsoy E+, *Arch Dermatol* 138, 467
(2001): Zucker DM+, *Gastroenterol Nurs* 24(4), 192 (with ribavirin)
(2000): Stafford-Fox V+, *Clin J Oncol Nurs* 4(4), 164
(1997): Brehler R+, *J Am Acad Dermatol* 36, 983 (passim)
(1995): Chang LW+, *Cutis* 56, 144
(1994): Czarnetzki BM+, *J Am Acad Dermatol* 30, 500
(1992): Tosti A+, *Dermatology* 184, 124
(1989): Olsen EA+, *J Am Acad Dermatol* 20, 395
(1987): Werter MJBP, *Ned Tijdschr Geneeskd* (Dutch) 131, 2081

Hair – alopecia areata
(1999): Kernland KH+, *Dermatology* 198, 418

Hair – curly
(2006): Tinio P+, *Skinmed* 5(1), 50 (with ribavirin)

Hair – hypertrichosis
(1996): Ariyoshi K+, *Am J Hematol* 53, 50 (eyebrows)
(1990): Berglund EF+, *South Med J* 83, 363
(1984): Foon KA+, *N Engl J Med* 19, 1259 (eyelashes)

Hair – pigmentation
(2004): Guillot B+, *Dermatology* 208(1), 49 (18%)
(1996): Fleming CJ+, *Br J Dermatol* 135, 337
(1995): Bernstein D+, *Am J Gastroenterol* 90, 1176 (canities)

Hair – straight
(2003): Lanigan SW, *Br J Dermatol* 148, 595 (with ribavirin)
(2002): Bessis D+, *Br J Dermatol* 147(2), 392

Eyes

Eyelashes – hypertrichosis
(2002): Misery L, *J Interferon Cytokine Res* 22, 881
(2000): Ozdogan M+, *J Interferon Cytokine Res* 20, 633

Retinopathy
(2006): *Prescrire Int* 15(82), 61
(2006): Okuse C+, *World J Gastroenterol* 12(23), 3756
(2005): Oishi A+, *Br J Ophthalmol* 89(11), 1542

Other

Asthenia
(2002): Goldberg JS+, *Cancer* 95(6), 1220 (2 cases)

Candidiasis (1%)

Chills
(2002): Alpsoy E+, *Arch Dermatol* 138, 467
(2000): Cornejo P+, *Arch Dermatol* 136, 429
(2000): Shenefelt PD+, *Arch Dermatol* 136, 837

Depression (5–15%)
(2006): Asnis GM+, *J Clin Gastroenterol* 40(4), 322
(2006): Camacho A+, *J Psychopharmacol* 20(5), 687
(2002): Bonaccorso S+, *J Clin Psychopharmacol* 22(1), 86
(2002): Castera L+, *Hepatology* 35(4), 978
(2002): Farah A, *J Clin Psychiatry* 63(2), 166
(2002): Herrine SK, *Ann Intern Med* 136(10), 747

(2002): Vega Palomares R+, *Gastroenterol Hepatol* 25(8), 483 (with ribavirin)
(2001): Bonaccorso S+, *Psychiatry Res* 105(1), 45
(2001): Debien C+, *Encephale* 27(4), 308 (5–15%)
(2001): Kraus MR+, *N Engl J Med* 345(5), 375
(2001): Maes M+, *Mol Psychiatry* 6(4), 475
(2001): Malik UR+, *Cancer* 92(6), 1664

Embolia cutis medicamentosa (Nicolau syndrome)
(2003): Reding EL+, *J Am Acad Dermatol* 48(3), 472 (passim)

Fever
(2002): Goldberg JS+, *Cancer* 95(6), 1220 (2 cases)
(2002): Wirth S+, *Hepatology* 36(5), 1280 (with ribavirin)

Headache
(2002): Goldberg JS+, *Cancer* 95(6), 1220 (1 case)

Hot flashes (1%)

Hypersensitivity
(2001): Beckman DB+, *Allergy* 56(8), 806

Hypertension
(2003): Al-Zahrani H+, *Leuk Lymphoma* 44(3), 471

Infections
(2002): Goldberg JS+, *Cancer* 95(6), 1220 (1 case)

Injection-site alopecia
(2000): Sparsa A+, *Rev Med Interne* 21(9), 756
(1999): Lang AM+, *Arch Dermatol* 135, 1127

Injection-site eczematous eruption
(2004): Guillot B+, *Dermatology* 208(1), 49 (39%)

Injection-site erythema
(2000): Sparsa A+, *Rev Med Interne* 21(9), 756
(1995): Chang LW+, *Cutis* 56, 144

Injection-site induration
(2000): Sparsa A+, *Rev Med Interne* 21(9), 756
(2000): Stafford-Fox V+, *Clin J Oncol Nurs* 4(4), 164
(1997): Siegel M, New York, NY (from Internet) (observation)
(1995): Chang LW+, *Cutis* 56, 144

Injection-site necrosis
(2000): Sparsa A+, *Rev Med Interne* 21(9), 756
(2000): Stafford-Fox V+, *Clin J Oncol Nurs* 4(4), 164
(1998): Krainick U+, *J Interferon Cytokine Res* 18, 823
(1997): Weinberg JM+, *Acta Derm Venereol* (Stockh) 77, 146
(1996): Konohana A+, *J Am Acad Dermatol* 35, 788
(1996): Kontochristopoulos G+, *J Hepatol* 25, 271
(1995): Shinohara K, *N Engl J Med* 333, 1222
(1994): Akiyama Y+, *Jpn J Dermatol* (Japanese) 104, 436
(1994): Tone T+, *Jpn J Dermatol* 104, 1047
(1993): Christian B+, *Presse Med* (French) 22, 783
(1993): Mihara K+, *Miyazakiikaishi* (Japanese) 17, 40
(1993): Nagai A+, *Int J Hematol* 58, 129
(1993): Oeda E+, *Am J Hematol* 44, 213
(1992): Orlow SJ+, *Arch Dermatol* 128, 566
(1991): Cnudde F+, *Int J Dermatol* 30, 147
(1989): Rasokat H+, *Dtsch Med Wochenschr* (German) 114, 158

Injection-site pruritus
(1989): Detmar U+, *Contact Dermatitis* 20, 149

Injection-site reactions
(2000): Stafford-Fox V+, *Clin J Oncol Nurs* 4(4), 164

Injection-site vasculitis
(1997): Christian MM+, *J Am Acad Dermatol* 37, 118

Myalgia/Myositis/Myopathy/Myotoxicity (71%) [L]; (69%) [K]
(2002): Alpsoy E+, *Arch Dermatol* 138, 467
(2002): Herrine SK, *Ann Intern Med* 136(10), 747
(2001): Karim A+, *Am J Med Sci* 322(4), 233
(2000): Shenefelt PD+, *Arch Dermatol* 136, 837
(1999): Spieth K+, *Arch Dermatol* 135, 1035
(1998): Dippel E+, *Arch Dermatol* 134, 880 (4 patients)
(1997): Brehler R+, *J Am Acad Dermatol* 36, 983 (passim)
(1984): Foon KA+, *N Engl J Med* 19, 1259 (passim)

Nephrotoxicity
(2002): Willson RA, *J Clin Gastroenterol* 35(1), 89 (with ribavirin)

(2001): Kintzel PE, *Drug Saf* 24(1), 19

Paresthesias (12%) [L]; (8%) [K]

Polyarteritis nodosa
(2001): *Drug & Ther Perspect* 17, 15

Polymyositis
(2002): Lee SW+, *J Korean Med Sci* 17(1), 141

Rhabdomyolysis
(2003): Gabrielli M+, *Am J Gastroenterol* 98(4), 940
(2001): van Londen GJ+, *J Clin Oncol* 19(17), 3794
(1995): Anderlini P+, *Cancer* 76, 678

Seizures
(2006): Kors C+, *J Eur Acad Dermatol Venereol* 20(4), 473

Sjøgren's (Sicca) syndrome
(1994): Lunel F, *Gastroenterol Clin Biol* (French) 19, 442

Suicidal ideation
(2003): Hosoda S+, *Seishin Shinkeigaku Zasshi* 105(6), 768
(2003): Schaefer M+, *Pharmacopsychiatry* 36 (Suppl 3), S203
(2003): Schafer M+, *Fortschr Neurol Psychiatr* 71(9), 469
(2002): Schaefer M+, *Prog Neuropsychopharmacol Biol Psychiatry* 26(4), 731
(2001): Ademmer K+, *Psychosomatics* 42(4), 365

Tremor
(2003): Tan EK+, *Neurology* 61(9), 1302

Vogt–Koyanagi–Harada disease
(2003): Sylvestre DL+, *J Viral Hepat* 10(6), 467 (with ribavirin)

INTERFERON BETA

Synonyms: rIFN-b; IFNB-1b; IFN-beta1b
Trade names: Avonex (Biogen); Betaseron (Berlex); Rebif (Merck)
Indications: Relapsing multiple sclerosis, cancers
Category: Immunomodulator; Interferon
Half-life: 10 hours

Reactions

Skin

Abscess

Adverse effects (sic)
(1999): Rice GP+, *Neurology* 52(9), 1893
(1998): Rio J+, *Neurologia* 13(9), 422

Allergic granulomatous angiitis (Churg–Strauss syndrome)
(1998): Mehta CL+, *J Am Acad Dermatol* 39(6), 1024

Allergic reactions (sic)
(1998): Cohen BA+, *Allergy Asthma Proc* 19(2), 85
(1997): Elgart GW+, *J Am Acad Dermatol* 37(4), 553
(1996): Neilley LK+, *Neurology* 46(2), 552

Basal cell carcinoma (<1%)

Bullae

Cellulitis

Clammy skin

Cyst (4%)

Dermatitis

Diaphoresis (23%)

Edema (generalized) (8%)

Erythema
(2000): Beghi E+, *Neurology* 54(2), 469 (local)

Erythema nodosum

Exanthems
(2002): Beaudet LD, Trois-Rivieres, Quebec (from Internet) (observation)

Exfoliative dermatitis

Facial edema

Furunculosis

Genital pruritus
Herpes simplex (2–3%)
Herpes zoster (3)
Hyperhidrosis
 (1997): Schwid SR+, Arch Neurol 54(9), 1169
 (1994): Connelly JF, Ann Pharmacother 28(5), 610
Induration
 (2001): Durieu C+, Ann Dermatol Venereol 128(12), 1336
 (1989): Glaspy JA+, Cancer 64(2), 409
Leukoderma
Lichenoid eruption
Livedo reticularis
 (2005): Gibbs MB+, J Am Acad Dermatol 52(6), 1009
Lupus erythematosus
 (2005): Crispin JC+, Lupus 14(6), 495
 (2000): Schmutz J+, Ann Dermatol Venereol 127(2), 237
 (1998): Nousari HC+, Lancet 352(9143), 1825 (subacute cutaneous)
Myxedema
 (2004): Kumar N+, Mult Scler 10(1), 85
Necrosis
 (2002): Yang CH+, Chang Gung Med J 25(11), 774
 (1999): Sasseville D+, J Cutan Med Surg 3(6), 320
 (1998): Weinberg JM, J Am Acad Dermatol 39(5 Pt 1), 807
 (1997): Albani C+, Minerva Med 88(6), 271
 (1997): Fruland JE+, J Am Acad Dermatol 37(3 Pt 1), 488
 (1997): Weinberg JM+, Acta Derm Venereol 77(2), 146
 (1995): Sheremata WA+, N Engl J Med 332(23), 1584
 (1995): Shinohara K, N Engl J Med 333(18), 1222
Nevi (3%)
Petechiae
Photosensitivity (<1%)
Pigmentation
Pruritus
 (2002): Beaudet LD, Trois-Rivieres, Quebec (from Internet) (observation)
Psoriasis
 (2005): Navne JE+, Ugeskr Laeger 167(32), 2903
 (1996): Webster GF+, J Am Acad Dermatol 34(2 Pt 2), 365
Raynaud's phenomenon
 (2000): De Broucker+, Ann Med Interne (Paris) 151(5), 424
Sarcoidosis
 (1987): Abdi EA+, Cancer 59(5), 896
Scleroderma
 (1999): Fortuno Y+, Med Clin (Barc) 113(12), 447 (9 cases)
 (1997): Elgart GW+, J Am Acad Dermatol 37(4), 553
Seborrhea
Spider angiomas
Squamous cell carcinoma
 (1997): Fruland JE+, J Am Acad Dermatol 37(3), 488
Telangiectasia
Ulcerations
 (2004): Inafuku H+, J Dermatol 31(8), 671
 (1999): Fortuno Y+, Med Clin (Barc) 113(12), 447 (9 cases)
Urticaria (5%)
 (2003): Mazzeo L+, Br J Dermatol 148(1), 172
Vasculitis
 (2004): Debat Zoguereh+, Rev Neurol (Paris) 160(11), 1081
Vesiculobullous eruption

Mucosal/ENT
Ageusia
Aphthous stomatitis
Balanitis
Cheilitis
Dysgeusia
Gingivitis

Glossitis
Mucosal bleeding (12–38%)
 (1988): Sperber SJ+, J Infect Dis 158(1), 166 (12.5–38%)
Oral candidiasis
Parosmia
Sialorrhea
Tongue disorder (sic)
Vaginitis (4%)
Xerostomia

Hair
Hair – alopecia (4%)
Hair – hirsutism

Other
Anaphylactoid reactions/Anaphylaxis
 (1999): Corona T+, Neurology 52(2), 425
Asthenia
 (2006): Gottesman MH+, Mult Scler 12(3), 271
 (2004): Festi D+, World J Gastroenterol 10(1), 12
 (2002): Exton MS+, Neuropsychobiology 45(4), 199
 (2002): Yang CH+, Chang Gung Med J 25(11), 774
 (2000): Gottberg K+, Mult Scler 6(5), 349
 (1998): Wadler S+, Cancer J Sci Am 4(5), 331
 (1997): Schwid SR+, Arch Neurol 54(9), 1169
 (1996): Huber S+, Schweiz Med Wochenschr 126(35), 1475 (31%)
 (1996): Neilley LK+, Neurology 46(2), 552
 (1991): Allen J+, J Clin Oncol 9(5), 783
 (1988): Schiller JH+, J Interferon Res 8(5), 581
 (1987): Grunberg SM+, Cancer Res 47(4), 1174
 (1987): Schiller JH+, Cancer Treat Rep 71(10), 945
Chills (21%)
 (1998): Mohr DC+, Mult Scler 4(6), 487
Death
 (2000): Beghi E+, Neurology 54(2), 469
Depression
 (2005): Patten SB+, Mult Scler 11(2), 175
 (2003): Goeb JL+, Clin Neuropharmacol 26(1), 5
 (2002): Lana-Peixoto MA+, Arq Neuropsiquiatr 60(3-B), 721
 (1999): Mohr DC+, Arch Neurol 56(10), 1263
 (1998): Mohr DC+, Mult Scler 4(6), 487
Embolia cutis medicamentosa (Nicolau syndrome)
 (2005): Reactions 1, 1058, 8
Fever
 (2004): Festi D+, World J Gastroenterol 10(1), 12
 (2002): Yang CH+, Chang Gung Med J 25(11), 774
 (1999): Garcia-Moreno JM+, Neurologia 14(4), 154
 (1998): Williams GJ+, J Interferon Cytokine 18(11), 967
 (1997): Munschauer FE+, Clin Ther 19(5), 883
 (1994): Connelly JF, Ann Pharmacother 28(5), 610
 (1991): Allen J+, J Clin Oncol 9(5), 783
 (1990): Fetell MR+, Cancer 65(1), 78
 (1990): Von Hoff+, J Interferon Res 10(5), 531
 (1990): Yung WK+, J Neurooncol 9(1), 29
 (1987): Grunberg SM+, Cancer Res 47(4), 1174
 (1987): Lillis PK+, Cancer Treat Rep 71(10), 965
 (1986): Rinehart J+, Cancer Res 46(10), 5364
 (1986): Sarna G+, Cancer Treat Rep 70(12), 1365
Fibrosis
 (1997): Elgart GW+, J Am Acad Dermatol 37(4), 553
Headache
Hypersensitivity (3%)
Infections (11%)
Injection-site atrophy
Injection-site burning
Injection-site ecchymoses (2%)
Injection-site edema
 (2004): Debat Zoguereh D+, Rev Neurol (Paris) 160(11), 1081

Injection-site erythema
  (2004): Debat Zoguereh D+, *Rev Neurol* (Paris) 160(11), 1081
  (1987): Grunberg SM+, *Cancer Res* 47(4), 1174
Injection-site hypersensitivity
Injection-site inflammation (3%)
Injection-site necrosis
  (1999): Radziwill AJ+, *J Neurol Neurosurg Psychiatry* 67(1), 115
Injection-site pain
  (2000): Gottberg K+, *Mult Scler* 6(5), 349
  (1996): Mohr DC+, *Mult Scler* 2(5), 222
Injection-site panniculitis
  (2002): Heinzerling L+, *Eur J Dermatol* 12(2), 194
Injection-site pruritus
  (2004): Debat Zoguereh D+, *Rev Neurol* (Paris) 160(11), 1081
Injection-site purpura (2%)
Injection-site reactions (sic) (4%)
  (2008): Conroy M+, *J Am Acad Dermatol* 59(2), S48
  (2002): Panitch H+, *Neurology* 59(10), 1496
Injection-site ulceration
  (2002): Yang CH+, *Chang Gung Med J* 25(11), 774
  (1997): Elgart GW+, *J Am Acad Dermatol* 37(4), 553
  (1997): Weinberg JM+, *Acta Derm Venereol* 77(2), 146
Lipoatrophy
  (2006): Beiske AG+, *J Neurol* 253(3), 377
Lipomatosis
Myalgia/Myositis/Myopathy/Myotoxicity (44%)
  (2002): Yang CH+, *Chang Gung Med J* 25(11), 774
  (1998): Williams GJ+, *J Interferon Cytokine Res* 18(11), 967
  (1997): Munschauer FE+, *Clin Ther* 19(5), 883
  (1994): Connelly JF, *Ann Pharmacother* 28(5), 610
  (1988): Schiller JH+, *J Interferon Res* 8(5), 581
  (1987): Grunberg SM+, *Cancer Res* 47(4), 1174
Nephrotoxicity
  (2005): Auty A+, *Can J Neurol Sci* 32(3), 366
Pain (52%)
  (2002): Heinzerling L+, *Eur J Dermatol* 12(2), 194 (52%)
Panniculitis
  (2002): Heinzerling L+, *Eur J Dermatol* 12(2), 194
Paresthesias
  (1998): Mohr DC+, *Mult Scler* 4(6), 487
Peyronie's disease
Rhabdomyolysis
  (2002): Lunemann JD+, *J Neurol Neurosurg Psychiatry* 72(2), 274
Seizures (2%)
  (2002): Dubisar BM+, *Pharmacotherapy* 22(11), 1504
Suicidal ideation
  (2002): Lana-Peixoto MA+, *Arq Neuropsiquiatr* 60(3), 721
Thrombophlebitis
  (1999): Fortuno Y+, *Med Clin* (Barc) 113(12), 447 (2 cases)
  (1997): Elgart GW+, *J Am Acad Dermatol* 37(4), 553
Tremor
Upper respiratory infection (31%)
Vertigo (35%)

INTERLEUKIN-2

(See ALDESLEUKIN)

IODIXANOL

Trade name: Visipaque (Amersham Health)
Indications: Angiocardiography
Category: Iodine-containing radiocontrast medium
Half-life: 2 hours
Clinically important, potentially hazardous interactions with: N/A

Reactions

Skin
Adverse effects (sic)
  (2001): Sutton AG+, *Am Heart J* 141(4), 677
Edema (<1%)
Erythema (2%)
Pruritus (<2%)
Rash (sic) (2%)
Urticaria (0.5%)

Mucosal/ENT
Dysgeusia (3.5%)
Parosmia (<1%)

Eyes
Visual disturbances

Other
Asthenia (1%)
Headache
  (1996): Poirier VC+, *Acad Radiol* 3 Suppl 3, S495 (2.5%)
Injection-site pain
Paresthesias (1%)
Vertigo (2%)

IOHEXOL

Trade name: Omnipaque (GE Healthcare)
Indications: Diagnostic aid in myelography, angiography and computerized tomography procedures
Category: Contrast agent
Half-life: variable
Clinically important, potentially hazardous interactions with: corticosteroids

Reactions

Skin
Diaphoresis
Pruritus (0.1%)
Purpura (0.1%)
Rash (sic)
Urticaria (0.3%)

Mucosal/ENT
Dysgeusia (1%)
Tinnitus

Eyes
Photophobia (2%)
Vision blurred (2%)

Other
Anxiety (0.3%)
Chest pain (1%)

Cough (0.2%)
Headache (18%)
  (1989): Sand T+, *Neuroradiology* 31(1), 49
  (1989): Sobel DF+, *Headache* 29(8), 519
  (1988): Nestvold K+, *Acta Radiol* 29(6), 637
  (1987): Sand T+, *Neuroradiology* 29(4), 385
  (1987): Simon JH+, *Radiology* 163(2), 455
Hypertension
Hypotension (0.7%)
Paresthesias (0.3%)
Somnolence (0.5%)
Vertigo (0.5%)
  (1988): Nestvold K+, *Acta Radiol* 29(6), 637

IOPROMIDE

Trade name: Ultravist (Berlex)
Indications: Arteriography, urography, body imaging
Half-life: ~2 hours
Clinically important, potentially hazardous interactions with: N/A

Reactions

Skin
Angioedema
Baboon syndrome
  (2007): Arnold AW+, *Dermatology* 214(1), 89
Edema
  (1995): Christensen J, *Acta Radiol* 36(1), 82
Erythema
  (1994): de Geeter P+, *Br J Radiol* 67(802), 958
Facial edema
  (2005): Mortele KJ+, *AJR Am J Roentgenol* 184(1), 31
Pruritus
Rash (sic)
  (1984): Steidle B+, *Dtsch Med Wochenschr* 109(34), 1275
Urticaria (0.8%)
  (2005): Mortele KJ+, *AJR Am J Roentgenol* 184(1), 31
  (1994): de Geeter P+, *Br J Radiol* 67(802), 958
  (1991): Gross-Fengels W+, *Med Klin* (Munich) 86(11), 561 (%)
  (1989): Broussel R, *Ann Radiol* (Paris) 32(4), 329

Mucosal/ENT
Dysgeusia
Tongue edema
  (1995): Christensen J, *Acta Radiol* 36(1), 82

Eyes
Vision blurred (0.1%)

Cardiovascular
Thrombosis

Other
Extravasation
  (1994): Newhouse JH+, *Invest Radiol* 29, S68
Headache
  (1994): Faykus MH+, *Invest Radiol* 29, S98 (4%)
  (1989): Neiss AC+, *Ann Radiol* (Paris) 32(1), 49
Hepatotoxicity
  (1998): Re G+, *J Toxicol Clin Toxicol* 36(3), 261
Hypersensitivity
  (1996): Schick E+, *Contact Dermatitis* 35(5), 312
Hypertension
Hypotension
Injection-site pain

  (1997): Justesen P+, *Cardiovasc Intervent Radiol* 20(4), 251
  (1994): de Geeter P+, *Br J Radiol* 67(802), 958
  (1984): Steidle B+, *Dtsch Med Wochenschr* 109(34), 1275
Nephrotoxicity
  (2005): Mueller C+, *Swiss Med Wkly* 135(19-2), 286 (mild)
Paresthesias
  (1997): Encina JL+, *Eur Radiol* 7, S115
  (1997): Justesen P+, *Cardiovasc Intervent Radiol* 20(4), 251
  (1997): Schmiedel E, *Aktuelle Radiol* 7(4), 183
  (1994): de Geeter P+, *Br J Radiol* 67(802), 958 (17%)
  (1994): Faykus MH+, *Invest Radiol* 29, S98
  (1994): Goldberg SN+, *Invest Radiol* 29, S76 (8%)
  (1993): Pugh ND+, *Clin Radiol* 47(2), 96
  (1989): Broussel R, *Ann Radiol* (Paris) 32(4), 329
  (1984): Steidle B+, *Dtsch Med Wochenschr* 109(34), 1275
Vertigo
  (1984): Steidle B+, *Dtsch Med Wochenschr* 109(34), 1275

IPODATE

Trade names: Bilivist; Oragrafin
Indications: Cholecystography
Category: Iodine-containing radiocontrast medium
Half-life: N/A

Reactions

Skin
Allergic reactions (sic) (<3%)
  (1986): Bigby M+, *JAMA* 256, 3358 (2.78%)
Exanthems
Pruritus
Purpura
Rash (sic)
Urticaria

Other
Anaphylactoid reactions/Anaphylaxis
Hypersensitivity
Serum sickness

IPRATROPIUM

Trade names: Alti-Ipratropium; Atrovent (Boehringer Ingelheim); Combivent (Boehringer Ingelheim); Duoneb (DEY); Novo-Ipramide
Indications: Bronchospasm
Category: Anticholinergic; Muscarinic antagonist
Half-life: 2 hours

Note: Combivent is albuterol and ipratropium

Reactions

Skin
Dermatitis
  (1988): Eedy DJ+, *Postgrad Med J* 64, 306
Exanthems
Miliaria profunda
  (1990): Saurat JH+, *Pediatr Dermatol* 7, 325
Pruritus (<1%)
Rash (sic) (1.2%)
Urticaria (<1%)

Mucosal/ENT
Dysgeusia (1%) (metallic taste)
(2002): Cuvelier A+, *Respir Care* 47(2), 159
(1980): Pakes GE+, *Drugs* 20, 237
Oral lesions (1–5%)
(1980): Pakes GE+, *Drugs* 20, 237
Oral ulceration (<1%)
(1987): High AS, *BMJ* 294, 375
(1986): Spencer PA, *BMJ* 292, 380
Stomatitis (<1%)
Xerostomia (3.2%)
(1995): Loesche WJ+, *J Am Geriatr Soc* 43(4), 401
(1980): Pakes GE+, *Drugs* 20, 237

Hair
Hair – alopecia (<1%)

Eyes
Mydriasis
(2006): Openshaw H, *Neurology* 67(5), 914

Other
Anaphylactoid reactions/Anaphylaxis
(1993): Bone WD+, *Chest* 103, 981
Death
(2003): Ringbaek T+, *Respir Med* 97(3), 264 (in patients with asthma and COPD)
Headache
Paresthesias (<1%)

IRBESARTAN

Trade names: Avalide (Bristol-Myers Squibb); Avapro (Bristol-Myers Squibb) (Sanofi-Aventis)
Indications: Hypertension
Category: Angiotensin II receptor antagonist
Half-life: 11–15 hours

Note: Avalide is irbesartan and hydrochlorothiazide (a sulfonamide)

Note: Avalide contains a sulfonamide which can be absorbed systemically. Sulfonamides can produce severe, possibly fatal, reactions such as toxic epidermal necrolysis and Stevens–Johnson syndrome

Reactions

Skin
Angioedema
(2002): Touraud JP+, *Ann Dermatol Venereol* 129(8), 1033
Dermatitis (<1%)
Eczema
(2002): Touraud JP+, *Ann Dermatol Venereol* 129(8), 1033 (2 cases)
Edema (1–10%)
Erythema (<1%)
Exanthems
(2006): Constable S+, *Br J Dermatol* 155(2), 491
Facial edema (<1%)
Lichenoid eruption
(2006): Pfab F+, *Allergy* 61(6), 786 (with hydrochlorothiazide)
Pemphigus herpetiformis
(2002): Viseux V+, *World Congress Dermatol* Poster, 0360
Pruritus (<1%)
Rash (sic) (1–10%)
Urticaria (<1%)

Mucosal/ENT
Oral lesions (<1%)

Eyes
Eyelid edema
(2002): Cohen PR, *J Drugs Dermatol* 1(3), 329

Other
Chills (<1%)
Cough
(2002): Coca A+, *Clin Ther* 24(1), 126
(2002): Touraud JP+, *Ann Dermatol Venereol* 129(8), 1033
Headache
Paresthesias (<1%)
Tremor (<1%)

IRINOTECAN

Synonyms: Camptothecin-11; CPT-11
Trade name: Camptosar (Pfizer)
Indications: Metastatic colorectal carcinoma
Category: Topoisomerase 1 inhibitor
Half-life: 6–10 hours
Clinically important, potentially hazardous interactions with: aprepitant, atazanavir, **St John's wort**

Reactions

Skin
Allergic reactions (sic) (9%)
(1997): Verschraegen CF+, *J Clin Oncol* 15, 625 (9%)
Diaphoresis (16%)
Edema (10.2%)
Exanthems
(2002): Liu CY, *Ann Pharmacother* 36(12), 1897
Hand–foot syndrome
(2004): Park SH+, *Oncology* 66(5), 353 (1 case)
(2003): Gerbrecht BM, *Cancer Nurs* 26(2), 161
(2002): Lin E+, *Oncology* (Huntingt) 16(12 Suppl 14), 31
Photosensitivity
(2002): Willey A+, *J Am Acad Dermatol* 47(3), 453
Pigmentation
(2002): Pui JC+, *J Drugs Dermatol* 1(2), 202
Pruritus
(2002): Liu CY, *Ann Pharmacother* 36(12), 1897
Pyogenic granuloma
(2002): Piguet V+, *Br J Dermatol* 147(6), 1270
Rash (sic) (<21%)
(1997): Verschraegen CF+, *J Clin Oncol* 15, 625 (21%)

Mucosal/ENT
Dysgeusia (metallic taste)
Mucositis (2%)
(2003): Mendez M+, *Clin Colorectal Cancer* 3(3), 174 (4 cases)
Oral ulceration
Sialorrhea
Stomatitis (<14%)
(2002): Bass AJ+, *J Clin Oncol* 20(13), 2995
(2000): Adjei AA+, *J Clin Oncol* 18, 1116
(1997): Verschraegen CF+, *J Clin Oncol* 15, 625 (14%)

Hair
Hair – alopecia (13–60.5%)
(2002): Kollmannsberger C+, *Br J Cancer* 87(7), 729 (2 cases)
(2001): Ulrich-Pur H+, *Ann Oncol* 12(9), 1269 (13%)
(1999): Takahashi Y+, *Gan To Kagaku Ryoho* (Japanese) 26, 1193

(1998): Berg D, *Oncol Nurs Forum* 25, 535
(1997): Verschraegen CF+, *J Clin Oncol* 15, 625 (48%)
(1996): Rougier P+, *Semin Oncol* 23, 34
(1995): Abigerges D+, *J Clin Oncol* 13, 210 (53%)
(1995): Catimel G+, *Ann Oncol* 6, 133
(1994): de Forni M+, *Cancer Res* 54, 4347
(1994): Sakata Y+, *Gan To Kagaku Ryoho* (Japanese) 21, 1039
    (40%)
(1994): Taguchi T+, *Gan To Kagaku Ryoho* (Japanese) 21, 1017
    (30%)
(1994): Taguchi T+, *Gan To Kagaku Ryoho* (Japanese) 21, 83
    (61%)
(1992): Fukuoka M+, *J Clin Oncol* 10, 16 (4%)
(1991): Negoro S+, *Gan To Kagaku Ryoho* (Japanese) 18, 1013
(1991): Takeuchi S+, *Gan To Kagaku Ryoho* (Japanese) 18, 1681
    (33%)
(1991): Takeuchi S+, *Gan To Kagaku Ryoho* (Japanese) 18, 579
    (33%)
(1990): Taguchi T+, *Gan To Kagaku Ryoho* (Japanese) 17, 115

Other
Asthenia
    (2002): Vaishampayan UN+, *Int J Radiat Oncol Biol Phys*
    53(3), 675
Chills (13.8%)
Death
    (2006): Schaaf LJ+, *Clin Cancer Res* 12(12), 3782
    (2003): Buckner JC+, *Cancer* 97(9 Suppl), 2352
    (2003): Mendez M+, *Clin Colorectal Cancer* 3(3), 174 (2 cases)
Fever
    (2002): Kollmannsberger C+, *Br J Cancer* 87(7), 729 (1 case)
Headache
Hypotension
    (2001): Blandizzi C+, *Toxicol Appl Pharmacol* 177(2), 149
Infections (sic) (3%)
    (2001): Ulrich Pur H+, *Ann Oncol* 12(9), 1269 (3%)
Neurotoxicity
    (2006): Hamberg P+, *J Natl Cancer Inst* 98(3), 219
    (2006): Kawahara M, *Expert Opin Drug Saf* 5(2), 303
Thrombophlebitis (1–10%)
Vertigo
    (2002): Liu CY, *Ann Pharmacother* 36(12), 1897

ISOCARBOXAZID

Trade names: Enerzer; Marplan (Oxford)
Indications: Depression
Category: Antidepressant; Monoamine oxidase (MAO) inhibitor
Half-life: N/A
**Clinically important, potentially hazardous interactions
with:** amitriptyline, amoxapine, bupropion, citalopram,
clomipramine, desipramine, doxepin, fluoxetine, fluvoxamine,
imipramine, meperidine, nefazodone, nortriptyline, paroxetine,
protriptyline, rizatriptan, sertraline, sibutramine, sumatriptan,
trimipramine, **tryptophan**, venlafaxine, zolmitriptan

Reactions

Skin
Diaphoresis
Exanthems (7%)
Peripheral edema (1–10%)
Photosensitivity (4%)
Pruritus (4%)
Rash (sic)
Telangiectasia

Mucosal/ENT
Tongue black
Xerostomia (1–10%)
    (1984): Zisook S, *J Clin Psychiatry* 45(7 Pt 2), 53

Other
Headache
    (1984): Zisook S, *J Clin Psychiatry* 45(7 Pt 2), 53
Myoclonus
    (1983): Davidson J+, *J Affect Disord* 5(2), 183
Vertigo
    (1984): Zisook S, *J Clin Psychiatry* 45(7 Pt 2), 53
    (1983): Davidson J+, *J Affect Disord* 5(2), 183

ISOETHARINE

Trade names: Arm-a-Med; Asthmalitan; Beta-2; Bronkomed;
Dey-Lute; Numotac
Indications: Bronchial asthma
Category: Adrenergic beta-receptor agonist
Half-life: N/A
**Clinically important, potentially hazardous interactions
with:** phenelzine

Reactions

Mucosal/ENT
Xerostomia (1–10%)

Other
Anaphylactoid reactions/Anaphylaxis
    (1982): Twarog FJ+, *JAMA* 248, 2030
Tremor

ISOFLURANE

Trade names: Aerrane; Floran; Forane (Baxter); Forene;
Forthane; Isofluran; Isoflurano; Isofor; Isorane; Lisorane; Sofloran;
Tensocold
Indications: Maintenance of general anesthesia
Category: Anesthetic, inhalation
Half-life: N/A
Onset of action: 7–10 minutes
**Clinically important, potentially hazardous interactions
with:** cisatracurium, doxacurium, muscle relaxants, pancuronium,
rapacuronium

Reactions

Skin
Shivering (post-operative)

Other
Death
    (2006): Ihtiyar E+, *Indian J Gastroenterol* 25(1), 41

ISONIAZID

Synonym: INH
Trade names: Cemidon; Diazid; Isotamine; Isozid; Nicotibine; Nicozid; PMS-Isoniazid; Rifamate (Sanofi-Aventis); Rifater (Sanofi-Aventis); Tibinide
Indications: Tuberculosis
Category: Antibiotic; Antimycobacterial
Half-life: 1–4 hours
Clinically important, potentially hazardous interactions with: insulin detemir, rifampin

Reactions

Skin

Acne
  (1988): Oliwiecki S+, *Clin Exp Dermatol* 13, 283
  (1988): Yamanaka M+, *Kekkaku* (Japanese) 63, 11
  (1982): Rosin MA+, *Southern Med J* 75, 81 (passim)
Acute generalized exanthematous pustulosis (AGEP)
  (1995): Moreau A+, *Int J Dermatol* 34, 263 (passim)
Angioedema (<1%)
  (1989): Yagi S+, *Kekkaku* (Japanese) 64, 407
Bullous dermatitis
  (2005): Trabelsi S+, *Therapie* 60(6), 599
  (1999): Scheid P+, *Allergy* 54, 294
Cutis laxa
  (1985): Koch SE+, *Pediatr Dermatol* 2, 282
Dermatitis
  (1993): Meseguer J+, *Contact Dermatitis* 28, 110 (systemic)
  (1986): Holdiness MR, *Contact Dermatitis* 15, 282
Dermatomyositis
Erythema multiforme (<1%)
  (1988): Hira SK+, *J Am Acad Dermatol* 19, 451 (in AIDS patients)
Exanthems (<1%)
  (1982): Rosin MA+, *Southern Med J* 75, 81 (passim)
Exfoliative dermatitis
  (1985): Holdiness MR, *Int J Dermatol* 24, 280
  (1982): Rosin MA+, *Southern Med J* 75, 81
Herpes zoster
Keratoacanthoma
Lichenoid eruption
  (2001): Sharma PK+, *J Dermatol* 28(12), 737
Lupus erythematosus
  (2002): Siddiqui MA+, *Am J Ther* 9(2), 163
  (1994): Yung RL+, *Rheum Dis Clin North Am* 20, 61
  (1992): Hofstra AH+, *Drug Metab Dispos* 20, 205
  (1992): Rubin RL+, *J Clin Invest* 90, 165
  (1992): Salazar-Paramo M+, *Ann Rheum Dis* 51, 1085
  (1992): Skaer TL, *Clin Ther* 14, 496
  (1991): Gatenby PA, *Autoimmunity* 11, 61
  (1990): Guleria R+, *Indian J Chest Dis Allied Sci* 32, 55
  (1989): Ueda Y+, *Kekkaku* (Japanese) 64, 613
  (1988): Jiang M, *Chung Kuo I Hsueh Ko Hsueh Yuan Hsueh Pao* (Chinese) 10, 379
  (1988): Umeki S, *Kekkaku* (Japanese) 63, 713
  (1986): Layer P+, *Dtsch Med Wochenschr* (German) 111, 1603
  (1985): Cush JJ+, *Am J Med Sci* 290, 36
  (1985): Holdiness MR, *Int J Dermatol* 24, 280
  (1985): Kale SA, *Postgrad Med* 77, 231
  (1985): Lovisetto P+, *Recenti Prog Med* (Italy) 76, 110
  (1985): Stratton MA, *Clin Pharm* 4, 657
  (1984): No Author, *Lancet* 2, 441
  (1984): Sim E+, *Lancet* 2, 422
  (1983): Escolar-Castellon F+, *Rev Clin Esp* (Spanish) 169, 209
  (1982): Grunwald M+, *Dermatologica* 165, 172
  (1982): Harmon CE+, *Clin Rheum Dis* 8, 121

  (1981): Reidenberg MM, *Arthritis Rheum* 24, 1004
  (1980): Agarwal MB+, *J Postgrad Med* 26, 263
  (1980): Condemi JJ, *Geriatrics* 35(3), 81
  (1980): Weinstein A, *Prog Clin Immunol* 4, 1
Peripheral edema
  (1999): Muratake T+, *Am J Psychiatry* 156, 660
  (1987): Schmutz JL+, *Ann Derm Venereol* (French) 114, 569
  (1983): Jorgensen J, *Int J Dermatol* 22, 44
  (1981): Meyrick Thomas RH+, *BMJ* 283, 287
Photosensitivity
  (1998): Lee AY+, *Photodermatol Photoimmunol Photomed* 14, 77 (lichenoid) (2 patients)
  (1987): Schmutz JL+, *Ann Dermatol Venereol* (French) 114, 569
Pruritus
Purpura
  (1992): Breathnach SM+, *Adverse Drug Reactions and the Skin* Blackwell, Oxford, 159 (passim)
  (1982): Rosin MA+, *Southern Med J* 75, 81 (passim)
  (1980): Miescher PA+, *Clin Haematol* 9, 505
Pustules
  (1993): Webster GF, *Clin Dermatol* 11, 541
  (1985): Yamasaki R+, *Br J Dermatol* 112, 504 (subcorneal)
Rash (sic) (<1%)
  (2000): Gordin F+, *JAMA* 283, 1445
Side effects (sic) (2%)
  (2003): Yee D+, *Am J Respir Crit Care Med* 167(11), 1472
  (1985): Holdiness MR, *Int J Dermatol* 24, 280 (2%)
Stevens–Johnson syndrome
  (2005): Pitche P+, *Med Trop* (Mars) 65(4), 359 (with rifampicin)
  (1992): Dukes CS+, *Trop Geogr Med* 44(4), 308
Striae
Toxic epidermal necrolysis (<1%)
  (2005): Pitche P+, *Med Trop* (Mars) 65(4), 359 (with rifampicin)
  (1990): Nanda A+, *Arch Dermatol* 126, 125
  (1983): Katoch K+, *Lepr India* 55, 133
Urticaria (1–5%)
  (1992): Breathnach SM+, *Adverse Drug Reactions and the Skin* Blackwell, Oxford, 159 (passim)
  (1982): Rosin MA+, *Southern Med J* 75, 81 (passim)
Vasculitis
  (1982): Rosin MA+, *Southern Med J* 75, 81 (passim)
Xanthoderma
  (2007): Haught JM+, *J Am Acad Dermatol* 57(6), 1051

Mucosal/ENT

Oral lesions
Oral ulceration
Tinnitus
  (1984): Snavely SR+, *Ann Intern Med* 101(1), 92
Xerostomia

Hair

Hair – alopecia
  (2001): Sharma PK+, *J Dermatol* 28(12), 737
  (1996): FitzGerald JM+, *Lancet* 347, 472

Eyes

Optic neuritis
  (2005): Noguera-Pons R+, *Ann Pharmacother* 39(12), 2131 (with etanercept)
Visual hallucinations
  (2006): Maalej S+, *Presse Med* 35(3 Pt 1), 425

Other

Anaphylactoid reactions/Anaphylaxis
  (2003): Crook MJ, *J Clin Pharmacol* 43(5), 545
Death
Gynecomastia
  (2003): Khanna P+, *Indian J Chest Dis Allied Sci* 45(4), 277

Hepatotoxicity
(2006): Aziz H+, *Curr Med Res Opin* 22(1), 217
(2005): Peters TS, *Toxicol Pathol* 33(1), 146
Hypersensitivity
(2001): Rebollo S+, *Contact Dermatitis* 45(5), 306
(1992): Dukes CS+, *Trop Geogr Med* 44, 308
Injection-site irritation
Myalgia/Myositis/Myopathy/Myotoxicity
(1989): Cronkright PJ+, *Ann Intern Med* 110, 945
Neurotoxicity
(2005): Mazzeo F+, *Pharmacol Res* 51(3), 269
Paresthesias
(1982): Porter IH, *Handbook of Clinical Neurology* 44, 648
Rhabdomyolysis (3%)
(2001): Panganiban LR+, *J Toxicol Clin Toxicol* 39(2), 143 (3%)
(1995): Blowey DL+, *Am J Emerg Med* 13(5), 543
Serum sickness
(1981): Simelaro J+, *J Am Osteopath Assoc* 80, 348

ISOPROTERENOL

Synonym: Isoprenaline
Trade names: Aerolone; Isopro; Isuprel (Hospira); Isuprel Mistometer; Isuprel Nebulimetro; Saventrine; Vapo-Iso
Indications: Bronchospasm, ventricular arrhythmias
Category: Adrenergic beta-receptor agonist; Catecholamine; Sympathomimetic
Half-life: 2.5–5 minutes
Clinically important, potentially hazardous interactions with: amitriptyline

Reactions

Skin
Diaphoresis (1–10%)
Edema
Pruritus
Rash (sic)
Urticaria

Mucosal/ENT
Oral lesions
Xerostomia (>10%)

Other
Death
Headache
Tremor
(1998): Takamasu T+, *Arerugi* 47(6), 573 (transient)

ISOSORBIDE

Trade name: Ismotic
Indications: Acute angle-closure glaucoma
Category: Diuretic
Half-life: 5–9.5 hours
Clinically important, potentially hazardous interactions with: sildenafil

Reactions

Skin
Rash (sic) (<1%)

Mucosal/ENT
Tinnitus

Eyes
Visual hallucinations
(1987): Rosenthal R, *Psychosomatics* 28(10), 555

Other
Headache
(2002): Kosmicki M+, *Pol Arch Med Wewn* 107(6), 509
(2000): Christiansen I+, *Cephalalgia* 20(5), 437
(2000): Vargas-Ayala G+, *Blood Press* 9(5), 283
(1999): Lewis BS+, *Cardiology* 91(1), 1 (19%)
(1998): Chen YH+, *Zhonghua Yi Xue Za Zhi (Taipei)* 61(10), 577
(1997): Glasser SP, *Am J Cardiol* 80(12), 1546 (28%)
(1996): Cleophas TJ+, *Angiology* 47(7), 679
(1996): Walker JM+, *Int J Cardiol* 53(2), 117 (40%)
(1995): Hutt V+, *Arzneimittelforschung* 45(2), 142
(1995): Kosoglou T+, *Clin Ther* 17(2), 241
Hypotension
(1996): Salerno F+, *Hepatology* 23(5), 1135
Suicidal ideation
(1987): Rosenthal R, *Psychosomatics* 28(10), 555

ISOSORBIDE DINITRATE

Synonyms: ISD; ISDN
Trade names: Apo-ISDN; Cedocard; Coradur; Dilatrate-SR (Schwarz); Isordil (Wyeth); Sorbitrate (AstraZeneca)
Indications: Angina pectoris
Category: Nitrate; Vasodilator
Half-life: 4 hours (oral)
Clinically important, potentially hazardous interactions with: sildenafil

Reactions

Skin
Diaphoresis
Edema (<1%)
(2002): Aquilina S+, *Clin Exp Dermatol* 27(8), 700
Exanthems
(2002): Aquilina S+, *Clin Exp Dermatol* 27(8), 700
Pallor
Peripheral edema
(1981): Rodger JC, *BMJ* 283, 1365

Mucosal/ENT
Xerostomia

Eyes
Visual hallucinations
(1987): Rosenthal R, *Psychosomatics* 28(10), 555

Other
Headache
(1996): Walker JM+, *Int J Cardiol* 53(2), 117 (40%)
(1995): Kosoglou T+, *Clin Ther* 17(2), 241
Hypotension
Suicidal ideation
(1987): Rosenthal R, *Psychosomatics* 28(10), 555

ISOSORBIDE MONONITRATE

Synonym: ISMN
Trade names: Imdur (Schering); Ismo; Monoket (Schwarz)
Indications: Angina pectoris
Category: Nitrate; Vasodilator
Half-life: ~4 hours
**Clinically important, potentially hazardous interactions
with:** sildenafil

Reactions

Skin
Diaphoresis
Edema (<1%)
Peripheral edema
  (1981): Rodger JC, *BMJ* 283, 1365
Pruritus (<1%)
Rash (sic) (<1%)

Other
Headache

ISOTRETINOIN

Synonym: 13-*cis*-retinoic acid
Trade names: Accutane (Roche); Amnesteem (Genpharm);
Isotrex; Roaccutan; Roaccutane; Roacutan; Roacuttan
Indications: Cystic acne
Category: Retinoid
Half-life: 10–20 hours
**Clinically important, potentially hazardous interactions
with:** acitretin, antacids, bexarotene, cholestyramine, co-
trimoxazole, corticosteroids, **fish oil supplements**, minocycline,
retinoids, tetracycline, vitamin A

Reactions

Skin
Acne (fulminans)
  (2002): Moroz B+, *World Congress Dermatol* Poster, 0119
  (1997): Tan BB+, *Clin Exp Dermatol* 22, 26
  (1996): Faverge B+, *Arch Pediatr* (French) 3, 188
  (1993): Bottomley WW+, *Acta Derm Venereol* (Stockh) 73, 74
  (1993): Lepagney ML+, *Ann Dermatol Venereol* (French)
    120, 917
  (1992): Choi EH+, *J Dermatol* 19, 378
  (1992): Hagler J+, *Int J Dermatol* 31, 199
  (1992): Jenkinson HA, *Br J Dermatol* 127, 62
  (1991): Elias LM+, *J Dermatol* 18, 366
  (1991): Joly P+, *Ann Dermatol Venereol* (French) 118, 369
  (1989): Rotoli M+, *G Ital Dermatol Venereol* (Italian) 124, 120
  (1988): Blanc D+, *Dermatologica* 177, 16
  (1985): Kellett JK+, *BMJ* 290, 820
  (1984): Darley CR+, *J R Soc Med* 77, 328
Acute febrile neutrophilic dermatosis (Sweet's syndrome)
  (2007): Ammar D+, *Ann Dermatol Venereol* 134(2), 151
  (2003): Gyorfy A+, *Med Pediatr Oncol* 40(2), 135
Angioedema
  (2006): Saray Y+, *J Eur Acad Dermatol Venereol* 20(1), 118
Bruising
  (1993): Green C, *Br J Dermatol* 128, 465
Cellulitis
  (1994): Boffa MJ+, *J Am Acad Dermatol* 31, 800

Desquamation (palms and soles) (5%)
  (1988): Shalita AR+, *Cutis* 42, 10
Diaphoresis
  (2000): Popescu C, Bucharest, Romania (from Internet)
    (observation)
  (1988): Rees JL+, *Br J Dermatol* 119, 79
  (1987): Kiistala R+, *Acta Derm Venereol* 67, 331 (increased
    number of active sweat glands)
Edema (subcutaneous, recurrent)
  (1999): Choquet-Kastylevsky G+, *Therapie* (French) 54, 263
  (1999): Graham BS+, *Arch Dermatol* 135, 349
Erythema multiforme
  (1988): Bigby M+, *J Am Acad Dermatol* 18, 543
Erythema nodosum
  (1997): Tan BB+, *Clin Exp Dermatol* 22, 26
  (1988): Bigby M+, *J Am Acad Dermatol* 18, 543
  (1985): Kellett JK+, *BMJ* 290, 820
Exanthems
  (1993): Litt JZ, Beachwood, OH (non-pruritic) (personal case)
    (observation)
  (1988): Bigby M+, *J Am Acad Dermatol* 18, 543
Exfoliative dermatitis (1–10%)
Facial edema (1–10%)
  (2006): Scheinfeld N+, *J Drugs Dermatol* 5(5), 467
Facial erythema
  (2005): Al-Mutairi N+, *J Drugs Dermatol* 4(3), 369
Facial scarring
  (1994): Katz BE+, *J Am Acad Dermatol* 30, 852
Fixed eruption
  (1988): Bigby M+, *J Am Acad Dermatol* 18, 543
Folliculitis
  (1990): Hughes BR+, *Br J Dermatol* 122, 683
Fragility
  (2000): *Prescrire Int* 7, 178 (from wax epilation)
  (1997): Litt JZ, Beachwood, OH (lips from wax epilation) (2
    personal cases) (observations)
  (1997): Woollons A+, *Br J Dermatol* 137, 389
  (1995): Holmes SC+, *Br J Dermatol* 132, 165
Granulation tissue
  (1991): Rodland O+, *Tidsskr Nor Laegeforen* (Norwegian)
    111, 2630
  (1985): Miller RA+, *J Am Acad Dermatol* 5, 888
  (1984): Robertson DB+, *Br J Dermatol* 111, 689
Herpes
  (1990): Joly P+, *Ann Dermatol Venereol* (French) 117, 860
Herpes simplex
  (2006): Yazici AC+, *J Eur Acad Dermatol Venereol* 20(1), 93
Keloid
  (2006): Dogan G, *Clin Exp Dermatol* 31(4), 535
  (1999): Ginarte M+, *Int J Dermatol* 38, 228
  (1997): Bernestein LJ+, *Arch Dermatol* 133, 111
  (1994): Katz BE+, *J Am Acad Dermatol* 30, 852
  (1988): Zachariae H, *Br J Dermatol* 118, 703
Keratolysis exfoliativa
Leukoderma
  (1988): Bigby M+, *J Am Acad Dermatol* 18, 543
Lichenoid eruption
  (2001): Boyd AS+, *Cutis* 68, 301
Melasma
  (1998): Thaler D, Monona, WI (from Internet) (observation)
  (1997): Verros CD, Tripolis, Greece (from Internet)
    (observation)
Miliaria
  (1986): Gupta AK+, *Cutis* 38, 275
Mycosis fungoides
  (1985): Molin L+, *Acta Derm Venereol* 65, 69
Nummular eczema
  (1987): Bettoli V+, *J Am Acad Dermatol* 16, 617

Pallor (1–10%)
Pemphigus
  (1995): Georgala S+, *Acta Derm Venereol* 75, 413
Photosensitivity (>10%)
  (2002): Carlin CS+, *J Cutan Med Surg* 6(2), 125
  (1991): Auffret N+, *J Am Acad Dermatol* 23, 321
  (1986): Ferguson J+, *Br J Dermatol* 115, 275
  (1986): Wong RC+, *J Am Acad Dermatol* 14, 1095
  (1985): Diffey BL+, *J Am Acad Dermatol* 12, 119
  (1983): McCormack LS+, *J Am Acad Dermatol* 9, 273
Pigmentation
  (2002): Carlin CS+, *J Cutan Med Surg* 6(2), 125
  (1988): Bigby M+, *J Am Acad Dermatol* 18, 543
Pityriasis rosea
  (1984): Helfman RJ+, *Cutis* 33, 297
Port-wine stain
  (2005): Hoque S+, *Clin Exp Dermatol* 30(5), 587
Pruritus (1–5%)
  (1994): Yee KC+, *Dermatology* 189, 117
  (1988): Shalita AR+, *Cutis* 42, 10
Pyoderma gangrenosum
  (2002): Moroz B+, *World Congress Dermatol* Poster
  (1997): Gangaram HP+, *Br J Dermatol* 136, 636
Pyogenic granuloma
  (2003): Turel A+, *J Eur Acad Dermatol Venereol* 17(5), 609
  (1992): Hagler J+, *Int J Dermatol* 31, 199 (fatal)
  (1988): Blanc D+, *Dermatologica* 177, 16
  (1984): Robertson DB+, *Br J Dermatol* 111, 689
  (1983): Campbell JP+, *J Am Acad Dermatol* 9, 708
  (1983): Exner JH+, *Arch Dermatol* 119, 808
  (1983): Spear KL+, *Mayo Clin Proc* 58, 509
  (1983): Valentic JP+, *Arch Dermatol* 119, 871
Rash (sic)
Telangiectasia
  (1994): Thompson D, *The Schoch Letter* 44, 17(#186)
    (observation)
Toxic epidermal necrolysis
  (1994): Rosen T, *Arch Dermatol* 130, 260
Urticaria
  (2006): Saray Y+, *J Eur Acad Dermatol Venereol* 20(1), 118
  (2000): Madnani N, Mumbai, India (from Internet) (observation)
  (1988): Bigby M+, *J Am Acad Dermatol* 18, 543
Varicosities
  (1994): Thompson D, *The Schoch Letter* 44, 47(#186)
    (observation)
Vasculitis
  (1990): Aractingi S+, *Lancet* 335, 362
  (1989): Dwyer JM+, *Lancet* 2, 494
  (1989): Reynolds P+, *Lancet* 2, 1216
  (1987): Epstein EH, *Arch Dermatol* 123, 1124
Xanthomas
  (1983): Shalita AR+, *J Am Acad Dermatol* 9, 629
  (1980): Dicken CH+, *Arch Dermatol* 116, 951
Xerosis (>10%)
  (2006): Scheinfeld N+, *J Drugs Dermatol* 5(5), 467
  (2005): Al-Mutairi N+, *J Drugs Dermatol* 4(3), 369
  (1997): Berger R, *The Schoch Letter* 47, 5
  (1988): Shalita AR+, *Cutis* 42, 10

Mucosal/ENT

Ageusia
  (1996): Halpern SM+, *Br J Dermatol* 134(2), 378
Cheilitis (>90%)
  (2006): Scheinfeld N+, *J Drugs Dermatol* 5(5), 467
  (2005): Al-Mutairi N+, *J Drugs Dermatol* 4(3), 369
  (2001): Önder M+, *J Dermatol Treat* 12, 115
  (1999): Graham BS+, *Arch Dermatol* 349
  (1997): Berger R, *The Schoch Letter* 47, 5
  (1997): Goulden V+, *Br J Dermatol* 137, 106

  (1988): Shalita AR+, *Cutis* 42, 10
Dysgeusia
  (1990): Heise E+, *Eur Arch Otorhinolaryngol* 247, 382
Mucosal denudation of lips
  (1999): Graham BS+, *Arch Dermatol* 349
Parosmia
  (1990): Heise E+, *Eur Arch Otorhinolaryngol* 247, 382
Tinnitus
Xerostomia (>10%)
  (2005): Al-Mutairi N+, *J Drugs Dermatol* 4(3), 369
  (2003): Bots CP+, *Ned Tijdschr Tandheelkd* 110(7), 295
  (1992): Breathnach SM+, *Adverse Drug Reactions and the Skin* Blackwell, Oxford, 259 (passim)
  (1987): Neely SM+, *Arch Intern Med* 147(3), 529

Hair

Hair – alopecia (16%)
  (2005): Al-Mutairi N+, *J Drugs Dermatol* 4(3), 369
  (2004): Fitch MH, Aiken, SC (from Internet) (observation)
  (2002): Hirsch R, Boston, MA (from Internet) (observation)
  (2000): Dintiman BJ, Fairfax, VA (from Internet) (4 observations)
  (2000): Frederickson KS, Novalo, CA (from Internet) (observation)
  (2000): Rehbein HM, Jacksonville, FL (from Internet) (2 observations)
  (1998): Litt JZ, Beachwood, OH (personal case) (observation)
  (1998): Thaler D, Monona, WI (from Internet) (observation)
  (1997): Berger R, *The Schoch Letter* 47, 5 (diffuse)
  (1997): Thaler D, Monona, WI (from Internet) (observation)
  (1994): Shelley WB+, *Cutis* 53, 237 (observation)
Hair – hirsutism
Hair – pili torti (curly hair)
  (2002): Spencer L, Crawforsville, IN (from Internet) (observation)
  (1996): van der Pijl JW+, *Lancet* 348, 622
  (1990): Bunker CB+, *Clin Exp Dermatol* 15, 143
  (1985): Hays SB+, *Cutis* 25, 466

Nails

Nails – brittle
  (2001): Önder M+, *J Dermatol Treat* 12, 115
Nails – elkonyxis
  (2005): Yung A+, *Br J Dermatol* 153(3), 671
Nails – growth
  (1994): Litt JZ, Beachwood, OH (personal case) (observation)
Nails – herpetic whitlow
  (2003): Stetson CL+, *Int J Dermatol* 42(6), 496
Nails – median canaliform dystrophy
  (1997): Dharmagunawardena B+, *Br J Dermatol*
  (1992): Bottomley WW+, *Br J Dermatol* 127, 447
  (1988): Bigby M+, *J Am Acad Dermatol* 18, 543
Nails – paronychia
  (1998): Lepine EM, Rock Hill, SC (from Internet) (observation)
  (1988): Bigby M+, *J Am Acad Dermatol* 18, 543
  (1986): DeRaeve L+, *Dermatologica* 172, 278
  (1984): Blumental G, *J Am Acad Dermatol* 10, 677
Nails – periungual hemorrhage
  (1997): Leal G, Fortaleza, Brazil (from Internet) (observation)

Eyes

Blepharoconjunctivitis
  (2001): Fraunfelder FT+, *Am J Ophthalmol* 132(3), 299
Corneal opacity
  (2004): Fraunfelder FW, *Drugs Today (Barc)* 40(1), 23
Keratitis
  (2004): Fraunfelder FW, *Drugs Today (Barc)* 40(1), 23
Myopia
  (2004): Fraunfelder FW, *Drugs Today* 40(1), 23
Ocular transient discomfort

(2004): Fraunfelder FW, *Drugs Today* (Barc) 40(1), 23
Optic edema
   (2005): Wenham CJ+, *Br J Hosp Med* (London) 66(11), 644
Photophobia
   (2004): Fraunfelder FW, *Drugs Today* (Barc) 40(1), 23
Vision impaired
   (2004): Fraunfelder FW, *Drugs Today* (Barc) 40(1), 23

Other
Abdominal pain
   (2005): Al-Mutairi N+, *J Drugs Dermatol* 4(3), 369
Chest pain
   (2007): Madan V+, *Br J Dermatol* 156(3), 590
Death
Depression
   (2002): Robusto O, *Acta Med Port* 15(4), 325
Gynecomastia
   (1994): Shelley WB+, *Cutis* 54, 149 (passim)
   (1992): Fluckiger R, *Schweiz Rundsch Med Prax* (German) 81, 1370
Headache
   (2005): Al-Mutairi N+, *J Drugs Dermatol* 4(3), 369
Myalgia/Myositis/Myopathy/Myotoxicity
   (1998): Heudes AM+, *Ann Dermatol Venereol* 125(2), 94
   (1996): Fiallo P+, *Arch Dermatol* 132, 1521
   (1986): Hodak E, *BMJ* 293, 425
Pseudoporphyria
   (1993): Riordan CA+, *Clin Exp Dermatol* 18, 69
Rhabdomyolysis
   (2001): Trauner MA+, *Dermatology Online Journal* 5, 2
   (2001): Zabawski E, Longwood, TX (from Internet) (observation)
   (1998): Heudes AM+, *Ann Dermatol Venereol* 125(2), 94

ISOXSUPRINE

Trade names: Duvadilan; Isoxine; Sincen; Vasodilan; Vasolan; Vasosuprina; Voxsuprine; Xuprin
Indications: Peripheral vascular disease, Raynaud's phenomenon
Category: Adrenergic beta-receptor agonist
Half-life: N/A

Reactions

Skin
Dermatitis

Other
Chest pain
   (1983): Evron S+, *J Perinat Med* 11(6), 272
Hypotension
   (2003): Raymajhi R+, *Kathmandu Univ Med J* (KUMJ) 1(2), 85

ISRADIPINE

Trade names: DynaCirc (Reliant); Dynacirc SRO; Lomir; Lomir SRO; Prescal; Vascal
Indications: Hypertension
Category: Calcium channel blocker
Half-life: 8 hours
Clinically important, potentially hazardous interactions with: epirubicin, imatinib

Reactions

Skin
Diaphoresis (<1%)
Edema (7.2%)
   (1992): Lopez LM+, *Ann Pharmacother* 26, 789
   (1992): Madias NE+, *Am J Hypertens* 5, 141
   (1991): Eisner GM+, *Am J Hypertens* 4, 154S
   (1991): Galloe AM+, *J Intern Med* 229, 447
   (1991): Schachter M, *J Clin Pharm Ther* 16, 79
   (1990): Vidt DG, *Cleve Clin J Med* 57, 677
Exanthems (1.5%)
   (1993): Blumenthal HL, Beachwood, OH (personal case) (observation)
   (1990): Fitton A+, *Drugs* 40, 31 (1.5%)
Peripheral edema
Pruritus (<6%)
   (1990): Zubair M+, *Drugs* 40 (Suppl 2), 26 (5.9%)
Rash (sic) (1.5%)
Urticaria (<1%)

Mucosal/ENT
Gingival hyperplasia/hypertrophy (<1%)
   (1998): Young PC+, *Cutis* 62(indu), 41
Oral lesions (6%)
   (1990): Zubair M+, *Drugs* 40 (Suppl 2), 26 (5.9%)
Xerostomia (<1%)

Other
Headache (9%)
   (2002): Flynn JT+, *Pediatr Nephrol* 17(9), 748 (9.5%)
Paresthesias (<1%)
Vertigo (9%)
   (2002): Flynn JT+, *Pediatr Nephrol* 17(9), 748 (9.5%)

ITRACONAZOLE

Trade names: Isox; Itranax; Sopronox; Sporacid; Sporal; Sporanox (Janssen) (Ortho); Sporanox 15 D
Indications: Onychomycosis, deep mycoses
Category: Antibiotic, triazole
Half-life: 21 hours
Clinically important, potentially hazardous interactions with: alfuzosin, alprazolam, amphotericin B, anisindione, antacids, aprepitant, astemizole, atorvastatin, bosentan, ciclesonide, cimetidine, clorazepate, conivaptan, dasatinib, dexamethasone, dicumarol, didanosine, eplerenone, erythromycin, ethotoin, fentanyl, fosamprenavir, fosphenytoin, **grapefruit juice**, HMG-CoA reductase inhibitors, imatinib, ixabepilone, lapatinib, lovastatin, mephenytoin, methylprednisolone, midazolam, pimozide, prednisolone, prednisone, quinidine, rifampin, rimonabant, sildenafil, simvastatin, sirolimus, solifenacin, temsirolimus, terfenadine, triazolam, vardenafil, vinblastine, vincristine, warfarin

Reactions

Skin
Acute generalized exanthematous pustulosis (AGEP)
   (1997): Park YM+, *J Am Acad Dermatol* 36, 794
   (1995): Heymann WR+, *J Am Acad Dermatol* 33, 130
Angioedema
   (1996): Foong H, Malaysia (from Internet) (observation)
Edema (<3.5%)
   (1994): Gupta AK+, *J Am Acad Dermatol* 30, 911

(1994): Rosen T, *Arch Dermatol* 130, 260
(1992): *Med Lett Drugs Ther* 34, 14
(1991): Diaz M+, *Chest* 100, 682
(1991): Sharkey PK+, *Antimicrob Agents Chemother* 35, 707
(1990): Denning DW+, *J Am Acad Dermatol* 23, 602 (2%)
(1990): Sharkey PK+, *J Am Acad Dermatol* 23, 577
(1990): Tucker RM+, *J Antimicrob Chemother* 26, 561
Erythema multiforme
(1998): Rademaker M+, *New Zealand Adverse Drug Reactions Committee*, April, 1998 (from Internet)
Exanthems (<3%)
(2005): Blumenthal H, Beachwood, OH (personal communication)
(1999): Burrow WH, Jackson, MS (from Internet) (observation)
(1999): Valentine MC, Everett, WA (from Internet) (observation) (2 cases)
(1998): Litt JZ, Beachwood, OH (personal case) (observation)
(1997): Blumenthal HL, Beachwood, OH (personal case) (observation)
(1997): Danby FW, Kingston, Ontario (2 cases) (from Internet) (observation)
(1996): Degreef H, *Cutis* 58, 90
(1994): Litt JZ, Beachwood, OH (2 personal cases) (observation)
(1991): Smith DE+, *AIDS* 5, 1367
(1990): Roseeuw D+, *Clin Exp Dermatol* 15, 101 (2.6%)
(1990): Tucker RM+, *J Am Acad Dermatol* 23, 593 (3%)
Facial rash (papular, id-like)
(1996): Thaler D, Monona, WI (2 cases) (from Internet) (observation)
Fixed eruption
(1997): Perry S, *The Schoch Letter* 47, 19
(1994): Litt JZ, Beachwood, OH (personal case) (observation)
Peripheral edema (4%)
(1998): N Z Medicines Adverse Reactions Committee (from Internet) (observation)
(1996): Tailor SA+, *Arch Dermatol* 132, 350 (with nifedipine)
Photosensitivity
(1996): Moreland A, *The Schoch Letter* 46, 19 (observation)
Phototoxicity
(1999): Gass M, Davis, CA (from Internet) (observation)
(1995): Epstein E Jr, *The Schoch Letter* 45, 28 (observation)
(1994): Milstein H, *The Schoch Letter* 44, 5 (observation)
Pruritus (<2.5%)
(2002): Faergemann J+, *Arch Dermatol* 138, 69
(1997): Gupta AK+, *J Am Acad Dermatol* 36, 789
(1994): Gupta AK+, *J Am Acad Dermatol* 30, 911 (0.7%)
(1992): Cleary JD+, *Ann Pharmacother* 26, 502
(1992): Lavrijsen AP+, *Lancet* 340, 251
(1991): De Beule K+, *Curr Ther Res* 49, 814
(1990): Tucker RM+, *J Antimicrob Chemother* 26, 561
(1989): Grant SM+, *Drugs* 39, 877 (0.6%)
Purpura
(1997): Kramer KE+, *J Am Acad Dermatol* 37, 994
Rash (sic) (1–<8.6%)
(2003): Gallin JI+, *N Engl J Med* 348(24), 2416
(1996): Odom R+, *J Am Acad Dermatol* 35, 110 (severe)
(1994): Gupta AK+, *J Am Acad Dermatol* 30, 911 (1.1%)
(1990): Sharkey PK+, *J Am Acad Dermatol* 23, 577
(1990): Tucker RM+, *J Am Acad Dermatol* 23, 593
(1990): Tucker RM+, *J Antimicrob Chemother* 26, 561
Side effects (sic)
(1999): Gupta AK+, *Dermatology* 199, 248
(1997): Gupta AK+, *J Am Acad Dermatol* 36, 789
Stevens–Johnson syndrome
Urticaria
(2002): Faergemann J+, *Arch Dermatol* 138, 69
(1999): Valentine MC, Everett, WA (from Internet) (observation)
(1997): Billon S, *The Schoch Letter* 47, 32 (observation)
(1996): Thaler D, Monona, WI (from Internet) (observation)

(1994): Litt JZ, Beachwood, OH (personal case) (observation)
(1993): Litt JZ, Beachwood, OH (personal case) (observation)
(1992): Piepponen T+, *J Antimicrob Chemother* 29, 195
Vasculitis
(1996): Odom R+, *J Am Acad Dermatol* 35, 110
Xanthoderma
(2007): Haught JM+, *J Am Acad Dermatol* 57(6), 1051

Mucosal/ENT

Tinnitus
Xerostomia
(1990): Tucker RM+, *J Am Acad Dermatol* 23, 593
(1990): Tucker RM+, *J Antimicrob Chemother* 26, 561

Hair

Hair – alopecia
(1995): Litt JZ, Beachwood, OH (personal case) (observation)
(1992): de Gans J+, *AIDS* 6, 185
(1986): Moller Heilesen A, *BMJ* 293, 823
Hair – alopecia areata
(2005): Spacek J+, *Mycoses* 48(3), 165

Nails

Nails – beading
(1994): Donker PD+, *Clin Exp Dermatol* 19, 404
Nails – onychocryptosis
(1995): Arenas R+, *Int J Dermatol* 34, 138

Other

Anaphylactoid reactions/Anaphylaxis
Death
(2002): Legras A+, *Am J Med* 113(4), 352 (with leflunomide)
Gynecomastia (<1%)
(1994): Gupta AK+, *J Am Acad Dermatol* 30, 911
Headache
Myalgia/Myositis/Myopathy/Myotoxicity (1%)
Neurotoxicity
(2005): Singh R+, *Diabetes Care* 28(1), 225
Rhabdomyolysis
(2004): Ferrari M+, *Respiration* 71(3), 289
(2003): Ruiz-Contreras J+, *Pediatr Infect Dis J* 22(11), 1024
(2002): Vlahakos DV+, *Transplantation* 73(12), 1962
(1995): Lees RS+, *N Engl J Med* 333(10), 664 (with lovastatin)
Serum sickness
(1998): Park H+, *Ann Pharmacother* 32, 1249

IVABRADINE

Trade name: Procoralan (Servier)
Indications: Chronic stable angina pectoris
Category: Cardiotonic agent
Half-life: 2 hours
Clinically important, potentially hazardous interactions with: azole antifungals (ketoconazole, etc.), ketoconazole, macrolide antibiotics, nefazodone, nelfinavir, ritonavir

Reactions

Eyes

Luminous phenomena (14.5%)
(2007): *Prescrire Int* 16(88), 53
(2007): Ruzyllo W+, *Drugs* 67(3), 393
(2006): Savelieva I+, *Adv Cardiol* 43, 79
Photopsia
Vision blurred (1–10%)

Other
Headache (2–5%)
Myalgia/Myositis/Myopathy/Myotoxicity (1–10%)
Vertigo (1–10%)

IVERMECTIN

Trade name: Stromectol (Merck)
Indications: Various infections caused by susceptible helmintic organisms
Category: Antihelmintic
Half-life: 16–35 hours
Clinically important, potentially hazardous interactions with: alprazolam, barbiturates, benzodiazepines, diazepam, midazolam, valproic acid

Reactions

Skin
Angioedema
    (2006): Olson BG+, *Pediatr Infect Dis J* 25(5), 466 (with praziquantel and albendazole)
Bullous dermatitis
    (1993): Burnham GM, *Trans R Soc Trop Med Hyg* 87, 313
Bullous pemphigoid
    (2001): Trindade P, Natal, Brazil (personal communication)
Burning
    (1999): Editorial, *Arch Dermatol* 135, 705
Dermatitis
    (1999): Editorial, *Arch Dermatol* 135, 705
Edema (10–53%)
    (1998): Jaramillo-Ayerbe F+, *Arch Dermatol* 134, 143
    (1995): Darge K+, *Trop Med Parasitol* 46, 206 (arms and legs) (10%)
    (1993): Burnham GM, *Trans R Soc Trop Med Hyg* 87, 313
    (1992): Chijioke CP+, *Trans R Soc Trop Med Hyg* 86, 284
    (1992): Collins RC+, *Am J Trop Med Hyg* 47, 156 (facial) (31.8%)
    (1992): Zea-Flores R+, *Trans R Soc Trop Med Hyg* 86, 663 (53%)
    (1991): Bryan RT+, *Lancet* 337, 304
    (1991): Guderian RH+, *Lancet* 337, 188 (leg)
Exanthems (1–34%)
    (1993): Burnham GM, *Trans R Soc Trop Med Hyg* 87, 313
    (1991): Whitworth JAG+, *Lancet* 337, 625 (1–5%)
    (1990): Ette EI+, *Drug Intell Clin Pharm* 24, 426 (34%)
Facial edema (1.2%)
    (1998): Jaramillo-Ayerbe F+, *Arch Dermatol* 134, 143
    (1993): Burnham GM, *Trans R Soc Trop Med Hyg* 87, 313
Peripheral edema
Pruritus (38%–71%)
    (2005): Nontasut P+, *Southeast Asian J Trop Med Public Health* 36(2), 442
    (1998): Jaramillo-Ayerbe F+, *Arch Dermatol* 134, 143
    (1995): Darge K+, *Trop Med Parasitol* 46, 206
    (1993): Burnham GM, *Trans R Soc Trop Med Hyg* 87, 313
    (1993): Kar SK+, *Acta Trop* 55, 21
    (1992): Chijioke CP+, *Trans R Soc Trop Med Hyg* 86, 284 (71.2%)
    (1992): Collins RC+, *Am J Trop Med Hyg* 47, 156 (34%)
    (1991): Bryan RT+, *Lancet* 337, 304
    (1991): Whitworth JAG+, *Lancet* 337, 625 (8%)
    (1990): Ette EI+, *Drug Intell Clin Pharm* 24, 426 (9.6%)
    (1989): Guderian RH+, *Eur J Epidemiol* 5, 294 (4%)
Pustules
Rash (sic) (1–93%)
    (1998): Jaramillo-Ayerbe F+, *Arch Dermatol* 134, 143
    (1993): Kar SK+, *Acta Trop* 55, 21

    (1991): Bryan RT+, *Lancet* 337, 304 (93%)
    (1991): Guderian RH+, *Lancet* 337, 188
    (1991): Whitworth JAG+, *Lancet* 337, 625 (8%)
    (1989): Guderian RH+, *Eur J Epidemiol* 5, 294 (4%)
Side effects (sic) (mild)
    (2002): *Prescrire Int* 11(61), 137
Urticaria (0.9–22.7%)
    (2006): Olson BG+, *Pediatr Infect Dis J* 25(5), 466 (with praziquantel and albendazole)

Other
Abdominal pain
    (2006): Olson BG+, *Pediatr Infect Dis J* 25(5), 466 (with praziquantel and albendazole)
Fever
    (2006): Olson BG+, *Pediatr Infect Dis J* 25(5), 466 (with praziquantel and albendazole)
    (2004): Pani SP+, *J Commun Dis* 36(4), 240
Headache
    (2004): Pani SP+, *J Commun Dis* 36(4), 240
Myalgia/Myositis/Myopathy/Myotoxicity (20%)
    (2004): Pani SP+, *J Commun Dis* 36(4), 240
    (1995): Darge K+, *Trop Med Parasitol* 46, 206 (20%)
    (1993): Kar SK+, *Acta Trop* 55, 21
Tremor

IXABEPILONE

Trade name: Ixempra (Bristol-Myers Squibb)
Indications: Breast cancer (advanced or metastatic)
Category: Epithilone
Half-life: 52 hours
Clinically important, potentially hazardous interactions with: amprenavir, atazanavir, clarithromycin, delavirdine, grapefruit juice, indinavir, itraconazole, ketoconazole, nefazodone, ritonavir, saquinavir, telithromycin, voriconazole

Note: Often prescribed along with capecitabine. Patients with diabetes may be at increased risk of severe neuropathy

Reactions

Skin
Edema (9%)
Erythema multiforme
Exfoliative dermatitis (2%)
Facial flushing
Hand–foot syndrome (8%) (with capecitabine 64%)
Pigmentation (2%)
Pruritus (6%)
Rash (sic) (9%)
Vasculitis

Mucosal/ENT
Dysgeusia (6%)
Dysphagia
Mucositis (29%)
Stomatitis (29%)

Hair
Hair – alopecia (48%)

Nails
Nail disorder (sic) (9%)

Eyes
Lacrimation (4%)

Other

Abdominal pain (13%)
Asthenia (56%)
Chest pain (5%)
Chills
Cough (2%)
Fever (8%)
Headache (11%)
Hypersensitivity (5%)
Hypotension
Infections
Insomnia (5%)
Myalgia/Myositis/Myopathy/Myotoxicity (49%)
Nephrotoxicity
Pain (8%)
Upper respiratory infection (6%)
Vertigo (7%)
Weight loss (6%)

JOJOBA OIL

Scientific names: *Buxus chinensis; Simmondsia chinensis*
Family: Simmondsiaceae
Trade and other common names: Coffeebush; Deer-nut;
Goat-nut; Pig-nut
Purported indications and other uses: Moisturizer in
cosmetics and hair care products, edible oil
Half-life: N/A
**Clinically important, potentially hazardous interactions
with:** N/A

Reactions

Skin

Dermatitis
(2006): Di Berardino+, *Contact Dermatitis* 55(1), 57
(1996): Wantke F+, *Contact Dermatitis* 34(1), 71

JUNIPER

Scientific names: *Juniperus communis; Juniperus oxycedrus;
Juniperus phoenicea; Juniperus virginiana*
Family: Cupressaceae
Trade and other common names: Baccae Juniperi; Cade Oil;
Enebro; Gemeiner Wachholder; Genevrier; Ginepro; Juniper Tar
Oil; Zimbro
Category: Anti-inflammatory
Purported indications and other uses: Cystitis, urethritis,
urinary tract infections, flatulent colic, rheumatism, arthritis, gout,
leucorrhea, blenorrhea, scrofula. **Topical:** joint pain, muscle pain,
neuralgia, chronic eczema. **Inhalant:** bronchitis, lung infections.
Condiment, flavor component (gin, Chartreuse, bitters), perfume
Half-life: N/A
**Clinically important, potentially hazardous interactions
with:** loop diuretics, spironolactone, thiazide diuretics,
triamterene

Reactions

Skin

Allergic reactions (sic)

Dermatitis
(1996): Meding B+, *Contact Dermatitis* 34(3), 185
Edema
Erythema
Sensitivity (sic)
(2001): *Int J Toxicol* 20, 41
Vesiculation

KANAMYCIN

Trade names: Kanamicina; Kanamycine; Kanamytrex; Kanescin;
Kannasyn; Kantrex; Randikan
Indications: Various infections caused by susceptible organisms
Category: Antibiotic, aminoglycoside
Half-life: 2–4 hours
**Clinically important, potentially hazardous interactions
with:** aldesleukin, atracurium, bumetanide, doxacurium,
ethacrynic acid, furosemide, methoxyflurane, non-depolarizing
muscle relaxants, pancuronium, polypeptide antibiotics,
rocuronium, succinylcholine, torsemide, vecuronium

Reactions

Skin

Burning
Dermatitis (systemic)
(1986): Holdiness MR, *Contact Dermatitis* 15, 282
Edema (>10%)
Erythema (<1%)
Exanthems
Photosensitivity (<1%)
Pruritus (1–10%)
Rash (sic) (1–10%)
Urticaria

Mucosal/ENT

Ototoxicity
(2002): de Jager P+, *Int J Tuberc Lung Dis* 6(7), 622
(1996): Voogt GR+, *S Afr J Commun Disord* 43, 3
(1988): Blagoveshchenskaia NS+, *Zh Vopr Neirokhir Im N N
Burdenko* (4), 56
Sialorrhea (<1%)

Other

Hypersensitivity
Injection-site irritation
Injection-site pain (<1%)
Nephrotoxicity
(2002): de Jager P+, *Int J Tuberc Lung Dis* 6(7), 622
Paresthesias
Phlebitis
Tremor

KAVA

Scientific name: *Piper methysticum*
Family: Piperaceae
Trade and other common names: Ava; Awa; Intoxicating Pepper; Kavosporal; Kew; Sakau; Tonga
Category: Anxiolytic
Purported indications and other uses: Psychosis, depression, headache, migraines, colds, rheumatism, cystitis, vaginal prolapse, otitis, abscesses, antistress, analgesic, local anesthetic, anticonvulsant
Half-life: N/A
Clinically important, potentially hazardous interactions with: alcohol, alprazolam, benzodiazepines, escitalopram, levodopa

Note: Products containing kava have been implicated in cases of severe liver toxicity. Serious adverse effects include hepatitis, cirrhosis and liver failure. At least one patient required a liver transplant. Kava has now been banned in many countries

Reactions

Skin
Adverse effects (sic)
  (2003): Bent S+, *Ann Intern Med* 138(6), 468
  (2002): Denham A+, *J Altern Complement Med* 8(3), 237
  (2002): Ernst E, *Ann Intern Med* 136(1), 42
  (2002): Haller CA+, *Adverse Drug React Toxicol Rev* 21(3), 143
  (2002): Stevinson C+, *Drug Saf* 25(4), 251
  (2000): Ernst E, *Br J Dermatol* 143(5), 923
Lymphocytic inflammation
Photosensitivity
Pigmentation (yellow)
Pruritus
Rash (sic)
Scaling
Seborrheic dermatitis
  (2000): Caro I, *Skin & Aging* 80
Urticaria
  (2005): Grace R, *J Am Acad Dermatol* 53(5), 906
Xerosis

Hair
Hair – pigmentation

Nails
Nails – pigmentation

Other
Death
  (2003): Gow PJ+, *Med J Aust* 178(9), 442
Hepatotoxicity
  (2006): Musch E+, *Dtsch Med Wochenschr* 131(21), 1214
  (2006): Teschke R, *Dtsch Med Wochenschr* 131(34-3), 1880 (with St John's wort)
Hypersensitivity
  (2000): Schmidt P+, *Contact Dermatitis* 42(6), 363
Oral numbness
Seizures
  (2003): Cairney S+, *Neuropsychopharmacology* 28(2), 389
Side effects (sic)
  (2001): Kava R, *Pac Health Dialog* 8(1), 115
  (2000): Ernst E, *Br J Dermatol* 143(5), 923
  (1999): Tinsley JA, *Minn Med* 82(5), 29
Vertigo
  (2001): Wheatley D, *Phytother Res* 15(6), 549

KETAMINE

Trade names: Calypsol; Ketalar (Monarch); Ketalin; Ketanest; Ketolar; Petar
Indications: Induction of anesthesia
Category: Anesthetic
Half-life: 2–3 hours
Clinically important, potentially hazardous interactions with: memantine

Reactions

Skin
Erythema
Exanthems
Pruritus
  (2001): Burstal R+, *Anaesth Intensive Care* 29(3), 246
  (2001): Subramaniam K+, *J Clin Anesth* 13(5), 339 (with morphine)
Rash (sic) (1–10%)

Mucosal/ENT
Sialorrhea (<1%)
  (2001): Green SM+, *Pediatr Emerg Care* 17(4), 244

Eyes
Nystagmus
  (2004): Launo C+, *Minerva Anestesiol* 70(10), 727–34
Photophobia
Visual hallucinations
  (2007): Webb AR+, *Anesth Analg* 104(4), 912

Other
Injection-site erythema
Injection-site pain (1–10%)
Seizures
  (2005): Agarwal A+, *Anesth Analg* 100(1), 85
Tremor (>10%)

KETOCONAZOLE

Trade names: Aquarius; Fungarest; Fungoral; Ketoderm; Ketoisidin; Nazoltec; Nizoral (McNeil) (Janssen)
Indications: Fungal infections
Category: Antibiotic, imidazole
Half-life: initial: 2 hours; terminal: 8 hours
Clinically important, potentially hazardous interactions with: alcohol, alfuzosin, almotriptan, alprazolam, amphotericin B, anisindione, anticoagulants, aprepitant, aripiprazole, astemizole, beclomethasone, benzodiazepines, bosentan, budesonide, chlordiazepoxide, ciclesonide, cimetidine, cinacalcet, clorazepate, conivaptan, cyclesonide, cyclosporine, dasatinib, dicumarol, didanosine, dofetilide, domperidone, eplerenone, erythromycin, eszopiclone, fentanyl, flunisolide, fluticasone, fosamprenavir, gastric alkanizers, HMG-CoA reductase inhibitors, imatinib, ivabradine, ixabepilone, methylprednisolone, midazolam, nevirapine, nisoldipine, non-sedating antihistamines, pimozide, prednisolone, prednisone, proton-pump inhibitors, rabeprazole, ramelteon, ranolazine, reboxetine, rifampin, rimonabant, ritonavir, saquinavir, sildenafil, solifenacin, sucralfate, sunitinib, tacrolimus, tadalafil, temsirolimus, tolterodine, triamcinolone, triazolam, vardenafil, vinblastine, vincristine, warfarin, zaleplon

Reactions

Skin

Allergic reactions (sic)
(1983): van Ketel WG, *Contact Dermatitis* 9, 313
Angioedema
(1994): Gonzalez-Delgado P+, *Ann Allergy* 73, 326
(1994): Gupta AK+, *J Am Acad Dermatol* 30, 677 (passim)
(1983): van Dijke CPH+, *BMJ* 287, 1673
Dermatitis
(1993): Lodi A+, *Contact Dermatitis* 29, 97
(1993): Valsecchi R+, *Contact Dermatitis* 29, 162
(1992): Santucci B+, *Contact Dermatitis* 27, 274
Eczema (generalized)
(1989): Garcia-Bravo B+, *Contact Dermatitis* 21, 346
Exanthems (1–9%)
(1985): Bradsher RW+, *Ann Intern Med* 103, 872 (2%)
(1985): Study Group, *Ann Intern Med* 103, 861 (9.7%)
(1984): Ford GP+, *Br J Dermatol* 111, 603 (5%)
(1984): Kahana M+, *Arch Dermatol* 120, 837
(1983): Dismukes WE+, *Ann Intern Med* 98, 13 (4%)
(1983): Rand R+, *Arch Dermatol* 119, 97
(1982): Heel RC+, *Drugs* 23, 1 (0.7%)
Exfoliative dermatitis
(1984): Parent D+, *Ann Dermatol Venereol* (French) 111,339
(1983): Rand R+, *Arch Dermatol* 119, 97
Fixed eruption
(1994): Gupta AK+, *J Am Acad Dermatol* 30, 677 (passim)
(1988): Bharija SC+, *Int J Dermatol* 27, 278
Hand–foot syndrome
(1994): Sella A+, *J Clin Oncol* 12(4), 683 (with doxorubicin)
Jarisch–Herxheimer reaction
Photosensitivity
(1988): Mohamed KN, *Clin Exp Dermatol* 13, 54
Pigmentation
(1992): Gallais V+, *Ann Dermatol Venereol* (French) 119, 471
(1990): Poizot-Martin I+, *Int Conf AIDS* 6, 357
(1985): Tucker WS+, *JAMA* 253, 2413
Pruritus (1–9%)
(1994): Gupta AK+, *J Am Acad Dermatol* 30, 677 (passim)
(1988): Mohamed KN, *Clin Exp Dermatol* 13, 54 (passim)
(1985): Study Group, *Ann Intern Med* 103, 861 (9.7%)
(1983): Rand R+, *Arch Dermatol* 119, 97 (1.5%)
(1982): Heel RC+, *Drugs* 23, 1 (1.7%)
Purpura
(1994): Gupta AK+, *J Am Acad Dermatol* 30, 677 (passim)
(1982): Heel RC+, *Drugs* 23, 1
Rash (sic) (1–3%)
(1994): Gupta AK+, *J Am Acad Dermatitis* 30, 677 (passim)
Urticaria (1–3%)
(1994): Gupta AK+, *J Am Acad Dermatol* 30, 677 (passim)
(1985): Bradsher RW+, *Ann Intern Med* 103, 872 (2%)
Vasculitis
(1982): Heel RC+, *Drugs* 23, 1
Xanthoderma
(2007): Haught JM+, *J Am Acad Dermatol* 57(6), 1051
Xerosis
(2002): Harris KA+, *J Urol* 168(2), 542
(1994): Gupta AK+, *J Am Acad Dermatol* 30, 677 (passim)
(1985): Study Group, *Ann Intern Med* 103, 861

Mucosal/ENT

Gingival hyperplasia/hypertrophy
(1988): Veraldi S+, *Int J Dermatol* 27, 730
Gingivitis
(1994): Gupta AK+, *J Am Acad Dermatol* 30, 677 (passim)
(1983): Dismukes WE+, *Ann Intern Med* 98, 13

Oral lesions (1–5%)
(1994): Gupta AK+, *J Am Acad Dermatol* 30, 677 (passim)
(1985): Study Group, *Ann Intern Med* 103, 861 (1–5%)
(1983): Dismukes WE+, *Ann Intern Med* 98, 13 (2%)
Oral lichenoid eruption
(1993): Ficarra G+, *Oral Surg Oral Med Oral Pathol* 76, 460
(1986): Markitziu A+, *Mykosen* (German) 29, 317
Oral pigmentation
(1991): Poizot-Martin I+, *Presse Med* (French) 20, 632
(1989): Langford A+, *Oral Surg Oral Med Oral Pathol* 67, 301 (in HIV-infected patients)
Stomatitis
(1994): Sella A+, *J Clin Oncol* 12(4), 683 (with doxorubicin)
Tongue pigmentation
(1982): Heel RC+, *Drugs* 23, 1

Hair

Hair – alopecia (<4%)
(1994): Gupta AK+, *J Am Acad Dermatol* 30, 677 (passim)
(1990): Venturoli S+, *J Clin Endocrinol Metab* 71, 335
(1985): Study Group, *Ann Intern Med* 103, 861 (3.7%)
(1982): Heel RC+, *Drugs* 23, 1 (0.2%)
Hair – trichoptilosis
(1993): Aljabre SH, *Int J Dermatol* 32, 150

Nails

Nails – pigmentation
(1985): Dreessen K, *Z Hautkr* (German) 60, 679 (black longitudinal bands)

Other

Anaphylactoid reactions/Anaphylaxis
(2005): Liu PY+, *Ann Pharmacother* 39(3), 547
(1994): Gupta AK+, *J Am Acad Dermatol* 30, 677 (passim)
(1983): van Dijke CPH+, *BMJ* 287, 1673
Asthenia
(2002): Harris KA+, *J Urol* 168(2), 542
Chills (1–3%)
Death
(2001): Duman D+, *Am J Med* 111(9), 737
(1994): Sella A+, *J Clin Oncol* 12(4), 683 (with doxorubicin)
Depression
(2002): Harris KA+, *J Urol* 168(2), 542
Gynecomastia (1–3%)
(1994): Gupta AK+, *J Am Acad Dermatol* 30, 677 (passim)
(1993): Thompson DF+, *Pharmacotherapy* 13, 37
(1982): Moncada B, *J Am Acad Dermatol* 7, 557
(1981): DeFelice R+, *Antimicrob Agents Chemo* 19, 1073
Headache
Hepatotoxicity
(2007): Stein CA+, *Invest New Drugs* 25(3), 277 (with lovastatin)
Hypersensitivity
(1994): Gonzalez-Delgado P+, *Ann Allergy* 73, 326
(1992): Verschueren GL+, *Contact Dermatitis* 26, 47
(1989): Garcia-Bravo B+, *Contact Dermatitis* 21, 346
Myalgia/Myositis/Myopathy/Myotoxicity
(1991): Garty BZ+, *Am J Dis Child* 145, 970
Paresthesias
(1994): Gupta AK+, *J Am Acad Dermatol* 30, 677 (passim)
Rhabdomyolysis
(2007): Akram K+, *Int J Cardiol* 118(1), e19 (with simvastatin)
(2007): Stein CA+, *Invest New Drugs* 25(3), 277 (with lovastatin)
(1999): Gilad R+, *Clin Neuropharmacol* 22(5), 295 (with simvastatin)
Suicidal ideation
(1991): Fisch RZ+, *Isr J Psychiatry Relat Sci* 28(1), 41
Tremor
(2003): Bulkowstein M+, *Vet Hum Toxicol* 45(5), 239

KETOPROFEN

Trade names: Alrheumat; Alrheumun; Aneol; Bi-Profenid; Gabrilen Retard; Keduril; Novo-Keto; Orudis (Sanofi-Aventis); Oruvail (Wyeth); Rhodis; Rhovail
Indications: Arthritis
Category: Non-steroidal anti-inflammatory
Half-life: 1.5–4 hours
Clinically important, potentially hazardous interactions with: aspirin, methotrexate, probenecid

Reactions

Skin

Allergic reactions (sic) (<1%)
Angioedema (<1%)
Bullous dermatitis (<1%)
Dermatitis
  (2007): Ota T+, *Contact Dermatitis* 56(1), 47 (contact)
  (2006): Diaz RL+, *Contact Dermatitis* 54(5), 239 (contact)
  (2006): Hindsen M+, *Contact Dermatitis* 54(3), 150 (contact)
    (photoallergic)
  (2004): Goossens A, *Photodermatol Photoimmunol Photomed* 20(3), 121
  (2004): Matthieu L+, *Contact Dermatitis* 50(4), 238 (contact)
  (2001): Preisz K+, *Orv Hetil* 142(51), 2841
  (2000): Bagheri H+, *Drug Saf* 22(5), 339
  (1998): Baudot S+, *Therapie* (French) 53, 137
  (1998): Horn HM+, *Contact Dermatitis* 38(6), 353 (contact)
  (1997): *Lakartidningen* (Swedish) 94, 2664
  (1996): Jeanmougin M+, *Ann Dermatol Venereol* (French) 123, 251
  (1996): Pigatto P+, *Am J Contact Dermat* 7, 220
  (1995): Gebhardt M+, *Z Rheumatol* (German) 54, 405
  (1995): Navarro LA+, *Contact Dermatitis* 32, 181
  (1994): Mastrolonardo M+, *Contact Dermatitis* 30, 110
  (1994): Oh VM, *BMJ* 309, 512
  (1993): Ophaswongse S+, *Contact Dermatitis* 29, 57
  (1990): Mozzanica N+, *Contact Dermatitis* 23, 336
  (1990): Tosti A+, *Contact Dermatitis* 23, 112
  (1990): Valsecchi R+, *Contact Dermatitis* 21, 345
  (1989): Lanzarini M+, *Contact Dermatitis* 21, 51
  (1989): Romaguera C+, *Contact Dermatitis* 20, 310
  (1987): Mozzanica N, *Contact Dermatitis* 17, 325
  (1985): Camarasa JG, *Contact Dermatitis* 12, 121
  (1983): Angelini G+, *Contact Dermatitis* 9, 234
  (1983): Valsecchi R+, *Contact Dermatitis* 9, 163
Diaphoresis (<1%)
  (1989): Roth DE+, *Med Clin North Am* 73, 1275
Eczema (<1%)
  (1990): Tosti A+, *Contact Dermatitis* 23, 112
  (1987): Mozzanica N, *Contact Dermatitis* 17, 325
Erythema multiforme (<1%)
Exanthems
Exfoliative dermatitis (<1%)
Facial edema (<1%)
Keratolysis exfoliativa
  (2006): Alvarez MT+, *Eur J Ophthalmol* 16(4), 582
Pemphigus (localized)
  (2001): Kanitakis J+, *Acta Derm Venereol* 81(4), 304
Peripheral edema (1–3%)
Photoallergic reaction
  (2000): Albes B+, *Dermatology* 201(2), 171
Photocontact dermatitis
  (2004): Matthieu L+, *Contact Dermatitis* 50(4), 238
Photosensitivity
  (2007): Ota T+, *Contact Dermatitis* 56(1), 47 (contact)

  (2006): Hindsen M+, *Contact Dermatitis* 54(3), 150
  (2004): Hindsen M+, *J Am Acad Dermatol* A(2), 215
  (2003): Durbize E+, *Contact Dermatitis* 48(3), 144
  (2002): Valenzuela N+, *Contact Dermatitis* 47(4), 237
  (2002): Vigan M+, *Ann Dermatol Venereol* 129(10), 1125 (11%)
  (2001): Kawada A+, *Contact Dermatitis* 44(6), 370
  (2001): Milpied-Homsi B, *Presse Med* 30(12), 605 (from gel)
  (2001): Sugiyama M+, *Am J Contact Dermat* 12(3), 180
  (2000): Albes B+, *Dermatology* 201(2), 171
  (2000): Bagheri H+, *Drug Saf* 22(5), 339
  (2000): Matsushita T+, *Photodermatol Photoimmunol Photomed* 17(1), 26 (from gel) (5 cases)
  (2000): Sugiura M+, *Contact Dermatitis* 43, 16 (4 cases)
  (1998): Baudot S+, *Therapie* (French) 53, 137
  (1998): Horn HM+, *Contact Dermatitis* 38(6), 353 (contact)
  (1998): Le Coz CJ+, *Contact Dermatitis* 38, 245
  (1997): Bastien M+, *Ann Dermatol Venereol* (French) 124, 523 (5 cases)
  (1997): Leroy D+, *Photodermatol Photoimmunol Photomed* 13, 93
  (1997): Mirande-Romero A+, *Contact Dermatitis* 37, 242 (connubial)
  (1996): Becker L+, *Acta Derm Venereol* 76(5), 337
  (1996): Jeanmougin M+, *Ann Dermatol Venereol* (French) 123, 251
  (1995): Nabeya R+, *Contact Dermatitis* 32, 52
  (1993): Ophaswongse S+, *Contact Dermatitis* 29, 57 (phototoxic and photoallergic)
  (1992): Serrano G+, *J Am Acad Dermatol* 27, 204 (passim)
  (1990): Black AK+, *Br J Dermatol* 123, 277
  (1990): Mozzanica N+, *Contact Dermatitis* 23, 336
  (1989): Roth DE+, *Med Clin North Am* 73, 1275
  (1987): Cusano F+, *Contact Dermatitis* 27, 108
  (1987): Cusano F+, *Contact Dermatitis* 27, 50
  (1985): Alomar A, *Contact Dermatitis* 12, 112
Pigmentation (<1%)
Pruritus (1–10%)
Psoriasis
  (1992): Shelley WB+, *Cutis* 51, 23 (observation)
Purpura (<1%)
  (1989): Roth DE+, *Med Clin North Am* 73, 1275
Rash (sic) (>10%)
Side effects (sic) (<1%)
  (1989): Le-Loet X, *Scand J Rheumatol* Suppl 83, 21 (0.7%)
Stevens–Johnson syndrome (<1%)
Toxic epidermal necrolysis (<1%)
  (1995): Tijhuis GJ+, *Dermatology* 190, 176
Urticaria (<1%)
  (2006): Asero R, *Ann Allergy Asthma Immunol* 97(2), 187
  (2003): Suzuki T+, *Contact Dermatitis* 48(5), 284 (contact)

Mucosal/ENT

Aphthous stomatitis
Dysgeusia (<1%)
Oral lesions
Oral mucosal paresthesias
  (2001): Passali D+, *Clin Ther* 23(9), 1508
Sialorrhea (<1%)
Stomatitis (<1%)
Tinnitus
Xerostomia (<1%)
  (2001): Passali D+, *Clin Ther* 23(9), 1508

Hair

Hair – alopecia (<1%)
  (1989): Roth DE+, *Med Clin North Am* 73, 1275

Other

Anaphylactoid reactions/Anaphylaxis (<1%)
  (2006): Castillo-Zamora C+, *Ther Drug Monit* 28(3), 458
  (1985): O'Brien WM+, *J Rheumatol* 12, 13

Embolia cutis medicamentosa (Nicolau syndrome)
  (2002): McGee AM+, *Br J Anaesth* 88(1), 139
Gynecomastia (<1%)
Headache
Hot flashes (<1%)
Myalgia/Myositis/Myopathy/Myotoxicity (<1%)
Paresthesias (<1%)
Pseudolymphoma
  (2001): Werth V, *Dermatology Times* 18
Pseudoporphyria
  (1992): Breathnach SM+, *Adverse Drug Reactions and the Skin*
    Blackwell, Oxford (passim)
  (1987): Taylor BJ+, *N Z Med J* 100, 322

KETOROLAC

Trade names: Acular (Allergan); Dolac; Kelac; Ketonic; Nodine;
Topadol; Toradol (Roche); Torolac; Torvin
Indications: Pain
Category: Analgesic, non-opioid; Non-steroidal anti-
inflammatory
Half-life: 2–8 hours
**Clinically important, potentially hazardous interactions
with:** aspirin, buprenorphine, methotrexate, probenecid,
salicylates

Reactions

Skin
Allergic reactions (sic)
  (2000): Reinhart DI, *Drug Saf* 22, 487
Angioedema
  (1994): Shapiro N, *J Oral Maxillofac Surg* 52, 626
Dermatitis (3–9%)
Diaphoresis (1–10%)
  (1990): Buckley MMT+, *Drugs* 39, 86
Edema (3–9%)
Exanthems (3–9%)
  (1990): Buckley MMT+, *Drugs* 39, 86
Excoriations
  (1994): Shelley WB+, *Cutis* 53, 235 (observation)
Exfoliative dermatitis (<1%)
Pruritus (3–9%)
Purpura (>1%)
  (1994): Shelley WB+, *Cutis* 54, 149 (palpable) (observation)
Rash (sic) (>1%)
Side effects (sic) (0.7%)
  (1990): Buckley MMT+, *Drugs* 39, 86
Stevens–Johnson syndrome (<1%)
Stinging (from topical)
  (2000): Shiuey Y+, *Ophthalmology* 107, 1512
Toxic epidermal necrolysis (<1%)
Urticaria
  (1990): Buckley MMT+, *Drugs* 39, 86

Mucosal/ENT
Aphthous stomatitis (<1%)
  (1990): Buckley MMT+, *Drugs* 39, 86
Dysgeusia
Stomatitis (>1%)
Tinnitus
Tongue edema (<1%)
Xerostomia
  (1990): Buckley MMT+, *Drugs* 39, 86

Other
Anaphylactoid reactions/Anaphylaxis (<1%)
Headache
Hypersensitivity
  (2000): Reinhart DI, *Drug Saf* 22, 487
Injection-site lichenoid reaction
  (2003): Vedamurthy M, Chennai, India (from Internet)
    (observation)
Injection-site pain (1–10%)
Myalgia/Myositis/Myopathy/Myotoxicity
Nephrotoxicity
  (2002): Galli G+, *G Ital Nefrol* 19(2), 199
Paresthesias
Vertigo
  (2002): Henderson SO+, *J Emerg Med* 23(3), 237

KETOTIFEN

Trade name: Zaditor (Novartis)
Indications: Allergic conjunctivitis
Category: Histamine H1 receptor antagonist
Half-life: 22 hours

Reactions

Skin
Allergic reactions (sic) (1–10%)
Dermatitis
  (1994): Niizeki H+, *Contact Dermatitis* 31(4), 266
Photosensitivity
Pityriasis rosea
  (1985): Wolf R+, *Dermatologica* 171, 355
Pruritus (1–10%)
  (2003): Sowunmi A, *Ann Trop Med Parasitol* 97(2), 103
Rash (sic) (1–10%)

Mucosal/ENT
Xerostomia
  (1982): Simons FE+, *Ann Allergy* 48(3), 145

Eyes
Ocular burning (1–10%)
  (2003): Ganz M+, *Adv Ther* 20(2), 79
Ocular stinging (1–10%)
Xerophthalmia (1–10%)

Other
Headache
  (2003): Ganz M+, *Adv Ther* 20(2), 79

L-CARNITINE

Trade names: Acetyl-L-carnitine; Aplegin; B(t)Factor; Carnitine; Carnitor; L-Carnipure; Levocarnitine; Propionyl-L-carnitine; Vitacarn; Vitamin B1
Indications: Improves lipid metabolism, red blood cell count, and antioxidant status, chronic fatigue syndrome, dementia, angina, post-MI cardioprotection, congestive heart failure, valproate toxicity, anorexia
Category: Food supplement
Half-life: N/A
Clinically important, potentially hazardous interactions with: None

Note: Mixed D, L-carnitine has been associated with myasthenic syndrome.

Reactions

None

L-METHYLFOLATE

Trade name: Deplin (PamLab)
Indications: Medicinal food for management of patients with low plasma and/or low red blood cell folate, antidepressant
Category: Dietary supplement ; Trimonoamine modulator
Clinically important, potentially hazardous interactions with: raltitrexed

Reactions

None

LABETALOL

Trade names: Abetol; Amipress; Hybloc; Ipolab; Labrocol; Normozide; Presolol; Salmagne; Trandate (Prometheus)
Indications: Hypertension
Category: Adrenergic beta-receptor antagonist; Antiarrhythmic class II
Half-life: 3–8 hours

Note: Normozide is labetalol and hydrochlorothiazide

Note: Cutaneous side effects of beta-receptor blockaders are clinically polymorphous. They apparently appear after several months of continuous therapy. Atypical psoriasiform, lichen planus-like, and eczematous chronic rashes are mainly observed. (1983): Hödl St, Z Hautkr (German) 1:58, 17

Reactions

Skin
Angioedema
  (1986): Ferree CE, Ann Intern Med 104, 729
Dermatitis
  (1990): Bause GS+, Contact Dermatitis 23, 51
Diaphoresis (<1%)
Eczema
Edema (<2%)
Exanthems (1–5%)
  (1989): Goa KL+, Drugs 37, 583
  (1984): Prichard BNC, Drugs 28 (Suppl 2), 51 (1–5%)
Exfoliative dermatitis
Facial edema
Lichen planus (bullous)
Lichenoid eruption
  (1982): Bertani E+, G Ital Dermatol Venereol (Italian) 117, 229
  (1980): Staughton R+, Lancet 2, 581
Lupus erythematosus
  (1984): Prichard BNC, Drugs 28 (Suppl 2), 51
  (1981): Brown RC+, Postgrad Med J 57, 189
Peripheral edema
Pigmentation (slate-gray)
Pityriasis rubra pilaris
Pruritus (1–10%)
  (1984): Prichard BNC, Drugs 28 (Suppl 2), 51 (1–5%)
Psoriasis (exacerbation)
  (1987): Savola J+, BMJ 295, 637 (induction)
  (1986): Czernielewski J+, Lancet 1, 808
  (1984): Arntzen N+, Acta Derm Venereol (Stockh) 64, 346
Purpura
Rash (sic) (<1%)
Raynaud's phenomenon (<1%)
Side effects (sic) (5.5%)
  (1982): Waal-Manning HJ+, Br J Clin Pharmacol 13 (Suppl 1), 65S
Urticaria
  (1986): Ferree CE, Ann Intern Med 104, 729
Xerosis

Mucosal/ENT
Dysgeusia (1–10%)
  (2000): Zervakis J+, Physiol Behav 68, 405
Xerostomia

Hair
Hair – alopecia (reversible)

Other
Anaphylactoid reactions/Anaphylaxis
  (1990): Bause GS+, Contact Dermatitis 23, 51
  (1986): Ferree CE, Ann Intern Med 104, 729
Headache
Hypersensitivity
Hypotension
  (2006): Jivraj S+, Can J Anaesth 53(7), 678
  (2000): Joye F, Presse Med 29(18), 1027
Myalgia/Myositis/Myopathy/Myotoxicity
  (1989): Willis J+, Ann Neurology 26, 456
  (1981): Teicher A+, BMJ 282, 1824
Paresthesias (7%)
  (1984): Prichard BNC, Drugs 28 (Suppl 2), 51 (scalp) (6%)
Peyronie's disease
Rhabdomyolysis
  (1990): Willis JK+, Pediatr Neurol 6(4), 275
Scalp tingling

LACTOBACILLUS

Scientific names: *Lactobacillus acidophilus; Lactobacillus amylovorus; Lactobacillus brevis; Lactobacillus bulgaricus; Lactobacillus casei; Lactobacillus crispatus; Lactobacillus delbrueckii; Lactobacillus fermentum; Lactobacillus gallinarum; Lactobacillus johnsonii; Lactobacillus paracasei; Lactobacillus plantarum; Lactobacillus reuteri; Lactobacillus rhamnosus; Lactobacillus salivarius; Lactobacillus sporogenes*
Family: Lactobacillaceae
Trade and other common names: Acidophilus; LAB (lactic acid bacteria); Lactobacillus GG; LC-1; Probiotics
Category: Immunomodulator; Probiotic
Purported indications and other uses: Oral: Acne, allergic rhinitis, atopic allergy, diarrhea, *Helicobacter pylori* infection, irritable bowel syndrome, rotavirus, ulcerative colitis, urinary tract infections. **Suppository:** vaginitis, urinary tract infections
Half-life: N/A

Reactions

None

LAMIVUDINE

Synonym: 3TC
Trade names: Combivir (GSK); Epivir (GSK); Trizivir (GSK)
Indications: HIV progression
Category: Antiretroviral; Nucleoside analog reverse transcriptase inhibitor
Half-life: 5–7 hours

Note: Combivir is lamivudine and zidovudine

Reactions

Skin
Acute generalized exanthematous pustulosis (AGEP)
  (1998): Aquilina C+, *Arch Intern Med* 158(19), 2160 (with zidovudine)
Angioedema
  (1996): Kainer MA+, *Lancet* 348, 1519
Dermatitis
  (2000): Smith KJ+, *Cutis* 65, 227
Exanthems
Pruritus
  (2000): Smith KJ+, *Cutis* 65, 227
Rash (sic) (9%)
Urticaria
  (1996): Kainer MA+, *Lancet* 348, 1519

Mucosal/ENT
Stomatopyrosis
  (2008): Moura MD+, *J Contemp Dent Pract* 9(1), 84 (with zidovudine and nevirapine)

Hair
Hair – alopecia
  (1994): Fong IW, *Lancet* 344, 1702

Nails
Nails – onychocryptosis
  (2001): James CW+, *Ann Pharmacother* 35(7), 881 (with ritonavir)
Nails – paronychia

(1998): Zerboni R+, *Lancet* 351, 1256

Other
Abdominal pain
  (2007): McMahon DK+, *HIV Clin Trials* 8(5), 269 (28%) (with zidovudine & indinavir)
Anaphylactoid reactions/Anaphylaxis
  (1996): Kainer MA+, *Lancet* 348(9040), 1519
Asthenia
  (2007): McMahon DK+, *HIV Clin Trials* 8(5), 269 (49%) (with zidovudine & indinavir)
Chills (1–10%)
Gynecomastia
  (2001): Manfredi R+, *Ann Pharmacother* 35(4), 438 (with savudine) (3 cases)
Headache
  (2007): McMahon DK+, *HIV Clin Trials* 8(5), 269 (28%) (with zidovudine & indinavir)
  (2006): Castillo SA+, *Drug Saf* 29(9), 811 (16%) (with abacavir)
Hypersensitivity
  (2002): Winston A+, *Int J STD AIDS* 13(3), 213
Myalgia/Myositis/Myopathy/Myotoxicity (8%)
Paresthesias (>10%)
Rhabdomyolysis
  (2005): Adani GL+, *Am J Transplant* 5(3), 634
  (2002): Yahagi K+, *Liver Transpl* 8(12), 1198
  (1997): Mendila M+, *Dtsch Med Wochenschr* 122(33), 1003
Vertigo
  (2006): Castillo SA+, *Drug Saf* 29(9), 811 (27%) (with abacavir)

LAMOTRIGINE

Synonyms: BW-430C; LTG
Trade name: Lamictal (GSK)
Indications: Epilepsy
Category: Anticonvulsant; Mood stabilizer
Half-life: 24 hours
Clinically important, potentially hazardous interactions with: oral contraceptives

Reactions

Skin
Acne (1.3%)
  (2004): Nielsen JN+, *J Clin Psychiatry* 65(12), 1720 (2 cases)
Acute generalized exanthematous pustulosis (AGEP)
  (2001): Wensween CA+, *Ned Tijdschr Geneeskd* 145(31), 1525
Adverse effects (sic)
  (2002): Hurley SC, *Ann Pharmacother* 36(5), 860
Angioedema (1–10%)
  (2001): Hebert AA+, *J Clin Psychiatry* 62(suppl 14), 22 (~1%)
Bullous dermatitis
  (1997): *Australian Adverse Drug Reactions Bulletin* 16(1), February
Diaphoresis (<1%)
Eczema (<1%)
Erythema (1–10%)
  (2001): Hebert AA+, *J Clin Psychiatry* 62(suppl 14), 22 (~10%)
Erythema multiforme
  (2006): Abdelmalek M+, *J Drugs Dermatol* 5(1), 76
  (2003): Berger Robin P, St. George, UT (from Internet) (observation)
  (2003): Ely HP, Grass Valley, CA (from Internet) (observation)
  (1997): *Australian Adverse Drug Reactions Bulletin* 16(1), February
Exanthems (1–10%)
  (2003): Warnock JK+, *Am J Clin Dermatol* 4(1), 21
  (2002): Rufo-Campos M, *Rev Neurol* 35, S74

(2001): Hebert AA+, *J Clin Psychiatry* 62(suppl 14), 22 (~10%)
(1997): *Australian Adverse Drug Reactions Bulletin* 16(1), February
(1997): Hyson C+, *Can J Neurol Sci* 24, 245
(1996): Dooley J+, *Neurology* 46, 240 (7%)
(1996): Li LM+, *Arq Neuropsiquiatr* 54, 47
(1995): Brodie MJ, *Can J Neurol Sci* 23, S6 (<5%)
(1995): Fitton A+, *Drugs* 50, 691
(1995): Makin AJ+, *BMJ* 311, 292
(1995): Tavernor SJ+, *Seizure* 4, 67
(1994): Tavernor SJ+, *Epilepsia* 35, 72

Facial edema (<1%)

Fixed eruption
(2001): Hsiao C-J+, *Br J Dermatol* 144, 1289

Hyperhidrosis
(2002): Gelisse P+, *Acta Neurol Scand* 105(3), 232 (withdrawal)

Lupus erythematosus
(2000): Sarzi-Puttini P+, *Lupus* 9(7), 555
(1997): Mackay FJ+, *Epilepsia* 38, 881

Petechiae (<1%)

Photosensitivity
(1999): Borowitz SM, *Pediatric Pharmacotherapy* 5, 3
(1999): Bozikas V+, *Am J Psychiatry* 156, 2015

Pruritus (3.1%)
(2001): Hebert AA+, *J Clin Psychiatry* 62(suppl 14), 22 (~1%)

Purpura
(2006): Amlie-Lefond CM+, *Pediatr Neurol* 35(3), 227 (localized)

Rash (sic) (10–20%)
(2007): Arif H+, *Neurology* 68(20), 1701
(2007): Lu W+, *Drug Metab Dispos* 35(7), 1050
(2006): Devulder J, *Acta Neurol Belg* 106(1), 15
(2006): Gelisse P+, *Rev Neurol* (Paris) 162(11), 1122
(2006): Ginsberg LD, *CNS Spectr* 11(5), 376 (13%)
(2006): Hirsch LJ+, *Epilepsia* 47(2), 318 (6%)
(2006): Ketter TA+, *J Clin Psychiatry* 67(3), 400
(2005): Ketter TA+, *J Clin Psychiatry* 66(5), 642
(2005): P-Codrea Tigaran S+, *Acta Neurol Scand* 111(3), 191 (6%)
(2005): Subuh Surja AA+, *J Clin Psychiatry* 66(3), 400
(2004): Pascual J+, *Headache* 244(10), 1024 (3 cases)
(2003): Choi H+, *Expert Opin Pharmacother* 4(2), 243
(2003): Feliciani C+, *Int J Immunopathol Pharmacol* 16(1), 89 (2 cases)
(2003): Naisbitt DJ+, *J Allergy Clin Immunol* 111(6), 1393
(2003): Vieta E+, *Actas Esp Psiquiatr* 31(2), 65
(2002): Anderson GD, *Epilepsia* 43(Suppl 3), 53 (10–20%)
(2002): Bowden CL, *Expert Opin Pharmacother* 3(10), 1513
(2002): Calabrese JR+, *J Clin Psychiatry* 63(11), 1012 (8.3%)
(2002): Huang CW+, *Kaohsiung J Med Sci* 18(11), 566
(2002): Hurley SC, *Ann Pharmacother* 36(5), 860
(2002): Labiner DM, *J Clin Psychiatry* 63(11), 1010
(2001): Eisenberg E+, *Neurology* 57, 505
(2000): Besag FM+, *Seizure* 9, 282
(2000): Husain AM+, *South Med J* 93, 335
(2000): Jurynczyk J+, *Neurol Neurochir Pol* (Polish) 34, 43
(2000): Messenheimer JA+, *Drug Saf* 22, 303
(2000): Messenheimer JA+, *Epilepsia* 41, 488
(2000): Parmeggiani L+, *J Child Neurol* 15, 15
(1999): Faught E+, *Epilepsia* 40, 1135
(1999): Gericke CA+, *Epileptic Disord* 1, 159
(1999): Guberman AH+, *Epilepsia* 40, 985
(1999): Matsuo F, *Epilepsia* 40, S30
(1998): Buzan RD+, *J Clin Psychiatry* 59, 87 (re-challenged)
(1998): Messenheimer JA, *Can J Neurol Sci* 25, S14
(1997): Mackay FJ+, *Epilepsia* 38, 881

Raynaud's phenomenon
(2000): Sarzi-Puttini P+, *Lupus* 9(7), 555

Stevens–Johnson syndrome (1–10%)
(2007): Hilas O+, *Am J Health Syst Pharm* 64(3), 273

(2007): Kocak S+, *Am J Clin Dermatol* 8(2), 107 (with valproic acid)
(2007): Matthews AM+, *J Clin Psychiatry* 68(4), 637
(2007): Shen YC+, *Int Clin Psychopharmacol* 22(4), 247 (with aripiprazole)
(2006): Hirsch LJ+, *Epilepsia* 47(2), 318 (1 case)
(2006): Wolf R+, *Int Arch Allergy Immunol* 141(3), 308
(2005): Fein JD+, *N Engl J Med* 352(16), 1696
(2005): Mockenhaupt M+, *Neurology* 64(7), 1134
(2003): Feliciani C+, *Int J Immunopathol Pharmacol* 16(1), 89
(2002): Bowden CL, *Expert Opin Pharmacother* 3(10), 1513
(2002): Calabrese JR+, *J Clin Psychiatry* 63(11), 1012 (1 case)
(2002): Huang CW+, *Kaohsiung J Med Sci* 18(11), 566
(2001): Hebert AA+, *J Clin Psychiatry* 62(suppl 14), 22 (~10%)
(2000): Popescu C, Bucharest, Romania (from Internet) (observation)
(2000): Yalcin B+, *J Am Acad Dermatol* 43, 898 (with valproic acid)
(1999): Bocquet H+, *Ann Dermatol Venereol* (French) 126, 46
(1999): Borowitz SM, *Pediatric Pharmacotherapy* 5, 3
(1999): Guberman AH+, *Epilepsia* 40, 985
(1999): Rzany B+, *Lancet* 353, 2190
(1998): *Drugs and Therapy Perspectives* 11, 11
(1998): Messenheimer J+, *Drug Saf* 18(4), 281
(1998): Schlienger RG+, *Epilepsia* 39, S22
(1998): Zachariae CO+, *Ugeskr Laeger* (Danish) 160, 6656
(1997): *Australian Adverse Drug Reactions Bulletin* 16(1), February
(1997): Knowles S+, *Curr Opin Pediatr* 9(4), 388
(1997): Mackay FJ+, *Epilepsia* 38, 881
(1997): Sachs B+, *Dermatology* 195, 60
(1996): Dooley J+, *Neurology* 46, 240 (7%)
(1995): Campistol J+, *Rev Neurol* (Spanish) 23, 1236
(1995): Duval X+, *Lancet* 345, 1301

Toxic epidermal necrolysis
(2008): Schwartz R+, *Arch Dermatol* 144(6), 724
(2006): Varghese SP+, *Pharmacotherapy* 26(5), 699
(2005): Mansouri P+, *Arch Dermatol* 141(6), 788 (with carbamazepine)
(2005): Rodriguez-Blanco I+, *Actas Dermosifiliogr* 96(2), 116
(2004): Haefliger IO+, *Klin Monatsbl Augenheilkd* 221(5), 395
(2004): Hashim N+, *Acta Derm Venereol* 84(1), 90 (with valproic acid)
(2004): Sladden M+, *Aust Fam Physician* 33(10), 829
(2003): Clennett S+, *J Wound Care* 12(4), 151
(2003): Feliciani C+, *Int J Immunopathol Pharmacol* 16(1), 89
(2003): Mayorga C+, *Ann Allergy Asthma Immunol* 91(1), 86
(2003): Sogut A+, *Acta Neurol Belg* 103(2), 95
(2002): Wirtzer A, Sherman Oaks, CA (from Internet) (observation)
(2001): Hebert AA+, *J Clin Psychiatry* 62(suppl 14), 22 (~1%)
(2001): Wensween CA+, *Ned Tijdschr Geneeskd* 145(31), 1525
(2000): Bhushan M+, *Clin Exp Dermatol* 25, 349
(2000): Fernandez-Calvo C+, *Rev Neurol* 31(12), 1162
(1999): *Actas Dermosifiliogr* (Spanish) 90, 612
(1999): Bocquet H+, *Ann Dermatol Venereol* (French) 126, 46
(1999): Borowitz SM, *Pediatric Pharmacotherapy* 5, 3
(1999): Rzany B+, *Lancet* 353, 2190
(1998): *Drugs and Therapy Perspectives* 11, 11
(1998): Page RL+, *Pharmacotherapy* 18, 392 (fatal)
(1998): Schlienger RG+, *Epilepsia* 39, S22
(1998): Zachariae CO+, *Ugeskr Laeger* (Danish) 160, 6656
(1997): *Australian Adverse Drug Reactions Bulletin* 16(1), February
(1997): Chaffin JJ+, *Ann Pharmacother* 31, 720 (suspected)
(1997): Fogh K+, *Seizure* 6, 63
(1997): Knowles S+, *Curr Opin Pediatr* 9(4), 388
(1997): Vukelic D+, *Dermatology* 195, 307
(1996): Sachs B+, *Lancet* 348, 1597
(1996): Sullivan JR+, *Australas J Dermatol* 37, 208
(1996): Wadelius M+, *Lancet* 348, 1041
(1995): Duval X+, *Lancet* 345, 1301

(1995): Sterker M+, *Int J Clin Pharmacol Ther* 33, 595
Urticaria (<1%)
Xerosis (<1%)

Mucosal/ENT

Dysgeusia (<1%)
  (2001): Avoni P+, *Neurology* 57(8), 1521 (3 cases)
Gingival hyperplasia/hypertrophy (<1%)
Gingivitis (<1%)
Oral ulceration (<1%)
Sialorrhea (<1%)
Stomatitis (<1%)
Vaginitis (4.1%)
Vulvovaginal candidiasis (<1%)
Xerostomia (1%)

Hair

Hair – alopecia (1.3%)
  (2006): Hillemacher T+, *Am J Psychiatry* 163(8), 1451
Hair – hirsutism (<1%)

Eyes

Conjunctivitis
  (2003): McDonald MA+, *Clin Experiment Ophthalmol* 31(6), 541
Diplopia
  (2008): Zaccara G+, *Seizure* nd, 182
Downbeat nystagmus
  (2005): Alkawi A+, *Epilepsy Res* 63(2–3), 85
Visual hallucinations
  (2006): Uher R+, *Am J Psychiatry* 163(4), 749

Other

Anaphylactoid reactions/Anaphylaxis
  (1999): Borowitz SM, *Pediatric Pharmacotherapy* 5, 3
Anticonvulsant hypersensitivity syndrome
  (2006): Chang CC+, *Prog Neuropsychopharmacol Biol Psychiatry* 30(4), 741
  (2006): Karande S+, *Indian J Med Sci* 60(2), 59
  (2006): Wolf R+, *Int Arch Allergy Immunol* 141(3), 308
  (2005): Jeandel PY+, *Presse Med* 34(7), 516
  (2005): Rahman M+, *Am J Psychiatry* 162(5), 1021
  (2004): Bavdekar SB+, *Ann Pharmacother* 38(10), 1648
  (2004): Papp Z+, *Orv Hetil* 145(32), 1665
  (2003): Bin-Nakhi HA+, *Med Princ Pract* 12(3), 197
  (2002): Beller TC+, *Allergy Asthma Proc* 23(6), 415
  (2002): Galindo PA+, *J Investig Allergol Clin Immunol* 12(4), 299
  (2002): Metin A+, *World Congress Dermatol* Poster, 0116
  (2002): Veyrac G+, *Therapie - Therapie* 57(3), 289
  (2000): Fervenza FC+, *Am J Kidney Dis* 36(5), 1034
Aseptic meningitis
  (2005): Kilfoyle DH+, *Epilepsia* 46(2), 327
Death
Headache
  (2006): Ginsberg LD, *CNS Spectr* 11(5), 376 (3%)
  (2003): Rocha FL+, *Int Clin Psychopharmacol* 18(2), 97
Hepatotoxicity
  (2006): Fix OK+, *Clin Gastroenterol Hepatol* 4(4), xxvi
Hot flashes (1–10%)
Hypersensitivity (1–10%)
  (2003): Feliciani C+, *Int J Immunopathol Pharmacol* 16(1), 89
  (2003): Naisbitt DJ+, *J Allergy Clin Immunol* 111(6), 1393
  (2002): Beller TC+, *Allergy Asthma Proc* 23(6), 415
  (2002): Monzon S+, *Contact Dermatitis* 47(6), 361
  (2001): Hebert AA+, *J Clin Psychiatry* 62(suppl 14), 22
  (2001): Lalanza J+, *Aten Primaria* 28(3), 213
  (2000): Schaub N+, *Allergy* 55, 191
  (1999): Borowitz SM, *Pediatric Pharmacotherapy* 5, 3
  (1999): Brown TS+, *Pediatr Dermatology* 16, 46
  (1999): Guberman AH+, *Epilepsia* 40, 985

(1999): Knowles SR+, *Drug Safety* 21, 489
(1999): Mylonakis E+, *Ann Pharmacol* 33, 557
(1999): Ronsdorf A+, *Schweiz Rundsch Med Prax* 88(41), 1660
(1998): Chapman MS+, *Br J Dermatol* 138, 710
(1998): Iannetti P+, *Epilepsia* 39, 502
(1998): Tugendhaft P+, *J Am Acad Dermatol* 38, 785 (phenytoin-like)
(1997): Jones D+, *J Am Acad Dermatol* 36, 1016 (phenytoin-like)
Myalgia/Myositis/Myopathy/Myotoxicity (>1%)
Paresthesias (>1%)
Porphyria
  (1996): Gregersen H+, *Ugeskr Laeger* (Danish) 158, 4091
Pseudolymphoma
  (1998): Pathak P+, *Neurology* 50, 1509
Rhabdomyolysis
  (1997): Chattergoon DS+, *Neurology* 49(5), 1442 (with valproic acid)
Seizures
  (2006): Hasan M+, *J Child Neurol* 21(9), 807 (exacerbation)
  (2006): Maiga Y+, *Rev Neurol* (Paris) 162(11), 1125 (exacerbation)
Tremor
  (2003): Das KB+, *J Child Neurol* 18(7), 479
  (2002): Gelisse P+, *Acta Neurol Scand* 105(3), 232 (withdrawal)
  (2002): Robillard M+, *Can J Psychiatry* 47(8), 767
  (2000): Messenheimer JA+, *Drug Saf* 22, 303
Vertigo
  (2008): Zaccara G+, *Seizure* nd, 182
  (2003): Rocha FL+, *Int Clin Psychopharmacol* 18(2), 97

LANREOTIDE

Trade names: Somatuline Autogel (Ipsen); Somatuline Depot (Ipsen); Somatuline LA (Ipsen)
Indications: Acromegaly, Carcinoid Syndrome, Thyrotrophic adenoma
Category: Hormone
Half-life: 2 hours (immediate release) 5 days (sustained release).
Clinically important, potentially hazardous interactions with: bromocriptine, cyclosporine, insulin

Reactions

Skin

Allergic reactions (SIC) (<1%)
Recall reaction
  (2007): Bauza A+, *Br J Dermatol* 157(5), 1061

Hair

Hair – alopecia
  (1999): Suliman M+, *J Endocrinol Invest* 22(6), 409

Other

Abdominal pain (7–19%)
  (2002): Caron P, *Ann Endocrinol (Paris)* 63(2 Pt 3), 2S19 (22%)
  (2000): Chanson P+, *Pituitary* 2(4), 269 (62%)
  (1996): Di Leo+, *Cancer* 78(1), 35 (79%)
Flatulence (~14%)
Headache (7%)
Hypertension (5%)
Injection-site erythema
  (2004): Antonijoan RM+, *J Pharm Pharmacol* 56(4), 471
Injection-site granuloma
  (2006): Caron P+, *Clin Endocrinol (Oxf* 64(2), 209
Injection-site induration
  (2006): Caron P+, *Clin Endocrinol (Oxf)* 64(2), 209

Injection-site inflammation
Injection-site nodules
  (2008): Debono M+, *J Clin Endocrinol Metab* 93(5), 1860
Injection-site pain (4%)
  (2000): Chanson P+, *Pituitary* 2(4), 269 (59%)
  (2000): Verhelst JA+, *Eur J Endocrinol* 143(5), 577 (9%)
Injection-site pruritus (<1%)
  (2004): Ashwell SG+, *Eur J Endocrinol* 150(4), 473
Injection-site reactions (6–22%)
  (2004): Ashwell SG+, *Eur J Endocrinol* 150(4), 473
Pain (7%)
  (2004): Ashwell SG+, *Eur J Endocrinol* 150(4), 473
Pancreatitis (fatal)
  (2006): Battaglia M+, *Scand J Urol Nephrol* 40(5), 423
Weight loss (5–11%)
  (1996): Di Leo+, *Cancer* 78(1), 35

LANSOPRAZOLE

Trade name: Prevacid (TAP)
Indications: Active duodenal ulcer
Category: Proton pump inhibitor
Half-life: 2 hours
Clinically important, potentially hazardous interactions with: eucalyptus, prednisone, sucralfate

Reactions

Skin
Acne (<1%)
Acute generalized exanthematous pustulosis (AGEP)
  (1997): Dewerdt S+, *Acta Derm Venereol* (Stockh) 77, 250
Dermatitis
  (2001): Vilaplana J+, *Contact Dermatitis* 44, 47 (with omeprazole)
Diaphoresis
  (2000): Natsch S+, *Ann Pharmacother* 34, 474
Edema (<1%)
  (2005): Severino G+, *Ann Pharmacother* 39(1), 162 (with imatinib)
Erythema multiforme
  (2005): Severino G+, *Ann Pharmacother* 39(1), 162
  (2004): Heaton NR+, *Clin Exp Dermatol* 29(6), 612
Erythroderma
  (1999): Cockayne SE+, *Br J Dermatol* 141, 173
Exanthems
  (2006): Selden ST, Chesapeake, VA (from Internet) (observation)
  (1996): Blumenthal HL, Beachwood, OH (personal case) (observation)
  (1996): Litt JZ, Beachwood, OH (personal case) (observation)
Facial edema
  (2002): Gonzalez P+, *Allergol Immunopathol* (Madr) 30(6), 342
  (2000): Natsch S+, *Ann Pharmacother* 34, 474
Lichenoid eruption
  (2000): Bong JL+, *BMJ* 320, 283
Lupus erythematosus
  (2005): Bracke A+, *Acta Derm Venereol* 85(4), 353 (2 cases)
Peripheral edema
  (2001): Brunner G+, *Dig Dis Sci* 46(5), 993
Pruritus (3–10%)
  (2000): Natsch S+, *Ann Pharmacother* 34, 474
Rash (sic) (3–10%)
Stevens–Johnson syndrome
  (2005): Severino G+, *Ann Pharmacother* 39(1), 162 (with imatinib)

Toxic epidermal necrolysis
  (2005): Severino G+, *Ann Pharmacother* 39(1), 162
  (2004): Heaton NR+, *Clin Exp Dermatol* 29(6), 612
Urticaria (<1%)
  (2002): Gonzalez P+, *Allergol Immunopathol* (Madr) 30(6), 342
  (2000): Gerson LB+, *Aliment Pharmacol* 14, 397 (1%)
  (2000): Natsch S+, *Ann Pharmacother* 34, 474

Mucosal/ENT
Dysgeusia (<1%)
Glossitis
  (1997): Greco S+, *Ann Pharmacother* 31, 1548
Stomatitis (<1%)
  (1997): Greco S+, *Ann Pharmacother* 31, 1548
Tongue black
  (1997): Greco S+, *Ann Pharmacother* 31, 1548
Xerostomia (<1%)

Hair
Hair – alopecia (<1%)
  (2000): Litt JZ, Beachwood, OH (personal case) (observation)

Other
Anaphylactoid reactions/Anaphylaxis
  (2006): Demirkan K+, *J Investig Allergol Clin Immunol* 16(3), 203 (3 cases)
  (2002): Gonzalez P+, *Allergol Immunopathol* (Madr) 30(6), 342
  (2000): Natsch S+, *Ann Pharmacother* 34, 474
Candidiasis (<1%)
Death
  (2004): Heaton NR+, *Clin Exp Dermatol* 29(6), 612
Gynecomastia (<1%)
  (2000): Comas A+, *Med Clin* (Barc) (Spanish) 114, 397
Headache
Hypersensitivity
  (2006): Perez Pimiento+, *J Allergy Clin Immunol* 117(3), 707
  (1999): Baudot S, *Therapie* (French) 54, 491
Myalgia/Myositis/Myopathy/Myotoxicity (<1%)
  (1998): Smith JD+, *Ann Pharmacother* 32, 196 (with eosinophilia)
Neurotoxicity
  (2005): Rajabally YA+, *Muscle Nerve* 31(1), 124
Paresthesias (<1%)

LANTHANUM

Trade name: Fosrenol (Shire)
Indications: Hyperphosphatemia in end-stage renal disease
Category: Chelator
Half-life: 53 hours
Clinically important, potentially hazardous interactions with: N/A

Reactions

Skin
Peripheral edema
  (2005): Finn WF+, *Curr Med Res Opin* 21(5), 657 (23.4%)

Other
Abdominal pain (17%)
Headache (21%)
Myalgia/Myositis/Myopathy/Myotoxicity
  (2005): Finn WF+, *Curr Med Res Opin* 21(5), 657 (20.8%)

LAPATINIB

Trade name: Tykerb (GSK)
Indications: Breast cancer
Category: Epidermal growth factor receptor (EGFR); Tyrosine kinase inhibitor
Half-life: 24 Hours
Clinically important, potentially hazardous interactions with: atazanavir, carbamazepine, clarithromycin, CYP3A4 inhibitors, dexamethasone, **grapefruit juice**, indinavir, itraconazole, nefazodone, nelfinavir, phenobarbital, phenytoin, rifabutin, rifampin, rifapentin, ritonavir, saquinavir, **St John's wort**, telithromycin, voriconazole. The concomitant use of strong CYP3A4 inducers should be avoided

Note: Lapitinib is used in conjunction with capecitabine

Reactions

Skin
Hand–foot syndrome (53%)
Inflammation (15%)
Rash (sic) (44%)
 (2006): Nelson MH+, *Ann Pharmacother* 40(2), 261
Xerosis (10%)

Mucosal/ENT
Stomatitis (14%)
Tinnitus (14%)

Hair
Depigmentation (21%)

Other
Abdominal pain (15%)
Asthenia (12%)
Insomnia
Pain (extremities) (12%)

LARONIDASE

Synonyms: TNX-901; E25; IGE-025; rhuMAb-E25
Trade name: Aldurazyme (Genzyme)
Indications: Mucopolysaccharidosis I
Category: Enzyme
Half-life: 1.5–3.6 hours
Clinically important, potentially hazardous interactions with: None

Reactions

Skin
Facial edema (9%)
Peripheral edema (9%)
Rash (sic) (36%)
Urticaria

Other
Anaphylactoid reactions/Anaphylaxis
Application-site pain (9%)
Application-site reactions (18%)
Chest pain (9%)
Fever
Headache
Hypersensitivity

Paresthesias (14%)
Upper respiratory infection

LATANOPROST

Trade name: Xalatan (Pfizer)
Indications: Glaucoma
Category: Prostaglandin analog
Half-life: 17 minutes

Reactions

Skin
Allergic reactions (sic) (1.1%)
Eczema (0.7%)
Erythema
 (2005): Ross EK+, *J Am Acad Dermatol* 53(6), 1095
Facial rash
 (1997): Rowe JA+, *Am J Ophthalmol* 124, 683
Hyperhidrosis
 (2005): Kumar H+, *Clin Experiment Ophthalmol* 33(6), 675
Irritation
 (1999): Hejkal TW+, *Semin Ophthalmol* 14, 114
Pruritus (0.2%)
 (2005): Ross EK+, *J Am Acad Dermatol* 53(6), 1095
 (1997): Crowe MA, Puyallup, WA (from Internet) (observation)
Rash (sic) (1–10%)
Toxic epidermal necrolysis
 (2005): Florez A+, *J Am Acad Dermatol* 53(5), 909 (with timolol & dorzolamide)

Eyes
Blepharitis (0.4%)
Choroidal detachment
 (2005): Pathanapitoon K+, *J Med Assoc Thai* 88(8), 1134
Conjunctival hyperemia
 (2005): Chiselita D+, *Oftalmologia* 49(3), 39
 (2005): Konstas AG+, *Ophthalmology* 112(2), 262
 (2003): Stewart WC+, *Am J Ophthalmol* 135(3), 314
 (2002): Eisenberg DL+, *Surv Ophthalmol* 47 Suppl 1, S105
 (2001): DuBiner H+, *Surv Opthalmol* 45(Suppl 4), S353–60
 (2001): Gandolfi S+, *Adv Ther* 18(3), 110
Eyelashes – hypertrichosis
 (2006): Elgin U+, *Eur J Ophthalmol* 16(2), 247
 (2006): Inoue K+, *Nippon Ganka Gakkai Zasshi* 110(8), 581
 (2005): Casson RJ+, *Am J Ophthalmol* 139(5), 932
 (2005): Chiselita D+, *Oftalmologia* 49(3), 39
 (2004): Tosti A+, *J Am Acad Dermatol* 51(5 Suppl), S149
 (2003): Costagliola C+, *Expert Opin Pharmacother* 4(10), 1775
 (2003): Herndon LW+, *Am J Ophthalmol* 135(5), 713
 (2003): Noecker RS+, *Am J Ophthalmol* 135(1), 55
 (2002): Eisenberg DL+, *Surv Ophthalmol* 47(Suppl 1), S105
 (2002): Johnstone MA+, *Surv Ophthalmol* 47(Suppl 1), S185
 (2002): Sugimoto M+, *Can J Ophthalmol* 37(6), 342
 (2001): Demitsu T+, *J Am Acad Dermatol* 44, 721 (77%)
 (2001): Strober BE+, *Cutis* 67, 109
 (1997): Johnstone MA, *Am J Ophthalmol* 124, 544
Eyelashes – pigmentation
 (2006): Inoue K+, *Nippon Ganka Gakkai Zasshi* 110(8), 581
 (2005): Chiselita D+, *Oftalmologia* 49(3), 39
 (2004): Grierson I+, *Jpn J Ophthalmol* 48(6), 602
 (2003): Costagliola C+, *Expert Opin Pharmacother* 4(10), 1775
 (1999): Hejkal TW+, *Semin Ophthalmol* 14, 114
 (1998): Reynolds A+, *Eye* 12, 741
 (1997): Johnstone MA, *Am J Ophthalmol* 124, 544
 (1997): Wand M, *Arch Ophthalmol* 115, 1206

Eyelashes – ptosis
  (2005): Casson RJ+, *Am J Ophthalmol* 139(5), 932
Eyelid burning (1.1%)
Eyelid edema (1–4%)
  (2001): Stewart WC+, *Am J Ophthalmol* 131(5), 631
Eyelid erythema (1–4%)
  (2006): Lai CH+, *Eur J Ophthalmol* 16(4), 627
Eyelid pain (0.4%)
Eyelid pigmentation
  (2006): Inoue K+, *Nippon Ganka Gakkai Zasshi* 110(8), 581
  (2003): Herndon LW+, *Am J Ophthalmol* 135(5), 713
  (2001): Wand M+, *Arch Ophthalmol* 119(4), 614
  (2000): Kook MS+, *Am J Ophthalmol* 129, 804
Eyelid pruritus (1.7%)
Eyelid stinging (0.4%)
Iris pigmentation
  (2006): *Jpn J Ophthalmol* 50(2), 96 (50%)
  (2006): Inoue K+, *Nippon Ganka Gakkai Zasshi* 110(8), 581
  (2005): Chiselita D+, *Oftalmologia* 49(3), 39
Macular edema
  (2005): Altintas O+, *Eur J Ophthalmol* 15(1), 158
Ocular edema
  (2005): Arcieri ES+, *Arch Ophthalmol* 123(2), 186
Ocular erythema
Ocular herpes simplex
  (2001): Morales J+, *Am J Ophthalmol* 132(1), 114 (2 cases)
Ocular pigmentation (5%)
  (2004): Grierson I+, *Jpn J Ophthalmol* 48(6), 602
  (2002): Novack GD+, *J Am Geriatr Soc* 50(5), 956
  (2002): Stjernschantz JW+, *Surv Ophthalmol* 47(Suppl 1), S162
  (2001): Aung T+, *Am J Ophthalmol* 131(5), 636
  (2001): Netland PA+, *Am J Ophthalmol* 132(4), 472 (5.2%)
  (2001): Stewart WC+, *Am J Ophthalmol* 131(5), 631
  (2000): Alm A+, *Acta Ophthalmol Scand* 78, 71
  (2000): Camras CB+, *J Glaucoma* 9, 95
  (1999): Hejkal TW+, *Semin Ophthalmol* 14, 114
  (1997): Bito LAZ, *Surv Ophthalmol* 41(Suppl 2), S1
  (1997): Wistrand JP+, *Surv Ophthalmol* 41(Suppl 2), S129
Ocular stinging
  (2004): Fechtner RD+, *Acta Ophthalmol Scand* 82(1), 42
Uveitis (1%)
  (2005): Cano Parra J+, *Arch Soc Esp Oftalmol* 80(3), 137
  (2003): Costagliola C+, *Expert Opin Pharmacother* 4(10), 1775
  (1999): Smith SL+, *Acta Ophthalmol Scand* 77(6), 668 (1%)
  (1998): Fechtner RD+, *Am J Ophthalmol* 126(1), 37

Other
Gynecomastia (0.2%)
Myalgia/Myositis/Myopathy/Myotoxicity (1–10%)

LAVENDER

Scientific names: *Lavandula angustifolia; Lavandula dentata; Lavandula spica; Lavandula vera*
Family: Lamiaceae
Trade and other common names: Alhucema; English Lavender; French Lavender; Spanish Lavender; Spike Lavender
Category: Anxiolytic
Purported indications and other uses: Restlessness, insomnia, loss of appetite, flatulence, colic, giddiness, nervous headache, migraine, toothache, sprains, neuralgia, rheumatism, acne, pimples, nausea, vomiting. Flavoring, fragrance, insect repellent
Half-life: N/A

Reactions

Skin
Dermatitis
  (2002): Schempp CM+, *Hautarzt* 53(2), 93
  (1999): Coulson IH+, *Contact Dermatitis* 41(2), 111

Other
Gynecomastia
  (2007): Dean CJ, *N Engl J Med* 356(24), 2543
  (2007): Henley DV+, *N Engl J Med* 356(5), 479
  (2007): Kalyan S, *N Engl J Med* 356(24), 2542

LEFLUNOMIDE

Trade name: Arava (Sanofi-Aventis)
Indications: Rheumatoid arthritis
Category: Disease-modifying antirheumatic; Tyrosine kinase inhibitor
Half-life: 14–15 days
Clinically important, potentially hazardous interactions with: warfarin

Reactions

Skin
Acne (1–10%)
Allergic reactions (sic) (2%)
  (2000): Smolen JS+, *Rheumatology* (Oxford) 39 (Suppl 1), 48
  (1999): Goldenberg MM, *Clin Ther* 21, 1837
  (1997): Silva Junior HT+, *Am J Med Sci* 313, 289
  (1995): Mladenovic V+, *Arthritis Rheum* 38, 1595
Bullous dermatitis
  (2003): Canonne-Courivaud D+, *Ann Dermatol Venereol* 130(4), 435
  (2000): Lepine G, Rock Hill, SC (6 months after starting drug) (from Internet) (observation)
Dermatitis (1–10%)
Dermatomyositis
  (2005): Gomez Rodriguez N+, *An Med Interna* 22(6), 300
Diaphoresis (1–10%)
Eczema (2%)
Erythema multiforme
  (2003): Fischer TW+, *Dermatology* 207(4), 386
Exfoliative dermatitis
  (2003): Bandyopadhyay D, *J Dermatol* 30(11), 845
Herpes (1–10%)
Herpes zoster
  (2006): Wolfe F+, *Rheumatology* (Oxford) 45(11), 1370
Lichenoid eruption
  (2004): Rivarola de Gutierrez E+, *Dermatology* 208(3), 232 (photodistributed)
  (2003): Canonne-Courivaud D+, *Ann Dermatol Venereol* 130(4), 435
Lupus erythematosus
  (2007): van Woerkom JM+, *Ann Rheum Dis* 66(8), 1026
  (2005): Chan SK+, *Clin Exp Dermatol* 30(6), 724
  (2005): Elias AR+, *Cutis* 76(3), 189
  (2005): Gensburger D+, *Ann Rheum Dis* 64(1), 153
  (2005): Goeb V+, *Rheumatology* (Oxford) 44(6), 823
  (2004): Kerr OA+, *Clin Exp Dermatol* 29(3), 319
Nodular eruption (1–10%)
Peripheral edema (1–10%)
Pigmentation (1–10%)
Pruritus (4%)

(2003): Canonne-Courivaud D+, *Ann Dermatol Venereol* 130(4), 435
Purpura (1–10%)
Rash (sic) (10%)
  (2006): Chan V+, *Pharmacoepidemiol Drug Saf* 15(7), 485
  (2006): Shastri V+, *Indian J Dermatol Venerol Leprol* 72(4), 286
  (2002): Hirohata S, *Nippon Rinsho* 60(12), 2357
  (2002): Sanders S+, *Am J Med Sci* 323(4), 190
  (2001): Cohen S+, *Arthritis Rheum* 44(9), 1984
  (2000): Emery P+, *Rheumatology* (Oxford) 39, 655
  (2000): Nousari HC+, *Arch Dermatol* 136, 1204
  (1999): Goldenberg MM, *Clin Ther* 21, 1837
  (1999): Smolen JS+, *Lancet* 353, 259
  (1997): Silva Junior HT+, *Am J Med Sci* 313, 289
  (1995): Mladenovic V+, *Arthritis Rheum* 38, 1595
Squamous cell carcinoma
  (2002): Shelley J (from Internet) (observation)
Stevens–Johnson syndrome
Toxic epidermal necrolysis
  (2006): Teraki Y+, *Int J Dermatol* 45(11), 1370
  (2003): Fischer TW+, *Dermatology* 207(4), 386
Ulcerations (1–10%)
  (2006): Jakob A+, *J Dtsch Dermatol* 4(4), 324
Urticaria (<1%)
Vasculitis (1–10%)
  (2003): Chan AT+, *Rheumatology* (Oxford) 42(3), 492
  (2001): Holm EA+, *Dermatology* 203(3), 258
Xerosis (2%)

Mucosal/ENT
Dysgeusia (1–10%)
Gingivitis (1–10%)
Oral candidiasis (3%)
Oral ulceration (3%)
Stomatitis (3%)
Vulvovaginal candidiasis (1–10%)
Xerostomia (1–10%)

Hair
Hair – alopecia (10%)
  (2007): van Woerkom JM+, *Ann Rheum Dis* 66(8), 1026
  (2002): Gottenberg JE+, *J Rheumatol* 29(8), 1806
  (2002): Hirohata S, *Nippon Rinsho* 60(12), 2357
  (2002): Sanders S+, *Am J Med Sci* 323(4), 190
  (2001): Cohen S+, *Arthritis Rheum* 44(9), 1984
  (2000): Emery P+, *Rheumatology* (Oxford) 39, 655
  (2000): Nousari HC+, *Arch Dermatol* 136, 1204
  (2000): Smolen JS+, *Rheumatology* (Oxford) 39 (Suppl 1), 48
  (1999): Goldenberg MM, *Clin Ther* 21, 1837
  (1999): Smolen JS+, *Lancet* 353, 259 (8%)
  (1997): Silva Junior HT+, *Am J Med Sci* 313, 289
  (1995): Mladenovic V+, *Arthritis Rheum* 38, 1595
Hair – alopecia areata
  (2002): Gottenberg JE+, *J Rheumatol* 29(8), 1806
Hair – pigmentation (1–10%)

Nails
Nails – changes (sic) (1–10%)

Other
Anaphylactoid reactions/Anaphylaxis (<1%)
Aseptic meningitis
  (2004): Cohen JD+, *Joint Bone Spine* 71(3), 243
Death
  (2002): Legras A+, *Am J Med* 113(4), 352 (with itraconazole)
Headache
Hepatotoxicity
  (2006): Sudarsanam TD+, *Postgrad Med J* 82(967), 313
Hypersensitivity

(2006): Shastri V+, *Indian J Dermatol Venerol Leprol* 72(4), 286
Infections (4%)
  (2006): Grover R+, *Rheumatology* (Oxford) 45(7), 918
  (2001): Cohen S+, *Arthritis Rheum* 44(9), 1984
Myalgia/Myositis/Myopathy/Myotoxicity (1–10%)
Nephrotoxicity
  (2003): Icardi A+, *Reumatismo* 55(2), 76 (rare)
Neurotoxicity
  (2005): Martin K+, *Ann Rheum Dis* 64(4), 649
Paresthesias (2%)
Rhabdomyolysis
  (2004): Rivarola de Gutierrez E+, *Dermatology* 208(3), 232
Tendinopathy/Tendon rupture (1–10%)

LEMON BALM

Scientific name: *Melissa officinalis*
Family: Labiatae
Trade and other common names: Balm mint; Blue balm; Dropsy plant; Garden balm; Melissa; Pharmaton; Sweet balm
Category: Carminative; Immunomodulator
Purported indications and other uses: Oral: Alzheimer's disease, anxiety, attention deficit disorder, colic, dementia, depression, hyperactivity, hyperthyroidism, insomnia, menstrual cramps, fevers, headache. **Topical:** genital herpes, herpes simplex, insect bites, insect repellent, muscle tension, skin irritation
Half-life: N/A

Reactions

None

LENALIDOMIDE

Synonym: CC-5013
Trade name: Revlimid (Celgene)
Indications: Transfusion-dependent anemia due to myeloplastic syndromes
Category: Immunomodulator; Thalidomide analog
Half-life: ~3 hours

Note: Lenalidomide is a major teratogen; it can also cause severe thrombocytopenia and neutropenia

Reactions

Skin
Acute febrile neutrophilic dermatosis (Sweet's syndrome)
  (2006): Hoverson AR+, *Arch Dermatol* 142(8), 1070
Diaphoresis (8%)
Erythema (5.4%)
Peripheral edema (20%)
Pruritus (42%)
Rash (sic) (36%)
  (2005): Rajkumar SV+, *Blood* 106(13), 4050 (6%)
Xerosis (14%)

Mucosal/ENT
Dysgeusia (6%)
Rhinitis (7%)
Stomatitis
Xerostomia (7%)

Other
Abdominal pain (12%)
Asthenia (31%)
  (2005): Rajkumar SV+, *Blood* 106(13), 4050 (15%)
Chest pain (5%)
Chills
Cough (20%)
Depression (5%)
Fever
Headache (20%)
Insomnia
Myalgia/Myositis/Myopathy/Myotoxicity (18%)
  (2005): Rajkumar SV+, *Blood* 106(13), 4050 (15%)
Upper respiratory infection (15%)
Vertigo (20%)

LETROZOLE

Trade name: Femara (Novartis)
Indications: Breast cancer
Category: Aromatase inhibitor
Half-life: ~2 days

Reactions

Skin
Diaphoresis (<5%)
Exanthems (5%)
Pruritus (2%)
Psoriasis (5%)
Rash (sic) (1–10%)
Toxic epidermal necrolysis
  (2006): Chia WK+, *Lancet Oncol* 7(2), 184
Vesiculation (5%)

Hair
Hair – alopecia (<5%)
  (2003): Carlini P+, *Ann Oncol* 14(11), 1689 (with triptorelin)

Other
Cardiac failure
  (2006): Scott LJ+, *Drugs* 66(3), 353
Headache
Hot flashes (6%)
  (2005): Mann BS+, *Clin Cancer Res* 11(16), 5671
Myalgia/Myositis/Myopathy/Myotoxicity
  (2005): Mann BS+, *Clin Cancer Res* 11(16), 5671
Osteoporosis
  (2006): Brufsky A, *Semin Oncol* 33(2), S13
  (2006): Forbes JF, *Semin Oncol* 33(2), S2
  (2006): McCloskey E, *Eur J Cancer* 42(8), 1044
  (2006): Mincey BA+, *Clin Breast Cancer* 7(2), 127
  (2006): Monnier A, *Cancer Treat Rev* 32(7), 532
  (2006): Perez EA+, *Oncology* (Williston Park) 20(9), 1029
  (2006): Scott LJ+, *Drugs* 66(3), 353

LEUCOVORIN

Synonyms: citrovorum factor; folinic acid
Trade names: Antrex; Citrec; Lederfolin; Leucovorin; Refolinin; Rescufolin; Rescuvolin
Indications: Overdose of methotrexate
Category: Adjuvant
Half-life: 15 minutes

Reactions

Skin
Erythema (<1%)
Pruritus (<1%)
Rash (sic) (<1%)
Urticaria (<1%)

Mucosal/ENT
Mucositis
  (2003): Tsalic M+, *Am J Clin Dermatol* 26(1), 103 (10%) (with fluorouracil)
Oral ulceration
  (2002): Xu D+, *Zhonghua Zhong Liu Za Zhi* 24(1), 93 (with fluorouracil)

Hair
Hair – alopecia
  (2001): Madnani N, Mumbai, India (from Internet) (observation)

Other
Anaphylactoid reactions/Anaphylaxis (<1%)
Death
  (2003): Tsalic M+, *Am J Clin* 26(1), 103 (2%) (with fluorouracil)
Hypersensitivity
Phlebitis
  (2002): Xu D+, *Zhonghua Zhong Liu Za Zhi* 24(1), 93 (with fluorouracil)

LEUPROLIDE

Synonym: leuprorelin acetate
Trade names: Carcinil; Eligard (Sanofi-Aventis); Enantone; Lucrin; Lupron (TAP); Procren Depot; Procrin; Tapros; Viadur (Bayer)
Indications: Prostate carcinoma, endometriosis
Category: Gonadotropin-releasing hormone agonist
Half-life: 3–4 hours

Reactions

Skin
Acne
Allergic granulomatous angiitis (Churg–Strauss syndrome)
  (2006): Sakamoto R+, *J Dermatol* 33(1), 43
Dermatitis (5%)
Dermatitis herpetiformis
  (2006): Yu SS+, *J Am Acad Dermatol* 54(2 Suppl), S58
  (2005): Grimwood RE+, *Cutis* 75(1), 49
Diaphoresis
Edema (1–10%)
Exanthems
Lupus erythematosus
  (1994): Fritzler MJ, *Lupus* 3, 455
Nodular eruption
  (2003): Saxby M, *BJU Int* 91(1), 125

Peripheral edema (4–12%)
  (1989): Crawford ED+, *N Engl J Med* 321, 419 (4%)
Photosensitivity
Pigmentation (<5%)
Pruritus (<5%)
Purpura (<1%)
Rash (sic) (1–10%)
Stickiness
  (2001): Sander HM, Austin, TX (from Internet) (observation)
Urticaria
Xerosis (<5%)

Mucosal/ENT
Dysgeusia (<5%)
Vaginitis

Hair
Hair – alopecia (<5%)
Hair – hypertrichosis (<1%)

Other
Depression
  (2003): Freeman MP+, *J Clin Psychiatry* 64(3), 341
Gynecomastia (7%)
Headache
Hot flashes (12–57%)
  (2002): Chu FM+, *J Urol* 168(3), 1199 (12–57%)
  (2002): Perez-Marreno R+, *Clin Ther* 24(11), 1902 (56.7%)
  (1993): Bressler LR+, *Ann Pharmacother* 27, 182
Injection-site granuloma
  (2006): Ferran M+, *Acta Derm Venereol* 86(5), 453
  (2006): Ouchi T+, *J Dermatol* 33(10), 719
  (2006): Sakamoto R+, *J Dermatol* 33(1), 43
  (2003): Saxby M, *BJU Int* 91(1), 125
  (2002): Whitaker IS+, *BJU Int* 90(3), 350
Injection-site inflammation (2%)
  (1989): Crawford ED+, *N Engl J Med* 321, 419 (2.1%)
Injection-site pruritus
  (1989): Crawford ED+, *N Engl J Med* 321, 419 (2.1%)
Injection-site reactions (24%)
  (2001): Fluker M+, *Fertil Steril* 75(1), 38 (24.4%)
Myalgia/Myositis/Myopathy/Myotoxicity
  (2002): Van Gerpen JA+, *J Am Geriatr Soc* 50(10), 1746
Osteoporosis
  (2006): Schlaff WD+, *Fertil Steril* 85(2), 314
Paresthesias (<5%)
Thrombophlebitis (2%)

LEVALBUTEROL

Synonym: R-albuterol
Trade name: Xopenex (Sepracor)
Indications: Bronchospasm
Category: Adrenergic beta-receptor agonist
Half-life: 3.3–4.0 hours

Reactions

Skin
Diaphoresis (<2%)

Eyes
Ocular pruritus (<2%)

Other
Chills (<2%)
Cough (1–4%)

Headache
Hypersensitivity
Myalgia/Myositis/Myopathy/Myotoxicity (<2%)
Pain (1–3%)
Paresthesias (<2%)
Tremor (~7%)

LEVAMISOLE

Trade names: Ascaridil; Decaris; Detrax 40; Ergamisol (Janssen); Ketrax; Solaskil; Termizole
Indications: Susceptible helmintic organism infections, colorectal carcinoma
Category: Antineoplastic; Immunomodulator
Half-life: 2–6 hours
Clinically important, potentially hazardous interactions with: alcohol, aldesleukin

Reactions

Skin
Angioedema (<1%)
Dermatitis (1–10%)
Edema (1–10%)
Erythema annulare
  (1989): Lioté F+, *Rev Rhum Mal Ostéoartic* (French) 56, 11
Erythema multiforme
Exanthems (2–10%)
  (1989): Lioté F I, *Rev Rhum Mal Ostéoartic* (French) 56, 11
  (1980): Miller B+, *Arthritis Rheum* 23, 172 (>10%)
Exfoliative dermatitis
Fixed eruption (<1%)
  (1994): Clavère P+, *Ann Dermatol Venereol* (French) 121, 238 (pigmented)
  (1991): Thankappen TP+, *Int J Dermatol* 30, 867 (0.88%)
Hemorrhage
  (1982): Papageorgiou P+, *J Clin Lab Immunol* 8, 121
Lichen planus
  (1980): Kirby JD+, *J R Soc Med* 73, 208 (passim)
Lichenoid eruption
  (1980): Kirby JD+, *J R Soc Med* 73, 208
Necrosis
  (2002): Kumar B+, *Clin Exp Dermatol* 27(1), 8
  (2002): Powell J+, *Clin Exp Dermatol* 27(1), 32
Pemphigus
  (1980): Mashkilleison NA, *Vestn Dermatol Venerol* (Russian) October, 46
Pruritus (<1%)
  (1992): Breathnach SM+, *Adverse Drug Reactions and the Skin* Blackwell, Oxford, 178 (passim)
  (1989): Lioté F+, *Rev Rhum Mal Ostéoartic* (French) 56, 11
  (1980): Kirby JD+, *J R Soc Med* 73, 208
Psoriasis
  (1980): Kirby JD+, *J R Soc Med* 73, 208 (passim)
Purpura
  (1999): Rongioletti F+, *Br J Dermatol* 140(5), 948
Rash (sic)
  (2005): Gupta R+, *Indian J Dermatol Venereol Leprol* 71(6), 428
  (1980): Husain Z+, *J Rheumatol* 7, 825
  (1980): Kinsella PL+, *J Rheumatol* 7, 288
  (1980): Miller B+, *Arthritis Rheum* 23, 172
Side effects (sic) (<20%)
Stevens–Johnson syndrome (<1%)
Urticaria (<1%)

(1992): Breathnach SM+, *Adverse Drug Reactions and the Skin*
Blackwell, Oxford, 178 (passim)
(1989): Lioté F+, *Rev Rhum Mal Ostéoartic* (French) 56, 11
Vasculitis
(1999): Rongioletti F+, *Br J Dermatol* 140(5), 948
(1989): Lioté F+, *Rev Rhum Mal Ostéoartic* (French) 56, 11
(1983): Ferlazzo B+, *Boll Ist Sieroter Milan* (Italian) 62, 107
(1980): Huskisson EC, *Agents Actions* Suppl 7, 55
Xerosis
(1980): Kirby JD+, *J R Soc Med* 73, 208

Mucosal/ENT

Dysgeusia (1–10%) (metallic taste)
Dysphagia
(2006): Wu VC+, *Medicine* (Baltimore) 85(4), 203 (51%)
Oral lesions (1–10%)
(1989): Lioté F+, *Rev Rhum Mal Ostéoartic* (French) 56, 11
(2.1%)
(1980): Miller B+, *Arthritis Rheum* 23, 172 (>10%)
Oral ulceration
Parosmia (<1%)
Stomatitis (1–10%)
(1980): Kinsella PL+, *J Rheumatol* 7, 288

Hair

Hair – alopecia (1–10%)
(1980): Kirby JD+, *J R Soc Med* 73, 208

Other

Anaphylactoid reactions/Anaphylaxis
Inappropriate secretion of antidiuretic hormone (SIADH)
(1992): Tweedy CR+, *N Engl J Med* 326(17), 1164
Infections (1–10%)
Myalgia/Myositis/Myopathy/Myotoxicity (1–10%)
Paresthesias (1–10%)

LEVETIRACETAM

Trade name: Keppra (UCB)
Indications: Partial onset seizures
Category: Anticonvulsant
Half-life: 7 hours
**Clinically important, potentially hazardous interactions
with:** carbamazepine

Reactions

Skin

Edema
(2003): Hawker K+, *Arch Neurol* 60(12), 1772
Fungal dermatitis (>1%)
Rash (sic) (>1%)
(2007): Arif H+, *Neurology* 68(20), 1701

Mucosal/ENT

Gingivitis (>1%)
Rhinitis
(2006): Glauser TA+, *Neurology* 66(11), 1654

Other

Abdominal pain
(2003): Cramer JA+, *Epilepsy Res* 56(2–3), 135
Asthenia (<22%)
(2007): Sirsi D+, *Expert Opin Drug Saf* 6(3), 241
(2006): Genton P+, *Acta Neurol Scand* 113(6), 387
(2006): Lambrechts DA+, *Seizure* 15(6), 434
(2006): Meco G+, *Clin Neuropharmacol* 29(5), 265

(2006): Ramael S+, *Epilepsia* 47(7), 1128 (11%)
(2005): Lagae L+, *Seizure* 14(1), 66
(2003): Abou-Khalil B+, *Seizure* 12(3), 141
(2003): Ben-Menachem E+, *Epilepsy Res* 53(1), 57 (22.6%)
(2003): Cramer JA+, *Epilepsy Res* 56(2–3), 135
(2003): Morrell MJ+, *Epilepsy Res* 54(2), 153
Cough
(2006): Glauser TA+, *Neurology* 66(11), 1654
Death
(2006): Skopp G+, *Arch Kriminol* 217(5-6), 161 (with
carbamazepine)
Depression
(2007): Mula M+, *Drug Saf* 30(7), 555
(2006): Wier LM+, *J Clin Psychiatry* 67(7), 1159
Headache (25%)
(2006): Genton P+, *Acta Neurol Scand* 113(6), 387
(2006): Lambrechts DA+, *Seizure* 15(6), 434
(2006): Ramael S+, *Epilepsia* 47(7), 1128 (8%)
(2006): Tsai JJ+, *Epilepsia* 47(1), 72 (11%)
(2003): Ben-Menachem E+, *Epilepsy Res* 53(1), 57 (25.8%)
(2003): Cramer JA+, *Epilepsy Res* 56(2–3), 135
Hepatotoxicity
(2006): Skopp G+, *Arch Kriminol* 217(5-6), 161 (with
carbamazepine)
Inappropriate secretion of antidiuretic hormone (SIADH)
(2005): Nasrallah K+, *Epilepsia* 46(6), 972
Infections (sic) (13–26%)
(2003): Ben-Menachem E+, *Epilepsy Res* 53(1), 57 (26.6%)
(2002): Boon P+, *Epilepsy Res* 48(1), 77
(2002): Glauser TA+, *Epilepsia* 43(5), 518
(2001): Nash EM+, *Am J Health Syst Pharm* 58(13), 1195
(2000): Cereghino JJ+, *Neurology* 55, 236
Neurotoxicity
(2005): Kapoor P+, *Electromyogr Clin Neurophysiol* 45(1), 15
Pain
(2002): Boon P+, *Epilepsy Res* 48(1), 77
Paresthesias (2%)
Somnolence
(2008): Zaccara G+, *Seizure* nd, 182
(2007): Sirsi D+, *Expert Opin Drug Saf* 6(3), 241
Suicidal ideation
(2007): Mula M+, *Epilepsy Behav* 11(1), 130 (4 cases)
Tremor
(2003): Cramer JA+, *Epilepsy Res* 56(2–3), 135
Vertigo (9–18%)
(2007): Sirsi D+, *Expert Opin Drug Saf* 6(3), 241
(2006): Genton P+, *Acta Neurol Scand* 113(6), 387
(2006): Lambrechts DA+, *Seizure* 15(6), 434
(2006): Ramael S+, *Clin Ther* 28(5), 734
(2006): Ramael S+, *Epilepsia* 47(7), 1128 (53%)
(2006): Tsai JJ+, *Epilepsia* 47(1), 72
(2003): Abou-Khalil B+, *Seizure* 12(3), 141
(2003): Ben-Menachem E+, *Epilepsy Res* 53(1), 57 (18%)
(2003): Cramer JA+, *Epilepsy Res* 56(2–3), 135
(2003): Ferrendelli JA+, *Epilepsy Behav* 4(6), 702 (9%)
(2003): Morrell MJ+, *Epilepsy Res* 54(2), 153

LEVOBETAXOLOL

Trade names: Betaxon (Alcon); L-betaxolol
Indications: Chronic open-angle glaucoma, ocular hypertension
Category: Adrenergic beta-receptor antagonist
Half-life: 20 hours

Reactions

Skin
Dermatitis (<2%)
Psoriasis (<2%)
Rash (sic)
Xerosis

Mucosal/ENT
Dysgeusia (<2%)
Tinnitus (<2%)

Hair
Hair – alopecia (<2%)

Eyes
Ocular transient discomfort (11%)

Other
Infections (<2%)
Tendinopathy/Tendon rupture (<2%)

LEVOBUNOLOL

Trade names: Betagan (Allergan); Bunolgan; Gotensin; Vistagan; Vistagen
Indications: Glaucoma, ocular hypertension
Category: Adrenergic beta-receptor antagonist
Half-life: N/A

Note: Peak effect: 1–7 days

Reactions

Skin
Dermatitis
 (2006): Hashimoto Y+, *J Dermatol* 33(7), 507
 (2001): Holdiness MR, *Am J Contact Dermat* 12(4), 217
 (1999): Erdmann S+, *Contact Dermatitis* 41, 44
 (1995): di Lernia V+, *Contact Dermatitis* 33, 57
 (1995): Koch P, *Contact Dermatitis* 33, 140
 (1995): Zucchelli V+, *Contact Dermatitis* 33, 66
 (1993): van der Meeren HL+, *Contact Dermatitis* 28, 41
 (1989): Schultheiss E, *Derm Beruf Umwelt* (German) 37, 185
Erythema
Lichen planus
 (1995): Beckman KA+, *Am J Ophthalmol* 120, 530
Pruritus (<1%)
Rash (sic) (<1%)
Urticaria

Hair
Hair – alopecia (1–10%)

Eyes
Ocular burning
 (1986): Ober M+, *Ophthalmologica* 192(3), 159
Ocular stinging
 (1986): Ober M+, *Ophthalmologica* 192(3), 159

Other
Headache
Hypersensitivity

LEVOBUPIVACAINE

Trade name: Chirocaine (Purdue)
Indications: Regional anesthesia for surgery, postoperative pain management
Category: Anesthetic, local
Half-life: 1.3 hours
Clinically important, potentially hazardous interactions with: None

Reactions

Skin
Angioedema
Diaphoresis (<1%)
Edema (<1%)
Erythema
Pigmentation (<1%)
Pruritus (3.7%)
Purpura (1.4%)
Rash (sic)
 (2003): Taylor R+, *Paediatr Anaesth* 13(2), 114
Shivering
 (2002): Cheng CR+, *Acta Anaesthesiol Sin* 40(1), 13
Urticaria

Mucosal/ENT
Tinnitus

Other
Anaphylactoid reactions/Anaphylaxis
Chills
Cough (1%)
Pain (7–18%)
Paresthesias (2%)
Seizures
 (2003): Breslin DS+, *Reg Anesth Pain Med* 28(2), 144
 (2003): Crews JC+, *Anesth Analg* 96(4), 1188
 (2003): Cumming C+, *Anaesthesia* 58(6), 610
 (2003): Dhileepan S+, *Anaesthesia* 58(6), 611
 (2002): Pirotta D+, *Anaesthesia* 57(12), 1187
Tremor (<1%)

LEVOCETIRIZINE

Trade names: Vozet; Xozal; Xusal; Xyzal (UCB Pharma)
Indications: Allergic rhinitis, chronic idiopathic urticaria
Category: Antihistamine
Half-life: 6–10 Hours
Clinically important, potentially hazardous interactions with: N/A

Reactions

Skin
Dermatitis
 (2006): Cusano F+, *Dermatology* 213(4), 353
Fixed eruption

(2005): Guptha SD+, *Indian J Dermatol Venereol Leprol* 71(5), 361
(2005): Mahajan VK+, *Int J Dermatol* 44(9), 796
Pruritus
Rash (SIC)
Urticaria
(2005): Kranke B+, *Dermatology* 210(3), 246

Mucosal/ENT
Nasopharyngitis (6%)
Rhinitis
Xerostomia (3%)

Other
Abdominal pain
Anaphylactoid reactions/Anaphylaxis
Asthenia (4%)
Cough
Fever
Headache
Hypersensitivity
Myalgia/Myositis/Myopathy/Myotoxicity
Seizures
Somnolence (5%)
Weight gain (0.5%)

LEVODOPA

Synonym: L-dopa
Trade names: Brocadopa; Dopaflex; Doparl; Eldopal; Levodopa-Woelm; Sinemet (Bristol-Myers Squibb)
Indications: Parkinsonism
Category: Dopamine precursor
Half-life: 1–3 hours
Clinically important, potentially hazardous interactions with: amisulpride, **kava**, MAO inhibitors, phenelzine, pyridoxine, sapropterin, selegiline, tetrabenazine, tranylcypromine, zuclopentixol acetate, zuclopentixol decanoate, zuclopentixol dihydrochloride

Note: Sinemet is carbidopa and levodopa

Reactions

Skin
Chromhidrosis (1–10%)
Diaphoresis
(1995): Sage JI+, *Ann Neurol* 37, 120
Exanthems
Hypomelanosis guttata
(2001): Mocci A, Panama City, Panama (from Internet) (observation)
Lupus erythematosus
(1985): Stratton MA, *Clin Pharm* 4, 657
Melanoma
(2002): Wobbes T+, *Ned Tijdschr Geneeskd* 146(27), 1286
(1997): Pfützner W+, *J Am Acad Dermatol* 37, 332
(1996): Kleinhans M+, *Hautarzt* (German) 47, 432
(1993): Weiner WJ+, *Neurology* 43, 674
(1992): Haider SA+, *Br J Ophthalmol* 76, 246
(1992): Sandyk R, *Int J Neurosci* 63, 137
(1989): Kande'l EI, *Zh Nevropatol Psikhiatr* (Russian) 89, 126
(1987): Morpurgo G+, *Eur J Cancer Clin Oncol* 23, 1213
(1985): Kochar AS, *Am J Med* 79, 119
(1985): Przybilla B+, *Acta Derm Venereol* (Stockh) 65, 556
(1985): Rampen FHJ, *J Neurol Neurosurg Psychiatry* 48, 585

(1984): Abramson DH+, *JAMA* 252, 1011
(1984): Rosin MA+, *Cutis* 33, 572
(1982): Van Rens GH+, *Ophthalmology* 89, 1464
(1980): Bernstein JE+, *Arch Dermatol* 116, 1041
(1980): Warner TF+, *J Cutan Pathol* 7, 50
Pemphigus
(1986): Pisani M+, *G Ital Dermatol Venereol* (Italian) 121, 39
Purpura
Rash (sic)
(1984): Goetz CG, *Clin Neuropharmacol* 7, 107
(1983): Goetz CG, *N Engl J Med* 309, 1387
Urticaria
Vitiligo
(1999): Sabate M+, *Ann Pharmacother* 33, 1228 (with tolcapone)

Mucosal/ENT
Ageusia
Anosmia
Dysgeusia
Glossopyrosis
Leukoplakia
Parosmia
Sialorrhea
Xerostomia (1–10%)

Hair
Hair – alopecia
Hair – pigmentation
(1989): Reynolds NJ+, *Clin Exp Dermatol* 14, 317

Nails
Nails – growth
(1984): Danial CR+, *J Am Acad Dermatol* 10, 250

Other
Delusions of parasitosis
(2005): Swick BL+, *J Am Acad Dermatol* 53(6), 1086
Headache
Hot flashes
Paresthesias
Phlebitis

LEVOFLOXACIN

Trade names: Levaquin (Ortho-McNeil); Quixin (Johnson & Johnson)
Indications: Various infections caused by susceptible organisms
Category: Antibiotic, quinolone
Half-life: 6–8 hours
Clinically important, potentially hazardous interactions with: zinc

Reactions

Skin
Acute generalized exanthematous pustulosis
(2005): Corral de la Calle M+, *Br J Dermatol* 152(5), 1076
Diaphoresis (0.1%)
Edema (0.1%)
Erythema
(2002): Famularo G+, *Ann Pharmacother* 36(9), 1380
(1992): Kanzaki H+, *Jpn J Antibiot* (Japanese) 45, 576
Erythema multiforme
Erythema nodosum (<3%)
Exanthems
(2000): Paily R, *J Dermatol* 27, 405

Exfoliative dermatitis
(2001): Sienkiewicz G, Johnson City, NY (from Internet) (observation)
Photosensitivity (<0.1%)
(2004): Viola G+, *Chem Biodivers* 1(5), 782
(2000): Boccumini LE+, *Ann Pharmacol* 34, 453
Phototoxicity
(2003): Dawe RS+, *Br J Dermatol* 149(6), 1232
(2001): Carbon C, *Therapie* 56(1), 35
Pigmentation
(2007): Lopez-Pestana A+, *Arch Dermatol* 143(11), 1441
Pruritus (1.6%)
(2006): Nelwan RH+, *Southeast Asian J Trop Med Public Health* 37(1), 126
Purpura (<0.5%)
(2002): Famularo G+, *Ann Pharmacother* 36(9), 1380
Rash (sic) (1.7%)
Side effects (sic)
(2002): Papastavros T+, *CMAJ* 167(2), 131 (with pyrazinamide) (14 cases)
Stevens–Johnson syndrome
Toxic epidermal necrolysis
(2005): Islam AF+, *Ann Pharmacother* 39(6), 1136 (fatal)
(2002): Digwood-Lettieri S+, *Pharmacotherapy* 22(6), 789
Urticaria (<0.5%)
(2001): Eisner J (from Internet) (personal reaction)
Vasculitis
(2006): Zaigraykin N+, *Isr Med Assoc J* 8(10), 726
(2003): Welsch MJ, *J Drugs Dermatol* 2, 193
(2002): Drayton G, Los Angeles, CA (from Internet) (observation)

Mucosal/ENT
Dysgeusia (0.2%)
Vaginitis (1.8%)
Xerostomia (<1%)

Other
Anaphylactoid reactions/Anaphylaxis
(2006): Sachs B+, *Drug Saf* 29(11), 1087
(2005): Takahama H+, *Int J Dermatol* 44(9), 789
(2001): *Drug & Ther Perspect* 17, 15
Candidiasis (0.3%)
Death
(2006): Sanchez Munoz LA+, *An Med Interna* 23(2), 102
(2004): Braun D+, *Joint Bone Spine* 71(6), 586 (from hypoglycemia)
(2003): Petitjeans F+, *Eur J Clin Pharmacol* 59(10), 779
(2001): Spahr L+, *J Hepatol* 35(2), 308
Delirium
(2006): Fernandez-Torre, *Clin Neurol Neurosurg* 108(6), 614
(2005): Hakko E+, *Clin Neurol Neurosurg* 107(2), 158
Headache
Hypersensitivity
(2003): *Prescrire Int* 12(63), 20
Injection-site reactions (sic)
Myalgia/Myositis/Myopathy/Myotoxicity (<0.5%)
(2003): Litt JZ, Beachwood, OH (personal case) (observation)
(2002): Papastavros T+, *CMAJ* 167(2), 131 (with pyrazinamide) (14 cases)
Nephrotoxicity
(2006): Zaigraykin N+, *Isr Med Assoc J* 8(10), 726
(2003): Ramalakshmi S+, *Am J Kidney Dis* 41(2), E7
(2002): Famularo G+, *Ann Pharmacother* 36(9), 1380
Paresthesias
Rhabdomyolysis
(2006): Korzets A+, *Nephrol Dial Transplant* 21(11), 3304
(2005): Hsiao SH+, *Ann Pharmacother* 39(1), 146

(2003): Petitjeans F+, *Eur J Clin Pharmacol* 59(10), 779
Seizures
(2007): Yamaguchi H+, *Chemotherapy* 53(2), 85
(2005): Bird SB+, *J Clin Psychopharmacol* 25(3), 287
(2005): Christie MJ+, *Ann Pharmacother* 39(5), 953
(2001): Kushner JM+, *Ann Pharmacother* 35(10), 1194
Tendinopathy/Tendon rupture
(2006): Beyer J+, *Br J Clin Pharmacol* 61(5), 609
(2006): Sanchez Munoz LA+, *An Med Interna* 23(2), 102
(2005): Alvarez Luque+, *Aten Primaria* 36(5), 286
(2005): Lado Lado FL+, *An Med Interna* 22(1), 28
(2005): Luthje P+, *Arch Orthop Trauma Surg* 125(2), 124
(2004): Braun D+, *Joint Bone Spine* 71(6), 586
(2004): Gomez Rodriguez+, *An Med Interna* 21(3), 154
(2004): Kahn F+, *Lakartidningen* 101(3), 190
(2004): Kowatari K+, *J Orthop Sci* 9(2), 186
(2003): *Prescrire Int* 12(63), 20
(2003): Bernacer L+, *Med Clin* (Barc) 120(2), 78
(2003): Cebrian P+, *Foot Ankle Int* 24(2), 122
(2003): de La Red G+, *Clin Rheumatol* 22(4–5), 367
(2003): Filippucci E+, *Reumatismo* 55(4), 267
(2003): Gold L+, *J Am Board Fam Pract* 16(5), 458
(2003): Leone R+, *Drug Saf* 26(2), 109
(2003): Litt JZ, Beachwood, OH (personal case) (observation)
(2003): Mathis AS+, *Ann Pharmacother* 37(7), 1014
(2003): Melhus A+, *Scand J Infect Dis* 35(10), 768
(2003): Tomas ME+, *Gastroenterol Hepatol* 26(1), 53
(2002): Aros C+, *Rev Med Chil* 130(11), 1277 (4 cases)
(2002): Greene BL, *Phys Ther* 82(12), 1224
(2001): Butler MW+, *Ir J Med Sci* 170(3), 198
(2001): Carbon C, *Therapie* 56(1), 35
(2001): Emmet S, Solana Beach, CA (Achilles; long-lasting) (from Internet) (observation)
(2001): Nuno Mateo FJ+, *Rev Clin Esp* 201(9), 539
(2000): Casado Burgos E+, *Med Clin* (Barc) (Spanish) 114, 319
(1999): Lewis JR I, *Ann Pharmacother* 33(7), 792 (Achilles, bilateral)
Tremor

LEVOLEUCOVORIN

Trade names: Antrex; FUSILEV (Spectrum pharmaceuticals); Leucovorin calcium
Indications: Antidote for folic acid antagonists, various cancersin combination with other medications
Category: Antidote; Chemotherapy modulating agent
Half-life: 4–8 hours

Reactions

Skin
Allergic reactions
Erythema
Pruritus
Rash (sic)
Urticaria

Other
Anaphylactoid reactions/Anaphylaxis
Wheezing

LEVOTHYROXINE

Synonyms: L-thyroxine sodium; T_4
Trade names: Berlthyrox; Droxine; Eferox; Eltroxin; Levo-T; Levothyroid (Forest); Levothyrox; Levoxyl (Monarch); Synthroid (Abbott); Thevier; Unithroid (Watson)
Indications: Hypothyroidism
Category: Thyroid hormone, synthetic
Half-life: 6–7 days
Clinically important, potentially hazardous interactions with: dicumarol, oral anticoagulants, raloxifene, **red rice yeast**, ritonavir, warfarin

Reactions

Skin

Acne
Allergic reactions (sic)
Angioedema
(1991): Levesque H+, *Lancet* 338, 393
(1990): Pandya AG+, *Arch Dermatol* 126, 1238
Dermatitis herpetiformis
Diaphoresis (<1%)
Nevi
Pruritus
(1990): Pandya AG+, *Arch Dermatol* 126, 1238
Rash (sic)
Urticaria
(2000): Drayton GE, Los Angeles, CA (from Internet) (observation)
(1994): Magner J+, *Thyroid* 4, 341 (from the blue dye)
(1990): Pandya AG+, *Arch Dermatol* 126, 1238
Xerosis

Hair

Hair – alopecia (<1%)

Other

Headache
Hypersensitivity
Myalgia/Myositis/Myopathy/Myotoxicity (<1%)
Tremor

LICORICE

Scientific names: *Glycyrrhiza glabra; Glycyrrhiza uralensis*
Family: Fabaceae; Leguminosae
Trade and other common names: Alcazuz; Gan Cao; Gan Zao; Orozuz; Reglisse; Subholz; Sweet Root
Category: Anti-inflammatory
Purported indications and other uses: Upper respiratory tract infection, gastric and duodenal ulcers, bronchitis, colic, dry cough, arthritis, lupus, sore throat, malaria, sores, abscesses, contact dermatitis. Flavoring in foods, beverages and tobacco
Half-life: N/A
Clinically important, potentially hazardous interactions with: alclometasone, **cascara**, digoxin, enalapril, hydrocortisone, oral contraceptives, prednisolone, **squill**

Reactions

Skin

Dermatitis
(1999): Nishioka K+, *Contact Dermatitis* 40(1), 56

Edema
(2000): Negro A+, *Ann Ital Med Int* 15(4), 296
(2000): Olukoga A+, *J R Soc Health* 120(2), 83

Eyes

Ocular adverse effects
(2004): Fraunfelder FW, *Am J Ophthalmol* 138(4), 639

Other

Hypertension
(2006): Breidthardt T+, *J Hum Hypertens* 20(6), 465
(2001): Brouwers AJ+, *Ned Tijdschr Geneeskd* 145(15), 744
Myalgia/Myositis/Myopathy/Myotoxicity
Rhabdomyolysis
(2005): van den Bosch AE+, *Neth J Med* 63(4), 146
(2003): Hussain RM, *Postgrad Med J* 79(928), 115
(2002): Firenzuoli F+, *Recenti Prog Med* 93(9), 482
(2002): Sardi A+, *Ann Ital Med Int* 17(2), 126
(1997): Barrella M+, *Ital J Neurol Sci* 18(4), 217
(1995): Berlango Jimenez A+, *An Med Interna* 12(1), 33
(1992): Caradonna P+, *Ultrastruct Pathol* 16(5), 529
(1989): Achar KN+, *Aust N Z J Med* 19(4), 365
(1988): Maresca MC+, *Minerva Med* 79(1), 55 (3 cases)
(1985): Ruggeri CS+, *Minerva Med* 76(14–15), 725
(1983): Corsi FM+, *Ital J Neurol Sci* 4(4), 493
(1983): Heidemann HT+, *Klin Wochenschr* 61(6), 303
(1982): Yokoyama F+, *Rinsho Shinkeigaku* 22(6), 552
(1980): Cumming AM+, *Postgrad Med J* 56(657), 526

LIDOCAINE

Synonym: lignocaine
Trade names: Anamantle HC (Doak); Anestacon; Dentipatch; DermaFlex; Dilocaine; ELA-Max (Ferndale); EMLA (AstraZeneca); Lidodan; Lidoderm (Endo); Lidoject-2; Octocaine; Xylocaine (AstraZeneca); Xylocard
Indications: Ventricular arrhythmias, topical anesthesia
Category: Anesthetic, local; Antiarrhythmic class IB
Half-life: terminal: 1.5–2 hours
Clinically important, potentially hazardous interactions with: amprenavir, antiarrhythmics, cimetidine, fosamprenavir, nilutamide

Reactions

Skin

Allergic reactions (sic)
(2002): Helfman M, *N Y State Dent J* 68(10), 24
Angioedema
(1987): Bricker SR+, *Anaesthesia* 42, 323
Bullous dermatitis
Dermatitis
(2006): Jovanovic M+, *Contact Dermatitis* 54(2), 124
(2005): Ismail F+, *Contact Dermatitis* 52(2), 111
(2003): Gammaitoni AR+, *J Clin Pharmacol* 43(2), 111
(2002): Kaufmann JM+, *J Drugs Dermatol* 1(2), 192
(2001): Breit S+, *Contact Dermatitis* 45(5), 296
(1999): Lodi A+, *Contact Dermatitis* 41(4), 221
(1998): Downs AM+, *Contact Dermatitis* 39, 33
(1997): Kawada A+, *Contact Dermatitis* 37(1), 45
(1996): Bassett IB+, *Australas J Dermatol* 37, 155
(1996): Bircher AJ+, *Contact Dermatitis* 34, 387
(1996): Whalen JD+, *Arch Dermatol* 132, 1256
(1995): Thakur BK+, *J Allergy Clin Immunol* 95, 776
(1994): Hardwick N+, *Contact Dermatitis* 30, 245
(1993): Duggan M+, *Contact Dermatitis* 28, 190
(1993): Handfield-Jones SE+, *Clin Exp Dermatol* 18, 342

(1990): Black RJ+, *Contact Dermatitis* 23, 117
(1989): Budde J+, *Derm Beruf Umwelt* (German) 37, 181
(1986): Curley KR, *Arch Dermatol* 122, 924
(1985): Fernandes-de-Corres L+, *Contact Dermatitis* 12, 114
(1983): Nurse DS+, *Contact Dermatitis* 9, 513
(1983): van Ketel WG+, *Contact Dermatitis* 9(6), 512
(1980): Chin TM+, *Int J Dermatol* 19, 147
Eczema
  (1990): Huwyler T+, *Schweiz Monatsschr Zahnmed* (German) 100, 751
  (1986): Curley KR, *Arch Dermatol* 122, 924
Edema (<1%)
  (2001): Breit S+, *Contact Dermatitis* 45(5), 296
Erythema
  (2006): Levy J+, *Can J Ophthalmol* 41(2), 204
  (2001): Breit S+, *Contact Dermatitis* 45(5), 296
Erythema multiforme
  (2008): Rodriguez-Carreon AA+, *Ann Pharmacother* 42(1), 127
  (1987): Arrowsmith JB+, *Ann Intern Med* 107, 693
Erythema nodosum
  (2008): Rodriguez-Carreon AA+, *Ann Pharmacother* 42(1), 127
Exanthems
  (2004): Chang MW, *Pediatrics* 113, 410 (with prilocaine)
  (2003): Gammaitoni AR+, *J Clin Pharmacol* 43(2), 111
Exfoliative dermatitis
  (1987): Arrowsmith JB+, *Ann Intern Med* 107, 693
Fixed eruption
  (1997): Garcia JC+, *J Investig Allergol Clin Immunol* 7, 127
  (1996): Kawada A+, *Contact Dermatitis* 35, 375
Lupus erythematosus
  (1988): Oliphant LD+, *Chest* 94, 427
Pigmentation
  (1987): Curley RK+, *Br Dent J* 162, 113
Pruritus (<1%)
  (2001): Breit S+, *Contact Dermatitis* 45(5), 296
Purpura
Rash (sic) (<1%)
Shivering (1–10%)
Stevens–Johnson syndrome
  (1987): Arrowsmith JB+, *Ann Intern Med* 107, 693
Toxicity (sic)
  (2006): Marra DE+, *Arch Dermatol* 142(8), 1024
Urticaria
  (2006): Jovanovic M+, *Contact Dermatitis* 54(2), 124
  (2004): Waton J+, *Contact Dermatitis* 51(5–6), 284
  (1980): Chin TM+, *Int J Dermatol* 19, 147

Mucosal/ENT

Stomatitis
  (1987): Arrowsmith JB+, *Ann Intern Med* 107, 693
Tinnitus
  (1999): Rump AF+, *Aviat Space Environ Med* 70(8), 769
  (1996): Chiang YY+, *Acta Anaesthesiol Sin* 34(4), 243
  (1985): Ruth RA+, *Arch Otolaryngol* 111(12), 799

Eyes

Eyelid edema
  (2006): Levy J+, *Can J Ophthalmol* 41(2), 204

Other

Anaphylactoid reactions/Anaphylaxis
  (2005): Li M+, *J Forensic Sci* 50(1), 169 (with Botox)
  (2001): Browne IM+, *Am J Obstet Gynecol* 185(5), 1253
  (1999): Bircher AJ+, *Aust Dent J* 44, 64
  (1984): Metzner HH+, *Dermatol Monatsschr* (German) 170, 648
  (1980): Agathos M, *Contact Dermatitis* 6, 236
Application-site edema
  (2001): Wahlgren CF+, *Plast Reconstr Surg* 107(3), 750
Application-site erythema

(2002): Gammaitoni AR+, *Am J Health Syst Pharm* 59(22), 2215
(2001): Wahlgren CF+, *Plast Reconstr Surg* 107(3), 750
Death
  (2005): Li M+, *J Forensic Sci* 50(1), 169 (with Botox)
  (2002): Kalin JR+, *J Forensic Sci* 47(5), 1135 (overdose)
  (2002): Nisse P+, *Acta Clin Belg* Suppl 1, 51
Embolia cutis medicamentosa (Nicolau syndrome)
  (1990): Wand A+, *Aktuel Dermatol* (German) 16, 128
Headache
Hypersensitivity
  (2007): Haugen RN+, *J Drugs Dermatol* 6(12), 1222
  (2006): Hickey JR+, *Contact Dermatitis* 54(4), 215
  (2003): Mackley CL+, *Arch Dermatol* 139(3), 343
  (1998): Marks JG+, *J Am Acad Dermatol* 38(6), 911
  (1996): Bircher AJ+, *Contact Dermatitis* 34, 387
  (1996): Whalen JD+, *Arch Dermatol* 132, 1256
  (1991): Klein CE+, *Contact Dermatitis* 25(1), 45
Injection-site pain
Injection-site phlebitis
Paresthesias (<1%)
  (2003): Dower JS Jr, *Dent Today* 22(2), 64
Seizures
  (2006): Dorf E+, *J Emerg Med* 31(3), 251
  (2005): Priya V+, *Acta Anaesthesiol Scand* 49(1), 124
  (2004): Ahmed SU+, *Anesth Analg* 99(2), 593 (with clonidine)
  (2004): Chang MW, *Pediatrics* 113, 410 (with prilocaine)
  (2002): DeToledo JC+, *Anesthesiology* 97(3), 737
  (2002): Yamashita S+, *J Pain Symptom Manage* 24(5), 543
Tremor

LINCOMYCIN

Trade names: Albiotic; Cillimicina; Cillimycin; Lincocin (Pfizer); Lincocine; Princol; Zumalin
Indications: Various infections caused by susceptible organisms
Category: Antibiotic, lincosamide
Half-life: 2–11.5 hours

Reactions

Skin

Acute generalized exanthematous pustulosis
  (2005): Otsuka A+, *J Dermatol* 32(11), 929
  (2003): Valois M+, *Contact Dermatitis* 48(3), 169
Allergic reactions (sic) (1–5%)
Angioedema
Dermatitis
  (1991): Vilaplana J+, *Contact Dermatitis* 24, 225
  (1985): Conde-Salazar L+, *Contact Dermatitis* 12, 59 (erythema multiforme-like)
Erythema multiforme
Exanthems
Exfoliative dermatitis
Photosensitivity
Pruritus
Pruritus ani et vulvae (<1%)
Purpura
Rash (sic) (<1%)
Stevens–Johnson syndrome (<1%)
Toxic epidermal necrolysis
  (2004): Ferchichi S+, *Ann Biol Clin (Paris)* 62(5), 578 (with NSAIDs)
Urticaria (<1%)
Vesiculobullous eruption

Mucosal/ENT

Glossitis (<1%)
Oral lesions
Stomatitis (<1%)
Tinnitus
Vaginitis (<1%)

Other

Anaphylactoid reactions/Anaphylaxis
Injection-site erythema
  (1990): Shen K, *Lancet* 336, 689
Serum sickness

LINDANE

Synonyms: Hexachlorocyclohexane; Gamma Benzene Hexachloride
Trade names: Aphtiria; Benhex Cream; Bicide; Bio-Well; Davesol; Delice; Elentol; G-Well; GAB; Gamabenceno; Gambex; Gamene; Gammalin; GBH; Herklin; Hexicid; Hexit; Jacutin; Kildane; Kwell; Kwildane; Lencid; Locion-V; Lorexane; PMS-Lindane; Quellada; Sacbexyl; Sarconyl; Scabecid; Scabene; Scabex; Scabi; Scabisan; Thinex; Varsan
Indications: Scabies, pediculosis capitis, pediculosis pubis
Category: Chemical; Scabicide
Half-life: 17–22 hours
Clinically important, potentially hazardous interactions with: oil-based hair dressings

Reactions

Skin

Acute generalized exanthematous pustulosis (AGEP)
  (2004): Juan WH+, *Dermatology* 209(3), 239
Adverse effects (sic)
  (2000): Hernandez Contreras N+, *Rev Cubana Med Trop* 52(3), 228 (2.54%)
  (1999): Hall RC+, *Psychosomatics* 40(6), 513
  (1995): Brown S+, *Clin Infect Dis* 20 (Suppl 1), S104
  (1981): Rasmussen JE, *J Am Acad Dermatol* 5(5), 507
Bullous dermatitis
  (1994): Bouree P+, *Bull Soc Fr Parasitol* 12, 75
Dermatitis
  (2005): Yu KJ+, *Contact Dermatitis* 52(2), 118 (ulcerative)
  (1990): Andersen KE, *Occupational Skin Disease* 2nd ed, 73–88
  (1983): *AMA Drug Evaluations* 5th ed, 1850
  (1983): Farkas J, *Derm Beruf Umwelt* (German) 31(6), 189
  (1983): Fiumara NJ+, *Am Fam Physician* 28(1), 137
Eczema
Erythema (2%)
  (1987): Bowerman JG+, *Pediatr Infect Dis* 6(3), 252 (2.6%)
  (1980): Smith DE+, *Cutis* 26(6), 618
Irritation (sic)
Non-Hodgkin's lymphoma
  (1998): Blair A+, *Am J Ind Med* 33(1), 82
Papulo-nodular lesions
  (2000): Hashimoto K+, *J Dermatol* 27(3), 181
Pruritus (2%)
  (2000): Hashimoto K+, *J Dermatol* 27(3), 181
  (1999): Revenga Arranz F+, *Rev Clin Esp* 199(2), 101
  (1998): Bowie C+, *Public Health* 112(4), 249
  (1990): Schultz MW+, *Arch Dermatol* 126(2), 167
  (1987): Bowerman JG+, *Pediatr Infect Dis* 6(3), 252 (2.6%)
Purpura
  (1981): Fagan JE, *Pediatrics* 67, 310

Toxicity (sic)
  (1999): Hall RC+, *Psychosomatics* 40(6), 513
Urticaria (0.16%)
  (1996): Shuster J, *Hosp. Pharm* 31, 370
  (1994): Fischer TF, *Ann Emerg Med* 24(5), 972

Other

Death
  (2003): Katsumata K+, *Intern Med* 42(4), 367
  (2000): Walker GJ+, *Cochrane Database Syst Rev* 3, CD00
  (1996): Lewis RJ, *Sax's Dangerous Properties of Industrial Materials* 9th ed, 338
  (1995): Aks SE+, *Ann Emerg Med* 26(5), 647
  (1995): Surber C+, *Hautarzt* (German) 46(8), 528
  (1994): Fischer TF, *Ann Emerg Med* 24(5), 972
  (1989): Vercel M+, *Cah Anesthesiol* 37(7), 543
  (1988): Sunder Ram Rao CV+, *Vet Hum Toxicol* 30(2), 132
  (1985): *American Hospital Formulary Service-Drug Information* 85, 1601
  (1984): Gosselin RE+, *Clinical Toxicology of Commercial Products* 5th ed, III–239
  (1983): Davies JE+, *Arch Dermatol* 119(2), 142
  (1982): Telch J+, *Can Med Assoc* 126(6), 662
  (1982): Telch J+, *Can Med Assoc* 127(9), 821
  (1980): Powell GM, *Cent Afr J Med* 26(7), 170
  (1980): Rasmussen JE, *Arch Dermatol* 116(11), 1226
Neurotoxicity
  (2006): *Prescrire Int* 15(82), 61
  (2006): Singal A+, *Am J Ther* 13(3), 277
Paresthesias
Rhabdomyolysis
  (1988): Sunder Ram Rao CV+, *Vet Hum Toxicol* 30(2), 132
  (1984): Jaeger U+, *Vet Hum Toxicol* 26(1), 11
Seizures
  (2002): Simpson WM Jr+, *Am Fam Physician* 65(8), 1599
  (2000): Cox R+, *J Miss Med Assoc* 41(8), 690
  (2000): Nordt SP+, *J Emerg Med* 18(1), 51
  (1995): Solomon BA+, *J Fam Pract* 40(3), 291
  (1994): Fischer TF, *Ann Emerg Med* 24(5), 972
  (1991): Ramchander V+, *West Indian Med J* 40(1), 41
  (1991): Tenenbein M, *J Am Geriatr Soc* 39(4), 394
  (1987): Friedman SJ, *Arch Dermatol* 123(8), 1056
  (1984): Jaeger U+, *Vet Hum Toxicol* 26(1), 11

LINEZOLID

Trade name: Zyvox (Pfizer)
Indications: Various infections caused by susceptible organisms
Category: Antibiotic, oxazolidinone
Half-life: 4–5 hours
Clinically important, potentially hazardous interactions with: amitriptyline, amoxapine, clomipramine, desipramine, desvenlafaxine, dextromethorphan, doxepin, fluoxetine, fluvoxamine, imipramine, meperidine, nortriptyline, paroxetine, protriptyline, sertraline, sibutramine, trazodone, tricyclic antidepressants, trimipramine, venlafaxine

Reactions

Skin

Adverse effects (sic) (4%)
  (2003): Birmingham MC+, *Clin Infect Dis* 36(2), 159 (4%)
Allergic reactions (sic) (4%)
  (2003): Birmingham MC+, *Clin Infect Dis* 36(2), 159 (4%)
Exanthems
  (2006): Borras-Blasco J+, *Int J Clin Pharmacol Ther* 44(7), 331 (generalized)

Fungal dermatitis (0.1–2%)
Pruritus
Rash (sic) (2%)
   (2005): Aneziokoro CO+, *J Chemother* 17(6), 643 (5%)

Mucosal/ENT
Candidal vaginitis (1–2%)
Dysgeusia (1–2%)
   (2002): Linden PK, *Drugs* 62(3), 425
Oral candidiasis (<1%)
Tongue pigmentation (<1%)

Eyes
Macular exanthems
   (2006): Borras-Blasco J+, *Int J Clin Pharmacol Ther* 44(7), 331
Optic neuropathy
   (2007): Narita M+, *Pharmacotherapy* 27(8), 1189
   (2006): Park IN+, *J Antimicrob Chemother* 58(3), 701
   (2006): Rucker JC+, *Neurology* 66(4), 595
   (2005): McKinley SH+, *J Neuroophthalmol* 25(1), 18 (2 cases)

Other
Headache
   (2006): Senneville E+, *Clin Ther* 28(8), 1155
Neurotoxicity
   (2006): Thai XC+, *Pharmacotherapy* 26(8), 1183

LINSEED

Scientific name: *Linum usitatissimum*
Family: Linaceae
Trade and other common names: alpha-linolenic acid;
Flaxseed; flaxseed oil; L-310; Igroco; Lini Semen; linseed oil; lint
bells; Salinum; winterlien
Category: Anti-inflammatory
Purported indications and other uses: Dry mouth,
menopause, osteoporosis, heart disease, catarrh, bronchitis,
furunculosis, pleuritic pains, constipation, high cholesterol, benign
prostatic hyperplasia, bladder inflammation, gastritis, enteritis,
irritable bowel syndrome. **Topical:** poultice for skin
inflammation. **Ophthalmologic:** oil used for removal of foreign
bodies from the eye.
Half-life: N/A

Reactions

Skin
Allergic reactions (sic)
Erythema
Irritation

Eyes
Eyelid edema

Other
Anaphylactoid reactions/Anaphylaxis
   (2003): Leon F+, *Allergol Immunopathol* (Madr) 31(1), 47 (seed)
   (1996): Alonso L+, *J Allergy Clin Immunol* 98(2), 469 (seed)
Fever

LIOTHYRONINE

Synonym: T_3 sodium
Trade names: Cynomel; Cytomel; T3; Tertroxin; Thyronine;
Trijodthyronin BC N; Triostat (King)
Indications: Hypothyroidism
Category: Thyroid hormone, synthetic
Half-life: 16–49 hours
**Clinically important, potentially hazardous interactions
with:** anticoagulants, dicumarol, warfarin

Reactions

Skin
Allergic reactions (sic)
Diaphoresis (<1%)
Rash (sic)
Urticaria
   (1994): Magner J+, *Thyroid* 4, 341 (from the blue dye)
   (1990): Pandya AG l, *Arch Dermatol* 126, 1238
Xerosis

Hair
Hair – alopecia (<1%)

Eyes
Vision blurred
   (2002): Serratrice J+, *Am J Ophthalmol* 134(6), 910

Other
Headache
   (2002): Serratrice J+, *Am J Ophthalmol* 134(6), 910
Hypersensitivity
Myalgia/Myositis/Myopathy/Myotoxicity (<1%)
Phlebitis (1%)
Tremor
Vertigo
   (2002): Serratrice J+, *Am J Ophthalmol* 134(6), 910

LISDEXAMFETAMINE

Trade name: Vyvanse (Shire)
Indications: Attention-deficit hyperactivity disorder (ADHD)
Category: CNS stimulant; Dextroamphetamine prodrug
Half-life: 1 Hour
**Clinically important, potentially hazardous interactions
with:** MAO inhibitors

Reactions

Skin
Angioedema
Rash (sic) (3%)
Stevens–Johnson syndrome
Toxic epidermal necrolysis
Urticaria

Mucosal/ENT
Dysgeusia
Xerostomia (5%)

Eyes
Vision blurred
Visual hallucinations

Other

Abdominal pain
  (2007): Biederman J+, *Clin Ther* 29(3), 450 (12%)
Anaphylactoid reactions/Anaphylaxis
Asthenia
Cardiac failure
Fever (2%)
Headache
  (2007): Biederman J+, *Clin Ther* 29(3), 450 (12%)
Hypersensitivity
Hypertension
Hypotension
Insomnia
  (2007): Biederman J+, *Clin Ther* 29(3), 450 (19%)
Seizures
Somnolence (2%)
Tremor
Vertigo (5%)
Weight loss
  (2007): Biederman J+, *Clin Ther* 29(3), 450 (9%)

LISINOPRIL

Trade names: Acerbon; Alapril; Apo-Lisinopril; Carace; Coric; Prinil; Prinivil (Merck); Prinzide (Merck); Tensopril; Vivatec; Zestoretic (AstraZeneca); Zestril (AstraZeneca)
Indications: Hypertension
Category: Angiotensin-converting enzyme inhibitor
Half-life: 12 hours
Clinically important, potentially hazardous interactions with: amiloride, **garlic**, spironolactone, tizanidine, triamterene

Note: Prinizide is lisinopril and hydrochlorothiazide; Zestoretic is lisinopril and hydrochlorothiazide

Reactions

Skin

Angioedema
  (2006): Piller LB+, *J Clin Hypertens* (Greenwich) 8(9), 649 (70%)
  (2001): Cohen EG+, *Ann Otol Rhinol Laryngol* 110(8), 701 (64 cases)
  (1999): Guo X+, *J Okla State Med Assoc* 92, 71
  (1999): Maestre ML+, *Rev Esp Anestesiol Reanim* (Spanish) 46, 88
  (1999): Neutel JM+, *Am J Ther* 6, 161
  (1997): Brown NJ+, *JAMA* 278, 232
  (1997): Pavletic AJ, *J Am Board Fam Pract* 10, 370
  (1996): Pillans PI+, *Eur J Clin Pharmacol* 51, 123
  (1995): Bauwens LJ+, *Ned Tijdschr Geneeskd* (Dutch) 139, 674
  (1995): Frontera Y+, *J Am Dent Assoc* 126, 217
  (1995): Kuo DC+, *J Emerg Med* 13, 327 (uvular)
  (1994): Krikorian RK+, *Chest* 106, 1922
  (1993): Soo Hoo GW+, *West J Med* 158, 412
  (1992): McElligott S+, *Ann Intern Med* 116, 426
  (1992): Nzerue MC, *Cent Afr J Med* 38(9), 391
  (1992): Shelley WB+, *Cutis* 49, 391 (tongue) (observation)
  (1990): Laher MS, *Drugs* 39 (Suppl 2), 55
  (1990): McAreavey D+, *Drugs* 40, 326 (0.4%)
  (1990): Orfan N+, *JAMA* 264, 1287
  (1988): Lancaster SG+, *Drugs* 35, 646 (0.6%)
  (1987): Rush JE+, *J Cardiovasc Pharmacol* 9, s99
Bullous dermatitis
  (1988): Barlow RJ+, *Clin Exp Dermatol* 13, 117
Diaphoresis (<1%)
Edema (1%)
Erythema (1%)

Exanthems (3%)
  (1990): Laher MS, *Drugs* 39 (Suppl 2), 55
  (1990): McAreavey D+, *Drugs* 40, 326 (3.2%)
  (1988): Barlow RJ+, *Clin Exp Dermatol* 13, 117
  (1988): Lancaster SG+, *Drugs* 35, 646 (3.2%)
Facial edema (<1%)
Kaposi's sarcoma
  (2004): Di Carlo, *Br J Dermatol* 150(1), 158
Lichenoid eruption
  (1992): Shelley WB+, *Cutis* 50, 182 (observation)
Lupus erythematosus
  (2001): Carter JD+, *South Med J* 94(11), 1122
Pemphigus
Pemphigus foliaceus
  (2004): Patterson CR+, *J Dermatolog Treat* 15(1), 60
  (2000): Ong CS+, *Australas J Dermatol* 41(4), 242
Peripheral edema (<1%)
  (1988): Uretsky BF+, *Am Heart J* 116, 480
Photosensitivity (<1%)
Pityriasis rosea
  (2006): Atzori L+, *Dermatology Online Journal* 12(1), 1 (with hydrochlorothiazide)
  (2004): Atzori L+, *J Eur Acad Dermatol Venereol* 18(6), 743
Pruritus (1.2%)
  (2000): Kalikhman ZM (from Internet) (observation)
Purpura
  (1993): Sztern B+, *Presse Med* (French) 22, 967
  (1988): Barlow RJ+, *Clin Exp Dermatol* 13, 117
Rash (sic) (1.5%)
  (1999): Horiuchi Y+, *J Dermatol* 26, 128
  (1989): Giles TD+, *J Am Coll Cardiol* 13, 1240
  (1988): Uretsky BF+, *Am Heart J* 116, 480
  (1987): Bolzano K+, *J Cardiovasc Pharmacol* 9, s43
  (1987): Rush JE+, *J Cardiovasc Pharmacol* 9, s99
Rosacea
  (1999): Oakley A, Hamilton, New Zealand (from Internet) (observation)
Stevens–Johnson syndrome
Telangiectasia
  (1999): Oakley A, Hamilton, New Zealand (from Internet) (observation)
Toxic epidermal necrolysis
Ulcerations (ischemic skin ulcer)
  (1987): Rush JE+, *J Cardiovasc Pharmacol* 9, s99
Urticaria (<1%)
  (1996): Pillans PI+, *Eur J Clin Pharmacol* 51, 123
  (1989): Cameron HA+, *J Human Hypertension* 3, 177
Vasculitis (<1%)
  (1988): Barlow RJ+, *Clin Exp Dermatol* 13, 117

Mucosal/ENT

Burning mouth syndrome
  (1992): Savino LB+, *Ann Pharmacother* 26(11), 1381
Dysgeusia
  (1988): Uretsky BF+, *Am Heart J* 116, 480
Tinnitus
Xerostomia (<1%)

Hair

Hair – alopecia (<1%)

Other

Anaphylactoid reactions/Anaphylaxis (<1%)
Cough
  (2005): Arslanagic A+, *Med Arh* 59(6), 346 (with amlodipine)
  (2004): Malacco E+, *Clin Ther* 26(6), 855 (7%)
  (2004): Wu SC+, *Heart Vessels* 19(1), 13 (30%)
  (2002): Lee TH, *Harv Heart Lett* 12(11), 8
  (2001): Adigun AQ+, *West Afr J Med* 20(1), 46–7

(2001): Lee SC+, *Hypertension* 38(2), 166
(2000): Ruszty L+, *Orv Hetil* 141(34), 1867
(1992): Os I+, *Tidsskr Nor Laegeforen* 112(27), 3429
(1992): Syvertsen JO+, *Tidsskr Nor Laegeforen* 112(27), 3432
(1991): Feder D+, *AMB Rev Assoc Med Bras* 37(3), 160
(1991): Woo J+, *Br J Clin Pract* 45(3), 178 (48%)
(1989): Cameron HA+, *J Hum Hypertens* 3 Suppl 1, 177
Headache
Hypotension
(2004): Kao CD+, *Ann Pharmacother* 38(11), 1840 (with tizanidine)
Myalgia/Myositis/Myopathy/Myotoxicity (0.5%)
Paresthesias (0.8%)
Tremor

LITHIUM

Trade names: Carbolith; Duralith; Eskalith (GSK); Hynorex Retard; Lithicarb; Lithizine; Lithobid (Solvay); Lithonate; Lithotabs; Priadel; Teralithe
Indications: Manic-depressive states
Category: Antipsychotic; Mood stabilizer
Half-life: 18–24 hours
Clinically important, potentially hazardous interactions with: aceclofenac, acetazolamide, acitretin, bendroflumethiazide, benzthiazide, chlorothiazide, chlorthalidone, **cocoa**, desvenlafaxine, etoricoxib, fluoxetine, **guarana**, haloperidol, hydrochlorothiazide, hydroflumethiazide, indapamide, insulin detemir, insulin glulisine, meperidine, mesoridazine, methotrexate, methyclothiazide, metolazone, olmesartan, pegfilgrastim, phenylbutazone, polythiazide, quinethazone, rocuronium, rofecoxib, sibutramine, thiazides, trichlormethiazide, valdecoxib

Note: An excellent review of the cutaneous conditions associated with lithium can be found in (1983): Sarantidis D+, *Br J Psychiatry* 143, 42

Reactions

Skin
Acne
(2004): Yeung CK+, *Am J Clin Dermatol* 5(1), 3 (passim)
(2001): Oztas P+, *Ann Pharmacother* 35(7), 961
(2000): Chan HH+, *J Affect Disord* 57(1-3), 107
(1991): Srebrnik A+, *Cutis* 48, 65
(1986): Remmer HI+, *J Clin Psychiatry* 47, 48
(1985): Albrecht G, *Hautarzt* (German) 36, 77 (passim)
(1984): Lambert D+, *Ann Med Interne Paris* (French) 135, 637
(1983): Sarantidis D+, *Br J Psychiatry* 143, 42 (11%)
(1982): Deandrea D+, *J Clin Psychopharmacol* 2, 199
(1982): Heng MCY, *Arch Dermatol* 118, 246
(1982): Heng MCY, *Br J Dermatol* 106, 107
(1982): Lambert D+, *Ann Dermatol Venereol* (French) 109, 19
(1980): Vestergaard P+, *Acta Psychiatrica Scand* 62, 193
Angioedema
(1985): Berova N+, *Dermatol Venerol* (Sofia) (Bulgarian) 24, 23
(1982): Lambert D+, *Ann Dermatol Venereol* (French) 109, 19
Atopic dermatitis (3%)
(1983): Sarantidis D+, *Br J Psychiatry* 143, 42 (3%)
Bullous dermatitis
(1987): McWhirter JD+, *Arch Dermatol* 123, 1122
Darier's disease
(1995): Rubin MB, *J Am Acad Dermatol* 32, 674
(1990): Milton GP, *J Am Acad Dermatol* 23, 926 (exacerbation)
(1986): Clark RD Jr+, *Psychosomatics* 27, 800 (exacerbation)

Dermatitis
(1980): Aldoroty N+, *Am J Psychiatry* 137, 870
Dermatitis herpetiformis
(1985): Albrecht G, *Hautarzt* (German) 36, 77 (passim)
(1983): Sarantidis D+, *Br J Psychiatry* 143, 42
(1982): Heng MCY, *Arch Dermatol* 118, 246
Eczema
(1980): Vestergaard P+, *Acta Psychiatrica Scand* 62, 193
Edema
(1984): Lambert D+, *Ann Med Interne Paris* (French) 135, 637
Erythema
(1996): Wakelin SH+, *Clin Exp Dermatol* 21, 296
Erythema multiforme
(1991): Balldin J+, *J Am Acad Dermatol* 24, 1015
Exanthems
(2004): Yeung CK+, *Am J Clin Dermatol* 5(1), 3 (passim)
(2003): Warnock JK+, *Am J Clin Dermatol* 4(1), 21
(1985): Albrecht G, *Hautarzt* (German) 36, 77 (passim)
(1983): Sarantidis D+, *Br J Psychiatry* 143, 42
(1982): Deandrea D+, *J Clin Psychopharmacol* 2, 199
(1982): Lambert D+, *Ann Dermatol Venereol* (French) 109, 19
(1980): Meinhold JM+, *J Clin Psychiatry* 41, 395
Exfoliative dermatitis (1%)
(1985): Albrecht G, *Hautarzt* (German) 36, 77 (passim)
(1983): Sarantidis D+, *Br J Psychiatry* 143, 42 (1%)
Follicular keratosis
(1996): Wakelin SH+, *Clin Exp Dermatol* 21, 296
(1982): Lambert D+, *Ann Dermatol Venereol* (French) 109, 19
Folliculitis
(2004): Yeung CK+, *Am J Clin Dermatol* 5(1), 3 (passim)
(1985): Hogan DJ+, *J Am Acad Dermatol* 13, 245 (passim)
(1983): Sarantidis D+, *Br J Psychiatry* 143, 42
Hidradenitis
(1997): Marinella MA, *Acta Derm Venereol* 77, 483
(1996): Blumenthal HL, Beachwood, OH (personal case) (observation)
(1995): Gupta AK+, *J Amer Acad Dermatol* 32, 382
(1981): Stamm T+, *Psychiatr Prax* (German) 8, 152
Ichthyosis (1%)
(1983): Sarantidis D+, *Br J Psychiatry* 143, 42 (1%)
Keratoderma
(1991): Labelle A+, *J Clin Psychopharmacol* 11, 149
Keratosis pilaris
(1985): Albrecht G, *Hautarzt* (German) 36, 77 (passim)
Lichen planus
(1994): Thompson DF+, *Pharmacotherapy* 14, 561
Lichen simplex chronicus
(1984): Shukla S+, *Am J Psychiatry* 141, 909
Linear IgA dermatosis
(2003): Avci O+, *J Am Acad Dermatol* 48(2), 299 (passim)
(2002): Cohen LM+, *J Am Acad Dermatol* 46, S32 (passim)
(1996): Tranvan A+, *J Am Acad Dermatol* 35, 865
(1987): McWhirter JD+, *Arch Dermatol* 123, 1122
Lupus erythematosus
(1994): Yung RL+, *Rheum Dis Clin North Am* 20, 61
(1985): Stratton MA, *Clin Pharm* 4, 657
(1982): Shukla VR+, *JAMA* 248, 921
(1981): Hess EV, *Arthritis Rheum* 24, 6
Morphea
(1982): Lambert D+, *Ann Dermatol Venereol* (French) 109, 19
Mycosis fungoides
(2001): Francis GJ+, *J Am Acad Dermatol* 44, 308
Myxedema
(1981): Kvetny J+, *Ugeskr Laeger* (Danish) 143, 1323
Papulo-nodular lesions (elbows)
Pigmentation ((fingers & toes)) (<1%)
Port-wine stain
(1987): Leung AK, *J Natl Med Assoc* 79, 877

Prurigo nodularis (1%)
  (1983): Sarantidis D+, *Br J Psychiatry* 143, 42 (1%)
Pruritus (<1%)
  (1985): Berova N+, *Dermatol Venerol* (Sofia) (Bulgarian) 24, 23
    (1–5%)
  (1984): Lambert D+, *Ann Med Interne Paris* (French) 135, 637
  (1983): Sarantidis D+, *Br J Psychiatry* 143, 42
  (1982): Lambert D+, *Ann Dermatol Venereol* (French) 109, 19
  (1980): Vestergaard P+, *Acta Psychiatrica Scand* 62, 193
Psoriasis (2%)
  (2007): Wachter T+, *Br J Dermatol*
  (2006): O'Brien M+, *J Drugs Dermatol* 5(5), 426
  (2005): Knijff EM+, *Bipolar Disord* 7(4), 388
  (2005): Yo MS+, *Ned Tijdschr Geneeskd* 149(6), 273
  (2004): Yeung CK+, *Am J Clin Dermatol* 5(1), 3 (passim)
  (2003): Akkerhuis GW+, *Am J Psychiatry* 160(7), 1355
  (2000): Chan HH+, *J Affect Disord* 57(1-3), 107
  (1997): Hanada K+, *Lancet* 350(9090), 1522
  (1996): Ockenfels HM+, *Arch Dermatol Res* 288, 173
  (1994): Dorevitch A, *Harefuah* (Hebrew) 127, 228
  (1993): Hermle L+, *Nervenarzt* (German) 64, 208
  (1992): Abel EA, *Semin Dermatol* 11, 269
  (1992): Hemlock C+, *Ann Pharmacother* 26, 211
  (1992): Rudolph RI, *J Am Acad Dermatol* 26, 135
  (1989): Sasaki T+, *J Dermatol* (Tokio) 16, 59 (exacerbation)
  (1988): Koo E+, *Orv Hetil* (Hungarian) 129, 1699
  (1988): Zirilli G+, *Minerva Psichiatr* (Italian) 29, 43
  (1987): Gupta MA+, *Gen Hosp Psychiatry* 9, 157
  (1986): Abel EA+, *J Am Acad Dermatol* 15, 1007 (exacerbation)
  (1986): Ghadirian AM+, *J Clin Psychiatry* 47, 212
  (1986): Holy B+, *Acta Univ Carol Med Praha* (Czech) 32, 217
  (1986): Pande AC+, *J Clin Psychiatry* 47, 330 (exacerbation)
  (1986): Segui-Montesinos J+, *Med Clin* (Barc) (Spanish) 86, 261
  (1985): Albrecht G, *Hautarzt* (German) 36, 77 (passim)
  (1984): Alvarez WA+, *Int J Psychosom* 31, 21
  (1984): Farber EM+, *J Am Acad Dermatol* 10, 511
  (1984): Fox BJ+, *J Assoc Military Dermatol* 10, 35 (exacerbation)
  (1984): Lambert D+, *Ann Med Interne Paris* (French) 135, 637
  (1984): Lin HN+, *Taiwan I Hsueh Hui Tsa Chih* (Chinese)
    83, 1064
  (1983): Hollander A, *Hautarzt* (German) 34, 487
  (1983): Sarantidis D+, *Br J Psychiatry* 143, 42 (2%)
  (1982): Deandrea D+, *J Clin Psychopharmacol* 2, 199
  (1982): Heng MCY, *Arch Dermatol* 118, 246 (exacerbation)
  (1982): Heng MCY, *Br J Dermatol* 106, 107 (exacerbation)
  (1982): Lambert D+, *Ann Dermatol Venereol* (French) 109, 19
    (exacerbation)
  (1982): Pincelli C+, *G Ital Dermatol Venereol* (Italian) 117, 113
  (1981): No Author, *Drug Ther Bull* 19, 68
  (1980): Bakris GL+, *Int J Psychiatry Med* 10, 327
  (1980): Thiers B, *J Am Acad Dermatol* 3, 101
Purpura
  (1984): Lambert D+, *Ann Med Interne Paris* (French) 135, 637
  (1982): Lambert D+, *Ann Dermatol Venereol* (French) 109, 19
Pustules
  (1993): Webster GF, *Clin Dermatol* 11, 541
  (1982): White SW, *J Am Acad Dermatol* 7, 660 (palms and soles)
Rash (sic) (1–10%)
  (1980): Bone S+, *Am J Psychiatry* 137:1, 103
Seborrheic dermatitis
  (1984): Lambert D+, *Ann Med Interne Paris* (French) 135, 637
  (1983): Sarantidis D+, *Br J Psychiatry* 143, 42
  (1982): Lambert D+, *Ann Dermatol Venereol* (French) 109, 19
Side effects (sic) (23–33%)
  (1985): Berova N+, *Dermatol Venerol* (Sofia) (Bulgarian) 24, 23
    (23%)
  (1983): Sarantidis D+, *Br J Psychiatry* 143, 42 (up to one-third)
  (1982): Lambert D+, *Ann Dermatol Venereol* (French) 109, 19
Subcorneal pustular dermatosis (Sneddon-Wilkinson)

Telangiectasia
  (1983): Brinkmann W+, *Z Hautkr* (German) 9, 681
Tinea
  (1997): Fearfield LA+, *Clin Exp Dermatol* 22, 57
Toxicoderma
  (1985): Lambert D, *Dermatologica* (French) 171, 209
Ulcerations (lower extremities)
  (1984): Lambert D+, *Ann Med Interne Paris* (French) 135, 637
Urticaria
  (1985): Berova N+, *Dermatol Venerol* (Sofia) (Bulgarian) 24, 23
  (1984): Lambert D+, *Ann Med Interne Paris* (French) 135, 637
  (1982): Lambert D+, *Ann Dermatol Venereol* (French) 109, 19
Vasculitis
  (1994): Blumenthal HL, Beachwood, OH (personal case)
    (observation)
  (1984): Lambert D+, *Ann Med Interne Paris* (French) 135, 637
  (1982): Lambert D+, *Ann Dermatol Venereol* (French) 109, 19
Verrucae
  (1982): White SW, *Int J Dermatol* 21, 107
Verrucous lesions
  (1984): Frenk E, *Z Hautkr* (German) 59, 97
Xerosis

Mucosal/ENT
Angular stomatitis (1%)
  (1983): Sarantidis D+, *Br J Psychiatry* 143, 42 (1%)
Dysgeusia (>10%)
Gingival hyperplasia/hypertrophy
Glossodynia
Lichenoid stomatitis
  (1995): Menni S+, *Ann Dermatol Venereol* (French) 122, 91
  (1991): Srebrnik A+, *Cutis* 48, 65
  (1985): Hogan DJ+, *J Am Acad Dermatol* 13, 245
Oral lichen planus
  (2005): Campisi G+, *J Oral Pathol Med* 34(2), 124
Oral ulceration
  (2000): Madinier I+, *Ann Med Interne* (Paris) (French) 151, 248
  (1985): Bar Nathan EA+, *Am J Psychiatry* 142, 1126
  (1985): Hogan DJ+, *J Am Acad Dermatol* 13, 245
Sialorrhea
  (2005): Boyce HW+, *J Clin Gastroenterol* 39(2), 89 (passim)
  (1982): Donaldson SR, *Am J Psychiatry* 139(10), 1350
Stomatitis
  (1985): Bar Nathan EA+, *Am J Psychiatry* 142, 1126
Stomatodynia
  (1985): Bar Nathan EA+, *Am J Psychiatry* 142, 1126
Tinnitus
Tongue geographic
  (1992): Patki AH, *Int J Dermatol* 31, 386
Vaginal ulceration
  (1991): Srebrnik A+, *Cutis* 48, 65
Xerostomia (<1%)
  (2005): Sajatovic M+, *Am J Geriatr Psychiatry* 13(4), 305
  (1987): Chacko RC+, *Hillside J Clin Psychiatry* 9(1), 79
  (1980): Bone S+, *Am J Psychiatry* 137:1, 103

Hair
Hair – abnormal texture
  (1985): McCreadle RG+, *Acta Psychiatr Scand* 72, 387
Hair – alopecia (10–19%)
  (2001): Francis GJ+, *J Am Acad Dermatol* 44, 308
  (2000): Mercke Y+, *Ann Clin Psychiatry* 12, 35 (12–19%)
  (1999): van dem Bent PM+, *Ned Tijdschr Geneeskd* (Dutch)
    143, 990
  (1998): Litt JZ, Beachwood, OH (personal case) (observation)
  (1996): McKinney PA+, *Ann Clin Psychiatry* 8, 183 (10%)
  (1991): Wagner KD+, *Psychosomatics* 32, 355
  (1986): Ghadirian AM+, *J Clin Psychiatry* 47, 212
  (1985): Albrecht G, *Hautarzt* (German) 36, 77 (passim)

(1984): Lambert D+, *Ann Med Interne Paris* (French) 135, 637
(1984): Mortimer PS+, *Int J Dermatol* 23, 603
(1983): Orwin A, *Br J Dermatol* 108, 503 (12%)
(1983): Shader RI, *J Clin Psychopharmacol* 3, 122
(1983): Yassa R+, *Can J Psychiatry* 28, 132
(1982): Dawber R+, *Br J Dermatol* 107, 125
(1982): Lambert D+, *Ann Dermatol Venereol* (French) 109, 19
(1982): Muniz CE+, *Psychosomatics* 23, 312
(1982): No Author, *Psychosomatics* 23, 563
Hair – alopecia areata (2%)
(1988): Silvestri A+, *Gen Hosp Psychiatry* 10, 46
(1983): Sarantidis D+, *Br J Psychiatry* 143, 42 (2%)
(1980): Vestergaard P+, *Acta Psychiatr Scand* 62, 193
Hair – brittle

Nails
Nails – Beau's lines (transverse nail bands)
(1988): Don PC+, *Cutis* 41, 20
Nails – dystrophy
(1988): Don PC+, *Cutis* 41, 20
(1982): Lambert D+, *Ann Dermatol Venereol* (French) 109, 19
Nails – onychomadesis
(1988): Don PC+, *Cutis* 41, 20
Nails – psoriasis
(1992): Rudolph RI, *J Am Acad Dermatol* 26, 135

Other
Asthenia
(2005): Sajatovic M+, *Am J Geriatr Psychiatry* 13(4), 305
Fever
(2003): Berry N+, *Pharmacotherapy* 23(2), 255 (with olanzapine)
Headache
(2005): Sajatovic M+, *Am J Geriatr Psychiatry* 13(4), 305
Infections
(2005): Sajatovic M+, *Am J Geriatr Psychiatry* 13(4), 305
Nephrotoxicity
(2006): van Gerven HA+, *Ned Tijdschr Geneeskd* 150(31), 1715
(2000): Markowitz GS+, *J Am Soc Nephrol* 11(8), 1439
(1998): Gabutti L+, *Ther Umsch* 55(9), 562 (1 case)
Neurotoxicity
(2007): Boker H+, *Psychiatr Prax* 34(1), 38 (with risperidone)
Pseudolymphoma
(1995): Magro CM+, *J Am Acad Dermatol* 32, 419
Rhabdomyolysis
(1991): Bateman AM+, *Nephrol Dial Transplant* 6(3), 203
(1982): Unger J+, *Acta Clin Belg* 39, 216 (overdose)
Seizures
(2006): Bellesi M+, *Neurol Sci* 26(6), 444
Somnambulism
(1999): Landry P+, *Int Clin Psychopharmacol* 14(3), 173
(1998): Landry P+, *Can J Psychiatry* 43(9), 957
(1986): Glassman JN+, *J Clin Psychiatry* 47(10), 523 (along with chlorpromazine, benztropine, and triazolam)
Tremor
Vertigo
(2005): Sajatovic M+, *Am J Geriatr Psychiatry* 13(4), 305
Weight gain
(2005): Ness-Abramof R+, *Drugs Today* (Barc) 41(8), 547

LODOXAMIDE

Trade name: Alomide (Alcon)
Indications: Non-infectious conjunctivitis
Category: Mast cell stabilizer
Half-life: N/A
Clinically important, potentially hazardous interactions with: N/A

Reactions

Skin
Rash (sic) (<1%)
Eyes
Blepharitis (<1%)
Corneal erosion (<1%)
Corneal ulcer (<1%)
Keratitis (<1%)
Keratopathy (<1%)
Lacrimation (1–5%)
Ocular burning (15%)
Ocular edema (<1%)
Ocular pain (<1%)
Ocular pruritus (1–5%)
Ocular stinging (15%)
Vision blurred (1–5%)
Other
Headache (1.5%)
Vertigo

LOMEFLOXACIN

Trade names: Logiflox; Maxaquin (Unimed); Ontop
Indications: Various infections caused by susceptible organisms
Category: Antibiotic, quinolone
Half-life: 4–6 hours
Clinically important, potentially hazardous interactions with: amiodarone, antacids, arsenic, bepridil, bismuth, bretylium, didanosine, disopyramide, erythromycin, NSAIDs, phenothiazines, procainamide, quinidine, sotalol, sucralfate, tricyclic antidepressants, zinc salts

Reactions

Skin
Allergic reactions (sic) (<1%)
Diaphoresis (<1%)
(1992): Crome P+, *Am J Med* 92 (Suppl 4A), 126S
(1992): Iravani A, *Am J Med* 92, 75S
Eczema
Edema (<1%)
Exanthems
Exfoliative dermatitis (<1%)
Facial edema (<1%)
Genital pruritus
(1992): Iravani A, *Am J Med* 92, 75S
Peripheral edema
Photosensitivity (2.4%)
(2006): Polimeni G+, *Drug Saf* 29(5), 449
(2006): Rafalsky V+, *Cochrane Database Syst Rev* 3
(2000): Ferguson J+, *J Antimicrob Chemother* 45, 503
(1998): Arata J+, *Antimicrob Agents Chemother* 42, 3141
(1998): Kimura M+, *Contact Dermatitis* 38, 180
(1996): Young AR+, *J Photochem Photobiol B* 32, 165
(1994): Cohen JB+, *Arch Dermatol* 130, 805 (following tanning bed)
(1994): Correia O+, *Arch Dermatol* 130, 808 (bullous)
(1994): Lowe NJ+, *Clin Pharmacol Ther* 56, 587
(1994): Poh-Fitzpatrick MB, *Arch Dermatol* 130, 261
(1993): Tozawa K+, *Hinyokika Kiyo* (Japanese) 39, 801
(1992): Crome P+, *Am J Med* 92 (Suppl 4A), 126S
(1992): Iravani A, *Am J Med* 92, 75S

(1992): Kurumaji Y+, *Contact Dermatitis* 26, 5
(1992): Rizk E, *Am J Med* 92, 130S (2.4%)
(1990): LeBel M+, *Antimicrob Agents Chemother* 34, 1254
Phototoxicity
  (2003): Leone R+, *Drug Saf* 26(2), 109
  (2000): Traynor NJ+, *Toxicol Vitr* 14, 275
  (1998): Martinez LJ+, *Photochem Photobiol* 67, 399
Pruritus (<1%)
  (1992): Cox CE, *Am J Med* 92, 82S
  (1992): Gotfried MH+, *Am J Med* 92, 108S
  (1992): Kemper P+, *Am J Med* 92, 98S
  (1992): Klimberg IW+, *Am J Med* 92, 121S
  (1992): Mouton Y+, *Am J Med* 92, 87S
  (1991): Wadworth AN+, *Drugs* 42, 1018
Purpura (<1%)
Pustules
  (1992): Mouton Y+, *Am J Med* 92, 87S
Rash (sic) (<1%)
  (1992): Crome P+, *Am J Med* 92 (Suppl 4A), 126S
  (1992): Gotfried MH+, *Am J Med* 92, 108S
  (1992): Iravani A, *Am J Med* 92, 75S
  (1992): Mouton Y+, *Am J Med* 92, 87S
  (1991): Wadworth AN+, *Drugs* 42, 1018
Stevens–Johnson syndrome
Toxic epidermal necrolysis
  (2003): Leone R+, *Drug Saf* 26(2), 109
Toxicoderma
  (1991): Wadworth AN+, *Drugs* 42, 1018
Urticaria (<1%)
  (1991): Wadworth AN+, *Drugs* 42, 1018
Vasculitis

Mucosal/ENT
Dysgeusia (<1%)
Tinnitus
Tongue pigmentation (<1%)
Vaginitis (<1%)
Vulvovaginal candidiasis
Xerostomia (<1%)
  (1992): Mant TG, *Am J Med* 92, 26S

Other
Chills (<1%)
Headache
Hypersensitivity
  (1991): Wadworth AN+, *Drugs* 42, 1018
Myalgia/Myositis/Myopathy/Myotoxicity (<1%)
Paresthesias (<1%)
  (1992): Crome P+, *Am J Med* 92 (Suppl 4A), 126S
Tendinopathy/Tendon rupture (many reports)
Tremor

LOMUSTINE

Synonym: CCNU
Trade names: Belustine; Cecenu; CeeNU (Bristol-Myers
Squibb); Lomeblastin; Lucostine; Lundbeck
Indications: Brain tumors, lymphomas, melanoma
Category: Alkylating agent; Nitrosourea
Half-life: 16–72 hours
**Clinically important, potentially hazardous interactions
with:** aldesleukin

Reactions

Skin
Acral erythema
  (1989): Oksenhendler E+, *Eur J Cancer Clin Oncol* 25, 1181
Neutrophilic eccrine hidradenitis
  (1996): Shear NH+, *J Am Acad Dermatol* 35, 819
Rash (sic) (1–10%)

Mucosal/ENT
Stomatitis (1–10%)

Hair
Hair – alopecia (<1%)

LOPERAMIDE

Trade names: Brek; Diar-Aid; Diarr-Eze; Diarstop-L; Imodium
(McNeil); Imossel; Lop-Dia; Loperhoe; Maalox (Novartis); Maalox
Anti-Diarrheal; Stopit; Vancotil
Indications: Diarrhea
Category: Opiate agonist
Half-life: 9–14 hours
**Clinically important, potentially hazardous interactions
with:** St John's wort

Reactions

Skin
Erythema nodosum
Exanthems
Fixed eruption
  (2005): Matarredona J+, *Med Clin (Barc)* 124(5), 198
Pruritus
Rash (sic)
Urticaria

Mucosal/ENT
Gingivitis
  (1990): DuPont HL+, *Am J Med* 88, 20S
Oral lesions (1.1%)
  (1990): DuPont HL+, *Am J Med* 88, 20S
Xerostomia
  (1990): DuPont HL+, *Am J Med* 88, 20S

Hair
Hair – alopecia
  (1993): Litt JZ, Beachwood, OH (personal case) (observation)

Other
Anaphylactoid reactions/Anaphylaxis
  (2007): Srinivasa MR+, *Allergy* 62(8), 965 (fatal)
Hypersensitivity

LORACARBEF

Trade names: Carbac; Lorabid (Monarch)
Indications: Various infections caused by susceptible organisms
Category: Cephalosporin, 2nd generation
Half-life: 60 minutes

Reactions

Skin
Erythema multiforme (<1%)
Exanthems
   (1992): Muller O+, *Infection* 20(3), 176
Pruritus (<1%)
Rash (sic) (1.2%)
   (1992): McCarty J, *Am J Med* 92(6A), 74S
   (1992): McCarty J+, *Clin Ther* 14(1), 30
   (1992): Muller O+, *Infection* 20(5), 301
Stevens–Johnson syndrome (<1%)
Urticaria (<1%)

Mucosal/ENT
Candidal vaginitis (1.3%)

Other
Candidiasis
Cough
   (1992): McCarty J, *Am J Med* 92(6A), 74S
Headache
   (1992): Dere WH+, *Clin Ther* 14(1), 41 (9%)
   (1992): Hyslop DL+, *Am J Med* 92(6A), 86S
   (1992): McCarty J+, *Am J Med* 92(6A), 80S
   (1992): Muller O+, *Infection* 20(5), 301
   (1992): Therasse DG, *Am J Med* 92(6A), 20S
   (1992): Zeckel ML, *Am J Med* 92(6A), 58S
   (1992): Zeckel ML+, *Clin Ther* 14(2), 214 (7%)
Serum sickness (<1%)

LORATADINE

Trade names: Alavert (Wyeth); Civeran; Claratyne; Claritin (Schering); Claritin-D (Schering); Claritine; Lisino; Lorastine; Velodan; Zeos
Indications: Allergic rhinitis, urticaria
Category: Histamine H1 receptor antagonist
Half-life: 3–20 hours

Reactions

Skin
Angioedema (>2%)
   (1989): Clissold SP+, *Drugs* 37, 42
Dermatitis (>2%)
Diaphoresis (>2%)
Erythema multiforme (>2%)
Exanthems
Fixed eruption
   (2003): Pionetti CH+, *Allergol Immunopathol* (Madr) 31(5), 291
   (2002): Ruiz-Genao DP+, *Br J Dermatol* 146(3), 528
Peripheral edema (>2%)
Photosensitivity (>2%)
Pruritus (>2%)
   (1989): Barenholtz HA+, *Drug Intell Clin Pharm* 23, 445
Purpura (>2%)
Rash (sic) (>2%)
Urticaria (>2%)
   (1992): Boner AL+, *Allergy* 47, 98
   (1989): Clissold SP+, *Drugs* 37, 42
Xerosis (>2%)

Mucosal/ENT
Dysgeusia (>2%)

Sialorrhea (>2%)
Stomatitis (>2%)
Tinnitus
Vaginitis (>2%)
Xerostomia (>10%)
   (1993): Pacor ML+, *Clin Ter 1993 Jun* 142(6), 529 (2%)
   (1992): Monroe EW+, *Arzneimittelforschung* (German) 42, 1119
   (1992): Olson OT+, *Arzneimittelforschung* (German) 42, 1227
   (1990): Del Carpio J+, *J Allergy Clin Immunology* 84, 741
   (1990): Irander K+, *Allergy* 45, 86
   (1990): Simons FE, *Clin Exp Allergy* 20, 19
   (1989): Barenholtz HA+, *Drug Intell Clin Pharm* 23, 445
   (1989): Bruttman G+, *J Allergy Clin Immunology* 83, 411
   (1988): Gutkowski A+, *J Allergy Clin Immunology* 81, 902

Hair
Hair – alopecia (>2%)
Hair – dry (>2%)

Other
Anaphylactoid reactions/Anaphylaxis (>2%)
Gynecomastia (>2%)
Headache
Myalgia/Myositis/Myopathy/Myotoxicity (>2%)
Paresthesias (>2%)

LORAZEPAM

Trade names: Apo-Lorazepam; Ativan (Wyeth) (Baxter); Durazolam; Laubeel; Merlit; Nu-Loraz; Punktyl; Tavor; Temesta; Titus
Indications: Anxiety, depression
Category: Benzodiazepine
Half-life: 10–20 hours
Clinically important, potentially hazardous interactions with: alcohol, amprenavir, barbiturates, chlorpheniramine, clarithromycin, CNS depressants, efavirenz, erythromycin, esomeprazole, imatinib, MAO inhibitors, narcotics, nelfinavir, phenothiazines, valproate

Reactions

Skin
Dermatitis (1–10%)
Diaphoresis (>10%)
Erythema multiforme
   (1991): Porteous DM+, *Arch Dermatol* 127, 741
Exanthems
Fixed eruption
   (1988): Jafferany M+, *Dermatologica* 177, 386
Pruritus
Purpura
Rash (sic) (>10%)
Stevens–Johnson syndrome
   (1991): Porteous DM+, *Arch Dermatol* 127, 741
Urticaria

Mucosal/ENT
Gingival lichenoid reaction
   (1986): Colvard MD+, *Periodont Case Rep* 8, 69
Sialopenia (>10%)
Sialorrhea (<1%)
Xerostomia (>10%)

Hair
Hair – alopecia

Hair – hirsutism

Other

Headache
Hypotension
 (1990): Ruff R+, *J Cardiothorac Anesth* 4(3), 314
Injection-site pain (>10%)
 (1981): Ameer B+, *Drugs* 21, 161 (7–52%)
Injection-site phlebitis (>10%)
 (1981): Clarke RSJ, *Drugs* 22, 26 (15%)
Paresthesias
Pseudolymphoma
 (1995): Magro CM+, *J Am Acad Dermatol* 32, 419
 (1988): Kardaun SH+, *Br J Dermatol* 118(4), 545
Rhabdomyolysis
 (1983): Cauana RJ+, *N C Med J* 44, 18 (with amitriptyline and
  perphenazine)
Tremor (1–10%)

LORCAINIDE

Trade name: Lorcainide (Janssen)
Indications: Ventricular arrhythmia
Category: Antiarrhythmic class 1c
Half-life: 8 Hours
**Clinically important, potentially hazardous interactions
with:** rifampin

Reactions

Skin

Diaphoresis
 (1984): Buss J+, *Dtsch Med Wochenschr* 109(48), 1829
 (1980): Meinertz T+, *Arzneimittelforschung* 30(9), 1593

Other

Anxiety
 (1984): Buss J+, *Dtsch Med Wochenschr* 109(48), 1829
Congestive heart failure
 (1989): Ravid S+, *J Am Coll* 14(5), 1326
Death
 (1995): Evers J+, *J Toxicol Clin Toxicol* 33(2), 157
 (1993): Cowley AJ+, *Int J Cardiol* 40(2), 161
Headache
 (1986): Vlay SC+, *Am Heart J* 111(3), 452
Hot flashes
 (1984): Buss J+, *Dtsch Med Wochenschr* 109(48), 1829
Hypotension
 (1985): Stroobandt R+, *Acta Cardiol* 40(6), 637
Inappropriate secretion of antidiuretic hormone (SIADH)
 (1984): Somani P+, *Am Heart J* 108(6), 1443
Insomnia
 (1987): Samanek M+, *Pediatr Cardiol* 8(1), 3
 (1984): Chesnie B+, *J Am Coll Cardiol* 3(6), 1531
 (1980): Meinertz T+, *Arzneimittelforschung* 30(9), 1593
Paresthesias
 (1985): Stroobandt R+, *Acta Cardiol* 40(6), 637
Restlessness
 (1984): Buss J+, *Dtsch Med Wochenschr* 109(48), 1829
Shock (fatal)
 (1995): Evers J+, *J Toxicol Clin Toxicol* 33(2), 157
Vertigo
 (1987): Samanek M+, *Pediatr Cardiol* 8(1), 3
 (1986): Vlay SC+, *Am Heart J* 111(3), 452
 (1984): Buss J+, *Dtsch Med Wochenschr* 109(48), 1829

LOSARTAN

Synonyms: DuP 753; MK 594
Trade names: Cozaar (Merck); Hyzaar (Merck)
Indications: Hypertension
Category: Angiotensin II receptor antagonist
Half-life: 2 hours

Note: Hyzaar is losartan and hydrochlorothiazide

Reactions

Skin

Angioedema (<1%)
 (2003): MacLean JA+, *Arch Intern Med* 163(12), 1488
 (2002): Abdi R+, *Pharmacotherapy* 22(9), 1173
 (2001): Chiu AG+, *Laryngoscope* 111(10), 1729 (3 cases)
 (1999): Rivera JO, *Ann Pharmacother* 33, 933
 (1999): Rupprecht R+, *Allergy* 54, 81
 (1998): van Rijnsoever EW+, *Arch Intern Med* 158, 2063
 (1996): *Med Sci Bull* 18, 6
 (1996): Boxer M, *J Allergy Clin Immunol* 98, 471
 (1995): Acker CG+, *N Engl J Med* 333, 1572
Dermatitis (<1%)
Diaphoresis (<1%)
Eczema
 (2005): Eastern J, N Caldwell, NJ (from Internet) (observation)
Edema (<1%)
Erythema (<1%)
Exanthems
Facial edema (<1%)
Lichenoid eruption
 (2005): Spencer L, Crawfordsville, IN (from Internet)
  (observation)
Photosensitivity (<1%)
Pruritus (<1%)
Purpura
 (2001): Brouard M+, *Br J Dermatol* 145(2), 362
 (1998): Bosch X, *Arch Intern Med* 158, 191
Rash (sic) (<1%)
Urticaria (<1%)
Xerosis (<1%)

Mucosal/ENT

Ageusia
 (2002): Ohkoshi N+, *Eur J Neurol* 9(3), 315
 (1996): Schlienger RG+, *Lancet* 347, 471
Aphthous stomatitis
 (1998): Goffin E+, *Clin Nephrol* 50, 197
Dysgeusia (<1%)
 (1998): Heeringa M+, *Ann Intern Med* 129, 72
Oral ulceration
 (2000): Madinier I+, *Ann Med Interne* (Paris) (French) 151, 248
Xerostomia (<1%)

Hair

Hair – alopecia (<1%)

Other

Anaphylactoid reactions/Anaphylaxis (<1%)
Headache
Myalgia/Myositis/Myopathy/Myotoxicity (1%)
Paresthesias (<1%)
 (1995): Ahmad S, *JAMA* 274, 1266
Pseudolymphoma
 (1999): Goldstein E, Toronto, ON (from Internet) (observation)
 (1997): Viraben R+, *Lancet* 350, 1366
Tremor (<1%)

LOTEPREDNOL

Synonym: loteprednol etabonate
Trade names: Alrex (Bausch & Lomb); Lotemax (Bausch & Lomb)
Indications: Ophthalmic inflammation, seasonal allergic conjunctivitis, rhinitis
Category: Corticosteroid, topical
Half-life: N/A
Clinically important, potentially hazardous interactions with: None

Reactions

Mucosal/ENT
Rhinitis (<15%)

Eyes
Conjunctivitis
Eyelid erythema
Keratoconjunctivitis
Ocular burning
Ocular edema
Ocular stinging
Photophobia
Visual disturbances
Xerophthalmia

Other
Headache (<15%)

LOVASTATIN

Trade names: Advicor (Kos); Altocor; Apo-Lovastatin; Lovalip; Mevacor (Merck); Mevinacor; Mevinolin; Nergadan; Rovacor; Taucor
Indications: Hypercholesterolemia
Category: HMG-CoA reductase inhibitor; Statin
Half-life: 1–2 hours
Clinically important, potentially hazardous interactions with: atazanavir, azithromycin, bosentan, cholestyramine, clarithromycin, cyclosporine, darunavir, delavirdine, erythromycin, fenofibrate, fosamprenavir, gemfibrozil, **grapefruit juice**, imatinib, itraconazole, **red rice yeast**, tacrolimus, telithromycin, tipranavir, verapamil

Reactions

Skin
Erythema
Erythema multiforme
Exanthems (<5%)
 (1988): Henwood JM+, Drugs 36, 429 (5%)
 (1988): Tobert JA+, Am J Cardiol 62 (Suppl), 28J (0.3%)
 (1987): Havel RJ+, Ann Intern Med 107, 609 (1%)
Lichenoid eruption
 (2004): Sebok B+, Acta Derm Venereol 84(3), 229
Lupus erythematosus
 (1994): Yung RL+, Rheum Dis Clin North Am 20, 61
 (1993): Ahmad S, Heart Dis Stroke 2, 262
 (1991): Ahmad S, Arch Intern Med 151, 1667
Pruritus (5.2%)
 (2002): Kashyap ML+, Am J Cardiol 89(6), 672 (with niacin)
 (1988): Tobert JA+, Am J Cardiol 62 (Suppl), 28J

Purpura
 (1999): Stein EA+, JAMA 281, 137
Rash (sic) (5.2%)
 (2002): Kashyap ML+, Am J Cardiol 89(6), 672 (with niacin)
 (1993): Krasovec M+, Dermatology 186, 248
 (1993): Merck Laboratories, The Lovastatin Study Groups I through IV 153, 1079
Stevens–Johnson syndrome
 (1998): Downs JR+, JAMA 279, 1615
Toxic epidermal necrolysis
Urticaria
Vasculitis

Mucosal/ENT
Dysgeusia (0.8%)
Hyposmia
 (1992): Weber R+, Laryngorhinootologie (German) 71, 483
Stomatitis
Xerostomia (>1%)

Hair
Hair – alopecia (>1%)

Other
Gynecomastia (1–10%)
 (1999): Stein EA+, JAMA 281, 137
Headache
 (2002): Kashyap ML+, Am J Cardiol 89(6), 672 (with niacin)
Hepatotoxicity
 (2007): Stein CA+, Invest New Drugs 25(3), 277 (with ketoconazole)
Hypersensitivity
Myalgia/Myositis/Myopathy/Myotoxicity (1–10%)
 (2005): Wortmann RL+, Am J Cardiol 95(8), 983 (low)
 (1995): Garnett WR, Am J Health Syst Pharm 52(15), 1639
 (1990): Kogan AD+, Postgrad Med J 66, 294
 (1989): Vaher VMG+, Lancet 2, 1098
Paresthesias (>1%)
Pseudolymphoma
 (1996): Magro CM+, Hum Pathol 27(2), 125
Rhabdomyolysis
 (2007): Stein CA+, Invest New Drugs 25(3), 277 (with ketoconazole)
 (2005): Wortmann RL+, Am J Cardiol 95(8), 983 (low)
 (2000): Davidson MH, Curr Atheroscler Rep 2(1), 14
 (1999): Bottorff M, Atherosclerosis 147(Suppl 1), S23
 (1999): Corsini A+, Pharmacol Ther 84, 413 (with cyclosporine, mibefradil or nefazodone)
 (1998): Reaven P+, Ann Intern Med 109, 597 (with nicotinic acid)
 (1998): Tobert JA+, Am J Cardiol 62, 28J (with gemfibrozil)
 (1998): Wong PW+, South Med J 91(2), 202 (with erythromycin)
 (1997): Chu PH+, Jpn Heart J 38(4), 541
 (1997): Grunden JW+, Ann Pharmacother 31(7), 859 (with azithromycin and clarithromycin)
 (1997): Hermida Lazcano I+, An Med Interne 14, 488
 (1997): Olbricht C+, Clin Pharmacol Ther 62(3), 311 (with cyclosporine)
 (1996): Ballantyne CM+, Am J Cardiol 78(5), 532
 (1996): Biesenbach G+, Wien Klin Wochenschr 108(11), 334
 (1995): Abdul-Ghaffar NU+, J Clin Gastroenterol 21(4), 340 (with gemfibrozil)
 (1995): Farmer JA+, Baillieres Clin Endocrinol Metab 9(4), 825
 (1995): Garnett WR, Am J Health Syst Pharm 52(15), 1639 (with cyclosporine, gemfibrozil or niacin)
 (1995): Lees RS+, N Engl J Med 333(10), 664 (with itraconazole)
 (1994): Alejandro DS+, J Am Soc Nephrol 5(2), 153 (with cyclosporine)
 (1994): Dallaire M+, CMAJ 150(12), 1991 (with danazol)
 (1993): Knoll RW+, Conn Med 57(9), 593 (with gemfibrozil)
 (1992): Chan PC+, Nephrol Dial Transplant 7(2), 93

(1992): Chrysanthopoulos C+, *BMJ* 304(6836), 1225 (with cholestyramine)
(1992): Hume AL, *Ann Pharmacother* 26(10), 1303
(1992): Wallace CS+, *Ann Pharmacother* 26(2), 190
(1991): Spach DH+, *West J Med* 154(2), 213 (with erythromycin)
(1991): Sylvain-Moore H+, *Heart Lung* 20(5 Pt 1), 464
(1990): *JAMA* 264(23), 2991 (with gemfibrozil)
(1990): Kogan AD+, *Postgrad Med J* 66(774), 294
(1990): Manoukian AA+, *Clin Chem* 36(12), 2145
(1990): Marais GE+, *Ann Intern Med* 112(3), 228 (with gemfibrozil)
(1990): Pierce LR+, *JAMA* 264(1), 71 (with gemfibrozil)
(1990): Tobert JA+, *Am J Cardiol* 65(Suppl), 23F
(1988): Corpier CL+, *JAMA* 260(2), 239 (cyclosporine)
(1988): Reaven P+, *Ann Intern Med* 109(7), 597
(1988): Tobert JA+, *Am J Cardiol* 62, 28J (with cyclosporine)

LOXAPINE

Trade names: Desconex; Loxapac; Loxitane (Watson)
Indications: Psychoses
Category: Antipsychotic, tricyclic
Half-life: 12–19 hours (terminal)

Reactions

Skin
Dermatitis
  (1992): Breathnach SM+, *Adverse Drug Reactions and the Skin* Blackwell, Oxford, 203 (passim)
Diaphoresis
Exanthems
Facial edema
Photosensitivity (<1%)
  (1991): Anon, *Drug Ther Bull* 29, 41
Pigmentation (<1%)
Pruritus (<1%)
  (1992): Breathnach SM+, *Adverse Drug Reactions and the Skin* Blackwell, Oxford, 203 (passim)
Purpura
Rash (sic) (1–10%)
Seborrhea
  (1992): Breathnach SM+, *Adverse Drug Reactions and the Skin* Blackwell, Oxford, 203 (passim)
Side effects (sic)
Urticaria

Mucosal/ENT
Xerostomia (>10%)

Hair
Hair – alopecia

Other
Gynecomastia (1–10%)
Headache
Myalgia/Myositis/Myopathy/Myotoxicity
  (1984): Thase ME+, *J Clin Psychopharmacol* 4, 46
Paresthesias
Rhabdomyolysis
  (1996): Meltzer HY+, *Neuropsychopharmacology* 15(4), 395
  (1984): Thase ME+, *J Clin Psychopharmacol* 4(1), 46 (with benztropine)

LUBIPROSTONE

Trade name: Amitiza (Takeda)
Indications: Constipation, Irritable bowel syndrome
Category: Chloride channel activator
Half-life: 0–1.4 hours

Reactions

Skin
Edema (~0.2%)
Hyperhidrosis (~0.2%)
Peripheral edema (4%)
Rash (sic) (~0.2%)
Urticaria (~0.2%)

Mucosal/ENT
Dysgeusia (~0.2%)
Sinusitis (5%)
Xerostomia (1%)

Other
Abdominal pain (7%)
Asthenia (2%)
Chest pain (1%)
Cough (1%)
Depression (1%)
Fever (1%)
Headache (13%)
Hypertension (1%)
Myalgia/Myositis/Myopathy/Myotoxicity (1%)
Pain (~0.2%)
Paresthesias (~0.2%)
Tremor (~0.2%)
Upper respiratory infection (4%)
Vertigo (~0.2%)

LUMIRACOXIB

Trade name: Prexige (Novartis)
Indications: Osteoarthritis
Category: COX-2 selective inhibitor
Half-life: 4 Hours
Clinically important, potentially hazardous interactions with: aspirin. other NSAIDs

Reactions

Skin
Angioedema
Exfoliative dermatitis
Peripheral edema (2%)
Stevens–Johnson syndrome
Toxic epidermal necrolysis

Mucosal/ENT
Nasopharyngitis (6.1%)

Other
Abdominal pain (1%)
Anaphylactoid reactions/Anaphylaxis
Asthenia (1.5%)
Cough (2%)
Headache (7.9%)

Hepatotoxicity
Hypertension
Insomnia (1%)
Myalgia/Myositis/Myopathy/Myotoxicity (1.5%)
Stroke
Vertigo (2%)

LUTROPIN ALFA

Trade name: Luveris (Merck)
Indications: Infertility
Category: Hormone modulator; Luteinizing hormone
Half-life: ~14 hours

Reactions

Skin
Edema
Erythema
Pruritus
Rash (sic)
Urticaria
Vesiculation
Xerosis

Hair
Hair – alopecia

Other
Abdominal pain (5–8%)
Asthenia (3%)
Chills
Fever
Gynecomastia
Headache (10%)
Injection-site edema
Injection-site irritation
Injection-site pain
Injection-site reactions (3–4%)
Paresthesias
Upper respiratory infection (1–2%)
Vertigo

LYCOPENE

Scientific names: *All-Trans-Lycopene; Psi-Psi-Carotene*
Trade and other common names: Carotenoid; Lyc-O-Mato; Lycovit (BASF)
Category: Antioxidant
Purported indications and other uses: Cancer (prevention), cardiovascular disease (prevention), asthma
Half-life: N/A

Note: Cooking increases bioavailability of lycopene. Major dietary sources are tomato paste, juice, and ketchup

Reactions

Skin
Pigmentation
   (2003): Saldana Chaparro RS+, *Ann Clin Biochem* 40(Pt 3), 280

MAFENIDE

Trade name: Sulfamylon
Indications: Second- and third-degree burns
Category: Antiseptic; Sulfonamide
Half-life: N/A
Clinically important, potentially hazardous interactions with: None

Note: Mafenide is a sulfonamide and can be absorbed systemically. Sulfonamides can produce severe, possibly fatal, reactions such as toxic epidermal necrolysis and Stevens–Johnson syndrome

Reactions

Skin
Allergic reactions (sic)
   (1995): McKenna SR+, *Burns* 21(4), 310
Bullous dermatitis
Burning
Dermatitis
   (1993): Sanz de Galdeano C+, *Contact Dermatitis* 28(4), 249
   (1992): Fernandez JC+, *Contact Dermatitis* 27(4), 262
Edema
Erythema
Excoriations
Facial edema
Pruritus (2.8%)
   (1993): Kucan JO+, *J Burn Care Rehabil* 14(2 Pt 1), 158
Rash (sic) (4.6%)
   (1993): Kucan JO+, *J Burn Care Rehabil* 14(2 Pt 1), 158

Other
Anaphylactoid reactions/Anaphylaxis
Application-site burning
Death
Hypersensitivity
   (1988): Perry AW+, *J Burn Care Rehabil* 9(2), 145
Pain
   (1993): Kucan JO+, *J Burn Care Rehabil* 14(2 Pt 1), 158
Porphyria

MAPROTILINE

Trade names: Delgian; Ludiomil (Novartis); Maprostad; Melodil; Mirpan; Nono-Maprotiline; Psymion; Retinyl
Indications: Depression, anxiety
Category: Antidepressant, tetracyclic; Muscarinic antagonist
Half-life: 27–58 hours

Reactions

Skin
Acne
   (1988): Warnock JK+, *Am J Psychiatry* 145, 425
   (1985): Oakley AM+, *Aust N Z J Med* 15, 256
   (1982): Ponte CD, *Am J Psychiatry* 139, 141
Diaphoresis (3–8%)
Edema
Erythema
Erythema multiforme
   (1990): Zukervar P+, *J Toxicol Clin Exp* 10, 169
Exanthems (1–9%)
   (1988): Warnock JK+, *Am J Psychiatry* 145, 425

Ichthyosis
(1991): Niederauer HH+, *Hautarzt* (German) 42, 455
Petechiae
Photosensitivity
(1989): KochP+, *Derm Beruf Umwelt* (German) 37, 203
(1988): Warnock JK+, *Am J Psychiatry* 145, 425
Pruritus
Purpura
(1988): Warnock JK+, *Am J Psychiatry* 145, 425
Rash (sic) (>10%)
Stevens–Johnson syndrome
(1990): Zukervar P+, *J Toxicol Clin Exp* 10, 169
Urticaria (4%)
(1988): Warnock JK+, *Am J Psychiatry* 145, 425
Vasculitis
(1985): Oakley AM+, *Aust N Z J Med* 15, 256

Mucosal/ENT
Dysgeusia
Sialorrhea
Stomatitis
Tinnitus
Tongue black
Xerostomia (20–40%)
(1981): Rafaelsen OJ+, *Acta Psychiatr Scand Suppl* 290, 364

Hair
Hair – alopecia
(2000): Mercke Y+, *Ann Clin Psychiatry* 12, 35
(1991): Niederauer HH+, *Hautarzt* (German) 42, 455

Other
Gynecomastia (<1%)
Headache
Tremor

MARAVIROC

Trade names: Celsentri; Selzentry (Pfizer)
Indications: HIV Infection
Category: Antiretroviral (CCR5 co-receptor antagonist)
Half-life: 14–18 hours
Clinically important, potentially hazardous interactions with: St John's wort

Reactions

Skin
Dermatitis (5%)
Folliculitis (5%)
Herpes (sic)
Pruritus (6%)
Rash (sic) (17%)
(2007): Ndegwa S, *Issues Emerg Health Technol* 110, 1

Mucosal/ENT
Stomatitis (4%)

Other
Abdominal pain (14%)
(2007): Ndegwa S, *Issues Emerg Health* 110, 1
Bronchitis
Cough (22%)
(2007): Ndegwa S, *Issues Emerg Health* 110, 1
Depression (6%)
Fever (21%)

(2007): Ndegwa S, *Issues Emerg Health* 110, 1
Hepatotoxicity
Hypersensitivity
Infections
Lipodystrophy (4.6%)
Myalgia/Myositis/Myopathy/Myotoxicity (5%)
(2007): Ndegwa S, *Issues Emerg Health* 110, 1
Pain (8%)
Paresthesias (8%)
Sleep disturbances (12%)
Upper respiratory infection (37%)
(2007): Ndegwa S, *Issues Emerg Health* 110, 1
Vertigo (14%)

MARIHUANA

Trade names: Marihuana; Marijuana
Indications: Nausea and vomiting, substance abuse drug
Category: Cannabinoid; Hallucinogen
Half-life: N/A
Clinically important, potentially hazardous interactions with: atazanavir

Note: Marihuana is the popular name for the dried flowering leaves of the hemp plant, *Cannabis sativa*. It contains tetrahydrocannabinols. It is also known as 'pot,' 'grass,' 'hashish,' 'marijuana,' etc.

Reactions

Skin
Allergic reactions (sic)
(2000): Perez JA, *J Emerg Med* 18, 260
Exanthems
Pruritus
Squamous syringometaplasia
(2000): Holdcroft A, *Br J Anaesth* 84(3), 419
Urticaria

Mucosal/ENT
Xerostomia
(1982): Weller RA+, *J Clin Psychiatry* 43(9), 362

Eyes
Visual hallucinations

Other
Anaphylactoid reactions/Anaphylaxis
Chest pain
(2002): Sidney S, *J Clin Pharmacol* 42(11 Suppl), 64S
Death
(2001): Gupta BD+, *Med Sci Law* 41(4), 349
Hypotension
(2002): Sidney S, *J Clin Pharmacol* 42(11 Suppl), 64S
Suicidal ideation
(2002): Fergusson DM+, *Addiction* 97(9), 1123

MAZINDOL

Trade names: Diestet; Liofindol; Solucaps; Teronac
Indications: Obesity
Category: Norepinephrine reuptake inhibitor
Half-life: 10 hours
**Clinically important, potentially hazardous interactions
with:** cocaine, fenfluramine, fluoxetine, fluvoxamine, lithium,
MAO inhibitors, paroxetine, phenelzine, sertraline,
tranylcypromine

Reactions

Skin
Diaphoresis
Edema
Exanthems
Rash (sic)
Urticaria

Mucosal/ENT
Dysgeusia
Xerostomia
  (1990): Griggs RC+, *Muscle Nerve* 13(12), 1169
  (1986): Vespignani H+, *Rev Electroencephalogr Neurophysiol Clin*
  16(3), 317

Other
Depression
  (1984): Rihmer Z+, *Am J Psychiatry* 141(11), 1497
Headache
  (1986): Iijima S+, *Sleep* 9(1 Pt 2), 265
Paresthesias
Vertigo

MDMA

Trade name: Ecstacy
Indications: N/A
Category: Amphetamine
Half-life: N/A

Note: 3,4-Methylenedioxymethamphetamine

Reactions

Skin
Acne
  (1998): Wollina U+, *Dermatology* 197(2), 171 (2 cases)
Diaphoresis
  (1999): Rochester JA+, *J Am Board Fam Pract* 12(2), 137
  (1998): Weinmann W+, *Forensic Sci Int* 91(2), 91
  (1988): Buchanan JF+, *Med Toxicol Adverse Drug Exp* 3(1), 1
Psoriasis
  (2004): Tan B+, *Australas J Dermatol* 45(3), 167 (guttate)
Rash (sic)

Mucosal/ENT
Oral ulceration
  (2003): Brazier WJ+, *Br Dent J* 194(4), 197
Xerostomia
  (2007): Brand HS+, *Ned Tijdschr Tandheelkd* 114(2), 104
  (2005): McGrath C+, *Br Dent J* 198(3), 159
  (1999): Milosevic A+, *Community Dent Oral Epidemiol* 27(4), 283

Other
Asthenia
  (1998): Vollenweider FX+, *Neuropsychopharmacology* 19(4), 241
Chills
Congestive heart failure
  (1993): Cregg MT+, *Ir Med J* 86(4), 118
Death
  (2005): Karlovsek MZ+, *Forensic Sci Int* 147, Suppl:S77
  (2005): McGrath C+, *Br Dent J* 198(3), 159
  (2005): O'Malley P, *Clin Nurse Spec* 19(2), 63
  (2003): Greene SL+, *Am J Emerg Med* 21(2), 121
  (2003): Schifano F+, *Hum Psychopharmacol* 18(7), 519 (202
  cases)
  (2003): Sticht G+, *Arch Kriminol* 211(3), 73
  (2003): Vuori E+, *Addiction* 98(3), 365 (4 cases) (with
  moclobemide)
  (2001): Braback L+, *Lakartidningen* 98(8), 817 (after one pill)
  (2001): Doyon S, *Curr Opin Pediatr* 13(2), 170
  (2001): Murray JB, *Psychol Rep* 88(3 Pt 1), 895
  (2001): Nielsen S+, *Ugeskr Laeger* 163(16), 2253
  (2001): Vickrey V, *Mich Med* 100(6), 53
  (2000): Carter N+, *Int J Legal Med* 113(3), 168
  (2000): Weir E, *CMAJ* 162(13), 1843
  (1999): de la Torre R+, *Lancet* 353(9152), 593
  (1999): Fineschi V+, *Forensic Sci Int* 104(1), 65
  (1999): Hedetoft C+, *Ugeskr Laeger* 161(50), 6907
  (1999): Lind J+, *Lancet* 354(9196), 2167
  (1999): Ramsey JD+, *Lancet* 354(9196), 2166
  (1999): Schwab M+, *Lancet* 352(9142), 1751
  (1999): Walubo A+, *Hum Exp Toxicol* 18(2), 119
  (1998): Byard RW+, *Am J Forensic Med Pathol* 19(3), 261 (5
  cases)
  (1998): Henry JA+, *Lancet* 352(9142), 1751
  (1998): Mueller PD+, *Ann Emerg Med* 32(3 Pt 1), 377
  (1998): Weinmann W+, *Forensic Sci Int* 91(2), 91
  (1997): Parr MJ+, *Med J Aust* 166(3), 136
  (1997): Thomasius R+, *Fortschr Neurol Psychiatr* 65(2), 49
  (1996): Burnat P+, *Presse Med* 25(26), 1208
  (1996): Dar KJ+, *Intensive Care Med* 22(9), 995
  (1996): Dowsett RP, *Med J Aust* 164(11), 700
  (1996): Fineschi V+, *Int J Legal Med* 108(5), 272
  (1996): McCauley JC, *Med J Aust* 164(1), 56
  (1996): Milroy CM+, *J Clin Pathol* 49, 149
  (1995): Nielsen JC+, *Ugeskr Laeger* 157(6), 724
  (1995): Squier MV+, *J Neurol Neurosurg Psychiatry* 58(6), 756
  (1994): Szukaj M, *Nervenarzt* 65(11), 802
  (1993): Cregg MT+, *Ir Med J* 86(4), 118
  (1992): Henry JA, *BMJ* 305, 5
  (1992): Henry JA+, *Lancet* 340, 284
  (1988): Buchanan JF+, *Med Toxicol Adverse Drug Exp* 3(1), 1
  (1988): Suarez RV+, *Am J Forensic Med Pathol* 9(4), 339
  (1987): Dowling GP+, *JAMA* 257(12), 1615 (5 cases)
Depression (37%)
  (2008): Brand HS+, *Br Dent J* 204(2), 77
  (2007): Brand HS+, *Ned Tijdschr Tandheelkd* 114(2), 104
  (2005): McGrath C+, *Br Dent J* 198(3), 159
  (2003): Verheyden SL+, *Hum Psychopharmacol* 18(7), 507 (37%)
  (2000): Morgan ML, *Psychopharmacol* (Berl) 152(3), 230
  (2000): Shannon M, *Pediatr Emerg Care* 16(5), 377
  (1999): Rochester JA+, *J Am Board Fam Pract* 12(2), 137
  (1998): Liberg JP+, *Tidsskr Nor Laegeforen* 118(28), 4384
  (1998): Pennings EJ+, *Ned Tijdschr Geneeskd* 142(35), 1942
  (1997): Williamson S+, *Drug Alcohol Depend* 44(2-3), 87
  (1993): Cregg MT+, *Ir Med J* 86(4), 118
Hypertension
  (1998): Vollenweider FX+, *Neuropsychopharmacology* 19(4), 241
Inappropriate secretion of antidiuretic hormone (SIADH)
  (2006): Wolff K+, *J Psychopharmacol* 20(3), 400
  (2002): Traub SJ+, *J Urban Health* 79(4), 549

(2001): Braback L+, *Lakartidningen* 98(8), 817 (fatal)
(1998): Pennings EJ+, *Ned Tijdschr Geneeskd* 142(35), 1942
(1994): Satchell SC+, *Br J Hosp Med* 51(9), 495
Myalgia/Myositis/Myopathy/Myotoxicity
Paresthesias
  (2000): Yates KM+, *N Z Med J* 113(1114), 315
Rhabdomyolysis
  (2004): Coco TJ+, *Curr Opin Pediatr* 16(2), 206
  (2003): Ben-Abraham R+, *Eur J Emerg Med* 10(4), 309
  (2003): Kunitz O+, *Anaesthesist* 52(6), 511
  (2002): Smith KM+, *Am J Health Syst Pharm* 59(11), 1067
  (2001): Halachanova V+, *Mayo Clin Proc* 76(1), 112
  (2001): Kalant H, *CMAJ* 165(7), 917
  (2001): Teter CJ+, *Pharmacotherapy* 21(12), 1486
  (1999): Fineschi V+, *Forensic Sci Int* 104(1), 65
  (1999): Hedetoft C+, *Ugeskr Laeger* 161(50), 6907
  (1999): Rochester JA+, *J Am Board Fam Pract* 12(2), 137
  (1998): Liberg JP+, *Tidsskr Nor Laegeforen* 118(28), 4384
  (1998): Ramcharan S+, *J Toxicol Clin Toxicol* 36(7), 727
  (1997): Cunningham M, *Intensive Crit Care Nurs* 13(4), 216
  (1997): Trkulja V+, *Lijec Vjesn* 119(5-6), 158
  (1997): Tsatsakis AM+, *Vet Hum Toxicol* 39(4), 241
  (1996): Dar KJ+, *Intensive Care Med* 22(9), 995
  (1996): Ellis AJ+, *Gut* 38(3), 454 (8 cases)
  (1996): Fineschi V+, *Int J Legal Med* 108(5), 272
  (1996): Gouzoulis-Mayfrank E+, *Nervenarzt* 67(5), 369
  (1996): Roebroek RM+, *Ned Tijdschr Geneeskd* 140(4), 205
  (1995): Lehmann ED+, *Postgrad Med J* 71(833), 186
  (1995): Nielsen JC+, *Ugeskr Laeger* 157(6), 724
  (1995): Steidle B+, *Rofo Fortschr Geb Roentgenstr Neuen Bildgeb Verfahr* 163(4), 353
  (1994): Forrest AR+, *Forensic Sci Int* 64(1), 57 (fatal)
  (1992): Henry JA+, *Lancet* 340(8816), 384 (7 fatal)
  (1992): Screaton GR+, *Lancet* 339(8794), 677
  (1992): Singarajah C+, *Anaesthesia* 47(8), 686
Seizures
  (2003): Ben-Abraham R+, *Eur J Emerg Med* 10(4), 309
Suicidal ideation
  (2000): Shannon M, *Pediatr Emerg Care* 16(5), 377
Tremor

MEADOWSWEET

Scientific names: *Filipendula ulmaria; Spiraea ulmaria*
Family: Rosaceae
Trade and other common names: Bridewort; Dolloff;
Dropwort; Meadow Queen; Meadow-Wart
Category: Anti-inflammatory; Diuretic
Purported indications and other uses: Colds, fevers, cough,
bronchitis, dyspepsia, heartburn, peptic ulcer, gout, rheumatic
disorders
Half-life: N/A
**Clinically important, potentially hazardous interactions
with:** salicylates

Reactions

Skin
  Rash (sic)

Other
  Hypersensitivity

MEBENDAZOLE

Trade names: Amycil; Bantenol; Helminzole; Lomper;
Mebensole; Mindol; Nemasol; Pantelmin; Revapole; Toloxim;
Vermicol; Vermox (Janssen)
Indications: Parasitic worm infestations
Category: Antibiotic, imidazole; Antihelmintic
Half-life: 1–12 hours
**Clinically important, potentially hazardous interactions
with:** theophylline

Reactions

Skin
  Allergic reactions (sic)
  Angioedema (<1%)
  Exanthems
    (1983): Seitz R+, *Z Gastroenterol* 21(7), 324
  Pruritus (<1%)
    (1991): Shikiya K+, *Kansenshogaku Zasshi* 65(6), 681
  Rash (sic) (<1%)
  Stevens–Johnson syndrome
    (2003): Chen KT+, *Am J Public Health* 93(3), 489
    (2000): Ajonuma LC+, *Trop Doc* 30, 57
  Urticaria

Mucosal/ENT
  Xerostomia

Hair
  Hair – alopecia
    (1993): Shcherbakov AM+, *Med Parazitol (Mosk)* (2), 14
    (1992): Breathnach SM+, *Adverse Drug Reactions and the Skin*
      Blackwell, Oxford, 177 (passim)
    (1985): Braithwaite PA+, *Aust N Z J Surg* 55(5), 519

Other
  Abdominal pain
    (2006): Canete R+, *Curr Med Res Opin* 22(11), 2131
    (1993): Teggi A+, *Antimicrob Agents Chemother* 37(8), 1679
  Headache
  Vertigo
    (1991): Shikiya K+, *Kansenshogaku Zasshi* 65(6), 681

MECAMYLAMINE

Trade names: Inversine (Targacept); Mevasine
Indications: Hypertension
Category: Ganglion blocker, peripheral; Nicotinic antagonist
Half-life: N/A
**Clinically important, potentially hazardous interactions
with:** alcohol, antibiotics, sulfonamides

Reactions

Skin
  Angioedema

Mucosal/ENT
  Glossitis
  Xerostomia

Other
  Abdominal pain
    (1984): Tennant FS Jr+, *NIDA Res Monogr* 49, 239
  Asthenia

(1984): Tennant FS+, *NIDA Res Monogr* 49, 239
Depression
Paresthesias
Seizures
Tremor
Vertigo

MECASERMIN

Trade name: Increlex (Tercica)
Indications: Growth failure in children with primary insulin growth factor 1 deficiency
Category: Hormone, polypeptide
Half-life: 5.8 hours
Clinically important, potentially hazardous interactions with: None

Reactions

Skin
Edema
  (2002): Mohamed-Ali V+, *Treat Endocrinol* 1(6), 399
Non-Hodgkin's lymphoma
  (1999): Reactions 1 #999, 9
Purpura (>5%)

Other
Headache (>5)
Hypotension
  (2002): Mohamed-Ali V+, *Treat Endocrinol* 1(6), 399
Injection-site pain
  (2002): Mohamed-Ali V+, *Treat Endocrinol* 1(6), 399
Lipohypertrophy (>5)
Myalgia/Myositis/Myopathy/Myotoxicity
  (2002): Mohamed-Ali V+, *Treat Endocrinol* 1(6), 399
Pain
  (2002): Mohamed-Ali V+, *Treat Endocrinol* 1(6), 399 (jaw)
Seizures (>5)
Vertigo

MECHLORETHAMINE

Synonyms: mustine; nitrogen mustard
Trade names: Mustargen; Mustine; Mustine Hydrochloride Boots
Indications: Hodgkin's disease, mycosis fungoides
Category: Alkylating agent
Half-life: <1 minute
Clinically important, potentially hazardous interactions with: aldesleukin, **vaccines**

Reactions

Skin
Acanthosis nigricans
  (1988): Schweitzer WJ+, *J Am Acad Dermatol* 19, 951
Angioedema
  (1981): Wilson KS+, *Ann Intern Med* 94, 823
Bullous dermatitis
  (2006): Freed J+, *J Drugs Dermatol* 5(1), 66
  (1990): Goday JJ+, *Contact Dermatitis* 22, 306
  (1981): Weiss RB+, *Ann Intern Med* 94, 66
Cellulitis

  (1981): Wilson KS+, *Ann Intern Med* 94, 823
Cyst
  (1991): Smith SP+, *J Am Acad Dermatol* 25, 940
Dermatitis
  (1999): Estève E+, *Arch Dermatol* 135, 1349
  (1991): Sheehan MP+, *J Pediatr* 119, 317
  (1988): Ramsay DL+, *J Am Acad Dermatol* 19, 684
  (1986): Mauduit G+, *Br J Dermatol* 115, 82
  (1985): Arrazola JM+, *Int J Dermatol* 24, 608
  (1985): Zachariae H, *Int J Clin Pharmacol Res* 5, 193
  (1984): Ramsay DL+, *Arch Dermatol* 120, 1585
  (1984): Vonderheid EC, *Int J Dermatol* 23, 180
  (1983): Bronner AK+, *J Am Acad Dermatol* 9, 645
  (1983): Nusbaum BP+, *Arch Dermatol* 119, 117
  (1983): Price NM+, *Cancer* 52, 2214
  (1982): Price NM+, *Arch Dermatol* 118, 234
  (1981): Halprin KM+, *Br J Dermatol* 105, 71
  (1981): Shelley WB, *Acta Derm Venereol* 61, 161
Erythema multiforme (<1%)
Exanthems (<1%)
Fungal dermatitis
  (1981): Shelley WB, *Acta Derm Venereol* 61, 164
Herpes zoster (>10%)
Pigmentation
  (1984): Vonderheid EC, *Int J Dermatol* 23, 180
  (1983): Bronner AK+, *J Am Acad Dermatol* 9, 645
  (1982): Price NM+, *Arch Dermatol* 118, 234
Pruritus
  (1981): Weiss RB+, *Ann Intern Med* 94, 66
  (1981): Wilson KS+, *Ann Intern Med* 94, 823
Purpura
  (1981): Weiss RB+, *Ann Intern Med* 94, 66
Rash (sic) (<1%)
Squamous cell carcinoma
  (1991): Smith SP+, *J Am Acad Dermatol* 25, 940
  (1982): Lee LA+, *J Am Acad Dermatol* 7, 590
Stevens–Johnson syndrome
  (1997): Newman JM+, *J Am Acad Dermatol* 36, 112
Urticaria
  (1981): Weiss RB+, *Ann Intern Med* 94, 66
  (1981): Wilson KS+, *Ann Intern Med* 94, 823
Xerosis
  (1984): Vonderheid EC, *Int J Dermatol* 23, 180

Mucosal/ENT
Dysgeusia (1–10%) (metallic taste)
Tinnitus

Hair
Hair – alopecia (1–10%)

Other
Anaphylactoid reactions/Anaphylaxis (1–10%)
  (1983): Bronner AK+, *J Am Acad Dermatol* 9, 645
Headache
Hypersensitivity (1–10%)
Injection-site extravasation (1–10%)
  (2000): Kassner E, *J Pediatr Oncol Nurs* 17, 135
Injection-site thrombophlebitis (1–10%)
  (1989): Kerker BJ+, *Semin Dermatol* 8, 173
  (1981): Wilson KS+, *Ann Intern Med* 94, 823

MECLIZINE

Trade names: Antivert (Pfizer); Antrizine; Bonamine; Bonine; Dizmiss; Dramamine II; Dramine; Meni-D; Nico-Vert; Peremesin; Postadoxin; Postafen; Suprimal; Vergon
Indications: Motion sickness
Category: Histamine H1 receptor antagonist
Half-life: 6 hours
Clinically important, potentially hazardous interactions with: alcohol, barbiturates, chloral hydrate, ethchlorvynol, paraldehyde, phenothiazines, zolpidem

Reactions

Skin
Angioedema (<1%)
Exanthems
   (2001): Litt JZ, Beachwood, OH (personal case) (observation)
Photosensitivity (<1%)
Rash (sic) (<1%)
Urticaria

Mucosal/ENT
Xerostomia (1–10%)

Eyes
Visual hallucinations
   (2004): Kuykendall JR+, *Ann Pharmacother* 38(11), 1968 (with metaxalone)

Other
Asthenia
Headache
Myalgia/Myositis/Myopathy/Myotoxicity (<1%)
Paresthesias (<1%)
Tremor

MECLOFENAMATE

Trade names: Kyroxan; Meclofenamate; Melvon; Movens
Indications: Arthritis
Category: Non-steroidal anti-inflammatory
Half-life: 2 hours
Clinically important, potentially hazardous interactions with: methotrexate

Reactions

Skin
Angioedema (<1%)
   (1984): Stern RS+, *JAMA* 252, 1433
Bullous dermatitis
Edema (>1%)
Erythema multiforme (<1%)
   (1985): Bigby M+, *J Am Acad Dermatol* 12, 866
   (1984): Stern RS+, *JAMA* 252, 1433
   (1983): Harrington T, *J Rheumatol* 10, 169
Erythema nodosum (<1%)
Erythroderma
   (1985): Bigby M+, *J Am Acad Dermatol* 12, 866
Exanthems (1–9%)
   (1992): Breathnach SM+, *Adverse Drug Reactions and the Skin* Blackwell, Oxford, 190 (passim)
   (1985): Bigby M+, *J Am Acad Dermatol* 12, 866 (3–9%)
   (1984): Stern RS+, *JAMA* 252, 1433

Exfoliative dermatitis (<1%)
   (1992): Breathnach SM+, *Adverse Drug Reactions and the Skin* Blackwell, Oxford, 190 (passim)
   (1984): Stern RS+, *JAMA* 252, 1433
Fixed eruption (<1%)
   (1992): Breathnach SM+, *Adverse Drug Reactions and the Skin* Blackwell, Oxford, 190 (passim)
   (1985): Bigby M+, *J Am Acad Dermatol* 12, 866
   (1984): Stern RS+, *JAMA* 252, 1433
Lupus erythematosus
Peripheral edema
Photosensitivity
   (1985): Bigby M+, *J Am Acad Dermatol* 12, 866
   (1984): Stern RS+, *JAMA* 252, 1433
Pruritus (1–10%)
   (1992): Breathnach SM+, *Adverse Drug Reactions and the Skin* Blackwell, Oxford, 190 (passim)
   (1985): Bigby M+, *J Am Acad Dermatol* 12, 866
   (1984): Stern RS+, *JAMA* 252, 1433
Psoriasis (exacerbation)
   (1983): Meyerhoff JO, *N Engl J Med* 309, 496
Purpura (>1%)
   (1992): Breathnach SM+, *Adverse Drug Reactions and the Skin* Blackwell, Oxford, 190 (passim)
   (1985): Bigby M+, *J Am Acad Dermatol* 12, 866
   (1984): Stern RS+, *JAMA* 252, 1433
   (1981): Rodriguez J, *Drug Intell Clin Pharm* 15, 999
Rash (sic) (3–9%)
   (1984): Stern RS+, *JAMA* 252, 1433
Stevens–Johnson syndrome (<1%)
Toxic epidermal necrolysis (<1%)
Urticaria (>1%)
   (1985): Bigby M+, *J Am Acad Dermatol* 12, 866
   (1984): Stern RS+, *JAMA* 252, 1433
Vasculitis
   (1992): Breathnach SM+, *Adverse Drug Reactions and the Skin* Blackwell, Oxford, 190 (passim)
   (1985): Bigby M+, *J Am Acad Dermatol* 12, 866
   (1984): Stern RS+, *JAMA* 252, 1433
Vesiculobullous eruption
   (1992): Breathnach SM+, *Adverse Drug Reactions and the Skin* Blackwell, Oxford, 190 (passim)
   (1984): Stern RS+, *JAMA* 252, 1433

Mucosal/ENT
Aphthous stomatitis
   (1996): Fetterman M, Hialeah, FL (from Internet) (observation)
Dysgeusia (<1%)
Oral ulceration
Stomatitis (1–3%)
Tinnitus
Xerostomia

Hair
Hair – alopecia (<1%)

Other
Headache
Hot flashes (<1%)
Hypersensitivity
   (1993): Fernandez-Rivas M+, *Ann Allergy* 71, 515
Paresthesias (<1%)
Porphyria
Serum sickness

MEDROXYPROGESTERONE

Trade names: Alti-MPA; Aragest 5; Clinofem; Depo-Provera (Pfizer); Gestapuran; Lunelle (Pfizer); Novo-Medrone; Perlutex; Premphase (Wyeth); Prempro (Wyeth); Progevera; Provera (Pfizer); Ralovera
Indications: Secondary amenorrhea, renal or endometrial carcinoma
Category: Progestogen
Half-life: 30 days
Clinically important, potentially hazardous interactions with: acitretin, dofetilide

Reactions

Skin
Acne (1–5%)
Allergic reactions (sic) (<1%)
Angioedema
Chloasma (1–10%)
Diaphoresis (<31%)
 (1990): Willemse PHB+, *Eur J Cancer* 26, 337 (31%)
Edema (>10%)
Erythema nodosum
Exanthems
Hemorrhage
Melasma (1–10%)
Mucha–Habermann disease
Peripheral edema
Photosensitivity
Pigmented purpuric eruption
 (2000): Tsao H+, *J Am Acad Dermatol* 43, 308
Pruritus (1–10%)
Rash (sic) (1–5%)
Scleroderma (<1%)
Striae
 (2000): Gupta M, *Br J Fam Plann* 26, 104
Urticaria
Xerosis (<1%)

Mucosal/ENT
Bromhidrosis (<1%)
Vaginitis (1–5%)
 (2006): Rager KM+, *ScientificWorldJournal* 6, 353

Hair
Hair – alopecia (1–5%)
Hair – hirsutism (<1%)
 (1984): Delanoe D+, *Lancet* 1, 276

Other
Anaphylactoid reactions/Anaphylaxis (<1%)
Gynecomastia (<1%)
Headache
Hot flashes
Injection-site necrosis
 (2000): Clark SM+, *Br J Dermatol* 143, 1356
Injection-site pain (>10%)
Osteoporosis
 (2006): Albertazzi P+, *Contraception* 73(6), 577
 (2006): Cromer BA+, *J Adolesc Health* 39(2), 296
Paresthesias (<1%)
Thrombophlebitis (1–10%)

MEFENAMIC ACID

Trade names: Dysman; Lysalgo; Mefac; Mefic; Parkemed; Ponstan; Ponstel (First Horizon); Ponstyl
Indications: Pain, dysmenorrhea
Category: Non-steroidal anti-inflammatory
Half-life: 3.5 hours
Clinically important, potentially hazardous interactions with: methotrexate

Reactions

Skin
Angioedema (<1%)
Bullous pemphigoid
 (1986): Shepherd AN+, *Postgrad Med J* 62, 67
Diaphoresis
Edema
Erythema multiforme (<1%)
 (1990): Sowden JM+, *Clin Exp Dermatol* 15, 387
 (1985): Ting HC+, *Int J Dermatol* 24, 587
Exanthems
 (1992): Breathnach SM+, *Adverse Drug Reactions and the Skin* Blackwell, Oxford, 190 (passim)
Exfoliative dermatitis
 (1992): Breathnach SM+, *Adverse Drug Reactions and the Skin* Blackwell, Oxford, 190 (passim)
Facial edema
Fixed eruption
 (2006): Teraki Y+, *Dermatology* 213(2), 83
 (2005): Dar NR+, *J Coll Physicians Surg Pak* 15(9), 562
 (2005): Rallis E+, *J Eur Acad Dermatol Venereol* 19(6), 753 (2 cases)
 (1998): Mahboob A+, *Int J Dermatol* 37, 833
 (1992): Long CC+, *Br J Dermatol* 126, 409
 (1991): Mohamed KN, *Aust N Z J Med* 21, 291
 (1990): Sowden JM+, *Clin Exp Dermatol* 15, 387
 (1986): Watson A+, *Australas J Dermatol* 27, 6
 (1986): Wilson CL+, *BMJ* 293, 1243
Photosensitivity
 (1997): O'Reilly FM+, American Academy of Dermatology Meeting, Poster #14
Pruritus (1–10%)
Purpura
Rash (sic) (>10%)
Stevens–Johnson syndrome (<1%)
 (1991): Chan JC+, *Drug Safety* 6, 230
Toxic epidermal necrolysis (<1%)
 (1991): Sakellariou G+, *Int J Artif Organs* 14, 634
 (1990): Black AK+, *Br J Dermatol* 123, 277
Urticaria (<1%)
 (1992): Breathnach SM+, *Adverse Drug Reactions and the Skin* Blackwell, Oxford, 190 (passim)
Vasculitis
 (1980): Malik S+, *Lancet* 2, 746

Mucosal/ENT
Glossitis
Oral ulceration
Sialorrhea
Xerostomia

Eyes
Visual disturbances
 (2006): Yokobori S+, *Pediatr Neurol* 34(3), 245 (with diclofenac)

Other
Anaphylactoid reactions/Anaphylaxis
  (1985): O'Brien WM+, *J Rheumatol* 12, 13
Headache
  (2006): Yokobori S+, *Pediatr Neurol* 34(3), 245 (with diclofenac)
Hot flashes (<1%)
Pseudoporphyria
  (1998): O'Hagan AH+, *Br J Dermatol* 139, 1131
Seizures
  (2006): Yokobori S+, *Pediatr Neurol* 34(3), 245 (with diclofenac)

MEFLOQUINE

Trade names: Lariam (Roche); Laricam; Mephaquin; Mephaquine
Indications: Malaria
Category: Antimalarial; Antiprotozoal
Half-life: 21–22 days

Reactions

Skin
Erythema
  (1992): Breathnach SM+, *Adverse Drug Reactions and the Skin*
    Blackwell, Oxford, 176 (passim)
Erythema multiforme
Exanthems (30%)
  (1999): Smith HR+, *Clin Exp Dermatol* 24, 249 (30%)
Exfoliative dermatitis
  (1993): Martin GJ+, *Clin Infect Dis* 16, 341
Facial rash
  (1991): Shlim DR, *JAMA* 266, 2560
Pruritus (4–10%)
  (1999): Smith HR+, *Clin Exp Dermatol* 24, 249 (4–10%)
  (1989): Sowunmi A+, *Lancet* 2, 313; 397
Psoriasis
  (1998): Potasman I+, *J Travel Med* 5, 156
Rash (sic) (1–10%)
  (2006): Chew HC+, *Am J Emerg Med* 24(5), 634
Stevens–Johnson syndrome
  (1999): Smith HR+, *Clin Exp Dermatol* 24, 249
  (1991): Van den Enden E+, *Lancet* 337, 683
Toxic epidermal necrolysis
  (1999): Smith HR+, *Clin Exp Dermatol* 24, 249 (fatal)
  (1997): McBride SR+, *Lancet* 349, 101
Urticaria
  (1999): Smith HR+, *Clin Exp Dermatol* 24, 249
Vasculitis
  (1999): Smith HR+, *Clin Exp Dermatol* 24, 249
  (1995): White AC+, *Ann Intern Med* 123, 894
  (1993): Scerri L+, *Int J Dermatol* 32, 517

Mucosal/ENT
Tinnitus

Hair
Hair – alopecia (<1%)

Other
Anaphylactoid reactions/Anaphylaxis
  (2006): Bavbek S+, *J Investig Allergol Clin Immunol* 16(5), 317
  (2003): Meyer P+, *Presse Med* 32(9), 408
Asthenia
  (2005): Murai Z+, *Orv Hetil* 146(3), 133
Death
Depression

  (2006): Soentjens P+, *J Travel Med* 13(3), 172 (passim)
  (2002): Dietz A+, *Pharmacopsychiatry* 35(5), 200
  (2002): van Riemsdijk MM+, *Clin Pharmacol Ther* 72(3), 294
Fever
  (2005): Adam I+, *Ann Trop Med Parasitol* 99(2), 111
Headache
Myalgia/Myositis/Myopathy/Myotoxicity (1–10%)
Seizures
  (2006): Soentjens P+, *J Travel Med* 13(3), 172 (passim)
  (2003): Meyer P+, *Presse Med* 32(9), 408
Suicidal ideation
  (2006): Jousset N+, *Presse Med* 35(5), 789
Vertigo
  (2005): Adam I+, *Ann Trop Med Parasitol* 99(2), 111 (25%)
  (2005): Murai Z+, *Orv Hetil* 146(3), 133

MELATONIN

Scientific name: *N-acetyl-5-methoxytryptamine*
Family: None
Trade and other common names: MEL; MLT
Category: Hormone
Purported indications and other uses: Jet lag, sleep disorders, Alzheimer's disease, free radical scavenger, chemotherapy adjunct, tinnitus, depression, migraine, cluster headache, hypertension, hyperpigmentation, osteoporosis, antioxidant. Skin protectant against sunburn
Half-life: N/A
Clinically important, potentially hazardous interactions with: acetaminophen, NSAIDs, setraline, warfarin

Reactions

Skin
Fixed eruption
  (2001): Morera AL+, *Actas Esp Psiquiatr* 29(5), 334 (2 cases)
  (1998): Bardazzi F+, *Acta Derm Venereol* 78(1), 69
Photosensitivity
  (1999): Haga HJ+, *Lupus* 8(4), 269

Other
Seizures
  (2001): Morera AL+, *Actas Esp Psiquiatr* 29(5), 334 (4 cases)

MELOXICAM

Trade name: Mobic (Boehringer Ingelheim)
Indications: Osteoarthritis
Category: COX-2 inhibitor; Non-steroidal anti-inflammatory
Half-life: 15–20 hours

Reactions

Skin
Adverse effects (sic) (18%)
  (1996): Huskisson EC+, *Br J Rheumatol* 35, 29 (18%)
Allergic reactions (sic) (<2%)
Angioedema (<2%)
  (2000): Quaratino D+, *Ann Allergy Asthma Immunol* 84, 613
Bullous dermatitis (<2%)
Edema (2–5%)
Erythema multiforme (<2%)
  (1999): Nikas SN+, *Am J Med* 107, 532

Exanthems (<2%)
(2004): Litt JZ, Beachwood, OH (from Internet) (observation)
(2004): Maffei K, Athens, GA (2 cases) (from Internet)
(observation)
(2000): Quaratino D+, *Ann Allergy Asthma Immunol* 84, 613
Facial edema
(2000): Quaratino D+, *Ann Allergy Asthma Immunol* 84, 613
Peripheral edema
(2004): Litt JZ, Beachwood, OH (from Internet) (observation)
(2002): Fleischmann R+, *Expert Opin Pharmacother* 3(10), 1501
Photosensitivity (<2%)
Pruritus (<2%)
(2004): Litt JZ, Beachwood, OH (from Internet) (observation)
(2001): Bunyaratavej N+, *J Med Assoc Thai* 84(Suppl 2), S542
(2%)
Psoriasis
(2006): Ilknur T+, *Eur J Dermatol* 16(4), 444
Purpura (<2%)
Rash (sic) (1–3%)
(2001): Bunyaratavej N+, *J Med Assoc Thai* 84, S542 (2%)
Stevens–Johnson syndrome (<2%)
Toxic epidermal necrolysis (<2%)
(2002): Eastern J, North Caldwell, NJ (from Internet)
(observation)
Urticaria (<2%)
(2004): Senna G+, *Allerg Immunol* (Paris) 36(6), 215
(2000): Quaratino D+, *Ann Allergy Asthma Immunol* 84, 613
Vasculitis (<2%)

Mucosal/ENT
Dysgeusia (<2%)
Ulcerative stomatitis (<2%)
Xerostomia (<2%)

Other
Anaphylactoid reactions/Anaphylaxis (<2%)
Headache
Hot flashes (<2%)
Hypersensitivity
(2001): Nettis E+, *Allergy* 56(8), 803
Paresthesias (<2%)
Tremor (<2%)

MELPHALAN

Trade name: Alkeran (GSK)
Indications: Multiple myeloma, carcinomas
Category: Alkylating agent
Half-life: 90 minutes
**Clinically important, potentially hazardous interactions
with:** aldesleukin, PEG-interferon

Reactions

Skin
Angioedema
(1983): Bronner AK+, *J Am Acad Dermatol* 9, 645
(1981): Weiss RB+, *Ann Intern Med* 94, 66
Dermatitis
(2002): Goon AT+, *Contact Dermatitis* 47(5), 309 (with
chlorambucil)
Eccrine squamous syringometaplasia
(1997): Valks R+, *Arch Dermatol* 133, 873
Edema
Exanthems (4%)
(1981): Harvey HA+, *Ann Intern Med* 94, 542

(1981): Weiss RB+, *Ann Intern Med* 94, 66
Petechiae
Pruritus (1–10%)
(1983): Bronner AK+, *J Am Acad Dermatol* 9, 645
Purpura
Rash (sic) (1–10%)
Scleroderma (localized)
(1998): Landau M+, *J Am Acad Dermatol* 39, 1011 (2 cases)
Toxicity (sic)
(2006): Cornett WR+, *J Clin Oncol* 24(25), 4196
Urticaria
(1983): Bronner AK+, *J Am Acad Dermatol* 9, 645
(1981): Harvey HA+, *Ann Intern Med* 94, 542
(1981): Weiss RB+, *Ann Intern Med* 94, 66
Vasculitis (1–10%)
(1986): Hannedouche T+, *Ann Med Intern* (Paris) (French)
137, 57
Vesiculation (1–10%)

Mucosal/ENT
Mucositis
(2002): Moreau P+, *Blood* 99(3), 731
Oral lesions
Oral mucositis
(2006): Grazziutti ML+, *Bone Marrow Transplant* 38(7), 501
(2006): Lilleby K+, *Bone Marrow Transplant* 37(11), 1031
(2006): Mori T+, *Bone Marrow Transplant* 38(9), 637
(2000): Wardley AM+, *Br J Haematol* 110, 292
Oral ulceration
Stomatitis (1–10%)

Hair
Hair – alopecia (1–10%)
(1992): Zaun H+, *Hautarzt* (German) 43, 215

Nails
Nails – Beau's lines (transverse nail bands)
(1992): Zaun H+, *Hautarzt* (German) 43, 215
(1983): James WD+, *Arch Dermatol* 119, 334
(1982): Jeanmougin M+, *Ann Dermatol Venereol* (French)
109, 169

Other
Anaphylactoid reactions/Anaphylaxis
(1983): Bronner AK+, *J Am Acad Dermatol* 9, 645
(1982): Dunagin WG, *Semin Oncol* 9, 14
Application-site edema
(1995): Vrouenraets BC+, *Melanoma Res* 5, 425
Death
(2001): Sanchorawala V+, *Bone Marrow Transplant* 28(7), 637
(14%)
Gynecomastia
(2000): Cohen JD+, *Presse Med* 29(35), 1936
Hypersensitivity (1–10%)
(1992): Weiss RB, *Semin Oncol* 19, 458
Inappropriate secretion of antidiuretic hormone (SIADH)
(1985): Greenbaum-Lefkoe B+, *Cancer* 55(1), 44
Injection-site edema
(1995): Vrouenraets BC+, *Melanoma Res* 5, 425
Rhabdomyolysis
(1997): Haier J+, *Langenbecks Arch Chir* 382(3), 128 (with TNF
alfa)
(1997): Hohenberger P+, *Chirurg* 68(9), 914 (with TNF alfa)

MEMANTINE

Trade names: Akatinol; Axura; Ebixa; Namenda (Forest)
Indications: Alzheimer's disease, Vascular dementia
Category: Adamantane; NMDA receptor antagonist
Half-life: 60–80 hours
Clinically important, potentially hazardous interactions with: amantadine, dextromethorphan, ketamine

Reactions

Skin
 Allergic reactions (sic) (<1%)
 Cellulitis (<1%)
 Dermatitis (<1%)
 Eczema (<1%)
 Exanthems (<1%)
 Peripheral edema (>2%)
 Pruritus (<1%)
 Rash (sic) (>1%)
 Ulcerations (<1%)
 Urticaria (<1%)

Mucosal/ENT
 Tinnitus

Hair
 Hair – alopecia (<1%)

Eyes
 Blepharitis
 Cataract
  (2004): Rossom R+, Am J Geriatr Pharmacother 2(4), 303
 Visual hallucinations
  (2007): Monastero R+, J Neurol Neurosurg Psychiatry 78(5), 546
   (3 cases)
  (2005): Menendez-Gonzalez M+, J Alzheimers Dis 8(3), 289

Other
 Abdominal pain
  (1992): Rabey JM+, J Neural Transm Park Dis Dement Section 4, 277
 Agitation
  (2005): Menendez-Gonzalez M+, J Alzheimers Dis 8(3), 289
 Asthenia (2%)
 Cough (4%)
 Depression (>2%)
 Headache (6%)
  (2004): Rossom R+, Am J Geriatr Pharmacother 2(4), 303
 Seizures
  (2005): Peltz G+, Am J Health Syst Pharm 2005 Feb 15;62(4), 420
 Vertigo (7%)
  (2004): Rossom R+, Am J Geriatr Pharmacother 2(4), 303
  (2002): Wilcock G+, Int Clin Psychopharmacol 17(6), 297 (7%)
  (1992): Rabey JM+, J Neural Transm Park Dis Dement Section 4, 277

MEPACRINE

(See QUINACRINE)

MEPENZOLATE

Trade names: Cantil; Trancolon
Indications: Peptic ulcer
Category: Muscarinic antagonist
Half-life: N/A
Clinically important, potentially hazardous interactions with: antacids, anticholinergics, arbutamine, digoxin, metoclopramide

Reactions

Skin
 Urticaria

Mucosal/ENT
 Ageusia
 Xerostomia

Other
 Anaphylactoid reactions/Anaphylaxis
 Headache
 Vertigo

MEPERIDINE

Trade names: Demerol (Sanofi-Aventis); Dolantin; Dolestine; Dolosal; Opistan; Pethidine; Petidin
Indications: Pain
Category: Opiate agonist
Half-life: 3–4 hours
Clinically important, potentially hazardous interactions with: acyclovir, **alcohol**, amphetamines, barbiturates, CNS depressants, fluoxetine, furazolidone, general anesthetics, isocarboxazid, linezolid, lithium, MAO inhibitors, moclobemide, phenelzine, phenobarbital, phenothiazines, rasagiline, ritonavir, selegiline, sibutramine, SSRIs, tranquilizers, tranylcypromine, tricyclic antidepressants, valacyclovir

Reactions

Skin
 Angioedema
 Diaphoresis
 Herpes
  (1986): Acalovschi I, Anaesthesia 41, 1271
 Necrotizing vasculitis
 Pruritus
  (1993): Riley RH, Anaesth Intensive Care 21, 474
  (1984): Saissy JM, Ann Fr Anesth Reanim (French) 3, 402
 Rash (sic) (<1%)
 Toxic epidermal necrolysis
 Urticaria (<1%)
  (2000): Anibarro B+, Allergy 55, 305

Mucosal/ENT
 Xerostomia (1–10%)

Eyes
 Visual hallucinations
  (2007): Huang SS+, J Formos Med Assoc 106(4), 323 (with tramadol)

Other
 Embolia cutis medicamentosa (Nicolau syndrome)

(1995): Faucher L+, *Pediatr Dermatol* 12, 187
Injection-site erythema
  (1993): Kundrotas L+, *Gastrointest Endosc* 39, 109
Injection-site pain (1–10%)
Injection-site scarring
  (1994): Danielsen AG+, *Ugeskr Laeger* (Danish) 156, 162
Injection-site ulceration
  (1994): Danielsen AG+, *Ugeskr Laeger* (Danish) 156, 162
Myalgia/Myositis/Myopathy/Myotoxicity
Tremor
Vertigo
  (2002): Henderson SO+, *J Emerg Med* 23(3), 237

MEPHENYTOIN

Trade names: Epilan-Gerot; Epilanex; Mesantoin (Novartis)
Indications: Partial seizures
Category: Antiepileptic, hydantoin
Half-life: 7 hours (for the active metabolite: 95–144 hours)
**Clinically important, potentially hazardous interactions
with:** chloramphenicol, cyclosporine, disulfiram, dopamine,
imatinib, itraconazole

Reactions

Skin
Acne
Angioedema
Bullous dermatitis
Dermatomyositis
Edema
Erythema multiforme
Exanthems (8–10%)
Exfoliative dermatitis
Lupus erythematosus
  (1989): Vivino FB+, *Arthritis Rheum* 32, 560
  (1980): Condemi JJ, *Geriatrics* 35(3), 81
Pigmentation
Pruritus
Purpura
Scleroderma
  (1990): May DG+, *Clin Pharmacol Ther* 28, 286
Side effects (sic)
Stevens–Johnson syndrome
Toxic epidermal necrolysis
Urticaria

Mucosal/ENT
Gingival hyperplasia/hypertrophy
Oral mucosal eruption
Stomatitis
  (1996): Meloni G+, *Lancet* 347, 1691

Hair
Hair – alopecia

Other
Polyarteritis nodosa

MEPHOBARBITAL

Trade names: Mebaral; Prominal
Indications: Epilepsy, anxiety
Category: Barbiturate
Half-life: 34 hours
**Clinically important, potentially hazardous interactions
with: alcohol**, anticoagulants, antihistamines, brompheniramine,
buclizine, chlorpheniramine, dicumarol, ethanolamine, imatinib,
warfarin

Reactions

Skin
Angioedema (<1%)
Exanthems
Exfoliative dermatitis (<1%)
Purpura
Rash (sic) (<1%)
Stevens–Johnson syndrome (<1%)
Urticaria

Other
Depression
  (1989): Hassler F, *Psychiatr Neurol Med Psychol (Leipz)*
    41(12), 737
Rhabdomyolysis
  (1990): Larpin R+, *Presse Med* 19(30), 1403
Serum sickness
Thrombophlebitis (<1%)

MEPROBAMATE

Trade names: Equagesic (Women First); Harmonin; Meditran;
Meditrara; Meprate; Meprospan; Miltaun; Miltown (MedPointe);
Neuramate; Praol; Probamyl; Urbilat; Visanon
Indications: Anxiety, insomnia
Category: Anxiolytic; Central muscle relaxant
Half-life: 10 hours

Reactions

Skin
Allergic reactions (sic)
Angioedema (<1%)
Bullous dermatitis (<1%)
Dermatitis (<1%)
Eczema
  (1981): Edwards JG, *Drugs* 22, 495 (passim)
Erythema multiforme (<1%)
Erythema nodosum (<1%)
Exanthems (2%)
  (1981): Edwards JG, *Drugs* 22, 495 (passim)
Exfoliative dermatitis
Fixed eruption (<1%)
  (1985): Kauppinen K+, *Br J Dermatol* 112, 575
  (1984): Boyle J+, *BMJ* 289, 802
  (1981): Edwards JG, *Drugs* 22, 495 (passim)
Lupus erythematosus
Pemphigus foliaceus
  (1980): Godard W+, *Ann Dermatol Venereol* (French) 107, 1213
Peripheral edema (<1%)
Petechiae

Photosensitivity
Pityriasis rosea
Pruritus (<1%)
Purpura (<1%)
 (1993): Pang BK+, *Ann Acad Med Singapore* 22, 870
 (1985): Ambriz-Fernandez R+, *Rev Invest Clin* (Spanish) 37, 347
 (1981): Edwards JG, *Drugs* 22, 495 (passim)
Rash (sic) (1–10%)
Side effects (sic) (2%)
Stevens–Johnson syndrome (<1%)
Toxic epidermal necrolysis (<1%)
Toxic erythema
Urticaria (2%)
 (1981): Edwards JG, *Drugs* 22, 495 (passim)
Vasculitis

Mucosal/ENT
Oral mucosal eruption
Oral ulceration
Stomatitis (<1%)
Xerostomia

Other
Anaphylactoid reactions/Anaphylaxis
Gynecomastia
Headache
Hypersensitivity
Paresthesias
Polyarteritis nodosa
Porphyria
 (1984): Magnus IA, *BMJ* 288, 1474
Rhabdomyolysis
 (1992): Bertran F+, *Therapie* 47(5), 444

MERCAPTOPURINE

Synonyms: 6-mercaptopurine; 6-MP
Trade names: Classen; Ismipur; Leukerin; Puri-Nethol; Purinethol (Gate)
Indications: Leukemias
Category: Antimetabolite; Antineoplastic
Half-life: triphasic: 45 minutes; 2.5 hours; 10 hours
Clinically important, potentially hazardous interactions with: aldesleukin, allopurinol, **influenza vaccines**, mycophenolate, olsalazine, **vaccines**

Reactions

Skin
Acral erythema
 (1991): Baack BR+, *J Am Acad Dermatol* 24, 457
Dermatitis (2%)
Edema
Exanthems (<1%)
 (1989): Present DH+, *Ann Intern Med* 111, 641 (0.5%)
Herpes zoster
 (1999): Korelitz BI+, *Am J Gastroenterology* 94, 424
Lichenoid eruption
Lupus erythematosus
Melanoma
 (2005): Glazier KD+, *J Clin Gastroenterol* 39(1), 21 (1 case)
Neoplasms
 (2006): Disanti W+, *Clin Gastroenterol Hepatol* 4(8), 1025
Palmar–plantar erythema
 (1986): Cox GJ+, *Arch Dermatol* 122, 1413

Peripheral edema
 (1987): Schmutz JL+, *Ann Dermatol Venereol* (French) 114, 569
Petechiae
Photo-recall
Photosensitivity
 (1987): Schmutz JL+, *Ann Dermatol Venereol* (French) 114, 569
Pigmentation (1–10%)
Pruritus
Purpura
Rash (sic) (1–10%)
 (2005): Glazier KD+, *J Clin Gastroenterol* 39(1), 21 (0.7%)
Toxic epidermal necrolysis
Urticaria
 (1985): Sparling R+, *Clin Lab Haematol* 7, 184
Vasculitis
 (1997): Andersen JM+, *Pharmacotherapy* 17, 173

Mucosal/ENT
Glossitis (<1%)
Mucositis (1–10%)
Oral lesions (1–5%)
 (1983): Bronner AK+, *J Am Acad Dermatol* 9, 645 (1–5%)
Stomatitis (1–10%)

Hair
Hair – alopecia
 (2005): Glazier KD+, *J Clin Gastroenterol* 39(1), 21 (1%)

Nails
Nails – loss

Other
Death
 (2005): Glazier KD+, *J Clin Gastroenterol* 39(1), 21 (1 case)
Fever
 (2005): Glazier KD+, *J Clin Gastroenterol* 39(1), 21 (1.4%)
Headache
 (2005): Glazier KD+, *J Clin Gastroenterol* 39(1), 21 (2.8%)
Lobular panniculitis
 (1997): Andersen JM+, *Pharmacotherapy* 17, 173
Serum sickness
 (1997): Andersen JM+, *Pharmacotherapy* 17, 173

MEROPENEM

Trade names: Meronem (AstraZeneca); Merrem I.V.
Indications: Aerobic and anaerobic infections, Febrile neutropenia
Category: Antibiotic, beta-lactam; Thienamycin
Half-life: 4–6 hours
Clinically important, potentially hazardous interactions with: oral contraceptives, probenecid, valproic acid

Reactions

Skin
Acute generalized exanthematous pustulosis (AGEP)
 (2003): Mysore V+, *J Dermatolog Treat* 14(1), 54
Angioedema
Dermatitis
 (2001): Yesudian PD+, *Contact Dermatitis* 45(1), 53 (occupational)
Diaphoresis
Erythema multiforme
Peripheral edema
Pruritus (1.2%)

Rash (sic) (1.9%)
  (2000): Feld R+, *J Clin Oncol* 18(21), 3690
  (2000): Lowe MN+, *Drugs* 60(3), 619
  (1999): Norrby SR+, *Scand J Infect Dis* 31(1), 3 (1.4%)
  (1995): Norrby SR+, *J Antimicrob Chemother* 36 Suppl A, 207
Stevens–Johnson syndrome
Toxic epidermal necrolysis
  (2002): Paquet P+, *Crit Care Med* 30(11), 2580
Ulcerations
Urticaria
  (2000): Kuo BI+, *Zhonghua Yi Xue Za Zhi* (Taipei) 63(5), 361

Mucosal/ENT
Glossitis
Oral candidiasis

Eyes
Vision blurred

Other
Abdominal pain
Adverse effects
  (2002): Hou F+, *Chin Med J* (Engl) 115(12), 1849
  (2001): Alvarez Lerma F+, *Antibiot Khimioter* 46(12), 42 (10%)
  (2001): Alvarez Lerma F+, *J Chemother* 13(1), 70 (10%)
  (1999): Bartoloni A+, *Drugs Exp Clin Res* 25(6), 243 (4%)
  (1997): Garau J+, *Eur J Clin Microbiol Infect Dis* 16(11), 789
    (17%)
Candidiasis
  (2003): Weinberger M+, *J Hosp Infect* 53(3), 183
Chest pain
Death
  (2002): Paquet P+, *Crit Care Med* 30(11), 2580
Depression
Fever
  (2004): Cheng AC+, *Antimicrob Agents Chemother* 48(5), 1763 (1
    case)
Headache (2.3%)
  (2004): Kuti JL+, *Clin Ther* 26(4), 493 (1 case)
Hypersensitivity
  (2004): Sodhi M+, *J Antimicrob Chemother* 54(6), 1155
Injection-site inflammation
Injection-site pain
  (2000): Lowe MN+, *Drugs* 60(3), 619
  (1999): Norrby SR+, *Scand J Infect Dis* 31(1), 3 (1%)
  (1995): Geroulanos SJ, *J Antimicrob Chemother* 36 Suppl A, 191
Injection-site reactions
  (1997): Hemsell DL+, *Clin Infect Dis* 24 Suppl 2, S222
Paresthesias
Seizures
  (2005): Coves-Orts FJ+, *Ann Pharmacother* 39(3), 533 (with
    valproic acid)
  (1999): Cunha BA, *Int J Antimicrob Agents* 11(2), 167 (0.1%)
  (1999): Norrby SR+, *Scand J Infect Dis* 31(1), 3 (0.8%)
Serum sickness
  (2003): Ralph ED+, *Clin Infect Dis* 36(11), E149
Vertigo

MESALAMINE

Synonyms: 5-aminosalicylic acid; 5-ASA; fisalamine; mesalazine
Trade names: Asacol (Procter & Gamble); Asacolitin; Canasa
(Axcan); Claversal; Mesalazine; Mesasal; Pentasa (Shire); Pentasa
SR; Quintasa; Rowasa (Solvay); Salofalk; Tidocol
Indications: Ulcerative colitis
Category: Aminosalicylate
Half-life: 0.5–1.5 hours

Reactions

Skin
Acne (1.2%)
Allergic granulomatous angiitis (Churg–Strauss syndrome)
  (2006): Sinico RA+, *Clin Exp Rheumatol* 24(2), S104
Allergic reactions (sic) (<1%)
  (1990): Boulain T+, *Gastroenterol Clin Biol* (French) 14, 288
  (1989): Brogden RN+, *Drugs* 38, 500
Baboon syndrome
  (2002): Gallo R+, *Contact Dermatitis* 46(2), 110
Diaphoresis (3%)
Eczema
Edema (1.2%)
Erythema
  (1990): Boulain T+, *Gastroenterol Clin Biol* 14, 288 (rectal)
Erythema nodosum
Exanthems
  (1991): LeGros V+, *BMJ* 302, 970
  (1988): Fardy JM+, *J Clin Gastroenterol* 10, 635
  (1988): Gron I+, *Ugeskr Laeger* (Danish) 150, 32
Facial edema
  (1990): Boulain T+, *Gastroenterol Clin Biol* 14, 288 (rectal
    application)
Folliculitis
  (1996): Lizasoain J+, *Am J Gastroenterol* 91, 819
Lichen planus
  (1991): Alstead EM+, *J Clin Gastroenterol* 13, 335
Lupus erythematosus
  (1997): Timsit MA+, *Rev Rhum Engl Ed* 64, 586
  (1992): Pent MT+, *BMJ* 305, 159
Peripheral edema (0.61%)
Photosensitivity
  (1999): Horiuchi Y+, *Am J Gastroenterol* 94, 3386
Pruritus (1.2%)
Psoriasis
Pustuloderma
  (2001): Gibbon KL+, *J Am Acad Dermatol* 45, S220–1
Pyoderma gangrenosum
Rash (sic) (3%)
  (1992): Giaffer MH+, *Aliment Pharmacol Ther* 6, 51
  (1992): Hautekeete ML+, *Gastroenterology* 103, 1925
  (1991): Lesur G+, *Gastroenterol Clin Biol* (French) 15, 457
Urticaria
Vasculitis
  (1994): Lim AG+, *BMJ* 308, 113
Xerosis

Mucosal/ENT
Dysgeusia
Mucocutaneous lymph node syndrome (Kawasaki
  syndrome)
  (1991): Waanders H+, *Am J Gastroenterol* 86, 219
Oral candidiasis
Oral lichenoid eruption
  (1991): Alstead EM+, *J Clin Gastroenterol* 13, 335

Oral ulceration
Tinnitus

Hair
Hair – alopecia (0.86%)
  (1997): Timsit MA+, *Rev Rhum Engl Ed* 64, 586
  (1995): Netzer P, *Schweiz Med Wochenschr* (German) 125, 2438
  (1991): Hadjigogos K, *Ital J Gastroenterol* (Italian) 23, 257
  (1989): Brogden RN+, *Drugs* 38, 500
  (1982): Kutty PK+, *Ann Intern Med* 97, 785

Nails
Nails – changes

Other
Headache
Hypersensitivity (<1%)
  (2001): Safer L+, *Gastroenterol Clin Biol* 25(1), 104 (following
    severe allergic reaction to sulfasalazine)
  (2001): Sule A+, *J Assoc Physicians India* 49, 1120
  (1996): Aparicio J+, *Am J Gastroenterol* 91, 620
  (1992): Hautekeete ML+, *Gastroenterology* 103, 1925
Myalgia/Myositis/Myopathy/Myotoxicity (3%)
  (2007): Persic M+, *Eur J Clin Pharmacol* 63(3), 315
Nephrotoxicity
  (1998): Mulder CJ+, *Mediators Inflamm* 7(3), 135
Paresthesias

MESNA

Trade names: Mesnex (Bristol-Myers Squibb); Mexan;
Uromitexan
Indications: Hemorrhagic cystitis induced by ifosfamide
Category: Prophylactic, urinary
Half-life: 24 minutes

Reactions

Skin
Allergic reactions (sic)
  (1991): D'Cruz D+, *Lancet* 338, 705
Angioedema
  (1998): Leal G, Fortaleza, Brazil (from Internet) (observation)
  (1992): Breathnach SM+, *Adverse Drug Reactions and the Skin*
    Blackwell, Oxford, 289
  (1992): Zonzits E+, *Arch Dermatol* 128, 80
Erythema
  (1992): Breathnach SM+, *Adverse Drug Reactions and the Skin*
    Blackwell, Oxford, 289
Exanthems
  (1998): Leal G, Fortaleza, Brazil (from Internet) (observation)
  (1992): Breathnach SM+, *Adverse Drug Reactions and the Skin*
    Blackwell, Oxford, 289
  (1992): Zonzits E+, *Arch Dermatol* 128, 80
Fixed eruption
  (1998): Leal G, Fortaleza, Brazil (from Internet) (observation) (2
    patients)
  (1992): Zonzits E+, *Arch Dermatol* 128, 80
Pruritus (<1%)
Rash (sic) (<1%)
Urticaria
  (1998): Leal G, Fortaleza, Brazil (from Internet) (observation)
  (1992): Breathnach SM+, *Adverse Drug Reactions and the Skin*
    Blackwell, Oxford, 289
  (1992): Zonzits E+, *Arch Dermatol* 128, 80
  (1988): Pratt CB+, *Drug Intell Clin Pharm* 22, 913

Mucosal/ENT
Dysgeusia (>17%)
Oral lesions
  (1988): Pralt CB+, *Drug Intell Clin Pharm* 22, 913
Oral ulceration
  (1992): Breathnach SM+, *Adverse Drug Reactions and the Skin*
    Blackwell, Oxford, 289

MESORIDAZINE

Trade names: Mesorin; Serentil (Boehringer Ingelheim)
Indications: Schizophrenia
Category: Antipsychotic, phenothiazine
Half-life: 24–48 hours
**Clinically important, potentially hazardous interactions
with:** antihistamines, arsenic, chlorpheniramine, dofetilide,
lithium, piperazine, quinolones, sparfloxacin

Reactions

Skin
Angioedema
Dermatitis
Eczema
Edema
Erythema
Exfoliative dermatitis
Lupus erythematosus
Peripheral edema
Photosensitivity (1–10%)
Pigmentation (blue-gray) (<1%)
Pruritus
Rash (sic) (1–10%)
Seborrhea
Urticaria
Xerosis

Mucosal/ENT
Hypertrophic papillae of tongue
Sialorrhea
Xerostomia

Hair
Hair – alopecia

Other
Anaphylactoid reactions/Anaphylaxis
Gynecomastia
Paresthesias
Tremor

METAMIZOLE

Synonym: Dipyrone
Trade names: Algopyrin; Analgin (BPG); Baralgin; Dipyrone;
Dolo-Tiaminol; Novalgin
Indications: Analgesic, antipyretic, anti-inflammatory
Category: Non-steroidal anti-inflammatory
Half-life: 2–10 hours

Note: Metamizole is banned in more than 30 countries, including
Japan, Australia, the USA, and the European Union

Reactions

Skin

Acute generalized exanthematous pustulosis
(2005): Schmutz JL+, *Ann Dermatol Venereol* 132(1), 100 (with pseudoephedrine)
(2003): Gonzalo-Garijo MA+, *Contact Dermatitis* 49(1), 47
Adverse effects (sic)
(2003): Borja JM+, *Allergy* 58(1), 84
Erythema multiforme
(2006): Hernandez-Salazar A+, *Arch Med Res* 37(7), 899
Erythema nodosum
(1994): Fernandes NC+, *Rev Inst Med Trop Sao Paulo* 36(6), 507
Erythroderma
(2004): Bernedo N+, *Contact Dermatitis* 50(5), 317
Exanthems
(2006): Hernandez-Salazar A+, *Arch Med Res* 37(7), 899
(2002): Herdeg C+, *Liver* 22(6), 507
(2001): Quinones Estevez D+, *Allergy* 56(3), 262
Fixed eruption
(2004): Ozkaya-Bayazit E, *Clin Exp Dermatol* 29(4), 419 (5 cases)
(2003): Ozkaya-Bayazit E+, *J Am Acad Dermatol* 49(6), 1003 (6%)
(2000): Ozkaya-Bayazit E+, *Eur J Dermatol* 10(4), 288 (9%)
(1999): Sempere Verdu E+, *Aten Primaria* 24(5), 304
(1998): Mahboob A+, *Int J Dermatol* 37(11), 833
(1994): Pinto Pereira LM, *West Indian Med J* 43(4), 146
(1984): Pandhi RK+, *Sex Transm Dis* 11(3), 164 (genitalia)
Lichen planus
(1982): Mashkilleison AL+, *Vestn Dermatol Venerol* (10), 40
Pemphigus
(1997): Brenner S+, *J Am Acad Dermatol* 36(3 Pt 1), 488
Toxic epidermal necrolysis
(1991): Saban J+, *Postgrad Med J* 67(784), 195
(1990): Arellano F+, *Rev Clin Esp* 186(6), 305
Toxicity (sic)
(2004): Bentur Y+, *J Toxicol Clin Toxicol* 42(3), 261 (16%)
Urticaria
(2006): Hernandez-Salazar A+, *Arch Med Res* 37(7), 899
(2006): Padilla Serrato MT+, *Rev Alerg Mex* 53(5), 179
(2002): Karakaya G+, *Allergol Immunopathol (Madr)* 30(5), 267

Mucosal/ENT

Xerostomia
(2002): Edwards JE+, *Cochrane Database Syst Rev* (4), CD003867

Eyes

Keratoconjunctivitis
(1988): Avisar R+, *Harefuah* 114(11), 543
Rhinoconjunctivitis
(1997): Anibarro B+, *Ann Allergy Asthma Immunol* 78(4), 345

Other

Anaphylactoid reactions/Anaphylaxis
(2005): Eckle T+, *Eur J Anaesthesiol* 22(10), 810
(2004): Etxaniz Alvarez A+, *Rev Esp Anestesiol Reanim* 51(7), 395
(2004): Hernandez C+, *Rev Esp Anestesiol Reanim* 51(3), 168
(2004): Molto L+, *Rev Esp Anestesiol Reanim* 51(3), 151
(2003): Janke C+, *Anaesthesist* 52(4), 321
(1999): Jaszczuk E+, *Przegl Lek* 56(2), 175
(1998): Andrade SE+, *J Clin Epidemiol* 51(12), 1357
(1986): Hoigne R+, *Agents Actions Suppl* 19, 189
(1983): Zoppi M+, *Schweiz Med Wochenschr* 113(47), 1768
Death
(2002): Hedenmalm K+, *Eur J Clin Pharmacol* 58(4), 265 (4 cases)
(1999): Jaszczuk E+, *Przegl Lek* 56(2), 175
(1998): Andrade SE+, *J Clin Epidemiol* 51(12), 1357
(1996): Mihajlovic G, *Srp Arh Celok Lek* 124(1–2), 44
(1994): Larregina A+, *Medicina (B Aires)* 54(1), 13
(1989): Berg PA+, *Dtsch Med Wochenschr* 114(11), 443
(1988): Vlakhov V+, *Vutr Boles* 27(2), 80
(1983): Shinar E+, *Isr J Med Sci* 19(3), 225
(1982): Hoerder U+, *Dtsch Med Wochenschr* 107(50), 1923
Fever
(2002): Bonkowsky JL+, *Pediatrics* 109(6), e98
(1998): Marquez JA+, *Sangre (Barc)* 43(5), 436
Gangrene
(1999): Cihan A+, *Dis Colon Rectum* 42(12), 1644
Hypersensitivity
(1999): Bellegrandi S+, *Allergy* 54(1), 88
Infections
(1998): Marquez JA+, *Sangre (Barc)* 43(5), 436
Injection-site pain
(2002): Edwards JE+, *Cochrane Database Syst Rev* (4), CD003867

METAXALONE

Trade name: Skelaxin (Elan)
Indications: Muscle spasm
Category: Central muscle relaxant
Half-life: 2–3 hours

Reactions

Skin

Dermatitis (<1%)
Fixed eruption
(2000): Mostow EN, Akron, OH (from Internet) (observation)
Pruritus
Rash (sic)
Urticaria

Eyes

Visual hallucinations
(2004): Kuykendall JR+, *Ann Pharmacother* 38(11), 1968 (with meclizine)

Other

Anaphylactoid reactions/Anaphylaxis (<1%)
Asthenia
(2004): Toth PP+, *Clin Ther* 26(9), 1355
Headache
Vertigo
(2004): Toth PP+, *Clin Ther* 26(9), 1355

METFORMIN

Trade names: Apo-Metformin; Avandamet; Diabex; Diaformin; Diformin; Gen-Metformin; Glucomet; Glucophage (Bristol-Myers Squibb); Glucovance (Bristol-Myers Squibb); Metaglip; Metforal; Metomin; Novo-Metformin
Indications: Diabetes
Category: Biguanide
Half-life: 6.2 hours

Note: Glucovance is metformin and glyburide

Note: Grinspan's syndrome: the triad of oral lichen planus, diabetes mellitus, and hypertension

Reactions

Skin
Eczema
Erythema (transient)
Exanthems
Grinspan's syndrome
 (1990): Lamey PJ+, *Oral Surg Oral Med Oral Pathol* 70, 184
Lichenoid eruption
Photosensitivity (1–10%)
Pruritus
Purpura
Rash (sic) (1–10%)
Urticaria (1–10%)
Vasculitis
 (2006): Ben Salem C+, *Ann Pharmacother* 40(9), 1685
 (1986): Klapholz L+, *BMJ* 293, 483

Mucosal/ENT
Dysgeusia (3%) (metallic taste)

Hair
Hair – alopecia
 (1999): Smith JG, Mobile, AL (from Internet) (2 observations)
 (1998): Klein AD, Statesboro, GA (from Internet) (observation)

Other
Death
 (2002): www.intellihealth.com (from Internet)
Hepatotoxicity
 (2005): Kutoh E, *Am J Geriatr Pharmacother* 3(4), 270
 (2002): Chitturi S+, *Semin Liver Dis* 22(2), 169
Nephrotoxicity
 (2006): Bjarnason NH+, *Ugeskr Laeger* 168(18), 1772
 (2006): Nyirenda MJ+, *Diabet Med* 23(4), 432

METHADONE

Trade names: Dolophine (Roxane); Eptadone; L-Polamidon; Mephenon; Metadon; Methadose
Indications: Pain, narcotic addiction
Category: Opiate agonist
Half-life: 15–25 hours
Clinically important, potentially hazardous interactions with: delavirdine, diazepam, erythromycin, fluconazole, fluvoxamine, **St John's wort**

Reactions

Skin
Angioedema
Cellulitis
 (1988): Naschitz JE+, *Harefuah* (Hebrew) 115, 271
Diaphoresis (<48%)
 (2004): Al-Adwani A+, *Addiction* 99(2), 259
 (2003): Caflisch C+, *Am J Psychiatry* 160(2), 386
 (1981): Langrod J+, *Int J Addict* 16(5), 947
Edema
 (2007): Kharlamb V+, *Am J Health Syst Pharm* 64(24), 2557
Exanthems
Facial edema
Pruritus (<1%)
Purpura
Rash (sic) (<1%)
 (2006): Lee MR+, *Australas J Dermatol* 47(2), 145

Urticaria (<1%)
Mucosal/ENT
Xerostomia (1–10%)
Other
Death
 (2005): Reith D+, *N Z Med J* 118(1209), U1293 (31 cases)
 (2003): Ballesteros MF+, *JAMA* 290(1), 40
 (2003): Gagajewski A+, *J Forensic Sci* 48(3), 668
 (2003): Grass H+, *Forensic Sci Int* 132(3), 195
 (2002): Buster MC+, *Addiction* 97(8), 993 (overdose)
 (2002): Caplehorn JR+, *Aust N Z J Public Health* 26(4), 358
 (2002): Ernst E+, *Aust N Z J Public Health* 26(4), 364
 (2002): Mikolaenko I+, *Am J Forensic Med Pathol* 23(3), 299 (101 cases)
 (2001): Vormfelde SV+, *Pharmacopsychiatry* 34(6), 217
Headache
Injection-site burning
Injection-site induration
Injection-site pain (1–10%)
Rhabdomyolysis
 (1990): Larpin R+, *Presse Med* 19(30), 1403
 (1983): Nanji AA+, *J Toxicol Clin Toxicol* 20(4), 353
Stroke
 (2006): Miller MA+, *J Emerg Med* 31(3), 305
Tremor
 (2001): Clark JD+, *Clin J Pain* 17(4), 375

METHAMPHETAMINE

Trade name: Desoxyn (Ovation)
Indications: Attention deficit disorder, obesity
Category: Amphetamine
Half-life: 4–5 hours
Clinically important, potentially hazardous interactions with: fluoxetine, fluvoxamine, MAO inhibitors, paroxetine, phenelzine, sertraline, tranylcypromine

Reactions

Skin
Acaraphobia
Diaphoresis (1–10%)
 (2006): Baylen CA+, *Addiction* 101(7), 933
Lichenoid eruption
 (1994): Deloach-Banta LJ, *Cutis* 53, 97
Nodular eruption
 (2002): Patatanian E+, *Pharmacotherapy* 22(9), 1157 (27 cases)
Pigmentation
Rash (sic) (<1%)
Toxic epidermal necrolysis
 (2002): Yung A+, *Australas J Dermatol* 43(1), 35
Urticaria (<1%)

Mucosal/ENT
Auditory hallucinations
 (2007): Yamamoto N+, *Psychiatry Clin Neurosci* 61(6), 691
Dysgeusia
Xerostomia (1–10%)
 (2006): Baylen CA+, *Addiction* 101(7), 933
 (2006): Donaldson M+, *Am J Health Syst Pharm* 63(21), 2078
 (2005): Saini T+, *Oral Health Prev Dent* 3(3), 189

Other
Anxiety
 (2006): Baylen CA+, *Addiction* 101(7), 933

Asthenia
  (2006): Baylen CA+, *Addiction* 101(7), 933
Death
  (2003): Ishigami A+, *J Med Invest* 50(1), 112 (2 cases)
  (2003): Nishida N+, *Med Sci Law* 43(3), 267
Delusions of parasitosis
  (1999): Gregg LJ, Tulsa, OK (from Internet) (2 observations)
Depression
  (2006): Baylen CA+, *Addiction* 101(7), 933
  (2004): London ED+, *Arch Gen Psychiatry* 61(1), 73
Gynecomastia
  (2002): Aguirre MA+, *J Rheumatol* 29(8), 1793
Headache
  (2006): Baylen CA+, *Addiction* 101(7), 933
Injection-site lipoatrophy
  (2002): Haas N+, *Pediatr Dermatol* 19(5), 432
Insomnia
  (2006): Baylen CA+, *Addiction* 101(7), 933
Myalgia/Myositis/Myopathy/Myotoxicity
  (2006): Baylen CA+, *Addiction* 101(7), 933
Neurotoxicity
  (2006): Gettig JP+, *J Sch Nurs* 22(2), 66
  (2006): Quinton MS+, *AAPS J* 8(2), E337
  (2006): Riddle EL+, *AAPS J* 8(2), E413
Polyarteritis nodosa
Rhabdomyolysis (43%)
  (1999): Richards JR+, *Am J Emerg Med* 17(7), 681 (43%)
  (1998): Kolecki P, *Pediatr Emerg Care* 14(6), 385
  (1998): Lan KC+, *J Formos Med Assoc* 97(8), 528
  (1994): Chan P+, *J Toxicol Clin Toxicol* 32(2), 147 (8 cases) (3 fatal)
  (1994): Sperling LS+, *Ann Intern Med* 121(12), 986
Stroke
  (2005): Ohta K+, *J Emerg Med* 28(2), 165
Tremor

METHANTHELINE

Trade name: Vagantin
Indications: Duodenal ulcer
Category: Muscarinic cholinergic agonist
Half-life: N/A
Clinically important, potentially hazardous interactions with: anticholinergics, arbutamine

Reactions

Skin
Dermatitis
  (1983): Przybilla B+, *Hautarzt* 34(9), 459
Exanthems
Exfoliative dermatitis
Urticaria
Xerosis

Mucosal/ENT
Ageusia
Dysgeusia
Sialopenia
Xerostomia

Other
Anaphylactoid reactions/Anaphylaxis

METHAZOLAMIDE

Trade name: Methazolamide
Indications: Glaucoma
Category: Carbonic anhydrase inhibitor; Diuretic
Half-life: ~14 hours

Reactions

Skin
Exanthems (<1%)
  (1998): Litt JZ, Beachwood, OH (personal case) (observation)
  (1993): Gandham SB+, *Arch Ophthalmol* 111, 370
Photosensitivity
Pruritus
Purpura
Rash (sic)
Stevens–Johnson syndrome
  (1998): Cotter JB, *Arch Ophthalmol* 116, 117
  (1997): Shirato S+, *Arch Ophthalmol* 115, 550
  (1995): Flach AJ+, *Ophthalmology* 102, 1677
Toxic epidermal necrolysis
Urticaria
  (1993): Gandham SB+, *Arch Ophthalmol* 111, 370
Vasculitis

Mucosal/ENT
Anosmia (<1%)
Dysgeusia (>10%) (metallic taste)
Tinnitus
Xerostomia (<1%)

Other
Hypersensitivity (<1%)
Paresthesias (<1%)

METHENAMINE

Trade names: Dehydral; Haiprex; Hip-Rex; Hipeksal; Hippramine; Hiprex (Sanofi-Aventis); Mandelamine; Prosed; Reflux; Urasal; Urised; Uroqid; Urotractan
Indications: Urinary tract infections
Category: Antibiotic
Half-life: 3–6 hours

Reactions

Skin
Dermatitis (systemic)
Edema
Erythema multiforme (<1%)
Exanthems (<1%)
Fixed eruption (<1%)
Photosensitivity
  (1994): Selvaag E+, *Photodermatol Photoimmunol Photomed* 10, 259
Pruritus (<1%)
Rash (sic) (3.5%)
Urticaria

Mucosal/ENT
Stomatitis

Other
Headache

METHICILLIN

Trade names: Estafcilina; Lucoperin; Mechicillin
Indications: Various infections caused by susceptible organisms
Category: Antibiotic, penicillin
Half-life: 30 minutes
**Clinically important, potentially hazardous interactions
with:** anticoagulants, cyclosporine, imipenem/cilastatin,
methotrexate, tetracycline

Reactions

Skin
Angioedema
Bullous dermatitis
Erythema multiforme
Erythema nodosum
Exanthems (29%)
  (1980): Fields DA, *West J Med* 133, 521
Exfoliative dermatitis
Hematomas
Jarisch–Herxheimer reaction
Pruritus
Psoriasis
Purpura
Rash (sic) (1–10%)
Stevens–Johnson syndrome
Toxic epidermal necrolysis
Urticaria
Vasculitis

Mucosal/ENT
Dysgeusia
Glossitis
Glossodynia
Oral candidiasis
Stomatitis
Stomatodynia
Tongue black
Vaginitis
Xerostomia

Other
Anaphylactoid reactions/Anaphylaxis
Hypersensitivity
Injection-site pain
Phlebitis (<1%)
Serum sickness (<1%)

METHIMAZOLE

Synonym: thiamazole
Trade names: Strumazol; Tapazole (Paladin); Thacapzol;
Thiamazol; Thyrozol; Unimazole
Indications: Hyperthyroidism
Category: Antithyroid, hormone modifier
Half-life: 4–13 hours
**Clinically important, potentially hazardous interactions
with:** anticoagulants, dicumarol, **myrrh**, warfarin

Reactions

Skin
Edema (<1%)
Erythema nodosum
Exanthems (1–15%)
  (1986): Shiroozu A+, *J Clin Endocrinol Metab* 63, 125 (5–15%)
Exfoliative dermatitis
Fixed eruption
  (1984): Chan HL, *Int J Dermatol* 23, 607
Lupus erythematosus (1–10%)
  (2002): Thong HY+, *Acta Derm Venereol* 82(3), 206
  (1995): Kawachi Y+, *Clin Exp Dermatol* 20, 345
  (1994): Sato-Matsumura KC+, *J Dermatol* 21, 501
  (1987): Sakata S+, *Jpn J Med* 26, 373
  (1981): Searles RP+, *J Rheumatol* 8, 498
  (1981): Takuwa N+, *Endocrinol Jpn* 28, 663
Pigmentation
  (2000): Drayton G, Los Angeles, CA (from Internet)
    (observation)
Pruritus (1–5%)
  (2004): Mikhail NE, *South Med J* 97(2), 178
  (1986): Shiroozu A+, *J Clin Endocrinol Metab* 63, 125 (2–3%)
Purpura (1%)
Rash (sic) (>10%)
Side effects (sic) (28% in high dosages)
Toxic epidermal necrolysis
  (2006): Ziora K+, *J Paediatr Child Health* 42(7-8), 472
Urticaria (>5%)
Vasculitis
  (2006): Bilu Martin D+, *Skinmed* 5(6), 302
  (2002): Thong HY+, *Acta Derm Venereol* 82(3), 206
  (1995): Kawachi Y+, *Clin Exp Dermatol* 20, 345

Mucosal/ENT
Ageusia (1–10%)
  (1982): Reck R+, *Fortschr Med* 100(11), 444
Dysgeusia
Oral ulceration
Sialadenitis
  (2002): Viseux V+, *Ann Dermatol Venereol* 129(1 Pt 1), 59
    (passim)

Hair
Hair – alopecia (<1%)

Other
Aplasia cutis congenita
  (1995): Vogt T+, *Br J Dermatol* 133, 994
  (1992): Martinez-Frias ML+, *Lancet* 339, 742
  (1985): Milham S, *Teratology* 32, 321
  (1984): Bachrach LK+, *Can Med Assoc J* 130, 1264
Headache
Hypersensitivity
  (2006): Ozaki N+, *Diabetes Care* 29(5), 1179
  (2005): Ozaki N+, *Thyroid* 15(12), 1333
Myalgia/Myositis/Myopathy/Myotoxicity
Paresthesias (<1%)
Polyarteritis nodosa
Scalp defects
  (1985): Milham S, *Teratology* 32, 321
Serum sickness
  (1983): Van Kuyk M+, *Acta Clin Belg* (French) 38, 68

METHOCARBAMOL

Trade names: Carbametin; Carxin; Delaxin; Lumirelax; Marbaxin; Miowas; Ortoton; Robaxin (Baxter) (Elkins-Sinn); Robinax; Robomol; Trolar
Indications: Muscle spasm, tetanus
Category: Central muscle relaxant
Half-life: 1–2 hours
Clinically important, potentially hazardous interactions with: ethanol

Reactions

Skin
Allergic reactions (sic) (1–10%)
Exanthems
Pruritus
Rash (sic)
Urticaria

Mucosal/ENT
Dysgeusia

Other
Anaphylactoid reactions/Anaphylaxis
Headache
Injection-site pain (<1%)
Thrombophlebitis (<1%)

METHOHEXITAL

Trade names: Brevimytal; Brevital; Brietal; Brietal Sodium
Indications: General anesthesia
Category: Barbiturate
Half-life: 4–8 minutes

Reactions

Skin
Angioedema
Erythema
Exanthems
Rash (sic)
Shivering
    (1996): Johns FR+, *J Oral Maxillofac Surg* 54(5), 578
Urticaria

Mucosal/ENT
Sialorrhea

Other
Anaphylactoid reactions/Anaphylaxis
Injection-site edema
Injection-site pain (18%)
Injection-site phlebitis
    (1981): Clark RSJ, *Drugs* 27, 26
Rhabdomyolysis
    (1990): Larpin R+, *Presse Med* 19(30), 1403
Thrombophlebitis (<1%)
Tremor

METHOTREXATE

Synonyms: amethopterin; MTX
Trade names: Farmitrexat; Lantarel; Ledertrexate; Maxtrex; Metex; Rheumatrex (Stada); Texate
Indications: Carcinomas, leukemias, lymphomas, psoriasis, rheumatoid arthritis
Category: Antimetabolite; Disease-modifying antirheumatic; Folic acid antagonist
Half-life: 3–10 hours
Clinically important, potentially hazardous interactions with: acitretin, aldesleukin, aminoglycosides, amiodarone, amoxicillin, ampicillin, aspirin, bacampicillin, bismuth, carbenicillin, chloroquine, cisplatin, cloxacillin, co-trimoxazole, dapsone, demeclocycline, dexamethasone, diclofenac, dicloxacillin, etodolac, etoricoxib, etretinate, fenoprofen, flurbiprofen, folic acid antagonists, haloperidol, hydrocortisone, ibuprofen, indomethacin, **influenza vaccines**, ketoprofen, ketorolac, lithium, magnesium trisalicylate, meclofenamate, mefenamic acid, methicillin, mezlocillin, minocycline, nabumetone, nafcillin, naproxen, NSAIDs, omeprazole, oxacillin, oxaprozin, oxytetracycline, paromomycin, penicillin g, penicillin V, penicillins, phenylbutazone, piperacillin, piroxicam, polypeptide antibiotics, prednisolone, prednisone, probenecid, procarbazine, rofecoxib, salicylates, salsalate, sapropterin, sulfadiazine, sulfamethoxazole, sulfapyridine, sulfasalazine, sulfisoxazole, sulindac, tetracycline, ticarcillin, tolmetin, trimethoprim, **vaccines**

Reactions

Skin
Acne
Acral erythema
    (2007): Varela CR+, *Pediatr Dermatol* 24(5), 541
    (2006): Kuruvila S+, *Indian J Dermatol Venereol Leprol* 72(6), 440 (bullous)
    (2005): Postovsky S+, *Pediatr Hematol Oncol* 22(2), 167 (2 cases)
    (2005): Werchniak AE+, *J Am Acad Dermatol* 52(5 Suppl 1), S93
    (2003): Feizy V+, *Dermatol Online J* 9(1), 14 (bullous variety – on soles)
    (2002): Morrell DS+, *J Pediatr Hematol Oncol* 24(3), 240
    (1999): Ikeda H+, *Ann Pharmacother* 33(5), 646
    (1999): Millot F+, *Pediatr Dermatol* 16(5), 398
    (1996): Hellier I+, *Arch Dermatol* 132, 590 (bullous variety)
    (1992): Wysocki M+, *Wiad Lek* 45(11–12), 462
    (1989): Kampmann KK+, *Cancer* 63, 2482
    (1983): Doyle LA+, *Ann Intern Med* 98, 611
Allergic reactions (sic)
    (2000): Postovsky S+, *Med Pediatr Oncol* 35, 131
Angiomas
    (2006): Kreitzer T+, *W V Med J* 102(1), 317
Bullous dermatitis
    (1987): Chang JC, *Arch Dermatol* 123, 990
    (1983): Reed KM+, *J Am Acad Dermatol* 8, 677
Burning (palms and soles)
Capillaritis
Carcinoma
Dermatitis
    (1999): Peters T+, *Acta Derm Venereol* 79(5), 391 (Exfoliative)
    (1996): Giordano N+, *Clin Exp Rheumatol* 14, 450
Dermatofibromas
    (2007): Huang PY+, *J Am Acad Dermatol* 57(5 Supp 1), S81 (multiple) (with prednisolone)
Eccrine squamous syringometaplasia
    (1997): Valks R+, *Arch Dermatol* 133, 873

Edema
  (2003): *Prescrire Int* 12(64), 59
Eosinophilic pustular folliculitis
  (2007): Laing ME+, *Photodermatol Photoimmunol Photomed* 23(2-3), 62
Erosion of psoriatic plaques
  (2003): Kazlow DW+, *J Am Acad Dermatol* 49, S197
  (1996): Pearce HP+, *J Am Acad Dermatol* 35, 835
  (1988): Kaplan DL+, *Int J Dermatol* 27, 59
  (1988): Shupack JL+, *JAMA* 259, 3594
  (1987): Ng HW+, *BMJ* 295, 752
  (1984): Lawrence CM+, *J Am Acad Dermatol* 11, 1059
  (1983): Reed KM+, *J Am Acad Dermatol* 8, 677
Erosions
  (1996): Zackheim HS+, *J Am Acad Dermatol* 34, 626
Erythema (>10%)
Erythema multiforme
  (1999): Goerttler E+, *J Am Acad Dermatol* 40, 702 (4 cases)
  (1989): Taylor SW+, *Gynecol Oncol* 33, 376
Erythroderma
  (2000): Alfaro J+, *Rev Med Chil* (Spanish) 128, 315
  (1996): Zackheim HS+, *J Am Acad Dermatol* 34, 626
Exanthems (15%)
  (2008): Mebazaa A+, *Ann Pharmacother* 42(1), 138
  (2003): Feizy V+, *Dermatol Online J* 9(1), 14
Folliculitis
Furunculosis
  (1996): Zackheim HS+, *J Am Acad Dermatol* 34, 626
Herpes simplex
  (1996): Vonderheid EC+, *J Am Acad Dermatol* 34, 470
Herpes zoster
  (2005): Kinder AJ+, *Rheumatology* (Oxford) 44(1), 61
Inflammation (reactivation)
Koebner phenomenon
  (2008): Yoon TY+, *J Dermatol* 35(3), 175
Lymphadenopathy
  (2006): Svensson AM+, *Int J Hematol* 83(1), 47
Lymphoma
  (2006): Chim CS+, *Haematologica* 91(8), ECR3
  (2006): Ikeda J+, *Int J Hematol* 83(4), 363
  (2006): Kennedy JW+, *J Hand Surg [AM]* 31(7), 1193
  (2006): Kojima M+, *Pathol Res Pract* 202(9), 679
Melanoma
  (1984): Wemmer U, *Z Hautkr* (German) 59, 665
Molluscum contagiosum
  (2007): Lim KS+, *Clin Exp Dermatol* 32(5), 591
Necrosis
  (1987): Harrison PV, *Br J Dermatol* 116, 867
  (1983): Reed KM+, *J Am Acad Dermatol* 8, 677
  (1982): Lawrence CM+, *Br J Dermatol* 107, 24
Nodular eruption
  (2004): Rivero MG+, *Rheumatology* (Oxford) 43(12), 1587
  (2001): Ahmed SS+, *Medicine* (Baltimore) 80(4), 271
  (1999): Dash S+, *J Rheumatol* 26(6), 1396
  (1999): Jang KA+, *J Dermatol* 26(7), 460
  (1998): Williams FM+, *J Am Acad Dermatol* 39, 359
  (1997): Falcini F+, *Arthritis Rheum* 40(1), 175
  (1996): Muzaffer MA+, *J Pediatr* 128, 698
  (1996): Smith MD, *J Rheumatol* 23, 2004
  (1995): Berris B+, *J Rheumatol* 22, 2359
  (1995): Das SK+, *J Assoc Physicians India* 43, 651
  (1994): Abu-Shakra M+, *J Rheumatol* 21, 934
  (1994): Karam NE+, *J Rheumatol* 21, 1960
  (1994): Smith MD, *J Rheumatol* 22, 1439
  (1992): Kerstens PJSM+, *J Rheumatol* 19, 867
  (1988): Segal R+, *Arthritis Rheum* 31, 1182
Non-Hodgkin's lymphoma
  (2006): Acero J+, *J Oral Maxillofac Surg* 64(4), 708

  (2006): Mackie GC+, *Clin Nucl Med* 31(5), 272
Photo-recall
  (2006): Kaya TI+, *J Eur Acad Dermatol Venereol* 20(3), 353 (with cytarabine)
  (2002): Thami GP+, *Postgrad Med J* 78(916), 116
  (2001): Camidge DR, *Am J Clin Oncol* 24(2), 211
  (2000): Kharfan Dabaja MA+, *Am J Clin Oncol* 23(5), 531
  (1995): Guzzo C+, *Photodermatol Photoimmunol Photomed* 11, 55 (sunburn)
Photosensitivity (5%)
  (2007): Bangert CA+, *Dermatol Ther* 20(4), 216 (passim)
  (2002): Thami GP+, *Postgrad Med J* 78(916), 116 (recall)
  (1996): Zackheim HS+, *J Am Acad Dermatol* 34, 626
  (1994): Oliver F, *The Schoch Letter* 44, 6 (observation)
  (1985): Neiman RA+, *J Rheumatol* 12, 354
Pigmentation (1–10%)
Pruritus (1–5%)
  (1998): Roenigk HH+, *J Am Acad Dermatol* 38, 478
Purpura
Radiodermatitis (reactivation)
Rash (sic) (1–3%)
  (2000): Emery P+, *Rheumatology* (Oxford) 39(6), 655
  (1995): Copur S+, *Anticancer Drugs* 6, 154
Raynaud's phenomenon
  (1988): Segal R+, *Arthritis Rheum* 31(9), 1182
Scabies (reactivation)
Side effects (sic)
  (1997): Kasteler JS+, *J Am Acad Dermatol* 36, 67 (passim)
  (1996): Furuya T+, *Rymachi* (Japanese) 36, 746
Squamous cell carcinoma
  (1989): Jensen DB+, *Acta Derm Venereol* (Stockh) 69, 274
Stevens–Johnson syndrome
  (2000): Hani N+, *Eur J Dermatol* 10(7), 548
  (1993): Cuthbert RJ+, *Ulster Med J* 62, 95
Sunburn (reactivation)
  (2000): Khan AJ+, *Cutis* 66, 379
  (1998): Roenigk HH+, *J Am Acad Dermatol* 38, 478
  (1987): Westwick TJ+, *Cutis* 39, 49
  (1986): Mallory SB+, *Pediatrics* 78, 514
  (1981): Korossy KS+, *Arch Dermatol* 117, 310
Telangiectasia
Toxic epidermal necrolysis (<1%)
  (2007): Gaigl Z+, *Eur J Dermatol* 17(2), 168
  (2000): Yang CH+, *Int J Dermatol* 39, 621 (with co-trimoxazole)
  (1999): Stone N+, *Clin Exp Dermatol* 24(4), 260
  (1997): Primka EJ+, *J Am Acad Dermatol* 36, 815 (fatal)
Toxicity (sic)
  (2006): Wessels JA+, *Arthritis Rheum* 54(4), 1087
Ulceration of psoriatic plaques
  (2003): *Prescrire Int* 12(64), 59
Ulcerations
  (2003): *Prescrire Int* 12(64), 59 (legs)
  (2003): Kazlow DW+, *J Am Acad Dermatol* 49(2), S197
  (2001): Del Pozo J+, *Eur J Dermatol* 11(5), 450 (knuckles)
  (2000): Montero LC+, *J Rheumatol* 27(9), 2290
  (1998): Ben-Amitai D+, *Ann Pharmacother* 32, 651
  (1998): Roenigk HH+, *J Am Acad Dermatol* 38, 478 (of psoriatic lesions)
  (1984): Lawrence CM+, *J Am Acad Dermatol* 11(6), 1059
Urticaria
  (2003): *Prescrire Int* 12(64), 59
  (1998): Roenigk HH+, *J Am Acad Dermatol* 38, 478
  (1995): al-Lamki Z+, *Med Pediatr Oncol* 24, 137
  (1983): Bronner AK+, *J Am Acad Dermatol* 9, 645
Vasculitis (>10%)
  (2000): Borcea A+, *Br J Dermatol* 143, 203 (urticarial)
  (1998): Halevy S+, *J Eur Acad Dermatol Venereol* 10, 81
  (1997): Torner O+, *Clin Rheumatol* 16, 108

(1995): Blanco R+, *Arthritis Rheum* 39, 1016
(1989): Fondevila CG+, *Br J Haematol* 72, 591
(1989): Jeurissen MEC+, *Clin Rheumatol* 8, 417
(1988): Segal R+, *Arthritis Rheum* 31(9), 1182
(1986): Navarro M+, *Ann Intern Med* 105, 471
(1984): Marks CR+, *Ann Intern Med* 100, 916

Mucosal/ENT

Aphthous stomatitis
(2003): Yoshida T+, *J Rheumatol* 30(9), 2082
Dysgeusia
(1988): Duhra P+, *Clin Exp Dermatol* 13, 126
Gingivitis (>10%)
Glossitis (>10%)
Mucositis
(2007): Bangert CA+, *Dermatol Ther* 20(4), 216 (passim)
(2005): Mazokopakis EE+, *Phytomedicine* 12(1-2), 25
(2005): Tonanont M+, *J Med Assoc Thai* 88(10), 1349 (6%)
(2000): Alfaro J+, *Rev Med Chil* (Spanish) 128, 315
Oral mucositis
(1997): Plevova P+, *J Natl Cancer Inst* 89, 326
(1996): Moe PJ, *Pediatr Hematol Oncol* 13, 313
(1996): Rask C+, *Pediatr Hematol Oncol* 13, 359
(1996): Zackheim HS+, *J Am Acad Dermatol* 34, 626
Oral ulceration
(2005): Deeming GM+, *Br Dent J* 2005 Jan 22;198(2), 83
(2003): *Prescrire Int* 12(64), 59
(2001): Litt JZ, Beachwood, OH (severe) (personal case)
(observation)
(2001): Werth V, *Dermatology Times* 15
(2000): Madinier I+, *Ann Med Interne* (Paris) (French) 151, 248
(1986): Barrett AP, *J Periodontol* 57, 318
Stomatitis (3-10%)
(1998): Roenigk HH+, *J Am Acad Dermatol* 38, 478 (ulcerative)
(1998): Zieglschmid ME+, *J Am Acad Dermatol* 38, 130
(1997): Kasteler JS+, *J Am Acad Dermatol* 36, 67 (passim)
(1996): Vonderheid EC+, *J Am Acad Dermatol* 34, 470
(1995): Zieglschmid-Adams ME+, *J Am Acad Dermatol* 32, 754
(1994): Montecucco C+, *Arthritis Rheum* 37, 777
Tinnitus

Hair

Hair – alopecia (1–6%)
(2007): Bangert CA+, *Dermatol Ther* 20(4), 216 (passim)
(2006): Weisman MH+, *Arthritis Rheum* 54(2), 607
(2000): Emery P+, *Rheumatology* (Oxford) 39, 655
(1998): Roenigk HH+, *J Am Acad Dermatol* 38, 478
(1998): Zieglschmid ME+, *J Am Acad Dermatol* 38, 130
(1997): Kasteler JS+, *J Am Acad Dermatol* 36, 67 (passim)
(1996): Zackheim HS+, *J Am Acad Dermatol* 34, 626
(1995): Zieglschmid-Adams ME+, *J Am Acad Dermatol* 32, 754
(1989): Fehlauer CS+, *J Rheumatol* 16, 307
(1988): Weinblatt ME+, *Arthritis Rheum* 31 (Suppl), s115
(1982): Bachman DM, *Arthritis Rheum* 25, s65
(1982): Bertino JR, *Med Pediatr Oncol* 10, 401
Hair – pigmented bands
(1983): Wheeland RG+, *Cancer* 51, 1356

Nails

Nails – discoloration
Nails – paronychia
(1983): Wantzin GL+, *Arch Dermatol* 119, 623
Nails – pigmentation
(1998): Malka N+, *Dermatology* 197(3), 276 (yellow)
(1981): Nixon DW+, *Cutis* 27, 181

Eyes

Optic neuropathy
(2005): Clare G+, *J Neuroophthalmol* 25(2), 109
(2002): Balachandran C+, *Clin Experiment Ophthalmol* 30(6), 440

Scotoma
(2006): Sbeity ZH+, *J Med Liban* 54(3), 164
Visual disturbances
(2004): Johansson B, *Acta Ophthalmol Scand* 2004 Oct;82(5), 625

Other

Anaphylactoid reactions/Anaphylaxis (1–10%)
(2006): Houtman PM+, *J Clin Rheumatol* 12(6), 321 (with etanercept)
(2003): *Prescrire Int* 12(64), 59
(2003): MacGinnitie AJ+, *Pediatr Allergy Immunol* 14(5), 409
(1996): Alkins SA+, *Cancer* 77, 2123
(1995): Lobelle C+, *Pediatr Hematol Oncol* 12, 213
Asthenia
(2007): Bangert CA+, *Dermatol Ther* 20(4), 216 (passim)
(2006): Weisman MH+, *Arthritis Rheum* 54(2), 607
Candidiasis
Cough
(2006): Weisman MH+, *Arthritis Rheum* 54(2), 607
Death
(2006): Kelly H+, *Obstet Gynecol* 107(2), 439
(2005): Kinder AJ+, *Rheumatology* (Oxford) 44(1), 61
Gynecomastia
(2007): Abe K+, *Mod Rheumatol* 17(6), 511
(2006): Pandhi D+, *Clin Exp Dermatol* 31(1), 138
(2004): Schmutz JL+, *Ann Dermatol Venereol* 131(11), 1024
(1995): Finger DR+, *J Rheumatol* 22, 796
(1995): Thomas E+, *J Rheumatol* 22, 2189
(1983): Del Paine DW+, *Arthritis Rheum* 26, 691
Headache
(2006): Weisman MH+, *Arthritis Rheum* 54(2), 607
Hepatotoxicity
(2007): Bangert CA+, *Dermatol Ther* 20(4), 216 (passim)
(2006): Berends MA+, *Aliment Pharmacol Ther* 24(5), 805
(2006): Boey O+, *Acta Clin Belg* 61(4), 166
(2006): Tilling L+, *Clin Drug Investig* 26(2), 55
(2005): Nieminen U+, *Duodecim - Duodecim* 121(24), 2680
(2005): Tonanont M+, *J Med Assoc Thai* 88(10), 1349 (6%)
(1998): Hakim NS+, *Int Surg* 83(3), 224
(1997): Cuellar ML+, *Rheum Dis Clin North Am* 23(4), 797
Hypersensitivity
(2007): Bangert CA+, *Dermatol Ther* 20(4), 216 (passim)
(2003): *Prescrire Int* 12(64), 59
Inappropriate secretion of antidiuretic hormone (SIADH)
(1988): Frahm H+, *Z Gesamte Inn Med* 43(15), 411
Infections (sic)
(2007): Bangert CA+, *Dermatol Ther* 20(4), 216 (passim)
Myalgia/Myositis/Myopathy/Myotoxicity
Nephrotoxicity
(2006): Widemann BC+, *Oncologist* 11(6), 694
(2004): Widemann BC+, *Cancer* 100(10), 2222 (%)
(2003): Kinoshita A+, *Cancer Chemother Pharmacol* 51(3), 256
(2003): Miyazaki J+, *Nippon Rinsho* 61(6), 973
(2002): Saland JM+, *Pediatr Nephrol* 17(10), 825
(2002): Sauer M+, *Pediatr Hematol Oncol* 19(2), 135
(2001): Kintzel PE, *Drug Saf* 24(1), 19
(2000): Abrey LE+, *J Clin Oncol* 18(17), 3144
(1999): Krackhardt A+, *Leuk Lymphoma* 35(5–6), 631
(1998): Kepka L+, *Leuk Lymphoma* 29(1–2), 205
(1998): Koch Nogueira PC+, *Pediatr Nephrol* 12(7), 572
(1997): Tesar V+, *Cas Lek Cesk* 136(7), 205
(1997): Widemann BC+, *J Clin Oncol* 15(5), 2125
Neurotoxicity
(2006): Haykin ME+, *J Neurooncol* 76(2), 153
(2006): Nakajima D+, *No To Hattatsu* 38(3), 195
Panniculitis
(2002): Nezondet-Chetaille AL+, *Joint Bone Spine* 69(3), 324
Peyronie's disease
(1992): Phelan MJI, *Br J Rheumatol* 31, 425

Porphyria cutanea tarda
  (1983): Malina L+, *Z Hautkr* (German) 58, 241
Pseudolymphoma
  (1997): Flipo RM+, *J Rheumatol* 24, 809
  (1995): Delaporte E+, *Ann Dermatol Venereol* (French) 122, 521
    (20 cases)
  (1994): Zimmer-Galler I+, *Mayo Clin Proc* 69, 258
  (1993): Kamel OW+, *N Engl J Med* 328, 1317
  (1993): Kerl H+, *Dermatology in General Medicine* McGraw-Hill,
    New York
  (1993): Shiroky JB+, *N Engl J Med* 329(22), 1657
  (1993): Taillan B+, *Rev Rhum Ed Fr* 60(3), 248
  (1992): Kingsmore SF+, *J Rheumatol* 19(9), 1462
  (1991): Ellman MH+, *J Rheumatol* 18(11), 1741
  (1991): Shiroky JB+, *J Rheumatol* 18(8), 1172
Stroke
  (2004): Rollins N+, *AJNR Am J Neuroradiol* 25(10), 1688
Tendinopathy/Tendon rupture
  (2001): Toverud EL+, *Med Pediatr Oncol* 37(2), 156
Vertigo
  (2005): Swale VJ+, *Clin Exp Dermatol* 30(3), 295

METHOXSALEN

Trade names: 8-MOP (Valeant); Geroxalen; Meladinine;
Oxsoralen (Valeant); Oxsoralon; Puvasoralen; Ultra-MOP
Indications: Psoriasis, vitiligo
Category: Psoralen; Repigmenting agent
Half-life: 1.1 hours
**Clinically important, potentially hazardous interactions
with: caffeine**, chloroquine, cyclosporine, fluoroquinolones,
phenothiazines, sulfonamides

Reactions

Skin

Acne
Acute generalized exanthematous pustulosis (AGEP)
  (2002): Morant C+, *Ann Dermatol Venereol* 129(2), 234
Basal cell carcinoma
  (1996): Stern RS+, *J Pediatr* 129, 915
  (1995): Gritiyarangsan P+, *Photodermatol Photoimmunol
    Photomed* 11, 174
Bowen's disease
Bullous dermatitis (with UVA)
  (1982): Stüttgen G, *Int J Dermatol* 21, 198
Bullous pemphigoid
  (1996): Perl S+, *Dermatology* 193, 245
Burning (1–10%)
  (1996): Geary P, *Burns* 22, 636
  (1991): Boucaud C+, *Presse Med* (French) 20, 1945
  (1982): Stüttgen G, *Int J Dermatol* 21, 198 (passim) (1–10%)
Carcinoma
  (1995): Halder RM+, *Arch Dermatol* 131, 734
  (1984): Halprin KM+, *Natl Cancer Inst Monogr* 66, 185
Dermatitis
  (1994): Korffmacher H+, *Contact Dermatitis* 30, 283
  (1991): Takashima A+, *Br J Dermatol* 124, 37
  (1980): Weissmann I+, *Br J Dermatol* 102, 113
Eczema
Edema (1–10%)
Ephelides (1–10%)
  (1995): Gritiyarangsan P+, *Photodermatol Photoimmunol
    Photomed* 11, 174
  (1995): Pierard GE+, *Dermatology* 190, 338
  (1984): Kietzmann E+, *Dermatologica* 168, 306

  (1983): Kanerva L+, *Dermatologica* 166, 281
  (1983): Kietzmann H+, *Ann Dermatol Venereol* (French) 110, 63
Erythema (1–10%)
Exanthems
  (2001): Ravenscroft J+, *J Am Acad Dermatol* 45, S2118–9
  (1986): Gisslen P+, *Photodermatol* 3, 308
Exfoliative dermatitis
Granuloma annulare
Herpes simplex
  (1982): Stüttgen G, *Int J Dermatol* 21, 198
Herpes zoster
  (1982): Stüttgen G, *Int J Dermatol* 21, 198
Hypomelanosis (1–10%)
Lichen planus
  (2003): Nanda S+, *J Dermatol* 30(2), 151
Lichen planus pemphigoides
  (2000): Kuramoto N+, *Br J Dermatol* 142(3), 509
Lupus erythematosus
  (1985): Bruze M+, *Acta Derm Venereol* (Stockh) 65, 31
Miliaria
Pemphigus
Photosensitivity
  (2001): Tanew A+, *J Am Acad Dermatol* 44, 638
  (1998): Clark SM+, *Contact Dermatitis* 38, 289
  (1992): Jeanmougin M+, *Ann Dermatol Venereol* (French)
    119, 277
  (1991): Boucaud C+, *Presse Med* (French) 20, 1945
  (1991): Takashima A+, *Br J Dermatol* 124, 37
  (1990): Cox NH+, *Clin Exp Dermatol* 15, 75
  (1989): Cox NH+, *Photodermatol* 6, 96
Phototoxicity
  (1997): Morison WL+, *J Am Acad Dermatol* 36, 183
  (1993): Calzavara-Pinton PG+, *J Am Acad Dermatol* 28, 657
  (1989): Morison WL, *Arch Dermatol* 125, 433 (topical)
  (1985): Berakha GJ+, *Ann Plast Surg* 14, 458
  (1984): Meffert H+, *Photodermatol* 1, 191
Pigmentation
  (1989): Weiss E+, *Int J Dermatol* 28, 188
  (1987): Bruce DR+, *J Am Acad Dermatol* 16, 1087
  (1986): MacDonald KJS+, *Br J Dermatol* 114, 395
Porokeratosis (actinic)
  (1988): Beiteke U+, *Photodermatol* 5, 274
  (1985): Hazen PG+, *J Am Acad Dermatol* 12, 1077
  (1980): Reymond JL, *Acta Derm Venereol* (Stockh) 60, 539
Prurigo
  (1982): Stüttgen G, *Int J Dermatol* 21, 198 (passim)
Pruritus (>10%)
  (1982): Stüttgen G, *Int J Dermatol* 21, 198 (passim)
Purpura
  (1981): Barriere H+, *Nouv Presse Med* (French) 10, 337
Rash (sic) (1–10%)
Scleroderma
Seborrheic dermatitis
  (1983): Tegner E, *Acta Derm Venereol* (Stockh) Suppl 107, 5
Squamous cell carcinoma
  (1998): Stern RS+, *Arch Dermatol* 134, 1582 (with UVA)
  (1986): Kahn JR+, *Clin Exp Dermatol* 11, 398
Urticaria
  (1994): Bech-Thomsen N+, *J Am Acad Dermatol* 31, 1063
Vasculitis
  (1981): Barriere H+, *Presse Med* (French) 10, 37
Verrucae
  (1982): Stüttgen G, *Int J Dermatol* 21, 198
Vitiligo
  (1983): Tegner E, *Acta Derm Venereol* (Stockh) Suppl 107, 5
Xerosis

Mucosal/ENT
Anosmia
(2003): Martin S+, *Photodermatol Photoimmunol Photomed*
19(4), 213
Cheilitis (1–10%)

Hair
Hair – hypertrichosis
(1983): Rampen FHJ, *Br J Dermatol* 109, 657

Nails
Nails – photo-onycholysis
(1990): Baran R+, *Ann Dermatol Venereol* (French) 117, 367
(1984): Balato N+, *Photodermatol* 1, 202
Nails – pigmentation
(1990): Trattner A+, *Int J Dermatol* 29, 310
(1989): Weiss E+, *Int J Dermatol* 28, 188
(1986): MacDonald KJS+, *Br J Dermatol* 114, 395
(1982): Naik RPC+, *Int J Dermatol* 21, 275

Other
Anaphylactoid reactions/Anaphylaxis
(2003): Park JY+, *Photodermatol Photoimmunol Photomed*
19(1), 37
(2001): Legat FJ+, *Br J Dermatol* 145(5), 821
Lymphoproliferative disease
(1989): Aschinoff R+, *J Am Acad Dermatol* 21, 1134
Pain
(1987): Norris PG+, *Clin Exp Dermatol* 12, 403
(1983): Tegner E, *Acta Derm Venereol* (Stockh) Suppl 107, 5
Tumors
(1988): Gupta AK+, *J Am Acad Dermatol* 19, 67
(1987): Henseler T+, *J Am Acad Dermatol* 16, 108

METHOXYFLURANE

Trade name: Penthrane (Abbott) (Ger)
Indications: Anesthesia
Category: Anesthetic, inhalation
Half-life: N/A
**Clinically important, potentially hazardous interactions
with:** cisatracurium, demeclocycline, doxacurium, doxycycline,
gentamicin, kanamycin, minocycline, neomycin, oxytetracycline,
pancuronium, rapacuronium, streptomycin, tetracycline

Reactions

Other
Hepatotoxicity
(1983): Delia JE+, *Int J Gynaecol Obstet* 21(1), 89
(1982): Zeana CD+, *Med Interne* 20(4), 295
Nephrotoxicity
(1996): Bosch T, *Anaesthesist* 45 Suppl 1, S41
(1995): Kharasch ED+, *Anesthesiology* 82(3), 689
(1987): Toomath RJ+, *N Z Med J* 100(836), 707
(1982): Mazzia VD, *Leg Med* 59

METHSUXIMIDE

Trade names: Celontin (Pfizer); Petinutin
Indications: Absence (petit-mal) seizures
Category: Antiepileptic, succinimide
Half-life: 2–4 hours

Reactions

Skin
Acanthosis nigricans
Erythema multiforme
Exanthems
Exfoliative dermatitis (<1%)
Lupus erythematosus (>10%)
Pruritus
Purpura
Rash (sic)
Stevens–Johnson syndrome (>10%)
Urticaria (<1%)

Mucosal/ENT
Gingival hyperplasia/hypertrophy
Oral ulceration

Hair
Hair – alopecia
Hair – hirsutism

Eyes
Periorbital edema

Other
Asthenia
(1983): Browne TR+, *Neurology* 33(4), 414
Headache
(1983): Browne TR+, *Neurology* 33(4), 414

METHYCLOTHIAZIDE

Trade names: Enduron-M; Thiazidil; Urimor
Indications: Hypertension
Category: Diuretic, thiazide
Half-life: N/A
**Clinically important, potentially hazardous interactions
with:** digoxin, lithium

Note: Methyclothiazide is a sulfonamide and can be absorbed
systemically. Sulfonamides can produce severe, possibly fatal,
reactions such as toxic epidermal necrolysis and Stevens–Johnson
syndrome

Reactions

Skin
Erythema multiforme
Exanthems
Photosensitivity (<1%)
Purpura
Rash (sic) (<1%)
Stevens–Johnson syndrome
Urticaria

Mucosal/ENT
Dysgeusia

Other

Anaphylactoid reactions/Anaphylaxis
Paresthesias (<1%)

METHYLDOPA

Trade names: Aldoclor (Merck); Aldomet; Aldoril; Amodopa; Densul; Dopamet; Equibar; Hydopa; Medimet; Nu-Medopa; Polinal; Presinol; Prodopa
Indications: Hypertension
Category: Adrenergic alpha-receptor agonist
Half-life: 1.7 hours
Clinically important, potentially hazardous interactions with: ephedrine

Note: Aldoril is methyldopa and hydrochlorothiazide

Reactions

Skin

Allergic granulomatous angiitis (Churg–Strauss syndrome)
Eczema
Edema
Erythema multiforme (<1%)
  (1985): Ting HC+, *Int J Dermatol* 24, 587
Erythema nodosum
Exanthems (3%)
  (1986): Gidseg G, *South Med J* 79, 389
Fixed eruption
Lichen planus
  (1994): Thompson DF+, *Pharmacotherapy* 14, 561
Lichenoid eruption
  (1986): Gonzalez JG+, *J Am Acad Dermatol* 15, 87
  (1982): Brooks SL, *J Oral Med* 37, 42
  (1982): Wiesenfeld D+, *Oral Surg Oral Med Oral Pathol* 54, 527
  (1980): *Med J Aust* 2, 130
Lupus erythematosus (<1%)
  (1995): Sakurai Y+, *Nippon Naika Gakkai Zasshi* (Japanese) 84, 2069
  (1994): Yung RL+, *Rheum Dis Clin North Am* 20, 61
  (1992): Skaer TL, *Clin Ther* 14, 496
  (1989): Nordstrom DM+, *Arthritis Rheum* 32, 205
  (1985): Cush JJ+, *Am J Med Sci* 290, 36
  (1985): Stratton MA, *Clin Pharm* 4, 657
  (1983): Homberg JC+, *J Pharmacol* (French) 14, 61
  (1982): Dupont A+, *BMJ* 2, 693
  (1981): Harrington TM+, *Chest* 79, 696
Papulovesicular eruption
Peripheral edema
Petechiae
Photosensitivity
  (1988): Vaillant L+, *Arch Dermatol* 124, 326
Pigmentation
  (1986): Brody HJ+, *Cutis* 38, 187
Pruritus
Purpura
Rash (sic) (<1%)
Seborrheic dermatitis
Stevens–Johnson syndrome
  (1985): Ting HC+, *Int J Dermatol* 24, 587
Toxic epidermal necrolysis
Urticaria
  (1986): Gidseg G, *S Med J* 79, 389
Vasculitis
  (1989): Matteson EL+, *Arthritis Rheum* 32, 356

Mucosal/ENT

Cheilitis
Glossodynia
Oral lichenoid eruption
  (1990): Espana A+, *Med Clin* (Barc) (Spanish) 94, 559
  (1988): Zain RB+, *Dent J Malays* 10, 15
  (1982): Brooks SL, *J Oral Med* 37, 42
Oral mucosal eruption
Oral ulceration
  (1980): McLellan GH+, *Clin Prevent Dent* 2, 18
Tongue black (<1%)
  (1986): Brody HJ+, *Cutis* 38, 137
Xerostomia (1–10%)

Hair

Hair – alopecia

Other

Gynecomastia (<1%)
Headache
Hepatotoxicity
  (2006): Phadnis SV+, *Aust N Z Obstet Gynaecol* 46(3), 256
  (2005): Fernandez-Marcote Menor EM+, *Rev Esp Enferm* 97(11), 840
  (2002): Chitturi S+, *Semin Liver Dis* 22(2), 169
Hypersensitivity
  (1993): Wolf R+, *Ann Allergy* 71, 166
Myalgia/Myositis/Myopathy/Myotoxicity
Nephrotoxicity
  (2006): Mazze RI, *Anesthesiology* 105(4), 843
Paresthesias (<1%)

METHYLPHENIDATE

Trade names: Centedrin; Concerta; Daytrana; Metadate CD (Celltech); Methylin (Mallinckrodt); Rilatine; Ritalin (Novartis); Rubifen
Indications: Attention deficit disorder, narcolepsy
Category: Amphetamine
Half-life: 2–4 hours
Clinically important, potentially hazardous interactions with: bupropion, cyclosporine, escitalopram, phenylbutazone, pimozide

Reactions

Skin

Angioedema
Diaphoresis
Erythema multiforme
Exanthems
Exfoliative dermatitis
Fixed eruption
  (1992): Cohen HA+, *Ann Pharmacother* 26, 1378 (scrotum)
Photosensitivity
Pruritus
Purpura
Rash (sic) (<1%)
Urticaria
Vasculitis

Mucosal/ENT

Sialorrhea
  (2003): Lavretsky H+, *J Clin Psychiatry* 64(12), 1410 (with citalopram)

Xerostomia
(2003): Lavretsky H+, *J Clin Psychiatry* 64(12), 1410 (with citalopram)
(1993): Pataki CS+, *J Am Acad Child Adolesc Psychiatry* 32, 1065

Hair
Hair – alopecia

Eyes
Eyelid edema

Other
Cardiotoxicity
(2006): *Prescrire Int* 15(84), 138
(2006): Langendijk PN+, *Ned Tijdschr Geneeskd* 150(31), 1713
Delusions of parasitosis
(1999): Eisner J (from Internet) (observation)
Depression
(2003): Gothelf D+, *J Clin Psychiatry* 64(10), 1163
Headache
(2006): McGough JJ+, *J Child Adolesc Psychopharmacol* 16(3), 351
Hypersensitivity (1–10%)
(1990): Calis KA+, *Clin Pharm* 9, 632
Injection-site abscess
Stroke
(2006): Thomalla G+, *World J Biol Psychiatry* 7(1), 56

METHYLPREDNISOLONE

Trade names: Advantan (Intendis); Medrol (Pharmacia); Solu-Medrol (Pharmacia)
Indications: Arthralgias, Asthma, Dermatoses, Ophthalmology, Rhinitis (many others)
Category: Corticosteroid, systemic
Half-life: N/A
Clinically important, potentially hazardous interactions with: aspirin, carbamazepine, clarithromycin, cyclosporine, daclizumab, erythromycin, itraconazole, ketoconazole, **live vaccines**, oral contraceptives, phenobarbital, rifampicin, rifampin, theophylline, troleandomycin, warfarin

Reactions

Skin
Acute generalized exanthematous pustulosis
(2001): Mussot-Chia+, *Ann Dermatol Venereol* 128(3), 241
Allergic reactions (sic)
(2003): Freymond N+, *Rev Med Interne* 24(10), 698
(2003): Ventura MT+, *Br J Dermatol* 148(1), 139
(1998): Vanpee D+, *Ann Emerg Med* 32(6), 754
Bruising
(1998): Dasgupta B+, *Br J Rheumatol* 37(2), 189
Dermatitis
(2004): Cahill J+, *Australas J Dermatol* 45(3), 192
(2000): Chew AL+, *Cutis* 65(5), 307
(1998): Corazza M+, *Contact Dermatitis* 38(6), 356
(1997): Balato N+, *Am J Contact Dermat* 8(1), 24
(1992): Aramoto Y+, *J Dermatol* 19(6), 375
Erythroderma
(1991): Fernandez de+, *Contact Dermatitis* 25(1), 68
Kaposi's sarcoma
(2004): Monti M+, *J Eur Acad Dermatol Venereol* 18(2), 191
Perioral dermatitis
(2001): Chow ET, *Australas J Dermatol* 42(1), 62
Pruritus

(2005): Hardy D, *Can J Anaesth* 52(2), 186 (with bupivacaine & epinephrine)
(2002): Mignogna MD+, *J Oral Pathol Med* 31(6), 339
Rash (sic)
(2004): Kuga A+, *Rinsho Shinkeigaku* 44(10), 691
(2001): Macchia PE+, *J Endocrinol Invest* 24(3), 152
Stevens–Johnson syndrome
(2002): Samimi SS+, *Pediatr Dermatol* 19(1), 52
Thinning
Urticaria
(2001): Borja JM+, *Allergy* 56(8), 791
(2001): Pollack B+, *Br J Dermatol* 144, 1228
(1996): Pizzuti P+, *Rev Rhum Engl Ed* 63(3), 223
(1990): Sieck JO+, *Br J Clin Pract* 44(12), 723

Mucosal/ENT
Dysgeusia
(2001): Macchia PE+, *J Endocrinol Invest* 24(3), 152
(1994): Chassard D+, *Presse Med* 23(11), 515
Dysphonia
(2006): Loeches-Yague B+, *Med Clin* (Barc) 126(2), 79
(2005): Hardy D, *Can J Anaesth* 52(2), 186 (with bupivacaine & epinephrine)

Hair
Hair – hypertrichosis

Eyes
Cataract
(2003): Nakamura T+, *Jpn J Ophthalmol* 47(3), 254 (with cyclosporine)
(1999): Marsh P+, *Ophthalmology* 106(4), 811
(1992): Yokota S+, *Ryumachi* 32(3), 215
Conjunctival ulceration
(1999): Zamir E+, *Ophthalmic Surg Lasers* 30(7), 565
Glaucoma
(1995): Katsushima H, *Nippon Ganka Gakkai Zasshi* 99(2), 238
(1992): Yokota S+, *Ryumachi* 32(3), 215
Ocular pain
Ocular pressure
(1999): Marsh P+, *Ophthalmology* 106(4), 811
Ophthalmitis
(2003): Mazur-Chlodek L+, *Klin Oczna* 105(3-4), 194
Periorbital urticaria
(1992): John GR+, *Am J Ophthalmol* 113(5), 588
Visual disturbances
(1991): Bettinelli A+, *Child Nephrol Urol* 11(1), 41

Other
Abdominal pain
(1994): Chassard D+, *Presse Med* 23(11), 515
Adverse effects
(2005): Chibane S+, *Rev Med Interne* 26(1), 20
(1992): Pozzi C+, *Nephron* 60(2), 235
Anaphylactoid reactions/Anaphylaxis
(2004): Saito R+, *Int J Urol* 11(3), 171
(2002): Burgdorff T+, *Ann Allergy Asthma Immunol* 89(4), 425
(2000): Young MF+, *J Neurol Neurosurg Psychiatry* 68(2), 255
(1999): Beynel P+, *Rev Mal Respir* 16(4), 529
(1999): Schonwald S, *Am J Emerg Med* 17(6), 583
(1997): Mace S+, *J Rheumatol* 24(6), 1191
(1997): van den Berg JS+, *J Neurol Neurosurg Psychiatry* 63(6), 813
(1996): Moreno-Ancillo A+, *J Allergy Clin Immunol* 97(5), 1169
(1993): Hopper JM+, *J Bone Joint Br* 75(3), 505 (with bupivacaine)
(1993): Watanabe I+, *Masui* 42(1), 112
(1991): Peces R+, *Nephron* 59(3), 497
(1990): Laine-Cessac P+, *Therapie* 45(6), 505
Asthenia

(2002): Mignogna MD+, *J Oral Pathol Med* 31(6), 339
Depression
  (2003): Antonijevic IA+, *Psychoneuroendocrinology* 28(6), 780
  (2002): Kulakowska A+, *Pol Merkuriusz Lek* 13(75), 200
  (1996): Naber D+, *Psychoneuroendocrinology* 21(1), 25
  (1993): Chrousos GA+, *JAMA* 269(16), 2110
Headache
  (2002): Mignogna MD+, *J Oral Pathol Med* 31(6), 339
Hepatotoxicity
  (2006): Topal F+, *Ann Pharmacother* 40(10), 1868
Hypersensitivity
  (2006): Sirvent AE+, *Nefrologia* 26(1), 128
  (2006): Venturini M+, *J Investig Allergol Clin Immunol* 16(1), 51
  (1996): Lopez-Serrano MC+, *J Investig Allergol Clin Immunol* 6(5), 324
Hypertension
  (2005): Chibane S+, *Rev Med Interne* 26(1), 20
  (2005): Hardy D, *Can J Anaesth* 52(2), 186 (with bupivacaine & epinephrine)
  (2003): Cortes-Hernandez J+, *Lupus* 12(4), 287
  (1992): Baethge BA+, *Ann Pharmacother* 26(3), 316
Hypotension
  (1998): Guillen EL+, *Am J Kidney Dis* 32(2), E4
Infections
  (2004): Kulig G+, *Przegl Lek* 61(8), 855
  (2004): Offidani M+, *Leuk Lymphoma* 45(8), 1617
  (2004): Tanaka Y, *Nippon Rinsho* 62(10), 1867
  (1994): Sayer HG+, *Blood* 84(4), 1328
  (1992): Baethge BA+, *Ann Pharmacother* 26(3), 316
Injection-site lipoatrophy
  (2000): Anderson B+, *Arch Intern Med* 151, 153
Lymphoproliferative disease
  (2002): Theate I+, *Eur J Haematol* 69(4), 248 (with methotrexate)
Myalgia/Myositis/Myopathy/Myotoxicity
  (2006): Lee HJ+, *Bone Marrow Transplant* 38(4), 299
  (2005): Qian T+, *Spinal Cord* 43(4), 199
  (2001): Odabas AR+, *Nephron* 87(1), 95
  (2000): Qian T+, *Med Hypotheses* 55(5), 452
Neurotoxicity
  (2004): Fodale V+, *Br J Anaesth* 92(2), 289 (with cisatracurium)
Osteoporosis
  (2004): Haugeberg G+, *Ann Rheum Dis* 63(8), 940
  (2003): de Deus RB+, *Nephron Clin Pract* 94(3), c69
Seizures
  (1996): Vaughn BV+, *Epilepsia* 37(12), 1175
  (1992): Baethge BA+, *Ann Pharmacother* 26(3), 316
  (1991): Bettinelli A+, *Child Nephrol Urol* 11(1), 41
Stroke
  (2006): Ziai WC+, *Arch Neurol* 63(11), 1643
Tendinopathy/Tendon rupture
  (2005): Chiou YM+, *Lupus* 14(4), 321
Vertigo
  (2005): Hardy D, *Can J Anaesth* 52(2), 186 (with bupivacaine & epinephrine)

METHYLTESTOSTERONE

Trade names: Android (Valeant); Androral; B; Enarmon; Estratest (Solvay); Metandren; Teston; Testotonic 'B'; Testovis; Testred (Valeant); Virilon; Viromone
Indications: Hypogonadism, impotence, metastatic breast cancer
Category: Androgen
Half-life: 2.5–3.5 hours
Clinically important, potentially hazardous interactions with: anticoagulants, cyclosporine, warfarin

Reactions

Skin
Acanthosis nigricans
  (1987): Shuttleworth D+, *Clin Exp Dermatol* 12, 288
Acne (>10%)
  (1992): Fryand O+, *Acta Derm Venereol* 72, 148
  (1990): Fuchs E+, *J Am Acad Dermatol* 23, 125
  (1989): Fryand O+, *Tidsskr Nor Laegeforen* (Norwegian) 109, 239
  (1989): Hartmann AA+, *Monatsschr Kinderheilkd* (German) 137, 466
  (1989): Heydenreich G, *Arch Dermatol* 125, 571 (fulminans)
  (1989): Scott MJ+, *Cutis* 44, 30
  (1989): von Muhlendahl KE+, *Dtsch Med Wochenschr* (German) 114, 712
  (1988): Traupe H+, *Arch Dermatol* 124, 414 (fulminans)
  (1987): Kiraly CL+, *Am J Dermatopathol* 9, 515
  (1984): Lamb DR, *Am J Sports Med* 12, 31
Dermatitis
  (1989): Holdiness MR, *Contact Dermatitis* 20, 3 (from patch)
Edema (>10%)
Exanthems
Furunculosis
  (1989): Scott MJ+, *Cutis* 44, 30
Lichenoid eruption
  (1989): Aihara M+, *J Dermatol* (Tokio) 16, 330
Lupus erythematosus
Pruritus
Psoriasis
  (1990): O'Driscoll JB+, *Clin Exp Dermatol* 15, 68
Purpura
Seborrhea
Seborrheic dermatitis
  (1989): Scott MJ+, *Cutis* 44, 30
Striae
  (1989): Scott MJ+, *Cutis* 44, 30
Urticaria

Mucosal/ENT
Stomatitis

Hair
Hair – alopecia
  (1989): Scott MJ+, *Cutis* 44, 30
Hair – hirsutism (1–10%) (in females)
  (1994): Castillo-Ceballos A+, *Med Clin* (Barc) (Spanish) 102, 78
  (1991): Bates GW+, *Clin Obstet Gynecol* 34, 848
  (1991): No Author, *Obstet Gynecol* 78, 474
  (1991): Parker LU+, *Cleve Clin J Med* 58, 43
  (1991): Urman B+, *Obstet Gynecol* 77, 595
  (1989): Scott MJ+, *Cutis* 44, 30

Eyes
Intraocular pressure increased
  (2006): Khurana RN+, *Am J Ophthalmol* 142(3), 494

Other
Anaphylactoid reactions/Anaphylaxis
Gynecomastia (<1%)
Headache
Hypersensitivity (<1%)
Injection-site pain
Paresthesias

METHYSERGIDE

Trade names: Deseril; Desernil; Deserril; Deseryl; Sansert (Novartis)
Indications: Vascular (migraine) headaches
Category: Hallucinogen; Psychotomimetic
Half-life: 10 hours
Clinically important, potentially hazardous interactions with: almotriptan, amprenavir, clarithromycin, delavirdine, efavirenz, erythromycin, indinavir, naratriptan, nelfinavir, ritonavir, rizatriptan, saquinavir, sibutramine, sumatriptan, troleandomycin, zolmitriptan

Reactions

Skin
Adverse effects (sic)
  (1991): Mylecharane EJ, *J Neurol* 238, S45
Collagen disease
Exanthems
Hypermelanosis
Lupus erythematosus
Orange-peel skin
Peripheral edema (1–10%)
Pruritus
Rash (sic) (1–10%)
Raynaud's phenomenon
Scleroderma
  (2005): Kluger N+, *Br J Dermatol* 153(1), 224
  (1984): Garcia de Quesada FJ I, *Med Clin* (Barc) (Spanish) 82, 604
  (1980): Graham JR, *Trans Am Clin Climatol Assoc* 92, 122
Telangiectasia
Urticaria

Hair
Hair – alopecia
  (1991): Mylecharane EJ, *J Neurol* 238, S45

Other
Cardiotoxicity
  (2006): *Prescrire Int* 15(85), 184
Headache
Myalgia/Myositis/Myopathy/Myotoxicity
Paresthesias

METIPRANOLOL

Trade names: Disorat; Metipranolol; OptiPranolol (Bausch & Lomb); Ripix; Turoptin
Indications: Open angle glaucoma, ocular hypertension
Category: Adrenergic beta-receptor antagonist
Half-life: N/A
Clinically important, potentially hazardous interactions with: beta-blockers, calcium channel blockers, reserpine

Reactions

Skin
Allergic reactions (sic)
Dermatitis
  (1988): de Groot AC+, *Contact Dermatitis* 18(2), 107
Psoriasis
  (1991): Steinkraus V+, *Dtsch Med Wochenschr* 116(47), 1814

Rash (sic)
Eyes
Blepharitis
Conjunctivitis
Epiphora
Eyelid burning
Eyelid dermatitis
Eyelid edema
Eyelid stinging
Ocular burning
  (1986): Ober M+, *Ophthalmologica* 192(3), 159
Ocular pain
Ocular stinging
  (1986): Ober M+, *Ophthalmologica* 192(3), 159
Uveitis
  (2005): Cano Parra J+, *Arch Soc Esp Oftalmol* 80(3), 137
  (1999): Kamalarajah S+, *Eye* 13(Pt 3a), 380
  (1998): Moorthy RS+, *Surv Ophthalmol* 42(6), 557
  (1997): Patel NP+, *Am J Ophthalmol* 123(6), 843
  (1997): Watanabe TM+, *Arch Ophthalmol* 115(3), 421
  (1996): Beck RW+, *Arch Ophthalmol* 114(10), 1181
  (1995): Burvenich H, *Bull Soc Belge Ophthalmol* 257, 63 (2 cases)
  (1994): KeBler C, *Arch Ophthalmol* 112(10), 1277
  (1994): Melles RB+, *Am J Ophthalmol* 118(6), 712 (2 cases)
  (1993): O'Connor GR, *Br J Ophthalmol* 77(8), 536
  (1993): Schultz JS+, *Arch Ophthalmol* 111(12), 1606
  (1991): Akingbehin T+, *Br J Ophthalmol* 75(9), 519
  (1991): Kinshuck D, *Br J Ophthalmol* 75(9), 575

Other
Asthenia
Cough
Depression
Headache
Myalgia/Myositis/Myopathy/Myotoxicity
Vertigo

METOCLOPRAMIDE

Trade names: Apo-Metoclop; Duraclamid; Emex; Gastrocil; Gastronerton; Maxeran; Maxolon; Mygdalon; Primperan; Reglan (Wyeth)
Indications: Gastroesophageal reflux
Category: Dopamine receptor antagonist
Half-life: 4–6 hours
Clinically important, potentially hazardous interactions with: mepenzolate, sertraline, venlafaxine, zuclopentixol acetate, zuclopentixol decanoate, zuclopentixol dihydrochloride

Reactions

Skin
Allergic reactions (sic)
  (1986): Bigby M+, *JAMA* 256, 3358
Angioedema
  (1983): Pinder RM+, *Drugs* 25, 451
Diaphoresis
  (2002): Fisher AA+, *Ann Pharmacother* 36(1), 67
Exanthems
  (1983): Pinder RM+, *Drugs* 25, 451
Rash (sic) (1–10%)
Urticaria
  (1983): Pinder RM+, *Drugs* 25, 451

Mucosal/ENT

Tongue pigmentation
  (1989): Alroe C+, *Med J Aust* 150, 724
Xerostomia (1–10%)

Eyes

Oculogyric crisis
  (2006): Hibbs AM+, *Pediatrics* 118(2), 746

Other

Abdominal pain
  (2006): Khan NU+, *J Emerg Med* 30(4), 411
Anaphylactoid reactions/Anaphylaxis
  (2006): Kerstan A+, *Ann Pharmacother* 40(10), 1889
Asthenia
  (2006): Hibbs AM+, *Pediatrics* 118(2), 746
Depression
  (1986): Weddington WW Jr+, *J Clin Psychiatry* 47(4), 208
Gynecomastia
  (1997): Madani S+, *J Clin Gastroenterol* 24, 79
Insomnia
  (1986): Weddington WW Jr+, *J Clin Psychiatry* 47(4), 208
Paresthesias
  (1997): du Bois A+, *Oncology* 54, 7
Porphyria
  (1997): Gorchein A, *Lancet* 350, 1104
  (1981): Doss M+, *Lancet* 2, 91
Suicidal ideation
  (1986): Weddington WW Jr+, *J Clin Psychiatry* 47(4), 208

METOLAZONE

Trade names: Barolyn; Diondel; Metenix 5; Normelan; Xuret; Zaroxolyn (Celltech)
Indications: Hypertension, edema
Category: Diuretic, thiazide
Half-life: 6–20 hours
Clinically important, potentially hazardous interactions with: digoxin, lithium

Note: Metolazone is a sulfonamide and can be absorbed systemically. Sulfonamides can produce severe, possibly fatal, reactions such as toxic epidermal necrolysis and Stevens–Johnson syndrome

Reactions

Skin

Edema (<2%)
Exanthems
Exfoliative dermatitis
Necrotizing arteritis
  (1982): Weinrauch LA+, *Cutis* 30(1), 83
Photosensitivity (<2%)
Pruritus (<2%)
Purpura (<1%)
Rash (sic) (<2%)
Stevens–Johnson syndrome
Toxic epidermal necrolysis
  (1991): Lacy JA, *Nutr Clin Pract* 6, 18
Urticaria (<2%)
Vasculitis
  (1991): Cox NH+, *Postgrad Med J* 67, 860
  (1982): Weinrauch LA+, *Cutis* 30, 83
Xerosis (<2%)

Mucosal/ENT

Dysgeusia (<2%)
Tinnitus
Xerostomia (<2%)

Eyes

Dyschromatopsia (<2%)

Other

Anaphylactoid reactions/Anaphylaxis (<2%)
Chills (1–10%)
Headache
Myalgia/Myositis/Myopathy/Myotoxicity
Paresthesias (<2%)
Seizures
Thrombosis
  (1988): Green ST+, *Scott Med J* 33(1), 211

METOPROLOL

Trade names: Beloc-Zoc; Betaloc; Betazok; Kenaprol; Lopressor (Novartis); Mycol; Prolaken; Ritmolol; Seloken-Zok; Selozok; Toprol XL (AstraZeneca)
Indications: Hypertension, angina pectoris
Category: Adrenergic beta-receptor agonist; Antiarrhythmic class II
Half-life: 3–4 hours
Clinically important, potentially hazardous interactions with: clonidine, epinephrine, propoxyphene, telithromycin, verapamil

Note: Lopressor HCT is metoprolol and hydrochlorothiazide

Note: Cutaneous side effects of beta-receptor blockaders are clinically polymorphic. They apparently appear after several months of continuous therapy. Atypical psoriasiform, lichen planus-like, and eczematous chronic rashes are mainly observed. (1983): Hödl St, *Z Hautkr* (German) 58, 17

Reactions

Skin

Angioedema
  (1994): Krikorian RK+, *Chest* 106, 1922
Diaphoresis
Eczema
  (1981): Neumann HAM+, *Dermatologica* 162, 330
Edema
Erythema multiforme
Exanthems (1%)
  (1986): Benfield P+, *Drugs* 31, 376 (1.5%)
Exfoliative dermatitis
Hyperkeratosis (palms and soles)
Lichen planus
  (2005): Meyer S+, *J Eur Acad Dermatol Venereol* 19(2), 236
Lichenoid eruption
  (1988): Kardaun SH+, *Br J Dermatol* 118, 545
  (1983): Hödl St, *Z Hautkr* (German) 58, 17
Lupus erythematosus
  (1981): Paladini G, *Int J Tissue React* 3, 95
Peripheral edema (1%)
Pigmentation
Pityriasis rubra pilaris
Prurigo
  (1983): Hödl St, *Z Hautkr* (German) 58, 17
Pruritus (1–5%)

(1994): Shelley WB+, *Cutis* 53, 39 (scalp) (observation)
(1986): Benfield P+, *Drugs* 31, 376
Psoriasis (induction and aggravation of)
  (2002): Litt JZ, Beachwood, OH (personal case) (observation)
    (induction of)
  (2002): Yilmaz MB+, *Angiology* 53(6), 737 (rare)
  (1993): Litt JZ, Beachwood, OH (personal case) (observation)
  (1988): Heng MCY+, *Int J Dermatol* 27, 619 (pustular,
    generalized)
  (1987): Altomare GF+, *G Ital Dermatol Venereol* (Italian)
    122, 531
  (1986): Abel EA+, *J Am Acad Dermatol* 15, 1007
  (1986): Czernielewski J+, *Lancet* 1, 808
  (1984): Arntzen N+, *Acta Derm Venereol* (Stockh) 64, 346
  (1981): Neumann HAM+, *Dermatologica* 162, 330
Purpura
Rash (sic) (<5%)
  (2002): Fisher AA+, *Cardiovasc Drugs Ther* 16(2), 161
Raynaud's phenomenon (<1%)
  (2002): Fisher AA+, *Cardiovasc Drugs Ther* 16(2), 161
  (1984): Eliasson K+, *Acta Med Scand* 215, 333
Scleroderma
  (1980): Graham JR, *Trans Am Clin Climatol Assoc* 92, 122
Toxic epidermal necrolysis
Urticaria
Xerosis

Mucosal/ENT
Dysgeusia
Oral lichenoid eruption
Tinnitus

Hair
Hair – alopecia
  (1981): Graeber CW+, *Cutis* 28, 633

Nails
Nails – dystrophy
Nails – pigmentation
Nails – transverse depression
  (1981): Graeber CW+, *Cutis* 28, 633

Eyes
Oculo-mucocutaneous syndrome
  (1982): Cocco G+, *Curr Ther Res* 31, 362
Visual hallucinations
  (2006): Sirois FJ, *Psychosomatics* 47(6), 537

Other
Gangrene (feet)
Headache
Hypotension
  (2002): Fisher AA+, *Cardiovasc Drugs Ther* 16(2), 161 (2 cases)
  (2000): Joye F, *Presse Med* 29(18), 1027
Paresthesias
Peyronie's disease
  (1981): Jones HA+, *Med J Aust* 2, 514
  (1981): Neumann HAM+, *Dermatologica* 162, 330
  (1981): Paladini G, *Int J Tissue React* 3, 95
Polymyositis
  (1991): Snyder S, *Ann Intern Med* 114, 96
Scalp tingling

METRONIDAZOLE

Trade names: Arilin; Ariline; Asuzol; Clont; Flagyl (Pfizer);
Fossyol; Helidac (Prometheus); Metrocream (Galderma);
Metrogel (Galderma); Metrolotion (Galderma); Milezzol; Nida
Gel; Noritate (Dermik); Novo-Nidazol; Otrozol; Protostat;
Rozagel; Rozex; Satric; Trikacide; Zadstat
Indications: Various infections caused by susceptible organisms,
rosacea
Category: Antibiotic, nitroimidazole
Half-life: 6–12 hours
**Clinically important, potentially hazardous interactions
with: alcohol,** anisindione, anticoagulants, astemizole, dicumarol,
disulfiram, fluorouracil, mycophenolate, warfarin

Reactions

Skin
Acute generalized exanthematous pustulosis (AGEP)
  (1999): Watsky KL, *Arch Dermatol* 135, 93
  (1994): Manders SM+, *Cutis* 54, 194 (with cefazolin)
Angioedema
Dermatitis
  (2002): Choudry K+, *Contact Dermatitis* 46(1), 60
  (1997): Vincenzi C+, *Contact Dermatitis* 36, 116
Erythema
Exanthems (1–5%)
  (1995): Litt JZ, Beachwood, OH (personal case) (observation)
Fixed eruption
  (2006): Nnoruka EN+, *Int J Dermatol* 45(9), 1062
  (2005): Jaffe P, Columbia, SC (from Internet) (observation)
  (2003): Sehgal VN+, *J Eur Acad Dermatol Venereol* 17(5), 607
  (2002): Short KA, (London) (England) March AAD Poster (4
    recurrences)
  (2002): Short KA+, *Clin Exp Dermatol* 27(6), 464
  (2002): Vila JB+, *Contact Dermatitis* 46(2), 122
  (2002): Walfish AE+, *Cutis* 69, 207 (doxycycline, in the same
    patient, also produced a fixed eruption)
  (2001): Gastaminza G+, *Contact Dermatitis* 44(1), 36
  (1998): Mahboob A+, *Int J Dermatol* 37, 833
  (1998): Thami GP+, *Dermatology* 196, 368
  (1990): Gaffoor PMA+, *Cutis* 45, 242
  (1990): Kanwar AJ+, *Dermatologica* 180, 277
  (1990): Mishra D+, *Int J Dermatol* 29, 740
  (1987): Shelley WB+, *Cutis* 39, 393
Linear IgA dermatosis
Pityriasis rosea
Pruritus (1–10%)
  (2001): Gastaminza G+, *Contact Dermatitis* 44(1), 36
  (1999): Kapoor K+, *Int J Clin Pharmacol Res* 19(3), 83
Rash (sic)
Stevens–Johnson syndrome
  (2006): Piskin G+, *Contact Dermatitis* 55(3), 192
  (2003): Chen KT+, *Am J Public Health* 93(3), 489
Toxic epidermal necrolysis
  (1999): Egan CA+, *J Am Acad Dermatol* 40, 458
  (1981): Titov RL, *Klin Med Mosk* (Russian) 59, 85
Urticaria
  (1999): Kapoor K+, *Int J Clin Pharmacol Res* 19(3), 83
  (1997): Blumenthal HL, Beachwood, OH (personal case)
    (observation)

Mucosal/ENT
Dysgeusia (<1%) (metallic taste)
  (1999): Kapoor K+, *Int J Clin Pharmacol Res* 19(3), 83
  (1997): Palop Larrea V+, *Aten Primaria* (Spanish) 20, 524
Dysphagia

(2005): Takase K+, *Rinsho Shinkeigaku* 45(5), 386
Glossitis
 (1999): Kapoor K+, *Int J Clin Pharmacol Res* 19(3), 83
 (1987): Shelley WB+, *Cutis* 39, 393
Oral mucosal eruption
Oral ulceration
Stomatitis
 (1987): Shelley WB+, *Cutis* 39, 393
Tinnitus
 (1994): Lawford R+, *Clin Infect Dis* 19(2), 346
Tongue furry (<1%)
 (1987): Shelley WB+, *Cutis* 39, 393
Vulvovaginal candidiasis (<1%)
Xerostomia (<1%)
 (1999): Kapoor K+, *Int J Clin Pharmacol Res* 19(3), 83

Other
Aseptic meningitis
 (2007): Khan S+, *Ann Intern Med* 146(5), 395
Candidiasis (exacerbation)
Disulfiram-like reaction
Gynecomastia
 (1985): Fagan TC+, *JAMA* 254, 3217
Headache
 (1999): Kapoor K+, *Int J Clin Pharmacol Res* 19(3), 83
Hypersensitivity (<1%)
 (2006): Garcia-Rubio I+, *Allergol Immunopathol* (Madr) 34(2), 70
Injection-site vasculitis
Neurotoxicity
 (2006): Hobson-Webb+, *J Child Neurol* 21(5), 429
Paresthesias
 (2005): Takase K+, *Rinsho Shinkeigaku* 45(5), 386
Serum sickness
 (1983): Weart CW+, *South Med J* 76, 410
Thrombophlebitis (<1%)

MEXILETINE

Trade names: Mexihexal; Mexilen; Mexitec; Mexitil (Boehringer Ingelheim)
Indications: Ventricular arrhythmias
Category: Antiarrhythmic class 1B
Half-life: 10–12 hours
Clinically important, potentially hazardous interactions with: caffeine

Reactions

Skin
Acute generalized exanthematous pustulosis (AGEP)
 (2001): Sasaki K+, *Eur J Dermatol* 11, 469
Diaphoresis (<1%)
Edema (3.8%)
Erythema
 (2005): Sekiguchi A+, *J Dermatol* 32(4), 278
Exanthems
 (2005): Sekiguchi A+, *J Dermatol* 32(4), 278
 (2001): Sasaki K+, *Eur J Dermatol* 11(5), 469
 (1997): Higa K+, *Pain* 73, 97
 (1996): Nagayama H+, *J Dermatol* 23, 899
 (1992): Habot B+, *Harefuah* (Hebrew) 123, 462
 (1991): Kikuchi K+, *Contact Dermatitis* 25, 70
 (1988): Kardaun SH+, *Br J Dermatol* 118, 545
 (1984): Ribera Pibernat M+, *Med Clin* (Barc) (Spanish) 83, 825
Exfoliative dermatitis (<1%)

Facial edema
 (2001): Sasaki K+, *Eur J Dermatil* 11(5), 469
Lupus erythematosus (<1%)
Pruritus
 (2005): Sekiguchi A+, *J Dermatol* 32(4), 278
 (1997): Higa K+, *Pain* 73, 97
Purpura
Rash (sic) (3.8%)
Stevens–Johnson syndrome (<1%)
Urticaria
 (1994): Yamazaki S+, *Br J Dermatol* 130, 538
 (1988): Kardaun SH+, *Br J Dermatol* 118, 545
Xerosis (<1%)

Mucosal/ENT
Dysgeusia (<1%)
 (2000): Zervakis J+, *Physiol Behav* 68, 405
Tinnitus
Xerostomia (2.8%)

Hair
Hair – alopecia (<1%)

Other
Congestive heart failure
 (1989): Ravid S+, *J Am Coll Cardiol* 14(5), 1326
Headache
Hot flashes (<1%)
Hypersensitivity
 (2005): Sekiguchi A+, *J Dermatol* 32(4), 278
 (2004): Seino Y+, *Diabet Med* 21(10), 1156
Paresthesias (3.8%)
Pseudolymphoma
 (1996): Magro CM+, *Hum Pathol* 27(2), 125
Tremor (12.6%)

MEZLOCILLIN

Trade name: Baypen
Indications: Various infections caused by susceptible organisms
Category: Antibiotic, penicillin
Half-life: 0.8–1.0 hours
Clinically important, potentially hazardous interactions with: anticoagulants, cyclosporine, demeclocycline, doxycycline, imipenem/cilastatin, methotrexate, minocycline, oxytetracycline, tetracycline

Reactions

Skin
Allergic reactions (sic)
 (1994): Pleasants RA+, *Chest* 106, 1124 (in patients with cystic fibrosis)
Angioedema
Bullous dermatitis
Dermatitis
 (1992): Keller K+, *Contact Dermatitis* 27, 348
Erythema multiforme
Erythema nodosum
Exanthems
Exfoliative dermatitis (<1%)
Hematomas
Jarisch–Herxheimer reaction
Jaundice
 (1992): Hargreaves JE+, *Clin Infect Dis* 15(1), 179

Pruritus
Rash (sic) (<1%)
Stevens–Johnson syndrome
Toxic epidermal necrolysis
Urticaria
Vasculitis

Mucosal/ENT
Dysgeusia
Glossitis
Glossodynia
Oral candidiasis
Stomatitis
Stomatodynia
Tongue black
Vaginitis
Xerostomia

Other
Anaphylactoid reactions/Anaphylaxis
Hypersensitivity
  (1992): Keller K+, *Contact Dermatitis* 27, 348
Injection-site pain
Nephrotoxicity
  (1986): Palla R+, *Clin Nephrol* 25(6), 315
  (1985): Cushner HM+, *Arch Intern Med* 145(7), 1204
Phlebitis
Serum sickness (<1%)
Thrombophlebitis

MIANSERIN

Trade names: Athimil (Hormoquimica); Bolvidon (Schering-Plough) (GSK); Lantanon (Schering-Plough); Lerivon (Schering-Plough); Miaxan (Orion Pharma); Norval (Schering-Plough) (GSK); Tetramide (Daiichi Sankyo); Tolvon (Schering-Plough)
Indications: Depression
Category: Antidepressant, tetracyclic
Half-life: 10 hours
Clinically important, potentially hazardous interactions with: codeine, diazepam, morphine, temazepam, zopiclone

Reactions

Skin
Edema
Rash (sic)

Mucosal/ENT
Xerostomia

Eyes
Vision blurred

Other
Hypertension
  (1997): Bottlender R+, *Nervenarzt* 68(7), 591
Seizures
Somnolence
Tremor
Vertigo

MICONAZOLE

Trade names: Aflorix; Aloid; Daktarin; Florid; Funcort; Fungoid Tincture; Lotrimin (Schering); Micotef; Miracol; Monazole-7; Monistat (Personal Products); Zole
Indications: Fungal infections
Category: Antibiotic, imidazole
Half-life: initial: 40 minutes; terminal: 24 hours
Clinically important, potentially hazardous interactions with: anisindione, anticoagulants, astemizole, dicumarol, vinblastine, vincristine, warfarin

Reactions

Skin
Angioedema (2%)
  (1983): Stevens DA, *Drugs* 26, 347 (2.4%)
Bullous dermatitis
  (1983): Stevens DA, *Drugs* 26, 347
Dermatitis
  (1996): Fernandez L+, *Contact Dermatitis* 34, 217
  (1995): Goday JJ+, *Contact Dermatitis* 32, 370
  (1991): Baes H, *Contact Dermatitis* 24, 89
  (1988): Perret CM+, *Contact Dermatitis* 19, 75
  (1988): Raulin C+, *Contact Dermatitis* 18, 76
  (1984): Aldridge RD+, *Contact Dermatitis* 10, 58
  (1983): Frenzel UH+, *Contact Dermatitis* 9, 74
  (1982): Foged EK+, *Contact Dermatitis* 8, 284
Erythema
Exanthems (2–87%)
  (1987): Verhagen C+, *Eur J Haematol* 38, 225 (28%)
  (1983): Stevens DA, *Drugs* 26, 347 (2.4%)
  (1980): Heel RC+, *Drugs* 19, 7 (3–8%)
Pruritus (2–36%)
  (1983): Stevens DA, *Drugs* 26, 347 (36%)
  (1980): Heel RC+, *Drugs* 19, 7 (2–21%)
Purpura (3–8%)
  (1980): Heel RC+, *Drugs* 19, 7 (3–8%)
Rash (sic) (9%)
Urticaria (2%)
  (1983): Stevens DA, *Drugs* 26, 347 (2.4%)
Xanthomas

Other
Anaphylactoid reactions/Anaphylaxis
Chills (>5%)
Injection-site pain (10%)
  (1980): Heel RC+, *Drugs* 19, 7 (0.5–2%)
Phlebitis (5–79%)
  (1983): Stevens DA, *Drugs* 26, 347 (35%)
  (1980): Heel RC+, *Drugs* 19, 7 (6–28%)

MIDAZOLAM

Trade names: Dormicum; Versed (Roche)
Indications: Preoperative sedation
Category: Benzodiazepine
Half-life: 1–4 hours
Clinically important, potentially hazardous interactions with: amprenavir, aprepitant, atazanavir, carbamazepine, chlorpheniramine, cimetidine, clarithromycin, clorazepate, CNS depressants, darunavir, delavirdine, dexamethasone, efavirenz, erythromycin, esomeprazole, fluconazole, fluoxetine, fosamprenavir, **grapefruit juice**, griseofulvin, imatinib, indinavir, itraconazole, ivermectin, ketoconazole, nelfinavir, nevirapine, phenobarbital, phenytoin, primidone, rifabutin, rifampin, ritonavir, roxithromycin, saquinavir, **St John's wort**, telithromycin, tipranavir

Reactions

Skin
Adverse effects
  (1993): Kundrotas L+, *Gastrointest Endosc* 39, 109
Angioedema
  (1992): Yakel DL+, *Crit Care Med* 20, 307
Edema
  (2006): Uchimura A+, *Masui* 55(1), 76
Exanthems
Facial edema
  (2006): Uchimura A+, *Masui* 55(1), 76
Peripheral edema (<1%)
Pruritus (<1%)
  (2006): Uchimura A+, *Masui* 55(1), 76
  (1989): Yates A+, *Anaesthesia* 44, 449
Rash (sic) (<1%)
Urticaria (<1%)
  (2004): McIlwain M+, *Pediatr Dent* 26(4), 359

Mucosal/ENT
Dysgeusia (<1%) (acid taste)
Sialorrhea (<1%)

Eyes
Eyelid edema
  (2006): Uchimura A+, *Masui* 55(1), 76
Periorbital edema
  (2004): McIlwain M+, *Pediatr Dent* 26(4), 359

Other
Anaphylactoid reactions/Anaphylaxis (<1%)
  (2006): Uchimura A+, *Masui* 55(1), 76
Chills
  (2004): Bergendahl HT+, *Acta Anaesthesiol Scand* 48(10), 1292
Depression
  (2002): Wenzel RR+, *J Am Soc Echocardiogr* 15(10 Pt 2), 1297 (6%)
Headache
Hypotension
  (2004): Choi YF+, *Emerg Med J* 21(6), 700 (19%)
  (2004): Jung HK+, *Korean J Gastroenterol* 43(2), 96
  (2003): Mitchell AR+, *Europace* 5(4), 391
  (2001): Kinoshita K+, *J Int Med Res* 29(4), 342
  (1990): Ruff R+, *J Cardiothorac Anesth* 4(3), 314
Injection-site pain (>10%)
  (1984): Dundee JW+, *Drugs* 28, 519 (26%)
Injection-site reactions (sic) (>10%)
Paresthesias

MIDODRINE

Trade names: Amatine; Gutron; Metligine; Midon; Proamatine (Shire)
Indications: Orthostatic hypotension, urinary incontinence
Category: Adrenergic alpha-receptor agonist
Half-life: ~3–4 hours

Reactions

Skin
Erythema multiforme
Pruritus (13%)
  (2004): Young TM+, *Ann Pharmacother* 38(11), 1868
  (1998): McClellan KJ+, *Drugs Aging* 12(1), 76
  (1993): Jankovic J+, *Am J Med* 95(1), 38 (scalp) (13.5%)
Rash (sic) (2.4%)
Xerosis (2%)

Mucosal/ENT
Aphthous stomatitis
Dysgeusia
  (2004): Young TM+, *Ann Pharmacother* 38(11), 1868
Parosmia
  (2004): Young TM+, *Ann Pharmacother* 38(11), 1868
Xerostomia (1–10%)

Hair
Hair – pili torti
  (1998): McClellan KJ+, *Drugs Aging* 12(1), 76
  (1989): McTavish D+, *Drugs* 38(5), 757

Other
Chills (5%)
Headache
Pain (5%)
Paresthesias (13–18%)
  (1998): McClellan KJ+, *Drugs Aging* 12(1), 76
  (1997): Cruz DN+, *Am J Kidney Dis* 30(6), 772
  (1993): Jankovic J+, *Am J Med* 95(1), 38 (scalp) (13.5%)

MIFEPRISTONE

Synonym: RU-486
Trade name: Mifeprex (Danco)
Indications: Medical termination of intrauterine pregnancy
Category: Corticosteroid antagonist; Progestogen antagonist
Half-life: ~20 hours

Reactions

Mucosal/ENT
Vaginitis (3%)

Other
Abdominal pain (89%)
  (2003): Piaggio G+, *Contraception* 68(6), 439
  (2002): Tang OS+, *Hum Reprod* 17(7), 1738 (89%) (with misoprostol)
Chills (3–38%)
  (2002): Tang OS+, *Hum Reprod* 17(7), 1738 (38%) (with misoprostol)
Fever (79%)
  (2002): Tang OS+, *Hum Reprod* 17(7), 1738 (79%) (with misoprostol)
Headache

Infections
(2001): DeHart RM+, *Ann Pharmacother* 35(6), 707

MIGLITOL

Trade name: Glyset (Pfizer)
Indications: Non-insulin dependent diabetes type II
Category: Alpha-glucosidase inhibitor
Half-life: ~2 hours

Reactions

Skin
Rash (sic) (1–10%)

Other
Abdominal pain
(2002): Drent ML+, *Diabetes Nutr Metab* 15(3), 152
(2000): Campbell LK+, *Ann Pharmacother* 34(11), 1291
(2000): Scott LJ+, *Drugs* 59(3), 521

MIGLUSTAT

Trade name: Zavesca (Actelion)
Indications: Gaucher's disease
Category: Glucosylceramide synthase inhibitor
Half-life: 6–7 hours

Reactions

Skin
Burning (hands & feet)

Mucosal/ENT
Xerostomia (8%)

Other
Abdominal pain (50%)
Headache (22%)
Neurotoxicity
(2005): *Prescrire Int* 14(79), 168 (19%)
Paresthesias (7%)
Tremor (~30%)
(2005): *Prescrire Int* 14(79), 168 (29%)
Vertigo (11%)

MILK THISTLE

Scientific names: *Carduus marainum; Silibum marianum*
Family: Asteraceae; Compositae
Trade and other common names: Holy Thistle; Lady's
Thistle; Marian Thistle; Mary Thistle; Silymarin
Category: Immunomodulator
Purported indications and other uses: Dyspepsia, liver
protectant, hepatitis, loss of appetite, spleen diseases, supportive
treatment for mushroom poisoning
Half-life: N/A

Reactions

Skin
Adverse effects (sic)

(2000): *Evid Rep Technol* p(21), 1
(1999): No Author, *Med J Aust* 170(5), 218
Allergic reactions (sic)
Diaphoresis
Rash (sic)
(2001): Saller R+, *Drugs* 61(14), 2035
Urticaria
(1990): Mironets VI+, *Vrach Delo* 7, 86

MINOCYCLINE

Trade names: Alti-Minocycline; Apo-Minocycline; Arestin;
Dynacin (Medicis); Mestacine; Minocin (Wyeth); Minoclir 50;
Minogalen; Minomycin; Mynocine; Solodyn (Medicis); Syn-
Minocycline
Indications: Various infections caused by susceptible organisms
Category: Antibiotic, tetracycline; Disease-modifying
antirheumatic
Half-life: 11–23 hours
**Clinically important, potentially hazardous interactions
with:** acitretin, aluminum salts, amoxicillin, ampicillin, antacids,
bacampicillin, bismuth, calcium, carbenicillin, cloxacillin, digoxin,
iron salts, isotretinoin, magnesium salts, methotrexate,
methoxyflurane, mezlocillin, nafcillin, oxacillin, penicillins,
piperacillin, ticarcillin, vitamin A, zinc, zinc salts

Reactions

Skin
Acute febrile neutrophilic dermatosis (Sweet's syndrome)
(2002): Khan Durani+, *Br J Dermatol* 147(3), 558
(1992): Thibault M-J1, *J Am Acad Dermatol* 27, 801
(1991): Mensing H+, *Dermatologica* 182, 43
Acute generalized exanthematous pustulosis (AGEP)
(1997): Yamamoto T+, *Acta Derm Venereol* (Stockh) 77, 168 (in
a patient with pustular psoriasis)
Angioedema
(1997): Shapiro LE+, *Arch Dermatol* 133, 1224
(1994): Levy SB, Chapel Hill, NC (reproducible) (personal case)
(observation)
(1993): Litt JZ, Beachwood, OH (personal case) (observation)
Cellulitis
(1994): Kaufmann D+, *Arch Intern Med* 154, 1983
(1989): Andreano JM+, *J Am Acad Dermatol* 20, 934
Elastolysis
(2000): Ho NC+, *Am J Med* 109(4), 340
Eosinophilic pustular folliculitis (Ofuji's disease)
(1989): Andreano JM+, *J Am Acad Dermatol* 20, 934
Erythema multiforme
(2003): Bamberg C+, *Hautarzt* 54(9), 864
(1987): Shoji A+, *Arch Dermatol* 123, 18
Erythema nodosum
(1990): Bridges AJ+, *J Am Acad Dermatol* 22, 959
Erythroderma
(2002): Murray C+, *World Congress Dermatol* Poster, 0120
Exanthems
(2002): Blumenthal HL, Beachwood, OH (personal case)
(observation)
(1996): Knowles SR+, *Arch Dermatol* 132, 934
(1995): Karofsky PS+, *Arch Pediatr Adolesc Med* 149, 217
(1995): Litt JZ, Beachwood, OH (2 personal cases, mother and
daughter) (observation)
(1994): Kaufmann D+, *Arch Intern Med* 154, 1983
Exfoliative dermatitis (<1%)
(1997): MacNeil M+, *J Am Acad Dermatol* 36, 347

(1996): Knowles SR+, *Arch Dermatol* 132, 934
(1989): Davies MG+, *BMJ* 298, 1523

Fixed eruption (<1%)
(2005): Monroe M+, *Dermatol Nurs* 17(2), 146
(1999): Correia O+, *Clin Exp Dermatol* 24, 137 (genital) (with doxycycline)
(1994): Chu P+, *J Am Acad Dermatol* 30, 802 (pigmentation)
(1992): Ridgway HB+, *Arch Dermatol* 128, 565
(1984): Bargman H, *J Am Acad Dermatol* 11, 900
(1983): LePaw MI, *J Am Acad Dermatol* 8, 263

Folliculitis
(1994): Kaufmann D+, *Arch Intern Med* 154, 1983 (pustular)
(1989): Andreano JM+, *J Am Acad Dermatol* 20, 934

Lichenoid eruption
(1993): Litt JZ, Beachwood, OH (personal case) (observation)

Livedo reticularis
(2005): Gibbs MB+, *J Am Acad Dermatol* 52(6), 1009
(2000): Schlienger RG+, *Dermatology* 200, 223
(1995): Elkayam O+, *Ann Rheum Dis* 55, 769

Lupus erythematosus
(2007): Benjamin RW+, *Pediatr Dermatol* 24(3), 246
(2007): Geddes R, *J Orthop Sports Phys Ther* 37(2), 65
(2006): Egger SS+, *Schweiz Rundsch Med Prax* 95(35), 1297
(2006): Leydet H+, *Rev Med Interne* 27(1), 72
(2004): van Steensel MA, *Med Hypotheses* 63(1), 31
(2003): Hill VA+, *Br J Dermatol* 148(5), 1056 (3 cases)
(2002): Marai I+, *Harefuah* 141(2), 151
(2001): Balestero S+, *Int J Dermatol* 40, 475
(2001): Gordon MM+, *J Rheumatol* 28(5), 1004
(2001): Graham LE+, *Clin Rheumatol* 20(1), 67
(2001): Lawson TM+, *Rheumatology (Oxford)* 40(3), 329
(2001): Marzo-Ortega H+, *J Rheumatol* 28(2), 377
(2000): Choi HK+, *Arthritis Rheum* 43, 2488
(2000): Colmegna I+, *J Rheumatol* 27, 1567
(2000): Dunphy J+, *Br J Dermatol* 142, 461
(2000): Schlienger RG+, *Dermatology* 200, 223 (57 cases)
(1999): Angulo JM+, *J Rheumatol* 26, 1420
(1999): Christodoulou CS+, *Chest* 115(5), 1471
(1999): Dadamessi I+, *Rev Med Interne* (French) 20, 930
(1999): Elkayam O+, *Semin Arthritis Rheum* 28, 392
(1999): Katz R, *Skin and Allergy News*, May, 13
(1999): Piette AM+, *Rev Med Interne* (French) 20, 869
(1999): Sturkenboom MC+, *Arch Intern Med* 159, 493
(1999): Thaler D, Monona, WI (from Internet) (observation)
(1999): Tournigand C+, *Lupus* 8, 773
(1998): Akin E+, *Pediatrics* 101, 926
(1998): Angulo JM+, *Semin Arthritis Rheum* 28, 187
(1998): Blumenthal HL, Beachwood, OH (personal case) (observation)
(1998): Knights SE+, *Clin Exp Dermatol* 16, 587
(1997): Crosson J+, *J Am Acad Dermatol* 36, 867
(1997): Emery P+, *J Rheumatol* 24, 1850
(1997): Farver DK, *Ann Pharmacother* 31, 1160
(1997): Golstein PE+, *Am J Gastroenterol* 92, 143
(1997): Hoefnagel JJ+, *Ned Tijdschr Geneeskd* 141, 1424
(1997): Pointud P, *J Rheumatol* 24, 1851
(1997): Singer SJ+, *JAMA* 277, 295
(1997): Wilde JL+, *Arch Dermatol* 133, 1344
(1996): Gough A+, *BMJ* 312, 169 (18 cases)
(1996): Hewack J, *Gastroenterology* 110, A1211
(1996): Knowles SR+, *Arch Dermatol* 132, 934
(1996): Masson C+, *J Rheumatol* 23, 2160
(1995): Bulgen DY, *Br J Rheumatol* 34, 398
(1995): Gendi NS+, *Br J Rheumatol* 34, 584
(1995): Gordon P+, *Br J Dermatol* 132, 120
(1994): Byrne PA+, *Br J Rheumatol* 33, 674
(1994): Inoue CN+, *Eur J Pediatr* 153, 540
(1994): Quilty B+, *Br J Rheumatol* 33, 1197
(1992): Matsuura T+, *Lancet* 340, 1553
(1984): Alston LL, *The Schoch Letter* 34, #8, Item 110

Lymphomatoid papulosis
(2004): Dukic R+, *Rev Med Interne* 25(5), 401

Nodular eruption (facial, blue-gray)
(1998): Dawe RS+, *Arch Dermatol* 134, 861

Ochronosis
(2004): Suwannarat P+, *Arthritis Rheum* 50(11), 3698 (5 cases)

Petechiae
(2000): Warshaw E, Minneapolis MN, *The Schoch Letter* 50, February #16

Photosensitivity (1–10%)
(2002): Thaler D, Monona, WI (from Internet) (observation)
(1996): Carrington PR, Little Rock, AR (from tanning bed) (from Internet) (observation)
(1996): Goulden V+, *Br J Dermatol* 134, 693
(1996): Uhlemann J, St. Charles, MO (from Internet) (observation)
(1996): Wegman A, Sydney, Australia (from Internet) (observation)
(1994): Litt JZ, Beachwood, OH (personal case) (observation)
(1990): Black AK+, *Br J Dermatol* 123, 277
(1985): Basler RSW, *Arch Dermatol* 121, 606

Phototoxicity
(2002): Sorkin M, Denver, CO (from Internet) (observation)
(2002): Zabawski E, Longview, TX (from Internet) (observation)

Pigmentation
(2007): Madan V+, *Br J Dermatol* 156(3), 590
(2006): Dodiuk-Gad RP+, *J Eur Acad Dermatol Venereol* 20(4), 435
(2006): Farady K, Austin, TX (from Internet) (observation)
(2006): Gerson DM+, *Cardiovasc Pathol* 15(3), 168
(2006): Holm AN+, *N Engl J* 355(20), e23
(2006): Kalia S+, *Can Fam Physician* 52, 595
(2006): Roberts G+, *J Rheumatol* 33(7), 1254
(2005): Ely EH, Grass Valley, CA (from Internet) (observation)
(2005): Rahman Z+, *J Cutan Pathol* 32(7), 516
(2004): Bloom E, Oakland, CA (from Internet) (observation)
(2004): Davidson D, Groton, CT (from Internet) (observation)
(2004): Mouton RW+, *Clin Exp Dermatol* 29(1), 8
(2004): Pandit S+, *Surgeon* 2(4), 236 (bone)
(2004): Patterson JW+, *Cutis* 74(5), 293
(2004): Sanchez AR+, *Int J Dermatol* 43(10), 709
(2004): Suwannarat P+, *Arthritis Rheum* 50(11), 3698
(2003): Bock GN, Stockton, CA (from Internet) (observation)
(2003): Cohen PR+, *Skin & Aging* August, 94
(2003): Condry PJ, Rochester, NY (from Internet) (observation)
(2003): Crowe MA, Tacoma, WA (from Internet) (observation)
(2003): Grasset L+, *Rev Med Interne* 24(5), 305
(2003): Gregg LJ, Tulsa, OK (from Internet) (observation)
(2003): Mitchell DF, Thomasville, GA (nuchal area – blue) (from Internet) (observation)
(2003): Nakamura S+, *Br J Dermatol* 148(5), 1073 (patient with atopic dermatitis)
(2003): Sienkiewicz G, Johnson City, NY (from Internet) (2 observations – slate-gray)
(2003): Stafford S, Mt Pleasant, SC (from Internet) (observation)
(2003): Thaler D, Monona, WI (from Internet) (observation)
(2002): Bloom E, Oakland, CA (shins) (from Internet) (observation)
(2002): Jaffe P, Columbia, SC (gray-black on lower legs) (from Internet) (observation)
(2002): Maffei KR, Athens, GA (from Internet) (observation)
(2002): Spencer LV, Crawfordsville, IN (from Internet) (observation)
(2002): Thaler D, Monona, WI (from Internet) (observation)
(2001): Assad SA+, *J Rheumatol* 28(3), 679 (extensive)
(2001): Bachelz H+, *Arch Dermatol* 137, 69 (grayish)
(2001): Bressack M, Merrillville, IN (bluish) (from Internet) (observation)
(2001): Ely H, Grass Valley, CA (from Internet) (observation)

(2001): Mocci A, Panama (deep blue spots on face) (from Internet) (observation)
(2001): Werth V, *Dermatology Times* 18 (shins, ankles, arms)
(2000): Chave TA+, *Ann R Coll Surg Engl* 82(5), 348
(2000): Gregg LJ, Tulsa, OK (from Internet) (observation)
(2000): Joseph WS+, *J Am Podiatr Med Assoc* 90, 268
(2000): Mouton RW, Poster Exhibit at University of Vienna clinical dermatology meeting (bluish)
(2000): Ozog DM+, *Arch Dermatol* 136, 1133 (7 cases; all with pemphigus or pemphigoid)
(1999): Aylesworth RJ, Rhinelander, WI (from Internet) (observation)
(1999): Drayton GE, Los Angeles, CA (from Internet) (observation)
(1999): Frederickson K, Novalo, CA (from Internet) (observation)
(1999): Gregg LJ, Tulsa, OK (from Internet) (observation)
(1999): Johnston AM+, *N Engl J Med* 340, 1597
(1999): Koester GA, Edmond, OK (from Internet) (observation)
(1999): Lycka BAS, Edmonton, Alberta (from Internet) (observation)
(1999): Messner E+, *J Clin Rheumatol* 5(5), 273
(1999): Pepper, M, *The Schoch Letter* 49, 25 Madison, WI (linear purple streaks of back)
(1998): Eisen D+, *Drug Saf* 18, 431
(1998): Greve B+, *Lasers Surg Med* 22, 223
(1998): Karrer S+, *Hautarzt* (German) 49, 219
(1998): Morrow GL+, *Am J Ophthalmol* 125, 396
(1998): Patel K+, *Br J Dermatol* 185, 560
(1998): Pavese P+, *Ann Med Interne (Paris)* 149(8), 521
(1998): Wasel NR+, *J Cutan Med Surg* 3, 105
(1998): Wood B+, *Br J Dermatol* 139, 562
(1997): Hoefnagel JJ+, *Ned Tijdschr Geneeskd* 141, 1424
(1997): Houck HE+, *Arch Dermatol* 133, 15
(1997): Rademaker M, New Zealand (eyelids) (from Internet) (observation)
(1997): Smith KC, Niagara Falls, Ontario (from Internet) (observation)
(1997): Wilde JL+, *Arch Dermatol* 133, 1344
(1996): Collins P+, *Br J Dermatol* 135, 317
(1996): Fleming CJ+, *Br J Dermatol* 134, 784
(1996): Goulden V+, *Br J Dermatol* 134, 693
(1996): Hardman CM+, *Clin Exp Dermatol* 21, 244
(1996): Knoell AG+, *Arch Dermatol* 132, 1251
(1996): Korbol M+, *J Am Podiatr Med Assoc* 76, 87
(1996): Tsao H+, *Arch Dermatol* 132, 1250
(1995): Hung PH+, *J Fam Pract* 41, 183
(1995): Meyer AJ+, *Arch Dermatol* 131, 1447
(1995): Poskitt L+, *Br J Dermatol* 132, 784
(1994): Miralles ES+, *J Dermatol* 21, 965
(1994): Siller GM+, *J Am Acad Dermatol* 30, 350
(1993): Dwyer CM+, *Br J Dermatol* 129, 158
(1993): Okada N+, *Br J Dermatol* 129, 403
(1993): Pepine M+, *J Am Acad Dermatol* 28, 295
(1993): Schofield JK+, *Br J Gen Pract* 43, 173
(1992): Altman DA+, *J Cutaneous Pathol* 19, 340 (in patients with bullous pemphigoid)
(1992): Fakhfakh AC+, *Ann Dermatol Venereol* (French) 119, 975
(1992): Ridgway HB+, *Arch Dermatol* 128, 565 (pseudo-mongolian)
(1991): Eady DJ+, *Clin Exp Dermatol* 16, 55
(1991): Leffell DJ, *J Am Acad Dermatol* 24, 501
(1990): Bamberger N+, *Ann Dermatol Venereol* (French) 117, 299
(1990): Black AK+, *Br J Dermatol* 123, 277
(1990): Bridges AJ+, *J Am Acad Dermatol* 22, 959
(1989): Cataldo E+, *J Mass Dent Soc* 38, 5
(1989): Layton AM+, *J Dermatol Treatment* 1, 9
(1989): Okada N+, *Br J Dermatol* 121, 247
(1988): Serwatka LM, *J Assoc Military Derm* 14, 10

(1987): Angeloni VL+, *Cutis* 40, 229
(1987): Argenyi ZB+, *J Cutaneous Pathol* 14, 176
(1987): Zijdenbos AM+, *Ned Tijdschr Geneeskd* (Dutch) 131, 999
(1986): Prigent F+, *Ann Dermatol Venereol* (French) 113, 227
(1986): Shum DT+, *Arch Dermatol* 122, 18
(1985): Basler RSW, *Arch Dermatol* 121, 606
(1985): Basler RSW+, *J Am Acad Dermatol* 12, 577
(1985): Butler JM+, *Clin Exp Dermatol* 10, 432
(1985): Gordon G, *Arch Dermatol* 121, 618
(1985): Liu TTT+, *Cutis* 35, 254
(1984): Wolfe ID+, *Cutis* 33, 457
(1983): Verret JL+, *Ann Dermatol Venereol* (French) 110, 777
(1983): White SW+, *Arch Dermatol* 119, 1
(1982): Ridgway HA, *Br J Dermatol* 107, 95
(1981): Leroy JP+, *Ann Dermatol Venereol* (French) 108, 871
(1981): Sato S+, *J Invest Dermatol* 77, 264
(1980): Fenske NA+, *J Am Acad Dermatol* 3, 308
(1980): Fenske NA+, *JAMA* 244, 1103
(1980): McGrae JD+, *Arch Dermatol* 116, 1262
(1980): Simons JJ+, *J Am Acad Dermatol* 3, 244

Pruritus (<1%)
(2000): Bachelz H+, *Arch Dermatol* 137, 69
(1998): Pavese P+, *Ann Med Interne (Paris)* 149(8), 521
(1996): Goulden V+, *Br J Dermatol* 134, 693
(1996): Montemarano AD+, *J Am Acad Dermatol* 34, 253

Purpura
(2003): D'Addario SF+, *J Drugs Dermatol* 2(3), 320
(2000): Warshaw E, Minneapolis MN, *The Schoch Letter* 50, February #16
(1995): Karofsky PS+, *Arch Pediatr Adolesc Med* 149, 217

Pustules (generalized)
(1999): Antunes A+, *Ann Dermatol Venereol* 126, 518

Rash (sic) (<1%)
(2000): Bachelz H+, *Arch Dermatol* 137, 69
(2000): Schlienger RG+, *Dermatology* 200, 223
(1997): Shapiro LE+, *Arch Dermatol* 133, 1224
(1995): Karofsky PS+, *Arch Pediatr Adolesc Med* 149, 217
(1994): Kaufmann D+, *Arch Intern Med* 154, 1983
(1994): Sitbon O+, *Arch Intern Med* 154, 1633

Raynaud's phenomenon
(2001): Gordon MM+, *J Rheumatol* 28(5), 1004
(1996): Hewack J, *Gastroenterology* 110, A1211

Stevens–Johnson syndrome
(1996): Knowles SR+, *Arch Dermatol* 132, 934
(1987): Shoji A+, *Arch Dermatol* 123, 18

Urticaria
(2005): Swain R, Mobile, AL (personal communication)
(2003): Tuckman DJ, Sun City, AZ (from Internet) (observation)
(2001): Bark J, Lexington, KY (from Internet) (observation)
(1997): Shapiro LE+, *Arch Dermatol* 133, 1224
(1996): Goulden V+, *Br J Dermatol* 134, 693
(1996): Knowles SR+, *Arch Dermatol* 132, 934
(1996): Ottuso P, *The Schoch Letter* 46, 37 Vero Beach, FL (from generic)
(1995): Wallis M, *The Schoch Letter* 45, 38 (from generic)
(1994): Litt JZ, Beachwood, OH (personal case) (observation)
(1993): Litt JZ, Beachwood, OH (2 personal cases) (observation)
(1990): Puyana J+, *Allergy* 45, 313

Vasculitis
(2002): Sakai H+, *Arerugi* 51(12), 1153
(2001): Schaffer JV+, *J Am Acad Dermatol* 44, 198 (necrotizing)
(2000): Choi HK+, *Arthritis Rheum* 43, 2488
(1999): Elkayam O+, *Semin Arthritis Rheum* 28, 392
(1999): Schrodt BJ, *Skin and Allergy News* April, 22 (2 cases)
(1999): Schrodt BJ+, *South Med J* 92, 502
(1998): Merkel PA, *Curr Opin Rheumatol* 10, 45

Mucosal/ENT
Esophagitis
(2004): Heidrich H, *Med Klin* (Munich) 99(7), 396

Gingival pigmentation (8%)
  (2005): LaPorta VN+, J Clin Periodontol 32(2), 119
  (1989): Berger RS+, J Am Acad Dermatol 21, 1300 (8%)
Glossitis
  (2004): Heidrich H, Med Klin (Munich) 99(7), 396
Oral pigmentation (7%)
  (2005): LaPorta VN+, J Clin Periodontol 32(2), 119
  (2004): Treister NS+, Oral Surg Oral Med Oral Pathol Oral Radiol Endod 97(6), 718 (2 cases)
  (2003): Ayangco L+, J Periodontol 74(5), 669
  (2003): Bradfield YS+, Arch Ophthalmol 121(1), 144
  (2003): Grasset L+, Rev Med Interne 24(5), 305
  (2002): Friedman IS+, Dermatol Surg 28(3), 205
  (2001): Werth V, Dermatology Times 18
  (1998): Cockings JM+, Aust Dent J 43, 14
  (1998): Morrow GL+, Am J Ophthalmol 125, 396
  (1998): Patel K+, Br J Dermatol 185, 560
  (1997): Eisen D, Lancet 349, 379
  (1997): Smith KC, Niagara Falls, Ontario (blue on lips) (from Internet) (observation)
  (1995): Odell EW+, Oral Surg Oral Med Oral Pathol Oral Radiol Endod 79, 459
  (1994): Chu P+, J Am Acad Dermatol 30, 802
  (1994): Siller GM+, J Am Acad Dermatol 30, 350
  (1989): Berger RS+, J Am Acad Dermatol 21, 1300 (7%)
  (1989): Regezi JA+, Oral Pathology WB Saunders, 166
  (1986): Beehner ME+, J Oral Maxillofac Surg 44, 582
  (1985): Salman RA+, J Oral Med 40, 154
  (1984): Fendrich P+, Oral Surg Oral Med Oral Pathol 58, 288
Oral ulceration
  (2000): Schlienger RG+, Dermatology 200, 223
Stomatitis
  (2004): Heidrich H, Med Klin (Munich) 99(7), 396
Tongue black
  (1995): Katz J+, Arch Dermatol 131, 620

Hair

Hair – alopecia
  (2000): Schlienger RG+, Dermatology 200, 223

Nails

Nails – photo-onycholysis
  (1987): Baran R+, J Am Acad Dermatol 17, 1012 (passim)
  (1981): Kestel JL, Cutis 28, 53
Nails – pigmentation (1–5%)
  (2005): LaPorta VN+, J Clin Periodontol 32(2), 119
  (2004): Sanchez AR+, Int J Dermatol 43(10), 709
  (2003): Grasset L+, Rev Med Interne 24(5), 305
  (2003): Mitchell DF, Thomasville, GA (from Internet) (observation)
  (2002): Kimyai-Asadi A+, J Drugs Dermatol 1(2), 197
  (2001): Gregg LJ, Tulsa, OK (from Internet) (observation)
  (2001): Werth V, Dermatology Times 18
  (1998): Morrow GL+, Am J Ophthalmol 125, 396
  (1995): Hung PH+, J Fam Pract 41, 183
  (1994): Mallon E+, Br J Dermatol 130, 794
  (1989): Berger RS+, J Am Acad Dermatol 21, 1300 (3–5%)
  (1988): Mooney E+, J Dermatol Surg Oncol 14, 1011
  (1987): Angeloni VL+, Cutis 40, 229
  (1985): Daniel CR III+, Dermatol Clin 3, 491 (longitudinal)
  (1985): Liu TTT+, Cutis 35, 254
  (1984): Wolfe ID+, Cutis 33, 457
  (1982): Litt JZ, Diagnosis 4, 23

Eyes

Conjunctival pigmentation
  (1981): Brothers DM+, Opthalmology 88, 1212
Scleral pigmentation
  (1998): Morrow GL+, Am J Ophthalmol 125, 396
  (1996): Sabroe RA+, Br J Dermatol 135(2), 314

  (1985): Liu TT+, Cutis 35, 254

Other

Anaphylactoid reactions/Anaphylaxis (<1%)
  (1996): Okano M+, Acta Derm Venereol (Stockh) 76, 164
Asthenia
  (2003): Grim SA+, Pharmacotherapy 23(12), 1659
  (1998): Pavese P+, Ann Med Interne (Paris) 149(8), 521
Candidiasis
DRESS syndrome
  (2008): Maubec E+, Dermatology 216(3), 200
  (2007): Favrolt N+, Rev Mal Respir 24(7), 892
Fever
  (2003): Grim SA+, Pharmacotherapy 23(12), 1659
Gynecomastia
  (1995): Davies JP+, Br J Clin Pract 49, 179
Headache
Hepatotoxicity
  (2006): Chamberlain MC+, J Pediatr Gastroenterol Nutr 42(2), 232
  (2004): Rikken NE+, Neth J Med 62(2), 62
  (2003): Abe M+, Intern Med 42(1), 48
  (2003): Bamberg C+, Hautarzt 54(9), 864
  (2000): Goldstein NS+, Am J Clin Pathol 114(4), 591
  (2000): Nietsch HH+, Am J Gastroenterol 95(10), 2993
  (1998): Bhat G+, J Clin Gastroenterol 27(1), 74
  (1998): Teitelbaum JE+, Arch Pediatr Adolesc Med 152(11), 1132
  (1997): Herzog D+, Dig Dis Sci 42(5), 1100
  (1996): Malcolm A+, Am J Gastroenterol 91(8), 1641
Hypersensitivity
  (2005): Trivin C+, Therapie 60(6), 590
  (2003): Grasset L+, Rev Med Interne 24(5), 305
  (2003): Roca B+, Intensive Care Med 29(2), 338
  (2002): Murray C+, World Congress Dermatol Poster, 0120
  (2002): Parc C+, Br J Ophthalmol 86(11), 1313
  (2002): Rahman Z+, Int J Dermatol 41(8), 530
  (2001): Bachelz H+, Arch Dermatol 137, 69
  (2001): Colvin JH+, Pediatr Dermatol 18(4), 295
  (2000): Gil P, Ann Dermatol Venereol 127(10), 841
  (1999): Antunes A+, Ann Dermatol Venereol 126, 518
  (1999): Clayton BD+, Arch Dermatol 135, 139
  (1999): Lupton JR+, Cutis 64, 91 (infectious-mononucleosis-like)
  (1999): Piette AM+, Rev Med Interne (French) 20, 869
  (1998): Dutz J, Vancouver, Canada (from Internet) (observation)
  (1998): Schlienger RG+, Epilepsia 39, S3 (passim)
  (1997): Hoefnagel JJ+, Ned Tijdschr Geneeskd (Dutch) 141, 1424
  (1997): MacNeil M+, J Am Acad Dermatol 36, 347
  (1997): Shapiro LE+, Arch Dermatol 133, 1224
  (1995): Parneix-Spake A+, Arch Dermatol 131, 490
  (1994): Sitbon O+, Arch Intern Med 154, 1633
Myalgia/Myositis/Myopathy/Myotoxicity
  (2007): Geddes R, J Orthop Sports Phys Ther 37(2), 65
  (2004): Narvaez J+, Am J Med 116(4), 282
  (2001): Gordon MM+, J Rheumatol 28(5), 1004
  (1998): Matteson EL+, J Rheumatol 25, 1653
  (1998): Pavese P+, Ann Med Interne (Paris) 149(8), 521
Nephrotoxicity
  (2003): Sethi S+, Am J Kidney Dis 42(2), E27
Paresthesias (<1%)
  (1994): Blanchard L, Schoch Letter 44, 6 (observation)
Polyarteritis nodosa
  (2007): Tehrani R+, J Clin Rheumatol 13(3), 146
  (2006): Abad S+, Arthritis Rheum 55(5), 831
  (2006): Katada Y+, Mod Rheumatol 16(4), 256
  (2005): Culver B+, Arthritis Rheum 53(3), 468
  (2003): Pelletier F+, Eur J Dermatol 13(4), 396
  (2001): Schaffer JV+, J Am Acad Dermatol 44, 198
  (1999): Schrodt BJ+, Pediatrics 103, 503
Pseudo-mongolian spot

(1992): Ridgway HB+, *Arch Dermatol* 128, 565
Rhabdomyolysis
  (2002): Rahman Z+, *Int J Dermatol* 41(8), 530
Serum sickness (3–5%)
  (2003): Grasset L+, *Rev Med Interne* 24(5), 305
  (2001): *Arch Dermatol* 137, 100 (2 cases)
  (1999): Elkayam O+, *Semin Arthritis Rheum* 28, 392
  (1998): Martinez JA+, *Med Clin* (Barc) (Spanish) 111, 198
  (1997): Blumenthal HL, Beachwood, OH (personal case)
    (observation)
  (1997): Hoefnagel JJ+, *Ned Tijdschr Geneeskd* (Dutch) 141, 1424
  (1997): Shapiro LE+, *Arch Dermatol* 133, 1224
  (1997): Zabawski E, Dallas, TX (from Internet) (observation)
  (1996): Harel L+, *Ann Pharmacother* 30, 481
  (1996): Levenson T+, *Allergy Asthma Proc* 17, 79
  (1990): Puyana J+, *Allergy* 45, 313
Upper respiratory infection
  (2006): NINDS NET-PD, *Neurology* 66(5), 664 (26%)

MINOXIDIL

Trade names: Alopexy; Apo-Gain; Hairgaine; Loniten (Par);
Lonolox; Lonoten; Minoximen; Regaine; Rogaine (topical) (Pfizer)
Indications: Hypertension, androgenetic alopecia
Category: Vasodilator
Half-life: 4.2 hours
**Clinically important, potentially hazardous interactions
with: alcohol**, guanethidine

Note: For topical reaction patterns, I have added a bracket [T]

Reactions

Skin
Acne
  (1985): Baral J, *J Am Acad Dermatol* 13, 1051 (scalp comedones)
Allergic reactions (sic) [T]
Bullous dermatitis (<1%)
  (1981): DiSantis DJ+, *Arch Intern Med* 141, 1515
Dermatitis (7.4%) [T]
  (2002): Suzuki K+, *Am J Contact* 13(1), 45
  (1998): Sanchez-Motilla J+, *Contact Dermatitis* 38, 283 (pustular)
  (1995): Ebner H+, *Contact Dermatitis* 32, 316
  (1992): Ruas E+, *Contact Dermatitis* 26, 57
  (1992): Veraldi S+, *Contact Dermatitis* 26, 211
  (1991): Wilson C+, *J Am Acad Dermatol* 24, 661
  (1988): Alomar A+, *Contact Dermatitis* 18, 51
  (1988): van Joost T, *Ned Tijdschr Geneeskd* (Dutch) 132, 1141
  (1987): Valsecchi R+, *Contact Dermatitis* 17, 58
  (1987): van der Willingen AH+, *Contact Dermatitis* 17, 44
  (1985): Degreef H+, *Contact Dermatitis* 13, 194
  (1985): Tosti A+, *Contact Dermatitis* 13, 275
Eczema
  (1992): Ruas E+, *Contact Dermatitis* 26, 57
  (1987): van der Willigen AH+, *Contact Dermatitis* 17, 44
Edema (>10%) [T]
Erythema [T]
Erythema multiforme
  (1981): DiSantis DJ+, *Arch Intern Med* 141, 1515
Erythroderma
  (1988): Ackerman BH+, *Drug Intell Clin Pharm* 22, 703
Exanthems
  (1988): Ackerman BH+, *Drug Intell Clin Pharm* 22, 703
  (1981): Campese VM, *Drugs* 22, 257
  (1981): DiSantis DJ+, *Arch Intern Med* 141, 1515
Folliculitis [T]
  (1996): Duvic M+, *J Am Acad Dermatol* 35, 74

Lupus erythematosus
  (1987): Tunkel AR+, *Arch Intern Med* 147, 599
  (1981): Mitas JA, *Arthritis Rheum* 24, 570
Peripheral edema (7%)
Pigmentation
Pruritus [T]
  (1996): Duvic M+, *J Am Acad Dermatol* 35, 74
  (1990): Colamarino R+, *Ann Intern Med* 113, 256
Pyogenic granuloma
  (1989): Baran R, *Dermatologica* 179(2), 76 (explosive, of the
    scalp)
Rash (sic) (<1%)
Seborrhea [T]
Stevens–Johnson syndrome (<1%)
  (1981): DiSantis DJ+, *Arch Intern Med* 141, 1515
Sunburn (<1%)
Urticaria
Xerosis

Mucosal/ENT
Anosmia
  (1993): Litt JZ, Beachwood, OH (personal case) (observation)
Dysgeusia [T]
  (1993): Litt JZ, Beachwood, OH (personal case) (observation)

Hair
Hair – alopecia [T]
  (1987): Olsen EA, *J Am Acad Dermatol* 16, 145
  (1983): Ingles RM+, *Int J Dermatol* 22, 120
Hair – hirsutism (in women) (100%)
  (1981): Campese VM, *Drugs* 22, 257 (100%)
Hair – hypertrichosis (80–100%)
  (2002): Litt JZ, Beachwood, OH (personal case) (observation)
  (1997): Peluso AM+, *Br J Dermatol* 136, 118
  (1995): Veyrac G+, *Therapie* (French) 50, 474 (in an infant)
  (1994): Gonzalez M+, *Clin Exp Dermatol* 19, 157 [T]
  (1990): Miwa LJ+, *Drug Intell Clin Pharm* 24, 365
  (1989): Rousseau C+, *Dermatologica* 179, 221
  (1988): Toriumi DN+, *Arch Otolaryngol Head Neck Surg* 114, 918
  (1985): Bencini PL+, *G Ital Dermatol Venereol* (Italian) 120, 137
  (1985): Lorette G+, *Ann Dermatol Venereol* (French) 112, 527
  (1984): Henkes J+, *Med Clin* (Barc) (Spanish) 83, 89
  (1983): Ingles RM+, *Int J Dermatol* 22, 120
  (1983): Wilkin JK+, *Cutis* 31, 61
  (1981): Campese VM, *Drugs* 22, 257 (100%)
  (1981): Nielsen PG, *Lakartidningen* (Swedish) 78, 1891
  (1980): Feldman HA+, *Curr Ther Res* 27, 205
  (1980): Ryckmanns F, *Hautarzt* (German) 31, 205
Hair – pigmentation
  (1989): Rebora A+, *J Am Acad Dermatol* 21, 1314
  (1983): Ingles RM+, *Int J Dermatol* 22, 120 (red)

Other
Anaphylactoid reactions/Anaphylaxis
  (2001): Blumenthal HL, Beachwood, OH (personal case)
    (observation)
Gynecomastia
Headache
Paresthesias
Polymyositis
  (1990): Colamarino R+, *Ann Intern Med* 113, 256
Tendinopathy/Tendon rupture [T]

MIRTAZAPINE

Trade name: Remeron (Organon)
Indications: Depression
Category: Adrenergic alpha-receptor agonist; Antidepressant, tetracyclic
Half-life: 20–40 hours

Reactions

Skin

Acne
Allergic reactions (sic)
(2003): Biswas PN+, J Psychopharmacol 17(1), 121 (3 cases)
Cellulitis
Diaphoresis
(2001): Demers JC+, Ann Pharmacother 35(10), 1217
(1999): Leinonen E+, Int Clin Psychopharmacol 14, 329
Edema (1–10%)
(2003): Biswas PN+, J Psychopharmacol 17(1), 121 (5 cases)
Exfoliative dermatitis
Facial edema
Herpes simplex
Peripheral edema (1–10%)
(2001): Kutscher EC+, Ann Pharmacother 35(11), 1494
Petechiae
Photosensitivity
Pruritus
Rash (sic) (1–10%)
(2003): Biswas PN+, J Psychopharmacol 17(1), 121 (20 cases)
Seborrhea
Ulcerations
Xerosis

Mucosal/ENT

Ageusia
Aphthous stomatitis
Dysgeusia
Glossitis (1–10%)
Oral candidiasis
Parosmia
Sialorrhea
Stomatitis
Tongue edema
Tongue pigmentation
Vaginitis
Xerostomia (25%)
(2001): Anttila SA+, CNS Drug Rev 7(3), 249
(1995): Montgomery SA, Int Clin Psychopharmacol 10, 37

Other

Asthenia
(2006): Freynhagen R+, Curr Med Res Opin 22(2), 257
(2003): Wan DD+, J Psychiatry Neurosci 28(1), 55
(2002): Beszlej A+, Psychiatr Pol 36(6), 115
Chills
Gynecomastia
(2006): Navarro-Gonzalez M+, Med Clin (Barc) 127(1), 37
(2005): Schmutz JL+, Ann Dermatol Venereol 132(2), 195
Headache
(2002): Beszlej A+, Psychiatr Pol 36(6), 115
Hepatotoxicity
(2002): Hui CK+, J Clin Gastroenterol 35(3), 270
Inappropriate secretion of antidiuretic hormone (SIADH)
(2006): Bavbek N+, Am J Kidney Dis 48(4), e61
Myalgia/Myositis/Myopathy/Myotoxicity (1–10%)

(2001): Jolliet P+, Eur Psychiatry 16(8), 503
Paresthesias
(2001): Ribeiro L+, Braz J Med Biol Res 34(10), 1303
Phlebitis
Rhabdomyolysis
(2006): Zink M+, J Clin Psychiatry 67(5), 835 (with risperidone)
(2005): Kuliwaba A, Aust N Z J Psychiatry 39(4), 312
(2004): Khandat AB+, Ann Pharmacother 38(7-8), 1321
(1998): Retz W+, Int Clin Psychopharmacol 13(6), 277
Tendinopathy/Tendon rupture
Thrombosis
(2006): Zink M+, J Clin Psychiatry 67(5), 835 (with risperidone)
Tremor (1–10%)
(2003): Ubogu EE+, Clin Neuropharmacol 26(2), 54
(2001): Demers JC+, Ann Pharmacother 35(10), 1217
Weight gain
(2005): Ness-Abramof R+, Drugs Today (Barc) 41(8), 547

MISOPROSTOL

Trade names: Arthrotec (Kaken); Cytotec (Pfizer); Symbol
Indications: Prevention of NSAID-induced ulcer
Category: Corticosteroid antagonist; Progestogen antagonist
Half-life: 20–40 minutes

Note: Arthrotec is diclofenac and misoprostol

Reactions

Skin

Dermatitis
Diaphoresis
Exanthems
(1987): Monk JP+, Drugs 33, 1
Rash (sic)
Shivering (17%)
(2002): Lumbiganon P+, BJOG 109(11), 1222
(2001): Elsheikh A+, Arch Gynecol Obstet 265(4), 204 (17.3%)
(2001): Gulmezoglu AM+, Lancet 358, 689
(2001): Li YT+, Zhonghua Yi Xue Za Zhi (Taipei) 64(12), 721 (33%)
(1999): Lumbiganon P+, Br J Obstet Gynaecol 106, 304

Mucosal/ENT

Dysgeusia
(2006): Parsons SM+, J Obstet Gynaecol Can 28(1), 20
(2004): Hamoda H+, Am J Obstet Gynecol 190(1), 55
Gingivitis
Tinnitus

Hair

Hair – alopecia

Other

Abdominal pain
(2006): Preutthipan S+, Fertil Steril 86(4), 990
(2006): Ruangchainikhom W+, J Med Assoc Thai 89(7), 928
(2006): Stojnic J+, Vojnosanit Pregl 63(6), 558
(2002): Tang OS+, Hum Reprod 17(7), 1738 (89%) (with mifepristone)
Anaphylactoid reactions/Anaphylaxis
(2002): Meuleman C+, Arch Mal Coeur Vaiss 95(12), 1230 (with diclofenac)
Chills
(2006): Derman RJ+, Lancet 368(9543), 1248
(2006): Parsons SM+, J Obstet Gynaecol Can 28(1), 20
(2005): Menakaya U+, J Obstet Gynaecol 25(6), 583

(2004): Nyende L+, *East Afr Med J* 81(4), 179
(2004): Vimala N+, *Contraception* 70(2), 117
(2002): Tang OS+, *Hum Reprod* 17(7), 1738 (38%) (with mifepristone)
Fever
(2006): Derman RJ+, *Lancet* 368(9543), 1248
(2006): Parsons SM+, *J Obstet Gynaecol Can* 28(1), 20
(2006): Preutthipan S+, *Fertil Steril* 86(4), 990 (7%)
(2006): Ruangchainikhom W+, *J Med Assoc Thai* 89(7), 928
(2006): Stojnic J+, *Vojnosanit Pregl* 63(6), 558
(2004): Nyende L+, *East Afr Med J* 81(4), 179
(2002): Tang OS+, *Hum Reprod* 17(7), 1738 (79%) (with mifepristone)
Gynecomastia
(1994): Garcia-Rodriguez LA+, *BMJ* 308, 503
Headache

MISTLETOE

Scientific names: *Phoradendron flavescens; Phoradendron leucarpum; Phoradendron macrophyllum; Phoradendron rubrum; Phoradendron serotinum; Phoradendron tomentosum; Viscum album*
Family: Loranthacae; Viscaceae
Trade and other common names: ABNOBA viscum; All-heal; Devil's fuge; Eurixor; Folia Visci; Helixor; Herbe de la Croix; Iscador (Weleda); Isorel (Novipharm); Lektinol; Lignum Crucis; Stipites Visci; VaQuFrF (Labor Hiscia); Vysorel
Category: Immunomodulator
Purported indications and other uses: Injected: adjuvant tumor therapy. **Oral:** abortifacient, arteriosclerosis, arthritis, asthma, colds, depression, headache, HIV infection, hypertension, hypotension, hysteria, labor pain, lumbago, metrorrhagia, muscle spasms, otitis, whooping cough, hemorrhoids, internal bleeding, gout, sleep disorders, amenorrhea, liver and gallbladder conditions
Half-life: N/A
Clinically important, potentially hazardous interactions with: bepridil, corticosteroids, digoxin, diltiazem, immunosuppressants, MAO inhibitors, **squill**, verapamil

Note: Purified extracts injected intramuscularly, subcutaneously or by intravenous infusion. Unless otherwise indicated, side effects listed are from injected preparations. The FDA considers *Viscum album* unsafe

Reactions

Skin
Adverse effects (sic)
(2005): Augustin M+, *Arzneimittelforschung* 55(1), 38 (12.8%)
(1999): Stein GM+, *Eur J Med Res* 4(5), 169
(1994): Stein G+, *Eur J Clin Phamacol* 47(1), 33
Allergic reactions (sic)
(2000): Büssing A, *Mistletoe: The Genus Viscum* Harwood Academic Publishers
(1994): Stein G+, *Eur J Clin Pharmacp;* 47(1), 33
(1991): Pichler WJ+, *Dtsch Med Wochenschr* (German) 116(35), 1333
Dermatitis
(2000): Büssing A, *Mistletoe: The Genus Viscum* Harwood Academic Publishers
Edema of lip
(1998): Hagenah W+, *Dtsch Med Wochenschr* (German) 123(34), 1001
Erythema
(2001): Hutt N+, *Allergol Immunopathol* (Madr) 29(5), 201

(1999): Stoss M+, *Arzneimittelforschung* 49(4), 366
(1999): van Wely+, *Am J Ther* 6(1), 37
Nodular eruption
(1998): Hagenah W+, *Dtsch Med Wochenschr* (German) 123(34), 1001
Pruritus
(1999): Stoss M+, *Arzneimittelforschung* 49(4), 366

Mucosal/ENT
Gingivitis
(1999): Gorter RW+, *Altern Ther Health Med* 5(6), 37
(1999): van Wely+, *Am J Ther* 6(1), 37

Other
Anaphylactoid reactions/Anaphylaxis (28%)
(2005): Bauer C+, *Ann Allergy Asthma Immunol* 94(1), 86 (1 case)
(2001): Hutt N+, *Allergol Immunopathol* (Madr) 29(5), 201
(1996): Friess H+, *Anticancer Res* 16(2), 915 (28%)
Chills
(2000): Büssing A, *Mistletoe: The Genus Viscum* Harwood Academic Publishers
(1995): Murray MT, *The Healing Power of Herbs* 253 Prima Publishing
Death (low incidence – accidental ingestion)
(1997): Krenzelok EP+, *Am J Emerg* 15(5), 516
(1996): Spiller HA+, *J Toxicol Clin Toxicol* 34(4), 405
(1995): Murray MT, *The Healing Power of Herbs* 253 Prima Publishing
(1986): Hall AH+, *Annals Emergency Med* 15, 1320
Injection-site edema
(1999): Stoss M+, *Arzneimittelforschung* 49(4), 366
Injection-site inflammation
(1999): Stein GM+, *Eur J Med Res* 4(5), 169
(1999): Stoss M+, *Arzneimittelforschung* (German) 49(4), 366
(1998): Gorter RW+, *Am J Ther* 5(3), 181
(1998): Stoss M I, *Nat Immun* 16(5), 185
(1995): Murray MT, *The Healing Power of Herbs* 253 Prima Publishing
(1990): Kast A+, *Schweiz Rundsch Med Prax* (German) 79(10), 291
Systemic reactions
(2005): Augustin M+, *Arzneimittelforschung* 55(1), 38 (3.3%)

MITHRAMYCIN

(See PLICAMYCIN)

MITOMYCIN

Synonyms: mitomycin-C; MTC
Trade names: Ametycine; Mitomycin; Mitomycin-C; Mitomycine; Mutamycin (Bristol-Myers Squibb)
Indications: Carcinomas
Category: Alkylating agent; Antibiotic, anthracycline
Half-life: 23–78 minutes
Clinically important, potentially hazardous interactions with: aldesleukin

Reactions

Skin
Angioedema
Bullous dermatitis
(1984): Ritch PS+, *Cancer* 54, 32
Dermatitis
(2006): Kureshi F+, *J Am Acad Dermatol* 55(2), 328

(1997): Gomez Torrrijos E+, *Allergy* 52, 687
(1993): Wahlberg JE+, *Lakartidningen* (Swedish) 90, 158
(1992): Vidal C+, *Dermatology* 184, 208
(1990): Colver GB+, *Br J Dermatol* 122, 217
(1987): Sala F+, *G Ital Dermatol Venereol* (Italian) 122, 265
(1984): Neild VJ+, *J R Soc Med* 77, 610
(1981): Nissenkorn I+, *J Urol* 126, 596

Edema
Erythema
Erythema multiforme
  (1984): Spencer HJ, *J Surg Oncol* 26, 47
Exanthems
  (1995): Echechipia S+, *Contact Dermatitis* 33, 432
  (1987): Sala F+, *G Ital Dermatol Venereol* (Italian) 122, 265
Exfoliative dermatitis
  (1987): Sala F+, *G Ital Dermatol Venereol* (Italian) 122, 265
  (1985): Bencini PL+, *Int J Dermatol* 24, 472
Hand–foot syndrome
  (2004): Rao S+, *Br J Cancer* 91(5), 839 (19.7%) (with
    capecitabine)
Necrosis
  (2000): Neulander EZ+, *J Urol* 164(4), 1306 (glans penis)
Palmar desquamation
  (1981): Nissenkorn I+, *J Urol* 126, 596
Photo-recall
  (2002): Stratman EJ, *J Am Acad Dermatol* 46(5), 797 (passim)
Photosensitivity
  (1981): Fuller B+, *Ann Intern Med* 94, 542
Pigmentation
  (1989): Kerker BJ+, *Semin Dermatol* 8, 173
Pityriasis rosea
  (1987): Sala F+, *G Ital Dermatol Venereol* (Italian) 122, 265
Pruritus (<1%)
Purpura
  (2001): Medina PJ+, *Curr Opin Hematol* 8(5), 286
Rash (sic) (<1%)
  (1981): Nissenkorn I+, *J Urol* 126, 596 (generalized)
Sarcoidosis
  (2001): Cuervo Pinna MA+, *An Med Interna* 18(12), 641
Ulcerations
  (1992): Ellsworth-Wolk J, *Oncol Nurs Forum* 19, 1554
Urticaria
  (1981): Weiss RB+, *Ann Intern Med* 94, 66

Mucosal/ENT

Mucositis
  (2004): Hofheinz RD+, *Br J Cancer* 91(5), 834 (3%) (with
    capecitabine)
Oral lesions (2–8%)
  (1987): Sala F+, *G Ital Dermatol Venereol* (Italian) 122, 265
  (1983): Bronner AK+, *J Am Acad Dermatol* 9, 645
Oral ulceration (1–10%)
  (1984): Spencer HJ, *J Surg Oncol* 26, 47
Stomatitis (>10%)

Hair

Hair – alopecia (1–10%)

Nails

Nails – pigmentation (purple) (1–10%)

Eyes

Corneal edema
  (2004): Pfister RR, *Cornea* 23(7), 744
Epiphora
  (2006): Khong JJ+, *Br J Ophthalmol* 90(7), 819
  (2004): Kopp ED+, *Br J Ophthalmol* 88(11), 1422
Keratitis

(2006): Kymionis GD+, *J Refract Surg* 22(5), 511
(2006): Poothullil AM+, *Semin Ophthalmol* 21(3), 161
Ocular stinging
  (2006): Poothullil AM+, *Semin Ophthalmol* 21(3), 161
Ocular toxicity
  (2006): Pirouzian A+, *Ophthalmologica* 220(6), 406
Xerophthalmia
  (2006): Kymionis GD+, *J Refract Surg* 22(5), 511

Other

Asthenia
  (2006): Feliu J+, *Cancer Chemother Pharmacol* 58(4), 527 (11%)
    (with docetaxel)
Death
  (2005): Meyer F+, *Chemotherapy* 51(1), 1 (2 cases)
Gangrene
  (2006): Kureshi F+, *J Am Acad Dermatol* 55(2), 328 (penile)
Infections
  (2004): Rao S+, *Br J Cancer* 91(5), 839 (2.3%) (with
    capecitabine)
Injection-site cellulitis (>10%)
Injection-site extravasation
  (2000): Kassner E, *J Pediatr Oncon Nurs* 17, 135
Injection-site necrosis (>10%)
  (1987): Aizawa H+, *Acta Derm Venereol* (Stockh) 67, 364
  (1987): Dufresne RG, *Cutis* 39, 197
  (1987): Sala F+, *G Ital Dermatol Venereol* (Italian) 122, 265
Injection-site thrombophlebitis
Nephrotoxicity
  (2001): Kintzel PE, *Drug Saf* 24(1), 19
Paresthesias (1–10%)
Thrombophlebitis (<1%)

MITOTANE

Synonym: o,p'-DDD
Trade name: Opeprim
Indications: Inoperable adrenocortical carcinoma
Category: Antineoplastic
Half-life: 18–159 days
**Clinically important, potentially hazardous interactions
with:** aldesleukin, spironolactone

Reactions

Skin

Acral erythema
  (1991): Baack BR+, *J Am Acad Dermatol* 24, 457
Angioedema (<1%)
Erythema multiforme
Exanthems (9–16%)
Pigmentation (16%)
Pruritus
Rash (sic) (15%)
Side effects (sic) (13–17%)
Urticaria
Vasculitis (<1%)

Hair

Hair – alopecia (16%)

Other

Myalgia/Myositis/Myopathy/Myotoxicity (1–10%)
Tremor (<1%)

MITOXANTRONE

Trade name: Novantrone (OSI)
Indications: Acute myelogenous leukemia, multiple sclerosis, prostate cancer
Category: Antibiotic, anthracycline; Antineoplastic
Half-life: median terminal: 75 hours
Clinically important, potentially hazardous interactions with: aldesleukin

Reactions

Skin
Allergic reactions (sic) (<1%)
Diaphoresis (1–10%)
Edema (>10%)
Erythema
Fungal dermatitis (>15%)
Necrosis
Petechiae (>10%)
Pigmentation (bluish)
Purpura (>10%)
Rash (sic) (<1%)
Ulcerations
Urticaria
Vitiligo
 (2001): Schmid-Wendtner M-H+, *Lancet* 358, 1575

Hair
Hair – alopecia (20–60%)
 (2004): Cohen BA+, *Neurology* 63(12 Suppl 6), S28

Other
Cardiotoxicity
 (2006): Murray TJ, *Expert Opin Drug Saf* 5(2), 265
Chills (1–10%)
Congestive heart failure
 (2006): Murray TJ, *Expert Opin Drug Saf* 5(2), 265
 (2004): Libersa C+, *Therapie* 59(1), 127
Death
 (2006): Murray TJ, *Expert Opin Drug Saf* 5(2), 265
Infections (>66%)
 (2004): Cohen BA+, *Neurology* 63(12 Suppl 6), S28

MIZORIBINE

Trade name: Bredinin
Indications: Rheumatoid arthritis, systemic lupus erythematosus, prevention of rejection in renal transplantation, lupus nephritis, nephrotic syndrome
Category: Immunosuppressant
Half-life: 6 hours

Reactions

Skin
Stevens–Johnson syndrome
 (2006): Matsushita K+, *Mod Rheumatol* 16(2), 113

Hair
Hair – alopecia
 (2006): Nozu K+, *Pediatr Int* 48(2), 152

Other
Hyperuricemia

 (2006): Goto M+, *Nippon Jinzo Gakkai Shi* 48(4), 365
 (2004): Tanaka H+, *Nihon Rinsho Meneki Gakkai Kaishi* 27(3), 171
 (2002): Kushihata S+, *Nippon Jinzo Gakkai Shi* 44(7), 543
 (1986): Ishikawa I+, *Nippon Jinzo Gakkai Shi* 28(10), 1353
Inappropriate secretion of antidiuretic hormone (SIADH)
 (2002): Fujino Y+, *Nephron* 92(4), 938
Nephrotoxicity
 (2002): Kushihata S+, *Nippon Jinzo Gakkai Shi* 44(7), 543
Pancreatitis
 (1997): Yutsudo Y+, *Ryumachi* 37(4), 564
Rhabdomyolysis
 (2005): Morimoto S+, *Am J Med Sci* 329(4), 211 (with Bezafibrate)

MOCLOBEMIDE

Trade names: Aurorix (Roche); Manerix (Roche)
Indications: Depression, social anxiety
Category: Antidepressant
Half-life: 2–4 hours
Clinically important, potentially hazardous interactions with: benzodiazepines, cimetidine, clomipramine, dextromethorphan, pethidine, selegiline, tyramine

Reactions

Skin
Allergic reactions (sic)
Angioedema
Pruritus
Rash (sic)
Urticaria

Mucosal/ENT
Xerostomia

Eyes
Vision blurred

Other
Agitation
Anaphylactoid reactions/Anaphylaxis
Anxiety
Confusion
Gynecomastia
Headache
 (1994): Moll E+, *Clin Neuropharmacol* 17(Suppl 1), S74
Hepatotoxicity
Hypertension
Hypotension
Insomnia
 (2003): Bonnet U, *CNS Drug Rev* 9(1), 97
 (1994): Moll E+, *Clin Neuropharmacol* 17(Suppl 1), S74
Seizures
Tremor
Vertigo
 (2003): Bonnet U, *CNS Drug Rev* 9(1), 97
 (1994): Moll E+, *Clin Neuropharmacol* 17(Suppl 1), S74

MODAFINIL

Trade names: Alertec; Provigil (Cephalon)
Indications: Narcolepsy
Category: Analeptic; CNS stimulant
Half-life: ~15 hours
**Clinically important, potentially hazardous interactions
with:** oral contraceptives

Reactions

Skin
Allergic reactions (sic) (>1%)
Diaphoresis (>1%)
Edema (>1%)
Erythema
Herpes simplex (1%)
Pruritus (>1%)
Psoriasis (>1%)
Rash (sic) (>1%)
Xerosis (1%)

Mucosal/ENT
Dysgeusia (>1%)
Gingivitis (1%)
Oral ulceration (1%)
Sialorrhea
Xerostomia (5%)

Other
Chills (2%)
Headache (28%)
    (2006): Greenhill LL+, *J Am Acad Child Adolesc Psychiatry*
       45(5), 503
    (2006): Swanson JM+, *J Clin Psychiatry* 67(1), 137
    (2006): Thase ME+, *CNS Spectr* 11(2), 93 (18%)
    (2006): Turner D, *Expert Rev Neurother* 6(4), 455
    (2005): Carter GT+, *Am J Hosp Palliat Care* 22(1), 55
    (2004): Rabkin JG+, *J Clin Psychiatry* 65(12), 1688
    (2003): Schwartz JR+, *Chest* 124(6), 2192 (28%)
Hot flashes
Myalgia/Myositis/Myopathy/Myotoxicity (>1%)
Paresthesias (3%)
    (2002): Nieves AV+, *Clin Neuropharmacol* 25(2), 111
Tremor (1%)
Vertigo
    (2006): Thase ME+, *CNS Spectr* 11(2), 93 (7%)
    (2002): Zifko UA+, *J Neurol* 249(8), 983 (3 cases)

MOEXIPRIL

Trade names: Uniretic (Schwarz); Univasc (Schwarz)
Indications: Hypertension
Category: Angiotensin-converting enzyme inhibitor
Half-life: 1 hour
**Clinically important, potentially hazardous interactions
with:** amiloride, spironolactone, triamterene

Note: Uniretic is moexipril and hydrochlorothiazide

Reactions

Skin
Adverse effects (sic)
    (1994): White WB+, *J Human Hypertens* 8, 917

Angioedema (<1%)
    (2001): Cohen EG+, *Ann Otol Rhinol Laryngol* 110(8), 701 (64
       cases)
Diaphoresis (<1%)
Exanthems (1.6%)
Pemphigus (<1%)
Pemphigus foliaceus
    (2000): Ong CS+, *Australas J Dermatol* 41(4), 242
Peripheral edema (1–10%)
    (1995): Drayer JIM+, *Am J Ther* 2, 525
Photosensitivity (<1%)
Pruritus (1–10%)
Rash (sic) (1.6%)
Urticaria (<1%)

Mucosal/ENT
Dysgeusia (<1%)
Xerostomia (<1%)

Hair
Hair – alopecia (1–10%)

Other
Anaphylactoid reactions/Anaphylaxis (<1%)
Cough
    (2005): Spinar J+, *Int J Cardiol* 100(2), 199 (2%)
    (2001): Adigun AQ+, *West Afr J Med* 20(1), 46–7
    (2001): Lee SC+, *Hypertension* 38(2), 166
Headache
Myalgia/Myositis/Myopathy/Myotoxicity (1.3%)

MOLINDONE

Trade name: Moban (Endo)
Indications: Schizophrenia
Category: Antipsychotic
Half-life: 1.5 hours
**Clinically important, potentially hazardous interactions
with:** paroxetine

Reactions

Skin
Allergic reactions (sic)
Edema
Peripheral edema
Photosensitivity (<1%)
Pigmentation (<1%)
Pruritus (<1%)
Rash (sic) (<1%)

Mucosal/ENT
Sialorrhea
Xerostomia (>10%)

Other
Gynecomastia (1–10%)
Hepatotoxicity
    (1985): Bhatia SC+, *Drug Intell Clin Pharm* 19(10), 744
Pain
    (1990): Sandyk R, *Ital J Neurol Sci* 11(6), 573 (leg)
Rhabdomyolysis
    (1986): Johnson SB+, *J Clin Psychiatry* 47(12), 607

MOMETASONE

Trade names: Elocon (Schering); Nasonex (Schering)
Indications: Dermatoses, rhinitis
Category: Corticosteroid, inhaled; Corticosteroid, topical
Half-life: 7 hours
Clinically important, potentially hazardous interactions with: live vaccines

Reactions

Skin
Acne
  (1998): Prakash A+, *Drugs* 55(1), 145
Atrophy
  (1993): Kecskes A+, *J Am Acad Dermatol* 29(4), 576
Burning
  (2002): Trangsrud AJ+, *Pharmacotherapy* 22(11), 1458
  (2000): Guenther LC+, *Clin Ther* 22(10), 1225 (with tazarotene)
  (1998): Onrust SV+, *Drugs* 56(4), 725
  (1998): Prakash A+, *Drugs* 55(1), 145
Erythema
  (2000): Guenther LC+, *Clin Ther* 22(10), 1225 (with tazarotene)
Folliculitis
  (1998): Prakash A+, *Drugs* 55(1), 145
Irritation
  (2000): Guenther LC+, *Clin Ther* 22(10), 1225 (with tazarotene)
  (1998): Onrust SV+, *Drugs* 56(4), 725
Pigmentation
Pruritus
  (2000): Guenther LC+, *Clin Ther* 22(10), 1225
Stinging
  (2002): Trangsrud AJ+, *Pharmacotherapy* 22(11), 1458
  (1998): Prakash A+, *Drugs* 55(1), 145
Telangiectasia
  (1993): Kecskes A+, *J Am Acad Dermatol* 29(4), 576
Xerosis
  (1998): Prakash A+, *Drugs* 55(1), 145

Mucosal/ENT
Oral candidiasis
  (2000): Bousquet J+, *Eur Respir J* 16(5), 808
  (1999): Bernstein DI+, *Respir Med* 93(9), 603

Eyes
Epiphora
  (2000): Magyar P+, *Orv Hetil* 141(25), 1407

Other
Headache
  (2002): Trangsrud AJ+, *Pharmacotherapy* 22(11), 1458
  (1999): Bernstein DI+, *Respir Med* 93(9), 603
  (1998): Onrust SV+, *Drugs* 56(4), 725

MONOSODIUM GLUTAMATE

Scientific name: *Monosodium glutamate*
Family: N/A
Trade and other common names: E620; MSG
Category: Food additive
Purported indications and other uses: Food additive, flavor enhancer
Half-life: N/A
Clinically important, potentially hazardous interactions with: bcg vaccine, MAO inhibitors

Note: The etiologic agent of Chinese Restaurant Syndrome

Reactions

Skin
Allergic granulomatous angiitis (Churg–Strauss syndrome)
  (2006): Chiu YK+, *J Am Acad Dermatol* 55(2), S1 (after BCG vaccine)
  (1991): Oliver AJ+, *Oral Surg Oral Med Oral Pathol* 71(5), 560
Angioedema
  (1993): Tarlo SM+, *Can Fam Physician* 39, 1119
  (1991): Oliver AJ+, *Oral Surg Oral Med Oral Pathol* 71(5), 560
  (1989): Montano Garcia ML, *Rev Alerg Mex* 36(3), 107
  (1988): Botey J+, *Allergol Immunopathol* (Madr) 16(6), 425
  (1987): Squire EN Jr, *Lancet* 1(8539), 988
Atopic dermatitis
  (1988): Botey J+, *Allergol Immunopathol* (Madr) 16(6), 425
  (1986): Sweatman MC+, *Clin Allergy* 16(4), 331
Burning
  (1987): Settipane GA, *N Engl Reg Allergy Proc* 8(1), 39
Diaphoresis
Edema
  (1986): Wilkin JK, *J Am Acad Dermatol* 15(2 Pt 1), 225
Sensitivity
  (2003): Prandota J, *Am J Ther* 10(1), 51
  (2000): Walker R+, *J Nutr* 130(4S Suppl), 1049S
Urticaria
  (2000): Simon RA, *J Nutr* 130(4S Suppl), 1063S (rare)
  (1998): Ehlers I+, *Allergy* 53(11), 1074
  (1993): Tarlo SM+, *Can Fam Physician* 39, 1119
  (1989): Montano Garcia ML, *Rev Alerg Mex* 36(3), 107
  (1988): Botey J+, *Allergol Immunopathol* (Madr) 16(6), 425

Mucosal/ENT
Rhinitis
  (2004): Pacor ML+, *Allergy* 59(2), 192 (8 cases)

Other
Anaphylactoid reactions/Anaphylaxis
  (1993): Tarlo SM+, *Can Fam Physician* 39, 1119
  (1989): Montano Garcia ML, *Rev Alerg Mex* 36(3), 107
Chest pain
Headache
  (2003): Millichap JG+, *Pediatr Neurol* 28(1), 9
  (2000): Strong FC 3rd, *Clin Exp Allergy* 30(5), 739
  (1997): Yang WH+, *J Allergy Clin Immunol* 99(6 Pt 1), 757
  (1996): Leira R+, *Rev Neurol* 24(129), 534
  (1991): Scopp AL, *Headache* 31(2), 107
Neurotoxicity
  (1982): Freed DL+, *Ann Allergy* 48(2), 96
Paresthesias
  (1997): Yang WH+, *J Allergy Clin Immunol* 99(6 Pt 1), 757
  (1987): Settipane GA, *N Engl Reg Allergy Proc* 8(1), 39
Tremor

MONTELUKAST

Trade name: Singulair (Merck)
Indications: Asthma
Category: Leukotriene receptor antagonist
Half-life: 2.7–5.5 hours
Clinically important, potentially hazardous interactions with: boswellia, prednisone

Reactions

Skin
Allergic granulomatous angiitis (Churg–Strauss syndrome)

(2007): Guilpain P+, *Presse Med* 36(5 Pt 2), 890
(2007): Zandman-Goddard G+, *Isr Med Assoc J* 9(1), 50
(2004): Boccagni C+, *Neurol Sci* 25(1), 21
(2004): Conen D+, *Swiss Med Wkly* 134(25–26), 377
(2004): Oberndorfer S+, *Neurologia* 19(3), 134
(2003): Michael AB+, *Age Ageing* 32(5), 551
(2002): Guilpain P+, *Rheumatology (Oxford)* 41(5), 535 (2 cases)
(2002): Jamaleddine G+, *Semin Arthritis Rheum* 31(4), 218
(2002): Mateo ML+, *Arch Bronconeumol* 38(1), 56
(2002): Perez de Llano LA+, *Arch Bronconeumol* 38(5), 251
(2000): *Can Fam Physician* 46, 86
(1999): *Prescrire Int* 8(43), 131
(1999): Franco J+, *Thorax* 54(6), 558
Angioedema
   (1998): Condry P, Webster, NY (from Internet) (observation)
Erythema nodosum
   (2000): Dellaripa PF+, *Mayo Clin Proc* 75(6), 643
Henoch–Schönlein purpura
   (2005): Khanna S+, *Indian J Gastroenterol* 24(2), 86
Pemphigus
   (2003): Cetkovska P+, *Clin Exp Dermatol* 28(3), 328
Peripheral edema
   (2000): Geller M, *Ann Intern Med* 132, 924
Rash (sic) (1.6%)
Urticaria (1.6%)
   (1998): Jaffe P, Columbia, SC (from Internet) (observation)
   (1998): Knorr B+, *JAMA* 279, 1181

Other
Cough
   (2001): Spector SL, *Ann Allergy Asthma Immunol* 86(6 Suppl 1), 18
Headache
   (2006): Ghosh G+, *Indian Pediatr* 43(9), 780 (10%)
Panniculitis
   (2000): Dellaripa PF+, *Mayo Clin Proc* 75(6), 643

MORICIZINE

Trade name: Ethmozine (Shire)
Indications: Ventricular arrhythmias
Category: Antiarrhythmic class 1c
Half-life: 3–4 hours
**Clinically important, potentially hazardous interactions
with:** diltiazem, warfarin

Reactions

Skin
Diaphoresis (2–5%)
Exanthems (<1%)
Pruritus (<2%)
Rash (sic) (<1%)
Urticaria (<2%)
Xerosis (<2%)

Mucosal/ENT
Dysgeusia (<2%)
Oral lesions
   (1990): Fitton A+, *Drugs* 40, 138
Tinnitus
Tongue edema (<2%)
Xerostomia (2–5%)
   (1990): Carnes CA+, *Drug Intell Clin Pharm* 24, 745 (2–5%)
   (1990): Fitton A+, *Drugs* 40, 138 (2%)

Eyes
Periorbital edema (1–10%)

Other
Congestive heart failure
   (1989): Ravid S+, *J Am Coll Cardiol* 14(5), 1326
Death
   (1992): Damle R+, *Ann Intern Med* 116(5), 375
   (1992): Nazari J+, *Pacing Clin Electrophysiol* 15(10 Pt 1), 1421
   (1992): Tonkin AM, *Med J Aust* 156(7), 488
Paresthesias (2–5%)
Thrombophlebitis (<2%)

MORPHINE

Trade names: Anamorph; Astramorph; Avinza (Ligand);
Contalgin; Duramorph (Baxter) (Elkins-Sinn); Epimorph;
Infumorph (Baxter); Kadian (aaiPharma); Morphine-HP; MOS;
Moscontin; MS Contin (Purdue); MS-IR; MS/S; MSIR Oral
(Purdue); MST Continus; OMS Oral; Oramorph SR; RMS;
Roxanol (aaiPharma); Sevredol; Statex
Indications: Severe pain, acute myocardial infarction
Category: Opiate agonist
Half-life: 2–4 hours
**Clinically important, potentially hazardous interactions
with:** buprenorphine, cimetidine, furazolidone, MAO inhibitors,
mianserin, pentazocine

Reactions

Skin
Acute generalized exanthematous pustulosis (AGEP)
   (2006): Kardaun SH+, *J Am Acad Dermatol* 55(2), S21
Diaphoresis
   (2003): Sayyid SS+, *Reg Anesth Pain Med* 28(2), 140
Edema
Exanthems
Pallor
Peripheral edema
Pruritus (5–65%)
   (2006): Chang KY+, *Acta Anaesthesiol Taiwan* 44(3), 153 (24%)
   (2006): Galea M, *Br J Anaesth* 97(3), 426
   (2006): Raffaeli W+, *Eur J Anaesthesiol* 23(7), 605
   (2005): Gambling D+, *Anesth Analg* 100(4), 1065
   (2005): Greenwald PW+, *Am J Emerg Med* 23(1), 35 (4%)
   (2005): Sfeir S+, *Middle East J Anesthesiol* 18(1), 133
   (2003): Charuluxananan S+, *Anesth Analg* 96(6), 1789
   (2003): Duale C+, *Br J Anaesth* 91(5), 690
   (2003): Murphy PM+, *Anesth Analg* 97(6), 1709
   (2003): Sayyid SS+, *Reg Anesth Pain Med* 28(2), 140
   (2002): Nakata K+, *J Clin Anesth* 14(2), 121
   (2001): Charuluxananan S+, *Anesth Analg* 93(1), 162
   (2001): Matsuda M+, *Masui* 50(10), 1096
   (2001): Mercadante S+, *Support Care Cancer* 9(6), 467
   (2001): Sakai T+, *Can J Anaesth* 48(8), 831
   (2001): Subramaniam K+, *J Clin Anesth* 13(5), 339 (with
      ketamine)
   (2000): Gunter JB+, *Paediatr Anaesth* 10, 167
   (2000): Yeh HM+, *Anesth Analg* 91, 172
   (1999): Joshi GP+, *Anesthesiology* 90(4), 1007
   (1998): Thangaturai D+, *Anaesthesia* 43, 1055 (62%)
   (1992): Cohen SE+, *Anesth Analg* 75(5), 747
   (1988): Gustafson LL+, *Drugs* 35, 597 (5–10%)
   (1986): Attia J+, *Anesthesiology* 65, 590 (20%)
Psoriasis
Rash (sic)

Mucosal/ENT
Xerostomia (>10%)
(2004): Andersen G+, *Eur J Pain* 8(3), 263
(2002): Andersen G+, *Palliat Med* 16(2), 107
(1989): White JD+, *BMJ* 298, 1222 (75%)

Other
Cardiotoxicity
(2006): Lotsch J+, *Clin Pharmacokinet* 45(11), 1051
Death
(2006): Lotsch J+, *Clin Pharmacokinet* 45(11), 1051
(2005): Reith D+, *N Z Med J* 118(1209), U1293 (33 cases)
(2002): Byard RW, *J Forensic Sci* 47(1), 202
Gynecomastia
Hypotension
(2005): Gambling D+, *Anesth Analg* 100(4), 1065
(1991): Randich A+, *Brain Res* 543(2), 256
Injection-site pain (>10%)
Rhabdomyolysis
(2002): Molia A+, *Therapie* 57(6), 595
(1985): Blain PG+, *Hum Toxicol* 4(1), 71
Vertigo
(2006): Vestergaard P+, *J Intern Med* 260(1), 76

MOXIFLOXACIN

Trade name: Avelox (Schering)
Indications: Various infections caused by susceptible organisms
Category: Antibiotic, quinolone
Half-life: 12 hours
Clinically important, potentially hazardous interactions with: amiodarone, arsenic, bepridil, bretylium, disopyramide, erythromycin, phenothiazines, procainamide, quinidine, sotalol, tricyclic antidepressants, zinc, ziprasidone

Reactions

Skin
Allergic reactions (sic)
Bullous dermatitis
(2004): Nori S+, *Arch Dermatol* 140(12), 1537
Burning
Desquamation (lips)
(2004): Nori S+, *Arch Dermatol* 140(12), 1537
Diaphoresis (<1%)
Edema
Exanthems
(2000): Litt JZ, Beachwood, OH (personal case; no pruritus)
Fixed eruption
(2001): Litt JZ, Beachwood, OH (personal case) (observation)
Peripheral edema (<1%)
Photosensitivity (<1%)
(2004): Viola G+, *Chem Biodivers* 1(5), 782
(2000): Balfour JA+, *Drugs* 59, 115
(2000): Stein GE+, *Inf Med* 17, 564
(2000): Traynor NJ+, *Toxicol Vitr* 14, 275
Pruritus (<1%)
Rash (sic) (<1%)
(2001): Culley CM+, *Am J Health-Syst Pharm* 58, 379
Toxic epidermal necrolysis
(2004): Nori S+, *Arch Dermatol* 140(12), 1537
Urticaria (<1%)
(2005): Bozkurt B+, *Allergol Immunopathol (Madr)* 33(1), 38 (1 case)
Xerosis (<1%)

Mucosal/ENT
Dysgeusia (>1%)
(2000): Stein GE+, *Inf Med* 17, 564
Glossitis (<1%)
Stomatitis (<1%)
Vaginitis (<1%)
(2000): Stein GE+, *Inf Med* 17, 564
Xerostomia (<1%)
(2001): Litt JZ, Beachwood, OH (personal case) (observation)

Eyes
Corneal ulcer
(2006): Walter K+, *Cornea* 25(7), 855

Other
Abdominal pain
(2004): Nori S+, *Arch Dermatol* 140(12), 1537
(2003): Carroll DN, *Pharmacotherapy* 23(11), 1517
Anaphylactoid reactions/Anaphylaxis
(2006): Sachs B+, *Drug Saf* 29(11), 1087
(2003): Ho DY+, *Ann Pharmacother* 37(7), 1018
(2001): Aleman A+, *J Allergy Clin Immunol* Feb, 107
Candidiasis (<1%)
Chills (<1%)
Headache
Hypersensitivity
(2004): Nori S+, *Arch Dermatol* 140(12), 1537
Myalgia/Myositis/Myopathy/Myotoxicity (<1%)
Paresthesias (<1%)
Tendinopathy/Tendon rupture
(2004): Burkhardt O+, *Scand J Infect Dis* 36(4), 315
Tremor (<1%)
Vertigo
(2003): Klossek JM+, *J Laryngol Otol* 117(1), 43

MUPIROCIN

Trade names: Bactoderm; Bactroban (GSK); Eismycin; Mupiderm
Indications: Secondarily infected traumatic skin lesions due to susceptible strains of *Staphylococcus aureus* and *Streptococcus pyogenes*, impetigo
Category: Antibiotic, topical
Half-life: N/A
Clinically important, potentially hazardous interactions with: None

Note: Also known as *pseudomonic acid*, mupirocin is an antibacterial agent produced by fermentation using the organism *Pseudomonas fluorescens*

Reactions

Skin
Allergic reactions (sic)
(1999): Mylotte JM+, *Infect Control Hosp Epidemiol* 20(11), 741 (intranasal)
(1995): Eedy DJ, *Contact Dermatitis* 32(4), 240
Burning
(1997): Bertino JS, *Am J Health Sys Pharm* 54(19), 2185 (of nose) (intranasal)
Cellulitis (<1%)
Dermatitis (<1%)
(1997): Zappi EG+, *J Am Acad Dermatol* 36(2 Pt 1), 266
Edema

(1997): Bertino JS, *Am J Health Syst Pharm* 54(19), 2185 (of nose) (intranasal)
Erythema
(1997): Bertino JS, *Am J Health Syst Pharm* 54(19), 2185 (of nose) (intranasal)
Pruritus (1–2.4%)
(1997): Bertino JS, *Am J Health Syst Pharm* 54(19), 2185 (of nose) (intranasal)
Rash (sic) (1.1%)
Stinging
(1997): Bertino JS, *Am J Health Syst Pharm* 54(19), 2185 (of nose) (intranasal)
Xerosis
(1997): Bertino JS, *Am J Health Syst Pharm* 54(19), 2185 (of nose) (intranasal)

Mucosal/ENT
Dysgeusia (3%) (intranasal)
Stomatitis (<1%)
Xerostomia (<1%) (intranasal)

Eyes
Blepharitis (<1%) (intranasal)

Other
Application-site burning (1–3.6%)
Cough (2%) (intranasal)
Headache
Vertigo (<1%)

MUROMONAB-CD3

Trade name: Orthoclone OKT 3 (Ortho-Biotech)
Indications: Reversal of acute allograft rejection in renal, cardiac and hepatic transplant patients
Category: Immunosuppressant; Monoclonal antibody
Half-life: N/A
Clinically important, potentially hazardous interactions with: N/A

Note: CRS is a clinical syndrome mostly experienced in patients following the first few doses of ORTHOCLONE. Symptoms diminish with successive doses but may reappear with increasing the amount of a dose or resuming treatment after a hiatus. Symptoms range from frequently reported mild "flu-like" symptoms to less frequently reported severe "shock-like" reactions (which may include cardiovascular and central nervous system manifestations). Symptoms include fever, chills, headache, tremor, nausea/vomiting, diarrhea, abdominal pain, malaise and muscle/joint aches and pains, and generalized weakness. Less frequently reported but serious and occasionally fatal adverse events include cardiorespiratory events (dyspnea, shortness of breath, bronchospasm/wheezing, tachypnea, respiratory arrest/failure/distress, cardiovascular collapse, cardiac arrest, angina/myocardial infarction, chest pain/tightness, tachycardia, hypertension, hypotension including profound shock, heart failure, pulmonary edema, adult respiratory distress syndrome, hypoxemia, apnea and arrhythmias) and neuro-psychiatric events.

Reactions

Skin
Diaphoresis (7%)
Edema (12%)
(1994): Shennib H+, *J Heart Lung Transplant* 13(3), 514
Herpes simplex
(1994): Jacobs U+, *Transplant Proc* 26(6), 3121 (Reactivation)
Kaposi's sarcoma

(1996): Besnard V+, *Dermatology* 193(2), 100
Pruritus (7%)
Rash (sic) (14%)
Shivering
(1996): Abdallah KA+, *Transplantation* 62(1), 145

Mucosal/ENT
Hearing loss
(2000): Hartnick CJ+, *Ann Otol Rhinol Laryngol* 109(1), 45
(1997): Hartnick CJ+, *Ann Otol Rhinol Laryngol* 106(8), 640
Tinnitus (1%)

Eyes
Conjunctivitis (<1%)
Photophobia (1%)
(1994): Gaughan WJ+, *Am J Kidney Dis* 24(3), 486
Uveitis
(2001): Gariano RF+, *Br J Ophthalmol* 85(4), 500
Vision loss
(1995): Jin DC+, *Nephrol Dial Transplant* 10(11), 2144
Visual hallucinations (<1%)

Other
Abdominal pain (6%)
Anaphylactoid reactions/Anaphylaxis
(2000): Berkowitz RJ+, *Pharmacotherapy* 20(1), 100
Aseptic meningitis
(1999): Thomas MC+, *Transplantation* 67(10), 1384
(1998): Uribe Roca MC+, *Neurologia* 13(2), 98
Asthenia (6%)
Cardiac arrest (<1%)
Cardiac failure (<1%)
Chest pain (9%)
Chills (43%)
(1994): Wagner FM+, *J Heart Lung Transplant* 13(3), 438
Confusion (6%)
Delirium
(2003): Pittock SJ+, *Transplantation* 75(7), 1058
Depression (3%)
Fever (77%)
(2006): Segovia J+, *Transplantation* 81(11), 1542
(1998): Whiting JF+, *Transplantation* 65(4), 577
(1995): Sosman JA+, *J Immunother Emphasis Tumor Immunol* 17(3), 171
(1994): Gaughan WJ+, *Am J Kidney Dis* 24(3), 486
(1994): Wagner FM+, *J Heart Lung Transplant* 13(3), 438
Headache (28%)
(1999): Quirce R+, *Rev Esp Med Nucl* 18(5), 363
(1996): Woodle ES+, *Clin Transplant* 10(4), 389
(1994): Gaughan WJ+, *Am J Kidney Dis* 24(3), 486
Hepatotoxicity (<1%)
(2002): Go MR+, *Transplantation* 73(12), 1957
Hypertension (19%)
(1994): Gaughan WJ+, *Am J Kidney Dis* 24(3), 486
Hypotension (25%)
(2006): Segovia J+, *Transplantation* 81(11), 1542
(1998): Whiting JF+, *Transplantation* 65(4), 577
(1995): Sosman JA+, *J Immunother Emphasis Tumor Immunol* 17(3), 171
(1994): Shennib H+, *J Heart Lung Transplant* 13(3), 514
Infections (sic)
(1995): Bock HA+, *Transplantation* 59(6), 830
(1994): Wagner FM+, *J Heart Lung Transplant* 13(3), 438
Mood changes (<1%)
Myalgia/Myositis/Myopathy/Myotoxicity
(1994): Gaughan WJ+, *Am J Kidney Dis* 24(3), 486
(1994): Shennib H+, *J Heart Lung Transplant* 13(3), 514
Nephrotoxicity

(1996): Wever PC+, *Eur J Clin Invest* 26(10), 873
Neurotoxicity
(2003): Pittock SJ+, *Transplantation* 75(7), 1058
Paranoia (<1%)
Seizures (1%)
(2001): Thaisetthawatkul P+, *J Child Neurol* 16(11), 825
(1997): Parizel PM+, *AJNR Am J Neuroradiol* 18(10), 1935
(1997): Seifeldin RA+, *Ann Pharmacother* 31(5), 586
(1994): Wagner FM+, *J Heart Lung Transplant* 13(3), 438
Somnolence (2%)
Tremor (14%)
Vertigo (6%)

MYCOPHENOLATE

Synonym: mycophenolate mofetil
Trade names: CellCept (Roche); Myfortic (Novartis)
Indications: Prophylaxis of organ rejection
Category: Immunosuppressant; TNF inhibitor
Half-life: 18 hours
**Clinically important, potentially hazardous interactions
with:** antacids, azathioprine, basiliximab, cholestyramine,
corticosteroids, cyclophosphamide, cyclosporine, daclizumab,
hemophilus B vaccine, mercaptopurine, metronidazole,
norfloxacin, tacrolimus, **vaccines**

Reactions

Skin

Acne (>10%)
(2007): Zwerner J+, *Dermatol Ther* 20(4), 229 (passim)
Bullous dermatitis
(2000): Rault R, *Ann Intern Med* 133, 921 (hands)
Carcinoma (non-melanoma) (4%)
Dermatitis herpetiformis (aggravation)
(2002): Gladstone GC, Worcester, MA (personal
correspondence)
Diaphoresis
Dyshidrosis
(2007): Zwerner J+, *Dermatol Ther* 20(4), 229 (passim)
Edema (12.2%)
Fixed eruption
(2006): Sontheimer R (from Internet) (observation)
Herpes simplex
(2000): Williams JV+, *Skin & Allergy News* September, 24
Herpes zoster
(2006): Jimenez-Perez M+, *Transplant Proc* 38(8), 2480
(2005): Shipkova M+, *Expert Opin Drug Metab Toxicol* 1(3), 505
Pemphigus
(2007): Scheinfeld N, *J Dermatolog Treat* 18(4), 243
Peripheral edema (28.6%)
Pruritus
(2002): Gladstone GC, Worcester, MA (personal
correspondence)
Rash (sic) (7.7%)
(2005): Levin N+, *Clin Neuropharmacol* 28(3), 152 (severe)
Toxicoderma
(2002): Hafraoui S+, *Gastroenterol Clin Biol* 26(1), 17 (2 cases)
Urticaria
(2007): Zwerner J+, *Dermatol Ther* 20(4), 229 (passim)

Mucosal/ENT

Gingival hyperplasia/hypertrophy
Gingivitis
Oral candidiasis (10.1%)

Oral ulceration
(2003): Schmutz JL+, *Ann Dermatol Venereol* 130(2), 241
(2003): van Gelder+, *Transplantation* 75(6), 788
(2001): Garrigue V+, *Transplantation* 72(5), 968

Hair

Hair – alopecia
(2001): Zierhut M+, *Ophthalmologe* 98(7), 647

Other

Abdominal pain
(2006): Kwinta-Rybicka J+, *Przegl Lek* 63, 44
(2005): Shipkova M+, *Expert Opin Drug Metab Toxicol* 1(3), 505
Asthenia
(2005): Galindo M+, *J Rheumatol* 32(1), 188
(2003): Lau CH+, *Clin Experiment Ophthalmol* 31(6), 487
Fever
(2007): Zwerner J+, *Dermatol Ther* 20(4), 229 (passim)
Headache
(2007): Zwerner J+, *Dermatol Ther* 20(4), 229 (passim)
(2003): Lau CH+, *Clin Experiment Ophthalmol* 31(6), 487
Hepatotoxicity
(2006): Loupy A+, *Transplantation* 82(4), 581
Hypersensitivity
(2005): Szyper-Kravitz M+, *Int Arch Allergy Immunol* 138(4), 334
Hypertension
(2007): Zwerner J+, *Dermatol Ther* 20(4), 229 (passim)
Infections (12–20%)
(2007): Zwerner J+, *Dermatol Ther* 20(4), 229 (passim)
(2006): Jimenez-Perez M+, *Transplant Proc* 38(8), 2480
(2005): Prokopenko EI+, *Ter Arkh* 77(1), 67
(2005): Shipkova M+, *Expert Opin Drug Metab Toxicol* 1(3), 505
(2002): Bernabeu-Wittel M+, *Eur J Clin Microbiol Infect Dis*
21(3), 173
Insomnia
(2007): Zwerner J+, *Dermatol Ther* 20(4), 229 (passim)
Myalgia/Myositis/Myopathy/Myotoxicity
(2007): Zwerner J+, *Dermatol Ther* 20(4), 229 (passim)
(2005): Galindo M+, *J Rheumatol* 32(1), 188
(2005): Shipkova M+, *Expert Opin Drug Metab Toxicol* 1(3), 505
(2002): Greiner K+, *Ophthalmologe* 99(9), 691
Neurotoxicity
(2007): Zwerner J+, *Dermatol Ther* 20(4), 229 (passim)
Paresthesias
Thrombophlebitis (1–10%)
Tremor (11%)
Vertigo
(2003): Lau CH+, *Clin Experiment Ophthalmol* 31(6), 487

MYRRH

Scientific names: *Commiphora abyssinica; Commiphora erythraea;
Commiphora habessinica; Commiphora kataf; Commiphora
madagascariensis; Commiphora molmol; Commiphora myrrh*
Family: Burseraceae
Trade and other common names: Bal; Balsamodendron;
Bdellium; Bol; Bola; Didin; Didthin; Heerabol; Mirazid; Mirra;
Morr
Category: Anti-inflammatory; Antihelmintic
Purported indications and other uses: Fascioliasis,
schistosomiasis, ulcers, eczema, catarrh, amenorrhea, gum
disease, aphthous stomatitis
Half-life: N/A
**Clinically important, potentially hazardous interactions
with:** methimazole, propylthiouracil

Reactions

Skin

Dermatitis
(2000): Anderson C+, *Phytother Res* 14(6), 452
(1999): Gallo R+, *Contact Dermatitis* 41(4), 230
(1998): Al-Suwaidan SN+, *Contact Dermatitis* 39(3), 137
(1993): Lee TY+, *Contact Dermatitis* 28(2), 89
(1993): Lee TY+, *Contact Dermatitis* 29(5), 279
Pruritus (0.5%)
(2001): Sheir Z+, *Am J Trop Med Hyg* 65(6), 700 (0.5%)
Side effects (sic)
(2001): Sheir Z+, *Am J Trop Med Hyg* 65(6), 700 (mild & transient)

Other

Abdominal pain (2%)
(2001): Sheir Z+, *Am J Trop Med Hyg* 65(6), 700 (2%)
Asthenia (2.5%)
(2001): Sheir Z+, *Am J Trop Med hyg* 65(6), 700 (2.5%)
Headache (0.5%)
(2001): Sheir Z+, *Am J Trop Med Hyg* 65(6), 700 (0.5%)
Rhabdomyolysis
(2004): Bianchi A+, *Ann Pharmacother* 38(7-8), 1222

NABILONE

Trade name: Cesamet (Valeant)
Indications: Nausea and vomiting
Category: Cannabinoid
Half-life: 2 hours
Clinically important, potentially hazardous interactions with: CNS depressants

Reactions

Mucosal/ENT

Xerostomia
(2006): Berlach DM+, *Pain Med* 7(1), 25
(1986): Pomeroy M+, *Cancer Chemother Pharmacol* 17(3), 285
(1983): George M+, *Biomed Pharmacother* 37(1), 24

Eyes

Vision blurred
(1985): Ward A+, *Drugs* 30(2), 127

Other

Abdominal pain
Anxiety
Asthenia
(1986): Pomeroy M+, *Cancer Chemother Pharmacol* 17(3), 285
(1983): Ahmedzai S+, *Br J Cancer* 48(5), 657 (57%)
Depression
Headache
Hypotension
(1986): Pomeroy M+, *Cancer Chemother Pharmacol* 17(3), 285
(1985): Ward A+, *Drugs* 30(2), 127
(1983): Ahmedzai S+, *Br J Cancer* 48(5), 657 (7%)
(1983): George M+, *Biomed Pharmacother* 37(1), 24
(1981): Einhorn LH+, *J Clin Pharmacol* 21(8–9 Suppl), 64S
Paranoia
Somnolence
Vertigo
(1987): Chan HS+, *Pediatrics* 79(6), 946
(1987): Niiranen A+, *Am J Clin Oncol* 10(4), 325
(1986): Dalzell AM+, *Arch Dis Child* 61(5), 502

(1986): Pomeroy M+, *Cancer Chemother Pharmacol* 17(3), 285
(1985): Niiranen A+, *Am J Clin Oncol* 8(4), 336
(1985): Ward A+, *Drugs* 30(2), 127
(1983): Ahmedzai S+, *Br J Cancer* 48(5), 657 (35%)
(1980): Steele N+, *Cancer Treat Rep* 64(2–3), 219

NABUMETONE

Trade names: Arthaxan; Consolan; Nabuser; Prodac; Relafen (GSK); Relif; Relifex; Unimetone
Indications: Arthritis
Category: Non-steroidal anti-inflammatory
Half-life: 22.5–30 hours
Clinically important, potentially hazardous interactions with: methotrexate

Reactions

Skin

Acne (<1%)
Adverse effects (sic)
(1990): Fletcher AP, *Drugs* 40 (Suppl 5), 43
Angioedema (<1%)
(1990): Jenner PN, *Drugs* 40 (Suppl 5), 80
Bullous dermatitis (<1%)
Diaphoresis (1–3%)
Edema (3–9%)
(1990): Munzel P+, *Drugs* 40 (Suppl 5), 62
Erythema
(1990): Alianti M+, *Clin Ter* (Italian) 133, 299
Erythema multiforme (<1%)
Exanthems (1.2%)
(1999): Litt JZ, Beachwood, OH (personal case) (observation)
(1988): Friedel HA+, *Drugs* 35, 504
Photosensitivity (<1%)
(1998): Litt JZ, Beachwood, OH (personal case) (observation)
(1994): Shelley WB+, *Cutis* 54, 70 (observation)
(1993): Litt JZ, Beachwood, OH (personal case) (observation)
(1989): Kaidbey KH+, *Arch Dermatol* 125, 783
(1988): Friedel HA+, *Drugs* 35, 504
Phototoxicity
(1989): Kaidbey KH+, *Arch Dermatol* 125, 783 and 824
Pruritus (3–9%)
(1999): Litt JZ, Beachwood, OH (personal case) (observation)
(1988): Friedel HA+, *Drugs* 35, 504
Rash (sic) (3–9%)
(1988): Friedel HA+, *Drugs* 35, 504
(1987): Jackson RE+, *Am J Med* 83, 115
(1987): Jenner PN+, *Am J Med* 83, 110
(1987): Mullen BJ, *Am J Med* 83, 70
Side effects (sic)
(1991): Riccieri V+, *Clin Ter* (Italian) 137, 185
Stevens–Johnson syndrome (<1%)
(1997): Sienkiewicz G, Johnson City, NY (from Internet) (observation)
Toxic epidermal necrolysis (<1%)
Urticaria (<1%)
Vasculitis (necrotizing)
(1990): Willkins RF, *Drugs* 40 (Suppl 5), 34
Xerosis
(1987): Mullen BJ, *Am J Med* 83, 70

Mucosal/ENT

Gingivitis (<1%)
Glossitis (<1%)
Oral ulceration

(1989): Lussier A+, *J Clin Pharmacol* 29, 225
Sialorrhea
Stomatitis (1–3%)
Tinnitus
Xerostomia (1–3%)

Hair

Hair – alopecia (<1%)
(1987): Mullen BJ, *Am J Med* 83, 70

Other

Anaphylactoid reactions/Anaphylaxis (<1%)
Headache
Hot flashes (<1%)
Hypersensitivity
(2006): Wyplosz B+, *Br J Clin Pharmacol* 61(4), 474
Myalgia/Myositis/Myopathy/Myotoxicity
Paresthesias (<1%)
Porphyria cutanea tarda (<1%)
Pseudolymphoma
(2001): Werth V, *Dermatology Times* 18
Pseudoporphyria
(2002): LaDuca JR+, *J Cutan Med Surg* 6(4), 320 (2 cases)
(2000): Antony F+, *Br J Dermatol* 142, 1067
(2000): Bergfeld W+, *Skin & Allergy News* December, 33
(2000): Cron RQ+, *J Rheumatol* 27(7), 1817
(1999): Aylesworth R, Rhinelander, WI (from Internet)
(observation)
(1999): Checketts SR+, *J Rheumatol* 26(12), 2703 (2 cases)
(1999): Krischer J+, *J Am Acad Dermatol* 40, 492
(1999): Magro CM+, *J Cutan Pathol* 26, 42
(1998): Varma S+, *Br J Dermatol* 138, 549

NADOLOL

Trade names: Apo-Nadolol; Corgard; Corzide (Monarch); Farmagard; Nadic; Solgol; Syn-Nadolol
Indications: Hypertension, angina pectoris
Category: Adrenergic beta-receptor antagonist; Antiarrhythmic class II
Half-life: 10–24 hours
Clinically important, potentially hazardous interactions with: clonidine, epinephrine, verapamil

Note: Corzide is nadolol and bendroflumethiazide

Note: Cutaneous side effects of beta-receptor blockaders are clinically polymorphous. They apparently appear after several months of continuous therapy. Atypical psoriasiform, lichen planus-like, and eczematous chronic rashes are mainly observed. (1983): Hödl St, *Z Hautkr* (German) 58, 17

Note: Bendroflumethiazide is a sulfonamide and can be absorbed systemically. Sulfonamides can produce severe, possibly fatal, reactions such as toxic epidermal necrolysis and Stevens–Johnson syndrome

Reactions

Skin

Bullous pemphigoid
(1984): Stage AH+, *Am J Obstet Gynecol* 150, 169
Diaphoresis (<1%)
(1980): Heel RC+, *Drugs* 20, 1 (0.6%)
Eczema
Edema (1–5%)
Erythema multiforme
Exanthems (<1%)

(1980): Heel RC+, *Drugs* 20, 1 (0.4%)
Exfoliative dermatitis
Facial edema (<1%)
Hyperkeratosis (palms and soles)
Lichenoid eruption
Lupus erythematosus
Pityriasis rubra pilaris
Pruritus (1–5%)
Psoriasis
(1988): Gold MH+, *J Am Acad Dermatol* 19, 837 (aggravation of)
(1988): Heng MCY+, *Int J Dermatol* 27, 619
(1986): Czernielewski J+, *Lancet* 1, 808
(1984): Arntzen N+, *Acta Derm Venereol* (Stockh) 64, 346
Pustules
(1991): Bernard P+, *Dermatologica* 182, 115
Rash (sic) (1–5%)
Raynaud's phenomenon (2%)
(1984): Eliasson K+, *Acta Med Scand* 215, 333
Scalp dermatitis
(1985): Shelley ED+, *Cutis* 35, 148
Toxic epidermal necrolysis
Urticaria
Xerosis

Mucosal/ENT

Dysgeusia
Gingivitis
(2002): Reynaert H, *J Hepatol* 37(2), 289
Oral lichenoid eruption
Oral mucosal eruption (<1%)
(1980): Heel RC+, *Drugs* 20, 1 (0.6%)
Tinnitus
Xerostomia (<1%)
(1980): Heel RC+, *Drugs* 20, 1

Hair

Hair – alopecia
(1985): Shelley ED+, *Cutis* 35, 148

Nails

Nails – dystrophy
Nails – pigmentation

Eyes

Oculo-mucocutaneous syndrome
(1982): Cocco G+, *Curr Ther Res* 31, 362

Other

Headache
Paresthesias (>5%)
Peyronie's disease

NAFARELIN

Trade names: Synarel (Pfizer); Synarela
Indications: Endometriosis
Category: Gonadotropin-releasing hormone agonist
Half-life: ~3 hours

Reactions

Skin

Acne (>10%)
Chloasma (<1%)
Edema (1–10%)
Exanthems (<1%)

Pruritus (1–10%)
Rash (sic) (1–10%)
Seborrhea (1–10%)
Urticaria (1–10%)

Mucosal/ENT
Sinusitis
  (2001): Heinig J+, *Eur J Obstet Gynecol Reprod Biol* 99(2), 266
Vaginitis

Hair
Hair – hirsutism (1–10%)

Other
Gynecomastia (<1%)
Hot flashes (>10%)
  (1997): Bergqvist A+, *Gynecol Endocrinol* 11(3), 187
Hypersensitivity (0.2%)
Myalgia/Myositis/Myopathy/Myotoxicity (>10%)
Paresthesias (<1%)

NAFCILLIN

Trade names: Nafcil (Merz); Vigopen
Indications: Various infections caused by susceptible organisms
Category: Antibiotic, penicillin
Half-life: 0.5–1.5 hours
Clinically important, potentially hazardous interactions
with: anticoagulants, cyclosporine, demeclocycline, doxycycline, imipenem/cilastatin, methotrexate, minocycline, oxytetracycline, tetracycline, warfarin

Reactions

Skin
Allergic reactions (sic)
  (1994): Pleasants RA+, *Chest* 106, 1124 (in patients with cystic fibrosis)
Angioedema
Bullous dermatitis
Erythema multiforme
Exanthems (10%)
Exfoliative dermatitis
Hematomas
Jarisch–Herxheimer reaction
Jaundice
  (1994): Schuman R+, *Am J Gastroenterol* 89(6), 952
Lupus erythematosus
  (2004): Blazes DL+, *Rheumatol Int* 24(4), 242
Necrosis
  (1980): Tilden SJ+, *Am J Dis Child* 134(11), 1046
Pruritus
Rash (sic) (1–32%)
  (2002): Maraqa NF+, *Clin Infect Dis* 34(1), 50 (32%)
Stevens–Johnson syndrome
Toxic epidermal necrolysis
Urticaria
Vasculitis

Mucosal/ENT
Dysgeusia
Glossitis
Glossodynia
Oral candidiasis
Stomatitis

Stomatodynia
Tongue black
Vaginitis
Xerostomia

Other
Anaphylactoid reactions/Anaphylaxis
Hepatotoxicity
  (1996): Presti ME+, *Dig Dis Sci* 41(1), 180
  (1993): Mazuryk H+, *Am J Gastroenterol* 88(11), 1960
  (1992): Lestico MR+, *Ann Pharmacother* 26(7–8), 985
Hypersensitivity (<1%)
Injection-site necrosis
  (1987): Dufresne RG, *Cutis* 39, 197
  (1980): Tilden SJ+, *Am J Dis Child* 134, 1046
Injection-site pain
Nephrotoxicity
  (1993): Guharoy SR+, *Ann Pharmacother* 27(2), 170
  (1992): Lestico MR+, *Ann Pharmacother* 26(7–8), 985
  (1984): Smith CR+, *Ann Intern Med* 101(4), 469 (28%)
Serum sickness
Thrombophlebitis (<1%)

NALBUPHINE

Trade names: Bufigen; Nalcryn SP; Nubain (Endo); Nubain SP
Indications: Moderate to severe pain
Category: Opiate agonist
Half-life: 5 hours
Clinically important, potentially hazardous interactions
with: CNS depressants, diazepam, pentobarbital, promethazine

Note: Nalbuphine contains sulfites

Reactions

Skin
Burning (<1%)
  (1995): Brenet O+, *Cah Anesthesiol* 43(3), 319
Clammy skin (9%)
Diaphoresis (9%)
Pruritus (<1%)
Urticaria (<1%)

Mucosal/ENT
Dysgeusia (<1%)
Xerostomia (4%)

Eyes
Vision blurred

Other
Depression (<1%)
Headache
Hypertension
  (1990): Blaise GA+, *Can J Anaesth* 37(7), 794
Injection-site pain
  (2001): Charuluxananan S+, *Anesth Analg* 93(1), 162
  (1995): van den Berg+, *Eur J Anaesthesiol* 12(5), 513
  (1989): Pugh GC+, *Br J Anaesth* 62(6), 601
Paresthesias
Vertigo (5%)
  (2001): Charuluxananan S+, *Anesth Analg* 93(1), 162

NALIDIXIC ACID

Trade names: Betaxina; Granexin; Mytacin; Nalidixin; Neggram; Nogram; Youdix
Indications: Various urinary tract infections caused by susceptible organisms
Category: Antibiotic, quinolone
Half-life: 6–7 hours
Clinically important, potentially hazardous interactions with: warfarin

Reactions

Skin
Angioedema (<1%)
Bullous dermatitis (<1%)
  (1981): Wolf A, *Z Hautkr* (German) 56, 109
Erythema multiforme (<1%)
Exanthems (>5%)
Exfoliative dermatitis
Lupus erythematosus
Photosensitivity (<1%)
  (1997): O'Reilly FM+, American Academy of Dermatology
    Meeting, Poster #14
  (1993): Wainwright NJ+, *Drug Saf* 9, 437
  (1990): Bilsland D+, *Br J Dermatol* 123, 548
  (1986): Ljunggren B+, *Photodermatol* 3, 26
  (1985): Epstein JH+, *Drugs* 30, 42
  (1982): Rosen K+, *Acta Derm Venereol* (Stockh) 62, 246
  (1981): Boisvert A+, *Drug Intell Clin Pharm* 15, 126
  (1981): Closas J+, *Rev Clin Esp* (Spanish) 162, 219
  (1980): Stern RS+, *Arch Dermatol* 116, 1269
Phototoxic bullous eruption
Pruritus (<1%)
Purpura
Rash (sic) (<1%)
Toxic epidermal necrolysis
Urticaria (<1%)
  (1985): Goolamali SK, *Postgrad Med J* 61, 925

Hair
Hair – alopecia

Other
Anaphylactoid reactions/Anaphylaxis
Headache
Paresthesias
Porphyria cutanea tarda
  (1992): Shelley WB+, *Advanced Dermatologic Diagnosis* WB
    Saunders, 414 (passim)
  (1983): Goldsman CI+, *Cleve Clin Q* 50, 151
Pseudoporphyria
  (1990): Bilsland D+, *Br J Dermatol* 123, 547
  (1984): Harber LC+, *J Invest Dermatol* 82, 207

NALMEFENE

Trade names: Cervene; Revex (Baxter)
Indications: Reversal of opioid depression, alcohol dependence, pathological gambling, pruritus of cholestasis
Category: Antidote; Opioid antagonist
Half-life: 10.8 Hours
Clinically important, potentially hazardous interactions with: flumazenil

Reactions

Skin
Pruritus (<1%)

Mucosal/ENT
Pharyngitis (<1%)
Xerostomia (<1%)

Other
Agitation (<1%)
  (1991): Fudala PJ+, *Clin Pharmacol Ther* 49(3), 300
Asthenia
  (2007): Karhuvaara S+, *Alcohol Clin Exp Res* 31(7), 1179
  (2005): Geer EB+, *Pituitary* 8(2), 115
Chills (1%)
Confusion (<1%)
  (2004): Anton RF+, *J Clin Psychopharmacol* 24(4), 421
Depression (<1%)
Fever (3%)
Headache (1%)
Hypertension (5%)
Hypotension (1%)
Insomnia
  (2007): Karhuvaara S+, *Alcohol Clin Exp* 31(7), 1179
  (2006): Grant JE+, *Am J Psychiatry* 163(2), 303
  (2004): Anton RF+, *J Clin Psychopharmacol* 24(4), 421
Pain (postoperative) (4%)
Somnolence (<1%)
Tremor (<1%)
Urinary retention (<1%)
Vertigo (3%)
  (2007): Karhuvaara S+, *Alcohol Clin Exp* 31(7), 1179
  (2006): Grant JE+, *Am J Psychiatry* 163(2), 303
  (2005): Geer EB+, *Pituitary* 8(2), 115
  (2004): Anton RF+, *J Clin Psychopharmacol* 24(4), 421
  (1986): Dixon R+, *Clin Pharmacol Ther* 39(1), 49

NALOXONE

Trade names: Nalpin; Narcan (Endo); Narcanti; Narcotan; Suboxone (Reckitt Benckiser); Talwin-NX (Sanofi-Aventis); Zynox
Indications: Narcotic overdose
Category: Opioid antagonist
Half-life: 1–1.5 hours
Clinically important, potentially hazardous interactions with: thioridazine

Reactions

Skin
Angioedema
  (1982): Smitz S+, *Ann Intern Med* 97, 788
Diaphoresis (1–10%)
  (2004): Buajordet I+, *Eur J Emerg Med* 11(1), 19
Exanthems
Pruritus
  (1982): Smitz S+, *Ann Intern Med* 97, 788
Rash (sic) (1–10%)
Urticaria
  (1982): Smitz S+, *Ann Intern Med* 97, 788

Mucosal/ENT
Xerostomia

(2000): Freye E+, *Arzneimittelforschung* 50(1), 24 (with tilidine)

Other

Asthenia
  (2000): Freye E+, *Arzneimittelforschung* 50(1), 24 (with tilidine)
Death
  (1997): Wang WS+, *Zhonghua Yi Xue Za Zhi (Taipei)* 60(4), 219
  (1989): Wride SR+, *Anaesth Intensive Care* 17(3), 374
Headache
  (2004): Buajordet I+, *Eur J Emerg Med* 11(1), 19
Hypertension
  (2003): Hasan RA+, *Ann Pharmacother* 37(11), 1587
  (1990): Olinger CP+, *Stroke* 21(5), 721
  (1990): Yealy DM+, *Ann Emerg Med* 19(8), 902
  (1989): Barsan WG+, *Crit Care Med* 17(8), 762
  (1987): Schoenfeld A+, *Arch Gynecol* 240(1), 45
  (1985): Levin ER+, *Am J Med Sci* 290(2), 70
  (1981): Pallasch TJ+, *Oral Surg Oral Med Oral Pathol* 52(6), 602
Hypotension
  (1990): Olinger CP+, *Stroke* 21(5), 721
  (1989): Barsan WG+, *Crit Care Med* 17(8), 762
Myoclonus
  (1990): Olinger CP+, *Stroke* 21(5), 721
  (1989): Barsan WG+, *Crit Care Med* 17(8), 762
Pain
  (2003): Koppert W+, *Pain* 106(1–2), 91
Seizures
  (2004): Buajordet I+, *Eur J Emerg Med* 11(1), 19
  (1996): Osterwalder JJ, *J Toxicol Clin Toxicol* 34(4), 409
  (1990): Olinger CP+, *Stroke* 21(5), 721
  (1990): Yealy DM+, *Ann Emerg Med* 19(8), 902
  (1989): Mariani PJ, *Am J Emerg Med* 7(1), 127
Tremor
  (2004): Buajordet I+, *Eur J Emerg Med* 11(1), 19

NALTREXONE

Trade names: Antaxone; Celupan; Nalorex; Nemexin; ReVia (Meda); Trexan; Vivitrex (Alkermes/Cephalon)
Indications: Substance abuse, opioid dependence, alcohol dependence
Category: Opioid antagonist
Half-life: 4 hours

Reactions

Skin

Acne (<1%)
Diaphoresis
Edema (<1%)
Exanthems
  (1988): Ganzalez JP+, *Drugs* 35, 192
Herpes simplex (<1%)
Herpes zoster (<1%)
Pruritus (<1%)
  (1997): Sullivan JR+, *Australas J Dermatol* 38(4), 196
  (1990): Abboud TK+, *Anesthesiol* 72, 233
Purpura
Rash (sic) (<10%)
  (1988): Gonzalez JP+, *Drugs* 35, 192
Seborrhea (<1%)
Tinea (<1%)

Mucosal/ENT

Tinnitus
Xerostomia (<1%)

Hair

Hair – alopecia (<1%)

Eyes

Eyelid edema (<1%)

Other

Asthenia
  (2004): Brune A+, *Hautarzt* 55(12), 1130
Chills (<10%)
Death (in ultrarapid detoxification)
Depression (<1%)
  (1996): Berg BJ+, *Drug Saf* 15(4), 274
  (1988): Gonzalez JP+, *Drugs* 35, 192
Headache
  (2006): Swainston Harrison T+, *Drugs* 66(13), 1741
  (2004): Brune A+, *Hautarzt* 55(12), 1130
Hot flashes
Injection-site reactions
  (2006): Swainston Harrison T+, *Drugs* 66(13), 1741
Myalgia/Myositis/Myopathy/Myotoxicity
Phlebitis (<1%)
Rhabdomyolysis
  (1999): Zaim S+, *Ann Pharmacother* 33(3), 312
Tremor
Vertigo
  (2004): Brune A+, *Hautarzt* 55(12), 1130

NAPROXEN

Trade names: Aleve; Anaprox; Apranax; Dymenalgit; Flanax; Laraflex; Naprelan; Naprogesic; Napron X; Naprosyn (Roche); Naprosyne; Naxen; Novo-Naprox; Nu-Naprox; Supradol; Synflex; Velsay
Indications: Pain, arthritis
Category: Non-steroidal anti-inflammatory
Half-life: 13 hours
Clinically important, potentially hazardous interactions with: boswellia, methotrexate, prednisolone

Reactions

Skin

Angioedema (<1%)
  (2000): Ghislain PD+, *Ann Med Interne* (Paris) 151, 227 (nuchal scalp)
  (1984): Stern RS+, *JAMA* 252, 1433
Baboon syndrome
  (2003): Wolf R+, *Dermatol Online J* 9(3), 2
Bullous dermatitis
  (2004): Leivo T+, *Br J Dermatol* 151(1), 232
  (1996): Gonzalo-Garijo MA+, *Allergol Immunopathol Madr* (Spanish) 24, 89
  (1990): Suarez SM+, *Arthritis Rheum* 33, 903
  (1989): Rivers JK+, *Med J Aust* 151, 167
  (1984): Stern RS+, *JAMA* 252, 1433
Diaphoresis (<3%)
  (1990): Todd PA+, *Drugs* 40, 91 (<3%)
  (1985): Bigby M+, *J Am Acad Dermatol* 12, 866
  (1982): Bailin PL+, *Clin Rheum Dis* 8, 493 (passim)
Edema (1–9%)
Erythema multiforme (<1%)
  (1985): Bigby M+, *J Am Acad Dermatol* 12, 866
  (1984): Stern RS+, *JAMA* 252, 1433
Erythema nodosum
  (1990): Todd PA+, *Drugs* 40, 91

Exanthems (1–14%)
(2002): Blumenthal HB, Beachwood, OH (personal case) (observation)
(1994): Shelley WB+, Cutis 55, 21 (observation)
(1990): Todd PA+, Drugs 40, 91
(1985): Bigby M+, J Am Acad Dermatol 12, 866 (1–5%)
(1984): Stern RS+, JAMA 252, 1433
Exfoliative dermatitis
Facial scarring
(2001): Wallace CA+, J Am Acad Dermatol 45, 746 (in children)
Fixed eruption
(2006): Nnoruka EN+, Int J Dermatol 45(9), 1062 (3%)
(2005): Ozkaya E+, J Am Acad Dermatol 53(1), 178
(2004): Leivo T+, Br J Dermatol 151(1), 232
(2004): Ozkaya-Bayazit E, Clin Exp Dermatol 29(4), 419
(2002): Li H+, Int J Dermatol 41(2), 96
(2001): Gonzalo MA+, Br J Dermatol 144(6), 1291
(2000): Ozkaya-Bayazit E+, Eur J Dermatol 10, 288
(1998): Leal G, Fortaleza, Brazil (from internet) (observation)
(1996): Enta T, Can Fam Physician 42, 1099
(1996): Gonzalo-Garijo MA+, Allergol Immunopathol Madr (Spanish) 24, 89
(1991): Shelley WB+, Cutis 48, 368 (observation)
(1990): Black AK+, Br J Dermatol 123, 277 (observation)
(1990): Todd PA+, Drugs 40, 91
(1987): Habbema L+, Dermatologica 174, 184
(1985): Bigby M+, J Am Acad Dermatol 12, 866
(1984): Stern RS+, JAMA 252, 1433
Lichen planus
(2006): Gunes AT+, Int J Dermatol 45(6), 709
(2002): Reed BR, Denver, CO (from Internet) (observation)
(1999): Acta Derm Venereol (Stockh) 79, 329 (bullous)
(1984): Heymann WR+, J Am Acad Dermatol 10, 299
Lichenoid eruption
(1996): Shelley WB+, Cutis 60, 20
(1990): Todd PA+, Drugs 40, 91
(1985): Bigby M+, J Am Acad Dermatol 12, 866
Linear IgA dermatosis
(2000): Bouldin MB+, Mayo Clin Proc 75(9), 967
Lupus erythematosus
(2004): Ting W+, Lupus 13(12), 941
(1992): Parodi A+, JAMA 268, 51
Peripheral edema
(2002): Bandyopadhyay P+, Int J Clin Pract 56(2), 145
Photosensitivity (<1%)
(2006): Bark J, Lexington, KY (from Internet) (observation)
(1999): Litt JZ, Beachwood, OH (personal case) (observation)
(1996): Becker L+, Acta Derm Venereol 76(5), 337
(1994): Berger TG+, Arch Dermatol 130, 609 (in HIV-infected)
(1991): Allen R+, J Rheumatol 18, 893
(1991): Lutzow-Holm C, Tidsskr Nor Laegeforen (Norwegian) 111, 2739
(1990): Suarez SM+, Arthritis Rheum 33, 903
(1990): Todd PA+, Drugs 40, 91
(1989): Kaidbey KH+, Arch Dermatol 125, 783
(1989): Rivers JK+, Med J Aust 151, 167
(1987): Sterling JC+, Br J Rheumatol 26, 210
(1986): Judd LE+, Arch Dermatol 122, 451
(1986): Mayou S+, Br J Dermatol 114, 519
(1986): Shelley WB+, Cutis 38, 169
(1986): Szczeklik A, Drugs 32 (Suppl 4), 148
(1985): Farr PM+, Lancet 1, 1166
(1983): Diffey BL+, Br J Rheumatol 22, 239
Phototoxicity
(1989): Kaidbey KH+, Arch Dermatol 125, 783
Pityriasis rosea
(1993): Yosipovitch G+, Harefuah (Hebrew) 124, 198; 247
Pruritus (3–17%)

(2002): Blumenthal HB, Beachwood, OH (personal case) (observation)
(1990): Todd PA+, Drugs 40, 91 (1–5%)
(1985): Bigby M+, J Am Acad Dermatol 12, 866 (14%)
(1982): Bailin PL+, Clin Rheum Dis 8, 493 (passim)
Purpura (<3%)
(1985): Bigby M+, J Am Acad Dermatol 12, 866
(1982): Bailin PL+, Clin Rheum Dis 8, 493 (passim)
Pustules
(1989): Grattan CEH, Dermatologica 179, 57
(1986): Page SR+, BMJ 293, 510
Pyogenic granuloma
(1994): Shelley WB+, Cutis 53, 36 (observation)
Rash (sic) (3–9%)
(2002): Bandyopadhyay P+, Int J Clin Pract 56(2), 145
(1995): Knulst AC+, Br J Dermatol 133, 647
Side effects (sic) (5–9%)
(1990): Todd PA+, Drugs 40, 91 (up to 9%)
(1985): Bigby M+, J Am Acad Dermatol 12, 866 (up to 5%)
Stevens–Johnson syndrome (<1%)
Toxic epidermal necrolysis (<1%)
(2005): Mansur AT+, Photodermatol Photoimmunol Photomed 21(2), 100
(2004): Ting W+, Lupus 13(12), 941
(1993): Correia O+, Dermatology 186, 32
Urticaria (1–5%)
(2003): Zembowicz A+, Arch Dermatol 139(12), 1577 (aspirin-induced)
(2002): Litt JZ, Beachwood, OH (personal case) (observation)
(1985): Bigby M+, J Am Acad Dermatol 12, 866 (1–5%)
(1984): Stern RS+, JAMA 252, 1433
Vasculitis
(1996): Lossos IS+, Harefuah (Hebrew) 130, 600
(1992): Jahangiri M+, Postgrad Med J 68, 766
(1992): Veraguth AJ+, Schweiz Med Wochenschr (German) 122, 923
(1990): Todd PA+, Drugs 40, 91 (1–5%) (necrotizing venulitis)
(1989): Singhal PC+, Ann Allergy 63, 107
(1985): Bigby M+, J Am Acad Dermatol 12, 866
(1980): Mordes JP, Arch Intern Med 140, 985
Vesiculobullous eruption
(1984): Stern RS+, JAMA 252, 1433

Mucosal/ENT
Aphthous stomatitis
(2001): Vincent L+, Ann Dermatol Venereol (French) 128(1), 57
Oral ulceration
(2000): Madinier I+, Ann Med Interne (Paris) (French) 151, 248
Salivary gland enlargement
(1995): Knulst AC+, Br J Dermatol 133, 647
Stomatitis (<3%)
Tinnitus
(1998): McKinnon BJ+, Mil Med 163(11), 792 (passim)
Xerostomia

Hair
Hair – alopecia (<1%)
(1990): Todd PA+, Drugs 40, 91 (<1%)
(1989): Barter AC, BMJ 298, 325
(1989): Barth JH, BMJ 298, 675

Other
Anaphylactoid reactions/Anaphylaxis (<1%)
(2005): Klote MM+, Allergy 60(2), 260
DRESS syndrome
(2006): Condat B+, Gastroenterol Clin Biol 30(1), 142 (with sulfasalazine)
(2006): Teo L+, Singapore Med J 47(3), 237
Headache

Hot flashes (<1%)
Hypersensitivity
   (2001): McMahon AD+, J Clin Epidemiol 54(12), 1271
Myalgia/Myositis/Myopathy/Myotoxicity (<1%)
Porphyria cutanea tarda
   (1992): Shelley WB+, Advanced Dermatologic Diagnosis WB
      Saunders, 414 (passim)
Pseudolymphoma
   (2001): Werth V, Dermatology Times 18
Pseudoporphyria
   (2002): Haber H, Cleveland, OH (Cleveland Dermatological
      Society)
   (2002): LaDuca JR+, J Cutan Med Surg 6(4), 320
   (2002): McNail S+, Arch Dermatol 138(12), 1607
   (2002): Schad SG+, Hautarzt 53(1), 51
   (2001): Maerker JM+, Hautarzt 52(11), 1026
   (2000): De Silva B+, Pediatr Dermatol 17, 480
   (1999): Al-Khenaizan S+, J Cutan Med Surg 3, 162
   (1995): Creemers MC+, Scand J Rheumatol 24, 185
   (1995): Girschick HJ+, Scand J Rheumatol 24, 108
   (1994): Lang BA+, J Pediatr 124, 639
   (1992): Cox NH+, Br J Dermatol 126, 86
   (1992): Petersen CS+, Ugeskr Laeger (Danish) 154, 1713
   (1991): Allen R+, J Rheumatol 18, 893
   (1991): Lutzow-Holm C, Tidsskr Nor Laegeforen 111(22), 2739
   (1990): Levy ML+, J Pediatr 117, 660
   (1990): Sternberg A, Acta Derm Venereol 70, 354
   (1990): Suarez SM+, Arthritis Rheum 33, 903
   (1990): Todd PA+, Drugs 40, 91
   (1989): Kaidbey KH+, Arch Dermatol 125, 783
   (1988): Diffey BL+, Clin Exp Dermatol 13, 207
   (1987): Burns DA, Clin Exp Dermatol 12, 296
   (1987): Nicholls D, N Z Med J 100, 427
   (1987): Shelley ED+, Cutis 40, 314
   (1987): Sterling JC+, Br J Rheumatol 26, 210
   (1987): Taylor BJ+, N Z Med J 100, 322
   (1986): Judd LE+, Arch Dermatol 122, 451
   (1986): Mayou S+, Br J Dermatol 114, 519
   (1985): Farr PM+, Lancet 1, 1166
   (1985): Howard AM+, Lancet 1, 819

NARATRIPTAN

Trade name: Amerge (GSK)
Indications: Acute migraine attacks
Category: 5-HT1 agonist; Serotonin receptor antagonist; Triptan
Half-life: 6 hours
**Clinically important, potentially hazardous interactions
with:** dihydroergotamine, ergotamine, methysergide, oral
contraceptives, rizatriptan, sibutramine, **St John's wort**,
sumatriptan, zolmitriptan

Reactions

Skin
Acne (<1%)
Allergic reactions (sic) (<1%)
Dermatitis (<1%)
Diaphoresis (<1%)
Edema (<1%)
Erythema (<1%)
Exanthems (<1%)
Folliculitis (<1%)
Photosensitivity (<1%)
Purpura (<1%)
Rash (sic) (<1%)

Sensitivity (sic) (<1)%
Urticaria (<1%)
Xerosis (<1%)
Mucosal/ENT
Dysgeusia (<1%)
Sialopenia (<1%)
Hair
Hair – alopecia (<1%)
Eyes
Ocular pigmentation (<1%)
Other
Asthenia
   (1999): Bomhof M+, Eur Neurol 42(3), 173
Headache
Paresthesias (2%)
Vertigo
   (1999): Bomhof M+, Eur Neurol 42(3), 173

NATALIZUMAB

Synonym: Antegren
Trade name: Tysabri (Bioglan) (Elan)
Indications: Multiple sclerosis
Category: Immunomodulator; Monoclonal antibody
Half-life: 11 days
**Clinically important, potentially hazardous interactions
with:** rilonacept

Note: Before Tysabri can be infused, all prescribers, patients, and
infusion sites must be enroled in the TOUCH Prescribing Program.
This is because of the increased risk of developing multifocal
leukoencephalopathy.

Reactions

Skin
Allergic reactions (sic) (7%)
   (2006): Polman CH+, N Engl J Med 354(9), 899 (9%)
Dermatitis (6%)
Pruritus (4%)
Rash (sic) (9%)
Mucosal/ENT
Vaginitis (8%)
Other
Anaphylactoid reactions/Anaphylaxis (0.8%)
Application-site reactions (22%)
Asthenia (24%)
   (2006): Polman CH+, N Engl J Med 354(9), 899 (27%)
Death
   (2006): Bartt RE, Curr Opin Neurol 19(4), 341
   (2006): Langer-Gould A+, Curr Neurol Neurosci Rep 6(3), 253
   (2005): Kleinschmidt-DeMasters BK+, N Engl J Med 353(4), 369
   (2005): Sandborn WJ+, N Engl J Med 353(18), 1912
   (2005): Schreiner B+, Nervenarzt 76(8), 999
Depression (17%)
Fever (<1%)
Headache (35%)
Hypersensitivity (<1%)
   (2006): Phillips JT+, Neurology 67(9), 1717
   (2006): Polman CH+, N Engl J Med 354(9), 899 (4%)
Hypotension (<1%)
Infections (sic) (2.1%)
Tremor (3%)

NATEGLINIDE

Trade name: Starlix (Novartis)
Indications: Type 2 diabetes
Category: Meglitinide
Half-life: 1.5 hours

Reactions

Skin
Eczema craquele
  (2004): Rosen RM, Tom's River, NJ (from Internet) (observation)
Exanthems
  (2002): Danby FW, Manchester, NH (from Internet)
    (observation)
Rash (sic)

Other
Vertigo
  (2001): Halas CJ, *Am J Health Syst Pharm* 58(13), 1200

NEBIVOLOL

Trade name: Nebilet (Menarini)
Indications: Hypertension
Category: Adrenergic beta-receptor antagonist
Half-life: 8 hours

Reactions

Skin
Dermatitis
  (2002): Fedele R+, *Allergy* 57(9), 864
Lichenoid eruption
  (2006): Bodmer M+, *Ann Pharmacother* 40(9), 1688

Other
Asthenia
  (1999): McNeely W+, *Drugs* 57(4), 633
  (1998): Mangrella M+, *Pharmacol Res* 38(6), 419
Headache
  (2002): Iakushin SS+, *Kardiologiia* 42(11), 36 (1 case)
  (1999): McNeely W+, *Drugs* 57(4), 633
  (1998): Mangrella M+, *Pharmacol Res* 38(6), 419
Myalgia/Myositis/Myopathy/Myotoxicity
Paresthesias
  (1999): McNeely W+, *Drugs* 57, 633
Vertigo
  (1999): McNeely W+, *Drugs* 57(4), 633
  (1998): Mangrella M+, *Pharmacol Res* 38(6), 419

NEDOCROMIL

Trade names: Alocril (Allergan); Mireze; Telavist; Tilade
(Monarch); Tilade Mint
Indications: Bronchial asthma, pruritus of allergic conjunctivitis
Category: Mast cell stabilizer
Half-life: 3.3 hours

Reactions

Skin
Rash (sic) (0.5%)

Mucosal/ENT
Dysgeusia (1–11.6%)
  (2002): Tauber J, *Adv Ther* 19(2), 73 (1.4%)
  (1995): Kjellman NI+, *Allergy* 50(21 Suppl), 14 (5%)
  (1993): Bailey CS+, *Eye* 7, 29
Rhinitis (7.3%)
Xerostomia (1%)

Eyes
Ocular burning (<3%)
  (2002): Tauber J, *Adv Ther* 19(2), 73 (2.7%)
  (1995): Kjellman NI+, *Allergy* 50(21 Suppl), 14
Ocular erythema
Ocular stinging
  (1995): Kjellman NI+, *Allergy* 50(21 Suppl), 14
  (1993): Bailey CS+, *Eye* 7, 29

Other
Abdominal pain (1.9%)
Asthenia (1%)
Cough (8.9%)
Headache
Tremor (<1%)
Upper respiratory infection (6.7%)

NEFAZODONE

Trade name: Serzone (Bristol-Myers Squibb)
Indications: Depression
Category: Antidepressant; Norepinephrine reuptake inhibitor
Half-life: 2–4 hours
**Clinically important, potentially hazardous interactions
with:** aprepitant, astemizole, buspirone, dasatinib, eszopiclone,
isocarboxazid, ivabradine, ixabepilone, lapatinib, MAO inhibitors,
phenelzine, pimozide, rimonabant, selegiline, sibutramine,
solifenacin, **St John's wort**, sumatriptan, temsirolimus, tramadol,
tranylcypromine, trazodone

Note: This drug has been withdrawn

Reactions

Skin
Acne (<1%)
Allergic reactions (sic) (<1%)
Burning
  (2000): Lerner V+, *J Clin Psychiatry* 61, 216
Cellulitis (<1%)
Eczema (<1%)
Exanthems (<1%)
Facial edema (<1%)
Peripheral edema (3%)
Photosensitivity (<1%)
Pruritus (2%)
Rash (sic) (2%)
Urticaria (<1%)
Vesiculobullous eruption (<1%)
Xerosis (<1%)

Mucosal/ENT
Ageusia (<1%)
Dysgeusia (2%)
Gingivitis (<1%)
Glossitis (<1%)
Oral candidiasis (<1%)

Oral ulceration (<1%)
Sialorrhea (<1%)
Stomatitis (<1%)
Vaginitis (2%)
Xerostomia (25%)
  (1996): Lader MH, *J Clin Psychiatry* 57 Suppl 2, 39

Hair
Hair – alopecia (<1%)
  (1998): Rademaker M, Hamilton, New Zealand (from Internet)
    (observation)
  (1997): Gupta S+, *J Fam Pract* 44, 20

Eyes
Amblyopia
  (1996): Lader MH, *J Clin Psychiatry* 57 Suppl 2, 39

Other
Asthenia
  (1996): Lader MH, *J Clin Psychiatry* 57 Suppl, 39
Death
  (2003): Edwards IR, *Lancet* 361, 1240 (11 cases)
Gynecomastia (<1%)
Headache
Infections (8%)
Myalgia/Myositis/Myopathy/Myotoxicity
Paresthesias (4%)
  (1999): Litt JZ, Beachwood, OH (personal case) (observation)
Rhabdomyolysis
  (2003): Skrabal MZ+, *South Med J* 96(10), 1034 (with
    simvastatin)
  (2002): Thompson M+, *Am J Psychiatry* 159(9), 1607 (with
    simvastatin)
  (1997): Jacobson RH+, *JAMA* 277(4), 296 (with simvastatin)
Vertigo
  (1996): Lader MH, *J Clin Psychiatry* 57 Suppl 2, 39

NELARABINE

Trade name: Arranon (GSK)
Indications: T-cell acute lymphoblastic leukemia, T-cell
lymphoblastic lymphoma
Category: Antineoplastic; Purine analog
Half-life: 0.5– 3 hours
**Clinically important, potentially hazardous interactions
with:** N/A

Note: Nelarabine is a pro-drug of Ara-G

Reactions

Skin
Edema (11%)
Peripheral edema (15%)
Petechiae (25%)

Mucosal/ENT
Dysgeusia (3%)
Stomatitis (8%)

Eyes
Vision blurred (4%)

Other
Abdominal pain (9%)
Asthenia (17%)
Chest pain (5%)
Cough (25%)

Depression (6%)
Headache (17%)
Hypotension (8%)
Infections (5%)
Myalgia/Myositis/Myopathy/Myotoxicity (13%)
Pain (11%)
Paresthesias (4%)
Seizures (6%)
Tremor (4%)
Vertigo (21%)

NELFINAVIR

Trade name: Viracept (Pfizer)
Indications: HIV infection
Category: Antiretroviral; Protease inhibitor, HIV
Half-life: 3.5–5 hours
**Clinically important, potentially hazardous interactions
with:** benzodiazepines, carbamazepine, chlordiazepoxide,
ciclesonide, clonazepam, clorazepate, dasatinib, diazepam,
dihydroergotamine, ergot alkaloids, eszopiclone, **eucalyptus**,
fentanyl, flurazepam, ivabradine, lapatinib, lorazepam,
methysergide, midazolam, oral contraceptives, oxazepam,
phenytoin, pimozide, quazepam, rifampin, sildenafil, solifenacin,
St John's wort, temazepam, temsirolimus

Note: Protease inhibitors cause dyslipidemia which includes elevated
triglycerides and cholesterol and redistribution of body fat centrally to
produce the so-called 'protease paunch,' breast enlargement, facial
atrophy, and 'buffalo hump'

Reactions

Skin
Allergic reactions (sic) (<1%)
Dermatitis (<1%)
Diaphoresis (<1%)
Exanthems
  (1998): Bourezane Y+, *Clin Infect Dis* 27(5), 1321 (with
    indinavir)
Hyperhidrosis
  (2000): Bonfanti P+, *J Acquir Immune Defic Syndr* 23(3), 236
Lichenoid eruption
  (1998): Bourezane Y+, *Clin Infect Dis* 27(5), 1321
Palmar erythema
  (1998): Bourezane Y+, *Clin Infect Dis* 27(5), 1321 (with
    indinavir)
Pruritus (<1%)
Rash (sic) (1–10%)
  (2001): Abraham PE+, *Ann Pharmacother* 35(5), 553
  (2000): Fortuny C+, *AIDS* 14, 335
Urticaria (<1%)
  (1998): Demoly P+, *J Allergy Clin Immunol* 102(5), 875
Vasculitis
  (1998): Bourezane Y+, *Clin Infect Dis* 27(5), 1321

Mucosal/ENT
Oral ulceration (<1%)

Other
Death
  (2002): Hare CB+, *Clin Infect Dis* 35(10), e111 (with
    simvastatin)
DRESS syndrome
  (1998): Bourezane Y+, *Clin Infect Dis* 27, 1321
Gynecomastia

(2001): Manfredi R+, *Ann Pharmacother* 35(4), 438
Headache
Hepatotoxicity
(2006): Brown LS+, *J Subst Abuse Treat* 30(4), 331
(2006): Mira JA+, *J Antimicrob Chemother* 58(1), 140
Hypersensitivity
(1999): Demoly P+, *J Allergy Clin Immunol* 104 (2 Pt 1), 504
Lipodystrophy
(2006): Scherpbier HJ+, *Pediatrics* 117(3), e528
Myalgia/Myositis/Myopathy/Myotoxicity (<1%)
Paresthesias (<1%)
Rhabdomyolysis
(2002): Hare CB+, *Clin Infect Dis* 35(10), e111 (with simvastatin)
Vertigo
(2006): Bates DE+, *Ann Pharmacother* 40(6), 1190 (with carbamazepine)

NEOMYCIN

Trade names: Cortosporin; Dexacine; Gemicina; Maxitrol (Falcon); Myciguent; Neomicina; Neomycine Diamant; Neosporin (Pfizer) (Monarch); Neosulf; Nivemycin; Poly-Pred
Indications: Various infections caused by susceptible organisms
Category: Antibiotic, aminoglycoside
Half-life: 3 hours
Clinically important, potentially hazardous interactions with: aldesleukin, aminoglycosides, atracurium, bumetanide, doxacurium, ethacrynic acid, furosemide, methoxyflurane, pancuronium, penicillin V, polypeptide antibiotics, rocuronium, succinylcholine, torsemide, vecuronium

Reactions

Skin
Allergic reactions (sic)
Angioedema
Bullous dermatitis
Dermatitis (1–10%)
(2006): Garcia-Rubio I+, *J Investig Allergol Clin Immunol* 16(4), 264
(2000): Hillen U+, *Hautarzt* 51, 239
(1999): Giordano-Labadie F+, *Contact Dermatitis* 40, 192 (2.6%) (in atopics)
(1999): Lestringant GG+, *Int J Dermatol* 38, 181 (5.1%)
(1998): Katsarou-Katsari A+, *J Eur Acad Dermatol Venereol* 11, 9
(1998): Kimura M+, *Contact Dermatitis* 39, 148
(1997): Dasaraju P+, *Clin Infect Dis* 25, 33
(1996): Sheretz EF, *Arch Dermatol* 132, 461
(1994): Fisher AA, *Cutis* 54, 300
(1993): Lipozencic J+, *Arh Hig Rada Toksikol* (Serbo-Croatian-Roman) 44, 173
(1991): Barros MA+, *Contact Dermatitis* 25, 156
(1991): Mariani R+, *Contact Dermatitis* 24, 227
(1990): Bouffioux B+, *Nouv Dermatol* (French) 9, 25
(1990): Grandinetti PJ+, *J Am Acad Dermatol* 23, 646
(1990): Smith IM+, *Clin Otolaryngol* 15, 155
(1989): Guin JD+, *Cutis* 43, 564
(1989): Massone L+, *Contact Dermatitis* 21, 344
(1988): Shupp DL+, *Cutis* 42, 528
(1987): Abdul-Gaffoor PM, *Indian J Dermatol* 32, 102
(1986): Bajaj AK+, *Int J Dermatol* 25, 103
(1986): Baldinger J+, *Ann Ophthalmol* 18, 95
(1986): Rebandel P+, *Contact Dermatitis* 15, 92
(1985): Fisher AA, *Cutis* 35, 315
(1985): Fraki JE+, *Acta Otolaryngol Stockh* 100, 414

(1985): Frenzel U+, *Phlebologie* (French) 38, 389
(1985): Szarmach H+, *Przegl Dermatol* (Polish) 72, 521 (disseminated)
(1984): Menne T+, *Hautarzt* (German) 35, 319
(1983): Macdonald RH+, *Clin Exp Dermatol* 8, 249
(1982): Fisher AA, *Ann Allergy* 49, 97
(1981): Fisher AA+, *Cutis* 28, 491
(1981): Gordon W, *S Afr Med J* 59, 212
(1981): LeRoy R+, *Derm Beruf Umwelt* (German) 29, 168
(1980): Epstein E, *Contact Dermatitis* 6, 219
Eczema
Erythema multiforme
(1986): Fisher AA, *Cutis* 37, 158
Exanthems
(1990): Bouffioux B+, *Nouv Dermatol* (French) 9, 25
Fixed eruption
(1985): Gomez B+, *Allergol Immunopathol Madr* (Spanish) 13, 87
Pruritus
Rash (sic) (1–10%)
Toxic epidermal necrolysis
Ulcerations
Urticaria (1–10%)

Hair
Hair – alopecia

Other
Anaphylactoid reactions/Anaphylaxis
(1986): Goh CL, *Australian J Dermatol* 27, 125
Hypersensitivity
(2001): Le Coz CJ, *Ann Dermatol Venereol* 128(12), 1359

NEPAFENAC

Trade name: Nevanac (Alcon)
Indications: Pain and inflammation associated with cataract surgery
Category: Non-steroidal anti-inflammatory
Half-life: N/A
Clinically important, potentially hazardous interactions with: None

Reactions

Mucosal/ENT
Sinusitis (1–4%)

Eyes
Conjunctival edema (1–5%)
Epiphora (1–5%)
Ocular hemorrhage (1–5%)
Ocular pain (1–5%)
Ocular pressure (5–10%)
Ocular pruritus (1–5%)
Photophobia (1–5%)
Vision blurred (5–10%)

Other
Headache (1–4%)

NESIRITIDE

Trade name: Natrecor (Scios)
Indications: Acutely decompensated congestive heart failure
Category: Hormone, polypeptide; Natriuretic
Half-life: 18 minutes

Reactions

Skin
  Diaphoresis (>1%)
  Pruritus (>1%)
  Rash (sic) (>1%)

Other
  Cough (>1%)
  Death
    (2006): Stampfli T+, *Rev Med Suisse* 2(50), 295
    (2005): Sackner-Bernstein JD+, *JAMA* 293(15), 1900
  Headache
  Hepatotoxicity
    (2006): Mallolas J, *AIDS Rev* 8(4), 238
  Nephrotoxicity
    (2006): Stampfli T+, *Rev Med Suisse* 2(50), 295
  Paresthesias (>1%)
  Phlebitis
  Tremor (>1%)

NEVIRAPINE

Trade name: Viramune (Boehringer Ingelheim)
Indications: HIV infections
Category: Antiretroviral; Non-nucleoside reverse transcriptase inhibitor
Half-life: 45 hours
Clinically important, potentially hazardous interactions with: ketoconazole, midazolam, **St John's wort**

Reactions

Skin
  Adverse effects (sic)
    (2001): *MMWR* 49, 1153
  Exanthems
    (2005): Pitche P+, *Ann Dermatol Venereol* 132(12 Pt 1), 970
    (2000): Barreiro P+, *AIDS* 14(14), 2153
    (2000): Palacios Munoz R+, *Rev Clin Esp* (Spanish) 200(11), 635
  Pruritus
  Rash (sic) (<48%)
    (2006): van Leth F+, *Ned Tijdschr Geneeskd* 150(31), 1719
    (2004): Patel SM+, *J Acquir Immune Defic Syndr* 35(2), 120 (8 cases)
    (2004): Steel-Duncan JC+, *West Indian Med J* 53(5), 356
    (2001): Barreiro P+, *Lancet* 356(9239), 392
    (2001): Bersoff-Matcha SJ+, *Clin Infect Dis* 32(1), 124
    (2001): Colebundrs R+, *Lancet* 357, 392
    (2001): Wong KH+, *Clin Infect Dis* 33(12), 2096
    (2000): Bardsley-Elliot A+, *Paediatr Drugs* 2(5), 373
    (1999): Anton P+, *AIDS* 13, 524
    (1998): Barner A+, *Lancet* 351, 1133
    (1998): Bourezane Y+, *Clin Infect Dis* 27, 1321
    (1998): Ho TT+, *AIDS* 12, 2082
    (1996): Luzuriaga K+, *J Infect Dis* 174, 713
    (1995): Havlir D+, *J Infect Dis* 171, 537 (48%)
  Stevens–Johnson syndrome (<1%)
    (2008): Jain V+, *Cornea* 27(3), 366
    (2008): Mason AR+, *Pediatr Dermatol* 25(1), 128
    (2007): Kra O+, *Bull Soc Pathol Exot* 100(2), 109
    (2006): Joao EC+, *Am J Obstet Gynecol* 194(1), 199 (1 case)
    (2005): Liechty CA+, *AIDS* 19(9), 993
    (2004): Hitti J+, *J Acquir Immune Defic Syndr* 36(3), 772 (1 case)
    (2004): Patel SM+, *J Acquir Immune Defic Syndr* 35(2), 120 (3 cases)
    (2003): Rotunda A+, *Acta Derm Venereol* 83(1), 1
    (2002): Dodi F+, *AIDS* 16(8), 1197 (2 cases)
    (2001): *MMWR* 49, 1153
    (2001): Fagot JP+, *AIDS* 15(14), 1843
    (2001): Metry DW+, *J Am Acad Dermatol* 44, 354
    (2001): Roujeau J-C+, *AIDS* 15, 1843
    (2000): Bardsley-Elliot A+, *Paediatr Drugs* 2(5), 373
    (2000): Garcia Fernandez D+, *Rev Clin Esp* (Spanish) 200, 179
    (1999): Wetterwald E+, *Br J Dermatol* 140, 980 (SJS/TEN overlap syndrome)
    (1998): McClain SA, SUNY Stony Brook, NY (from Internet) (observation)
    (1998): Warren KJ+, *Lancet* 351–567
  Toxic epidermal necrolysis
    (2004): Claes P+, *Eur J Intern Med* 15(4), 255
    (2001): Cattelan AM+, *J Infect* 43(4), 246 (2 cases)
    (2001): Fagot JP+, *AIDS* 15(14), 1843
    (2001): Roujeau J-C+, *AIDS* 15, 1843
    (1999): Descamps V+, *Lancet* 353, 1855
    (1999): Phan TG+, *Australas J Dermatol* 40, 153
    (1999): Wetterwald E+, *Br J Dermatol* 140, 980 (SJS/TEN overlap syndrome)
  Toxicity (sic)
    (2006): Taiwo BO, *Int J STD AIDS* 17(6), 364

Mucosal/ENT
  Dysgeusia
    (2008): Moura MD+, *J Contemp Dent Pract* 9(1), 84 (with zidovudine and lamivudine)
  Gingivitis (1–3%)
  Stomatopyrosis
    (2008): Moura MD+, *J Contemp Dent Pract* 9(1), 84 (with zidovudine and lamivudine)
  Ulcerative stomatitis (4%)
  Xerostomia
    (2008): Moura MD+, *J Contemp Dent Pract* 9(1), 84 (with zidovudine and lamivudine)

Other
  Death
    (2005): *AIDS Patient Care STDS* 2005 Mar;19(3), 202
  DRESS syndrome
    (2005): Fields KS+, *J Drugs Dermatol* 4(4), 510
    (2005): Pitche P+, *Ann Dermatol Venereol* 132(12 Pt 1), 970
    (2001): Claudio GA+, *Arch Intern Med* 161(20), 2501
    (2001): Lanzafame M+, *Scand J Infect Dis* 33(6), 475
    (2000): Sissoko D+, *Presse Med* (French) 29, 1041
    (1998): Bourezane Y+, *Clin Infect Dis* 27(5), 1321
  Fever
    (2004): Patel SM+, *J Acquir Immune Defic Syndr* 35(2), 120 (11 cases)
  Headache
  Hepatotoxicity
    (2006): Drummond NS+, *Antivir Ther* 11(3), 393
    (2006): Haas DW+, *Clin Infect Dis* 43(6), 783
    (2006): Lyons F+, *HIV Med* 7(4), 255
    (2006): Maida I+, *J Acquir Immune Defic Syndr* 42(2), 177
    (2006): van Leth F+, *Ned Tijdschr Geneeskd* 150(31), 1719
  Hypersensitivity
    (2006): Drummond NS+, *Antivir Ther* 11(3), 393
    (2006): Littera R+, *AIDS* 20(12), 1621
    (2005): Martin AM+, *AIDS* 19(1), 97

(2001): Wit FW+, *AIDS* 15(18), 2423
(2000): Podzamczer D+, *AIDS* 14, 331
Lipodystrophy
　(2000): Lewis RH+, *J Acquir Immune Defic Syndrom* 23, 355
　(1999): Aldeen T+, *AIDS* 13, 865
Myalgia/Myositis/Myopathy/Myotoxicity (1–10%)
Paresthesias (2%)

NIACIN

Synonym: nicotinic acid
Trade names: Advicor (Kos); Apo-Nicotinamide; I; IV; Nia-Bid; Niac; Niacels; Niacor (Upsher-Smith); Niaspan (Merck); Nicobid; Nicobion; Nicotinex; Nicovital; Pepeom Amide; Slo-Niacin (Upsher-Smith); Vitamin B$_3$
Indications: Hyperlipidemia
Category: Vitamin
Half-life: 45 minutes
Clinically important, potentially hazardous interactions with: atorvastatin, selenium

Reactions

Skin

Acanthosis nigricans (8%)
　(2002): Burrall BA, Sacramento, CA (from Internet) (observation)
　(2002): Eisner J, Mt. Vernon, WA (from Internet) (observation)
　(2002): Liss WA, Pleasanton, CA (from Internet) (observation)
　(2002): Marmelzat, JA, Los Angeles, CA (from Internet) (observation)
　(1994): McKenney JM+, *JAMA* 271, 672
　(1994): Stals H+, *Dermatology* 189, 203
　(1993): Stone OJ, *Med Hypotheses* 40, 154
　(1992): Coates P+, *Br J Dermatol* 126, 412
　(1990): Audicana M+, *Contact Dermatitis* 22, 60
　(1990): Brown G+, *N Engl J Med* 323, 1289 (8.3%)
　(1989): Larmi E, *Int J Dermatol* 28, 609
　(1989): Ylipieti S+, *Contact Dermatitis* 21, 105
　(1981): Elgart ML, *J Am Acad Dermatol* 5, 709
Dermatitis
　(1995): Bilbao I+, *Contact Dermatitis* 33, 435
Erythema
　(1995): Fisher AA, *Cutis* 55, 132
Exanthems (<3%)
　(1997): Blumenthal HL, Beachwood, OH (personal case) (observation)
　(1997): Litt JZ, Beachwood, OH (2 personal cases) (observation)
　(1990): Brown G+, *N Engl J Med* 323, 1289 (2.8%)
Fixed eruption (<1%)
　(1992): de la Hoz-Caballer B+, *Med Clin* (Barc) (Spanish) 98, 357
Ichthyosis
Keratoses
Pigmentation
　(1992): Breathnach SM+, *Adverse Drug Reactions and the Skin* Blackwell, Oxford, 265 (passim)
Pruritus (1–5%)
　(2005): Ely EH, Grass Valley, CA (from Internet) (observation)
　(2005): Litt JZ, Beachwood, OH (personal case) (observation)
　(2002): Kashyap ML+, *Am J Cardiol* 89(6), 672 (with lovastatin)
　(1997): Blumenthal HL, Beachwood, OH (personal case) (observation)
　(1997): Jungnickel PW+, *J Gen Intern Med* 12, 591
　(1994): Fivenson DP+, *Arch Dermatol* 130, 753
　(1994): McKenney JM+, *JAMA* 271, 672

(1992): Breathnach SM+, *Adverse Drug Reactions and the Skin* (Oxford) 265 (passim)
　(1992): Whelan AM+, *J Fam Pract* 34, 165 (passim)
Rash (sic) (<1%)
　(2005): Alisky JM, *Nutr Neurosci* 8(5-6), 327
　(2002): Kashyap ML+, *Am J Cardiol* 89(6), 672 (with lovastatin)
　(1994): McKenney JM+, *JAMA* 271, 672
　(1992): Breathnach SM+, *Adverse Drug Reactions and the Skin* Blackwell, Oxford, 265 (passim)
　(1988): Figge HL+, *Pharmacotherapy* 8, 287
Scaling
　(1992): Breathnach SM+, *Adverse Drug Reactions and the Skin* Blackwell, Oxford, 265 (passim)
Urticaria
　(1995): Fisher AA, *Cutis* 55, 132
Xerosis

Mucosal/ENT

Burning mouth syndrome
　(1988): Haustein UF, *Contact Dermatitis* 19, 225
Gingivitis
　(1998): Leighton RF I, *Chest* 114, 1472
Xerostomia

Eyes

Exophthalmos
　(1995): Fraunfelder FW+, *Br J Ophthalmol* 79(1), 54
Eyelid edema
　(1995): Fraunfelder FW+, *Br J Ophthalmol* 79(1), 54
Eyelid pigmentation
　(1995): Fraunfelder FW+, *Br J Ophthalmol* 79(1), 54
Maculopathy
　(2006): Dajani HM+, *Can J Ophthalmol* 41(2), 197
Ocular adverse effects
　(2004): Fraunfelder FW, *Am J Ophthalmol* 138(4), 639
Periorbital edema
　(1995): Fraunfelder FW+, *Br J Ophthalmol* 79(1), 54
Punctate keratitis
　(1995): Fraunfelder FW+, *Br J Ophthalmol* 79(1), 54
Vision blurred
　(1995): Fraunfelder FW+, *Br J Ophthalmol* 79(1), 54

Other

Anaphylactoid reactions/Anaphylaxis
Asthenia
　(2004): Zhao XQ+, *Am J Cardiol* 93(3), 307 (9%) (with simvastatin)
Headache
　(2002): Kashyap ML+, *Am J Cardiol* 89(6), 672 (with lovastatin)
Hypotension
　(2006): Mularski RA+, *Clin Toxicol* (Phila) 44(1), 81
Myalgia/Myositis/Myopathy/Myotoxicity
　(2004): Zhao XQ+, *Am J Cardiol* 93(3), 307 (5%) (with simvastatin)
　(1994): Gharavi AG+, *Am J Cardiol* 74, 841
　(1989): Goldstein MR, *Am J Med* 87, 248
　(1989): Litin SC+, *Am J Med* 86, 481
Paresthesias (1–10%)
　(1997): Jungnickel PW+, *J Gen Intern Med* 12, 591
　(1992): Whelan AM+, *J Fam Pract* 34, 165 (passim)
Sjøgren's (Sicca) syndrome
　(1995): Fraunfelder FW+, *Br J Ophthalmol* 79(1), 54

NIACINAMIDE

Synonyms: nicotinamide; vitamin B$_3$
Trade name: Niacinamide
Indications: Prophylaxis and treatment of pellagra
Category: Vitamin
Half-life: 45 minutes
Clinically important, potentially hazardous interactions with: primidone

Reactions

Skin
Acanthosis nigricans
  (1984): Papa CM, *Arch Dermatol* 120, 281
Pruritus (1–5%)
  (1981): Zackheim HS+, *J Am Acad Dermatol* 4, 736
  (1980): Bures FA, *J Am Acad Dermatol* 3, 530
Rash (sic)

Other
Hepatotoxicity
  (2000): Knip M+, *Diabetologia* 43(11), 1337 (high doses)
Paresthesias (1–10%)

NICARDIPINE

Trade names: Antagonil; Cardene (Roche); Dagan; Loxen; Nicardal; Nicodel; Ranvil; Ridene; Rydene
Indications: Angina, hypertension
Category: Calcium channel blocker
Half-life: 2–4 hours
Clinically important, potentially hazardous interactions with: epirubicin, imatinib

Reactions

Skin
Allergic reactions (sic)
Edema (1%)
Exanthems
Peripheral edema (7.1%)
  (1998): Knowles S+, *J Am Acad Dermatol* 38, 201 (passim)
  (1990): Webster J+, *Br J Clin Pharmacol* 29, 587P (leg)
Rash (sic) (1.2%)
  (1998): Knowles S+, *J Am Acad Dermatol* 38, 201 (passim)
  (1985): Deedwania PC+, *Clin Pharmacol Ther* 37, 190
  (1985): Gelman JS+, *Am J Cardiol* 56, 232
Side effects (sic)
  (1993): Kitamura K+, *J Dermatol* 20, 279 (psoriasiform)
Urticaria
  (1983): Brodmerkel GJ, *Ann Intern Med* 99, 415
  (1983): Fisher JR+, *Ann Intern Med* 98, 671
  (1982): Grunwald Z, *Drug Intell Clin Pharm* 16, 492

Mucosal/ENT
Gingival hyperplasia/hypertrophy (<1%)
  (2004): Maguin B+, *Rev Stomatol Chir Maxillofac* 105(4), 219
  (1997): Pascual-Castroviejo I+, *Neurologia* 12(1), 37
Tinnitus
Xerostomia (1.4%)

Other
Erythromelalgia
  (1989): Drenth JH, *BMJ* 298, 1582

  (1989): Levesque H+, *BMJ* 298, 1252
Headache
Myalgia/Myositis/Myopathy/Myotoxicity (1%)
  (1998): Knowles S+, *J Am Acad Dermatol* 38, 201 (passim)
Paresthesias (1%)

NICORANDIL

Trade names: Adancor; Angicor; Corflo (Wockhardt); Dancor; Ikorel; Korandil (Sun Pharma); Nicoran (Torrent); Nikoril; Zynicor (Cadila Healthcare)
Indications: Angina pectoris prophylaxis and treatment
Category: Potassium channel activator
Half-life: N/A
Clinically important, potentially hazardous interactions with: tadalafil

Reactions

Skin
Allergic reactions (sic)
  (1990): Kinoshita M+, *Cardiovasc Drugs Ther* 4(4), 1075 (mild)
Edema
Ulcerations
  (2007): McKenna DJ+, *Br J Dermatol* 156(2), 394 (legs)
  (2006): *Prescrire Int* 15(81), 19 (anal)
  (2006): Biggins J+, *J Wound Care* 15(5), 197 (anal)
  (2006): Claeys A+, *Br J Dermatol* 155(2), 494 (anal; vulvar)
  (2006): Toquero L+, *Colorectal Dis* 8(8), 717 (anal) (6 cases)

Mucosal/ENT
Aphthous stomatitis
  (2001): O'Mahony P, *Age Ageing* 30(1), 90
  (2000): Boulinguez S+, *Presse Med* 29(33), 1828 (5%)
  (2000): Gupta A+, *Age Ageing* 29(4), 372
  (2000): Haas C+, *Presse Med* 29(38), 2092
  (1999): Shotts RH+, *Oral Surg Oral Med Oral Pathol Oral Radiol Endod* 87(6), 706 (3 cases)
  (1998): Agbo-Godeau S+, *Lancet* 352(9140), 1598
  (1998): Roussel S+, *Rev Stomatol Chir Maxillofac* 99(4), 207
Oral ulceration
  (2006): *Prescrire Int* 15(81), 19
  (2005): Webster K+, *Br Dent J* 198(10), 619
  (2004): Healy CM+, *Heart* 90(7), e38
  (2004): O'Sullivan EM, *J Ir Dent Assoc* 50(4), 157
  (2003): Boulinguez S+, *J Oral Pathol Med* 32(8), 482
  (2003): Farah CS+, *Aust Fam Physician* 32(6), 452
  (2001): O'Mahony P, *Age Ageing* 30(1), 90
  (2001): Pemberton MN+, *Oral Surg Oral Med Oral Pathol Oral Radiol Endod* 92(1), 2
  (2001): Scully C+, *Oral Surg Oral Med Oral Pathol Oral Radiol Endod* 91(2), 189
  (2000): Boulinguez S+, *Presse Med* 29(33), 1828
  (2000): Gupta A+, *Age Ageing* 29(4), 372
  (2000): Markham A+, *Drugs* 60(4), 955
  (1999): Marquart-Elbaz C+, *Ann Dermatol Venereol* 126(8–9), 587
  (1999): Shotts RH+, *Oral Surg Oral Med Oral Pathol Oral Radiol Endod* 87(6), 706
  (1999): Vincent S+, *Therapie* 54(2), 260
  (1998): Agbo-Godeau S+, *Lancet* 352(9140), 1598
  (1998): Cribier B+, *Br J Dermatol* 138(2), 372
  (1998): Desruelles F+, *Br J Dermatol* 138(4), 712
  (1998): Roussel S+, *Rev Stomatol Chir Maxillofac* 99(4), 207
  (1997): Boulinguez S+, *Presse Med* 26(12), 558
Perianal ulcerations
  (2006): *Prescrire Int* 15(81), 19

(2006): Cooke NS+, *Br J Dermatol* 154(1), 199
(2005): Katory M+, *Dis Colon Rectum* 48(7), 1442
(2005): Malik R+, *Br J Dermatol* 152(4), 809
(2005): Wong T+, *Br J Dermatol* 152(6), 1360
(2004): Katory M+, *Colorectal Dis* 6(6), 527
(2004): Passeron T+, *Br J Dermatol* 150(2), 394
(2004): Renwick AA+, *ANZ J Surg* 74(12), 1128
(2004): Watson A+, *Colorectal Dis* 6(5), 330
(2002): Vella M+, *Lancet* 360(9349), 1979
(2002): Watson A+, *Lancet* 360(9332), 546
Tongue ulceration
(2004): Jang HS+, *Br J Dermatol* 151(4), 939
(2000): Haas C+, *Presse Med* 29(38), 2092

Other
Asthenia
Headache
(2003): Udaykumar P+, *JIACM* 4(3), 205 (5%)
(2000): Markham A+, *Drugs* 60(4), 955
(1995): Witchitz S+, *Cardiovasc Drugs Ther* 9 Suppl 2, 237
(1993): Raftery EB+, *Eur Heart J* 14 Suppl B, 35
(1993): Roland E, *Eur Heart J* 14 Suppl B, 48
(1992): Krumenacker M+, *J Cardiovasc Pharmacol* 20 Suppl 3, S93
(1990): Hughes LO+, *Am J Cardiol* 66(7), 679
(1990): Kinoshita M+, *Cardiovasc Drugs Ther* 4(4), 1075 (5–34%)
(1989): Camm AJ+, *Am J Cardiol* 63(21), 61J
Vertigo
(2003): Udaykumar P+, *JIACM* 4(3), 205
(1989): Camm AJ+, *Am J Cardiol* 63(21), 61J

NICOTINE

Trade names: Exodus; Habitrol Patch (Novartis); Nicabate; Nicoderm (GSK); Nicolan; Nicorette (GSK); Nicorette Plus; Nicotinell-TTS; Nicotrans; Nicotrol (Pfizer); Nikofrenon; Stubit
Indications: Aid to smoking cessation
Category: Alkaloid
Half-life: varies with the delivery system
Clinically important, potentially hazardous interactions with: horsetail

Note: Smoking cessation therapy has various delivery systems. These include: transdermal patches, chewing gum, nasal spray, inhaler, and oral forms

Reactions

Skin
Carcinoma
(2003): Taybos G, *Am J Med Sci* 326(4), 179
Dermatitis
(1993): Farm G, *Contact Dermatitis* 29, 214
Diaphoresis (1–3%)
Edema
Erythema (>10%)
Keratoses
(2003): Taybos G, *Am J Med Sci* 326(4), 179
Melanosis
(2003): Taybos G, *Am J Med Sci* 326(4), 179
Pigmentation
(2003): Taybos G, *Am J Med Sci* 326(4), 179
Pruritus (>10%)
Rash (sic)
Urticaria
Vasculitis
(1996): Van der Klauw MM+, *Br J Dermatol* 134, 361

Mucosal/ENT
Dysgeusia
Gingivitis
(2003): Taybos G, *Am J Med Sci* 326(4), 179
Sialorrhea (>10%)
Stomatitis (>10%)
(2003): Taybos G, *Am J Med Sci* 326(4), 179
Tinnitus
Tongue black
(2003): Taybos G, *Am J Med Sci* 326(4), 179
Xerostomia (1–3%)

Other
Application-site burning
Application-site erythema
Application-site pruritus
Headache
Hypersensitivity (<1%)
Myalgia/Myositis/Myopathy/Myotoxicity (1–10%)
Paresthesias
Tremor

NIFEDIPINE

Trade names: Adalat (Bayer); Adalate; Apo-Nifed; Aprical; Calcilat; Coracten; Corogal; Corotrend; Nifecor; Nu-Nifed; Pidilat; Procardia (Pfizer)
Indications: Angina, hypertension
Category: Calcium channel blocker
Half-life: 2–5 hours
Clinically important, potentially hazardous interactions with: epirubicin, **grapefruit juice**, imatinib, rifampin, ritonavir

Reactions

Skin
Acute generalized exanthematous pustulosis (AGEP)
(1995): Moreau A+, *Int J Dermatol* 34, 263 (passim)
(1991): Roujeau J-C+, *Arch Dermatol* 127, 1333
Angioedema (<1%)
(1998): Knowles S+, *J Am Acad Dermatol* 38, 201 (passim)
(1989): Stern R+, *Arch Intern Med* 149, 829
Bullous dermatitis
(1989): Stern R+, *Arch Intern Med* 149, 829
(1987): Alcalay J+, *Dermatologica* 175, 191
Dermatitis (<2%)
Diaphoresis (<2%)
(1989): Stern R+, *Arch Intern Med* 149, 829
(1983): Lewis JG, *Drugs* 25, 196
Edema
(2003): Ioulios P+, *Dermatol Online J* 9(5), 6 (passim)
(1983): Lewis JG, *Drugs* 25, 196
Erysipelas
(1988): Leibovici V+, *Cutis* 41, 367
(1983): Lewis JG, *Drugs* 25, 196
Erythema
(1998): Knowles S+, *J Am Acad Dermatol* 38, 201 (passim)
(1992): Gonzalez-Castro U+, *Med Clin* (Barc) (Spanish) 98, 759
Erythema multiforme
(1998): Knowles S+, *J Am Acad Dermatol* 38, 201 (passim)
(1997): Springuel P, *Can Med Assoc J* 156, 90
(1989): Stern R+, *Arch Intern Med* 149, 829
(1986): Myrhed M+, *Acta Pharmacol Toxicol* 58, 133
Erythema nodosum
(1998): Knowles S+, *J Am Acad Dermatol* 38, 201 (passim)

(1989): Stern R+, *Arch Intern Med* 149, 829
Exanthems (1%)
  (1998): Knowles S+, *J Am Acad Dermatol* 38, 201 (passim)
  (1995): Litt JZ, Beachwood, OH (personal case) (observation)
  (1992): Parish LC+, *Cutis* 49, 113 (morbilliform)
  (1989): Stern R+, *Arch Intern Med* 149, 829
  (1987): Alcalay J+, *Dermatologica* 175, 191
  (1985): Findlay GH, *S Afr Med J* 68, 176
  (1983): Lewis JG, *Drugs* 25, 196 (1%)
  (1982): Grunwald Z, *Drug Intell Clin Pharm* 16, 492
  (1980): Antman E+, *N Engl J Med* 302, 1269 (1%)
Exfoliative dermatitis (<1%)
  (1994): Mohammed KN, *Ann Pharmacother* 28, 967
  (1993): Collins P, *Br J Dermatol* 129, 630 (passim)
  (1989): Reynolds HJ+, *Br J Dermatol* 121, 401
  (1989): Stern R+, *Arch Intern Med* 149, 829
  (1984): Scoble JE+, *Clin Nephrol* 21, 302
Facial edema (1%)
Fixed eruption
  (1993): Litt JZ, Beachwood, OH (personal case) (observation)
  (1987): Alcalay J+, *Dermatologica* 175, 191
  (1986): Alcalay J+, *BMJ* 292, 450
Lichenoid eruption
  (1989): Reynolds HJ+, *Br J Dermatol* 121, 401
  (1988): Leibovici V+, *Cutis* 41, 367
  (1984): Scoble JE+, *Clin Nephrol* 21, 302
Lupus erythematosus
  (2003): Gubinelli E+, *J Cutan Med Surg*
  (1998): Callen JP, Academy '98 Meeting
  (1997): Crowson AN+, *Hum Pathol* 28, 67
Pemphigoid nodularis
  (2000): Ameen M+, *Br J Dermatol* 142, 575
Pemphigus foliaceus
  (1993): Kim S-C+, *Acta Derm Venereol* (Stockh) 73, 210
Pemphigus vulgaris
  (1999): Brenner S+, *J Eur Acad Dermatol Venereol* 13(2), 123
Peripheral edema
  (2006): Poole-Wilson PA+, *Cardiovasc Drugs Ther* 20(1), 45
  (2002): No author, *Medscape Primary Care* 4
  (1996): Tailor SA+, *Arch Dermatol* 132, 350 (with itraconazole)
  (1994): Mohammed KN, *Ann Pharmacother* 28, 967
  (1991): Salmasi AM+, *Int J Cardiol* 30, 303
  (1989): Williams SA+, *Eur J Clin Pharmacol* 37, 333
  (1985): Findlay GH, *S Afr Med J* 68, 176
  (1982): Grunwald Z, *Drug Intell Clin Pharm* 16, 492
Photosensitivity
  (2004): Mittal A, Udaipur, India (from Internet) (observation)
  (1996): Seggev JS+, *J Allergy Clin Immunol* 97, 852
  (1991): Zenarola P+, *Dermatologica* 182, 196
  (1990): Guarrera M+, *Photodermatology* 7, 25
  (1988): Zlotogorski A, *Dermatologica* 177, 249
  (1986): Thomas SE+, *BMJ* 292, 992
Prurigo nodularis
  (1992): Shelley WB+, *Cutis* 50, 179 (observation)
Pruritus (<2%)
  (1998): Knowles S+, *J Am Acad Dermatol* 38, 201 (passim)
  (1993): Collins P, *Br J Dermatol* 129, 630 (passim)
  (1989): Stern R+, *Arch Intern Med* 149, 829
Purpura (<2%)
  (1990): Regazzini R+, *Chron Derm* (Italian) 21, 225
  (1989): Oren R+, *Drug Intell Clin Pharm* 23, 88
  (1985): Findlay GH, *S Afr Med J* 68, 176
Rash (sic) (<3%)
  (1998): Knowles S+, *J Am Acad Dermatol* 38, 201 (passim)
  (1989): Stern R+, *Arch Intern Med* 149, 829
Side effects (sic)
  (1993): Kitamura K+, *J Dermatol* 20, 279 (psoriasiform)
Stevens–Johnson syndrome
  (1998): Knowles S+, *J Am Acad Dermatol* 38, 201 (passim)

(1993): Collins P, *Br J Dermatol* 129, 630 (passim)
(1989): Stern R+, *Arch Intern Med* 149, 829
Telangiectasia
  (1994): Shelley WB+, *Cutis* 53, 40 (observation)
  (1993): Collins P, *Br J Dermatol* 129, 630 (photodistribution)
  (1992): Tsele E+, *Lancet* 339, 365
Toxic epidermal necrolysis
  (1998): Knowles S+, *J Am Acad Dermatol* 38, 201 (passim)
  (1993): Collins P, *Br J Dermatol* 129, 630 (passim)
Ulcerations
  (1999): Luca S+, *Minerva Cardioangiol* 47, 219
Urticaria (<1%)
  (1999): Luca S+, *Minerva Cardioangiol* 47, 219 (legs)
  (1998): Knowles S+, *J Am Acad Dermatol* 38, 201 (passim)
  (1991): Zenarola P+, *Dermatologica* 182, 196
  (1989): Stern R+, *Arch Intern Med* 149, 829
  (1988): Toner M+, *Chest* 93, 1320
  (1986): Myrhed M+, *Acta Pharmacol Toxicol* 58, 133
Vasculitis
  (1989): Oren R+, *Drug Intell Clin Pharm* 23, 88
  (1987): Alcalay J+, *Dermatologica* 175, 191
  (1985): Brenner S+, *Harefuah* (Hebrew) 108, 139

Mucosal/ENT
Anosmia
  (2003): Kharoubi S+, *Presse Med* 32(27), 1269
Dysgeusia (<1%)
  (1985): Levenson JL+, *Ann Intern Med* 102(1), 135
Gingival hyperplasia/hypertrophy (6–10%)
  (2005): Torrezan PR+, *Rev Assoc Med Bras* 51(4), 200 (with cyclosporine)
  (2002): Prisant LM+, *J Clin Hypertens* (Greenwich) 4(4), 310 (with calcium channel blockers)
  (2001): Uzel MI+, *J Periodontol* 72(7), 921
  (2000): Das SJ+, *Cytokine* 12(10), 1566
  (2000): James JA+, *J Clin Periodontol* 27, 109 (with cyclosporine)
  (1999): Ellis JS+, *J Periodontol* 70, 63 (6.3%)
  (1999): Naidoo LC+, *Spec Care Dentist* 19(1), 29
  (1998): Bokor-Bratic M+, *Med Pregl* (Serbo-Croatian [Roman]) 51, 445
  (1998): Desai P+, *J Can Dent Assoc* 64, 263
  (1998): Knowles S+, *J Am Acad Dermatol* (2), 201
  (1998): Nakayama J+, *Eur J Dermatol* 8(8), 563 (with cyclosporine)
  (1998): Nakou M+, *J Periodontol* 69, 664
  (1998): Nohl F+, *Ther Umsch* (German) 55, 573
  (1998): Santi E+, *Int J Periodontics Restorative Dent* 18(1), 80
  (1997): Jackson C+, *N Y State Dent J* 63, 46
  (1997): Slezak R, *J West Soc Periodontal Periodontal Abstr* 45, 105
  (1997): Thomason JM+, *Clin Oral Investig* 1, 35
  (1997): Westbrook P+, *J Periodontol* 68, 645
  (1996): Abitbol TE+, *N Y State Dent J* 63, 34
  (1996): Ciantar M, *Dent Update* 23, 374
  (1996): Darbar UR+, *J Clin Periodontol* 23, 941
  (1996): Deen-Duggins L+, *Quintessence Int* 27, 163 (4 cases)
  (1996): Neumann C+, *Eur J Med Res* 1(6), 273
  (1996): Saito K+, *J Periodontol Res* 31, 545
  (1995): Harel-Raviv M+, *Oral Surg Oral Med Oral Pathol Oral Radiol Endod* 79, 715
  (1995): Nery EB+, *J Periodontol* 66, 572
  (1995): O'Valle F+, *J Clin Periodontol* 22(8), 591 (with cyclosporine)
  (1995): Ramsdale DR+, *Br Heart J* 73, 115
  (1995): Silverstein LH+, *J Oral Implantol* 21, 116
  (1995): Thomason JM+, *J Periodontol* 66(8), 742 (with cyclosporine)
  (1995): Wynn RL, *Gen Dent* 43, 218
  (1994): Henderson JS+, *Miss Dent Assoc J* 50, 12
  (1994): Shelley WB+, *Cutis* 53, 282 (passim)
  (1993): King GN+, *J Clin Periodontol* 20, 286

(1993): Kychakova SI+, *Stomatologiia (Mosk)* 72(3), 23
(1993): Morisaki I+, *J Periodontal Res* 28, 396
(1993): Shoieb MA+, *Egypt Dent J* 39(4), 555
(1993): Steele RM+, *Arch Intern Med* 120, 663
(1993): Thomason JM+, *J Clin Periodontol* 20(1), 37 (with cyclosporine)
(1992): Barclay S+, *J Clin Periodontol* 19(5), 311
(1992): Bhatia RS, *J Assoc Physicians India* 40(7), 486
(1992): Burkes EJ+, *J Tenn Dent Assoc* 72(2), 35
(1992): Ellis JS+, *Lancet* 339(8806), 1382
(1992): Hancock RH+, *J Clin Periodontol* 19, 12
(1992): Katz J+, *Ann Dent* 51(1), 5
(1991): Akimoto Y+, *J Nihon Univ Sch Dent* 33(3), 174
(1991): Gonzalez-Jaranay M+, *Rev Eur Odontoestomatol* 3(2), 127
(1991): Gupta AK+, *J Assoc Physicians India* 39(6), 506
(1991): Nishikawa SJ+, *J Periodontol* 62, 30
(1991): Wynn RL, *Gen Dent* 39, 240
(1990): Katayama H+, *Aichi Gakuin Daigaku Shigakkai Shi* 28(2), 697
(1990): Sanz Cantalapiedra R+, *Aten Primaria* 7(2), 160
(1990): Tagawa T+, *Int J Oral Maxillofac Surg* 19(2), 72
(1989): Veraldi S+, *Clin Exp Dermatol* 14, 93
(1989): Yusof WZ, *J Can Dent Assoc* 55(5), 389
(1988): Boisnic S+, *Ann Dermatol Venereol* (French) 115, 373
(1988): Zlotogorski A, *Dermatologica* 177, 249
(1986): Bencini PL+, *G Ital Dermatol Venereol* (Italian) 121, 29
(1986): Jones CM, *Br Dent J* 160, 416
(1985): Bencini PL+, *Acta Derm Venereol* (Stockh) 65, 362
(1985): Lucas RM+, *J Periodontol* 56, 211
(1984): Lederman D+, *Oral Surg Oral Med Oral Pathol* 57, 620
(1984): Ramon Y+, *Int J Cardiol* 5, 195
Parosmia
Sialadenitis
(2002): Viseux V+, *Ann Dermatol Venereol* 129(1), 59 (passim)
Tinnitus
Xerostomia (<3%)

Hair
Hair – alopecia (1%)
(1998): Knowles S+, *J Am Acad Dermatol* 38, 201 (passim)
(1993): Collins P, *Br J Dermatol* 129, 630 (passim)
(1989): Reynolds HJ+, *Br J Dermatol* 121, 401
(1989): Stern R+, *Arch Intern Med* 149, 829
Hair – pigmentation
(1989): Stern R+, *Arch Intern Med* 149, 829

Nails
Nails – dystrophy
(1989): Stern R+, *Arch Intern Med* 149, 829

Eyes
Periorbital edema (1%)
(1985): Tordjman K+, *Am J Cardiol* 55, 1445

Other
Asthenia
(2006): Poole-Wilson PA+, *Cardiovasc Drugs Ther* 20(1), 45
Chills (2%)
Depression
(2002): Patalia AH+, *J Assoc Physicians India* 50, 1432
Erythromelalgia (<0.5%)
(1989): Stern R+, *Arch Intern Med* 149, 829
(1987): Alcalay J+, *Dermatologica* 175, 191
(1983): Brodmerkel GJ, *Ann Intern Med* 99, 415
(1983): Fisher JR+, *Ann Intern Med* 98, 671
Gynecomastia (<1%)
(1995): Marcos-Olea JL+, *Aten Primaria* (Spanish) 16, 115
(1993): Braunstein GD, *N Engl J Med* 328(7), 490
(1988): Zlotogorski A, *Dermatologica* 177, 249
(1986): Clyne CAC, *BMJ* 292, 380

Headache
Hypotension
(2006): Poole-Wilson PA+, *Cardiovasc Drugs Ther* 20(1), 45
Myalgia/Myositis/Myopathy/Myotoxicity (<1%)
Paresthesias (<3%)
(1982): Macdonald JB, *BMJ* 285, 1744
Tremor (2–8%)

NILUTAMIDE

Synonym: RU-23908
Trade names: Anandron (Sanofi-Aventis); Nilandron (Sanofi-Aventis)
Indications: Metastatic prostate cancer, androgen-independent prostate cancer
Category: Antiandrogen; Antineoplastic
Half-life: N/A
Clinically important, potentially hazardous interactions with: alcohol, aminophylline, aspirin, chlordiazepoxide, diazepam, lidocaine, phenytoin, propranolol, theophylline, warfarin

Reactions

Skin
Diaphoresis (6%)
Edema (2%)
Peripheral edema (<2%)
Pruritus (2%)
Rash (sic) (5%)
Urticaria
Xerosis (5%)

Mucosal/ENT
Xerostomia (2%)

Hair
Hair – alopecia

Eyes
Cataract (2%)
Ocular toxicity (sic)
(1987): Brisset JM+, *Br J Ophthalmol* 71(8), 639
(1986): Harnois C+, *Br J Ophthalmol* 70(6), 471
Photophobia (2%)
Visual disturbances
(2005): Nakabayashi M+, *BJU Int* 96(6), 783
(1997): Dijkman GA+, *Ann Pharmacother* 31(12), 1550
(1993): Harris MG+, *Drugs Aging* 3(1), 9
(1993): Janknegt RA, *Cancer* 72(12), 3874
(1991): Boccardo F+, *Cancer Detect Prev* 15(6), 501 (27%)
(1991): Decensi A+, *Eur J Cancer* 27(9), 1100 (30%)
(1991): Decensi AU+, *J Urol* 146(2), 377
(1991): Du Plessis, *Urology* 37(2), 20
(1986): Harnois C+, *Br J Ophthalmol* 70(6), 471

Other
Abdominal pain (10%)
Asthenia (19%)
Cardiac failure (3%)
Chest pain (1–10%)
Cough (2%)
(2002): van der Drift MA+, *Ned Tijdschr Geneeskd* 146(4), 145
(1992): Jonville AP+, *Therapie* 47(5), 393
(1988): Seigneur J+, *Chest* 93(5), 1106
Death

(1996): Marty F+, *Gastroenterol Clin Biol* 20(8-9), 710
(1993): Pescatore P+, *Gastroenterol Clin Biol* 17(6-7), 499
Depression (9%)
(1997): Maroy B+, *Therapie* 52(1), 79
Fever (1–10%)
(2002): van der Drift MA+, *Ned Tijdschr Geneeskd* 146(4), 145
(1992): Jonville AP+, *Therapie* 47(5), 393
(1988): Seigneur J+, *Chest* 93(5), 1106
Gynecomastia (10%)
Headache (<3%)
Hepatotoxicity (1%)
(2003): Edouard A+, *Gastroenterol Clin Biol* 27(12), 1170 (fatal fulminating)
(1996): Marty F+, *Gastroenterol Clin Biol* 20(8-9), 710 (fatal fulminating)
(1993): Pescatore P+, *Gastroenterol Clin Biol* 17(6-7), 499 (fatal fulminating)
(1992): Gomez JL+, *Am J Med* 92(5), 563
(1991): Hammel P+, *Gastroenterol Clin Biol* 15(6-7), 557
Hot flashes (28%)
Hypertension (5%)
Pain (27%)
Paresthesias (3%)
Upper respiratory infection (8%)
Vertigo (10%)

NIMESULIDE

Trade names: Ainex; Aulin; Donulide; Edrigyl; Eskaflam; Heugan; Lusemin; Mesulid; Nemil-OS; Nimulid; Nise; Novolid; Novolid S
Indications: Pain, Arthopathies
Category: COX-2 inhibitor; Non-steroidal anti-inflammatory; Sulfonamide
Half-life: N/A
Clinically important, potentially hazardous interactions with: N/A

Note: Sulfamethoxazole is a sulfonamide and can be absorbed systemically. Sulfonamides can produce severe, possibly fatal, reactions such as toxic epidermal necrolysis and Stevens–Johnson syndrome

Reactions

Skin
Acute generalized exanthematous pustulosis
(2006): Teixeira M+, *Dermatol Online J* 12(6), 20
Angioedema
(2000): Mangalvedhekar SS+, *J Assoc Physicians India* 48(5), 548
Fixed eruption
(2005): Malheiro D+, *Allergol Immunopathol* (Madr) 33(5), 285
(2002): Sarkar R+, *Pediatr Dermatol* 19(6), 553
(2000): Cordeiro MR+, *Contact Dermatitis* 43(5), 307
Photosensitivity
(2001): Tursen U+, *Int J Dermatol* 40(12), 767 (lichenoid)
Pityriasis rosea
(2006): Atzori L+, *Dermatol Online J* 12(1), 1
Pruritus
(2002): Sarkar R+, *Pediatr Dermatol* 19(6), 553 (passim)
Purpura
(2002): Sarkar R+, *Pediatr Dermatol* 19(6), 553 (passim)
(2000): Kanwar AJ+, *Dermatology* 201(4), 376
Rash (sic)
(2002): Sarkar R+, *Pediatr Dermatol* 19(6), 553 (passim)
Toxic pustuloderma

(2002): Lateo S+, *Br J Dermatol* 147(3), 624
Urticaria
(2005): Asero R, *Clin Exp Allergy* 35(6), 713
(2002): Nettis E+, *Allergy* 57(5), 442 (137 cases)
(2000): Asero R, *Ann Allergy Asthma Immunol* 85(2), 156
(1998): Asero R, *Ann Allergy Asthma Immunol* 81(3), 237
Vasculitis
(2006): Polimeni G+, *Drug Saf* 29(5), 449 (3 cases)

Mucosal/ENT
Stomatitis
(1992): Valsecchi R+, *Dermatology* 185(1), 74 (bullous)

Other
Abdominal pain
Headache
Hepatotoxicity
(2006): Lapeyre-Mestre M+, *Fundam Clin Pharmacol* 20(4), 391
(2006): Polimeni G+, *Drug Saf* 29(5), 449 (3 cases)
(2006): Sanchez-Matienzo D+, *Clin Ther* 28(8), 1123
(2004): Castaneda Hernandez G+, *Gac Med Mex* 140(6), 679
(2004): Quadranti P, *Schweiz Rundsch Med Prax* 93(43), 1785
(2003): Ozgur O+, *Turk J Gastroenterol* 14(3), 208
(2003): Papaioannides D+, *Indian J Gastroenterol* 22(6), 239
(2002): Boelsterli UA, *Drug Saf* 25(9), 633
(2002): Boelsterli UA, *Int J Clin Pract Suppl* 128, 30
(2002): Dumortier J+, *Gastroenterol Clin Biol* 26(4), 415
(2002): Gallego Rojo FJ+, *Rev Esp Enferm Dig* 94(1), 41
(2002): Macia MA+, *Clin Pharmacol Ther* 72(5), 596
(2001): Sbeit W+, *Ann Pharmacother* 35(9), 1049
(2000): Andrade RJ+, *J Hepatol* 32(1), 174 (fatal)
(2000): Ferreiro C+, *Gastroenterol Hepatol* 23(9), 428
(2000): Perez-Moreno J+, *Gastroenterol Hepatol* 23(10), 498
(2000): Rodrigues de Oliveira J+, *Gastroenterol Clin Biol* 24(5), 592
(2000): Schattner A+, *J Intern Med* 247(1), 153 (fatal)
(2000): Tejos S+, *Rev Med Chil* 128(12), 1349
(1999): Romero Gomez M+, *Med Clin* (Barc) 113(9), 357 (3 cases)
(1999): Romero-Gomez M+, *Liver* 19(2), 164
(1999): Weiss P, *Isr Med Assoc J* 1(3), 221
(1999): Weiss P+, *Isr Med Assoc J* 1(2), 89
(1998): Van Steenbergen W+, *J Hepatol* 29(1), 135 (6 cases)
Nephrotoxicity
(2004): Benini D+, *Pediatr Nephrol* 19(2), 232
(2004): Magnani C+, *Eur J Obstet Gynecol Reprod Biol* 116(2), 244
(2002): Van der Niepen P+,, *Nephrol Dial Transplant* 17(2), 315
(2000): Balasubramaniam J, *Lancet* 355(9203), 575
(1997): Apostolou T+, *Nephrol Dial Transplant* 12(7), 1493
Seizures
(2004): Sienaert P+, *J ECT* 20(1), 52
Vertigo

NIMODIPINE

Trade names: Admon; Nimotop (Bayer); Periplum; Vasotop
Indications: Subarachnoid hemorrhage
Category: Calcium channel blocker
Half-life: 3 hours
Clinically important, potentially hazardous interactions with: epirubicin, imatinib

Reactions

Skin
Acne (<1%)

Acute generalized exanthematous pustulosis (AGEP)
  (1999): Zabawski E+, Dallas, TX (from Internet) (observation)
Allergic reactions (sic)
  (2002): Nucera E+, *Contact Dermatitis* 47(4), 246
Diaphoresis (<1%)
Edema (2%)
Exanthems (2.4%)
  (1989): Langley MS+, *Drugs* 37, 669
Peripheral edema
Pruritus (<1%)
Purpura
Rash (sic) (3%)

Hair
Hair – alopecia
  (1995): Daghfous R+, *Therapie* (French) 50, 590

Other
Headache
Hypotension
  (2004): Gerloni R+, *Eur J Emerg Med* 11(5), 295

NISOLDIPINE

Trade names: Baymycard; Sular (First Horizon); Syscor
Indications: Hypertension
Category: Calcium channel blocker
Half-life: 7–12 hours
**Clinically important, potentially hazardous interactions
with:** cyclosporine, epirubicin, **grapefruit juice**, imatinib,
ketoconazole

Reactions

Skin
Acne (<1%)
Angioedema
Cellulitis (<1%)
Diaphoresis (<1%)
Edema
  (2003): White WB+, *Am J Hypertens* 16(9 Pt 1), 739
Exanthems (<1%)
  (1988): Friedel HA+, *Drugs* 36, 682 (0.7%)
Exfoliative dermatitis (<1%)
Facial edema (<1%)
Herpes simplex (<1%)
Herpes zoster (<1%)
Peripheral edema (22%)
  (2003): Pepine CJ+, *Am J Cardiol* 91(3), 274
  (2001): Lenz TL+, *Pharmacotherapy* 21(8), 898 (4 cases) (with
    amlodipine)
  (1998): Hoglund C+, *Int J Clin Pract* 52(4), 221
  (1997): *Eur Heart J* 18(1), 31
  (1997): Opie LH+, *Am J Hypertens* 10(3), 250
  (1997): Ruddy TD+, *Cardiovasc Drugs Ther* 11(4), 581
Petechiae (<1%)
Photosensitivity
Pigmentation (<1%)
Pruritus (<1%)
Pustules (<1%)
Rash (sic) (2%)
Side effects (sic)
  (1993): Kitamura K+, *J Dermatol* 20, 279
Ulcerations (<1%)
Urticaria (<1%)

Xerosis (<1%)
Mucosal/ENT
Dysgeusia (<1%)
Gingival hyperplasia/hypertrophy (<1%)
Glossitis (<1%)
Oral ulceration (<1%)
Vaginitis (<1%)
Xerostomia (<1%)

Hair
Hair – alopecia (<1%)

Other
Chest pain
  (2001): Lenz TL+, *Pharmacotherapy* 21(8), 898
Chills (<1%)
Gynecomastia (<1%)
Headache
  (2003): Pepine CJ+, *Am J Cardiol* 91(3), 274
  (2003): White WB+, *Am J Hypertens* 16(9 Pt 1), 739
  (1998): Hoglund C+, *Int J Clin Pract* 52(4), 221
  (1997): Ruddy TD+, *Cardiovasc Drugs Ther* 11(4), 581
Hypersensitivity
Paresthesias (<1%)
Tremor (<1%)
Vertigo
  (2003): White WB+, *Am J Hypertens* 16(9 Pt 1), 739

NITAZOXANIDE

Trade names: Alinia (Romark); Cryptaz
Indications: Diarrhea caused by *Cryptosporidium parvum* or
Giardia lamblia (in children)
Category: Antiprotozoal
Half-life: N/A

Reactions

Skin
Diaphoresis (<1%)
Pruritus (<1%)
Mucosal/ENT
Rhinitis (<1%)
Salivary gland enlargement (<1%)

Eyes
Scleral pigmentation (pale-yellow) (<1%)

Other
Abdominal pain
  (2002): Stockis A+, *Int J Clin Pharmacol Ther* 40(5), 221
  (1999): Rodriguez-Garcia R+, *Rev Gastroenterol Mex* 64(3), 122
Infections (<1%)
Vertigo (<1%)

NITISINONE

Trade name: Orfadin (Rare Disease Therapeutics)
Indications: Hereditary tyrosinemia
Category: Tyrosine catabolism inhibitor
Half-life: 54 hours

Reactions

Skin
Exanthems (1%)
Exfoliative dermatitis (1%)
Pruritus (1%)
Rash (sic)
Xerosis (1%)

Hair
Hair – alopecia (1%)

Eyes
Blepharitis (1%)
Conjunctivitis (2%)
Ocular stinging (1%)

Other
Death
Infections (<1%)
Porphyria (1%)
Seizures (<1%)

NITRAZEPAM

Trade names: Alodorm; Eunoctin; Hypnotex; Mogadon (Roche); Pacisyn; Pelson; Remnos; Somnite
Indications: Insomnia
Category: Benzodiazepine; CNS depressant
Half-life: 14–48 hours
Clinically important, potentially hazardous interactions with: erythromycin

Reactions

Mucosal/ENT
Dysphagia
(1992): Lim HC+, *Brain Dev* 14(5), 309
Sialorrhea
(1986): Wyllie E+, *N Engl J Med* 314(1), 35

Eyes
Visual hallucinations
(1996): Tokinaga N+, *Psychiatry Clin Neurosci* 50(6), 337 (with erythromycin)

Other
Abdominal pain
Anticonvulsant hypersensitivity syndrome
(2006): Kwong KL+, *J Paediatr Child Health* 42(7-8), 474
Confusion
Death
(1999): Rintahaka PJ+, *Epilepsia* 40(4), 492
Headache
Mood changes (sic)
Rhabdomyolysis
(1998): Yotsuyanagi T+, *Clin Exp Dermatol* 23(3), 113
Somnolence
Vertigo

NITROFURANTOIN

Trade names: Furadantin (First Horizon); Furadantina; Furadoine; Furalan; Furan; Furobactina; Infurin; Macrobid (Procter & Gamble); Macrodantin (Procter & Gamble); Nephronex; Novo-Furan; Urofuran
Indications: Various urinary tract infections caused by susceptible organisms
Category: Antibiotic
Half-life: 20–60 minutes

Reactions

Skin
Acute febrile neutrophilic dermatosis (Sweet's syndrome)
(1999): Retief CR+, *Cutis* 63, 177
Adverse effects (sic)
(2004): Karpman E+, *J Urol* 172(2), 448 (2–3%)
Angioedema (<0.1%)
(1982): Penn RG+, *BMJ* 284, 1440
(1981): Chisholm JC+, *J Nat Med Assoc* 73, 59 (passim)
Bullous dermatitis
Dermatitis
Eczema
Erythema multiforme
(1990): Chan HL+, *Arch Dermatol* 126, 43
(1986): Chapman JA, *Ann Allergy* 56, 16
Erythema nodosum
(1981): Chisholm JC+, *J Nat Med Assoc* 73, 59
Exanthems (1–5%)
(2002): Blumenthal HL, Beachwood, OH (personal case) (observation)
(1984): Paver R+, *Current Ther* 25, 55
(1983): Swinyer LJ, *Dermatol Clin* 1, 417
(1980): Calderwood SB+, *Surgical Clin N Amer* 60, 65
(1980): Holmberg L+, *Am J Med* 69, 733 (28%)
Exfoliative dermatitis
(1984): Paver R+, *Current Ther* 25, 55
(1983): Swinyer LJ, *Dermatol Clin* 1, 417
Fixed eruption
(1985): Kauppinen K+, *Br J Dermatol* 112, 575
Lupus erythematosus
(2006): Salle V+, *Rev Med Interne* 27(4), 344
(1986): Chapman JA, *Annals Allergy* 56, 16
(1985): Stratton MA, *Clin Pharm* 4, 657
(1981): Fleck RM, *Pennsylvania Med* 84, 36
Photosensitivity
(1987): Australian Drug Evaluation Committee, 61 (Oct 15)
Pruritus (<1%)
(1987): Australian Drug Evaluation Committee, 61 (Oct 15)
(1981): Chisholm JC+, *J Nat Med Assoc* 73, 59 (passim)
Purpura
(1984): Paver R+, *Current Ther* 25, 55
(1983): Swinyer LJ, *Dermatol Clin* 1, 417
Rash (sic) (<1%)
(1982): Penn RG+, *BMJ* 284, 1440
Reticular hyperplasia
Stevens–Johnson syndrome
(2005): Shilad A+, *Obstet Gynecol* 105(5 Pt 2), 1254 (1 case)
Toxic epidermal necrolysis
(1993): Stables GI+, *Br J Dermatol* 128, 357
(1984): Kauppinen K+, *Acta Derm Venereol* (Stockh) 64, 320
(1983): Swinyer LJ, *Dermatol Clin* 1, 417
Urticaria (0.4%)
(1999): Litt JZ, Beachwood, OH (personal case) (observation)

(1996): Blumenthal HL, Beachwood, OH (personal case) (observation)
(1983): Griffin JP, *Practitioner* 227, 1283
(1983): Swinyer LJ, *Dermatol Clin* 1, 417
(1982): Schneider RE, *Clin Ther* 4, 390

Mucosal/ENT
Sialadenitis
(2002): Viseux V+, *Ann Dermatol Venereol* 129(1 Pt 1), 59 (passim)
Xerostomia

Hair
Hair – alopecia
(1983): No Author, *Lakartidningen* (Swedish) 80, 4040
(1983): Swinyer LJ, *Dermatol Clin* 1, 417

Other
Anaphylactoid reactions/Anaphylaxis
(1987): Australian Drug Evaluation Committee, 61 (Oct 15)
(1982): Penn RG+, *BMJ* 284, 1440
(1980): Calderwood SB+, *Surg Clin N Amer* 60, 65
Chills
(2006): Williams EM+, *Pharmacotherapy* 26(5), 713
Death
(2004): Karpman E+, *J Urol* 172(2), 448 (3 cases)
Headache
Hepatotoxicity
(2007): Koulaouzidis A+, *Ann Hepatol* 6(2), 119
(2006): Peedikayil MC+, *Ann Pharmacother* 40(10), 1888
(2006): Salle V+, *Rev Med Interne* 27(4), 344
Hypersensitivity
Myalgia/Myositis/Myopathy/Myotoxicity
Panniculitis (nodular nonsuppurative)
(1987): Sanford RG+, *Arthritis Rheum* 30, 1076
Paresthesias (1–10%)
(2003): Lacerna RA+, *J Am Geriatr Soc* 51(12), 1822 (with pyridoxine)
Pseudolymphoma
(1993): Kerl H+, *Dermatology in General Medicine* McGraw-Hill New York

NITROFURAZONE

Trade names: Actin-N; Furacept; Furacin (Pharma Pac, Quality Care, Roberts, Southwood); Furacine; Nigermex; Nitrofurazone (Taro); Rafuzone
Indications: Second- and third-degree burns, skin grafting
Category: Antibiotic, nitrofuran
Half-life: N/A
Clinically important, potentially hazardous interactions with: None

Reactions

Skin
Allergic reactions (sic)
Depigmentation (skin & eyelashes)
Dermatitis
(2006): Prieto A+, *Contact Dermatitis* 54(2), 126
(1999): Guijarro SC+, *Am J Contact Dermat* 10(4), 226
(1995): Conde-Salazar L+, *Contact Dermatitis* 32(5), 307
(1994): Ballmer-Weber BK+, *Contact Dermatitis* 31(4), 274
(1990): Lo JS+, *Dermatol Clin* 8(1), 165
(1986): Bajaj AK+, *Int J Dermatol* 25(2), 103
(1985): Ancona A, *Contact Dermatitis* 13(1), 35
(1981): Burkhart CG, *Cutis* 27(6), 630 (pustular)

Edema (~1%)
Pruritus (~1%)
Rash (sic) (~1%)

NITROGLYCERIN

Synonyms: glyceryl trinitrate; nitroglycerol; NTG
Trade names:
Buccal tablets
Lingual aerosol: Nitrolingual (First Horizon)
Oral capsules: Nitrocap; Nitrocine; Nitroglyn; Nitrospan
Oral tablets: Klavikordal; Niong; Nitronet; Nitrong
Parenteral: Nitro-Bid; Nitroject; Nitrol; Nitrostat (Pfizer); Tridil
Sublingual tablets: Nitrostat (Pfizer)
Topical ointment: Nitrol; Nitrong; Nitrostat (Pfizer)
Topical transdermal systems: Deponit; Minitran (3M); Nitrocine; Nitrodisc; Nitrodur; Transderm-Nitro (Various pharmaceutical companies.)
Indications: Acute angina
Category: Nitrate; Vasodilator
Half-life: 1–4 minutes
Clinically important, potentially hazardous interactions with: acetylcysteine, alteplase, sildenafil

Reactions

Skin
Allergic reactions (sic) (<1%)
Angioedema
(1998): Rademaker M+, *New Zealand Adverse Drug Reactions Committee*, April, 1998 (from Internet)
Cyanosis
Dermatitis (to topical systems) (<1%)
(2006): Ramey JT+, *Allergy Asthma Proc* 27(3), 273
(2000): McKenna KE, *Contact Dermatitis* 42, 246
(1999): Machet L+, *Dermatology* 198, 106
(1994): de la Fuente-Prieto R+, *Ann Allergy* 72, 344
(1992): Torres V+, *Contact Dermatitis* 26, 53
(1991): Kanerva L+, *Contact Dermatitis* 24, 356
(1991): Laine R+, *Duodecim* (Finnish) 107, 41
(1990): Vaillant L+, *Contact Dermatitis* 23, 142
(1989): Carmichael AJ+, *Contact Dermatitis* 21, 113
(1989): Di Landro A+, *Contact Dermatitis* 21, 115
(1989): Holdiness MR, *Contact Dermatitis* 20, 3
(1988): Apted J, *Med J Aust* 148, 482
(1988): Niedner R, *Hautarzt* (German) 39, 761
(1987): Gupta AK+, *Arch Dermatol* 123, 295
(1987): Harari Z+, *Dermatologica* 174, 249
(1987): Topaz O+, *Ann Allergy* 59, 365
(1986): Schrader BJ+, *Pharmacotherapy* 6, 83
(1986): Weickel R+, *Hautarzt* (German) 37, 511
(1985): Fischer RG+, *South Med J* 78, 1523
(1984): Fisher AA, *Cutis* 34, 526
(1984): Letendre PW+, *Drug Intell Clin Pharm* 18, 69
(1984): Rosenfeld AS+, *Am Heart J* 108, 1061
(1983): Camarasa JG+, *Contact Dermatitis* 9, 320
Diaphoresis (<1%)
Eczema
(1989): Carmichael AJ+, *Contact Dermatitis* 21, 113
(1987): Topaz O+, *Ann Allergy* 59, 365
Edema
Erythema (to transdermal delivery system)
(2002): Barrios V+, *Rev Clin Esp* 202(7), 379 (3%)
(1990): Hogan JD+, *J Am Acad Dermatol* 22, 811
Erythema multiforme
(2001): Silvestre JF+, *Contact Dermatitis* 45(5), 299

Erythroderma
Exanthems
Exfoliative dermatitis (1–10%)
Facial flushing
  (2006): Ramey JT+, *Allergy Asthma Proc* 27(3), 273
Irritation
  (2002): Barrios V+, *Rev Clin Esp* 202(7), 379 (10%)
Pallor
Peripheral edema (<1%)
Purpura
  (1989): Nishioka K+, *J Dermatol* 16, 220 (pigmented)
Rash (sic) (1–10%)
Rosacea (exacerbation)
  (1980): Wilkin JK, *Arch Dermatol* 116, 598
Urticaria
  (2006): Ramey JT+, *Allergy Asthma Proc* 27(3), 273

Mucosal/ENT

Ageusia
  (1989): Ewing RC+, *Clin Pharm* 8(2), 146
Burning mouth syndrome
Oral burn (from sublingual)
Xerostomia (<1%)

Other

Anaphylactoid reactions/Anaphylaxis (from perianal
  application)
  (1999): Pietroletti R+, *Am J Gastroenterol* 94, 292
Headache
  (2006): Ramey JT+, *Allergy Asthma Proc* 27(3), 273
  (2006): Schoonman GG+, *Cephalalgia* 26(7), 816
  (2003): Bujold E+, *Am J Obstet Gynecol* 189(4), 1070 (42%)
  (2002): Barrios V+, *Rev Clin Esp* 202(7), 379 (80%)
Hypotension
  (2006): Ramey JT+, *Allergy Asthma Proc* 27(3), 273
  (1994): Ma SX+, *Life Sci* 55(21), 1595
Systemic reactions
  (2002): Barrios V+, *Rev Clin Esp* 202(7), 379 (4%)

NITROPRUSSIDE

Synonym: Sodium nitroferricyanide
Trade name: Nitropress (Hospira)
Indications: Hypertensive crises, congestive heart failure,
erectile dysfunction
Category: Vasodilator
Half-life: minutes
**Clinically important, potentially hazardous interactions
with:** N/A

Reactions

Skin

Diaphoresis (1–10%)
Rash (sic)

Mucosal/ENT

Tinnitus (1–10%)

Other

Application-site irritation
Asthenia (1–10%)
Death
Headache (1–10%)
Hypertension
  (1981): Gelman S+, *Anesthesiology* 54(1), 90

  (1980): Ward CF+, *Anesthesiology* 52(6), 525
Hypotension
  (2002): Thomas JE+, *Stroke* 33(2), 486
  (1993): Brock G+, *J Urol* 150(3), 864 (3 cases)
Nephrotoxicity
  (1987): Reid GM+, *Am J Nephrol* 7(4), 313

NIZATIDINE

Trade names: Apo-Nizatidine; Axid (Reliant); Calmaxid;
Gastrax; Nizax; Nizaxid; Panaxid; Tazac; Zanizal
Indications: Duodenal ulcer, Gastroesophageal Reflux Disease
(GERD)
Category: Histamine H2 receptor antagonist
Half-life: 1–2 hours

Reactions

Skin

Acne (<1%)
Allergic reactions (sic) (<1%)
Dermatitis
Diaphoresis (1%)
  (1988): Price AH+, *Drugs* 36, 521 (1%)
  (1987): Cloud ML, *Scand J Gastroenterol* 22, 39
Edema
Exanthems
Exfoliative dermatitis
Pruritus (1.7%)
  (1988): Price AH+, *Drugs* 36, 521
  (1987): Cloud ML, *Scand J Gastroenterol* 22, 39
Rash (sic) (1.9%)
  (1987): Cloud ML, *Scand J Gastroenterol* 22, 39
Urticaria (<1%)
  (1988): Price AH+, *Drugs* 36, 521 (0.5%)
Vasculitis
Xerosis (<1%)

Mucosal/ENT

Xerostomia (1.4%)

Other

Gynecomastia
  (1987): Cloud ML, *Scand J Gastroenterol* 22, 39
Headache
Myalgia/Myositis/Myopathy/Myotoxicity (1.7%)
Paresthesias (<1%)
Pseudolymphoma
  (1995): Magro CM+, *J Am Acad Dermatol* 32, 419
Serum sickness

NORFLOXACIN

Trade names: Barazan; Chibroxin (Merck); Chibroxine;
Chibroxol; Lexinor; Noroxin (Shire) (Roberts); Noroxine;
Oranor; Utinor; Zoroxin
Indications: Various urinary tract infections caused by
susceptible organisms, conjunctivitis
Category: Antibiotic, quinolone
Half-life: 2.3–4 hours
**Clinically important, potentially hazardous interactions
with:** amiodarone, arsenic, bepridil, bretylium, ciprofibrate,
disopyramide, erythromycin, mycophenolate, phenothiazines,
procainamide, quinidine, sotalol, tricyclic antidepressants

Reactions

Skin

Acute febrile neutrophilic dermatosis (Sweet's syndrome)
 (2004): Aguiar-Bujanda D+, QJM 97(1), 55
Angioedema
Bullous dermatitis
 (1993): Ramsey B+, Br J Dermatol 129, 500
Dermatitis
 (1998): Silvestre JF+, Contact Dermatitis 39, 83
Diaphoresis (<1%)
Edema
Erythema (<1%)
Erythema multiforme
Exanthems (0.2%)
 (1988): Wolfson JS+, Ann Intern Med 108, 238
 (1985): Holmes B+, Drugs 30, 482 (0.2%)
Exfoliative dermatitis
Fixed eruption
 (1997): Fenandez-Rivas M, Allergy 52, 477
Photosensitivity
Phototoxicity
 (2000): Traynor NJ+, Toxicol Vitr 14, 275
 (1998): Martinez LJ+, Photochem Photobiol 67, 399
 (1994): Fujita H+, Photodermatol Photoimmunol Photomed 10, 202
 (1993): Ferguson J+, Br J Dermatol 128, 285
Pruritus (<1%)
 (1985): Holmes B+, Drugs 30, 482 (0.2%)
Pustules
 (1992): Allegue F+, Med Clin (Barc) (Spanish) 99, 274
Rash (sic) (<1%)
Stevens–Johnson syndrome
 (1992): Kubo-Shimasaki A+, Rinsho Ketsueki (Japanese) 33, 823
Subcorneal pustular dermatosis (Sneddon-Wilkinson)
 (1988): Shelley ED+, Cutis 42(1), 24
Toxic epidermal necrolysis
 (2005): Sahin MT+, Ann Pharmacother 39(4), 768
 (1993): Correia O+, Dermatology 186, 32
Toxic pustuloderma
 (1993): Tsuda S+, Acta Derm Venereol (Stockh) 73, 382 (passim)
Urticaria
Vasculitis

Mucosal/ENT

Dysgeusia (<1%) (bitter taste)
Stomatitis
Tinnitus
Vulvovaginal candidiasis
 (2002): Menday AP, Int J Antimicrob Agents 20(4), 297
Xerostomia (<1%)

Nails

Nails – photo-onycholysis
 (1987): Baran R+, J Am Acad Dermatol 17, 1012
 (1986): Baran R+, Dermatologica 173, 185

Eyes

Ocular stinging (from ophthalmic solution)
Visual hallucinations
 (1996): Rataboli PV+, J Assoc Physicians India 44(7), 504

Other

Anaphylactoid reactions/Anaphylaxis
Headache
Myalgia/Myositis/Myopathy/Myotoxicity
 (2001): Guis S+, J Rheumatol 28, 1405
Paresthesias

Rhabdomyolysis
 (2001): Guis S+, J Rheumatol 28, 1405
 (1996): Blain H+, Rev Med Interne 17(10), 859 (with ciprofibrate)
Tendinopathy/Tendon rupture (<1%)
 (2005): Cano Valles B+, Aten Primaria 36(7), 404
 (2003): van der Linden PD+, Arch Intern Med 163(15), 1801
 (2001): van der Linden PD+, Arthritis Rheum 45(3), 235
 (1983): Bailey RR+, N Z Med J 96, 590
Vertigo
 (2005): Otsubo T+, Pharmacopsychiatry 38(1), 30

NORTRIPTYLINE

Trade names: Allegron; Apo-Nortriptyline; Aventyl (Ranbaxy); Noritren; Norpress; Nortrilen; Pamelor (Mallinckrodt); Paxtibi; Vividyl
Indications: Depression
Category: Antidepressant, tricyclic
Half-life: 28–31 hours
Clinically important, potentially hazardous interactions with: amprenavir, arbutamine, clonidine, epinephrine, fluoxetine, formoterol, guanethidine, isocarboxazid, linezolid, MAO inhibitors, phenelzine, quinolones, sparfloxacin, tranylcypromine

Reactions

Skin

Acne
Allergic reactions (sic) (<1%)
Diaphoresis (1–10%)
Edema
Erythema
Exanthems
Petechiae
Photosensitivity (<1%)
Phototoxicity
Pruritus
Purpura
Rash (sic)
Urticaria
Vasculitis
Xerosis

Mucosal/ENT

Dysgeusia (>10%)
Stomatitis
Tinnitus
Tongue black
 (1990): Vitiello B+, Clin Pharm 9, 421
Tongue edema
Vaginitis
Xerostomia (>10%)
 (2006): Haggstram FM+, Pulm Pharmacol Ther 19(3), 205
 (2002): Hammack JE+, Pain 98(1), 195
 (2001): Pomara N+, Prog Neuropsychopharmacol Biol Psychiatry 25(5), 1035
 (1999): Marraccini RL+, Int J Geriatr Psychiatry 14(12), 1014
 (1998): Pollock BG+, Am J Psychiatry 155(8), 1110
 (1981): Rafaelsen OJ+, Acta Psychiatr Scand Suppl 290, 364

Hair

Hair – alopecia (<1%)

Other

Gynecomastia (<1%)

Paresthesias
Seizures
  (2006): Endo G+, *Seishin Shinkeigaku Zasshi* 108(8), 792
Tremor
Vertigo
  (2005): Otsubo T+, *Pharmacopsychiatry* 38(1), 30
  (2002): Hammack JE+, *Pain* 98(1), 195

NYSTATIN

Trade names: Biofanal; Candio-Hermal; Mestatin; Moronal; Mycolog-11 (Bristol-Myers Squibb); Mycostatin (Bristol-Myers Squibb); Nistaquim; Nyaderm; Nystacid; Nystan; Nystex; Oranyst; Pedi-Dri
Indications: Candidiasis
Category: Antimycobacterial
Half-life: N/A

Reactions

Skin
Acute generalized exanthematous pustulosis (AGEP)
  (2003): Poszepczynska-Guigne E+, *Ann Dermatol Venereol* 130(4), 439
  (1999): Przybilla B+, *Hautarzt* (German) 50, 136
  (1998): Rosenberger A+, *Hautarzt* (German) 49, 492
  (1997): Kuchler A+, *Br J Dermatol* 137, 808 (3 cases)
Dermatitis (<1%)
  (1994): Fisher AA, *Cutis* 54, 300
  (1993): Hills RJ+, *Contact Dermatitis* 28, 48
  (1991): Quirce S+, *Contact Dermatitis* 25(3), 197 (generalized)
  (1990): de Groot AC+, *Dermatologic Clinics* 8, 153
  (1987): Lechner T+, *Mykosen* (German) 30, 143
  (1985): Lang E+, *Contact Dermatitis* 12, 182
Eczema
  (1987): Lechner T+, *Mykosen* (German) 30, 143
Erythema multiforme
  (1991): Garty BZ, *Arch Dermatol* 127, 741
Erythroderma
  (1980): Pareek SS, *Br J Dermatol* 103, 679
Exanthems
  (1991): Quirce S+, *Contact Dermatitis* 25, 197
Fixed eruption
  (1980): Pareek SS, *Br J Dermatol* 103, 679
Linear IgA dermatosis
  (1999): Stuber E+, *Z Gastroenterol* 37(6), 519
Pruritus
  (1987): Lechner T+, *Mykosen* (German) 30, 143
Rash (sic)
Stevens–Johnson syndrome (<1%)
  (1991): Garty BZ, *Arch Dermatol* 127, 741
Urticaria

Mucosal/ENT
Tongue edema
  (1991): Quirce S+, *Contact Dermatitis* 25, 197
Vaginitis
  (2001): Dan M, *Am J Obstet Gynecol* 185(1), 254

Other
Hypersensitivity (<1%)
  (2001): Barranco R+, *Contact Dermatitis* 45(1), 60

OCTREOTIDE

Trade names: Sandostatin (Novartis); Sandostatina; Sandostatine
Indications: Diarrhea
Category: GABA receptor agonist
Half-life: 1.5 hours

Reactions

Skin
Allergic granulomatous angiitis (Churg–Strauss syndrome)
  (2001): Rideout DJ+, *Clin Nucl Med* 26, 650 (buttock)
Allergic reactions (sic)
Cellulitis (1–4%)
Diaphoresis
Edema (1–10%)
Exanthems
  (1990): Saltz L+, *Proc Am Soc Clin Oncol* 9, 97
Petechiae (1–4%)
Pruritus (1–4%)
Purpura (1–4%)
Rash (sic) (<1%)
Raynaud's phenomenon (1–4%)
Urticaria (1–4%)

Mucosal/ENT
Vaginitis (1–4%)
Xerostomia

Hair
Hair – alopecia (<1%)
  (1995): Nakauchi Y+, *Endocr J* 42, 385
  (1991): Jonsson A+, *Ann Intern Med* 115, 913

Other
Anaphylactoid reactions/Anaphylaxis
Gynecomastia (1–4%)
Headache
Hepatotoxicity
  (2006): Feenstra J+, *Eur J Endocrinol* 154(6), 805 (with pegvisomant)
Injection-site erythema (1%)
Injection-site granuloma
  (2001): Rideout DJ+, *Clin Nucl Med* 26(7), 650
Injection-site pain (7.5%)
Injection-site reactions (sic)
Thrombophlebitis (1–4%)

OFLOXACIN

Trade names: Bactocin; Exocine; Flobasin; Floxan; Floxil; Floxin (Ortho-McNeil); Floxstat; Ocuflox (Allergan); Oflocet; Oflocin; Tabrin; Taravid
Indications: Various infections caused by susceptible organisms
Category: Antibiotic, quinolone
Half-life: 4–8 hours
Clinically important, potentially hazardous interactions with: amiodarone, arsenic, bepridil, bretylium, disopyramide, erythromycin, phenothiazines, procainamide, quinidine, sotalol, tricyclic antidepressants, zinc

Reactions

Skin

Acute febrile neutrophilic dermatosis (Sweet's syndrome)
  (2005): Ozdemir D+, *J Infect* 162, 162
Angioedema
  (1987): Jüngst G+, *Drugs* 34 (Suppl 1), 144
  (1987): Monk JP, *Drugs* 33, 346
Bullous dermatitis
Dermatitis
  (2000): Litt JZ, Beachwood, OH (personal case) (observation)
  (1987): Monk JP, *Drugs* 33, 346
Diaphoresis
Edema (<1%)
Erythema multiforme
Erythema nodosum
Exanthems
  (1994): Shelley WB+, *Cutis* 54, 146 (observation)
  (1994): Shelley WB+, *Cutis* 55, 22 (observation)
  (1993): Litt JZ, Beachwood, OH (personal case) (observation)
  (1987): Jüngst G+, *Drugs* 34 (Suppl 1), 144
  (1987): Monk JP, *Drugs* 33, 346
  (1986): Baran R+, *Dermatologica* 173, 185
Exfoliative dermatitis
Fixed eruption
  (1996): Kawada A+, *Contact Dermatitis* 34, 427
  (1994): Kawada A+, *Contact Dermatitis* 31, 182
Petechiae
Photosensitivity (<1%)
  (2002): Trisciuoglio D+, *Toxicol In Vitro* 16(4), 449
  (1994): Fujita H+, *Photodermatol Photoimmunol Photomed* 10, 202
  (1993): Scheife RT+, *Int J Dermatol* 32, 413
  (1990): Przybilla G+, *Dermatologica* 181, 98
  (1988): Halkin H, *Rev Infect Dis* 10 (Suppl 1), 258
  (1987): Jensen T+, *J Antimicrob Chemother* 20, 585
  (1987): Jüngst G+, *Drugs* 34 (Suppl 1), 144
  (1986): Baran R+, *Dermatologica* 173, 185
Phototoxicity
  (2000): Traynor NJ+, *Toxicol Vitr* 14, 275
  (1998): Martinez LJ+, *Photochem Photobiol* 67, 399
Pigmentation
Pruritus (1–3%)
  (2000): Litt JZ, Beachwood, OH (personal case) (observation)
  (1987): Jüngst G+, *Drugs* 34 (Suppl 1), 144
  (1987): Monk JP, *Drugs* 33, 346
Pruritus ani et vulvae (1–3%)
Purpura
Rash (sic) (1–10%)
  (1988): Kromann-Andersen B+, *J Antimicrob Chemother* 22 (Suppl C), 143
Side effects (sic) (0.4%)
  (1988): Fostini R+, *Drug Exp Clin Res* 14, 393
  (1987): Monk JP, *Drugs* 33, 346
Stevens–Johnson syndrome
Toxic epidermal necrolysis
  (2001): Melde LM, *Ann Pharmacother* 35, 1388
Toxic pustuloderma
  (1993): Tsuda S+, *Acta Derm Venereol* (Stockh) 73, 382
Urticaria (<1%)
  (1987): Jüngst G+, *Drugs* 34 (Suppl 1), 144
  (1987): Monk JP, *Drugs* 33, 346
Vasculitis (<1%)
  (1996): Pipek R+, *Am J Med Sci* 311, 82
  (1989): Huminer D+, *BMJ* 299, 303
  (1989): Pace JL+, *BMJ* 299, 658
  (1987): Jüngst G+, *Drugs* 34 (Suppl 1), 144

Mucosal/ENT

Dysgeusia (1–3%)
  (1995): Dark DS+, *Infections in Medicine* October, 551
Oral mucosal eruption
  (1987): Jüngst G+, *Drugs* 34 (Suppl 1), 144
  (1987): Monk JP, *Drugs* 33, 346
Parosmia
Tinnitus
Vaginitis (1–10%)
Xerostomia (1–3%)

Nails

Nails – photo-onycholysis
  (1987): Baran R+, *J Am Acad Dermatol* 17, 1012
  (1986): Baran R+, *Dermatologica* 173, 185

Eyes

Visual hallucinations
  (1986): Davies BI+, *Pharm Weekbl Sci* 8(1), 53

Other

Anaphylactoid reactions/Anaphylaxis
  (2006): Sachs B+, *Drug Saf* 29(11), 1087
  (2003): Ho DY+, *Ann Pharmacother* 37(7), 1018
  (1987): Jüngst G+, *Drugs* 34 (Suppl 1), 144
  (1987): Monk JP, *Drugs* 33, 346
Candidiasis
  (1987): Jüngst G+, *Drugs* 34 (Suppl 1), 144
Chills (<1%)
Death
  (2001): Melde SL, *Ann Pharmacother* 35(11), 1388
Headache
Hypersensitivity
  (1999): Desai C+, *J Assoc Physicians India* 47, 349
Injection-site pain (1–10%)
Myalgia/Myositis/Myopathy/Myotoxicity (<1%)
Neurotoxicity
  (2007): Guven EO+, *Int Urol Nephrol* 39(2), 647
Paresthesias (<1%)
Rhabdomyolysis
  (2005): Hsiao SH+, *Ann Pharmacother* 39(1), 146
  (1999): Baril L+, *Clin Infect Dis* 29(6), 1598
Serum sickness
Tendinopathy/Tendon rupture (<1%)
  (9999):
  (2006): Vaucher N+, *Presse Med* 35(9), 1271
  (2004): Aouam K+, *Therapie* 59(6), 653
  (2003): van der Linden PD+, *Arch Intern Med* 163(15), 1801
  (2001): van der Linden PD+, *Arthritis Rheum* 45(3), 235
  (1999): van der Linden PD+, *Br J Clin Pharmacol* 48(3), 433
  (1992): Ribard P+, *J Rheumatol* 19(9), 1479

OLANZAPINE

Synonym: LY170053
Trade name: Zyprexa (Lilly)
Indications: Psychotic disorders
Category: Antipsychotic; Muscarinic antagonist
Half-life: 21–54 hours
Clinically important, potentially hazardous interactions with: eszopiclone

Reactions

Skin

Acute generalized exanthematous pustulosis

(2006): Christen S+, *Acta Medica* (Hradec Kralove) 49(1), 75

Angioedema
(2001): Biswasl PN+, *J Psychopharmacol* 15(4), 265

Dermatitis (<1%)

Diaphoresis (>1%)

Eczema (<1%)

Edema
(2006): Deshauer D+, *Can Fam Physician* 52, 620

Exanthems (<1%)

Facial edema (<1%)

Peripheral edema (3%)
(2003): Ng B+, *Int Clin Psychopharmacol* 18(1), 57 (3%)
(2000): Yovtcheva SP+, *Gen Hosp Psychiatry* 22, 290

Photosensitivity (<1%)

Pigmentation (<1%)
(2004): Jhirwal OP+, *Int J Dermatol* 43(10), 778

Pruritus (>1%)

Psoriasis
(2003): Latini A+, *Eur J Dermatol* 13(4), 404 (2 cases)
(2000): Ascari-Raccagni A+, *J Eur Acad Dermatol Venereol* 14(4), 315

Pustules
(1999): Adams BB+, *J Am Acad Dermatol* 41, 851

Rash (sic) (>2%)
(2001): Street JS+, *Int J Geriatr Psychiatry* 16(Suppl 1), S62
(1999): Green B, *Curr Med Res Opin* 15, 79 (2%)

Seborrhea (<1%)

Ulcerations (<1%)

Urticaria (<1%)

Vasculitis
(2006): Papaioannides D+, *Int J Low Extrem Wounds* 5(2), 116

Vesiculobullous eruption (2%)

Xanthomas
(2006): Sinnott BP+, *Endocr Pract* 12(2), 183
(2003): Chang HY+, *Arch Dermatol* 139(8), 1045

Xerosis (<1%)

Mucosal/ENT

Aphthous stomatitis (<1%)

Auditory hallucinations
(2005): Chou KL+, *Clin Neuropharmacol* 28(5), 215

Dysgeusia (<1%)

Gingivitis (<1%)

Glossitis (<1%)

Oral candidiasis (<1%)

Oral ulceration (<1%)

Sialorrhea (<1%)
(2006): Hori T+, *Prog Neuropsychopharmacol Biol Psychiatry* 30(4), 758 (with fluvoxamine)
(2004): Cheng-Shannon J+, *J Child Adolesc Psychopharmacol* 14(3), 372
(1998): Perkins DO+, *Am J Psychiatry* 155, 993

Stomatitis (<1%)

Tongue black
(2006): Tamam L+, *Mt Sinai J Med* 73(6), 891

Tongue edema (<1%)
(1997): Litt JZ, Beachwood, OH (personal case) (observation)

Tongue pigmentation (<1%)

Vaginitis (>1%)

Xerostomia (13%)
(2006): Brown EB+, *J Clin Psychiatry* 67(7), 1025
(2003): Corya SA+, *J Clin Psychiatry* 64(11), 1349 (with fluoxetine)
(2003): Tohen M+, *Am J Psychiatry* 160(7), 1263
(2002): Tohen M+, *Arch Gen Psychiatry* 59(1), 62 (with lithium)
(1999): Green B, *Curr Med Res Opin* 15, 79 (7%)
(1998): Bever KA+, *Am J Health Syst Pharm* 55, 1003

Hair

Hair – alopecia (<1%)
(2002): Leung M+, *Can J Psychiatry* 47(9), 891
(2000): Mercke Y+, *Ann Clin Psychiatry* 12, 35

Hair – hirsutism (<1%)

Eyes

Oculogyric crisis
(2006): Desarkar P+, *Aust N Z J Psychiatry* 40(4), 374
(2006): Rosenhagen MC+, *J Clin Psychopharmacol* 26(4), 431

Visual hallucinations
(2005): Chou KL+, *Clin Neuropharmacol* 28(5), 215

Other

Candidiasis (<1%)

Coma
(2005): Bhanji NH+, *Can J Psychiatry* 50(2), 126

Death
(2004): *Prescrire Int* 13(74), 226
(2002): Meatherall R+, *J Forensic Sci* 47(4), 893
(1999): Wyderski RJ+, *Ann Pharmacother* 33(7–8), 787

Delirium
(2006): Lim CJ+, *Ann Pharmacother* 40(1), 135

Fever
(2003): Berry N+, *Pharmacotherapy* 23(2), 255 (with lithium)

Gynecomastia

Headache
(2003): Corya SA+, *J Clin Psychiatry* 64(11), 1349 (with fluoxetine)

Hepatotoxicity
(2006): Ozcanli T+, *Prog Neuropsychopharmacol Biol Psychiatry* 30(6), 1163

Hypersensitivity
(2001): Raz A+, *Am J Med Sci* 321(2), 156

Hypotension
(2006): Fleischhaker C+, *J Child Adolesc Psychopharmacol* 16(3), 308

Myalgia/Myositis/Myopathy/Myotoxicity (>1%)
(2006): Waring WS+, *Hum Exp Toxicol* 25(12), 735
(2001): Rosebraugh CJ+, *Ann Pharmacother* 35(9), 1020

Rhabdomyolysis
(2005): Baumgart U+, *Pharmacopsychiatry* 38(1), 36
(2001): Rosebraugh CJ+, *Ann Pharmacother* 35(9), 1020
(2000): Shuster J, *Nursing* 30(9), 87
(1999): Marcus EL+, *Ann Pharmacother* 33(6), 697
(1999): Wyderski RJ+, *Ann Pharmacother* 33(7–8), 787
(1996): Meltzer HY+, *Neuropsychopharmacology* 15(4), 395

Seizures
(2005): Bhanji NH+, *Can J Psychiatry* 50(2), 126
(2004): Gazdag G+, *Ideggyogy Sz* 57(11–12), 385 (40%)
(2003): Bonelli RM, *Ann Pharmacother* 37(1), 149
(2003): Reuther LO+, *Ugeskr Laeger* 165(14), 1447
(1999): Wyderski RJ+, *Ann Pharmacother* 33(7–8), 787

Somnambulism
(2001): Kolivakis TT+, *Am J Psychiatry* 158(7), 1158

Stroke
(2004): *Prescrire Int* 13(74), 226

Tremor (1–10%)
(2006): Fleischhaker C+, *J Child Adolesc Psychopharmacol* 16(3), 308
(2002): Tohen M+, *Arch Gen Psychiatry* 59(1), 62 (with lithium)
(2001): Ishigooka J+, *Psychiatry Clin Neurosci* 55(4), 353

Vertigo
(2003): Hwang JP+, *J Clin Psychopharmacol* 23(2), 113

Weight gain
(2006): Fleischhaker C+, *J Child Adolesc Psychopharmacol* 16(3), 308
(2006): Schwetschenau KH, *J Manag Care Pharm* 12(3), 260
(2005): Ness-Abramof R+, *Drugs Today* (Barc) 41(8), 547

OLMESARTAN

Trade name: Benicar (Sankyo)
Indications: Hypertension
Category: Angiotensin II receptor antagonist
Half-life: ~13 hours
**Clinically important, potentially hazardous interactions
with: ephedra, garlic, ginseng,** lithium

Reactions

Skin
Angioedema
 (2007): Nykamp D+, *Ann Pharmacother* 41(3), 518
Facial edema
Lichen planus
 (2006): Sontheimer RD, Oklahoma City, OK (from Internet)
  (observation)
Lichenoid eruption
 (2006): Sontheimer R (from Internet) (observation)
Peripheral edema (>0.5)
Rash (sic) (0.5%)

Other
Cough (0.7%)
Myalgia/Myositis/Myopathy/Myotoxicity (>0.5%)
Pain (>0.5%)
Upper respiratory infection (>1%)
Vertigo (3%)
 (2003): Brousil JA+, *Clin Ther* 25(4), 1041 (3%)
 (2003): Gardner SF+, *Ann Pharmacother* 37(1), 99

OLOPATADINE

Trade name: Patanol (Alcon)
Indications: Pruritus due to allergic conjunctivitis
Category: Histamine H1 receptor antagonist
Half-life: 3 hours

Reactions

Skin
Burning
 (2003): Ganz M+, *Adv Ther* 20(2), 79
Pruritus

Mucosal/ENT
Dysgeusia

Eyes
Eyelid burning (<5%)
Eyelid edema (<5%)
Eyelid stinging (<5%)

Other
Headache
 (2003): Ganz M+, *Adv Ther* 20(2), 79

OLSALAZINE

Trade name: Dipentum (Celltech)
Indications: Ulcerative colitis
Category: Aminosalicylate
Half-life: 0.9 hours
**Clinically important, potentially hazardous interactions
with:** azathioprine, mercaptopurine

Reactions

Skin
Acne
 (1990): Zinberg J+, *Am J Gastroenterol* 85, 562
Exanthems (0.4%)
 (1994): Shelley WB+, *Cutis* 53, 240 (observation)
 (1991): Wadworth AN+, *Drugs* 41, 647
Lupus erythematosus
 (1997): Gunnarsson I+, *Scand J Rheumatol* 26, 65
Pallor
Pruritus (1.1%)
 (1993): Ferry GD+, *J Pediatr Gastroenterol Nutr* 17(1), 32
Rash (sic) (2.3%)
 (1993): Ferry GD+, *J Pediatr Gastroenterol Nutr* 17(1), 32
 (1990): *Drug Ther Bull* 28, 57
Urticaria (4.3%)
 (1987): Meyers S+, *Gastroenterology* 93, 1255

Mucosal/ENT
Stomatitis (1%)
Tinnitus

Eyes
Myopia
 (1992): Doman DB+, *Am J Gastroenterol* 87(11), 1684

Other
Fever
 (1993): Ferry GD+, *J Pediatr Gastroenterol Nutr* 17(1), 32
Headache
 (1993): Ferry GD+, *J Pediatr Gastroenterol Nutr* 17(1), 32
Nephrotoxicity
 (2000): Stein RB+, *Drug Saf* 23(5), 429

OMALIZUMAB

Trade name: Xolair (Genentech) (Novartis)
Indications: Asthma
Category: Immunomodulator; Monoclonal antibody
Half-life: 26 days
**Clinically important, potentially hazardous interactions
with:** None

Reactions

Skin
Allergic reactions (sic)
 (2008): Barry PJ+, *J Allergy Clin Immunol* 121(3), 785
Dermatitis (2%)
Edema
 (2003): Nayak A+, *Allergy Asthma Proc* 24(5), 323
Erythema
 (2003): Nayak A+, *Allergy Asthma Proc* 24(5), 323
Pruritus (2%)
Rash (sic)

(2003): Nayak A+, *Allergy Asthma Proc* 24(5), 323
Urticaria (7%)
(2003): Berger W+, *Ann Allergy Asthma Immunol* 91(2), 182 (5%)

Mucosal/ENT
Sinusitis (16%)
(2004): Bang LM+, *BioDrugs* 18(6), 415
(2004): Bang LM+, *Treat Respir Med* 3(3), 183
Tongue edema

Other
Anaphylactoid reactions/Anaphylaxis (45%)
(2007): *Prescrire Int* 16(91), 179 (passim)
(2007): Limb SL+, *J Allergy Clin Immunol*
(2007): Price KS+, *Allergy Asthma Proc* 28(3), 313 (2 cases)
(2006): Dreyfus DH+, *Ann Allergy Asthma Immunol* 96(4), 624
(2006): Price K, *American Academy Allergy Asthma Immunology* (poster)
(2005): Lanier BQ, *Allergy Asthma Proc* 26(6), 435
Asthenia (3%)
Headache (15%)
(2004): Bang LM+, *BioDrugs* 18(6), 415
(2004): Bang LM+, *Treat Respir Med* 3(3), 183
(2003): Berger W+, *Ann Allergy Asthma Immunol* 91(2), 182
Hypersensitivity
Injection-site burning
Injection-site erythema
Injection-site induration
Injection-site pruritus
Injection-site purpura
Injection-site reactions (sic) (45%)
(2004): Bang LM+, *BioDrugs* 18(6), 415
(2004): Bang LM+, *Treat Respir Med* 3(3), 183
Injection-site urticaria
Pain (7%)
Serum sickness
(2007): Pilette C+, *J Allergy Clin Immunol* 120(4), 972
Upper respiratory infection (20%)
(2004): Bang LM+, *BioDrugs* 18(6), 415
(2004): Bang LM+, *Treat Respir Med* 3(3), 183
(2003): Berger W+, *Ann Allergy Asthma Immunol* 91(2), 182
Vertigo (3%)

OMEGA-3 FATTY ACIDS

Scientific names: *docosahexaenoic acid (DHA); eicosapentaenoic acid (EPA); Omega-3 fatty acids*
Family: N/A
Category: Anti-inflammatory; Lipid regulator
Purported indications and other uses: Albuminuria, anorexia nervosa, hypertension, lupus erythematosus, macular degeneration, osteoarthritis, otitis media, psoriasis
Half-life: N/A
Clinically important, potentially hazardous interactions with: N/A

Reactions

Skin
Malignant melanoma
(1997): Veierod MB+, *Int J Cancer* 71(4), 600
Rash (sic)

Mucosal/ENT
Dysgeusia
(2002): Carroll DN+, *Ann Pharmacother* 36(12), 1950

(1992): Zakaria B+, *Fortschr Med* 110(10), 178

Eyes
Glaucoma
(2004): Kang JH+, *Am J Clin Nutr* 79(5), 755

Other
Abdominal pain
Hypersensitivity
Lymphoid hyperplasia
(1988): Ogden P+, *Ann Intern Med* 109(10), 843

OMEPRAZOLE

Trade names: Antra; Audazol; Gastroloc; Inhibitron; Logastric; Losec; Mopral; Omed; Ozoken; Parizac; Prilosec (AstraZeneca); Ulsen
Indications: Duodenal ulcer, Gastroesophageal Reflux Disease (GERD)
Category: Proton pump inhibitor
Half-life: 0.5–1 hour
Clinically important, potentially hazardous interactions with: eucalyptus, methotrexate, prednisone

Reactions

Skin
Angioedema (<1%)
(2002): Odeh M+, *Postgrad Med J* 78(916), 114 (passim)
(1994): Bowlby HA+, *Pharmacotherapy* 14, 119
(1992): Haeney MR, *BMJ* 305, 870
Baboon syndrome
(2003): Wolf R+, *Dermatol Online J* 9(3), 2 (with clarithromycin and amoxicillin)
Bullous dermatitis
(1995): Stenier C+, *Br J Dermatol* 133, 343
Bullous pemphigoid
(1991): Chosidow O+, *Ann Dermatol Venereol* (French) 118, 45
(1990): Joly P+, *Gastroenterol Clin Biol* (French) 14, 682
Burning
(1984): Blanchi A+, *Gastroenterol Clin Biol* (French) 8, 943
Contact dermatitis
(2007): Conde-Salazar L+, *Contact Dermatitis* 56(1), 44
(2006): Kamann S+, *Hautarzt* 57(11), 1016
Dermatitis
(2002): Odeh M+, *Postgrad Med J* 78(916), 114 (passim)
Dermatomyositis
(2006): Pan Y+, *Br J Dermatol* 154(3), 557
Diaphoresis (<1%)
(1989): Delchier JC+, *Gut* 30, 1173
Eczema
(1985): Classen M+, *Dtsch Med Wochenschr* (German) 110, 628 (scalp)
Edema (1–10%)
(2000): Natsch S+, *Ann Pharmacother* MH(4), 474 (1–10%)
(1989): Danish Omeprazole Study Group, *BMJ* 298, 645
Erythema
(1984): Blanchi A+, *Gastroenterol Clin Biol* (French) 8, 943
Erythema multiforme (<1%)
Erythema nodosum
(1996): Ricci RM+, *Cutis* 57, 434
Erythroderma
(1999): Cockayne SE+, *Br J Dermatol* 141, 173
Exanthems
(1991): Langman MSJ, *BMJ* 303, 481
Exfoliative dermatitis

(1998): Rebuck JA+, *Pharmacotherapy* 18, 877
(1995): Epelde-Gonzalo FD+, *Ann Pharmacother* 29, 82
Facial edema
   (2002): Gonzalez P+, *Allergol Immunopathol* (Madr) 30(6), 342
Fixed eruption
   (1999): Kepekci Y+, *Int J Clin Pharmacol Ther* 37, 307 (hands)
Furunculosis
   (1998): West BC+, *Clin Infect Dis* 26, 1234
Lichen planus
   (1997): Litt JZ, Beachwood, OH (personal case) (observation)
   (1986): Pounder RE+, *Scand J Gastroenterol* 21, 108
   (1984): Sharma BK+, *Gut* 25, 957
Lichen spinulosus
   (2002): Odeh M+, *Postgrad Med J* 78(916), 114 (passim)
   (1989): Lee ML+, *Med J Aust* 150, 410
Lichenoid eruption
   (2006): Kamann S+, *Hautarzt* 57(11), 1016
   (2000): Bong JL+, *BMJ* 320, 283
Lupus erythematosus
   (2006): Sontheimer RD, Oklahoma City, OK (3 cases) (from
     Internet) (observation)
   (1994): Sivakumar K+, *Lancet* 344, 619
Pemphigus (exacerbation)
   (1992): Cox NH, *Lancet* 340, 857
   (1991): Chosidow D+, *Ann Dermatol Venereol* (French) 118, 45
Peripheral edema (<1%)
   (2002): Chan FK+, *N Engl J Med* 347(26), 2104 (with diclofenac)
   (2001): Brunner G+, *Dig Dis Sci* 46(5), 993
Pityriasis rosea
   (1996): Buckley C, *Br J Dermatol* 135, 660
Pruritus (1–10%)
   (2000): Natsch S+, *Ann Pharmacother* 34, 474
   (1994): Bowlby HA+, *Pharmacotherapy* 14, 119
   (1989): Danish Omeprazole Study Group, *BMJ* 298, 645
   (1989): Lee ML+, *Med J Aust* 150, 410
   (1987): Bertaccini G+, *Clin Ter* (Italian) 121, 201
   (1987): Klinkenberg-Knol EC+, *Lancet* 1, 349
   (1986): Bardhan KD+, *J Clin Gastroenterol* 8, 408
   (1986): Rinetti M+, *Drugs Exp Clin Res* 12, 701
Psoriasis
   (1984): Blanchi A+, *Gastroenterol Clin Biol* (French) 8, 943
Purpura
Rash (sic) (1.5%)
   (2002): Odeh M+, *Postgrad Med J* 78(916), 114 (passim)
   (1989): Delchier JC+, *Gut* 30, 1173
   (1989): Lauritsen K+, *Aliment Pharmacol Ther* 3, 59
   (1988): Hirschowitz BI+, *Gastroenterol* 94, A188
   (1986): Bardhan KD+, *J Clin Gastroenterol* 8, 408
Stevens–Johnson syndrome (<1%)
Toxic epidermal necrolysis (<1%)
   (2006): Casacci M+, *Eur J Dermatol* 16(6), 699
   (2002): Odeh M+, *Postgrad Med J* 78(916), 114 (passim)
   (1992): Cox NH, *Lancet* 340, 857
Urticaria (1–10%)
   (2002): Gonzalez P+, *Allergol Immunopathol* (Madr) 30(6), 342
   (2002): Odeh M+, *Postgrad Med J* 78(916), 114 (passim)
   (1994): Bowlby HA+, *Pharmacotherapy* 14, 119
   (1994): Schneider S+, *Gastroenterol Clin Biol* (French) 18, 534
   (1993): Litt JZ, Beachwood, OH (personal case) (observation)
   (1992): Haeney MR, *BMJ* 305, 870
Vasculitis
   (2006): Kamann S+, *Hautarzt* 57(11), 1016
   (2002): Odeh M+, *Postgrad Med J* 78(916), 114 (passim)
Xerosis (<1%)
   (2005): Chen CY+, *World J Gastroenterol* 11(20), 3112
   (1988): Marks IN+, *S Afr Med J* (Suppl), 54

Mucosal/ENT
Dysgeusia (1–10%)
   (1996): Markitziu A+, *Scand J Gastroenterol* 31, 624
Oral candidiasis
   (1995): Anderson PC, *Arch Dermatol* 131, 966
   (1993): Mosimann F, *Transplantation* 56, 492
   (1992): Larner AJ+, *Gut* 33, 860
Tinnitus
Xerostomia (1–10%)
   (1995): Teare JP+, *Scand J Gastroenterol* 30(3), 216
   (1985): Classen M+, *Dtsch Med Wochenschr* (German) 110, 628

Hair
Hair – alopecia (<1%)
   (2002): Litt JZ, Beachwood, OH (observation)
   (1999): Litt JZ, Beachwood, OH (2 personal cases)
     (observations)
   (1997): Borum ML+, *Am J Gastroenterol* 92, 1576
   (1994): Bowlby HA+, *Pharmacotherapy* 14, 119 (passim)
Hair – pigmentation

Eyes
Periorbital edema
   (2000): Natsch S+, *Ann Pharmacother* 34, 474

Other
Abdominal pain
   (2005): Colls BM+, *N Z Med J* 118(1208), U1263
Anaphylactoid reactions/Anaphylaxis
   (2006): Kamann S+, *Hautarzt* 57(11), 1016
   (2002): Gonzalez P+, *Allergol Immunopathol* (Madr) 30(6), 342
   (2000): Natsch S+, *Ann Pharmacother* 34, 474
   (1999): Galindo PA1, *Ann Allergy Asthma Immunol* 82, 52
Cough
   (2003): Howaizi M+, *Ann Pharmacother* 37(11), 1607
Fever
   (2005): Colls BM+, *N Z Med J* 118(1208), U1263
Gynecomastia
   (2006): Kamann S+, *Hautarzt* 57(11), 1016
   (2000): Hugues FC+, *Ann Med Interne* (Paris) (French) 151, 10
     (passim)
   (1998): N Z Medicines Adverse Reactions Committee (from
     Internet) (observation) (3 cases)
   (1995): Carvajal A+, *Am J Gastroenterol* 90, 1028
   (1995): Durand JM+, *Ann Med Interne* (Paris) (French) 146, 195
   (1994): Garcia-Rodriguez LA+, *BMJ* 308, 503
   (1994): Lindquist M+, *BMJ* 305, 451
   (1994): Pedrosa M+, *Med Clin* (Barc) (Spanish) 102, 435
   (1991): Convens C+, *Lancet* 338, 1153
   (1991): Santucci L+, *N Engl J Med* 324, 635
Headache
Myalgia/Myositis/Myopathy/Myotoxicity (1–10%)
Paresthesias (<1%)
   (1986): Rinetti M+, *Drugs Exp Clin Res* 12, 701
   (1984): Blanchi A+, *Gastroenterol Clin Biol* (French) 8, 943
Tremor (<1%)

ONDANSETRON

Trade names: Emeset; Oncoden; Zofran (GSK); Zofron
Indications: Nausea and vomiting
Category: 5-HT3 antagonist; Serotonin type 3 receptor antagonist
Half-life: 4 hours
Clinically important, potentially hazardous interactions with: eucalyptus

Reactions

Skin
Angioedema
Exanthems
Fixed eruption
 (2000): Bernard S+, *Dermatology* 201, 184 (similar fixed
  eruption from acetaminophen)
 (1995): Iglesias ME+, *Dermatology* 191, 270
Pruritus (5%)
Rash (sic) (<1%)
Urticaria
 (2005): Bousquet PJ+, *Allergy* 60(4), 543

Mucosal/ENT
Dysgeusia
 (2000): Robbins L, *Headache* 11, 275
Sialopenia (1–5%)
Xerostomia (1–10%)
 (1994): Ahn MJ+, *Am J Clin Oncol* 17, 150
 (1991): Milne RJ+, *Drugs* 41, 574

Hair
Hair – alopecia

Other
Anaphylactoid reactions/Anaphylaxis
 (2001): Weiss KS, *Arch Intern Med* 161(18), 2263
 (1998): Ross AK+, *Anesth Analg* 87, 779
 (1991): Milne RJ+, *Drugs* 41, 574
Chills (5–10%)
Headache
Hypersensitivity (<1%)
 (1996): Kataja V+, *Lancet* 347, 584
Injection-site burning
Injection-site erythema
Injection-site pain
Injection-site reactions (sic) (4%)
Paresthesias (2%)
Porphyria
 (1992): DeWet M+, *S Afr Med J* 82, 480

ORAL CONTRACEPTIVES

Trade names: Alesse (Wyeth); Aviane (Barr); Brevicon
(Watson); Demulen (Pfizer); Desogen (Organon); Estrostep
(Pfizer); Evra (Johnson & Johnson); Genora; Intercon; Levlen
(Berlex); Levlite (Berlex); Levora (Watson); Lo/Ovral (Wyeth);
Loestrin (Barr); Lunelle (Pfizer); Mircette (Organon); Modicon
(Ortho); Necon (Watson); NEE; Nelova; Nordette (Monarch);
Norethin; Norinyl (Watson); Ortho Tri-Cyclen (Ortho-McNeil);
Ortho-Cept (Ortho-McNeil); Ortho-Cyclen (Ortho-McNeil);
Ortho-Novum (Ortho-McNeil); Ovcon (Warner Chilcott); Ovral
(Wyeth); Tri-Levlen (Berlex); Tri-Norinyl (Watson); Triphasil
(Wyeth); Trivora (Watson); Yasmin (Berlex); Zovia (Watson)
Indications: Prevention of pregnancy
Category: Hormone
Half-life: N/A

**Clinically important, potentially hazardous interactions
with:** anticonvulsants, aprepitant, beclomethasone, bosentan,
budesonide, **cigarette smoking**, danazol, efavirenz, flunisolide,
fluticasone, hydrocortisone, insulin detemir, lamotrigine, **licorice**,
methylprednisolone, modafinil, nelfinavir, prednisolone,
prednisone, rifabutin, rifampin, ritonavir, **saw palmetto**,
selegiline, **St John's wort**, theophylline, triamcinolone,
troleandomycin, tuberculostatics, zolmitriptan

Reactions

Skin
Acanthosis nigricans
Acne
 (1987): Kovacs G+, *Australasian J Dermatol* 28, 86
 (1984): van der Meeren HL+, *Ned Tijdschr Geneeskd* (Dutch)
  128, 1333
 (1981): Scholz C+, *Zentralbl Gynakol* (German) 103, 1158
Acute febrile neutrophilic dermatosis (Sweet's syndrome)
 (2002): Saez M+, *Dermatology* 204(1), 84
 (1991): Tefany FJ+, *Aust J Dermatol* 32, 55
Angioedema
 (2000): Bouillet L+, *Presse Med* (French) 29, 640
 (1990): Borradori L+, *Dermatologica* 181, 78
Bullous dermatitis
 (1981): Honeyman JF+, *Arch Dermatol* 117, 264
Chloasma
 (1987): Kovacs G+, *Australasian J Dermatol* 28, 86
Cold urticaria
 (1983): Burns MR+, *Ann Intern Med* 98, 1025
Dermatitis herpetiformis
Eczema
 (1988): Edman B, *Acta Derm Venereol* 68, 402 (palmar)
Edema
Erythema
Erythema multiforme
Erythema nodosum
 (1981): Touboul JL+, *Nouv Presse Med* (French) 10, 712
 (1980): Beaucaire G+, *Sem Hôp* (French) 56, 1426
 (1980): Salvatore MA+, *Arch Dermatol* 116, 557
Exanthems
 (1981): Scholz C+, *Zentralbl Gynakol* (German) 103, 1158
Fixed eruption
Fox–Fordyce disease
Herpes genitalis
 (1981): Scholz C+, *Zentralbl Gynakol* (German) 103, 1158
Herpes gestationis
 (1989): Kemper T+, *Akt Dermatol* (German) 15, 121
Lichenoid eruption
Livedo reticularis (Sneddon's syndrome)
 (1991): Berchtold B+, *Hautarzt* (German) 42, 328
Lupus erythematosus
 (2001): Kakehasi AM+, *Arq Neuropsiquiatr* 59(3), 609
 (1994): Hess EV+, *Curr Opin Rheumatology* 6, 474
 (1994): Strom BL+, *Am J Epidemiol* 140, 632
 (1994): Yung RL+, *Rheum Dis Clin North Am* 20, 61
 (1993): Arden NK+, *Lupus* 2, 381
 (1991): Furukawa F+, *J Dermatology* (Tokio) 18, 56
 (1990): Franceschi S+, *Tumori* (Italian) 76, 439
 (1990): Zanetti R+, *Int J Epidemiol* 19, 522
 (1989): Beaumont V+, *Clin Physiol Biochem* 7, 263
 (1989): Iskander MK+, *J Rheumatol* 16, 850
 (1988): Mathur AK+, *J Rheumatology* 15, 1042
 (1986): Asherson RA+, *Arthritis Rheum* 29, 1535
 (1982): Jungers P+, *Arthritis Rheum* 25, 618
 (1982): Jungers P+, *Nouv Presse Med* (French) 11, 3765
 (1980): Condemi JJ, *Geriatrics* 35(3), 81

(1980): Garovich M+, *Arthritis Rheum* 23, 1396
Melanoma
  (1992): Le MG+, *Cancer Causes Control* 3, 199
  (1985): Bork K, *Hautarzt* (German) 36, 542
  (1985): Gallagher RP+, *Br J Cancer* 52, 901
  (1985): Green A+, *Med J Aust* 142, 446
  (1985): Quencez E+, *Ann Dermatol Venereol* (French) 112, 341
Melasma
  (1985): Lutfi RJ+, *J Clin Endocrinol Metab* 61, 28
  (1981): Witkiewicz IM+, *Ned Tijdschr Geneeskd* (Dutch) 125, 609
Mucha–Habermann disease
Perioral dermatitis
  (1989): Ehlers G, *Hautarzt* (German) 20, 287
Photosensitivity
  (1994): Litt JZ, Beachwood, OH (personal case) (observation)
  (1989): Boonstra H+, *Photodermatol* 6, 55
  (1988): Neumann R, *Photodermatol* 5, 40
Pigmentation
  (1981): Granstein RD+, *J Am Acad Dermatol* 5, 1
  (1981): Scholz C+, *Zentralbl Gynakol* (German) 103, 1158
  (1980): Hertz RS+, *J Am Dent Assoc* 100, 713
Pruritus (<1%)
Psoriasis
  (1981): Scholz C+, *Zentralbl Gynakol* (German) 103, 1158
Purpura
  (1983): McShane PM+, *Am J Obstet Gynecol* 145, 762
Seborrhea
  (1981): Scholz C+, *Zentralbl Gynakol* (German) 103, 1158
    (seborrheic dermatitis)
Spider angiomas
Stevens–Johnson syndrome
Telangiectasia
  (1983): Wilkin JK+, *J Am Acad Dermatol* 8, 468
Urticaria
  (1981): Scholz C+, *Zentralbl Gynakol* (German) 103, 1158
Varicosities

Mucosal/ENT

Gingival hyperplasia/hypertrophy
Oral pigmentation
  (1980): Hertz RS+, *J Am Dent Assoc* 100, 713 (gingival)

Hair

Hair – alopecia
  (1989): Burke KE, *Postgrad Med* 85, 52
  (1987): Kovacs G+, *Australasian J Dermatol* 28, 86
  (1982): Hauser GA+, *Int J Tissue React* 4, 159
  (1981): Scholz C+, *Zentralbl Gynakol* (German) 103, 1158
Hair – alopecia areata
Hair – hirsutism
  (1994): Burdova M+, *Ceska Gynekol* (Czech) 59, 62
  (1987): Kovacs G+, *Australasian J Dermatol* 28, 86
  (1981): Scholz C+, *Zentralbl Gynakol* (German) 103, 1158

Other

Application-site reactions (sic) (92%)
  (2002): Sibai BM+, *Fertil Steril* 77(2 Suppl 2), S19 (patch) (92%)
Candidiasis
  (1983): Lebherz TB+, *Clin Ther* 5, 409
Depression
  (2001): Freeman MP, *JAMA* 286(6), 671
Porphyria cutanea tarda
  (2001): Emri G+, *Orv Hetil* 142(47), 2635
  (1992): McKenna KE+, *Br J Dermatol* 127, 401
  (1983): Doss M, *Dtsch Med Wochenschr* (German) 108, 1857
  (1983): Zaumseil RP+, *Zentralbl Gynakol* (German) 105, 527
  (1982): Zaumseil RP+, *Z Gesamte In Med* (German) 37, 703
  (1981): Fiedler H+, *Dermatol Monatsschr* (German) 167, 481

Porphyria variegata
Pseudoporphyria
  (2003): Silver EA+, *Arch Dermatol* 139, 227
Thrombophlebitis
  (1985): Taylor F, *Aust Fam Physician* 14(8), 744
Tremor
  (2001): Chetty M+, *Ther Drug Monit* 23(5), 556 (with chlorpromazine)

ORLISTAT

Trade name: Xenical (Roche)
Indications: Obesity, weight reduction
Category: Lipase inhibitor
Half-life: 1–2 hours
Clinically important, potentially hazardous interactions with: cyclosporine, warfarin

Reactions

Skin

Dermatitis
Lichenoid eruption
  (2006): Sergeant A+, *Br J Dermatol* 154(5), 1020
Nodular eruption
Rash (sic) (4.3%)
Xerosis

Mucosal/ENT

Gingivitis (4.1%)
Vaginitis (3.8%)
  (2006): Acharya NV+, *Int J Obes* (Lond) 30(11), 1645

Other

Abdominal pain
  (2006): Acharya NV+, *Int J Obes* (Lond) 30(11), 1645
Asthenia
  (2006): Acharya NV+, *Int J Obes* (Lond) 30(11), 1645
Headache
Hepatotoxicity
  (2006): Umemura T+, *Am J Med* 119(8), e7
Myalgia/Myositis/Myopathy/Myotoxicity (4.2%)
Tendinopathy/Tendon rupture

ORPHENADRINE

Trade names: Banflex (Forest); Biorfen; Biorphen; Disipal; Distalene; Flexojet; Flexon; Myolin; Norflex (3M); Norgesic; Opheryl; Orfenace; Prolongatum
Indications: Painful musculoskeletal conditions
Category: Central muscle relaxant; Muscarinic antagonist
Half-life: 14 hours

Reactions

Skin

Exanthems
Fixed eruption
  (1998): Mahboob A+, *Int J Dermatol* 37, 833
Pigmentation
Pruritus
Rash (sic) (1–10%)
Urticaria

Mucosal/ENT
Xerostomia

Other
Anaphylactoid reactions/Anaphylaxis
Embolia cutis medicamentosa (Nicolau syndrome)
Headache
Hypersensitivity
Paresthesias

OSELTAMIVIR

Trade name: Tamiflu (Roche)
Indications: Influenza infection
Category: Antiviral; Neuraminidase inhibitor
Half-life: 6–10 hours

Reactions

Skin
Rash (sic)
(2005): Kaji M+, *J Infect Chemother* 11(1), 41
(2003): Li L+, *Chin Med J* (Engl) 116(1), 44
Toxic epidermal necrolysis
(2006): *Prescrire Int* 15(85), 182

Other
Anaphylactoid reactions/Anaphylaxis
(2008): Hirschfeld G+, *Allergy* 63(2), 243
Confusion
(2006): *Prescrire Int* 15(85), 182
Cough
(2002): Bowles SK+, *J Am Geriatr Soc* 50(4), 608
Death
(2006): *Prescrire Int* 15(85), 182
Delirium
(2007): *Prescrire Int* 16(91), 200
(2006): *Prescrire Int* 15(85), 182
Myalgia/Myositis/Myopathy/Myotoxicity
(2001): McNicholl IR+, *Ann Pharmacother* 35(1), 57
Neurotoxicity
(2006): *Prescrire Int* 15(85), 182 (fatal)
Seizures
(2007): *Prescrire Int* 16(91), 200
(2006): *Prescrire Int* 15(85), 182
Suicidal ideation
(2007): *Prescrire Int* 16(91), 200
(2006): *Prescrire Int* 15(85), 182
Upper respiratory infection
(2001): McNicholl IR+, *Ann Pharmacother* 35(1), 57

OXACILLIN

Trade names: Bactocill; Bristopen; Oxacillin; Prostaphlin; Stapenor
Indications: Various infections caused by susceptible organisms
Category: Antibiotic, penicillin
Half-life: 23–60 minutes
Clinically important, potentially hazardous interactions with: anticoagulants, cyclosporine, demeclocycline, doxycycline, imipenem/cilastatin, methotrexate, minocycline, oxytetracycline, tetracycline

Reactions

Skin
Angioedema
Bullous dermatitis
Erythema multiforme
Erythema nodosum
Exanthems
Exfoliative dermatitis
Hematomas
Jarisch–Herxheimer reaction
Necrosis
(1980): Tilden SJ+, *Am J Dis Child* 134, 1046
Pruritus
(1998): Siegfried EC+, *J Am Acad Dermatol* 39, 797 (passim)
Rash (sic) (1–22%)
(2002): Maraqa NF+, *Clin Infect Dis* 34(1), 50 (22%)
Stevens–Johnson syndrome
(1982): Sukovatykh TN+, *Pediatriia* (Russian) May, 76
Toxic epidermal necrolysis
Urticaria
(1998): Siegfried EC+, *J Am Acad Dermatol* 39, 797 (passim)
Vasculitis
(2001): Koutkia P+, *Diagn Microbiol Infect Dis* 46(5), 993

Mucosal/ENT
Dysgeusia
Glossitis
Glossodynia
Oral candidiasis
Stomatitis
Stomatodynia
Tongue black
Tongue furry
Vaginitis
Xerostomia

Other
Anaphylactoid reactions/Anaphylaxis (0.04%)
(1998): Siegfried EC+, *J Am Acad Dermatol* 39, 797 (passim)
Hypersensitivity
Injection-site pain
Phlebitis
Serum sickness (<1%)
Thrombophlebitis

OXALIPLATIN

Trade names: Eloxatin (Sanofi-Aventis); Heloxatin
Indications: Metastatic carcinoma of the colon or rectum (in combination with fluorouracil)
Category: Alkylating agent; Antineoplastic
Half-life: 391 hours
Clinically important, potentially hazardous interactions with: None

Reactions

Skin
Allergic reactions (sic) (3%)
Angioedema
(2007): Lee MY+, *Support Care Cancer* 15(1), 89
Diaphoresis (2–5%)
(2005): Mis L+, *Ann Pharmacother* 39(5), 966

(2003): Brandi G+, *Br J Cancer* 89(3), 477

Edema (10%)
(2006): Saif MW, *Expert Opin Drug* 5(5), 687
(2003): Brandi G+, *Br J Cancer* 89(3), 477

Erythema
(2006): Saif MW, *Expert Opin Drug* 5(5), 687
(2003): Brandi G+, *Br J Cancer* 89(3), 477
(2003): Thomas RR+, *Cancer* 97(9), 2301

Exanthems (2–5%)

Facial flushing
(2006): Saif MW, *Expert Opin Drug* 5(5), 687

Hand–foot syndrome (1%)

Peripheral edema (5%)

Photo-recall
(2001): Camidge R, *Clin Oncol* 13(3), 236
(2001): Chan RT+, *Clin Oncol* 13(1), 55

Pruritus (2–5%)
(2006): Saif MW, *Expert Opin Drug* 5(5), 687
(2003): Brandi G+, *Br J Cancer* 89(3), 477
(2003): Thomas RR+, *Cancer* 97(9), 2301

Purpura (2–5%)

Rash (sic) (5%)
(2006): Saif MW, *Expert Opin Drug* 5(5), 687
(2004): Gowda A+, *Oncology (Williston Park)* 18(13), 1671

Urticaria
(2000): Petit-Laurent F+, *Gastroenterol Clin Biol* 24(8), 851

Xerosis (2–5%)

Mucosal/ENT
Dysgeusia (5%)
Gingivitis (2–5%)
Mucositis (2%)
Rhinitis (6%)
Stomatitis (14%)
(2000): Haller DG, *Oncology* 14(12), 15

Tongue edema
(2006): Saif MW, *Expert Opin Drug* 5(5), 687

Xerostomia (2–5%)

Hair
Hair – alopecia (3%)

Eyes
Conjunctivitis (2–5%)

Epiphora
(2004): Gowda A+, *Oncology (Williston Park)* 18(13), 1671
(2003): Brandi G+, *Br J Cancer* 89(3), 477

Ocular stinging
(2002): Wilson RH+, *J Clin Oncol* 20(7), 1767

Ocular toxicity
(2006): O'Dea D+, *Clin J Oncol Nurs* 10(2), 227

Vision blurred
(2004): Gowda A+, *Oncology (Williston Park)* 18(13), 1671

Vision loss
(2006): O'Dea D+, *Clin J Oncol Nurs* 10(2), 227

Other
Abdominal pain
(2005): Mis L+, *Ann Pharmacother* 39(5), 966

Anaphylactoid reactions/Anaphylaxis
(2007): Lee MY+, *Support Care Cancer* 15(1), 89
(2006): Sagawa T+, *Gan To Kagaku Ryoho* 33(13), 2093
(2006): Saif MW, *Expert Opin Drug Saf* 5(5), 687
(2005): Gonzalez-Mahave I+, *J Investig Allergol Clin Immunol* 15(1), 75
(2005): Maindrault-Goebel F+, *Eur J Cancer* 41(15), 2262
(2001): Alliot C+, *Clin Oncol (R Coll Radiol)* 13(3), 236
(2001): Arotcarena R+, *Gastroenterol Clin Biol* 25(2), 206
(1999): Larzilliere I+, *Am J Gastroenterol* 94(11), 3387

(1999): Medioni J+, *Ann Oncol* 10(5), 610
(1998): Tournigand C+, *Eur J Cancer* 34(8), 1297

Asthenia (61%)
(2006): Saif MW, *Expert Opin Drug* 5(5), 687
(2003): Mancuso A+, *Anticancer Res* 23(2C), 1917
(1998): Gerard B+, *Anticancer Drugs* 9(4), 301 (with 5FU)

Chest pain
(2005): Mis L+, *Ann Pharmacother* 39(5), 966

Chills
(2006): Saif MW, *Expert Opin Drug* 5(5), 687
(2005): Mis L+, *Ann Pharmacother* 39(5), 966

Cough (11%)

Death

Depression (2–5%)

Extravasation
(2003): Kretzschmar A+, *J Clin Oncol* 21(21), 4068

Fever (25%)
(2006): Saif MW, *Expert Opin Drug* 5(5), 687
(2004): Gowda A+, *Oncology (Williston Park)* 18(13), 1671
(2003): Thomas RR+, *Cancer* 97(9), 2301
(2000): Ulrich-Pur H+, *Oncology* 59(3), 187

Headache
(2006): Saif MW, *Expert Opin Drug* 5(5), 687

Hepatotoxicity
(2006): Arotcarena R+, *Gastroenterol Clin Biol* 30(11), 1313

Hot flashes (2–5%)

Hypersensitivity
(2007): Edmondson DA+, *Am J Ther* 14(1), 116
(2006): de Vries RS+, *Ann Oncol* 17(11), 1723
(2006): Herrero T+, *J Investig Allergol Clin Immunol* 16(5), 327
(2006): Hewitt MR+, *Clin Colorectal Cancer* 6(2), 114
(2006): Saif MW, *Expert Opin Drug Saf* 5(5), 687 (12%)
(2006): Siu SW+, *Ann Oncol* 17(2), 259
(2005): Bonosky K+, *Clin J Oncol Nurs* 9(3), 325
(2005): Mis L+, *Ann Pharmacother* 39(5), 966
(2005): Ng CV, *Ann Pharmacother* 39(6), 1114 (2 cases)
(2004): Bhargava P+, *Cancer* 100(1), 211
(2004): Gowda A+, *Oncology (Williston Park)* 18(13), 1671 (19%)
(2004): Lim KH+, *Anticancer Drugs* 15(6), 605
(2003): Brandi G+, *Br J Cancer* 89(3), 477 (13%)
(2003): Lenz G+, *Anticancer Drugs* 14(9), 731
(2003): Thomas RR+, *Cancer* 97(9), 2301
(2002): Meyer L+, *J Clin Oncol* 20(4), 1146
(2002): Wilson RH+, *J Clin Oncol* 20(7), 1767 (to cold)

Hypotension
(2005): Mis L+, *Ann Pharmacother* 39(5), 966

Injection-site edema

Injection-site erythema

Injection-site extravasation

Injection-site necrosis

Injection-site pain
(2002): Wilson RH+, *J Clin Oncol* 20(7), 1767

Injection-site reactions (sic)
(2003): Fracasso PM+, *Gynecol Oncol* 90(1), 177 (3 cases)

Myalgia/Myositis/Myopathy/Myotoxicity (2–5%)

Neurotoxicity (48%)
(2006): Arotcarena R+, *Gastroenterol Clin Biol* 30(11), 1313
(2006): Fracasso PM+, *Gynecol Oncol* 103(2), 523
(2006): Kiernan MC+, *Curr Med Chem* 13(24), 2901
(2006): Mitchell PL+, *Clin Colorectal Cancer* 6(2), 146
(2006): Pasetto LM+, *Crit Rev Oncol Hematol* 59(2), 159
(2006): Pietrangeli A+, *Eur Neurol* 56(1), 13
(2006): Shirao K+, *Jpn J Clin Oncol* 36(5), 295
(2006): Susman E, *Lancet Oncol* 7(4), 288
(2005): Cersosimo RJ, *Ann Pharmacother* 39(1), 128
(2004): Leonard GD+, *Anticancer Drugs* 15(7), 733

Pain (14%)

(2003): Mancuso A+, *Anticancer Res* 23(2C), 1917
Paresthesias
  (2006): Pasetto LM+, *Crit Rev Oncol* 59(2), 159
  (2002): Gamelin E+, *Semin Oncol* 29(5), 21
  (2002): Wilson RH+, *J Clin Oncol* 20(7), 1767
  (1998): Gerard B+, *Anticancer Drugs* 9(4), 301 (with 5FU)
  (1990): Extra JM+, *Cancer Chemother Pharmacol* 25(4), 299
Upper respiratory infection (7%)
  (2005): Mis L+, *Ann Pharmacother* 39(5), 966
Vertigo (7%)
  (2006): Saif MW, *Expert Opin Drug* 5(5), 687

OXAPROZIN

Trade names: Daypro (Pfizer); Deflam; Duraprox
Indications: Arthritis
Category: Non-steroidal anti-inflammatory
Half-life: 42–50 hours
Clinically important, potentially hazardous interactions with: methotrexate

Reactions

Skin
Angioedema (<1%)
Diaphoresis (<1%)
Edema (<1%)
Erythema
Erythema multiforme (<1%)
  (1986): Todd PA+, *Drugs* 32, 291
Exanthems
  (1995): Litt JZ, Beachwood, OH (personal case) (observation)
  (1994): Litt JZ, Beachwood, OH (personal case) (observation)
  (1994): Shelley WB+, *Cutis* 54, 72 (eczematous eruption)
    (observation)
  (1983): Hubsher JA+, *Clin Pharmacol Ther* 33, 267
Exfoliative dermatitis (<1%)
Fixed eruption
  (1999): Blumenthal HL, Beachwood, OH (personal case)
    (observation)
Linear IgA dermatosis
  (1999): Abate KL+, *Arch Dermatol* 135, 81 (off-center fold)
Photosensitivity (<1%)
Phototoxicity
  (1995): Shelley WB+, *Cutis* 55, 143 (observation)
  (1986): Todd PA+, *Drugs* 32, 291
Pruritus (1–10%)
  (1994): Shelley WB+, *Cutis* 53, 284 (observation)
Purpura
Rash (sic) (>10%)
  (1983): Kahn SB+, *J Clin Pharmacol* 23, 139
Stevens–Johnson syndrome (<1%)
  (1998): Bell MJ+, *J Rheumatol* 25, 2027
Toxic epidermal necrolysis
  (1999): Carucci JA+, *Int J Dermatol* 38, 233
  (1999): Egan CA+, *J Am Acad Dermatol* 40, 458
  (1998): Paul CD+, *J Burn Care Rehabil* 19, 321 (fatal)
Urticaria (<1%)
  (1997): Hicks A, Houston, TX (from Internet) (observation)
    (Note: Person is not a physician)
Vasculitis
  (1999): Reed BR, Denver, CO (from Internet) (observation)

Mucosal/ENT
Dysgeusia
Stomatitis (<1%)

Tinnitus

Hair
Hair – alopecia

Other
Anaphylactoid reactions/Anaphylaxis (<1%)
Death
Headache
Pseudolymphoma
  (2001): Werth V, *Dermatology Times* 18
Pseudoporphyria
  (2002): LaDuca JR+, *J Cutan Med Surg* 6(4), 320 (3 cases)
  (1999): Al-Khenaizan S+, *J Cutan Med Surg* 3, 162
  (1996): Ingrish G+, *Arch Dermatol* 132, 1519
  (1996): Jaffe PG, Columbia, SC (from Internet) (observation)
Serum sickness (<1%)

OXAZEPAM

Trade names: Adumbran; Apo-Oxazepam; Azutranquil; Durazepam; Murelax; Novoxapam; Oxpam; Praxiten; Serax (Mayne); Serepax; Zapex
Indications: Anxiety, depression
Category: Benzodiazepine
Half-life: 3–6 hours
Clinically important, potentially hazardous interactions with: amprenavir, chlorpheniramine, clarithromycin, efavirenz, esomeprazole, imatinib, nelfinavir

Reactions

Skin
Dermatitis (1–10%)
Diaphoresis (>10%)
Edema
Erythema multiforme
  (1986): McAlpine C, *BMJ* 293, 510
Exanthems
Fixed eruption
  (1996): Krischer J, *Arch Dermatol* 132, 718
Pruritus
Purpura
Rash (sic) (>10%)
Toxic epidermal necrolysis
  (2001): van der Meer JB+, *Clin Exp Dermatol* 26(8), 654
Urticaria

Mucosal/ENT
Sialopenia (>10%)
Sialorrhea (1–10%)
Tongue furry
Xerostomia (>10%)

Other
DRESS syndrome
  (2004): Cordel N+, *Ann Dermatol Venereol* 131(12), 1059
Headache
Paresthesias
Tremor

OXCARBAZEPINE

Synonym: GP 47680
Trade name: Trileptal (Novartis)
Indications: Partial epileptic seizures
Category: Anticonvulsant; Mood stabilizer
Half-life: 1–2.5 hours

Reactions

Skin
Acne
Allergic reactions (sic) (2%)
  (1994): Dam M, *Epilepsia* 35, S23
  (1993): Beran RG, *Epilepsia* 34, 163
Angioedema
Dermatitis
Diaphoresis (3%)
Eczema
Edema (2%)
Erythema multiforme
Exanthems
  (2003): Warnock JK+, *Am J Clin Dermatol* 4(1), 21
  (1999): Ruble R+, *CNS Drugs* 12, 215
Facial rash (sic)
Folliculitis
Genital pruritus
Lupus erythematosus
Photosensitivity
Purpura (2%)
Rash (sic) (<6%)
  (2007): Arif H+, *Neurology* 68(20), 1701
  (2006): Wagner KD+, *Am J Psychiatry* 163(7), 1179
  (1993): Friis ML+, *Acta Neurol Scand* 84, 224 (6%)
Sensitivity
  (1991): Watts D+, *Neurol Neurosurg Psychiatry* 54, 376
Stevens–Johnson syndrome
Toxic epidermal necrolysis
Vitiligo

Mucosal/ENT
Dysgeusia (5%)
Gingival hyperplasia/hypertrophy
Oral ulceration
  (2003): Misra UK+, *Postgrad Med J* 79(938), 703
Stomatitis
Ulcerative stomatitis
Vaginitis (2%)
Xerostomia (3%)

Hair
Hair – alopecia

Eyes
Diplopia
  (2006): Kothare SV+, *Pediatr Neurol* 35(4), 235
  (2006): Sagawa M+, *Leukemia* 20(9), 1566
  (2006): Wagner KD+, *Am J Psychiatry* 163(7), 1179

Other
Asthenia
  (2006): Martinez W+, *Epilepsy Behav* 9(3), 448
  (2006): Sagawa M+, *Leukemia* 20(9), 1566
DRESS syndrome
  (2004): Bosdure E+, *Arch Pediatr* 11(9), 1073
Headache
  (2006): Martinez W+, *Epilepsy Behav* 9(3), 448

Hot flashes (2%)
Hypersensitivity
  (2006): Romano A+, *Curr Pharm Des* 12(26), 3373
  (2006): Seitz CS+, *Ann Allergy Asthma* 97(5), 698
  (2001): *Prescrire Int* 10(56), 170
Inappropriate secretion of antidiuretic hormone (SIADH)
  (2002): Cilli AS+, *J Clin Psychiatry* 63(8), 742
  (1994): Van Amelsvoort T+, *Epilepsia* 35(1), 181
Infections (2%)
Myalgia/Myositis/Myopathy/Myotoxicity
  (2006): Kothare SV+, *Pediatr Neurol* 35(4), 235
Seizures
  (2006): Grosso S+, *Eur J Neurol* 13(10), 1142
Tremor (4–6%)
Vertigo
  (2006): Davids E+, *Prog Neuropsychopharmacol Biol Psychiatry* 30(6), 1033
  (2006): Kothare SV+, *Pediatr Neurol* 35(4), 235
  (2006): Martinez W+, *Epilepsy Behav* 9(3), 448
  (2006): Sagawa M+, *Leukemia* 20(9), 1566
  (2006): Wagner KD+, *Am J Psychiatry* 163(7), 1179

OXILAN

Trade name: Ioxilan (Guerbet)
Indications: Contrast imaging
Category: Diagnostic aid
Half-life: 102 min (women); 137 min (men)

Reactions

Skin
Diaphoresis (<0.5%)
Edema (<0.5%)
Facial edema (<0.5%)
Peripheral edema (<0.5%)
Pruritus (<0.5%)
Rash (sic) (0.8%)
Urticaria (0.8%)

Mucosal/ENT
Dysgeusia (<0.5%)
Dysphagia (<0.5%)

Eyes
Amblyopia (<0.5%)
Conjunctivitis (<0.5%)
Nystagmus (<0.5%)

Other
Asthenia (<0.5%)
Chest pain (<0.5%)
Chills (0.6%)
Fever (1.7%)
Headache (3.6%)
Hypertension (1.1%)
Hypotension (0.9%)
Pain (<0.5%)
Paresthesias (<0.5%)
Vertigo (<0.5%)

OXYBUTYNIN

Trade names: Albert (Oxybutynin); Cystrin; Ditropan (Ortho-McNeil); Dridase; Novitropan; Oxyban; Tropax
Indications: Neurogenic bladder, urinary incontinence
Category: Anticholinergic; Muscarinic antagonist
Half-life: 1–2.3 hours
Clinically important, potentially hazardous interactions with: anticholinergics, arbutamine

Reactions

Skin
Allergic reactions (sic) (<1%)
  (1993): Jonville AP+, *Arch Fr Pediatr* (French) 50, 27
  (1992): Jonville AP+, *Therapie* (French) 47, 389
Erythema multiforme
  (1992): Jonville AP+, *Therapie* (French) 47, 389
Pruritus (18%)
  (2001): Ho C, *Issues Emerg Health Technol* 24, 1 (18%)
Rash (sic) (1–10%)
Urticaria
Xerosis (6%)
  (1998): Arango Toro O+, *Actas Urol Esp* (Spanish) 22, 124 (6%)

Mucosal/ENT
Sialopenia (42%)
  (1998): Arango Toro O+, *Actas Urol Esp* (Spanish) 22, 124 (42%)
  (1995): Loesche WJ+, *J Am Geriatr Soc* 43, 401
Xerostomia (7–94%)
  (2006): Abrams P+, *Int J Urol* 13(6), 692
  (2006): Anderson RU+, *Int Urogynecol J Pelvic Floor Dysfunct* 17(5), 502
  (2006): Corcos J+, *BJU Int* 97(3), 520
  (2006): Davila GW+, *Urol Clin North Am* 33(4), 455
  (2005): Armstrong RB+, *Int Urol Nephrol* 37(2), 247 (28%)
  (2004): Ethans KD+, *J Spinal Cord Med* 27(3), 214
  (2003): Homma Y+, *BJU Int* 92(7), 741 (53.7%)
  (2002): Dmochowski RR+, *J Urol* 168(2), 580 (7%)
  (2002): Youdim K+, *Urology* 59(3), 428
  (2001): Crandall C, *J Womens Health Gend Based Med* 10(8), 735
  (2001): Davila GW+, *J Urol* 166(1), 140 (67–94%)
  (2001): Harvey MA+, *Am J Obstet Gynecol* 185, 56
  (2001): Ho C, *Issues Emerg Health Technol* 24, 1
  (2000): Versi E+, *Obstet Gynecol* 95, 718
  (1999): Gupta SK+, *J Clin Pharmacol* 39(3), 289
  (1998): Arango Toro O+, *Actas Urol Esp* 22(2), 124
  (1997): Hooper P+, *Br J Urol* 80(3), 414
  (1995): Loesche WJ+, *J Am Geriatr Soc* 43(4), 401

Other
Anhidrosis
Application-site pruritus (10%)
  (2002): Dmochowski RR+, *J Urol* 168(2), 580 (10.8%)
Headache
Hot flashes (1–10%)

OXYCODONE

Trade names: Endocodone; OxyContin (Purdue); OxyIR (Purdue); Percocet (Endo); Roxicodone (aaiPharma); Supeudol; Tylox (Ortho-McNeil)
Indications: Pain
Category: Opiate agonist
Half-life: 4.6 hours
Clinically important, potentially hazardous interactions with: cimetidine, clonazepam

Note: Oxycodone is often combined with acetaminophen (Percocet, Roxicet, Tylox) or aspirin (Percodan, Roxiprin)

Reactions

Skin
Baboon syndrome
  (2003): Wolf R+, *Dermatol Online J* 9(3), 2
Diaphoresis
Pruritus
  (2003): *Prescrire Int* 12(65), 83
  (1999): Hale ME+, *Clin J Pain* 15, 179
  (1999): Salzman RT+, *J Pain Symptom Manage* 18, 271
Rash (sic) (<1%)
Urticaria (<1%)

Mucosal/ENT
Xerostomia (1–10%)

Eyes
Visual hallucinations
  (2003): Moore TA, *Am J Geriatr Psychiatry* 11(4), 470 (musical)

Other
Death
  (2005): Wolf BC+, *J Forensic Sci* 50(1), 192 (with alprazolam) (18 cases)
  (2003): Burrows DL+, *J Forensic Sci* 48(3), 683 (with clonazepam)
Headache
Injection-site pain (1–10%)

OXYMORPHONE

Synonym: 14-hydroxy-dihydromorphinone
Trade names: Numorphan (Endo); Opana (Endo)
Indications: Pain (moderate to severe)
Category: Analgesic; Opiate agonist
Half-life: 1.3 ± 7.0 hours
Clinically important, potentially hazardous interactions with: N/A

Reactions

Skin
Allergic reactions (<1%)
Dermatitis (sic) (<1%)
Diaphoresis (1–10%)
Edema (<1%)
Facial edema
Pruritus (8%)
Rash (sic) (<1%)
Urticaria (<1%)

Mucosal/ENT
Xerostomia (1–10%)

Eyes
Diplopia
Miosis
Vision blurred

Other
Abdominal pain (<1%)
Asthenia
Confusion
Depression (<1%)
Fever (14.2%)
Headache (6.8%)
Hypersensitivity (<1%)
Hypertension (<1%)
Hypotension (1–10%)
Injection-site reactions (1–10%)
Somnolence
Vertigo

OXYTETRACYCLINE

Trade names: Aknin; Cotet; Macocyn; Oxacycle; Oxitraklin; Oxy; Rorap; Terramycin (Pfizer); Terramycine; Uri-Tet
Indications: Various infections caused by susceptible organisms
Category: Antibiotic, tetracycline
Half-life: 6–10 hours
Clinically important, potentially hazardous interactions with: amoxicillin, ampicillin, antacids, bacampicillin, calcium, carbenicillin, cloxacillin, digoxin, methotrexate, methoxyflurane, mezlocillin, nafcillin, oxacillin, penicillins, piperacillin, ticarcillin

Reactions

Skin
Angioedema
Dermatitis
Exanthems
Exfoliative dermatitis (<1%)
Fixed eruption
  (1985): Gomez B+, *Allergol Immunopathol Madr* (Spanish) 13, 87
  (1981): Shukla SR, *Dermatologica* 163, 160
Lupus erythematosus
Photosensitivity (1–10%)
  (1987): Santucci B+, *G Ital Dermatol Venereol* (Italian) 122
  (1982): Hawk JL, *Clin Exp Dermatol* 7, 341
Pigmentation
Pruritus (<1%)
Purpura
Pustules
Sensitivity (sic)
  (1997): Rudzki E+, *Contact Dermatitis* 37, 136
Urticaria
Vasculitis

Mucosal/ENT
Oral lesions
Tongue black

Nails
Nails – pigmentation (<1%)

Other
Anaphylactoid reactions/Anaphylaxis (<1%)
Hypersensitivity (<1%)
Paresthesias (<1%)
Porphyria cutanea tarda
  (1982): Hawk JL, *Clin Exp Dermatol* 7, 341
Thrombophlebitis (<1%)

PACLITAXEL

Trade names: Abraxane; Paclimer; Paxene; Taxol (Bristol-Myers Squibb)
Indications: Breast cancer and metastatic carcinoma of the ovary
Category: Taxane
Half-life: 5–17 hours

Reactions

Skin
Acral erythema
  (1996): de Argila D+, *Dermatology* 192, 377
  (1995): Zimmerman GC+, *Arch Dermatol* 131, 202
Allergic reactions (sic) (15%)
  (2002): Cantu MG+, *J Clin Oncol* 20(5), 1232 (15%)
  (2002): Feher O+, *Head Neck* 24(3), 228
  (2001): Ansell SM+, *Cancer* 91(8), 1543
  (2001): Hurwitz CA+, *J Pediatr Hematol Oncol* 23(5), 277
  (2001): Sakai H+, *Cancer Chemother Pharmacol* 48(6), 499 (with cisplatin)
  (1995): Link CJ+, *Invest New Drugs* 13, 261
Angioedema
  (1990): Weiss RB+, *J Clin Oncol* 8, 1263
Desquamation (7%)
  (2003): Formenti SC+, *J Clin Oncol* 21(5), 864 (7%)
Edema (21%)
  (2003): Kupfer I+, *J Am Acad Dermatol* 48(2), 279
Erythema
  (2003): Kuhnt T+, *Strahlenther Onkol* 179(10), 673
  (2003): Kupfer I+, *J Am Acad Dermatol* 48(2), 279
  (2001): Robinson JB+, *Gynecol Oncol* 82(3), 550
  (1995): Berghmans T+, *Support Care Cancer* 3, 203
  (1995): Zimmerman GC+, *Arch Dermatol* 131, 202
Exanthems (<1%)
  (2003): Lin XG+, *Ai Zheng* 22(4), 411 (with cisplatin)
  (1990): Weiss RB+, *J Clin Oncol* 8, 1263
Fixed eruption
  (2000): Baykal C+, *Eur J Gynaecol Oncol* 21, 190
  (1996): Young PC+, *J Am Acad Dermatol* 34, 313 (bullous)
Folliculitis
  (2003): Belda-Iniesta C+, *J Natl Cancer Inst* 95(5), 410
Hand–foot syndrome
  (2006): Blum JL+, *J Clin Oncol* 24(27), 4384 (with capecitabine)
  (2004): Drayton G, Los Angeles, CA (from Internet) (observation)
  (2004): Feng JF+, *Ai Zheng* 23(12), 1704 (with fluorouracil)
  (1999): Villalona-Calero MA+, *J Clin Oncol* 17(6), 1915 (with capecitabine)
  (1994): Zimmerman GC+, *J Natl Cancer Inst* 86, 557
  (1993): Vukelja SJ+, *J Natl Cancer Inst* 85, 1423
Lupus erythematosus
  (2007): Adachi A+, *J Dermatol* 34(7), 473 (2 cases)
Photo-recall (<1%)
  (2004): Kundak I+, *Tumori* 90(2), 256 (with carboplatin)
  (1996): McCarty MJ+, *Med Pediatr Oncol* 27, 185
  (1995): Phillips KA+, *J Clin Oncol* 13, 305
  (1995): Schweitzer VG+, *Cancer* 76, 1069

(1994): Meehan JL+, *J Natl Cancer Inst* 86, 1250
(1994): Shenkier T+, *J Clin Oncol* 12, 439
(1993): Raghavan VT+, *Lancet* 341, 1354

Photosensitivity
(2005): Cohen AD+, *J Dermatolog Treat* 16(1), 19 (with trastuzumab)
(2000): Mermershtain W+, *Ann Oncol* 11(suppl 4), 28 (with trastuzumab) (3 cases)

Pigmentation
(2003): Kupfer I+, *J Am Acad Dermatol* 48(2), 279

Pruritus (<1%)
(2001): Robinson JB+, *Gynecol Oncol* 82(3), 550
(1995): Freilich RJ+, *J Natl Cancer Inst* 87, 933
(1990): Weiss RB+, *J Clin Oncol* 8, 1263

Purpura
Pustules
(1997): Weinberg JM+, *Int J Dermatol* 36, 559

Rash (sic) (12%)
(2006): Yamamoto N+, *Anticancer Res* 26(1B), 777

Recall reaction
(1996): du Bois A+, *Gynecol Oncol* 60, 94
(1994): Meehan JL+, *J Natl Cancer Inst* 86, 1250

Scleroderma
(2003): De Angelis R+, *Clin Rheumatol* 22(1), 49
(2003): Kupfer I+, *J Am Acad Dermatol* 48(2), 279
(2002): Lauchli S+, *Br J Dermatol* 147(3), 619

Stevens–Johnson syndrome
(2004): Hiraki A+, *Anticancer Res* 24(2C), 1135 (1 case)

Toxicity (sic)
(2003): Ellerbroek N+, *Breast J* 9(2), 74

Urticaria
(2005): Feldweg AM+, *Gynecol Oncol* 96(3), 824
(2002): Lehoczky O+, *Orv Hetil* 143(38), 2189
(1990): Weiss RB+, *J Clin Oncol* 8, 1263

Mucosal/ENT

Mucocutaneous reactions (sic)
(1996): Payne JY+, *South Med J* 89, 542

Mucositis (>10%)
(2006): Langer CJ+, *Cancer Invest* 24(2), 164 (with cisplatin)
(2003): Kuhnt T+, *Strahlenther Onkol* 179(10), 673
(2002): Feher O+, *Head Neck* 24(3), 228

Oral lesions (3–8%)
(1990): McGuire WP+, *Ann Intern Med* 111, 273 (3–8%)

Ototoxicity
(2006): Ozguroglu M+, *Int J Gynecol Cancer* 16 Suppl 1, 394 (with carboplatin)

Stomatitis (2–39%)
(2006): Izquierdo MA+, *Eur J Cancer* 42(12), 1789 (with docetaxel)
(2003): Formenti SC+, *J Clin Oncol* 21(5), 864 (2%)
(2001): Miglietta L+, *Oncology* 60(2), 116

Hair

Hair – alopecia (87 – 100%)
(2006): Hatori S+, *Gan To Kagaku Ryoho* 33(9), 1257 (76%)
(2004): Mizuiri H+, *Gan To Kagaku Ryoho* 31(12), 2043
(2003): Emoto T+, *Gan To Kagaku Ryoho* 30(6), 809 (50%)
(2003): Leyland-Jones B+, *J Clin Oncol* 21(21), 3965 (with trastuzumab)
(2002): *Lancet* 360(9332), 505 (with carboplatin)
(2002): Iwamoto S+, *Gan To Kagaku Ryoho* 29(6), 917
(2002): Sehouli J+, *Gynecol Oncol* 85(2), 321 (with carboplatin)
(2001): Rohl J+, *Gynecol Oncol* 81(2), 201
(2001): Sakai H+, *Cancer Chemother Pharmacol* 48(6), 499 (with cisplatin)
(2000): Oettle H+, *Anticancer Drugs* 11(8), 635
(1997): Jiang Z+, *Chung Hua Chung Liu Tsa Chih* (Chinese) 19, 445

(1995): Lemenager M+, *Lancet* 346, 371
(1990): McGuire WP+, *Ann Intern Med* 111, 273 (total) (100%) (between days 14 and 21; reversible)

Hair – alopecia areata
(2003): Motl SE+, *Pharmacotherapy* 23(1), 104 (recurrent) (with caboplatin)

Nails

Nails – changes (sic)
(1998): Luftner D+, *Ann Oncol* 9, 1139

Nails – leukonychia
(2002): Lehoczky O+, *J Obstet Gynaecol* 22(6), 694 (with carboplatin)

Nails – Mees' lines
(1995): Link CJ+, *Invest New Drugs* 13, 261 (2 cases)

Nails – paronychia
(2003): Albares MP+, *Dermatol Online J* 9(3), 16

Nails – pigmentation (2%)
(1998): Auvinet M+, *Rev Med Interne* (French) 19, 353

Nails – subungual hyperkeratosis
(2006): Tejera A+, *Actas Dermosifiliogr* 97(8), 536 (with capecitabine)

Nails – thickening
(1995): Link CJ+, *Invest New Drugs* 13, 261 (2 cases)

Other

Abdominal pain
(2006): Armstrong DK+, *Gynecol Oncol* 103(2), 391

Anaphylactoid reactions/Anaphylaxis
(1999): Smith ME, *Oncol Nurs Forum* 26, 516
(1997): Ciesielski-Carlucci C+, *Am J Clin Oncol* 20(4), 373 (with cisplatin)
(1995): Rowinsky EK+, *N Engl J* 332(15), 1004

Asthenia
(2006): Green MR+, *Ann Oncol* 17(8), 1263
(2006): Izquierdo MA+, *Eur J Cancer* 42(12), 1789 (with docetaxel)
(2006): Koizumi W+, *Anticancer Res* 26(5B), 3797
(2006): Markman M+, *Gynecol Oncol* 101(3), 436 (8%)
(2003): Formenti SC+, *J Clin Oncol* 21(5), 864 (10%)
(2003): Leyland-Jones B+, *J Clin Oncol* 21(21), 3965 (with trastuzumab)
(2003): Takahashi H+, *Gan To Kagaku Ryoho* 30(5), 653

Cardiotoxicity
(2006): Ruiz-Casado A+, *Clin Transl Oncol* 8(1), 60
(2006): Salvatorelli E+, *J Pharmacol Exp Ther* 318(1), 424

Congestive heart failure
(2004): Libersa C+, *Therapie* 59(1), 127

Death
(2006): Davies AM+, *J Clin Oncol* 24(33), 5242
(2006): Jang JS+, *J Invasive Cardiol* 18(5), 205 (stent)
(2006): Ostoros G+, *Int J Gynecol Cancer* 16 Suppl 1, 391
(2006): Tomasello L+, *Anticancer Res* 26(6C), 4775
(2004): Kloover JS+, *Br J Cancer* 90(2), 304
(2001): Fidias P+, *Clin Cancer Res* 7(12), 3942
(2001): Hurwitz CA+, *J Pediatr Hematol Oncol* 23(5), 277

Hypersensitivity (2–41%)
(2005): Feldweg AM+, *Gynecol Oncol* 96(3), 824
(2004): Kloover JS+, *Br J Cancer* 90(2), 304
(2003): Formenti SC+, *J Clin Oncol* 21(5), 864 (2%)
(2002): Denman JP+, *J Clin Oncol* 20(11), 2760
(2002): Kobierski J+, *Ginekol Pol* 73(11), 1015
(2002): Kwon JS+, *Gynecol Oncol* 84(3), 420
(2002): Lehoczky O+, *Orv Hetil* 143(38), 2189
(2002): Myers JS, *Clin J Oncol Nurs* 6(3), 177
(2001): Kintzel PE, *Ann Pharmacother* 35(9), 1114
(2001): Koppler H+, *Onkologie* 24(3), 283
(2001): Robinson JB+, *Gynecol Oncol* 82(3), 550 (with carboplatin)
(2001): Szebeni J+, *Int Immunopharmacol* 1(4), 721

(2001): Yamada Y+, *Ann Oncol* 12(8), 1133 (15%)
(1998): Borovik R+, *Harefuah* (Hebrew) 134, 605
(1998): Lokich J+, *Ann Oncol* 9, 573
(1998): Tsavaris NB+, *Cancer Chemother Pharmacol* 42, 509
(1995): Del Priore G+, *Gynecol Oncol* 56, 316
(1994): Uziely B+, *Ann Oncol* 5, 474
(1993): Peereboom DM+, *J Clin Oncol* 11, 885
Inappropriate secretion of antidiuretic hormone (SIADH)
(2005): Yokoyama Y+, *Eur J Gynaecol Oncol* 26(5), 531
Infections (sic) (3–22%)
(2006): Yamamoto N+, *Anticancer Res* 26(1B), 777
(2003): Formenti SC+, *J Clin Oncol* 21(5), 864 (22%)
(2003): Kuhnt T+, *Strahlenther Onkol* 179(10), 673
(2002): Souglakos J+, *Cancer* 95(6), 1326 (3%)
(2001): Fidias P+, *Clin Cancer Res* 7(12), 3942 (8.8%)
Injection-site cellulitis (>10%)
Injection-site extravasation (>10%)
(2002): Barutca S+, *Support Care Cancer* 10(7), 563
(1997): Herrington JD+, *Pharmacotherapy* 17, 163
(1995): Berghmans T+, *Support Care Cancer* 3, 203
(1995): Raymond E+, *Rev Med Interne* (French) 16, 141
Injection-site pain (>10%)
Injection-site reactions (sic) (13%)
(2003): Leyland-Jones B+, *J Clin Oncol* 21(21), 3965 (with
trastuzumab)
Myalgia/Myositis/Myopathy/Myotoxicity (19–60%)
(2006): Izquierdo MA+, *Eur J Cancer* 42(12), 1789 (with
docetaxel)
(2005): Ansari TN+, *J Coll Physicians Surg Pak* 15(4), 200
(2003): Garrison JA+, *Oncology* (Huntingt) 17(2), 271
(2003): Leyland-Jones B+, *J Clin Oncol* 21(21), 3965 (with
trastuzumab)
(2002): Cantu MG+, *J Clin Oncol* 20(5), 1232 (19%)
(2002): Hasegawa K+, *Gan To Kagaku Ryoho* 29(4), 569
(2001): Ishikawa H+, *Int J Clin Oncol* 6(3), 128
(1999): Markman M+, *Gynecol Oncol* 72, 100
(1999): Villalona-Calero MA+, *J Clin Oncol* 17(6), 1915 (with
capecitabine)
(1998): Savarese D+, *J Clin Oncol* 16, 3918
(1997): Jiang Z+, *Chung Hua Chung Liu Tsa Chih* (Chinese)
19, 445
Nephrotoxicity
(2006): Ozguroglu M+, *Int J Gynecol Cancer* 16 Suppl 1, 394
(with carboplatin)
Neurotoxicity
(2006): Bamias A+, *BMC Cancer* 6, 228 (with carboplatin)
(2006): Bell J+, *Gynecol Oncol* 102(3), 432 (with carboplatin)
(2006): Green MR+, *Ann Oncol* 17(8), 1263
(2006): Izquierdo MA+, *Eur J Cancer* 42(12), 1789 (with
docetaxel)
(2006): Koizumi W+, *Anticancer Res* 26(5B), 3797
(2006): Lachkar S+, *Rev Mal Respir* 23(1 Pt 1), 73
(2006): Le T+, *Gynecol Oncol* 102(1), 49 (15%)
(2006): Markman M+, *Gynecol Oncol* 101(3), 436 (21%)
(2006): Melli G+, *Neurobiol Dis* 24(3), 525
(2006): Yamamoto N+, *Anticancer Res* 26(1B), 777
(2005): Kahl BS+, *Cancer Invest* 23(1), 13
Pain
(2006): Blum JL+, *J Clin Oncol* 24(27), 4384 (with capecitabine)
(2003): Emoto T+, *Gan To Kagaku Ryoho* 30(6), 809
(2003): Formenti SC+, *J Clin Oncol* 21(5), 864 (17%)
Paresthesias (>10%)
(2003): Leyland-Jones B+, *J Clin Oncol* 21(21), 3965 (with
trastuzumab)
Seizures
(2004): Cronk M+, *J Natl Cancer Inst* 96(6), 487
Thrombosis
(2006): Feres F+, *Catheter Cardiovasc Interv* 68(1), 83 (stent)
Tumor lysis syndrome

(2006): Yahata T+, *Gynecol Oncol* 103(2), 752
Vertigo
(2003): Takahashi H+, *Gan To Kagaku Ryoho* 30(5), 653

PALIFERMIN

Trade name: Kepivance (Amgen)
Indications: Severe oral mucositis in cancer patients
Category: Keratinocyte growth factor
Half-life: 4.5 hours
**Clinically important, potentially hazardous interactions
with:** heparin

Reactions

Skin
Edema
(2006): Blazar BR+, *Blood* 108(9), 3216
Erythema (32%)
(2004): Spielberger R+, *N Engl J Med* 351(25), 2590
Pruritus (35%)
(2004): Spielberger R+, *N Engl J Med* 351(25), 2590
Rash (sic) (62%)
(2006): Blazar BR+, *Blood* 108(9), 3216
(2006): Keefe D+, *Support Care Cancer* 14(6), 580
(2004): Spielberger R+, *N Engl J Med* 351(25), 2590
Toxicity (sic)
(2005): Siddiqui MA+, *Drugs* 65(15), 2139

Mucosal/ENT
Dysgeusia (16%)
(2005): Siddiqui MA+, *Drugs* 65(15), 2139
(2004): Spielberger R+, *N Engl J Med* 351(25), 2590
Gingival hyperplasia/hypertrophy
(2001): Das SJ+, *J Periodontol* 72(6), 745
Oral mucositis
(2006): Keefe D+, *Support Care Cancer* 14(6), 580
Tongue edema (17%)
(2004): Spielberger R+, *N Engl J Med* 351(25), 2590
Tongue pigmentation (17%)

Other
Fever (39%)
Hypertension (~12%)
Infections
(2006): Blazar BR+, *Blood* 108(9), 3216
Pain (16%)
(2006): Blazar BR+, *Blood* 108(9), 3216
Paresthesias (12%)

PALIPERIDONE

Trade name: Invega (Janssen)
Indications: Schizophrenia
Half-life: ~23 hours
**Clinically important, potentially hazardous interactions
with:** N/A

Note: Paliperidone is the active metabolite of risperidone

Reactions

Skin
Angioedema (tongue)

Edema

Mucosal/ENT
Xerostomia

Eyes
Vision blurred

Other
Abdominal pain
Anaphylactoid reactions/Anaphylaxis
Anxiety
Confusion
Cough
Fever
Headache (~5%)
Hypertension
Somnolence
Tremor

PALIVIZUMAB

Trade name: Synagis (MedImmune)
Indications: Prophylaxis of serious lower respiratory tract disease caused by RSV in pediatric patients
Category: Immunomodulator; Monoclonal antibody
Half-life: 18 days

Reactions

Skin
Eczema (>1%)
Erythema
Fungal dermatitis (>1%)
Rash (sic) (25.6%)
Seborrhea (>1%)

Mucosal/ENT
Oral candidiasis (>1%)

Other
Anaphylactoid reactions/Anaphylaxis
  (2002): Medscape Medical News
Fever
  (2004): Fenton C+, *Paediatr Drugs* 6(3), 177
Infections
Injection-site bruising (1–3%)
  (1999): Scott LJ+, *Drugs* 58, 305 (1–3%)
Injection-site edema (1–3%)
  (1999): Scott LJ+, *Drugs* 58, 305 (1–3%)
Injection-site erythema (1–3%)
  (1999): Scott LJ+, *Drugs* 58, 305 (1–3%)
  (1998): *Pediatrics* 102, 531
Injection-site induration (1–3%)
  (1999): Scott LJ+, *Drugs* 58, 305 (1–3%)
Injection-site pain (1–8.5%)
  (1999): Scott LJ+, *Drugs* 58, 305 (1–3%)
Injection-site reactions (sic)
  (2004): Fenton C+, *Paediatr Drugs* 6(3), 177
  (1999): Sandritter T, *J Pediatr Health Care* 13, 191

PALONOSETRON

Trade names: Aloxi (MGI); Onicit
Indications: Antiemetic (for cancer chemotherapy)
Category: 5-HT3 antagonist; Serotonin type 3 receptor antagonist
Half-life: 40 hours

Reactions

Skin
Dermatitis (<1%)
Pruritus (8–22%)
Rash (sic) (6%)

Mucosal/ENT
Xerostomia (<1%)

Other
Abdominal pain
  (2005): Tonini G+, *Expert Opin Drug Metab Toxicol* 1(1), 143 (%)
Asthenia
  (2005): Tonini G+, *Expert Opin Drug Metab Toxicol* 1(1), 143 (%)
Fever
  (2006): Mechanick JI+, *J Spinal Cord Med* 29(4), 406
  (2006): Sauter M+, *Am J Kidney Dis* 47(6), 1075
Headache (9%)
  (2005): Tonini G+, *Expert Opin Drug Metab Toxicol* 1(1), 143 (9%)
  (2004): Stoltz R+, *J Clin Pharmacol* 44(5), 520
Hot flashes (<15)
Nephrotoxicity
  (2006): Bergner R+, *Onkologie* 29(11), 534
  (2006): Perez EA+, *Oncology (Williston Park)* 20(9), 1029
  (2006): Tanvetyanon T+, *Ann Oncol* 17(6), 897
Paresthesias
Vertigo (1%)
  (2005): Tonini G+, *Expert Opin Drug Metab Toxicol* 1(1), 143 (1%)

PAMIDRONATE

Trade name: Aredia (Novartis)
Indications: Hypercalcemia, Paget's disease
Category: Bisphosphonate
Half-life: 1.6 hours

Reactions

Skin
Angioedema (<1%)
Edema (1%)
Exanthems (1%)
  (1984): Mantalen CA+, *BMJ* 288, 828 (1.2%)
Rash (sic) (<1%)

Mucosal/ENT
Dysgeusia (<1%)
Stomatitis (1%)
Tinnitus
  (1995): Reid IR+, *Calcif Tissue Int* 56(6), 584

Eyes
Conjunctivitis
  (2003): Frauenfelder FW+, *Am J Opthalmol* 135, 219
  (2003): Frauenfelder FW+, *N Engl J Med* 348, 1187

(1994): Macarol V+, *Am J Ophthalmol* 118(2), 220
Ocular stinging
(2003): Frauenfelder FW+, *N Engl J Med* 348, 1187
Scleritis
(2006): Benderson D+, *Clin Lymphoma Myeloma* 7(2), 145
Uveitis
(2002): Margarita, C, *Medication-Induced Uveitis in Diagnosis and Treatment of Uveitis* Saunders. p. 859
(2001): Fraunfelder FT+, *Calcium Regulating Agents in Drug-Induced Ocular Side Effects* Butterworth Heinemann. p. 482
(1996): Stewart GO+, *Aust N Z J Med* 26(3), 414
(1995): O'Donnell NP+, *Br J Clin Pract* 49(5), 272
(1994): Ghose K+, *Aust N Z J Med* 24(3), 320
(1994): Macarol V+, *Am J Ophthalmol* 118(2), 220 (7 cases)
(1993): Siris ES, *Lancet* 341(8842), 436
Visual disturbances
(2004): Coleman CI+, *Pharmacotherapy* 24(6), 799 (rare)

Other
Asthenia
(2003): Rosen LS+, *Cancer* 98(8), 1735
Candidiasis
Fever
(2005): Akerkar SM+, *Indian J Med Sci* 59(4), 165
(1989): Gallacher SJ+, *Lancet* 2(8653), 42
Headache
Hypersensitivity (<1%)
Injection-site reactions (sic) (4%)
(2001): Body JJ, *Semin Oncol* 28(4 Suppl 11), 49
Myalgia/Myositis/Myopathy/Myotoxicity (1%)
(2005): Akerkar SM+, *Indian J Med Sci* 59(4), 165
Nephrotoxicity
(2006): Bergner R+, *Onkologie* 29(11), 534
(2003): Banerjee D+, *Am J Kidney Dis* 41(5), E18
(2003): Perazella MA, *Am J Med Sci* 325(6), 349
(2002): Lockridge L+, *Am J Kidney Dis* 40(1), E2
(2001): Janssen van Doorn K+, *Nephron* 89(4), 467
(2001): Markowitz GS+, *J Am Soc Nephrol* 12(6), 1164

PANCRELIPASE

Trade names: Cotazym (Organon); Creon (Solvay); Ilozyme; Ku-Zyme; Lipram; Pancoate; Pancrease (Ortho-McNeil); Panokase (Breckenridge); Protilase; Ultrase (Axcan); Viokase (Axcan); Zymase
Indications: Pancreatic insufficiency, Steatorrhea
Category: Enzyme
Half-life: N/A
Clinically important, potentially hazardous interactions with: None

Reactions

Skin
Dermatitis
Peripheral edema
Rash (sic) (rare)

Mucosal/ENT
Oral mucosal irritation

Other
Abdominal pain

PANCURONIUM

Trade names: Alpax; Bromurex; Curon-B; Panconium; Panslan
Indications: Anesthesia adjunct, neuromuscular blockade, muscle relaxant
Category: Non-depolarizing neuromuscular blocker
Half-life: 89–161 minutes
Clinically important, potentially hazardous interactions with: aminoglycosides, cortisone, cyclopropane, enflurane, gentamicin, halothane, hydrocortisone, isoflurane, kanamycin, methoxyflurane, neomycin, piperacillin, prednisolone, prednisone, streptomycin, tobramycin

Reactions

Skin
Burning
Edema
Erythema
(1989): Patriarca G+, *Br J Anaesth* 62(2), 210
Pruritus
Rash (sic)

Mucosal/ENT
Sialorrhea

Other
Anaphylactoid reactions/Anaphylaxis
(1998): Sanchez-Guerrero IM+, *Eur J Anaesthesiol* 15(5), 613
(1990): Moneret-Vautrin DA+, *Br J Anaesth* 64(6), 743
(1989): Patriarca G+, *Br J Anaesth* 62(2), 210
(1986): Bonnet MC+, *Cah Anesthesiol* 34(3), 253
(1985): Conil C+, *Ann Fr Anesth Reanim* 4(2), 241
(1985): Galletly DC+, *Anaesthesia* 40(4), 329
(1985): Moneret-Vautrin DA+, *Anesth Analg* 64(9), 944
(1984): Mishima S+, *Anesth Analg* 63(9), 865
(1984): Pappagallo S+, *Minerva Anestesiol* 50(9), 481
Hypersensitivity
(1983): Nagao H+, *Br J Anaesth* 55(3), 253
Myalgia/Myositis/Myopathy/Myotoxicity
(1994): Giostra E+, *Chest* 106(1), 210
(1993): De Smet, *Rev Neurol* 149(10), 573
(1993): Miyoshi T+, *Rinsho Shinkeigaku* 33(6), 620
Rhabdomyolysis
(1993): Clavelou P+, *Ann Fr Anesth Reanim* 12(3), 326

PANITUMUMAB

Synonym: ABX-EGF
Trade name: Vectibix (Amgen)
Indications: Metastatic colorectal carcinoma (to reduce progression of)
Category: Monoclonal antibody
Half-life: ~7.5 days
Clinically important, potentially hazardous interactions with: N/A

Reactions

Skin
Acne (57%)
(2005): Segaert S+, *Ann Oncol* 16(9), 1425
(2005): Segaert S+, *J Dtsch Dermatol Ges* 3(8), 599
Eczema
(2005): Segaert S+, *Ann Oncol* 16(9), 1425

(2005): Segaert S+, *J Dtsch Dermatol* 3(8), 599
Erythema (65%)
Exfoliative dermatitis (25%)
Fissures (20%)
  (2005): Segaert S+, *Ann Oncol* 16(9), 1425
Peripheral edema (12%)
Photosensitivity
Pigmentation
  (2005): Segaert S+, *Ann Oncol* 16(9), 1425
Pruritus (57%)
Rash (sic) (22%)
  (2006): Gibson TB+, *Clin Colorectal Cancer* 6(1), 29
  (2006): Saif MW+, *Clin Colorectal Cancer* 6(2), 118 (90%)
Telangiectasia
  (2005): Segaert S+, *Ann Oncol* 16(9), 1425
Xerosis (10%)
  (2005): Segaert S+, *Ann Oncol* 16(9), 1425
  (2005): Segaert S+, *J Dtsch Dermatol* 3(8), 599

Mucosal/ENT
Oral mucositis (6%)
Stomatitis (7%)

Hair
Hair – changes (sic)
  (2005): Segaert S+, *Ann Oncol* 16(9), 1425
  (2005): Segaert S+, *J Dtsch Dermatol* 3(8), 599

Nails
Nails – changes
  (2005): Segaert S+, *J Dtsch Dermatol* 3(8), 599
Nails – paronychia (25%)
  (2005): Segaert S+, *Ann Oncol* 16(9), 1425
Nails – pyogenic granulomas
  (2005): Segaert S+, *Ann Oncol* 16(9), 1425

Eyes
Conjunctivitis (4%)
Eyelashes – hypertrichosis
Eyelid irritation (1%)
Lacrimation (2%)
Ocular toxicity
Toxicity (sic) (9%)

Other
Abdominal pain (25%)
Asthenia (26%)
Cough (14%)
Injection-site reactions (4%)

PANTOPRAZOLE

Trade name: Protonix (Wyeth)
Indications: Esophagitis associated with Gastroesophageal Reflux Disease (GERD)
Category: Proton pump inhibitor
Half-life: 1 hour
Clinically important, potentially hazardous interactions with: allopurinol, **eucalyptus**

Reactions

Skin
Abscess (<1%)
Acne (<1%)
Allergic reactions (sic) (<1%)

Angioedema (<1%)
Dermatitis (<1%)
Diaphoresis (<1%)
  (2000): Natsch S+, *Ann Pharmacother* 34, 474
Eczema (<1%)
Edema (<1%)
Erythema multiforme (<1%)
Exanthems (<1%)
Facial edema (<1%)
  (2002): Gonzalez P+, *Allergol Immunopathol* (Madr) 30(6), 342
Fungal dermatitis (<1%)
Herpes simplex (<1%)
Herpes zoster (<1%)
Lichenoid eruption (<1%)
  (2000): Bong JL+, *BMJ* 320, 283
Lupus erythematosus (discoid)
  (2001): Correia O+, *Clin Exp Dermatol* 26(5), 455
Peripheral edema
  (2001): Brunner G+, *Dig Dis Sci* 46(5), 993
  (1994): Brunner G, *Aliment Pharmacol Ther* 8, 59
Photosensitivity
  (2001): Correia O+, *Clin Exp Dermatol* 26(5), 455
Phototoxicity
  (2001): Correia O+, *Clin Exp Dermatol* 26, 455
Pruritus (<1%)
  (2000): Natsch S+, *Ann Pharmacother* 34, 474
Rash (sic) (<1%)
  (2000): Avner DL, *Clin Ther* 22(10), 1169
  (1992): Muller P+, *Z Gastroenterol* 30, 771
Stevens–Johnson syndrome (<1%)
Toxic epidermal necrolysis (<1%)
Ulcerations (<1%)
Urticaria (<1%)
  (2002): Gonzalez P+, *Allergol Immunopathol* (Madr) 30(6), 342
  (2000): Natsch S+, *Ann Pharmacother* 34, 474
Vasculitis
  (2006): Jacobs-Kosmin D+, *J Rheumatol* 33(3), 629
Xerosis (<1%)

Mucosal/ENT
Aphthous stomatitis (<1%)
Balanitis (<1%)
Dysgeusia (<1%)
Gingivitis (<1%)
Glossitis (<1%)
Oral candidiasis (<1%)
Rhinitis
  (2006): Miner PB Jr+, *Clin Ther* 28(5), 725 (2 cases)
Sialorrhea (<1%)
Stomatitis (<1%)
Tongue edema
  (2000): Natsch S+, *Ann Pharmacother* 34, 474
Tongue pigmentation (<1%)
Vaginitis (<1%)
Xerostomia (<1%)

Hair
Hair – alopecia (<1%)

Other
Anaphylactoid reactions/Anaphylaxis (<1%)
  (2004): Kollmeier AP+, *J Allergy Clin Immunol* 114(4), 975
  (2002): Fardet L+, *Am J Gastroenterol* 97(6), 1578
  (2002): Gonzalez P+, *Allergol Immunopathol* (Madr) 30(6), 342
  (2002): Kaatz M+, *Allergy* 57(2), 184
  (2000): Natsch S+, *Ann Pharmacother* 3(4), 474
Asthenia

(2004): Ra A+, *Ann Pharmacother* 38(1), 41
Fever
  (2004): Ra A+, *Ann Pharmacother* 38(1), 41
Headache
  (2006): Miner PB+, *Clin Ther* 28(5), 725 (1 case)
Hypersensitivity
  (2004): Ra A+, *Ann Pharmacother* 38(1), 41
Infections (1–10%)
Myalgia/Myositis/Myopathy/Myotoxicity (<1%)
Paresthesias (<1%)
Thrombophlebitis (<1%)
Tremor (<1%)

PANTOTHENIC ACID

Synonym: Vitamin B$_5$
Trade name: Dexol
Indications: Vitamin B complex malabsorption
Category: Vitamin
Half-life: N/A

Reactions

Skin
Dermatitis
  (1998): Stables GI+, *Contact Dermatitis* 38(4), 236
  (1988): Jeanmougin M+, *Contact Dermatitis* 18(4), 240
  (1987): Keilig W, *Derm Beruf Umwelt* 35(6), 206
  (1985): Gollhausen R+, *Contact Dermatitis* 13(1), 38
  (1904): van Ketel WG, *Contact Dermatitis* 10(1), 48
  (1981): Ippen H, *Derm Beruf Umwelt* 29(2), 45
Exanthems
Pruritus
Urticaria
  (2000): Schalock PC+, *Contact Dermatitis* 43(4), 223

Other
Chest pain
  (2001): Debourdeau PM+, *Ann Pharmacother* 35(4), 424 (with vitamin H)

PAPAVERINE

Trade names: Angioverin; Genabid; Optenyl; Pameion; Papaverine 60; Papaverini; Pavabid; Pavagen; Pavased; Pavatine
Indications: Peripheral and cerebral ischemia
Category: Opium alkaloid; Vasodilator, peripheral
Half-life: 0.5–2 hours
Clinically important, potentially hazardous interactions with: reboxetine

Reactions

Skin
Diaphoresis (<1%)
Exanthems
Fixed eruption
  (1994): Kirby KA+, *Urology* 43, 886
Pruritus (<1%)
Pyogenic granuloma
  (1990): Summers JL, *J Urol* 143, 1227
Rash (sic)
Toxic epidermal necrolysis

(1989): Simochkina ZA+, *Vrach Delo* (Russian) October, 91
Urticaria

Mucosal/ENT
Xerostomia (<1%)

Other
Headache
Hypotension
  (2006): Madhusudan Reddy KR+, *J Neurosurg Anesthesiol* 18(3), 221
Injection-site thrombophlebitis (<1%)

PARA-AMINOSALICYLIC ACID (PAS)

(See AMINOSALICYLATE SODIUM)

PARAMETHADIONE

Trade name: Paradione
Indications: Absence (petit-mal) seizures
Category: Antiepileptic, oxazolidinedione
Half-life: 12–24 hours

Reactions

Skin
Acne
Erythema multiforme
Exanthems
Exfoliative dermatitis
Lupus erythematosus
Pruritus

Mucosal/ENT
Gingivitis
Oral mucosal eruption

Hair
Hair – alopecia

Other
Paresthesias

PARICALCITOL

Trade name: Zemplar (Abbott)
Indications: Secondary hyperparathyroidism associated with renal failure
Category: Vitamin D receptor agonist
Half-life: N/A
Clinically important, potentially hazardous interactions with: digitalis (with overdose of paricalcitol)

Reactions

Skin
Edema
  (1999): Goldenberg MM, *Clin Ther* 21(3), 432
Peripheral edema (7%)

Mucosal/ENT

Dysgeusia
(2001): Lindberg J+, *Clin Nephrol* 56(4), 315
Xerostomia (3%)
(1999): Goldenberg MM, *Clin Ther* 21(3), 432

Other

Chills (5%)
(1999): Goldenberg MM, *Clin Ther* 21(3), 432
Fever
(1999): Goldenberg MM, *Clin Ther* 21(3), 432
Vertigo
(1999): Goldenberg MM, *Clin Ther* 21(3), 432

PAROMOMYCIN

Trade names: Gabbroral; Gabroral; Humagel; Humatin (Monarch) (Sanofi-Aventis); Sinosid
Indications: Intestinal amebiasis
Category: Antibiotic, aminoglycoside
Half-life: N/A
Clinically important, potentially hazardous interactions with: methotrexate, succinylcholine

Reactions

Skin

Exanthems (<1%)
Pruritus (<1%)

Mucosal/ENT

Ototoxicity
(1992): Scott JA+, *Trans R Soc Trop Med Hyg* 86(6), 617

Other

Abdominal pain
(1995): Tan WW+, *Ann Pharmacother* 29(1), 22

PAROXETINE

Trade names: Aropax 20; Paxil (GSK)
Indications: Depression
Category: Antidepressant; Selective serotonin reuptake inhibitor
Half-life: 21 hours
Clinically important, potentially hazardous interactions with: amitriptyline, amphetamines, aprepitant, astemizole, clarithromycin, dexibuprofen, dextroamphetamine, diethylpropion, digitalis, digoxin, duloxetine, erythromycin, isocarboxazid, linezolid, MAO inhibitors, mazindol, methamphetamine, molindone, phendimetrazine, phenelzine, phentermine, phenylpropanolamine, pseudoephedrine, risperidone, selegiline, sibutramine, **St John's wort**, sumatriptan, sympathomimetics, tranylcypromine, trazodone, troleandomycin

Reactions

Skin

Acne (<1%)
Allergic reactions (sic) (<1%)
(1998): Beauquier B+, *Encephale* (French) 24, 62
Angioedema (<1%)
(1996): Mithani H+, *J Clin Psychiatry* 57, 486
Dermatitis (<1%)

Diaphoresis (11.2%)
(2005): Marcy TR+, *Ann Pharmacother* 39(4), 748
(2004): Velez LI+, *Ann Pharmacother* 38(2), 269 (with alcohol)
(2003): Denys D+, *J Clin Psychopharmacol* 23(6), 568
(2003): Wade A+, *Int Clin Psychopharmacol* 18(3), 133
(1998): Stein MB+, *JAMA* 280, 708
(1997): Kiev A+, *J Clin Psychiatry* 58(4), 146
(1997): Litt JZ, Beachwood, OH (personal case) (observation)
(1992): Boyer WF+, *J Clin Psychiatry* 53, 61
(1991): Dechant KL+, *Drugs* 41, 225
(1990): Sindrup SH+, *Pain* 42, 135
(1985): Laursen AL+, *Acta Psychiatr Scand* 71, 249
Eczema
Edema (<1%)
Erythema multiforme
(2000): Altman, EA, New York, NY (from Internet) (observation)
Erythema nodosum (<1%)
Exanthems (<1%)
(2006): Mera MT+, *Allergol Immunopathol (Madr)* 34(3), 125
(2002): Sannicandro TJ+, *Pharmacotherapy* 22(4), 516
Facial edema (<1%)
Furunculosis (<1%)
Melanoma (<1%)
Peripheral edema (<1%)
Photosensitivity (<1%)
(2002): Vilaplana J+, *Contact Dermatitis* 47(2), 118
(2001): Richard MA+, *Ann Dermatol Venereol* 128, 759
Pigmentation (<1%)
Pruritus (<1%)
(2002): Sannicandro TJ+, *Pharmacotherapy* 22(4), 516
(1991): Dechant KL+, *Drugs* 41, 225
Psoriasis
(2002): Osborne SF+, *Am J Psychiatry* 159(12), 2113
Purpura (<1%)
Rash (sic) (1.7%)
Toxic epidermal necrolysis
(2000): Nelson RA+, Nashville, TN (Poster exhibit #16 from Academy 2000)
Urticaria (<1%)
Vasculitis
(2006): Welsh JP+, *J Drugs Dermatol* 5(10), 1012 (urticarial)
(2001): Margolese HC+, *Am J Psychiatry* 158(3), 497
Xerosis (<1%)

Mucosal/ENT

Ageusia (<1%)
(1997): Litt JZ, Beachwood, OH (personal case) (observation)
Anosmia
(1997): Litt JZ, Beachwood, OH (personal case) (observation)
Aphthous stomatitis (<1%)
Dysgeusia (2.4%)
(1998): Litt JZ, Beachwood, OH (personal case) (observation)
Gingivitis (<1%)
Glossitis (<1%)
Oral ulceration
Sialorrhea (<1%)
Stomatitis (<1%)
Tinnitus
Tongue edema (<1%)
(1996): Mithani H+, *J Clin Psychiatry* 57, 486
Vaginitis
Vulvovaginal candidiasis (<1%)
Xerostomia (18.1%)
(2005): *Med Lett Drugs Ther* 47(1204), 23
(1998): Stein MB+, *JAMA* 280, 708
(1997): Kiev A+, *J Clin Psychiatry* 58(4), 146 (27%)
(1992): Boyer WF+, *J Clin Psychiatry* 53, 61

(1992): Claghorn JL, *J Clin Psychiatry* 53, 33
(1992): Fabre LF, *J Clin Psychiatry* 53, 40
(1992): Shrivastava RK+, *J Clin Psychiatry* 53, 48
(1992): Smith WT+, *J Clin Psychiatry* 53, 36
(1991): Dechant KL+, *Drugs* 1, 225
(1991): Dunbar GC+, *Br J Psychiatry* 159, 394
(1990): Cohn JB+, *Psychopharmacol Bull* 26, 185
(1990): Sindrup SH+, *Pain* 42, 135

Hair

Hair – alopecia (<1%)
(2000): Umansky L+, *Harefuah* (Hebrew) 138, 547 ('massive')

Eyes

Glaucoma
(2004): Levy J+, *Can J Ophthalmol* 39(7), 780
Vision impaired
(2007): Terao T+, *Prog Neuropsychopharmacol Biol Psychiatry* 31(1), 295

Other

Agitation
(2007): Terao T+, *Prog Neuropsychopharmacol Biol Psychiatry* 31(1), 295
Asthenia
(1997): Kiev A+, *J Clin Psychiatry* 58(4), 146
Candidiasis
Chills
(2007): Terao T+, *Prog Neuropsychopharmacol Biol Psychiatry* 31(1), 295
(2004): Jagestedt M+, *Lakartidningen* 101(18), 1618 (with buspirone)
Cough
(2000): Hamel H+, *Presse Med* (French) 29, 1045
Death
(2006): Gambassi G+, *Aging Clin Exp Res* 18(3), 266 (with clozapine)
(2004): Farah RE+, *Ann Pharmacother* 38(9), 1435 (with clozapine)
Depression
(2004): Jick H+, *JAMA* 292(3), 338
Fever
(2004): Jagestedt M+, *Lakartidningen* 101(18), 1618 (with buspirone)
Headache
(2007): Terao T+, *Prog Neuropsychopharmacol Biol Psychiatry* 31(1), 295
(2004): Detke MJ+, *Eur Neuropsychopharmacol* 14(6), 457
(2003): Denys D+, *J Clin Psychopharmacol* 23(6), 568
(2003): Wade A+, *Int Clin Psychopharmacol* 18(3), 133
(1997): Kiev A+, *J Clin Psychiatry* 58(4), 146
Hypertension
(2005): Hendrix Y+, *Ned Tijdschr Geneeskd* 149(16), 888 (with sumatriptan)
Inappropriate secretion of antidiuretic hormone (SIADH)
(2006): Kubota T+, *J Anesth* 20(2), 126
(2006): Saegusa T+, *Gan To Kagaku Ryoho* 33(13), 2053 (with cisplatin)
(2006): Tanii H+, Ishii T+, *Am J Kidney Dis* 48(1), 155
(2004): Malik AR+, *Can J Psychiatry* 49(11), 785
(2003): Fabian TJ+, *J Geriatr Psychiatry Neurol* 16(3), 160
(2002): Arinzon ZH+, *Ann Pharmacother* 36(7-8), 1175
(1999): Odeh M+, *J Clin Pharmacol* 39(12), 1290
(1998): Leung VP+, *Pharmacopsychiatry* 31(1), 32
(1996): Christensen O+, *Ugeskr Laeger* 158(48), 6920
(1996): Flint AJ+, *Am J Psychiatry* 153(1), 134
(1996): Liu BA+, *CMAJ* 155(5), 519
(1996): van Campen JP+, *Ann Pharmacother* 30(12), 1499
Lymphedema
Mania

(2001): Ramasubbu R, *Acta Psychiatr Scand* 104(3), 236
Myalgia/Myositis/Myopathy/Myotoxicity (1–10%)
Paresthesias (3.8%)
Suicidal ideation
(2006): Apter A+, *J Child Adolesc Psychopharmacol* 16(1–2), 77
(2006): Aursnes I+, *BMC Psychiatry* 6, 55 (11 cases)
(2006): Lenzer J, *BMJ* 332(7551), 1175
Tremor (1–10%)
(2007): Terao T+, *Prog Neuropsychopharmacol Biol Psychiatry* 31(1), 295
(2004): Jagestedt M+, *Lakartidningen* 101(18), 1618 (with buspirone)

PEG-INTERFERON

Trade name: PEG-Intron (Schering)
Indications: Chronic hepatitis C
Category: Immunomodulator; Interferon
Half-life: ~40 hours
Clinically important, potentially hazardous interactions with: ACE inhibitors, melphalan, warfarin, zidovudine

Reactions

Skin

Abscess (~1%)
Angioedema (~1%)
Dermatitis (7%)
Diaphoresis (6%)
Eczema
(2007): Veldt BJ+, *J Clin Gastroenterol* 41(4), 432
Exanthems
(2003): Meller S+, *Hautarzt* 54(10), 992
Fixed eruption
(2003): Sidhu-Malik NK+, *J Drugs Dermatol* 2(5), 570 (with ribavirin)
Granuloma annulare
Nummular eczema
(2005): Shen Y+, *Arch Dermatol* 141(1), 102 (with ribavirin)
(2004): Moore MM+, *Arch Dermatol* 140(2), 215 (with ribavirin)
Pruritus (12%)
(2006): Lee H+, *Korean J Hepatol* 12(1), 31 (with ribavirin)
Psoriasis (~1%)
(2005): Kartal ED+, *Chemotherapy* 51(2-3), 167 (with ribavirin)
(2005): Ketikoglou I+, *Eur J Dermatol* 15(2), 107
Purpura
Rash (sic) (6%)
Rosacea fulminans
(2006): Bettoli V+, *Acta Derm Venereol* 86(3), 258 (with ribavirin)
(2003): Jensen SL+, *J Drugs Dermatol* 2(5), 554 (with ribavirin)
Sarcoidosis
(2007): Perez-Gala S+, *J Eur Acad Dermatol Venereol* 21(3), 393 (with ribavirin)
(2006): Benali S+, *Gastroenterol Clin Biol* 30(4), 615 (2 cases)
(2006): Bruch-Gerharz D+, *Hautarzt* 57(4), 317
(2006): Sanchez-Ruano JJ+, *Gastroenterol Hepatol* 29(3), 150 (with ribavirin)
(2005): Guilabert A+, *Br J Dermatol* 152(2), 377
(2005): Hurst EA+, *Arch Dermatol* 141(7), 865 (with ribavirin)
(2005): Ramos-Casals M+, *Medicine (Baltimore)* 84(2), 69
(2004): Alfageme Michavila I+, *Arch Bronconeumol* 40(1), 45 (with ribavirin)
(2004): Blank E, *Schoch Letter* 52(4), 15 (with ribavirin)
Urticaria (~1%)

Vesiculation
(2003): Gallina K+, J Drugs Dermatol 2(1), 63
Vitiligo
(2006): Tinio P+, Skinmed 5(1), 50 (with ribavirin)
(2006): Tomasiewicz K+, Adv Ther 23(1), 139 (with ribavirin)
Xerosis (11%)

Mucosal/ENT
Dysgeusia (1–10%)
Tinnitus
(2004): Formann E+, Am J Gastroenterol 99(5), 873
Tongue black
(2006): Gurguta C+, Am J Gastroenterol 101(1), 197 (with ribavirin)

Hair
Hair – alopecia (22%)
(2006): Demirturk N+, Eur J Dermatol 16(5), 579 (rare) (with ribavirin)
(2004): Bagheri H+, Pharmacotherapy 24(11), 1546 (with ribavirin)
Hair – alopecia areata
(2006): Demirturk N+, Eur J Dermatol 16(5), 579 (with ribavirin)

Eyes
Eyelashes – hypertrichosis
(2005): Howaizi M, J Gastroenterol Hepatol 20(12), 1945
Ocular toxicity
(2006): Avila MP+, Arq Bras Oftalmol 69(2), 255 (with ribavirin)
Retinopathy
(2006): Andrade RJ+, Antivir Ther 11(4), 491 (15%) (with ribavirin)
(2006): Avila MP+, Arq Bras Oftalmol 69(2), 255 (with ribavirin)
(2006): Okuse C+, World J Gastroenterol 12(23), 3756 (5 cases) (with ribavirin)
Vision blurred
(2004): Bagheri H+, Pharmacotherapy 24(11), 1546 (with ribavirin)

Other
Anaphylactoid reactions/Anaphylaxis (~1%)
Asthenia
(2005): Mukherjee S+, J Gastroenterol Hepatol 20(2), 198 (with ribavirin)
Cough (6%)
Death
(2006): Helbling B+, J Viral Hepat 13(11), 762 (2 cases) (with ribavirin)
Depression (16–29%)
(2005): Raison CL+, J Clin Psychiatry 66(1), 41 (39%) (with ribavirin)
(2004): Bagheri H+, Pharmacotherapy 24(11), 1546 (with ribavirin)
(2003): Alvarado Y+, Cancer Chemother Pharmacol 51(1), 81
(2002): Fried MW+, N Engl J Med 347(13), 975 (with ribavirin)
Embolia cutis medicamentosa (Nicolau syndrome)
(2005): Sonntag M+, Hautarzt 56(10), 968
Headache
(2002): Gupta SK+, J Clin Pharmacol 42(10), 1109
Hypersensitivity (~1%)
Injection-site necrosis
(2005): Dalmau J+, J Am Acad Dermatol 53(1), 62
Injection-site pain (2%)
Injection-site reactions
(2004): Bagheri H+, Pharmacotherapy 24(11), 1546 (with ribavirin)
Myalgia/Myositis/Myopathy/Myotoxicity (38–42%)
(2001): Perry CM+, Drugs 61(15), 2263
Nephrotoxicity

(2006): Alves Couto C+, Liver Int 26(10), 1294 (with ribavirin)
Pain (12%)
Vogt–Koyanagi–Harada disease
(2003): Sylvestre DL+, J Viral Hepat 10(6), 467 (with ribavirin)

PEGAPTANIB

Trade name: Macugen (Eyetech) (Pfizer)
Indications: Age-related macular degeneration (AMD), neovascular
Category: Vascular endothelial growth factor antagonist
Half-life: 10 (±4) days
Clinically important, potentially hazardous interactions with: none

Reactions

Skin
Angioedema
(2007): Steffensmeier AC+, Am J Ophthalmol 143(3), 512
Dermatitis (1–5%)
Urticaria
(2007): Steffensmeier AC+, Am J Ophthalmol 143(3), 512

Mucosal/ENT
Otitis (1–5%)

Eyes
Blepharitis (6–10%)
Cataract (10–40%)
(2006): Prescrire Int 15(84), 127
(2006): D'Amico DJ+, Ophthalmology 113(6), 992
Conjunctival hemorrhage (10–40%)
Conjunctivitis (6–10%)
Corneal edema (10–40%)
Endophthalmitis (<1%)
(2006): Prescrire Int 15(84), 127
(2006): D'Amico DJ+, Ophthalmology 113(6), 992
(2005): Maberley D, Issues Emerg Health Technol 76, 1
(2004): Gragoudas ES+, N Engl J Med 351(27), 2805 (1.3%)
Eyelid irritation (1–5%)
Meibomianitis (1–5%)
Mydriasis (1–5%)
Ocular edema (1–5%)
Ocular hypertension
(2006): Prescrire Int 15(84), 127 (transient, 15%)
Ocular inflammation
(2006): Hughes MS+, Ophthalmic Surg Lasers Imaging 37(6), 446
(2005): Doggrell SA, Expert Opin Pharmacother 6(8), 1421
Ocular pain (10–40%)
Ocular pressure (10–40%)
Ophthalmitis (1–5%)
Photopsia (6–10%)
Punctate keratitis (10–40%)
Retinal detachment (<1–10%)
(2006): Prescrire Int 15(84), 127
(2006): D'Amico DJ+, Ophthalmology 113(6), 992
(2006): Dhalla MS+, Am J Ophthalmol 141(4), 752
(2006): Singh RP+, Am J Ophthalmol 142(1), 160
(2004): Gragoudas ES+, N Engl J Med 351(27), 2805 (0.6%)
Vision blurred (10–40%)
Visual disturbances (10–40%)

Other
Anaphylactoid reactions/Anaphylaxis
(2007): Steffensmeier AC+, Am J Ophthalmol 143(3), 512

Chest pain (1–5%)
Headache (6–10%)
Hypertension (10–40%)
Vertigo (1–5%)

PEGASPARGASE

Synonym: NSC-644954
Trade name: Oncaspar (Enzon)
Indications: Acute lymphoblastic leukemia
Category: Antineoplastic
Half-life: 5.7 days
Clinically important, potentially hazardous interactions with: N/A

Reactions

Skin
Allergic reactions (>5%)
  (2003): Agrawal NR+, *Cancer* 98(1), 94
  (2003): Graham ML, *Adv Drug Deliv Rev* 55(10), 1293
  (1998): Graham ML+, *Bone Marrow Transplant* 21(9), 879
Angioedema (1–5%)
Diaphoresis
Edema (>5%)
Erythema (<1%)
Facial edema (<1%)
Peripheral edema
Petechiae (<1%)
Pruritus (<1%)
Purpura (<1%)
Rash (sic) (1 5%)
  (1998): Sikorska-Fic B+, *Wiad Lek* 51, 233
Urticaria (1–5%)

Mucosal/ENT
Tongue edema

Other
Abdominal pain (1–5%)
Anaphylactoid reactions/Anaphylaxis (1–5%)
Asthenia
Chest pain (<1%)
Chills (1–5%)
Cough (<1%)
Fever (>5%)
Headache (1–5%)
Hypertension (<1%)
Hypotension (>5%)
Injection-site edema
Injection-site pain
Myalgia/Myositis/Myopathy/Myotoxicity (1–5%)
Pain
Paresthesias (1–5%)
Seizures (1–5%)
  (2002): Rathi B+, *Pediatr Neurosurg* 37(4), 203
  (1997): Bushara KO+, *Pediatr Neurol* 17(2), 185
Upper respiratory infection (<1%)
Vertigo (<1%)

PEGFILGRASTIM

Synonym: G-CSF (PEG Conjugate)
Trade name: Neulasta (Amgen)
Indications: Myelosuppressive chemotherapy, decreases incidence of infection
Category: Colony stimulating factor; Hematopoietic
Half-life: 15–80 hours
Clinically important, potentially hazardous interactions with: lithium

Reactions

Skin
Acute febrile neutrophilic dermatosis (Sweet's syndrome)
  (2005): Draper BK+, *J Am Acad Dermatol* 52(5), 901
Allergic reactions (sic) (<1%)
Peripheral edema
Pyoderma gangrenosum
  (2006): Miall FM+, *Br J Haematol* 132(1), 115
  (2006): White LE+, *Skinmed* 5(2), 96
Rash (sic) (<1%)
Urticaria (<1%)

Mucosal/ENT
Dysgeusia
Mucositis
Stomatitis

Hair
Hair – alopecia

Other
Anaphylactoid reactions/Anaphylaxis (<1%)
Asthenia
  (2006): Hatzimichael E+, *Clin Lab Haematol* 28(6), 416
Headache
  (2006): Hatzimichael E+, *Clin Lab Haematol* 28(6), 416
Injection-site reactions
  (2006): *Prescrire Int* 15(85), 189
Myalgia/Myositis/Myopathy/Myotoxicity
  (2006): Hosing C+, *Br J Haematol* 133(5), 533

PEGVISOMANT

Synonyms: B2036-PEG; G120K-PEG; Trovert
Trade name: Somavert (Pfizer)
Indications: Acromegaly
Category: Growth hormone analog
Half-life: N/A
Clinically important, potentially hazardous interactions with: insulin, latex, opioids, oral hypoglycemics

Reactions

Skin
Edema
Peripheral edema (4–8%)
Pruritus

Mucosal/ENT
Sinusitis (8%)

Other
Abdominal pain

Acromegaloid features
   (2006): Maffei P+, *Ann Intern Med* 145(4), 310
Anaphylactoid reactions/Anaphylaxis
Chest pain (4%)
Headache
   (2007): Schreiber I+, *Eur J Endocrinol* 156(1), 75 (%)
Hepatotoxicity
   (2006): Feenstra J+, *Eur J Endocrinol* 154(6), 805 (with octreotide)
Hypersensitivity
Infections (23%)
Injection-site reactions (sic) (8–14%)
   (2007): Schreiber I+, *Eur J Endocrinol* 156(1), 75 (%)
Lipohypertrophy
   (2007): Marazuela M+, *Ann Intern Med* 147(10), 741
   (2006): Maffei P+, *Ann Intern Med* 145(4), 310
Pain (8%)
Paresthesias
Vertigo (8%)

PEMETREXED

Trade name: Alimta (Lilly)
Indications: Malignant pleural mesothelioma
Category: Folic acid antagonist
Half-life: 3.5 hours
Clinically important, potentially hazardous interactions with: nephrotoxic drugs, NSAIDs, probenecid

Reactions

Skin
Adverse effects (sic) (53%)
   (2000): John W+, *Cancer* 88(8), 1807 (53%)
   (2000): Miller KD+, *Ann Oncol* 11(1), 101
Allergic reactions (sic)
Desquamation (22%)
Peripheral edema
Photo-recall
   (2006): Barlesi F+, *Lung Cancer* 54(3), 423
   (2005): Hureaux J+, *Lung Cancer* 50(2), 255
Pressure necrosis
Pruritus
Purpura
Rash (sic) (42%)
   (2003): Martin M+, *Ann Oncol* 14(8), 1246
   (2001): Miles DW+, *Eur J Cancer* 37(11), 1366 (42%)
   (1999): Cripps C+, *Ann Oncol* 10(10), 1175
Vasculitis
   (2006): Lopes G+, *Lung Cancer* 51(2), 247 (urticaral)

Mucosal/ENT
Aphthous stomatitis
Gingivitis
Mucositis (5–17%)
   (2004): Calvert AH+, *Oncology (Williston Park)* 18(13 Suppl 8), 13
   (2001): Miles DW+, *Eur J Cancer* 37(11), 1366 (5%)
   (2001): Pivot X+, *Br J Cancer* 85(5), 649 (17.1%)
Stomatitis (5%)
   (2006): Sweeney CJ+, *J Clin Oncol* 24(21), 3451
   (2006): von der Masse H+, *Ann Oncol* 17(10), 1533 (with gemcitabine)
   (2003): Martin M+, *Ann Oncol* 14(8), 1246 (5%)
   (1999): Cripps C+, *Ann Oncol* 10(10), 1175

Eyes
Eyelid edema
   (2006): Kurata T+, *Lung Cancer* 54(2), 241

Other
Abdominal pain
   (1999): Cripps C+, *Ann Oncol* 10(10), 1175
Asthenia (6–10%)
   (2006): Sweeney CJ+, *J Clin Oncol* 24(21), 3451
   (2003): Martin M+, *Ann Oncol* 14(8), 1246 (10%)
   (2003): Scagliotti GV+, *J Clin Oncol* 21(8), 1556 (6.3%)
Chest pain
Chills
Cough
Death
   (1999): Cripps C+, *Ann Oncol* 10(10), 1175
Depression (14%)
Fever
   (1999): Cripps C+, *Ann Oncol* 10(10), 1175
Headache
Hepatotoxicity
   (2006): Brandes JC+, *Cancer Invest* 24(3), 283
Hypersensitivity (2%)
Infections
   (2004): Calvert AH+, *Oncology (Williston Park)* 18(13 Suppl 8), 13
   (2001): Miles DW+, *Eur J Cancer* 37(11), 1366
Pain
Paresthesias
Rhabdomyolysis
   (2006): Ceribelli A+, *Lancet Oncol* 7(4), 353
Seizures
Vertigo

PEMIROLAST

Trade names: Alamast (Johnson & Johnson); Alegysal
Indications: Pruritus of allergic conjunctivitis
Category: Mast cell stabilizer
Half-life: 4.5 hours

Reactions

Skin
Allergic reactions (sic)

Eyes
Ocular burning
Ocular stinging (<5%)
Xerophthalmia

PEMOLINE

Trade names: Betanamin; Cylert (Abbott); Tradon
Indications: Attention deficit disorder, narcolepsy
Category: Amphetamine
Half-life: 9–14 hours
Clinically important, potentially hazardous interactions with: pimozide

Note: Pemoline has been withdrawn

Reactions

Skin
Exanthems (<1%)
  (1992): Zürcher K and Krebs A, *Cutaneous Drug Reactions*
    Karger, 280
Rash (sic) (>10%)

Other
Delusions of parasitosis
  (2005): Krauseneck T+, *Psychopathology* 38(2), 103
Headache
Hepatotoxicity
  (2001): Safer DJ+, *J Am Acad Child Adolesc Psychiatry* 40(6), 622
  (1998): Adcock KG+, *Ann Pharmacother* 32(4), 422
  (1998): Hochman JA+, *Pediatrics* 101(1 Pt 1), 106
  (1998): Marotta PJ+, *J Pediatr* 132(5), 894
  (1998): Rosh JR+, *Pediatrics* 101(5), 921
  (1997): McCurry L+, *Am J Psychiatry* 154(5), 713
  (1997): Shevell M, *Pediatr Neurol* 16(4), 353
  (1997): Shevell M+, *Pediatr Neurol* 16(1), 14
  (1996): Sterling MJ+, *Am J Gastroenterol* 91(10), 2233
  (1995): Berkovitch M+, *Clin Pharmacol Ther* 57(6), 696
  (1990): Elitsur Y, *J Pediatr Gastroenterol Nutr* 11(1), 143
  (1990): Nehra A+, *Gastroenterology* 99(5), 1517
  (1990): Pratt DS+, *J Pediatr Gastroenterol Nutr* 10(2), 239
  (1984): Patterson JF, *South Med J* 77(7), 938
Hypotension
  (2000): Bohringer CH+, *Anesth Analg* 91(5), 1131
Rhabdomyolysis
  (1988): Briscoe JG+, *Med Toxicol Adverse Drug Exp* 3(1), 72

PENBUTOLOL

Trade names: Betapresin; Betapressin; Levatol (Schwarz)
Indications: Hypertension
Category: Adrenergic beta-receptor antagonist
Half-life: 5 hours
**Clinically important, potentially hazardous interactions
with:** clonidine, epinephrine, verapamil

Note: Cutaneous side effects of beta-receptor blockaders are
clinically polymorphous. They apparently appear after several months
of continuous therapy. Atypical psoriasiform, lichen planus-like, and
eczematous chronic rashes are mainly observed. (1983): Hödl St, *Z
Hautkr* (German) 1:58, 17

Reactions

Skin
Allergic reactions (sic) (1–5%)
  (1985): Marone C+, *Curr Med Res Opin* 9, 417 (1–5%)
Diaphoresis (1.6%)
Exanthems (1–5%)
  (1985): Marone C+, *Curr Med Res Opin* 9, 417 (1–5%)
Peripheral edema
Pruritus
Psoriasis
Purpura
Rash (sic)

Mucosal/ENT
Dysgeusia

Hair
Hair – alopecia

Nails
Nails – pigmentation

Other
Headache
Paresthesias
Peyronie's disease

PENCICLOVIR

Trade name: Denavir (Novartis)
Indications: Herpes simplex (recurrent)
Category: Antiviral
Half-life: N/A
**Clinically important, potentially hazardous interactions
with:** N/A

Reactions

Skin
Pigmentation
Pruritus
Rash (sic) (0.1%)
Urticaria

Mucosal/ENT
Dysgeusia (0.2%)
Parosmia

Other
Headache (5.3%)
Pain
Paresthesias

PENICILLAMINE

Trade names: Artamin; D-Penamine; Depen (MedPointe);
Distamine; Kelatin; Pendramine
Indications: Wilson's disease, rheumatoid arthritis
Category: Antidote; Chelator; Disease-modifying antirheumatic
Half-life: 1.7–3.2 hours
**Clinically important, potentially hazardous interactions
with:** aluminum hydroxide, antacids, ascorbic acid, bone marrow
suppressants, chloroquine, cytotoxic agents, **food**, gold,
hydroxychloroquine, iron, magnesium, primaquine, probenecid

Note: For excellent reviews of many of the cutaneous manifestations
caused by penicillamine see (1983): Levy RS+, *J Am Acad Dermatol* 8,
548 and (1981): Sternlieb I+, *J Rheumatol* 8 (Suppl 7), 149

Reactions

Skin
Anetoderma
Atrophy
  (1982): Bailin PL+, *Clin Rheum Dis* 8, 493 (passim)
Bullous dermatitis
  (1996): Bialy-Golan A+, *J Am Acad Dermatol* 35, 732 (passim)
  (1982): Fulton RA+, *Br J Dermatol* 107 (Suppl 22), 95
Bullous pemphigoid
  (1998): Weller R+, *Ann Pharmacother* 32, 1368
  (1996): Weller R+, *Clin Exp Dermatol* 21, 121
  (1989): Rasmussen HB+, *J Cutan Pathol* 16, 154
  (1987): Brown MD+, *Arch Dermatol* 123, 1119

(1986): Gall Y+, *Ann Dermatol Venereol* (French) 113, 55

Cicatricial pemphigoid
   (1985): Shuttleworth D+, *Clin Exp Dermatol* 10, 392

Cutis laxa
   (2005): Rosen LB+, *Cutis* 76(1), 49
   (2004): Pinter R+, *Am J Med Genet A* 128(3), 294
   (2000): Hill VA+, *Br J Dermatol* 142(3), 560
   (2000): Werth V, *Dermatology Times* 18
   (1994): Amichai B+, *Isr J Med Sci* 30, 667
   (1983): Harpey JP+, *Lancet* 2, 858
   (1983): Levy RS+, *J Am Acad Dermatol* 8, 548
   (1982): Bailin PL+, *Clin Rheum Dis* 8, 493 (passim)

Cyst

Dermatitis
   (1993): De Moor A+, *Contact Dermatitis* 29, 155 (eyedrops)
   (1990): Coenraads PJ+, *Contact Dermatitis* 23, 371

Dermatomyositis
   (1992): Kolsi R+, *Rev Rhum Mal Osteoartic* (French) 59, 341
   (1991): Wilson CL+, *Int J Dermatol* 30, 148
   (1988): Grasedyck K, *Z Rheumatol* 47 Suppl 1, 17
   (1987): Carroll CG+, *J Rheumatol* 14, 995
   (1987): Carroll GJ+, *J Rheumatol* 14(5), 995
   (1984): Halla JT+, *Am J Med* 77(4), 719
   (1983): Doyle DR+, *Ann Intern Med* 98, 327
   (1983): Levy RS+, *J Am Acad Dermatol* 8, 548
   (1983): Lund HI+, *Scand J Rheumatol* 12, 350
   (1982): Bailin PL+, *Clin Rheum Dis* 8, 493 (passim)
   (1981): Major GA, *J R Soc Med* 74, 393
   (1980): Wojnarowska F, *J R Soc Med* 73, 884

Edema of lip (1–10%)
   (1999): Hsu HL+, *Taiwan Erh Ko I Hsueh Tsa Chih* 40, 448 (lip)

Ehlers–Danlos syndrome
   (1982): Bailin PL+, *Clin Rheum Dis* 8, 493 (passim)
   (1982): Yung CW+, *J Am Acad Dermatol* 6, 317 (passim)

Elastosis perforans serpiginosa
   (2005): Becuwe C+, *Dermatology* 210(1), 60
   (2005): Rath N+, *Indian J Dermatol Venereol Leprol* 71(3), 182
   (2005): Rosen LB+, *Cutis* 76(1), 49
   (2002): Deguti MM+, *Am J Gastroenterol* 97(8), 2153
   (2001): Danby FW, Manchester, NH (from Internet)
      (observation)
   (2000): Hill VA+, *Br J Dermatol* 142, 560
   (2000): Werth V, *Dermatology Times* 18
   (1997): Iozumi K+, *J Dermatol* 24(7), 458
   (1994): Amichai B+, *Isr J Med Sci* 30, 667
   (1994): Ratnavel RC+, *Dermatology* 189, 81
   (1994): Wilhelm KP+, *Hautarzt* (German) 45, 45
   (1989): Sahn EE+, *J Am Acad Dermatol* 20, 279
   (1989): Sahn EE+, *J Am Acad Dermatol* 20(5 Pt 2), 979
   (1988): Grasedyck K, *Z Rheumatol* 47 Suppl 1, 17
   (1988): van Joost T+, *Ned Tijdschr Geneeskd* (Dutch) 132, 501
   (1986): Price RG+, *Am J Dermatopathol* 8, 314
   (1985): Meyrick-Thomas RHM+, *Clin Exp Dermatol* 10, 386
   (1984): Venencie PY+, *Ann Med Interne* (Paris) (French) 135, 642
   (1983): Levy RS+, *J Am Acad Dermatol* 8, 548
   (1983): Rosenblum GA, *J Am Acad Dermatol* 8, 718
   (1982): Bailin PL+, *Clin Rheum Dis* 8, 493 (passim)
   (1982): Essigman WK, *Ann Rheum Dis* 41, 617
   (1982): Gloor M+, *Hautarzt* (German) 33, 291
   (1982): Raymond JL+, *J Cutan Pathol* 9, 352
   (1981): Bardach H+, *Wien Klin Wochenschr* (German) 93, 117
   (1981): Gebhart W+, *Am J Dermatopathol* 3(1), 33
   (1981): Hashimoto K+, *J Am Acad Dermatol* 4(3), 300

Epidermolysis bullosa
   (1982): Bailin PL+, *Clin Rheum Dis* 8, 493 (passim)
   (1982): Yung CW+, *J Am Acad Dermatol* 6, 317 (passim)

Epidermolysis bullosa acquisita
   (2003): Cetkovska P+, *J Am Acad Dermatol* 49(6), 1157

Erythema multiforme (1–5%)

Erythema nodosum (<1%)
   (1983): Grauer JL+, *Presse Med* (French) 12, 1997

Exanthems
   (1999): Hsu HL+, *Taiwan Erh Ko I Hsueh Tsa Chih* 40, 448
   (1983): Levy RS+, *J Am Acad Dermatol* 8, 548
   (1982): Bailin PL+, *Clin Rheum Dis* 8, 493 (passim)
   (1982): Egeland T+, *J Oral Pathol* 11, 183
   (1981): Walshe JM, *J Rheumatol* 8 (Suppl 7), 155
   (1980): Stein HB+, *Ann Intern Med* 92, 24

Exfoliative dermatitis

Facial edema
   (1996): Bialy-Golan A+, *J Am Acad Dermatol* 35, 732 (passim)

Fragility
   (1981): Shaw M+, *Clin Exp Dermatol* 6, 429

Graft-versus-host reaction
   (1998): Jappe U+, *Hautarzt* (German) 49, 126 (passim)

Grover's disease
   (1997): Zvulunov A+, *Int J Dermatol* 36(6), 476

Lichen planus
   (1994): Thompson DF+, *Pharmacotherapy* 14, 561
   (1986): Weismann K+, *Ugeskr Laeger* (Danish) 148, 456
   (1981): Powell FC+, *Lancet* 2, 525

Lichenoid eruption
   (1983): Levy RS+, *J Am Acad Dermatol* 8, 548
   (1983): Powell FC+, *J Am Acad Dermatol* 9, 540
   (1982): Bailin PL+, *Clin Rheum Dis* 8, 493 (passim)
   (1982): Powell FC+, *Br J Dermatol* 107, 616
   (1981): Seehafer JR+, *Arch Dermatol* 117, 140
   (1981): Van Hecke E+, *Arch Dermatol* 117, 676

Lupus erythematosus
   (2000): Lin HC+, *J Microbiol Immunol Infect* 33, 202
   (1996): Bialy-Golan A+, *J Am Acad Dermatol* 35, 732 (passim)
   (1995): Barthel HR+, *Dtsch Med Wochenschr* (German) 120, 1253
   (1994): Borg AA, *Clin Rheumatol* 13, 522
   (1994): Fritzler MJ, *Lupus* 3, 455
   (1994): Yung RL+, *Rheum Dis Clin North Am* 20, 61
   (1993): Donnelly S+, *Br J Rheumatol* 32, 251
   (1992): Rubin RL+, *J Clin Invest* 90, 165
   (1992): Skaer TL, *Clin Ther* 14, 496
   (1991): Chin GL+, *J Rheumatol* 18, 947
   (1991): Weinstein A, *Arthritis Rheum* 34, 1343
   (1990): Enzenauer RJ+, *Arthritis Rheum* 33, 1582
   (1990): Suda M+, *Nippon Jinzo Gakkai Shi* (Japanese) 32, 1235
   (1990): Tsankov NK+, *Int J Dermatol* 29, 571
   (1988): Grasedyck K, *Z Rheumatol* 47 Suppl 1, 17
   (1987): Hobbs RN+, *Ann Rheum Dis* 46, 408
   (1987): Lopez-Guerra N+, *Med Clin* (Barc) (Spanish) 88, 552
   (1985): Kalina P+, *Bratisl Lek Listy* (Slovak) 84, 336
   (1985): Lovisetto P+, *Recenti Prog Med* (Italian) 76, 110
   (1985): Stratton MA, *Clin Pharm* 4, 657
   (1984): Clerc C+, *Ann Dermatol Venereol* (French) 135, 420
   (1983): Levy RS+, *J Am Acad Dermatol* 8, 548
   (1982): Bailin PL+, *Clin Rheum Dis* 8, 493 (passim)
   (1982): Chalmers A+, *Ann Intern Med* 97, 659
   (1982): Egeland T+, *J Oral Pathol* 11, 183
   (1982): Yung CW+, *J Am Acad Dermatol* 6, 317 (passim)
   (1981): Hughes GR+, *Arthritis Rheum* 24, 1070
   (1981): Thorvaldsen J, *Dermatologia* 162, 277
   (1981): Walshe JM, *J Rheumatol* 7, 155
   (1980): Condemi JJ, *Geriatrics* 35(3), 81

Morphea
   (1989): Liddle BJ, *Ann Rheum Dis* 48, 963
   (1981): Bernstein RM+, *Ann Rheum Dis* 40, 42

Papular lesions
   (1985): Thomas RHM+, *Clin Exp Dermatol* 10, 386

Pemphigus
   (2004): Sugita K+, *J Dermatolog Treat* 15(4), 214

(2004): Szegedi A+, *Acta Derm Venereol* 84(4), 318
(2000): Shapiro M+, *J Am Acad Dermatol* 42, 297
(2000): Werth V, *Dermatology Times* 18
(1999): Jan V+, *Ann Dermatol Venereol* (French) 126, 153
(1997): Brenner S+, *J Am Acad Dermatol* 36, 919
(1997): Haimowitz JE+, PA, American Academy of Dermatology
   Meeting (SF) (gross and microscopic)
(1995): Ciompi ML+, *Rheumatol Int* 15, 95
(1993): Brenner S+, *Clin Dermatol* 11, 501
(1993): Jones E+, *J Am Acad Dermatol* 28, 655
(1992): Bauer-Vinassac D+, *Scand J Rheumatol* 21, 17
(1991): Korman NJ+, *J Invest Dermatol* 96, 273
(1991): Wolf R+, *Dermatologica* 182(4), 207
(1990): Black AK+, *Br J Dermatol* 123, 277
(1990): Broggini M+, *Minerva Med* 81(3), 197
(1990): Wouters EA+, *Acta Clin Belg* (French) 45, 1
(1989): Civatte J, *Dermatol Monatsschr* (German) 175, 1
(1989): Marti-Huguet T+, *Arch Ophthalmol* 107, 1115
(1988): Blanken R+, *Acta Derm Venereol* (Stockh) 68, 456
(1988): Buckley C+, *Ir J Med Sci* 157, 267
(1988): Grasedyck K, *Z Rheumatol* 47 Suppl 1, 17
(1988): Savill JS+, *Clin Nephrol* 29(5), 267
(1987): Enjolras O+, *Ann Dermatol Venereol* (French) 114, 25
(1987): Kind P+, *Hautarzt* (German) 38, 548
(1987): Walton S+, *Clin Exp Dermatol* 12, 275
(1986): Civatte J, *Bull Soc Fr Dermatol Syphiligr* (French)
   170, 1057
(1986): Dijkstra JW, *J Am Acad Dermatol* 14, 687
(1986): Kay A, *Br J Rheumatol* 25(2), 193
(1986): Peyri J+, *J Am Acad Dermatol* 14, 681 (cicatricial)
(1986): Steen VD+, *Ann Intern Med* 104, 699
(1986): Tholen S, *Z Hautkr* (German) 61, 719
(1985): Ho VC+, *J Rheumatol* 12, 583
(1985): Lever LR+, *Br J Dermatol* 113, 88
(1985): Piette-Brion B+, *Dermatologica* (French) 170, 297
(1985): Shuttleworth D+, *Br J Dermatol* 113, 89
(1985): Shuttleworth D+, *Clin Exp Dermatol* 10, 392 (cicatricial)
(1985): Velthuis PJ+, *Br J Dermatol* 112, 615
(1984): Hashimoto K+, *Arch Dermatol* 120, 762
(1984): Stein HB+, *Clin Invest Med* 7(1), 73
(1984): Venencie PY+, *Ann Med Interne* (Paris) (French)
   135, 642
(1983): Doutre MS+, *Rev Rhum Mal Osteoartic* (French) 50, 167
(1983): Kaplan RP+, *Clin Dermatol* 1, 42
(1983): Levy RS+, *J Am Acad Dermatol* 8, 548
(1983): Tinozzi CC, *G Ital Dermatol Venereol* (Italian) 118, 45
(1982): Barety M+, *Therapie* (French) 37, 471
(1982): Benito-Urbino S+, *Rev Clin Esp* (Spanish) 166, 249
(1982): Fye KH+J, *Rheumatol* 9, 331
(1982): Ruocco V+, *Arch Dermatol Res* 274, 123
(1982): Ruocco V+, *Dermatologica* 164, 236
(1982): Yung CW+, *J Am Acad Dermatol* 6, 317 (pemphigus
   syndrome)
(1982): Zone J+, *JAMA* 247, 2705
(1981): Livden JK+, *Scand J Rheumatol* 10, 95
(1981): Santa-Cruz DJ+, *Am J Dermatopathol* 3, 85
(1981): Troy JL+, *J Am Acad Dermatol* 4, 547
(1981): Trunnell TN+, *Cutis* 27, 402 (pemphigus-like)
(1980): Chouvet B+, *Dermatologica* (French) 160, 297
(1980): Trau H+, *Arch Dermatol* 116, 721

Pemphigus erythematodes (Senear–Usher)
(1990): Willemsen MJ+, *Int J Dermatol* 29, 193
(1985): Amerian ML+, *Int J Dermatol* 24, 16
(1985): Gibson LE+, *J Am Acad Dermatol* 12, 883
(1984): Amerian ML+, *J Am Acad Dermatol* 10, 215
(1982): Yung CW+, *J Am Acad Dermatol* 6, 317
(1980): Keilhauer A+, *Z Hautkr* (German) 55, 948

Pemphigus foliaceus
(2005): Nagao K+, *Clin Exp Dermatol* 30(1), 43
(2000): Elston DM+, *Cutis* 66, 375

(2000): Werth V, *Dermatology Times* 18
(1999): Toth GG+, *Br J Dermatol* 141, 583
(1998): Brenner S+, *J Am Acad Dermatol* 39, 137
(1997): McGovern TW+, *Arch Dermatol* 133, 499
(1997): Peñas PF+, *J Am Acad Dermatol* 37, 121
(1995): Brenner S+, American Academy of Dermatology
   Meeting, New Orleans (observation)
(1993): Zillikens D+, *Hautarzt* (German) 44, 167
(1986): Kohn SR, *Arch Dermatol* 122, 17 (fatal)
(1985): Bahmer FA+, *Arch Dermatol* 121, 665
(1984): Knezevic W+, *Aust N Z J Med* 14, 50
(1983): Brenner S+, *Harefuah* (Hebrew) 104, 94
(1982): Kohn SR, *Dermatologic Capsule and Comment* 4, 11
(1981): Matkaluk RM+, *Arch Dermatol* 117, 156

Pemphigus herpetiformis
(1988): Weltfriend S+, *Hautarzt* (German) 39, 587
(1980): Morioka S+, *J Dermatol* 7, 425

Peripheral edema (1–10%)

Pruritus (44–50%)
(1982): Bailin PL+, *Clin Rheum Dis* 8, 493 (passim)
(1982): Yung CW+, *J Am Acad Dermatol* 6, 317 (passim)

Pseudoxanthoma elasticum
(2005): Rath N+, *Indian J Dermatol Venereol Leprol* 71(3), 182
(2000): Werth V, *Dermatology Times* 18
(1998): Coatesworth AP+, *J Clin Pathol* 51, 169
(1992): Bolognia JL+, *Dermatology* (Basel) 184, 12
(1992): Narron GH+, *Ann Plast Surg* 29, 367
(1991): Buckley C+, *Clin Exp Dermatol* 16, 310
(1990): Dalziel KL+, *Br J Dermatol* 123, 305
(1988): Burge S+, *Clin Exp Dermatol* 13, 255
(1987): Dootson G+, *Clin Exp Dermatol* 12, 66
(1986): Light N+, *Br J Dermatol* 114, 381
(1905): Bentley-Phillips B, *J R Soc Med* 78, 787
(1985): Meyrick-Thomas RH+, *Clin Exp Dermatol* 10, 386

Psoriasis
(1987): Forgie JC+, *BMJ* 294, 1101
(1986): Daunt SON+, *Br J Rheumatol* 25, 74
(1983): Levy RS+, *J Am Acad Dermatol* 8, 548
(1981): Sternlieb I+, *J Rheumatol* 8, 149

Purpura
(1983): Trice JM+, *Arch Intern Med* 143, 1487
(1982): Bailin PL+, *Clin Rheum Dis* 8, 493 (passim)
(1982): Speth PA+, *J Rheumatol* 9, 812

Rash (sic) (44–50%)
(2003): Corrigan JJ Jr+, *Haemophilia* 9(1), 64
(2000): Shannon MW+, *Ann Pharmacother* 34, 15
(1991): Barash J+, *Clin Exp Dermatol* 9, 541
(1982): Kean WF+, *J Am Geriatr Soc* 30, 94
(1982): Smith PJ+, *Br Med J (Clin Res Ed)* 285, 595

Scleroderma
(2002): Dourmishev LA+, *J Eur Acad Dermatol Venereol*
   16(5), 538
(1992): Natsuda H+, *Intern Med* 31(2), 244
(1991): Bourgeois P+, *Baillieres Clin Rheumatol* 5, 13
(1987): Miyagawa S+, *Br J Dermatol* 116, 95
(1981): Bernstein RM+, *Ann Rheum Dis* 40, 42

Stevens–Johnson syndrome
(1996): Kammler H-J, Jena, Germany (from Internet)
   (observation)

Toxic epidermal necrolysis (<1%)
(1984): Chan HL+, *J Am Acad Dermatol* 10, 973
(1981): Ward K+, *Ir J Med Sci* 150, 252

Transient acantholytic dermatosis (Grover's disease)
(1997): Zvulunov A+, *Int J Dermatol* 36(6), 476

Urticaria (44–50%)
(1983): Levy RS+, *J Am Acad Dermatol* 8, 548

Vasculitis
(1998): Merkel PA, *Curr Opin Rheumatol* 10, 45
(1986): Gall Y+, *Ann Dermatol Venereol* (French) 113, 55

(1983): Banfi G+, *Nephron* 33, 56
(1983): Curran JJ+, *J Rheumatol* 10, 344
(1982): Bailin PL+, *Clin Rheum Dis* 8, 493 (passim)
Vesiculation
(1992): Godar JM+, *Arch Dermatol* 128, 977
Wrinkling (sic)
(1983): Levy RS+, *J Am Acad Dermatol* 8, 548
Xerosis
(1982): Yung CW+, *J Am Acad Dermatol* 6, 317 (passim)

Mucosal/ENT
Ageusia (12%)
(2002): ter Borg EJ+, *Neth J Med* 60(10), 402
(1982): Yung CW+, *J Am Acad Dermatol* 6, 317 (passim)
Aphthous stomatitis
(1983): Levy RS+, *J Am Acad Dermatol* 8, 548
Bromhidrosis
(1996): Bialy-Golan A+, *J Am Acad Dermatol* 35, 732 (passim)
Dysgeusia (metallic taste)
(1996): Bialy-Golan A+, *J Am Acad Dermatol* 35, 732 (passim)
(1988): Grasedyck K, *Z Rheumatol* 47 Suppl 1, 17 (5–30%)
(1986): Steen VD+, *Ann Intern Med* emic(ug), 699
(1985): Bodenheimer HC+, *Hepatology* 5(6), 1139
(1984): Gutierrez Fuentes JA+, *Rev Clin Esp* 172(3), 149
(1983): Levy RS+, *J Am Acad Dermatol* 8, 548
(1982): Kean WF+, *J Am Geriatr Soc* 30, 94
(1980): Stein HB+, *Ann Intern Med* 92, 24
Gingivitis
Glossitis
Hypogeusia (25–33%)
Mucocutaneous reactions (sic)
(1982): Halla JT+, *Am J Med* 72, 423
Mucosal lesions (pemphigus-like)
(1981): Eisenberg E+, *Oral Surg Oral Med Oral Pathol* 51, 409
Mucosal ulceration
(1981): Eisenberg E+, *Oral Surg* 51, 409
Oral lichenoid eruption
(1984): Blasberg B+, *J Rheumatol* 11, 348
Oral ulceration
(2000): Madinier I+, *Ann Med Interne* (Paris) (French) 151, 248
(1996): Bialy-Golan A+, *J Am Acad Dermatol* 35, 732 (passim)
(1982): Egeland T+, *J Oral Pathol* 11, 183
(1980): Stein HB+, *Ann Intern Med* 92, 24
Stomatitis
(1996): Bialy-Golan A+, *J Am Acad Dermatol* 35, 732 (passim)
(1982): Yung CW+, *J Am Acad Dermatol* 6, 317 (passim)
(1981): Sternlieb I+, *J Rheumatol* 8 (Suppl 7), 149 (passim)
(1980): Stein HB+, *Ann Intern Med* 92, 24
Tinnitus

Hair
Hair – alopecia
(1988): Grasedyck K, *Z Rheumatol* 47 Suppl 1, 17 (1–2%)
(1983): Levy RS+, *J Am Acad Dermatol* 8, 548
(1981): Sternlieb I+, *J Rheumatol* 8 (Suppl 7), 149
Hair – hirsutism
(1990): Rose BI+, *J Reprod Med* 35, 43
(1983): Levy RS+, *J Am Acad Dermatol* 8, 548

Nails
Nails – dystrophy
(1987): Brown MD+, *Arch Dermatol* 123, 1119 (passim)
Nails – elkonyxis (punched-out appearance of the nail at lunulae)
(1989): Bjellerup M, *Acta Derm Venereol* (Stockh) 69, 339
Nails – leukonychia
Nails – longitudinal ridges
Nails – onychoschizia
(1989): Bjellerup M, *Acta Derm Venereol* (Stockh) 69, 339

Nails – pigmentation
(1991): Ichikawa Y+, *Tokai J Exp Clin Med* 16, 203
(1989): Bjellerup M, *Acta Derm Venereol* (Stockh) 69, 339
(1983): Ilchyshyn A+, *Acta Derm Venereol* (Stockh) 63, 534

Other
Death
Gynecomastia
(1994): Desautels JE, *Can Assoc Radiol J* 45, 143 (gigantism)
(1985): Kahl LE+, *J Rheumatol* 12, 990
(1982): Reid DM+, *BMJ* 285, 1083
Hypersensitivity
(1999): Hsu HL+, *Taiwan Erh Ko I Hsueh Tsa Chih* 40, 448
(1994): Chan CY+, *Am J Gastroenterol* 89, 442
Nephrotoxicity
(2007): Bienaime F+, *Am J Kidney Dis* 50(5), 821
(2004): Ohno I+, *Nippon Rinsho* 62(10), 1919
Polymyositis
(2002): Dourmishev LA+, *J Eur Acad Dermatol Venereol* 16(5), 538
(1996): Bialy-Golan A+, *J Am Acad Dermatol* 35, 732 (passim)
(1991): Santos JC+, *Clin Exp Dermatol* 16, 76
(1987): Carroll GJ+, *J Rheumatol* 14(5), 995
(1986): Takahashi K+, *Arthritis Rheum* 29(4), 560
(1985): Leden I+, *Scand J Rheumatol* 14(1), 90
Serum sickness
(1996): Bialy-Golan A+, *J Am Acad Dermatol* 35, 732 (passim)
Sjøgren's (Sicca) syndrome
(1996): Bialy-Golan A+, *J Am Acad Dermatol* 35, 732 (passim)

PENICILLIN G

Trade names: Benzylpenicillin; Crystapen (Britannia); Megacillin; Novopen-G
Indications: Anthrax, cellulitis, endocarditis, infections, otitis media, rheumatic fever, respiratory infections, septicemia
Category: Antibiotic, penicillin
Half-life: 4 hours
Clinically important, potentially hazardous interactions with: estrogens, methotrexate, phenindione, probenecid, sulfinpyrazone, warfarin

Reactions

Skin
Angioedema
Dermatitis
Edema
Exfoliative dermatitis
Jarisch–Herxheimer reaction
(2008): Berger EM+, *J Drugs Dermatol* 7(6), 583
(2007): Gurses C+, *Epileptic Disord* 9(1), 51
(2005): See S+, *Ann Pharmacother* 39(12), 2128
(2002): Silberstein P+, *J Clin Neurosci* 9(6), 689
(2000): Cooper PJ+, *J Infect Dis* 181(1), 203
(1999): Vecsei AK+, *Wien Klin Wochenschr* 111(10), 410
(1998): Myles TD+, *Obstet Gynecol* 92(5), 859
(1998): van Voorst Vader PC, *Dermatol Clin* 16(4), 699
(1997): Coxon RE+, *QJM* 90(3), 213
(1996): Fekade D+, *N Engl J Med* 335(5), 311
(1996): Remick DG+, *J Infect Dis* 174(3), 627
(1996): Rodriguez AC+, *J Obstet Gynecol Neonatal Nurs* 25(5), 383
(1994): Emmanouilides CE+, *Clin Infect Dis* 18(6), 1004
(1994): Zifko U+, *J Neurol Neurosurg Psychiatry* 57(7), 865
(1993): Borgnolo G+, *Trop Geogr Med* 45(2), 66

(1992): Gebrehiwot T+, *Ethiop Med J* 30(3), 175
(1989): Kosbab R+, *Dermatol Monatsschr* 175(11), 685
(1988): Weber K+, *Ann N Y Acad Sci* 539, 324
(1987): Melkert PW, *Trop Geogr Med* 39(1), 92 (fatal)
(1985): Loveday C+, *Genitourin Med* 61(1), 27
(1983): Perine PL+, *Am J Trop Med Hyg* 32(5), 1096
Linear IgA dermatosis
(1993): Combemale P+, *Ann Dermatol Venereol* 120(11), 847
Rash (sic)
(2003): Zdziarski P, *Pol Merkuriusz Lek* 14(79), 50
(1996): Markowitz M+, *Pediatrics* 97(6 Pt 2), 981
Urticaria
(2006): Padilla Serrato MT+, *Rev Alerg Mex* 53(5), 179

Mucosal/ENT
Tongue black

Other
Abdominal pain
Anaphylactoid reactions/Anaphylaxis
(2007): Linares T+, *J Investig Allergol Clin Immunol* 17(1), 50
(2007): Schafer JA+, *Pharmacotherapy* 27(4), 542
(1991): *Lancet* 337(8753), 1308
Chills
Embolia cutis medicamentosa (Nicolau syndrome)
(2006): Luton K+, *Int J Dermatol* 45(11), 1326
Fever
Hepatotoxicity
(2001): Andrade RJ+, *Ann Pharmacother* 35(6), 783
(1997): Bauer TM+, *J Hepatol* 26(2), 429
Hypersensitivity
(2003): Scala E+, *Allergy* 58(5), 439
(1990): Prieto Lopez C+, *Allergol Immunopathol (Madr)*
18(3), 141
Lipoatrophy
(1996): Kayikcioglu A+, *J Pediatr* 129(1), 166
Myalgia/Myositis/Myopathy/Myotoxicity
Nephrotoxicity
(2000): Adlam D+, *J Infect* 40(1), 102
Seizures
Serum sickness
Thrombosis

PENICILLIN V

Trade names: Abbocillin; Apo-Pen; Diistaquaine V-K; Novapen-VK; Ospen; Penbeta; Phenoxymethylpenicillin
Indications: Cellulitis, endocarditis, erysipelas, oral infections, otitis media, rheumatic fever, scarlet fever, tonsillitis
Category: Antibiotic, penicillin
Half-life: 4 hours
Clinically important, potentially hazardous interactions with: estrogens, methotrexate, neomycin, phenindione, probenecid, sulfinpyrazone, warfarin

Reactions

Skin
Angioedema
Exanthems
(1981): Rockl H, *Hautarzt 1981 Sep* 32(9), 467
Exfoliative dermatitis
Rash (sic)
Toxic epidermal necrolysis
(2001): Robak E+, *J Med* 32(1–2), 31 (with aminophenazone & paracetamol)

Urticaria
Vasculitis
(1981): Rockl H, *Hautarzt 1981 Sep* 32(9), 467

Mucosal/ENT
Tongue black

Other
Anaphylactoid reactions/Anaphylaxis
(1990): Guberman D, *Harefuah* 118(7), 392
Chills
Fever
(1985): Drapkin MS+, *Arch Surg* 120(11), 1321
Hypersensitivity
(2003): Schindler C+, *Chemotherapy* 49(1–2), 90
Nephrotoxicity
Seizures
Serum sickness
(1995): Martin J+, *N Z Med J* 108(997), 123
(1990): Heckbert SR+, *Am J Epidemiol* 132(2), 336

PENTAGASTRIN

Trade names: Gastrodiagnost; Peptavlon (Wyeth)
Category: Diagnostic aid; Polypeptide hormone
Half-life: 10 minutes

Reactions

Skin
Angioedema
(1985): Arnved J+, *Lancet* 2, 1068
Diaphoresis
Exanthems
Pruritus
Purpura
(1985): Arnved J+, *Lancet* 2, 1068
Rash (sic)
Urticaria

Other
Hypersensitivity
Injection-site pain
Paresthesias

PENTAMIDINE

Trade names: NebuPent (Astellas); Pentacarinat; Pentam-300 (Astellas)
Indications: *Pneumocystis carinii* infection, trypanosomiasis
Category: Antiprotozoal
Half-life: 9.1–13.2 hours (IM); 6.5 hours (IV)
Clinically important, potentially hazardous interactions with: adefovir, amisulpride, insulin detemir, insulin glulisine, sparfloxacin

Note: The rate of adverse side effects is increased in patients with AIDS

Reactions

Skin
Bullous dermatitis
Edema

Erythema
Exanthems (1–15%)
(1992): Breathnach SM+, *Adverse Drug Reactions and the Skin*
    Blackwell, Oxford, 179 (passim)
(1990): Leoung GS+, *N Engl J Med* 323, 769 (0.25%)
(1990): Monk JP+, *Drugs* 39, 741
(1990): Soo Hoo GW+, *Ann Intern Med* 113, 195 (1–5%)
(1989): Berger TG+, *Ann Intern Med* 110, 1035
(1988): Leen CLS+, *Lancet* 2, 1250
(1988): Sattler FR+, *Ann Intern Med* 109, 280 (15%)
(1987): Goa KL+, *Drugs* 33, 242 (1.5%)
(1984): Gordon FM+, *Ann Intern Med* 100, 495 (3%)
(1984): Kovacs JA+, *Ann Intern Med* 100, 663 (6%)
Jarisch–Herxheimer reaction (<1%)
(1987): Goa KL+, *Drugs* 33, 242
Pruritus
(1989): Berger TG+, *Ann Intern Med* 110, 1035
(1988): Leen CLS+, *Lancet* 2, 1250
Purpura
Rash (sic) (1–47%)
(1993): Dohn M+, *Int Conf AIDS* 9, 372
(1988): Leen CL+, *Lancet* 2, 1250
(1984): Gordin FM+, *Ann Intern Med* 100, 495
Side effects (sic)
(1989): Berger TG+, *Ann Intern Med* 110, 1035
Stevens–Johnson syndrome (0.2%)
Toxic epidermal necrolysis
(1988): Leen CLS+, *Lancet* 2, 1250 (passim)
(1987): Goa KL+, *Drugs* 33, 242
(1985): Heng MCY, *Br J Dermatol* 113, 597
Ulcerations
(1985): Gottlieb JR+, *Plast Reconstr Surg* 76, 630
Urticaria
(1993): Belsito DV, *Contact Dermatitis* 29, 158 (contact)
(1992): Breathnach SM+, *Adverse Drug Reactions and the Skin*
    Blackwell, Oxford, 179 (passim)
(1988): Leen CLS+, *Lancet* 2, 1250
Vasculitis
Xerosis

Mucosal/ENT
Ageusia
Anosmia
Dysgeusia (1.7%) (metallic taste)
(2002): Lai A Fat E+, *Int J Dermatol* 41, 796
Gingivitis
Xerostomia
(1995): Costa JM+, *Rev Soc Bras Med Trop* 28(4), 405

Other
Headache
Injection-site calcification
(1987): Goa KL+, *Drugs* 33, 242
Injection-site irritation
(1996): Andersen JM, *Am J Health Syst Pharm* 53, 185
(1996): Herrero-Ambrosio A+, *Am J Health Syst Pharm* 53, 2881
Injection-site pain
(2002): Lai A Fat E+, *Int J Dermatol* 41, 796
Injection-site reactions (sic) (>10%)
(1992): Jones RS+, *Clin Infect Dis* 15, 561
Injection-site ulceration
(1991): Bolognia JL, *Dermatologica* 183, 221
Myalgia/Myositis/Myopathy/Myotoxicity (<5%)
Phlebitis
Rhabdomyolysis
(2004): Hauben M+, *Br J Clin Pharmacol* 58(6), 675
(2003): Delobel P+, *J Antimicrob Chemother* 51(5), 1319
(2003): Lightburn E+, *Med Trop (Mars)* 63(1), 35
(1985): Sensakovic JW+, *Arch Intern Med* 145(12), 2247

PENTAZOCINE

Trade names: Fortral; Fortwin; Liticon; Ospronim; Pentafen;
Sosegon; Susevin; Talacen; Talwin (Hospira)
Indications: Pain
Category: Opiate agonist
Half-life: 2–3 hours
**Clinically important, potentially hazardous interactions
with:** cimetidine, morphine

Reactions

Skin
Calcification
(1990): Furner BB, *J Am Acad Dermatol* 694 (passim)
Cellulitis
(1992): Breathnach SM+, *Adverse Drug Reactions and the Skin*
    Blackwell, Oxford, 212 (passim)
Dermatitis
Diaphoresis
Exanthems
(1987): Pedragosa R+, *Arch Dermatol* 123, 297
Facial edema
Generalized eruption (sic)
(1992): Breathnach SM+, *Adverse Drug Reactions and the Skin*
    Blackwell, Oxford, 212 (passim)
Pigmentation (surrounding ulcers)
(1990): Furner BB, *J Am Acad Dermatol* 694 (passim)
Pruritus (<1%)
Rash (sic) (1–10%)
Scleroderma
(2000): D'Cruz D, *Toxicol Lett* 112 and 421
(1991): Bourgeois P+, *Baillieres Clin Rheumatol* 5, 13
Sclerosis
(1980): Palestine RF+, *J Am Acad Dermatol* 2, 47
Toxic epidermal necrolysis (<1%)
(1987): Pedragosa R+, *Arch Dermatol* 123, 297 (passim)
Ulcerations
(2005): Prasad HR+, *Int J Dermatol* 44(11), 910
(1992): Breathnach SM+, *Adverse Drug Reactions and the Skin*
    Blackwell, Oxford, 212 (passim)
(1990): Furner BB, *J Am Acad Dermatol* 694
(1980): Palestine RF+, *J Am Acad Dermatol* 2, 47
Urticaria

Mucosal/ENT
Dysgeusia
Tinnitus
Xerostomia (1–10%)

Other
Embolia cutis medicamentosa (Nicolau syndrome)
(1983): Bockers M+, *Med Welt* (German) 34, 1450
Injection-site calcification
(1991): Magee KL+, *Arch Dermatol* 127, 1591
(1986): Hertzman A+, *J Rheumatol* 13, 210
Injection-site fibrosis
Injection-site granuloma
(1982): Menon PA, *J Assoc Military Dermatol* 2, 65
Injection-site induration
(1996): Bellman B+, *Arch Dermatol* 132, 1365
(1996): Gillum P, Oklahoma City, OK (from Internet)
    (observation)
(1984): Choucair AK+, *Neurology* 34, 524
(1983): Adams EM+, *Arch Intern Med* 143, 2203
Injection-site pain
Injection-site pigmentation

(1980): Palestine RF+, *J Am Acad Dermatol* 2, 47
Injection-site scleroderma
    (2004): Ho J+, *Dermatol Surg* 30(9), 1252
Lipogranulomas
Panniculitis (chronic)
    (1992): Breathnach SM+, *Adverse Drug Reactions and the Skin*
       Blackwell, Oxford, 212 (passim)
Paresthesias
Phlebitis
    (1992): Breathnach SM+, *Adverse Drug Reactions and the Skin*
       Blackwell, Oxford, 212 (passim)

PENTOBARBITAL

Trade names: Medinox Mono; Mintal; Nova Rectal;
Pentobarbitone; Prodromol; Sombutol
Indications: Insomnia, sedation
Category: Barbiturate
Half-life: 15–50 hours
Clinically important, potentially hazardous interactions
with: alcohol, anticoagulants, antihistamines, brompheniramine,
buclizine, chlorpheniramine, dicumarol, ethanolamine, imatinib,
nalbuphine, warfarin

Reactions

Skin
Acne
Angioedema (<1%)
Bullous dermatitis
Erythema multiforme
Exanthems
Exfoliative dermatitis (<1%)
Fixed eruption
Herpes simplex (activation)
Lupus erythematosus
Necrosis
Photosensitivity
Pruritus
Purpura
Rash (sic) (<1%)
Stevens–Johnson syndrome (<1%)
Toxic epidermal necrolysis
Urticaria
Vasculitis

Mucosal/ENT
Oral ulceration

Other
Headache
Hypersensitivity
Injection-site pain (1–10%)
Injection-site reactions (sic) (<1%)
Porphyria
Porphyria variegata
Rhabdomyolysis
    (1990): Larpin R+, *Presse Med* 19(30), 1403
Thrombophlebitis (<1%)

PENTOSAN

Synonym: PPS
Trade name: Elmiron (Ortho-McNeil)
Indications: Bladder pain, interstitial cystitis
Category: Analgesic, urinary
Half-life: 4.8 hours

Reactions

Skin
Allergic reactions (sic) (<1%)
Photosensitivity (<1%)
Pruritus (<1%)
Purpura (<1%)
Rash (sic) (1–10%)
Urticaria (<1%)

Mucosal/ENT
Gingivitis (<1%)
Oral ulceration (<1%)

Hair
Hair – alopecia (1–10%)

Other
Headache
    (2005): Nickel JC+, *J Urol* 173(4), 1252

PENTOSTATIN

Trade name: Nipent (SuperGen)
Indications: Hairy-cell leukemia
Category: Antimetabolite; Antineoplastic
Half-life: 5–15 hours
Clinically important, potentially hazardous interactions
with: aldesleukin, clofazimine

Reactions

Skin
Acne (<3%)
Adverse effects (sic) (17%)
Allergic granulomatous angiitis (Churg–Strauss syndrome)
    (2002): Sironi M+, *Histopathology* 40(5), 483
Allergic reactions (sic) (>10%)
Bullous dermatitis (3–10%)
Dermatitis (<1%)
Diaphoresis (3–10%)
Eczema (3–10%)
Erythema
Erythroderma
    (1999): Ghura HS+, *BMJ* 319, 549
Exanthems (3–10%)
    (1997): Greiner D+, *J Am Acad Dermatol* 36, 950
    (1989): O'Dwyer PJ+, *Cancer Chemother Pharmacol* 23, 173
Exfoliative dermatitis (<3%)
Facial edema (<3%)
Herpes simplex (3–10%)
Herpes zoster (3–10%)
    (2000): Kurzrock R, *Semin Oncol* 27(2 Suppl 5), 64
    (1999): Kurzrock R+, *J Clin Oncol* 17(10), 3117
    (1999): Ribeiro P+, *Cancer* 85(1), 65
Peripheral edema (3–10%)

Petechiae (3–10%)
Photosensitivity (<3%)
Pigmentation (3–10%)
Pruritus (3–10%)
Psoriasis (<3%)
Purpura (<3%)
  (1999): Leach JW+, *Am J Hematol* 61, 268
Rash (sic) (26%)
  (2000): Kraut EH, *Semin Oncol* 27(2 Suppl 5), 27
  (1992): Shimoyama M+, *Jpn J Clin Oncol* 22(6), 406
Recall reaction
  (1989): Kerker BJ+, *Semin Dermatol* 8, 173
  (1985): Camisa C+, *J Am Acad Dermatol* 12, 1108
Seborrhea (3–10%)
Urticaria (<1%)
Xerosis (3–10%)

Mucosal/ENT
Dysgeusia (<3%)
Gingivitis (<3%)
Leukoplakia (<3%)
Stomatitis (1–10%)
Tinnitus
Vaginitis (<3%)

Hair
Hair – alopecia (<3%)

Eyes
Conjunctivitis
  (1996): Monfardini S+, *Oncology* 53(2), 163 (7%)
Keratoconjunctivitis
  (1996): Spiers AS, *Haematologia (Budap)* 27(2), 55

Other
Anaphylactoid reactions/Anaphylaxis (<3%)
Candidiasis (<3%)
Fever
  (1999): Kurzrock R+, *J Clin Oncol* 17(10), 3117
  (1999): Ribeiro P+, *Cancer* 85(1), 65
  (1992): Kane BJ+, *Ann Pharmacother* 26(7–8), 939
  (1992): Shimoyama M+, *Jpn J Clin Oncol* 22(6), 406
Gynecomastia (<3%)
Headache
Hepatotoxicity
  (2000): Ho AD+, *Semin Oncol* 27(2 Suppl 5), 52 (3%)
  (2000): Margolis J+, *Semin Oncol* 27(2 Suppl 5), 9
  (1999): Sanchez M+, *Br J Haematol* 105(1), 316
  (1996): Spiers AS, *Haematologia (Budap)* 27(2), 55
Infections
  (2000): Ho AD+, *Semin Oncol* 27(2 Suppl 5), 52 (10%)
  (1996): Spiers AS, *Haematologia (Budap)* 27(2), 55
  (1992): Kane BJ+, *Ann Pharmacother* 26(7–8), 939
Injection-site bleeding (<3%)
Injection-site inflammation (<3%)
Myalgia/Myositis/Myopathy/Myotoxicity (>10%)
Nephrotoxicity
  (2001): Kintzel PE, *Drug Saf* 24(1), 19
Paresthesias (3–10%)
Thrombophlebitis (3–10%)

PENTOXIFYLLINE

Trade names: Apo-Pentoxifylline; Artal; Azupentat; Elorgan; Hemovas; Pentoxi; Pentoxil (Upsher-Smith); Pexal; Torental; Trental (Sanofi-Aventis)
Indications: Peripheral vascular disease, intermittent claudication
Category: Vasodilator, peripheral; Xanthine alkaloid
Half-life: 0.4–0.8 hours
Clinically important, potentially hazardous interactions with: ceftobiprole

Reactions

Skin
Allergic reactions (sic)
  (1986): Bigby M+, *JAMA* 256, 3358
Angioedema (<1%)
  (1994): Samlaska CP+, *J Am Acad Dermatol* 30, 603 (passim)
Diaphoresis
Edema (<1%)
Exanthems
Pruritus (<1%)
  (1994): Samlaska CP+, *J Am Acad Dermatol* 30, 603 (passim)
Purpura
Rash (sic) (<1%)
Urticaria

Mucosal/ENT
Dysgeusia (<1%)
Dysphagia
  (1997): Fetterman M, Miami, FL (from Internet) (observation)
  (1997): Puritz E, Smithtown, NY (from Internet) (observation)
Sialorrhea (<1%)
Xerostomia (<1%)
  (1996): Huizinga TW+, *Ann Rheum Dis* 55(11), 833
  (1994): Samlaska CP+, *J Am Acad Dermatol* 30, 603 (passim)

Nails
Nails – brittle (<1%)

Other
Aseptic meningitis
  (2002): Mathian A+, *Neurology* 59(9), 1468
Headache
Paresthesias
  (1994): Samlaska CP+, *J Am Acad Dermatol* 30, 603 (passim)
Serum sickness
  (1986): Panwalker AP+, *Drug Intell Clin Pharm* 20, 953
Tremor

PEPLOMYCIN

Trade name: Peplomycin (Nihon Kayaku)
Indications: Chemotherapy
Category: Antibiotic, anthracycline
Half-life: N/A

Reactions

Skin
Scleroderma
  (2004): Asano Y+, *Br J Dermatol* 150(6), 1213
Stevens–Johnson syndrome
  (2004): Umebayashi Y+, *J Dermatol* 31(10), 802

Hair

Hair – alopecia
   (1999): Kishi K+, *Radiology* 213, 173 (transient)

Eyes

Conjunctivitis
   (2004): Umebayashi Y+, *J Dermatol* 31(10), 802

PEPPERMINT

Scientific name: *Mentha piperita*
Family: Labiatae
Trade and other common names: Aludrox; brandy mint; Colpermin; Enteroplant (peppermint and caraway oils); menthol; PCC
Category: Analgesic; Carminative; Vasodilator, peripheral
Purported indications and other uses: Dyspepsia, regress pancreatic, mammary, and liver tumors, irritable bowel syndrome, colonic spasm, colic, nausea, vomiting, biliary disorders, common cold, dysmenorrhoea, anxiolytic. **Topical:** pain, itching, inflammations, headaches, toothache, pruritus, urticaria, mosquito repellant. **Vapor:** bronchial catarrh, fever, influenza. Flavoring, cosmetics, toothpaste, mouthwash
Half-life: N/A
Clinically important, potentially hazardous interactions with: cisapride

Reactions

Skin

Adverse effects (sic)
   (1999): Madisch A+, *Arzneimittelforschung* 49(11), 925
   (1996): May B+, *Arzneimittelforschung* 46(12), 1149
Allergic reactions (sic)
Burning (anal)
   (1987): Weston CF, *Postgrad Med J* 63(742), 717
Dermatitis
   (2002): Schempp CM+, *Hautarzt* 53(2), 93
   (1994): Wilkinson SM+, *Contact Dermatitis* 30(1), 42
   (1984): Mooller NE+, *Acta Pharmacol Toxicol* (Copenh) 55(2), 139 (occupational)
Lichenoid eruption
   (1995): Morton CA+, *Contact Dermatitis* 32(5), 281
Perioral dermatitis
   (1995): Sainio EL+, *Contact Dermatitis* 33(2), 100
Rash (sic)
   (1997): Liu JH+, *J Gastroenterol* 32(6), 765
Sensitivity
   (2001): Nair B, *Int J Toxicol* 20, 61
   (1995): Morton CA+, *Contact Dermatitis* 32(5), 281

Mucosal/ENT

Burning mouth syndrome
   (1995): Morton CA+, *Contact Dermatitis* 32(5), 281
Cheilitis
   (1995): Sainio EL+, *Contact Dermatitis* 33(2), 100
   (1984): Hausen BM, *Dtsch Med Wochenschr* 109(8), 300
Gingivitis
   (1995): Sainio EL+, *Contact Dermatitis* 33(2), 100
Glossitis
   (1995): Sainio EL+, *Contact Dermatitis* 33(2), 100
Oral ulceration
   (1999): Moghadam BK+, *Cutis* 64(2), 131 (mouthwash abuse)
   (1995): Morton CA+, *Contact Dermatitis* 32(5), 281
Stomatitis

   (1995): Rogers SN+, *Dent Update* 22(1), 36
   (1995): Sainio EL+, *Contact Dermatitis* 33(2), 100

Other

Hypersensitivity
   (1995): Sainio EL+, *Contact Dermatitis* 33(2), 100
Side effects (sic)
   (1998): Belanger JT, *Altern Med Rev* 3(6), 448
   (1982): Jaffe G+, *J Int Med Res* 10(6), 437
Toxicity (sic)
   (2001): Lazutka JR+, *Food Chem Toxicol* 39(5), 485

PERFLUTREN

Trade names: Definity (DuPont); Optison (Amersham)
Indications: Echocardiogram imaging
Category: Radiographic contrast medium
Half-life: 1.3 minutes

Reactions

Skin

Diaphoresis (<0.5%)
Erythema (0.7%)
Exanthems (<0.5%)
Hematomas (<0.5%)
Pruritus (<0.5%)
Rash (sic) (<0.5%)
Urticaria (<0.5%)
Xerosis (<0.5%)

Mucosal/ENT

Dysgeusia (<0.5%)
Rhinitis (<0.5%)
Tongue disorder (sic) (<0.5%)
Xerostomia (<0.5%)

Eyes

Conjunctivitis (<0.5%)
Visual disturbances (<0.5%)

Other

Abdominal pain (<0.5%)
Application-site reactions (sic) (0.6%)
Asthenia (<0.5%)
Chest pain (0.8%)
Cough (<0.5%)
Death
Fever (<0.5%)
Headache (2.3%)
Hypertension (<0.5%)
Hypotension (<0.5%)
Pain (<0.5%)
Paresthesias (<0.5%)
Vertigo (0.6%)

PERGOLIDE

Trade names: Celance; Parkotil; Pergolide; Permax (Lilly)
Indications: Parkinsonism
Category: Dopamine receptor agonist; Ergot alkaloid
Half-life: 27 hours

Reactions

Skin

Acne
Diaphoresis (2.1%)
Edema (1.6%)
  (2005): Bianchi M+, *Clin Neuropharmacol* 28(5), 245
Exanthems
Facial edema (1.1%)
  (1993): Garcia-Escrig M+, *Medicina Clinica* (Spanish) 101, 275
Peripheral edema (1–10%)
  (2000): Varsano S+, *Respiration* 67(5), 580
Pigmentation
Pruritus
Rash (sic) (3.2%)
Seborrhea
Ulcerations
Urticaria
Vasculitis
  (2002): Serratrice J+, *Rev Med Interne* 23(9), 800
  (1989): Horn TD+, *Arch Dermatol* 125, 1512
Xerosis

Mucosal/ENT

Dysgeusia (1.6%)
Gingivitis (<1%)
Tinnitus
Xerostomia (1–10%)

Hair

Hair – alopecia
  (1988): Factor SA+, *J Neurol Neurosurg Psychiatry* 51(4), 529
Hair – hirsutism

Other

Chest pain
  (1988): Ahlskog JE+, *Mayo Clin Proc* 63(10), 969
Chills (1–10%)
Erythromelalgia
  (1989): Horn TD+, *Arch Dermatol* 125, 1512
  (1984): Monk BE+, *Br J Dermatol* 111, 97 (on shins)
Fever
  (1991): Lamberts SW+, *J Clin Endocrinol Metab* 72(3), 635
Fibrosis
  (2004): Agarwal P+, *Mov Disord* 19(6), 699
  (2000): Mondal BK+, *Int J Clin Pract* 54(6), 403
Hypotension
  (1991): Pezzoli G+, *Clin Ter* 136(1), 39
  (1990): Kando JC+, *DICP* 24(5), 543
Myalgia/Myositis/Myopathy/Myotoxicity (<1%)
Paresthesias (1.6%)
Tremor (1–10%)
Vertigo
  (1988): Ahlskog JE+, *Mayo Clin Proc* 63(10), 969

PERINDOPRIL

Trade names: Aceon (Solvay); Acertil; Coversum; Coversyl; Prexum
Indications: Hypertension
Category: Angiotensin-converting enzyme inhibitor
Half-life: 1.5–3 hours

Reactions

Skin

Allergic reactions (sic) (1.3%)
  (1993): Desche P+, *Am J Cardiol* 71, 61E
Angioedema (<1%)
  (2001): Cohen EG+, *Ann Otol Rhinol Laryngol* 110(8), 701 (64 cases)
  (1998): Lapostolle F+, *Am J Cardiol* 81, 523 (lingual)
Diaphoresis (0.3–1%)
Edema (3.9%)
Erythema (0.3–1%)
Exanthems
Facial edema (<1%)
Herpes simplex (0.3–1%)
Palmar–plantar pustulosis
  (1995): Eriksen JG+, *Ugeskr Laeger* (Danish) 157, 3335
Pemphigus foliaceus
  (2000): Ong CS+, *Australas J Dermatol* 41(4), 242
Pruritus (1–10%)
Psoriasis (<1%)
Purpura (<0.1%)
Rash (sic) (1–10%)
  (1991): Dratwa M+, *J Cardiovasc Pharmacol* 18, S40
Xerosis (0.3–1%)

Mucosal/ENT

Dysgeusia (<1%)
Vaginitis (0.3–1%)
Xerostomia (0.3–1%)

Other

Anaphylactoid reactions/Anaphylaxis (<1%)
  (1998): Speirs C+, *Br J Clin Pharmacol* 46, 63
Chills (<1%)
Cough
  (2007): Tumanan-Mendoza BA+, *J Clin Epidemiol* 60(6), 547
  (2005): Bavanandan S+, *Med J Malaysia* 60(2), 158 (14%)
  (2005): Tsuruoka S+, *J Clin Pharmacol* 45(11), 1319
  (2004): Guo W+, *Am J Ther* 11(3), 199 (8%)
  (2004): Neutel JM+, *Am J Cardiovasc Drugs* 4(5), 335 (7%)
  (2002): Ragot S+, *Arch Mal Coeur Vaiss* 95(7–8), 738
  (2002): Simpson D+, *Drugs* 62(9), 1367
  (2001): Adigun AQ+, *West Afr J Med* 20(1), 46
  (2001): Clark LT, *Am J Cardiol* 88(7), 36i
  (2001): Hurst M+, *Drugs* 61(6), 867
  (2001): Lee SC+, *Hypertension* 38(2), 166
  (2000): Lee YJ+, *Diabetes Care* 23(3), 427
  (1990): Brown CL, *J Hum Hypertens* 4 Suppl 4, 51
  (1989): Santoni JP+, *Arch Mal Coeur Vaiss* 82 Spec No 1, 87
Headache
Myalgia/Myositis/Myopathy/Myotoxicity (<1%)
Paresthesias (2.3%)

PERPHENAZINE

Trade names: Apo-Perphenzine; Decentan; Etrafon; Fentazin; Leptopsique; Peratsin; Perphenan; Triavil; Trilafon (Schering); Trilifan Retard; Triomin
Indications: Psychotic disorders, nausea and vomiting
Category: Antipsychotic, phenothiazine
Half-life: 9 hours
Clinically important, potentially hazardous interactions with: sparfloxacin

Note: Etrafon and Triavil are combinations of perphenazine and amitriptyline

Reactions

Skin

Acute febrile neutrophilic dermatosis (Sweet's syndrome)
  (2004): Mecca P+, *J Cutan Pathol* 31(2), 189 (with citalopram and amoxapine) (photodistributed)
Angioedema
Dermatitis
Diaphoresis
Eczema
Erythema
Exanthems
Exfoliative dermatitis
Lupus erythematosus
  (1988): Steen VD+, *Arthritis Rheum* 31, 923
  (1986): Gupta MA+, *J Am Acad Dermatol* 14, 638
Peripheral edema
Photosensitivity
Pigmentation (blue-gray) (<1%)
Pruritus
Purpura
Rash (sic) (1–10%)
Seborrhea
Urticaria
Xerosis

Mucosal/ENT

Sialorrhea
Tinnitus
Xerostomia

Other

Anaphylactoid reactions/Anaphylaxis
Congestive heart failure
  (2003): Ansari A+, *Tex Heart Inst J* 30(1), 76
Gynecomastia
Headache
Pseudolymphoma
  (1995): Magro CM+, *J Am Acad Dermatol* 32, 419
Rhabdomyolysis
  (1983): Caruana RJ+, *N C Med J* 44, 18 (with lorazepam and amitriptyline)
  (1983): Lefkowitz D+, *J Neurol Neurosurg Psychiatry* 46(2), 183 (with amitriptyline)

PHELLODENDRON

Scientific names: *Phellodendron amurense; Phellodendron chinense; Phellodendron wilsonii*
Family: Rutaceae
Trade and other common names: Amur Cork-tree; Chuan huangbo; Cortex Phellodendri; Guan huangbo; Huang Bai; Nexrutine (Next Pharma); phellamurin. Ingredient in Oren-gedoku-to, zhi bai kuncao tang and Shangke Wangshui
Category: COX-2 selective inhibitor; Immunosuppressant
Purported indications and other uses: anti-inflammatory, muscle and joint pain, gastroenteritis, abdominal pain, diarrhea, gastric ulcers, thrush, cholera, night sweats, fever, nocturnal emissions, dysentery, jaundice, leukorrhea, weakness and edema of legs, consumptive fever. **Topical:** sores, skin infection with local redness and swelling, eczema with itching, periodontal disease (in dentifrice)
Half-life: N/A
Clinically important, potentially hazardous interactions with: aspirin, cyclosporine, NSAIDs

Reactions

Skin

Edema

PHENAZOPYRIDINE

Trade names: Azodine; Baridium; Eridium; Geridium; Phenazo; Prodium; Pyridiate; Pyridium (Warner Chilcott); Pyronium; Sedural; Urodine; Urogesic; Urohman; Uropyridin
Indications: Urinary urgency, dysuria
Category: Analgesic, urinary
Half-life: N/A

Reactions

Skin

Allergic reactions (sic) (<1%)
  (1986): Bigby M+, *JAMA* 256, 3358 (0.88%)
Edema
Exanthems (<1%)
Pigmentation (<1%)
Pruritus
Rash (sic) (<1%)

Nails

Nails – pigmentation
  (1997): Amit G+, *Ann Intern Med* 127, 1137

Other

Anaphylactoid reactions/Anaphylaxis
Headache

PHENDIMETRAZINE

Trade names: Bontril (Amarin); Obesan-X
Indications: Obesity
Category: Amphetamine
Half-life: 5–12.5 hours
**Clinically important, potentially hazardous interactions
with:** cyclobenzaprine, fluoxetine, fluvoxamine, MAO inhibitors, paroxetine, phenelzine, sertraline, tranylcypromine

Note: Phendimetrazine has been withdrawn in the European Union and some other countries

Reactions

Skin
Diaphoresis
Rash (sic)
   (1998): Markowitz GS+, *Clin Nephrol* 50(4), 252 (with phentermine)
Urticaria

Mucosal/ENT
Dysgeusia
Xerostomia

Other
Death
   (1989): Kintz P+, *Forensic Sci Int 1989 Feb* 40(2), 153
Headache
   (1993): Kokkinos J+, *Stroke* 24(2), 310
Nephrotoxicity
   (1998): Markowitz GS+, *Clin Nephrol* 50(4), 252 (with phentermine)
Rhabdomyolysis
   (2006): Kwiker D+, *Am J Ther* 13(2), 175
Stroke
   (1993): Kokkinos J+, *Stroke* 24(2), 310

PHENELZINE

Trade names: Nardelzine; Nardil (Pfizer)
Indications: Depression
Category: Antidepressant; Monoamine oxidase (MAO) inhibitor; Muscarinic antagonist
Half-life: N/A
**Clinically important, potentially hazardous interactions
with:** amitriptyline, amoxapine, amphetamines, bupropion, citalopram, clomipramine, cyproheptadine, desipramine, dextroamphetamine, dextromethorphan, diethylpropion, dopamine, doxepin, entacapone, **ephedra**, ephedrine, epinephrine, fluoxetine, fluvoxamine, **ginseng**, imipramine, levodopa, mazindol, meperidine, methamphetamine, nefazodone, nortriptyline, paroxetine, phendimetrazine, phentermine, phenylephrine, propoxyphene, protriptyline, pseudoephedrine, rizatriptan, sertraline, sibutramine, sumatriptan, sympathomimetics, tramadol, tricyclic antidepressants, trimipramine, **tryptophan**, venlafaxine, zolmitriptan

Reactions

Skin
Angioedema
Diaphoresis
   (1985): Levy AB+, *Can J Psychiatry* 30, 434

Edema
Exanthems
Lupus erythematosus
Peripheral edema
Photosensitivity
   (1988): Case JD+, *Photodermatology* 5, 101
Pruritus (13%)
Rash (sic)
Telangiectasia
Urticaria

Mucosal/ENT
Glossitis
   (1992): Zürcher K+, *Cutaneous Drug Reactions* Karger, Basel
   (passim)
Tinnitus
   (1981): Glass RM+, *J Clin Psychopharmacol* 1(3), 152
Tongue black
Xerostomia (1–10%)

Other
Headache
Inappropriate secretion of antidiuretic hormone (SIADH)
   (1989): Giese AA+, *J Clin Psychopharmacol* 9(4), 309
Rhabdomyolysis
   (1984): Linden CH+, *Ann Emerg Med* 13(12), 1137
Tremor
Vertigo
   (2004): Birkenhager TK+, *J Clin Psychiatry* 65(11), 1505 (21%)

PHENINDAMINE

Trade name: Nolahist
Indications: Allergic rhinitis, urticaria, angioedema
Category: Histamine H1 receptor antagonist
Half-life: N/A

Reactions

Skin
Angioedema
Dermatitis
Diaphoresis
Erythema
Lupus erythematosus
Photosensitivity
Purpura
Rash (sic)
Urticaria

Mucosal/ENT
Xerostomia

PHENOBARBITAL

Synonyms: phenobarbitone; phenylethylmalonylurea
Trade names: Alepsal; Barbilixir; Barbita; Barbital; Gardenal; Luminal (Sanofi-Aventis); Luminaletten; Phenaemal; Phenobarbitone; Solfoton
Indications: Insomnia, seizures
Category: Anticonvulsant; Barbiturate
Half-life: 2–6 days
Clinically important, potentially hazardous interactions with: alcohol, anticoagulants, antihistamines, betamethasone, brompheniramine, buclizine, buprenorphine, chlorpheniramine, darunavir, dasatinib, delavirdine, dexamethasone, dicumarol, ethanolamine, fluconazole, flunisolide, fosamprenavir, hydrocortisone, imatinib, **influenza vaccines**, lapatinib, meperidine, methylprednisolone, midazolam, prednisolone, prednisone, solifenacin, telithromycin, temsirolimus, teniposide, triamcinolone, warfarin

Reactions

Skin

Acne
  (1992): Hesse S+, *Ann Dermatol Venereol* (French) 119, 655
Acute generalized exanthematous pustulosis (AGEP)
  (1996): Wolkenstein P+, *Contact Dermatitis* 35, 234
Allergic reactions (sic)
  (1987): Pigatto PD, *Contact Dermatitis* 16, 279
Angioedema (<1%)
Bullous dermatitis
  (1990): Dunn C+, *Cutis* 45, 43 (in coma)
Depigmentation
  (1992): Mion N+, *Ann Dermatol Venereol* (French) 119, 927
Diaphoresis
  (2006): Tanabe Y, *No To Shinkei* 58(8), 687
Edema
  (2006): Tanabe Y, *No To Shinkei* 58(8), 687
Erythema multiforme
  (1994): Shelley WB+, *Cutis* 53, 162 (observation)
  (1994): Stewart MG+, *Otolaryngol Head Neck Surg* 111, 236
  (1990): Salomon D+, *Br J Dermatol* 123, 797
  (1988): Shear NH+, *J Clin Invest* 82, 1826
  (1986): Palomeque A+, *An Esp Pediatr* (Spanish) 34, 328
Erythroderma
  (1993): Sakai C+, *Intern Med* 32, 182
Exanthems
  (2001): Hebert AA+, *J Clin Psychiatry* 62 (suppl 14), 22
  (1997): Hyson C+, *Can J Neurol Sci* 24, 245
  (1988): Shear NH+, *J Clin Invest* 82, 1826
  (1986): Savich RD+, *Ill Med J* 169, 232
  (1984): Fernandez de Corres L+, *Contact Dermatitis* 11, 319
Exfoliative dermatitis (<1%)
  (1993): Sakai C+, *Intern Med* 32, 182
  (1986): Savich RD+, *Ill Med J* 169, 232
Fixed eruption
  (2002): Hashizume H+, *J Immunol* 168(10), 5359
  (1998): Mahboob A+, *Int J Dermatol* 37, 833
  (1989): Shiohara T+, *Arch Dermatol* 125, 1371
  (1987): Savchak VI, *Vestn Dermatol Venerol* (Russian) 6, 62
Graft-versus-host reaction
  (1998): Jappe U+, *Hautarzt* (German) 49, 126 (passim)
Herpes simplex (activation)
Lupus erythematosus
Necrosis
Pemphigus
  (1986): Dourmishev AL+, *Dermatologica* 173, 256

Peripheral edema
  (1982): Stadler R+, *Hautarzt* (German) 33, 276
Photosensitivity
Pigmentation
  (2006): Tanabe Y, *No To Shinkei* 58(8), 687
Pruritus
  (1994): Sigl B, *Hautarzt* (German) 45, 409
Purpura
Pustules (generalized)
  (1991): Kleier RS+, *Arch Dermatol* 127, 1361
Rash (sic) (<1%)
  (2007): Arif H+, *Neurology* 68(20), 1701
Stevens–Johnson syndrome (<1%)
  (2005): Mockenhaupt M+, *Neurology* 64(7), 1134
  (1999): Duncan KO, *J Am Acad Dermatol* 40, 493 (at sites of radiation therapy)
  (1999): Rzany B+, *Lancet* 353, 2190
  (1995): Labandiera-Garcia J, *An Med Interna* (Spanish) 12, 569
  (1995): Wolkenstein P+, *Arch Dermatol* 131, 544
  (1994): Koukoulis A+, *An Med Interna* (Spanish) 11, 311
  (1993): Leenutaphong V+, *Int J Dermatol* 32, 428
  (1992): Lleonart R+, *Med Clin* (Barc) (Spanish) 99, 474
  (1985): Avery JK, *J Tenn Med Assoc* 78, 764
  (1985): de Rego JA+, *Hillside J Clin Psychiatry* 7, 141
  (1982): Brahams D, *Lancet* 2, 1474
  (1982): Oles KS+, *Clin Pharm* 1, 565
Toxic epidermal necrolysis
  (2004): Vincenzi B+, *J Clin Oncol* 22(22), 4649
  (2000): Devidal R+, *Therapie* 55, 225 (2 cases)
  (1999): Rzany B+, *Lancet* 353, 2190
  (1996): Blum L+, *J Am Acad Dermatol* 34, 1088
  (1995): Wolkenstein P+, *Arch Dermatol* 131, 544
  (1994): Errani A+, *Br J Dermatol* 131, 586
  (1994): Shelley WB+, *Cutis* 53, 162 (observation)
  (1993): Correia O I, *Dermatology* 186, 32
  (1993): Leenutaphong V+, *Int J Dermatol* 32, 428
  (1989): Dominguez-Perez F+, *Rev Esp Anestesiol Reanim* (Spanish) 36, 350
  (1988): Shear NH+, *J Clin Invest* 82, 1826
  (1987): Teillac D+, *Arch Fr Pediatr* (French) 44, 583
  (1985): de Rego JA+, *Hillside J Clin Psychiatry* 7, 141
  (1984): Chan HL, *J Am Acad Dermatol* 10, 973
Toxicoderma
  (1998): Arima M+, *Jpn Circ J* 62, 132
Urticaria
Vasculitis

Mucosal/ENT
Gingival hyperplasia/hypertrophy
  (2002): Sinha S+, *J Neurol Neurosurg Psychiatry* 73(5), 601
Oral ulceration
Xerostomia

Hair
Hair – poliosis
  (1992): Mion N+, *Ann Dermatol Venereol* (French) 119, 927

Nails
Nails – hypoplasia
  (1991): Thakker JC+, *Indian Pediatr* 28, 73
  (1990): Holder M+, *Monatsschr Kinderheilkr* (German) 138, 34

Other
Anticonvulsant hypersensitivity syndrome
  (2005): Ito T+, *Rinsho Shinkeigaku* 45(7), 495
  (2004): Bavdekar SB+, *Ann Pharmacother* 2004 Oct;38(10), 1648
  (2004): Papp Z+, *Orv Hetil* 145(32), 1665
  (2002): Galindo PA+, *J Investig Allergol Clin Immunol* 12(4), 299
  (2002): Kaur S+, *Pediatr Dermatol* 19(2), 142
  (1997): Morkunas AR+, *Crit Care Clin* 13(4), 727

(1995): Vittorio CC+, *Arch Intern Med* 155(21), 2285
Death
DRESS syndrome
  (2007): Giordano N+, *Clin Exp Rheumatol* 25(2), 339
  (2004): Allam JP+, *Eur J Dermatol* 14(5), 339
  (2003): Baruzzi A+, *Clin Neuropharmacol* 26(4), 177
  (2001): Lachgar T+, *Allerg Immunol* (Paris) 33(4), 173
  (1997): Descamps V+, *Br J Dermatol* 137, 605
Headache
Hypersensitivity (<1%)
  (2004): Criado PR+, *J Dermatol* 31(12), 1009
  (2002): Metin A+, *World Congress Dermatol* Poster, 0116
  (1999): Moss DM+, *J Emerg Med* 17, 503
  (1998): Chapman MS+, *Br J Dermatol* 138, 710
  (1998): Schlienger RG+, *Epilepsia* 39, S3 (passim)
  (1997): Morkunas AR+, *Crit Care Clin* 13, 727
  (1992): Nagata T+, *Jpn J Clin Oncol* 22, 421
  (1984): Fonseca JC+, *Med Cutan Ibero Lat Am* (Spanish) 12, 187
Injection-site bullous eruption
  (1987): Haroun M+, *Cutis* 39, 233
Injection-site pain (>10%)
Injection-site thrombophlebitis (>10%)
Pain
  (2006): Tanabe Y, *No To Shinkei* 58(8), 687
Porphyria cutanea tarda
Porphyria variegata
Rhabdomyolysis
  (1990): Larpin R+, *Presse Med* 19(30), 1403

PHENOLPHTHALEIN

Trade names: Agoral; Alophen; Bom-Bon; Bonomint; Caroid; Correctol; Darmol; Doxidan; Easylax; Espotabs; Evac-U-Gen; Ex-Lax (Novartis); Feen-A-Mint; Medilax; Phenolax; Prulet; Purganol; Ruguletts; Trilax
Indications: Constipation
Category: Stimulant laxative
Half-life: N/A

Reactions

Skin
Angioedema
Bullous dermatitis
Diaphoresis
Erythema annulare
Erythema multiforme
  (1992): Breathnach SM+, *Adverse Drug Reactions and the Skin*
    Blackwell, Oxford, 344
Exanthems
Exfoliative dermatitis
Fixed eruption
  (1997): Blumenthal HL, Beachwood, OH (personal case)
    (observation)
  (1993): Zanolli MD+, *Pediatrics* 91, 1199
  (1991): Smoller BR+, *J Cutan Pathol* 18, 13
  (1990): Gaffoor PMA+, *Cutis* 45, 242
  (1987): Stroud MB+, *Arch Dermatol* 123, 1227
  (1986): Kanwar AJ+, *Dermatologica* 172, 315
  (1985): Kauppinen K+, *Br J Dermatol* 112, 575
  (1984): Chan HL, *Int J Dermatol* 23, 607
Lupus erythematosus
  (1992): Breathnach SM+, *Adverse Drug Reactions and the Skin*
    Blackwell, Oxford, 344
Perianal irritation

Pigmentation
Pruritus
Stevens–Johnson syndrome
Toxic epidermal necrolysis
  (1997): Artymowicz RJ+, *Ann Pharmacother* 31, 1157
  (1986): Kar PK+, *J Indian Med Assoc* 84, 189
Urticaria

Mucosal/ENT
Oral mucosal fixed eruption
Oral pigmentation
Oral ulceration

Nails
Nails – discoloration
  (1984): Daniel CR+, *J Am Acad Dermatol* 10, 250

PHENOXYBENZAMINE

Trade names: Dibenyline; Dibenzyline (Wellspring); Dibenzyran
Indications: Pheochromocytoma
Category: Adrenergic alpha-receptor antagonist
Half-life: 24 hours
Clinically important, potentially hazardous interactions with: epinephrine

Reactions

Skin
Allergic reactions (sic)
Dermatitis
  (1998): Sommer S+, *Contact Dermatitis* 38(6), 352

Mucosal/ENT
Xerostomia (1–10%)
  (1981): Kedia KR+, *Urology* 18(6), 620

Other
Asthenia
  (1981): Kedia KR+, *Urology* 18(6), 620
Death
  (2006): Vaidyanathan S+, *Spinal Cord* 44(3), 188
Hypotension
  (2005): Pan DL+, *Zhonghua Yi Xue Za Zhi* 85(20), 1403
  (2002): O'Blenes SB+, *J Thorac Cardiovasc Surg* 123(5), 1012
  (1984): Ghostine SY+, *J Neurosurg* 60(6), 1263
Vertigo
  (2006): Vaidyanathan S+, *Spinal Cord* 44(3), 188
  (2002): Te AE, *Clin Ther* 24(6), 851

PHENSUXIMIDE

Trade name: Milontin
Indications: Petit mal seizures
Category: Anticonvulsant
Half-life: 5–12 hours

Reactions

Skin
Erythema multiforme (<1%)
Lupus erythematosus
Pruritus
Purpura

(1980): Miescher PA+, *Clin Haematol* 9, 505
Rash (sic)
Stevens–Johnson syndrome

Mucosal/ENT
Gingival hyperplasia/hypertrophy
Oral ulceration

Hair
Hair – alopecia
Hair – hirsutism

Eyes
Periorbital edema

PHENTERMINE

Trade names: Adipex-P (Gate); Behapront; Diminex; Ionamin (Celltech); Minobese-Forte; Panbesy; Panbesyl; Redusa; Umine; Zantryl
Indications: Obesity
Category: Amphetamine
Half-life: 19–24 hours
Clinically important, potentially hazardous interactions with: fluoxetine, fluvoxamine, MAO inhibitors, paroxetine, phenelzine, sertraline, tranylcypromine

Reactions

Skin
Diaphoresis (<1%)
Peripheral edema
Photo-recall
(2006): Ash RB+, *Breast J* 12(2), 186
Purpura
Radiodermatitis
(2006): Ash RB+, *Breast J* 12(2), 186
Rash (sic)
Raynaud's phenomenon
(1990): Aeschlimann A+, *Scand J Rheumatol* 19, 87
Urticaria
Vasculitis
(2006): White RE, Rock Hell, SC (from Internet) (observation)

Mucosal/ENT
Dysgeusia
Xerostomia
(2006): Kim KK+, *Yonsei Med J* 47(5), 614

Hair
Hair – alopecia (<1%)

Eyes
Optic neuropathy
(2005): Chan JW, *Eye* 19(11), 1238

Other
Abdominal pain
(2003): Comay D+, *Can J Gastroenterol* 17(12), 719
Chest pain
(2001): Caccitolo JA+, *J Thorac Cardiovasc Surg* 122(4), 656
Death
(1999): Strother J+, *Arch Pathol Lab Med* 123(6), 539 (with fenfluramine)
(1997): Dillon KA+, *JAMA* 278(16), 1320 (with fenfluramine)
(1997): Mark EJ+, *N Engl J Med* 337(9), 602 (with fenfluramine)
(1984): Levine B+, *J Forensic Sci* 29(4), 1242

Depression
(1983): Douglas A+, *Int J Obes* 7(6), 591
Headache
(1983): Douglas A+, *Int J Obes* 7(6), 591
Hypertension
(2005): Stephens LC+, *Anaesth Intensive Care* 33(4), 525
(2004): Horton MR+, *Crit Rev Comput Tomogr* 45(5–6), 335
(2002): Tomita T+, *Chest 2002 Feb* 121(2), 649 (with fenfluramine)
(2000): Imoberdorf R+, *Ther Umsch* 57(8), 522
(2000): Teramae CY+, *Mayo Clin Proc* 75(5), 456 (13%) (with fenfluramine)
(1999): Strother J+, *Arch Pathol Lab Med* 123(6), 539 (with fenfluramine)
(1998): Goldstein SE+, *Harefuah* 135(11), 489 (with fenfluramine)
(1998): Wolf I+, *Harefuah* 135(11), 515 (with fenfluramine)
(1997): Dillon KA+, *JAMA* 278(16), 1320 (with fenfluramine)
(1983): Douglas A+, *Int J Obes* 7(6), 591
Myalgia/Myositis/Myopathy/Myotoxicity (<1%)
Nephrotoxicity
(1998): Markowitz GS+, *Clin Nephrol* 50(4), 252 (with phendimetrazine)
Tremor

PHENTOLAMINE

Trade names: Regitin; Regitine (Novartis); Rogitene; Rogitine
Indications: Hypertensive episodes in pheochromocytoma
Category: Adrenergic alpha-receptor antagonist
Half-life: 19 minutes

Reactions

Skin
Rash (sic)
(2006): Mizuno J+, *Masui* 55(2), 169

Mucosal/ENT
Rhinitis
(2002): Ugarte F+, *Int J Impot Res* 14 Suppl 2, S48

Other
Headache
(2002): Ugarte F+, *Int J Impot Res* 14 Suppl 2, S48
Hypertension
(1994): Zorgniotti AW, *Int J Impot Res* 6(1), 37

PHENYLBUTAZONE

Trade names: Butatab; Butazolidine; Butazone
Indications: Ankylosing spondylitis, gouty arthritis, osteoarthritis, rheumatoid arthritis
Category: Non-steroidal anti-inflammatory
Half-life: 54–99 hours
Clinically important, potentially hazardous interactions with: anticoagulants, antidiabetics, barbiturates, chlorpheniramine, corticosteroids, digoxin, lithium, methotrexate, methylphenidate, phenytoin, rifampin, sulfonamides

Reactions

Skin
Acne
Acute febrile neutrophilic dermatosis (Sweet's syndrome)
(2008): Levang J+, *Ann Dermatol Venereol* 135(4), 291
Angioedema
(2001): Das J+, *Indian J Dermatol Venereol Leprol* 67(5), 238
(1984): Diez Gomez ML+, *Allergol Immunopathol* (Madrid)
12(3), 179
Bullae
Contact dermatitis
(1995): Kerre S+, *Contact Dermatitis* 33(3), 213
(1991): Nayar M+, *Contact Dermatitis* 25(4), 263
(1982): Brandao FM+, *Contact Dermatitis* 8(4), 264
(1980): Varga M+, *Orv Hetil* 121(11), 625
Dermatomyositis
(1987): Curran JJ+, *J Rheumatol* 14(2), 397
Edema
Erythema multiforme
(1992): Stampien TM+, *Am Fam Physician* 46(4), 1171
(1985): Leroy D+, *Photodermatol* 2(3), 176
Erythroderma
(1986): Giam YC+, *Ann Acad Med Singapore* 15(1), 118 (2 cases)
Exanthems
Exfoliative dermatitis
Fixed eruption
(2001): Das J+, *Indian J Dermatol Venereol Leprol* 67(5), 238
Lupus erythematosus
(1984): Wollina U, *Z Gesamte Inn Med* 39(5), 69
Pemphigus
(1989): Civatte J, *Dermatol Monatsschr* 175(1), 1
Photosensitivity
Pruritus
Psoriasis
(1983): Reshad H+, *Br J Dermatol* 109(1), 111
Purpura
Rash (sic)
Sarcoidosis
Stevens–Johnson syndrome
(1985): Bigby M+, *J Am Acad Dermatol* 12(5 Pt 1), 866
Toxic epidermal necrolysis
(1987): Guillaume JC+, *Arch Dermatol* 123(9), 1166
(1986): Giam YC+, *Ann Acad Med Singapore* 15(1), 118 (4 cases)
(1985): Bigby M+, *J Am Acad Dermatol* 12(5 Pt 1), 866
Urticaria
(2001): Das J+, *Indian J Dermatol Venereol Leprol* 67(5), 238
(1984): Diez Gomez ML+, *Allergol Immunopathol* (Madrid)
12(3), 179
Vasculitis
(1986): Giam YC+, *Ann Acad Med Singapore* 15(1), 118 (2 cases)
(1985): Leung AC+, *Arch Intern Med* 145(4), 685

Mucosal/ENT
Dysgeusia
Gingival ulceration
Glossitis
Oral ulceration
Salivary gland enlargement
Sialadenitis
(2008): Levang J+, *Ann Dermatol Venereol* 135(4), 291
(2002): Viseux V+, *Ann Dermatol Venereol* 129(1 Pt 1), 59
(1982): Speed BR+, *Aust N Z J Med* 12(3), 261 (7 cases)
Stomatitis
Xerostomia

Other
Anaphylactoid reactions/Anaphylaxis
Embolia cutis medicamentosa (Nicolau syndrome)
(1985): Razinskas G+, *Z Hautkr* 60(20), 1639
Gynecomastia
Hepatotoxicity
(1981): Benjamin SB+, *Hepatology* 1(3), 255
Hypersensitivity
(2005): Lim YL+, *Singapore Med J* 46(12), 714
(1981): Benjamin SB+, *Hepatology* 1(3), 255
Polyarteritis nodosa
Serum sickness
(2000): Sanchez G+, *J Investig Allergol Clin Immunol* 10(3), 170

PHENYLEPHRINE

Trade names: Dionephrine; Dura-Vent; Neo-Synephrine;
Novahistine; Prefrin Liquifilm; Prolex-D; Rynatan (MedPointe);
Tussi-12D (MedPointe)
Indications: Nasal congestion, glaucoma, hypotension
Category: Adrenergic alpha-receptor agonist; Sympathomimetic
Half-life: 2.5 hours
Clinically important, potentially hazardous interactions
with: furazolidone, MAO inhibitors, phenelzine, tranylcypromine

Reactions

Skin
Dermatitis
(2004): Yamamoto A+, *Clin Exp Dermatol 2004 Mar* 29(2), 200
(2002): Erdmann SM+, *Am J Contact Dermat* 13(1), 37
(2002): Narayan S+, *Am J Contact* 13(4), 208
(1997): Mancuso G+, *Contact Dermatitis* 36, 110
(1997): Marcos ML+, *Contact Dermatitis* 37, 189
(1995): Thomas P+, *Contact Dermatitis* 32, 249
(1993): Wilkinson SM+, *Contact Dermatitis* 29, 100
(1991): Anibarro B+, *Contact Dermatitis* 25, 323
(blepharoconjunctivitis)
(1991): Bardazzi F+, *Contact Dermatitis* 24, 56
(1991): Okamoto H+, *Cutis* 47, 357
(1990): Zucchi A+, *G Ital Dermatol Venereol* (Italian) 125, 155
(1986): Ducombs G+, *Contact Dermatitis* 15, 107
(1984): Camarasa JG, *Contact Dermatitis* 10, 182
(1983): Hanna C+, *Am J Ophthalmol* 95, 703
Erythroderma
(2002): Gonzalo-Garijo MA+, *Allergol Immunopathol* (Madr)
30(4), 239
Pallor
Stinging (from nasal or ophthalmic preparations) (1–10%)

Eyes
Blepharoconjunctivitis
(1999): Resano A+, *J Invest Allergol Clin Immunol* 9, 55
(1998): Rafael M+, *Contact Dermatitis* 39, 143
(1998): Thomas P+, *Contact Dermatitis* 38, 41
(1998): Wigger-Alberti W+, *Allergy* 53, 217
Conjunctivitis
(2003): Ventura MT+, *Immunopharmacol Immunotoxicol*
25(4), 529 (53.8%)
Ocular allergy (sic)
(2003): Ventura MT+, *Immunopharmacol Immunotoxicol*
25(4), 529
Periorbital dermatitis
(1997): Moreno-Ancillo M+, *Ann Allergy Asthma Immunol* 78, 569
(1997): Ockenfels HM+, *Dermatology* 195, 119
(1983): Rarber KA, *Contact Dermatitis* 9, 274

Periorbital edema
(1998): Blum A+, *Hautarzt* (German) 49, 651
Visual hallucinations
(2006): Jimenez-Jimenez FJ+, *Rev Neurol* 43(10), 603 (with scopolamine & atropine)

Other
Headache
Hypersensitivity
(2007): Dewachter P+, *Acta Anaesthesiol Scand* 51(5), 637
(1991): Quirce Gancedo S+, *Med Clin* (Barc) (Spanish) 96, 317
Hypertension
(1993): Hopson JR+, *Herz* 18(3), 164
Injection-site reactions (sic)
Paresthesias
Tremor

PHENYLPROPANOLAMINE

Synonym: PPA
Trade names: Acutrim; BC Cold Powder; Control; Dex-a-Diet; Dexatrim; Diet Gum; Genex; Maigret-50; Phenoxine; Phenyldrine; Prolamine; Propagest; Propandrine; Rhindecon; Spray-U-Thin; St. Joseph Aspirin-Free Cold Tablets (McNeil); Stay Trim; Unitrol; Westrim
Indications: Nasal decongestion, anorexiant
Category: Adrenergic alpha-receptor agonist
Half-life: 3–4 hours
Clinically important, potentially hazardous interactions with: caffeine, cocoa, ephedra, ephedrine, fluoxetine, fluvoxamine, furazolidone, **guarana,** paroxetine, sertraline, tranylcypromine

Reactions

Skin
Fixed eruption
(2000): Heikkila H+, *Br J Dermatol* 142(4), 845
Pallor

Mucosal/ENT
Xerostomia

Other
Death
(1984): Logie AW+, *Br Med J* 289(6445), 591
(1983): Mueller SM, *N Engl J* 308(11), 653
Depression
Rhabdomyolysis
(1983): Blewitt GA+, *JAMA* 249(22), 3017
(1983): Hampel G+, *Hum Toxicol* 2(2), 197
(1983): Rumpf KW+, *JAMA* 250(16), 2112
(1982): Swenson RD+, *JAMA* 248(10), 1216
Tremor

PHENYTOIN

Synonyms: diphenylhydantoin; DPH; phenytoin sodium
Trade names: Di-Hydran; Dilantin (Pfizer); Diphenylan; Epanutin; Fenytoin; Phenhydan; Phenytek; Pyoredol; Zentropil
Indications: Grand mal seizures
Category: Antiarrhythmic class Ib; Antiepileptic, hydantoin
Half-life: 7–42 hours (dose dependent)
Clinically important, potentially hazardous interactions with: amprenavir, aprepitant, beclomethasone, buprenorphine, calcium, chloramphenicol, cimetidine, clobazam, clorazepate, cyclosporine, darunavir, dasatinib, delavirdine, dexamethasone, diazoxide, disulfiram, dopamine, fluconazole, flunisolide, fluoxetine, fosamprenavir, **ginkgo biloba,** hydrocortisone, imatinib, indinavir, **influenza vaccines,** isoniazid, isradipine, itraconazole, lapatinib, meperidine, methylprednisolone, midazolam, nelfinavir, nilutamide, phenylbutazone, posaconazole, prednisolone, prednisone, **primrose,** ritonavir, **sage,** saquinavir, solifenacin, **St John's wort,** sucralfate, telithromycin, temsirolimus, teniposide, ticlopidine, tizanidine, triamcinolone, uracil/tegafur, vigabatrin

Note: An excellent overview of cutaneous reactions to phenytoin can be found in (1988): Silverman AK+, *J Am Acad Dermatol* 18, 721

Note: About 19% of patients receiving phenytoin develop skin reactions (1983): Rapp RP+, *Neurosurg* 13, 272. They typically develop 10 to 14 days following the start of treatment

Note: The fetal hydantoin syndrome (FHS) – children whose mothers receive phenytoin during pregnancy are born with FHS. The main features of this syndrome are mental and growth retardation, unusual facies, digital and nail hypoplasia, and coarse scalp hair. Occasionally neonatal acne will be present

Reactions

Skin
Acne
(1993): Shah M+, *Eur J Dermatol* 3, 576
(1990): Grunwald MH+, *Int J Dermatol* 29, 559
(1983): Greenwood R+, *Br Med J Clin Res Ed* 287, 1669
(1980): Stankler L+, *Br J Dermatol* 103, 453 (neonatal)
Acute generalized exanthematous pustulosis (AGEP)
(2001): Burrow W, Jackson, MS (from Internet) (observation)
(1995): Moreau A+, *Int J Dermatol* 34, 263 (passim)
Angioedema
(1992): Schlaifer D+, *Eur J Hematol* 48, 274
Bullous dermatitis
(1988): Baird BJ+, *Int J Dermatol* 27, 170
Dermatomyositis
(1998): Dimachkie MM+, *J Child Neurol* 13, 577
Eosinophilic fasciitis
(1980): Buchanan RR+, *J Rheumatol* 7, 733
Epidermolysis bullosa
(1982): Bergfeld WF+, *J Am Acad Dermatol* 7, 275
Erythema multiforme
(2001): Bravo F, Lima, Peru (from Internet) (observation)
(1999): Marinella MA, *Ann Pharmacother* 33, 748
(1999): Micali G+, *Pharmacotherapy* 19, 223 (with cranial irradiation)
(1995): Rodriguez-Castellanos M+, *Arch Dermatol* 131, 620
(1990): Giroud M+, *Therapie* (French) 45, 23
(1988): Delattre JY+, *Neurology* 38, 194
(1988): Shear NH+, *J Clin Invest* 82, 1826
(1986): Green ST, *Clin Neuropharmacol* 9, 561
(1985): Tucker MS+, *J Am Osteopath Assoc* 85, 511
Erythroderma

(1996): Chopra S+, *Br J Dermatol* 134, 1109
(1991): Yamashina T+, *Nippon Shokakibyo Gakkai Zasshi* (Japanese) 88, 1269
(1983): Lillie MA+, *Arch Dermatol* 119, 415

Exanthems (6–71%)
  (2004): Scheinfeld N, *Expert Opin Drug Saf* 3(6), 655
  (2004): Singh G+, *J Neurol Neurosurg Psychiatry* 75(2), 331 (3 cases)
  (2003): Misra UK+, *Postgrad Med J* 79(938), 703 (with carbamazepine)
  (2001): Hebert AA+, *J Clin Psychiatry* 62, 22
  (2000): Cohen AD+, *Isr Med Assoc J* 1, 95
  (1997): Hyson C+, *Can J Neurol Sci* 24, 245
  (1996): Leong KP+, *Asian Pac J Allergy Immunol* 14, 65 (71.4%)
  (1992): Tone T+, *J Dermatol* 19, 27
  (1991): Pelekanos J+, *Epilepsia* 32, 554
  (1988): Shear NH+, *J Clin Invest* 82, 1826
  (1984): Chadwick D+, *J Neurol Neurosurg Psychiatry* 47, 642 (6%)
  (1983): Rapp RP+, *Neurosurgery* 13, 272

Exfoliative dermatitis
  (2004): Scheinfeld N, *Expert Opin Drug Saf* 3(6), 655
  (2002): ten Holder SM+, *Ann Pharmacother* 36(1), 130
  (1997): Westhoven GS+, *Arch Dermatol* 133, 494
  (1996): Leong KP+, *Asian Pac J Allergy Immunol* 14, 65 (2.4%)
  (1996): Sigurdsson V+, *J Am Acad Dermatol* 35, 53
  (1989): Danno K+, *J Dermatol* (Tokio) 16, 392
  (1985): Matson JR+, *Hum Pathol* 16, 94
  (1983): Rapp RP+, *Neurosurgery* 13, 272

Fixed eruption
  (2004): Scheinfeld N, *Expert Opin Drug Saf* 3(6), 655
  (2002): ten Holder SM+, *Ann Pharmacother* 36(1), 130
  (1997): Chan HL+, *J Am Acad Dermatol* 36, 259
  (1988): Baird BJ+, *Int J Dermatol* 27, 170 (bullous)

Hand–foot syndrome
  (2003): Scheinfeld N, *Dermatol Online J* 9(3), 6

Heel pad thickening

Kaposi's varicelliform eruption
  (2006): Ajith C+, *Int J Dermatol* 45(12), 1452

Lichen planus
  (1991): MacLeod SP+, *Br Dent J* 171, 237

Lichenoid eruption
  (1992): Tone T+, *J Dermatol* 19, 27

Linear IgA dermatosis
  (2004): Scheinfeld N, *Expert Opin Drug Saf* 3(6), 655
  (2003): Avci O+, *J Am Acad Dermatol* 48(2), 299 (passim)
  (2003): Tran D+, *Australas J Dermatol* 44(4), 284
  (2002): Cohen LM+, *J Am Acad Dermatol* 46(2), S32 (passim)
  (2000): Mofid MZ+, *J Burn Care Rehabil* 21(3), 246 (with vancomycin)
  (1998): Acostamadiedo JM+, *J Am Acad Dermatol* 38, 352
  (1994): Kuechle MK+, *J Am Acad Dermatol* 30, 187

Lupus erythematosus
  (2003): Scheinfeld N, *Dermatol Online J* 9(3), 6
  (2002): Ross S+, *Clin Exp Dermatol* 27(6), 474
  (1993): Drory VE+, *Clin Neuropharmacol* 16, 19 (passim)
  (1988): Jiang M, *Chung Kuo I Hsueh Ko Hsueh Yuan Hsueh Pao* (Chinese) 10, 379
  (1985): Lovisetto P+, *Recenti Prog Med* (Italian) 76, 84
  (1984): Wollina U, *Z Gesamte Int Med* (German) 39, 69
  (1982): Gleichman H, *Arthritis Rheum* 25, 1387
  (1981): Grossman J+, *Arthritis Rheum* 24, 927

Lupus syndrome
  (2004): Scheinfeld N, *Expert Opin Drug Saf* 3(6), 655

Lymphoma (<1%)
  (1995): Abbondazo SL+, *Am J Surg Pathol* 19(6), 675
  (1985): Wolf R+, *Arch Dermatol* 121, 1181

Mycosis fungoides
  (2004): Scheinfeld N, *Expert Opin Drug Saf* 3(6), 655

(1991): Rijlaarsdam U+, *J Am Acad Dermatol* 24(2 Pt 2), 216 (with carbamazepine)
(1990): Souteyrand P+, *Curr Probl Dermatol* 19, 176
(1988): Cooke LE+, *Clin Pharm* 7(2), 153
(1985): Wolf R+, *Arch Dermatol* 121, 1181
(1982): Rosenthal CH+, *Cancer* 49, 2305
(1981): Adams JD, *Australas J Dermatol* 22(1), 28

Necrosis
  (2001): Bravo F, Lima, Peru (from Internet) (observation)

Pemphigus
  (1988): Seghal VN+, *Int J Dermatol* 27, 258

Peripheral edema
  (2002): Kaur S+, *Pediatr Dermatol* 19(1), 93

Pigmentation
  (2004): Scheinfeld N, *Expert Opin Drug Saf* 3(6), 655
  (1990): Ono T+, *J Dermatol* 17(11), 684

Pruritus
  (2003): Misra UK+, *Postgrad Med J* 79(938), 703 (with carbamazepine)
  (2002): Coplin WM+, *Neurol Res* 24(8), 842
  (1997): Litt JZ, Beachwood, OH (personal case) (observation)
  (1985): Rubinstein N+, *Int J Dermatol* 24, 54

Pseudoacanthosis nigricans

Purple glove syndrome
  (2006): Sonohata M+, *J Orthop Sci* 11(4), 409
  (2004): Scheinfeld N, *Expert Opin Drug Saf* 3(6), 655
  (2001): Endoh T+, *No To Hattatsu* 33(5), 442
  (2000): Schmutz J+, *Ann Dermatol Venereol* (French) 127, 548
  (2000): Yoshikawa H+, *J Child Neurol* 15(11), 762
  (1998): Cadenbach A+, *Dtsch Med Wochenschr* (German) 123, 318
  (1994): Helfaer MA+, *J Neurosurg Anesthesiol* 6, 48

Purpura

Pustules
  (1993): O'Brien TJ+, *Australas J Dermatol* 34, 128
  (1991): Kleier RS, *Arch Dermatol* 127, 1361

Rash (sic) (1–10%)
  (2007): Arif H+, *Neurology* 68(20), 1701
  (2006): Ajith C+, *Int J Dermatol* 45(12), 1452
  (2001): Aihara M+, *Br J Dermatol* 144(6), 1231
  (1999): Mamon HJ+, *Epilepsia* 40, 341 (with cranial radiation)
  (1987): Maguire JH+, *Br J Clin Pharmacol* 24, 554

Reticular hyperplasia

Rhinophyma
  (2000): Jaramillo MJ+, *Br J Plast Surg* 53(6), 521

Scleroderma

Sezary syndrome
  (1994): Doyle MF+, *Acta Hematol* 92, 204

Stevens–Johnson syndrome (14%)
  (2006): Powell N+, *Postgrad Med J* 82(968), e10
  (2005): Lin MS+, *Intern Med J* 35(3), 188
  (2005): Mockenhaupt M+, *Neurology* 64(7), 1134
  (2004): Gomez-Criado MS+, *Rev Neurol* 38(11), 1056
  (2004): Scheinfeld N, *Expert Opin Drug Saf* 3(6), 655
  (2004): Singh G+, *J Neurol Neurosurg Psychiatry* 75(2), 331 (1 case)
  (2003): Camartin C+, *Schweiz Rundsch Med Prax* 92(9), 393
  (2001): Eralp Y+, *Am J Clin Oncol* 24(4), 347
  (2000): Madnani NA, Mumbai, India (from Internet) (observation)
  (1999): DeToledo JC+, *Ther Drug Monit* 21(1), 137
  (1999): Khafaga YM+, *Acta Oncol* 38, 111 (with cranial irradiation)
  (1999): Ruble R+, *CNS Drugs* 12, 215
  (1999): Rzany B+, *Lancet* 353, 2190
  (1996): Cockey G+, *Am J Clin Oncol* 19, 32 (with irradiation of brain)
  (1996): Leong KP+, *Asian Pac J Allergy Immunol* 14, 65 (14.3%)

(1995): Borg M+, *Australas Radiol* 39, 42 (with irradiation of brain)
(1995): Cockey GH+, *Am J Clin Oncol* 19, 32
(1995): Wolkenstein P+, *Arch Dermatol* 131, 544
(1994): Marti J+, *An Med Interna* (Spanish) 11, 621
(1993): Janinis J+, *Eur J Cancer* 29A, 478 (with cranial irradiation)
(1993): Leenutaphong V+, *Int J Dermatol* 32, 428
(1993): Schlienger RG+, *Schweiz Rundsch Med Prax* (German) 82, 888
(1992): Tone T+, *J Dermatol* 19, 27
(1989): Kelly DF+, *Neurosurgery* 25, 976
(1988): Delattre JY+, *Neurology* 38, 194 (with cranial irradiation)
(1988): Shear NH+, *J Clin Invest* 82, 1826
(1985): Burge SM+, *J Am Acad Dermatol* 13, 665
(1985): de Rego JA+, *Hillside J Clin Psychiatry* 7, 141
(1985): Maiche A+, *Lancet* 2, 45 (with radiation therapy)
(1985): Tucker MS+, *J Am Osteopath Assoc* 85(8), 511
(1982): Oles KS+, *Clin Pharm* 1, 565
(1980): Livingston S+, *Am Fam Physician* 22(2), 123

Toxic dermatitis (sic)
Toxic epidermal necrolysis (2%)
(2007): Fernandez FA+, *Actas Dermosifiliogr* 98(7), 483
(2006): Rodriguez G+, *J Am Acad Dermatol* 55(5), S96 (mother and fetus)
(2005): Lin MS+, *Intern Med J* 35(3), 188
(2004): Aguiar D+, *J Neurooncol* 66(3), 345
(2004): Gomez-Criado MS+, *Rev Neurol* 38(11), 1056
(2004): Scheinfeld N, *Expert Opin Drug Saf* 3(6), 655
(2002): Schummer W+, *J Neurosurg Anesthesiol* 14(3), 229
(2002): ten Holder SM+, *Ann Pharmacother* 36(1), 130
(2000): Cohen AD+, *Isr Med Assoc J* 1, 95 (2 patients)
(2000): Moussala M+, *J Fr Ophtalmol* (French) 23, 229
(1999): Cohen AD+, *Isr Med Assoc J* 1, 95 (2 cases)
(1999): Egan CA+, *J Am Acad Dermatol* 40, 458 (3 cases)
(1999): Ruble R+, *CNS Drugs* 12, 215
(1999): Rzany B+, *Lancet* 353, 2190
(1997): Jester BA+, American Academy of Dermatology Meeting (SF), Poster #163
(1997): Redondo Bellon P, *Rev Neurol* 25, S309
(1997): Sapadin A+, American Academy of Dermatology Meeting (SF), Poster #111 (with radiation)
(1996): Creamer JD+, *Clin Exp Dermatol* 21, 116
(1996): Frangogiannis NG+, *South Med J* 89, 1001
(1996): Leong KP+, *Asian Pac J Allergy Immunol* 14, 65 (2.4%)
(1995): Pion IA+, *N Engl J Med* 333, 1609
(1993): Janinis J+, *Eur J Cancer* 29A, 478
(1993): Leenutaphong V+, *Int J Dermatol* 32, 428
(1992): Tone T+, *J Dermatol* 19, 27
(1991): Rowe JE+, *Int J Dermatol* 30, 747
(1989): Kelly DF+, *Neurosurgery* 25, 976
(1989): Renfro L+, *Int J Dermatol* 28, 441
(1988): Dreyfuss DA+, *Ann Plast Surg* 20, 146
(1987): Birchall N+, *J Am Acad Dermatol* 16, 368
(1985): Burge SM+, *J Am Acad Dermatol* 13, 665
(1985): Muhar U, *Pediatr Dermatology* 3, 54
(1985): Sherertz EF+, *J Am Acad Dermatol* 12, 178
(1984): Chan HL, *J Am Acad Dermatol* 10, 973
(1984): Smith DA+, *J Am Acad Dermatol* 10, 106 (followed by universal depigmentation)
(1983): Schmidt D+, *Epilepsia* 24, 440 (fatal)
(1982): Peterson KA+, *Md State Med J* 31, 53
(1981): Spechler SJ+, *Ann Intern Med* 95, 455

Urticaria
(2004): Singh G+, *J Neurol Neurosurg Psychiatry* 75(2), 331 (1 case)
(1995): Rodriguez-Castellanos M+, *Arch Dermatol* 131, 620

Vasculitis (2%)
(2004): Scheinfeld N, *Expert Opin Drug Saf* 3(6), 655
(2002): ten Holder SM+, *Ann Pharmacother* 36(1), 130
(1999): Holt P, *N Z Med J* 112, 100

(1996): Leong KP+, *Asian Pac J Allergy Immunol* 14, 65 (2.4%)
(1996): Parry RG+, *Nephrol Dial Transplant* 11, 357
(1993): Drory VE+, *Clin Neuropharmacol* 16, 19 (passim)
(1984): Smith DA+, *J Am Acad Dermatol* 10(1), 106
(1983): Yermakov VM+, *Hum Pathol* 14, 182

Verrucae
(1998): Kayal JD+, *Cutis* 61, 101

Mucosal/ENT

Ageusia
(1998): Henkin RI, *Lancet* 352, 68
(1998): Zeller JA+, *Lancet* 351, 1101

Dysgeusia
(2004): Baumann CR+, *Br J Clin Pharmacol* 58(6), 678

Gingival hyperplasia/hypertrophy (>10%)
(2004): Scheinfeld N, *Expert Opin Drug* 3(6), 655
(2004): Soga Y+, *Life Sci* 74(7), 827
(2003): Jaiarj N, *J Mass Dent Soc* 52(3), 16
(2003): Takada K+, *J Periodontal Res* 38(5), 477
(2002): Prasad VN+, *J Indian Soc Pedod Prev Dent* 20(2), 73
(2001): Brunet L+, *Eur J Clin Invest* 31(9), 781
(2001): Uzel MI+, *J Periodontol* 72(7), 921
(2000): Sharma S+, *N Engl J Med* 342(5), 325
(1999): Kamali F+, *J Periodontal Res* 34, 145
(1999): Trevisol-Bittencourt PC+, *Arq Neuropsiquiatr* 57(3B), 784
(1999): Wood WH, San Jose, CA (from Internet) (observation)
(1998): Desai P+, *J Can Dent Assoc* 64, 263
(1998): Garzino-Demo P+, *Minerva Somatol* (Italian) 47, 387
(1998): Mattson JS+, *J Am Dent Assoc* 129, 78
(1998): Meraw SJ+, *Mayo Clin Proc* 73, 1196
(1997): Casetta I+, *Neuroepidemiology* 16(6), 296 (40%)
(1997): Huang JS+, *Kaohsiung J Med Sci* 13(3), 141
(1997): Iacopino AM+, *J Periodontol* 68, 73
(1997): Mattioli A, *Minerva Stomatol* (Italian) 46, 525
(1997): Newland JR, *J Gt House Dent Soc* 69, 3
(1997): Silverstein LH+, *Gen Dent* 45, 371
(1996): Ball DE+, *J Periodontol* 67(6), 597
(1996): Hayakawa I+, *Quintessence Int* 27, 235
(1996): Saito K+, *J Periodontal Res* 31, 545
(1996): Seymour RA+, *J Clin Periodontol* 23(3 Pt 1), 165
(1995): McLaughlin WS+, *J Clin Periodontol* 22(12), 942
(1995): Moghadam BKH+, *Cutis* 56, 46 (passim)
(1995): Perlik F+, *Ther Drug Monit* 17(5), 445
(1994): Tigaran S, *Acta Neurol Scand* 90(5), 367
(1993): Lipton JM+, *J Indiana Dent Assoc* 72, 18
(1992): Romanos GE+, *J Oral Pathol Med* 21(6), 256
(1992): Thomason JM+, *Community Dent Oral Epidemiol* 20(5), 288
(1991): Brown RS+, *Oral Surg Oral Med Oral Pathol* 71(5), 565
(1991): Dahllof G+, *Swed Dent J* 15(3), 139
(1991): Hassell TM+, *Crit Rev Oral Biol Med* 2, 103
(1990): Hall WB, *Compendium* (Suppl) 14, 502
(1990): Kinane DF+, *Arch Oral Biol* 35(7), 561
(1990): Levratti E+, *Minerva Ortognatod* 8(2), 103
(1990): Penarrocha-Diago M+, *J Periodontol* 61(9), 571
(1989): Backman K+, *Scand J Dent Res* 97, 222
(1989): Dooley G+, *J N Z Soc Periodontol* 68, 19
(1989): Pugliesi NS+, *Rev Faculdade Odontol FZL* 1(2), 97
(1987): Norris JF+, *Int J Dermatol* 26, 602
(1987): Stinnett E+, *J Am Dent Assoc* 114, 814

Hypogeusia
(2004): Baumann CR+, *Br J Clin Pharmacol* 2004 Dec;58(6), 678

Mucocutaneous eruption
(1992): Tone T+, *J Dermatol* 19, 27

Mucocutaneous lymph node syndrome (Kawasaki syndrome)

Oral ulceration
(2003): Misra UK+, *Postgrad Med J* 79(938), 703 (with carbamazepine)

(2004): Scheinfeld N, *Expert Opin Drug Saf* 3(6), 655
(2002): Lifshitz AY, Israel (solitary in infant) (from Internet)
(observation)
(1998): Cooke LE+, *Clin Pharm* 7, 153
(1997): Gigli GL+, *Int J Neurosci* 87, 181
(1995): Wolkenstein P+, *Arch Dermatol* 131, 544
(1994): Rijlaarsdam JU+, *Semin Dermatol* 13(3), 187
(1993): Kerl H+, *Dermatology in General Medicine* McGraw-Hill
New York
(1993): Sigal M+, *Ann Dermatol Venereol* (French) 120, 175
(1992): Braddock SW+, *J Am Acad Dermatol* 27, 337
(1992): D'Incan M+, *Arch Dermatol* 128, 1371
(1992): Harris DW+, *Br J Dermatol* 127, 403
(1991): Rijlaarsdam U+, *J Am Acad Dermatol* 24(2), 216
(1989): Torne R+, *Am J Dermatopathol* 11(6), 544
(1988): Cooke LE+, *Clin Pharm* 7, 153
(1988): Silverman AK+, *J Am Acad Dermatol* 18, 721
(1985): Brodell RT, *Dermatol Clin* 3, 719
(1985): Wolf R+, *Arch Dermatol* 121(9), 1181
(1983): Rapp RP+, *Neurosurgery* 13, 272
(1982): Rosenthal CJ+, *Cancer* 49, 2305
(1981): Adams JD, *Australas J Dermatol* 22, 28
(1980): Vellucci A+, *Clin Ter* (Italian) 94, 229
Rhabdomyolysis
(2005): Santos-Calle FJ+, *Int J Clin Pharmacol Ther* 43(9), 436
(1989): Korman LB+, *Clin Pharm* 8(7), 514
(1986): Engel JN+, *Am J Med* 81, 928
Serum sickness
(1981): Menitove JE+, *Am J Hematol* 10, 277
Sjøgren's (Sicca) syndrome
(1996): Chakravarty K+, *Br J Rheumatol* 35, 1033
Somnolence
(2007): Kemper EM+, *Ned Tijdschr Geneeskd* 151(2), 138
Thrombophlebitis (<1%)
Thrombosis
(2006): Garcia-Fuster MJ+, *Med Clin* (Barc) 126(10), 397

PHYSOSTIGMINE

Synonyms: Eserine salicylates; Physostigmine salicylates;
Physostigmine sulfate
Trade names: Antilirium; Isopto Eserine
Indications: Miotic in glaucoma treatment, reverses toxic CNS
effects caused by anticholinergic drugs
Category: Cholinesterase inhibitor
Half-life: 15–40 minutes
**Clinically important, potentially hazardous interactions
with:** bethanechol, corticosteroids, galantamine, methacholine,
succinylcholine

Note: Antilirium is a derivative of the Calabar bean, and its active
moiety, physostigmine, is also known as eserine.
Note: Physostigmine is used to reverse the effect upon the nervous
system caused by clinical or toxic dosages of drugs and herbs capable
of producing the anticholinergic syndrome.
Some of the drugs responsible are: amitriptyline, amoxapine,
atropine, benztropine, biperiden, clidinium, cyclobenzaprine,
desipramine, doxepin, hyoscyamine, imipramine, lorazepam,
maprotiline, nortriptyline, protriptyline, propantheline, scopolamine,
trimipramine. Some herbals that can elicit the anticholinergic
syndrome are black henbane, deadly nightshade, Devil's apple, Jimson
weed, Loco seeds or weeds, Matrimony vine, night blooming
jessamine, stinkweed.

Reactions

Skin
Diaphoresis (>10%)
Erythema (1–10%)
(1995): Walter K+, *Br J Clin Pharmacol* 39(1), 59 (from
transdermal patch)

Mucosal/ENT
Sialorrhea (>10%)

Eyes
Epiphora (>10%)
Ocular burning (1–10%)
Ocular stinging (>10%)

Other
Death
Seizures (1–10%)
(1994): Amital D+, *Biol Psychiatry* 36(7), 498

PHYTONADIONE

Synonyms: phylloquinone; phytomenadione; vitamin K_1
Trade names: Kaywan; Konakion; Mephyton; Phytomenadione;
Vitak; Vitamin K (Abbott)
Indications: Coagulation disorders
Category: Vitamin
Half-life: 2–4 hours
**Clinically important, potentially hazardous interactions
with:** warfarin

Reactions

Skin
Allergic reactions (sic)
(1999): Wong DA+, *Australas J Dermatol* 40, 147
(1990): Pigatto PD+, *Contact Dermatitis* 22, 307
Dermatitis
(2006): Ruiz-Hornillos FJ+, *Contact Dermatitis* 55(4), 246
(2005): Serra-Baldrich E+, *Contact Dermatitis* 53(3), 174
(1999): Drayton G, Los Angeles, CA (from Internet)
(observation)
(1995): Bruynzeel I+, *Contact Dermatitis* 32, 78
(1995): Guy C+, *Therapie* (French) 50, 483
(1988): Dinis A+, *Contact Dermatitis* 18, 170
(1982): Camarasa JG+, *Contact Dermatitis* 8, 268
(1980): Romaguera C+, *Contact Dermatitis* 6, 355
Diaphoresis (<1%)
Eczema
(1992): Lee MM+, *Arch Dermatol* 128, 257
(1988): Sanders MN+, *J Am Acad Dermatol* 19, 699
Erythema (annular)
(1986): Kay MH+, *Cutis* 37, 445
Exanthems
(1987): Finkelstein H+, *J Am Acad Dermatol* 16, 540
Rash (sic)
Scleroderma
(1995): Morell A+, *Int J Dermatol* 34, 201
(1994): Guidetti MS+, *Contact Dermatitis* 31, 45
(1992): Fitzpatrick JE, *Dermatol Clin* 10, 19
(1989): Pujol RM+, *Cutis* 43, 365
(1988): Brunskill NJ+, *Clin Exp Dermatol* 13, 276
(1987): Finkelstein H+, *J Am Acad Dermatol* 16, 540
(1985): Janin-Mercier A+, *Arch Dermatol* 121, 1421
(1982): Rommel A+, *Ann Pediatr* (Paris) (French) 29, 64

(1981): Jean-Pastor MJ+, *Therapie* (French) 36, 369
Urticaria
  (1993): Ford G, *J Paediatr Child Health* 29, 241
  (1988): Sanders MN+, *J Am Acad Dermatol* 19, 699
  (1987): Mosser C+, *Ann Dermatol Venereol* (French) 114, 243
Vasculitis

Mucosal/ENT
Dysgeusia (<1%)

Other
Anaphylactoid reactions/Anaphylaxis (<1%)
  (2002): Riegert-Johnson DL+, *Ann Allergy Asthma Immunol*
    89(4), 400 (14 cases)
  (2001): Riegert-Johnson DL+, *Bone Marrow Transplant*
    28(12), 1176
Embolia cutis medicamentosa (Nicolau syndrome)
  (2003): Reding EL+, *J Am Acad Dermatol* 48(3), 472 (passim)
Headache
Hypersensitivity (<1%)
  (1998): Keogh GC+, *Cutis* 61, 81 (eczematous)
Injection-site eczematous eruption
  (1996): Moreau-Cabarrot A+, *Ann Dermatol Venereol* (French)
    123, 177
  (1995): Keltz M+, American Academy of Dermatology Meeting,
    New Orleans (observation)
  (1994): Giudetti MS+, *Contact Dermatitis* 31, 45
  (1989): Allue-Bellosta L+, *Rev Clin Esp* (Spanish) 185, 217
  (1988): Joyce JP+, *Arch Dermatol* 124, 27
  (1988): Tsuboi R+, *J Am Acad Dermatol* 18, 386
  (1987): Finkelstein H+, *J Am Acad Dermatol* 16, 540
Injection-site erythema
  (1995): Keltz M+, American Academy of Dermatology Meeting,
    New Orleans (observation)
  (1993): Lemlich G+, *J Am Acad Dermatol* 28, 345
  (1992): Breathnach SM+, *Adverse Drug Reactions and the Skin*
    Blackwell, Oxford, 265 (passim)
Injection-site induration (Texier's syndrome) (<1%)
  (2001): Jaffe PG, Columbia, SC (from Internet) (observation)
  (1999): Chung JY+, *Cutis* 63, 33 (2 cases)
  (1996): Bourrat E+, *Ann Dermatol Venereol* (French) 123, 634 (6
    cases)
  (1996): Pang BK+, *Australas J Dermatol* 37, 44
  (1995): Keltz M+, American Academy of Dermatology Meeting,
    New Orleans (observation)
  (1994): Shelley WB+, *Cutis* 52, 203 (passim)
  (1993): Lemlich G+, *J Am Acad Dermatol* 28, 345
  (1993): Long CC+, *BMJ* 307, 336
  (1992): Tuppal R+, *J Am Acad Dermatol* 27, 105
  (1989): Pujol RM+, *Cutis* 43, 365
  (1988): Brunskill NJ+, *Clin Exp Dermatol* 13, 276
  (1988): Joyce JP+, *Arch Dermatol* 124, 27
  (1988): Tsuboi R+, *J Am Acad Dermatol* 18, 386
Injection-site scleroderma
  (1998): Alonso-Llamazares J+, *J Am Acad Dermatol* 38(2 Pt
    2), 322

PILOCARPINE

Trade names: Adsorbocarbine; Akarpine; Diocarpine; Isopto
Pilocarpine; Liocarpina; Miocarpine; Ocusert Pilo (Akorn); Pilo
Grin; Pilogel; Pilopine (Alcon); Pilopt; Salagen (MGI); Sno Pilo;
Spersacarpine; Storzine; Vistacarpin
Indications: Glaucoma, miosis induction, xerostomia
Category: Miotic; Muscarinic cholinergic agonist
Half-life: N/A
**Clinically important, potentially hazardous interactions
with:** galantamine

Reactions

Skin
Burning (1–10%)
  (1996): Rattenbury JM+, *Ann Clin Biochem* 33, 456
Dermatitis
  (2001): Holdiness MR, *Am J Contact Dermat* 12(4), 217
  (1993): Cusano F+, *Contact Dermatitis* 29, 99
  (1991): Helton J+, *Contact Dermatitis* 25, 133
  (1991): Ortiz FJ+, *Contact Dermatitis* 25, 203
Diaphoresis (<1%)
  (2006): Chainani-Wu N+, *Spec Care Dentist* 26(4), 164
  (2003): Tsifetaki N+, *Ann Rheum Dis* 62(12), 1204
Edema (4%)
Photosensitivity
  (1991): Helton J+, *Contact Dermatitis* 25, 133
Pruritus
Rash (sic)
Stinging (1–10%)
Urticaria
  (1997): LeGrys VA+, *Pediatr Pulmonol* 24, 296

Mucosal/ENT
Dysgeusia (2%)
Sialorrhea (<1%)

Eyes
Cataract
  (2006): Maldonado MJ+, *Ophthalmology* 113(8), 1283
Ocular cicatricial pemphigoid
  (2000): Plotkin A+, *Arch Dermatol* 136, 113

Other
Chills
Headache
  (2003): Tsifetaki N+, *Ann Rheum Dis* 62(12), 1204
Hypersensitivity (1–10%)
Myalgia/Myositis/Myopathy/Myotoxicity (1%)

PIMECROLIMUS

Synonym: ASM981
Trade name: Elidel (Novartis)
Indications: Atopic dermatitis
Category: Immunomodulator; Macrolactam
Half-life: N/A

Reactions

Skin
Burning
  (2005): Ashcroft DM+, *BMJ* 330(7490), 516
  (2002): Wahn U+, *Pediatrics* 110(1 Pt 1), e2 (10.5%)
Dermatitis
  (2007): Shaw DW+, *J Am Acad Dermatol* 56(2), 342
  (2006): Andersen KE+, *Contact Dermatitis* 55(6), 354 (oleyl
    alcohol)
Edema
  (2006): Richter B+, *Cochrane Database Syst Rev* (4), CD006060
Herpes simplex (1.2%)
  (2007): Langley RG+, *Dermatology* 215 (Suppl 1), 27
Molluscum contagiosum (1.2%)
  (2007): Goksugur N+, *Pediatr Dermatol* 24(5), E63
Peripheral edema
  (2006): Boden G+, *Expert Opin Investig Drugs* 15(3), 243
  (2006): Johansen OE+, *Tidsskr Nor Laegeforen* 126(15), 1928

(2006): Majima T+, *Endocr J* 53(3), 325
Rosacea
  (2006): El Sayed F+, *J Am Acad Dermatol* 54(3), 548
  (2006): Hughes PS, *J Am Acad Dermatol* 54(3), 546
Tinea
  (2008): Rallis E+, *Mycoses* 51(1), 71
  (2004): Crawford KM+, *Skinmed* 3(6), 352

Eyes

Macular edema
  (2006): Ryan EH Jr+, *Retina* 26(5), 562

Other

Application-site burning (8–26%)
Application-site irritation (0.9%)
  (2003): Allen BR+, *Arch Dis Child* 88(11), 969 (5 cases)
Application-site pruritus (0.6%)
Application-site reactions (sic) (2.1%)
Cardiac arrest
  (2006): Boden G+, *Expert Opin Investig Drugs* 15(3), 243
  (2006): Holleman F+, *Ned Tijdschr Geneeskd* 150(7), 358
Cough
  (2002): Wahn U+, *Pediatrics* 110(1 Pt 1), e2
Headache
Infections (5.4%)
  (2002): Wahn U+, *Pediatrics* 110(1 Pt 1), e2 (12.4%)
Upper respiratory infection (19.4%)

PIMOZIDE

Trade names: Frenal; Neurap; Orap (Gate); Pimodac
Indications: Tourette's syndrome, schizophrenia
Category: Antipsychotic
Half-life: 50 hours
**Clinically important, potentially hazardous interactions
with:** amphetamines, aprepitant, astemizole, atazanavir,
azithromycin, azole antifungals, clarithromycin, darunavir,
dirithromycin, erythromycin, fluoxetine, fosamprenavir,
grapefruit juice, imatinib, indinavir, itraconazole, ketoconazole,
methylphenidate, nefazodone, nelfinavir, pemoline,
phenothiazines, protease inhibitors, quinidine, ritonavir,
saquinavir, sertraline, sparfloxacin, telithromycin, thioridazine,
tipranavir, tricyclic antidepressants, troleandomycin,
voriconazole, zileuton, ziprasidone

Reactions

Skin

Diaphoresis
Exanthems
Facial edema (1–10%)
Photosensitivity
  (1991): Opler LA+, *J Clin Psychiatry* 52, 221
Pigmentation
  (1991): Opler LA+, *J Clin Psychiatry* 52, 221
Pruritus
Rash (sic) (8.3%)
Urticaria

Mucosal/ENT

Dysgeusia
Sialorrhea (13.8%)
  (1987): Shapiro AK+, *Pediatrics* 79, 1032
Xerostomia (>10%)
  (1991): Opler LA+, *J Clin Psychiatry* 52, 221
  (1990): Sandor P+, *J Clin Psychopharmacol* 10, 197

(1987): Shapiro AK+, *Pediatrics* 79, 1032

Eyes

Periorbital edema

Other

Death
  (2001): Glassman AH+, *Am J Psychiatry* 158(11), 1774
Depression
  (1997): Bloch M+, *J Clin Psychiatry* 58(10), 433
Gynecomastia (>10%)
Headache
Myalgia/Myositis/Myopathy/Myotoxicity (2.7%)
Tremor

PINDOLOL

Trade names: Alti-Pindolol; Apo-Pindol; Barbloc; Durapindol;
Gen-Pindolol; Nonspi; Pinbetol; Pinden; Syn-Pindol; Visken
(Novartis); Vypen
Indications: Hypertension
Category: Adrenergic beta-receptor antagonist
Half-life: 3–4 hours
**Clinically important, potentially hazardous interactions
with:** clonidine, epinephrine, verapamil

Note: Cutaneous side effects of beta-receptor blockaders are
clinically polymorphous. They apparently appear after several months
of continuous therapy. Atypical psoriasiform, lichen planus-like, and
eczematous chronic rashes are mainly observed. (1983): Hödl St, *Z
Hautkr* (German) 1:58, 17

Reactions

Skin

Diaphoresis (2%)
Eczema
Edema (6%)
Erythema multiforme
Exanthems
Exfoliative dermatitis
Hyperkeratosis (palms and soles)
Lichenoid eruption
Lupus erythematosus
Peripheral edema
Pityriasis rubra pilaris
Pruritus (1–5%)
Psoriasis
  (1986): Abel EA+, *J Am Acad Dermatol* 15, 1007
  (1986): Czernielewski J+, *Lancet* 1, 808
  (1984): Arntzen N+, *Acta Derm Venereol* (Stockh) 64, 346
Purpura
Rash (sic) (1–10%)
Raynaud's phenomenon
  (1984): Eliasson K+, *Acta Med Scand* 215, 333
Toxic epidermal necrolysis
Urticaria
Xerosis

Mucosal/ENT

Dysgeusia
Oral lichenoid eruption

Hair

Hair – alopecia

Nails
Nails – dystrophy

Eyes
Oculo-mucocutaneous syndrome
(1982): Cocco G+, *Curr Ther Res* 31, 362

Other
Hypotension
(1982): Gonasun LM+, *Am Heart J* 104(2 Pt 2), 482
Myalgia/Myositis/Myopathy/Myotoxicity
(1980): Uusitupa M+, *BMJ* 1, 183
Paresthesias (3%)
Peyronie's disease

PIOGLITAZONE

Trade name: Actos (Takeda)
Indications: Type 2 diabetes
Category: Thiazolidinedione
Half-life: 3–7 hours
**Clinically important, potentially hazardous interactions
with:** gemfibrozil

Reactions

Skin
Angioedema
(2002): Shadid S+, *Diabetes Care* 25(2), 405
Edema (4–11%)
(2005): *Prescrire Int* 14(78), 133
(2005): Belcher G+, *Diabetes Res Clin Pract* 70(1), 53
(2005): Bongartz T+, *Rheumatology (Oxford)* 44(1), 126
(2005): Charbonnel BH+, *Diabet Med* 22(4), 399
(2005): Kahara T+, *Endocr J* 52(3), 373
(2003): Mudaliar S+, *Endocr Pract* 9(5), 406
(2002): *Prescrire Int* 11(62), 170
(2001): Chilcott J+, *Clin Ther* 23(11), 1792 (11.7%)
(2001): Toyota T, *Nippon Rinsho* 59(11), 2211

Eyes
Dyschromatopsia
(2003): Muller T+, *J Neurol* 250(1), 101

Other
Cardiac failure
(2005): *Prescrire Int* 14(78), 133
Headache
Hepatotoxicity
(2005): *Prescrire Int* 14(78), 133
(2004): Arotcarena R+, *Gastroenterol Clin Biol* 28(6–7), 610
(2004): Farley-Hills E+, *BMJ* 329(7463), 429
(2004): Marcy TR+, *Ann Pharmacother* 38(9), 1419 (5 cases)
(2002): Pinto AG+, *Ann Intern Med* 137(10), 857
Myalgia/Myositis/Myopathy/Myotoxicity (5.4%)

PIPECURONIUM

Trade name: Arduan (Organon)
Indications: Adjunct to general anesthesia
Category: Non-depolarizing neuromuscular blocker
Half-life: 2–3 hours
**Clinically important, potentially hazardous interactions
with:** anesthetics (inhalational), antibiotics, gentamicin,
magnesium salts, quinidine, succinylcholine

Reactions

Skin
Rash (sic) (<1%)
Urticaria (<1%)

Mucosal/ENT
Dysphagia
(1995): El Mikatti N+, *Br J Anaesth* 74(1), 16

Eyes
Diplopia
(1995): El Mikatti N+, *Br J Anaesth* 74(1), 16
Ptosis
(1995): El Mikatti N+, *Br J Anaesth* 74(1), 16

PIPERACILLIN

Trade names: Avocin; Ivacin; Picillin; Pipcil; Piperilline; Pipracil
(Wyeth); Pipril; Piprilin; Pitamycin; Zosyn (Wyeth)
Indications: Various infections caused by susceptible organisms
Category: Antibiotic, penicillin
Half-life: 0.6–1.2 hours
**Clinically important, potentially hazardous interactions
with:** anisindione, anticoagulants, atracurium, cisatracurium,
demeclocycline, dicumarol, doxacurium, doxycycline,
imipenem/cilastatin, methotrexate, minocycline, non-depolarizing
muscle relaxants, oxytetracycline, pancuronium, rapacuronium,
reteplase, tetracycline, warfarin

Note: Zosyn is piperacillin and tazobactam

Reactions

Skin
Acute febrile neutrophilic dermatosis (Sweet's syndrome)
(2008): Cholongitas E+, *Am J Dermatopathol* 30(2), 203
Acute generalized exanthematous pustulosis (AGEP)
(2005): Grieco T+, *J Am Acad Dermatol* 52(4), 732 (with
tazobactam)
(2003): Mysore V+, *J Dermatolog Treat* 14(1), 54
Allergic reactions (sic) (2–4%)
(1994): Pleasants RA+, *Chest* 106, 1124 (in patients with cystic
fibrosis)
(1984): Holmes B+, *Drugs* 28, 375
Angioedema
(2005): Mazzeo F+, *Pharmacol Res* 51(3), 269
Bullous dermatitis
Edema
Erythema nodosum
Exanthems (56%)
(2002): Romano A+, *Int Arch Allergy Immunol* 129(2), 169
(1993): Warrington RJ+, *J Allergy Clin Immunol* 92, 626
(1985): Mead GM+, *Lancet* 2, 499 (56%)
(1985): No Author, *Lancet* 2, 723
(1984): Holmes B+, *Drugs* 28, 375
Exfoliative dermatitis
Jarisch–Herxheimer reaction (<1%)
Photo-recall
(2001): Krishnan RS+, *J Am Acad Dermatol* 44, 1045 (with
tobramycin & ciprofloxacin)
Pruritus
Purpura
(2000): Yata Y+, *Ann Hematol* 79(10), 593
Rash (sic) (1%)

Stevens–Johnson syndrome
 (1995): Cheriyan S+, *Allergy Proc* 16, 85
Toxic epidermal necrolysis
Urticaria
 (2002): Romano A+, *Int Arch Allergy Immunol* 129(2), 169
 (1995): Moscato G+, *Eur Respir J* 8, 467
 (1984): Holmes B+, *Drugs* 28, 375
Vasculitis
Vesiculation

Mucosal/ENT
Glossodynia
Oral candidiasis
Stomatodynia
Tinnitus
Vaginitis

Other
Anaphylactoid reactions/Anaphylaxis (<1%)
 (2007): Rank MA+, *Allergy* 62(8), 964
Candidiasis
DRESS syndrome
 (2006): Fahim S+, *Cutis* 77(6), 353 (with tazobactam)
Headache
Hypersensitivity (<1%)
 (2006): Fahim S+, *Cutis* 77(6), 353
 (2002): Romano A+, *Allergy* 57(5), 459
 (1998): Cabanes R+, *Allergy* 53, 819
 (1995): Behbahani R+, *Ann Pharmacother* 29(9), 936
Injection-site pain (2%)
 (1984): Holmes B+, *Drugs* 28, 375
Injection-site phlebitis (2%)
 (1984): Holmes B+, *Drugs* 28, 375
Nephrotoxicity
 (2006): Mannaerts L+, *Ned Tijdschr Geneeskd* 150(14), 804
Paresthesias
 (2006): Lambourne J+, *Ann Pharmacother* 40(5), 977
Seizures
 (2002): Bassilios N+, *Clin Nephrol* 58(4), 327
Serum sickness
Thrombophlebitis (<1%)

PIRBUTEROL

Trade names: Exirel; Maxair (3M); Spirolair; Zeisin Autohaler
Indications: Asthma, bronchospasm
Category: Adrenergic beta-receptor agonist
Half-life: 2–3 hours

Reactions

Skin
Edema
Pruritus
Purpura (<1%)
Rash (sic)

Mucosal/ENT
Dysgeusia (1–10%)
Glossitis
Xerostomia

Hair
Hair – alopecia

Other
Headache
Paresthesias (<1%)
Tremor
 (1980): Brandon ML, *Ann Allergy* 45(1), 8 (mild)

PIROXICAM

Trade names: Antiflog; Apo-Piroxicam; Baxo; Doblexan; Felden; Feldene (Pfizer); Larapam; Nu-Pirox; Rogal; Sotilen; Zunden
Indications: Arthritis
Category: Non-steroidal anti-inflammatory
Half-life: 50 hours
Clinically important, potentially hazardous interactions with: methotrexate, ritonavir

Reactions

Skin
Allergic reactions (sic)
 (2001): Trujillo MJ+, *Allergol Immunopathol* (Madr) 29(4), 133 (with thimerosal)
Angioedema (<1%)
 (1987): Gerber D, *Drug Intell Clin Pharm* 21, 707 (passim)
Bullous dermatitis
 (1985): Guillaume JC+, *Ann Dermatol Venereol* (French) 112, 807
Dermatitis
 (1995): Valsecchi R+, *Contact Dermatitis* 32, 63
 (1993): Ophaswongse S+, *Contact Dermatitis* 29, 57
 (1993): Valsecchi R+, *Contact Dermatitis* 29, 167
 (1992): Green C+, *Contact Dermatitis* 27, 261 (to the gel)
 (1990): Serrano G+, *J Am Acad Dermatol* 23, 479
Diaphoresis (<1%)
 (1987): Gerber D, *Drug Intell Clin Pharm* 21, 707 (passim)
Dyshidrosis
 (1985): Braunstein BL, *Cutis* 35, 485
Edema (>1%)
Erythema (<1%)
Erythema annulare centrifugum
 (1985): Hogan DJ+, *J Am Acad Dermatol* 13, 840
Erythema multiforme (<1%)
 (1991): Lisi P+, *Ann Ital Dermatol Clin Sper* 45, 193
 (1987): Gerber D, *Drug Intell Clin Pharm* 21, 707 (passim)
 (1986): Penso D, *J Am Acad Dermatol* 14, 275
 (1986): Stern RS, *J Am Acad Dermatol* 14, 276
 (1985): Bigby M+, *J Am Acad Dermatol* 12, 866
 (1985): Guillaume JC+, *Ann Dermatol Venereol* (French) 112, 807
 (1985): O'Brien WM+, *J Rheumatol* 12, 13
 (1984): Brogden RN+, *Drugs* 28, 292
 (1984): Duro JC+, *J Rheumatol* 11, 554
 (1984): Stern RS+, *JAMA* 252, 1433
 (1982): Bertail MA, *Ann Dermatol Venereol* (French) 109, 261
 (1982): Faure M, *Ann Dermatol Venereol* (French) 109, 255
Erythroderma
 (1993): Sangla I+, *Rev Neurol* (Paris) (French) 149, 217
 (1985): Guillaume JC+, *Ann Dermatol Venereol* (French) 112, 807
Exanthems (>5%)
 (1994): Litt JZ, Beachwood, OH (personal case) (observation)
 (1991): Lisi P+, *Ann Ital Dermatol Clin Sper* 45, 193
 (1987): Gerber D, *Drug Intell Clin Pharm* 21, 707 (passim)
 (1985): Bigby M+, *J Am Acad Dermatol* 12, 866 (2.4%)
 (1985): Guillaume JC+, *Ann Dermatol Venereol* (French) 112, 807
 (1984): Brogden RN+, *Drugs* 28, 292 (0.8%)
 (1984): Stern RS+, *JAMA* 252, 1433
 (1982): Faure M+, *Ann Dermatol Venereol* (French) 109, 255
Exfoliative dermatitis (<1%)

(1987): Gerber D, *Drug Intell Clin Pharm* 21, 707 (passim)
Fixed eruption
(2006): Ozkaya E, *Eur J Dermatol* 16(5), 591
(2003): Montoro J+, *Allergol Immunopathol* (Madr) 31(1), 53
(2002): Tanaka S, *Contact Dermatitis* 46(3), 174
(1998): Leal G, Fortaleza, Brazil (from Internet) (observation) (2 cases)
(1995): Ordoqui E+, *Allergy* 50, 741
(1994): Ordoqui E+, *J Allergy Clin Immunology* 93, 242
(1993): Gastaminza G+, *Contact Dermatitis* 28, 43
(1993): No Author, *Dermatology* 186, 164
(1990): de la Hoz B+, *Int J Dermatol* 29, 672
(1990): Stubb S+, *J Am Acad Dermatol* 22, 1111
(1989): Shiohara T+, *Arch Dermatol* 125, 1371
(1989): Valsecchi R+, *J Am Acad Dermatol* 21, 1300
Lichenoid eruption
(1993): Veraldi S+, *Eur J Dermatol* 3, 156
(1992): Vaillant L+, *Ann Dermatol Venereol* (French) 119, 936
(1991): Lisi P+, *Ann Ital Dermatol Clin Sper* 45, 193
(1985): Guillaume JC+, *Ann Dermatol Venereol* (French) 112, 807
(1984): Stern RS+, *JAMA* 252, 1433
Linear IgA dermatosis
(2003): Avci O+, *J Am Acad Dermatol* 48(2), 299 (passim)
(2001): Plunkett RW+, *J Am Acad Dermatol* 45(5), 691
(1998): Camilleri M+, *J Eur Acad Dermatol Venereol* 10, 70
Lupus erythematosus
(1991): Roura M+, *Dermatologica* 182, 56
Pemphigus
(1985): Guillaume JC+, *Ann Dermatol Venereol* (French) 112, 807
(1985): Piette-Brion B+, *Dermatologica* 170(6), 297 (with penicillamine)
(1983): Martin RL, *N Engl J Med* 309, 795
Pemphigus foliaceus
(1984): Brogden RN+, *Drugs* 28, 292
Peripheral edema
(2002): Pertusa Martinez S+, *Aten Primaria* 30(9), 589
Petechiae (<1%)
Photosensitivity (<1%)
(2001): Trujillo MJ+, *Allergol Immunopathol* (Madr) 29(4), 133 (with thimerosal)
(1998): Valentine M, Everett, WA (from Internet) (observation)
(1998): Varela P+, *Acta Med Port* (Portuguese) 11, 997
(1998): Varela P+, *Contact Dermatitis* 38, 229
(1996): Becker L+, *Acta Derm Venereol* 76(5), 337
(1996): Stingeni L+, *Contact Dermatitis* 34, 60
(1995): Gebhardt M+, *Z Rheumatol* (German) 54, 405
(1995): Mammen L+, *Am Fam Physician* 52, 575
(1994): Sassolas B+, *Clin Exp Dermatol* 19, 189
(1993): Hariya T+, *J Dermatol Sci* 5, 165
(1993): Youn JI+, *Clin Exp Dermatol* 18, 52
(1992): Goncalo M+, *Contact Dermatitis* 27, 287
(1992): Izekawa Z+, *J Invest Dermatol* 98, 918
(1992): Serrano G+, *J Am Acad Dermatol* 26, 545
(1992): Torinuki W, *Tohoku J Exp Med* 167, 267
(1991): de Castro JL+, *Contact Dermatitis* 24, 187
(1991): Roura M+, *Dermatologica* 182, 56
(1990): Black AK+, *Br J Dermatol* 123, 277
(1990): Serrano G+, *J Am Acad Dermatol* 23, 479
(1989): Cirne de Castro JL+, *J Am Acad Dermatol* 20, 706
(1989): De la Cuadra J+, *Contact Dermatitis* 21, 349
(1989): Kaidbey KH+, *Arch Dermatol* 125, 783
(1989): Sunohara A, *Photodermatol* 6, 188
(1987): Figueiredo A+, *Contact Dermatitis* 17, 73
(1987): Gerber D, *Drug Intell Clin Pharm* 21, 707 (passim)
(1987): Halasz CL, *Cutis* 39, 37
(1987): Magana-Garcia M+, *Rev Invest Clin* (Spanish) 39, 177
(1987): Morison WL+, *J Am Acad Dermatol* 17, 698
(1986): Kochevar IE+, *Arch Dermatol* 122, 1283
(1986): McKerrow KJ+, *J Am Acad Dermatol* 15, 1237
(1985): Bigby M+, *J Am Acad Dermatol* 12, 866

(1985): Braunstein BL, *Cutis* 35, 485
(1985): Guillaume JC+, *Ann Dermatol Venereol* (French) 112, 807
(1985): Serrano G+, *J Am Acad Dermatol* 11, 113
(1985): Weigand DA, *J Am Acad Dermatol* 12, 373
(1984): Brogden RN+, *Drugs* 28, 292
(1984): Stern RS+, *JAMA* 252, 1433
(1983): Diffey BL+, *Br J Rheumatol* 22, 239
(1983): Fjellner B, *Acta Derm Venereol* (Stockh) 63, 557
(1982): Faure M+, *Ann Dermatol Venereol* (French) 109, 255
Pruritus (1–10%)
(1991): Lisi P+, *Ann Ital Dermatol Clin Sper* 45, 193
(1987): Gerber D, *Drug Intell Clin Pharm* 21, 707 (passim)
(1984): Brogden RN+, *Drugs* 28, 292
(1984): Stern RS+, *JAMA* 252, 1433
Purpura (<1%)
(1987): Gerber D, *Drug Intell Clin Pharm* 21, 707 (passim)
(1984): Brogden RN+, *Drugs* 28, 292
Rash (sic) (>10%)
Side effects (sic) (46.9%)
(1987): Gerber D, *Drug Intell Clin Pharm* 21, 707 (passim)
Stevens–Johnson syndrome (<1%)
(1995): Katoh N+, *J Dermatol* 22, 677
(1985): Guillaume JC+, *Ann Dermatol Venereol* (French) 112, 807
Toxic dermatitis (sic)
(1991): Chosidow O+, *Ann Dermatol Venereol* (French) 118, 903
Toxic epidermal necrolysis (<1%)
(2002): Correia O+, *Arch Dermatol* 138, 29 (2 cases)
(1996): Blum L+, *J Am Acad Dermatol* 34, 1088
(1993): Correia O+, *Dermatology* 186, 32
(1991): Lisi P+, *Ann Ital Dermatol Clin Sper* 45, 193
(1990): Black AK+, *Br J Dermatol* 123, 277
(1987): Gerber D, *Drug Intell Clin Pharm* 21, 707 (passim)
(1987): Guillaume JC+, *Arch Dermatol* 123, 1166
(1986): Penso D+, *J Am Acad Dermatol* 14, 275 (letter)
(1986): Szczeklik A, *Drugs* 32 (Suppl 4), 148
(1985): Coscojuela C+, *Med Cutan Ibero Lat Am* (Spanish) 13, 291
(1985): Guillaume JC+, *Ann Dermatol Venereol* (French) 112, 807
(1982): Faure M+, *Ann Dermatol Venereol* (French) 109, 255
Urticaria (<1%)
(1991): Lisi P+, *Ann Ital Dermatol Clin Sper* 45, 193
(1987): Gerber D, *Drug Intell Clin Pharm* 21, 707 (passim)
(1985): Serrano G+, *J Am Acad Dermatol* 11, 113
(1984): Stern RS+, *JAMA* 252, 1433
(1982): Torras H+, *Med Cutan Ibero Lat Am* (Spanish) 10, 351
Vasculitis (<1%)
(1985): Bigby M+, *J Am Acad Dermatol* 12, 866
(1985): Guillaume JC+, *Ann Dermatol Venereol* (French) 112, 807
(1984): Stern RS+, *JAMA* 252, 1433
Vesiculation (<1%)
(1986): Stern RS, *J Am Acad Dermatol* 14, 276 (letter)
(1984): Stern RS+, *JAMA* 252, 1433

Mucosal/ENT
Aphthous stomatitis
(2004): Lisi P+, *J Am Acad Dermatol* 50(4), 648
(2001): Vincent L+, *Ann Dermatol Venereol* 128(1), 57
(1991): Siegel MA+, *J Am Dent Assoc* 122, 75
Oral mucosal fixed eruption
(2003): Montoro J+, *Allergol Immunopathol* (Madr) 31(1), 53
Oral ulceration
(1987): Gerber D, *Drug Intell Clin Pharm* 21, 707 (passim)
Stomatitis (>1%)
Tinnitus
(1998): Carbone PP+, *Cancer Epidemiol Biomarkers Prev* 7(10), 907
(1986): Vernick DM+, *Am J Otol* 7(2), 97 (2 cases)
Xerostomia (<1%)

Hair

Hair – alopecia
  (1987): Gerber D, *Drug Intell Clin Pharm* 21, 707
  (1985): Bigby M+, *J Am Acad Dermatol* 12, 866
  (1984): Stern RS+, *JAMA* 252, 1433

Other

Anaphylactoid reactions/Anaphylaxis (<1%)
Death
  (2002): Correia O+, *Arch Dermatol* 138, 29
Embolia cutis medicamentosa (Nicolau syndrome)
  (2005): Lee DP+, *Int J Dermatol* 44(12), 1069
Headache
Hot flashes (<1%)
Paresthesias
  (1987): Gerber D, *Drug Intell Clin Pharm* 21, 707
Pseudoporphyria
  (2000): De Silva B+, *Pediatr Dermatol* 17, 480
Serum sickness (<1%)

PLICAMYCIN

Synonym: mithramycin
Trade names: Mithracin; Mithraline
Indications: Paget's disease, malignant testicular tumors
Category: Antibiotic
Half-life: 1 hour
**Clinically important, potentially hazardous interactions
with:** aldesleukin, ceftobiprole

Reactions

Skin

Exanthems
Petechiae (1–10%)
Purpura (10%)
Seborrheic keratoses (inflammation of)
  (1987): Johnson TM+, *J Am Acad Dermatol* 17, 192
Toxic epidermal necrolysis

Mucosal/ENT

Dysgeusia (metallic taste)
Oral lesions (1–15%)
  (1989): Kerker BJ+, *Semin Dermatol* 8, 173 (1–5%)
Stomatitis (>10%)

Other

Injection-site cellulitis (1–10%)
Injection-site erythema (1–10%)
Injection-site pain (1–10%)

PNEUMOCOCCAL VACCINE

Trade names: PCV (Lederle); PncOMP (Merck); Pneumovax II
(Sanofi-Aventis); Pnu-Immune (Lederle); PPV (Lederle); Prevenar
(Wyeth)
Indications: Prevention of bacteremia, meningitis, pneumonia,
respiratory tract infections, otitis media, sinusitis
Category: Vaccine
Half-life: N/A

Reactions

Skin

Dermatitis
  (2003): Holdiness MR+, *South Med J* 96(1), 64
Facial edema
  (2002): Kikuchi Y+, *Clin Nephrol* 58(1), 68
Peripheral edema
  (2002): Kikuchi Y+, *Clin Nephrol* 58(1), 68
Petechiae
  (2003): Holdiness MR+, *South Med J* 96(1), 64
Pityriasis rosea
  (2003): Sasmaz S+, *J Dermatol* 30(3), 245
Pruritus
  (2003): Holdiness MR+, *South Med J* 96(1), 64
Rash (sic)
  (2006): *Prescrire Int* 15(86), 227
  (2004): Wise RP+, *JAMA* 292(14), 1702
Urticaria
  (2006): *Prescrire Int* 15(86), 227
  (2005): Ghaffar F, *Expert Opin Drug Saf* 4(4), 631
  (2004): Wise RP+, *JAMA* 292(14), 1702
  (2003): Holdiness MR+, *South Med J* 96(1), 64
  (2002): Black S+, *Eur J Pediatr* 161 Suppl 2, S127

Eyes

Photophobia
  (2005): Hasan S+, *J Natl Med Assoc* 97(2), 284
Uveitis
  (2002): Kikuchi Y+, *Clin Nephrol* 58(1), 68
Visual disturbances
  (2002): Kikuchi Y+, *Clin Nephrol* 58(1), 68

Other

Anaphylactoid reactions/Anaphylaxis
  (2004): Wise RP+, *JAMA* 292(14), 1702
  (2001): Ponvert C+, *Vaccine* 19(32), 4588
Asthenia
  (2005): de Aristegui Fernandez J+, *Vaccine* 23(16), 1917 (20%)
  (2004): Socan M+, *Vaccine* 22(23–24), 3087
  (2000): Suda T, *Nihon Kokyuki Gakkai Zasshi* 38(11), 836
Fever
  (2006): *Prescrire Int* 15(86), 227
  (2006): Shao PL+, *J Formos Med Assoc* 105(7), 542
  (2005): de Aristegui Fernandez J+, *Vaccine* 23(16), 1917 (7%)
  (2005): Ghaffar F, *Expert Opin Drug Saf* 4(4), 631
  (2005): Jackson LA+, *Vaccine* 23(28), 3697
  (2004): Socan M+, *Vaccine* 22(23–24), 3087
  (2004): Wise RP+, *JAMA* 292(14), 1702
  (2002): *Prescrire Int* 11(57), 7
  (2002): Black S+, *Eur J Pediatr* 161 Suppl 2, S127
  (2002): D'heilly S+, *Am J Infect Control* 30(5), 261
  (2002): Darkes MJ+, *Paediatr Drugs* 4(9), 609
  (2002): Shinefield H+, *Pediatr Infect Dis J* 21(3), 182
  (2000): Suda T, *Nihon Kokyuki Gakkai Zasshi* 38(11), 836
Headache
  (2005): Hasan S+, *J Natl Med Assoc* 97(2), 284
Hypersensitivity
  (2002): Kikuchi Y+, *Clin Nephrol* 58(1), 68
Injection-site edema
  (2005): Ghaffar F, *Expert Opin Drug Saf* 4(4), 631
  (2004): Socan M+, *Vaccine* 22(23–24), 3087
  (2002): Black S+, *Eur J Pediatr* 161 Suppl 2, S127
  (2002): D'heilly S+, *Am J Infect Control* 30(5), 261 (23%)
  (2002): Shinefield H+, *Pediatr Infect Dis J* 21(3), 182
  (2000): Suda T, *Nihon Kokyuki Gakkai Zasshi* 38(11), 836
Injection-site erythema
  (2005): de Aristegui Fernandez J+, *Vaccine* 23(16), 1917 (40%)

(2005): Ghaffar F, *Expert Opin Drug Saf* 4(4), 631
(2005): Hasan S+, *J Natl Med Assoc* 97(2), 284
(2004): Socan M+, *Vaccine* 22(23–24), 3087
(2002): Black S+, *Eur J Pediatr* 161 Suppl 2, S127
(2002): D'heilly S+, *Am J Infect Control* 30(5), 261 (23%)
(2002): Shinefield H+, *Pediatr Infect Dis J* 21(3), 182
(2000): Suda T, *Nihon Kokyuki Gakkai Zasshi* 38(11), 836
Injection-site induration
(2005): de Aristegui Fernandez J+, *Vaccine* 23(16), 1917 (32%)
(2005): Ghaffar F, *Expert Opin Drug Saf* 4(4), 631
(2005): Hasan S+, *J Natl Med Assoc* 97(2), 284
Injection-site inflammation
(2002): Darkes MJ+, *Paediatr Drugs* 4(9), 609
Injection-site pain
(2005): Ghaffar F, *Expert Opin Drug Saf* 4(4), 631
(2005): Hasan S+, *J Natl Med Assoc* 97(2), 284
(2002): D'heilly S+, *Am J Infect Control* 30(5), 261 (23%)
(2000): Suda T, *Nihon Kokyuki Gakkai Zasshi* 38(11), 836
Injection-site reactions
(2006): *Prescrire Int* 15(86), 227
(2006): Jackson LA+, *Vaccine* 24(2), 151
(2005): Ghaffar F, *Expert Opin Drug Saf* 4(4), 631
(2005): Jackson LA+, *Vaccine* 23(28), 3697
(2005): Lin PL+, *Pediatrics* 116(1), 160
(2004): Wise RP+, *JAMA* 292(14), 1702
(2002): *Prescrire Int* 11(57), 7
Myalgia/Myositis/Myopathy/Myotoxicity
(2004): Socan M+, *Vaccine* 22(23–24), 3087
Paresthesias
Seizures
(2005): Ghaffar F, *Expert Opin Drug Saf* 4(4), 631
(2004): Wise RP+, *JAMA* 292(14), 1702
Serum sickness
(2006): Hengge UR+, *Int J STD AIDS* 17(3), 210
(2004): Wise RP+, *JAMA* 292(14), 1702

POLYPODIUM LEUCOTOMOS

Synonym: Polypodiaceae
Trade names: Anapsos; Calagualine; Calagula; Difur; Fernblock; Heliocare; Polypodium leucotomos
Indications: Oral and topical photoprotection, vitiligo, psoriasis, dermatitis, arthritis
Category: Anti-inflammatory; Antioxidant
Half-life: N/A

Note: It is the first oral agent effective in reducing side effects of PUVA treatment

Reactions

Skin
Pruritus
(1983): Pineiro Alvarez B, *Med Cutan Ibero Lat Am* 11(1), 65

POLYTHIAZIDE

Trade names: Drenusil; Minizide (Pfizer); Nephril; Renese (Pfizer)
Indications: Hypertension, edema
Category: Adrenergic alpha-receptor agonist; Diuretic, thiazide
Half-life: N/A
Clinically important, potentially hazardous interactions with: digoxin, lithium

Note: Minizide is prazosin and polythiazide

Note: Polythiazide is a sulfonamide and can be absorbed systemically. Sulfonamides can produce severe, possibly fatal, reactions such as toxic epidermal necrolysis and Stevens–Johnson syndrome

Reactions

Skin
Exanthems
Photosensitivity (<1%)
Purpura
Rash (sic) (<1%)
Urticaria
Vasculitis

Other
Paresthesias

PORFIMER

Synonym: CL-184116
Trade name: Photofrin (Axcan)
Indications: Esophageal (and other) cancers, Barrett's esophagus
Category: Antineoplastic; Photosensitizer
Half-life: 13–21 days
Clinically important, potentially hazardous interactions with: N/A

Reactions

Skin
Allergic reactions (>10%)
Edema (1–10%)
(1992): Wilson BD+, *Arch Dermatol* 128(12), 1597
Nodular eruption (1–10%)
Photosensitivity (10–80%)
(2006): *Prescrire Int* 15(82), 58 (50%)
(2005): Yamaguchi S+, *Oncology* 69(2), 110 (48%)
(2001): Moriwaki SI+, *Photodermatol Photoimmunol Photomed* 17(5), 241
(1996): Mimura S+, *Lasers Surg Med* 19(2), 168
(1995): Baas P+, *Lasers Surg Med* 16(4), 359
(1995): Tsukagoshi S, *Gan To Kagaku Ryoho* 22(9), 1271
Pigmentation (1–10%)
(1995): Tsukagoshi S, *Gan To Kagaku Ryoho* 22(9), 1271
Urticaria
(2000): Karasic DS+, *Ann Pharmacother* 34(10), 1208
(1997): Koehler IK, *Lasers Surg Med* 20(1), 97
Wrinkling (1–10%)

Mucosal/ENT
Dysphagia (24%)

Hair

Hair – hypertrichosis (1–10%)

Other

Abdominal pain (20%)
Asthenia (1–10%)
Candidiasis (1–10%)
Cardiac failure (6–7%)
Chest pain (5–22%)
Cough (7%)
Fever
Hypertension (6–7%)
Hypotension (6–7%)
Pain
  (1992): Wilson BD+, *Arch Dermatol* 128(12), 1597

POSACONAZOLE

Synonym: SCH 56592.
Trade name: Noxafil (Schering)
Indications: *Aspergillus* and *Candida* infection prophylaxis in immunocompromised patients
Category: Antifungal, triazole
Half-life: ~37 hours
Clinically important, potentially hazardous interactions with: cimetidine, phenytoin, rifabutin

Reactions

Skin

Allergic reactions (sic)
Edema (9%)
Herpes simplex (15%)
Peripheral edema (15%)
Pruritus (11%)
Rash (19%)

Mucosal/ENT

Dysgeusia (~2%)
Mucositis (17%)

Eyes

Vision blurred (~2%)

Other

Abdominal pain (27%)
Asthenia (8%)
Cough (24%)
Fever (45%)
Headache (28%)
  (2005): Torres HA+, *Lancet Infect Dis* 5(12), 775
Hypertension (18%)
Hypotension (14%)
Myalgia/Myositis/Myopathy/Myotoxicity (16%)
Tremor (~2%)
Upper respiratory infection (7%)
Vertigo (11%)

POTASSIUM IODIDE

Synonyms: KI; Lugol's solution; strong iodine solution
Trade names: Jodatum; Jodid; Kalium; Kie; SSKI (Upsher-Smith); Thyroid-Block
Indications: Hyperthyroidism, erythema nodosum, sporotrichosis
Category: Antihyperthyroid; Antimycobacterial
Half-life: N/A
Clinically important, potentially hazardous interactions with: ACE inhibitors, potassium-sparing diuretics, spironolactone, triamterene

Reactions

Skin

Acne (1–10%)
Angioedema (1–10%)
Bullous pemphigoid
  (1994): Piletta P+, *Br J Dermatol* 131, 145
Dermatitis (systemic)
  (2004): Sicherer SH, *J Allergy Clin Immunol* 114(6), 1395
Dermatitis herpetiformis
  (1989): Zone JJ+, *Immunol Ser* 46, 565
Diaphoresis
Exanthems
  (1981): Farkas J, *Dermatol Monatsschr* (German) 167, 579
Iododerma
  (1996): Alpay K+, *Pediatr Dermatol* 13, 51
  (1990): Soria C +, *J Am Acad Dermatol* 22, 418 (vegetating)
  (1989): Romanenko VN+, *Vestn Dermatol Venerol* (Russian) 12, 60
  (1987): O'Brien TJ, *Australas J Dermatol* 28, 119
  (1986): Raznatovskii IM+, *Vestn Dermatol Venerol* (Russian) 10, 71
  (1985): Stone OJ, *Int J Dermatol* 24, 565
  (1985): Wilkin JK+, *Cutis* 36, 335
  (1981): Huang TY+, *Ann Allergy* 46, 264
Lupus erythematosus
Psoriasis
Purpura
Rash (sic)
Urticaria (1–10%)
Vasculitis
  (1987): Eeckhout E+, *Acta Derm Venereol* (Stockh) 67, 362
  (1981): Zone JJ, *Arch Dermatol* 117, 758

Mucosal/ENT

Dysgeusia (1–10%) (metallic taste)
Gingivitis
Sialorrhea
Stomatodynia

Other

Anaphylactoid reactions/Anaphylaxis
  (2004): Sicherer SH, *J Allergy Clin Immunol* 114(6), 1395
Paresthesias
Serum sickness

PRAMIPEXOLE

Trade name: Mirapex (Pfizer) (Boehringer Ingelheim)
Indications: Parkinsonism
Category: Dopamine receptor agonist
Half-life: ~8 hours

Reactions

Skin
Adverse effects (sic) (2%)
Allergic reactions (sic) (>1%)
Diaphoresis (>1%)
Edema (5%)
Peripheral edema (5%)
  (2000): Tan EK+, *Arch Neurol* 57, 729
Pruritus (>1%)
Rash (sic) (>1%)
Vasculitis
  (2004): Famularo G+, *Clin Exp Rheumatol* 22(6), 785

Mucosal/ENT
Dysgeusia (>1%)
Sialorrhea (>1%)
Xerostomia (7%)
  (2006): Montplaisir J+, *Eur J Neurol* 13(12), 1306 (2%)
  (1998): Dooley M+, *Drugs Aging* 12, 495

Hair
Hair – alopecia
  (2006): Katz KA+, *J Am Acad Dermatol* 55(5), S103

Eyes
Dyschromatopsia
  (2003): Muller T+, *J Neurol* 250(1), 101

Other
Asthenia
  (2006): Montplaisir J+, *Eur J Neurol* 13(12), 1306 (9%)
Headache
  (2006): Montplaisir J+, *Eur J Neurol* 13(12), 1306 (4%)
Inappropriate secretion of antidiuretic hormone (SIADH)
  (2005): Tomita M+, *Nippon Jinzo Gakkai Shi* 47(5), 531
Myalgia/Myositis/Myopathy/Myotoxicity (>1%)
Nephrotoxicity
  (2004): Famularo G+, *Clin Exp Rheumatol* 22(6), 785
Paresthesias (>1%)
Vertigo
  (2006): Montplaisir J+, *Eur J Neurol* 13(12), 1306 (8%)

PRAMLINTIDE

Trade name: Symlin (Amlin)
Indications: Diabetes, Adjunct to insulin treatment
Category: Amylinomimetic; Protein analog
Half-life: 48 minutes
Clinically important, potentially hazardous interactions with: acarbose, acetaminophen, **alcohol**, anticholinergic agents, atropine, miglitol

Reactions

Skin
Allergic reactions (sic) (6%)
Diaphoresis

Other
Abdominal pain (8%)
Asthenia (7%)
Coma
Cough (6%)
Headache (13%)
Injection-site edema
Injection-site pain
Injection-site pruritus
Seizures
Tremor
Vertigo (5–6%)

PRANLUKAST

Trade names: Azlaire (Schering-Plough); Onon (Ono Pharmaceuticals)
Indications: Bronchial asthma and allergic rhinitis
Category: Leukotriene receptor antagonist
Half-life: 1.5 hours

Reactions

Skin
Allergic granulomatous angiitis (Churg–Strauss syndrome)
  (2007): Guilpain P+, *Presse Med* 36(5 Pt 2), 890
  (2005): Shimbo J+, *Clin Rheumatol* 24(6), 661
  (2003): Garcia-Marcos L+, *Drug Saf* 26(7), 483
  (2003): Katsura T+, *Ann Intern Med* 139(5 Pt 1), 386
  (2003): Kobayashi S+, *Clin Rheumatol* 22(6), 491
  (2000): Baba K+, *Arerugi* 49(6), 512
  (1999): Kinoshita M+, *J Allergy Clin Immunol* 103(3 Pt 1), 534
Edema (leg)
  (2004): Obase Y+, *Respiration* 71(3), 225

Other
Fever
  (2001): Takahashi N+, *Intern Med* 40(8), 791
Hypersensitivity
  (1998): Schurman SJ+, *Chest* 114(4), 1220
Nephrotoxicity
  (1998): Schurman SJ+, *Chest* 114(4), 1220
Vertigo
  (2004): Obase Y+, *Respiration* 71(3), 225

PRANOPROFEN

Trade name: Niflan (Mitsubishi Tanabe Pharma)
Indications: Pain, inflammation
Category: Non-steroidal anti-inflammatory
Half-life: N/A

Reactions

Other
Anaphylactoid reactions/Anaphylaxis
  (2007): Shirai T+, *Intern Med* 46(6), 315

PRAVASTATIN

Trade names: Elisor; Lipostat; Pravachol (Bristol-Myers Squibb); Pravasin; Pravasine; Selectin; Selektine; Selipran
Indications: Hypercholesterolemia
Category: HMG-CoA reductase inhibitor; Statin
Half-life: ~2–3 hours
Clinically important, potentially hazardous interactions with: azithromycin, ciprofibrate, clarithromycin, cyclosporine, darunavir, erythromycin, gemfibrozil, imatinib, **red rice yeast**

Reactions

Skin

Allergic reactions (sic)
  (1994): de Boer EM+, *Contact Dermatitis* 30, 238
Angioedema
Dermatomyositis
  (2005): Zuech P+, *Rev Med Interne* 26(11), 897
  (1992): Schalke BB+, *N Engl J Med* 327, 649
Eczema (generalized)
  (1993): Krasovec M+, *Dermatology* 186, 248
Erythema multiforme
Exanthems
Ichthyosis
  (2007): Sparsa A+, *J Eur Acad Dermatol Venereol* 21(4), 549
Lichenoid eruption
  (2006): Pua VS+, *Australas J Dermatol* 47(1), 57
  (1998): Keough GC+, *Cutis* 61, 98
  (1997): Anthony JL, Montgomery, AL (from Internet) (observation)
Lupus erythematosus
Photosensitivity
Pruritus
  (1992): Yoshimura N+, *Transplantation* 53, 94
  (1991): Malini PL+, *Clin Ther* 13, 500
Purpura
Rash (sic) (1–10%)
  (1992): Betteridge DJ+, *BMJ* 304, 1335
  (1992): Jungnickel PW+, *Clin Pharm* 11, 677
  (1991): *Med Lett Drugs Ther* 33, 18
  (1991): Crepaldi G+, *Arch Intern Med* 151, 146
  (1991): McTavish D+, *Drugs* 42, 65
  (1991): Raasch RH, *Drug Intell Clin Pharm* 25, 388
  (1990): Hunninghake DB+, *Atherosclerosis* 85, 81 (3.4%)
Stevens–Johnson syndrome
Toxic epidermal necrolysis
Urticaria
Vasculitis

Mucosal/ENT

Dysgeusia (<1%)
Stomatitis

Hair

Hair – alopecia
  (1999): Oakley A, Hamilton, New Zealand (from Internet) (observation)
Hair – broken-off patches of scalp hair (greenish)
  (1998): Fixler R, Cincinnati, OH (personal communication) (observation)

Other

Abdominal pain
  (2006): Tsigrelis C+, *World J Gastroenterol* 12(43), 7055
Anaphylactoid reactions/Anaphylaxis
Gynecomastia

  (1999): Aerts J+, *Presse Med* (French) 28, 787
Headache
Hypersensitivity
Myalgia/Myositis/Myopathy/Myotoxicity (2.7%)
  (2005): Alayli G+, *Ann Pharmacother* 39(7-8), 1358 (with colchicine)
  (2003): Litt JZ, Beachwood, OH (personal case) (observation)
  (2002): Sinzinger H, *Wien Klin Wochenschr* 114(21), 943
  (2002): Wilhelmi M+, *Cardiovasc Drugs Ther* 16(5), 471
  (2001): Rehbein H, Jacksonville, FL (from Internet) (observation)
  (1995): Garnett WR, *Am J Health Syst Pharm* 52(15), 1639
  (1992): Schalke BB+, *N Engl J Med* 327, 649
Paresthesias
Polymyositis
  (2004): Takagi A+, *Rinsho Shinkeigaku* 44(1), 25
Porphyria cutanea tarda
  (1994): Perrot JL+, *Ann Dermatol Venereol* (French) 121, 817
Rhabdomyolysis
  (2007): Schindler C+, *Clin Ther* 29(1), 172
  (2006): Biggs MJ+, *J Heart Lung Transplant* 25(3), 356
  (2005): Andrejak M+, *Therapie* 60(3), 299
  (2004): Graham DJ+, *JAMA* 292(21), 2585 (low risk)
  (2002): Cohen LH, *Ned Tijdschr Geneeskd* 146(9), 440
  (2002): Sica DA+, *Am J Geriatr Cardiol* 11(1), 48
  (2002): Sica DA+, *Curr Opin Nephrol Hypertens* 11(2), 123
  (2002): Wilhelmi M+, *Cardiovasc Drugs Ther* 16(5), 471
  (2001): Borrego FJ+, *Nefrologia* 21(3), 309
  (1999): Takei A+, *Psychiatry Clin Neurosci* 53(4), 539
  (1998): Kamiuchi K+, *Nihon Rinsho Meneki Gakkai Kaishi* 21(1), 48
  (1996): Ballantyne CM+, *Am J Cardiol* 78(5), 532
  (1996): Hino I+, *Arthritis Rheum* 39(7), 1259
  (1995): Farmer JA+, *Baillieres Clin Endocrinol Metab* 9(4), 825
  (1995): Garnett WR, *Am J Health Syst Pharm* 52(15), 1639 (with either cyclosporine, erythromycin, gemfibrozil or niacin)
  (1995): Rosenberg AD+, *Anesth Analg* 81(5), 1089
  (1993): Decoulx E+, *Ann Cardiol Angeiol (Paris)* 42(5), 267
  (1992): Raimondeau J+, *Presse Med* 21(14), 663 (with fenofibrate)

PRAZEPAM

Trade names: Centrax; Demetrin; Lysanxia; Prazene; Sedapran; Trepidan
Indications: Anxiety, depression
Category: Benzodiazepine
Half-life: 30–100 hours

Reactions

Skin

Dermatitis (1–10%)
Diaphoresis (>10%)
Exanthems
Facial edema
Peripheral edema
Pruritus
Purpura
Rash (sic) (>10%)
Urticaria

Mucosal/ENT

Gingivitis
Sialopenia (>10%)
Sialorrhea (1–10%)
Xerostomia (>10%)

Hair
Hair – alopecia
Hair – hirsutism

Other
Paresthesias

PRAZIQUANTEL

Trade names: Biltricide; Cisticid; Distocide; Flukacide; Kalcide; Prazite; Tecprazin; Teniken
Indications: Helmintic infections
Category: Antihelmintic
Half-life: 0.8–1.5 hours
Clinically important, potentially hazardous interactions with: dexamethasone

Reactions

Skin
Angioedema
  (2006): Olson BG+, *Pediatr Infect Dis J* 25(5), 466 (with ivermectin and albendazole)
Diaphoresis (1–10%)
Edema
  (1995): Stelma FF+, *Am J Trop Med Hyg* 53, 167
Pruritus (<1%)
Rash (sic) (<1%)
Urticaria (<1%)
  (2006): Olson BG+, *Pediatr Infect Dis J* 25(5), 466 (with ivermectin and albendazole)
  (1996): Jaoko WG+, *East Afr Med J* 73, 499
  (1995): Stelma FF+, *Am J Trop Med Hyg* 53, 167

Other
Abdominal pain
  (2006): Olson BG+, *Pediatr Infect Dis J* 25(5), 466 (with ivermectin and albendazole)
  (2004): Raso G+, *Trans R Soc Trop Med Hyg* 98(1), 18
Anaphylactoid reactions/Anaphylaxis
  (2007): Shen C+, *Am J Trop Med Hyg* 76(3), 603
Fever
  (2006): Olson BG+, *Pediatr Infect Dis J* 25(5), 466 (with ivermectin and albendazole)
Headache
Vertigo
  (2004): Raso G+, *Trans R Soc Trop Med Hyg* 98(1), 18

PRAZOSIN

Trade names: Alti-Prazosin; Apo-Prazo; Duramipress; Eurex; Hypovase; Minipress (Pfizer); Minizide (Pfizer); Nu-Prazo; Peripress; Pratisol; Pressin
Indications: Hypertension
Category: Adrenergic alpha-receptor antagonist
Half-life: 2–4 hours
Clinically important, potentially hazardous interactions with: epinephrine

Note: Minizide is prazosin and polythiazide

Reactions

Skin
Angioedema
  (1983): Ruzicka T+, *Lancet* 1, 473
Diaphoresis (<1%)
Edema (1–4%)
Exanthems (1–5%)
Lichen planus (<1%)
Lichenoid eruption
Lupus erythematosus
Pruritus (<1%)
Rash (sic) (1–4%)
  (1983): Stanaszek WF+, *Drugs* 25, 339
Urticaria
  (1983): Ruzicka T+, *Lancet* 1, 473

Mucosal/ENT
Tinnitus
Xerostomia (1–4%)
  (1983): Stanaszek WF+, *Drugs* 25, 339

Hair
Hair – alopecia (<1%)

Eyes
Visual hallucinations

Other
Anaphylactoid reactions/Anaphylaxis
  (1983): Ruzicka T+, *Lancet* 1, 473
Headache
Myalgia/Myositis/Myopathy/Myotoxicity
Paresthesias (<1%)

PREDNICARBATE

Trade name: Dermatop (Dermik)
Indications: Dermatoses
Category: Corticosteroid, topical
Half-life: N/A
Clinically important, potentially hazardous interactions with: live vaccines

Reactions

Skin
Allergic reactions (sic)
  (1999): Stingeni L+, *Contact Dermatitis* 40(5), 286
  (1990): Lubach D+, *Hautarzt* 41(1), 43
Bullous dermatitis
  (1999): Lew DB+, *Pediatr Dermatology* 16, 146
Burning
  (2004): Gupta AK+, *J Drugs Dermatol* 3(5), 553
Dermatitis
  (2004): Gupta AK+, *J Drugs Dermatol* 3(5), 553
  (2000): Chew AL+, *Cutis* 65, 307
  (1995): Bircher AJ+, *Acta Derm Venereol* 75, 490
  (1991): Dunkel FG+, *Contact Dermatitis* 24(1), 59
  (1991): Dunkel FG+, *Contact Dermatitis* 25(2), 97
  (1991): Senff H+, *Hautarzt* 42(1), 53
Edema
  (2004): Gupta AK+, *J Drugs Dermatol* 3(5), 553
Erythema multiforme
  (1999): Lew DB+, *Pediatr Dermatol* 16, 146
Folliculitis

(2004): Gupta AK+, *J Drugs Dermatol* 3(5), 553
Genital edema
  (1998): Miranda-Romero+, *Contact Dermatitis* 38(4), 228
Lupus erythematosus
  (2006): Sanchez-Perez J+, *Contact Dermatitis* 55(4), 247
Pruritus
  (2004): Gupta AK+, *J Drugs Dermatol* 3(5), 553
  (1999): Lew DB+, *Pediatr Dermatology* 16, 146
Rash (sic)
  (2004): Gupta AK+, *J Drugs Dermatol* 3(5), 553
Scaling
  (2004): Gupta AK+, *J Drugs Dermatol* 3(5), 553
Urticaria
  (2004): Gupta AK+, *J Drugs Dermatol* 3(5), 553

Other

Anaphylactoid reactions/Anaphylaxis
  (1995): Jacqz-Aigrain E+, *Arch Pediatr* (French) 2, 353
Pain
  (2004): Gupta AK+, *J Drugs Dermatol* 3(5), 553
Paresthesias
  (2004): Gupta AK+, *J Drugs Dermatol* 3(5), 553
Vertigo
  (2004): Gupta AK+, *J Drugs Dermatol* 3(5), 553

PREDNISOLONE

Trade names: Blephamide (Allergan); Delta-Cortef (Pharmacia); Hydeltrasol (Merck); Inflamase (Novartis); Pediapred (UCB); Prelone (Teva)
Indications: Arthralgias, Asthma, Dermatoses, Ophthalmology (many others)
Category: Corticosteroid, systemic
Half-life: N/A
Clinically important, potentially hazardous interactions with: aluminum, carbamazepine, carbimazole, cyclosporine, daclizumab, diuretics, etoposide, etretinate, **grapefruit juice**, indomethacin, isoniazid, itraconazole, ketoconazole, **licorice**, **live vaccines**, methotrexate, naproxen, oral contraceptives, pancuronium, phenobarbital, phenytoin, rifampicin, theophylline, troleandomycin

Reactions

Skin

Acanthosis nigricans (sic)
  (2000): Ozerdem U+, *Am J Ophthalmol* 130(2), 240
Acne
  (2004): Escher JC, *Eur J Gastroenterol Hepatol* 16(1), 47
  (2003): Richardus JH+, *Lepr Rev* 74(4), 319
Acute generalized exanthematous pustulosis
  (2006): Buettiker U+, *Dermatology* 213(1), 40
Allergic reactions
  (2000): Bircher AJ+, *Dermatology* 200(4), 349
  (1999): Burova K+, *Br J Dermatol* 141(3), 597
Atrophy
Bruising
  (2001): Walsh LJ+, *Thorax* 56(4), 279
Dermatitis
  (2000): Bircher AJ+, *Dermatology* 200(4), 349
  (2000): Harris A+, *Australas J Dermatol* 41(2), 124
  (1998): Isaksson M+, *Am J Contact Dermat* 9(2), 136
Dermatofibromas
  (2007): Huang PY+, *J Am Acad Dermatol* 57(5 Suppl 1), S81
    (multiple) (with methotrexate)

Erythema
  (1999): Alexiou C+, *Laryngorhinootologie* 78(10), 573
  (1998): Alexiou C+, *Arch Otolaryngol Head Neck Surg* 124(11), 1260
Erythema multiforme
  (2004): Sen P+, *Ann Acad Med Singapore* 33(6), 793 (recurrence)
  (1999): Lew DB+, *Pediatr Dermatol* 16(2), 146
Exanthems
  (2005): Padial A+, *Allergy* 60(5), 665
  (2000): Bircher AJ+, *Dermatology* 200(4), 349
  (2000): Chew AL+, *Cutis* 65(5), 307
Kaposi's sarcoma
  (2004): Elliott AM+, *J Infect Dis* 190(5), 869
  (2001): Sato-Matsumura KC+, *Br J Dermatol* 145(4), 633
  (1997): Halpern SM+, *Br J Dermatol* 137(1), 140 (with azathioprine)
Pruritus
  (1999): Alexiou C+, *Laryngorhinootologie* 78(10), 573
  (1998): Alexiou C+, *Arch Otolaryngol Head Neck Surg* 124(11), 1260
Psoriasis
  (2006): Elston GE+, *Clin Exp Dermatol* 31(1), 133 (pustular) (generalized)
Squamous cell carcinoma
  (1999): Ahuja M+, *Am J Kidney Dis* 34(3), 521 (with azathioprine)
Stevens–Johnson syndrome
  (2003): Jo DS+, *Pediatr Nephrol* 18(9), 959
Thinning
  (2003): Schou AJ+, *J Pediatr Endocrinol* 16(7), 973
Toxicoderma
  (1996): Mathelier-Fusade P+, *Ann Dermatol Venereol* 123(8), 453
Urticaria
  (2005): Padial A+, *Allergy* 60(5), 665

Hair

Hair – hypertrichosis

Eyes

Cataract
  (2003): Richardus JH+, *Lepr Rev* 74(4), 319
  (2001): Walsh LJ+, *Thorax* 56(4), 279
  (1998): Dasgupta B+, *Br J Rheumatol* 37(2), 189
Chorioretinopathy
  (2004): Koyama M+, *Ophthalmologica* 218(2), 107
  (1997): Wakakura M+, *Jpn J Ophthalmol* 41(3), 180
Diplopia
  (1997): Brocq O+, *Presse Med* 26(6), 271
Glaucoma
  (2003): Richardus JH+, *Lepr Rev* 74(4), 319
  (1995): Kong L+, *Yan Ke Xue Bao* 11(1), 53
Ocular burning
Ocular pain
Ocular pressure
  (2004): Tham CC+, *Am J Ophthalmol* 137(1), 198
  (2000): Ozerdem U+, *Am J Ophthalmol* 130(2), 240
Ocular stinging
Vision blurred
  (2000): Ozerdem U+, *Am J Ophthalmol* 130(2), 240

Other

Adverse effects (sic)
  (2004): Gotzsche PC+, *Cochrane Database Syst Rev* f(3), CD00
Anaphylactoid reactions/Anaphylaxis
  (2005): Erdmann SM+, *J Am Board Fam Pract* 18(2), 143
Candidiasis
  (2002): Tanaka H+, *Pediatr Int* 44(6), 702
  (2001): Walsh LJ+, *Thorax* 56(4), 279
Depression

(2002): Fauchais AL+, *Rev Med Interne* 23(10), 828
(1998): Dasgupta B+, *Br J Rheumatol* 37(2), 189
(1988): Braunig P+, *Nervenarzt* 59(10), 596

Headache
(1998): Sharma VK+, *Pediatr Dermatol* 15(4), 313

Hypertension
(1998): Dasgupta B+, *Br J Rheumatol* 37(2), 189
(1995): Sato A+, *Am J Hypertens* 8(8), 823

Infections
(2004): Lamb SR+, *Clin Exp Dermatol* 29(3), 254
(2003): Kunisada M+, *Int J Dermatol* 42(9), 710
(2003): Richardus JH+, *Lepr Rev* 74(4), 319
(2002): Han BG+, *Yonsei Med J* 43(5), 686
(2001): Polnau U+, *Z Rheumatol* 60(1), 41
(2001): Yasumi M+, *Rinsho Ketsueki* 42(8), 601
(2000): Hovi L+, *Bone Marrow Transplant* 26(9), 999
(2000): Maeno Y+, *Respirology* 5(4), 393
(1999): Ahuja M+, *Am J Kidney Dis* 34(3), 521 (with azathioprine)
(1999): Matsuda K+, *J Gastroenterol* 34(3), 390
(1998): Matsuno O+, *Am J Trop Med Hyg* 59(1), 42 (with melphalan)
(1998): Yagi T+, *Kekkaku* 73(9), 557
(1996): Gallardo D+, *Bone Marrow Transplant* 18(6), 1135

Lipomatosis
(2000): Jalladeau E+, *Rev Neurol* (Paris) 156(5), 517

Myalgia/Myositis/Myopathy/Myotoxicity
(2003): Kumar S, *Neurol India* 51(4), 554
(2001): Walsh LJ+, *Thorax* 56(4), 279

Osteoporosis
(2005): Griffith JF+, *Radiology* 235(1), 168 (0.6–13%)
(2005): Schoon EJ+, *Clin Gastroenterol Hepatol* 3(2), 113
(2005): Vestergaard P+, *J Intern Med* 257(4), 374
(2005): Yee CS+, *Ann Rheum Dis* 64(1), 111
(2004): Shimojima Y+, *Clin Rheumatol* 23(3), 262
(2004): Tobias JH+, *Aliment Pharmacol Ther* 20(9), 951
(2004): Yonemura K+, *Am J Kidney Dis* 43(1), 53
(2003): de Deus RB+, *Nephron Clin Pract* 94(3), c69
(2003): Loddenkemper K+, *Clin Exp Rheumatol* 21(1), 19
(2003): Mirzaei S+, *J Asthma* 40(3), 251
(2002): Jones NP+, *Eye* 16(5), 587
(2002): Tsugeno H+, *Osteoporos Int* 13(8), 650
(2002): Walsh LJ+, *Am J Respir Crit Care Med* 166(5), 691
(2001): Haugeberg G+, *Scand J Gastroenterol* 36(7), 759
(2001): Inoue T+, *Endocr J* 48(1), 11
(2001): Rau R, *Z Rheumatol* 60(6), 485
(2001): Ugur A+, *Transplantation* 71(5), 645
(2001): Walsh LJ+, *Thorax* 56(4), 279
(2000): Jardinet D+, *Rheumatology* (Oxford) 39(4), 389
(2000): Lezhnina MB+, *Klin Med* (Mosk) 78(9), 28
(2000): Yonemura K+, *Calcif Tissue Int* 66(2), 123
(1999): Ebeling PR+, *J Bone Miner Res* 14(3), 342
(1999): Matsuda K+, *J Gastroenterol* 34(3), 390
(1999): Reginster JY+, *Osteoporos Int* 9(1), 75
(1998): Boot AM+, *Gut* 42(2), 188
(1998): Dasgupta B+, *Br J Rheumatol* 37(2), 189
(1998): Pearce G+, *Br J Rheumatol* 37(3), 292
(1998): Pearce G+, *J Clin Endocrinol Metab* 83(3), 801
(1997): Rizzato G+, *Respir Med* 91(8), 449
(1996): Villareal MS+, *Ann Allergy Asthma Immunol* 76(4), 369

Side effects (sic)
(2004): Potter JM+, *Ther Drug Monit* 26(4), 408
(2001): Macchia PE+, *J Endocrinol Invest* 24(3), 152
(2000): Eastell R+, *Osteoporos Int* 11(4), 331
(2000): Ozaki D+, *J Nippon Med Sch* 67(4), 271

Toxicity (sic)
(2000): Hiraoka M+, *Kidney Int* 58(3), 1247

Tumors
(2000): de Bono JS+, *Ann Oncol* 11(6), 749

Vertigo
(1998): Sharma VK+, *Pediatr Dermatol* 15(4), 313

PREDNISONE

Trade names: Deltasone (Pharmacia); Meticorten (Schering)
Indications: Arthralgias, Asthma, Dermatoses, Ophthalmology (many others)
Category: Corticosteroid, systemic
Half-life: N/A
Clinically important, potentially hazardous interactions with: aluminum, aminophylline, aspirin, chlorambucil, cimetidine, clarithromycin, cyclophosphamide, cyclosporine, dicumarol, diuretics, docetaxel, estrogens, **grapefruit juice**, indomethacin, itraconazole, ketoconazole, lansoprazole, **live vaccines**, methotrexate, montelukast, omeprazole, oral contraceptives, pancuronium, phenobarbital, phenytoin, ranitidine, rifampicin, rifampin, timolol, tolbutamide, vitamin A

Reactions

Skin
Acanthosis nigricans
(1980): Gottlieb NL+, *JAMA* 243, 1260
Acne
Allergic reactions (sic)
(1999): Alexiou C+, *Laryngorhinootologie* (German) 78, 573
Atrophy
Bruising
Cellulitis
(2004): Lafleur L+, *Cutis* 74(3), 165
Dermatitis
(2003): Levine A+, *J Pediatr Gastroenterol Nutr* 36(2), 248
(2000): Chew AL+, *Cutis* 65, 307
(2000): Harris A+, *Australas J Dermatol* 41, 124
Dermatofibromas
(2002): Massone C+, *Int J Dermatol* 41(5), 279
Diaphoresis
(1999): Alexiou C+, *Laryngorhinootologie* (German) 78, 573
Eczema
(2000): Bircher AJ+, *Dermatology* 200(4), 349
Edema
Erythema
(1999): Alexiou C+, *Laryngorhinootologie* (German) 78, 573
Linear hypopigmentation
(1980): Gottlieb L+, *Arch Dermatol* 140, 1507
Lymphoma
(2004): Cohen Y+, *Eur J Haematol* 73(2), 134
Pruritus
(1999): Alexiou C+, *Laryngorhinootologie* (German) 78, 573
Purpura
(1990): Capewell S+, *BMJ* 300, 1548
Rash (sic)
(2003): Prasad GV+, *Clin Transplant* 17(2), 135
Sensitivity
(2000): Bircher AJ+, *Dermatology* 200(4), 349
Squamous cell carcinoma
(2003): Hernandez G+, *Oral Oncol* 39(1), 87
(2002): Preciado DA+, *Head Neck* 24(4), 319
Staphylococcal scalded skin syndrome
(1998): Shirin S+, *Cutis* 62, 223 (in an adult)
Thinning
(1990): Capewell S+, *BMJ* 300, 1548
Toxicoderma
(1996): Mathelier-Fusade P+, *Ann Dermatol Venereol* 123(8), 453

Urticaria
(1990): Ashford RF+, *Postgrad Med J* 56, 437

Mucosal/ENT
Leukoplakia
(2003): Hernandez G+, *Oral Oncol* 39(1), 87

Hair
Hair – hypertrichosis

Eyes
Cataract
(2004): Matas AJ+, *Ann Surg* 240(3), 510
(2001): Ghodsi Z+, *Transfusion* 41(12), 1464
Chorioretinopathy
(2002): Bandello F+, *Eur J Ophthalmol* 12(2), 123
Glaucoma
(2000): Derzko-Dzulynsky L+, *Am J Ophthalmol* 129(6), 807
Uveitis
(2003): Zamani M+, *Am J Ophthalmol* 135(6), 891
Vision impaired

Other
Adverse effects (sic)
(2004): Caporali R+, *Ann Intern Med* 141(7), 493
(2003): Gladman DD+, *J Rheumatol* 30(9), 1955
(2003): Proven A+, *Arthritis Rheum* 49(5), 703
(2002): Khumalo NP+, *Arch Dermatol* 138(3), 385
Anaphylactoid reactions/Anaphylaxis
(1995): Jacqz-Aigrain E+,, *Arch Pediatr* (French) 2, 353
Asthenia
(2004): Miozzari M+, *Nephrol Dial Transplant* 19(10), 2615
Depression
(2004): Ros LT, *Afr J Med Med Sci* 33(3), 263
Headache
(2004): Miozzari M+, *Nephrol Dial Transplant* 19(10), 2615
(2003): Prasad GV+, *Clin Transplant* 17(2), 135
Hypertension
(2007): Fardet L+, *Br J Dermatol* 157(1), 142
(2005): Sinclair DB+, *Pediatr Neurol* 32(5), 300
(2001): Szymanik-Grzelak H+, *Pol Merkuriusz Lek* 10(58), 259
Infections
(2004): Arend SM+, *Eur J Clin Microbiol Infect Dis* 23(8), 638
   (with infliximab)
(2004): Uzuka T+, *No Shinkei Geka* 32(2), 127
(2003): Casals DS+, *J Dermatol* 30(4), 332
(2003): Prasad GV+, *Clin Transplant* 17(2), 135
(2003): Yoo SS+, *J Dermatol* 30(5), 405
(2000): Hovi L+, *Bone Marrow Transplant* 26(9), 999
Lipodystrophy
(2007): Fardet L+, *Br J Dermatol* 157(1), 142
Lipomatosis
(2002): ter Borg EJ+, *Ned Tijdschr Geneeskd* 146(2), 67
Myalgia/Myositis/Myopathy/Myotoxicity
(2007): Fardet L+, *Br J Dermatol* 157(1), 142
(2004): Miozzari M+, *Nephrol Dial Transplant* 19(10), 2615
Osteoporosis
(2005): Ton FN+, *J Bone Miner* 20(3), 464
(2003): Bianchi ML+, *Osteoporos Int* 14(9), 761
(2003): Boyanov M+, *Clin Rheumatol* 22(4-5), 318
(2003): Conn DL+, *Curr Opin Rheumatol* 15(3), 193
(2003): Crawford BA+, *J Clin Endocrinol Metab* 88(7), 3167
(2003): de Deus RB+, *Nephron Clin Pract* 94(3), c69
(2003): Emkey R+, *Arthritis Rheum* 48(4), 1102
(2003): Frediani B+, *Bone* 33(4), 575
(2003): Gulati S+, *Am J Kidney Dis* 41(6), 1163
(2003): Oliveri B+, *Joint Bone Spine* 70(1), 46
(2003): Prasad GV+, *Clin Transplant* 17(2), 135
(2003): van Everdingen AA+, *Clin Exp Rheumatol* 21(2), 155
(2002): Koc S+, *Blood* 100(1), 48

(2002): Solomon DH+, *Arthritis Rheum* 46(12), 3136
(2002): van Everdingen AA+, *Ann Intern Med* 136(1), 1
(2001): Kroot EJ+, *Arthritis Rheum* 44(6), 1254
(2001): Szymanik-Grzelak H+, *Pol Merkuriusz Lek* 10(58), 259
(2000): Garey KW+, *Chest* 118(6), 1826
(2000): Lespessailles E+, *Joint Bone Spine* 67(2), 119
(2000): Monier-Faugere MC+, *J Am Soc Nephrol* 11(6), 1093
(1996): Villareal MS+, *Ann Allergy Asthma Immunol* 76(4), 369
Side effects (sic)
(2003): Lande MB+, *Pediatr Nephrol* 18(4), 342
(2002): Joly P+, *N Engl J Med* 346(5), 321
(2001): Macchia PE+, *J Endocrinol Invest* 24(3), 152
Tendinopathy/Tendon rupture
(2002): Khurana R+, *Respirology* 7(2), 161
Vertigo

PREGABALIN

Trade name: Lyrica (Pfizer)
Indications: Neuropathy, Post-herpetic neuralgia, Partial epilepsy
Category: Anticonvulsant; GABA analog
Half-life: 6 hours

Reactions

Skin
Abscess
Allergic granulomatous angiitis (Churg–Strauss syndrome)
Angioedema
Atrophy
Cellulitis
Eczema
Edema (2%)
Exfoliative dermatitis
Lichenoid eruption
Peripheral edema (9%)
(2005): *Prescrire Int* 14(80), 203
(2005): Frampton JE+, *Drugs* 65(1), 111
(2005): Freynhagen R+, *Pain* 115(3), 254
Petechiae
Photosensitivity
Pigmentation
Pruritus
Purpura
Pustules
Stevens–Johnson syndrome
Ulcerations
Urticaria
Vesiculobullous eruption
Xerosis

Mucosal/ENT
Ageusia
Aphthous stomatitis
Balanitis
Dysgeusia
Dysphagia
Oral ulceration
Otitis
Parosmia
Tinnitus
Tongue edema
Xerostomia (5%)

Hair
Hair – alopecia
Hair – hirsutism

Eyes
Amblyopia
Blepharitis
Conjunctivitis
Diplopia (9%)
Iritis
Keratoconjunctivitis
Miosis
Mydriasis
Nystagmus
Ocular atrophy
Ocular hemorrhage
Photophobia
Ptosis
Uveitis
Vision blurred (6%)
Vision loss

Other
Abdominal pain
Anaphylactoid reactions/Anaphylaxis
Asthenia (5%)
  (2008): Zaccara G+, *Seizure* nd, 182
  (2005): Gil-Nagel Rein A+, *Rev Neurol* 40(10), 609
Chest pain (2%)
Chills
Coma
Fever
Headache (7%)
Hypotension
Infections (7%)
Myalgia/Myositis/Myopathy/Myotoxicity
Myoclonus
  (2001): Huppertz HJ+, *Epilepsia* 42(6), 790
Pain (5%)
Paresthesias
Somnolence
  (2008): Zaccara G+, *Seizure* nd, 182
Suicidal ideation
Thrombophlebitis
Tremor (1%)
Vertigo (4%)
  (2008): Zaccara G+, *Seizure* nd, 182
  (2006): Hamandi K+, *Seizure* 15(2), 73
  (2006): van Seventer R+, *Curr Med Res Opin* 22(2), 375 (6%)
  (2005): *Prescrire Int* 14(80), 203
  (2005): Beydoun A+, *Neurology* 64(3), 475
  (2005): Frampton JE+, *Drugs* 65(1), 111
  (2005): Freynhagen R+, *Pain* 115(3), 254
  (2005): Gil-Nagel Rein A+, *Rev Neurol* 40(10), 609
  (2005): Hadj Tahar A, *Issues Emerg Health Technol* 67, 1
  (2005): Richter RW+, *J Pain* 6(4), 253
  (2005): Warner G+, *CNS Drugs* 19(3), 265
  (2004): Lesser H+, *Neurology* 63(11), 2104
  (2004): Pande AC+, *J Clin Psychopharmacol* 24(2), 141
  (2003): Feltner DE+, *J Clin Psychopharmacol* 23(3), 240
  (2003): Pande AC+, *Am J Psychiatry* 160(3), 533
Weight gain
  (2007): Ben-Menachem, *Epilepsia* 48, 42

PRIMAQUINE

Synonym: prymaccone
Trade names: Neo-Quipenyl; Palum; Primaquine (Sanofi-Aventis)
Indications: Malaria
Category: Antimalarial; Antiprotozoal
Half-life: 4–10 hours
Clinically important, potentially hazardous interactions with: penicillamine

Reactions

Skin
Angioedema
Exanthems (5%)
Pallor
Pruritus (<1%)
Psoriasis
Urticaria

Other
Cough
  (1995): Fryauff DJ+, *Lancet* 346(8984), 1190

PRIMIDONE

Trade names: Midone; Mylepsin; Mysoline (Xcel); PMS Primidone; Prysoline; Sertan
Indications: Seizures
Category: Anticonvulsant; Barbiturate
Half-life: 10–12 hours
Clinically important, potentially hazardous interactions with: alcohol, anticoagulants, antihistamines, brompheniramine, buclizine, chlorpheniramine, dexamethasone, dicumarol, ethanolamine, imatinib, midazolam, niacinamide, warfarin

Reactions

Skin
Acne
Allergic reactions (sic)
  (1984): Steffan MA+, *Contact Dermatitis* 10, 184
Erythema multiforme (<1%)
  (2002): Krivo JM, Franklin Square, NY (from Internet)
  (observation)
Exanthems (1–5%)
  (1980): Marghescu S+, *Fortschr Med* (German) 98, 723
Exfoliative dermatitis
Lupus erythematosus (<1%)
  (1994): Yung RL+, *Rheum Dis Clin North Am* 20, 61
  (1993): Drory VE+, *Clin Neuropharmacol* 16, 19 (passim)
  (1980): Condemi JJ, *Geriatrics* 35(3), 81
Rash (sic) (<1%)
  (2007): Arif H+, *Neurology* 68(20), 1701
Toxic epidermal necrolysis
  (1985): Muhar U+, *Pediatr Dermatol* 3, 54
Urticaria
  (1984): Steffan MA+, *Contact Dermatitis* 10, 184

Mucosal/ENT
Gingival hyperplasia/hypertrophy
Mucocutaneous syndrome

Other

Anticonvulsant hypersensitivity syndrome
  (2002): Kaur S+, *Pediatr Dermatol* 19(2), 142
Hypersensitivity
  (2002): Krivo JM, Franklin Square, NY (from Internet)
    (observation)
  (1998): Schlienger RG+, *Epilepsia* 39, S3 (passim)
Rhabdomyolysis
  (1990): Larpin R+, *Presse Med* 19(30), 1403

PROBENECID

Trade names: Bencid; Benecid; Benuryl; Panuric; Probalan;
Procid; Solpurin; Urocid
Indications: Gouty arthritis
Category: Uricosuric
Half-life: 6–12 hours (dose-dependent)
Clinically important, potentially hazardous interactions
with: amphotericin B, benzodiazepines, doripenem, ertapenem,
furosemide, glibenclamide, ketoprofen, ketorolac, methotrexate,
NSAIDs, pemetrexed, penicillamine, penicillin g, penicillin V,
salicylates, sulfamethoxazole, sulfonamides

Reactions

Skin

Allergic reactions (sic)
Dermatitis
Erythema multiforme
  (1985): Ting HC+, *Int J Dermatol* 24, 587
Exanthems
Pruritus (1–10%)
Rash (sic) (1–10%)
Urticaria (1–5%)

Mucosal/ENT

Gingivitis (1–10%)

Hair

Hair – alopecia

Other

Anaphylactoid reactions/Anaphylaxis (<1%)
Hypersensitivity
  (1998): Myers KW+, *Ann Allergy Asthma Immunol* 80, 416 (in
    AIDS)
Nephrotoxicity

PROCAINAMIDE

Trade names: Amisalen; Biocoryl; Procan (Pfizer); Procan SR;
Procanbid (Pfizer); Promine; Pronestyl; Rhythmin; Ritmocamid
Indications: Ventricular arrhythmias
Category: Antiarrhythmic class 1a
Half-life: 2.5–4.5 hours
Clinically important, potentially hazardous interactions
with: abarelix, amisulpride, arsenic, astemizole, ciprofloxacin,
enoxacin, gatifloxacin, imidapril, lomefloxacin, moxifloxacin,
norfloxacin, ofloxacin, quinolones, rocuronium, sparfloxacin

Reactions

Skin

Angioedema (<1%)
  (1985): Ponte CD+, *Drug Intell Clin Pharm* 19, 139
Dermatitis (6%)
  (1985): Gorsulowsky DC+, *J Am Acad Dermatol* 12, 245 (6%)
Eczema
Exanthems (1–8%)
  (1999): Numata T+, *Sangyo Ika Daigaku Zasshi* (Japanese)
    21, 235
  (1985): Gorsulowsky DC+, *J Am Acad Dermatol* 12, 245 (8%)
  (1984): Christensen DJ+, *Ann Intern Med* 100, 918
Lichen planus
  (1988): Sherertz EF, *Cutis* 42, 51
Lupus erythematosus (>10%)
  (2002): Siddiqui MA+, *Am J Ther* 9(2), 163 (passim)
  (1998): Kameda H+, *Br J Rheumatol* 37, 1236
  (1998): Ohtani Y+, *Nihon Kokyuki Gakkai Zasshi* (Japanese)
    36, 535
  (1997): Yung R+, *Arthritis Rheum* 40, 1436
  (1996): Miyasaka N, *Intern Med* 35, 527
  (1995): Finger DR+, *J Rheumatol* 22, 574
  (1995): Muramatsu M+, *Nippon Naika Gakkai Zasshi* (Japanese)
    84, 1736
  (1995): Panine VV+, American Academy of Dermatology
    Meeting, New Orleans (observation)
  (1995): Price EJ+, *Drug Saf* 12(4), 283
  (1995): Rubin RL+, *J Immunol* 154, 2483
  (1994): Cohen MG, *J Rheumatol* 21, 578
  (1993): McDonald E+, *Hosp Pract Off ED* 28, 95
  (1992): Klimas NG+, *Am J Med Sci* 303, 99
  (1992): Rubin RL, *Clin Biochem* 25, 223
  (1992): Rubin RL+, *J Clin Invest* 90, 165
  (1992): Skaer TL, *Clin Ther* 14, 496
  (1992): Stevens MB, *Hosp Pract Off Ed* 27, 27
  (1990): Pauls JD+, *Mol Immunol* 27, 701
  (1989): Adams LE+, *J Lab Clin Med* 113, 482
  (1989): Asherson RA+, *Ann Rheum Dis* 48, 232
  (1989): Mohindra SK+, *Crit Care Med* 17, 961
  (1989): Nichols CJ+, *Ophthalmology* 96, 1535
  (1989): Turgeon PW+, *Ophthalmology* 96, 68
  (1989): Vivino FB+, *Arthritis Rheum* 32, 560
  (1988): Agudelo CA+, *J Rheumatol* 15, 1431
  (1988): Forrester J+, *J Rheumatol* 15, 1384
  (1988): Hess E, *N Engl J Med* 318, 1460
  (1988): No Author, *J Tenn Med Assoc* 81, 579
  (1988): Sheretz EF, *Cutis* 42, 51
  (1988): Totoritis MC+, *N Engl J Med* 318, 1431
  (1988): Uetrecht JP, *Chem Res Toxicol* 1, 133
  (1987): Craft JE+, *Arthritis Rheum* 30, 689
  (1987): Shoenfeld Y+, *J Clin Immunol* 7, 410
  (1986): Harle JR+, *Ann Med Interne Paris* (French) 137, 599
  (1986): Jackson C+, *Clin Exp Rheumatol* 4, 290
  (1986): Reidenberg MM+, *Angiology* 37, 968
  (1986): Rubin RL+, *Am J Med* 80, 999
  (1986): Vitas B+, *Lijec Vjesn* (Serbo-Croatian-Roman) 108, 137
  (1986): Weisbart RH+, *Ann Intern Med* 104, 310
  (1985): Amadio P+, *Ann Intern Med* 102, 419
  (1985): Cush JJ+, *Am J Med Sci* 290, 36
  (1985): Epstein A+, *Arthritis Rheum* 28, 158
  (1985): Gorsulowsky DC+, *J Am Acad Dermatol* 12, 245 (>5%)
  (1985): Kale SA, *Postgrad Med* 77, 231
  (1985): Lovisetto P+, *Recenti Prog Med* (Italian) 76, 110
  (1985): Rubin RL+, *Clin Immunol Immunopathol* 36, 49
  (1985): Stratton MA, *Clin Pharm* 4, 657
  (1985): Totoritis MC+, *Postgrad Med* 78, 149
  (1984): Browning CA+, *Am J Cardiol* 53, 376
  (1984): Goldberg SK+, *Am J Med* 76, 146

(1984): Tan EM+, *Allergy Clin Immunol* 74, 631
(1984): Wollina U, *Z Gesamte Inn Med* (German) 39, 69
(1982): Chokron R+, *Nouv Presse Med* (French) 11, 2568
(1982): Gupta AK+, *Indian J Dermatol* 27, 112
(1982): Harmon CE+, *Clin Rheum Dis* 8, 121
(1982): Hess EV, *Arthritis Rheum* 25, 857
(1982): Tannen RH+, *Immunol Commun* 11, 33
(1981): Edwards RL+, *Arch Intern Med* 141, 1688
(1981): Gonzalez ER, *JAMA* 246, 1634
(1981): Hess EV, *Arthritis Rheum* 24, vi
(1981): Reidenberg MM, *Arthritis Rheum* 24, 1004
(1981): Schoen RT+, *Am J Med* 71, 5
(1981): Sheikh TK+, *Am J Clin Pathol* 75, 755
(1981): Tan EM+, *Arthritis Rheum* 24, 1064
(1981): Uetrecht JP+, *Arthritis Rheum* 24, 994
(1980): Ahmad S, *Circulation* 61, 865
(1980): Chubick A, *Adv Intern Med* 26, 467
(1980): Condemi JJ, *Geriatrics* 35(3), 81
(1980): Dixon JA+, *J Rheumatol* 7, 544
(1980): Seligmann H+, *Harefuah* (Hebrew) 99, 166
(1980): Weinstein A, *Prog Clin Immunol* 4, 1
Pruritus (<1%)
Purpura
  (1984): Christensen DJ+, *Ann Intern Med* 100, 918
Rash (sic) (<1%)
Urticaria (1–5%)
  (1988): Knox JP+, *Cutis* 42, 469
Vasculitis
  (1988): Knox JP+, *Cutis* 42, 469
  (1984): Ekenstam E+, *Arch Dermatol* 120, 484

Mucosal/ENT
Dysgeusia (3–4%) (bitter taste)
  (2000): Zervakis J+, *Physiol Behav* 68, 405
Oral mucosal eruption (2%)
  (1985): Gorsulowsky DC+, *J Am Acad Dermatol* 12, 245 (2%)

Other
Chills (<1%)
Congestive heart failure
  (1992): Hook BG+, *Pacing Clin Electrophysiol* 15(3), 324
Myalgia/Myositis/Myopathy/Myotoxicity (<1%)
  (1986): Lewis CA+, *BMJ* 292, 593
Pseudolymphoma
  (1996): Magro CM+, *Hum Pathol* 27(2), 125
Sjøgren's (Sicca) syndrome
Tremor (<1%)

PROCARBAZINE

Trade names: Matulane (Sigma-Tau); Natulan
Indications: Hodgkin's disease, lymphomas
Category: Alkylating agent
Half-life: 60 minutes
**Clinically important, potentially hazardous interactions
with:** aldesleukin, methotrexate

Note: Disulfiram-like reactions include headache, respiratory
difficulties, nausea, vomiting, sweating, thirst, hypotension, and
flushing

Reactions

Skin
Allergic reactions (sic) (<1%)
Angioedema
Dermatitis (<1%)

Diaphoresis
Edema
Exanthems (4–9%)
  (1980): Andersen E+, *Scand J Haematol* 24, 149 (9%)
Exfoliative dermatitis
Fixed eruption
  (1988): Giguere JK+, *Med Pediatr Oncol* 16, 378
Herpes zoster
Petechiae
Photosensitivity
Pigmentation (1–10%)
Pruritus (<1%)
Purpura
Rash (sic)
Toxic epidermal necrolysis
  (1980): Andersen E+, *Scand J Haematol* 24, 149
Urticaria (9%)
  (1980): Andersen E+, *Scand J Haematol* 24, 149 (9%)

Mucosal/ENT
Oral lesions (1–5%)
  (1983): Bronner AK+, *J Am Acad Dermatol* 9, 645 (1–5%)
Stomatitis (>10%)
Xerostomia

Hair
Hair – alopecia (1–10%)

Other
Disulfiram-like reaction
Gynecomastia
Headache
Hypersensitivity (2%)
Myalgia/Myositis/Myopathy/Myotoxicity (<1%)
Paresthesias (>10%)

PROCHLORPERAZINE

Trade names: Compazine (GSK); Edisylate; Novamin; Novomit;
Pasotomin; Prorazin; Stella; Stemetil; Tementil; Vertigon
Indications: Psychotic disorders
Category: Antipsychotic, phenothiazine; Muscarinic antagonist
Half-life: 23 hours
**Clinically important, potentially hazardous interactions
with:** antihistamines, arsenic, chlorpheniramine, dofetilide,
piperazine, quinine, quinolones, sparfloxacin

Reactions

Skin
Diaphoresis
Eczema
Erythema
Exanthems
Exfoliative dermatitis
Fixed eruption (<1%)
  (1984): Reilly GD+, *Acta Derm Venereol* (Stockh) 64, 270
Lupus erythematosus
Peripheral edema
Photosensitivity (1–10%)
  (1997): O'Reilly FM+, American Academy of Dermatology
      Meeting, Poster #14
  (1988): Rasmussen HB+, *Ugeskr Laeger* (Danish) 150, 930
Phototoxicity
Pigmentation (<1%) (blue-gray)

Pruritus (1–10%)
Purpura
Rash (sic) (1–10%)
Seborrhea
Toxic epidermal necrolysis
  (1986): Mérot Y+, *Arch Dermatol* 122, 455
Urticaria
Xerosis

Mucosal/ENT

Lip ulceration
  (1984): Reilly GD+, *Acta Derm Venereol* (Stockh) 64, 270
Sialorrhea
Tongue pigmentation
  (1989): Alroe C+, *Med J Aust* 150, 724
Xerostomia (>10%)

Other

Anaphylactoid reactions/Anaphylaxis (1–10%)
Gynecomastia (1–10%)
Headache
Seizures
  (2000): Muniz AE, *South Med J* 93(6), 629
Tremor

PROCYCLIDINE

Trade names: Apricolin; Kemadren; Kemadrin (Monarch); Onservan; Procyclid
Indications: Parkinsonism
Category: Muscarinic antagonist
Half-life: N/A
Duration of action: 4 hours
Clinically important, potentially hazardous interactions with: anticholinergics, arbutamine

Reactions

Skin

Photosensitivity (1–10%)
Rash (sic) (<1%)
Urticaria
Xerosis (>10%)

Mucosal/ENT

Xerostomia (>10%)

PROGESTINS

Generic names:
  Hydroxyprogesterone
    Trade names: Delta-Lutin; Duralutin; Hylutin; Pro-Depo; Prodrox
  Medroxyprogesterone
    Trade names: Curretab; Provera (Pfizer)
  Megestrol
    Trade name: Megace
  Norethindrone
    Trade names: Aygestin (Barr); Micronor; Norlutin; Norlutate; Nor-QD
  Norgestrol
    Trade name: Ovrette
  Progesterone
    Trade names: Gesterol 50; Progestaject
Category: Progestogen
Half-life: N/A
Clinically important, potentially hazardous interactions with: acitretin, dofetilide

Reactions

Skin

Acne
  (2003): Cohen EB+, *Ned Tijdschr Geneeskd* 147(43), 2137 (implant)
  (1995): Freeman EW+, *JAMA* 274, 51
Acute generalized exanthematous pustulosis (AGEP)
  (1998): Kuno Y+, *Acta Derm Venereol* 78, 383
Angioedema
Dermatitis
  (2001): Izu K+, *J UOEH* 23(4), 431
Diaphoresis (31%)
  (1990): Willemse PHB+, *Eur J Cancer* 26, 337 (31%)
Edema
Erythema multiforme
  (2005): Suzuki R+, *Br J Dermatol* 152(2), 370
  (1985): Wojnarowska F+, *J R Soc Med* 78, 407
Erythema nodosum
Exanthems
Hemorrhage
Melasma
Peripheral edema
Pruritus
Rash (sic)
Telangiectasia
Urticaria
  (1995): Shelley WB+, *Cutis* 55, 282 (observation)
  (1994): Shelley WB+, *Cutis* 55, 21 (observation)
  (1994): Yee KC+, *Br J Dermatol* 130, 121

Hair

Hair – alopecia
Hair – hirsutism

Other

Anaphylactoid reactions/Anaphylaxis
Gynecomastia (painful)

PROMAZINE

Trade names: Liranol; Prazine; Protactyl; Savamine; Talofen
Indications: Psychotic disorders, schizophrenia
Category: Antipsychotic, phenothiazine
Half-life: 24 hours
**Clinically important, potentially hazardous interactions
with:** sparfloxacin

Reactions

Skin
Dermatitis
Edema
Exanthems
Photosensitivity (1–10%)
Phototoxicity
    (1997): Eberlein-Konig B+, *Dermatology* 194(2), 131 (16%)
    (1985): Chignell CF+, *Environ Health Perspect* 64, 103
    (1985): Motten AG+, *Photochem Photobiol* 42, 9
Pigmentation (<1%) (slate-gray)
Purpura
Rash (sic) (1–10%)
Urticaria
Xerosis

Mucosal/ENT
Xerostomia

Other
Gynecomastia
Hypotension
    (1990): Hu OY+, *Biopharm Drug Dispos* 11(7), 557–68
Vertigo
    (1990): Hu OY+, *Biopharm Drug Dispos* 11(7), 557–68

PROMETHAZINE

Trade names: Anergan; Atosil; Bonnox; Closin; Goodnight;
Histantil; Pentazine; Phenazine; Phenergan (Wyeth); Prometh-50;
Prothiazine; Pyrethia
Indications: Allergic rhinitis, urticaria
Category: Antipsychotic, phenothiazine; Histamine H1 receptor
antagonist
Half-life: 10–14 hours
**Clinically important, potentially hazardous interactions
with:** antihistamines, arsenic, chlorpheniramine, dofetilide,
nalbuphine, piperazine, quinolones, sparfloxacin, zaleplon

Reactions

Skin
Allergic reactions (sic) (<1%)
Angioedema (<1%)
Bullous dermatitis (<1%)
Dermatitis
    (1997): Varela P, Porto, Portugal (from Internet) (observation)
Diaphoresis
Eczema
Erythema multiforme
    (1986): Dikland WJ+, *Pediatr Dermatol* 3, 135
    (1986): Fisher AA, *Cutis* 37, 158
Exanthems
Fixed eruption

    (1984): Chan HL, *Int J Dermatol* 23, 607
Jaundice
Lupus erythematosus
Photosensitivity (<1%)
    (1997): Varela P, Porto, Portugal (from Internet) (observation)
    (1991): Bergner T+, *J Allergy Clin Immunol* 87, 278
    (1988): Menz J+, *J Am Acad Dermatol* 18, 1044
    (1982): Rosen K+, *Acta Derm Venereol* 62, 246
    (1982): Torinuki W+, *Tohoku J Exp Med* 138, 223
Pigmentation
Purpura
Rash (sic) (<1%)
    (1991): Blanc VF+, *Can J Anaesth* 38, 54
Stevens–Johnson syndrome
Toxic epidermal necrolysis (<1%)
Urticaria
    (1994): Myers P+, *Arch Ophthalmol* 112, 734
    (1988): Mills PJ, *Anaesthesia* 43, 66 (with temazepam)

Mucosal/ENT
Oral ulceration
Tinnitus
Xerostomia (1–10%)
    (1991): Blanc VF+, *Can J Anaesth* 38, 54

Other
Anaphylactoid reactions/Anaphylaxis
    (1988): Mills PJ, *Anaesthesia* 43, 66 (with temazepam)
Chills
Embolia cutis medicamentosa (Nicolau syndrome)
    (1995): Faucher L+, *Pediatr Dermatol* 12, 187
Gynecomastia
Headache
Hypersensitivity
    (1996): Palop V+, *Aten Primaria* (Spanish) 18, 47
Injection-site reactions (sic)
Myalgia/Myositis/Myopathy/Myotoxicity (<1%)
Paresthesias (<1%)

PROPAFENONE

Trade names: Arythmol; Norfenon; Normorytmin; Rythmex;
Rythmol (Reliant); Rytmonorm
Indications: Ventricular arrhythmias
Category: Antiarrhythmic class 1c
Half-life: 10–32 hours
**Clinically important, potentially hazardous interactions
with:** digoxin, fosamprenavir, **grapefruit juice**, ritonavir,
tipranavir

Reactions

Skin
Acne (1%)
Acute generalized exanthematous pustulosis
    (2005): Huang YM+, *Int J Dermatol* 44(3), 256
Diaphoresis (1%)
Edema (<1%)
Exanthems
Lupus erythematosus (<1%)
    (1986): Guindo J+, *Ann Intern Med* 104, 589
Pruritus (<1%)
Psoriasis
    (2005): Capella GL, *Ann Dermatol Venereol* 132(4), 370
Purpura (<1%)

Rash (sic) (1–3%)
Urticaria

Mucosal/ENT
Dysgeusia (3–23%)
  (2000): Zervakis J+, *Physiol Behav* 68, 405
Oral lesions (>5%)
Parosmia (<1%)
Tinnitus
Xerostomia (2%)

Hair
Hair – alopecia (<1%)

Other
Congestive heart failure
  (1990): Lange H+, *Am J Cardiol* 65(7), 458
  (1989): Ravid S+, *J Am Coll Cardiol* 14(5), 1326
Death
  (2004): Holzki J+, *Paediatr Anaesth* 14(3), 265
Headache
Hypotension
  (2002): Zaidenstein R+, *Pharmacoepidemiol Drug Saf* 11(3), 235
Injection-site pain (28–90%)
  (2004): Agarwal A+, *Anesth Analg* 98(3), 683 (28–90%)
  (2004): Basaranoglu G, *Anaesthesia* 59(2), 189
  (2004): Kunitz O+, *Anasthesiol Intensivmed Notfallmed Schmerzther* 39(1), 10
  (2003): Yoshimura Y+, *Masui* 52(11), 1204
Paresthesias (<1%)
Seizures
  (2004): Puranik S+, *Eur J Anaesthesiol* 21(1), 72
Tremor (<1%)

PROPANTHELINE

Trade names: Bropantil; Corrigast; Ercoril; Ercotina; Norproban; Propantel; Propantheline
Indications: Peptic ulcer
Category: Muscarinic antagonist
Half-life: 1.6 hours
Clinically important, potentially hazardous interactions with: anticholinergics, arbutamine, digoxin

Reactions

Skin
Allergic reactions (sic)
Dermatitis
  (1996): Jansen T+, *Dtsch Med Wochenschr* (German) 121, 41
  (1983): Przybilla B+, *Hautarzt* (German) 34, 459 (from antiperspirant)
  (1982): Gall H+, *Derm Beruf Umwelt* (German) 30, 55 (from antiperspirant)
Diaphoresis (>10%)
Exanthems
Rash (sic) (<1%)
Urticaria
Xerosis (>10%)

Mucosal/ENT
Ageusia
Dysgeusia
Sialopenia
Xerostomia (>10%)
  (1993): Ahmed T+, *Bone Marrow Transplant* 12(2), 131

(1986): Hassan M+, *Am J Gastroenterol* 81(5), 334

Other
Anaphylactoid reactions/Anaphylaxis
Headache

PROPOFOL

Trade name: Diprivan (AstraZeneca)
Indications: Induction and maintenance of anesthesia
Category: Anesthetic, general
Half-life: initial: 40 minutes; terminal: 3 days
Clinically important, potentially hazardous interactions with: zinc

Reactions

Skin
Allergic reactions (sic)
  (1988): Jamieson V+, *Anaesthesia* 43, 70
Edema (<1%)
Exanthems (6%)
  (1987): Boittiaux P+, *Ann Fr Anesth Reanim* (French) 6, 324 (6.6%)
  (1987): Coursange F+, *Ann Fr Anesth Reanim* (French) 6, 258 (6.6%)
Fixed eruption (1%)
Pruritus (>1%)
  (1987): Coursange F+, *Ann Fr Anesth Reanim* (French) 6, 258
Rash (sic) (5%)
Raynaud's phenomenon
  (1999): Gilston A, *Anaesthesia* 54, 307
Urticaria
  (1988): Aitken HA, *Anaesthesia* 43, 170
  (1987): Coursange F+, *Ann Fr Anesth Reanim* (French) 6, 258

Mucosal/ENT
Dysgeusia (<1%)
  (2007): Erden V+, *Eur J Anaesthesiol* 24(6), 516
Sialorrhea (>1%)
Tinnitus
Xerostomia (<1%)

Hair
Hair – pigmentation
  (1994): Motsch J+, *Eur J Anaesthesiol* 11, 499 (passim)
  (1992): Bublin JG+, *J Clin Pharm Ther* 17, 297

Other
Anaphylactoid reactions/Anaphylaxis (1–10%)
  (2003): Hofer KN+, *Ann Pharmacother* 37(3), 398
  (2001): Girgis Y, *Anaesthesia* 56(10), 1016
  (2001): Knoarzewski W+, *Anaesthesia* 56(5), 497 (fatal) (with fentanyl)
  (2001): Lewis S+, *Anaesthesia* 56(11), 1128
  (2001): Tsai MH+, *J Formos Med Assoc* 100(6), 424
  (2000): Ducart AR+, *J Cardiothorac Vasc Anesth* 14(2), 200
Cardiac failure
  (2007): Zarovnaya EL+, *Epilepsia* 48(5), 1002
  (2006): Fudickar A+, *Curr Opin Anaesthesiol* 19(4), 404
Cough
  (2002): Maile CJ, *Anaesthesia* 57(2), 202
  (2001): Aly EE, *Anaesthesia* 56(10), 1016
Death
  (2006): Fudickar A+, *Curr Opin Anaesthesiol* 19(4), 404
  (2006): Merz TM+, *Anesth Analg* 103(4), 1050
  (2002): Kang TM, *Ann Pharmacother* 36(9), 1453

(2002): Mertes PM+, *Anaesthesia* 57(8), 821 (with fentanyl)
(2001): Cannon ML+, *J Neurosurg* 95(6), 1053
(2001): Girgis Y, *Anaesthesia* 56(10), 1016

Hypotension
(2006): Frank LR+, *Am J Emerg Med* 24(5), 599 (6 cases)

Injection-site erythema (<1%)

Injection-site necrosis
(2006): Roth W+, *Paediatr Anaesth* 16(8), 887

Injection-site pain (>10%)
(2005): Auerswald K+, *Anasthesiol Intensivmed Notfallmed Schmerzther* 40(5), 259
(2005): Maleck WH+, *Anesth Analg* 100(6), 1858
(2004): Ayuso MA+, *Rev Esp Anestesiol Reanim* 51(9), 531 (27%)
(2004): Schaub E+, *Anesth Analg* 99(6), 1699
(2003): Dubey PK+, *Clin J Pain* 19(2), 121
(2003): Morishima T+, *Anesth Analg* 96(2), 631
(2003): Pellegrini M+, *Br J Anaesth* 90(3), 375
(2003): Roehm KD+, *Anaesthesia* 58(2), 165
(2002): Cheong MA+, *Anesth Analg* 95(5), 1293
(2002): Davies AF+, *Anaesthesia* 57(6), 557
(2002): Grauers A+, *Acta Anaesthesiol Scand* 46(4), 361
(2002): Huang YW+, *Acta Anaesthesiol Scand* 46(8), 1021
(2002): Kang TM, *Ann Pharmacother* 36(9), 1453
(2002): Lembert N+, *Ann Fr Anesth Reanim* 21(4), 263
(2002): Memis D+, *Anesth Analg* 95(3), 606
(2002): Piper SN+, *Anasthesiol Intensivmed Notfallmed Schmerzther* 37(9), 528
(2002): Suzuki S+, *Masui* 51(2), 140
(2002): White PF, *Anesth Analg* 94(4), 1042
(2001): Gupta S+, *Anaesthesia* 56(10), 1016
(2001): Larsen B+, *Anaesthesist* 50(11), 842
(2001): Larsen R+, *Anaesthesist* 50(9), 676
(2001): Liljeroth E+, *Acta Anaesthesiol Scand* 45(7), 839
(2001): Tsubokura H+, *Masui* 50(11), 1196
(2000): Levecque JP+, *Can J Anaesth* (French) 47, 291
(2000): Picard P+, *Anesth Analg* 90, 963
(2000): Pickford A+, *Pediatr Anaesth* 10, 129
(1998): Nathanson MH+, *Anaesthesia* 53, 608
(1998): Ozturk E+, *Anesthesiology* 89, 1041
(1998): Tan CH+, *Anaesthesia* 53, 468
(1988): Langley MS+, *Drugs*

Injection-site pruritus (<1%)

Myalgia/Myositis/Myopathy/Myotoxicity (>1%)

Myoclonus
(2005): Nimmaanrat S, *J Med Assoc Thai* 88(12), 1955

Phlebitis

Rhabdomyolysis
(2007): Sabsovich I+, *Am J Crit Care* 16(1), 82
(2007): Zarovnaya EL+, *Epilepsia* 48(5), 1002
(2005): Liolios A+, *Anesth Analg* 100(6), 1804
(2004): Casserly B+, *Am J Kidney Dis* 44(6), e98
(2002): Kang TM, *Ann Pharmacother* 36(9), 1453
(2001): Cannon ML+, *J Neurosurg* 95(6), 1053
(1998): Hanna JP+, *Neurology* 50(1), 301

Seizures
(2005): Manikandan S+, *Anesth Analg* 100(5), 1468
(2003): Reuther LO+, *Ugeskr Laeger* 165(14), 1447

PROPOLIS

Scientific name: *Propolis*
Family: None
Trade and other common names: Bee Glue; Bee Propolis; Hive Dross; Propolis Balsam; Propolis Resin; Propolis Wax; Russian Penicillin
Category: Immunomodulator
Purported indications and other uses: Tuberculosis, bacterial, fungal and protozoal infections, nasopharyngeal carcinoma, duodenal ulcer, *Helicobacter pylori* infection, cold, wound cleansing, mouth rinse, genital herpes. Ingredient in cosmetics
Half-life: N/A

Reactions

Skin

Allergic reactions (sic)
(2002): Junghans V+, *Am J Contact Dermat* 13(2), 87
(2001): Callejo A+, *Allergy* 56(6), 579
(1996): Bellagrandi S+, *J Am Acad Dermatol* 35(4), 644 (in HIV-positive patient)
(1988): Hausen BM+, *Contact Dermatitis* 19(4), 296
(1988): Slezak R, *Prakt Zubn Lek* 36(7), 208
(1987): Blanken R+, *Ned Tijdschr Geneeskd* 131(26), 1121
(1987): Rudzki E+, *Przegl Dermatol* 19(4), 296

Dermatitis
(2006): Lee SY+, *J Drugs Dermatol* 5(5), 458
(2005): Black RJ, *Clin Exp Dermatol* 30(1), 91
(2005): Walgrave SE+, *Dermatitis* 16(4), 209
(2004): Giusti F+, *Contact Dermatitis* 51(5-6), 255 (5.9%)
(2004): Ting PT+, *J Drugs Dermatol* 3(6), 685
(2003): Lombardi C+, *Allerg Immunol* (Paris) 35(2), 52
(2002): Henschel R+, *Contact Dermatitis* 47(1), 52
(2002): Lieberman HD+, *J Am Acad Dermatol* 46, S30
(2001): Teraki Y+, *Br J Dermatol* 144(6), 1277 (granulomatous)
(2000): Tumova L+, *Ceska Slov Farm* 49(6), 285
(1998): Burdock GA, *Food Chem Toxicol* 36(4), 347
(1998): Downs AM+, *Contact Dermatitis* 38(6), 359 (occupational)
(1998): Thomas P+, *Arch Dermatol* 134(4), 511
(1997): Silvani S+, *Contact Dermatitis* 37(1), 48 (in patients with psoriasis)
(1990): Hegyi E+, *Hautarzt* 41(12), 675 (0.64%)
(1990): Raton JA+, *Contact Dermatitis* 22(3), 183
(1988): Schuler TM+, *Hautarzt* 39(3), 139 (6 patients)
(1987): Angelini G+, *Contact Dermatitis* 17(4), 251 (in psoriasis)
(1987): Cirasino L+, *Contact Dermatitis* 16(2)
(1987): Frosch PJ, *Z Haut* 62(23), 1631
(1987): Hausen BM+, *Contact Dermatitis* 17(3), 163
(1987): Kleinhaus D, *Contact Dermatitis* 17(3), 187 (airborne)
(1987): Trevisan G+, *Contact Dermatitis* 16(1), 48
(1985): Ayala F+, *Contact Dermatitis* 12(3), 181
(1985): Machackova J, *Contact Dermatitis* 13(1), 43
(1985): Rudzki E+, *Contact Dermatitis* 13(3), 198
(1985): Tosti A+, *Contacr Dermatitis* 12(4), 227
(1984): Bedello PG+, *G Ital Deramtol Venereol* 119(6), 431
(1984): Pincelli C+, *Contact Dermatitis* 11(1), 49
(1984): Valsecchi R+, *Contact Dermatitis* 11(5), 317
(1983): Kokelj F+, *Contact Dermatitis* 9(6), 518
(1983): Melli MC+, *Contact Dermatitis* 9(5), 427 (in a bee-keeper)
(1983): Monti M+, *Contact Dermatitis* 9(2), 163 (occupational and cosmetic)
(1983): Rudzki E+, *Contact Dermatitis* 9(1), 40
(1983): Takahashi M+, *Contact Dermatitis* 9(6) (from honeybee royal jelly)
(1982): Monti M+, *G Ital Dermatol Venereol* 117(2), 119

(1982): Proserpio G, *G Ital Dermatol Venereol* 117(5), 316
Eczema (vulval)
  (2005): Black RJ, *Clin Exp Dermatol* 30(1), 91
Erythroderma
  (2001): Horiuchi Y, *Br J Dermatol* 145, 691
Sensitivity (sic)
  (1988): Nakamura T, *Contact Dermatitis* 18(5), 313
  (1987): Young E, *Contact Dermatitis* 16(1), 49
  (1980): Bogdaszewska-Czabanowska J+, *Przegl Dermatol* 67(6), 747

Mucosal/ENT
Cheilitis
  (1996): Bellegrandi S+, *J Am Acad Dermatol* 35, 644
Mucositis
  (1990): Hay KD+, *Oral Surg Oral Med Oral Pathol* 70, 584
Oral lesions
  (2006): Brailo V+, *Med Oral Patol Oral Cir Bucal* 11(4), E303
Oral ulceration
  (1990): Hay KD+, *Oral Surg Oral Med Oral Pathol* 70, 584
Stomatitis
  (1996): Bellegrandi S+, *J Am Acad Dermatol* 35, 644

Other
Hypersensitivity
  (1987): Rudzki E+, *Pol Tyg Lek* (Polish) 42(2), 40
  (1984): Tosti A+, *G Ital Dermatol Venereol* 119(5)

PROPOXYPHENE

Trade names: Algafan; Antalvic; Darvocet-N (aaiPharma); Darvon (Lilly); Darvon Compound (aaiPharma); Develin; Dolotard; Doloxene; Liberan; Parvon
Indications: Pain
Category: Opiate agonist
Half-life: 8–24 hours
Clinically important, potentially hazardous interactions with: alcohol, alprazolam, carbamazepine, metoprolol, phenelzine, ritonavir, warfarin

Note: Darvocet is propoxyphene and acetaminophen; Darvon Compound is propoxyphene and aspirin

Reactions

Skin
Acute generalized exanthematous pustulosis (AGEP)
  (2000): Machet L+, *Acta Derm Venereol* 80(3), 224
Diaphoresis
Exanthems
Facial edema
Pruritus
Rash (sic) (<1%)
Urticaria (<1%)

Mucosal/ENT
Perianal ulcerations
  (1984): Laplanche G+, *Ann Dermatol Venereol* (French) 111, 347 (from suppositories)
Xerostomia (1–10%)

Eyes
Miosis
  (2004): Zacny JP+, *Drug Alcohol Depend* 73(2), 133

Other
Death
  (2006): Barkin RL+, *Am J Ther* 13(6), 534

Injection-site nodules
  (1987): Pedragosa R+, *Arch Dermatol* 123, 297
Injection-site pain (1–10%)
Seizures
  (2006): Barkin RL+, *Am J Ther* 13(6), 534
Vertigo
  (2006): Kamal-Bahl SJ+, *Am J Geriatr Pharmacother* 4(3), 219
  (2006): Marraffa JM+, *Clin Pharmacol Ther* 79(3), 282

PROPRANOLOL

Trade names: Acifol; Apsolol; Betabloc; Cinlol; Detensol; Inderal (Wyeth); Inderalici; Inderex; Inderide (Wyeth); Novo-Pranol; Prosin; Sinal; Tesnol
Indications: Hypertension, angina pectoris
Category: Adrenergic beta-receptor antagonist; Antiarrhythmic class II
Half-life: 2–6 hours
Clinically important, potentially hazardous interactions with: cimetidine, clonidine, epinephrine, **eucalyptus,** haloperidol, insulin, insulin detemir, insulin glargine, insulin glulisine, nilutamide, terbutaline, verapamil

Note: Inderide is propranolol and hydrochlorothiazide

Note: Cutaneous side effects of beta-receptor blockaders are clinically polymorphous. They apparently appear after several months of continuous therapy. Atypical psoriasiform, lichen planus-like, and eczematous chronic rashes are mainly observed. (1983): Hödl St, *Z Hautkr* (German) 58, 17

Reactions

Skin
Acne
Angioedema
  (1983): Hannaway PJ+, *N Engl J Med* 308, 1536
Bullous dermatitis
Dermatitis
  (1994): Valsecchi R+, *Contact Dermatitis* 30, 177 (occupational)
  (1990): Rebandel P+, *Contact Dermatitis* 23, 199
Diaphoresis
Eczema
  (1981): van Joost T+, *Arch Dermatol* 117, 600
Edema
Erythema (systemic)
Erythema multiforme
Exanthems (<1%)
  (2004): Litt JZ, Beachwood, OH (personal case) (observation)
Exfoliative dermatitis
Fixed eruption
  (2006): Zaccaria E+, *Acta Derm Venereol* 86(4), 371
Hyperkeratosis (palms and soles)
Lichenoid eruption
  (1991): Massa MC+, *Cutis* 48, 41
  (1980): Hawk JLM, *Clin Exp Dermatol* 5, 93
Lupus erythematosus
  (1982): Hughes GRV, *BJM* 284, 1358
Necrosis
Pemphigus
  (1982): Ruocco V+, *Arch Dermatol Res* 274, 123
  (1980): Godard W+, *Ann Dermatol Venereol* (French) 107, 1213
Peripheral edema
Photosensitivity
Phototoxicity
  (1992): Shelley WB+, *Cutis* 50, 182 (observation)

Pruritus
  (2004): Litt JZ, Beachwood, OH (personal case) (observation)
Psoriasis
  (1993): Halevy S+, J Am Acad Dermatol 29, 504
  (1992): Raychaudhuri SP+, J Am Acad Dermatol 27, 787
  (1990): Halevy S+, Arch Dermatol Res 283, 472
  (1988): Heng MCY+, Int J Dermatol 27, 619
  (1987): Altomare GF+, G Ital Dermatol Venereol (Italian) 122, 531
  (1987): Savola J+, BMJ 295, 637
  (1986): Abel EA+, J Am Acad Dermatol 15, 1007
  (1986): Czernielewski J, Lancet 1, 808 (exacerbation)
  (1985): Hu C-H+, Arch Dermatol 121, 1326
  (1984): Arntzen K+, Acta Derm Venereol (Stockh) 64, 346
  (1983): Kaur S+, Indian Heart J 35, 181
Purpura
Rash (sic) (1–10%)
Raynaud's phenomenon (59%)
  (1981): Lancet 2(8246), 539
Sclerosis
  (1980): Graham JR, Trans Am Clin Climatol Assoc 92, 122
Stevens–Johnson syndrome
  (1990): Zukervar P+, J Toxicol Clin Exp (French) 10, 169
  (1989): Mukul+, J Assoc Physicians India 37, 797
Toxic epidermal necrolysis
Toxicoderma
  (1981): Danilov LN, Vestn Dermatol Venerol (Russian) January, 42
Urticaria
  (1983): Hannaway PJ+, N Engl J Med 308, 1536
  (1983): Oliver R, Cent Afr J Med 29, 91
Xerosis

Mucosal/ENT
Cheilitis
Dysgeusia
  (2000): Zervakis J+, Physiol Behav 68, 405
Oral ulceration
  (1980): Hawk JLM, Clin Exp Dermatol 5, 93
Tongue pigmentation
Xerostomia

Hair
Hair – alopecia
  (1994): Friedman M, J Fam Pract 39, 114
  (1983): Hödl ST, Z Hautkr (German) 58, 17.
  (1982): England JRF+, Aust Fam Physician 11, 225
Hair – alopecia areata
  (2001): Vinson RP, El Paso, TX (from a single dose) (from Internet) (observation)

Nails
Nails – discoloration
Nails – pitting (psoriasiform)
Nails – thickening
  (1983): Hödl ST, Z Hautkr (German) 58, 17.

Eyes
Vision impaired
  (2006): Finsterer J+, South Med J 99(7), 768

Other
Anaphylactoid reactions/Anaphylaxis
  (1983): Hannaway PJ+, N Engl J Med 308, 1536
Cardiac arrest
  (2006): Sandroni C+, Acta Anaesthesiol Scand 50(6), 759
Headache
Hypertension
  (1985): Schroeder JS+, Acta Pharmacol Toxicol (Copenh) 57 Suppl 2, 55

Hypotension
  (2000): Joye F, Presse Med 29(18), 1027
Myalgia/Myositis/Myopathy/Myotoxicity
  (2006): Finsterer J+, South Med J 99(7), 768
  (1980): Uuisitupa M+, BMJ 1, 183
Paresthesias
Peyronie's disease
  (1981): Neumann HAM+, Dermatologica 162, 330
Serum sickness
  (1983): Yen MC+, Postgrad Med 74, 291
Somnambulism
  (1986): Pradalier A+, Therapie 41(4), 318

PROPYLTHIOURACIL

Trade names: Propacil; Propycil; Propyl-Thyracil (Paladin); Tiotil
Indications: Hyperthyroidism
Category: Antithyroid, hormone modifier
Half-life: 1–5 hours
Clinically important, potentially hazardous interactions with: anticoagulants, dicumarol, **myrrh**, warfarin

Reactions

Skin
Acne
  (1980): Vasily DB+, JAMA 243, 458
Acute febrile neutrophilic dermatosis (Sweet's syndrome)
  (2005): Boulenger-Vazel A+, Ann Dermatol Venereol 132(1), 27
  (1999): Miller RM+, Br J Dermatol 141(5), 943
Adverse effects (sic)
  (1982): Pacini F+, J Endocrinol Invest 5, 403
Angioedema (1%)
  (1980): Vasily DB+, JAMA 243, 458
Dermatitis
  (1993): Elias AN+, J Am Acad Dermatol 29, 78
Edema (<1%)
Erythema nodosum
  (1985): Keren G+, Isr J Med Sci 21, 62
Exanthems (3–5%)
  (1987): Wing SS+, Can Med Assoc J 136, 121
  (1982): Gammeltoft M+, Acta Dermatol Venereol (Stockh) 62, 171 (3–5%)
  (1980): Vasily DB+, JAMA 243, 458
Exfoliative dermatitis (<1%)
Lichenoid eruption
Lupus erythematosus (1–20%)
  (1994): Sato-Matsumura KC+, J Dermatol 21, 501
  (1992): Skaer TL, Clin Ther 14, 496
  (1991): Alarcon-Segovia D+, Baillieres Clin Rheumatol 5, 1
  (1989): Horton RC+, Lancet 2, 568
  (1987): Wing SS+, Can Med Assoc J 136, 121 (20% ANA)
  (1985): Bulvik S+, Harefuah (Hebrew) 109, 13
  (1983): Berkman EM+, Transfusion 23, 135
  (1981): Searles RP+, J Rheumatol 8, 498
  (1981): Takuwa N+, Endocrinol (Jpn) 28, 663
  (1980): Condemi JJ, Geriatrics 35(3), 81
Lupus syndrome
  (2006): Aycan Z+, Turk J Pediatr 48(2), 162
  (2002): Yamada A+, Intern Med 41(12), 1204
Photosensitivity
  (1997): Ohtsuka M+, Eur Resp J 10, 1405
Pigmentation
Pruritus (<1%)
  (2006): Aycan Z+, Turk J Pediatr 48(2), 162

(1980): Vasily DB+, *JAMA* 243, 458
Purpura
  (1987): Wing SS+, *Can Med Assoc J* 136, 121
Pyoderma gangrenosum
  (2006): Gungor K+, *J Endocrinol Invest* 29(6), 575
  (2005): Boulenger-Vazel A+, *Ann Dermatol Venereol* 132(1), 27
  (2004): Hong SB+, *Dermatology* 208(4), 339
  (1999): Darben T+, *Australas J Dermatol* 40, 144
Rash (sic) (>10%)
Rosacea
  (1980): Vasily DB+, *JAMA* 243, 458
Subcorneal pustular dermatosis (Sneddon-Wilkinson)
  (2005): Boulenger-Vazel+, *Ann Dermatol Venereol* 132(1), 27
Ulcerations
  (2002): Helfgott SM+, *N Engl J Med* 347(2), 122
  (1987): Wing SS+, *Can Med Assoc J* 136, 121
Urticaria (<1%)
  (2006): Aycan Z+, *Turk J Pediatr* 48(2), 162
  (1980): Vasily DB+, *JAMA* 243, 458
Vasculitis (<1%)
  (2007): Gao Y+, *Int Immunopharmacol* 7(1), 55
  (2007): Yu F+, *Am J Kidney Dis* 49(5), 607
  (2006): Aloush V+, *Semin Arthritis Rheum* 36(1), 4
  (2006): Aycan Z+, *Turk J Pediatr* 48(2), 162
  (2006): Pillinger MH+, *Semin Arthritis Rheum* 36(1), 1
  (2006): Sheen YS+, *Arch Dermatol* 142(7), 879
  (2006): Zhao MH+, *Kidney Int* 69(8), 1477
  (2005): Wisniewski P+, *Pol Merkur Lekarski* 19(113), 674
  (2003): Jacobs EM+, *Neth J Med* 61(9), 296
  (2002): Helfgott SM+, *N Engl J Med* 347(2), 122
  (2002): Poomthavorn P+, *J Med Assoc Thai* 85(Suppl 4), S1295
  (2000): Lopez-Marina V+, *Med Clin* (Barc) (Spanish) 114, 398
  (2000): Morita S+, *Endocr J* 47(4), 467
  (2000): Otsuka S+, *Br J Dermatol* 142(4), 828
  (2000): Wang LH+, *J Formos Med Assoc* 99(8), 642
  (1999): Gunton JE+, *J Clin Endocrinol Metab* 84(1), 13
  (1998): Harper L+, *Nephrol Dial Transplant* 13, 455
  (1998): Merkel PA, *Curr Opin Rheumatol* 10, 45
  (1998): Miller RM+, *Australas J Dermatol* 39, 96
  (1997): Fujii A+, *Ryumachi* 37(6), 788
  (1997): Kitahara T+, *Clin Nephrol* 47, 336
  (1997): Yarman S+, *Int J Clin Pharm Ther* 35, 282
  (1993): Dolman KM+, *Lancet* 342, 651
  (1992): Stankus SJ+, *Chest* 102, 1595
  (1992): Wolf D+, *Cutis* 49, 253
  (1987): Carrasco MD+, *Arch Intern Med* 147, 1677
  (1987): Wing SS+, *Can Med Assoc J* 136, 121
  (1986): Gleisner A+, *Rev Child Pediatr* (Spanish) 57, 64
  (1985): Cox NH+, *Clin Exp Dermatol* 10, 292
  (1982): Gammeltoft M+, *Acta Dermatol Venereol* (Stockh) 62, 171
  (1982): Reidy TJ+, *South Med J* 75, 1297
  (1980): Vasily DB+, *JAMA* 243, 458
Vesiculation (in newborn)
  (1980): Vasily DB+, *JAMA* 243, 458

Mucosal/ENT
Ageusia (1–10%)
Dysgeusia (1–10%) (metallic taste)
  (1993): Elias AN+, *J Am Acad Dermatol* 29, 78
  (1991): Tauveron I+, *Therapie* 46(5), 410
Epistaxis
  (2006): Akarsu E+, *Mt Sinai J Med* 73(7), 1021
Oral lesions
Oral ulceration
Ototoxicity
  (2004): Sano M+, *ORL J Otorhinolaryngol Relat Spec* 66(5), 281
Tinnitus
  (2004): Thamprajamchit S+, *Endocr Pract* 10(5), 432

Hair
Hair – alopecia (<1%)
  (1997): Ohtsuka M+, *Eur Resp J* 10, 1405
  (1980): Vasily DB+, *JAMA* 243, 458
Hair – poliosis
  (1980): Vasily DB+, *JAMA* 243, 458

Nails
Nails – lichen planus
  (2007): Saito M+, *J Dermatol* 34(10), 696

Other
Cough
  (2006): Aycan Z+, *Turk J Pediatr* 48(2), 162
  (2003): Ohwada R+, *Intern Med* 42(10), 1026
Fever
  (2006): Aycan Z+, *Turk J Pediatr* 48(2), 162
Gangrene
  (2006): Farah RE+, *Ann Pharmacother* 40(6), 1211
Headache
Hepatotoxicity
  (2006): Benyounes M+, *World J Gastroenterol* 12(38), 6232 (1–33%)
Hypersensitivity
  (2006): Aycan Z+, *Turk J Pediatr* 48(2), 162
  (1999): Chastain MA+, *J Am Acad Dermatol* 41, 757
  (1991): Fong PC+, *Horm Res* 35, 132
Myalgia/Myositis/Myopathy/Myotoxicity
Nephrotoxicity
  (2002): Winters MJ+, *Pediatr Nephrol* 17(4), 257
  (1997): Kato H+, *Nippon Jinzo Gakkai Shi* 39(5), 517
Paresthesias (<1%)

PROTAMINE SULFATE

Indications: Heparin overdose
Category: Heparin antagonist
Half-life: 2 hours
Clinically important, potentially hazardous interactions with: None

Reactions

Skin
Adverse effects (sic)
  (1993): Cormack JG+, *Coron Artery Dis* 4(5), 420
Allergic reactions (sic)
  (2002): Lee AY+, *Acta Derm Venereol* 82(2), 114
  (2000): Ralley FE+, *J Cardiothorac Vasc Anesth* 14(6), 710
  (1999): Bollinger ME+, *J Allergy Clin Immunol* 104(2), 462
  (1999): Petays T+, *Duodecim* 115(5), 517 (immediate)
  (1999): Porsche R+, *Heart Lung* 28(6), 418
  (1995): Hughes C+, *CRNA* 6, 172
  (1995): Hynynen M+, *Duodecim* 111(20), 1969
  (1994): Pharo GH+, *Anesth Analg* 78(1), 181
  (1993): Sticco SL, *CRNA* 4(3), 144
  (1986): Bruni S+, *Diabetes Care* 9(5), 552
  (1983): Watson RA+, *Urology* 22(5), 493
  (1982): Sanchez MB+, *Lancet* 1(8283), 1243
Angioedema
  (1999): Bollinger ME+, *J Allergy Clin Immunol* 104(2), 462
  (1993): Kim R, *Del Med J* 65(1), 17
  (1991): Roelofse JA+, *Anesth Prog* 38, 99
Erythema
  (1992): Neidhart PP+, *Eur Heart J* 13(6), 856
Exanthems

(1989): Weiss ME+, *N Engl J Med* 320(14), 886
Rash (sic)
  (1991): Weiss ME+, *Clin Rev Allergy* 9(3), 339
  (1990): Weiss ME+, *Clin Exp Allergy* 20(6), 713
Urticaria
  (1993): Kim R, *Del Med J* 65(1), 17
  (1991): Weiss ME+, *Clin Rev Allergy* 9(3), 339
  (1990): Weiss ME+, *Clin Exp Allergy* 20(6), 713
  (1989): Weiss ME+, *N Engl J Med* 320(14), 886
  (1988): Gottschlich GM+, *Ann Allergy* 61(4), 277 (passim)

Other

Anaphylactoid reactions/Anaphylaxis
  (2006): Kudoh O+, *Masui* 55(5), 605
  (2005): Lee S+, *Masui* 54(9), 1043
  (2003): Panos A+, *Eur J Cardiothorac* 24(2), 325
  (2002): Lee AY+, *Acta Derm Venereol* 82(2), 114
  (2002): Viaro F+, *Chest* 122(3), 1061
  (2000): Peng CH+, *Acta Anaesthesiol Sin* 38(2), 97
  (1999): Ravi R+, *Heart Dis* 1(5), 289
  (1997): Abe K+, *Can J Anaesth* 44(6), 662 (2 cases)
  (1996): Takenoshita M+, *Anesthesiology* 84(1), 233
  (1995): Hruby M+, *Rozhl Chir* 74(6), 282
  (1994): Dykewicz MS+, *J Allergy Clin Immunol* 93(1), 117 (2 cases)
  (1993): Kim R, *Del Med J* 65(1), 17
  (1993): Mezt S, *Anesthesiology* 79(3), 617
  (1992): Neidhart PP+, *Eur Heart J* 13(6), 856
  (1991): Hobbhahn J+, *Anaesthesist* 40(7), 365
  (1991): Hobbhahn J+, *Anaesthesist* 40(8), 421
  (1991): Roelofse JA+, *Anesth Prog* 38, 99
  (1991): Vincent GM+, *Cathet Cardiovasc Diagn* 23(3), 164
  (1989): Gupta SK+, *J Vasc Surg* 9(2), 342 (11 cases)
  (1989): Kambam JR+, *Can J Anaesth* 36(4), 463 (2 cases)
  (1989): Zhang ZY+, *Proc Chin Med Sci Peking Union Med Coll* 4(2), 117
  (1988): Gottschlich GM+, *Ann Allergy* 61(4), 277 (passim)
  (1988): Oswald-Mammosser M+, *Rev Fr Allergol* (French) 28, 173
  (1988): Shikuma LR+, *Drug Intell Clin Pharm* 22(3), 211
  (1985): Horrow JC, *Int Anesthesiol Clin* 23(3), 133
  (1985): Mingi CL+, *Ma Zui Xue Za Zhi* 23(4), 220
  (1985): Sharath MD+, *J Thorac Cardiovasc Surg* 90(1), 86
  (1985): Weiler JM+, *J Allergy Clin Immunol* 75(2), 297
  (1985): Westaby S+, *Br Heart J* 53(5), 574
  (1984): Holland CL+, *Clin Cardiol* 7(3), 157 (4 cases)
  (1984): Stewart WJ+, *Circulation* 70(5), 788 (patient allergic to fish)
  (1984): Walker WS+, *Br Heart J* 52(1), 112 (2 patients)
  (1983): Best N+, *Br J Anaesth* 55(11), 1149
  (1983): Vierthaler LD+, *J Kans Med Soc* 84(9), 454
  (1982): Vontz FK+, *Am Surg* 48(10), 549
  (1981): Doolan L+, *Anaesth Intensive Care* 9(2), 147 (3 cases)
  (1981): Knape JT+, *Anesthesiology* 55(3), 324 (patient allergic to fish)
  (1980): Moorthy SS+, *Anesth Analg* 59(1), 77
Death
  (2005): Welsby IJ+, *Anesthesiology* 102(2), 308
  (2003): Panos A+, *Eur J Cardiothorac Surg* 24(2), 325
  (2002): Kimmel SE+, *Anesth Analg* 94(6), 1402
  (2000): Hakala T+, *Ann Chir Gynaecol* 89(2), 150
  (2000): Peng CH+, *Acta Anaesthesiol Sin* 38(2), 97
  (1991): Hobbhahn J+, *Anaesthesist* 40(7), 365
  (1991): Weiss ME+, *Clin Rev Allergy* 9(3), 339
  (1989): Gupta SK+, *J Vasc Surg* 9(2), 342 (11 cases)
  (1988): Gottschlich GM+, *Ann Allergy* 61(4), 277 (passim)
  (1984): Holland CL+, *Clin Cardiol* 7(3), 157 (4 cases)
  (1984): Just-Viera JO+, *Am Surg* 50(1), 52
  (1984): Stewart WJ+, *Circulation* 70(5), 788 (patient allergic to fish)

Headache
Hypersensitivity
  (2005): Raap U+, *Contact Dermatitis* 53(1), 57
  (2003): Comunale ME+, *J Cardiothorac Vasc Anesth* 17(3), 309
  (2003): Gruchalla RS, *J Allergy Clin Immunol* 111(2), S548
  (2002): Madsen CS+, *Ugeskr Laeger* 164(36), 4187
  (1993): Kim R, *Del Med J* 65(1), 17
  (1992): Hulshof MM+, *Br J Dermatol* 127(3), 286 (granulomatous)
  (1991): Kollner A+, *Dtsch Med Wochenschr* 116(33), 1234
  (1989): Lindblad B, *Eur J Vasc Surg* 3, 195
  (1986): Tsuji Y+, *Kyobu Geka* 39(12), 973
  (1984): Campbell FW+, *Anesthesiology* 61(6), 761
Hypertension
  (2005): Ocal A+, *Tohoku J Exp* 207(1), 51
  (2001): Boigner H+, *Paediatr Anaesth* 11(6), 729
Hypotension
  (2005): Lee S+, *Masui* 54(9), 1043
  (2003): Seifert HA+, *Anesth Analg* 97(2), 383
  (2002): Viaro F+, *Chest* 122(3), 1061
Rhabdomyolysis
  (1999): Lobato EB+, *Anesthesiology* 91(1), 303

PROTEIN C CONCENTRATE (HUMAN)

Trade name: Ceprotin (Baxter)
Indications: Congenital protein C deficiency
Category: Anticoagulant glycoprotein
Half-life: 5–15 hours
Clinically important, potentially hazardous interactions with: N/A

Reactions

Skin

Allergic reactions (sic)
  (2003): *Prescrire Int* 12(63), 11
Angioedema
Diaphoresis
Hyperhidrosis
Pruritus
Rash (sic)
Urticaria

Other

Anaphylactoid reactions/Anaphylaxis
Fever
Headache
Hypersensitivity
Hypotension
Infections (sic)
Injection-site burning
Restlessness
Vertigo

PROTRIPTYLINE

Trade names: Concordin; Triptil; Vivactil (Odyssey)
Indications: Depression
Category: Antidepressant, tricyclic
Half-life: 54–92 hours
**Clinically important, potentially hazardous interactions
with:** amprenavir, arbutamine, clonidine, epinephrine,
formoterol, guanethidine, isocarboxazid, linezolid, MAO
inhibitors, phenelzine, quinolones, sparfloxacin, tranylcypromine

Reactions

Skin
Acne
Allergic reactions (sic) (<1%)
Angioedema
Dermatitis (3%)
Diaphoresis (1–10%)
Edema
Erythema
Exanthems
Petechiae
Photosensitivity (<1%)
Phototoxicity
  (1980): Kochevar IE, *Toxicol App Pharmacol* 54, 258
Pruritus (1–5%)
Purpura
Rash (sic)
Urticaria
Vasculitis
Xerosis

Mucosal/ENT
Dysgeusia (>10%)
Glossitis
Oral mucosal eruption
Stomatitis
Tinnitus
Tongue black
Xerostomia (>10%)

Hair
Hair – alopecia (<1%)

Other
Death
Gynecomastia (<1%)
Headache
Paresthesias
Rhabdomyolysis
Tremor

PSEUDOEPHEDRINE

Trade names: Allegra-D (Sanofi-Aventis); Balminil; Benadryl
(Pfizer); Bromfed (Muro); Deconsal; Eltor 120; Entex (Andrx);
Maxiphed; Robidrine; Robitussin-CF (Wyeth); Sudafed (Pfizer);
Trinalin (Schering)
Indications: Nasal congestion
Category: Adrenergic alpha-receptor agonist
Half-life: 9–16 hours
**Clinically important, potentially hazardous interactions
with:** bromocriptine, fluoxetine, fluvoxamine, furazolidone, MAO
inhibitors, paroxetine, phenelzine, rasagiline, sertraline,
tranylcypromine

Reactions

Skin
Acute generalized exanthematous pustulosis (AGEP)
  (2005): Schmutz JL+, *Ann Dermatol Venereol* 132(1), 100 (with
    metamizole)
  (2004): Padial MA+, *Br J Dermatol* A(1), 139
Angioedema
  (1997): Rademaker M, Hamilton, New Zealand (3 personal
    cases) (observation)
  (1993): Cavanah DK+, *Ann Intern Med* 119, 302
Baboon syndrome
  (2000): Sanchez TS+, *Contact Dermatitis* 42, 312
Dermatitis
  (1998): Downs AM+, *Contact Dermatitis* 39, 33
  (1998): Vega F+, *Allergy* 53, 218
  (1991): Tomb RR+, *Contact Dermatitis* 24, 86
Diaphoresis (1–10%)
  (2001): Pederson KJ+, *Can J Cardiol* 17(5), 599 (with bupropion)
Eczema
  (1991): Tomb RR+, *Contact Dermatitis* 24, 86
Erythema multiforme
  (2002): Fontaine JF+, *Allerg Immunol* (Paris) 34(7), 230
Erythroderma
  (2003): Millard TP+, *Contact Dermatitis* 49(5), 263
  (2002): Gonzalo-Garijo MA+, *Allergol Immunopathol* (Madr)
    30(4), 239
Exanthems
  (1995): Rochina A+, *J Invest Allergol Clin Immunol* 5, 235
  (1994): Shelley WB+, *Cutis* 52, 203 (observation)
  (1993): Cavanah DK+, *Ann Intern Med* 119, 302 (generalized)
Exfoliative dermatitis
  (1993): Cavanah DK+, *Ann Intern Med* 119, 302
Fixed eruption
  (2001): Cowen E, *Dermatology Online Journal* 7, 23C
  (2001): Cowen E, *Dermatology Online Journal* 7, 24C
    (disseminated bullous)
  (1998): Anibarro B+, *Allergy* 53, 902
  (1998): Hindioglu U+, *J Am Acad Dermatol* 38, 499 (non-
    pigmenting solitary)
  (1998): Litt JZ, Beachwood, OH (personal case) (observation)
  (1998): Vidal C+, *Ann Allergy Asthma Immunol* 80, 309 (non-
    pigmenting)
  (1997): Garcia Ortiz JC+, *Allergy* 52, 229 (non-pigmenting)
  (1996): Alanko K+, *J Am Acad Dermatol* 35, 647
  (1996): Quan MB+, *Int J Dermatol* 35, 367 (non-pigmenting)
  (1994): Hauken M, *Ann Intern Med* 120, 442
  (1994): Krivda SJ+, *J Am Acad Dermatol* 31, 291 (non-
    pigmenting)
  (1994): Shelley WB+, *Cutis* 53, 116 (observation)
  (1994): Shelley WB+, *Cutis* 54, 240 (observation)
  (1988): Camisa C, *Cutis* 41, 339

(1987): Shelley WB+, *J Am Acad Dermatol* 17, 403 (non-pigmenting)

Pallor

Toxic erythema

(1999): Oakley A (from Internet) (2 observations)

Urticaria

(1997): Rademaker M, Hamilton, New Zealand (3 personal cases) (observation)

(1994): Shelley WB+, *Cutis* 54, 375 (observation)

Mucosal/ENT

Tinnitus

Xerostomia

(2002): Xiao Z+, *Zhonghua Nei Ke Za Zhi* 41(8), 547 (1%)

Other

Headache

Tremor

(2005): Lopez Lois G+, *An Pediatr (Barc)* 62(4), 378

PSORALENS

Trade names: 8-MOP (Valeant); Oxsoralen (Valeant); Trisoralen (Valeant)
Indications: Vitiligo
Category: Psoralen
Half-life: 2 hours

Reactions

Skin

Acne

Basal cell carcinoma

(2002): Katz KA+, *J Invest Dermatol* 118(6), 1038

(1999): Hannuksela-Svahn A+, *J Am Acad Dermatol* 40, 694

Bowen's disease

Bullous pemphigoid (with UVA)

(1996): George PM, *Photodermatol Photoimmunol Photomed* 11, 185

(1996): Perl S+, *Dermatology* 193, 245

(1994): Fryer EJ+, *J Am Acad Dermatol* 30, 651 (passim)

(1990): Bastian P+, *Ann Dermatol Venereol* 117(10), 734

(1989): Weber PJ+, *Arch Dermatol* 125, 690

(1985): Grunwald MH+, *J Am Acad Dermatol* 13, 224

(1982): Stüttgen G, *Int J Dermatol* 21, 198

Burning (1–10%)

(2000): Al-Qattan MM, *Burns* 26(7), 653 (children)

(1996): Nettelblad H+, *Burns* 22, 633

(1982): Stüttgen G, *Int J Dermatol* 21, 198 (passim)

Dermatitis

(1998): Adams SP, *Can Fam Physician* 44, 503

(1994): Finkelstein E+, *Int J Dermatol* 33, 116

(1994): Korffmacher H+, *Contact Dermatitis* 30, 283

(1993): Leopold JC+, *Am J Dis Child* 147, 311

(1991): Takashima A+, *Br J Dermatol* 124, 37

(1990): Fleming D+, *Allergy Proc* 11, 125

(1990): Moller H, *Photodermatol Photoimmunol Photomed* 7, 43

(1985): Lembo G+, *Photodermatol* 2, 119

(1984): Goitre M, *G Ital Dermatol Venereol* (Italian) 119, 435

(1983): Heskel NS+, *Contact Dermatitis* 9(4), 278

Eczema

(1994): Korffmacher H+, *Contact Dermatitis* 30, 283

Edema (1–10%)

Ephelides (1–10%)

(1993): Sheehan MP+, *Br J Dermatol* 129, 431 (PUVA)

(1984): Kietzmann E+, *Dermatologica* 168, 306

(1983): Kanerva L+, *Dermatologica* 166, 281

(1983): Kietzmann H+, *Ann Dermatol Venereol* (French) 110, 63

Erythema

(2000): Yeo UC+, *Br J Dermatol* 142, 733

Folliculitis

Granuloma annulare

Herpes simplex

(1993): Sheehan MP+, *Br J Dermatol* 129, 431 (PUVA)

(1982): Stüttgen G, *Int J Dermatol* 21, 198

Herpes zoster

(1982): Stüttgen G, *Int J Dermatol* 21, 198

Hypomelanosis (1–10%)

Keratoacanthoma

Lichen planus

(1980): Dupre A+, *Ann Dermatol Venereol* (French) 107, 557

Lichen planus pemphigoides

(2000): Kuramoto N+, *Br J Dermatol* 142(3), 509

Lupus erythematosus

(1991): Lehmann P, *J Am Acad Dermatol* 24, 515 (discoid)

(1985): Bruze M+, *Acta Derm Venereol* (Stockh) 65, 31

Melanoma

(1999): Lindelof B, *Drug Saf* 20, 289

(1994): Reseghetti A+, *Dermatology* 189, 75

(1980): Forrest JB+, *J Surg Oncol* 13, 337

Miliaria

Pemphigus

(1980): Lutowiecka-Wranicz A+, *Przegl Dermatol* (Polish) 67, 641

Pemphigus foliaceus

(1998): Aghassi D+, *Arch Dermatol* 134(10), 1300

Pemphigus vulgaris

(1994): Fryer EJ+, *J Am Acad Dermatol* 30, 651

Photosensitivity

(2001): Tanew A+, *J Am Acad Dermatol* 44, 638

(1998): Clark SM+, *Contact Dermatitis* 38, 289

(1991): Takashima A+, *Br J Dermatol* 124, 37

(1990): Moller H, *Photodermatol Photoimmunol Photomed* 7, 43

(1986): Jeanmougin M, *Biochimie* (French) 68, 891

(1986): Lerman S, *Ophthalmology* 93, 304

(1986): Morliere P, *Biochimie* (French) 68, 849

(1982): Haudenschild-Falb E+, *Ther Umsch* (German) 39, 178

(1982): Kavli G+, *Acta Derm Venereol* 62, 435

(1982): Weiss W+, *Dermatol Monatsschr* (German) 168, 116

(1981): Bleehen SS, *Br J Dermatol* 105, 23

(1980): Dupre A+, *Ann Dermatol Venereol* (French) 107, 557

(1980): Heidbreder G, *Z Hautkr* (German) 55, 84

Phototoxicity

(2005): Nimkulrat P+, *J Med Assoc Thai* 88(10), 1406

(2001): Snellman E+, *Br J Dermatol* 144, 490

(2001): Voss A+, *Arch Dermatol* 137, 383 (fatal)

(1997): Morison WL, *Arch Dermatol* 133, 1609

(1997): Morison WL+, *J Am Acad Dermatol* 36, 183

(1997): Neumann NJ+, *Acta Derm Venereol* 77, 385

(1990): Ljunggren B, *Arch Dermatol* 126, 1334

(1989): Morison WL, *Arch Dermatol* 125, 433 (topical)

(1986): Lowe NJ, *Br J Dermatol* 115, 86

(1986): Toback AC+, *Dermatol Clin* 4, 223

(1983): Kavli G+, *Contact Dermatitis* 9, 257

(1980): Barth J+, *Z Arztl Fortbild Jena* (German) 74, 789

(1980): Kornhauser A, *Ann N Y Acad Sci* 346, 398

(1980): Wolska H+, *Przegl Dermatol* (Polish) 67, 439

Pigmentation

(1994): Burrows NP+, *Clin Exp Dermatol* 19, 380

(1993): Poskitt BL+, *J R Soc Med* 86, 665

(1990): Trattner A+, *Int J Dermatol* 29, 310

(1989): Weiss E+, *Int J Dermatol* 28, 188

(1987): Bruce DR+, *J Am Acad Dermatol* 16, 1087

(1986): MacDonald KJS+, *Br J Dermatol* 114, 395

(1985): Rodighiero G, *Farmaco Prat* 40, 173

(1983): Farber EM+, *Arch Dermatol* 119, 426

(1981): No Author, *Br Med J Clin Red Ed* 283, 335
Porokeratosis (actinic)
  (1988): Beiteke U+, *Photodermatology* 5, 274
  (1985): Hazen PG+, *J Am Acad Dermatol* 12, 1077
  (1980): Reymond JL, *Acta Derm Venereol* (Stockh) 60, 539
Prurigo
  (1982): Stüttgen G, *Int J Dermatol* 21, 198 (passim)
Pruritus (>10%)
  (1990): Roelandts R+, *Photodermatol Photoimmunol Photomed* 7, 141
  (1982): Stüttgen G, *Int J Dermatol* 21, 198 (passim)
Psoriasis
Rash (sic) (1–10%)
Rosacea
  (1989): McFadden JP+, *Br J Dermatol* 121, 413
Scleroderma
Seborrheic dermatitis
  (1983): Tegner E, *Acta Derm Venereol* (Stockh) Suppl 107, 5
Squamous cell carcinoma
  (2002): Katz KA+, *J Invest Dermatol* 118(6), 1038
  (1986): Kahn JR+, *Clin Exp Dermatol* 11, 398
Urticaria
  (1994): Bech-Thomsen N+, *J Am Acad Dermatol* 31, 1063
Vasculitis
  (1981): Barriere H+, *Presse Med* (French) 10, 37
Verrucae
  (1982): Stüttgen G, *Int J Dermatol* 21, 198
Vesiculation
  (1993): Sheehan MP+, *Br J Dermatol* 129, 431 (PUVA)
  (1991): No Author, *Ned Tijdschr Geneeskd* (Dutch) 135, 1764
Vitiligo
  (1983): Tegner E, *Acta Derm Venereol* (Stockh) 107 (Suppl), 5

Mucosal/ENT
Cheilitis (1–10%)

Hair
Hair – hypertrichosis
  (1992): Shelley WB+, *Advanced Dermatologic Diagnosis* WB Saunders, 725 (passim)
  (1983): Rampen FHJ, *Br J Dermatol* 109, 657

Nails
Nails – photo-onycholysis
  (2002): Baran R+, *Photodermatol Photoimmunol Photomed* 18(4), 202
Nails – pigmentation
  (1990): Trattner A+, *Int J Dermatol* 29, 310
  (1989): Weiss E+, *Int J Dermatol* 28, 188
  (1986): MacDonald KJS+, *Br J Dermatol* 114, 395
  (1982): Naik RPC+, *Int J Dermatol* 21, 275

Other
Anaphylactoid reactions/Anaphylaxis
  (2003): Park JY+, *Photodermatol Photoimmunol Photomed* 19(1), 37
  (2001): Legat FJ+, *Br J Dermatol* 145(5), 821
Lymphoproliferative disease
  (1989): Aschinoff R+, *J Am Acad Dermatol* 21, 1134
Pain
  (1993): Burrows NP+, *Br J Dermatol* 129, 504
  (1987): Norris PG+, *Clin Exp Dermatol* 12, 403
  (1983): Tegner E, *Acta Derm Venereol* (Stockh) Suppl 107, 5
Tumors (for the most part malignant)
  (2004): McKenna KE, *Photodermatol Photoimmunol Photomed* 20(6), 289
  (1995): Weinstock MA+, *Arch Dermatol* 131, 701
  (1994): Altman JS+, *J Am Acad Dermatol* 31, 505
  (1994): Lever LR+, *Clin Exp Dermatol* 19, 443 (malignant)
  (1994): Lewis FM+, *Lancet* 344, 1157

(1993): Lindelof B+, *Br J Dermatol* 129, 39
(1990): Young AR, *J Photochem Photobiol B* 6, 237
(1989): Hannuksela M+, *J Am Acad Dermatol* 21, 813
(1989): Stern RS+, *Carcinog Compr Surv* 11, 85
(1988): Gupta AK+, *J Am Acad Dermatol* 19, 67
(1987): Henseler T+, *J Am Acad Dermatol* 16, 108
(1983): Farber EM+, *Arch Dermatol* 119, 426
(1983): Shafrir A, *Harefuah* (Hebrew) 104, 364
(1981): No Author, *Br Med J Clin Red Ed* 283, 335
(1980): Brown FS+, *J Am Acad Dermatol* 2, 393
(1980): Halprin KM, *J Am Acad Dermatol* 2, 334
(1980): Halprin KM, *J Am Acad Dermatol* 2, 432

PYRAZINAMIDE

Trade names: Braccopril; Dipimide; Isopas; Lynamide; Pirilene; Pyrazide; Pyrazinamide (Clonimel); Rifater (Sanofi-Aventis); Rozide; Tebrazid; Zinastat
Indications: Tuberculosis
Category: Antibiotic
Half-life: 9–10 hours
Clinically important, potentially hazardous interactions with: rifampin

Reactions

Skin
Acne (<1%)
Erythema multiforme
  (1996): Perdu D I, *Allergy* 51, 340
Exanthems
  (1990): Goday J+, *Contact Dermatitis* 22, 181
Fixed eruption
  (1990): Goday J+, *Contact Dermatitis* 22, 181
Peripheral edema
  (1983): Jorgensen J, *Int J Dermatol* 22, 44
Photoallergic reaction
  (2001): Maurya V+, *Int J Tuberc Lung Dis* 5(11), 1075
Photosensitivity (<1%)
  (1999): Choonhakarn C+, *J Am Acad Dermatol* 40, 645 (lichenoid)
Pruritus (<1%)
Purpura
Rash (sic) (<1%)
  (2003): Yee D+, *Am J Respir Crit Care Med* 167(11), 1472
  (2000): Gordin F+, *JAMA* 283, 1445
  (1998): Olivier C+, *Arch Pediatr* (French) 5, 289
  (1998): Radal M+, *Rev Mal Respir* (French) 15, 305 (3 cases)
Side effects (sic)
  (2002): Papastavros T+, *CMAJ* 167(2), 131 (with levofloxacin) (14 cases)
Urticaria

Mucosal/ENT
Oral lesions
Tinnitus

Other
Death
  (2003): Castro KG+, *Chest* 123(3), 967 (with rifampin)
  (2002): Medinger A, *Chest* 121(5), 1710 (with rifampin)
  (2002): No authors, *JAMA* 288(23), 2967 (with rifampin)
  (2002): No authors, *MMWR Morb Mortal* 51(44), 998
  (2001): No authors, *Can Commun Dis Rep* 27(13), 114 (with rifampin)
  (2001): No authors, *JAMA* 286(12), 1445 (with rifampin)

(2001): No authors, *MMWR Morb Mortal Wkly Rep* 50(34), 733
(with rifampin)
Hepatotoxicity
 (2006): Cook PP+, *Clin Infect Dis* 43(3), 271 (6%) (with
 rifampin)
 (2006): Yew WW+, *Respirology* 11(6), 699
Hypersensitivity
Myalgia/Myositis/Myopathy/Myotoxicity (1–10%)
 (2002): Papastavros T+, *CMAJ* 167(2), 131 (with levofloxacin)
 (14 cases)
Porphyria cutanea tarda (<1%)
Rhabdomyolysis
 (1991): Namba S+, *Jpn J Med* 30(5), 468

PYRIDOXINE

Synonym: vitamin B_6
Trade names: B(6)-Vicotrat; Beesix; Benadon; Godabion B6;
Hexa-Betalin; Nestrex
Indications: Pyridoxine deficiency
Category: Vitamin
Half-life: 15–20 days
**Clinically important, potentially hazardous interactions
with:** levodopa

Reactions

Skin
Acne
 (1991): Sherertz EF, *Cutis* 48, 119
Allergic reactions (sic) (<1%)
Bullous dermatitis
 (1984): Ruzicka T+, *Hautarzt* (German) 35, 197
Dermatitis
 (2001): Bajaj AK+, *Contact Dermatitis* 44(3), 184 (occupational)
 (1990): Camarasa JG+, *Contact Dermatitis* 23, 115
 (1985): Yoshikawa K+, *Contact Dermatitis* 12, 55
 (1983): Fujita M+, *Contact Dermatitis* 9, 61
Fixed eruption
Photosensitivity
 (2001): Bajaj AK+, *Contact Dermatitis* 44(3), 184 (occupational)
 (1998): Murata Y+, *J Am Acad Dermatol* 39, 314 (2 cases)
 (1996): Morimoto K+, *J Am Acad Dermatol* 35(2), 304
 (1996): Tanaka M+, *J Dermatol* 23, 708
Purpura
Rosacea fulminans
 (2001): Jansen T+, *J Eur Acad Dermatol Venereol* 15(5), 484
Toxic epidermal necrolysis
 (1980): Andriushchenko OM+, *Klin Med Mosk* (Russian) 58, 101
Vasculitis
 (1984): Ruzicka T+, *Hautarzt* (German) 35, 197
Vesiculation
 (1986): Friedman MA+, *J Am Acad Dermatol* 14, 915

Hair
Hair – pigmentation

Other
Hypersensitivity
Injection-site burning
Injection-site pain
Paresthesias (<1%)
 (2003): Lacerna RA+, *J Am Geriatr Soc* 51(12), 1822 (with
 nitrofurantoin)
Porphyria cutanea tarda

(1992): Shelley WB+, *Advanced Dermatologic Diagnosis* WB
Saunders, 414 (passim)
Pseudoporphyria
 (1984): Baer RL+, *J Am Acad Dermatol* 10, 527

PYRILAMINE

Trade name: Pyrilamine
Indications: Allergic rhinitis
Category: Histamine H1 receptor antagonist
Half-life: N/A

Reactions

Skin
Angioedema
Dermatitis
Diaphoresis
Lupus erythematosus
Photosensitivity
Purpura
Rash (sic)
Urticaria

Mucosal/ENT
Stomatitis
Tinnitus
Xerostomia

Other
Anaphylactoid reactions/Anaphylaxis
Gynecomastia
Paresthesias

PYRIMETHAMINE

Trade names: Daraprim (GSK); Erbaprelina; Fansidar (Roche);
Malocide; Pirimecidan
Indications: Malaria
Category: Antimalarial; Antiprotozoal
Half-life: 80–95 hours
**Clinically important, potentially hazardous interactions
with:** dapsone

Note: Fansidar is pyrimethamine and sulfadoxine

Reactions

Skin
Acute generalized exanthematous pustulosis (AGEP)
 (1995): Moreau A+, *Int J Dermatol* 34, 263 (passim)
Angioedema
 (1992): Breathnach SM+, *Adverse Drug Reactions and the Skin*
 Blackwell, Oxford, 176 (passim)
Bullous dermatitis
 (1992): Breathnach SM+, *Adverse Drug Reactions and the Skin*
 Blackwell, Oxford, 176 (passim)
 (1989): Caumes E+, *Presse Med* (French) 18, 1708
Dermatitis (<1%)
Erythema multiforme (<1%)
 (1993): Sturchler D+, *Drug Saf* 8, 160
 (1991): Porteous DM+, *Arch Dermatol* 127, 740 (in HIV+
 patients)
 (1987): Hellgren U+, *Br Med J Clin Res Ed* 295, 365

(1986): Miller KD+, *Am J Trop Med Hyg* 35, 451
Exanthems
  (2002): Thong BY+, *Ann Allergy Asthma Immunol* 88(5), 527
    (with dapsone)
  (1989): Ortel B+, *Dermatologica* 178, 39 (papular)
  (1987): Groth H+, *Schweiz Rundsch Med Prax* (German) 76, 570
Exfoliative dermatitis
  (1987): Elsas T+, *Tidsskr Nor Laegeforen* (Norwegian) 107, 1231
  (1986): Langtry JA+, *Br Med J Clin Res Ed* 292, 1107
Fixed eruption
  (2006): Nnoruka EN+, *Int J Dermatol* 45(9), 1062
  (1988): Tham SN+, *Singapore Med J* 29, 300
Lichenoid eruption
  (1989): Zain RB, *Southeast Asian J Trop Med Public Health* 20, 253
    (oral)
  (1980): Cutler TP, *Clin Exp Dermatol* 5, 253
Lymphoma
  (1997): Costello JM+, *N Z Med J* 86, 430
Photosensitivity (>10%)
  (1992): Breathnach SM+, *Adverse Drug Reactions and the Skin*
    Blackwell, Oxford, 176 (passim)
  (1989): Ortel B+, *Dermatologica* 178, 39
Pigmentation (<1%)
  (2002): Ozturk R+, *J Dermatol* 29(7), 443
  (1991): Poizot-Martin I+, *Presse Med* (French) 20, 632
  (1990): Poizot-Martin I+, *Int Conf AIDS* 6, 357
Pruritus
  (1987): Groth H+, *Schweiz Rundsch Med Prax* (German) 76, 570
Purpura
Pustules
Rash (sic) (<1%)
Stevens–Johnson syndrome (1–10%)
  (2006): Gimnig JE+, *Am J Trop Med Hyg* 74(5), 738 (%) (with
    sulfadoxine)
  (2005): Oduro-Boatey C+, *Trop Doct* 35(2), 118
  (1997): Teira R+, *Scand J Infect Dis* 29(6), 595 (with sulfadoxine)
  (1995): Caumes E+, *Clin Infect Dis* 21, 656
  (1993): Schlienger RG+, *Schweiz Rundsch Med Prax* (German)
    82, 888
  (1993): Sturchler D+, *Drug Saf* 8, 160
  (1992): Breathnach SM+, *Adverse Drug Reactions and the Skin*
    Blackwell, Oxford, 176 (passim)
  (1991): Porteous DM+, *Arch Dermatol* 127, 740 (in HIV+
    patients)
  (1990): Thiel HJ+, *Klin Monatsbl Augenheilkd* (German) 197, 142
  (1989): Ortel B+, *Dermatologica* 178, 39
  (1989): Phillips-Howard PA+, *Lancet* 2, 803
  (1988): Mimoun G+, *Bull Soc Ophtalmol Fr* (French) 88, 961
  (1987): Hellgren U+, *Br Med J Clin Res Ed* 295, 365
  (1987): Lenox-Smith I, *J Infect* 14, 90 (fatal)
  (1987): Lyn PC+, *Med J Aust* 146, 335
  (1986): Bamber MG+, *J Infect* 13, 31 (fatal)
  (1986): Gascon-Brustenga J+, *Med Clin* (Barc) (Spanish) 87, 821
  (1986): Jeffrey RF, *Postgrad Med J* 62(731), 893 (with sulfadoxine)
  (1986): Miller KD+, *Am J Trop Med Hyg* 35, 451
  (1985): Adams SJ+, *Postgrad Med J* 61, 263
  (1985): Clareus BW+, *Lakartidningen* (Swedish) 82, 4211
  (1983): Ligthelm RJ+, *Ned Tijdschr Geneeskd* (Dutch) 127, 1735
  (1982): Hornstein OP+, *N Engl J Med* 307, 1529
Toxic dermatitis (sic)
  (1995): Piketty C+, *Presse Med* (French) 24, 1710
Toxic epidermal necrolysis (<1%)
  (2006): Gimnig JE+, *Am J Trop Med Hyg* 74(5), 738 (%) (with
    sulfadoxine)
  (1998): Moussala M+, *J Fr Ophtalmol* (French) 21, 72
  (1998): Schmidt-Westhausen A+, *Oral Dis* 4, 90
  (1995): Caumes E+, *Clin Infect Dis* 21, 656
  (1993): Sturchler D+, *Drug Saf* 8, 160

(1992): Breathnach SM+, *Adverse Drug Reactions and the Skin*
  Blackwell, Oxford, 176 (passim)
(1991): Kimura S+, *Jpn J Med* 30, 553
(1990): Ward DJ+, *Burns* 16, 97
(1988): *Morb Mortal Wkly Rep* 37, 571
(1988): Phillips-Howard PA+, *Br Med J Clin Res Ed* 296, 1605
(1988): Raviglione MC+, *Arch Intern Med* 148, 2683 (fatal)
(1987): Hellgren U+, *Br Med J Clin Res Ed* 295, 365
(1986): Miller KD+, *Am J Trop Med Hyg* 35, 451
Urticaria
Vasculitis

Mucosal/ENT
Dysgeusia
Glossitis (<1%) (atrophic)
Tinnitus
Xerostomia (<1%)

Hair
Hair – alopecia

Other
Anaphylactoid reactions/Anaphylaxis (<1%)
Asthenia
  (2006): Fanello CI+, *Trop Med Int Health* 11(5), 589 (with
    sulfadoxine)
Death
Hypersensitivity (>10%)
  (2002): Thong BY+, *Ann Allergy Asthma Immunol* 88(5), 527
    (with dapsone)
Lymphoproliferative disease
Vertigo
  (2006): Fanello CI+, *Trop Med Int Health* 11(5), 589 (with
    sulfadoxine)

QUAZEPAM

Trade names: Doral (MedPointe); Oniria; Pamerex; Quazium;
Quiedorm; Selepam; Temodal
Indications: Insomnia
Category: Benzodiazepine
Half-life: 25–41 hours
**Clinically important, potentially hazardous interactions
with:** amprenavir, chlorpheniramine, clarithromycin, efavirenz,
esomeprazole, imatinib, indinavir, nelfinavir, ritonavir

Reactions

Skin
Dermatitis (1–10%)
Diaphoresis (>10%)
Pruritus
  (1991): Roth T+, *J Clin Psychiatry* 52 Suppl 38–41
Purpura
Rash (sic) (>10%)
  (1991): Roth T+, *J Clin Psychiatry* 52 Suppl 38–41
Urticaria

Mucosal/ENT
Dysgeusia
Oral ulceration
Sialopenia (>10%)
Sialorrhea (1–10%)
Xerostomia (1–5%)
  (1991): Roth T+, *J Clin Psychiatry* 52 Suppl 38–41

Hair

Hair – alopecia

Hair – hirsutism

Other

Headache

Paresthesias

QUETIAPINE

Trade name: Seroquel (AstraZeneca)
Indications: Psychotic disorders, schizophrenia
Category: Antipsychotic; Mood stabilizer
Half-life: ~6 hours

Reactions

Skin

Angioedema

(1999): Drayton G, Los Angeles, CA (patient is also allergic to sulfa) (from Internet) (observation)

Diaphoresis (1–10%)

Edema

Erythema multiforme

(2006): Lin GL+, *J Clin Psychopharmacol* 26(6), 668

Facial edema (<1%)

Peripheral edema

(2005): Rozzini L+, *Drugs Aging* 22(2), 183

Photosensitivity (<1%)

Rash (sic) (4%)

Xerosis (<1%)

Mucosal/ENT

Gingivitis (<1%)

Glossitis (<1%)

Oral ulceration (<1%)

Sialorrhea (<1%)

(2007): Allen S+, *Prim Care Companion J Clin Psychiatry* 9(3), 233

Stomatitis (<1%)

Tongue edema (<1%)

Xerostomia (7–14%)

(2006): Bellino S+, *J Clin Psychiatry* 67(7), 1042

(2006): Thase ME+, *J Clin Psychopharmacol* 26(6), 600

(2004): Denys D+, *J Clin Psychiatry* 65(8), 1040

(2001): Mullen J+, *Clin Ther* 23(11), 1839 (14.5%)

(2000): Matheson AJ+, *CNS Drugs* 14(2), 157

Other

Asthenia

(2005): Beszlej JA+, *Psychiatr Pol* 39(2), 293 (10.5%)

Candidiasis (<1%)

Headache

Hypotension

(2006): Miodownik C+, *Expert Rev Neurother* 6(7), 983

Inappropriate secretion of antidiuretic hormone (SIADH)

(2006): van den Heuvel OA+, *Ned Tijdschr Geneeskd* 150(35), 1944

Myalgia/Myositis/Myopathy/Myotoxicity (<1%)

(2003): Fountoulakis KN+, *Br J Psychiatry* 182, 81

Paresthesias (1%)

Rhabdomyolysis

(2006): Himmerich H+, *J Clin Psychopharmacol* 26(6), 676

Somnolence

(2006): Tariot PN+, *Am J Geriatr Psychiatry* 14(9), 767

Thrombophlebitis (<1%)

Vertigo

(2006): Bellino S+, *J Clin Psychiatry* 67(7), 1042

(2006): Potkin SG+, *Schizophr Res* 85(1–3), 254

(2006): Thase ME+, *J Clin Psychopharmacol* 26(6), 600

Weight gain

(2005): Ness-Abramof R+, *Drugs Today* (Barc) 41(8), 547

QUINACRINE

Trade name: Atabil
Indications: Various infections caused by susceptible helminths
Category: Antibiotic; Antimalarial
Half-life: 4–10 hours

Reactions

Skin

Dermatitis

Erythema dyschromicum perstans

Erythema nodosum

(1981): Bauer F, *J Am Acad Dermatol* 4, 239

Exanthems

(1981): Bauer F, *J Am Acad Dermatol* 4, 239 (eczematous) (80%)

Exfoliative dermatitis (8%)

(1981): Bauer F, *J Am Acad Dermatol* 4, 239 (8%)

Fixed eruption

Hypomelanosis

Keratoderma

Lichenoid eruption (12%)

(1981): Bauer F, *J Am Acad Dermatol* 4, 239 (12%)

Ochronosis

Photosensitivity

(1997): Hindson C, *The Schoch Letter* 47, 53

Pigmentation

(2002): Furukawa H+, *Nippon Rinsho* 60(8), 1649 (yellow)

(1982): Sokol RJ+, *Pediatrics* 69, 232 (yellow)

(1981): Koranda FC, *J Am Acad Dermatol* 4, 650

(1981): Zuehlke RL+, *Int J Dermatol* 20, 57

Pruritus (<1%)

Squamous cell carcinoma

Urticaria

Xanthoderma

(2007): Haught JM+, *J Am Acad Dermatol* 57(6), 1051

Mucosal/ENT

Oral pigmentation

(2004): Martin TJ+, *Br J Oral Maxillofac Surg* 42(4), 351

(2000): Kleinegger CL+, *Oral Surg Oral Med Oral Pathol Oral Radiol Endod* 90, 189

Hair

Hair – alopecia (80%)

(1981): Bauer F, *J Am Acad Dermatol* 4, 239 (eczematous) (80%)

Nails

Nails – changes (sic)

Nails – pigmentation (ala nasi) (blue-gray)

(2000): Kleinegger CL+, *Oral Surg Oral Med Oral Pathol Oral Radiol Endod* 90, 189

Other

Rhabdomyolysis

(2005): Creel N+, *J Drugs Dermatol* 4(2), 225

QUINAPRIL

Trade names: Accupril (Pfizer); Accuprin; Accupro; Acuitel; Acupril; Asig; Korec; Quinazil
Indications: Hypertension
Category: Angiotensin-converting enzyme inhibitor
Half-life: 1–2 hours
Clinically important, potentially hazardous interactions with: amiloride, spironolactone, triamterene

Reactions

Skin
Angioedema (<1%)
 (2001): Cohen EG+, *Ann Otol Rhinol Laryngol* 110(8), 701 (64 cases)
 (1997): Sigler C+, *Arch Dermatol* 113, 972
 (1996): Boxer M, *J Allergy Clin Immunol* 98, 471
 (1995): Maier C, *Anaesthesist* (German) 44, 875
 (1994): Cosano L+, *Med Clin* (Barc) (Spanish) 102, 275
 (1993): Mendez-Mora JL+, *Med Clin* (Barc) (Spanish) 101, 76
 (1992): Materson BJ, *Am J Cardiol* 69, 46C
 (1989): Sedman AJ+, *Angiology* 40 (4 Pt 2), 360
Bullous dermatitis
 (1998): Sienkiewicz G, Johnson City, NY (from Internet) (observation)
Diaphoresis (<1%)
 (1991): Morant J+, *Arzneimittel-Kompendium der Schweiz* (German) Basel, Documed, 1990
 (1989): Frank GJ+, *Angiology* 40 (4 Pt 2), 405
 (1989): Maclean D, *Angiology* 40 (4 Pt 2), 370
Edema
 (1989): Frank GJ, *Cardiology* 76 (Suppl 2), 56
 (1989): Frank GJ+, *Angiology* 40 (4 Pt 2), 405
Exanthems
 (1991): Morant J+, *Arzneimittel-Kompendium der Schweiz* (German) Basel, Documed, 1990
Exfoliative dermatitis (<1%)
Facial edema
 (1989): Sedman AJ+, *Angiology* 40 (4 Pt 2), 360
Pemphigus (<1%)
Pemphigus foliaceus
 (2000): Ong CS+, *Australas J Dermatol* 41(4), 242
Pemphigus vulgaris
 (2000): Ong CS+, *Australas J Dermatol* 41(4), 242
Peripheral edema
 (1992): Bahena JH+, *Clin Ther* 14, 527
 (1991): Wadworth AN+, *Drugs* 41, 378
Photosensitivity (<1%)
 (1989): Maclean D, *Angiology* 40 (4 Pt 2), 370
Pruritus (<1%)
 (1991): Cetnarowski-Cropp AB, *Drug Intell Clin Pharm* 25, 499
 (1991): Morant J+, *Arzneimittel-Kompendium der Schweiz* (German) Basel, Documed, 1990
 (1990): Frishman WH, *Clin Cardiol* 13 (Suppl 7), VII19
 (1990): Swartz RD+, *J Clin Pharmacol* 30, 1136
 (1989): Frank GJ, *Cardiology* 76 (Suppl 2), 56
 (1989): Frank GJ+, *Angiology* 40 (4 Pt 2), 405
 (1989): Maclean D, *Angiology* 40 (4 Pt 2), 370
Rash (sic) (1.2%)
 (1992): Materson BJ, *Am J Cardiol* 69, 46C
 (1989): Frank GJ, *Cardiology* 76 (Suppl 2), 56
 (1989): Frank GJ+, *Angiology* 40 (4 Pt 2), 405
 (1989): Maclean D, *Angiology* 40 (4 Pt 2), 370
 (1989): Taylor SH, *Angiology* 40 (4 Pt 2), 382
Urticaria (<1%)
Vasculitis (<1%)

Mucosal/ENT
Dysgeusia
 (1991): Cetnarowski-Cropp AB, *Drug Intell Clin Pharm* 25, 499
 (1989): Taylor SH, *Angiology* 40 (4 Pt 2), 382
Xerostomia (<1%)

Hair
Hair – alopecia (<1%)

Other
Cough
 (2007): Gliddon AE+, *Arthritis Rheum* 56(11), 3837
 (2004): Unnikrishnan D+, *J Am Med Dir Assoc* 5(2), 107
 (2002): Culy CR+, *Drugs* 62(2), 339 (2–4%)
 (2001): Adigun AQ+, *West Afr J Med* 20(1), 46
 (2001): Lee SC+, *Hypertension* 38(2), 166
 (1989): Just PM, *Pharmacotherapy* 9(2), 82
 (1987): Ollivier JP+, *Presse Med* 16(16), 759
Headache
Hypersensitivity
Myalgia/Myositis/Myopathy/Myotoxicity (1.5%)
Paresthesias (<1%)

QUINESTROL

Trade name: Estrovis
Indications: Atrophic vaginitis, menopausal symptoms
Category: Estrogen
Half-life: 120 hours

Reactions

Skin
Angioedema
Chloasma (<1%)
Edema (<1%)
Erythema
Melasma (<1%)
Peripheral edema (>10%)
Photosensitivity
Rash (sic) (<1%)
Urticaria

Other
Gynecomastia (>10%)
Thrombophlebitis

QUINETHAZONE

Trade names: Aquamox; Hydromox
Indications: Hypertension, edema
Category: Diuretic, thiazide
Half-life: N/A
Clinically important, potentially hazardous interactions with: digoxin, lithium

Note: Quinethazone is a sulfonamide and can be absorbed systemically. Sulfonamides can produce severe, possibly fatal, reactions such as toxic epidermal necrolysis and Stevens–Johnson syndrome

Reactions

Skin
Bullous dermatitis (<1%)
Exanthems
Photosensitivity (<1%)
Pruritus
Purpura
Rash (sic) (<1%)
Urticaria
Vasculitis

Mucosal/ENT
Xerostomia

Eyes
Dyschromatopsia

Other
Hypersensitivity
Paresthesias

QUINIDINE

Trade names: Cardine; Cin-Quin; Gluquine; Kinidin; Quinalan; Quinate; Quini Durules; Quinora
Indications: Tachycardia, atrial fibrillation
Category: Antiarrhythmic class Ia; Antimalarial; Antiprotozoal
Half-life: 6–8 hours
Clinically important, potentially hazardous interactions with: abarelix, amiloride, amiodarone, amisulpride, amprenavir, anisindione, anticoagulants, aripiprazole, arsenic, astemizole, celiprolol, ciprofloxacin, delavirdine, dicumarol, digoxin, duloxetine, enoxacin, fosamprenavir, gatifloxacin, itraconazole, lomefloxacin, moxifloxacin, norfloxacin, ofloxacin, pimozide, pipecuronium, quinolones, ranolazine, ritonavir, rocuronium, **senna**, sparfloxacin, **squill**, tipranavir, vecuronium, verapamil, voriconazole, warfarin

Reactions

Skin
Acne
  (1981): Burkhart CG, Arch Dermatol 117, 603
Acute generalized exanthematous pustulosis (AGEP)
  (1995): Moreau A+, Int J Dermatol 34, 263 (passim)
  (1991): Roujeau J-C+, Arch Dermatol 127, 1333
Allergic reactions (sic) (1%)
  (1986): Bigby M+, JAMA 256, 3358 (1.34%)
Angioedema (<1%)
Bullous dermatitis
Dermatitis
  (1985): Fowler JF, Contact Dermatitis 13, 280
  (1981): Wahlberg JE+, Contact Dermatitis 7, 27 (occupational)
Eczema
Erythema multiforme
  (1989): Alanko K, Acta Derm Venereol (Stockh) 69, 223
Exanthems
  (1990): Lou CP+, Postgrad Med J 66, 406
  (1985): Bruce S+, J Am Acad Dermatol 12, 332
  (1982): Holt RJ, Drug Intell Clin Pharm 16, 615
  (1980): Harrison DC+, Am Heart J 100, 1046 (16.6%)
Exfoliative dermatitis (<1%)
  (1996): Sigurdsson V+, J Am Acad Dermatol 35, 53
  (1987): Bellogini GC+, Minerva Cardioangiol (Italian) 35, 457

  (1985): Bruce S+, J Am Acad Dermatol 12, 332
Fixed eruption
  (2007): Muso Y+, J Dermatol 34(6), 385 (2 cases) (tonic water)
Granuloma annulare
  (1991): Ross EV+, J Assoc Military Dermatol XVII (1), 16
Lichen planus
  (1994): Thompson DF+, Pharmacotherapy 14, 561
  (1985): Bruce S+, J Am Acad Dermatol 12, 332 (passim)
  (1985): Rebondy JP+, Ann Dermatol Venereol (French) 112, 989
  (1980): Maltz BL+, Int J Dermatol 19, 96
Lichenoid eruption
  (1988): de Larrard G+, Ann Dermatol Venereol (French) 115, 1172
  (1987): Jeanmougin M+, Ann Dermatol Venereol (French) 114, 1397 (photosensitive)
  (1982): Berger TC+, Cutis 29, 595
  (1981): Haim S+, Harefuah (Hebrew) 101, 310
Livedo reticularis (<1%)
  (2005): Gibbs MB+, J Am Acad Dermatol 52(6), 1009
  (1989): Manzi S+, Arch Dermatol 125, 417 (photosensitive)
  (1985): Bruce S+, J Am Acad Dermatol 12, 332 (photosensitive)
Lupus erythematosus (<1%)
  (1996): Rich MW, Postgrad Med 100, 299
  (1995): Alloway JA+, Semin Arthritis Rheum 24, 315
  (1994): Yung RL+, Rheum Dis Clin North Am 20, 61
  (1992): Rubin RL, Clin Biochem 25, 223
  (1992): Rubin RL+, J Clin Invest 90, 165
  (1992): Skaer TL, Clin Ther 14, 496
  (1991): Alarcon-Segovia D+, Baillieres Clin Rheumatol 5, 1
  (1991): Tebas P+, Rev Clin Esp (Spanish) 189, 123
  (1989): Cohen MG, Geriatric Med Today 8, 95
  (1988): Cohen MG+, Ann Intern Med 108, 369
  (1988): Schmid FR, Ann Intern Med 109, 247
  (1988): Webb J+, Med J Aust 149, 53
  (1987): Sukenik S+, Isr J Med Sci 23, 1232
  (1986): Bar-El Y+, Am Heart J 111, 1209
  (1985): Amadio P+, Ann Intern Med 102, 419
  (1985): Gastineau DA+, Arch Intern Med 145, 1926
  (1985): Krainin MJ+, Arch Intern Med 145, 1740
  (1985): Lavie CJ+, Arch Intern Med 145, 446
  (1985): McCormack GD+, Semin Arthritis Rheum 15, 73
  (1985): Rebondy JP+, Ann Dermatol Venereol (French) 112, 989
  (1985): Stratton MA, Clin Pharm 4, 657
  (1984): West SG+, Ann Intern Med 100, 840
  (1982): Chagnon A+, Nouv Presse Med (French) 11, 2020
  (1981): Barrier J+, Nouv Presse Med (French) 10, 2991
  (1980): Condemi JJ, Geriatrics 35(3), 81
Palmar–plantar desquamation
  (1988): De Larrard G+, Ann Dermatol Venereol (French) 115, 1172
Photosensitivity (<1%)
  (1992): Schürer NY+, Photodermatol Photoimmunol Photomed 9, 78
  (1991): Schürer NY+, Hautarzt (German) 42, 158
  (1990): Fertin C+, Nouv Dermatol (French) 9, 446
  (1989): Rosen C, Semin Dermatol 8, 149
  (1988): De Larrard G+, Ann Dermatol Venereol (French) 115, 1172
  (1987): Bonnetblanc JM+, Ann Dermatol Venereol (French) 114, 957 (lichenoid)
  (1987): Ferguson J+, Br J Dermatol 117, 631
  (1987): Wolf R+, Dermatologica 174, 285 (lichenoid and eczematous)
  (1986): Jeanmougin M+, Ann Dermatol Venereol (French) 113, 985
  (1986): Ljunggren B+, Photodermatol 3, 26
  (1985): Armstrong RB+, Arch Dermatol 121, 525
  (1985): Bonnetblanc JM+, Ann Dermatol Venereol (French) 112, 671
  (1985): Rebondy JP+, Ann Dermatol Venereol (French) 112, 989

(1984): Fisher DA, *Arch Dermatol* 120, 298
(1983): Lang PS, *J Am Acad Dermatol* 9, 124
(1983): Marx JL+, *Arch Dermatol* 119, 39
(1982): Berger TC+, *Cutis* 29, 595 (lichenoid)
Pigmentation (<1%)
  (1996): Conroy EA+, *Cutis* 57, 425
  (1996): Messina JL+, *J Geriatr Dermatol* 4, 198
  (1995): Rippis G+, American Academy of Dermatology Meeting,
    New Orleans (observation)
  (1986): Mahler R+, *Arch Dermatol* 122, 1062
Pruritus (<1%)
  (1985): Bruce S+, *J Am Acad Dermatol* 12, 332 (passim)
  (1982): Holt RJ, *Drug Intell Clin Pharm* 16, 615
Psoriasis (<1%)
  (1998): Smith KC, Niagara Falls, Canada (from Internet)
    (observation)
  (1993): Brenner S+, *Arch Dermatol* 129, 1331
  (1986): Abel EA+, *J Am Acad Dermatol* 15, 1007
  (1983): Harwell WB, *J Am Acad Dermatol* 9, 278
Purpura (1%)
  (1993): Kaufman DW+, *Blood* 82, 2714
  (1991): Salom IL, *JAMA* 266, 1220 (letter)
  (1988): Reid DM+, *Ann Intern Med* 108, 206
  (1981): Barrier J+, *Nouv Presse Med* (French) 10, 2991
  (1981): Conri C+, *Nouv Presse Med* (French) 7, 3361
  (1980): Miescher PA+, *Clin Haematol* 9, 505
Pustules
Rash (sic) (1–10%)
Side effects (sic) (1%)
Subcorneal pustular dermatosis (Sneddon-Wilkinson)
  (2005): Boulenger-Vazel A+, *Ann Dermatol Venereol* 132(1), 27
Toxic epidermal necrolysis
  (2000): Adornato MC, *N Y State Dent J* 66, 38
Urticaria (<1%)
  (1985): Bruce S+, *J Am Acad Dermatol* 12, 332
Vasculitis (<1%)
  (1990): Zax RH+, *Arch Dermatol* 126, 69
  (1989): Cohen MG, *Geriatric Med Today* 8, 99
  (1988): Quin J+, *Med J Aust* 148, 145 (allergic granulomatous)
  (1985): Shalit M+, *Arch Intern Med* 145, 2051

Mucosal/ENT

Dysgeusia (>10%) (bitter taste)
Oral mucosal eruption
  (1988): De Larrard G+, *Ann Dermatol Venereol* (French)
    115, 1172
Oral pigmentation
  (1988): Birek C+, *Oral Surg Oral Med Oral Pathol* 66, 59
Oral ulceration
Tinnitus

Hair

Hair – alopecia
  (1988): de Larrard G+, *Ann Dermatol Venereol* (French)
    115, 1172

Eyes

Uveitis

Other

Congestive heart failure
  (1997): Choy AM+, *Circulation* 96(7), 2149
  (1992): Hook BG+, *Pacing Clin Electrophysiol* 15(3), 324
Headache
Hypersensitivity
Lymphoproliferative disease
  (1987): Gay RG+, *Am J Med* 82, 143
Myalgia/Myositis/Myopathy/Myotoxicity (<1%)
Polymyositis

(1995): Alloway JA+, *Semin Arthritis Rheum* 24, 315
Porphyria
Pseudoporphyria
  (1992): Petersen CS+, *Ugeskr Laeger* (Danish) 154, 1713
Sjøgren's (Sicca) syndrome (<1%)
  (1983): Naschitz JE+, *J Toxicol Clin Toxicol* 20, 367
Tremor (2%)

QUININE

Trade names: Adaquin; Chinine; Formula-Q; Genin; M-KYA; Q-Vel; Quinoctal; Quinsan; Quinsul; Quiphile
Indications: Malaria, nocturnal leg cramps
Category: Antimalarial; Antiprotozoal
Half-life: 8–14 hours
Clinically important, potentially hazardous interactions with: anisindione, anticoagulants, astemizole, atorvastatin, dicumarol, warfarin

Reactions

Skin

Acne
  (1981): Burkhart CC, *Arch Dermatol* 117, 603
Acral erythema
  (2000): Abreu-Gerke L+, *Hautarzt* 51(5), 332
Acral necrosis
  (2002): Agarwal N+, *J Postgrad Med* 48(3), 197
  (2000): Abreu-Gerke L+, *Hautarzt* 51(5), 332
Angioedema (<1%)
Bullous dermatitis
Dermatitis
  (1994): Dias M+, *Contact Dermatitis* 30, 121
  (1994): Isaksson M+, *Acta Derm Venereol* 74, 286
  (1994): Tapadinhas C+, *Contact Dermatitis* 31, 127 (from hair
    lotion)
Diaphoresis
Eczema
Erythema
Erythema multiforme (<1%)
  (2000): Abreu-Gerke L+, *Hautarzt* 51(5), 332 (passim)
Exanthems (1–5%)
  (2000): Abreu-Gerke L+, *Hautarzt* 51(5), 332 (passim)
Exfoliative dermatitis
Facial edema
Fixed eruption
  (2003): Asero R, *J Allergy Clin Immunol* 111(1), 198
  (2003): Kubota Y, *Arerugi* 52(4), 447
  (2000): Litt JZ, Beachwood, OH (personal case) (observation)
  (1993): Litt JZ, Beachwood, OH (from quinine water) (personal
    case) (observation)
  (1990): Gaffoor PMA+, *Cutis* 45, 242 (passim)
Lichen planus
  (1994): Litt JZ, Beachwood, OH (personal case) (observation)
  (1986): Dawson TAJ, *Clin Exp Dermatol* 11, 670
  (1986): Meyrick-Thomas RH+, *Clin Exp Dermatol* 11, 97
    (photosensitive distribution)
Lichenoid eruption
  (1995): Dawson TA, *BMJ* 310, 738
  (1989): Tan SV+, *Clin Exp Dermatol* 14, 335
  (1987): Ferguson J+, *Br J Dermatol* 117, 631
Livedo reticularis (photosensitive)
  (1988): Diffey BL+, *Br J Dermatol* 118, 679
Lupus erythematosus
  (1996): Rosa-Re D+, *Ann Rheum Dis* 55, 559

Ochronosis
  (1986): Bruce S+, *J Am Acad Dermatol* 15, 357
Photosensitivity
  (2005): Nacher M+, *Trop Doct* 35(2), 117
  (2000): Abreu-Gerke L+, *Hautarzt* 51(5), 332 (passim)
  (1998): Rademaker M, Hamilton, New Zealand (from Internet)
    (observation)
  (1995): Dawson TA, *BMJ* 310, 738
  (1995): Delmas A+, *Presse Med* (French) 24, 1707
  (1994): Isaksson M+, *Acta Derm Venereol* 74, 286
  (1994): Litt JZ, Beachwood, OH (personal case) (observation)
  (1994): Okun MM+, *Clin Exp Dermatol* 19, 246 (mycosis
    fungoides-like)
  (1994): Wagner GH+, *Br J Dermatol* 131, 734 (from tonic water)
  (1992): Fitzpatrick JE, *Dermatol Clin* 10, 19
  (1992): Ljunggren B+, *Contact Dermatitis* 26, 1
  (1990): Guzzo C+, *Photodermatol Photoimmunol Photomed*
    7, 166
  (1988): Diffey BL+, *Br J Dermatol* 118, 679
  (1987): Ferguson J+, *Br J Dermatol* 117, 631
  (1986): Dawson TAJ, *Clin Exp Dermatol* 11, 670 (lichenoid)
  (1986): Ljunggren B+, *Arch Dermatol* 122, 909
  (1986): Ljunggren B+, *Photodermatol* 3, 26
  (1984): Jeanmougin M+, *Ann Dermatol Venereol* (French) 11, 565
Pigmentation
  (2005): Rosen T+, *Cutis* 75(2), 114
  (1999): Rosen T+, Houston, TX (personal case) (observation)
  (1994): Litt JZ, Beachwood, OH (personal case) (observation)
  (1986): Bruce S+, *J Am Acad Dermatol* 15, 357 (from injections)
  (1986): Mahler R+, *Arch Dermatol* 122, 1062
Pruritus (<1%)
  (2000): Abreu-Gerke L+, *Hautarzt* 51(5), 332 (passim)
Psoriasis
  (1998): Smith KC, Niagara Falls, Canada (from Internet)
    (observation)
Purpura
  (2001): *Ann Intern Med* 135(12), S
  (2001): Medina PJ+, *Curr Opin Hematol* 8(5), 286
  (2000): Abreu-Gerke L+, *Hautarzt* 51(5), 332 (passim)
  (1993): Kaufman DW+, *Blood* 82, 2714
  (1985): Ambriz-Fernandez R+, *Rev Invest Clin* (Spanish) 37, 347
  (1980): Miescher PA+, *Clin Haematol* 9, 505
Rash (sic) (<1%)
  (1993): Siderov J, *J Am Geriatr Soc* 41, 498
Raynaud's phenomenon
  (2002): Agarwal N+, *J Postgrad Med* 48(3), 197
Stevens–Johnson syndrome
  (1986): Gascon-Brustenga J+, *Med Clin* (Barc) (Spanish) 87, 821
Toxic epidermal necrolysis (<1%)
Urticaria
  (2000): Abreu-Gerke L+, *Hautarzt* 51(5), 332 (passim)
Vasculitis
  (1992): Price EJ+, *Br J Clin Pract* 46, 138
  (1991): Harland CC+, *BMJ* 302, 295
  (1990): Mathur S+, *BMJ* 300, 613
Vitiligo
  (1998): Rademaker M, Hamilton, New Zealand (following
    photosensitivity) (from Internet) (observation)

Mucosal/ENT
Oral mucosal eruption
Oral ulceration
Tinnitus
  (2007): Gunawan CA+, *Acta Med Indones* 39(1), 27
  (1994): Karbwang J+, *Southeast Asian J Trop Med Public Health*
    25(2), 397
  (1993): Bodenhamer JE+, *J Emerg Med* 11(3), 279 (passim)
  (1991): Bruchfeld J+, *Trop Med Parasitol* 42(2), 153
  (1991): Bruchfeld J+, *Trop Med Parasitol* 42(4), 386

  (1990): Roche RJ+, *Br J Clin Pharmacol* 29(6), 780
  (1986): Bateman DN+, *Adverse Drug React Acute Poisoning Rev*
    5(4), 215

Nails
Nails – photo-onycholysis
  (1989): Tan SV+, *Clin Exp Dermatol* 14, 335

Eyes
Vision loss
  (2007): Lundorff T+, *Ugeskr Laeger* 169(43), 3677

Other
Death
  (2003): Morrison LD+, *Vet Hum Toxicol* 45(6), 303
DRESS syndrome
  (2006): Greco M+, *Ann Dermatol Venereol* 133(4), 354 (with
    thiamine)
Headache
Hypersensitivity (<1%)
  (1998): Schattner A, *Am J Med* 104–488
Nephrotoxicity
  (2006): Lim AK+, *Intern Med J* 36(7), 465 (with atorvastatin)
Porphyria
Rhabdomyolysis
  (2006): Lim AK+, *Intern Med J* 36(7), 465 (with atorvastatin)

QUINUPRISTIN/DALFOPRISTIN

Synonyms: pristinamycin; RP59500
Trade name: Synercid (Monarch)
Indications: Serious life-threatening bacterial infections
Category: Antibiotic, streptogramin
Half-life: 1.3–1.5 hours

Reactions

Skin
Acute febrile neutrophilic dermatosis (Sweet's syndrome)
  (2003): Choi HS+, *Korean J Intern Med* 18(3), 187
Allergic reactions (sic) (<1%)
Diaphoresis (<1%)
Exanthems (<1%)
Peripheral edema (<1%)
Pruritus (1.5%)
Rash (sic) (2–4%)
  (2001): Allington DR+, *Clin Ther* 23(1), 24 (2.5–4.6%)
Ulcerations (<1%)
Urticaria (<1%)

Mucosal/ENT
Oral candidiasis (<1%)
Stomatitis (<1%)
Vaginitis (<1%)

Other
Anaphylactoid reactions/Anaphylaxis (<1%)
Candidiasis (<1%)
Injection-site edema (17.3%)
  (2001): Allington DR+, *Clin Ther* 23(1), 24
Injection-site extravasation (42%)
  (2001): Allington DR+, *Clin Ther* 23(1), 24
Injection-site pain (40%)
  (2001): Allington DR+, *Clin Ther* 23(1), 24
  (2000): Delgado G+, *Pharmacotherapy* 20(12), 1469
Injection-site reactions (sic) (13.4%)
Myalgia/Myositis/Myopathy/Myotoxicity (<1–5%)

(2006): Gupte G+, *Pediatr Infect Dis J* 25(3), 281
(2003): Carver PL+, *Pharmacotherapy* 23(2), 159
(2002): Linden PK, *Drugs* 62(3), 425
(2001): Allington DR+, *Clin Ther* 23(1), 24
(2001): Manzella JP, *Am Fam Physician* 64(11), 1863
(2001): Olsen KM+, *Clin Infect Dis* 32(4), 83
(2000): Delgado G+, *Pharmacotherapy* 20(12), 1469
Paresthesias (<1%)
Phlebitis (<1%)
Thrombophlebitis (2.4%)
(2001): Allington DR+, *Clin Ther* 23(1), 24
Tremor (<1%)

RABEPRAZOLE

Synonym: pariprazole
Trade name: Aciphex (Eisai) (Janssen)
Indications: Gastroesophageal reflux disease (GERD)
Category: Proton pump inhibitor
Half-life: 1–2 hours
**Clinically important, potentially hazardous interactions
with:** digoxin, ketoconazole, simvastatin

Reactions

Skin
Allergic reactions (sic) (<1%)
Diaphoresis (<1%)
Edema
Facial edema (<1%)
Herpes zoster (<1%)
Peripheral edema (<1%)
Photosensitivity (<1%)
Pigmentation (<1%)
Pruritus (<1%)
Psoriasis (<1%)
Purpura
Rash (sic) (<1%)
Urticaria (<1%)
Xerosis (<1%)

Mucosal/ENT
Gingivitis (<1%)
Glossitis (<1%)
Oral ulceration
Stomatitis (<1%)
(2003): Stoecker WV, MO (from Internet) (observation)
Tongue edema
(2003): Stoecker WV, MO (from Internet) (observation)
Xerostomia (<1%)

Hair
Hair – alopecia (<1%)

Other
Chills (<1%)
Gynecomastia (<1%)
Headache
(2002): Robinson M+, *Aliment Pharmacol Ther* 16(3), 445
Hypersensitivity
(2006): Perez Pimiento AJ+, *J Allergy Clin Immunol* 117(3), 707
Myalgia/Myositis/Myopathy/Myotoxicity (<1%)
(2006): Clark DW+, *Eur J Clin Pharmacol* 62(6), 473
Nephrotoxicity
(2005): Geevasinga N+, *Nephrology (Carlton)* 10(1), 7

Paresthesias (<1%)
Rhabdomyolysis
(2002): Bourlon S+, *Therapie* 57(6), 597 (with domperidone)
Thrombophlebitis (<1%)
Tremor (<1%)

RALOXIFENE

Synonym: Keoxifene
Trade name: Evista (Lilly)
Indications: Osteoporosis
Category: Selective estrogen receptor modulator (SERM)
Half-life: 27.7 hours
**Clinically important, potentially hazardous interactions
with:** cholestyramine, levothyroxine

Reactions

Skin
Capillaritis
(2005): Erbagci Z+, *Saudi Med J* 26(2), 314
Diaphoresis (3.1%)
Edema
Peripheral edema (3–5%)
(2000): Eriksen EF, *Ugeskr Laeger* (Danish) 162, 4182
(1999): Cummings SR+, *JAMA* 281, 2189
(1999): Ettinger B+, *JAMA* 282, 637 (5%)
Rash (sic) (5.5%)
Vitiligo
(2002): Litt JZ, Beachwood, OH (personal case) (observation)
(after 3 weeks of raloxifene, patient developed leukoderma over exposed areas of chest and forearms after sun exposure)

Mucosal/ENT
Vaginitis (4.3%)

Other
Hot flashes (5–24%)
(2006): Uray IP+, *Expert Opin Investig Drugs* 15(12), 1583
(2004): Morii H, *Clin Calcium* 14(10), 100
(2003): Kung AW+, *J Clin Endocrinol Metab* 88(7), 3130 (5.6%)
(2002): Kinsinger LS+, *Ann Intern Med* 137(1), 59
(2001): Seeman E, *J Bone Miner Metab* 19, 65 (4.6%)
(2000): Eriksen EF, *Ugeskr Laeger* (Danish) 162, 4182
(2000): Snyder KR+, *Am J Health Syst Pharm* 57, 1669
(1999): Ettinger B+, *JAMA* 282, 637 (10%)
(1999): Scott JA+, *Am Fam Physician* 60, 1131
(1998): Walsh BW+, *JAMA* 279, 1445 (22%)
Infections (~2%)
Myalgia/Myositis/Myopathy/Myotoxicity (7.7%)
(2006): Land SR+, *JAMA* 295(23), 2742
Stroke
(2006): Barrett-Connor E+, *N Engl J Med* 355(2), 125
Thrombosis
(2006): Barrett-Connor E+, *N Engl J Med* 355(2), 125
(2006): Uray IP+, *Expert Opin Investig Drugs* 15(12), 1583

RALTEGRAVIR

Trade name: Isentress (Merck)
Indications: HIV-1 Infections
Category: Antiretroviral; Integrase inhibitor
Half-life: 9 hours
**Clinically important, potentially hazardous interactions
with:** atazanavir, **St John's wort**

Reactions

Skin
Herpes simplex
Pruritus (4%)

Other
Abdominal pain
Asthenia
Headache (2%)
  (2006): Markowitz M+, *J Acquir Immune Defic Syndr* 43(5), 509
Hepatotoxicity
Lipodystrophy
Nephrotoxicity

RALTITREXED

Trade name: Tomudex (AstraZeneca)
Indications: Colorectal neoplasms (advanced)
Category: Antimetabolite; Antineoplastic; Folate analogue
Half-life: Terminal: up to 198 Hours
**Clinically important, potentially hazardous interactions
with:** folic acid/folates, L-methylfolate

Reactions

Skin
Cellulitis (1–10%)
Diaphoresis (1–10%)
Edema (9–10%)
Exfoliative dermatitis (1–10%)
Pruritus (14%)
Rash (sic) (14%)

Mucosal/ENT
Dysgeusia (1–10%)
Mucositis (12–48%)
Pharyngitis (1–10%)
Stomatitis (12–48%)
Xerostomia (1–10%)

Hair
Hair – alopecia (1–10%)

Eyes
Conjunctivitis (1–10%)

Other
Abdominal pain (18%)
Asthenia (47%)
Chills (1–10%)
Congestive heart failure (2%)
Cough (1–10%)
Depression (1–10%)
Fever (2–23%)
Flatulence (1–10%)

Headache (1–10%)
Hypersensitivity (<1%)
Infections (1–10%)
Insomnia (1–10%)
Myalgia/Myositis/Myopathy/Myotoxicity (1–10%)
Pain (1–10%)
Sepsis (1–10%)
Weight loss (1–10%)

RAMELTEON

Trade name: Rozerem (Takeda)
Indications: Insomnia
Category: Melatonin receptor agonist
Half-life: 1–2.6 hours
**Clinically important, potentially hazardous interactions
with:** **alcohol**, fluconazole, fluvoxamine, ketoconazole, rifampin

Reactions

Mucosal/ENT
Dysgeusia (2%)

Other
Asthenia (4%)
  (2006): Borja NL+, *Clin Ther* 28(10), 1540 (4%)
  (2005): McGechan A+, *CNS Drugs* 19(12), 1057 (4%)
Depression (2%)
Headache (7%)
  (2006): Borja NL+, *Clin Ther* 28(10), 1540 (7%)
Infections (1%)
Myalgia/Myositis/Myopathy/Myotoxicity (2%)
Upper respiratory infection (3%)
Vertigo (5%)
  (2006): Borja NL+, *Clin Ther* 28(10), 1540 (5%)
  (2005): McGechan A+, *CNS Drugs* 19(12), 1057 (5%)

RAMIPRIL

Trade names: Altace (Monarch); Delix; Hytren; Pramace;
Quark; Ramace; Triatec; Tritace; Unipril
Indications: Hypertension
Category: Angiotensin-converting enzyme inhibitor
Half-life: 3–17 hours
**Clinically important, potentially hazardous interactions
with:** amiloride, spironolactone, triamterene

Reactions

Skin
Acne
  (1987): Predel HG+, *Am J Cardiol* 59, 143D
Angioedema (0.3%)
  (2007): Roper AJ+, *J Laryngol Otol* 121(8), e11
  (2007): Serratrice J+, *Rev Neurol* (Paris) 163(2), 241
  (2002): Kaur S+, *J Dermatol* 29(6), 336
  (2001): Cohen EG+, *Ann Otol Rhinol Laryngol* 110(8), 701 (64 cases)
  (1995): Epeldo-Gonzalo F+, *Ann Pharmacother* 29, 431
  (1990): Todd PA+, *Drugs* 39, 110
Dermatitis (<1%)
Diaphoresis (<1%)
  (1988): Zabludowski J+, *Curr Med Res Opin* 11, 93

(1987): Walter U+, *Am J Cardiol* 59, 125D
Edema (<1%)
  (1990): Todd PA+, *Drugs* 39, 110
Erythema (circumscribed)
  (1987): Predel HG+, *Am J Cardiol* 59, 143D
Erythema multiforme (<1%)
Exanthems
  (1990): Todd PA+, *Drugs* 39, 110
Facial xerosis (sic)
  (1987): Fukiyama K+, *Am J Cardiol* 59, 121D
Lichen planus pemphigoides
  (2006): Zhu YI+, *Int J Dermatol* 45(12), 1453
  (1997): Ogg GS+, *Br J Dermatol* 136, 412
Pemphigus (<1%)
  (1996): Vignes S+, *Br J Dermatol* 135, 657
Pemphigus foliaceus
  (2000): Ong CS+, *Australas J Dermatol* 41(4), 242
Photosensitivity (<1%)
  (2000): Wagner SN+, *Contact Dermatitis* 43(4), 245 (with
    hydrochlorothiazide)
  (1994): Shelley WB+, *Cutis* 53, 39 (observation)
  (1993): Shelley WB+, *Cutis* 52, 81 (observation)
Pruritus (<1%)
  (1990): Todd PA+, *Drugs* 39, 110
  (1987): Predel HG+, *Am J Cardiol* 59, 143D
  (1987): Walter U+, *Am J Cardiol* 59, 125D
Purpura (<1%)
Rash (sic) (<1%)
  (1990): Janka HU+, *Arzneimittelforschung* (German) 40, 432
  (1990): Todd PA+, *Drugs* 39, 110
  (1987): Ball SG+, *Am J Cardiol* 59, 23D
  (1987): Walter U+, *Am J Cardiol* 59, 125D
Stevens–Johnson syndrome
  (2003): Oskay T+, *Int J Dermatol* 42(7), 580
Urticaria (<1%)
Vasculitis (<1%)
  (2004): Gupta S+, *J Drugs in Dermatol* 3(1), 81

Mucosal/ENT
Ageusia (<1%)
Dysgeusia (<1%)
  (1990): Todd PA+, *Drugs* 39, 110
Sialorrhea (<1%)
Tinnitus
Xerostomia (<1%)

Hair
Hair – alopecia (1–10%)

Other
Anaphylactoid reactions/Anaphylaxis (<1%)
Cough
  (2006): Lacourciere Y+, *Am J Hypertens* 19(1), 104 (10%)
  (2005): Chu CS+, *Kaohsiung J Med Sci* 21(11), 511 (15%)
  (2005): Sharpe N, *Cardiovasc Drugs Ther* 19(3), 197 (4%)
  (2004): Kumar NS+, *J Assoc Physicians India* 52, 454
  (2001): Adigun AQ+, *West Afr J Med* 20(1), 46
  (2001): Lee SC+, *Hypertension* 38(2), 166
  (1998): Singh NP+, *J Assoc Physicians India* 46(5), 448 (24%)
  (1991): Carre A+, *J Cardiovasc Pharmacol* 18, S141
  (1989): Just PM, *Pharmacotherapy* 9(2), 82
  (1989): McEwan JR+, *BMJ* 299(6690), 13
Headache
Hypersensitivity (<1%)
Hypotension
  (2005): Chu CS+, *Kaohsiung J Med Sci* 21(11), 511 (2%)
Nephrotoxicity
  (2007): Chen JP, *Heart Lung* 36(4), 298
Paresthesias (<1%)

(1987): Walter U+, *Am J Cardiol* 59, 125D
Tremor (<1%)
Vertigo
  (2005): Chu CS+, *Kaohsiung J Med Sci* 21(11), 511 (6%)
  (1991): Carre A+, *J Cardiovasc Pharmacol* 18, S141

RANIBIZUMAB

Trade name: Lucentis (Genentech)
Indications: Wet, age-related macular degeneration
Category: Recombinant humanized monoclonal antibody
Half-life: 9 days
**Clinically important, potentially hazardous interactions
with:** N/A

Reactions

Mucosal/ENT
Sinusitis

Eyes
Blepharitis
Cataract
Conjunctival hemorrhage
Conjunctival hyperemia
Endophthalmitis
  (2006): Heier JS+, *Ophthalmology* 113(4), 642
Epiphora
Intraocular pressure increased
Iridocyclitis
  (2006): Heier JS+, *Ophthalmology* 113(4), 642
  (2006): Rosenfeld PJ+, *Ophthalmology* 113(4), 632
Maculopathy
Ocular injection-site reactions
  (2006): Rosenfeld PJ+, *Ophthalmology* 113(4), 632
Ocular pain
Ocular pruritus
Ocular xerosis
Retinal vein occlusion
  (2006): Heier JS+, *Ophthalmology* 113(4), 642
Subretinal fibrosis
Vision blurred
Visual disturbances
Vitreous floaters

Other
Cough
Headache
Hypertension
Upper respiratory infection

RANITIDINE

Trade names: Apo-Ranitidine; Axoban; Azantac; Nu-Ranit; Raniben; Raniplex; Ranisen; Sostril; Zantab; Zantac (GSK); Zantac-C; Zantic
Indications: Duodenal ulcer
Category: Histamine H2 receptor antagonist
Half-life: 2.5 hours
Clinically important, potentially hazardous interactions with: alfentanil, **devil's claw**, fentanyl, prednisone

Note: Ranitidine is present in mother's milk in relatively large amounts. It is thought that gynecomastia develops as a result of ranitidine blocking the androgen receptors at the end organs

Reactions

Skin
Acute generalized exanthematous pustulosis (AGEP)
  (2003): Martinez MB+, *Contact Dermatitis* 49(1), 47
  (1996): Sawhney RA+, *Int J Dermatol* 35, 826
Angioedema (<1%)
Dermatitis
  (2003): Ryan PJ+, *Contact Dermatitis* 48(2), 67
  (1988): Romaguera C+, *Contact Dermatitis* 18, 177
  (1987): Alomar A+, *Contact Dermatitis* 17, 54
  (1984): Goh CL+, *Contact Dermatitis* 4, 252
  (1983): Rycroft RJ, *Contact Dermatitis* 9, 456 (occupational)
Eczema
  (1992): Juste S+, *Contact Dermatitis* 27, 339
  (1988): Romaguera C+, *Contact Dermatitis* 18, 177
Erythema multiforme
Exanthems
  (2007): Okamoto O+, *J Dermatol* 34(1), 74
  (1993): Devuyst O+, *Acta Clin Belg* 48, 109
  (1989): Grant SM+, *Drugs* 37, 801
  (1988): Haboubi N+, *Br Med J Clin Res Ed* 296, 897
  (1984): Khandheria BK, *JAMA* 253, 3252
Fixed eruption
  (1990): Black AK+, *Br J Dermatol* 123, 277
Hemorrhage
  (2006): Oldfield V+, *BioDrugs* 20(3), 197
Lichenoid eruption
  (1996): Horiuchi Y+, *J Dermatol* 23, 510
Lupus erythematosus
  (1999): Crowson AN+, *J Cutan Pathol* 26, 95 (subacute cutaneous)
Papuloerythroderma
  (2007): Fujii K, *J Dermatol* 34(10), 736
Photosensitivity
  (2000): Kondo S+, *Dermatology* 201, 71
  (1995): Todd P+, *Clin Exp Dermatol* 20, 146
Pruritus (<1%)
  (1985): Classen M+, *Dtsch Med Wochenschr* (German) 110, 628
Psoriasis
  (1991): Andersen M, *Ugeskr Laeger* (Danish) 153, 132
Purpura
  (1989): Gafter U+, *Gastroenterol* 84, 560
  (1987): Gafter U+, *Ann Intern Med* 106, 477
Pustules
Rash (sic) (1–10%)
  (1988): Haboubi N+, *Br Med J Clin Res Ed* 296, 897
Stevens–Johnson syndrome
  (2001): Lin C-C+, *Gastroenterol Hepatol* 16, 481
Toxic epidermal necrolysis
  (2000): Velez A+, *J Am Acad Dermatol* 42, 305
  (1995): Miralles ES+, *J Am Acad Dermatol* 32, 133

Urticaria
  (1997): Sancho Calabuig A+, *Aten Primaria* 20, 396
  (1989): Grant SM+, *Drugs* 37, 801
  (1984): Khandheria BK, *JAMA* 253, 3252
  (1983): Picardo M+, *Contact Dermatitis* 4, 327
Vasculitis
  (1988): Haboubi N+, *BMJ* 296, 897
Xerosis

Mucosal/ENT
Dysgeusia
  (1985): Classen M+, *Dtsch Med Wochenschr* (German) 110, 628
Rhinitis
  (2006): Martinez AJ+, *J Investig Allergol Clin Immunol* 16(2), 142

Hair
Hair – alopecia
  (1995): Shelley WB+, *Cutis* 55, 148 (observation)

Other
Anaphylactoid reactions/Anaphylaxis
  (2008): Oliva A+, *J Med Case Reports* A, 232
  (2007): Thurot-Guillou C+, *Eur J Dermatol* A(2), 170
  (2006): Demirkan K+, *J Investig Allergol Clin Immunol* 16(3), 203 (2 cases)
  (2003): Kaneko K+, *J Anesth* 17(3), 199
  (1993): Lazaro M+, *Allergy* 48, 385
  (1993): Powell JA+, *Anaesth Intensive Care* 21, 702
Gynecomastia (>1%)
  (1994): Garcia-Rodriguez LA+, *BMJ* 308, 503
  (1984): Bianchi Porro G+, *It J Gastroenterol* (Italian) 16, 56
  (1982): Tosi S+, *Lancet* 2, 160
Headache
Hepatotoxicity
  (2001): Fisher AA+, *Drug Saf* 24(1), 39
Hypersensitivity
  (2006): Oldfield V+, *BioDrugs* 20(3), 197
  (1996): Gonzalo-Garijo MA+, *Allergy* 51, 659
Injection-site burning
Injection-site pain
Myalgia/Myositis/Myopathy/Myotoxicity
Porphyria
  (1988): Bhadoria DP+, *J Assoc Physicians India* 36, 295
  (1988): Pratap D+, *J Assoc Physicians India* 36, 237
  (1988): Tripathi SK, *J Assoc Physicians India* 36, 680
Pseudolymphoma
  (1995): Magro CM+, *J Am Acad Dermatol* 32, 419
  (1988): Kardaun SH+, *Br J Dermatol* 118(4), 545

RANOLAZINE

Trade name: Ranexa (CV Therapeutics)
Indications: Angina
Category: Anti-ischemic; Fatty acid oxidation inhibitor
Half-life: 7 hours
Clinically important, potentially hazardous interactions with: cyclosporine, diltiazem, dofetilide, erythromycin, grapefruit, ketoconazole, quinidine, ritonavir, simvastatin, sotalol, thioridazine, verapamil, ziprasidone

Note: Ranolazine is contraindicated in patients with existing QTc prolongation, and in patients with liver disease

Reactions

Skin
Peripheral edema

Mucosal/ENT
Tinnitus (<2%)
Xerostomia (<2%)

Eyes
Vision blurred (<1%)

Other
Abdominal pain (<2%)
Asthenia
  (2004): Chaitman BR+, *JAMA* 291, 309
Headache (3%)
Hypotension (<1%)
Paresthesias (<1%)
Somnolence
Tremor (<1%)
Vertigo
  (2004): Chaitman BR+, *JAMA* 291, 309

RAPACURONIUM

Trade name: Raplon (Organon)
Indications: To facilitate tracheal intubation
Category: Non-depolarizing neuromuscular blocker
Half-life: ~22 days
**Clinically important, potentially hazardous interactions
with:** aminoglycosides, cyclopropane, enflurane, halothane,
isoflurane, methoxyflurane, piperacillin

Note: This drug has been withdrawn

Reactions

Skin
Diaphoresis (~1%)
Edema
Erythema
  (1999): Abouleish EI+, *Br J Anaesth* 83, 862
Exanthems (>1%)
Peripheral edema (~1%)
Pruritus
Purpura (~1%)
Rash (sic) (~1%)
Urticaria (~1%)

Mucosal/ENT
Sialorrhea (~1%)
  (2000): Meakin GH+, *Anesthesiology* 92, 1002

Other
Injection-site pain (~1%)
Injection-site reactions (sic) (~1%)
  (1999): Onrust SV+, *Drugs* 58, 887
Myalgia/Myositis/Myopathy/Myotoxicity (~1%)
Thrombophlebitis (~1%)

RASAGILINE

Trade names: Agilect; Azilect (Teva)
Indications: Parkinsonism
Category: Monoamine oxidase B inhibitor
Half-life: 0.6–2.0 hours
**Clinically important, potentially hazardous interactions
with:** ciprofloxacin, dextromethorphan, entacapone, fluoxetine
fluvoxamine, MAO inhibitors, meperidine, pethidine,
pseudoephedrine, SSRIs, theophylline

Reactions

Skin
Allergic reactions (sic)
Dermatitis (1%)
Melanoma (<1%)
Rash (sic)
Vesiculobullous eruption (1%)

Mucosal/ENT
Rhinitis (3%)
Xerostomia (3%)

Hair
Hair – alopecia

Eyes
Conjunctivitis (3%)
Visual hallucinations

Other
Abdominal pain (>1%)
Asthenia (2%)
Asthma
Chest pain
Depression (5%)
Fever (3%)
Headache (14%)
Hypotension (5%)
Rhabdomyolysis
Stroke (<1%)
Vertigo (2%)
Weight loss

RASBURICASE

Trade names: Elitek (Sanofi-Aventis); Fasturtec; Uricozyme
Indications: Hyperuricemia (associated with tumor lysis
syndrome)
Category: Antimetabolite; Urate oxidase
Half-life: 18 hours
**Clinically important, potentially hazardous interactions
with:** N/A

Reactions

Skin
Allergic reactions (sic) (<1%)
  (2001): Patte C+, *Semin Hematol* 38(4), 9
Cellulitis (~1%)
Edema (<1%)
  (2001): Pui CH+, *Leukemia* 15(10), 1505 (%)
Rash (sic) (13%)

(2002): Brant JM, *Clin J Oncol Nurs* 6(1), 12
(2002): Goldman S+, *38th Annual Meeting of the Proceedings of the ASCO 21, 399a*
(2001): Easton J+, *Paediatr Drugs* 3(6), 433
(1998): Lascombes F+, *Blood* 92(10 Suppl 1), 237B
(1997): Landman-Parker J+, *Med Pediatr Oncol* 29(5), 339
(1997): Schaison G+, *Proceedings Am Assoc Cancer Res* 38, 223
Urticaria

Mucosal/ENT
Mucositis (2–15%)
(2002): Brant JM, *Clin J Oncol Nurs* 6(1), 12
(2002): Pui C-H+, *38th Annual Meeting of the Proceedings of the ASCO 21, 370a*

Other
Abdominal pain (20%)
Anaphylactoid reactions/Anaphylaxis (<1%)
Chest pain (~1%)
Fever (46%)
Headache
Hot flashes (~1%)
Hypersensitivity (<1%)
(2002): Goldman S+, *38th Annual Meeting of the Proceedings of the ASCO 21, 399a*
(2001): Pui C-H, *Leukemia* 15, 1505 (%)
(2001): Pui C-H+, *J Clin Oncol* 19, 697
(1998): Lascombes F+, *Blood* 92(10 Suppl 1), 237B
Infections (~1%)
Myalgia/Myositis/Myopathy/Myotoxicity (<1%)
(2001): Pui CH+, *Leukemia* 15(10), 1505 (%)
Pain
(2002): Pui C-H+, *38th Annual Meeting of the Proceedings of the ASCO 21, 370a*
Paresthesias (~1%)
Seizures (~1%)
Thrombophlebitis (~1%)

RASPBERRY LEAF

Scientific name: *Rubus idaeus*
Family: Rosaceae
Trade and other common names: Braamboss; Bramble of Mount Ida; Hindberry; Hindebar; Raspis
Category: Food supplement
Purported indications and other uses: Astringent, stimulant, gargle for sore throat, mouth ulcers, bleeding gums, diarrhea, morning sickness, to shorten labor, menstrual complaints, respiratory tract infections, fever, dysmenorrhea, menorrhagia, rash
Half-life: N/A
Clinically important, potentially hazardous interactions with: atropine, codeine, theophylline

Reactions

Skin
Allergic reactions (sic)

REBOXETINE

Trade names: Davedax; Edronax (Pharmacia & Upjohn); Integrex; Irenor; Norebox; Prolift; Solvex; Vestra
Indications: Clinical depression, Panic Disorder
Category: Antidepressant; Noradrenaline reuptake inhibitor
Half-life: 13 hours
Clinically important, potentially hazardous interactions with: bosentan, ketoconazole, MAO inhibitors, papaverine

Reactions

Skin
Diaphoresis (1.1%)
(2006): Taner E+, *Adv Ther* 23(6), 974
(2005): Eker SS+, *Turk Psikiyatri Derg* 16(3), 153
(2004): Rubio G+, *J Affect Disord* 81(1), 67
(2003): Carvalhal AS+, *J Clin Psychiatry* 64(4), 421
(2003): Fava M+, *J Clin Psychopharmacol* 23(4), 365
(2000): Kasper S+, *Expert Opin Pharmacother* 1(4), 771
(2000): Scates AC+, *Ann Pharmacother* 34(11), 1302
(2000): Versiani M+, *J Clin Psychopharmacol* 20(1), 28
Rash (sic)
Shivering
(2003): Carvalhal AS+, *J Clin Psychiatry* 64(4), 421

Mucosal/ENT
Xerostomia
(2006): Langworth S+, *J Clin Psychopharmacol* 26(2), 121
(2006): Taner E+, *Adv Ther* 23(6), 974
(2005): Eker SS+, *Turk Psikiyatri Derg* 16(3), 153
(2004): Rubio G+, *J Affect Disord* 81(1), 67
(2003): Fava M+, *J Clin Psychopharmacol* 23(4), 365
(2002): Versiani M+, *J Clin Psychiatry* 63(1), 31
(2000): Aguglia E, *Int J Geriatr Psychiatry* 15(9), 784
(2000): Kasper S+, *Expert Opin Pharmacother* 1(4), 771
(2000): Scates AC+, *Ann Pharmacother* 34(11), 1302
(2000): Versiani M+, *J Clin Psychopharmacol* 20(1), 28

Eyes
Vision blurred
(2000): Versiani M+, *J Clin Psychopharmacol* 20(1), 28

Other
Headache
(2006): Taner E+, *Adv Ther* 23(6), 974
(2005): Eker SS+, *Turk Psikiyatri Derg* 16(3), 153
(2003): Fava M+, *J Clin Psychopharmacol* 23(4), 365
(2000): Aguglia E, *Int J Geriatr Psychiatry* 15(9), 784
Hypertension
Inappropriate secretion of antidiuretic hormone (SIADH)
(2003): Abdelrahman N+, *Eur J Clin Pharmacol* 59(2), 177
Insomnia (1.3%)
(2003): Carvalhal AS+, *J Clin Psychiatry* 64(4), 421
(2003): Fava M+, *J Clin Psychopharmacol* 23(4), 365
(2002): Stahl SM+, *J Clin Psychopharmacol* 22(4), 388
(2002): Versiani M+, *J Clin Psychiatry* 63(1), 31
(2000): Aguglia E, *Int J Geriatr Psychiatry* 15(9), 784
(2000): Scates AC+, *Ann Pharmacother* 34(11), 1302
(2000): Versiani M+, *J Clin Psychopharmacol* 20(1), 28
Mania
(2001): Vieta E+, *J Clin Psychiatry* 62(8), 655
Paresthesias (0.8%)
Seizures
Somnolence
(2005): Eker SS+, *Turk Psikiyatri Derg* 16(3), 153
(2005): Ratner S+, *J Am Acad Child Adolesc Psychiatry* 44(5), 428
Vertigo (0.8%)
Weight loss
(2005): Lu TY+, *Br J Clin Pharmacol* 60(2), 218

RED CLOVER

Scientific name: *Trifolium pratense*
Family: Leguminosae
Trade and other common names: Coumestrol; Cow Clover; Cowgrass; Meadow Clover; Menoflavon (Pascoe); Pavine Clover; Promensil (Novogen); Purple Clover; Three-Leaved Grass
Category: Phytoestrogen
Purported indications and other uses: Menopausal symptoms, hot flashes, muscle spasms, hypercholesterolemia, breast pain, osteoporosis, diuretic, expectorant, mild antispasmodic, sedative, blood purifier, bladder infections, liver disorders. Ointment for acne, eczema, psoriasis and other rashes
Half-life: N/A
Clinically important, potentially hazardous interactions with: conjugated estrogens, heparin, ticlopidine, warfarin

Reactions

None

RED RICE YEAST

Scientific name: *Monascus purpureus*
Family: Monascaceae
Trade and other common names: Cholestin (Pharmanex); Hong Qu; Red Koji; Xuezhikang; Zhi Tai
Category: HMG-CoA reductase inhibitor
Purported indications and other uses: Hypercholesterolemia, indigestion, diarrhea, improved circulation. In foodstuff
Half-life: N/A
Clinically important, potentially hazardous interactions with: atorvastatin, cerivastatin, cyclosporine, fluvastatin, **grapefruit juice**, levothyroxine, lovastatin, pravastatin, simvastatin, **St John's wort**

Note: Red yeast rice is the product of fermentation with *Monascus purpureus* yeast. Red yeast that is not fermented correctly may contain the nephrotoxin, citrinin.

Reactions

Other
Abdominal pain
Anaphylactoid reactions/Anaphylaxis
  (1999): Wigger-Alberti W+, *Allergy* 54(12), 1330
Headache
Myalgia/Myositis/Myopathy/Myotoxicity
  (2003): Smith DJ+, *South Med J* 96(12), 1265
Rhabdomyolysis
  (2002): Prasad GV+, *Transplantation* 74(8), 1200
Vertigo

REGADENOSON

Trade name: Lexiscan (Baxter)
Indications: Radionuclide myocardial perfusion imaging
Category: Adenosine A2A receptor agonist; Diagnostic aid
Half-life: Immediate: 30 minutes; Terminal: 2 hours

Reactions

Mucosal/ENT
Dysgeusia (5%)

Other
Abdominal pain (5%)
Fever (5%)
Headache
  (2008): Leaker BR+, *J Nucl Cardiol* 15(3), 329 (45%)
Hypotension (7%)
Vertigo (8%)
  (2008): Leaker BR+, *J Nucl Cardiol* 15(3), 329 (53%)

REPAGLINIDE

Trade name: Prandin (Novo Nordisk)
Indications: Non-insulin dependent diabetes type II
Category: Meglitinide
Half-life: 1 hour
Clinically important, potentially hazardous interactions with: clarithromycin, erythromycin, gemfibrozil, **grapefruit juice**

Reactions

Skin
Allergic reactions (sic) (2%)

Other
Anaphylactoid reactions/Anaphylaxis (<1%)
Headache
  (2004): Plosker GL+, *Pharmacoeconomics* 22(6), 389
Hepatotoxicity
  (2005): Lopez-Garcia F+, *Diabetes Care* 28(3), 752
  (2004): Nan DN+, *Ann Intern Med* 141(10), 823
Paresthesias (3%)
Upper respiratory infection
  (2004): Plosker GL+, *Pharmacoeconomics* 22(6), 389

RESERPINE

Trade names: Anserpin; Inerpin; Novo-Reserpine; Resa; Reserfia; Sedaraupin; Ser-Ap-Es (Novartis); Serpalan; Serpasil (Novartis); Serpasol; Serpatabs; Tionsera
Indications: Hypertension
Category: Rauwolfia alkaloid
Half-life: 50–100 hours
Clinically important, potentially hazardous interactions with: metipranolol, tetrabenazine

Note: Ser-Ap-Es is reserpine, hydralazine and hydrochlorothiazide

Reactions

Skin
Bullous dermatitis
  (1994): Watanabe S+, *Reg Anesth* 19, 59 (following intravenous block)
Edema
Exanthems
Lupus erythematosus (exacerbation)
Peripheral edema (1–10%)

Pruritus
Purpura
Rash (sic) (<1%)
Toxic epidermal necrolysis
Urticaria

Mucosal/ENT
Sialorrhea
Xerostomia (>10%)

Other
Depression
  (1996): Webster J+, *J Cardiovasc Pharmacol* 27 Suppl 3, S49
Gynecomastia
Headache

RESVERATROL

Scientific names: *3,4',5-trihydroxystilbene; trans-resveratrol-3-O-glucuronide; trans-resveratrol-3-sulfate*
Family: N/A
Trade and other common names: Kojo-kon; Protykin Resveratrol (Natrol); Resveratrol Antioxidant Protection (Source Naturals)
Category: Immunomodulator; Phytoestrogen
Purported indications and other uses: Cancers, dermal wound healing, atherosclerosis, herpes simplex, cholesterol-lowering, heart disease, skin cancers
Half-life: N/A
Clinically important, potentially hazardous interactions with: aspirin, warfarin

Reactions

Skin
Dermatitis
  (2003): Gallo R+, *Contact Dermatitis* 48(3), 176

RETAPAMULIN

Trade name: Altabax (GSK)
Indications: Impetigo, Bacterial skin infections
Category: Pleuromutilin antibacterial
Half-life: N/A
Clinically important, potentially hazardous interactions with: N/A

Reactions

Skin
Dermatitis (contact) (<1%)
Eczema (in children) (1%)
Pruritus (in children) (1.5%)

Mucosal/ENT
Nasopharyngitis (1.2%)

Other
Application-site erythema (<1%)
Application-site irritation (1.6%)
Application-site pain (<1%)
Application-site pruritus (in children) (1.9%)
Fever (1.2%)
Headache (1.2%)

RETEPLASE

Synonyms: recombinant plasminogen activator; r-PA
Trade name: Retavase (Centocor)
Indications: Acute myocardial infarction
Category: Fibrinolytic
Half-life: 13–16 minutes
Clinically important, potentially hazardous interactions with: abciximab, aspirin, bivalirudin, dipyridamole, piperacillin, salicylates

Reactions

Skin
Allergic reactions (sic) (<1%)
Purpura

Other
Anaphylactoid reactions/Anaphylaxis (<1%)
Headache
Injection-site bleeding (1–10%)

RIBAVIRIN

Synonyms: RTCA; tribavirin
Trade names: Copegus; Rebetol (Schering); Rebetron (Schering); Viramid; Virazid; Virazole (Valeant)
Indications: Respiratory syncytial viral infections
Category: Antiviral, nucleoside analog
Half-life: 24 hours
Clinically important, potentially hazardous interactions with: zidovudine

Note: Rebetron is interferon and ribavirin

Reactions

Skin
Eczema
  (2004): Vazquez-Lopez F+, *Br J Dermatol* 150(5), 1046 (with interferon-alfa)
  (2002): Dereure O+, *Br J Dermatol* 147(6), 1142
Erythema multiforme
Exanthems
  (2003): Okai T+, *J Clin Gastroenterol* 36(3), 283
  (2002): Farady KK, Austin, TX (from Internet) (observation)
  (1990): Janai HK+, *Pediatr Infect Dis J* 9, 209 (0.5%)
Fixed eruption
  (2003): Sidhu-Malik NK+, *J Drugs Dermatol* 2(5), 570
Herpes simplex (activation)
Lichenoid eruption
  (2005): Armour K+, *Australas J Dermatol* 46(1), 21 (with PEG-interferon alfa-2a)
Nummular eczema
  (2005): Shen Y+, *Arch Dermatol* 141(1), 102 (with PEG-interferon)
  (2004): Moore MM+, *Arch Dermatol* 140(2), 215
Photosensitivity
  (2002): Castillo R+, *World Congress Dermatol* Poster, 0091
  (2002): Dereure O+, *Br J Dermatol* 147(6), 1142
  (1999): Stryjek-Kaminska D+, *Am J Gastroenterol* 94, 1686
Pigmentation
  (2003): Willems M+, *Br J Dermatol* 149(2), 390
Pruritus (>10%)

(2006): Lee H+, *Korean J Hepatol* 12(1), 31 (with peg-interferon)

(1999): Stryjek-Kaminska D+, *Am J Gastroenterol* 94, 1686

Psoriasis

(2005): Kartal ED+, *Chemotherapy* 51(2-3), 167 (with Peg-Interferon)

Rash (sic) (<10%)

(2001): Karim A+, *Am J Med Sci* 322(4), 233

Rosacea fulminans

(2006): Bettoli V+, *Acta Derm Venereol* 86(3), 258 (with peg-interferon)

(2003): Jensen SL+, *J Drugs Dermatol* 2(5), 554 (with PEG-interferon alfa-2B)

Sarcoidosis

(2007): Perez-Gala S+, *J Eur Acad Dermatol Venereol* 21(3), 393 (with peg-interferon)

(2006): Perera GK+, *Clin Exp Dermatol* 31(3), 387 (with interferon-alpha)

(2006): Sanchez-Ruano JJ+, *Gastroenterol Hepatol* 29(3), 150 (with interferon alfa)

(2005): Bolukbas C+, *Acta Gastroenterol Belg* 68(4), 432 (with interferon alfa)

(2005): Hurst EA+, *Arch Dermatol* 141(7), 865 (with peg-interferon)

(2005): Ramos-Casals M+, *Medicine (Baltimore)* 84(2), 69 (60%) (with interferon alfa)

(2004): Alfageme Michavila I+, *Arch Bronconeumol* 40(1), 45 (with PEG-interferon)

(2004): Blank E, *Schoch Letter* 52(4), 15 (with PEG-interferon)

(2004): Rogers CJ+, *J Am Acad Dermatol* 50(4), 649 (with Interferon alfa)

(2004): Salvio A+, *Ann Ital Med Sci* 19(1), 58 (with Interferon alfa)

(2003): Tahan V+, *Dig Dis Sci* 48(1), 169

(2002): Cogrel O+, *Br J Dermatol* 146(2), 320

(2002): Gitlin N, *Eur J Gastroenterol Hepatol* 14(8), 883 (with interferon)

(2002): Wendling J+, *Arch Dermatol* 138, 546 (2 cases)

(2000): Savoye G+, *Gastroenterol Clin Biol* 24(6-7), 679 (with Interferon alfa)

Transient acantholytic dermatosis (Grover's disease)

(2000): Antunes I+, *Br J Dermatol* 142, 1257

Urticaria

(1999): Stryjek-Kaminska D+, *Am J Gastroenterol* 94, 1686

Vitiligo

(2006): Tinio P+, *Skinmed* 5(1), 50 (with peg-interferon)

(2006): Tomasiewicz K+, *Adv Ther* 23(1), 139 (with peg-interferon)

Mucosal/ENT

Dysgeusia (1–10%)

Oral lichen planus

(2005): Nagao Y+, *Int J Mol Med* 15(2), 237 (with interferon)

Tinnitus

(2004): Formann E+, *Am J Gastroenterol* 99(5), 873

Tongue black

(2006): Gurguta C+, *Am J Gastroenterol* 101(1), 197 (with Peg-interferon)

Hair

Hair – alopecia (>10%)

(2006): Demirturk N+, *Eur J Dermatol* 16(5), 579 (rare) (with peg-interferon)

(2004): Bagheri H+, *Pharmacotherapy* 24(11), 1546 (with PEG-interferon alfa-2b)

(2001): Zucker DM+, *Gastroenterol Nurs* 24(4), 192

Hair – alopecia areata

(2006): Demirturk N+, *Eur J Dermatol* 16(5), 579 (with peg-interferon)

Hair – hypertrichosis

(2002): Misery L, *J Interferon Cytokine Res* 22(8), 881 (with interferon)

Eyes

Blepharospasm

(2005): Girard C+, *Br J Dermatol* 152(1), 182 (with interferon alfa)

Ocular toxicity

(2006): Avila MP+, *Arq Bras Oftalmol* 69(2), 255 (with peg-interferon)

Retinopathy

(2006): Andrade RJ+, *Antivir Ther* 11(4), 491 (15%) (with peg-interferon)

(2006): Avila MP+, *Arq Bras Oftalmol* 69(2), 255 (with peg-interferon)

(2006): Okuse C+, *World J Gastroenterol* 12(23), 3756 (5 cases) (with peg-interferon)

Vision blurred

(2004): Bagheri H+, *Pharmacotherapy* 24(11), 1546 (with PEG-interferon alfa-2b)

Other

Asthenia

(2005): Mukherjee S+, *J Gastroenterol Hepatol* 20(2), 198 (with PEG-interferon alfa-2b)

Cough

(2001): Karim A+, *Am J Med Sci* 322(4), 233

Death

(2006): Helbling B+, *J Viral Hepat* 13(11), 762 (2 cases) (with peg-interferon)

Depression

(2005): Raison CL+, *J Clin Psychiatry* 66(1), 41 (39%) (with PEG-interferon alfa)

(2004): Bagheri H+, *Pharmacotherapy* 24(11), 1546 (with PEG-interferon alfa-2b)

(2002): Fried MW+, *N Engl J Med* 347(13), 975 (with PEG-interferon)

(2002): Vega Palomares R+, *Gastroenterol Hepatol* 25(8), 483 (with interferon)

(2001): Karim A+, *Am J Med Sci* 322(4), 233

Fever

(2002): Wirth S+, *Hepatology* 36(5), 1280 (with interferon)

Headache

Hepatotoxicity

(2006): Chaves J+, *Clin Infect Dis* 42(8), e72

Injection-site reactions

(2004): Bagheri H+, *Pharmacotherapy* 24(11), 1546 (with PEG-interferon alfa-2b)

Myalgia/Myositis/Myopathy/Myotoxicity (>10%)

Nephrotoxicity

(2006): Alves Couto C+, *Liver Int* 26(10), 1294 (with peg-interferon)

(2002): Willson RA, *J Clin Gastroenterol* 35(1), 89 (with interferon alfa)

Vogt–Koyanagi–Harada disease

(2003): Sylvestre DL+, *J Viral Hepat* 10(6), 467

RIBOFLAVIN

Synonyms: Lactoflavin; Vitamin B$_2$; Vitamin G
Trade name: Riobin
Indications: Riboflavin deficiency
Category: Vitamin
Half-life: 66–84 minutes

Reactions

Skin

Acne
Allergic reactions (sic)
Angioedema
Ichthyosis
  (1985): Spirov G+, *Dermatol Venereol* (Sofia) 24, 50
Urticaria

Other

Anaphylactoid reactions/Anaphylaxis
  (2001): Ou LS+, *Ann Allergy Asthma Immunol* 87(5), 430

RIFABUTIN

Trade name: Mycobutin (Pfizer)
Indications: Prevention of disseminated *Mycobacterium avium* infection
Category: Antibiotic, rifamycin
Half-life: 45 hours
Clinically important, potentially hazardous interactions with: amiodarone, anisindione, anticoagulants, azithromycin, corticosteroids, cyclosporine, dapsone, delavirdine, dicumarol, fosamprenavir, lapatinib, midazolam, oral contraceptives, ritonavir, solifenacin, tacrolimus, temsirolimus, voriconazole

Reactions

Skin

Lupus erythematosus
  (1997): Berning SE+, *Lancet* 349, 1521
Pigmentation
  (1995): Smith JF+, *Clin Infect Dis* 21, 1515
  (1990): Siegal FP+, *AIDS* 4(5), 433
Rash (sic) (11%)
Urticaria

Mucosal/ENT

Ageusia
  (1993): Morris JT+, *Ann Intern Med* 119, 171
Aphthous stomatitis
  (1990): Siegal FP+, *AIDS* 4(5), 433
Dysgeusia (3%)

Eyes

Corneal opacity
  (2002): Ponjavic V+, *Acta Ophthalmol Scand* 80(5), 553
Macular edema
  (2002): Vaudaux JD+, *J Antimicrob Chemother* 49(2), 421
Ocular toxicity
  (2006): Boyer SP+, *Optometry* 77(10), 494
  (1997): Le Saux N+, *Pediatr Infect Dis J* 16(7), 716
Uveitis
  (2005): Cano Parra J+, *Arch Soc Esp Oftalmol* 80(3), 137
  (2005): Olesen HH+, *Pediatr Infect Dis J* 24(11), 1023
  (2005): Skolik S+, *Ocul Immunol Inflamm* 13(6), 483
  (2004): Mulliez P+, *Rev Mal Respir* 21(5 Pt 1), 1004
  (2001): Bhagat N+, *Ophthalmology* 108(4), 750
  (2000): Khan MA+, *Eye* 14 (Pt 3A), 344
  (1999): Schaller UC+, *Ophthalmologe* 96(4), 267
  (1998): Johnson TM+, *J Pediatr Ophthalmol Strabismus* 35(2), 119
  (1998): Moorthy RS+, *Surv Ophthalmol* 42(6), 557
  (1998): Ramon PM+, *Rev Mal Respir* 15(2), 204
  (1997): Arevalo JF+, *Ophthalmic Surg Lasers* 28(4), 321
  (1997): Saran BR, *Ann Pharmacother* 31(11), 1405

  (1996): Diemer PR+, *Klin Monatsbl Augenheilkd* 209(1), 40
  (1996): Nichols CW, *Clin Infect Dis* 22 Suppl 1, S43
  (1996): Petrowski JT, *J Am Optom Assoc* 67(11), 693
  (1996): Schimkat M+, *Ger J Ophthalmol* 5(4), 195
  (1996): Zenone T+, *Scand J Infect Dis* 28(3), 325
  (1995): Chevalley GF+, *Klin Monatsbl Augenheilkd* 206(5), 388
  (1995): Dunn AM+, *Pediatr Infect Dis J* 14(3), 246
  (1995): Frau E+, *J Fr Ophtalmol* 18(6–7), 435
  (1995): Gioulekas J+, *Aust N Z J Ophthalmol* 23(4), 319
  (1995): Rifai A+, *Arch Ophthalmol* 113(6), 707
  (1995): Tseng AL+, *Ann Pharmacother* 29(11), 1149
  (1994): *MMWR Morb Mortal Wkly Rep* 43(35), 658
  (1994): Havlir D+, *Ann Intern Med 1994 Oct 1* 121(7), 510
  (1994): Jacobs DS+, *Am J Ophthalmol* 118(6), 716
  (1994): Saran BR+, *Arch Ophthalmol* 112(9), 1159
  (1990): Siegal FP+, *AIDS* 4(5), 433
Visual disturbances
  (2002): Ponjavic V+, *Acta Ophthalmol Scand* 80(5), 553
  (1996): Chaknis MJ+, *Am J Ophthalmol* 122(4), 580

Other

Headache
Inappropriate secretion of antidiuretic hormone (SIADH)
  (2001): Chitre MM+, *Pharmacotherapy* 21(4), 493
Myalgia/Myositis/Myopathy/Myotoxicity (2%)
Paresthesias (<1%)

RIFAMPIN

Synonym: rifampicin
Trade names: Abrifam; Corifam; Ramicin; Rifadin (Sanofi-Aventis); Rifaldin; Rifamed; Rimactane (Novartis); Rimpin; Rimycin; Rofact
Indications: Tuberculosis
Category: Antibiotic, rifamycin
Half-life: 3–5 hours
Clinically important, potentially hazardous interactions with: amiodarone, amprenavir, anisindione, antacids, anticoagulants, aprepitant, atazanavir, atovaquone, beclomethasone, buprenorphine, corticosteroids, cortisone, cyclosporine, dapsone, darunavir, delavirdine, dexamethasone, dicumarol, digoxin, eszopiclone, flunisolide, fosamprenavir, halothane, imatinib, isoniazid, itraconazole, ketoconazole, lapatinib, lorcainide, methylprednisolone, midazolam, nelfinavir, nifedipine, oral contraceptives, phenylbutazone, prednisone, protease inhibitors, pyrazinamide, ramelteon, ritonavir, saquinavir, solifenacin, sunitinib, tacrolimus, telithromycin, temsirolimus, tipranavir, triamcinolone, triazolam, voriconazole, warfarin, zaleplon

Reactions

Skin

Acne
  (1990): Mimouni A+, *Drug Intell Clin Pharm* 24, 947
  (1985): Holdiness MR, *Int J Dermatol* 24, 280
Acute generalized exanthematous pustulosis
  (2006): Azad A+, *Intern Med J* 36(9), 619
Allergic reactions (sic)
Angioedema
  (1989): Holdiness MR, *Med Toxicol Adv Drug Exp* 4, 444 (72%)
Bullous dermatitis (<1%)
Burning
  (2003): Dogra S+, *Acta Derm Venereol* 83(1), 56
Dermatitis

(1991): Guerra L+, *Contact Dermatitis* 25, 328
(1986): Holdiness MR, *Contact Dermatitis* 15, 282
(1986): Milpied B+, *Contact Dermatitis* 14, 252
Dermatomyositis
(1987): Camus JP+, *Ann Med Interne* (Paris) 138(7), 524
Diaphoresis (1–10%)
Erythema multiforme (<1%)
(1990): Mimouni A+, *Drug Intell Clin Pharm* 24, 947
(1988): Hira SK+, *J Am Acad Dermatol* 19, 451 (in AIDS patients)
Exanthems (1–5%)
(1998): Zimmerli W+, *JAMA* 279, 1537
(1989): Wurtz RM+, *Lancet* 1, 955 (in AIDS patients)
(1985): Holdiness MR, *Int J Dermatol* 24, 280
Exfoliative dermatitis
(1987): Goldin HM+, *Ann Intern Med* 107, 789
Facial edema
Fixed eruption
(2001): Goel A+, *Indian J Lepr* 73(2), 159 (bullous, necrotizing)
(2000): Jaiswal AK+, *Lepr Rev* 71, 217
(1998): John SS, *Lepr Rev* 69, 397
(1993): Pavithran K, *Indian J Lepr* 65, 339
(1990): Mimouni A+, *Drug Intell Clin Pharm* 24, 947
(1985): Naik RPC+, *Indian J Lepr* 57, 648
Linear IgA dermatosis
(2003): Avci O+, *J Am Acad Dermatol* 48(2), 299 (passim)
(2002): Cohen LM+, *J Am Acad Dermatol* 46, S32 (passim)
(1994): Kuechle MK+, *J Am Acad Dermatol* 30, 187
Lupus erythematosus
(2001): Patel GK+, *Clin Exp Dermatol* 26(3), 260
Pemphigus
(2004): Goldberg I+, *Skinmed* 3(5), 294
(1995): Hoss DM+, *Arch Dermatol* 131, 647
(1993): Tsankov NK+, *Int J Dermatol* 32, 401 (passim)
(1987): Honeybourne D+, *Br J Clin Pract* 41, 937
(1986): Miyagawa S+, *Br J Dermatol* 114, 729 (exacerbation)
(1984): Lee CW+, *Br J Dermatol* 111, 619 (foliaceus)
(1982): Ruocco V+, *Arch Dermatol Res* 274, 123
Pemphigus vulgaris
(2004): Goldberg I+, *Skinmed* 3(5), 294
Pruritus (1–62%)
(1995): Hoss DM+, *Arch Dermatol* 131, 647
(1995): Walker-Renard P, *Ann Pharmacother* 29, 267
(1993): Tsankov NK+, *Int J Dermatol* 32, 401 (passim)
(1989): Holdiness MR, *Med Toxicol Adv Drug Exp* 4, 444 (62%)
(1987): Goldin HM+, *Ann Intern Med* 107, 789
Purpura (<1%)
(1980): Miescher PA+, *Clin Haematol* 9, 505
Rash (sic) (1–5%)
(2000): Gordin F+, *JAMA* 283, 1445
(1995): Chaisson RE, *Infections in Medicine* 12, 48
Red man syndrome
(1995): Dayavathi+, *J Assoc Physicians India* 43, 724
(1992): Gupta M+, *Indian Pediatr* 29, 1315
(1989): Holdiness MR, *Med Toxicol Adv Drug Exp* 4, 444
(1988): Gross DJ+, *Cutis* 42, 175 (red/orange person syndrome)
(1986): Bolan G+, *Pediatrics* 77, 633
(1980): Meisel S+, *Ann Intern Med* 92, 262
Side effects (sic) (5%)
(1985): Holdiness MR, *Int J Dermatol* 24, 280 (5%)
Stevens–Johnson syndrome
(2005): Pitche P+, *Med Trop* (Mars) 65(4), 359 (8 cases) (with isoniazid)
(1994): Marfatia YS, *Arch Dermatol* 130, 1074 (passim)
(1993): Tsankov NK+, *Int J Dermatol* 32, 401 (passim)
(1988): Hira SK+, *J Am Acad Dermatol* 19, 451 (in AIDS patients)
Toxic epidermal necrolysis
(2005): Pitche P+, *Med Trop* (Mars) 65(4), 359 (8 cases) (with isoniazid)
(1996): Blum L+, *J Am Acad Dermatol* 34, 1088

(1994): Marfatia YS, *Arch Dermatol* 130, 1074 (passim)
(1990): Prazuck T+, *Scand J Infect Dis* 22, 629
(1987): Guillaume JC+, *Arch Dermatol* 123, 1166
(1987): Okano M+, *J Am Acad Dermatol* 17, 303
Urticaria
(1997): Sharma VK+, *Lepr Rev* 68, 331
(1987): Grob JJ+, *Contact Dermatitis* 16(5), 284
(1987): Gupta CM+, *Lepr Rev* 58, 308
(1985): Holdiness MR, *Int J Dermatol* 24, 280
Vasculitis
(1995): Hoss DM+, *Arch Dermatol* 131, 647
(1990): Chan CH+, *Tubercle* 71, 297
(1989): Iredale JP+, *Chest* 96, 215

Mucosal/ENT
Glossodynia
Mucosal bleeding
Oral mucosal eruption
Stomatitis (<1%)

Hair
Hair – alopecia areata
(2001): McMillen R+, *J Am Acad Dermatol* 44(1), 142 (in 2 sisters)

Other
Anaphylactoid reactions/Anaphylaxis
(1999): Garcia F+, *Allergy* 54, 527 (to topical)
(1999): Magnan A+, *J Allergy Clin Immunol* 103, 954
(1998): Erel F+, *Ann Allergy Asthma Immunol* 81, 257
(1995): Cardot E+, *J Allergy Clin Immunol* 95, 1
(1989): Piazza I, *Allergologia* 12, 96 (suppl)
(1989): Wurtz RM+, *Lancet* 1, 955 (in AIDS patients)
Death
(2003): Castro KG+, *Chest* 123(3), 967 (with pyrazinamide)
(2002): Medinger A, *Chest* 121(5), 1710 (with pyrazinamide)
(2002): No authors, *JAMA* 288(23), 2967 (with pyrazinamide)
(2002): No authors, *MMWR Morb Mortal* 51(44), 998 (with pyrazinamide)
(2001): No authors, *Can Commun Dis Rep* 27(13), 114 (with pyrazinamide)
(2001): No authors, *JAMA* 286(12), 1445 (with pyrazinamide)
(2001): No authors, *MMWR Morb Mortal Wkly Rep* 50(34), 733 (with pyrazinamide)
Headache
Hepatotoxicity
(2006): Cook PP+, *Clin Infect Dis* 43(3), 271 (6%) (with pyrazinamide)
(1999): Gallieni M+, *Int J Artif Organs* 22(7), 477
Hypersensitivity
(2006): Buergin S+, *Int Arch Allergy Immunol* 140(1), 20
Injection-site erythema
(1988): Fan-Havard P+, *Clin Pharm* 7, 616
Myalgia/Myositis/Myopathy/Myotoxicity
Nephrotoxicity
(2006): Jover-Saenz A+, *Enferm Infecc Microbiol Clin* 24(1), 64
(1999): Gallieni M+, *Int J Artif Organs* 22(7), 477
Porphyria
(1985): Holdiness MR, *Int J Dermatol* 24, 280
(1982): Igual JP+, *Presse Med* (French) 11, 2846
Porphyria cutanea tarda
(1980): Millar JW, *Br J Dis Chest* 74, 405
Serum sickness
(1994): Parra FM+, *Ann Allergy* 73, 123
Vertigo
(2005): Danby FW, Manchester, NH (from Internet) (observation)
(2005): Verma S, Baroda, India (from Internet) (observation)

RIFAPENTINE

Trade name: Priftin (Sanofi-Aventis)
Indications: Tuberculosis
Category: Antibiotic, rifamycin
Half-life: 14–17 hours
Clinically important, potentially hazardous interactions with: amiodarone, anisindione, anticoagulants, corticosteroids, cyclosporine, dicumarol, indinavir, ritonavir, solifenacin, tacrolimus, warfarin

Reactions

Skin
Acne (1–10%)
Peripheral edema (<1%)
Pigmentation (<1%)
Pruritus (1–10%)
Purpura (<1%)
Rash (sic) (1–10%)
Urticaria (<1%)

Other
Headache

RIFAXIMIN

Trade name: Xifaxan (Salix)
Indications: Travelers' diarrhea (caused by non-invasive strains of *E. coli*)
Category: Antibiotic, rifamycin
Half-life: ~5 hours
Clinically important, potentially hazardous interactions with: None

Reactions

Skin
Allergic reactions
Angioedema
Clammy skin (<2%)
Dermatitis
Diaphoresis (<2%)
Pruritus
Rash (sic)
Sunburn
Urticaria
  (2002): Tursi A+, *Dig Liver Dis* 34(7), 510

Mucosal/ENT
Ageusia (<2%)
Cheilitis (0.3%)
Dysgeusia (<2%)
Gingival lesions (<2%)
Tinnitus (<2%)

Other
Abdominal pain (7.2%)
  (2005): Paik YH+, *Yonsei Med J* 46(3), 399
Asthenia (<2%)
Chest pain (<2%)
Fever
Headache (9.7%)
Hot flashes (<2%)

Hypersensitivity
Myalgia/Myositis/Myopathy/Myotoxicity (<2%)
Pain (<2%)
Vertigo

RILONACEPT

Trade name: Arcalyst (Regeneron)
Indications: Cryopyrin-Associated Periodic Syndromes (CAPS) including Familial cold autoinflammatory syndrome (FCAS), Muckle-Wells syndrome (MWS)
Category: Fusion protein; Interleukin-1 inhibitor
Clinically important, potentially hazardous interactions with: anti-tnf agents, **live vaccines**, natalizumab

Note: CAPS are characterized by life-long, recurrent symptoms of rash, fever/chills, joint pain, eye redness/pain, and fatigue. Intermittent, disruptive exacerbations or flares can be triggered at any time by exposure to cooling temperatures, stress, exercise, or other unknown stimuli.

Reactions

Mucosal/ENT
Sinusitis (9%)

Other
Chills
Cough (9%)
Fever
Headache
Injection-site reactions (48%)
Upper respiratory infection (26%)

RILUZOLE

Trade name: Rilutek (Sanofi-Aventis)
Indications: Amyotrophic lateral sclerosis (ALS)
Category: Neuromuscular blocker (in ALS)
Half-life: N/A

Reactions

Skin
Allergic granulomatous angiitis (Churg–Strauss syndrome)
Cellulitis
Eczema (1.6%)
Edema
Exfoliative dermatitis
Facial edema
Peripheral edema (3%)
Petechiae
Photosensitivity
Pruritus
Purpura

Mucosal/ENT
Dysgeusia
Dysphagia
  (2001): Debove C+, *Amyotroph Lateral Scler Other Motor Neuron Disord* 2(3), 153
Gingival bleeding
Glossitis

Oral candidiasis (0.6%)
Stomatitis (1%)
Tongue pigmentation
Vulvovaginal candidiasis
Xerostomia (3.5%)

Hair
Hair – alopecia (1%)

Other
Abdominal pain (2%)
  (2004): Siniscalchi A, *Clin Ter* 155(1), 25
  (2000): Pongratz D+, *J Neurol Sci* 180(1), 82 (2.5%)
Asthenia (5%)
  (2004): Siniscalchi A, *Clin Ter* 155(1), 25
  (2002): Lacomblez L+, *Therapie* 57(1), 65
  (2002): Mohammadi B+, *Muscle Nerve* 26(4), 539
  (2000): Pongratz D+, *J Neurol Sci* 180(1), 82 (5.8%)
  (2000): Roch-Torreilles I+, *Therapie* 55(2), 303
  (1997): Wagner ML+, *Ann Pharmacother* 31(6), 738
  (1996): Bryson HM+, *Drugs* 52(4), 549
  (1996): Clark W+, *J Clin Pharm Ther* 21(6), 373
  (1996): Lacomblez L+, *Lancet* 347(9013), 1425
  (1996): Lacomblez L+, *Neurology* 47(6), S242
  (1994): Bensimon G+, *N Engl J Med* 330(9), 585
Candidiasis
Chills
Headache
  (1999): Le Liboux+, *J Clin Pharmacol* 39(5), 480
Hypersensitivity
  (2006): Sorenson EJ, *Neurology* 67(12), 2260
Injection-site reactions (sic)
Paresthesias (circumoral)
  (2004): Siniscalchi A, *Clin Ter* 155(1), 25
  (1997): Wagner ML+, *Ann Pharmacother* 31(6), 738
  (1996): Bryson HM+, *Drugs* 52(4), 549
Phlebitis (1%)
Vertigo
  (2004): Siniscalchi A, *Clin Ter* 155(1), 25
  (2000): North WA+, *Ann Pharmacother* 34(3), 322
  (1997): Wagner ML+, *Ann Pharmacother* 31(6), 738
  (1996): Bryson HM+, *Drugs* 52(4), 549
  (1996): Lacomblez L+, *Lancet* 347(9013), 1425

RIMANTADINE

Trade names: Flumadine (Forest); Ruflual
Indications: Various infections caused by influenza virus
Category: Adamantane; Antiviral
Half-life: 25–30 hours

Reactions

Skin
Edema (pedal) (1–10%)
Rash (sic) (1%)
  (1989): Hayden FG+, *N Engl J Med* 321, 1696 (1%)

Mucosal/ENT
Ageusia (<0.3%)
Dysgeusia
Parosmia (<0.3%)
Stomatitis
Xerostomia (1.6%)

Other
Headache

(1999): Fong TL+, *Am J Gastroenterol* 94(4), 990
Vertigo
  (1999): Fong TL+, *Am J Gastroenterol* 94(4), 990

RIMONABANT

Synonym: SR 141716
Trade name: Acomplia (Sanofi-Aventis)
Indications: Obesity
Category: CB1 Cannabinoid receptor antagonist
Half-life: N/A
**Clinically important, potentially hazardous interactions
with:** clarithromycin, itraconazole, ketoconazole, nefazodone,
ritonavir, telithromycin

Note: Not approved in the USA

Reactions

Skin
Diaphoresis
Pruritus

Eyes
Visual hallucinations

Other
Anxiety
  (2007): Patel PN+, *Am J Health Syst Pharm* 64(5), 481
  (2006): *Prescrire Int* 15(84), 123
  (2005): Despres JP+, *N Engl J Med* 353(20), 2121
Asthenia
Depression
  (2007): Patel PN+, *Am J Health Syst Pharm* 64(5), 481
  (2006): *Prescrire Int* 15(84), 123
  (2005): Despres JP+, *N Engl J Med* 353(20), 2121
Insomnia
Memory Loss
Mood changes
  (2007): Padwal RS+, *Lancet* 369(9555), 71
Myalgia/Myositis/Myopathy/Myotoxicity
Paresthesias
Tendinopathy/Tendon rupture
Upper respiratory infection
Vertigo
  (2007): Patel PN+, *Am J Health Syst Pharm* 64(5), 481
  (2006): *Prescrire Int* 15(84), 123

RISEDRONATE

Trade name: Actonel (Procter & Gamble)
Indications: Paget's disease of bone, postmenopausal
osteoporosis
Category: Bisphosphonate
Half-life: terminal: 220 hours

Reactions

Skin
Edema
Facial edema
  (2005): Barrera BA+, *Osteoporos Int* 16(12), 1989 (6 cases)
Peripheral edema (8.2%)
Pruritus (3.0%)

Rash (sic) (11.5%)
Stevens–Johnson syndrome
   (2005): Barrera BA+, *Osteoporos Int* 16(12), 1989 (1 case)
Urticaria
   (2002): Gordon MS+, *Endocr Pract* 8(3), 202

Mucosal/ENT
Glossitis (<1%)
Tongue edema
   (2005): Barrera BA+, *Osteoporos Int* 16(12), 1989

Eyes
Conjunctivitis
   (2003): Frauenfelder FW+, *N Engl J Med* 348, 1187
Scleritis
   (2005): Barrera BA+, *Osteoporos Int* 16(12), 1989
   (2002): Vinas G+, *Med Clin (Barc)* 118(15), 598

Other
Headache
   (2004): Ogura Y+, *J Bone Miner Metab* 22(2), 120
   (1998): Mitchell DY+, *Pharm Res* 15(2), 228
Myalgia/Myositis/Myopathy/Myotoxicity (6.6%)
Paresthesias (2.1%)
Tendinopathy/Tendon rupture (3.0%)

RISPERIDONE

Trade name: Risperdal (Janssen)
Indications: Psychotic disorders
Category: Antipsychotic; Mood stabilizer
Half-life: 3–30 hours
Clinically important, potentially hazardous interactions with: clozapine, paroxetine

Reactions

Skin
Acne (<1%)
Allergic reactions (sic) (<1%)
   (1998): Terao T+, *J Clin Psychiatry* 59, 82
Angioedema
   (2001): Kores Plesnicar B+, *Eur Psychiatry* 16(8), 506
   (1995): Cooney C+, *BMJ* 311, 1204
Bullous dermatitis (<1%)
Bullous pemphigoid
   (1996): Wijeratne C+, *Am J Psychiatry* 153, 735
Dermatitis
Diaphoresis (<1%)
Edema
   (2006): Feroz-Nainar C+, *Autism* 10(3), 308
   (2001): Ravasia S, *Can J Psychiatry* 46(5), 453
   (1996): Baldassano CF+, *J Clin Psychiatry* 57, 422 (generalized)
Exfoliative dermatitis (0.1–1%)
Furunculosis (<1%)
Hyperkeratosis (<1%)
Lichenoid eruption (<1%)
Peripheral edema (16%)
   (2001): Hwang JP+, *J Clin Psychopharmacol* 21(6), 583 (16.4%)
Photosensitivity (1–10%)
   (1998): Almond DS+, *Postgrad Med J* 74, 252
Pigmentation (1%)
Pruritus (<1%)
Psoriasis (<1%)
Purpura (<1%)
Rash (sic) (5%)

Seborrhea
Ulcerations (<1%)
Urticaria (<0.1%)
   (2007): Mishra B+, *Br J Clin Pharmacol* 64(4), 558 (giant) (recurrent)
Verrucae (<1%)
Xerosis (2%)

Mucosal/ENT
Dysgeusia (<1%)
Dysphagia
   (2003): Stewart JT, *Dysphagia* 18(4), 274
   (2001): Nair S+, *Gen Hosp Psychiatry* 23(4), 231
Gingivitis (<1%)
Sialopenia (5%)
Sialorrhea (2%)
   (2007): Panagiotidis PT+, *Schizophr Res* 93(1-3), 410
   (2006): Kontaxakis VP+, *Eur Arch Psychiatry Clin Neurosci* 256(6), 350 (with clozapine)
   (2006): Luby J+, *J Child Adolesc Psychopharmacol* 16(5), 575
   (2005): Boyce HW+, *J Clin Gastroenterol* 39(2), 89 (passim)
   (2005): Duran JC+, *Int Psychogeriatr* 17(4), 591
   (2001): Buitelaar JK+, *J Clin Psychiatry* 62(4), 239
   (2001): Gajwani P+, *Psychosomatics* 42(3), 276
Stomatitis (<1%)
Tinnitus
Tongue edema (<1%)
Tongue pigmentation (<1%)
Xerostomia (1–18%)
   (2002): McCracken JT+, *N Engl J Med* 347(5), 314 (18%)
   (2001): Hodge CH+, *Vet Hum Toxicol* 43(6), 339 (2 cases)
   (2001): Mullen J+, *Clin Ther* 23(11), 1839 (6.9%)

Hair
Hair – alopecia (<1%)
   (2000): Mercke Y+, *Ann Clin Psychiatry* 12, 35
Hair – hypertrichosis (<1%)

Other
Anaphylactoid reactions/Anaphylaxis
Death
Delirium
   (2006): *Prescrire Int* 15(85), 183
Depression (14%)
   (2003): Fleischhacker WW+, *J Clin Psychiatry* 64(10), 1250 (14%)
   (2003): Nishimura M+, *No To Hattatsu* 35(6), 473
   (2003): Zalsman G+, *J Child Adolesc Psychopharmacol* 13(3), 319
Gynecomastia (1–10%)
   (2005): Mendhekar DN+, *Indian J Med Sci* 59(8), 361 (unilateral)
   (1999): Benazzi F, *Pharmacopsychiatry* 32, 41
Headache
Inappropriate secretion of antidiuretic hormone (SIADH)
   (1997): Whitten JR+, *Ann Clin Psychiatry* 9(3), 181
Injection-site pain
   (2005): Pinninti NR+, *J Clin Psychiatry* 66(5), 656
Myalgia/Myositis/Myopathy/Myotoxicity (<1%)
Neurotoxicity
   (2007): Boker H+, *Psychiatr Prax* 34(1), 38 (with lithium)
Osteoporosis
   (2005): Wyszogrodzka-Kucharska A+, *Psychiatr Pol* 39(6), 1173
Paresthesias (<1%)
Rhabdomyolysis
   (2006): Zink M+, *J Clin Psychiatry* 67(5), 835 (with mirtazapine)
   (2004): Webber MA+, *J Psychopharmacol* 18(3), 432 (with simvastatin)
   (2002): Giner V+, *J Intern Med* 251(2), 177 (with cerivastatin)
   (1997): Whitten JR+, *Ann Clin Psychiatry* 9(3), 181

(1996): Meltzer HY+, *Neuropsychopharmacology* 15(4), 395

Seizures
(2003): Reuther LO+, *Ugeskr Laeger* 165(14), 1447
(1997): Whitten JR+, *Ann Clin Psychiatry* 9(3), 181

Somnolence
(2006): Kontaxakis VP+, *Eur Arch Psychiatry Clin Neurosci* 256(6), 350 (with clozapine)
(2005): Duran JC+, *Int Psychogeriatr* 17(4), 591

Thrombophlebitis (<1%)

Thrombosis
(2006): Zink M+, *J Clin Psychiatry* 67(5), 835 (with mirtazapine)

Tremor (14%)
(2006): Fleischhaker C+, *J Child Adolesc Psychopharmacol* 16(3), 308 (5%)
(2002): McCracken JT+, *N Engl J Med* 347(5), 314 (14%)

Tumors
(2006): Szarfman A+, *Pharmacotherapy* 26(6), 748 (pituitary)

Weight gain
(2006): Fleischhaker C+, *J Child Adolesc Psychopharmacol* 16(3), 308
(2005): Ness-Abramof R+, *Drugs Today* (Barc) 41(8), 547

RITODRINE

Trade name: Pre-Par
Indications: Preterm labor
Category: Adrenergic beta2-receptor agonist; Tocolytic
Half-life: 1.3–12 hours

Reactions

Skin
Diaphoresis (1–14%)
Erythema (10–15%)
Erythema multiforme
(1988): Beitner O+, *Drug Intell Clin Pharm* 22, 724
Exanthems
(1995): del Pozo Hernando LJ+, *Med Clin* (Barc) 105(7), 277
Pustules (in a pregnant woman with psoriasis)
(1998): D'Incan M+, *J Eur Acad Dermatol Venereol* 11, 91
Rash (sic) (1–3%)
(2001): Yamada T+, *Arch Gynecol Obstet* 264(4), 218
Toxic epidermal necrolysis
(1998): Claessens N+, *Dermatology* 196(4), 461
Urticaria
Vasculitis
(2004): Cobeta-Garcia JC+, *Ann Pharmacother* 38(1), 66
(1991): Bosnyak S+, *Am J Obstet Gyn* 165, 427

Eyes
Glaucoma
(2006): Leung DY+, *Acta Obstet Gynecol Scand* 85(2), 251
(2005): Guvendag Guven ES+, *Acta Obstet Gynecol Scand* 84(5), 489

Other
Anaphylactoid reactions/Anaphylaxis (1–3%)
Chest pain
(2001): Kagabu M+, *J Obstet Gynaecol Res* 27(6), 337
(1992): *N Engl J Med* 327(5), 308
Chills (3–10%)
Headache
Hepatotoxicity
(1999): Castro Fernandez M+, *Med Clin* (Barc) 113(6), 239
(1998): Ceriani R+, *Ital J Gastroenterol Hepatol* 30(3), 315
(1996): De Arcos F+, *Acta Obstet Gynecol Scand* 75(4), 340

Rhabdomyolysis
(2002): Matsuda Y+, *J Perinat Med* 30(6), 514
Tremor (>10%)

RITONAVIR

Trade name: Norvir (Abbott)
Indications: HIV infection
Category: Antiretroviral; Protease inhibitor, HIV
Half-life: 3–5 hours
Clinically important, potentially hazardous interactions with: alfentanil, alfuzosin, alprazolam, amiodarone, amprenavir, aprepitant, astemizole, atazanavir, bepridil, buprenorphine, bupropion, carbamazepine, chlordiazepoxide, ciclesonide, clozapine, conivaptan, cyclosporine, dasatinib, diazepam, dihydroergotamine, ergot alkaloids, estazolam, eszopiclone, etravirine, ezetimibe, fentanyl, flecainide, flurazepam, fluticasone, halazepam, ivabradine, ixabepilone, ketoconazole, lapatinib, levothyroxine, meperidine, methysergide, midazolam, nifedipine, oral contraceptives, phenytoin, pimozide, piroxicam, propafenone, propoxyphene, quazepam, quinidine, ranolazine, rifabutin, rifampin, rifapentine, rimonabant, saquinavir, sildenafil, simvastatin, solifenacin, **St John's wort**, tadalafil, temsirolimus, triazolam, vardenafil, voriconazole, zolpidem

Note: Protease inhibitors cause dyslipidemia which includes elevated triglycerides and cholesterol and redistribution of body fat centrally to produce the so-called 'protease paunch,' breast enlargement, facial atrophy, and 'buffalo hump'

Reactions

Skin
Acne (<2%)
Allergic granulomatous angiitis (Churg–Strauss syndrome)
(2002): Kawsar M+, *Int J STD AIDS* 13(4), 273
Allergic reactions (sic) (<2%)
Angioedema
Bullous dermatitis (<2%)
Dermatitis (<2%)
Diaphoresis (1–10%)
Eczema (<2%)
Edema
Exanthems (<2%)
(2005): Calista D+, *Eur J Dermatol* 15(2), 97 (with lopinavir)
(1997): Bachmeyer C+, *Dermatology* 195, 301 (2 HIV patients)
Facial edema (<2%)
Folliculitis (<2%)
Peripheral edema (<2%)
Photosensitivity (<2%)
Pruritus (<2%)
Psoriasis (<2%)
Rash (sic) (1–10%)
Seborrhea (<2%)
Stevens–Johnson syndrome
Urticaria (<2%)
Xanthomas
(2004): Geyer AS+, *Arch Dermatol* 140(5), 617
Xerosis (<2%)

Mucosal/ENT
Ageusia (<2%)
Cheilitis (<2%)
(2000): Bonfanti P+, *J Acquir Immune Defic Syndr* 23(3), 236

Dysgeusia (10.3%)
Gingivitis (<2%)
Macroglossia
    (2005): Vritsali E+, J Oral Pathol Med 34(1), 56 (with lopinavir)
Oral candidiasis (<2%)
Oral ulceration (<2%)
Parosmia (<2%)
Xerostomia (<2%)

Hair
Hair – alopecia
    (2002): Ginarte M+, AIDS 16(12), 1695 (with indinavir)

Nails
Nails – onychocryptosis
    (2001): James CW+, Ann Pharmacother 35(7), 881 (with
        indinavir)

Other
Anaphylactoid reactions/Anaphylaxis
Gynecomastia
    (2001): Manfredi R+, Ann Pharmacother 35(4), 438
    (2000): Bonfanti P+, J Acquir Immune Defic Syndr 23(3), 236
Headache
Hypertension
    (2006): Crane HM+, AIDS 20(7), 1019 (with lopinavir)
Lipodystrophy
    (2002): Reid S, Can Adv Drug Reaction Newsletter 12, 5
    (2001): van der Valk M+, AIDS 15(7), 847
Myalgia/Myositis/Myopathy/Myotoxicity (1–10%)
Nephrotoxicity
    (1998): Deray G+, Presse Med 27(35), 1801 (13%)
Paresthesias (2.6%)
    (2001): Scully C+, Oral Dis 7(4), 205 (circumoral) (passim)
Rhabdomyolysis
    (2003): Mah Ming JB+, AIDS Patient Care STDS 17(5), 207 (with
        clarithromycin, atorvastatin and lopinavir)
    (2002): Cheng CH+, Am J Health Syst Pharm 59(8), 728
Seizures
    (2003): Reuther LO+, Ugeskr Laeger 165(14), 1447
Thrombophlebitis
    (2000): Bonfanti P+, J Acquir Immune Defic Syndr 23(3), 236

RITUXIMAB

Trade name: Rituxan (Genentech)
Indications: Non-Hodgkin's lymphoma
Category: Immunosuppressant; Monoclonal antibody
Half-life: 60 hours (after first infusion)

Reactions

Skin
Angioedema (>10%)
    (2003): Fierro MT+, J Am Acad Dermatol 49, 281 (passim)
Dermatitis
    (2006): Scheinfeld N, Dermatol Online J 12(1), 3
Diaphoresis
    (1999): Dillman RO, Cancer Metastasis Rev 18(4), 465
Exanthems
    (2002): Lowndes S+, Ann Oncol 13(12), 1948
Herpes zoster
    (2006): Antoniu SA, Expert Opin Investig Drugs 15(9), 1115
    (2006): Cabanillas F+, Ann Oncol 17(9), 1424
    (2006): El Tal AK+, J Am Acad Dermatol 55(3), 449 (reactivation)

    (2003): Martinelli G+, Br J Haematol 123(2), 271 (with
        chlorambucil) (2 cases)
Kaposi's sarcoma
    (2005): Clifford KS+, J Am Acad Dermatol 53(1), 155
Necrosis
    (2006): Pearlman AN+, Ear Nose Throat J 85(7), 431 (nasal)
Paraneoplastic pemphigus
    (2006): Scheinfeld N, Dermatol Online J 12(1), 3
Peripheral edema
Pruritus (10%)
    (2006): Tamminga RY+, Pediatr Blood Cancer 47(5 Suppl), 714
    (2002): Salopek TG+, J Am Acad Dermatol 47(5), 785
Rash (sic) (10%)
    (2006): Penalver FJ+, Ann Hematol 85(6), 400
    (1999): Dillman RO, Cancer Metastasis Rev 18(4), 465
Stevens–Johnson syndrome
    (2006): El Tal AK+, J Am Acad Dermatol 55(3), 449
    (2006): Scheinfeld N, Dermatol Online J 12(1), 3
    (2002): Lowndes S+, Ann Oncol 13(12), 1948
Toxic epidermal necrolysis
    (2006): Scheinfeld N, Dermatol Online J 12(1), 3
Urticaria (10%)
    (2006): Errante D+, Ann Oncol 17(11), 1720
    (2003): Fierro MT+, J Am Acad Dermatol 49, 281 (passim)

Mucosal/ENT
Mucocutaneous reactions
    (2006): Scheinfeld N, Dermatol Online J 12(1), 3
Orogenital ulceration
    (2002): Lowndes S+, Ann Oncol 13(12), 1948
Otitis
    (2006): Cabanillas F+, Ann Oncol 17(9), 1424 (3 cases)
Perianal ulcerations
    (2003): Martinelli G+, Br J Haematol 123(2), 271 (with
        chlorambucil)
Rhinitis
    (2003): Rehwald U+, Blood 101(2), 420
Sinusitis
    (2006): Cabanillas F+, Ann Oncol 17(9), 1424 (16 cases)

Other
Anaphylactoid reactions/Anaphylaxis
    (2006): Biswas G+, J Assoc Physicians India 54, 29
Application-site reactions (sic)
    (2006): Biswas G+, J Assoc Physicians India 54, 29
    (2006): Solal-Celigny P, Leuk Res 30 Suppl 1, S16
    (2003): Plosker GL+, Drugs 63(8), 803
    (2002): Motto DG+, Isr Med Assoc J 4(11), 1006
Cardiotoxicity
    (2006): Scheinfeld N, Dermatol Online J 12(1), 3
Chills (10%)
    (2006): Antoniu SA, Expert Opin Investig Drugs 15(9), 1115
    (2003): Prescrire Int 12(66), 125
    (2003): Boye J+, Ann Oncol 14(4), 520
    (2003): Fierro MT+, J Am Acad Dermatol 49, 281 (passim)
    (2003): Rehwald U+, Blood 101(2), 420
    (2002): Salopek TG+, J Am Acad Dermatol 47(5), 785
Death
    (2006): Herishanu Y+, Clin Lymphoma Myeloma 6(5), 407
    (2006): Iyer A+, Arch Pathol Lab Med 130(10), 1557
    (2006): Perceau G+, Br J Dermatol 155(5), 1053
    (2006): Scheinfeld N, Dermatol Online J 12(1), 3
    (2006): Seifert G+, Haematologica 91(6 Suppl), ECR23
    (2003): Sirvent-Von Bueltzingsloewen A+, Med Pediatr Oncol
        40(6), 408
    (2001): Huhn D+, Blood 98(5), 1326
    (2001): Suzan F+, N Engl J Med 345(13), 1000
Fever
    (2006): Cabanillas F+, Ann Oncol 17(9), 1424 (2 cases)

(2006): Penalver FJ+, *Ann Hematol* 85(6), 400
(2006): Tamminga RY+, *Pediatr Blood Cancer* 47(5 Suppl), 714
(2004): Vieira CA+, *Transplantation* 77(4), 542
(2003): *Prescrire Int* 12(66), 125
(2003): Boye J+, *Ann Oncol* 14(4), 520
(2003): Fierro MT+, *J Am Acad Dermatol* 49, 281 (passim)
(2003): Rehwald U+, *Blood* 101(2), 420
Headache
Hepatotoxicity
(2006): Iyer A+, *Arch Pathol Lab Med* 130(10), 1557
(2006): Ozgonenel B+, *Am J Hematol* 81(4), 302
(2006): Sera T+, *Intern Med* 45(11), 721 (reactivation)
Hypersensitivity
(2003): Hellerstedt B+, *Ann Oncol* 14(12), 1792
Hypotension
(2006): Biswas G+, *J Assoc Physicians India* 54, 29
Infections
(2006): Biehn SE+, *Hematol Oncol* 24(4), 234
(2006): Cabanillas F+, *Ann Oncol* 17(9), 1424 (18 cases)
(2006): El Tal AK+, *J Am Acad Dermatol* 55(3), 449
(2002): Motto DG+, *Isr Med Assoc J* 4(11), 1006
Injection-site burning
(2005): Fink-Puches R+, *J Am Acad Dermatol* 52(5), 847
Injection-site edema
(2006): Perez-Gala S+, *Arch Dermatol* 142(11), 1516 (2 cases)
Injection-site erythema
(2005): Fink-Puches R+, *J Am Acad Dermatol* 52(5), 847
Injection-site pain
(2005): Fink-Puches R+, *J Am Acad Dermatol* 52(5), 847
Injection-site pruritus
(2006): Perez-Gala S+, *Arch Dermatol* 142(11), 1516
Injection-site reactions (sic)
(2002): Meo P+, *Recenti Prog Med* 93(7), 421
(2002): Motto DG+, *Isr Med Assoc J* 4(11), 1006
(2001): Stasi R+, *Blood* 98(4), 952
(2001): Wood AM, *Am J Health Syst Pharm* 58(3), 215
Myalgia/Myositis/Myopathy/Myotoxicity (7%)
Nephrotoxicity
(2006): Scheinfeld N, *Dermatol Online J* 12(1), 3
Serum sickness
(2007): Finger E+, *J Clin Rheumatol* 13(2), 94
(2007): Todd DJ+, *J Rheumatol* 34(2), 430
(2006): Schutgens RE, *Br J Haematol* 135(2), 147
(2006): Tamminga RY+, *Pediatr Blood Cancer* 47(5 Suppl), 714
(2005): Catuogno M+, *Rheumatology* (Oxford) 44(3), 406
(2002): Herishanu Y, *Am J Hematol* 70(4), 329
(2001): D'Arcy CA+, *Arthritis Rheum* 44, 1717
Upper respiratory infection
(2006): Antoniu SA, *Expert Opin Investig Drugs* 15(9), 1115

RIVASTIGMINE

Trade name: Exelon (Novartis)
Indications: Alzheimer's disease and dementia
Category: Cholinesterase inhibitor
Half-life: 1–2 hours
**Clinically important, potentially hazardous interactions
with:** galantamine

Reactions

Skin
Allergic reactions (sic) (~1%)
Bullous dermatitis (~1%)
Cellulitis (~1%)
Clammy skin (~1%)

Dermatitis (~1%)
Diaphoresis (10%)
Edema (~1%)
Exanthems (~1%)
  (2001): Monastero R+, *Am J Med* 111(7), 583
Exfoliative dermatitis (~1%)
Facial edema (~1%)
Herpes simplex (~1%)
Peripheral edema (~2%)
Psoriasis (~1%)
Purpura (~1%)
Rash (sic) (~2%)
Ulcerations (~1%)
Urticaria (~1%)

Mucosal/ENT
Ageusia (~1%)
Dysgeusia (~1%)
Gingivitis (~1%)
Glossitis (~1%)
Sialorrhea (~1%)
Ulcerative stomatitis (~1%)
Vaginitis (~1%)
Xerostomia (~1%)

Hair
Hair – alopecia (~1%)

Eyes
Periorbital edema (~1%)

Other
Headache
Hot flashes (~1%)
Infections (~2%)
Myalgia/Myositis/Myopathy/Myotoxicity (20%)
Paresthesias (~1%)
Thrombophlebitis (<2%)
Tremor (4%)
  (2004): Emre M+, *N Engl J Med* 351(24), 2509 (10%)
Vertigo
  (2006): Potkin SG+, *Drugs Aging* 23(3), 241 (10%)

RIZATRIPTAN

Synonym: MK462
Trade name: Maxalt (Merck)
Indications: Migraine
Category: 5-HT1 agonist; Serotonin receptor agonist; Triptan
Half-life: 2–3 hours
**Clinically important, potentially hazardous interactions
with:** dihydroergotamine, ergot-containing drugs, isocarboxazid,
MAO inhibitors, methysergide, naratriptan, phenelzine,
propanolol, sibutramine, **St John's wort**, sumatriptan,
tranylcypromine, zolmitriptan

Reactions

Skin
Diaphoresis (<1%)
Facial edema (<1%)
Pruritus (<1%)

Mucosal/ENT
Tongue edema
Xerostomia (<5%)

Other
Asthenia
  (2002): Wellington K+, *Drugs* 62(10), 1539
  (2001): Gobel H+, *Headache* 41(3), 264
  (2000): Pascual J+, *Cephalalgia* 20(5), 455
  (1999): Bomhof M+, *Eur Neurol* 42(3), 173
  (1999): Dooley M+, *Drugs* 58(4), 699
  (1998): Block GA+, *Headache* 38(10), 764
  (1998): Teall J+, *Headache* 38(4), 281
  (1997): Gijsman H+, *Cephalalgia* 17(6), 647
Chest pain
  (2002): Wellington K+, *Drugs* 62(10), 1539
  (1999): Dooley M+, *Drugs* 58(4), 699
Chills (<1%)
Headache
Hot flashes (1–10%)
Myalgia/Myositis/Myopathy/Myotoxicity (<1%)
Nephrotoxicity
  (2006): Fulton JA+, *Clin Toxicol (Phila)* 44(2), 177
Paresthesias
Vertigo
  (2003): Christie S+, *Eur Neurol* 49(1), 20 (6.7%)
  (2002): Wellington K+, *Drugs* 62(10), 1539
  (2001): Gobel H+, *Headache* 41(3), 264
  (2000): Pascual J+, *Cephalalgia* 20(5), 455
  (2000): Silberstein SD, *Neurology* 55(9 Suppl 2), S25
  (1999): Bomhof M+, *Eur Neurol* 42(3), 173
  (1999): Dooley M+, *Drugs* 58(4), 699
  (1998): Teall J+, *Headache* 38(4), 281
  (1997): Gijsman H+, *Cephalalgia* 17(6), 647

ROCURONIUM

Synonym: ORG 946
Trade names: Esmeron; Zemuron (Organon)
Indications: Adjunct to general anesthesia
Category: Non-depolarizing neuromuscular blocker
Half-life: 1–2 minutes
Clinically important, potentially hazardous interactions with: aminoglycosides, bacitracin, clindamycin, lithium, procainamide, quinidine, tetracycline, vancomycin

Reactions

Skin
Edema (<1%)
Rash (sic) (<1%)

Other
Anaphylactoid reactions/Anaphylaxis
  (2005): Bhananker SM+, *Anesth Analg* 101(3), 819
  (2005): Brozovic G+, *Eur J Anaesthesiol* 22(1), 72
  (2005): Harboe T+, *Anesthesiology* 102(5), 897
  (2005): Santiveri Papiol X+, *Rev Esp Anestesiol Reanim* 52(5), 307
  (2004): Bermejo Alvarez MA+, *Rev Esp Anestesiol Reanim* 51(9), 562
  (2004): Mertes PM+, *Ann Fr Anesth Reanim* 23(12), 1133
  (2003): Kierzek G+, *Eur J Anaesthesiol* 20(2), 169
  (2003): Louvier N+, *Ann Fr Anesth Reanim* 22(1), 54
  (2003): Mertes PM+, *Anesthesiology* 99(3), 536
  (2003): Thomas R+, *Anaesthesia* 58(2), 196
  (2002): Baillard C+, *Br J Anaesth* 88(4), 600 (2 cases; one fatal)
  (2002): Joseph P+, *Ann Fr Anesth Reanim* 21(3), 221
  (2001): Booij LH+, *Br J Anaesth* 87(5), 805
  (2001): Laake JH+, *Acta Anaesthesiol Scand* 45(10), 1196 (29 cases)

  (2001): Laxenaire MC+, *Br J Anaesth* 87(4), 549
  (2001): Rose M+, *Br J Anaesth* 86(5), 678 (24 cases)
  (2000): Allen SJ+, *Anaesthesia* 55(12), 1223
  (2000): Donnelly T, *Br J Anaesth* 84(5), 696
  (2000): Heier T+, *Acta Anaesthesiol Scand* 44(7), 775 (3 cases)
  (2000): Laxenaire MC+, *Br J Anaesth* 85(2), 325
  (2000): Matthey P+, *Can J Anaesth* 47(9), 890
  (1999): Barthelet Y+, *Ann Fr Anesth Reanim* 18(8), 896 (4 cases)
  (1996): Yee R+, *Anaesth Intensive Care* 24(5), 601
Hypertension (>1%)
Hypotension (>1%)
Injection-site pain
  (2005): Mahajan R+, *Can J Anaesth* 52(1), 111
  (2005): Memis D+, *Can J Anaesth* 52(4), 437
  (2005): Park JT+, *Yonsei Med J* 46(6), 765
  (2004): Mencke T+, *Acta Anaesthesiol Scand* 48(10), 1245 (32.5%)
  (2003): Blunk JA+, *Eur J Anaesthesiol* 20(3), 245
  (2003): Chiarella AB+, *Br J Anaesth* 90(3), 377
  (2003): Turan A+, *Anaesth Intensive Care* 31(3), 277
  (2000): Cheong KF+, *Br J Anaesth* 84(1), 106
  (1998): Ti LK+, *Br J Anaesth* 81(3), 487
  (1997): Borgeat A+, *Br J Anaesth* 79(3), 382
  (1997): Joshi GP+, *Anesth Analg* 84(1), 228
  (1996): Robertson EN, *Anaesthesia* 51(1), 93
  (1995): Lockey D+, *Anaesthesia* 50(5), 474
  (1995): Moorthy SS+, *Anesth Analg* 80(5), 1067
Injection-site pruritus (<1%)

ROFECOXIB

Trade name: Vioxx (Merck)
Indications: Osteoarthritis, acute pain
Category: COX-2 inhibitor; Non-steroidal anti-inflammatory
Half-life: 17 hours
Clinically important, potentially hazardous interactions with: anisindione, anticoagulants, dicumarol, lithium, methotrexate, tizanidine, warfarin

Note: This drug has been withdrawn

Reactions

Skin
Abrasion (<2%)
Allergic reactions (sic) (<2%)
Angioedema
  (2006): Downing A+, *Br J Clin Pharmacol* 62(4), 496
  (2002): Kumar NP+, *Postgrad Med J* 78(921), 439
  (2001): Kelkar PS+, *J Rheumatol* 28(11), 2553
  (2000): Medicines Control Agency and Committee on Safety of Medicines Reports (5 cases)
Atopic dermatitis (<2%)
Basal cell carcinoma (<2%)
Bullous dermatitis (<2%)
Cellulitis (<2%)
Dermatitis (<2%)
Diaphoresis (<2%)
Edema (3.7%)
  (2006): Valat JP+, *Presse Med* 35(9 Spec No 1), 1S25
  (2002): Carder KR+, *Pediatr Dermatol* 19(4), 353 (palms & soles)
  (2000): Medicines Control Agency and Committee on Safety of Medicines Reports (101 cases)
Erythema (<2%)
  (2000): Wright WL, Castro Valley, CA (from Internet) (observation) (after the second day)

Exanthems
  (2000): Blumenthal HL, Beachwood, OH (personal case)
    (observation)
Fixed eruption
  (2002): Nederost ST+, Cutis 70, 125
  (2001): Kaur C+, Dermatology 203(4), 351 (with sulfonamides)
  (2000): Conners RC, Greenwich, CT (personal communication)
Fungal dermatitis (<2%)
Granuloma annulare
  (2000): Rotman H, Houston, TX (personal communication)
    (observation)
Hematomas
  (2005): Khan FY+, Saudi Med J 26(2), 336 (with enoxaparin)
Herpes simplex (<2%)
Herpes zoster (<2%)
Leg ulceration
  (2003): Smith KJ+, Int J Dermatol 42(5), 389
Neutrophilic dermatosis
  (2003): Smith KJ+, Int J Dermatol 42(5), 389
Nodular eruption
  (2003): Smith KJ+, Int J Dermatol 42(5), 389
Peripheral edema (6%)
  (2006): Zhang J+, JAMA 296(13), 1619
  (2003): Smith KJ+, Int J Dermatol 42(5), 389
  (2001): Litt JZ, Beachwood, OH (2 personal cases)
  (2000): Litt JZ, Beachwood, OH (personal case)
Photosensitivity
  (2001): Klein AD, Statesboro, GA (from Internet) (observation)
  (2000): Valentine M, Everett, WA (from Internet) (observation)
  (1999): Gregg LJ, Tulsa, OK (from Internet) (observation)
Phototoxicity
  (2001): Klein AD, Statesboro, GA (from Internet) (observation)
Pruritus (<2%)
  (2004): Klein AD, Streetsboro, GA (not allergic to celecoxib)
    (from Internet) (observation)
Psoriasis
  (2003): Clark DW+, Arch Dermatol 139(9), 1223
Purpura
  (2001): Litt JZ, Beachwood, OH (personal case)
  (2000): Litt JZ, Beachwood, OH (personal case)
Rash (sic) (<2%)
Stevens–Johnson syndrome
  (2005): La Grenade L+, Drug Saf 28(10), 917 (17 cases)
  (2004): Goldberg D+, Cornea, 2004 Oct 23(7), 736 (1 case)
  (2003): Layton D+, Br J Clin Pharmacol 55(2), 166 (1 case)
Toxic epidermal necrolysis
  (2005): La Grenade L+, Drug Saf 28(10), 917 (17 cases)
Urticaria (<2%)
  (2004): Klein AD, Streetsboro, GA (not allergic to celecoxib)
    (from Internet) (observation)
  (2002): Nettis E+, Ann Allergy Asthma 88(3), 331
  (2001): Kelkar PS+, J Rheumatol 28(11), 2553
  (2000): Wright WL, Castro Valley, CA (from Internet) (2
    observations, after the second day)
Vasculitis
  (2003): Lillicrap MS+, Rheumatology (Oxford) 42(10), 1267
  (2003): Palop-Larrea V+, Ann Pharmacother 37(11), 1731
  (2002): Reed BR, Denver, CO (from Internet) (observation)
Wrinkling (sic)
  (2002): Carder KR+, Pediatr Dermatol 19(4), 353 (aquagenic –
    palms & soles)
Xerosis (<2%)

Mucosal/ENT
Aphthous stomatitis (<2%)
Auditory hallucinations
  (2007): Sabolek M+, Psychiatr Prax 34(4), 200
Oral mucosal eruption
  (2004): Bagan JV+, Oral Dis 10(6), 401
Oral ulceration (<2%)
Tinnitus
  (2001): Litt JZ, Beachwood, OH (personal case)
Xerostomia (<2%)

Hair
Hair – alopecia (<2%)

Nails
Nails – changes (sic) (<2%)

Eyes
Visual hallucinations
  (2007): Sabolek M+, Psychiatr Prax 34(4), 200

Other
Congestive heart failure
  (2006): Valat JP+, Presse Med 35(9 Spec No 1), 1S25
Death
  (2005): Graham DJ+, Lancet 365(9458), 475 (27%)
  (2002): Kumar NP+, Postgrad Med J 78(921), 439
  (2001): Weaver J+, Am J Gastroenterol 96(12), 3449
Headache
Hypertension
  (2006): Valat JP+, Presse Med 35(9 Spec No 1), 1S25
  (2006): Zhang J+, JAMA 296(13), 1619
Myalgia/Myositis/Myopathy/Myotoxicity (<2%)
  (2003): Smith KJ+, Int J Dermatol 42(5), 389
Nephrotoxicity
  (2006): Zhang J+, JAMA 296(13), 1619
  (2001): Papaioannides D+, Int Urol Nephrol 33(4), 609
  (2001): Woywodt A+, J Rheumatol 28(9), 2133
Paresthesias (<2%)
Pseudoporphyria
  (2004): Markus R+, J Am Acad Dermatol 50(4), 647
Tendinopathy/Tendon rupture (<2%)
Thrombosis
  (2006): Baron JA+, Gastroenterology 131(6), 1674
  (2006): Valat JP+, Presse Med 35(9 Spec No 1), 1S25
Vertigo (2%)
  (2003): Bannwarth B+, Drug Saf 26(1), 49 (2.1%)

ROMIPLOSTIM

Trade name: Nplate (Amgen)
Indications: Thrombocytopenic purpura, myelodysplastic syndromes
Category: Recombinant thrombopoeitin
Half-life: 1 to 34 Days (mean=3.5 Days)

Reactions

Other
Abdominal pain (11%)
Asthenia
Confusion
Fever
Headache
Insomnia (16%)
Myalgia/Myositis/Myopathy/Myotoxicity (14%)
Paresthesias (6%)
Vertigo (17%)

ROPINIROLE

Trade name: Requip (GSK)
Indications: Parkinsonism
Category: Dopamine receptor agonist
Half-life: ~6 hours
**Clinically important, potentially hazardous interactions
with:** warfarin

Reactions

Skin
Basal cell carcinoma (>1%)
Cellulitis (<1%)
Dermatitis (<1%)
Diaphoresis (6%)
Eczema (<1%)
Edema (<1%)
Exanthems (<1%)
Fungal dermatitis (<1%)
Furunculosis (<1%)
Herpes simplex (<1%)
Herpes zoster (<1%)
Hyperkeratosis (<1%)
Hypertrophy (<1%)
Peripheral edema (<1%)
Photosensitivity (<1%)
Pigmentation (<1%)
Pruritus (<1%)
Psoriasis (<1%)
Purpura (<1%)
Rash (sic) (>1%)
   (1999): Ondo W, *Mov Disord* 14(1), 138
Ulcerations (<1%)
Urticaria (<1%)

Mucosal/ENT
Balanitis (<1%)
Gingivitis (>1%)
Glossitis (<1%)
Sialorrhea (>1%)
Stomatitis (<1%)
Tongue edema (<1%)
Ulcerative stomatitis (<1%)
Vulvovaginal candidiasis (<1%)
Xerostomia (5%)

Hair
Hair – alopecia (<1%)

Other
Asthenia
   (2006): *Prescrire Int* 15(85), 173
   (2004): Adler CH+, *Neurology* 62(8), 1405
Gynecomastia (<1%)
Headache
   (2004): Trenkwalder C+, *J Neurol Neurosurg Psychiatry* 75(1), 92
Hypotension
   (2006): *Prescrire Int* 15(85), 173
   (2003): Etminan M+, *Drug Saf* 26(6), 439
Paresthesias (5%)
Peyronie's disease (<1%)
Thrombophlebitis (<1%)
Tremor (6%)
Vertigo

(2003): Etminan M+, *Drug Saf* 26(6), 439
(2003): Im JH+, *J Neurol* 250(1), 90
(1999): Kuzel MD, *Am J Health Syst Pharm* 56(3), 217
(1998): Brooks DJ+, *Clin Neuropharmacol* 21(2), 101

ROSEMARY

Scientific name: *Rosmarinus officinalis*
Family: Lamiaceae; Labiatae
Trade and other common names: Compass weed; Polar plant; Rusmari
Category: Antibacterial; Antifungal
Purported indications and other uses: Oral: dyspepsia, flatulence, gout, cough, headache, loss of appetite, high blood pressure. **Topical:** alopecia areata, circulatory disturbances, toothache, eczema, musculoskeletal pain. Culinary spice, fragrance component, insect repellent
Half-life: N/A
**Clinically important, potentially hazardous interactions
with:** N/A

Reactions

Skin
Dermatitis
   (2005): Inui S+, *J Dermatol* 32(8), 667
   (2003): Armisen M+, *Contact Dermatitis* 48(1), 52
   (1997): Fernandez L+, *Contact Dermatitis* 37(5), 248
   (1997): Hjorther AB+, *Contact Dermatitis* 37(3), 99
Erythema
Photosensitivity
   (2003): Armisen M+, *Contact Dermatitis* 48(1), 52

Mucosal/ENT
Cheilitis
   (2001): Guin JD, *Contact Dermatitis* 45(1), 63

Other
Seizures
   (1999): Burkhard PR+, *J Neurol* 246(8), 667

ROSIGLITAZONE

Trade names: Avandamet (GSK); Avandia (GSK)
Indications: Type 2 diabetes
Category: Thiazolidinedione
Half-life: 3.5 hours
**Clinically important, potentially hazardous interactions
with:** grapefuit juice, pomegranate

Reactions

Skin
Edema (4.8%)
   (2006): Kahn SE+, *N Engl J Med* 355(23), 2427
   (2006): Karalliedde J+, *J Am Soc Nephrol* 17(12), 3482
   (2006): Ko GT+, *Adv Ther* 23(5), 799 (peripheral)
   (2005): *Prescrire Int* 14(78), 133
   (2004): Le Feuvre C, *Ann Endocrinol* (Paris) 65(1 Suppl), S26
   (2004): Le Feuvre C, *Presse Med* 33(11), 735
   (2004): Singh N, *J Cardiovasc Pharmacol Ther* 9(1), 21 (2 patients)
   (2002): *Prescrire Int* 11(62), 170
   (2002): Kuschel U+, *Med Klin* 97(9), 553
   (2001): Werner AL+, *Pharmacotherapy* 21(9), 1082

Exanthems
(1999): Rehbein HM, Jacksonville, FL (from Internet) (observation)
Exfoliative dermatitis
(2000): Vinson RP, El Paso, TX (from Internet) (observation)
Facial edema
(2002): Niemeyer NV+, *Pharmacotherapy* 22(7), 924
Peripheral edema
(2006): Johansen OE+, *Tidsskr Nor Laegeforen* 126(15), 1928 (3 cases)
(2006): Karalliedde J+, *J Am Soc Nephrol* 17(12), 3482
(2006): Ko GT+, *Adv Ther* 23(5), 799 (7%)
(2006): Ryan EH+, *Retina* 26(5), 562
(2002): Niemeyer NV+, *Pharmacotherapy* 22(7), 924

Eyes

Blindness
(2005): Colucciello M, *Arch Ophthalmol* 123(9), 1273
Macular edema
(2006): Kendall C+, *CMAJ* 174(5), 623
(2006): Ryan EH+, *Retina* 26(5), 562
(2006): Sivagnanam G, *CMAJ* 175(3), 276
(2005): Colucciello M, *Arch Ophthalmol* 123(9), 1273
Proptosis
(2005): Levin F+, *Arch Ophthalmol* 123(1), 119

Other

Cardiac failure
(2007): Home PD+, *N Engl J Med* 357(1), 28
(2005): *Prescrire Int* 14(78), 133
(2004): Le Feuvre C, *Ann Endocrinol* (Paris) 65(1 Suppl), S26
(2004): Le Feuvre C, *Presse Med* 33(11), 735
(2004): Marceille JR+, *Pharmacotherapy* 24(10), 1317
Congestive heart failure
(2004): Singh N, *J Cardiovasc Pharmacol Ther* 9(1), 21 (2 patients)
Headache
Hepatotoxicity
(2006): Su DH+, *Diabet Med* 23(1), 105
(2005): Menees SB+, *J Clin Gastroenterol* 39(7), 638
(2004): Marcy TR+, *Ann Pharmacother* 38(9), 1419
(2000): Al-Salman J+, *Ann Intern Med* 132(2), 121
(2000): Forman LM+, *Ann Intern Med* 132(2), 118
Lipomatosis
(2004): Mafong DD+, *AIDS* 18(12), 1742
Myalgia/Myositis/Myopathy/Myotoxicity
(2007): Kennie N+, *Ann Pharmacother* 41(3), 521
Nephrotoxicity
(2006): Castledine C+, *Nephrol Dial Transplant* 21(7), 1994
Weight gain
(2006): Kahn SE+, *N Engl J Med* 355(23), 2427

ROSUVASTATIN

Trade name: Crestor (AstraZeneca)
Indications: Hypercholesterolemia, Mixed dyslipidemia
Category: HMG-CoA reductase inhibitor; Statin
Half-life: ~19 hours
Clinically important, potentially hazardous interactions with: ciprofibrate, cyclosporine, gemfibrozil, warfarin

Reactions

Skin

Peripheral edema (>2%)
Pruritus (>1%)
Rash (sic) (>2%)

Mucosal/ENT

Rhinitis (2.2%)
Sinusitis (2%)

Other

Abdominal pain (>2%)
Asthenia (2.7%)
Cough (>2%)
Depression (>2%)
Headache (6%)
Infections
Myalgia/Myositis/Myopathy/Myotoxicity (2.8%)
(2007): Dedhia V+, *J Assoc Physicians India* (India) 55, 152 (with fenofibrate)
(2007): Kasliwal R+, *Drug Saf* 30(2), 157
(2006): Glueck CJ+, *Clin Ther* 28(6), 933 (1 case)
(2005): Samman A+, *J Heart Lung Transplant* 24(8), 1008
(2004): Davidson MH, *Expert Opin Drug Saf* 3(6), 547
(2004): Shepherd J+, *Am J Cardiol* 94(7), 882
Nephrotoxicity
(2005): Alsheikh-Ali AA+, *Circulation* 111(23), 3051
(2004): *Prescrire Int* 13(72), 132
Pain (>2%)
Paresthesias (>2%)
Rhabdomyolysis
(2007): *Prescrire Int* 16(88), 68
(2005): Alsheikh-Ali AA+, *Circulation* 111(23), 3051
(2005): Blumenthal H, Beachwood, OH (personal communication)
(2005): Ireland JH+, *Ann Intern Med* 142(11), 949 (with fenofibrate)
(2004): Davidson MH, *Expert Opin Drug Saf* 3(6), 547
(2004): Wooltorton E, *CMAJ* 171(2), 129
Vertigo (>2%)

ROTAVIRUS VACCINE

Trade names: Rotarix (GSK); RotaTeq (Merck)
Indications: Prevention of rotavirus gastroenteritis
Half-life: N/A
Clinically important, potentially hazardous interactions with: N/A

Note: Rotarix origin is monovalent human live attenuated, RotaTeq origin is pentavalent bovine live. Only currently licensed forms of the vaccine are considered here

Reactions

Skin

Dermatitis
Rash (sic)

Mucosal/ENT

Rhinitis

Other

Abdominal pain
(2006): Vesikari T+, *Vaccine* 24(22), 4821
Asthenia
Cough
Fever
(2007): Block SL+, *Pediatrics* 119(1), 11
(2006): Bhandari N+, *Vaccine* 24(31-3), 5817
(2006): Vesikari T+, *Pediatr Infect Dis J* 25(2), 118
Myalgia/Myositis/Myopathy/Myotoxicity
Upper respiratory infection

ROTIGOTINE

Trade name: Neupro (Schwarz)
Indications: Parkinsonism
Category: Dopamine receptor agonist
Half-life: 5–7 Hours
Clinically important, potentially hazardous interactions with: N/A

Reactions

Skin
Allergic reactions (sic)
Diaphoresis
Exanthems
Peripheral edema
Pruritus
Purpura
Rash (sic) (2%)

Mucosal/ENT
Sialorrhea
Tinnitus
Xerostomia

Eyes
Photopsia
Visual disturbances (3%)
Visual hallucinations (2%)
  (2001): Metman LV+, *Clin Neuropharmacol* 24(3), 163

Other
Application-site dermatitis (contact)
Application-site pruritus
  (2007): LeWitt PA+, *Neurology* 68(16), 1262
Application-site reactions (37%)
  (2007): LeWitt PA+, *Neurology* 68(16), 1262
  (2007): Splinter MY, *Ann Pharmacother* 41(2), 285
  (2007): Watts RL+, *Neurology* 68(4), 272 (44%)
  (2003): The Parkinson Study Group, *Arch Neurol* 60(12), 1721
Asthenia
  (2007): Watts RL+, *Neurology* 68(4), 272 (33%)
  (2003): The Parkinson Study Group, *Arch Neurol* 60(12), 1721
Cardiac failure
Confusion
Fever
Headache (14%)
Hypertension
Insomnia (10%)
  (2003): The Parkinson Study Group, *Arch Neurol* 60(12), 1721
Paranoia
Paresthesias
Vertigo (18%)
  (2007): Watts RL+, *Neurology* 68(4), 272 (19%)
  (2003): The Parkinson Study Group, *Arch Neurol* 60(12), 1721
Weight gain

ROXATIDINE

Trade name: Roxit (Noristan)
Indications: Gastric and duodenal ulcers
Category: Histamine H2 receptor antagonist
Half-life: 5–6 hours
Clinically important, potentially hazardous interactions with: None

Reactions

Skin
Erythema multiforme
  (2000): Horiuchi Y, *J Dermatol* 27(5), 352
Erythroderma
  (2005): Igawa K+, *Clin Exp Dermatol* 30(3), 304
Lichenoid eruption
  (2002): Greve B+, *Lasers Surg Med* 31(1), 23
  (1996): Horiuchi Y+, *J Dermatol* 23, 510
Pruritus
Rash (sic)
  (1995): Brandstatter G+, *Clin Ther* 17(3), 467
  (1988): Inoue M, *Drugs* 35, 114

Other
Headache (27%)
  (1995): Brandstatter G+, *Clin Ther* 17(3), 467
Myalgia/Myositis/Myopathy/Myotoxicity
Vertigo (27%)
  (1995): Brandstatter G+, *Clin Ther* 17(3), 467

ROXITHROMYCIN

Trade names: Biaxsig (Aventis); Romicin (Pacific); Ruclid; Rulid (Roussel-Uclaf); Ruxid; Surlid
Indications: Respiratory tract, urinary and soft tissue infections
Category: Antibiotic, macrolide
Half-life: 8–15 hours
Clinically important, potentially hazardous interactions with: digoxin, disopyramide, ergot alkaloids, gemfibrozil, midazolam, simvastatin, terfenadine, theophylline, warfarin

Reactions

Skin
Adverse effects
  (2004): Akcay A+, *Ann Pharmacother* 38(4), 721
  (2000): Hatipoglu ON+, *Yonsei Med J* 41(3), 340 (6.6%)
  (1998): Moniot-Ville N+, *J Int Med Res* 26(3), 144
  (1998): Tatsis G+, *J Antimicrob Chemother* 41 Suppl B, 69 (3%)
  (1994): Markham A+, *Drugs* 48(2), 297 (4%)
  (1992): De Vlieger A+, *Diagn Microbiol Infect Dis* 15(4 Suppl), 123S
  (1992): Marsac JH, *Diagn Microbiol Infect Dis* 15(4 Suppl), 81S (4%)
Allergic granulomatous angiitis (Churg–Strauss syndrome)
  (1998): Dietz A+, *Laryngorhinootologie* 77(2), 111
Angioedema
Baboon syndrome
  (2002): Amichai B+, *Clin Exp Dermatol* 27(6), 523
Erythema
  (2001): Easton-Carter KL+, *Pharmacotherapy* 21(7), 867
Fixed eruption
  (1998): Kruppa A+, *Dermatology* 196(3), 335
Pruritus
Purpura
Rash (sic)
  (2001): Easton-Carter KL+, *Pharmacotherapy* 21(7), 867
  (1995): Durant J+, *Infection* 23 Suppl 1, S33
Urticaria
  (2002): Gurvinder SK+, *Allergy* 57(3), 262
  (1998): Kruppa A+, *Dermatology* 196(3), 335

Mucosal/ENT
Dysgeusia
Parosmia

Nails
Nails – pigmentation
  (1995): Dawn G+, *Dermatology* 191(4), 342

Other
Abdominal pain
  (1998): Sprinz E+, *J Antimicrob Chemother* 41 Suppl B, 85
  (1995): Durant J+, *Infection* 23 Suppl 1, S33
Asthenia
  (1996): Muller O, *J Antimicrob Chemother* 37 Suppl C, 83
Headache
  (1996): Muller O, *J Antimicrob Chemother* 37 Suppl C, 83
Hypersensitivity
  (1998): Kruppa A+, *Dermatology* 196(3), 335
Infections
  (2002): Perez-Castrillon JL+, *Ann Pharmacother* 36(11), 1808
Paresthesias

RUE

Scientific names: *Ruta chalepensis; Ruta corsica; Ruta graveolens; Ruta montana*
Family: Rutaceae
Trade and other common names: Country man's treacle; Herb of grace; Herbygrass; ruda
Category: Antispasmodic
Purported indications and other uses: Hysteria, coughs, croup, colic, flatulence, mild stomachic, insomnia, abdominal cramps, nervous headache, giddiness, hysteria, palpitation, abortifacient, cysticide, vermifuge, insecticide. **Topical:** irritant, rubefacient for eczemas, psoriasis and rheumatic pain, sciatica, headache, chronic bronchitis. Flavoring in alcoholic beverages, salads, meats and cheeses
Half-life: N/A

Reactions

Skin
Bullous dermatitis
  (1999): Schempp CM+, *Hautarzt* 50(6), 432
Clammy skin
Dermatitis
Edema
Erythema
  (1985): Brener S+, *Contact Dermatitis* 12(4), 230
  (1983): Heskel NS+, *Contact Dermatitis* 9(4), 278
Photosensitivity
  (1999): Schempp CM+, *Hautarzt* 50(6), 432
  (1999): Wessner D+, *Contact Dermatitis* 41(4), 232
  (1995): Ortiz-Frutos FJ+, *Contact Dermatitis* 33(4), 284
  (1990): Ena P+, *Contact Dermatitis* 22(1), 63
  (1989): Goncalo S+, *Contact Dermatitis* 21(3), 200
  (1985): Brener S+, *Contact Dermatitis* 12(4), 230
  (1983): Gawkrodger DJ+, *Contact Dermatitis* 9(3), 224
  (1983): Heskel NS+, *Contact Dermatitis* 9(4), 278
Vesiculation
  (1985): Brener S+, *Contact Dermatitis* 12(4), 230
  (1983): Heskel NS+, *Contact Dermatitis* 9(4), 278

Other
Death
Seizures

SACCHARIN

Trade names: Saccharin; Sweet 'n Low
Indications: Sugar substitute
Category: Sweetening agent
Half-life: N/A

Note: Saccharin is a sulfonamide and can be absorbed systemically. Sulfonamides can produce severe, possibly fatal, reactions such as toxic epidermal necrolysis and Stevens–Johnson syndrome

Reactions

Skin
Dermatitis
  (1989): Birbeck J, *N Z Med J* 102, 24
Exanthems
Fixed eruption
Photosensitivity
Pruritus
  (1989): Birbeck J, *N Z Med J* 102, 24
Sensitivity (sic)
Urticaria
  (1989): Birbeck J, *N Z Med J* 102, 24

Mucosal/ENT
Dysgeusia

SALMETEROL

Trade names: Advair (GSK); Salmeter; Serevent (GSK); Serobid; Zantirel
Indications: Asthma
Category: Adrenergic beta2-receptor agonist
Half-life: 3–4 hours

Reactions

Skin
Angioedema
Eczema
  (1997): Leal GB, Fortaleza, Brazil (from Internet) (observation)
Exanthems
Pruritus
Rash (sic) (1–3%)
  (1994): D'Alonzo GE+, *JAMA* 271, 1412
  (1991): Hatton MQ+, *Lancet* 337, 1169
Urticaria (1–3%)
  (1991): Hatton MQF+, *Lancet* 337, 1169

Mucosal/ENT
Oral candidiasis
  (2002): Beeh KM+, *Pneumologie* 56(2), 91

Other
Death
  (2006): Currie GP+, *Drug Saf* 29(8), 647
  (2006): Dekhuijzen PN, *Ned Tijdschr Geneeskd* 150(16), 889
  (2006): Donohue JF+, *J Fam Pract* Suppl, 1
  (2006): Lang DM, *Cleve Clin J Med* 73(11), 973
  (2006): Martinez FD, *Clin Rev Allergy Immunol* 31(2–3), 269
  (2006): Salpeter SR+, *Ann Intern Med* 144(12), 904
  (2003): *Prescrire Int* 12(66), 142
Headache
Hypersensitivity (<1%)
Infections (2–12%)

(2000): Beeh KM+, *Pneumologie* (German) 54, 225 (2.7%)
Myalgia/Myositis/Myopathy/Myotoxicity (1–3%)
Paresthesias
Tremor (1–10)
  (2001): Shrewsbury S+, *Ann Allergy Asthma Immunol* 87(6), 465
  (5.7%)
  (2000): Beeh KM+, *Pneumologie* (German) 54, 225

SALSALATE

Synonyms: disalicylic acid; salicylic acid
Trade names: Argesic-SA; Artha-G; Atisuril; Disalgesic;
Marthritic; Mono-Gesic (Schwarz); Nobegyl; Salflex; Salgesic;
Salina; Umbradol
Indications: Arthritis
Category: Non-steroidal anti-inflammatory; Salicylate
Half-life: 7–8 hours
**Clinically important, potentially hazardous interactions
with:** methotrexate

Reactions

Skin
Angioedema
Dermatitis
Exanthems
Lichenoid eruption
  (2001): Powell MI+, *J Am Acad Dermatol* 45, 616
Pruritus
Purpura
Rash (sic) (1–10%)
Urticaria
  (1986): Chudwin DS+, *Ann Allergy* 57, 133

Mucosal/ENT
Tinnitus
  (1989): Montrone F+, *J Int Med Res* 17(4), 316

Nails
Nails – onychoschizia
  (2001): Powell MI+, *J Am Acad Dermatol* 45, 616

Other
Anaphylactoid reactions/Anaphylaxis (1–10%)
Hypertension
  (2002): Phillips BB+, *Ann Pharmacother* 36(4), 624

SAPROPTERIN

Trade name: Kuvan (BioMarin)
Indications: Phenylketonuria
Category: Enzyme
Half-life: 6.7 hours
**Clinically important, potentially hazardous interactions
with:** levodopa, methotrexate

Reactions

Skin
Rash (sic)

Other
Abdominal pain
Confusion

Cough
Fever
Headache
Upper respiratory infection
  (2007): Levy HL+, *Lancet* 370(9586), 504

SAQUINAVIR

Trade name: Invirase (Roche)
Indications: Advanced HIV infection
Category: Antiretroviral; Protease inhibitor, HIV
Half-life: 12 hours
**Clinically important, potentially hazardous interactions
with:** alprazolam, astemizole, clindamycin, darunavir, dasatinib,
dihydroergotamine, eplerenone, ergot derivatives, fentanyl,
garlic, ixabepilone, ketoconazole, lapatinib, methysergide,
midazolam, phenytoin, pimozide, rifampin, ritonavir, sildenafil,
solifenacin, **St John's wort**, temsirolimus

Note: Protease inhibitors cause dyslipidemia which includes elevated
triglycerides and cholesterol and redistribution of body fat centrally to
produce the so-called 'protease paunch,' breast enlargement, facial
atrophy, and 'buffalo hump'

Reactions

Skin
Acne (<2%)
Bullous dermatitis
Dermatitis (<2%)
Diaphoresis (<2%)
Eczema (<2%)
Erythema (<2%)
Erythema multiforme
  (1998): Garat H+, *Ann Dermatol Venereol* (French) 125, 42
Exanthems (<2%)
Fixed eruption
  (2000): Smith KJ+, *Cutis* 66, 29 (2 cases)
Folliculitis (<2%)
Furunculosis
Herpes simplex (<2%)
Herpes zoster (<2%)
Papulovesicular eruption
  (2000): Smith KJ+, *Cutis* 66, 29 (2 cases)
Photosensitivity (<2%)
  (1997): Winter AJ+, *Genitourin Med* 73, 323
Pigmentation (<2%)
  (2000): Smith KJ+, *Cutis* 66, 29 (2 cases)
Pruritus
  (2000): Smith KJ+, *Cutis* 66, 29 (2 cases)
Psoriasis
  (2000): Bonfanti P+, *J Acquir Immune Defic Syndr* 23(3), 236
Rash (sic) (1.3%)
Seborrheic dermatitis (<2%)
Stevens–Johnson syndrome
Ulcerations (<2%)
Urticaria (<2%)
Verrucae (<2%)
Xerosis (<2%)
  (2000): Bonfanti P+, *J Acquir Immune Defic Syndr* 23(3), 236

Mucosal/ENT
Cheilitis (<2%)
Dysgeusia (<2%)
Gingivitis (<2%)

Glossitis (<2%)
Oral ulceration (2.5%)
Stomatitis (<2%)
Tongue lesions
   (1998): Ruscin JM+, *Ann Pharmacother* 32, 1248
Xerostomia (<2%)

Hair

Hair – alopecia
Hair – changes (sic) (<2%)

Other

Candidiasis (<2%)
Gynecomastia
   (2000): Bonfanti P+, *J Acquir Immune Defic Syndr* 23(3), 236
   (1999): Donovan B+, *Int J STD AIDS* 10, 49
Headache
Lipodystrophy
   (2002): Reid S, *Can Adv Drug Reaction Newsletter* 12, 5
Paresthesias (2.6%)

SARGRAMOSTIN

(See GRANULOCYTE COLONY-STIMULATING FACTOR [GCSF])

SARSAPARILLA

Scientific names: *Smilax aristolochiaefolia; Smilax febrifuga; Smilax glabra; Smilax japicanga; Smilax officinalis; Smilax ornata; Smilax regelii; Smilax rotundifolia*
Family: Smilacaceae
Trade and other common names: Greenbriar; Horsebrier; jupicanga; khao yen; Round-leaf; Salsaparrilha; saparna; smilace; smilax; zarzaparilla
Category: Anti-inflammatory; Immunomodulator
Purported indications and other uses: blood purifier, general tonic, gout, syphilis, gonorrhea, rheumatism, wounds, arthritis, fever, cough, scrofula, hypertension, digestive disorders, psoriasis, skin diseases, cancer
Half-life: N/A
Clinically important, potentially hazardous interactions with: digoxin

Reactions

None

SAW PALMETTO

Scientific names: *Sabal serrulata; Serenoa repens; Serenoa serrulata*
Family: Arecaceae; Palmae
Trade and other common names: American Dwarf Palm Tree; Cabbage Palm; Ju-Zhong; Palmier Nain; Sabal Fructus
Category: 5-alpha-reductase inhibitor; Anti-inflammatory; Hormone modulator
Purported indications and other uses: Benign prostatic hyperplasia, diuretic, sedative, prostate cancer (with other herbs), aphrodisiac, hair growth, colds, coughs, sore throat, asthma, chronic bronchitis, migraine
Half-life: N/A
Clinically important, potentially hazardous interactions with: oral contraceptives, warfarin

Reactions

Skin

Adverse effects (sic)
   (2002): Ernst E, *Ann Intern Med* 136(1), 42
   (2002): Mattsson K+, *Lakartidningen* 99(50), 5095
   (2002): Wilt T+, *Cochrane Database Syst Rev* imed(3), CD00
Hemorrhage
   (2001): Cheema P+, *J Intern Med* 250(2), 167
Sensitization
   (2002): Sinclair RD+, *Australas J Dermatol* 43(4), 311

Other

Hepatotoxicity
   (2006): Jibrin I+, *South Med J* 99(6), 611

SCOPOLAMINE

Trade names: Isopto Hyoscine Ophthalmic; Scopace; Scopase; Scopoderm-TTS; Transderm-Scop Patch (Novartis); Transdermal-V
Indications: Nausea and vomiting, excess salivation
Category: Anticholinergic; Muscarinic antagonist
Half-life: 8 hours
Clinically important, potentially hazardous interactions with: anticholinergics, arbutamine

Note: Systemic adverse effects have been reported following ophthalmic administration

Reactions

Skin

Allergic reactions (sic)
   (2001): Decraene T+, *Contact Dermatitis* 45(5), 309
Dermatitis (transdermal patch and ophthalmic)
   (2006): Nachum Z+, *Clin Pharmacokinet* 45(6), 543 (10%)
   (1990): Hogan DJ+, *J Am Acad Dermatol* 22, 811
   (1989): Gordon CR+, *BMJ* 298(6682), 1220
   (1989): Holdiness MR, *Contact Dermatitis* 20, 3
   (1988): van der Willigen AH+, *J Am Acad Dermatol* 18, 146
   (1985): Clissold SP+, *Drugs* 29, 189
   (1985): Trozak DJ, *J Am Acad Dermatol* 13, 247
   (1984): Fisher AA, *Cutis* 34, 526
Edema (<1%) (ophthalmic)
Erythema
   (2006): Nachum Z+, *Clin Pharmacokinet* 45(6), 543
Erythema multiforme

(1986): Fisher AA, *Cutis* 37, 158; 262
Exanthems
  (1985): Clissold SP+, *Drugs* 29, 189 (transdermal patch)
Fixed eruption
  (1981): Kanwar AJ+, *Dermatologica* 162, 378
Photosensitivity (1–10%)
Rash (sic) (<1%)
Urticaria
Xerosis (>10%)

Mucosal/ENT
Oral lesions (>5%)
  (1985): Clissold SP+, *Drugs* 29, 189 (transdermal patch) (>5%)
Xerostomia (>60%)
  (2006): Nachum Z+, *Clin Pharmacokinet* 45(6), 543 (50%)
  (2002): Kranke P+, *Anesth Analg* 95(1), 133
  (1989): Parrott AC, *Aviat Space Environ Med* 60(1), 1
  (1985): Clissold SP+, *Drugs* 29, 189 (transdermal patch) (66%)
  (1985): van Marion WF+, *Clin Pharmacol Ther* 38(3), 301
  (1981): Price NM+, *Clin Pharmacol Ther* 29, 414

Eyes
Dilated pupils
  (2006): Firth AY+, *Dev Med Child Neurol* 48(2), 137
Reduced visual acuity
  (2006): Firth AY+, *Dev Med Child Neurol* 48(2), 137
Vision blurred
  (1989): Parrott AC, *Aviat Space Environ Med* 60(1), 1
Visual hallucinations
  (2006): Jimenez-Jimenez FJ+, *Rev Neurol* 43(10), 603 (with
    atropine & phenylephrine)

Other
Anaphylactoid reactions/Anaphylaxis
  (1995): Manhart AR+, *J Toxicol Clin Toxicol* 33, 189 (fatal)
  (1994): Watanabe F+, *J Toxicol Clin Toxicol* 32, 593 (fatal)
Death
Headache
  (2006): Nachum Z+, *Clin Pharmacokinet* 45(6), 543
Injection-site irritation (>10%)
Vertigo
  (2002): Kranke P+, *Anesth Analg* 95(1), 133

SECOBARBITAL

Synonym: quinalbarbitone
Trade names: Immenoctal; Novo-Secobarb; Secanal; Seconal
(Ranbaxy)
Indications: Insomnia
Category: Barbiturate
Half-life: 15–40 hours
**Clinically important, potentially hazardous interactions
with: alcohol**, anticoagulants, antihistamines, brompheniramine,
buclizine, chlorpheniramine, dicumarol, ethanolamine, imatinib,
warfarin

Reactions

Skin
Angioedema (<1%)
Exanthems
Exfoliative dermatitis (<1%)
Purpura
Rash (sic) (<1%)
Stevens–Johnson syndrome (<1%)
Urticaria

Other
Headache
Hypersensitivity
Injection-site pain (>10%)
Rhabdomyolysis
  (1990): Larpin R+, *Presse Med* 19(30), 1403
Serum sickness
Thrombophlebitis (<1%)

SECRETIN

Trade name: Secretin-Ferring (Ferring)
Indications: Diagnosis of gastrinoma (Zollinger–Ellison
syndrome)
Category: Hormone, polypeptide
Half-life: N/A

Reactions

Skin
Allergic reactions (sic)
Urticaria

Other
Injection-site reactions (sic)

SELEGILINE

Synonyms: deprenyl; L-deprenyl
Trade names: Apo-Selegiline; Carbex; Eldeprine; Eldepryl
(Somerset); Emsam; Jumex; Movergan; Novo-Selegiline; Plurimen
Indications: Parkinsonism
Category: Antidepressant; Monoamine oxidase B inhibitor
Half-life: 9 minutes
**Clinically important, potentially hazardous interactions
with:** carbidopa, citalopram, doxepin, **ephedra**, ephedrine,
escitalopram, fluoxetine, fluvoxamine, levodopa, meperidine,
moclobemide, nefazodone, oral contraceptives, paroxetine,
sertraline, venlafaxine

Reactions

Skin
Diaphoresis
Peripheral edema
Photosensitivity
Rash (sic)

Mucosal/ENT
Dysgeusia
Oral ulceration
  (2003): *Prescrire Int* 12(67), 179
Stomatitis
  (2003): *Prescrire Int* 12(67), 179
Tinnitus
Xerostomia (>10%)
  (1988): Golbe LI+, *Clin Neuropharmacol* 11, 45

Hair
Hair – alopecia
Hair – hypertrichosis (facial)

Other

Application-site reactions (sic)
(2006): Amsterdam JD+, *J Clin Psychopharmacol* 26(6), 579
(15%)
(2006): Feiger AD+, *J Clin Psychiatry* 67(9), 1354
(2002): Bodkin JA+, *Am J Psychiatry* 159(11), 1869
Death
(2002): *Prescrire Int* 11(60), 108
Headache
Paresthesias
Seizures
(2006): Baumann P+, *J Clin Psychopharmacol* 26(6), 679
Tremor

SELENIUM

Trade names: Bio-Active Selenium (Solaray); Exsel Shampoo; Head & Shoulders Intensive Treatment Dandruff Shampoo (Procter & Gamble); Selenate; Selenite; selenium dioxide; selenium sulfide; selenocysteine; SelenoMax (Source Naturals); selenomethionine; Selsun Blue (Chattem); Selsun Shampoo (Chattem); Vpak51
Indications: Anticancer (stomach, colorectal, lung, prostate), arthritis, asthma, heart disease, HIV inhibitor. Treatment of dandruff, fungal infections (tinea versicolor), and seborrhea
Category: Antioxidant; Trace element
Half-life: 12–41 hours; Selenomethionine: 252 days, Selinite: 102 days
Clinically important, potentially hazardous interactions with: cholesterol-lowering drugs, cisplatin, clozapine, dimercaprol, niacin, oral corticosteroids, simvastatin

Note: Selenium is an essential component of glutathione peroxidase. Inadequate concentrations of dietry selenium account, in part, for Keshan disease (a fatal cardiomyopathy)

Reactions

Skin

Adverse effects (sic)
(1994): Yang G+, *J Trace Elem Electrolytes Health Dis* 8(3–4), 159
(chronic exposure)
(1989): Stacchini A+, *J Trace Elem Electrolytes Health Dis*
3(4), 193
Allergic reactions (sic)
Carcinoma
(2001): Vinceti M+, *Rev Environ Health* 16(4), 233 (chronic exposure)
(2000): Vinceti M+, *J Clin Epidemiol* 53(10), 1062 (chronic exposure)
(2000): Vinceti M+, *Sci Total Environ* 250(1–3), 1 (chronic exposure)
(1999): Barceloux DG, *J Toxicol Clin Toxicol* 37(2), 145 (deficiency)
(1997): Foster LH+, *Crit Rev Food Sci Nutr* 37(3), 211 (deficiency)
Dermatitis
(2001): Vinceti M+, *Rev Environ Health* 16(4), 233 (chronic exposure)
Diaphoresis
Erythema chronicum persistans
(2003): Smith S, Louisville, KY (from Internet) (observation)
Lupus erythematosus (from deficiency)
Melanoma

(1998): Vinceti M+, *Cancer Epidemiol Biomarkers Prev* 7(10), 853
(chronic exposure)
Photosensitivity
Pruritus
Rash (sic)
Scleroderma (deficiency)

Mucosal/ENT

Dysgeusia (metallic taste)
Sialorrhea

Hair

Hair – alopecia
(2001): Vinceti M+, *Rev Environ Health* 16(4), 233 (chronic exposure)
(1996): Whanger P+, *Ann Clin Lab Sci* 26(2), 99 (chronic exposure)
Hair – brittle
(1994): Yang G+, *J Trace Elem Electrolytes Health Dis* 8(3–4), 159 (chronic exposure)
Hair – changes (sic)
(1999): Barceloux DG, *J Toxicol Clin Toxicol* 37(2), 145 (chronic exposure)
(1997): Hathcock JN, *Am J Clinical Nutrition* 66, 427
Hair – pigmentation

Nails

Nails – brittle
(1997): Hathcock JN, *Am J Clinical Nutrition* 66, 427
(1996): Whanger P+, *Ann Clin Lab Sci* 26(2), 99 (chronic exposure)
(1995): Yang GQ+, *Biomed Environ Sci* 8(3), 187 (deficiency)
(1994): Yang G+, *J Trace Elem Electrolytes Health Dis* 8(3–4), 159 (chronic exposure)
Nails – loss
(2001): Vinceti M+, *Rev Environ Health* 16(4), 233 (chronic exposure)
Nails – paronychia
Nails – white streaking

Other

Death (overdose)
Infections
Myalgia/Myositis/Myopathy/Myotoxicity
Paresthesias
Tremor

SENNA

Scientific names: *Cassia acutifolia; Cassia angustifolia; Cassia obtusifloia; Cassia senna; Cassia tora; Senna alexandrina; Senna obtusifolia; Senna tora*
Family: Caesalpiniaceae; Fabaceae
Trade and other common names: Agiolax; Agoral (Numark); Alesandrian; Black-Draught (Monticello); Cassia leaf; Ex-Lax (Novartis); Fletcher's Castoria (Mentholatum); Gentlax ; Glysennid; Goldline Senna; Herbal Trim Tea; Khartoum senna; Laci Le Beau Corp; Manevac; Perdiem (Novartis); PMS-Sennosides; Prodiem Plus (Novartis); Riva-Senna; Senexon; Senna alexxandrina; Senna Lax; Senna-Gen; Sennatab; Senokot; Senolax; Super Dieter's Tea; X-Prep
Category: Stimulant laxative
Purported indications and other uses: Laxative, cathartic, cholagogue, purgative
Half-life: N/A
Clinically important, potentially hazardous interactions with: digoxin, quinidine, **squill**

Note: Part used: Leaves and/or seed pods

Reactions

Skin
 Acute generalized exanthematous pustulosis (AGEP)
  (2003): Bonnetblanc JM+, *Ann Dermatol Venereol* 130(1 Pt 1), 59
 Adverse effects (sic)
  (1996): Sykes NP, *J Pain Symptom Manage* 11(6), 363
  (1993): Passmore AP+, *Pharmacology* 47, 249
  (1988): Jagjivan B+, *Br J Radiol* 61(729), 853
 Allergic reactions (sic)
  (1991): Marks GB+, *Am Rev Respir Dis* 144(5), 1065
 Bullous dermatitis
  (2003): Spiller HA+, *Ann Pharmacother* 37(5), 636
 Dermatitis
  (2001): Leventhal JM+, *Pediatrics* 107(1), 178
 Edema
 Erythema multiforme
  (2006): Sugita K+, *Int J Dermatol* 45(9), 1123
 Exfoliative dermatitis
  (2003): Spiller HA+, *Ann Pharmacother* 37(5), 636
 Pruritus
 Rash (sic)
 Side effects (sic)

Eyes
 Rhinoconjunctivitis (occupational exposure)

Other
 Death (from abuse)

SERMORELIN

Trade names: Geref (Merck); Gerel
Category: Growth hormone-releasing hormone analog
Half-life: ~12 minutes
Clinically important, potentially hazardous interactions with: aspirin, drugs affecting pituitary secretion of somatotropin, glucocorticoids, indomethacin, insulin

Reactions

Skin
 Pallor
 Pruritus
 Urticaria

Mucosal/ENT
 Dysgeusia
 Dysphagia

Other
 Injection-site edema
 Injection-site erythema
 Injection-site pain
 Vertigo

SERTACONAZOLE

Trade name: Ertaczo Cream (Ortho)
Indications: Tinea pedis
Category: Antibiotic, imidazole
Half-life: N/A

Reactions

Skin
 Burning
 Dermatitis
  (1995): Goday JJ+, *Contact Dermatitis* 32(6), 370
 Desquamation
 Erythema
 Pigmentation
 Pruritus
 Tenderness (2%)
 Vesiculation
 Xerosis

Other
 Application-site reactions (sic)

SERTRALINE

Trade names: Atruline; Zoloft (Pfizer)
Indications: Depression, panic disorders, obsessive compulsive disorders
Category: Antidepressant; Selective serotonin reuptake inhibitor
Half-life: 24–26 hours
Clinically important, potentially hazardous interactions with: amphetamines, astemizole, clarithromycin, dextroamphetamine, diethylpropion, erythromycin, isocarboxazid, linezolid, MAO inhibitors, mazindol, methamphetamine, metoclopramide, phendimetrazine, phenelzine, phentermine, phenylpropanolamine, pimozide, pseudoephedrine, selegiline, sibutramine, **St John's wort**, sumatriptan, sympathomimetics, tranylcypromine, trazodone, troleandomycin, zolmitriptan

Reactions

Skin
 Acne (<1%)

Acute generalized exanthematous pustulosis (AGEP)
  (2001): Thedenat B+, *Dermatology* 203(1), 87
Allergic reactions (sic)
  (1998): Beauquier B+, *Encephale* (French) 24, 62
  (1991): Guthrie SK, *Drug Intell Clin Pharm* 25, 952
Angioedema
  (2001): Adson DE+, *Ann Pharmacother* 35(11), 1375
  (1994): Gales BJ+, *Am J Hosp Pharm* 51, 118
Bullous dermatitis (<1%)
  (2004): Kirkup ME+, *Br J Dermatol* 150(1), 164
Dermatitis (<1%)
Diaphoresis (8.4%)
  (2002): Ahmed A, *Am J Geriatr Psychiatry* 10(4), 484
  (2002): Fisher AA+, *Ann Pharmacother* 36(1), 67
  (2000): Henney JE, *JAMA* 283, 596
  (1991): Guthrie SK, *Drug Intell Clin Pharm* 25, 952
  (1990): Reimherr FW+, *J Clin Psychiatry* 51, 18
  (1988): Doogan DP+, *J Clin Psychiatry* 49, 46
Edema (<1%)
Erythema
Erythema multiforme (<1%)
  (1994): Gales BJ+, *Am J Hosp Pharm* 51, 118
Exanthems (<1%)
  (2000): Fernandes B+, *Contact Dermatitis* 42, 287
  (2000): Kittay SA (from Internet) (observation)
  (1999): Blumenthal HL, Beachwood, OH (personal case) (observation)
  (1998): Litt JZ, Beachwood, OH (personal case) (observation)
Fixed eruption
  (1997): Sawada KY, Wheat Ridge, CO (from Internet) (observation)
Lupus erythematosus
  (1998): Hill VA+, *J R Army Med Corps* 144, 109
Necrosis
  (2004): Kirkup ME+, *Br J Dermatol* 150(1), 164
Photosensitivity (<1%)
Pigmentation (<1%)
Pruritus (<1%)
  (1999): Blumenthal HL, Beachwood, OH (personal case) (observation)
Purpura (<1%)
Rash (sic) (2.1%)
Stevens–Johnson syndrome
  (1999): Jan V+, *Acta Derm Venereol* 79, 401
Urticaria (<1%)
Xerosis (<1%)

Mucosal/ENT
Aphthous stomatitis (<1%)
Balanitis (<1%)
Bromhidrosis (<1%)
Dysgeusia
Gingival hyperplasia/hypertrophy (<1%)
Glossitis (<1%)
Sialorrhea (<1%)
Stomatitis (<1%)
Tinnitus
Tongue edema (<1%)
Tongue ulceration (<1%)
Vaginitis (atrophic)
Xerostomia (16.3%)
  (2004): Chung MY+, *Hum Psychopharmacol* 19(7), 489 (19.6%)
  (2000): Brady K+, *JAMA* 283, 1837
  (1992): Berman H+, *Hosp Community Psychiatry* 43, 671
  (1991): Guthrie SK, *Drug Intell Clin Pharm* 25, 952
  (1990): Reimherr FW+, *J Clin Psychiatry* 51, 18
  (1988): Doogan DP+, *J Clin Psychiatry* 49, 46

Hair
Hair – abnormal texture (<1%)
Hair – alopecia (<1%)
  (2006): Hedenmalm K+, *Pharmacoepidemiol Drug Saf* 15(10), 719 (27 cases)
  (1996): Bourgeois JA, *J Clin Psychopharmacol* 16, 91
Hair – hirsutism (<1%)

Eyes
Periorbital edema (<1%)

Other
Death
  (2002): Musshoff F+, *Arch Kriminol* 210(1), 51
  (2001): Fartoux-Heymann L+, *J Hepatol* 35(5), 683
  (2001): Gillespie JA, *Ann Pharmacother* 35(12), 1671
  (2001): Hoehns JD+, *Ann Pharmacother* 35(7), 862 (with clozapine)
Gynecomastia (<1%)
  (1994): Hall MJ, *Am J Psychiatry* 151(9), 1395
Headache
Inappropriate secretion of antidiuretic hormone (SIADH)
  (1997): Bouman WP+, *Am J Psychiatry* 154(4), 580
  (1996): Bradley ME+, *Pharmacotherapy* 16(4), 680
  (1996): Goldstein L+, *Am J Psychiatry* 153(5), 732
  (1996): Kessler J+, *N Engl J Med* 335(7), 524
  (1996): Liu BA+, *CMAJ* 155(5), 519 (11.7%)
  (1995): Bluff DD+, *Ann Intern Med* 123(10), 811
  (1995): Jackson C+, *Am J Psychiatry* 152(5), 809
  (1995): Thornton SL+, *Am J Psychiatry* 152(5), 809
  (1994): Doshi D+, *Am J Psychiatry* 151(5), 779
  (1994): Llorente MD+, *J Clin Psychiatry* 55(12), 543
  (1993): Crews JR+, *Am J Psychiatry* 150(10), 1564
Mania
  (2003): Mendhekar DN+, *Acta Psychiatr Scand* 108(1), 70
  (2001): Ramasubbu R, *Acta Psychiatr Scand* 104(3), 236
  (1994): Ghaziuddin M, *Am J Psychiatry* 151(6), 944
Paresthesias (2%)
  (2006): Ozalp E+, *Prog Neuropsychopharmacol Biol Psychiatry* 30(7), 1337
Seizures
  (1996): Goldstein L+, *Am J Psychiatry* 153(5), 732
Tremor (1–10%)
  (2002): No Author, *Prescrire Int* 11(59), 69

SEVOFLURANE

Trade names: Sevorane; Ultane (Abbott)
Indications: Induction and maintenance of general anesthesia
Category: Anesthetic, inhalation
Half-life: 15–23 hours
Clinically important, potentially hazardous interactions with: N/A

Reactions

Skin
Pruritus (~1%)
Rash (sic) (~1%)
Shivering (6%)

Mucosal/ENT
Dysgeusia
Sialorrhea (4%)
Xerostomia (~1%)

Eyes
Amblyopia (~1%)
Conjunctivitis (~1%)

Other
Asthenia (~1%)
Cough (5%)
Fever (1%)
Headache (1%)
Hepatotoxicity
  (2005): Jang Y+, *Paediatr Anaesth* 15(12), 1140
Hypertension (~1%)
Hypotension (~1%)
  (2005): Nagata S+, *Radiat Med* 23(6), 427
Pain (~1%)
Rhabdomyolysis
  (2002): Vorrakitpokatorn P+, *J Med Assoc Thai* 85, S884
Seizures
  (2006): Poon KS+, *Acta Anaesthesiol Taiwan* 44(2), 123
  (2006): Ruffmann C+, *Expert Rev Neurother* 6(4), 575
  (2002): Kuczkowski KM, *Anaesthesia* 57(12), 1234
Stroke
  (2005): Nagata S+, *Radiat Med* 23(6), 427

SIBERIAN GINSENG

Scientific names: *Acanthopanax senticosus; Eleutherococcus senticosus*
Family: Araliaceae
Trade and other common names: Ciwuija; Devil's root; Eleuthero; Ezoukogi; Medexport; Shigoka; Taiga Wurzel; Touch-me-not
Category: Immunomodulator
Purported indications and other uses: Alzheimer's disease, anaphylaxis, arthritis, colds, depression, fatigue, flu, impotence, infertility, menopause, multiple sclerosis, osteoporosis, perimenopause, PMS, stress
Half-life: N/A
Clinically important, potentially hazardous interactions with: antihypertensives, digoxin

Reactions

Other
Headache

SIBUTRAMINE

Trade name: Meridia (Abbott)
Indications: Obesity
Category: Norepinephrine antagonist; Serotonin antagonist
Half-life: 1.1 hours
Clinically important, potentially hazardous interactions with: desvenlafaxine, dextromethorphan, dihydroergotamine, **ephedra**, ergot, fluoxetine, fluvoxamine, isocarboxazid, linezolid, lithium, MAO inhibitors, meperidine, methysergide, naratriptan, nefazodone, paroxetine, phenelzine, rizatriptan, sertraline, sumatriptan, tranylcypromine, **tryptophan**, venlafaxine, verapamil, zolmitriptan

Reactions

Skin
Acne (1.0%)
Allergic reactions (sic) (1.5%)
Diaphoresis (2.5%)
Edema (2%)
Herpes simplex (1.3%)
Peripheral edema (>1%)
Pruritus (>1%)
Rash (sic) (3.8%)
Xerosis
  (2003): Fanghanel G+, *Adv Ther* 20(2), 101

Mucosal/ENT
Dysgeusia (2.2%)
Vulvovaginal candidiasis (1.2%)
Xerostomia (17.2%)
  (2005): Milano W+, *Adv Ther* 22(1), 25
  (2005): Violante-Ortiz R+, *Adv Ther* 22(6), 642
  (2004): Kaya A+, *Biomed Pharmacother* 58(10), 582
  (2003): Appolinario JC+, *Arch Gen Psychiatry* 60(11), 1109
  (2001): Bray GA, *Rev Endocr Metab Disord* 2(4), 403
  (2001): Scheen AJ, *Rev Med Liege* 56(9), 656

Other
Asthenia
  (2001): Bray GA, *Rev Endocr Metab Disord* 2(4), 403
Death
  (2002): London, *Reuters Health Information* 3-26-02 (2 cases)
Headache
  (2005): Martinez D+, *Sleep Med* 6(5), 467
  (2004): Gomis Barbara R, *Rev Med Univ Navarra* 48(2), 63
  (2004): Kaya A+, *Biomed Pharmacother* 58(10), 582
  (2003): Fanghanel G+, *Adv Ther* 20(2), 101
Hepatotoxicity
  (2005): Chounta A+, *Ann Intern Med* 143(10), 763
Hypertension
  (2005): Violante-Ortiz R+, *Adv Ther* 22(6), 642
  (2004): Gomis Barbara R, *Rev Med Univ Navarra* 48(2), 63
Myalgia/Myositis/Myopathy/Myotoxicity (1.9%)
Paresthesias (2.0%)
Vertigo
  (2004): Ning G+, *Zhonghua Yi Xue Za Zhi* 84(15), 1243 (3%)

SILDENAFIL

Trade name: Viagra (Pfizer)
Indications: Erectile dysfunction, Hypertension
Category: Phosphodiesterase type 5 inhibitor
Half-life: 4 hours
Clinically important, potentially hazardous interactions with: amprenavir, amyl nitrite, atazanavir, delavirdine, erythromycin, fosamprenavir, indinavir, isosorbide dinitrate, isosorbide mononitrate, itraconazole, ketoconazole, nelfinavir, nitrates, nitroglycerin, ritonavir, saquinavir

Reactions

Skin
Allergic reactions (sic) (<2%)
Dermatitis (<2%)
Diaphoresis (<2%)
  (2004): Deveci S+, *Int J Urol* 11(11), 989
Edema (<2%)

Exfoliative dermatitis (<2%)
(2002): Smith JG, Mobile, AL (from Internet) (observation)
Facial edema (<2%)
Fixed eruption (urticarial)
(1998): Reed BR, Denver, CO (from Internet) (observation)
Genital edema (<2%)
Herpes simplex (<2%)
Lichenoid eruption
(2005): Antiga E+, J Dermatol 32(12), 972
(2000): Goldman BD, Cutis 66, 282
Peripheral edema (<2%)
Photosensitivity (<2%)
Pruritus (<2%)
Rash (sic) (2%)
Ulcerations (<2%)
Urticaria (<2%)

Mucosal/ENT
Gingivitis (<2%)
Glossitis (<2%)
Rhinitis
(2003): Berman JR+, J Urol 170(6 Pt 1), 2333
Stomatitis (<2%)
Tinnitus
(2007): Buranakitjaroen P+, J Med Assoc Thai 90(6), 1100
(2002): Hamzavi J+, Wien Klin Wochenschr 114(1-2), 54
Xerostomia (<2%)

Eyes
Dyschromatopsia (3–11%) (blue-green vision)
(2003): Prescrire Int 12(65), 98
(2002): Coelho OR, Int J Impot Res 14, S54
(2002): Laties A+, Prog Retin Eye Res 21(5), 485
(1998): Craig D+, Cleveland Clinic Foundation 52, 963 (11%)
Macular infarction
(2005): Quiram P+, Graefes Arch Clin Exp Ophthalmol 243(4), 339
Ocular pigmentation (<2%)
Optic neuropathy
(2006): Bella AJ+, Can J Urol 13(5), 3233
(2006): Gorkin L+, Int J Clin Pract 60(4), 500 (%)
(2005): Egan RA+, Arch Ophthalmol 123(5), 709
(2005): Gruhn N+, Acta Ophthalmol Scand 83(1), 131
(2005): Pomeranz HD+, J Neuroophthalmol 25(1), 9 (7 cases)
(2003): Prescrire Int 12(65), 98
(2003): Gandhi JS, Ophthalmology 110(9), 1860
(2002): Boshier A+, Int J Clin Pharmacol Ther 40(9), 422
(2002): Dheer S+, J Assoc Physicians India 50, 265
(2002): Pomeranz HD+, Ophthalmology 109(3), 584
(2001): Cunningham AV+, J Neuroophthalmol 21(1), 22
(2000): Egan R+, Arch Ophthalmol 118(2), 291
Vision loss
(2005): Med Lett Drugs Ther 47(1211), 49
Visual disturbances
(2006): Fava M+, J Clin Psychiatry 67(2), 240 (3%)
Visual hallucinations
(2006): Sharma RK+, Am J Kidney Dis 48(1), 128 (1 case)
Visual halos
(2002): Potter MJ+, Ophthalmology 109(5), 823

Other
Death
(2002): Dumestre-Toulet V+, Forensic Sci Int 126(1), 71
Gynecomastia (<2%)
Headache (4–19%)
(2006): Blonde L, Curr Med Res Opin 22(11), 2111 (5%)
(2006): de L Figuerola M+, Cephalalgia 26(5), 617
(2006): Heymann WR, J Am Acad Dermatol 55(3), 501
(2006): Oliver JJ+, Hypertension 48(4), 622

(2005): Sunwoo S+, Int J Impot Res 17(1), 71 (2.6%)
(2005): Woodall T, Rock Hill, SC (from Internet) (observation)
(2004): DeBusk RF+, Am J Cardiol 93(2), 147
(2004): Deveci S+, Int J Urol 11(11), 989
(2003): Berman JR+, J Urol 170(6 Pt 1), 2333
(2003): Carson CC, Expert Opin Pharmacother 4(3), 397
(2003): Govier F+, Clin Ther 25(11), 2709 (8.8%)
(2003): Raina R+, Urology 62(6), 1103
(2003): Stroberg P+, Clin Ther 25(11), 2724 (4.5%)
(2002): Becher E+, Int J Impot Res 14, S33
(2002): Coelho OR, Int J Impot Res 14, S54 (19%)
(2002): Glina S+, Int J Impot Res 14, S27
Hypotension
(2006): Nieminen T+, Clin Drug Investig 26(11), 667 (with tamsulosin)
Myalgia/Myositis/Myopathy/Myotoxicity (<2%)
(2006): Heymann WR, J Am Acad Dermatol 55(3), 501
(2006): Oliver JJ+, Hypertension 48(4), 622
Paresthesias (<2%)
Seizures
(2002): Gilad R+, BMJ 325(7369), 869
Stroke
(2006): Habek M+, Clin Neuropharmacol 29(3), 165

SIMVASTATIN

Trade names: Denan; Lipex; Liponorm; Lodales; Simovil; Sivastin; Vytorin; Zocor (Merck); Zocord
Indications: Hypercholesterolemia
Category: HMG-CoA reductase inhibitor; Statin
Half-life: 1.9 hours
Clinically important, potentially hazardous interactions with: amiodarone, atazanavir, azithromycin, bosentan, ciprofibrate, clarithromycin, clopidogrel, cyclosporine, darunavir, delavirdine, diltiazem, erythromycin, fosamprenavir, fusidic acid, gemfibrozil, **grapefruit juice**, imatinib, itraconazole, rabeprazole, ranolazine, **red rice yeast**, ritonavir, roxithromycin, selenium, **St John's wort**, tacrolimus, telithromycin, tipranavir, verapamil, warfarin

Note: Vytorin is a combination of ezetimibe and simvastatin

Reactions

Skin
Acute generalized exanthematous pustulosis
(2003): Oskay T+, Clin Exp Dermatol 28(5), 558
Angioedema
Dermatomyositis
(2004): Vasconcelos OM+, Muscle Nerve 30(6), 803
(1995): Hill C+, Aust N Z J Med 25(6), 745
(1994): Khattak FH+, Br J Rheumatol 32(2), 199
Diaphoresis
(1991): Scott RS+, N Z Med J 104, 493
Eczema
(1995): Proksch E, Hautarzt (German) 46, 76
(1993): Feldmann R+, Dermatology 186, 272
(1993): Krasovec M+, Dermatology 186, 248
(1991): Steyn K+, S Afr Med J 79, 639
Eosinophilic fasciitis
(2001): Choquet-Kastylevsky G+, Arch Intern Med 161(11), 1456
Erythema multiforme
(1993): Feldmann R+, Dermatology 186, 272
Erythema nodosum
Exanthems
(1991): McDowell IF+, Br J Clin Pharmacol 31, 340

Lichen planus
  (1991): Steyn K+, *S Afr Med J* 79, 639
Lichen planus pemphigoides
  (2003): Stoebner PE+, *Ann Dermatol Venereol* 130(2 Pt 1), 187
Lichenoid eruption
  (1994): Roger D+, *Clin Exp Dermatol* 19, 88
Lupus erythematosus
  (2000): Ahmad A+, *Tenn Med* 93(1), 21
  (1998): Hanson J+, *Lancet* 352, 1070
  (1998): Khosia R+, *South Med J* 91, 873
  (1992): Bannwarth B+, *Arch Intern Med* 152, 1093
Lupus syndrome
  (2004): Noel B+, *Dermatology* 208(3), 276
Peripheral edema
  (1991): Borland Y+, *Nephron* 57, 365
Petechiae
  (1997): Horiuchi Y+, *J Dermatol* 24, 549
Photo-recall
  (1995): Abadir R+, *Clin Oncol R Coll Radiol* 7, 325
Photosensitivity
  (2002): Hare CB+, *Clin Infect Dis* 35(10), e111
  (2002): Holme SA+, *Photodermatol Photoimmunol Photomed* 18(6), 313
  (1998): Granados MT+, *Contact Dermatitis* 38, 294
  (1995): Morimoto K+, *Contact Dermatitis* 33, 274
  (1991): Brocard JJ+, *Schweiz Med Wochenschr* (German) 121, 977
Pruritus
  (1993): Feldmann R+, *Dermatology* 186, 272
  (1991): Steyn K+, *S Afr Med J* 79, 639
Purpura
  (1998): Koduri PR, *Lancet* 352, 2020
  (1998): McCarthy LJ+, *Lancet* 352, 1284
  (1991): Steyn K+, *S Afr Med J* 79, 639
Pustules
Rash (sic) (1–10%)
  (2001): Coverman M, *The Schoch Letter* 51, 23 (with atorvastatin)
  (1993): Feldmann R+, *Dermatology* 186, 272
  (1990): Ziegler O+, *Cardiology* 77 (Suppl 4), 50
Rosacea
  (1991): Brocard JJ+, *Schweiz Med Wochenschr* (German) 121, 977
Stevens–Johnson syndrome
Toxic epidermal necrolysis
Urticaria
Vasculitis

Mucosal/ENT

Cheilitis
  (1998): Mehregan DR+, *Cutis* 62, 197
Dysgeusia (<1%)
  (1991): Saito Y+, *Arterioscler Thromb* 11, 816

Hair

Hair – alopecia
  (1999): Litt JZ, Beachwood, OH (personal case) (observation)
  (1998): Robb-Nicholson C, *Harv Womens Health Watch* 5, 8 (anecdote)
  (1997): Shelley WB+, *Cutis* 60, 20 (observation)
  (1995): Litt JZ, Beachwood, OH (personal case) (observation)
  (1994): Litt JZ, Beachwood, OH (personal case) (observation)

Other

Anaphylactoid reactions/Anaphylaxis
Asthenia (9%)
  (2004): Zhao XQ+, *Am J Cardiol* 93(3), 307 (9%) (with niacin)
Death
  (2002): Hare CB+, *Clin Infect Dis* 35(10), e111 (with nelfinavir)

  (2001): Federman DG+, *South Med J* 94(10), 1023
  (2000): Weise WJ+, *Am J Med* 108(4), 351
Gynecomastia
Headache
Hepatotoxicity
  (2006): Alla V+, *J Clin Gastroenterol* 40(8), 757 (2 cases)
  (2006): Ricaurte B+, *Ann Pharmacother* 40(4), 753 (with amiodarone)
Hypersensitivity
Myalgia/Myositis/Myopathy/Myotoxicity (1–10%)
  (2007): Boltan DD+, *Am J Cardiol* 99(8), 1171 (fatal)
  (2006): Baker SK+, *Muscle Nerve* 34(4), 478 (Rippling disease)
  (2004): Zhao XQ+, *Am J Cardiol* 93(3), 307 (5%) (with niacin)
  (2003): Litt JZ, Beachwood, OH (personal case) (observation)
  (2003): Olsson AG+, *Clin Ther* 25(1), 119 (2.4%)
  (2003): Rogge N+, *Schweiz Rundsch Med Prax* 92(20), 965
  (2002): Hsu WC+, *Clin Neuropharmacol* 25(5), 266 (with colchicine)
  (2002): Litt JZ, Beachwood, OH (personal observation)
  (2002): Sinzinger H, *Wien Klin Wochenschr* 114(21), 943
  (2002): Udawat H+, *J Assoc Physicians India* 50, 439
  (2001): Litt JZ, Beachwood, OH (personal case)
  (2001): Rehbein H, Jacksonville, FL (from Internet) (observation)
  (1998): Galper JB, *Am J Cardiol* 81(2), 259
  (1995): Garnett WR, *Am J Health Syst Pharm* 52(15), 1639
  (1994): al-Jubouri MA+, *BMJ* 308, 588
  (1991): Deslypere JP+, *Ann Intern Med* 114, 342
  (1990): Bilheimer DW, *Cardiology* 77 (Suppl 4), 58
Paresthesias
Polymyositis
  (2003): Riesco-Eizaguirre G+, *Rev Neurol* 37(10), 934
Porphyria cutanea tarda
  (1994): Perrot JL+, *Ann Dermatol Venereol* (French) 121, 817
Rhabdomyolysis
  (2007): Akram K+, *Int J Cardiol* 118(1), e19 (with ketoconazole)
  (2007): Molden E+, *Pharmacotherapy* 27(4), 603 (with erythromycin and Clarithromycin)
  (2006): Ricaurte B+, *Ann Pharmacother* 40(4), 753 (with amiodarone)
  (2006): Ronaldson KJ+, *Drug Saf* 29(11), 1061
  (2006): Schreiber DH+, *J Emerg Med* 31(2), 177
  (2005): Andrejak M+, *Therapie* 60(3), 299
  (2005): Finsterer J+, *South Med J* 98(8), 827
  (2005): Sochman J+, *Int J Cardiol* 99(1), 145
  (2005): Tong J+, *Bone Marrow Transplant* 36(8), 739 (with cyclosporine)
  (2004): Baker SK+, *Muscle Nerve* 30(6), 799 (with colchicine)
  (2004): Bhatia V, *J Postgrad Med* 50(3), 234 (with amoxicillin)
  (2004): Graham DJ+, *JAMA* 292(21), 2585 (low risk)
  (2004): Havens-Verkler J+, *J Emerg Nurs* 30(1), 9
  (2004): Ho MR+, *Am J Emerg Med* 22(3), 234
  (2004): Jamil S+, *Heart* 90(1), e3
  (2004): Kahri AJ+, *Ann Pharmacother* 38(4), 719 (with clarithromycin)
  (2004): Moro H+, *AIDS Patient Care STDS* 18(12), 687 (with fluconazole)
  (2004): Roten L+, *Ann Pharmacother* 38(6), 978 (with amiodarone)
  (2004): Trieu J+, *Clin Nucl Med* 29(12), 803 (with clarithromycin)
  (2004): Webber MA+, *J Psychopharmacol* 18(3), 432 (with risperidone)
  (2003): Andreou ER+, *Can J Clin Pharmacol* 10(4), 172 (with danazol)
  (2003): Chiffoleau A+, *Therapie* 58(2), 168 (with verapamil and cyclosporine)
  (2003): de Denus S+, *Am J Health Syst Pharm* 60(17), 1791 (with amiodarone)
  (2003): Gumprecht J+, *Med Sci Monit* 9(9), CS89 (with cyclosporine)
  (2003): Pinilla Moraza J+, *Rev Clin Esp* 203(12), 615

(2003): Shaukat A+, *Ann Pharmacother* 37(7), 1032 (with fluconazole)
(2003): Skrabal MZ+, *Am J Health Syst Pharm* 60(6), 578
(2003): Skrabal MZ+, *South Med J* 96(10), 1034 (with nefazodone)
(2003): Wratchford P+, *Am J Health Syst Pharm* 60(7), 698
(2003): Yuen SL+, *Med J Aust* 179(3), 172 (with fusidic acid)
(2002): Cheng CH+, *Am J Health Syst Pharm* 59(8), 728
(2002): Hare CB+, *Clin Infect Dis* 35(10), e111 (with nelfinavir)
(2002): Rhodes CA+, *Clin Nucl Med* 27(11), 793
(2002): Thompson M+, *Am J Psychiatry* 159(9), 1607 (with nefazodone)
(2001): Borrego FJ+, *Nefrologia* 21(3), 309
(2001): Federman DG+, *South Med J* 94(10), 1023 (with gemfibrozil)
(2001): Kanathur N+, *Tenn Med* 94(9), 339 (with diltiazem)
(2001): Lee AJ, *Ann Pharmacother* 35(1), 26 (with clarithromycin)
(2001): Peces R+, *Nephron* 89(1), 117 (with diltiazem)
(2001): Reed BR, Denver, CO (from internet) (observation)
(2001): Stirling CM+, *Nephrol Dial Transplant* 16(4), 873
(2000): Al Shohaib, *Am J Nephrol* 20(3), 212
(2000): Davidson MH, *Curr Atheroscler Rep* 2(1), 14
(2000): Kusus M+, *Am J Med Sci* 320(6), 394 (with cyclosporine, digoxin and verapamil)
(2000): Oldemeyer JB+, *Cardiology* 94(2), 127 (with gemfibrozil)
(2000): Weise WJ+, *Am J Med* 108(4), 351
(1999): Bottorff M, *Atherosclerosis* 147(Suppl 1), S23
(1999): Corsini A+, *Pharmacol Ther* 84, 413 (with either cyclosporine, mibefradil or nefazodone)
(1999): Gilad R+, *Clin Neuropharmacol* 22(5), 295 (with ketoconazole)
(1999): Mogyorosi A+, *J Intern Med* 246(6), 599 (with warfarin)
(1997): Jacobson RH+, *JAMA* 277(4), 296 (with nefazodone)
(1997): Tal A+, *South Med J* 1997 May; 90(5), 546 (with gemfibrozil)
(1996): Ballantyne CM+, *Am J Cardiol* 78(5), 532
(1996): van Puijenbroek EP+, *J Intern Med* 240(6), 403 (with gemfibrozil)
(1995): Farmer JA+, *Baillieres Clin Endocrinol Metab* 9(4), 825
(1995): Garnett WR, *Am J Health Syst Pharm* 52(15), 1639 (with either cyclosporine, erythromycin, gemfibrozil or niacin)
(1995): Meier C+, *Schweiz Med Wochenschr* 125(27), 1342 (with cyclosporine)
(1992): Blaison G+, *Rev Med Interne* 13(1), 61 (with cyclosporine)
(1992): Dromer C+, *Rev Rhum Mal Osteoartic* 59(4), 281
Tendinopathy/Tendon rupture
(2005): Daghfous R+, *Tunis Med* 83(5), 253
(2001): Chazerain P+, *Joint Bone Spine* 68(5), 430

SINCALIDE

Trade name: Kinevac (Bracco)
Indications: Diagnostic aid for: gall bladder function, pancreatic function, accelerating transit of barium meal
Category: Diagnostic aid; Hormone; Polypeptide
Half-life: 6 hours
Clinically important, potentially hazardous interactions with: N/A

Reactions

Skin
  Allergic reactions (sic) (<1%)
  Diaphoresis ((<1%)
  Rash (sic) ((<1%)

Other
  Abdominal pain (~20%)
    (1995): Teitelbaum DH+, *J Pediatr Surg* 30(7), 1082
  Headache (<1%)
  Hypertension (<1%)
  Hypotension (<1%)
  Paresthesias (<1%)
  Vertigo (2%)

SINECATECHINS

Trade name: Veregen
Indications: Condylomata acuminata
Category: Immunomodulator

Reactions

Other
  Application-site burning
  Application-site edema
  Application-site erythema
  Application-site pain
  Application-site pruritus

SIROLIMUS

Synonym: Rapamycin
Trade name: Rapamune (Wyeth)
Indications: Prophylaxis of organ rejection in renal transplants
Category: Antibiotic, macrolide; Immunosupressant; Non-calcineurin inhibitor
Half-life: 62 hours
Clinically important, potentially hazardous interactions with: cyclosporine, **hemophilus B vaccine**, itraconazole, **St John's wort**, telithromycin, voriconazole

Reactions

Skin
  Abscess (3–20%)
  Acne (20–31%)
    (2008): Lubbe J+, *Dermatology* 216(3), 239
    (2006): Mahe E+, *J Am Acad Dermatol* 55(1), 139 (45%)
    (2005): Mahe E+, *Transplantation* 79(4), 476 (46%)
    (2001): Reitamo S+, *Br J Dermatol* 145(3), 438 (13%) (with cyclosporine)
    (2000): Kahan BD, *Lancet* 356(9225), 194
    (2000): Vasquez EM, *Am J Health Syst Pharm* 57, 437
  Angioedema
    (2007): Mahe E+, *Dermatology* 214(3), 205
    (2005): Mahe E+, *Transplantation* 79(4), 476 (15%)
  Carcinoma
    (2004): Montalbano M+, *Transplantation* 78(2), 264
  Cellulitis (3–20%)
  Dermatitis
    (2004): Montalbano M+, *Transplantation* 78(2), 264 (25%)
  Dermatitis herpetiformis (aggravation)
    (2002): Gladstone GC, Worcester, MA (personal correspondence)
  Diaphoresis (3–20%)
  Edema (16–24%)
    (2007): Augustine JJ+, *Drugs* 67(3), 369
    (2006): Buhaescu I+, *Ther Drug Monit* 28(5), 577

(2005): Mahe E+, *Transplantation* 79(4), 476 (55%)
(2004): Montalbano M+, *Transplantation* 78(2), 264 (5–57%)
Facial edema (3–20%)
(2004): Montalbano M+, *Transplantation* 78(2), 264 (2%)
Fissures
(2005): Mahe E+, *Transplantation* 79(4), 476 (11%)
Folliculitis
(2005): Mahe E+, *Transplantation* 79(4), 476 (26%)
Fungal dermatitis (3–20%)
Hidradenitis
(2005): Mahe E+, *Transplantation* 79(4), 476 (12%)
Hypertrophy (3–20%)
Peripheral edema (54–64%)
Pruritus (3–20%)
(2002): Gladstone GC, Worcester, MA (personal
correspondence)
Purpura (3–20%)
(2002): Hardinger KL+, *Transplantation* 74(5), 739
Rash (sic) (10–20%)
(2000): Vasquez EM, *Am J Health Syst Pharm* 57, 437
Scrotal edema
Ulcerations (3–20%)
Vasculitis
(2005): Nagarajan S+, *Pediatr Transplant* 9(1), 97
(2002): Hardinger KL+, *Transplantation* 74(5), 739

Mucosal/ENT
Aphthous stomatitis (9%)
(2005): Mahe E+, *Transplantation* 79(4), 476 (60%)
(2001): Reitamo S+, *Br J Dermatol* 145(3), 438 (9%) (with
cyclosporine)
Dysgeusia
(1999): Watson CJ+, *Transplantation* 67, 505
Gingival hyperplasia/hypertrophy (3–20%)
Gingivitis (3–20%)
(2005): Mahe E+, *Transplantation* 79(4), 476 (20%)
Oral candidiasis (3–20%)
Oral ulceration (3–20%)
(2005): Kuypers DR, *Drug Saf* 28(2), 153
(2004): Montalbano M+, *Transplantation* 78(2), 264 (24%)
(2003): Fairbanks KD+, *Liver Transpl* 9(10), 1079
Stomatitis (3–20%)
Tinnitus (3–20%)

Hair
Hair – hirsutism (3–20%)

Nails
Nails – onychopathy
(2006): Mahe E+, *Ann Dermatol Venereol* 133(6-7), 531
(2005): Mahe E+, *Transplantation* 79(4), 476 (74%)
Nails – periungual infections
(2005): Mahe E+, *Transplantation* 79(4), 476 (16%)

Eyes
Eyelid edema (40%)
(2001): Mohaupt MG+, *Transplantation* 72(1), 162 (40%)

Other
Abdominal pain
(2005): Nagarajan S+, *Pediatr Transplant* 9(1), 97
Asthenia
(2006): Champion L+, *Ann Intern Med* 144(7), 505 (20 cases)
Chills (3–20%)
Cough
(2006): Champion L+, *Ann Intern Med* 144(7), 505 (23 cases)
Death
(2007): Burzotta F+, *Am J Cardiol* 99(3), 364 (1 case)
Depression (3–20%)

Fever
(2006): Champion L+, *Ann Intern Med* 144(7), 505 (16 cases)
Headache
Hepatotoxicity
(2004): Neff GW+, *Ann Pharmacother* 38(10), 1593
Hot flashes
(2001): Reitamo S+, *Br J Dermatol* 145(3), 438 (12%) (with
cyclosporine)
Infections
(2002): *Prescrire Int* 11(62), 165
Myalgia/Myositis/Myopathy/Myotoxicity
(2003): Josef F+, *Transplantation* 76(12), 1773
Nephrotoxicity
(2007): Cho ME+, *Am J Kidney Dis* 49(2), 310
(2006): Pallet N+, *Nephrol Ther* 2(4), 183
Paresthesias (3–20%)
Serum sickness (from stent)
(2007): Rana JS+, *Ann Allergy Asthma Immunol* 98(2), 201
Thrombophlebitis (3–20%)
Thrombosis
(2007): Kastrati A+, *N Engl J Med* 356(10), 1030
(2004): Montalbano M+, *Transplantation* 78(2), 264
Tremor (21–31%)
(1999): Groth CG+, *Transplantation* 67, 1036
Upper respiratory infection (20–26%)

SITAGLIPTIN

Synonym: MK0431
Trade name: Januvia (Merck)
Indications: Adjunct to diet and exercise to lower blood sugar in
Type 2 diabetes mellitus
Category: Dipeptidyl peptidase (DPP-4) inhibitor
Half-life: 12.4 hours
**Clinically important, potentially hazardous interactions
with:** N/A

Reactions

Mucosal/ENT
Nasopharyngitis

Other
Abdominal pain (2.3%)
Headache
Upper respiratory infection

SITAXENTAN

Synonym: Sitaxsentan
Trade name: Thelin (Encysize)
Indications: Pulmonary arterial hypertension
Half-life: 10 hours
**Clinically important, potentially hazardous interactions
with:** warfarin

Reactions

Skin
Peripheral edema (9%)
(2005): Widlitz AC+, *Expert Rev Cardiovasc Ther* 3(6), 985

Mucosal/ENT

Rhinitis
  (2005): Widlitz AC+, *Expert Rev Cardiovasc Ther* 3(6), 985

Other

Abdominal pain (>2%)
Chest pain
  (2005): Widlitz AC+, *Expert Rev Cardiovasc Ther* 3(6), 985
Headache (15%)
  (2005): Widlitz AC+, *Expert Rev Cardiovasc Ther* 3(6), 985
Hepatotoxicity
  (2007): Benza RL+, *J Heart Lung Transplant* 26(1), 63
  (2007): Wittbrodt ET+, *Ann Pharmacother* 41(1), 100
Myalgia/Myositis/Myopathy/Myotoxicity (>2%)
Vertigo (>2%)

SMALLPOX VACCINE

Trade name: Dryvax (Wyeth)
Indications: Prevention of smallpox (variola)
Category: Vaccine
Half-life: ~5 years
Clinically important, potentially hazardous interactions with: corticosteroids

Reactions

Skin

Acne
Allergic reactions (sic)
Basal cell carcinoma
  (1988): Ribeiro R+, *Med Cutan Ibero Lat Am* 16(2), 137
Bullous dermatitis
Carcinoma
  (1980): Gecht ML, *JAMA* 244(15), 1675
Dermatitis
  (2004): Gaertner EM+, *Arch Pathol Lab Med* 128(10), 1173
  (2004): Greenberg RN+, *Clin Infect Dis* 38(7), 958
Dermatofibrosarcoma protuberans
  (2003): Green JJ+, *J Am Acad Dermatol* 48, S54 (in scar)
Eczema
  (2003): Wharton M+, *MMWR Recomm Rep* 52(RR-7), 1
Eczema vaccinatum
Erythema
  (2004): Greenberg RN+, *Clin Infect Dis* 38(7), 958
Erythema multiforme
  (2004): Chopra A+, *Mayo Clin Proc* 79(9), 1193
Erythema nodosum
Exanthems
  (2004): Greenberg RN+, *Clin Infect Dis* 38(7), 958
Exfoliative dermatitis
Folliculitis
  (2005): Oh RC, *Mil Med* 170(2), 133 (2 cases)
  (2004): Greenberg RN+, *Clin Infect Dis* 38(7), 958
Herpes simplex
  (1982): Mintz L, *JAMA* 247(19), 2704 (recurrent) (at site)
Herpes zoster
Histiocytoma
  (1981): Slater DN+, *Br J Dermatol* 105(2), 215
Jadassohn–Borst epithelioma
Kaposi's varicelliform eruption
Keratoacanthoma
Lichen vaccinatus
Lupus erythematosus (discoid)

  (1987): Lupton GP, *J Am Acad Dermatol* 17, 688 (in vaccination scar)
Melanoma
Photosensitivity
Pigmentation
Pruritus
  (2004): Greenberg RN+, *Clin Infect Dis* 38(7), 958
Purpura
  (1981): Burke PJ+, *Pa Med* 84(9), 49
Pyogenic granuloma
Rash (sic)
  (2002): Frey SE+, *N Engl J Med* 346, 1265 (site other than vaccination site)
Scar
  (2006): Waibel KH+, *Int J Dermatol* 45(6), 764 (exaggerated)
Side effects (sic) (0.01%)
Stevens–Johnson syndrome
  (2004): Chopra A+, *Mayo Clin Proc* 79(9), 1193
  (2003): Wharton M+, *MMWR Recomm Rep* 52(RR-7), 1
Toxic epidermal necrolysis
Urticaria
  (2004): Greenberg RN+, *Clin Infect Dis* 38(7), 958
Vaccinia
  (2004): Kelly CD+, *J Clin Microbiol* 42(3), 1373
  (2003): Miller JR+, *Emerg Infect Dis* 9(12), 1649
  (2003): Wharton M+, *MMWR Recomm Rep* 52(RR-7), 1
  (1988): Landthaler M+, *Hautarzt* 39, 322
  (1980): Kanra G+, *Cutis* 26, 267 (vulva from 7–month-old daughter's vaccination)
Vaccinia gangrenosum
Vaccinia necrosum
  (1982): *MMWR Morb Mortality Wkly Rep* 31(36), 501
  (1981): Funk EA+, *South Med J* 74(3), 383

Eyes

Blepharitis
  (2004): Fillmore GL+, *Ophthalmology* 111(11), 2086
Conjunctivitis
  (2004): Fillmore GL+, *Ophthalmology* 111(11), 2086
Corneal opacity
  (2004): Fillmore GL+, *Ophthalmology* 111(11), 2086
Eyelid pruritus
  (2004): Fillmore GL+, *Ophthalmology* 111(11), 2086
Iritis
  (2004): Fillmore GL+, *Ophthalmology* 111(11), 2086
Keratouveitis
  (1994): Lee SF+, *Am J Ophthalmol* 117(4), 480 (autoinoculation)
Periorbital edema
  (2004): Fillmore GL+, *Ophthalmology* 111(11), 2086
Photophobia
  (2005): McMahon AW+, *Vaccine* 2005 Jan 19;23(9), 1097

Other

Chills
  (2002): Frey SE+, *N Engl J Med* 346, 1265
Death
  (2006): Kretzschmar M+, *PLoS Med* 3(8), e272
  (2003): *MMWR Morb Mortal Wkly Rep* 52(39), 933 (2 cases)
Fever
Headache
  (2005): Sejvar J+, *Headache* 45(1), 87 (108 cases)
  (2004): Greenberg RN+, *Clin Infect Dis* 38(7), 958
Injection-site pain
  (2002): Frey SE+, *N Engl J Med* 346, 1265
Injection-site pyoderma
  (2003): Wharton M+, *MMWR Recomm Rep* 52(RR-7), 1
Myalgia/Myositis/Myopathy/Myotoxicity
  (2002): Frey SE+, *N Engl J Med* 346, 1265

Paresthesias
(2004): Greenberg RN+, *Clin Infect Dis* 38(7), 958
Suicidal ideation
(2006): Murali H+, *Sleep* 29(8), 1025 (1 case)
Tremor
(2006): Murali H+, *Sleep* 29(8), 1025 (1 case)
Tumors

SODIUM CROMOGLYCATE

(See CROMOLYN)

SODIUM OXYBATE

Synonyms: Gamma Hydroxybutyrate; GHB
Trade name: Xyrem (Orphan Medical)
Indications: Cataplexy (in patients with narcolepsy)
Category: Anesthetic, general
Half-life: 0.3–1 hour
Clinically important, potentially hazardous interactions with: alcohol, hypnotics, sedatives

Note: Sodium oxybate is a class of drugs that are also known as: 'Designer' drugs; Party drugs; Club drugs; Recreational drugs; 'Rave' drugs; Fantasy drugs; Date rape drugs; abuse drugs

Reactions

Skin
Diaphoresis
(2001): Bowles TM+, *Pharmacotherapy* 21(2), 254 (following withdrawal)
(2001): Dyer JE+, *Ann Emerg Med* 37(2), 147 (following withdrawal)
(2000): Craig K+, *J Emerg Med* 18(1), 65 (following withdrawal)

Mucosal/ENT
Sialorrhea
Sinusitis

Other
Death
(2002): Smith KM+, *Am J Health Syst Pharm* 59(11), 1067
(2001): Dyer JE+, *Ann Emerg Med* 37(2), 147 (following withdrawal)
(2001): Kalasinsky KS+, *J Forensic Sci* 46(3), 728
(2001): Nini A+, *Harefuah* 140(12), 1148
(2001): Okun MS+, *J Pharm Pharm Sci* 4(2), 167
(2001): Persson SA+, *Lakartidningen* 98(38), 4026
(2000): Timby N+, *Am J Med* 108(6), 518
(1998): Li J+, *Ann Emerg Med* 31(6), 729
(1995): Ferrara SD+, *J Forensic Sci* 40(3), 501 (also taking IV heroin)
Depression
Infections
Pain
Porphyria
Rhabdomyolysis
Seizures
(2002): Smith KM+, *Am J Health Syst Pharm* 59(11), 1067
(1998): Hovda KE+, *Tidsskr Nor Laegeforen* 118(28), 4390
(1998): Kam PC+, *Anaesthesia* 53(12), 1195
(1997): Galloway GP+, *Addiction* 92(1), 89
(1995): Steele MT+, *Mo Med* 92(7), 354
(1992): Adornato BT+, *West J Med* 157(4), 471
(1991): Dyer JE, *Am J Emerg Med* 9(4), 321

Tremor
(2001): Dyer JE+, *Ann Emerg Med* 37(2), 147 (following withdrawal)
(2000): Craig K+, *J Emerg Med* 18(1), 65 (following withdrawal)
(1998): Hovda KE+, *Tidsskr Nor Laegeforen* 118(28), 4390 (following withdrawal)
(1997): Galloway GP+, *Addiction* 92(1), 89 (following withdrawal)
Upper respiratory infection

SOLIFENACIN

Trade name: Vesicare (GSK)
Indications: Overactive bladder
Category: Muscarinic antagonist
Half-life: 45–68 hours
Clinically important, potentially hazardous interactions with: atazanavir, carbamazepine, clarithromycin, indinavir, itraconazole, ketoconazole, nefazodone, nelfinavir, phenobarbital, phenytoin, rifabutin, rifampin, rifapentine, ritonavir, saquinavir, **St John's wort**, troleandomycin, voriconazole

Reactions

Skin
Lichenoid eruption
(2007): Shalders K+, *Clin Exp Dermatol*

Mucosal/ENT
Xerostomia (11–27%)
(2005): *Med Lett Drugs Ther* 47(1204), 23
(2005): Simpson D+, *Drugs Aging* 22(12), 1061
(2004): Chapple CR+, *BJU Int* 93(3), 303
(2004): Sand PK, *J Am Acad Nurse Pract* 16(10), 8
(2004): Smulders RA+, *J Clin Pharmacol* 44(9), 1023

Eyes
Vision blurred (4–5%)
(2005): Simpson D+, *Drugs Aging* 22(12), 1061
Xerophthalmia (0.3–1.6%)

Other
Abdominal pain (1.2–1.9%)
Asthenia (1–2.1%)
Cough (0.2–1.1%)
Depression (0.8–1.2%)
Hypertension (0.5–1.4%)
Vertigo (1.9%)

SOMATROPIN

Trade names: Genotropin (Pfizer); Growject BC; Humatrope (Lilly); Norditropin (Novo Nordisk); Norditropin Simplexx; Nutropin (Genentech); Nutropin AQ; Saizen (Merck); Scitropin; Serostim (Merck); Tev-Tropin (Teva)
Indications: Growth failure, growth hormone deficiency, short stature (in Turner's syndrome), muscle wasting (in HIV positive patients)
Category: Growth hormone analog
Half-life: 0.4 hours (IV); 3 hours (subcutaneous)
Clinically important, potentially hazardous interactions with: glucocorticoids, insulin detemir, insulin glulisine

Reactions

Skin
Acanthosis nigricans
  (1999): Downs AM+, *Br J Dermatol* 141(2), 390
Edema (11.4%)
  (2002): Bryant J+, *J Endocrinol* 175(2), 545
Lupus erythematosus
  (2001): Bae YS+, *Lupus* 10(6), 448 (flare)
Peripheral edema (18.2%)
Pruritus
Rash (sic)
Urticaria

Mucosal/ENT
Rhinitis (11.4%)

Other
Asthenia
Cough
Death (in critically ill patients)
  (2004): Mills JL+, *J Pediatr* 144(4), 430
  (2004): Vliet GV+, *J Pediatr* 144(1), 129
  (2000): Osterziel KJ+, *N Engl J Med* 342(2), 134
  (2000): Van den Berge G, *N Engl J Med* 342(2), 135
  (1999): Takala J+, *N Engl J Med* 341(11), 785
Gynecomastia
  (1998): Sullivan DH+, *J Gerontol A Biol Sci Med Sci* 53(3), M183
Headache (6.8%)
Injection-site inflammation
Injection-site pain
Myalgia/Myositis/Myopathy/Myotoxicity (9.1%)
Pain (13.6%)
Paresthesias (13.6%)

SORAFENIB

Synonym: BAY 43-9006
Trade name: Nexavar (Bayer)
Indications: Advanced renal cell carcinoma
Category: Tyrosine kinase inhibitor
Half-life: 25–48 hours
Clinically important, potentially hazardous interactions with: doxorubicin, warfarin

Reactions

Skin
Acne (1–10%)
  (2007): Alexandrescu DT+, *Clin Exp Dermatol* 32(1), 71
Actinic keratoses
  (2006): Lacouture ME+, *Clin Exp Dermatol* 31(6), 783
    (inflammation of)
Desquamation (40%)
Eczema (<1%)
Eruptive facial cysts
  (2008): Autier J+, *Arch Dermatol* 144(7), 886
Erythema (>10%)
Erythema multiforme (<1%)
Exfoliative dermatitis (1–10%)
Folliculitis (<1%)
Hand–foot syndrome (30%)
  (2008): Autier J+, *Arch Dermatol* 144(7), 886 (60%)
  (2008): Chu D+, *Acta Oncol* 47(2), 176
  (2007): Yang CH+, *Br J Dermatol*

  (2004): Ahmad T+, *Clin Cancer Res* 10(18 Pt 2), 6388S
Hyperkeratosis
  (2008): Autier J+, *Arch Dermatol* 144(7), 886
Pruritus (19%)
  (2002): Hotte SJ+, *Curr Pharm Des* 8(25), 2249
Rash (sic) (40%)
  (2002): Hotte SJ+, *Curr Pharm Des* 8(25), 2249
Seborrheic dermatitis
  (2007): Yang CH+, *Br J Dermatol*
Side effects (71%)
  (2005): Awada A+, *Br J Cancer* 92(10), 1855
  (2005): Kupsch P+, *Clin Colorectal Cancer* 5(3), 188
  (2005): Strumberg D+, *J Clin Oncol* 23(5), 965
Squamous cell carcinoma
  (2008): Hong DS+, *Arch Dermatol* 144(6), 779
Urticaria (<1%)
Vasculitis
  (2006): Chung NM+, *Arch Dermatol* 142(11), 1510
Xerosis (11%)

Mucosal/ENT
Angular stomatitis
  (2007): Yang CH+, *Br J Dermatol*
Cheilitis
  (2002): Hotte SJ+, *Curr Pharm Des* 8(25), 2249
Dysphagia (1–10%)
Glossodynia (1–10%)
Mucositis (1–10%)
Rhinorrhea (<1%)
Stomatitis (1–10%)
  (2008): Autier J+, *Arch Dermatol* 144(7), 886
Tinnitus (<1%)
Xerostomia (1–10%)

Hair
Hair – alopecia (27%)
  (2008): Autier J+, *Arch Dermatol* 144(7), 886 (44%)

Nails
Nails – splinter hemorrhages
  (2008): Autier J+, *Arch Dermatol* 144(7), 886 (70%)

Other
Abdominal pain (11%)
  (2002): Hotte SJ+, *Curr Pharm Des* 8(25), 2249
Asthenia (37%)
  (2005): Strumberg D+, *J Clin Oncol* 23(5), 965
Cough (13%)
Depression (1–10%)
Gynecomastia (<1%)
Headache (10%)
Hematotoxicity
Hypersensitivity (<1%)
Hypertension (17%)
Infections (<1%)
Myalgia/Myositis/Myopathy/Myotoxicity
Neurotoxicity (2–40%)
  (2005): Kupsch P+, *Clin Colorectal Cancer* 5(3), 188
Pain (>10%)
  (2005): Awada A+, *Br J Cancer* 92(10), 1855 (64%)

SOTALOL

Trade names: Beta-Cardone; Betades; Betapace (Berlex); Cardol; Sotacor; Sotahexal; Sotalex
Indications: Ventricular arrhythmias
Category: Adrenergic beta-receptor antagonist; Antiarrhythmic class III
Half-life: 7–18 hours
Clinically important, potentially hazardous interactions with: abarelix, amisulpride, arsenic, astemizole, ciprofloxacin, enoxacin, gatifloxacin, lomefloxacin, moxifloxacin, norfloxacin, ofloxacin, quinolones, ranolazine, sparfloxacin

Reactions

Skin
Cold extremities
Diaphoresis (<1%)
  (1995): Schmutz JL+, *Dermatology* 190, 86
Edema (5%)
Exanthems
Irritation (sic)
Lichenoid eruption
  (1994): O'Brien TJ+, *Australas J Dermatol* 35, 93
Peripheral edema
Photosensitivity (<1%)
Pruritus (1–10%)
Psoriasis
  (1988): Heng MCY+, *Int J Dermatol* 27, 619
  (1986): Czernielewski J+, *Lancet* 1, 808
  (1984): Arntzen N+, *Acta Derm Venereol* (Stockh) 64, 346
Rash (sic) (3%)
Raynaud's phenomenon (<1%)
Scleroderma
  (1988): Ahmad N+, *Scott Med J* 33, 210
Thickening
Urticaria
Vasculitis
  (1998): Rustmann WC+, *J Am Acad Dermatol* 38, 111

Mucosal/ENT
Dysgeusia
Xerostomia (<1%)

Hair
Hair – alopecia (<1%)

Other
Cardiotoxicity
  (2006): Kim RJ+, *Pacing Clin Electrophysiol* 29(11), 1219 (9%)
Headache
Hypotension
  (2000): Joye F, *Presse Med* 29(18), 1027
Injection-site extravasation (<1%)
Myalgia/Myositis/Myopathy/Myotoxicity
Paresthesias (3%)
Phlebitis (<1%)

SPARFLOXACIN

Trade names: Spara; Sparlox; Torospar; Zagam
Indications: Community-acquired pneumonia
Category: Antibiotic, quinolone
Half-life: 16–30 hours
Clinically important, potentially hazardous interactions with: amiodarone, amisulpride, amitriptyline, amoxapine, arsenic, bepridil, bretylium, calcium, chlorpromazine, clomipramine, desipramine, disopyramide, doxepin, erythromycin, fluphenazine, imipramine, iron salts, magnesium, mesoridazine, nortriptyline, perphenazine, phenothiazines, pimozide, procainamide, prochlorperazine, promazine, promethazine, protriptyline, quinidine, sotalol, sucralfate, thioridazine, tricyclic antidepressants, trifluoperazine, trimipramine, zinc salts

Reactions

Skin
Acne (<1%)
Allergic reactions (sic) (<1%)
Angioedema (<1%)
Bullous dermatitis (<1%)
Cellulitis (<1%)
Dermatitis (<1%)
Diaphoresis (<1%)
Edema (<1%)
Erythema nodosum
Exanthems (<1%)
Exfoliative dermatitis (<1%)
Facial edema (<1%)
Fixed eruption
  (2001): Sharma R, Aligarh, India (recurrence with ciprofloxacin) (from Internet) (observation)
Furunculosis (<1%)
Herpes simplex (<1%)
Lichenoid eruption
  (1998): Hamanaka H+, *J Am Acad Dermatol* 38, 945
Peripheral edema (<1%)
Petechiae (<1%)
Photosensitivity (3.6%)
  (2006): Rafalsky V+, *Cochrane Database Syst Rev* 3
  (2005): Mahajan VK+, *Australas J Dermatol* 46(2), 104
  (2000): Schentag JJ, *Clin Ther* 22, 372
  (1999): Hamanaka H, *J Dermatol Sci* 21, 27
  (1999): Lipsky BA+, *Clin Ther* 21, 148
  (1998): Hamanaka H+, *J Am Acad Dermatol* 38, 945
  (1997): Burrow WH, Jackson, MS (from Internet) (observation)
  (1996): Tokura Y+, *Arch Dermatol Res* 288, 45
  (1995): Hamanaka H+, *Jpn J Dermatol* 105, 601
  (1995): Hiramoto T+, *Rinsho Dermatol* (Japanese) 37, 1681
Phototoxicity (7.9%)
  (2003): Dawe RS+, *Br J Dermatol* 149(6), 1232
  (2001): Lubasch A+, *Eur Respir J* 2001 Apr 17(4), 641
  (2000): Pierfitte C+, *Br J Clin Pharmacol* 49, 609
  (1999): Blondeau JM, *Clin Ther* 21, 6
  (1996): Tokura Y+, *Arch Dermatol Res* 288, 45
Pigmentation (<1%)
  (2003): Dawe RS+, *Br J Dermatol* 149(6), 1232
Pruritus (3.3%)
Purpura
Pustules (<1%)
Rash (sic) (1.1%)
Stevens–Johnson syndrome
Toxic epidermal necrolysis

Urticaria (<1%)
Vasculitis
Xerosis (<1%)

Mucosal/ENT

Anosmia
Dysgeusia (1.4%)
 (1999): Lipsky BA+, *Clin Ther* 21, 148
Gingivitis (<1%)
Oral candidiasis (<1%)
Oral ulceration (<1%)
Stomatitis (<1%)
Tongue disorder (<1%)
Vaginitis (<1%)
Vulvovaginal candidiasis (2.8%)
Xerostomia (1.4%)

Hair

Hair – alopecia (<1%)

Nails

Nails – photo-onycholysis
 (2005): Mahajan VK+, *Australas J Dermatol* 46(2), 104
Nails – pigmentation
 (2005): Guptha SD+, *Indian J Dermatol Venereol Leprol* 71(1), 47

Eyes

Corneal opacity
 (2004): Gokhale NS, *Indian J Ophthalmol* 52(1), 79

Other

Anaphylactoid reactions/Anaphylaxis (<1%)
Headache
Hypersensitivity
Myalgia/Myositis/Myopathy/Myotoxicity (<1%)
Paresthesias (<1%)
Serum sickness
Tendinopathy/Tendon rupture

SPECTINOMYCIN

Trade names: Spectam; Trobicin (Pfizer)
Indications: Gonorrhea
Category: Antibiotic
Half-life: 1–3 hours

Reactions

Skin

Dermatitis
 (1994): Dal-Monte A+, *Contact Dermatitis* 31, 204
  (occupational)
 (1991): Vilaplana J+, *Contact Dermatitis* 24, 225
Exanthems
Pruritus (<1%)
Rash (sic) (<1%)
Urticaria (<1%)

Mucosal/ENT

Oral lesions

Other

Anaphylactoid reactions/Anaphylaxis
 (1983): Bender BS+, *South Med J* 76(11), 1456
Chills
Hypersensitivity
Injection-site induration

Injection-site pain (<1%)
 (1990): Novak E+, *Antimicrob Agents Chemother* 34(12), 2342
 (1990): Novak E+, *Clin Ther* 12(3), 269
 (1990): Peters GR+, *Int J Clin Pharmacol Ther Toxicol* 28(9), 361
Vertigo
 (1990): Novak E+, *Antimicrob Agents Chemother* 34(12), 2342
 (1990): Novak E+, *Clin Ther* 12(3), 269
 (1990): Peters GR+, *Int J Clin Pharmacol Ther Toxicol* 28(9), 361

SPIRONOLACTONE

Trade names: Aldactazide (Pfizer); Aldactone (Pfizer); Aldopur; Almatol; Diram; Merabis; Novo-Spiroton; Osiren; Spiroctan; Tensin
Indications: Hyperaldosteronism, hirsutism, hypertension
Category: Aldosterone antagonist; Diuretic
Half-life: 78–84 minutes
Clinically important, potentially hazardous interactions with: ACE inhibitors, **alcohol**, amiloride, barbiturates, benazepril, captopril, cyclosporine, enalapril, fosinopril, **juniper**, lisinopril, mitotane, moexipril, narcotics, NSAIDs, potassium chloride, potassium iodide, quinapril, ramipril, trandolapril, triamterene

Note: Aldactazide is spironolactone and hydrochlorothiazide

Reactions

Skin

Bullous pemphigoid
 (2002): Modeste AB+, *Ann Dermatol Venereol* 129(1), 56
 (1997): Grange F+, *Ann Dermatol Venereol* 124(10), 700
Chloasma
 (1988): Hughes BR+, *Br J Dermatol* 118, 687
Dermatitis
 (1996): Corazza M+, *Contact Dermatitis* 35, 365
 (1994): Aguirre A+, *Contact Dermatitis* 30, 312
 (1994): Balato N+, *Contact Dermatitis* 31, 203
 (1994): Fernandez-Vozmediano JM+, *Contact Dermatitis* 30, 118
 (1993): Vincenzi C+, *Contact Dermatitis* 29, 277 (from anti-acne cream)
 (1984): Klijn J, *Contact Dermatitis* 10, 105
Diaphoresis
Eczema
 (1994): Balato N+, *Contact Dermatitis* 31, 203
 (1994): Fernandez-Vozmediano JM+, *Contact Dermatitis* 30, 118
Erythema
Erythema annulare centrifugum
 (1987): Carsuzaa F+, *Ann Dermatol Venereol* (French) 114, 375
Erythema multiforme
 (1986): Greenberger PA+, *N Engl Reg Allergy Proc* 7, 343
Exanthems (<5%)
 (1994): Gupta AK+, *Dermatol* 189, 402
 (1988): Hughes BR+, *Br J Dermatol* 118, 687 (9.3%)
 (1986): Wathen CG+, *Lancet* 1, 919
Facial edema
 (1998): Lubbos HG+, *Arch Dermatol* 134, 1163
Graft-versus-host reaction
 (1998): Jappe U+, *Hautarzt* (German) 49, 126 (passim)
Lichen planus
Lichenoid eruption
 (1998): Clark C+, *Clin Exp Dermatol* 23, 43
 (1994): Schon MP+, *Acta Derm Venereol* 74, 476
Lupus erythematosus
 (2002): Boye T+, *World Congress Dermatol* Poster, 0088
 (1987): Leroy D+, *Ann Dermatol Venereol* (French) 114, 1237

Melasma
(2000): Shaw JC, *J Am Acad Dermatol* 43, 498
Necrotizing vasculitis
Pemphigus
(2002): Karam A+, *World Congress Dermatol* Poster, 0328
(1997): Grange F+, *Ann Dermatol* (French) 124, 700
Photosensitivity
Pigmentation
(1988): Hughes BR, *Dermatology Times* June, 10 (chloasma-like)
(1988): Hughes BR+, *Br J Dermatol* 118, 687 (chloasma-like)
(1983): Luderschmidt C, *Dtsch Med Wochenschr* (German) 108, 1922
Pruritus
(2003): Hussain S+, *Nephrol Dial Transplant* 18(11), 2364
(1988): Hughes BR, *Dermatology Times* June, 10
(1986): Wathen CG+, *Lancet* 1, 919
Purpura
Rash (sic) (1–10%)
(1988): Hughes BR, *Dermatology Times* June, 10
Raynaud's phenomenon
Side effects (sic)
Urticaria
(1988): Helfer EL+, *J Clin Endocrinol Metab* 66, 208
Vasculitis
(1984): Phillips GWL+, *BMJ* 288, 368
Xerosis (40%)
(2000): Shaw JC, *J Am Acad Dermatol* 43, 498
(1988): Hughes BR, *Dermatology Times* June, 10
(1988): Hughes BR+, *Br J Dermatol* 118, 687 (40%)

Mucosal/ENT

Ageusia
Oral lichen planus
(1990): Lamey PJ+, *Oral Surg Oral Med Oral Pathol* 70, 184
Xerostomia
(2003): Hussain S+, *Nephrol Dial Transplant* 18(11), 2364

Hair

Hair – alopecia
(1988): Helfer EL+, *J Clin Endocrinol Metab* 66, 208
Hair – hirsutism

Other

Anaphylactoid reactions/Anaphylaxis
Chills
Congestive heart failure
(2000): Vanpee D+, *Aging* (Milano) 12(4), 315
DRESS syndrome
(2004): Ghislain PD+, *Acta Derm Venereol* 84(1), 65
Gynecomastia (<1%)
(2006): Williams EM+, *Clin Cardiol* 29(4), 149 (2%)
(2005): Fukuchi K+, *Clin Nucl Med* 30(2), 105
(2003): Hussain S+, *Nephrol Dial Transplant* 18(11), 2364
(2001): Yamamoto S, *Intern Med* 40(6), 550
(2000): Hugues FC+, *Ann Med Interne* (Paris) (French) 151, 10 (passim)
(1994): *BMJ* 308, 503
(1994): Dove F, *Hosp Pract Off Ed* 29, 27
(1993): Thompson DF+, *Pharmacotherapy* 13, 37
(1988): Hughes BR+, *Br J Dermatol* 118, 687
Headache
Paresthesias

SQUILL

Scientific names: *Drimia indica; Drimia maritima; Scilla indica; Scilla maritima; Urginea indica; Urginea maritima; Urginea scilla*
Family: Liliaceae
Trade and other common names: European Squill; Indian Squill; Mediterranean Squill; Red Squill; Sea Onion; Sea Squill; White Squill
Category: Diuretic
Purported indications and other uses: Arrhythmias, asthma, edema, bronchitis, whooping cough, abortifacient. Also used as a rodenticide
Half-life: N/A
Clinically important, potentially hazardous interactions with: digoxin, **ginger**, **ginseng**, hawthorn, **licorice**, **mistletoe**, quinidine, **senna**
Note: Squill is unsafe for self-medication

Reactions

Skin

Dermatitis
Rash (sic)
Urticaria

Eyes

Visual disturbances

Other

Asthenia
Death
(1995): Tuncok Y+, *J Toxicol Clin Toxicol* 33(1), 83
Depression
Headache
Seizures
(1995): Tuncok Y+, *J Toxicol Clin Toxicol* 33(1), 83

ST JOHN'S WORT

Scientific names: *Hypericum perforatum; Kira (Lichtwer); Quanterra Emotional Balance (Warner Lambert)*
Family: Hypericaceae
Trade and other common names: Amber; Demon Chaser; Fuga Daemonum; Goatweed; Hardhay; Hypereikon; Hypericum; Johns Wort; Klamath Weed; Rosin Rose; Tipton Weed
Category: Anxyolytic
Purported indications and other uses: Depression, dysthymic disorder, fatigue, insomnia, loss of appetite, anxiety, obsessive-compulsive disorders, mood disturbances, migraine headaches, neuralgia, fibrositis, sciatica, palpitations, exhaustion, headache, muscle pain, vitiligo, diuretic, bruises, abrasions, first-degree burns, hemorrhoids
Half-life: 24–48 hours
Clinically important, potentially hazardous interactions with: alprazolam, amitriptyline, amprenavir, atazanavir, bosentan, buspirone, carbamazepine, citalopram, cyclosporine, digoxin, eplerenone, escitalopram, etoposide, fenfluramine, fexofenadine, fluoxetine, fluvoxamine, fosamprenavir, **ginkgo biloba**, imatinib, indinavir, irinotecan, loperamide, methadone, midazolam, naratriptan, nefazodone, nelfinavir, nevirapine, oral contraceptives, paroxetine, phenobarbitone, phenprocoumon, phenytoin, quinolones, raltegravir, reserpine, ritonavir, rizatriptan, saquinavir, sertraline, simvastatin, sirolimus, solifenacin, SSRIs, sumatriptan, tacrolimus, temsirolimus, tetracyclines, theophylline, tricyclic antidepressants, warfarin, zolmitriptan

Reactions

Skin
Adverse effects (sic)
  (2002): Ernst E, *Ann Intern Med* 136(1), 42
  (2002): Haller CA+, *Adverse Drug React Toxicol Rev* 21(3), 143
Allergic reactions (sic)
  (1994): Woelk H+, *J Geriatr Psychiatry Neurol* 7 (Suppl 1), S34
Erythroderma
  (2000): Holme SA+, *Br J Dermatol* 143(5), 1127
Irritation
Photo-recall
  (2006): Putnik K+, *Radiat Oncol* 1, 32
Photosensitivity
  (2004): *Prescrire Int* 13(73), 187
  (2001): Pribitkin ED+, *Arch Facial Plast Surg* 3(2), 127
  (2000): Lane-Brown MM, *Med J Aust* 172(6), 302
  (2000): Schulz V, *Schweiz Rundsch Med Prax* 89(50), 2131
  (1999): Gulick RM+, *Ann Intern Med* 130, 510
  (1997): Brockmoller J+, *Pharmacopsychiatry* 30, 94
  (1997): Golsch S+, *Hautarzt* (German) 48, 249
Phototoxicity
  (2005): Beattie PE+, *Br J Dermatol* 153(6), 1187
Pruritus
  (1997): Golsch S+, *Hautarzt* 48, 249

Mucosal/ENT
Xerostomia
  (1997): *Med Lett Drugs Ther* 39, 107

Hair
Hair – alopecia
  (2001): Parker V+, *Can J Psychiatry* 46(1), 77

Other
Hepatotoxicity
  (2006): Teschke R, *Dtsch Med Wochenschr* 131(34-3), 1880 (with Kava)
Hypersensitivity
Paresthesias
  (1998): Ernst E+, *Eur J Clin Pharmacol* 54, 589
Side effects (sic)
  (1999): Tinsley JA, *Minn Med* 82(5), 29

STANOZOLOL

Trade names: Menabol; Stromba; Winstrol (Ovation)
Indications: Hereditary angioedema
Category: Anabolic steroid
Half-life: N/A
Clinically important, potentially hazardous interactions with: anticoagulants, warfarin

Reactions

Skin
Acne (>10%)
  (1995): Helfman T+, *J Am Acad Dermatol* 32, 254
Edema
Exanthems
Folliculitis
  (1995): Helfman T+, *J Am Acad Dermatol* 32, 254
Pigmentation (1–10%)
Rosacea
  (1995): Helfman T+, *J Am Acad Dermatol* 32, 254
Seborrheic dermatitis

  (1995): Helfman T+, *J Am Acad Dermatol* 32, 254
Urticaria

Hair
Hair – alopecia (in women)
Hair – hirsutism (in women)
  (1995): Helfman T+, *J Am Acad Dermatol* 32, 254
  (1987): Sheffer AL+, *J Allergy Clin Immunol* 80, 855

Other
Chills (1–10%)
Death
  (2001): Fineschi V+, *Arch Pathol Lab Med* 125(2), 253 (abuse)
  (1999): Sullivan ML+, *J Emerg Med* 17(5), 851 (abuse)
Gynecomastia (>10%)
  (1995): Helfman T+, *J Am Acad Dermatol* 32, 254
Hepatotoxicity
  (2002): Stimac D+, *J Clin Gastroenterol* 35(4), 350 (abuse)
  (2000): Segal S+, *J Am Acad Dermatol* 43(3), 558
Hypersensitivity
Hypertension
  (1999): Sullivan ML+, *J Emerg Med* 17(5), 851 (abuse)
  (1990): Tully MP+, *DICP* 24(12), 1234
Nephrotoxicity
  (1999): Habscheid W+, *Dtsch Med Wochenschr* 124(36), 1029
  (1994): Yoshida EM+, *CMAJ* 151(6), 791 (abuse)

STAR ANISE (Chinese)

Scientific name: *Illicium verum*
Family: Illiciaceae
Trade and other common names: Anisi stellati fructus; Badiana; Chinese anise; Eight-horned anise
Category: Antimycobacterial; Insecticide
Purported indications and other uses: Bronchitis, colic, cough, flatulence, menstrual complaints, respiratory tract inflammation. Culinary spice, fragrance component in cosmetics
Half-life: N/A

Note: Star anise preparations are sometimes contaminated with highly poisonous Japanese star anise (*Illicium anisatum*)
Star anise contains a compound used in the manufacture of Tamiflu

Reactions

Skin
Dermatitis
Erythema
Scaling
Sensitization

Other
Seizures
  (2002): Gil Campos M+, *An Esp Pediatr* 57(4), 366

STAVUDINE

Synonym: d4T
Trade name: Zerit (Bristol-Myers Squibb)
Indications: Human immunodeficiency virus (HIV)
Category: Antiretroviral; Nucleoside analog reverse transcriptase inhibitor
Half-life: 1.44 hours

Reactions

Skin
Allergic reactions (sic) (9%)
Diaphoresis (19%)
Neutrophilic eccrine hidradenitis
  (1998): Krischer J+, *J Dermatol* 25, 199
Rash (sic) (~40%)

Other
Chills (50%)
Death
  (2001): Hwang SW+, *Singapore Med J* 42(6), 247 (2 cases) (with didanosine)
Gynecomastia
  (2001): Aquilina C+, *Int J STD AIDS* 12(7), 481 (with didanosine)
  (2001): Manfredi R+, *Ann Pharmacother* 35(4), 438 (with didanosine)
  (2001): Manfredi R+, *Ann Pharmacother* 35(4), 438 (with lamivudine) (3 cases)
  (1998): Melbourne KM+, *Ann Pharmacother* 32, 1108
Headache
Lipoatrophy
  (2004): McComsey GA+, *Clin Infect Dis* 38(2), 263
  (2001): Lichtenstein KA+, *AIDS* 15(11), 1389
Lipodystrophy
  (2002): Bernasconi E+, *J Acquir Immune Defic Syndr* 31(1), 50
  (2002): Reid S, *Can Adv Drug Reaction Newsletter* 12, 5
  (2001): Aquilina C+, *Int J STD AIDS* 12(7), 481 (with didanosine)
  (2001): Arpadi SM+, *J Acquir Immune Defic Syndr* 27(1), 30
  (2001): Bogner JR+, *J Acquir Immune Defic Syndr* 27(3), 237
  (2001): van der Valk M+, *AIDS* 15(7), 847
  (1999): Ruel M+, *Ann Med Interne* (Paris) (French) 150, 269
Myalgia/Myositis/Myopathy/Myotoxicity (32%)
  (2000): Miller KD+, *Ann Intern Med* 133, 192
Paresthesias

STREPTOKINASE

Trade names: Kabikinase (Pfizer); Streptase (AstraZeneca)
Indications: Pulmonary embolism, acute myocardial infarction
Category: Fibrinolytic
Half-life: 83 minutes
Clinically important, potentially hazardous interactions with: bivalirudin

Reactions

Skin
Allergic reactions (sic) (4.4%)
  (2003): Janousek S, *Vnitr Lek* 49(11), 880
  (2001): Toquero J+, *Rev Esp Cardiol* 54(10), 1225
  (1998): Stephens MB+, *Postgrad Med* 103, 89
  (1997): Cannas S+, *G Ital Cardiol* (Italian) 27, 278
Angioedema (>10%)
  (1994): Cooper JP+, *Postgrad Med J* 70, 592

Diaphoresis (1–10%)
Exanthems (1–5%)
  (1990): Goa KL+, *Drugs* 39, 693
Hematomas
  (2006): Cakici N+, *Anadolu Kardiyol Derg* 6(4), 380
Pruritus (1–10%)
Purpura
Rash (sic) (1–10%)
Urticaria (1–5%)
  (1990): Goa KL+, *Drugs* 39, 693
Vasculitis
  (1994): Penswick J+, *BMJ* 309, 378
  (1991): Patel A+, *J Am Acad Dermatol* 24, 652
  (1988): Davidson JR+, *Clin Exp Rheumatol* 6, 381
  (1988): Ong AC+, *Int J Cardiology* 21, 71
  (1988): Sorber WA+, *Cutis* 42(1), 57
  (1986): Manoharan A+, *Aust N Z J Med* 16, 815
  (1985): Thompson RF+, *Clin Pharm* 4, 383

Mucosal/ENT
Stomatitis (following local application)
Tongue edema (with hemorrhagic swelling)

Eyes
Periorbital edema (>10%)

Other
Anaphylactoid reactions/Anaphylaxis (<1%)
  (2003): Janousek S, *Vnitr Lek* 49(11), 880
  (1993): Hohage H+, *Wien Klin Wochenschr* (German) 105, 176
Headache
Injection-site bleeding
  (1990): Goa KL+, *Drugs* 39, 693 (3%)
Injection-site phlebitis
Rhabdomyolysis
  (1999): Emmett LM+, *Clin Nucl Med* 24(12), 991
  (1995): Bennett D, *BMJ* 311(7018), 1472
Serum sickness
  (1995): Creamer JD+, *Clin Exp Dermatol* 20, 468
  (1994): Proctor BD+, *N Engl J Med* 330, 576
  (1991): Patel A+, *J Am Acad Dermatol* 24, 652
  (1984): Alexopoulos D+, *Eur Heart J* 5, 1010
  (1982): Totty WG+, *Am J Roentgenol* 138, 143

STREPTOMYCIN

Trade name: Streptomycin (Pfizer)
Indications: Tuberculosis
Category: Antibiotic, aminoglycoside
Half-life: 2–5 hours
Clinically important, potentially hazardous interactions with: aldesleukin, aminoglycosides, atracurium, bumetanide, doxacurium, ethacrynic acid, furosemide, methoxyflurane, non-depolarizing muscle relaxants, pancuronium, polypeptide antibiotics, rocuronium, succinylcholine, torsemide, vecuronium

Reactions

Skin
Acute generalized exanthematous pustulosis (AGEP)
  (1995): Moreau A+, *Int J Dermatol* 34, 263 (passim)
Allergic reactions (sic)
Angioedema (<1%)
Bullous dermatitis (<1%)
Dermatitis
  (1988): Holdiness MR, *Contact Dermatitis* 15, 282

(1983): Fisher AA, *Cutis* 32, 314
Eczema
Edema
Erythema multiforme (<1%)
  (1988): Hira SK+, *J Am Acad Dermatol* 19, 451 (in AIDS patient)
  (1985): Holdiness MR, *Int J Dermatol* 24, 280 (1–5%)
  (1985): Ting HC+, *Int J Dermatol* 24, 587
Erythema nodosum (<1%)
Exanthems (>5%)
Exfoliative dermatitis
  (1992): Matsuzawa Y+, *Kekkaku* (Japanese) 67, 413
  (1986): Sehgal VN+, *Dermatologica* 173, 278
  (1985): Holdiness MR, *Int J Dermatol* 24, 280
Fixed eruption (<1%)
Follicular pustular eruption
  (1981): Kushimoto H+, *Arch Dermatol* 117, 444
Jarisch–Herxheimer reaction
  (1992): Playford RJ+, *Gut* 33(1), 132 (with co-trimoxazole)
Lichenoid eruption
Lupus erythematosus
  (1993): Toyoshima M+, *Kekkaku* (Japanese) 68, 319
  (1986): Layer P+, *Dtsch Med Wochenschr* (German) 111, 1603
  (1980): Agarwal MB+, *J Postgrad Med* 26, 263
  (1980): Condemi JJ, *Geriatrics* 35(3), 81
Photosensitivity
Pruritus (<1%)
Purpura
Pustules
  (1981): Kushimoto H+, *Arch Dermatol* 117, 444
Rash (sic) (<1%)
Stevens–Johnson syndrome
  (1988): Hira SK+, *J Am Acad Dermatol* 19, 451 (in AIDS patient)
  (1985): Holdiness MR, *Int J Dermatol* 24, 280
  (1982): Sarkar SK+, *Tubercle* 63, 137
Toxic epidermal necrolysis
  (2005): Hmouda H+, *Ann Pharmacother* 39(1), 165
  (1994): *Drug Facts and Comparisons* 1926
  (1988): Fesenko IP+, *Vrach Delo* (Russian) April, 93
  (1980): Jain VK+, *Indian J Chest Dis Allied Sci* 22, 73
Toxic erythema
  (1981): Kushimoto H+, *Arch Dermatol* 117, 444
Urticaria
Vasculitis

Mucosal/ENT
Cheilitis (2%)
Glossitis (2%)
Oral mucosal eruption
Oral ulceration
Ototoxicity
  (2006): Lima ML+, *Rev Inst Med Trop Sao Paulo* 48(2), 99
  (2002): de Jager P+, *Int J Tuberc Lung Dis* 6(7), 622
Stomatitis
Tinnitus
Tongue black

Hair
Hair – hypertrichosis
  (1992): Shelley WB+, *Advanced Dermatologic Diagnosis* WB
    Saunders, 725 (passim)

Other
Anaphylactoid reactions/Anaphylaxis
  (2002): Romano A+, *Allergy* 57(11), 1087
DRESS syndrome
  (2004): Passeron T+, *Acta Derm Venereol* 84(1), 92
Embolia cutis medicamentosa (Nicolau syndrome)
  (2003): Reding EL+, *J Am Acad Dermatol* 48(3), 472

Headache
Injection-site granuloma
Injection-site reactions (sic)
Nephrotoxicity
  (2002): de Jager P+, *Int J Tuberc Lung Dis* 6(7), 622
Paresthesias (<1%)
Rhabdomyolysis
  (1992): Nakahara Y+, *Nippon Jinzo Gakkai Shi* 34(11), 1233
Tremor (<1%)

STREPTOZOCIN

Trade name: Zanosar (Gensia)
Indications: Carcinoma of the pancreas, carcinoid tumor, Hodgkin's disease
Category: Alkylating agent
Half-life: 35 minutes
Clinically important, potentially hazardous interactions with: aldesleukin

Reactions

Skin
Edema
Exanthems
Pruritus
Purpura
Toxic epidermal necrolysis

Other
Injection-site erythema
Injection-site necrosis
  (1987): Dufresne RG, *Cutis* 39, 197
Injection-site pain (1–10%)
Nephrotoxicity
  (2001): Kintzel PE, *Drug Saf* 24(1), 19
  (1988): Hricik DE+, *Am J Med* 84(1), 153

SUCCIMER

Synonyms: dimercaptosuccinic acid; DMSA
Trade name: Chemet (Sanofi-Aventis)
Indications: Heavy metal poisoning
Category: Chelator
Half-life: 2 days
Clinically important, potentially hazardous interactions with: other chelating agents

Reactions

Skin
Exanthems (11%)
Pruritus (11%)
Rash (sic) (<11%)
  (2000): *Pediatr Res* 48(5), 593 (3.5%)
  (1991): Grandjean P+, *Ugeskr Laeger* 153(41), 2897

Mucosal/ENT
Dysgeusia (metallic) (21%)
Mucocutaneous eruption (11%)

Nails
Nails – dystrophy

(1987): Thomas G+, *J Toxicol Clin Exp* 7(4), 285

Other
Abdominal pain (16%)
Candidiasis (16%)
Chills (16%)
Cough (1%)
Fever (16%)
Headache (16%)
Pain (3%)
Paresthesias (13%)
Vertigo

SUCCINYLCHOLINE

Synonym: suxamethonium
Trade name: Anectine (Sabex)
Indications: Skeletal muscle relaxation during general anesthesia
Category: Cholinesterase inhibitor; Depolarizing muscle relaxant
Half-life: N/A
Clinically important, potentially hazardous interactions with: amikacin, aminoglycosides, galantamine, gentamicin, kanamycin, neomycin, paromomycin, physostigmine, pipecuronium, streptomycin, tobramycin, vancomycin, vecuronium

Reactions

Skin
Dermatitis
  (1996): Delgado J+, *Contact Dermatitis* 35, 120
Erythema (<1%)
Exanthems
Pruritus (<1%)
Rash (sic) (<1%)
Urticaria

Mucosal/ENT
Sialorrhea (1–10%)

Other
Anaphylactoid reactions/Anaphylaxis
  (2002): Joly V+, *Anesthesiology* 97(1), 269
  (1999): Porter JM+, *Ir J Med Sci* 168, 99
  (1999): Villas Martinez F+, *J Investig Allergol Clin Immunol* 9, 126
  (1998): Tresch K+, *Ann Fr Anesth Reanim* (French) 17, 1181
  (1990): Moneret-Vautrin DA+, *Br J Anaesth* 64(6), 743
  (1981): Moneret-Vautrin DA+, *Clin Allergy* 11, 175 (13 cases)
Hypersensitivity
  (1983): Yamaya R+, *Masui* (Japanese) 32, 1464
Myalgia/Myositis/Myopathy/Myotoxicity (<1%)
  (2006): Hassani M+, *Middle East J Anesthesiol* 18(5), 929
  (2006): Kettler RE, *Anesthesiology* 105(1), 222
  (2006): Sakuraba S+, *Acta Anaesthesiol Belg* 57(3), 253
  (2003): Kararmaz A+, *Acta Anaesthesiol Scand* 47(2), 180
  (2003): Schreiber JU+, *Anesth Analg* 96(6), 1640
  (2002): Amornyotin S+, *J Med Assoc Thai* 85, S969
  (1996): van den Berg AA+, *Anaesth Intensive Care* 24, 116
  (1990): Shoji S, *Nippon Rinsho* (Japanese) 48, 1517
Rhabdomyolysis
  (2005): Escudero A+, *Rev Esp Anestesiol Reanim* 52(3), 184
  (2001): Gronert GA, *Anesthesiology* 94(3), 523
  (2000): Le Puura+, *Acta Anaesthesiol Belg* 51(1), 51

(2000): Matthews JM, *Anesth Analg* 91(6), 1552
(2000): Shaaban MJ+, *Middle East J Anesthesiology* 15(6), 681
(1996): Fiacchino F, *Anesthesiology* 84(2), 480
(1996): Pedrozzi NE+, *Pediatr Neurol* 15(3), 254 (2 cases)
(1996): Perret D+, *Ann Fr Anesth Reanim* 15(8), 1193
(1996): Takamatsu F+, *Masui* 45(11), 1406
(1995): Friedman S+, *Anesth Analg* 81(2), 422
(1995): Schulte-Sasse U, *HNO* 43(11), 676
(1994): Sullivan M+, *Can J Anaesth* 41(6), 497
(1993): Bhave CG+, *J Postgrad Med* 39(3), 157
(1992): Bakshi KK, *J Assoc Physicians India* 40(8), 549
(1991): Gokhale YA+, *J Assoc Physicians India* 39(12), 968
(1987): Lee SC+, *J Oral Maxillofac Surg* 45(9), 789 (with enflurane)
(1987): Lee SC+, *Ma Zui Xue Za Zhi* 25(2), 97
(1985): Hawker F+, *Anaesth Intensive Care* 13(2), 208
(1985): Sodano R+, *Minerva Anestesiol* 51(3), 109
(1984): Blumberg A+, *Schweiz Med Wochenschr* 114(30), 1068 (2 cases)
(1984): Hool GJ+, *Anaesth Intensive Care* 12(4), 360
(1981): Lewandowski KB, *Br J Anaesth* 53(9), 981

SUCRALFATE

Trade names: Antepsin; Carafate (Axcan); Sucrabest; Sulcrate; Ulcar; Ulcogant; Ulcyte; Urbal
Indications: Duodenal ulcer
Category: Chelator
Half-life: N/A
Clinically important, potentially hazardous interactions with: ciprofloxacin, clorazepate, ketoconazole, lansoprazole, lomefloxacin, phenytoin, sparfloxacin, tetracycline

Note: Sucralfate use can lead to symptoms of aluminium toxicity

Reactions

Skin
Angioedema
Exanthems
  (1984): Brogden RN+, *Drugs* 17, 233
Facial edema
Pruritus (<0.5%)
Rash (sic) (<0.5%)
Urticaria

Mucosal/ENT
Xerostomia (<1%)
  (1982): Garnett WR, *Clin Pharm* 1(4), 307 (1%)
  (1981): Ishimori A, *J Clin Gastroenterol* 3(Supp 2), 169 (%)

Other
Headache
Nephrotoxicity
  (2001): Hemstreet BA, *Ann Pharmacother* 35(3), 360

SUCRALOSE

Trade name: Splenda (McNeil)
Indications: Weight reduction
Half-life: 2–5 hours
Clinically important, potentially hazardous interactions with: N/A

Reactions

Other
Migraine
  (2007): Hirsch AR, *Headache* 47(3), 447
  (2006): Bigal ME+, *Headache* 46(3), 515
  (2006): Patel RM+, *Headache* 46(8), 1303

SUFENTANIL

Trade name: Sufenta (Akorn)
Indications: Epidural and general anesthesia
Category: Anesthetic, general; Opiate agonist
Half-life: 152 minutes
Clinically important, potentially hazardous interactions with: cimetidine

Reactions

Skin
Clammy skin (<1%)
Erythema
Pruritus
  (2005): Fournier R+, *Reg Anesth Pain Med* 30(3), 249
  (2004): Waxler B+, *Can J Anaesth* 51(7), 685
  (2003): Eriksson SL+, *Eur J Obstet Gynecol Reprod Biol* 110(2), 131 (85%) (with bupivacaine)
  (2002): Yazigi A+, *J Clin Anesth* 14(3), 183
  (2001): Hubler M+, *Eur J Anaesthesiol* 18(7), 450
  (2000): Abouleish AE+, *Can J Anaesth* 47(12), 1171
  (1999): Lau WC+, *Anesth Analg* 89(4), 889
  (1999): Lo WK+, *Singapore Med J* 40(10), 639
Rash (sic) (<1%)
Urticaria (<1%)

Other
Chills

SULFACETAMIDE

Trade names: Ak-Sulf; Albucid; Antebor; Blephamide (Allergan); Cetasil; Colirio Sulfacetamido Kriya; Covosulf; Dansemid; Dayto-Sulf; Diosulf; I-Sulfacet; Klaron (Dermik); Lersa; Novacet; Ocu-Sulf; Ophthacet; Optamide; Optin; Optisol; Ovace (Healthpoint); Plexion (Medicis); Prontamid; Rosula (Doak); Sodium Sulfacetamide; Spectro-Sulf; Spersacet; Storz-Sulf; Sulf-10; Sulfac; Sulfacel-15; Sulfacet Sodium (Dermik); Sulfacet-R (Dermik); Sulfair; Sulfamide; Sulfex; Sulphacalre; Vasocidin (Novartis); Vasosulf (Novartis)
Indications: Infectious conjunctivitis, acne vulgaris, seborrheic dermatitis
Category: Antibiotic, sulfonamide
Half-life: 7–13 hours
Clinically important, potentially hazardous interactions with: anticoagulants, cyclosporine, silver salts

Reactions

Skin
Allergic reactions (sic)
  (2002): Smith JG, Mobile, AL (Klaron & Sulfacet-R) (from Internet) (observations 2 cases)

  (2000): Blumenthal HL, Beachwood, OH (Novacet Lotion) (personal case) (observation)
Dermatomyositis
Edema
Erythema
Erythema multiforme
  (1985): Genvert GI+, *Am J Ophthalmol* 99(4), 465 (topical)
Exfoliative dermatitis (1–10%)
Lupus erythematosus – dermatomyositis
Photosensitivity
Pruritus
Stevens–Johnson syndrome (1–10%)
Toxic epidermal necrolysis (1–10%)
  (2003): Spencer L, Crawfordsville, IN (from Internet) (observation) (from topical Silvadene)

Eyes
Corneal opacity
  (1984): Tabbara KF+, *Am J Ophthalmol* 98(3), 378
Keratopathy
  (1986): Grossniklaus HE+, *Ophthalmology* 93(2), 260
Ocular burning
Ocular stinging

Other
Death
Hypersensitivity
Infections

SULFADIAZINE

Trade names: Coptin; Microsulfon
Indications: Various infections caused by susceptible organisms
Category: Antibiotic, sulfonamide
Half-life: 17 hours
Clinically important, potentially hazardous interactions with: anticoagulants, cyclosporine, methotrexate

Note: Sulfadiazine is a sulfonamide and can be absorbed systemically. Sulfonamides can produce severe, possibly fatal, reactions such as toxic epidermal necrolysis and Stevens–Johnson syndrome

Reactions

Skin
Allergic reactions (sic)
  (1991): de la Hoz Caballer B+, *J Allergy Clin Immunol* 88, 137
Erythema multiforme
  (1983): Lockhart SP+, *Burns Incl Therm Inj* 10, 9
Exanthems
  (1984): Finland M+, *JAMA* 251, 1467
Exfoliative dermatitis
Fixed eruption (12%)
  (2004): Tornero P+, *Contact Dermatitis* 51(2), 57
  (1991): Thankappen TP+, *Int J Dermatol* 30, 867 (12.4%)
Lupus erythematosus
Photosensitivity (>10%)
Pigmentation
  (1985): Dupuis LL+, *J Am Acad Dermatol* 12, 1112
Pruritus (>10%)
Purpura
Rash (sic) (>10%)
Stevens–Johnson syndrome (1–10%)
  (1999): Carrion-Carrion C+, *Ann Pharmacother* 33, 379 (fatal) (in AIDS patient)
Toxic epidermal necrolysis (1–10%)

(1993): Correia O+, *Dermatology* 186, 32
Urticaria
  (2005): Chen QK+, *World J Gastroenterol* 11(16), 2462 (2 cases)

Mucosal/ENT
Sialadenitis
  (1997): Anibarro B+, *Ann Pharmacother* 31(1), 59
Stomatitis
Tinnitus

Eyes
Periorbital edema

Other
Anaphylactoid reactions/Anaphylaxis
  (2001): Stephens R+, *Br J Anaesth* 87(2), 306 (with
    chlorhexidine)
Chills
Death
DRESS syndrome
  (2005): Michel F+, *Joint Bone Spine* 72(1), 82
Hypersensitivity
  (2005): Orita M+, *Nippon Shokakibyo Gakkai Zasshi* 102(5), 600
  (2001): Morand JJ+, *Ann Dermatol Venereol* 128(12), 1351
  (1987): Volckaert A+, *Acta Clin Belg* 42, 381
  (1985): Jia XM, *Chung Hua Cheng Hsing Shao Shang Wai Ko Tsa
    Chih* (Chinese) 1, 232
Nephrotoxicity
  (2006): Hyvernat H+, *Presse Med* 35(3 Pt 1), 423
  (2000): Crespo M+, *Clin Nephrol* 54(1), 68
Serum sickness (<1%)

SULFADOXINE

Trade names: Cryodoxin; Fansidar (Roche); Malocide; Methipox
Indications: Malaria
Category: Antibiotic, sulfonamide; Antimalarial
Half-life: 5–8 days

Note: Fansidar is sulfadoxine and pyrimethamine (this combination is
almost always prescribed)

Note: Sulfadoxine is a sulfonamide and can be absorbed systemically.
Sulfonamides can produce severe, possibly fatal, reactions such as
toxic epidermal necrolysis and Stevens–Johnson syndrome

Reactions

Skin
Bullous dermatitis
  (1985): Hernborg A, *Lancet* 1, 1072
Erythema multiforme (<1%)
  (1993): Sturchler D+, *Drug Saf* 8, 160
  (1989): Ortel B+, *Dermatologica* 178, 39
  (1986): Miller KD+, *Am J Trop Med Hyg* 35, 451
Exanthems
  (1987): Groth H+, *Schweiz Rundsch Med Prax* (German) 76, 570
Exfoliative dermatitis
  (1987): Elsas T+, *Tidsskr Nor Laegeforen* (Norwegian) 107, 1231
  (1987): Zitelli BJ+, *Ann Intern Med* 106, 393
  (1986): Langtry JA+, *Br Med J Clin Res Ed* 292, 1107
Fixed eruption
  (2006): Nnoruka EN+, *Int J Dermatol* 45(9), 1062
Lupus erythematosus
Necrosis (<1%)
Photosensitivity (>10%)
  (1989): Ortel B+, *Dermatologica* 178, 39
  (1985): Hernborg A, *Lancet* 1, 1072 (passim)

Pruritus
  (1987): Groth H+, *Schweiz Rundsch Med Prax* (German) 76, 570
Purpura
  (1985): Hernborg A, *Lancet* 1, 1072 (passim)
Pustules
Rash (sic) (<1%)
Stevens–Johnson syndrome (1–10%)
  (2006): Gimnig JE+, *Am J Trop Med Hyg* 74(5), 738 (%) (with
    pyrimethamine)
  (2005): Oduro-Boatey C+, *Trop Doct* 35(2), 118
  (1997): Teira R+, *Scand J Infect Dis* 29(6), 595 (with
    pyrimethamine)
  (1993): Sturchler D+, *Drug Saf* 8, 160
  (1990): Thiel HJ+, *Klin Monatsbl Augenheilkd* (German) 197, 142
  (1989): Ortel B+, *Dermatologica* 178, 39
  (1989): Phillips-Howard PA+, *Lancet* 2, 803
  (1987): Hellgren U+, *Br Med J Clin Res Ed* 295, 365
  (1987): Lenox-Smith I, *J Infect* 14, 90 (fatal)
  (1986): Bamber MG+, *J Infect* 13, 31 (fatal)
  (1986): Gascon-Brustenga J+, *Med Clin* (Barc) (Spanish) 87, 821
  (1986): Jeffrey RF, *Postgrad Med J* 62, 893
  (1986): Miller KD+, *Am J Trop Med Hyg* 35, 451
  (1986): Steffen R+, *Lancet* 1, 610
  (1985): Adams SJ+, *Postgrad Med J* 61, 263
  (1985): Clareus BW+, *Lakartidningen* (Swedish) 82, 4211
  (1985): Hernborg A, *Lancet* 2, 1072
  (1985): Navin TR+, *Lancet* 1, 1332
  (1983): Ligthelm RJ+, *Ned Tijdschr Geneeskd* (Dutch) 127, 1735
  (1982): Aberer W+, *Hautarzt* (German) 33, 484
  (1982): Hornstein OP+, *N Engl J Med* 307, 1529
  (1982): Olsen VV+, *Lancet* 2, 994
Toxic epidermal necrolysis
  (2006): Gimnig JE+, *Am J Trop Med Hyg* 74(5), 738 (%) (with
    pyrimethamine)
  (2000): Moussala M+, *J Fr Ophtalmol* (French) 23, 229
  (1998): Moussala M+, *J Fr Ophtalmol* (French) 21, 72
  (1998): Schmidt-Westhausen A+, *Oral Dis* 4, 90
  (1993): Correia O+, *Dermatology* 186, 32
  (1993): Sturchler D+, *Drug Saf* 8, 160
  (1991): Kimura S+, *Jpn J Med* 30, 553
  (1990): Ward DJ+, *Burns* 16, 97
  (1989): Caumes E+, *Presse Med* (French) 18, 1708 (fatal)
  (1988): No Author, *JAMA* 260, 2193 (fatal)
  (1988): No Author, *Morb Mortal Wkly Rep* 37, 571 (fatal)
  (1988): Raviglione MC+, *Arch Intern Med* 148, 2863 (fatal)
  (1986): Miller KD+, *Am J Trop Med Hyg* 35, 451
  (1984): Chan HL, *J Am Acad Dermatol* 10, 973
  (1983): Ghinelli F+, *Acta Biomed Ateneo Parmense* (Italian)
    54, 363
Urticaria

Mucosal/ENT
Ageusia
Glossitis (>10%)
Oral lichenoid eruption
  (1989): Zain RB, *Southeast Asian J Trop Med Public Health* 20, 253
Oral ulceration
  (1985): Hernborg A, *Lancet* 1, 1072
Stomatitis
  (1985): Hernborg A, *Lancet* 1, 1072 (passim)
Tinnitus
Urogenital ulceration
  (1985): Hernborg A, *Lancet* 1, 1072

Eyes
Periorbital edema

Other
Anaphylactoid reactions/Anaphylaxis
Asthenia

(2006): Fanello CI+, *Trop Med Int Health* 11(5), 589 (with pyrimethamine)
Death
Hypersensitivity (>10%)
Tremor (>10%)
Vertigo
(2006): Fanello CI+, *Trop Med Int Health* 11(5), 589 (with pyrimethamine)

SULFAMETHOXAZOLE

Trade names: Bactrim (Women First); Septra (Monarch); Sinomin; Urobak
Indications: Various infections caused by susceptible organisms
Category: Antibiotic, sulfonamide; Folic acid antagonist
Half-life: 7–12 hours
Clinically important, potentially hazardous interactions with: anticoagulants, cyclosporine, methotrexate, probenecid, warfarin

Note: Sulfamethoxazole is commonly used in conjunction with trimethoprim (see co-trimoxazole)

Note: Sulfamethoxazole is a sulfonamide and can be absorbed systemically. Sulfonamides can produce severe, possibly fatal, reactions such as toxic epidermal necrolysis and Stevens–Johnson syndrome

Reactions

Skin
Acute febrile neutrophilic dermatosis (Sweet's syndrome)
(1996): Walker DC+, *J Am Acad Dermatol* 34, 918
(1989): Cobb MW, *J Am Acad Dermatol* 21, 339 (passim)
(1986): Su WPD+, *Cutis* 37, 167
Acute generalized exanthematous pustulosis (AGEP)
(2003): Anliker MD+, *J Investig Allergol Clin Immunol* 13(1), 66 (with co-trimoxazole)
(1995): Moreau A+, *Int J Dermatol* 34, 263 (passim)
Allergic reactions (sic)
(2004): Karpman E+, *J Urol* 172(2), 448
(2002): Choquet-Kastylevsky G+, *Curr Allergy Asthma Rep* 2(1), 16
Angioedema (1–5%)
(1988): Fihn SD+, *Ann Intern Med* 108, 350 (1–5%)
Bullous dermatitis
(1989): Caumes E+, *Presse Med* (French) 18, 1708
Dermatitis
(1989): Atahan IL+, *Br J Radiol* 62, 1107 (at previously irradiated area)
(1987): Vukelja SJ+, *Cancer Treat Rep* 71, 668 (at previously irradiated area)
(1984): Shelley WB+, *J Am Acad Dermatol* 11, 53 (at site of previous sunburn)
Erythema multiforme
(1997): Rieder MJ+, *Pediatr Infect Dis J* 16, 1028 (70% in children with HIV)
(1991): Tilden ME+, *Arch Ophthalmol* 109, 67
(1990): Chan HL+, *Arch Dermatol* 126, 43
(1989): Alanko K+, *Acta Derm Venereol* (Stockh) 69, 223
(1988): Hira SK+, *J Am Acad Dermatol* 19, 451
(1988): Platt R+, *J Infect Dis* 158, 474
(1987): Penmetcha M, *BMJ* 295, 556
(1987): Schöpf E, *Infection* 15 (Suppl 5P), S254
(1985): Heer M+, *Gastroenterology* 88, 1954
(1982): Brettle RP+, *J Infect* 4, 149
Erythema nodosum

Erythroderma
Exanthems (1–5%)
(1998): Hattori N+, *J Dermatol* 25, 269
(1997): Caumes E+, *Arch Dermatol* 133, 465
(1995): Hertl M+, *Br J Dermatol* 132, 215
(1995): Wolkenstein P+, *Arch Dermatol* 131, 544
(1994): Litt JZ, Beachwood, OH (personal case) (observation)
(1993): Agarwal BR+, *Indian Pediatr* 30, 1026
(1993): Litt JZ, Beachwood, OH (personal case) (observation)
(1993): Malnick SDH+, *Ann Pharmacotherapy* 27, 1139
(1990): Medina I+, *N Engl J Med* 323, 776 (47% in AIDS patients)
(1988): DeRaeve L+, *Br J Dermatol* 119, 521 (in AIDS patient)
(1988): Fihn SD+, *Ann Intern Med* 108, 350 (1–5%)
(1988): Sattler FR+, *Ann Intern Med* 109, 280 (44% in AIDS patients)
(1988): Weinke T+, *Dtsch Med Wochenschr* (German) 113, 1129 (25% in AIDS patients)
(1987): Goa KL+, *Drugs* 33, 242 (65% in AIDS patients)
(1987): Schöpf E, *Infection* 15 (Suppl 5P), S254
(1986): Sonntag MR+, *Schweiz Med Wochenschr* (German) 116, 142
(1985): DeHovitz JA+, *Ann Intern Med* 103, 479
(1985): Maayan S+, *Arch Intern Med* 145, 1607
(1984): Gordon FM+, *Ann Intern Med* 100, 495 (51% in AIDS patients)
(1984): Kovacs JA+, *Ann Intern Med* 100, 663 (29% in AIDS patients)
(1983): Mitsuyasu R+, *N Engl J Med* 308, 1535 (69% in AIDS patients)
(1982): Goetz MB+, *JAMA* 247, 3118
(1980): Fennell RS+, *Clin Pediatr* 19, 124
Exfoliative dermatitis
(1990): Ponte CD+, *Drug Intell Clin Pharm* 24, 140 (feet)
Fixed eruption
(2007): *Prescrire Int* 16(87), 21 (with trimethoprim)
(2006): Rasi A+, *Dermatol Online J* 12(6), 12 (with trimethoprim)
(2004): Tornero P+, *Contact Dermatitis* 51(2), 57
(1997): Gruber F+, *Clin Exp Dermatol* 22, 144
(1996): Sharma VK+, *J Dermatol* 23, 530
(1995): Wolkenstein P+, *Arch Dermatol* 131, 544
(1993): Oleaga JM+, *Contact Dermatitis* 29, 155
(1993): Ramam M+, *Indian Pediatr* 30, 110 (in an infant)
(1992): Lim JT+, *Ann Acad Med Singapore* 21, 408
(1991): Jain VK+, *Ann Dent* 50, 9 (oral mucous membrane)
(1991): Smoller BR+, *J Cutan Pathol* 18, 13
(1990): Gaffoor PMA+, *Cutis* 45, 242 (genitalia)
(1989): Basomba A+, *J Allergy Clin Immunol* 84, 409
(1989): Bharija SC+, *Australas J Dermatol* 30, 43
(1989): Gupta R, *Indian J Dermatol* 55, 181 (in an infant)
(1989): Varsano I+, *Dermatologica* 178, 232
(1988): Baird BJ+, *Int J Dermatol* 27, 170 (bullous and generalized)
(1988): Bharija SC+, *Dermatologica* 176, 108 (in an infant)
(1987): Amir J+, *Drug Intell Clin Pharm* 21, 41
(1987): Hughes BR+, *Br J Dermatol* 116, 241
(1987): Van Voorhees A+, *Am J Dermatopathol* 9, 528
(1986): Kanwar AJ+, *Dermatologica* 172, 230
(1985): Gomez B+, *Allergol Immunopathol Madr* (Spanish) 13, 87
(1984): Pandhi RK+, *Sex Transm Dis* 11, 164
(1982): Gibson JR, *BMJ* 284, 1529
(1980): Talbot MD, *Practitioner* 224, 823
Lichenoid eruption
(1994): Berger TG+, *Arch Dermatol* 130, 609
Linear IgA dermatosis
(2003): Avci O+, *J Am Acad Dermatol* 48(2), 299 (passim)
(1994): Kuechle MK+, *J Am Acad Dermatol* 30, 187
Lupus erythematosus
(1985): Stratton MA, *Clin Pharm* 4, 657
Photo-recall

(1990): Leslie MD+, *Br J Radiol* 63, 661
(1987): Vukelja SJ+, *Cancer Treat Rep* 71, 668 (at previously irradiated area)
(1984): Shelley WB+, *J Am Acad Dermatol* 11, 53 (at site of previous sunburn)

Photosensitivity (>10%)
(1994): Berger TG+, *Arch Dermatol* 130, 609 (in HIV-infected) (4 cases)
(1994): Shelley WB+, *Cutis* 53, 162 (observation)
(1987): Schöpf E, *Infection* 15 (Suppl 5P), S254
(1986): Chandler MJ, *J Infect Dis* 153, 1001

Pruritus (10%)
(1997): Caumes E+, *Arch Dermatol* 133, 465
(1997): Thaler D, Monona, WI (from Internet) (observation)
(1996): Litt JZ, Beachwood, OH (personal case) (observation)
(1990): Medina I+, *N Engl J Med* 323, 776 (1–5%)
(1987): Colebunders R+, *Ann Intern Med* 107, 599 (4% in AIDS patients)
(1986): Sher MR, *J Allergy Clin Immunol* 77, 133
(1984): Kramer BS+, *Cancer* 53, 329

Pruritus ani et vulvae
(1981): *Modern Medicine* 49, 111

Psoriasis

Purpura
(1993): Kaufman DW+, *Blood* 82, 2714
(1989): Saxena SK, *J Assoc Physicians India* 37, 479

Pustules
(1994): Spencer JM+, *Br J Dermatol* 130, 514
(1990): Guy C+, *Nouv Dermatol* (French) 9, 540
(1989): Grattan CEH, *Dermatologica* 179, 57 (passim)
(1986): Macdonald KJS+, *BMJ* 293, 1279

Rash (sic) (>10%)
(2006): Hemstreet BA+, *Pharmacotherapy* 26(4), 551 (with trimethoprim)
(1995): Williams JW+, *JAMA* 273, 1015
(1993): Malnick SD+, *Ann Pharmacother* 27, 1139

Side effects (sic) (2%)
(1994): Roudier C+, *Arch Dermatol* 130, 1383 (48% in AIDS patients)

Stevens–Johnson syndrome (1–10%)
(2006): Hemstreet BA+, *Pharmacotherapy* 26(4), 551 (with trimethoprim)
(1997): Douglas R+, *Clin Infect Dis* 25, 1480
(1997): Rieder MJ+, *Pediatr Infect Dis J* 16, 1028 (10% in children with HIV)
(1996): Caumes E, *Rev Mal Respir* (French) 13, 101
(1996): McCarty J, Fort Worth, TX (from Internet) (observation)
(1995): Kuper K+, *Ophthalmologe* (German) 92, 823
(1995): Sharma VK+, *Pediatr Dermatol* 12, 178
(1995): Wolkenstein P+, *Arch Dermatol* 131, 544
(1994): Shelley WB+, *Cutis* 53, 159 (observation)
(1993): Litt JZ, Beachwood, OH (personal case) (observation)
(1990): Chan HL+, *Arch Dermatol* 126, 43
(1988): Platt R+, *J Infect Dis* 158, 474
(1985): Heer M+, *Gastroenterology* 88, 1954
(1982): Brettle RP+, *J Infect* 4, 149

Toxic epidermal necrolysis (1–10%)
(2002): Nassif A+, *J Invest Dermatol* 118(4), 728
(2001): See S+, *Ann Pharmacother* 35(6), 694
(2000): Moussala M+, *J Fr Ophtalmol* (French) 23, 229
(1996): Caumes E, *Rev Mal Respir* 13, 101
(1996): Rehbein H, Jacksonville, FL (from Internet) (observation)
(1995): Sharma VK+, *Pediatr Dermatol* 12, 178
(1995): Wolkenstein P+, *Arch Dermatol* 131, 544 (7 cases)
(1993): Correia O+, *Dermatology* 186, 32
(1990): Chan HL+, *Arch Dermatol* 126, 43
(1990): Kobza Black A+, *Br J Dermatol* 123, 277
(1990): Roujeau JC+, *Arch Dermatol* 126, 37
(1990): Ward DJ+, *Burns* 16, 97

(1989): Carmichael AJ+, *Lancet* 2, 808
(1989): Whittington RM, *Lancet* 2, 574
(1988): De Raeve L+, *Br J Dermatol* 119, 521 (passim)
(1987): Guillaume JC+, *Arch Dermatol* 123, 1166
(1987): Schöpf E, *Infection* 15 (Suppl 5P), S254
(1986): Miller KD+, *Am J Trop Med Hyg* 33, 451
(1986): Revuz J, *J Dermatol Paris* 153
(1986): Roman O+, *Rev Pediatr Obstet Ginecol Pediatr* (Romanian) 35, 261
(1984): Fong PH+, *Singapore Med J* 25, 184
(1984): Westly ED+, *Arch Dermatol* 120, 721
(1983): Petersen P+, *Ugeskr Laeger* (Danish) 145, 3345
(1982): Ortiz JE+, *Ann Plast Surg* 9, 249

Urticaria
(2006): Batioglu F+, *Cutan Ocul Toxicol* 25(4), 281 (with trimethoprim)
(1994): Blumenthal HL, Beachwood, OH (personal case) (observation)
(1993): Litt JZ, Beachwood, OH (personal case) (observation)
(1991): Greenberger PA, *JAMA* 265, 458
(1987): Schöpf E, *Infection* 15 (Suppl 5P), S254
(1985): Goolamali SK, *Postgrad Med J* 61, 925
(1985): Maayan S+, *Arch Intern Med* 145, 1607
(1984): Kramer BS+, *Cancer* 53, 329
(1981): Abi-Mansur P+, *Am J Gastroenterol* 76, 356

Vasculitis (<1%)
(1989): Verne-Pignatelli J+, *Postgrad Med J* 65, 51
(1987): Schöpf E, *Infection* 15 (Suppl 5P), S254

Mucosal/ENT

Aphthous stomatitis
(1981): *J Antimicrob Chemother* 7, 179

Dysgeusia
(1988): Fischl MA+, *JAMA* 259, 1185

Glossitis

Mucocutaneous syndrome
(1982): Brettle RP+, *J Infect* 4, 149

Oral mucosal eruption
(1991): Tilden ME+, *Arch Ophthalmol* 109, 67
(1988): Fihn SD+, *Ann Intern Med* 108, 350 (1–5%)

Oral ulceration
(1987): Hughes WT+, *N Engl J Med* 316, 1627
(1981): Orenstein WA+, *Am J Med Sci* 282, 27

Stomatitis

Tongue black
(1993): Blumenthal HL, Beachwood, OH (personal case) (observation)

Tongue ulceration
(1981): *J Antimicrob Chemother* 7, 179

Vaginitis
(1985): Wong ES+, *Ann Intern Med* 102, 302

Eyes

Visual disturbances
(2006): Batioglu F+, *Cutan Ocul Toxicol* 25(4), 281 (with trimethoprim)

Other

Abdominal pain
(2003): Floris-Moore MA+, *Ann Pharmacother* 37(12), 1810 (with trimethoprim)

Anaphylactoid reactions/Anaphylaxis
(2006): Hemstreet BA+, *Pharmacotherapy* 26(4), 551 (with trimethoprim)
(2003): Schuster C+, *Allergy* 58(10), 1072 (with celecoxib)
(1988): Arnold PA+, *Drug Intell Clin Pharm* 22, 43
(1985): Gossius G+, *Scand J Infect Dis* 16, 373

Death

Hypersensitivity

(2006): Mohammedi I+, *Rev Med Interne* 27(6), 499 (with trimethoprim)
(1998): Chen D, Chicagi, IL (from Internet) (observation)
(1997): Hicks ME+, *Ann Pharmacother* 31, 1259
(1993): Marinac JS+, *Clin Infect Dis* 16, 178
(1993): Martin GJ+, *Clin Infect Dis* 16, 175
(1993): Mathelier-Fusade P+, *Presse Med* (French) 22, 1363
(1993): Mehta J+, *J Assoc Physicians India* 41, 235
Nephrotoxicity
(1998): Schwarz A+, *Int J Clin Pharmacol Ther* 36(3), 164
Pseudolymphoma
Rhabdomyolysis
(2006): Walker S+, *Am J Med Sci* 331(6), 339 (with trimethoprim)
Serum sickness (<1%)
(1988): Platt R+, *J Infect Dis* 158, 474
Tremor
(2003): Floris-Moore MA+, *Ann Pharmacother* 37(12), 1810 (with trimethoprim)

SULFASALAZINE

Synonym: salicylazosulfapyridine
Trade names: Azulfidine (Pfizer); Colo-Pleon; Salazopyrin; Salisulf; Saridine; SAS-500; Sulfazine; Ulcol
Indications: Inflammatory bowel disease, ulcerative colitis, rheumatoid arthritis
Category: Aminosalicylate; Disease-modifying antirheumatic; Sulfonamide
Half-life: 5–10 hours
Clinically important, potentially hazardous interactions with: cholestyramine, methotrexate

Note: Sulfasalazine is a sulfonamide and can be absorbed systemically. Sulfonamides can produce severe, possibly fatal, reactions such as toxic epidermal necrolysis and Stevens–Johnson syndrome

Reactions

Skin

Acute generalized exanthematous pustulosis (AGEP)
(1999): Kawaguchi M+, *J Dermatol* 26, 359
(1998): Mitchell D, Thomasville, GA (from Internet) (observation)
(1993): Marce S+, *Presse Med* (French) 22, 271
(1993): Wainwright NJ+, *Drug Saf* 9, 437
Adverse effects (sic)
(1993): Gran JT+, *Scand J Rheumatol* 22, 229
Angioedema
(1990): Donovan S+, *Br J Rheumatol* 29, 201
(1990): Petterson T+, *Br J Rheumatol* 29, 239
Bullous dermatitis
Bullous pemphigoid
(2001): Vaccaro M+, *Dermatology* 203(2), 194
Dermatitis
(2001): Lau G+, *Forensic Sci Int* 122(2), 79
(1989): Challier P+, *Presse Med* (French) 18, 778
Diaphoresis
(1986): Farr M+, *Drugs* 32 (Suppl 1), 49
Eczema
Erythema multiforme
(1987): Penmetcha M, *BMJ* 295, 556
(1986): Garcia e Silva L, *Acta Med Port* (Portuguese) 7, 71
(1985): Heer M+, *Gastroenterology* 88, 1954
(1985): Hernborg A, *Lancet* 2, 1072

(1985): Huff JC, *Dermatol Clin* 3, 141
(1982): Hornstein OP+, *N Engl J Med* 307, 1529
Erythema nodosum
(1986): Areias E+, *Ann Dermatol Venereol* (French) 113, 197
Erythroderma
(1984): Sala F+, *Cronica Dermatol* (Italian) 15, 209
Exanthems (2–23%)
(1995): Wolkenstein P+, *Arch Dermatol* 131, 544
(1994): Akahoshi K+, *J Gastroenterol* 29, 772
(1992): Bodokh I+, *Presse Med* (French) 21, 630
(1991): Hertzberger-ten-Cate R+, *Clin Exp Rheumatol* 9, 85
(1990): Donovan S+, *Br J Rheumatol* 29, 201 (4.1%)
(1990): Gupta AK+, *Arch Dermatol* 126, 487 (23%)
(1990): Petterson T+, *Br J Rheumatol* 29, 239
(1989): Alanko K+, *Acta Derm Venereol* (Stockh) 69, 223
(1989): Gremse DA+, *J Pediatr Gastroenterol Nutr* 9, 261
(1988): Williams HJ+, *Arthritis Rheum* 31, 702 (7%)
(1986): Farr M+, *Drugs* 32 (Suppl 1), 49
(1986): Poland GA+, *Am J Med* 81, 707
(1985): Maayan S+, *Arch Intern Med* 145, 1607
(1984): Iwatsuki K+, *Arch Dermatol* 120, 964
(1984): Peppercorn MA, *Ann Intern Med* 101, 377
(1984): Purdy BH+, *Ann Intern Med* 100, 512
(1982): Goetz MB+, *JAMA* 247, 3118
(1980): Fennell RS+, *Clin Pediatr* 19, 124
Exfoliative dermatitis
(1990): Donovan S+, *Br J Rheumatol* 29, 201
(1984): Sala F+, *Cronica Dermatol* (Italian) 15, 209
Fixed eruption
(1996): Kawada A+, *Contact Dermatitis* 34, 155
(1988): Bharija SC+, *Dermatologica* 176, 108
(1987): Hughes BR+, *Br J Dermatol* 116, 241
(1987): Kanwar AJ+, *Dermatologica* 174, 104
(1986): Kanwar AJ+, *Dermatologica* 172, 230
(1982): Gibson JR, *BMJ* 284, 1529
(1980): Talbot MD, *Practitioner* 224, 823
Lichen planus
(1995): Kaplan S+, *J Rheumatol* 22, 191
(1991): Alstead EM+, *J Clin Gastroenterol* 13, 335
Lupus erythematosus
(2002): Angelova I+, *World Congress Dermatol* Poster, 0083 (patient has psoriasis)
(2002): Siddiqui MA+, *Am J Ther* 9(2), 163 (passim)
(2002): Tsai WC+, *Clin Rheumatol* 21(4), 339
(2000): Chebli JM+, *Arq Gastroenterol* 37(4), 224
(2000): Gunnarsson I+, *Rheumatology* (Oxford) 39(8), 886
(1997): Gunnarsson I+, *Br J Rheumatol* 36, 1089
(1996): Khattak FH+, *Br J Rheumatol* 35, 104
(1995): Veale DJ+, *Br J Rheumatol* 34, 383
(1994): Borg AA+, *Clin Rheumatol* 13, 522
(1994): Bray VJ+, *J Rheumatol* 21, 2157
(1994): Caulier M+, *J Rheumatol* 21, 750
(1994): Fritzler MJ, *Lupus* 3, 455
(1994): Mongey AB+, *Br J Rheumatol* 33, 789
(1994): Walker EM+, *Br J Rheumatol* 33, 175
(1993): Siam AR+, *J Rheumatol* 20, 207
(1993): Wildhagen K+, *Clin Rheumatol* 12, 265
(1992): Skaer TL, *Clin Ther* 14, 496
(1991): Alarcon-Segovia D+, *Baillieres Clin Rheumatol* 5, 1
(1989): Deboever G+, *Am J Gastroenterol* 84, 85
(1989): Sugimoto M+, *Nippon Naika Gakkai Zasshi* (Japanese) 78, 583
(1988): Clementz GL+, *Am J Med* 84, 535
(1987): Hobbs RN+, *Ann Rheum Dis* 46, 408
(1985): Lovisetto P+, *Recenti Prog Med* (Italian) 76, 110
(1985): Stratton MA, *Clin Pharm* 4, 657
(1983): Vanheule BA+, *Eur J Pediatr* 140, 66
(1982): Carr-Locke DL, *Am J Gastroenterol* 77, 614
(1980): Crisp AJ+, *J R Soc Med* 73, 60
(1980): Rouleau L+, *Union Med Can* (French) 109, 1326

Necrosis
    (1988): Krakamp B+, *Med Klin* (German) 83, 611
Photosensitivity (10%)
    (2006): Duparc A+, *Presse Med* 35(7–8), 1138
    (1999): Bouyssou-Gauthier ML, *Dermatology* 198, 388
    (1994): Shelley WB+, *Cutis* 53, 240 (observation)
    (1986): Amos RS+, *BMJ* 293, 420 (1–5%)
    (1986): Chandler MJ, *J Infect Dis* 153, 1001
Pigmentation
    (1992): Gabazza EC+, *Am J Gastroenterol* 87, 1654 (orange-yellow)
Pruritus (10%)
    (1993): Gran JT+, *Scand J Rheumatol* 22, 229
    (1990): Donovan S+, *Br J Rheumatol* 29, 201
    (1990): Peppercorn MA, *Ann Intern Med* 112, 50 (1–5%)
    (1987): Colebunders R+, *Ann Intern Med* 107, 599
    (1986): Farr M+, *Drugs* 32 (Suppl 1), 49
    (1986): Sher MR, *J Allergy Clin Immunol* 77, 133
    (1984): Kramer BS+, *Cancer* 53, 329
Pruritus ani et vulvae
    (1981): *Modern Medicine* 49, 111
Psoriasis
    (1991): Bliddal H+, *Clin Rheumatol* 10, 178
Purpura
    (1989): Gremse DA+, *J Pediatr Gastroenterol Nutr* 9, 261
Pustules
    (1994): Gallais V+, *Ann Dermatol Venereol* (French) 121, 11
Rash (sic) (>10%)
    (2003): Fischetti F+, *Minerva Med* 94(6), 437
    (2000): Jung JH+, *Clin Exp Rheumatol* 18, 245
    (1999): Besnard M+, *Arch Pediatr* 6, 643
    (1994): McCarthy C+, *Ir J Med Sci* 163, 238
    (1993): Koski JM, *Clin Exp Dermatol* 11, 169
    (1992): Brooks H+, *Clin Rheumatol* 11, 566
    (1992): Giaffer MH+, *Aliment Pharmacol Ther* 6, 51 (10 cases))
    (1989): Gyssens IC+, *Ned Tijdschr Geneeskd* (Dutch) 133, 1608
    (1989): Scott DL+, *J Rheumatol* Suppl 16, 17
    (1986): Bax DE+, *Ann Rheum Dis* 45, 139
    (1984): Farr M+, *Clin Rheumatol* 3, 473
    (1984): Purdy BH+, *Ann Intern Med* 100, 512
Raynaud's phenomenon
    (1984): Ahmad J+, *J Assoc Physicians India* 32(4), 370
    (1984): Peppercorn MA, *Ann Intern Med* 101, 377
    (1980): Reid J+, *Postgraduate Med J* 56, 106
Side effects (sic) (5%)
    (1986): Amos RS+, *BMJ* 293, 420 (5.5%)
Stevens–Johnson syndrome (<1%)
    (2007): Fuentes-Paez G+, *Ann Ophthalmol* (Skokie) 39(2), 152
    (2007): Fuentes-Paez G+, *Compr Ther* 33(2), 99
    (2003): Borras-Blasco J+, *Ann Pharmacother* 37(9), 1241
    (2001): Martin L+, *Rev Pneumol Clin* 57(4), 297
Toxic epidermal necrolysis (1–10%)
    (2001): Martin L+, *Rev Pneumol Clin* 57(4), 297
    (1995): Jullien D+, *Arthritis Rheum* 38, 573
    (1987): Guillaume JC+, *Arch Dermatol* 123, 1166
    (1985): Curley RK+, *Br Med J Clin Res Ed* 290, 471 (fatal)
    (1985): Heng MCY, *Br J Dermatol* 113, 597
    (1984): Peppercorn MA, *Ann Intern Med* 101, 377
    (1981): Hensen E, *Tijdschr Ziekenverpl* (Dutch) 34, 563
    (1981): Hensen EJ+, *Lancet* 2, 151
    (1980): Maddocks JL+, *J R Soc Med* 73, 587
Urticaria (1–5%)
    (2002): Liss WA, Pleasanton, WA (from Internet) (observation)
    (2000): Jung JH+, *Clin Exp Rheumatol* 18, 245
    (1989): Alanko K+, *Acta Derm Venereol* (Stockh) 69, 223
    (1986): Amos RS+, *BMJ* 293, 420 (1–5%)
    (1986): Farr M+, *Drugs* 32 (Suppl 1), 49
    (1985): Maayan S+, *Arch Intern Med* 145, 1607
    (1984): Kramer BS+, *Cancer* 53, 329

    (1984): Peppercorn MA, *Ann Intern Med* 101, 377
    (1984): Purdy BH+, *Ann Intern Med* 100, 512
    (1981): Abi-Mansur P+, *Am J Gastroenterol* 76, 356
Vasculitis
    (2000): Chebli JM+, *Arq Gastroenterol* 37(4), 224
    (1995): Laversuch CJ+, *Br J Rheumatol* 34(5), 435
Xerosis
    (1990): Donovan S+, *Br J Rheumatol* 29, 201

Mucosal/ENT
Aphthous stomatitis
    (1981): *J Antimicrob Chemother* 7, 179
Cheilitis
    (1986): Farr M+, *Drugs* 32 (Suppl 1), 49
Dysgeusia
    (1991): Marcus RW, *J Rheumatol* 18, 634
Glossitis
Hypogeusia
Mucocutaneous reactions (6%)
    (1990): Donovan S+, *Br J Rheumatol* 29, 201 (6.3%)
    (1986): Farr M+, *Drugs* 32 (Suppl 1), 49 (5.5%)
Oral mucosal eruption (<1%)
    (1990): Petterson T+, *Br J Rheumatol* 29, 239
    (1986): Amos RS+, *BMJ* 293, 420 (0.3%)
    (1984): Iwatsuki K+, *Arch Dermatol* 120, 964
Oral ulceration
    (1987): Hughes WT+, *N Engl J Med* 316, 1627
    (1986): Farr M+, *Drugs* 32 (Suppl 1), 49
    (1981): Orenstein WA+, *Am J Med Sci* 282, 27
Stomatitis
    (1993): Gran JT+, *Scand J Rheumatol* 22, 229
Tongue ulceration
    (1981): *J Antimicrob Chemother* 7, 179
Vaginitis
    (1985): Wong ES+, *Ann Intern Med* 102, 302
Xerostomia
    (1990): Donovan S+, *Br J Rheumatol* 29, 201

Hair
Hair – alopecia
    (1988): Fich A+, *J Clin Gastroenterol* 10, 466
    (1987): Codeluppi P+, *Dig Dis Sci* 32, 221
    (1986): Breen EG+, *BMJ* 292, 802
    (1986): Farr M+, *Drugs* 32 (Suppl 1), 49
    (1983): Taffet SL+, *Dig Dis Sci* 28, 833
    (1981): Attar A+, *Gastroenterology* 80, 1102

Eyes
Conjunctival pigmentation
    (2007): Fuentes-Paez G+, *Ann Ophthalmol* (Skokie) 39(2), 152
    (2007): Fuentes-Paez G+, *Compr Ther* 33(2), 99
Glaucoma
    (2007): Lee GC+, *Clin Experiment Ophthalmol* 35(1), 55
Periorbital edema

Other
Anaphylactoid reactions/Anaphylaxis
    (1990): Donovan S+, *Br J Rheumatol* 29, 201
    (1988): Arnold PA+, *Drug Intell Clin Pharm* 22, 43
    (1985): Gossius G+, *Scand J Infect Dis* 16, 373
Asthenia
    (2006): Combe B+, *Ann Rheum Dis* 65(10), 1357
    (2003): Fischetti F+, *Minerva Med* 94(6), 437
Death
    (2001): Lau G+, *Forensic Sci Int* 122(2), 79
    (2000): Chebli JM+, *Arq Gastroenterol* 37(4), 224
DRESS syndrome
    (2006): Bejia I+, *Joint Bone Spine* 73(6), 764
    (2006): Bourguignon R+, *Rev Med Liege* 61(9), 643
    (2006): Condat B+, *Gastroenterol Clin Biol* 30(1), 142

(2006): Teo L+, *Singapore Med J* 47(3), 237
(2005): Descloux E+, *Intensive Care Med* 31(12), 1727
(2005): Michel F+, *Joint Bone Spine* 72(1), 82
(2001): Descamps V+, *Arch Dermatol* 137, 301
(2001): Queyrel V+, *Rev Med Interne* 22(6), 582
(1998): Tohyama M+, *Arch Dermatol* 134, 1113
Fever
(2003): Fischetti F+, *Minerva Med* 94(6), 437
Headache
(2006): Combe B+, *Ann Rheum Dis* 65(10), 1357
(2006): Duparc A+, *Presse Med* 35(7–8), 1138
(2003): Fischetti F+, *Minerva Med* 94(6), 437
Hepatotoxicity
(2006): Duparc A+, *Presse Med* 35(7–8), 1138
(2006): Kampmann P+, *Ugeskr Laeger* 168(39), 3331
(2004): Petrov AV, *Lik Sprava* (1), 60
(2003): Fischetti F+, *Minerva Med* 94(6), 437
Hypersensitivity (1–5%)
(2003): Kunisaki Y+, *Intern Med* 42(2), 203
(2000): Marino C+, *Arthritis Care Res* 13(5), 335
(1998): Tohyama M+, *Arch Dermatol* 134, 1113
(1997): Otero S+, *Gastroenterol Hepatol* (Spanish) 20, 416
(1995): Tolia V, *Am J Gastroenterol* 87, 1029
(1992): Leroux JL+, *Clin Exp Rheumatol* 10, 427
(1987): Ackerman Z+, *Postgrad Med J* 63, 55
(1984): Korelitz BI+, *J Clin Gastroenterol* 6, 27
Lymphoproliferative disease
(1989): Lafeuillade A+, *Presse Med* (French) 18, 1709
Myalgia/Myositis/Myopathy/Myotoxicity
(1994): Norden DK+, *Am J Gastroenterology* 89, 801
Nephrotoxicity
(2006): Avdeev VG+, *Ter Arkh* 78(1), 77
Pseudolymphoma
(1994): Gallais V+, *Ann Dermatol Venereol* (French) 121, 11
Serum sickness (<1%)
(1992): Brooks H+, *Clin Rheumatol* 11, 566
(1990): Petterson T+, *Br J Rheumatol* 29, 239

SULFINPYRAZONE

Trade names: Antazone; Antiran; Anturan; Anturane (Novartis); Anturano; Enturen; Falizal; Novopyrazone
Indications: Gouty arthritis
Category: Sulfonamide
Half-life: 2–7 hours
Clinically important, potentially hazardous interactions
with: anisindione, anticoagulants, ceftobiprole, dicumarol, penicillin g, penicillin V, warfarin

Note: Sulfinpyrazone is a sulfonamide and can be absorbed systemically. Sulfonamides can produce severe, possibly fatal, reactions such as toxic epidermal necrolysis and Stevens–Johnson syndrome

Reactions

Skin
Dermatitis (1–10%)
Edema
Exanthems (<3%)
Purpura
Rash (sic) (1–10%)

Other
Nephrotoxicity
(1998): Walls M+, *Am J Med Sci* 315(5), 319
(1986): Boelaert J+, *J Cardiovasc Pharmacol* 8(2), 386

(1984): Boelaert J+, *Arch Intern Med* 144(3), 648
(1984): Docci D+, *Nephron* 37(3), 213
(1984): Prior C+, *Acta Med Austriaca* 11(2), 55
(1983): Docci D+, *Clin Nephrol* 20(1), 53
(1983): Lijnen P+, *Clin Nephrol* 19(3), 143
(1983): Perez Mijares R+, *Clin Nephrol* 19(1), 54
(1982): Boelaert J+, *Am Heart J* 104(1), 174
(1982): Keidar S+, *Clin Nephrol* 17(5), 266
(1982): Mayrhofer EF+, *Dtsch Med Wochenschr* 107(27), 1057
(1982): Scherrer JJ+, *S D J Med* 35(4), 17
(1981): Boelaert J+, *N Engl J Med* 305(19), 1154
(1981): Butler AL, *N Engl J Med* 305(2), 106
(1981): Howard T+, *Am Heart J* 102(2), 294

SULFISOXAZOLE

Trade names: Isoxazine; Novo-Soxazole; Oxazole; Pediazole (Abbott); Sulfazin; Sulfazole; Sulizole; Thiazin; Urazole
Indications: Various infections caused by susceptible organisms
Category: Antibiotic, sulfonamide
Half-life: 3–7 hours
Clinically important, potentially hazardous interactions
with: anticoagulants, cyclosporine, methotrexate, warfarin

Note: Sulfisoxazole is a sulfonamide and can be absorbed systemically. Sulfonamides can produce severe, possibly fatal, reactions such as toxic epidermal necrolysis and Stevens–Johnson syndrome

Reactions

Skin
Allergic reactions (sic) (3%)
Angioedema (<1%)
Bullous dermatitis (<1%)
Eczema
Erythema multiforme (<1%)
(1987): Penmetcha M, *BMJ* 295, 556
(1985): Heer M+, *Gastroenterology* 88, 1954
(1985): Hernborg A, *Lancet* 2, 1072
Erythema nodosum
Exanthems (1–5%)
(1985): Maayan S+, *Arch Intern Med* 145, 1607
(1982): Goetz MB+, *JAMA* 247, 3118
(1980): Fennell RS+, *Clin Pediatr* 19, 124
Exfoliative dermatitis
Fixed eruption (<1%)
(1988): Bharija SC+, *Dermatologica* 176, 108
(1987): Hughes BR+, *Br J Dermatol* 116, 241
(1986): Kanwar AJ+, *Dermatologica* 172, 230
(1982): Gibson JR, *BMJ* 284, 1529
(1980): Talbot MD, *Practitioner* 224, 823
Linear IgA dermatosis
(1981): Safai B+, *J Am Acad Dermatol* 4, 435
Lupus erythematosus
Photosensitivity (>10%)
(1986): Chandler MJ, *J Infect Dis* 153, 1001
(1981): Flach AJ+, *Arch Ophthalmol* 100, 1206 (from topical application)
(1981): Flach AJ+, *Arch Ophthalmol* 99, 609 (from topical application)
Phototoxicity
(1982): Flach AJ+, *Arch Ophthalmol* 100, 1286 (from topical application)
Pruritus (1–10%)
(1987): Colebunders R+, *Ann Intern Med* 107, 599
(1986): Sher MR, *J Allergy Clin Immunol* 77, 133

(1984): Kramer BS+, *Cancer* 53, 329

Pruritus ani et vulvae
  (1981): *Modern Medicine* 49, 111

Purpura
  (1980): Miescher PA+, *Clin Haematol* 9, 505

Pustules

Rash (sic) (>10%)

Side effects (sic) (2%)

Stevens–Johnson syndrome (1–10%)
  (1983): Fischer PR+, *Am J Dis Child* 137, 914

Toxic epidermal necrolysis (1–10%)
  (1995): Raymond F+, *Arch Pediatr* (French) 2, 494
  (1990): Jacqz-Aigrain E+, *Lancet* 336, 1010
  (1989): Alanko K+, *Acta Derm Venereol* (Stockh) 69, 223

Urticaria
  (1985): Maayan S+, *Arch Intern Med* 145, 1607
  (1984): Kramer BS+, *Cancer* 53, 329
  (1981): Abi-Mansur P+, *Am J Gastroenterol* 76, 356

Vasculitis (<1%)

Mucosal/ENT

Aphthous stomatitis
  (1981): *J Antimicrob Chemother* 7, 179

Dysgeusia
  (1988): Fischl MA+, *JAMA* 259, 1185

Glossitis

Oral psoriasis

Oral ulceration
  (1987): Hughes WT+, *N Engl J Med* 316, 1627
  (1981): Orenstein WA+, *Am J Med Sci* 282, 27

Stomatitis

Tinnitus

Tongue ulceration
  (1981): *J Antimicrob Chemother* 7, 179

Vaginitis
  (1985): Wong ES+, *Ann Intern Med* 102, 302

Hair

Hair – alopecia

Eyes

Periorbital edema

Other

Anaphylactoid reactions/Anaphylaxis
  (1988): Arnold PA+, *Drug Intell Clin Pharm* 22, 43
  (1985): Gossius G+, *Scand J Infect Dis* 16, 373

Headache

Hypersensitivity

Myalgia/Myositis/Myopathy/Myotoxicity

Serum sickness (<1%)

SULFITES

Scientific names: *Ammonium bisulfite [AB]; potassium bisulfite [PB]; potassium metabisulfite [PM]; sodium bisulfite [SB]; sodium metabisulfite [SM]; sodium sulfite [SS]; sulfur dioxide [SD]*

Family: N/A

Category: Trace element

Purported indications and other uses: Food additive, drug additive, sanitary agent

Half-life: N/A

Clinically important, potentially hazardous interactions with: aspirin, NSAIDs

Reactions

Skin

Adverse effects (sic)
  (1992): Miyata M+, *CMAJ* 147(9), 1333
  (1990): Fazio T+, *Food Addit Contam* 7(4), 433

Allergic reactions (sic)
  (2002): Naftalin LW+, *Dent Clin North Am* 46(4), 733 (in local anesthetics)
  (2001): Campbell JR+, *Anesth Prog* 48(1), 21 (in lidocaine)
  (1999): Langevin PB, *Chest* 116(4), 1140 (in propofol)
  (1996): Bellido J+, *Allergy* 51(3), 196 (SM in fish)
  (1996): Gall H+, *Allergy* 51(7), 516 (SM in beer)
  (1994): Hassoun S+, *Allerg Immunol* (Paris) 26(5), 184, 187

Angioedema
  (1993): Belchi-Hernandez J+, *Ann Allergy* 71(3), 230
  (1990): Sokol WN+, *Ann Allergy* 65(3), 233 (SM)

Dermatitis
  (2001): Lee A+, *Contact Dermatitis* 44(2), 127 (SM)
  (2000): Sanchez-Perez J+, *Contact Dermatitis* 42(3), 176 (SM in antihemorrhoidal cream)
  (1999): Tucker SC+, *Contact Dermatitis* 40(3), 164 (MS in Trimovate)
  (1997): Nagayama H+, *J Dermatol* 24(10), 675 (SB in Tathion eye drops)
  (1996): Pambor M, *Contact Dermatitis* 35(1), 48 (AB in bleaching cream)
  (1995): Jacobs MC+, *Contact Dermatitis* 33(1), 65 (SM)
  (1994): Bonneau JC, *Allerg Immunol* (Paris) 26(9), 324
  (1994): Vena GA+, *Contact Dermatitis* 31(3), 172 (PM, SB, SS)
  (1993): Lodi A+, *Contact Dermatitis* 29(2), 97 (SS in antifungal cream)

Eczema
  (1998): Agard C+, *Rev Mal Respir* 15(4), 537

Edema
  (1997): Nagayama H+, *J Dermatol* 24(10), 675 (SB in Tathion eye drops)
  (1992): Hyndiuk RA+, *Lens Eye Toxic Res* 9(3–4), 331 (in intraocular epinephrine)

Erythema
  (1997): Nagayama H+, *J Dermatol* 24(10), 675 (SB in Tathion eye drops)

Facial edema
  (2003): Vally H+, *Addict Biol* 8(1), 3

Lichen planus

Pruritus
  (2003): Vally H+, *Addict Biol* 8(1), 3

Rash (sic)
  (1998): Arai Y+, *Arerugi* 47(11), 1163 (16.7%) (in foods)
  (1995): Lester MR, *J Am Coll Nutr* 14(3), 229

Sensitivity
  (2002): Harrison DA+, *Contact Dermatitis* 46(5), 310 (SM in clobetasone)
  (2002): Vally H+, *Thorax* 57(7), 569
  (1999): Heshmati S+, *Contact Dermatitis* 41(3), 166 (SM in hydrocortisone cream)
  (1991): Frick WE+, *J Asthma* 28(3), 221

Urticaria
  (1998): Arai Y+, *Arerugi* 47(11), 1163 (36.7%) (in foods)
  (1993): Belchi-Hernandez J+, *Ann Allergy* 71(3), 230
  (1993): Wuthrich B, *Ann Allergy* 71(4), 379 (in foods)
  (1993): Wuthrich B+, *Dermatology* 187(4), 290
  (1990): Sokol WN+, *Ann Allergy* 65(3), 233 (SM)

Vasculitis
  (1993): Wuthrich B, *Ann Allergy* 71(4), 379 (in foods)

Mucosal/ENT

Burning mouth syndrome

(1996): Levanti C+, *Acta Derm Venereol* 76(2), 158 (SM)
Rhinitis
(2004): Pacor ML+, *Allergy* 59, 192 (6 cases)
(2003): Vally H+, *Addict Biol* 8(1), 3
(1996): Miltgen J+, *Rev Pneumol Clin* 52(6), 363 (PM)

Eyes
Eyelid dermatitis
(2006): Seitz CS+, *Contact Dermatitis* 55(4), 249 [SM]
Rhinoconjunctivitis
(1993): Valero AL+, *Allergol Immunopathol (Madr)* 21(6), 221 (SB, SM)

Other
Abdominal pain
Anaphylactoid reactions/Anaphylaxis
(2000): Reus KE+, *Ned Tijdschr Geneeskd* 144(38), 1836 (in foods)
(1996): Miltgen J+, *Rev Pneumol Clin* 52(6), 363 (PM)
(1993): Wuthrich B+, *Dermatology* 187(4), 290
(1992): Smolinske SC, *J Toxicol Clin Toxicol* 30(4), 597 (in local anesthetics, gentamicin, metoclopramide, doxycycline, vitamin B complex)
(1991): Soulat JM+, *Cah Anesthesiol* 39(4), 257 (in local anesthetic with epinephrine)
(1983): Schwartz HJ, *J Allergy Clin Immunol* 71, 487
(1982): Twarog FJ+, *JAMA* 248, 2030 (in isoetharine)
(1981): Stevenson DD+, *J Allergy Clin Immunol* 68, 26
Asthenia
Cough
(2003): Vally H+, *Addict Biol* 8(1), 3
Death
(1986): *FDA Fed Reg* 51, 25021 25026
(1984): *FDA Drug Bull* 14, 24
Headache
(2003): Vally H+, *Addict Biol* 8(1), 3
Hot flashes
Hypersensitivity
(2003): Stormont JM+, *Ann Allergy Asthma Immunol* 91(3), 314
(1998): Arai Y+, *Arerugi* 47(11), 1163 (36.7%) (in foods)
(1996): Sonneville A, *Allerg Immunol (Paris)* 28(7), 246 (in E 220– E 227)
(1995): Hallstrom H, *Lakartidningen* 92(4), 295
Seizures
(1992): Meisel SB+, *Ann Pharmacother* 26(12), 1515 (SB in morphine)

SULINDAC

Trade names: Aflodac; Algocetil; APO-Sulin; Arthrocine; Clinoril; Mobilin; Novo-Sundac; Sulene; Sulic; Suloril
Indications: Arthritis
Category: Non-steroidal anti-inflammatory
Half-life: 7.8–16.4 hours
Clinically important, potentially hazardous interactions with: methotrexate, warfarin

Reactions

Skin
Angioedema (<1%)
Dermatitis
(1991): Renaut JJ, *Allerg Immunol Paris* (French) 23, 365
Diaphoresis
Edema
Erythema
(1991): Renaut JJ, *Allerg Immunol Paris* (French) 23, 365

Erythema multiforme (<1%)
(1987): Jeanmougin M+, *Ann Dermatol Venereol* (French) 114, 1400
(1985): Bigby M+, *J Am Acad Dermatol* 12, 866
(1985): O'Brien WM+, *J Rheumatol* 12, 13
(1984): Stern RS+, *JAMA* 252, 1433
(1982): Park GD+, *Arch Intern Med* 142, 1292
(1981): Husain Z+, *J Rheumatol* 8, 176
(1981): Maguire FW, *Del Med J* 53, 193
(1980): Russell IJ, *Ann Intern Med* 92, 716
Exanthems (1–5%)
(1993): Litt JZ, Beachwood, OH (personal case) (observation)
(1991): Hyson CP+, *Arch Intern Med* 151, 387
(1987): Jeanmougin M+, *Ann Dermatol Venereol* (French) 114, 1400
(1985): Bigby M+, *J Am Acad Dermatol* 12, 866
(1984): Stern RS+, *JAMA* 252, 1433
(1982): Park GD+, *Arch Intern Med* 142, 1292
(1981): Dhand A+, *Gastroenterology* 80, 585
(1980): Russell IJ, *Ann Intern Med* 92, 716
Exfoliative dermatitis (<1%)
Exfoliative erythroderma
(1984): Stern RS+, *JAMA* 252, 1433
Facial erythema
Fixed eruption (<1%)
(1987): Jeanmougin M+, *Ann Dermatol Venereol* (French) 114, 1400
(1986): Bruce DR+, *Cutis* 38, 323
(1985): Bigby M+, *J Am Acad Dermatol* 12, 866
(1984): Aram H, *Int J Dermatol* 23, 421
(1984): Stern RS+, *JAMA* 252, 1433
Jaundice
Lichen planus
(1983): Hamburger J+, *BMJ* 287, 1258
Pernio
(1981): Reinertsen JL, *Arthritis Rheum* 24, 1215
Photosensitivity (<1%)
(1987): Jeanmougin M+, *Ann Dermatol Venereol* (French) 114, 1400
(1984): Stern RS+, *JAMA* 252, 1433
Phototoxicity
Pruritus (1–10%)
(1987): Jeanmougin M+, *Ann Dermatol Venereol* (French) 114, 1400
(1985): Bigby M+, *J Am Acad Dermatol* 12, 866
(1984): Stern RS+, *JAMA* 252, 1433
(1982): Park GD+, *Arch Intern Med* 142, 1292
(1980): Russell IJ, *Ann Intern Med* 92, 716
Purpura (<1%)
(1987): Jeanmougin M+, *Ann Dermatol Venereol* (French) 114, 1400
(1984): Stern RS+, *JAMA* 252, 1433
Rash (sic) (>10%)
Raynaud's phenomenon
(1981): Reinertsen JL, *Arthritis Rheum* 24, 1215 (passim)
Stevens–Johnson syndrome (<1%)
(1993): Awaya N+, *Ryumachi* (Japanese) 33, 432
(1983): Klein SM+, *J Rheumatol* 10, 512
(1981): Husain Z+, *J Rheumatol* 8, 176
(1981): Maguire FW, *Del Med J* 53, 193
(1980): Levitt L+, *JAMA* 243, 1262
Toxic epidermal necrolysis (<1%)
(1990): Hovde O, *Tidsskr Nor Laegeforen* (Norwegian) 110, 2537
(1988): Small RE+, *Clin Pharm* 7, 766
(1987): Ikeda N+, *Z Rechtsmed* (German) 98, 141
(1987): Jeanmougin M+, *Ann Dermatol Venereol* (French) 114, 1400
(1986): Rodt SA+, *Tidsskr Nor Laegeforen* (Norwegian) 106, 2982

(1985): Bigby M+, *J Am Acad Dermatol* 12, 866
(1985): Chevrant-Breton JC, *Therapie* (French) 40, 67
(1985): Heng MCY, *Br J Dermatol* 113, 597
(1984): Stern RS+, *JAMA* 252, 1433
(1983): Klein SM+, *J Rheumatol* 10, 512
(1982): Park GD+, *Arch Intern Med* 142, 1292
(1980): Levitt L+, *JAMA* 243, 1262
(1980): Russell IJ, *Ann Intern Med* 92, 716
Urticaria (<1%)
  (1987): Jeanmougin M+, *Ann Dermatol Venereol* (French) 114, 1400
  (1985): Bigby M+, *J Am Acad Dermatol* 12, 866
  (1984): Stern RS+, *JAMA* 252, 1433
  (1981): Burrish G+, *Ann Emerg Med* 10, 154
Vasculitis (<1%)

Mucosal/ENT
Ageusia (<1%)
Aphthous stomatitis
Dysgeusia (<1%)
Glossitis (<1%)
Oral lichenoid eruption
  (1983): Hamburger J+, *BMJ* 287, 1258
Oral mucosal eruption (3%)
  (1985): Bigby M+, *J Am Acad Dermatol* 12, 866
Oral mucosal erythema
Oral ulceration
Rectal mucosal ulceration
  (2002): Cruz-Correa M+, *Gastroenterology* 122(3), 641
Stomatitis (<1%)
  (1991): Renaut JJ, *Allerg Immunol Paris* (French) 23, 365
Tinnitus
Xerostomia
  (1980): Smith F+, *JAMA* 244, 269

Hair
Hair – alopecia (<1%)

Other
Anaphylactoid reactions/Anaphylaxis (<1%)
  (1991): Hyson CP+, *Arch Intern Med* 151, 387
  (1985): O'Brien WM+, *J Rheumatol* 12, 13
  (1981): Burrish G+, *Ann Emerg Med* 10, 154
  (1980): Smith F+, *JAMA* 244, 269
Death
Gynecomastia
  (1983): Kapoor A, *JAMA* 250, 2284
Headache
Hepatotoxicity
  (2006): Lapeyre-Mestre M+, *Fundam Clin Pharmacol* 20(4), 391
  (2006): Sanchez-Matienzo D+, *Clin Ther* 28(8), 1123 (6–10%)
Hot flashes (<1%)
Hypersensitivity (<1%) (potentially fatal)
Pain (sic)
  (1984): Stern RS+, *JAMA* 252, 1433
Paresthesias (<1%)
Pseudolymphoma
  (2000): Werth V, *Dermatology Times* 18
Serum sickness
  (1984): Stern RS+, *JAMA* 252, 1433

SUMATRIPTAN

Trade names: Imigrane; Imitrex (GSK)
Indications: Migraine attacks
Category: 5-HT1 agonist; Serotonin receptor agonist; Triptan (topical)
Half-life: 2.5 hours
Clinically important, potentially hazardous interactions with: citalopram, dihydroergotamine, ergot-containing drugs, escitalopram, fluoxetine, fluvoxamine, isocarboxazid, MAO inhibitors, methysergide, naratriptan, nefazodone, paroxetine, phenelzine, rizatriptan, sertraline, sibutramine, **St John's wort**, tranylcypromine, venlafaxine, zolmitriptan

Reactions

Skin
Angioedema
  (1995): Dachs R+, *Am J Med* 99, 684
Burning (1–10%)
Diaphoresis (1.6%)
Erythema (<1%)
Exanthems
Photosensitivity (<1%)
Pruritus (<1%)
Rash (sic) (<1%)
Raynaud's phenomenon (<1%)
Sensitivity (sic)
  (1994): Black P+, *N Z Med J* 107, 20
Urticaria
  (1996): Pradalier A+, *Cephalalgia* 16, 280

Mucosal/ENT
Dysgeusia (<1%)
  (2006): Cady R+, *Expert Opin Pharmacother* 7(11), 1503
  (2005): *Prescrire Int* 14(76), 45
  (2004): Natarajan S+, *Headache* 44(10), 969 (17%)
  (2003): Dahlof C, *Neurology* 61(8), S31
  (2001): Hershey AD+, *Headache* 41, 693
Glossodynia
Parosmia (<1%)
Xerostomia

Eyes
Vision loss
  (2005): *Prescrire Int* 14(76), 45

Other
Anaphylactoid reactions/Anaphylaxis
Asthenia
  (2004): Landy S+, *Int J Clin Pract* 58(10), 913
Chest pain
  (2006): Cady R+, *Expert Opin Pharmacother* 7(11), 1503 (4%)
Headache
Hot flashes (>10%)
Hypertension
  (2005): *Prescrire Int* 14(76), 45
  (2005): Hendrix Y+, *Ned Tijdschr Geneeskd* 149(16), 888 (with paroxetine)
Injection-site burning
  (2006): Winner P+, *Clin Ther* 28(10), 1582 (5%)
Injection-site reactions (sic) (10–58%)
  (2006): Wendt J+, *Clin Ther* 28(4), 517 (43%)
  (1991): Multiple authors, *N Engl J Med* 325, 316 (10–20%)
Myalgia/Myositis/Myopathy/Myotoxicity (1.8%)
  (2007): Winner P+, *Mayo Clin Proc* 82(1), 61
Paresthesias (13.5%)

(2006): Cady R+, *Expert Opin Pharmacother* 7(11), 1503 (42%)
(2006): Wendt J+, *Clin Ther* 28(4), 517 (10%)
(2005): Sheftell FD+, *Clin Ther* 27(4), 407
(2004): Landy S+, *Int J Clin Pract* 58(10), 913
Stroke
(2005): *Prescrire Int* 14(76), 45
Vertigo
(2007): Winner P+, *Mayo Clin Proc* 82(1), 61
(2006): Wendt J+, *Clin Ther* 28(4), 517 (10%)
(2004): Landy S+, *Int J Clin Pract* 58(10), 913

SUNITINIB

Synonym: Synonym: SU11248
Trade name: Sutent (Pfizer)
Indications: Gastrointestinal stromal tumor, Metastatic renal cell carcinoma
Category: Tyrosine kinase inhibitor
Half-life: 40–60 hours
Clinically important, potentially hazardous interactions with: ketoconazole, rifampin

Note: [G] = treated for Gastrointestinal tumor; [R] = treated for Metastatic renal cell carcinoma

Reactions

Skin
Bullous dermatitis
  (2006): Faivre S+, *J Clin Oncol* 24(1), 25 (7%) ([R])
Edema
  (2006): Faivre S+, *J Clin Oncol* 24(1), 25
Hand-foot syndrome (12–14%)
Peripheral edema (17%) [R]
Pigmentation
  (2006): Faivre S+, *J Clin Oncol* 24(1), 25 (yellow) (30–33%)
Pyoderma gangrenosum
  (2008): ten Freyhaus+, *Br J Dermatol* 159(1), 242
Rash (sic) (14–38%)
Side effects (sic)
  (2005): Robert C+, *Lancet Oncol* 6(7), 491
Xerosis (17%) [R]

Mucosal/ENT
Dysgeusia (21–43%)
Glossodynia (15%) [R]
Mucositis (29–53%)
Stomatitis
  (2006): Faivre S+, *J Clin Oncol* 24(1), 25 (29–53%)

Hair
Hair – alopecia (5–12%)
Hair – pigmentation
  (2006): Faivre S+, *J Clin Oncol* 24(1), 25 (yellow) (7%) ([G])

Eyes
Epiphora (6%) [R]
Periorbital edema (7%) [R]

Other
Abdominal pain (20–33%)
Asthenia (22%) [G]
Cardiotoxicity
  (2007): Chu TF+, *Lancet* 370(9604), 2011
Cough (8–17%)
Fever (15–18%)
Headache (13–25%)

Hypertension
  (2006): Faivre S+, *J Clin Oncol* 24(1), 25 (15–28%)
Myalgia/Myositis/Myopathy/Myotoxicity (14–17%)
Neurotoxicity (10%) [R]
Pain (18%) [R]
Seizures
Vertigo (16%) [R]

TACRINE

Synonym: THA
Trade name: Cognex (First Horizon)
Indications: Dementia of Alzheimer's disease
Category: Cholinesterase inhibitor
Half-life: 1.5–4 hours
Clinically important, potentially hazardous interactions with: fluvoxamine, galantamine, ibuprofen

Reactions

Skin
Acne (<1%)
Basal cell carcinoma
Bullous dermatitis
Cellulitis
Cyst
Dermatitis (<1%)
Desquamation
Diaphoresis
Eczema
Edema (<1%)
Exanthems (7%)
Facial edema (<1%)
Furunculosis (<1%)
Herpes simplex (<1%)
Herpes zoster (<1%)
Melanoma (<1%)
Necrosis (<1%)
Peripheral edema (<1%)
Petechiae
Pruritus (7%)
Psoriasis (<1%)
Purpura (2%)
Rash (sic) (7%)
  (1998): Estadieu MC+, *Therapie* 53(1), 67
Seborrhea
Squamous cell carcinoma
Ulcerations (<1%)
Urticaria (7%)
Xerosis (<1%)

Mucosal/ENT
Dysgeusia (<1%)
Gingivitis (<1%)
Glossitis (<1%)
Sialorrhea (<1%)
Stomatitis (<1%)
Xerostomia (<1%)

Hair
Hair – alopecia (<1%)

Other
Headache

Hepatotoxicity
(2001): Michel BF+, *Rev Neurol (Paris)* 157(11), 1365 (33%)
(1999): *Prescrire Int* 8(39), 16
(1998): Blackard WG Jr+, *J Clin Gastroenterol* 26(1), 57
(1998): Estadieu MC+, *Therapie* 53(1), 67
(1998): Gracon SI+, *Alzheimer Dis Assoc Disord* 12(2), 93
(1997): Samuels SC+, *Drug Saf* 16(1), 66
(1995): Woo JK+, *Geriatrics* 50(5), 50
Myalgia/Myositis/Myopathy/Myotoxicity (9%)
Myoclonus
(1998): Abilleira S+, *J Neurol Neurosurg Psychiatry* 64(2), 281
Paresthesias (<1%)
Tremor (1–10%)

TACROLIMUS

Synonym: FK506
Trade names: Prograf (Astellas); Protopic (Astellas)
Indications: Prophylaxis of organ rejection, atopic dermatitis (topical)
Category: Calcineurin inhibitor; Immunosuppressant; Macrolactam
Half-life: ~8.7 hours
Clinically important, potentially hazardous interactions with: amiodarone, beta-blockers, caspofungin, cyclosporine, **dairy products**, danazol, erythromycin, etoricoxib, **grapefruit juice**, **hemophilus B vaccine**, HMG-CoA reductase inhibitors, ibuprofen, immunosuppressants, ketoconazole, lovastatin, mycophenolate, peanuts, potassium, potassium-sparing diuretics, rifabutin, rifampin, rifapentine, simvastatin, **St John's wort**, telithromycin, **vaccines**

Reactions

Skin
Angioedema
(2003): Lykavieris P+, *Transplantation* 75(1), 152
Burning (46%)
(2005): Ashcroft DM+, *BMJ* 330(7490), 516
(2005): Hanifin JM+, *J Am Acad Dermatol* 53(2 Suppl 2), S186
(2005): Harper J+, *J Invest Dermatol* 124(4), 695
(2004): Lampropoulos CE+, *Rheumatology* (Oxford) 43(11), 1383
(2004): Pascual JC+, *Skin Therapy Lett* 9(9), 1
(2002): Rozycki TW+, *J Am Acad Dermatol* 46, 27
(2002): Russell JJ, *Am Fam Physician* 66(10), 1899
(2001): Goldman D, *J Am Acad Dermatol* 44, 995 (transient, localized)
(2000): Reitamo S+, *Arch Dermatol* 136, 999 (46.8%)
(1999): Ruzicka R+, *Arch Dermatol* 135, 574
(1998): Alaiti S+, *J Am Acad Dermatol* 38, 69
Dermatitis
(2007): Shaw DW+, *J Am Acad Dermatol* 56(2), 342
Diaphoresis (>3%)
Edema (>10%)
Erythema (12%)
(2005): Hanifin JM+, *J Am Acad Dermatol* 53(2 Suppl 2), S186
(2001): Bohannon JS, Midlothian, VA (facial) (from topical) (following wine) (from Internet) (observation)
(2000): Reitamo S+, *Arch Dermatol* 136, 999 (12.3%)
Exanthems (4%)
(2001): Takamatsu Y+, *Bone Marrow Transplant* 28(4), 421 (with cyclosporine)
(2000): Reitamo S+, *Arch Dermatol* 136, 999 (4.1%)
Exfoliative dermatitis

(2004): Lampropoulos CE+, *Rheumatology* (Oxford) 43(11), 1383
Folliculitis (10%)
(2006): Singalavanija S+, *J Med Assoc Thai* 89(11), 1915 (2%)
(2000): Reitamo S+, *Arch Dermatol* 136, 999 (10.8%)
Graft-versus-host reaction
(2004): Tamaki H+, *Int J Hematol* 80(3), 291
(2003): Bunetel L+, *J Periodontol* 74(4), 552
Herpes simplex (13%)
(2005): Joseph MA+, *Cornea* 24(4), 417
(2005): Lonsdale-Eccles AA+, *Clin Exp Dermatol* 30(1), 95 (vulva)
(2004): Furue M+, *J Dermatol* 31(4), 277
(2000): Reitamo S+, *Arch Dermatol* 136, 999 (13%)
Irritation
(2002): Rozycki TW+, *J Am Acad Dermatol* 46(1), 27
Kaposi's sarcoma
(2006): Chua R+, *Heart Lung Circ* 15(5), 340
(2006): Schmutz JL+, *Ann Dermatol Venereol* 133(3), 303 (from topical)
Kaposi's varicelliform eruption
(2004): Miyake-Kashima M+, *Cornea* 23(2), 190
Lentigo
(2005): Hickey JR+, *Br J Dermatol* 152(1), 152
Melanoma
(2005): Hickey JR+, *Br J Dermatol* 152(1), 152 (3 cases)
Molluscum contagiosum
(2004): Wilson LM+, *Australas J Dermatol* 45(3), 184
Nevi
(1999): Reed BR, Denver, CO (from Internet) (observation)
Peripheral edema (26%)
Photosensitivity (>3%)
Pigmentation
(2007): Kim YJ+, *J Am Acad Dermatol* 57(5 Suppl 1), S125
(2005): Lan CC+, *Br J Dermatol* 153(3), 498
(2002): Phillips R, Melbourne, Australia (from Internet) (observation)
Pruritus (25–36%)
(2007): Madan V+, *Dermatol Ther* 20(4), 239 (passim)
(2005): Hanifin JM+, *J Am Acad Dermatol* 53(2 Suppl 2), S186
(2004): Pascual JC+, *Skin Therapy Lett* 9(9), 1
(2002): Russell JJ, *Am Fam Physician* 66(10), 1899
(2000): Emre S+, *Transpl Int* 13, 73
(2000): Reitamo S+, *Arch Dermatol* 136, 999 (25.3%)
Purpura
(1996): Nash RA+, *Blood* 88, 3634
Pustules (6%)
(2000): Reitamo S+, *Arch Dermatol* 136, 999 (6.3%)
Rash (sic) (24%)
(2007): Madan V+, *Dermatol Ther* 20(4), 239 (passim)
Rosacea
(2004): Antille C+, *Arch Dermatol* 140(4), 457
(2003): Bernard LA+, *Arch Dermatol* 139(2), 229 (granulomatous)
Squamous cell carcinoma
(2001): Otley CC+, *Arch Dermatol* 137, 459
Urticaria
(2001): Takamatsu Y+, *Bone Marrow Transplant* 28(4), 421 (with cyclosporine)

Mucosal/ENT
Dysphagia (>3%)
(2001): Hernandez G+, *Oral Surg Oral Med Oral Pathol Oral Radiol Endod* 92(5), 526
Gingival hyperplasia/hypertrophy
(2007): Madan V+, *Dermatol Ther* 20(4), 239 (passim)
(2006): de Oliveira Costa F+, *J Periodontol* 77(6), 969
(2000): Schmutz J+, *Ann Dermatol Venereol* (French) 127, 646
(1998): Basile C+, *Nephrol Dial Transplant* 13, 2980

Oral candidiasis (>3%)
Oral pigmentation
  (2005): Fricain JC+, *Dermatology* 210(3), 229
  (2004): Shen JT+, *J Am Acad Dermatol* 50(2), 326
Oral ulceration
  (2001): Hernandez G+, *Oral Surg Oral Med Oral Pathol Oral Radiol Endod* 92(5), 526
  (2001): Macario-Barrel A+, *Ann Dermatol Venereol* 128(12), 1327
Ototoxicity
  (2006): Norman K+, *Transpl Int* 19(7), 601
Tinnitus
  (1999): Min DI+, *Pharmacotherapy* 19(7), 891

Hair

Hair – alopecia (>3%)
  (1999): Ushigome H+, *Transplant Proc* 31, 2885 (2 cases)
  (1998): Shapiro R+, *Transplantation* 65, 1284
  (1997): Talbot D+, *Transplantation* 64, 1631
Hair – hirsutism
  (2007): Madan V+, *Dermatol Ther* 20(4), 239 (passim)
Hair – hypertrichosis
  (2005): Prats Caelles I+, *Pediatr Dermatol* 22(1), 86
  (1994): Yamamoto S+, *J Dermatol Sci* 7, S47

Eyes

Vision loss
  (2004): Tamaki H+, *Int J Hematol* 80(3), 291

Other

Abdominal pain
  (2007): Madan V+, *Dermatol Ther* 20(4), 239 (passim)
Anaphylactoid reactions/Anaphylaxis (<1%)
  (2001): Takamatsu Y+, *Bone Marrow Transplant* 28(4), 421 (with cyclosporine)
Application-site burning
  (2006): Singalavanija S+, *J Med Assoc Thai* 89(11), 1915 (21%)
  (1997): Ruzicka T+, *N Engl J Med* 337, 816
Application-site erythema
  (2006): Singalavanija S+, *J Med Assoc Thai* 89(11), 1915
Application-site infections
  (2006): Singalavanija S+, *J Med Assoc Thai* 89(11), 1915 (3%)
Application-site pruritus
  (2006): Hebert AA+, *Cutis* 78(5), 357
  (2006): Pacor ML+, *Allergy Asthma Proc* 27(6), 527 (transient)
  (2006): Singalavanija S+, *J Med Assoc Thai* 89(11), 1915 (9%)
Headache
  (2005): Gonzalez-Lama Y+, *Inflamm Bowel Dis* 11(1), 8 (1 case)
  (2005): Hanifin JM+, *J Am Acad Dermatol* 53(2 Suppl 2), S186
Hepatotoxicity
  (2007): Madan V+, *Dermatol Ther* 20(4), 239 (passim)
  (2000): Emre S+, *Transpl Int* 13(s), 73
Human papilloma virus reactivation
  (2007): Bilenchi R+, *Br J Dermatol* 156(2), 405
Hypertension (49%)
  (2007): Madan V+, *Dermatol Ther* 20(4), 239 (passim)
  (2000): Yanik G+, *Bone Marrow Transplant* 26(2), 161
Inappropriate secretion of antidiuretic hormone (SIADH)
  (2003): Azuma T+, *Int J Hematol* 78(3), 268
Infections (>10%)
  (2005): Hanifin JM+, *J Am Acad Dermatol* 53(2 Suppl 2), S186
Myalgia/Myositis/Myopathy/Myotoxicity (>3%)
Nephrotoxicity
  (2007): Tse KC+, *Lupus* 16(1), 46 (1 case)
  (2006): Boger CA+, *Am J Transplant* 6(8), 1963
  (2006): Borrows R+, *Ther Drug Monit* 28(2), 269 (6 cases)
  (2006): Dittrich K+, *Pediatr Nephrol* 21(7), 958
  (2006): Froud T+, *Cell Transplant* 15(7), 613
  (2006): Ruddock B, *Issues Emerg Health Technol* 88, 1

  (2006): Ueno T+, *Transplant Proc* 38(6), 1762
  (2005): McLaughlin GE+, *Nephrol Dial Transplant* 20(7), 1471
  (2004): Kuypers DR+, *Clin Pharmacol Ther* 75(5), 434
  (2003): Flechner SM, *Transplant Proc* 35(3 Suppl), 118S
  (2002): Barone GW+, *JOP* 3(2), 49
  (2002): Bolley R+, *Transplantation* 73(6), 1009
  (2002): Khanna A+, *Kidney Int* 62(6), 2257
  (2002): Lytton SD+, *Clin Exp Immunol* 127(2), 293
  (2001): Morales JM+, *Nephrol Dial Transplant* 16 Suppl 1, 121
  (2001): Pescovitz MD+, *Am J Kidney Dis* 38(4 Suppl 2), S16
  (2001): Venkataramanan R+, *J Clin Pharmacol* 41(5), 542
  (2001): Wondimu B+, *Int J Paediatr Dent* 11(6), 424
  (2000): de Mattos AM+, *Am J Kidney Dis* 35(2), 333
  (2000): Emre S+, *Transpl Int* 13(s), 73
  (2000): Yanik G+, *Bone Marrow Transplant* 26(2), 161
  (1999): Finn WF, *Ren Fail* 21(3–4), 319
  (1999): Soccal PM+, *Transplantation* 68(1), 164
  (1999): Zoppo A+, *Transplantation* 68(8), 1211
  (1998): Heering P+, *Clin Transplant* 12(5), 465
  (1998): Solez K+, *Transplantation* 66(12), 1736
  (1997): Duddridge M+, *Ann Rheum Dis* 56(11), 690
  (1997): Filler G+, *Nephrol Dial Transplant* 12(8), 1668
  (1997): Katari SR+, *Clin Transplant* 11(3), 237
  (1997): Katari SR+, *Transplant Proc* 29(1–2), 311
Neurotoxicity
  (2007): Kaczmarek I+, *J Heart Lung Transplant* 26(1), 89
  (2006): Froud T+, *Cell Transplant* 15(7), 613
  (2001): Wondimu B+, *Int J Paediatr Dent* 11(6), 424
  (2000): Emre S+, *Transpl Int* 13(s), 73
Pain
  (2002): Malat GE+, *Pediatr Transplant* 6(5), 435
Paresthesias (40%)
  (1997): Sandborn WJ, *Am J Gastroenterol* 92, 876
  (1996): *Arch Dermatol* 132, 419
Seizures (<10%)
  (2004): Tamaki H+, *Int J Hematol* 80(3), 291
  (2000): Yanik G+, *Bone Marrow Transplant* 26(2), 161
Tremor (>10%)
  (2000): Yanik G+, *Bone Marrow Transplant* 26(2), 161
Tumors
  (2007): Levi Z+, *Am J Transplant* 7(2), 476 (facial)

TADALAFIL

Trade name: Cialis (Lilly-ICOS)
Indications: Erectile dysfunction
Category: Phosphodiesterase type 5 inhibitor
Half-life: 17.5 hours
Clinically important, potentially hazardous interactions with: alpha-ii-blockers, doxazosin, ketoconazole, nicorandil, nitrates, ritonavir

Reactions

Skin

Diaphoresis (<2%)
Erythema multiforme
  (2005): Woodall T, Rock Hill, SC (from Internet) (observation)
Facial edema (<2%)
Pruritus (<2%)
Rash (sic) (<2%)

Mucosal/ENT

Xerostomia (<2%)

Eyes

Dyschromatopsia (<2%)

Eyelid edema (<2%)
  (2004): Chandeclerc ML+, *South Med J* 97(11), 1142
Eyelid pain (<2%)
Optic neuropathy
  (2006): Bella AJ+, *Can J Urol* 13(5), 3233
  (2005): Bollinger K+, *Arch Ophthalmol* 123(3), 400
  (2005): Egan RA+, *Arch Ophthalmol* 123(5), 709
  (2005): Escaravage GK+, *Arch Ophthalmol* 123(3), 399

Other
Asthenia (<2%)
Headache (4–15%)
  (2007): Goldstein I+, *J Sex Med* 4(1), 166 (5%)
  (2007): Segraves RT+, *J Clin Psychopharmacol* 27(1), 62
  (2006): Buvat J+, *J Sex Med* 3(3), 512
  (2006): Dinn RB+, *Cephalalgia* 26(11), 1344
  (2006): Guo YL+, *Int J Urol* 13(6), 721
  (2006): Martin-Morales A+, *Actas Urol Esp* 30(8), 791
  (2006): Morgentaler A+, *J Sex Med* 3(3), 492
  (2006): Yip WC+, *Asian J Androl* 8(6), 685
  (2006): Zhu XW+, *Zhonghua Nan Ke Xue* 12(5), 421 (11 cases)
  (2004): Eardley I+, *BJU Int* 94(6), 871
  (2003): Govier F+, *Clin Ther* 25(11), 2709 (11.2%)
  (2003): Stroberg P+, *Clin Ther* 25(11), 2724 (4.8%)
  (2002): Brock GB+, *J Urol* 168(4), 1332
  (2002): Porst H, *Int J Impot Res* 14, S57
  (2002): Tejada Saenz de I+, *Diabetes Care* 25(12), 2159
  (2001): Padma-Nathan H+, *Int J Impot Res* 13(1), 2
Myalgia/Myositis/Myopathy/Myotoxicity (1–4%)
  (2004): Eardley I+, *BJU Int* 94(6), 871
  (2002): Porst H, *Int J Impot Res* 14, S57
Pain (1–3%)
Paresthesias (<2%)
Vertigo (<2%)
  (2006): Gonzalez RR+, *Expert Opin Drug Metab Toxicol* 2(4), 609
  (2006): Guo YL+, *Int J Urol* 13(6), 721
  (2006): Yip WC+, *Asian J Androl* 8(6), 685
  (2006): Zhu XW+, *Zhonghua Nan Ke Xue* 12(5), 421 (11 cases)

TAMOXIFEN

Trade names: Apo-Tamox; Bilim; Istubol; Kessar; Mamofen; Nolvadex (AstraZeneca); Novofen; Tamaxin; Tamofen; Tamoxan; Taxus; Valodex
Indications: Advanced breast cancer
Category: Selective estrogen receptor modulator (SERM)
Half-life: 7 days
Clinically important, potentially hazardous interactions with: black cohosh, dong quai, ginseng

Reactions

Skin
Dermatomyositis
  (1982): Harris AL+, *BMJ* 284, 1674
Diaphoresis
  (1986): Buchanan RB+, *J Clin Oncology* 4, 1326
  (1980): Pritchard KI+, *Cancer Treat Rep* 64, 787
Edema (2–6%)
  (1986): Buchanan RB+, *J Clin Oncology* 4, 1326
Exanthems (3%)
  (1999): Descamps V+, *Ann Dermatol Venereol* (French) 126, 716
  (1980): Pritchard KI+, *Cancer Treat Rep* 64, 787
Lupus erythematosus
  (2005): Fumal I+, *Dermatology* 210(3), 251
Peripheral edema

Photo-recall
  (2006): Kundranda MN+, *Am J Clin Oncol* 29(6), 637
  (2004): Singer EA+, *Breast J* 10(2), 170
  (1999): Bostrom A+, *Acta Oncol* 38, 955
  (1992): Parry BR, *Lancet* 340, 49
Pruritus
  (1980): Pritchard KI+, *Cancer Treat Rep* 64, 787
Pruritus ani et vulvae
  (1980): Pritchard KI+, *Cancer Treat Rep* 64, 787
Purpura
Radiodermatitis
  (2006): Kundranda MN+, *Am J Clin Oncol* 29(6), 637
Rash (sic) (1–10%)
Recall reaction
  (2006): Kundranda MN+, *Am J Clin Oncol* 29(6), 637
Sarcoma
  (2006): ACOG, *Obstet Gynecol* 107(6), 1475 (uterine)
  (2006): Arenas M+, *Int J Gynecol Cancer* 16(2), 861 (uterine) (3 cases)
  (2006): Atallah D+, *Obstet Gynecol* 108(3 Pt 2), 762 (uterine)
  (2006): Botsis D+, *Int J Gynecol Pathol* 25(2), 173 (uterine)
  (2006): Liu IF+, *Taiwan J Obstet Gynecol* 45(2), 167 (uterine)
  (2006): Mouridsen HT, *Curr Med Res Opin* 22(8), 1609
  (2006): Oztekin O+, *Int J Gynecol Cancer* 16(4), 1694 (endometrial)
  (2006): Uray IP+, *Expert Opin Investig Drugs* 15(12), 1583 (uterine)
Urticaria
Vasculitis
  (2006): Baptista MZ+, *J Clin Oncol* 24(21), 3504
  (1994): Rzany B+, *J Am Acad Dermatol* 30, 509
  (1990): Drago F+, *Ann Intern Med* 112, 965
Xerosis (7%)

Mucosal/ENT
Dysgeusia
Vaginal pruritus
Xerostomia (7%)

Hair
Hair – alopecia
  (2001): Puglisi F+, *Ann Intern Med* 134(12), 1154 (total)
  (1993): Litt JZ, Beachwood, OH (personal case) (observation)
  (1980): Pritchard KI+, *Cancer Treat Rep* 64, 787
Hair – hirsutism
  (1980): Pritchard KI+, *Cancer Treat Rep* 64, 787
Hair – hypertrichosis
Hair – pigmentation
  (1995): Hampson JP+, *Br J Dermatol* 132, 483

Eyes
Cataract
  (2003): Parkkari M+, *Acta Ophthalmol Scand* 81(5), 495 (7%)
Keratopathy
  (2006): Zinchuk O+, *Arch Ophthalmol* 124(7), 1046
Maculopathy
  (2003): Parkkari M+, *Acta Ophthalmol Scand* 81(5), 495
Ocular allergy (sic)
  (2003): Parkkari M+, *Acta Ophthalmol Scand* 81(5), 495
Ocular toxicity
  (2006): Muftuoglu O+, *Eye Contact Lens* 32(5), 228
  (2005): Cronin BG+, *Int Ophthalmol* 26(3), 101

Other
Depression
  (2001): Day R+, *J Natl Cancer Inst* 93(21), 1615
Headache
Hepatotoxicity
  (2007): Osman KA+, *Expert Opin Drug Saf* 6(1), 1 (40%)

(2006): Ahmed MH+, *Pathology* 38(3), 270
(2006): Liu CL+, *Anticancer Drugs* 17(6), 709

Hot flashes
(2007): Coates AS+, *J Clin Oncol* 25(5), 486
(2006): Garreau JR+, *Am J Surg* 192(4), 496 (35%)
(2006): Land SR+, *JAMA* 295(23), 2742
(2006): Sestak I+, *J Clin Oncol* 24(24), 3991
(2006): Uray IP+, *Expert Opin Investig Drugs* 15(12), 1583
(2003): Goetz MP+, *J Natl Cancer Inst* 95(23), 1734
(2002): Kinsinger LS+, *Ann Intern Med* 137(1), 59
(2001): Vogel NE+, *Ned Tijdschr Geneeskd* 145(22), 1041

Myalgia/Myositis/Myopathy/Myotoxicity
(1982): Harris AL+, *BMJ* 284, 1674

Stroke
(2006): Chlebowski RT+, *Clin Breast Cancer* 6 Suppl 2, S58
(2006): Mouridsen HT, *Curr Med Res Opin* 22(8), 1609
(2006): Uray IP+, *Expert Opin Investig Drugs* 15(12), 1583

Thrombophlebitis
(1996): Zimmet S, *The Schoch Letter* 46, 22 (#86) (observation)

Thrombosis
(2007): Coates AS+, *J Clin Oncol* 25(5), 486
(2007): Cuzick J+, *J Natl Cancer inst* 99(4), 272
(2007): Osman KA+, *Expert Opin Drug Saf* 6(1), 1
(2006): Pritchard KI+, *Drugs* 66(13), 1727
(2006): Uray IP+, *Expert Opin Investig Drugs* 15(12), 1583

TAMSULOSIN

Trade name: Flomax (Boehringer Ingelheim)
Indications: Benign prostatic hypertrophy
Category: Adrenergic alpha-receptor antagonist
Half-life: 9–13 hours
Clinically important, potentially hazardous interactions with: vardenafil

Reactions

Skin
Angioedema
Eczema
(2000): Frederickson KS, Novalo, CA (from Internet) (observation)
Erythema multiforme
(1999): Reed BR, Denver, CO (from Internet) (observation)
Pruritus
Rash (sic)

Mucosal/ENT
Rhinitis
(2003): Wilt TJ+, *Cochrane Database Syst Rev* sses(1), CD00

Eyes
Floppy iris syndrome
(2007): Chadha V+, *Br J Ophthalmol* 91(1), 40 (57%)
(2007): Oshika T+, *Am J Ophthalmol* 143(1), 150 (43%)
(2007): Shapiro BL+, *Am J Ophthalmol* 143(2), 351
(2006): Allen D+, *J Cataract Refract Surg* 32(11), 1899
(2006): Arshinoff SA, *J Cataract Refract Surg* 32(4), 559
(2006): Bendel RE+, *J Cataract Refract Surg* 32(10), 1603
(2006): Cheung CM+, *J Cataract Refract Surg* 32(8), 1336 (35%)
(2006): Lawrentschuk N+, *BJU Int* 97(1), 2
(2006): Lim LA+, *J Cataract Refract Surg* 32(10), 1777
(2006): Nguyen DQ+, *BJU Int* 97(1), 197
(2006): Parssinen O+, *Invest Ophthalmol Vis Sci* 47(9), 3766
(2005): Chang DF+, *J Cataract Refract Surg* 31(4), 664 (2%)
(2005): Kershner RM, *J Cataract Refract Surg* 31(12), 2239
(2005): Nguyen DQ+, *J Cataract Refract Surg* 31(12), 2240

Other
Headache
Hypotension
(2006): Nieminen T+, *Clin Drug Investig* 26(11), 667 (with sildenafil)
Seizures
(2006): Ivanez V+, *Epilepsia* 47(10), 1741
Vertigo
(2006): Rahardjo D+, *Int J Urol* 13(11), 1405 (6%)
(2005): Lucas MG+, *BJU Int* 95(3), 354 (10%)
(2003): Wilt TJ+, *Cochrane Database Syst Rev* sses(1), CD00

TARTRAZINE

Synonyms: Acid Yellow T; Acilan Yellow GG; Cake Yellow; Tartar Yellow S; Wool Yellow
Trade names: E102; FD&C yellow No.5
Category: Food additive
Half-life: N/A

Note: Tartrazine intolerance has been estimated to affect between 0.01% and 0.1% of the population. Adverse reactions are most common in people who are sensitive to aspirin. Banned in Norway and Austria

Reactions

Skin
Adverse effects (sic)
(1986): Stevenson DD+, *J Allergy Clin Immunol* 78(1 Pt 2), 182
(1982): Rosenhall L, *Eur J Respir Dis* 63(5), 410
(1981): Neumann CJ+, *Am J Hosp Pharm* 38(6), 790, 792
Allergic reactions (sic)
(2000): Bhatia MS, *J Clin Psychiatry* 61(7), 473
(1989): Pollock I+, *BMJ* 299(6700), 649
(1988): McLean JD, *Can J Psychiatry* 33(4), 331
(1987): Pohl R+, *Am J Psychiatry* 144(2), 237 (in antidepressents)
(1982): MacCara ME, *Can Med Assoc J* 126(8), 910
Angioedema
(1996): Jimenez-Aranda GS+, *Rev Alerg Mex* (Spanish) 43(6), 152
(1992): Novembre E+, *Pediatr Med Chir* (Italian) 14(1), 39 (passim)
(1989): Hong SP+, *Yonsei Med J* 30(4), 339
(1989): Montano Garcia ML, *Rev Alerg Mex* (Spanish) 36(3), 107
(1989): Montano Garcia ML+, *Rev Alerg Mex* (Spanish) 36(1), 15
(1985): Collins-Williams C, *J Asthma* 22(3), 139 (aspirin intolerance)
(1984): Diez Gomez ML+, *Allergol Immunopathol* (Madr) (Spanish) 12(3), 179
(1981): Alvarez Cuesta E+, *Allergol Immunopathol* (Madr) (Spanish) 9(1), 45
(1980): Makol GM+, *Ariz Med* 37(2), 79
Atopic dermatitis
(2001): Worm M+, *Clin Exp Allergy* 31(2), 265
(1992): Devlin J+, *Arch Dis Child* 67(6), 709
Dermatitis
(1990): Dipalma JR, *Am Fam Physician* 42(5), 1347
Edema
(1989): Pachor ML+, *Oral Surg Oral Med Oral Pathol* 67(4), 393
Fixed eruption
(1997): Orchard DC+, *Australas J Dermatol* 38(4), 212
Photosensitivity
Pruritus
(1981): Alvarez Cuesta E+, *Allergol Immunopathol* (Madr) (Spanish) 9(1), 45
Purpura
(1999): Kalinke DU+, *Hautarzt* (German) 50(1), 47

(1993): Wuthrich B, *Ann Allergy* 71(4), 379
(1990): Dipalma JR, *Am Fam Physician* 42(5), 1347
(1985): Parodi G+, *Dermatologica* 171(1), 62
(1981): Alvarez Cuesta E+, *Allergol Immunopathol* (Madr) (Spanish) 9(1), 45
Rash (sic)
(1995): Thuvander A, *Lakartidningen* (Swedish) 92(4), 296
Urticaria (often related to aspirin intolerance)
(1996): Jimenez-Aranda GS+, *Rev Alerg Mex* (Spanish) 43(6), 152
(1993): Wuthrich B, *Ann Allergy* 71(4), 379
(1992): Novembre E+, *Pediatr Med Chir* (Italian) 14(1), 39
(1990): Dipalma JR, *Am Fam Physician* 42(5), 1347
(1989): Baumgardner DJ, *Postgrad Med* 85(6), 265
(1989): Hong SP+, *Yonsei Med J* 30(4), 339
(1989): Montano Garcia ML, *Rev Alerg Mex* (Spanish) 36(3), 107
(1989): Montano Garcia ML+, *Rev Alerg Mex* (Spanish) 36(1), 15
(1989): Wilson N+, *Clin Exp Allergy* 19(3), 267
(1987): Settipane GA, *N Engl Reg Allergy Proc* 8(1), 39 (aspirin intolerance)
(1986): Chudwin DS+, *Ann Allergy* 57(2), 133 (aspirin intolerance)
(1986): Simon RA, *N Engl Reg Allergy Proc* 7(6), 533
(1986): Warrington RJ+, *Clin Allergy* 16(6), 527
(1985): Collins-Williams C, *J Asthma* 22(3), 139 (aspirin intolerance)
(1985): Podell RN, *Postgrad Med* 78(8), 83, 87, 92
(1984): Diez Gomez ML+, *Allergol Immunopathol* (Madr) (Spanish) 12(3), 179
(1984): Royal College of Physicians and the British Nutrition Foundation, *J Royal College of Physicians of London* 18(2)
(1982): Ortolani C+, *Ann Allergy* 48(1), 50
(1982): Warin RP+, *Br Med J (Clin Res Ed)* 284(6327), 1443
(1981): Alvarez Cuesta E+, *Allergol Immunopathol* (Madr) (Spanish) 9(1), 45
(1981): Juhlin L, *Br J Dermatology* 104, 369
(1981): Wuthrich B+, *Schweiz Med Wochenschr* 111(39), 1445 (6.1%)
(1980): Makol GM+, *Ariz Med* 37(2), 79
(1980): Valverde E+, *Clin Allergy* 10(6), 691
Vasculitis
(1999): Kalinke DU+, *Hautarzt* (German) 50(1), 47
(1993): Wuthrich B, *Ann Allergy* 71(4), 379
(1990): Dipalma JR, *Am Fam Physician* 42(5), 1347

Mucosal/ENT

Gingival hyperplasia/hypertrophy
(1989): Pachor ML+, *Oral Surg Oral Med Oral Pathol* 67(4), 393
Rhinitis
(2004): Pacor ML+, *Allergy* 59(2), 192 (2 cases)

Other

Anaphylactoid reactions/Anaphylaxis
(1993): Wuthrich B, *Ann Allergy* 71(4), 379
(1989): Montano Garcia ML, *Rev Alerg Mex* (Spanish) 36(3), 107
(1981): Desmond RE+, *Ann Allergy* 46(2), 81
(1981): Schneiweiss F, *Ann Allergy* 46(5), 294
(1980): Kallos P+, *Med Hypotheses* 6(5), 487
Asthenia
Depression
(1992): Novembre E+, *Pediatr Med Chir* (Italian) 14(1), 39
Hypersensitivity
(1995): Sakakibara H+, *Nihon Kyobu Shikkan Gakkai Zasshi* (Japanese) 33, 106
(1995): Thuvander A, *Lakartidningen* (Swedish) 92(4), 296
(1980): Weliky N+, *Clin Allergy* 10(4), 375
Paresthesias
(1981): Alvarez Cuesta E+, *Allergol Immunopathol* (Madr) (Spanish) 9(1), 45
Serum sickness

TEA TREE

Scientific names: *Melaleuca alternifolia; Melaleuca cajeputi; Melaleuca dissitifolia; Melaleuca linafolia*
Family: Myrtaceae
Trade and other common names: Amber Gold; Australian Tea Tree; Burnaid; Cajuput; Dessert Essence; Melasol; New Zealand Manuka,; New Zealand Ti-Tree; Teatree oil
Category: Antiseptic
Purported indications and other uses: Gram-negative and Gram-positive bacteria, acne, vaginal infection, burns, onychomycosis, tinea pedis, bruises, insect bites, skin infections, mouthwash, genital herpes, antiperspirant, gingivitis, disinfectant, scabies
Half-life: N/A
Clinically important, potentially hazardous interactions with: colophony, turpentine

Reactions

Skin

Adverse effects (sic)
(2002): Haller CA+, *Adverse Drug React Toxicol Rev* 21(3), 143
Allergic reactions (sic)
(2002): Haller CA+, *Adverse Drug React Toxicol Rev* 21(3), 143
(2000): Ernst E+, *Forsch Komplementarmed Klass Naturheilkd* 7(1), 17
(2000): Thomson KF+, *Br J Dermatol* 142, 84
(2000): Varma S+, *Contact Dermatitis* 42(5), 309
(1997): Hackzell-Bradley M+, *Lakartidningen* 94(47), 4359
(1994): Selvaag E+, *Contact Dermatitis* 31(2), 124
(1993): de Groot AC+, *Contact Dermatitis* 28(5), 309
Burning
(2002): Groppo FC+, *Int Dent J* 52(6), 433
Dermatitis
(2005): Hartford O+, *Cutis* 76(3), 178
(2005): Willcox M, *Nurs Times* 101(11), 32
(2003): Perrett CM+, *Clin Exp Dermatol* 28(2), 167
(2002): Schempp CM+, *Hautarzt* 53(2), 93
(2001): Fritz TM+, *Ann Dermatol Venereol* 128(2), 123 (7 cases)
(2000): Khanna M+, *Am J Contact Dermat* 11(4), 238
(1999): Bruynzeel DP, *Trop Med Int Health* 4(9), 630
(1999): Greig JE+, *Contact Dermatitis* 41(6), 354
(1999): Hausen BM+, *Am J Contact Dermat* 10(2), 68
(1998): Rubel DM+, *Australas J Dermatol* 39(4), 244
(1998): Wolner-Hanssen P+, *Lakartidningen* 95(30), 3309
(1997): Bhushan M+, *Contact Dermatitis* 36(2), 117
(1997): Kranke B, *Hautarzt* 48(3), 203
(1996): De Groot AC, *Contact Dermatitis* 35(5), 304
(1994): Knight TE+, *J Am Acad Dermatol* 30(3), 423
(1994): van der Valk PG+, *Ned Tijdschr Geneeskd* 138(16), 823 (4 cases)
(1992): de Groot AC+, *Contact Dermatitis* 27(4), 279
(1991): Apted JH, *Australas J Dermatol* 32(3), 177
Eczema
(2002): Dharmagunawardena B+, *Contact Dermatitis* 47(5), 288
Erythema multiforme
(2000): Khanna M+, *Am J Contact Dermat* 11(4), 238
Inflammation
(1999): Syed TA+, *Trop Med Int Health* 4(4), 284 (4 cases) (with butenafine)
Linear IgA dermatosis
(2003): Perrett CM+, *Clin Exp Dermatol* 28(2), 167
Pruritus
(1998): Wolner-Hanssen P+, *Lakartidningen* 95(30), 3309
Rash (sic)
Sensitization

(1999): Hausen BM+, *Am J Contact Dermat* 10(2), 68
Toxicity (sic)
(1995): Carson CF+, *J Toxicol Clin Toxicol* 33(2), 193

Other
Depression
(1994): Villar D+, *Vet Hum Toxicol* 36(2), 139 (ingested)
Gynecomastia
(2007): Dean CJ, *N Engl J Med* 356(24), 2543
(2007): Henley DV+, *N Engl J Med* 356(5), 479
(2007): Kalyan S, *N Engl J Med* 356(24), 2542
Hypersensitivity
(2003): Mozelsio NB+, *Allergy Asthma Proc* 24(1), 73
(2001): Fritz TM+, *Ann Dermatol Venereol* 128(2), 123 (7 cases)
Side effects (sic)
(2000): Ernst E, *Br J Dermatol* 143(5), 923
Tremor
(1994): Villar D+, *Vet Hum Toxicol* 36(2), 139

TEGASEROD

Trade name: Zelnorm (Novartis)
Indications: Irritable bowel syndrome
Category: 5-HT4 agonist; Serotonin type 4 receptor agonist
Half-life: 11±5 hours
Clinically important, potentially hazardous interactions with: None

Reactions

Skin
Diaphoresis
Facial edema
Pruritus
Raynaud's phenomenon
(2003): Bertoli R+, *Eur J Clin Pharmacol* 58(10), 717

Mucosal/ENT
Oral vesiculation

Other
Abdominal pain
(2007): Kale-Pradhan PB+, *Pharmacotherapy* 27(2), 267
(2006): Muller-Lissner S+, *Am J Gastroenterol* 101(11), 2558 (%)
(2004): Schoenfeld P, *Aliment Pharmacol Ther* 20, 25
(2002): Fidelholtz J+, *Am J Gastroenterol* 97(5), 1176
(2002): Tougas G+, *Aliment Pharmacol Ther* 16(10), 1701 (7%)
Depression
Headache (12%)
(2007): Kale-Pradhan PB+, *Pharmacotherapy* 27(2), 267
(2006): Muller-Lissner S+, *Am J Gastroenterol* 101(11), 2558 (%)
(2006): Quigley EM+, *Clin Gastroenterol Hepatol* 4(5), 605
(2004): Nyhlin H+, *Scand J Gastroenterol* 39(2), 119
(2004): Schoenfeld P, *Aliment Pharmacol Ther* 20, 25
(2003): Kellow J+, *Gut* 52(5), 671 (12%)
(2002): Tougas G+, *Aliment Pharmacol Ther* 16(10), 1701 (8%)
Pain
Vertigo (4%)

TELBIVUDINE

Trade name: Tyzeka (Novartis)
Indications: Hepatitis B (chronic)
Category: Nucleoside analog reverse transcriptase inhibitor
Half-life: ~15 hours
Clinically important, potentially hazardous interactions with: N/A

Reactions

Skin
Rash (sic) (4%)

Other
Abdominal pain (12%)
Asthenia (>5%)
Cough (7%)
Fever (4%)
Headache (11%)
Myalgia/Myositis/Myopathy/Myotoxicity (3%)
Upper respiratory infection (>5%)
Vertigo (4%)

TELITHROMYCIN

Synonyms: HMR 3647; RU-647; RU-66647
Trade name: Ketek (Sanofi-Aventis)
Indications: Community-acquired pneumonia, chronic bronchitis
Category: Antibiotic, macrolide
Half-life: 10–13 hours
Clinically important, potentially hazardous interactions with: atorvastatin, carbamazepine, cisapride, cyclosporine, digoxin, dihydroergotamine, ergotamine, hexobarbital, ixabepilone, lapatinib, lovastatin, metoprolol, midazolam, phenobarbital, phenytoin, pimozide, rifampin, rimonabant, simvastatin, sirolimus, tacrolimus, temsirolimus, triazolam, warfarin

Reactions

Skin
Angioedema (<2%)
(2007): Bottenberg MM+, *Ann Allergy Asthma Immunol* 98(1), 89
Diaphoresis
Eczema (<2%)
Erythema multiforme (<2%)
Facial edema (<2%)
Pruritus (<2%)
Rash (sic) (<2%)
Urticaria (<2%)
Vasculitis (<2%)

Mucosal/ENT
Dysgeusia (1.6%)
(2005): Kasbekar N+, *Am J Health Syst Pharm* 62(9), 905
Glossitis (<2%)
Stomatitis (<2%)
Vulvovaginal candidiasis (<2%)
Xerostomia (<2%)

Eyes
Vision blurred
Visual disturbances

Other

Abdominal pain (<2%)
Anaphylactoid reactions/Anaphylaxis (<2%)
  (2007): Bottenberg MM+, *Ann Allergy Asthma Immunol* 98(1), 89
Asthenia (<2%)
Candidiasis (<2%)
Headache (4%)
  (2005): Kasbekar N+, *Am J Health Syst Pharm* 62(9), 905
  (2003): *Prescrire Int* 12(63), 8
Hepatotoxicity
  (2006): *Ann Intern Med* 144(6), 142
  (2006): Bertino JS, *Ann Intern Med* 145(6), 472
  (2006): Clay KD+, *Ann Intern Med* 144(6), 415 (3 cases)
  (2005): Peters TS, *Toxicol Pathol* 33(1), 146
Hypersensitivity (<2%)
  (2007): Bottenberg MM+, *Ann Allergy Asthma Immunol.* 98(1), 89
Myalgia/Myositis/Myopathy/Myotoxicity (<2%)
Nephrotoxicity
  (2004): Tintillier M+, *Am J Kidney Dis* 44(2), e25
Paresthesias (<2%)
Tremor (<2%)
Vertigo (2–6%)
  (2005): Kasbekar N+, *Am J Health Syst Pharm* 62(9), 905
  (2003): *Prescrire Int* 12(63), 8

TELMISARTAN

Trade name: Micardis (Boehringer Ingelheim)
Indications: Hypertension
Category: Angiotensin II receptor antagonist
Half-life: 24 hours

Reactions

Skin

Allergic reactions (sic) (<1%)
Angioedema (>0.3%)
  (2003): Borazan A+, *Allergy* 58(5), 454
Dermatitis (>0.3%)
Diaphoresis (>0.3%)
Eczema (>0.3%)
Edema
  (2001): Lacourciere Y+, *J Hum Hypertens* 15(11), 763
Fungal dermatitis (>0.3%)
Peripheral edema (1%)
Pruritus (>0.3%)
Rash (sic) (>0.3%)

Mucosal/ENT

Xerostomia (>0.3%)

Other

Asthenia
  (2005): Kulkarni RB+, *J Indian Med Assoc* 103(3), 187
  (2004): Jayaram S+, *J Indian Med Assoc* 102(9), 525
  (2003): Ingino C+, *J Int Med Res* 31(6), 561
Cough
  (2006): Williams B+, *J Hypertens* 24(1), 193 (%)
  (2004): Chen JH+, *Int J Clin Pract.* Suppl. (145), 29 (8%)
  (2002): Amerena J+, *J Int Med Res* 30(6), 543 (0.8%) (with
    enalapril)
  (2002): White WB, *J Clin Hypertens* (Greenwich) 4(4), 20
  (2001): Dunselman PH+, *Int J Cardiol* 77(2-3), 131 (3%)
  (2001): Sharpe M+, *Drugs* 61(10), 1501
Headache
  (2003): Ingino C+, *J Int Med Res* 31(6), 561

  (2002): Buranakitjaroen P+, *J Med Assoc Thai* 85(9), 968
Myalgia/Myositis/Myopathy/Myotoxicity (1%)
Paresthesias (>0.3%)
Vertigo
  (2005): Kulkarni RB+, *J Indian Med Assoc* 103(3), 187
  (2004): Jayaram S+, *J Indian Med Assoc* 102(9), 525
  (2002): Buranakitjaroen P+, *J Med Assoc Thai* 85(9), 968

TEMAZEPAM

Trade names: Apo-Temazepam; Cerepax; Euhypnos; Lenal;
Levanxene; Normison; Nu-Temazepam; Planum; Restoril
(Mallinckrodt); Temazepam
Indications: Insomnia, anxiety
Category: Benzodiazepine
Half-life: 8–15 hours
**Clinically important, potentially hazardous interactions
with:** amprenavir, chlorpheniramine, clarithromycin, efavirenz,
esomeprazole, imatinib, mianserin, nelfinavir

Reactions

Skin

Adverse effects (sic)
  (1984): Stricker BH, *Ned Tijdschr Geneeskd* (Dutch) 128, 870
Bullous dermatitis
  (1999): Verghese J+, *Acad Emerg Med* 6, 1071
Dermatitis (1–10%)
Diaphoresis (>10%)
Exanthems
Fixed eruption
  (1988): Archer CB+, *Clin Exp Dermatol* 13, 336
Lichenoid eruption
  (1986): Norris P+, *BMJ* 293, 510
Pruritus
Purpura
Rash (sic) (>10%)
Urticaria

Mucosal/ENT

Dysgeusia
Sialopenia (>10%)
Sialorrhea (1–10%)
Xerostomia (1.7%)

Eyes

Visual hallucinations
  (2006): Iraqi A+, *J Am Geriatr Soc* 54(10), 1627

Other

Anaphylactoid reactions/Anaphylaxis
  (1988): Mills PJ, *Anaesthesia* 43, 66
Headache
Paresthesias
Tremor (<1%)

TEMOZOLOMIDE

Trade name: Temodar (Schering)
Indications: Anaplastic astrocytoma
Category: Alkylating agent; Antineoplastic
Half-life: 1.8 hours

Reactions

Skin
Allergic reactions
 (2004): Sipos L+, *Ideggyogy Sz* 57(11-12), 394
Edema
 (2003): Hwu W-J, *J Drugs Dermatol* 2, 53 (with thalidomide)
Hand–foot syndrome
 (2007): Kanat O+, *J Postgrad Med* 53(2), 146
Kaposi's sarcoma
 (2006): Ganiere V+, *Nat Clin Pract Oncol* 3(6), 339
Peripheral edema (11%)
Pruritus (8%)
Rash (sic) (8%)
 (2004): Chua SL+, *Neuro-oncol* 6(1), 38 (14%) (with doxorubicin)
 (2003): Hwu W-J, *J Drugs Dermatol* 2, 53 (with thalidomide)

Hair
Hair – alopecia
 (2005): Daponte A+, *Anticancer Res* 25(2B), 1441 (14%) (with cisplatin)

Other
Asthenia
 (2005): Daponte A+, *Anticancer Res* 25(2B), 1441 (11%) (with cisplatin)
 (2003): Talbot SM+, *Cancer* 98(9), 1942
Death
 (2007): Grewal J+, *N Engl J Med* 356(15), 1591
 (2007): Soetekouw PM+, *Ned Tijdschr Geneeskd* 151(4), 253
Fever
 (2006): Ganiere V+, *Nat Clin Pract Oncol* 3(6), 339
Headache
 (2006): Ganiere V+, *Nat Clin Pract Oncol* 3(6), 339
Hepatotoxicity
 (2007): Chheda MG+, *Neurology* 68(12), 955 (reactivation)
Infections
 (2006): Ganiere V+, *Nat Clin Pract Oncol* 3(6), 339
 (2003): Hwu W-J, *J Drugs Dermatol* 2, 53 (with thalidomide)
Myalgia/Myositis/Myopathy/Myotoxicity (5%)
Paresthesias (9%)
Tremor
 (2003): Hwu W-J, *J Drugs Dermatol* 2, 53 (with thalidomide)

TEMSIROLIMUS

Synonym: CCI-779
Trade name: Torisel (Wyeth)
Indications: Renal cell carcinoma, other cancers
Category: Analog of sirolimus; mTOR inhibitor
Half-life: 13–25 Hours
**Clinically important, potentially hazardous interactions
with:** atazanavir, carbamazepine, clarithromycin, dexamethasone, indinavir, itraconazole, ketoconazole, nefazodone, nelfinavir, phenobarbital, phenytoin, rifabutin, rifampicin, rifampin, ritonavir, saquinavir, **St John's wort**, telithromycin, voriconazole

Reactions

Skin
Acne (10%)
 (2004): Raymond E+, *J Clin Oncol* 22(12), 2336
Exanthems
 (2005): Chan S+, *J Clin Oncol* 23(23), 5314 (51%)
 (2004): Raymond E+, *J Clin Oncol* 22(12), 2336
Follicular dermatitis
 (2005): Margolin K+, *Cancer* 104(5), 1045
Peripheral edema
 (2007): Hudes G+, *N Engl J Med* 356(22), 2271
Pruritus (19%)
 (2005): Boni JP+, *Clin Pharmacol Ther* 77(1), 76
Rash (sic) (47%)
 (2007): Hudes G+, *N Engl J Med* 356(22), 2271
 (2006): Duran I+, *Br J Cancer* 95(9), 1148
 (2005): Chan S+, *J Clin Oncol* 23(23), 5314
 (2005): Margolin K+, *Cancer* 104(5), 1045
 (2004): Raymond E+, *J Clin Oncol* 22(12), 2336
 (2003): Punt CJ+, *Ann Oncol* 14(6), 931
Xerosis (11%)

Mucosal/ENT
Dysgeusia (20%)
Mucositis (30%)
 (2005): Chan S+, *J Clin Oncol* 23(23), 5314 (70%)
 (2004): Raymond E+, *J Clin Oncol* 22(12), 2336
 (2003): Punt CJ+, *Ann Oncol* 14(6), 931 (fatal)
Pharyngitis (12%)
Rhinitis (10%)
Stomatitis
 (2005): Chang SM+, *Invest New Drugs* 23(4), 357
 (2005): Margolin K+, *Cancer* 104(5), 1045
 (2004): Chang SM+, *Invest New Drugs* 22(4), 427
 (2004): Raymond E+, *J Clin Oncol* 22(12), 2336
 (2003): Punt CJ+, *Ann Oncol* 14(6), 931

Nails
Nail disorder (sic) (14%)

Eyes
Conjunctivitis (7%)

Other
Abdominal pain (21%)
Asthenia (30%)
 (2006): Duran I+, *Br J Cancer* 95(9), 1148 (78%)
 (2005): Chan S+, *J Clin Oncol* 23(23), 5314
 (2005): Margolin K+, *Cancer* 104(5), 1045
 (2004): Raymond E+, *J Clin Oncol* 22(12), 2336
Chest pain (16%)
Chills (8%)
Cough (26%)
 (2006): Duran I+, *Eur J Cancer* 42(12), 1875
Depression (4%)
 (2005): Chan S+, *J Clin Oncol* 23(23), 5314 (10%)
Fever (24%)
Headache (15%)
Hypersensitivity (9%)
 (2006): Duran I+, *Eur J Cancer* 42(12), 1875
Hypertension (7%)
Infections (20%)
Insomnia (12%)
Myalgia/Myositis/Myopathy/Myotoxicity (8%)
Pain (28%)
Somnolence
 (2005): Chan S+, *J Clin Oncol* 23(23), 5314 (6%)

Thrombophlebitis (1%)
Upper respiratory infection (7%)

TENECTEPLASE

Trade name: TNKase (Genentech)
Indications: Acute myocardial infarction
Category: Fibrinolytic
Half-life: 90–130 minutes
Clinically important, potentially hazardous interactions with: bivalirudin

Reactions

Skin
Angioedema (<1%)
Hematomas (local) (12%)
Livedo reticularis (<1%)
Purple glove syndrome (<1%)
Purpura
Rash (sic) (<1%)
Urticaria (<1%)

Other
Anaphylactoid reactions/Anaphylaxis (<1%)
Gangrene (<1%)
Rhabdomyolysis (<1%)

TENIPOSIDE

Synonyms: VM-26; PTG; EPT
Trade name: Vumon (Bristol-Myers Squibb)
Indications: Acute lymphocytic leukemia, Non-Hodgkin's lymphoma, Small cell lung cancer
Category: Antineoplastic; Topoisomerase 2 inhibitor
Half-life: 45 minutes
Clinically important, potentially hazardous interactions with: phenobarbital, phenytoin

Reactions

Skin
Facial edema
(1988): Nolte H+, *Am J Pediatr Hematol Oncol* 10(4), 308
Rash (sic)
(1986): de Vries EG+, *Cancer Treat Rep* 70(5), 595
Urticaria
(1988): Nolte H+, *Am J Pediatr Hematol Oncol* 10(4), 308

Mucosal/ENT
Mucositis
(1991): Schwartsmann G+, *Eur J Cancer* 27(12), 1637
Stomatitis (3%)

Hair
Hair – alopecia (31%)
(1992): Smit EF+, *Semin Oncol* 19(2 Suppl 6), 35
(1992): Smit EF+, *Semin Oncol* 19(2 Suppl 6), 40
(1992): Tummarello D+, *Eur J Cancer* 28A(6–7), 1081
(1991): Schwartsmann G+, *Eur J Cancer* 27(12), 1637
(1990): Pfeiffer P+, *Gynecol Oncol* 37(2), 230 (75%)
(1986): Bork E+, *J Clin Oncol* 4(4), 524

Eyes
Ocular hemorrhage
(1982): Razon-Veronesi S, *Tumori* 68(3), 253

Other
Allergic reactions (5–15%)
(1992): Wysocki M+, *Wiad Lek* 45(3–4), 91
(1985): Hayes FA+, *Cancer Treat Rep* 69(4), 439
Anaphylactoid reactions/Anaphylaxis
(1989): Siddall SJ+, *Lancet* 1(8634), 394
(1984): Koster B+, *Klin Padiatr* 196(3), 178 (2 cases)
Cardiac failure
(1982): Razon-Veronesi S, *Tumori* 68(3), 253
Death
(1995): Postmus PE+, *J Clin Oncol* 13(3), 660
(1992): Smit EF+, *Semin Oncol* 19(2 Suppl 6), 35
(1988): Cerny T+, *Eur J Cancer Clin Oncol* 24(11), 1791
Headache
Hepatotoxicity (2%)
Hypersensitivity (2–11%)
(1991): Kellie SJ+, *Cancer* 67(4), 1070
(1989): Carstensen H+, *Lancet* 2(8653), 55
(1988): Nolte H+, *Am J Pediatr Hematol Oncol* 10(4), 308
(1986): O'Dwyer PJ+, *J Clin Oncol* 4(8), 1262
Hypertension
(1987): Shimizu H+, *Am J Pediatr Hematol Oncol* 9(3), 239
(1982): Razon-Veronesi S, *Tumori* 68(3), 253
Hypotension
(1991): McLeod HL+, *Cancer Chemother Pharmacol* 29(2), 150
(1988): Nolte H+, *Am J Pediatr Hematol Oncol* 10(4), 308
Injection-site phlebitis
Nephrotoxicity (2%)
(1981): Habibi B+, *Lancet* 1(8235), 1423

TENOFOVIR

Synonyms: PMPA; TDF
Trade name: Viread (Gilead)
Indications: Management of HIV Infections in combination with at least two other antiretroviral agents
Category: Antiretroviral; Nucleotide analog reverse transcriptase inhibitor
Half-life: 12.0–14.4 hours
Clinically important, potentially hazardous interactions with: acyclovir, cidofovir, didanosine, valganciclovir

Reactions

Skin
Lichenoid eruption
(2004): Woolley IJ+, *AIDS* 18(13), 1857
Purpura
Rash (sic)

Other
Abdominal pain
(2002): Fung HB+, *Clin Ther* 24(10), 1515
Asthenia
(2002): Fung HB+, *Clin Ther* 24(10), 1515
Chills
Headache
(2002): Fung HB+, *Clin Ther* 24(10), 1515
Hypersensitivity
(2007): Lockhart SM+, *AIDS* 21(10), 1370
Nephrotoxicity
(2007): Gitman MD+, *Expert Opin Drug Saf* 6(2), 155

(2007): Gupta Samir K, *AIDS Read* 17(2), 102
(2007): Sax PE+, *AIDS Read* 17(2), 90, 99
(2006): Cirino CM+, *AIDS* 20(12), 1671
(2006): de la Prada F+, *Nefrologia* 26(5), 626
(2006): Gatanaga H+, *AIDS Res Hum Retroviruses* 22(8), 744
(2006): Izzedine H+, *J Infect Dis* 194(11), 1481
(2006): Lanzafame M+, *Clin Infect Dis* 42(11), 1656
(2006): Mathew G+, *J Gen Intern Med* 21(11), C3
(2006): Scott JD+, *HIV Clin Trials* 7(2), 55
(2006): Valle R+, *Adv Chronic Kidney Dis* 13(3), 314
(2005): Antoniou T+, *HIV Med* 6(4), 284 (4%)
(2005): Fine DM, *AIDS Read* 15(7), 362
(2005): Izzedine H+, *Am J Kidney Dis* 45(5), 804
(2005): Padilla S+, *AIDS Patient Care STDS* 19(7), 421 (%)
(2004): Barrios A+, *AIDS* 18(6), 960
(2004): Hansen AB+, *Scand J Infect Dis* 36(5), 389
(2004): James CW+, *Pharmacotherapy* 24(3), 415
(2004): Rifkin BS+, *Am J Med* 117(4), 282
(2003): Perazella MA, *Am J Med Sci* 325(6), 349
(2002): Coca S+, *Am J Med Sci* 324(6), 342
(2002): Verhelst D+, *Am J Kidney Dis* 40(6), 1331
Neurotoxicity (3%)
  (2004): *Prescrire Int* 13(73), 180 (3%)
Pain (fingers or toes)
Paresthesias
Rhabdomyolysis
  (2003): Callens S+, *J Infect* 47(3), 262
Tremor

TERAZOSIN

Trade names: Heitrin; Hitrin; Hytrin (Abbott); Hytrine; Hytrinex; Itrin; Vicard
Indications: Hypertension, benign prostatic hypertrophy
Category: Adrenergic alpha-receptor antagonist
Half-life: 12 hours
Clinically important, potentially hazardous interactions with: vardenafil

Reactions

Skin
Diaphoresis (>1%)
Edema (1–10%)
Exanthems
  (1998): Hernandez-Cano N+, *Lancet* 352, 202 (generalized)
  (1998): Rosen R (following PUVA) (from Internet) (observation)
Facial edema (>1%)
Lichenoid eruption
  (2008): Koh MJ+, *Br J Dermatol* 158(2), 426
  (1993): Shelley WB+, *Cutis* 52, 88 (observation)
Peripheral edema (5.5%)
Phototoxicity
  (1993): Shelley WB+, *Cutis* 52, 259 (observation)
Pruritus (>1%)
  (1998): Hernandez-Cano N+, *Lancet* 352, 202
Rash (sic) (>1%)

Mucosal/ENT
Tinnitus
Xerostomia (1–10%)

Other
Anaphylactoid reactions/Anaphylaxis
Headache
Myalgia/Myositis/Myopathy/Myotoxicity (>1%)
Paresthesias (2.9%)

TERBINAFINE

Trade name: Lamisil (Novartis)
Indications: Fungal infections of the skin and nails
Category: Antimycobacterial
Half-life: 22–26 hours
Clinically important, potentially hazardous interactions with: carbamazepine

Reactions

Skin
Acute generalized exanthematous pustulosis (AGEP)
  (2006): Bajaj V+, *Acta Derm Venereol* 86(5), 448
  (2005): Beltraminelli HS+, *Br J Dermatol* 152(4), 780
  (2005): Greco M+, *Eur J Dermatol* 15(2), 116
  (2003): Lombardo M+, *J Am Acad Dermatol* 49(1), 158
  (2003): Saissi EH+, *Ann Dermatol Venereol* 130(6-7), 612
  (2003): Taberner R+, *Eur J Dermatol* 13(3), 313
  (2001): Rogalski C+, *Hautarzt* 52(5), 444
  (2000): Hall AP+, *Australas J Dermatol* 41, 42
  (1998): Condon CA+, *Br J Dermatol* 138, 709
  (1997): Kempinaire A+, *J Am Acad Dermatol* 37, 653
  (1996): Dupin N+, *Arch Dermatol* 132, 1253 (2 cases)
Allergic reactions (sic) (1–10%)
  (1989): Savin R, *Clin Exp Dermatol* 14, 116
Angioedema
  (1997): Hall M+, *Arch Dermatol* 133, 1213
Baboon syndrome
  (2001): Weiss JM+, *Hautarzt* 52(12), 1104
Bullous pemphigoid
  (2003): Aksakal BA+, *Ann Pharmacother* 37(11), 1625
Dermatitis (1–10%)
Desquamation
  (1995): Wachs F+, *Arch Dermatol* 131, 960 (passim)
Eczema (<1%)
  (1997): Hall M+, *Arch Dermatol* 133, 1213 (0.2%)
  (1990): Villars V+, *J Dermatol Treat* 1, 33
Erythema multiforme
  (1998): Gupta AK+, *Br J Dermatol* 138, 529 (5 patients)
  (1997): Hall M+, *Arch Dermatol* 133, 1213
  (1995): Todd P+, *Clin Exp Dermatol* 20, 247
  (1995): Tramaloni S+, *Therapie* (French) 50, 594
  (1994): Carstens J+, *Acta Derm Venereol* (Stockh) 74, 391
  (1994): McGregor JM+, *Br J Dermatol* 131, 587
  (1994): Rzany B+, *J Am Acad Dermatol* 30, 509
Erythroderma
  (1998): Gupta AK+, *Br J Dermatol* 138, 529
  (1996): Mitchell D, Charleston, SC (from Internet) (observation)
  (1990): Villars V+, *J Dermatol Treat* 1, 33
Exanthems
  (2001): Weiss JM+, *Hautarzt* 52(12), 1104
  (1999): Valentine MC, Everett, WA (from Internet) (observation)
  (1997): Sidhu JS, Malaysia (from Internet) (observation)
  (1995): Hofmann H+, *Arch Dermatol* 131, 919
  (1995): Wachs F+, *Arch Dermatol* 131, 960 (passim)
  (1990): Villars V+, *J Dermatol Treat* 1, 33
Fixed eruption
  (2006): Nakano N+, *J Dermatol* 33(11), 753
  (2001): Weiss JM+, *Hautarzt* 52(12), 1104
  (1995): Munn SE+, *Br J Dermatol* 133, 815
Hemorrhage
  (2006): Tan C+, *Clin Exp Dermatol* 31(1), 153
Lichenoid eruption
  (2004): Teraki Y+, *Dermatology* 208(1), 81
  (2002): McCarty JR, Fort Worth, TX (from Internet) (3 observations)

Lupus erythematosus
  (2008): Hivnor CM+, *Cutis* 81(2), 156
  (2007): de Langen-Wouterse JJ+, *Ned Tijdschr Geneeskd*
    151(6), 367
  (2006): Amitay-Layish I+, *Harefuah* 145(7), 480
  (2006): Cetkovska P+, *Int J Dermatol* 45(3), 320
  (2006): Farhi D+, *Dermatology* 212(1), 59
  (2006): Moller M+, *Ugeskr Laeger* 168(50), 4427
  (2006): Pallotta P+, *Rheumatology* (Oxford) 45(1), 116
  (2006): Terrab Z+, *Ann Dermatol Venereol* 133(5 Pt 1), 463
  (2005): Zabawski E, Crawfordsville, IN (from Internet)
    (observation)
  (2004): Matthes T+, *Hautarzt* 55(7), 653
  (2004): McKay DA+, *Acta Derm Venereol* 84, 472
  (2004): McKellar G+, *Rheumatology* (Oxford) 43(2), 249
  (2003): Hill VA+, *Br J Dermatol* 148, 1056 (subacute)
  (2001): Bonsmann G+, *J Am Acad Dermatol* 44, 925 (subacute
    cutaneous) (4 cases)
  (2001): Callen JP, *Arch Dermatol* 137, 1196
  (2000): Callen JP, *Skin & Allergy News* March, 23 (subacute)
  (2000): Gruchalla RS, *Lancet* 356, 1505
  (2000): Reed BR, Denver, CO (personal communication) (from a
    meeting presented by Callen JP, Louisville, KY) (4 cases)
  (1999): *Ann Dermatol Venereol* (French) 126, 463
  (1999): Phillips R+, *Dermatol Online J* 5(2), 9
  (1999): Poster Exhibit #239, AAD Meeting, March 1999
    (reported by ED and WB Shelley) (3 patients)
  (1998): Brooke R+, *Br J Dermatol* 139, 1132
  (1998): Holmes S+, *Br J Dermatol* 139, 1133
  (1998): Murphy M+, *Br J Dermatol* 138, 708
  (1997): Crowson AN+, *Hum Pathol* 28, 67 (subacute cutaneous)
Peripheral edema
  (1997): Hall M+, *Arch Dermatol* 133, 1213
Photosensitivity
  (1998): Litt JZ, Beachwood, OH (personal case) (observation)
  (1997): Sidhu JS, Malaysia (from Internet) (observation)
Pigmentation
  (2005): Breuer K+, *Hautarzt* 56(11), 1056 (Face)
Pityriasis rosea
  (1998): Gupta AK+, *Br J Dermatol* 138, 529
Pruritus (<2.8%)
  (2005): Gupta AK+, *J Drugs Dermatol* 4(3), 302
  (2001): Chambers WM+, *Eur J Gastroenterol Hepatol* 13, 1115
  (1998): Litt JZ, Beachwood, OH (personal case) (observation)
  (1997): Hall M+, *Arch Dermatol* 133, 1213 (0.3%)
  (1995): Wachs F+, *Arch Dermatol* 131, 960 (passim)
  (1990): Villars V+, *J Dermatol Treat* 1, 33
Psoriasis
  (2007): Kim BS+, *J Korean Med Sci* 22(1), 167
  (2003): Szepietowski JC, *Acta Dermatovenerol Croat* 11(1), 17
  (2000): Le Guyadec T+, *Ann Dermatol Venereol* (French)
    127, 279
  (1999): Pauluzzi P+, *Acta Derm Venereol* 79(5), 389 (inverse)
  (1998): Gupta AK+, *Br J Dermatol* 138, 529 (2 patients)
  (1998): Papa CA+, *J Am Acad Dermatol* 39, 115
  (1998): Wilson NJ+, *Br J Dermatol* 139, 168
  (1997): Gupta AK+, *J Am Acad Dermatol* 36, 858
  (1995): Gupta AK+, unpublished findings
  (1995): Wachs F+, *Arch Dermatol* 131, 960 (erythema annulare
    centrifugum-like [sic])
Pustules
  (1999): Bennett ML+, *Int J Dermatol* 38, 596
Rash (sic) (5.6%)
  (2006): Danielsen AG+, *Ugeskr Laeger* 168(44), 3825
  (2005): Gupta AK+, *J Drugs Dermatol* 4(3), 302
  (1995): Haroon TS+, *Br J Dermatol* 135, 86
Side effects (sic) (2.7%)
  (1990): Villars V+, *J Dermatol Treat* 1, 33
Stevens–Johnson syndrome

  (2006): Terrab Z+, *Ann Dermatol Venereol* 133(5 Pt 1), 463
  (1999): Rosen R (from Internet) (observation)
  (1994): Rzany B+, *J Am Acad Dermatol* 30, 509
Toxic epidermal necrolysis
  (1996): White SI+, *Br J Dermatol* 134, 188
  (1994): Carstens J+, *Acta Derm Venereol* (Stockh) 74, 391
  (1993): Beutler M+, *BMJ* 307, 26
Toxicoderma
  (1997): Hall M+, *Arch Dermatol* 133, 1213
Urticaria (<1.1%)
  (2005): Ginsburg BC, Birmingham, AL (from Internet)
    (observation)
  (2005): Gupta AK+, *J Drugs Dermatol* 4(3), 302
  (1998): Gupta AK+, *Br J Dermatol* 138, 529
  (1998): Rademaker M+, *New Zealand Adverse Drug Reactions
    Committee*, April, 1998 (from Internet)
  (1997): Billon S, *The Schoch Letter* 47, 32 (observation)
  (1997): Hall M+, *Arch Dermatol* 133, 1213 (0.3%)
  (1995): Wachs F+, *Arch Dermatol* 131, 960 (passim)
  (1990): Savin RC, *J Am Acad Dermatol* 23, 807
  (1990): Villars V+, *J Dermatol Treat* 1, 33
Xanthoderma
  (2007): Haught JM+, *J Am Acad Dermatol* 57(6), 1051

Mucosal/ENT

Ageusia
  (2005): Doty RL+, *Laryngoscope* 115(11), 2035
  (2003): Gregg LJ, Tulsa, OK (from Internet) (observation)
  (2003): Wood WH, San Jose, CA (from Internet) (observation)
  (2000): Schmutz JL+, *Ann Dermatol Venereol* (French) 127, 341
    (persistent)
  (1999): Private Patient Query (from Internet)
  (1999): Villota Hoyos R+, *Aten Primaria* (Spanish) 23, 102
  (1998): Bong JL+, *Br J Dermatol* 139, 747
  (1997): Hall M+, *Arch Dermatol* 133, 1213 (0.3%)
  (1996): Stricker BH+, *Br J Clin Pharmacol* 42(3), 313
  (1995): Haroon TS+, *Br J Dermatol* 135, 86
  (1995): Martinez-Yelamos S+, *Med Clin* (Barc) (Spanish) 105, 276
  (1994): Cribier B+, *Ann Dermatol Venereol* (French) 121, 15
  (1993): Dekker PJ, *Ned Tijdschr Geneeskd* 137(12), 616
  (1993): Stricker BHC, *Ned Tijdschr Geneeskd* 137, 617
  (1993): van Damme PA, *Ned Tijdschr Geneeskd* 137(12), 617
  (1992): Back D, *Lancet* 340, 252
  (1992): Juhlin L, *Lancet* 339, 1483
  (1992): Ottervanger JP+, *Lancet* 340, 728
  (1992): Stricker BH+, *Ned Tijdschr Geneeskd* 136(49), 2438 (7
    cases)
Anosmia
  (1993): Beutler M+, *BMJ* 307, 26
Aphthous stomatitis
  (1998): Litt JZ, Beachwood, OH (personal case) (observation)
Dysgeusia (<2.8%) (metallic taste)
  (2005): Danby FW, Manchester, NH (from Internet)
    (observation)
  (2005): Ginsburg BC, Birmingham, AL (from Internet)
    (observation)
  (2005): Gupta AK+, *J Drugs Dermatol* 4(3), 302
  (2001): Gupta AK+, *Dermatology* 202(3), 235
  (2001): Lemont H+, *J Am Podiatr Med Assoc* 91(10), 540
  (2000): Duxbury AJ+, *Br Dent J* 188, 295 (persistent)
  (2000): Marmelzat J, Los Angeles, CA (from Internet)
    (observation)
  (1999): Marmelzat J, Los Angeles, CA (lasted for 6 months)
    (from Internet) (observation)
  (1997): Danby FW, Kingston, Ontario (from Internet)
    (observation)
  (1997): Hall M+, *Arch Dermatol* 133, 1213 (0.4%)
  (1997): Marmelzat J, Los Angeles, CA (from Internet)
    (observation)
  (1997): Sidhu JS, Malaysia (from Internet) (observation)

(1993): Beutler M+, *BMJ* 307, 26
(1992): Ottervanger JP+, *Lancet* 340, 728
Gingivitis
(1998): Gupta AK+, *J Am Acad Dermatol* 38, 765
Hypogeusia
(1992): Ottervanger JP+, *Lancet* 340, 728
Hyposmia
(1999): Villota Hoyos R+, *Aten Primaria* (Spanish) 23, 102
Parosmia
(1997): Hall M+, *Arch Dermatol* 133, 1213 (0.02%)
Sialadenitis
(2004): Abecassis S+, *J Am Acad Dermatol* 51(5), 827
Sinusitis
(2006): Tavakkol A+, *Am J Geriatr Pharmacother* 4(1), 1 (4%)
Stomatitis
(1998): Gupta AK+, *J Am Acad Dermatol* 38, 765
Tongue pigmentation
(1992): Ottervanger JP+, *Lancet* 340, 728

Hair
Hair – alopecia (1–10%)
(2001): Richert B+, *Br J Dermatol* 145(5), 842
Hair – alopecia areata
(1990): Del Palacio Hernanz A+, *Clin Exp Dermatol* 15, 210

Nails
Nails – onychocryptosis
(2000): Weaver TD+, *Cutis* 66, 211
(1995): Arenas R+, *Int J Dermatol* 34, 138

Eyes
Dyschromatopsia (green vision)
(1996): Gupta AK+, *Arch Dermatol* 132, 845

Other
Abdominal pain
(2005): Gupta AK+, *J Drugs Dermatol* 4(3), 302
Anaphylactoid reactions/Anaphylaxis
Asthenia
(2006): Nikkels AF+, *Am J Clin Dermatol* 7(5), 327
Death
(2005): Gupta AK+, *J Drugs Dermatol* 4(3), 302 (rare)
Depression
(2001): Richert B+, *Br J Dermatol* 145(5), 842
DRESS syndrome
(2004): Abecassis S+, *J Am Acad Dermatol* 51(5), 827
Fever
(2006): Nikkels AF+, *Am J Clin Dermatol* 7(5), 327
Headache
Hepatotoxicity
(2007): Kim BS+, *J Korean Med Sci* 22(1), 167
(2007): Perveze Z+, *Liver Transpl* 13(1), 162
(2004): Agca E+, *Ann Pharmacother* 38(6), 1088
(2003): Ajit C+, *Am J Med Sci* 325(5), 292
(2003): Zapata Garrido AJ+, *Ann Hepatol* 2(1), 47
(1998): Gupta AK+, *Clin Exp Dermatol* 23(2), 64
(1997): Shiloah E+, *Harefuah* 133(1-2), 11
(1996): Lazaros GA+, *J Hepatol* 24(6), 753
(1996): Vantaux P+, *Gastroenterol Clin Biol* 20(4), 402
Hypersensitivity
(1998): Gupta AK+, *Australas J Dermatol* 39, 171
(1998): Schlienger RG+, *Epilepsia* 39, S3 (passim)
(1997): Gupta AK+, *J Am Acad Dermatol* 36, 1018
(1996): Gupta AK+, London, Ontario (observation)
(1996): Marmelzat J, Los Angeles, CA (from Internet) (observation)
(1996): Uhleman J, St. Charles, MO (from Internet) (observation)
Rhabdomyolysis
(2006): Gallego Peris A+, *Med Clin* (Barc) 127(20), 799

Serum sickness
(1995): Kruczynski K+, *Can J Clin Pharmacol* 2, 1
Sjøgren's (Sicca) syndrome
(2004): Abecassis S+, *J Am Acad Dermatol* 51(5), 827

TERBUTALINE

Trade names: Ataline; Brethine (aaiPharma); Bricanyl (AstraZeneca); Brothine; Bucaril; Butaline; Convon; Respirol; Vacanyl
Indications: Bronchospasm
Category: Adrenergic beta2-receptor agonist; Tocolytic
Half-life: 11–16 hours
Clinically important, potentially hazardous interactions with: beta-blockers, epinephrine, insulin detemir, propranolol, sympathomimetics

Reactions

Skin
Dermatitis (irritant)
(1988): Eedy DJ+, *Postgrad Med J* 64, 306
Diaphoresis (1–10%)
Exanthems
(1996): Drugge R, Stamford, CT (from Internet) (observation)
Pruritus
(1996): Drugge R, Stamford, CT (from Internet) (observation)
Urticaria
Vasculitis
(1988): Enat R+, *Ann Allergy* 61, 275

Mucosal/ENT
Dysgeusia (1–10%)
Oral ulceration
(1987): High S, *BMJ* 294, 375
Xerostomia (1–10%)

Other
Headache
Rhabdomyolysis
(1989): Blake PG+, *Nephron* 53(1), 76

TERCONAZOLE

Synonym: triaconazole
Trade names: Fungistat; Gyno-Terazol; Terazol (Ortho-McNeil); Tercospor
Indications: Vulvovaginal candidiasis
Category: Antibiotic, triazole
Half-life: N/A

Reactions

Skin
Pruritus (2.3%)
Toxic epidermal necrolysis
(1998): Searles GE+, *J Cutan Med Surg* 3, 85 (from vaginal suppository)

Mucosal/ENT
Vulvovaginal burning (1–10%)

Other
Chills

Fever
   (1994): Hyder SS+, *South Med J* 87(7), 762
Headache

TERFENADINE

Trade names: Alergist; Allerplus; Cyater; Ferdin; Teldane;
Teldanex; Triludan
Category: Histamine H1 receptor antagonist
Half-life: 16–22 hours
**Clinically important, potentially hazardous interactions
with:** amisulpride, aprepitant, astemizole, darunavir, **devil's
claw**, erythromycin, **grapefruit juice**, roxithromycin,
troleandomycin

Note: This drug has been withdrawn

Reactions

Skin
Angioedema (<1%)
   (1986): Stricker BHC+, *BMJ* 293, 536
Atopic dermatitis (exacerbation)
   (1986): Goodfield MJD+, *BMJ* 293, 1103
Diaphoresis
Exanthems
   (1986): Stricker BHC+, *BMJ* 293, 536
Exfoliative dermatitis
   (1986): Stricker BHC+, *BMJ* 293, 536
Fixed eruption
   (1994): Gani F+, *Ann Allergy* 72, 76
Lupus erythematosus
   (2006): Farhi D+, *Dermatology* 212(1), 59
Photosensitivity (<1%)
   (1994): Berger TG+, *Arch Dermatol* 130, 609 (in HIV-infected) (2
      cases)
   (1994): Shelley WB+, *Cutis* 53, 121 (observation)
   (1986): Fenton D+, *BMJ* 293, 823
   (1986): Stricker BHC+, *BMJ* 293, 536
Pruritus
Psoriasis (exacerbation)
   (1990): Navaratnam AE+, *Clin Exp Dermatol* 15, 78
   (1988): Harrison PV+, *Clin Exp Dermatol* 13, 275
Purpura
Rash (sic) (<1%)
Side effects (sic)
   (1995): McClintock AD+, *N Z Med J* 108, 208
Urticaria
   (1986): Stricker BHC+, *BMJ* 293, 536

Mucosal/ENT
Oral mucosal eruption
   (1990): McTavish D+, *Drugs* 39, 552
Stomatitis
Xerostomia (1–10%)
   (1990): McTavish D+, *Drugs* 39, 552

Hair
Hair – alopecia
   (1993): Shelley WB+, *Cutis* 52, 81 (observation)
   (1992): Frazier CA, *N C Med J* 53, 390
   (1985): Jones SK+, *BMJ* 291, 940

Other
Anaphylactoid reactions/Anaphylaxis
Gynecomastia
Myalgia/Myositis/Myopathy/Myotoxicity (<1%)

Paresthesias (<1%)
Pseudolymphoma
   (1995): Magro CM+, *J Am Acad Dermatol* 32, 419

TERIPARATIDE

Trade name: Forteo (Lilly)
Indications: Postmenopausal osteoporosis
Category: Parathyroid hormone analog
Half-life: 1 hour
**Clinically important, potentially hazardous interactions
with:** digoxin

Reactions

Skin
Allergic reactions (sic)
Diaphoresis
Rash (sic)

Mucosal/ENT
Dysgeusia (<2%)
Rhinitis

Other
Asthenia
Cough
Depression
Headache
   (2005): *Prescrire Int* 14(75), 5
   (2004): Brixen KT+, *Basic Clin Pharmacol Toxicol* 94(6), 260
   (2004): Cappuzzo KA+, *Ann Pharmacother* 38(2), 294
Injection-site edema
Injection-site erythema
Injection-site pain (<2%)
Pain
Paresthesias (<2%)
Vertigo
   (2004): Brixen KT+, *Basic Clin Pharmacol Toxicol* 94(6), 260
   (2004): Cappuzzo KA+, *Ann Pharmacother* 38(2), 294

TESTOLACTONE

Synonym: delta-1-testolactone
Trade name: Teslac (Bristol-Myers Squibb)
Indications: Advanced disseminated breast carcinoma
Category: Androgen; Antineoplastic; Aromatase inhibitor
Half-life: N/A
**Clinically important, potentially hazardous interactions
with:** anticoagulants

Reactions

Skin
Angioedema
Exanthems
Peripheral edema

Mucosal/ENT
Glossitis

Hair
Hair – alopecia

Other
Abdominal pain
(1993): Feuillan PP+, *J Clin Endocrinol Metab* 77(3), 647
Asthenia
Headache
(1993): Feuillan PP+, *J Clin Endocrinol Metab* 77(3), 647
Hypertension
Paresthesias

TESTOSTERONE

Trade names: Andro-L.A; Androderm (Watson); AndroGel (Unimed); Andronaq; Delatest; Delatestryl (Savient); depAndro; Duratest; Malogen; Testandro; Testex; Testim (Auxilium); Testoderm (Ortho-McNeil); Testopel
Indications: Androgen replacement, hypogonadism, postpartum breast pain
Category: Androgen
Half-life: 10–100 minutes
Clinically important, potentially hazardous interactions with: anisindione, anticoagulants, cyclosporine, dicumarol, warfarin

Reactions

Skin
Acne (>10%)
(2006): Kalantaridou SN+, *Semin Reprod Med* 24(2), 106
(1998): Kwon PS+, *Arch Dermatol* 134, 376
(1995): Tabata N+, *J Am Acad Dermatol* 33, 676 (infantile)
(1992): Fyrand O+, *Acta Derm Venereol* 72, 148
(1990): Fuchs E+, *J Am Acad Dermatol* 23, 125
(1989): Fyrand O+, *Tidsskr Nor Laegeforen* (Norwegian) 109, 239
(1989): Hartmann AA+, *Monatsschr Kinderheilkd* (German) 137, 466
(1989): Heydenreich G, *Arch Dermatol* 125, 571 (fulminans)
(1989): Scott MJ+, *Cutis* 44, 30
(1989): von Muhlendahl KE+, *Dtsch Med Wochenschr* (German) 114, 712
(1988): Traupe H+, *Arch Dermatol* 124, 414 (fulminans)
(1987): Kiraly CL+, *Am J Dermatopathol* 9, 515
(1984): Lamb DR, *Am J Sports Med* 12, 31
Carcinoma
(2006): Dizon DS+, *Gynecol Obstet Invest* 62(4), 226 (ovarian)
Dermatitis (4%)
(1998): Buckley DA+, *Contact Dermatitis* 39, 91 (from patch)
(1989): Holdiness MR, *Contact Dermatitis* 20, 3 (from patch)
Edema (1–10%)
Exanthems
(2001): McGriff NJ+, *Pharmacotherapy* 21(11), 1425
Folliculitis
(1998): Kwon PS+, *Arch Dermatol* 134, 376
Furunculosis
(1989): Scott MJ+, *Cutis* 44, 30
Lichenoid eruption
(1989): Aihara M+, *J Dermatol* (Tokio) 16, 330
Lupus erythematosus
Peripheral edema
Pruritus
(2001): McGriff NJ+, *Pharmacotherapy* 21(11), 1425
Psoriasis
(1990): O'Driscoll JB+, *Clin Exp Dermatol* 15, 68
Rash (sic) (2%)
Seborrhea (<1%)
Seborrheic dermatitis
(1989): Scott MJ+, *Cutis* 44, 30
Striae
(1989): Scott MJ+, *Cutis* 44, 30
Urticaria

Mucosal/ENT
Stomatitis

Hair
Hair – alopecia (<1%)
(1989): Scott MJ+, *Cutis* 44, 30
Hair – hirsutism (1–10%)
(2006): Kalantaridou SN+, *Semin Reprod Med* 24(2), 106
(2004): Hernandez-Nunez A+, *J Eur Acad Dermatol Venereol* 18(2), 208 (oral, 2 cases)
(1994): Castillo-Ceballos A+, *Med Clin* (Barc) (Spanish) 102, 78
(1991): Bates GW+, *Clin Obstet Gynecol* 34, 848
(1991): No Author, *Obstet Gynecol* 78, 474
(1991): Parker LU+, *Cleve Clin J Med* 58, 43
(1991): Urman B+, *Obstet Gynecol* 77, 595
(1989): Scott MJ+, *Cutis* 44, 30

Eyes
Intraocular pressure increased
(2006): Khurana RN+, *Am J Ophthalmol* 142(3), 494 (with estogen)

Cardiovascular
Atherosclerosis
(2007): Hak AE+, *Maturitas* 56(2), 153

Other
Anaphylactoid reactions/Anaphylaxis (<1%)
Application-site bullae (12%)
Application-site burning (3%)
Application-site erythema (7%)
Application-site induration (3%)
Application-site pruritus (37%)
Application-site vesicles (6%)
Gynecomastia (<1%)
Headache
Hypersensitivity (<1%)
Injection-site pain
(2002): Amory JK+, *J Androl* 23(1), 84
Paresthesias (<1%)

TETRABENAZINE

Trade names: Nitoman (Lifehealth LTD); Xenazine
Indications: Hyperkinetic movement disorders: Huntington's chorea, hemiballismus, senile chorea, Tourette syndrome, and tardive dyskinesia
Category: Central Monoamine-Depleting Agent
Clinically important, potentially hazardous interactions with: antipsychotics, cyclic antidepressants, levodopa, MAO inhibitors, reserpine

Reactions

Mucosal/ENT
Dysphagia (1%)
Sialorrhea
(1982): Jankovic J, *Ann Neurol* 11(1), 41

Eyes
Vision blurred (1%)

Other
Anxiety (10%)
  (1997): Jankovic J+, *Neurology* 48(2), 358 (10.3%)
  (1988): Jankovic J+, *Neurology* 38(3), 391
  (1982): Jankovic J, *Ann Neurol* 11(1), 41
Asthenia
Confusion (2%)
Depression (15%)
  (2007): Kenney C+, *Mov Disord* 22(2), 193 (7.6%)
  (2006): Kenney C+, *Clin Neuropharmacol* 29(5), 259 (15.1%)
  (1999): Schreiber W+, *J Neurol Neurosurg Psychiatry* 67(4), 550
  (1997): Jankovic J+, *Neurology* 48(2), 358 (15%)
  (1988): Jankovic J+, *Neurology* 38(3), 391
  (1984): Jankovic J+, *Neurology* 34(5), 688
Disorientation
Headache (1%)
Hypotension
  (1982): Jankovic J, *Ann Neurol* 11(1), 41
Insomnia (11%)
  (1997): Jankovic J+, *Neurology* 48(2), 358 (11%)
  (1988): Jankovic J+, *Neurology* 38(3), 391
  (1982): Jankovic J, *Ann Neurol* 11(1), 41
Memory Loss (2%)
Paranoia (1%)
Paresthesias (1%)
Restlessness
  (1982): Jankovic J, *Ann Neurol* 11(1), 41
Somnolence (37%)
  (2007): Kenney C+, *Mov Disord* 22(2), 193 (25%)
  (2006): Kenney C+, *Clin Neuropharmacol* 29(5), 259 (27.4%)
  (1997): Jankovic J+, *Neurology* 48(2), 358 (36.5%)
  (1984): Jankovic J+, *Neurology* 34(5), 688
  (1982): Jankovic J, *Ann Neurol* 11(1), 41
Suicidal ideation
  (2006): *Neurology* 66(3), 366
Tremor (3%)
Vertigo (1%)

TETRACYCLINE

Trade names: Apo-Tetra; Economycin; Florocycline; Helidac (Prometheus); Steclin; Sumycin (Par); Teflin; Teline; Tetramig; Topicycline (Topical); Zorbenal-G
Indications: Various infections caused by susceptible organisms
Category: Antibiotic, tetracycline
Half-life: 6–11 hours
Clinically important, potentially hazardous interactions with: acitretin, aluminum hydroxide, amoxicillin, ampicillin, antacids, bacampicillin, betamethasone, bismuth, **bromelain**, calcium, carbenicillin, cholestyramine, cloxacillin, corticosteroids, **dairy products**, dicloxacillin, didanosine, digoxin, **food**, iron, isotretinoin, methicillin, methotrexate, methoxyflurane, mezlocillin, nafcillin, oxacillin, penicillins, piperacillin, retinoids, rocuronium, sucralfate, ticarcillin, vitamin A, zinc

Reactions

Skin
Acne
Allergic granulomatous angiitis (Churg–Strauss syndrome)
Angioedema
  (1997): Shapiro LE+, *Arch Dermatol* 133, 1224
Bullous dermatitis
Dermatitis
Diaphoresis
Eczema
Erythema multiforme
  (1988): Lewis-Jones MS+, *Clin Exp Dermatol* 13, 245
  (1987): Curley RK+, *Clin Exp Dermatol* 12, 124
  (1987): Leroy D+, *Photodermatol* 4, 52 (photodistributed)
  (1987): Shoji A+, *Arch Dermatol* 123, 18
  (1983): Albengres E+, *Therapie* (French) 38, 577
Exanthems
  (1993): Chaffins ML+, *J Am Acad Dermatol* 28, 988
Exfoliative dermatitis (<1%)
Fixed eruption (15%)
  (2005): Monroe M+, *Dermatol Nurs* 17(2), 146
  (2003): Marmelzat J, Los Angeles, CA (from Internet) (observation)
  (1998): Leal G, Fortaleza, Brazil (pulsating) (from Internet) (observation)
  (1998): Mahboob A+, *Int J Dermatol* 37, 833
  (1994): Bielan B, *Dermatol Nurs* 6, 198
  (1991): Thankappen TP+, *Int J Dermatol* 30, 867 (15.9%)
  (1990): Gaffoor PMA+, *Cutis* 45, 242
  (1988): Chan HL+, *Ann Acad Med Singapore* 17, 514
  (1986): Sehgal VH+, *Genitourin Med* 62, 56 (genital)
  (1985): Chan HL+, *J Am Acad Dermatol* 13, 302
  (1985): Dodds PR+, *J Urol* 133, 1044 (balanitis)
  (1985): Kauppinen K+, *Br J Dermatol* 112, 575
  (1985): Pandhi RK+, *Australas J Dermatol* 26, 88
  (1984): Chan HL, *Int J Dermatol* 23, 607
  (1984): Kanwar AJ+, *J Dermatol* 11, 383
  (1984): Pandhi RK+, *Sex Transm Dis* 11, 164 (male genitalia)
  (1982): Kanwar AJ+, *Dermatologica* 164, 115
  (1982): Murray VK+, *J Periodontol* 53(4), 267
  (1981): Bhargava NC+, *Int J Dermatol* 20, 435
  (1981): Fiumara NJ+, *Sex Transm Dis* 8, 23 (penile)
  (1981): Fiumara NJ+, *Sex Transm Dis* 8, 258
Jarisch–Herxheimer reaction
  (1992): Gebrehiwot T+, *Ethiop Med J* 30(3), 175
  (1985): Teklu B+, *Trans R Soc Trop Med Hyg* 79(1), 74
  (1983): Perine PL+, *Am J Trop Med Hyg* 32(5), 1096
Lichenoid eruption
Lupus erythematosus
  (1999): Sturkenboom MCJM+, *Arch Int Med* 159, 493
  (1985): Stratton MA, *Clin Pharm* 4, 657
  (1980): Condemi JJ, *Geriatrics* 35(3), 81
Lymphoepithelioma
Photosensitivity (1–10%)
  (1997): Shapiro LE+, *Arch Dermatol* 133, 1224
  (1993): Wainwright NJ+, *Drug Saf* 9, 437
  (1989): Rosen C, *Semin Dermatol* 8, 149
Phototoxicity
  (2002): Sorkin M, Denver, CO (from Internet) (observation)
  (1995): Smith EL+, *Br J Dermatol* isor(ug), 316
  (1980): Stern RS+, *Arch Dermatol* 116, 1269
Pigmentation
  (2006): Adisen E+, *Int J Dermatol* 45(10), 1245
  (2001): Dereure O, *Am J Clin Dermatol* 2(4), 253
  (1983): White SW+, *Arch Dermatol* 119, 1
  (1981): Granstein RD+, *J Am Acad Dermatol* 5, 1 (blue-black)
Pruritus (<1%)
  (1995): Nowakowski J+, *J Am Acad Dermatol* 32, 223
Pruritus ani et vulvae
Psoriasis (exacerbation)
  (1990): Bergner T+, *J Am Acad Dermatol* 23, 770
  (1988): Tsankov N+, *J Am Acad Dermatol* 19, 629
Purpura
Pustules
Rash (sic)
  (1997): Shapiro LE+, *Arch Dermatol* 133, 1224

Stevens–Johnson syndrome
(1997): Shoji T+, J Am Acad Dermatol 37, 337
(1993): Leenutaphong V+, Int J Dermatol 32, 428
(1985): Burge SM+, J Am Acad Dermatol 13, 665
Sunburn (exaggerated)
Toxic epidermal necrolysis
(1993): Leenutaphong V+, Int J Dermatol 32, 428
(1989): Davies MG+, BMJ 298, 1523
(1988): Gimova EK+, Sov Med (Russian) 6, 119
(1987): Curley RK+, Clin Exp Dermatol 12, 124
(1985): Burge SM+, J Am Acad Dermatol 13, 665
(1985): Tatnall FM+, Br J Dermatol 113, 629
(1984): Chan HL, J Am Acad Dermatol 10, 973
Urticaria
(2000): Yap LM+, Australas J Dermatol 41(3), 181
(1997): Shapiro LE+, Arch Dermatol 133, 1224
Vasculitis
Verrucae (flat)

Mucosal/ENT
Cheilitis
Gingivitis
Glossitis
Mucocutaneous syndrome
Mucosal membrane pigmentation
Oral mucosal fixed eruption
(1982): Murray VK+, J Periodontology 53, 267
Oral ulceration
(1996): Nordt SP, Ann Pharmacother 30(5), 547
Tinnitus
(1984): Snavely SR+, Ann Intern Med 101(1), 92
Tongue black
Vaginitis

Hair
Hair – straight
(2004): Rehbein H, Jacksonville, FL (from Internet) (observation)

Nails
Nails – discoloration (<1%)
(1980): Hendricks AA, Arch Dermatol 116, 438 (yellow lunulae)
Nails – photo-onycholysis
(2002): Rudolph RI, Wyomissing, PA (from Internet) (observation)
(1990): Baran R+, Ann Dermatol Venereol 117(5), 367
(1987): Baran R+, J Am Acad Dermatol 17, 1012
(1983): Ibsen HH+, Acta Derm Venereol 63, 555

Eyes
Conjunctival pigmentation
(1981): Brothers DM+, Ophthalmology 88, 1212
Ocular pigmentation
(2006): Lapid-Gortzak R+, Cornea 25(8), 969

Other
Anaphylactoid reactions/Anaphylaxis (<1%)
Candidiasis
Headache
Hypersensitivity (<1%)
(1997): Shapiro LE+, Arch Dermatol 133, 1224
Paresthesias (<1%)
(1996): Sorkin M, The Schoch Letter 45(5), 18 (observation)
(1994): Blanchard L,, The Schoch Letter 44, 6 (observation)
Porphyria cutanea tarda
(1992): Shelley WB+, Advanced Dermatologic Diagnosis WB Saunders, 414 (passim)
Pseudoporphyria
Serum sickness
(1997): Shapiro LE+, Arch Dermatol 133, 1224
Thrombophlebitis (<1%)

THALIDOMIDE

Trade names: Contergan; Distaval; Kevadon; Thalomid (Celgene)
Indications: Graft-versus-host reactions, recalcitrant aphthous stomatitis
Category: Antiemetic; Immunosuppressant; TNF modulator
Half-life: 8.7 hours

Note: Thalidomide is a potent teratogen, an agent that causes congenital malformations and developmental abnormalities if introduced during gestation. Some of these teratogenic side effects of thalidomide include fetal limb growth retardation (arms, legs, hands, feet), ingrown genitalia, absence of lung, partial/total loss of hearing or sight, malformed digestive tract, heart, kidney, and stillborn infant.

Reactions

Skin
Adverse effects (sic)
(2003): Okafor MC, Pharmacotherapy 23(4), 481
Bullous dermatitis (5%)
Burning
(1989): Gutierrez-Rodriguez O+, J Rheumatol 16, 158
Dermatitis
Desquamation
(2006): Olencki T+, Invest New Drugs 24(4), 321 (with interleukin-2)
Diaphoresis
Edema
(2007): Rosenbach M+, Dermatol Ther 20(4), 175 (passim)
(2006): Abgrall JF+, Haematologica 91(8), 1027
(2005): Moschella SL, Skinmed 4(1), 19
(2004): Strupp C+, Eur J Haematol 72(1), 52 (2 cases)
(2003): Hwu W-J, J Drugs Dermatol 2, 53 (with temozolomide)
(2000): Oliver SJ+, Clin Immunol 97(2), 109
(1997): Duran McKinster C, Skin and Allergy News August, 37
(1996): Tseng S+, J Am Acad Dermatol 35, 969 (passim)
(1989): Grinspan D+, J Am Acad Dermatol 20, 1060
(1984): Gutierrez-Rodriguez O, Arthritis Rheum 27, 1118
Erythema
(2005): Moschella SL, Skinmed 4(1), 19
(1989): Gutierrez-Rodriguez O+, J Rheumatol 16, 158
Erythema multiforme
(2003): Hall VC+, J Am Acad Dermatol 48(4), 548 (3 cases) (with dexamethasone)
Erythema nodosum
(2000): Gardener-Merwin JM+, Ann Rheum Dis 53, 828
(1988): Viraben R+, Dermatologica 176, 107
Erythroderma
(1996): Tseng S+, J Am Acad Dermatol 35, 969 (passim)
(1994): Bielsa I+, Dermatology (Basel) 189, 178
Exanthems
(2000): Camisa C+, Arch Dermatol 136, 1442
(1999): Burrow WH, Jackson, MS (from Internet) (observation)
(1991): Williams I+, Lancet 337, 436 (37% in AIDS patients)
Exfoliative dermatitis
(2005): Patt YZ+, Cancer 103(4), 749
(2003): Hall VC+, J Am Acad Dermatol 48(4), 548 (3 cases) (with dexamethasone)
(1996): Tseng S+, J Am Acad Dermatol 35, 969 (passim)
(1988): Salafia A+, Int J Lepr Other Mycobact Dis 56, 625
Exfoliative erythroderma
(2005): Moschella SL, Skinmed 4(1), 19
Facial erythema (1–5%)
(1989): Gutierrez-Rodriguez O+, J Rheumatol 16, 158
Nodular eruption

(2000): Bahl S+, *Skin and Aging*, May, 41

Palmar erythema
(1996): Tseng S+, *J Am Acad Dermatol* 35, 969 (passim)

Peripheral edema
(2000): Camisa C+, *Arch Dermatol* 136, 1442
(2000): Gardener-Merwin JM+, *Ann Rheum Dis* 53, 828

Pruritus
(2007): Rosenbach M+, *Dermatol Ther* 20(4), 175 (passim)
(1996): Tseng S+, *J Am Acad Dermatol* 35, 969 (passim)
(1989): Gutierrez-Rodriguez O+, *J Rheumatol* 16, 158

Psoriasis
(2006): Varma K+, *Br J Dermatol* 154(4), 789
(2003): Dobson CM+, *Br J Dermatol* 149(2), 432

Purpura
(2005): Moschella SL, *Skinmed* 4(1), 19
(1996): Tseng S+, *J Am Acad Dermatol* 35, 969 (passim)

Pustuloderma
(1999): Rua-Figuero I+, *Lupus* 8, 248

Rash (sic) (11–50%)
(2007): Rosenbach M+, *Dermatol Ther* 20(4), 175 (passim)
(2006): Bringhen S+, *Expert Opin Investig Drugs* 15(12), 1565
(2006): Olencki T+, *Invest New Drugs* 24(4), 321 (with interleukin-2)
(2005): Patt YZ+, *Cancer* 103(4), 749 (20%)
(2004): Wang TE+, *World J Gastroenterol* 10(5), 649
(2003): Hwu W-J, *J Drugs Dermatol* 2, 53 (with temozolomide)
(2003): Matthews SJ+, *Clin Ther* 25(2), 342
(2003): Okafor MC, *Pharmacotherapy* 23(4), 481
(2002): Baughman RP+, *Chest* 122(1), 227
(2002): Steins MB+, *Blood* 99(3), 834
(2002): Tosi P+, *Haematologica* 87(4), 408 (11%)
(2001): Rajkumar SV, *Oncology (Huntingt)* 15(7), 867
(2001): Singhal S+, *BioDrugs* 15(3), 163 (30%)
(2000): Gardener-Merwin JM+, *Ann Rheum Dis* 53, 828
(2000): Oliver SJ+, *Clin Immunol* 97(2), 109
(2000): Rajkumar SV, *Oncology (Huntingt)* 14(12), 11
(1997): Haslett P+, *Infect Med* 14, 393
(1997): Jacobson JM+, *New Engl J Med* 336, 1487 (>50%)
(1993): Holm AL+, *Arch Dermatol* 129, 1548 (passim)
(1986): Hamza MH, *Clin Rheumatol* 5, 365

Stevens–Johnson syndrome
(2001): Clark TE+, *Drug Saf* 24(2), 87

Toxic epidermal necrolysis
(2003): Hall VC+, *J Am Acad Dermatol* 48(4), 548 (3 cases) (with dexamethasone)
(2001): Diggle GE, *Int J Clin Pract* 55(9), 627
(2000): Rajkumar SV+, *N Engl J Med* 343(13), 972
(1999): Horowitz SB+, *Pharmacotherapy* 19, 1177

Toxic pustuloderma
(1997): Darvay A+, *Clin Exp Dermatol* 22, 297

Ulcerations
(2001): Schlossberg H+, *Bone Marrow Transplant* 27, 229 (serious)

Urticaria (3%)
(2005): Moschella SL, *Skinmed* 4(1), 19

Vasculitis
(2007): Yildirim ND+, *Jpn J Clin Oncol* 37(9), 704
(1996): Tseng S+, *J Am Acad Dermatol* 35, 969 (passim)

Xerosis
(2007): Rosenbach M+, *Dermatol Ther* 20(4), 175 (passim)
(2002): Bariol C+, *J Gastroenterol Hepatol* 17(2), 135
(2000): Bahl S+, *Skin and Aging* May, 41
(2000): Oliver SJ+, *Clin Immunol* 97(2), 109
(1989): Gutierrez-Rodriguez O+, *J Rheumatol* 16, 158

Mucosal/ENT

Xerostomia
(2002): Bariol C+, *J Gastroenterol Hepatol* 17(2), 135
(2000): Bahl S+, *Skin and Aging* May, 41

(1999): Monastirli A+, *Skin Pharmacol Appl Skin Physiol* 12(6), 305
(1996): Huizinga TW+, *Ann Rheum Dis* 55(11), 833
(1996): Tseng S+, *J Am Acad Dermatol* 35, 969 (passim)
(1994): Gardener-Merwin JM+, *Ann Rheum Dis* 53, 828
(1989): Grinspan D+, *J Am Acad Dermatol* 20, 1060
(1989): Gutierrez-Rodriguez O+, *J Rheumatol* 16, 158

Hair

Hair – alopecia
(1989): Gutierrez-Rodriguez O+, *J Rheumatol* 16, 158

Nails

Nails – brittle
(1996): Tseng S+, *J Am Acad Dermatol* 35, 969 (passim)

Eyes

Corneal abnormalities
(2005): Srinivasan S+, *Cornea* 24(1), 103

Cardiovascular

Ischemia
(2007): Martino M+, *Eur J Haematol* 78(1), 35 (3 cases)

Other

Abdominal pain
(2005): Cuadrado MJ+, *Am J Med* 118(3), 246

Agitation
(2007): Lazzerini M+, *Aliment Pharmacol Ther* 25(4), 419

Asthenia
(2007): Martino M+, *Eur J Haematol* 78(1), 35 (2 cases)
(2006): Bringhen S+, *Expert Opin Investig Drugs* 15(12), 1565
(2006): Chan JK+, *Gynecol Oncol* 103(3), 919 (65%)
(2006): Olencki T+, *Invest New Drugs* 24(4), 321 (with interleukin-2)
(2005): Lin AY+, *Cancer* 103(1), 119 (81%)
(2004): Offidani M+, *Eur J Haematol* 72(6), 403 (20%)
(2004): Strupp C+, *Eur J Haematol* 72(1), 52 (8 cases)

Chills
(2006): Olencki T+, *Invest New Drugs* 24(4), 321 (with interleukin-2)

Death
(2001): Diggle GE, *Int J Clin* 55(9), 627

Fever
(2006): Olencki T+, *Invest New Drugs* 24(4), 321 (with interleukin-2)

Gynecomastia
(2002): Pulik M+, *Am J Hematol* 70(3), 265

Headache
(2007): Rosenbach M+, *Dermatol Ther* 20(4), 175 (passim)

Hepatotoxicity
(2006): Hanje AJ+, *Pharmacotherapy* 26(7), 1018

Hypersensitivity
(2005): Moschella SL, *Skinmed* 4(1), 19
(2002): Kane S+, *J Clin Gastroenterol* 35(2), 149

Hypotension
(2007): Rosenbach M+, *Dermatol Ther* 20(4), 175 (passim)

Infections
(2007): Martino M+, *Eur J Haematol* 78(1), 35 (2 cases)
(2003): Hwu W-J, *J Drugs Dermatol* 2, 53 (with temozolomide)

Mood changes
(2007): Rosenbach M+, *Dermatol Ther* 20(4), 175 (passim)

Neurotoxicity
(2006): Chan JK+, *Gynecol Oncol* 103(3), 919 (71%)
(2006): Durk HA, *Onkologie* 29(12), 582
(2005): Cuadrado MJ+, *Am J Med* 118(3), 246 (27%)
(2005): Fleming FJ+, *Neuromuscul Disord* 15(2), 172 (4 cases)
(2005): Moschella SL, *Skinmed* 4(1), 19
(2005): Tosi P+, *Eur J Haematol* 74(3), 212 (75%)
(2004): Briani C+, *Neurology* 62(12), 2288

(2004): Offidani M+, *Eur J Haematol* 72(6), 403 (39%)
(2004): Strupp C+, *Eur J Haematol* 72(1), 52 (2 cases)
(2004): Wang TE+, *World J Gastroenterol* 10(5), 649
(2003): Foldyna D+, *Vnitr Lek* 49(11), 859 (41%)
(2003): Matthews SJ+, *Clin Ther* 25(2), 342
(2003): Okafor MC, *Pharmacotherapy* 23(4), 481
(2002): Grover JK+, *Ann Oncol* 13(10), 1636
(1992): Awofeso N, *Trop Doct* 22(3), 139
Paresthesias
(2005): Moschella SL, *Skinmed* 4(1), 19
(2005): Tosi P+, *Eur J Haematol* 74(3), 212
(2004): Nguyen YT+, *J Am Acad Dermatol* A(2), 235
(2002): Baughman RP+, *Chest* 122(1), 227
(2000): Bahl S+, *Skin and Aging*, May, 41
(2000): Ordi-Ros J+, *J Rheumatol* 27, 1429
(1999): Duong DJ, *Arch Dermatol* 135, 1079
(1998): Lee JB+, *J Am Acad Dermatol* 39, 835
Seizures
(2005): Moschella SL, *Skinmed* 4(1), 19
Somnolence
(2007): Lazzerini M+, *Aliment Pharmacol Ther* 25(4), 419
(2007): Rosenbach M+, *Dermatol Ther* 20(4), 175 (passim)
(2003): Matthews SJ+, *Clin Ther* 25(2), 342
Thrombosis
(2007): Prince HM+, *Leuk Lymphoma* 48(1), 46 (3%)
(2006): Anscher MS+, *Int J Radiat Oncol Biol Phys* 66(2), 477
(2006): Bennett CL+, *JAMA* 296(21), 2558
(2006): Bringhen S+, *Expert Opin Investig Drugs* 15(12), 1565
(2006): Doss DS, *Clin J Oncol Nurs* 10(4), 514 (with dexamethasone)
(2006): Durk HA, *Onkologie* 29(12), 582
(2006): Harousseau JL, *Future Oncol* 2(5), 577 (with dexamethasone)
(2006): Ikhlaque N+, *Am J Hematol* 81(6), 420
(2006): Miller KC+, *Leuk Lymphoma* 47(11), 2339
(2006): Olencki T+, *Invest New Drugs* 24(4), 321 (with interleukin-2)
Tremor
(2005): Chiruka S+, *Am J Hematol* 78(1), 81
(2005): Tosi P+, *Eur J Haematol* 74(3), 212
(2003): Hwu W-J, *J Drugs Dermatol* 2, 53 (with temozolomide)
(1999): Duong DJ+, *Arch Dermatol* 135(9), 1079
Vertigo
(2007): Lazzerini M+, *Aliment Pharmacol Ther* 25(4), 419
(2007): Rosenbach M+, *Dermatol Ther* 20(4), 175 (passim)
(2006): Durk HA, *Onkologie* 29(12), 582
(2005): Moschella SL, *Skinmed* 4(1), 19
(2005): Tosi P+, *Eur J Haematol* 74(3), 212
(2003): Foldyna D+, *Vnitr Lek* 49(11), 859 (47%)
(2002): Baughman RP+, *Chest* 122(1), 227
(2002): Crouch RB+, *Australas J Dermatol* 43(4), 278

THALLIUM

Indications: For diagnostic use in myocardial perfusion imaging
Category: Radioactive element [Tl]
Half-life: 73.1 hours
Clinically important, potentially hazardous interactions with: None

Reactions

Skin
Acute generalized exanthematous pustulosis (AGEP)
(2004): Aziz Jalali MH+, *J Eur Acad Dermatol Venereol* 18(3), 321
Pruritus

Rash (sic)

Mucosal/ENT
Sialorrhea
(2005): Freudenreich O, *Drugs Today (Barc)* 41(6), 411

Hair
Hair – alopecia
(2007): Ammendola A+, *Neurol Sci* 28(4), 205
(2007): Goel A+, *Natl Med J India* 20(4), 182
(2006): Jha S+, *J Assoc Physicians India* 54, 53
(2004): Saha A+, *Occup Environ Med* 61(7), 640
(1998): Huang J+, *Zhonghua Yi Xue Za Zhi* 78(8), 610
(1995): Herrero F+, *J Toxicol Clin Toxicol* 33(3), 261
(1994): Meggs WJ+, *J Toxicol Clin Toxicol* 32(6), 723
(1994): Tabandeh H+, *Am J Ophthalmol* 117(2), 243
(1993): Feldman J+, *Pediatr Dermatol* 10(1), 29
(1983): Majoos FL+, *S Afr Med J* 64(9), 328

Nails
Nails – dystrophy
(2004): Saha A+, *Occup Environ Med* 61(7), 640
Nails – Mees' lines
(1998): Huang J+, *Zhonghua Yi Xue Za Zhi* 78(8), 610
(1995): Herrero F+, *J Toxicol Clin Toxicol* 33(3), 261

Eyes
Conjunctivitis
Lens opacities
(1994): Tabandeh H+, *Am J Ophthalmol* 117(2), 243
Ophthalmoplegia
(1994): Tabandeh H+, *Am J Ophthalmol* 117(2), 243
Optic neuropathy
(1994): Tabandeh H+, *Am J Ophthalmol* 117(2), 243
Ptosis
(1994): Tabandeh H+, *Am J Ophthalmol* 117(2), 243
Retinopathy
(1997): Schmidt D+, *Int Ophthalmol* 21(3), 143
Vision blurred
Visual hallucinations
(2006): Tsai YT+, *Neurotoxicology* 27(2), 291

Other
Abdominal pain
(2006): Jha S+, *J Assoc Physicians India* 54, 53
(1998): Huang J+, *Zhonghua Yi Xue Za Zhi* 78(8), 610
(1995): Herrero F+, *J Toxicol Clin Toxicol* 33(3), 261
(1983): Majoos FL+, *S Afr Med J* 64(9), 328
Anaphylactoid reactions/Anaphylaxis
Anxiety
(2006): Tsai YT+, *Neurotoxicology* 27(2), 291
Chills
Confusion
(2006): Tsai YT+, *Neurotoxicology* 27(2), 291
Death
(2004): Sharma AN+, *Am J Forensic Med Pathol* 25(2), 156
(1994): Tabandeh H+, *Am J Ophthalmol* 117(2), 243
Delirium
(2006): Jha S+, *J Assoc Physicians India* 54, 53
Depression
(2006): Tsai YT+, *Neurotoxicology* 27(2), 291
Fever
Hypertension
(1994): Meggs WJ+, *J Toxicol Clin Toxicol* 32(6), 723
Hypotension
Paresthesias
(1995): Herrero F+, *J Toxicol Clin Toxicol* 33(3), 261
Tremor

THEOPHYLLINE

(See AMINOPHYLLINE)
Clinically important, potentially hazardous interactions with: arformoterol, **bcg vaccine**, carbimazole, cimetidine, erythromycin, nilutamide

THIABENDAZOLE

Synonym: tiabendazole
Trade name: Triasox
Indications: Various infections caused by susceptible helminths
Category: Antibiotic, imidazole; Antihelmintic
Half-life: 1.2 hours

Reactions

Skin
Angioedema
Dermatitis
  (1994): Mancuso G, *Contact Dermatitis* 31, 207
  (1993): Izu R+, *Contact Dermatitis* 28, 243 (photoaggravated)
Erythema multiforme (<1%)
  (2003): Johnson-Reagan L+, *Allergy* 58(5), 445 (similar eruptions
    in 2 siblings)
  (1988): Humphreys F+, *Br J Dermatol* 118, 855
  (1988): Kardaun SH+, *Br J Dermatol* 118, 545
Exanthems (>5%)
  (1982): Sanchez del Rio J+, *Actas Dermosifiliogr* (Spanish) 73, 125
Fixed eruption (<1%)
  (1982): Sanchez del Rio J+, *Actas Dermosifiliogr* 73(3–4), 125
Jarisch–Herxheimer reaction
Perianal rash
Pruritus (<1%)
Psoriasis (exacerbation)
Rash (sic) (1–10%)
Stevens–Johnson syndrome (1–10%)
  (2003): Johnson-Reagan L+, *Allergy* 58(5), 445 (similar eruptions
    in 2 siblings)
Toxic epidermal necrolysis (<1%)
  (1993): Correia O+, *Dermatology* 186, 32
Urticaria (1–5%)

Mucosal/ENT
Dry mucous membranes
Tinnitus
Xerostomia

Eyes
Dyschromatopsia (<1%)

Other
Anaphylactoid reactions/Anaphylaxis
Headache
Hypersensitivity (<1%)
Paresthesias
Sjøgren's (Sicca) syndrome
  (1995): Bion E+, *J Hepatol* 23, 672
  (1983): Rex D+, *Gastroenterology* 85(3), 718

THIAMINE

Synonym: vitamin B$_1$
Trade names: Actamin; Beneuril; Betabion; Betalin; Betamin; Betaxin; Bewon; Biamine; Thiamilate; Tiamina; Vitantial
Indications: Thiamine deficiency
Category: Vitamin
Half-life: N/A

Reactions

Skin
Allergic reactions (sic)
Angioedema (<1%)
Dermatitis
  (1989): Ingemann-Larsen A+, *Contact Dermatitis* 20, 387
Diaphoresis
Eczema
Exanthems
  (1980): Kolz R+, *Hautarzt* (German) 31, 657
Pruritus (<1%)
Purpura
  (1989): Nishioka K+, *J Dermatol* 16, 220
  (1980): Nishioka K+, *Clin Exp Dermatol* 5, 213
Rash (sic) (<1%)
Urticaria
Vasculitis
  (1989): Nishioka K+, *J Dermatol* 16, 220

Other
Anaphylactoid reactions/Anaphylaxis
  (2000): Johri S+, *Am J Emerg Med* 18(5), 642
  (1998): Morinville V+, *Schweiz Med Wochenschr* 128, 1743
  (1997): Fernandez M+, *Allergy* 52, 958
DRESS syndrome
  (2006): Greco M+, *Ann Dermatol Venereol* 133(4), 354 (with
    quinine)
Injection-site reactions (sic)
Paresthesias (<1%)

THIMEROSAL

Trade names: Aeroaid; Curativ; Merseptyl; Mersol; Merthiolate; Topicaldermo; Vitaseptol
Indications: Antiseptic, bacteriostatic, fungistatic
Category: Antiseptic
Half-life: N/A

Reactions

Skin
Allergic reactions (sic)
  (2001): Suneja T+, *J Am Acad Dermatol* 45(1), 23
  (2001): Trujillo MJ+, *Allergol Immunopathol* (Madr) 29(4), 133
    (with piroxicam)
  (2000): Kiec-Swierczynska M+, *Int J Occup Med Environ Health*
    13(3), 179
  (1997): Rees S+, *Br Dent J* 183, 395 (in health care workersr)
  (1997): Wray D, *Br Dent J* 183, 316 (in health care workers)
  (1995): Barbaud A+, *Ann Dermatol Venereol* 122(3), 129
  (1993): Pirker C+, *Contact Dermatitis* 29(3), 152
  (1992): Wonk WK+, *Contact Dermatitis* 26(3), 195
Atopic dermatitis
  (1999): Patrizi A+, *Contact Dermatitis* 40(2), 94
  (1998): Romaguera C+, *Contact Dermatitis* 39(6), 277

Dermatitis
(2006): Laxmisha C+, *J Eur Acad Dermatol Venereol* 20(10), 1370
(2001): Suneja T+, *J Am Acad Dermatol* 45(1), 23
(2000): Kiec-Swierczynska M+, *Int J Occup Med Environ Health* 13(3), 179
(2000): Schafer MP+, *Contact Dermatitis* 43(3), 150
(2000): Westphal GA+, *Int Arch Occup Environ Health* 73(6), 384
(1999): Lebrec H+, *Cell Biol Toxicol* 15(1), 57
(1999): McKenna KE, *Contact Dermatitis* 40(3), 158
(1999): Sertoli A+, *Am J Contact Dermat* 10(1), 18
(1998): Ramsay HM+, *Contact Dermatitis* 39(4), 205
(1998): Romaguera C+, *Contact Dermatitis* 39(6), 277
(1998): Santucci B+, *Contact Dermatitis* 38(6), 325
(1997): Luka RE+, *J Allergy Clin Immunol* 100(1), 138
(1995): Aberer W+, *Contact Dermatitis* 32(6), 367
(1995): Schafer T+, *Contact Dermatitis* 32(2), 114
(1995): Zenarola P+, *Contact Dermatitis* 32(2), 107 (systemic)
(1994): Meding B+, *Contact Dermatitis* 30(3), 129
(1994): Wantke F+, *Contact Dermatitis* 30(2), 115
(1994): Zemstov A+, *Contact Dermatitis* 30(1), 57 (bullous)
(1991): Oritz FJ+, *Contact Dermatitis* 25(3), 203
(1990): Landa A+, *Contact Dermatitis* 22(5), 290
(1990): Wekkeli M+, *Contact Dermatitis* 22(5), 295
(1989): Seidenari S+, *G Ital Dermatol Venereol* 124(7–8), 335
(1987): Bardazzi F+, *Contact Dermatitis* 16(5), 298
(1987): Smith JM+, *Practitioner* 231, 579
(1987): Tosti A+, *Contact Dermatitis* 15, 187
(1987): Tosti A+, *G Ital Dermatol Venereol* 122(10), 543
(1986): Melino M+, *Contact Dermatitis* 14(2), 125
(1986): Moeller H, *Acta Derm Venereol* (Stockh) 57(6), 509 (3.7%)
(1986): Novak M+, *Contact Dermatitis* 15(5), 309 (in infants)
(1985). Fisher AA, *Cutis* 36(3), 209
(1985): Whittington CV, *Contact Dermatitis* 13(3), 186 (eye cream)
(1984): Miller JR, *West J Med* 140(5), 791 (contact lens solution)
(1984): Stolman LP+, *N Engl J Med* 311(23), 1521 (contact lens)
(1982): Rietschel RL+, *Arch Dermatol* 118(3), 147 (contact lens)
(1981): Fisher AA, *Cutis* 27(6), 580 (merthiolate)
(1980): Miranda A+, *Actas Dermatosifiliogr* 71(7–8), 301
(1980): Moller H, *Int J Dermatol* 19(1), 29
(1980): Sertoli A+, *Contact Dermatitis* 6(4), 292 (soft contact lens)
Eczema
(1999): Patrizi A+, *Contact Dermatitis* 40(2), 94
(1998): Romaguera C+, *Contact Dermatitis* 39(6), 277
Exanthems
(2005): Lee-Wong M+, *Ann Allergy Asthma Immunol* 94(1), 90
Lichen planus
(2001): Scalf LA+, *Am J Contact Dermat* 12(3), 146
Lichenoid eruption
(1984): Lindemayr H+, *Hautarzt* 35, 192
Photoallergic reaction
(1993): de la Cuadra J, *Ann Dermatol Venereol* 120(1), 37 (with piroxicam)
(1991): de Castro JL+, *Contact Dermatitis* 24(3), 187 (with piroxicam)
(1989): de la Cuadra J+, *Contact Dermatitis* 21(5), 349 (with piroxicam)
Photosensitivity
(2001): Trujillo MJ+, *Allergol Immunopathol* (Madr) 29(4), 133 (with piroxicam)
Urticaria
(1987): Lohiya G+, *West J Med* 147(3), 341
(1984): Lindemayr H+, *Hautarzt* 35, 192

Mucosal/ENT
Cheilitis
(1999): Kanthraj GR+, *Contact Dermatitis* 40(5), 285

Eyes
Conjunctivitis (allergic contact)
(1998): *Allergy* 53(3):333
(1988): Tosti A+, *Contact Dermatitis* 18(5), 268 (eye drops)
(1980): van Ketel WG+, *Contact Dermatitis* 6(5), 321 (soft contact lens)
Eyelid dermatitis
(1999): Wolfe, S, Statesville, NC (from Internet) (observation)
(1990): de Groot AC+, *Contact Dermatitis* 23(3), 168 (from contact lens fluid)

Other
Hypersensitivity (local)
(2007): Fagundes A+, *Acta Trop* 101(1), 25
(2006): Zoller L+, *Contact Dermatitis* 55(4), 227
(2001): Ball LK+, *Pediatrics* 107(5):1147
(2001): van't Veen AJ, *Drugs* 61(5), 565
(1994): van't Veen AJ+, *Contact Dermatitis* 31(5), 293
(1991): Aberer W, *Contact Dermatitis* 24(1), 6
(1991): Noel I+, *Lancet* 338(8768), 705 (in hepatitis B vaccine)
(1991): Osawa J+, *Contact Dermatitis* 24(3), 178
(1990): Rietschel RL+, *Dermatol Clin* 8(1), 161
(1989): Tosti A+, *Contact Dermatitis* 20(3), 173
(1980): Forstrom L+, *Contact Dermatitis* 6(4), 241
Injection-site pain
(1984): Lindemayr H+, *Hautarzt* 35, 192
Injection-site urticaria
(1988): Bork K, *Cutaneous Side Effects Of Drugs* WB Saunders, 114
Systemic reactions (sic)
(1986): Tosti A+, *Contact Dermatitis* 15(3), 187

THIOGUANINE

Synonyms: TG; 6-TG; 6-thioguanine; tioguanine
Trade name: Lanvis
Indications: Leukemias
Category: Antimetabolite; Antineoplastic
Half-life: 11 hours
Clinically important, potentially hazardous interactions with: aldesleukin, **vaccines**

Reactions

Skin
Exanthems
(1988): Zimm S+, *J Clin Oncol* 6, 696
Malignancies
(1997): Zackheim HS+, *J Am Acad Dermatol* 30, 452 (nonmelanoma)
Palmar erythema
(1988): Shall L+, *Br J Dermatol* 119, 249
Petechiae
Photosensitivity (<1%)
(1988): Zimm S+, *J Clin Oncol* 6, 696
Pruritus
(1999): Silvis NG+, *Arch Dermatol* 135, 433
Psoriasis
(1999): Silvis NG+, *Arch Dermatol* 135, 433
Purpura
Rash (sic) (1–10%)

Mucosal/ENT
Oral lesions
Stomatitis (1–10%)
Xerostomia

(1999): Silvis NG+, *Arch Dermatol* 135, 433

Hair

Hair – alopecia
  (1999): Murphy FP+, *Arch Dermatol* 135, 1495
  (1988): Zimm S+, *J Clin Oncol* 6, 696

Eyes

Vision loss
  (2006): Chaudhry IA+, *Eur J Ophthalmol* 16(4), 651

Other

Hepatotoxicity
  (2006): Vora A+, *Lancet* 368(9544), 1339
Infections
  (2006): Vora A+, *Lancet* 368(9544), 1339

THIOPENTAL

Trade names: Anesthal; Hypnostan; Intraval; Nesdonal; Sodipental; Thiopental (Baxter); Trapanal
Indications: Induction of anesthesia
Category: Barbiturate
Half-life: 3–12 hours
Clinically important, potentially hazardous interactions with: ethanol, ethanolamine

Reactions

Skin

Angioedema
Bullous dermatitis
  (1987): Saiag P+, *Ann Dermatol Venereol* (French) 114, 1440
Erythema (<1%)
Erythema multiforme
Exanthems (3%)
  (1987): Boittiaux P+, *Ann Fr Anesth Reanim* (French) 6, 324
    (3.3%)
Exfoliative dermatitis
Fixed eruption
  (1995): Bremang JA+, *Can J Anaesth* 42, 628
  (1990): Desmeules H, *Anesth Analg* 70, 216 (non-pigmenting)
  (1987): Saiag P+, *Ann Dermatol Venereol* (French) 114, 1440
Hypomelanosis
Pruritus (<1%)
Purpura
Rash (sic)
Shivering (27%)
  (1987): Boittiaux P+, *Ann Fr Anesth Reanim* (French) 6, 324
    (27%)
Stevens–Johnson syndrome
Toxic epidermal necrolysis
  (1987): Saiag P+, *Ann Dermatol Venereol* (French) 114, 1440
Urticaria

Other

Anaphylactoid reactions/Anaphylaxis (<1%)
  (2001): Garvey LH+, *Acta Anaesthesiol Scand* 45(10), 1204
  (1993): Seymour DG, *JAMA* 270, 2503 (letter)
  (1992): Breathnach SM+, *Adverse Drug Reactions and the Skin*
    Blackwell, Oxford, 193 (passim)
  (1988): Cheema AL+, *J Allergy Clin Immunol* 81, 220
Headache
Inappropriate secretion of antidiuretic hormone (SIADH)
  (1998): Frere T+, *Gastroenterol Clin Biol* 22(8-9), 727
Injection-site necrosis
Injection-site pain (>10%)

Injection-site phlebitis (6%)
  (1981): Clark RSJ, *Drugs* 22, 26 (6%)
Porphyria
  (1993): Harrison GG+, *Anaesthesia* 48, 1008–1010
Rhabdomyolysis
  (1990): Larpin R+, *Presse Med* 19(30), 1403
Thrombophlebitis (<1%)

THIORIDAZINE

Trade names: Aldazine; Apo-Thioridazine; Calmaril; Dazine; Mellaril (Novartis); Melleril; Ridazin; Thinin; Thioril
Indications: Psychotic disorders
Category: Antipsychotic, phenothiazine
Half-life: 21–25 hours
Clinically important, potentially hazardous interactions with: amisulpride, antihistamines, arsenic, chlorpheniramine, darifenacin, dofetilide, duloxetine, epinephrine, **evening primrose**, naloxone, pimozide, piperazine, quinolones, ranolazine, sparfloxacin, zaleplon

Reactions

Skin

Acanthosis nigricans
Angioedema (<1%)
Dermatitis
Erythema multiforme
  (1985): Rees TD, *J Periodontol* 56, 480
Exanthems
Exfoliative dermatitis
Lichenoid eruption
  (2004): Llambrich A+, *Photodermatol Photoimmunol Photomed*
    20(2), 108
Lupus erythematosus
Peripheral edema
Photosensitivity (1–10%)
  (1987): Röhrborn W+, *Contact Dermatitis* 17, 241
Phototoxicity
Pigmentation (<1%) (blue-gray)
Purpura
Rash (sic) (1–10%)
  (1981): Georgotas A+, *Psychopharmacology* 73, 292
Seborrhea
Toxic epidermal necrolysis
  (1987): Harnar TJ+, *J Burn Care Rehabil* 8, 554
Urticaria
Vasculitis
  (2002): Greenfield JR+, *Br J Dermatol* 147(6), 1265 (confirmed
    on re-challenge)
Xerosis

Mucosal/ENT

Oral mucosal eruption
  (1985): Rees TD, *J Periodontol* 56, 480
Xerostomia
  (1981): Georgotas A+, *Psychopharmacology* 73, 292

Hair

Hair – alopecia
Hair – hypertrichosis

Eyes

Retinopathy
  (2003): Hadden PW+, *Clin Experiment Ophthalmol* 31(6), 533

(1985): Taylor F, *Aust Fam Physician* 14(8), 744

Other

Anaphylactoid reactions/Anaphylaxis
Death
  (2001): Glassman AH+, *Am J Psychiatry* 158(11), 1774
  (2000): Timell AM, *Ann Clin Psychiatry* 12(3), 147 (4 cases)
Gynecomastia
Headache
Hypersensitivity
Inappropriate secretion of antidiuretic hormone (SIADH)
  (1986): Ananth J+, *Int J Psychiatry Med* 16(4), 401
Lymphoproliferative disease
  (1992): Aguilar JL+, *Arch Dermatol* 128, 121
Paresthesias
Porphyria
  (1985): Kamal S+, *Union Med Can* (French) 114, 330
Pseudolymphoma
  (1988): Kardaun SH+, *Br J Dermatol* 118, 545
Tremor

THIOTEPA

Synonym: TSPA
Trade name: Thioplex (Amgen)
Indications: Breast, ovarian and bladder carcinomas
Category: Alkylating agent
Half-life: 109 minutes
Clinically important, potentially hazardous interactions with: aldesleukin

Reactions

Skin

Allergic reactions (sic) (1–10%)
Angioedema
  (1992): Breathnach SM+, *Adverse Drug Reactions and the Skin*
    Blackwell, Oxford, 292 (passim)
  (1987): Lee M+, *J Urol* 138, 143
  (1985): Levine N+, *Cancer Treat Rev* 5, 67
  (1981): Weiss RB+, *Ann Intern Med* 94, 66
Bruising
Eccrine squamous syringometaplasia
  (1997): Valks R+, *Arch Dermatol* 133, 873
Leukoderma
Pigmentation (1–10%)
  (1992): Breathnach SM+, *Adverse Drug Reactions and the Skin*
    Blackwell, Oxford, 292 (passim)
  (1989): Horn TD+, *Arch Dermatol* 125, 524
Pruritus (1–10%)
  (1992): Breathnach SM+, *Adverse Drug Reactions and the Skin*
    Blackwell, Oxford, 292 (passim)
  (1987): Lee M+, *J Urol* 138, 143
  (1985): Levine N+, *Cancer Treat Rev* 5, 67
  (1981): Weiss RB+, *Ann Intern Med* 94, 66
Rash (sic) (1–10%)
Urticaria (3%)
  (1992): Breathnach SM+, *Adverse Drug Reactions and the Skin*
    Blackwell, Oxford, 292 (passim)
  (1987): Lee M+, *J Urol* 138, 143
  (1985): Levine N+, *Cancer Treat Rev* 5, 67
  (1981): Weiss RB+, *Ann Intern Med* 94, 66

Mucosal/ENT

Stomatitis (<1%)

Hair

Hair – alopecia (1–10%)
  (2002): de Jonge ME+, *Bone Marrow Transplantation* 30(9), 593
    (permanent) (with carboplatin and cyclophosphamide)

Other

Anaphylactoid reactions/Anaphylaxis (<1%)
Inappropriate secretion of antidiuretic hormone (SIADH)
  (1999): Sica S+, *Bone Marrow Transplant* 24(5), 571
Injection-site pain (>10%)

THIOTHIXENE

Synonym: tiotixene
Trade names: Navane (Pfizer); Orbinamon
Indications: Psychotic disorders
Category: Antipsychotic
Half-life: >24 hours

Reactions

Skin

Diaphoresis (14%)
Exanthems (14%)
  (1994): Shelley WB+, *Cutis* 54, 71 (observation)
Palmar erythema
  (1982): Matsuoka LY, *J Am Acad Dermatol* 7, 405
Peripheral edema
Photosensitivity (1–10%)
Pigmentation (blue-gray) (<1%)
Pruritus
Rash (sic) (1–10%)
Raynaud's phenomenon
  (1991): McCance-Katz EF, *J Clin Psychiatry* 52, 89
Seborrheic dermatitis
  (1984): Binder RL+, *J Clin Psychiatry* 45, 125
  (1983): Binder RL+, *Arch Dermatol* 119, 473
Sensitivity (sic)
  (1982): Matsuoka LY, *J Am Acad Dermatol* 7, 405
Telangiectasia
  (1982): Matsuoka LY, *J Am Acad Dermatol* 7, 405
Urticaria

Mucosal/ENT

Dysgeusia
  (2000): Heymann WR, *Cutis* 66, 25
Sialorrhea
Tongue black
  (2000): Heymann WR, *Cutis* 66, 25
Xerostomia
  (2000): Heymann WR, *Cutis* 66, 25
  (1987): Sarai K+, *Pharmacopsychiatry* 20, 38

Hair

Hair – alopecia

Other

Anaphylactoid reactions/Anaphylaxis
Gynecomastia
Paresthesias

TIAGABINE

Trade name: Gabitril (Cephalon)
Indications: Partial seizures
Category: Anticonvulsant; Mood stabilizer
Half-life: 7–9 hours

Reactions

Skin

Acne (>1%)
Allergic reactions (sic) (<1%)
Carcinoma (<1%)
Dermatitis (<1%)
Diaphoresis (<1%)
Eczema (<1%)
Edema (<1%)
Exanthems (<1%)
Exfoliative dermatitis (<1%)
Facial edema (<1%)
Furunculosis (<1%)
Herpes simplex (<1%)
Herpes zoster (<1%)
Neoplasms (benign) (<1%)
Nodular eruption (<1%)
Peripheral edema (<1%)
Petechiae (<1%)
Photosensitivity (<1%)
Pigmentation (<1%)
Pruritus (2%)
Psoriasis (<1%)
Rash (sic) (5%)
  (2007): Arif H+, *Neurology* 68(20), 1701
Stevens–Johnson syndrome
Ulcerations (<1%)
Urticaria (<1%)
Vesiculobullous eruption (<1%)
Xerosis (<1%)

Mucosal/ENT

Ageusia (<1%)
Dysgeusia (<1%)
Gingival hyperplasia/hypertrophy (<1%)
Gingivitis (<1%)
Glossitis (<1%)
Oral ulceration (2%)
Parosmia (<1%)
Sialorrhea (<1%)
Stomatitis (<1%)
Ulcerative stomatitis (<1%)
Vaginitis (<1%)
Xerostomia (>1%)
  (2006): Schwartz TL+, *Expert Opin Pharmacother* 7(14), 1977

Hair

Hair – alopecia (<1%)
Hair – hirsutism (<1%)

Other

Asthenia
  (2006): Schwartz TL+, *Expert Opin Pharmacother* 7(14), 1977
  (2002): Pereira J+, *Cochrane Database Syst Rev* (3), CD00
  (2001): Schachter SC, *Expert Opin Pharmacother* 2(1), 179
  (2000): Kozik A, *Neurol Neurochir Pol* 34, 17
Depression

  (2007): Mula M+, *Drug Saf* 30(7), 555
  (2001): Kalvianen R, *Epilepsia* 42(Suppl 3), 46
  (2000): Kozik A, *Neurol Neurochir Pol* 34, 17
Gynecomastia (<1%)
Headache
  (2006): Schwartz TL+, *Expert Opin Pharmacother* 7(14), 1977
  (2001): Schachter SC, *Expert Opin Pharmacother* 2(1), 179
Infections
  (2001): Schachter SC, *Expert Opin Pharmacother* 2(1), 179
Myalgia/Myositis/Myopathy/Myotoxicity (>1%)
Myoclonus
  (2007): Vollmar C+, *Neurology* 68(4), 310
Paresthesias (4%)
Thrombophlebitis (<1%)
Tremor (>1%)
  (2002): Pereira J+, *Cochrane Database Syst Rev* (3), CD00
  (2001): Kalvianen R, *Epilepsia* 42(Suppl 3), 43
  (2000): Fakhoury T+, *Seizure* 9, 431 (31%)
Vertigo
  (2006): Schwartz TL+, *Expert Opin Pharmacother* 7(14), 1977
  (2002): Pereira J+, *Cochrane Database Syst Rev* (3), CD00
  (2001): Arroyo S+, *Rev Neurol* 32(11), 1041
  (2001): Crawford P+, *Epilepsia* 42(4), 531
  (2001): Schachter SC, *Expert Opin Pharmacother* 2(1), 179
  (2000): Kozik A, *Neurol Neurochir Pol* 34, 17

TICARCILLIN

Trade names: Ticar (GSK); Timentin
Indications: Various infections caused by susceptible organisms
Category: Antibiotic, penicillin
Half-life: 1.0–1.2 hours
Clinically important, potentially hazardous interactions with: anticoagulants, ceftobiprole, cyclosporine, demeclocycline, doxycycline, methotrexate, minocycline, oxytetracycline, tetracycline

Note: Timentin is Ticarcillin + Clavulanic acid

Reactions

Skin

Allergic reactions (sic)
  (1994): Pleasants RA+, *Chest* 106, 1124 (in patients with cystic fibrosis)
Angioedema
Bullous dermatitis
Erythema multiforme
Erythema nodosum
Exanthems
  (1980): Brogden RN+, *Drugs* 20, 325 (1%)
Exfoliative dermatitis
Hematomas
Jarisch–Herxheimer reaction (<1%)
Pruritus
Purpura
Rash (sic) (<1%)
Stevens–Johnson syndrome
Toxic epidermal necrolysis
Urticaria
Vasculitis

Mucosal/ENT

Dysgeusia
Glossitis

Glossodynia
Oral candidiasis
Stomatitis
Stomatodynia
Tongue black
Vaginitis
Xerostomia

Other
Anaphylactoid reactions/Anaphylaxis (<1%)
Hypersensitivity (<1%)
  (1986): Croydon EA+, *J Antimicrob Chemother* 17, 233 (2%)
Injection-site erythema
  (1986): Croydon EA+, *J Antimicrob Chemother* 17, 233
Injection-site pain
  (1986): Croydon EA+, *J Antimicrob Chemother* 17, 233
  (1980): Brogden RN+, *Drugs* 20, 325
Injection-site phlebitis
  (1986): Croydon EA+, *J Antimicrob Chemother* 17, 233
  (1985): Sanders CV+, *Am J Med* 79(5B), 96
  (1980): Brogden RN+, *Drugs* 20, 325
Injection-site reactions
  (1986): Croydon EA+, *J Antimicrob Chemother* 17, 233 (5%)
Serum sickness
Thrombophlebitis (<1%)

TICLOPIDINE

Trade names: Anagregal; Panaldine; Ticlid (Roche); Ticlidil;
Ticlodix; Ticlodone; Tiklid; Tiklyd
Indications: To reduce risk of thrombotic stroke
Category: Antiplatelet, thienopyridine
Half-life: 24 hours
**Clinically important, potentially hazardous interactions
with:** alteplase, **dong quai**, fondaparinux, **garlic, ginger,
ginseng, horse chestnut (bark, flower, leaf, seed)**, phenytoin,
red clover

Reactions

Skin
Acute generalized exanthematous pustulosis (AGEP)
  (2000): Cannavò SP+, *Br J Dermatol* 142, 577
Angioedema (<1%)
  (1999): Chassany O+, *Presse Med* (French) 28, 18
Dermatitis
  (1998): Ceylan C+, *Am J Hematol* 59, 260
Diaphoresis (<2%)
  (1984): Stiegler H+, *Dtsch Med Wochenschr* (German) 109, 1240
    (1.7%)
Erythema
  (1990): McTavish D+, *Drugs* 40, 238
Erythema multiforme (<1%)
  (1999): Yosipovitch G+, *J Am Acad Dermatol* 41, 473
Erythema nodosum (<1%)
Exanthems (1–11.9%)
  (2000): Prost C+, *Presse Med* (French) 29, 303
  (1999): Yosipovitch G+, *J Am Acad Dermatol* 41, 473
  (1997): Litt JZ, Beachwood, OH (personal case) (observation)
  (1990): McTavish D+, *Drugs* 40, 238 (7%)
  (1989): Hass WK+, *N Engl J Med* 321, 501 (11.9%)
  (1987): Saltiel E+, *Drugs* 34, 222 (1–5%)
Exfoliative dermatitis (<1%)
Facial erythema
  (1999): Yosipovitch G+, *J Am Acad Dermatol* 41, 473

Fixed eruption
  (2002): Borras-Blasco J+, *Ann Pharmacother* 36(2), 344
  (2001): Garcia CM+, *Contact Dermatitis* 44, 40
  (1999): Yosipovitch G+, *J Am Acad Dermatol* 41, 473
Hematomas (2%)
  (1984): Stiegler H+, *Dtsch Med Wochenschr* (German) 109, 1240
    (2.7%)
Lichen planus
  (2005): Kurokawa I+, *Int J Dermatol* 44(5), 436
Lupus erythematosus (positive ANA) (<1%)
  (2006): Ohtake T+, *Nephrol Dial Transplant* 21(7), 1992
  (2006): Reich A+, *Int J Dermatol.* 2006 Sep 45(9), 1112
  (2002): Spiera RF+, *Arch Intern Med* 162(19), 2240 (4 cases)
Petechiae (2%)
  (1984): Stiegler H+, *Dtsch Med Wochenschr* (German) 109, 1240
    (1.7%)
Pruritus (1.3%)
  (1999): Yosipovitch G+, *J Am Acad Dermatol* 41, 473
  (1990): McTavish D+, *Drugs* 40, 238
  (1987): Saltiel E+, *Drugs* 34, 222
Purpura (1–5%)
  (2006): Makkar K+, *Ann Pharmacother* 40(6), 1204
  (2006): Matsuda N+, *Rinsho Shinkeigaku* 46(10), 693
  (2003): Turken O+, *Acta Haematol* 109(1), 40
  (2001): Medina PJ+, *Curr Opin Hematol* 8(5), 286
  (2001): Naseer N+, *Heart Dis* 3(4), 221
  (2001): Yang CW+, *Ren Fail* 23(6), 851 (2 cases)
  (2000): Chemnitz JM+, *Med Klin* (German) 95, 96
  (2000): Tsai H-M+, *Ann Intern Med* 132, 794
  (1999): Bennett CL+, *Ann Intern Med* 159, 2524
  (1999): Chen DK+, *Arch Intern Med* 159, 311
  (1999): Elangovan L, *Arch Int Med* 159, 1624
  (1999): Mauro M+, *Blood* 94, 1–646a
  (1999): Steinhubl SR+, *JAMA* 281, 806
  (1998): Bennett CL+, *Ann Intern Med* 128, 541
  (1998): Bennett CL+, *Lancet* 352, 1036
  (1998): Jamar S+, *Acta Cardiol* 53, 285
  (1998): Mukamal KJ+, *Ann Intern Med* 129, 837
  (1998): Muszkat M+, *Pharmacotherapy* 18, 1352
  (1997): Kupfer Y+, *N Engl J Med* 337, 1245
  (1996): Wysowski DK+, *JAMA* 276, 952
  (1991): Page Y+, *Lancet* 337, 774
  (1990): McTavish D+, *Drugs* 40, 238 (1–5%)
  (1990): Takishita S+, *N Engl J Med* 323, 1487
  (1989): Hass WK+, *N Engl J Med* 321, 501 (4%)
  (1984): Stiegler H+, *Dtsch Med Wochenschr* (German) 109, 1240
    (1–5%)
  (1982): de Fraiture WH+, *Ned Tijdschr Geneeskd* (Dutch)
    126, 1051
Rash (sic) (5.1%)
  (2006): Makkar K+, *Ann Pharmacother* 40(6), 1204 (with
    clopidogrel)
  (2005): Grabowski M+, *Pol Arch Med Wewn.* 114(4), 974
  (1999): Quinn MJ+, *Circulation* 100, 1667
  (1999): Whetsel TR+, *Pharmacotherapy* 19, 228
Side effects (sic) (8%)
  (1984): Stiegler H+, *Dtsch Med Wochenschr* (German) 109, 1240
    (8%)
Stevens–Johnson syndrome (<1%)
Toxic erythema
  (1999): Hsi DH+, *N Engl J Med* 340, 1212
Urticaria (1–5%)
  (1999): Yosipovitch G+, *J Am Acad Dermatol* 41, 473
  (1990): McTavish D+, *Drugs* 40, 238
  (1989): Hass WK+, *N Engl J Med* 321, 501 (2%)
  (1987): Saltiel E+, *Drugs* 34, 222 (1–5%)
Vasculitis (<1%)
  (2001): Pintor E+, *Rev Esp Cardiol* 54(1), 114

Mucosal/ENT
 Tinnitus

Other
 Asthenia
  (2003): Turken O+, *Acta Haematol* 109(1), 40
 Death
  (2006): Patel TN+, *J Invasive Cardiol* 18(7), E211
 Erythromelalgia
  (1999): Yosipovitch G+, *J Am Acad Dermatol* 41, 473
 Fever
  (2006): Matsuda N+, *Rinsho Shinkeigaku* 46(10), 693
  (2005): Elikowski W+, *Pol Arch Med Wewn* 114(2), 773
 Headache
 Nephrotoxicity
  (2006): Matsuda N+, *Rinsho Shinkeigaku* 46(10), 693
 Septic–toxic shock
  (2005): Grabowski M+, *Pol Arch Med Wewn* 114(4), 974
 Serum sickness

TIGECYCLINE

Trade name: Tygacil (Wyeth)
Indications: Complicated skin or intra-abdominal infections
Category: Antibiotic, tetracycline
Half-life: 36 hours
Clinically important, potentially hazardous interactions with: warfarin

Reactions

Skin
 Allergic reactions (sic) (<2%)
 Diaphoresis
 Peripheral edema
 Pruritus
 Rash (sic)
 Urticaria
  (2006): Nord CE+, *Antimicrob Agents Chemother* 50(10), 3375
   (1 case)

Mucosal/ENT
 Dysgeusia
 Vaginitis (<2%)
 Xerostomia (<2%)

Other
 Abdominal pain
  (2006): Doan TL+, *Clin Ther* 28(8), 1079 (6%)
 Asthenia
 Chills (<2%)
 Cough
 Fever
  (2006): Doan TL+, *Clin Ther* 28(8), 1079 (6%)
 Headache
  (2006): Doan TL+, *Clin Ther* 28(8), 1079 (8%)
  (2004): Zhanel GG+, *Drugs* 64(1), 63
 Infections
  (2006): Doan TL+, *Clin Ther* 28(8), 1079 (7%)
 Injection-site edema (<2%)
 Injection-site inflammation (<2%)
 Injection-site pain (<2%)
 Injection-site phlebitis (<2%)
 Injection-site reactions (<2%)
  (2006): Doan TL+, *Clin Ther* 28(8), 1079 (8%)

 Pain
 Vertigo

TILUDRONATE

Trade name: Skelid (Sanofi-Aventis)
Indications: Paget's Disease of the bone
Category: Bisphosphonate
Half-life: 150 hours
Clinically important, potentially hazardous interactions with: indomethacin

Reactions

Skin
 Diaphoresis (<1%)
 Edema (3%)
 Pruritus (<1%)
 Rash (sic) (3%)
 Stevens–Johnson syndrome (<1%)

Mucosal/ENT
 Dysphagia
 Rhinitis (5%)
 Sinusitis (5%)
 Xerostomia (<1%)

Eyes
 Cataract (3%)
 Conjunctivitis (3%)
 Glaucoma (3%)

Other
 Abdominal pain (<1%)
 Asthenia (<1%)
 Chest pain (3%)
 Cough (3%)
 Death
  (1999): Zojer N+, *Drug Saf* 21(5), 389
 Hypertension (<1%)
 Nephrotoxicity
  (1999): Zojer N+, *Drug Saf* 21(5), 389
  (1991): Dumon JC+, *Bone Miner* 15(3), 257
 Paresthesias (4%)
 Vertigo (<1%)

TIMOLOL

Trade names: Apo-Timol; Aquanil; Betimol; Blocadren (Merck); CoSopt (Merck); Dispatim; Nu-Timolol; Tenopt; Tiloptic; Timacor; Timoptic (ophthalmic) (Merck); Timoptol
Indications: Hypertension
Category: Adrenergic beta-receptor antagonist
Half-life: 2–2.7 hours
Clinically important, potentially hazardous interactions with: clonidine, epinephrine, ergot, prednisone, verapamil

Note: CoSopt is timolol and dorzolamide; Timolide is timolol and hydrochlorothiazide. Dorzolamide and hydrochlorothiazide are sulfonamides and can be absorbed systemically. Sulfonamides can produce severe, possibly fatal, reactions such as toxic epidermal necrolysis and Stevens–Johnson syndrome

Note: Cutaneous side-effects of beta-receptor blockaders are clinically polymorphous. They apparently appear after several months of continuous therapy. Atypical psoriasiform, lichen planus-like, and eczematous chronic rashes are mainly observed. (1983): Hödl St, *Z Hautkr* (German) 1:58, 17

Reactions

Skin

Angioedema
Dermatitis (eyedrops)
  (2006): Kalavala M+, *Contact Dermatitis* 54(6), 345
  (2001): Holdiness MR, *Am J Contact Dermat* 12(4), 217
  (1993): Corazza M+, *Contact Dermatitis* 28, 188
  (1993): O'Donnell BF+, *Contact Dermatitis* 28, 121
  (1991): Kubota K+, *Br J Clin Pharmacol* 31, 471
  (1986): Fernandez-Vozmediano JM+, *Contact Dermatitis* 14, 252
  (1986): Romaguera C+, *Contact Dermatitis* 14, 248
Diaphoresis
Eczema
  (1991): Cameli N+, *Contact Dermatitis* 25, 129
Edema (0.6%)
Erythema multiforme
Erythroderma
  (1997): Shelley WB+, *J Am Acad Dermatol* 37, 799
  (1993): Shelley WB+, *Cutis* 51, 330 (observation)
Exanthems
Exfoliative dermatitis
Hyperkeratosis (palms and soles)
Lichenoid eruption
  (2004): Mullins RJ+, *Australas J Dermatol* 45(2), 151 (with dorzolamide)
Lupus erythematosus
  (1994): Cohen MG, *J Rheumatol* 21, 578
  (1992): Zamber RW+, *J Rheumatol* 19, 977
Pemphigus
  (1987): Fiore PM+, *Arch Ophthalmol* 105, 1660
Photosensitivity
Pigmentation
Pityriasis rubra pilaris
Pruritus (1–5%)
  (1996): Lazarov A+, *Cutis* 58, 363 (from eye drops)
Psoriasis
  (1992): Germain ML+, *Therapie* (French) 47, 447
  (1989): Puig L+, *Am J Ophthalmol* 108, 455
  (1987): Savola J+, *BMJ* 295, 637 (also aggravation of psoriasis)
  (1986): Czernielewski J+, *Lancet* 1, 808
  (1984): Arntzen N+, *Acta Derm Venereol* (Stockh) 64, 346
Purpura
Rash (sic) (1–10%)
Raynaud's phenomenon
  (1990): Meuche C+, *Fortschr Ophthalmol* 87(1), 45
  (1984): Eliasson K+, *Acta Med Scand* 215, 333
Toxic epidermal necrolysis
  (2005): Florez A+, *J Am Acad Dermatol* 53(5), 909 (with dorzolamide & latanoprost)
Urticaria
Xerosis

Mucosal/ENT

Dysgeusia
Oral lichenoid eruption
Tinnitus
Xerostomia (19%)
  (1998): LeBlanc RP, *Ophthalmology* 105, 1960
  (1997): Schuman JS+, *Arch Ophthalmol* 115, 847 (19.4%)
  (1996): Schuman JS, *Surv Ophthalmol* 41, S27

Hair

Hair – alopecia (1–10%)
  (2004): Litt JZ, Beachwood, OH (eye drops) (observation)
  (1990): Fraunfelder FT+, *JAMA* 263, 1493

Nails

Nails – dystrophy
Nails – pigmentation
  (1981): Feiler-Ofry V, *Ophthalmologica* (Basel) 182, 153

Eyes

Conjunctival hyperemia
  (2006): Hollo G+, *Eur J Ophthalmol* 16(6), 816 (6%)
  (2006): Hoy SM+, *Drugs Aging* 23(7), 587 (with travoprost)
  (2006): Konstas AG+, *Arch Ophthalmol* 124(11), 1553
  (2002): Higginbotham EJ+, *Arch Ophthalmol* 120(10), 1286
Conjunctivitis
  (1991): Cameli N+, *Contact Dermatitis* 25, 129
Eyelid dermatitis
  (2000): Quiralte J+, *Contact Dermatitis* 42, 245
  (1995): Koch P, *Contact Dermatitis* 33, 140
  (1988): Kanzaki T+, *Contact Dermatitis* 19, 388
Ocular allergy
  (1998): LeBlanc RP, *Ophthalmology* 105, 1960
  (1996): Schuman JS, *Surv Ophthalmol* 41, S27
Ocular burning
  (2003): Hommer A+, *Br J Ophthalmol* 87(5), 592 (with unoprostone, brimonidine, or dorzolamide)
  (1998): LeBlanc RP, *Ophthalmology* 105, 1960
  (1997): Schuman JS+, *Arch Ophthalmol* 115, 847 (41.9%)
  (1996): Schuman JS, *Surv Ophthalmol* 41, S27
Ocular itching
  (2006): Konstas AG+, *Arch Ophthalmol* 124(11), 1553
Ocular lichenoid eruption
  (2004): Mullins RJ+, *Australas J Dermatol* 45(2), 151
Ocular pemphigoid
  (1992): Shelley WB+, *Advanced Dermatologic Diagnosis* WB Saunders, 554 (passim)
Ocular stinging
  (2006): Konstas AG+, *Arch Ophthalmol* 124(11), 1553
  (2004): Fechtner RD+, *Acta Ophthalmol Scand* 82(1), 42 (with dorzolamide)
  (2003): Hommer A+, *Br J Ophthalmol* 87(5), 592 (with unoprostone, brimonidine, or dorzolamide)
  (1998): LeBlanc RP, *Ophthalmology* 105, 1960
  (1997): Schuman JS+, *Arch Ophthalmol* 115, 847 (41.9%)
  (1996): Schuman JS, *Surv Ophthalmol* 41, S27
Oculo-mucocutaneous syndrome
  (1982): Cocco G+, *Curr Ther Res* 31, 362

Other

Anaphylactoid reactions/Anaphylaxis
Headache
Myalgia/Myositis/Myopathy/Myotoxicity
Paresthesias (<1%)
Peyronie's disease

TINIDAZOLE

Trade names: Fasigyn; Tindamax (Presutti)
Indications: Amebiasis, giardiasis, trichomoniasis
Category: Antibiotic, nitroimidazole
Half-life: 12-14 hours
Clinically important, potentially hazardous interactions with: None

Reactions

Skin
Angioedema
  (1983): Okhrimovich LM+, *Vrach Delo* L(8), 100
Burning
Diaphoresis
Fixed eruption
  (1998): Thami GP+, *Dermatology* 196(3), 368
  (1990): Kanwar AJ+, *Dermatologica* 180(4), 277
  (1990): Mishra D+, *Int J Dermatol* 29(10), 740
  (1988): Jafferany M+, *Int J Dermatol* 27(4), 279
  (1987): Jafferany M+, *J Pak Med Assoc* 37(5), 136
Pruritus
Rash (sic)
Urticaria
Vasculitis
  (1983): Okhrimovich LM+, *Vrach Delo* L(8), 100

Mucosal/ENT
Dysgeusia (metallic/bitter taste) (4.5%)
  (2006): Canete R+, *Curr Med Res Opin* 22(11), 2131
Oral candidiasis
Sialorrhea
Stomatitis
Tongue furry
Tongue pigmentation
Xerostomia

Other
Abdominal pain
Asthenia (2%)
Candidiasis
Depression
Fever
Headache (1.3%)
  (2006): Canete R+, *Curr Med Res Opin* 22(11), 2131
Myalgia/Myositis/Myopathy/Myotoxicity
Paresthesias
Seizures
Vertigo (2%)

TINZAPARIN

Trade name: Innohep (Pharmion)
Indications: Acute symptomatic deep vein thrombosis
Category: Heparin, low molecular weight
Half-life: 3–4 hours
**Clinically important, potentially hazardous interactions
with:** butabarbital

Reactions

Skin
Abscess (<1%)
Allergic reactions (sic)
Angioedema (<1%)
Bullous dermatitis (1–10%)
Cellulitis (<1%)
Exanthems (<1%)
Necrosis (1%)
Neoplasms
Pruritus (1–10%)
Purpura (<1%)

  (1996): Simpson HK+, *Haemostasis* 26, 90
Rash (sic) (1%)
Urticaria (<1%)

Mucosal/ENT
Epistaxis
  (1996): Simpson HK+, *Haemostasis* 26(2), 90 (2 cases)

Hair
Hair – alopecia
  (2003): Sarris W+, *Am J Kidney Dis* 41(5)

Eyes
Ocular hemorrhage
  (1996): Simpson HK+, *Haemostasis* 26(2), 90 (1 case)

Other
Anaphylactoid reactions/Anaphylaxis (In sulfite-sensitive
  people)
Headache
Hypersensitivity
Infections
Injection-site bleeding
  (2002): Wong NN, *Heart Dis* 4, 331
Injection-site hematoma (16%)
Injection-site pain
Phlebitis
Thrombophlebitis
Thrombosis
  (2007): Hull RD+, *Am J Med* 120(1), 72 (5%)

TIOPRONIN

Trade names: Acadione; Captimer; Thiola (Mission)
Indications: Cystinuria
Category: Antiurilithic
Half-life: N/A

Reactions

Skin
Angioedema (14%)
  (1988): Sigaud M+, *Rev Rhum Mal Osteoartic* (French) 55, 467
  (14.5%)
Bullous pemphigoid
  (1988): Nakajima H+, *Nippon Hifuka Gakkai Zasshi* (Japanese)
  98, 803
Dermatitis
  (1995): Romano A+, *Contact Dermatitis* 33, 269
Edema
Elastosis perforans serpiginosa
Erythema
  (1990): Sany J+, *Rev Rhum Mal Osteoartic* (French) 57, 105
Erythema multiforme
  (1988): Nakajima H+, *Nippon Hifuka Gakkai Zasshi* (Japanese)
  98, 803
Exanthems (14%)
  (1988): Sigaud M+, *Rev Rhum Mal Osteoartic* (French) 55, 467
  (14.5%)
  (1984): Shichiri M+, *Arch Intern Med* 144, 89
Lichenoid eruption
  (1994): Pierard E+, *J Am Acad Dermatol* 31, 665
  (1990): Kurumaji Y+, *J Dermatol* (Tokio) 17, 176
  (1988): Kawabe Y+, *J Dermatol* (Tokio) 15, 434 (bullous)
Lupus erythematosus
  (1986): Katayama I+, *J Dermatol* (Tokio) 13, 151
Pemphigus (5%)

(1994): Verdier-Sevrain S+, *Br J Dermatol* 130, 238
(1990): Meunier L+, *Ann Dermatol Venereol* (French) 117, 959
(1990): Sany J+, *Rev Rhum Mal Osteoartic* (French) 57, 105
(1988): Sigaud M+, *Rev Rhum Mal Osteoartic* (French) 55, 467
     (5.8%)
(1987): Enjolras O+, *Ann Dermatol Venereol* (French) 114, 25
Pemphigus erythematodes
  (1982): Alinovi A+, *Acta Derm Venereol* (Stockh) 62, 452
Pemphigus foliaceus
  (1983): Lucky PA+, *J Am Acad Dermatol* 8, 667
Pemphigus vulgaris
  (1984): Trotta F+, *Scand J Rheumatol* 13(1), 93
Photosensitivity (1%)
  (1988): Sigaud M+, *Rev Rhum Mal Osteoartic* (French) 55, 467
     (1.5%)
Pityriasis rosea (5%)
  (1990): Sany J+, *Rev Rhum Mal Osteoartic* (French) 57, 105
  (1988): Sigaud M+, *Rev Rhum Mal Osteoartic* (French) 55, 467
     (5.8%)
Pruritus
Rash (sic)
Side effects (sic) (27%)
  (1988): Sigaud M+, *Rev Rhum Mal Osteoartic* (French) 55, 467
     (27.5%)
Toxic epidermal necrolysis
Urticaria
Wrinkling (sic)

Mucosal/ENT
Ageusia
  (1989): Mordini M+, *Minerva Med* 80(9), 1019
Dysgeusia
Hypogeusia
Mucocutaneous reactions (sic)
  (1990): Sany J+, *Rev Rhum Mal Osteoartic* (French) 57, 105
     (32.8%)
Oral lesions (4%)
  (1988): Sigaud M+, *Rev Rhum Mal Osteoartic* (French) 55, 467
     (4.4%)
  (1984): Shichiri M+, *Arch Intern Med* 144, 89
Oral ulceration
  (2000): Madinier I+, *Ann Med Interne* (Paris) (French) 151, 248
Parosmia
Stomatitis
  (1990): Sany J+, *Rev Rhum Mal Osteoartic* (French) 57, 105
  (1988): Sigaud M+, *Rev Rhum Mal Osteoartic* (French) 55, 467
Xerostomia

Hair
Hair – alopecia
  (1990): Sany J+, *Rev Rhum Mal Osteoartic* (French) 57, 105
Hair – hypertrichosis
  (1993): Arnaud M+, *Joint Bone Spine Dis* 60, 548

Other
Myalgia/Myositis/Myopathy/Myotoxicity
  (1988): Menkes CJ+, *Presse Med* (French) 17, 1156
Polymyositis
  (1999): Cacoub B+, *Presse Med* (French) 28, 911

TIOTROPIUM

Trade name: Spiriva (Boehringer Ingelheim)
Indications: Bronchospasm (associated with COPD)
Category: Anticholinergic; Muscarinic antagonist
Half-life: 5–6 days
**Clinically important, potentially hazardous interactions
with:** None

Reactions

Skin
Allergic reactions (sic) (1–3%)
Angioedema (<1%)
Edema (5%)
Herpes zoster (1–3%)
Lichenoid eruption
  (2007): Perez-Perez L+, *Dermatology* 214(1), 97
Lupus erythematosus
  (2005): Pham HC+, *Arch Dermatol* 141(7), 911
Photosensitivity
  (2007): Perez-Perez L+, *Dermatology* 214(1), 97
Pruritus
Rash (sic) (4%)
Urticaria

Mucosal/ENT
Rhinitis (6%)
Sinusitis (11%)
Stomatitis (1–3%)
Xerostomia (10–16%)
  (2006): Kesten S+, *Chest - Chest* 130(6), 1695
  (2006): Kesten S+, *Chest* 130(6), 1695
  (2005): Koumis T+, *Clin Ther* 27(4), 377
  (2004): Gross NJ, *Chest* 126(6), 1946 (10–16%)
  (2002): Casaburi R+, *Eur Respir J* 19(2), 217 (16%)
  (2002): Hansel TT+, *Drugs Today* (Barc) 38(9), 585 (10–15%)
  (2002): Hvizdos KM+, *Drugs* 62(8), 1195 (10–16%)
  (2002): Shukla VK, *Issues in Emerging Health Technologies* 35, 1
  (2001): Barnes PJ, *Expert Opin Investig Drugs* 10(4), 733 (~10%)
  (2000): Casaburi R+, *Chest* 118(5), 1294 (9.3%)
  (2000): van Noord JA+, *Thorax* 55(4), 289 (14.7%)

Eyes
Cataract (1–3%)

Other
Abdominal pain (5%)
Candidiasis (4%)
Chest pain (7%)
Cough (>3%)
Depression (1–3%)
Hypersensitivity
Infections
Myalgia/Myositis/Myopathy/Myotoxicity (4%)
Paresthesias (1–3%)
Upper respiratory infection (41%)
  (2006): Kesten S+, *Chest* 130(6), 1695

TIPRANAVIR

Trade name: Aptivus (Boehringer Ingelheim)
Indications: Antiretroviral treatment of HIV-1
Category: Protease inhibitor, HIV; Sulfonamide
Half-life: 4.8–6.0 hours
**Clinically important, potentially hazardous interactions
with:** amiodarone, bepridil, dihydroergotamine, ergotamine,
etravirine, flecainide, lovastatin, midazolam, pimozide,
propafenone, quinidine, rifampin, simvastatin, **St John's wort**,
triazolam

Reactions

Skin
Exanthems (<2%)
Herpes simplex (<2%)
Herpes zoster (<2%)
Pruritus (<2%)
Rash (sic) (2%)

Other
Asthenia (1.5%)
Cough (0.8%)
Depression (2%)
Fever (4.6%)
Headache (3.1%)
Hepatotoxicity (with ritonavir)
Hypersensitivity (<2%)
Lipoatrophy (<2%)
Lipodystrophy (<2%)
Lipohypertrophy (<2%)
Myalgia/Myositis/Myopathy/Myotoxicity (<2%)
Neurotoxicity (<2%)
Vertigo

TIROFIBAN

Trade name: Aggrastat (Merck)
Indications: Acute coronary syndrome
Category: Antiplatelet; Glycoprotein IIb / IIIa inhibitor
Half-life: 2 hours
**Clinically important, potentially hazardous interactions
with:** fondaparinux, NSAIDs

Reactions

Skin
Diaphoresis (2%)
Edema (2%)
Rash (sic) (<1%)
Urticaria (<1%)

TIXOCORTOL

Trade name: Rectovalone (not available in USA)
Indications: Infections, ulcerative colitis
Category: Corticosteroid
Half-life: N/A
**Clinically important, potentially hazardous interactions
with: live vaccines**

Reactions

Skin
Allergic reactions (sic)
  (2001): Devos SA+, *Contact Dermatitis* 44(6), 362
  (2001): Isaksson M, *Drug Saf* 24(5), 369
  (2000): Bircher AJ+, *Dermatology* 200(4), 349
  (2000): Isaksson M+, *Contact Dermatitis* 42(1), 27
  (2000): Jonker MJ+, *Contact Dermatitis* 42(6), 330
  (1999): Isaksson M+, *Am J Contact Dermat* 10(1), 31
  (1997): de Groot AC+, *Ned Tijdschr Geneeskd* 141(32), 1559
  (1996): Rasanen L+, *Br J Dermatol* 135(6), 931
  (1995): Bircher AJ+, *ORL J Otorhinolaryngol Relat Spec* 57(1), 54
  (1995): Lepoittevin JP+, *Arch Dermatol* 131(1), 31
  (1993): Fedler R+, *Hautarzt* 44(2), 91
  (1990): Bircher AJ, *Contact Dermatitis* 22(4), 237
  (1989): Dooms-Goossens AE+, *J Am Acad Dermatol* 21(3), 538
  (1988): Camarasa JG+, *Contact Dermatitis* 19(2), 147
Dermatitis
  (2006): Mimesh S+, *Dermatitis* 17(3), 137
  (2000): English JS, *Clin Exp Dermatol* 25(4), 261
  (2000): Isaksson M+, *Acta Derm Venereol* 80(1), 33
  (1998): Lutz ME+, *J Am Acad Dermatol* 38(5), 691
  (1997): Vestergaard L+, *Ugeskr Laeger* (Danish) 159, 5662
  (1984): Boujnah-Khouadja A+, *Contact Dermatitis* 11(2), 83
Eczema
  (1987): Foussereau J+, *Presse Med* 16(17), 832
Sensitivity
  (2000): Bircher AJ+, *Dermatology* 200(4), 349
  (1998): Gibson-Smith B+, *Contact Dermatitis* 38(6), 351

Mucosal/ENT
Stomatitis
  (1993): Callens A+, *Contact Dermatitis* 29(3), 161

Other
Hypersensitivity
  (2002): Le Coz CJ, *Ann Dermatol Venereol* 129(3), 348
  (1998): Khoo BP+, *Am J Contact Dermat* 9(2), 87
  (1998): Lutz ME+, *J Am Acad Dermatol* 38(5), 691
  (1996): Bircher AJ+, *Br J Dermatol* 135(2), 310
  (1995): Goldsmith PC+, *Contact Dermatitis* 33(6), 429
  (1993): Lauerma AI+, *Contact Dermatitis* 28(1), 10
  (1991): Lauerma AI, *Contact Dermatitis* 24(2), 123
  (1984): Boujnah-Khouadja AE+, *Contact Dermatitis* 11(2), 83 (6
    cases)

TIZANIDINE

Trade names: Sirdalud; Ternalax; Ternelin; Zanaflex (Acorda)
Indications: Muscle spasticity, multiple sclerosis
Category: Adrenergic alpha2-receptor agonist
Half-life: 2.5 hours
**Clinically important, potentially hazardous interactions
with:** ciprofloxacin, fluvoxamine, lisinopril, phenytoin, rofecoxib

Reactions

Skin
Acne (<1%)
Allergic reactions (sic) (<1%)
Cellulitis (<1%)
Diaphoresis (>1%)
Edema (<1%)
Exanthems (<1%)
Exfoliative dermatitis (<1%)

Herpes simplex (<1%)
Herpes zoster (<1%)
Pallor
  (2004): Tanaka H+, *No To Hattatsu* 36(6), 455
  (2000): Johnson TR+, *J Child Neurol* 15(12), 818 (with lisinopril)
Petechiae (<1%)
Pruritus (1–10%)
Purpura (<1%)
Rash (sic) (1–10%)
Ulcerations (>1%)
Urticaria (<1%)
Xerosis (<1%)

Mucosal/ENT
Vulvovaginal candidiasis (<1%)
Xerostomia (49%)
  (2004): Chou R+, *J Pain Symptom Manage* 28(2), 140
  (2002): Saper JR+, *Headache* 42(6), 470 (23%)
  (2000): Taricco M+, *Cochrane Database Syst Rev* (2), CD00
  (1997): Nance PW+, *Arch Neurol* 54(6), 731
  (1997): Wagstaff AJ+, *Drugs* 53(3), 435
  (1994): Iakhno NN+, *Ter Arkh* 66(10), 10
  (1994): Nance PW+, *Neurology* 44(11), S44
  (1994): Wallace JD, *Neurology* 44(11), S60
  (1992): Fogelholm R+, *Headache* 32(10), 509
  (1988): Bass B+, *Can J Neurol Sci* 15(1), 15
  (1987): Lapierre Y+, *Can J Neurol Sci* 14(3), 513
  (1987): Stien R+, *Acta Neurol Scand* 75(3), 190

Hair
Hair – alopecia (<1%)

Eyes
Visual hallucinations
  (1994): Wallace JD, *Neurology* 44(11), S60

Other
Asthenia
  (2002): Saper JR+, *Headache* 42(6), 470 (19%)
  (1997): Nance PW+, *Arch Neurol* 54(6), 731
  (1994): Nance PW+, *Neurology* 44(11), S44
  (1994): Wallace JD, *Neurology* 44(11), S60
Candidiasis (<1%)
Hepatotoxicity
  (1999): Afonso Perez+, *Med Clin* (Barc) 112(12), 478
  (1996): de Graaf+, *J Hepatol* 25(5), 772
Hypotension
  (2004): Kao CD+, *Ann Pharmacother* 38(11), 1840 (with lisinopril)
Paresthesias (>1%)
Tremor (1–10%)
Vertigo
  (1997): Nance PW+, *Arch Neurol* 54(6), 731
  (1994): Wallace JD, *Neurology* 44(11), S60

TOBRAMYCIN

Trade names: AKTob Ophthalmic; Oftalmotrisol-T; TOBI (Chiron); Tobra; TobraDex (Alcon); Tobrex
Indications: Various serious infections caused by susceptible organisms, superficial ocular infections
Category: Antibiotic, aminoglycoside
Half-life: 2–3 hours
Clinically important, potentially hazardous interactions with: adefovir, aldesleukin, aminoglycosides, atracurium, bumetanide, doxacurium, ethacrynic acid, furosemide, neuromuscular blockers, pancuronium, polypeptide antibiotics, rocuronium, succinylcholine, torsemide, vecuronium

Note: TobraDex is tobramycin and dexamethasone

Reactions

Skin
Eczema
Erythema multiforme
  (1983): Ansel J+, *Arch Dermatol* 119, 1006
Exanthems
  (2006): Garcia-Rubio I+, *J Investig Allergol Clin Immunol* 16(4), 264
  (2002): Spigarelli MG+, *Pediatr Pulmonol* 33(4), 311
  (1991): Karp S+, *Cutis* 47, 331
Exfoliative dermatitis
  (1991): Karp S+, *Cutis* 47, 331
Photo-recall
  (2001): Krishnan RS I, *J Am Acad Dermatol* 44, 1045 (ultraviolet) (with piperacillin & ciprofloxacin)
Pruritus (<1%)
Purpura
Rash (sic) (<1%)
  (2002): Spigarelli MG+, *Pediatr Pulmonol* 33(4), 311
Side effects (sic)
Urticaria

Mucosal/ENT
Sialorrhea
Tinnitus
  (2002): *Prescrire Int* 11(62), 177

Eyes
Blepharitis
  (2005): Gonzalez-Mendiola MR+, *Allergy* 60(4), 527
Conjunctivitis
  (2005): Gonzalez-Mendiola MR+, *Allergy* 60(4), 527
Eyelid dermatitis (<1%)
  (2002): Litt JZ, Beachwood, OH (personal observation)
  (1998): Litt JZ, Beachwood, OH (personal case) (observation)
  (1995): Caraffini S+, *Contact Dermatitis* 32, 186
  (1990): Menendez Ramos F+, *Contact Dermatitis* 22, 305
Eyelid edema (from ophthalmic preparations) (<1%)

Other
Cough
  (2005): Scheinberg P+, *Chest* 127(4), 1420
Headache
Hepatotoxicity
  (2007): Nisly SA+, *Ann Pharmacother* 41(12), 2061
Hypersensitivity
  (2007): Santos RP+, *BMC Pediatr* 7, 11
  (2002): Spigarelli MG+, *Pediatr Pulmonol* 33(4), 311
  (1995): Schretlen-Doherty JS+, *Ann Pharmacother* 29, 704
Injection-site pain

Nephrotoxicity
  (2006): Cannella CA+, *Am J Health Syst Pharm* 63(19), 1858
  (2006): Izquierdo MJ+, *Clin Nephrol* 66(6), 464
  (2006): Laporta R+, *J Heart Lung transplant* 25(5), 608
  (2006): Patrick BN+, *Ann Pharmacother* 40(11), 2037
  (1996): Prins JM+, *Antimicrob Agents Chemother* 40(11), 2494
Paresthesias (<1%)
Tremor (<1%)

TOCAINIDE

Trade name: Tonocard (AstraZeneca)
Indications: Ventricular arrhythmias
Category: Antiarrhythmic class 1B
Half-life: 11–14 hours

Reactions

Skin
Allergic reactions (sic)
  (1987): Arrowsmith JB+, *Ann Intern Med* 107, 693
  (1985): Coulter DM+, *N Z Med J* 98, 553
Clammy skin
Diaphoresis (<1%)
Erythema multiforme (<1%)
Exanthems
  (1988): Dunn JM+, *Drug Intell Clin Pharm* 22, 142
Exfoliative dermatitis (<1%)
Lupus erythematosus (<1%)
  (1994): Gelfand MS+, *South Med J* 87, 839
  (1988): Oliphant LD+, *Chest* 94, 427
Pallor (<1%)
Pruritus (<1%)
Rash (sic) (0.5–8.4%)
Stevens–Johnson syndrome (<1%)
Vasculitis (<1%)

Mucosal/ENT
Dysgeusia (8.4%)
Gingivitis
  (1988): Dunn JM+, *Drug Intell Clin Pharm* 22, 142
Parosmia (<1%)
Stomatitis (<1%)
Tinnitus
Xerostomia (<1%)

Hair
Hair – alopecia (<1%)

Other
Congestive heart failure
  (1989): Ravid S+, *J Am Coll Cardiol* 14(5), 1326
Headache
Hypersensitivity (<1%)
Myalgia/Myositis/Myopathy/Myotoxicity (<1%)
Paresthesias (3.5–9%)

TOCILIZUMAB

Trade name: Actemra (Roche)
Indications: Rheumatoid arthritis, Juvenile idiopathic arthritis, Castleman's disease
Category: Anti-interleukin-6 receptor monoclonal antibody

Reactions

Other
Anaphylactoid reactions/Anaphylaxis
  (2008): Yokota S+, *Lancet* 371(9617), 998
Asthenia
Cardiac failure
Headache
Hypersensitivity
Hypertension
Infections
  (2008): Smolen JS+, *Lancet* 371, 987
  (2007): Nishimoto N+, *Ann Rheum Dis* 66(9), 1162
  (2006): Ding C+, *Rev Recent Clin Trials* 1(3), 193
Nephrotoxicity
  (2007): Matsuyama M+, *Intern Med* 46(11), 771
Upper respiratory infection

TOLAZAMIDE

Trade names: Diabewas; Diadutos; Norglycin; Tolanase; Tolinase (Pfizer); Tolisan
Indications: Non-insulin dependent diabetes type II
Category: Sulfonylurea
Half-life: 7 hours
Clinically important, potentially hazardous interactions with: phenylbutazones

Note: Tolazamide is a sulfonamide and can be absorbed systemically. Sulfonamides can produce severe, possibly fatal, reactions such as toxic epidermal necrolysis and Stevens–Johnson syndrome

Reactions

Skin
Dermatitis
Diaphoresis
Eczema
  (1985): Frosch PJ+, *Contact Dermatitis* 13, 272
Erythema (0.4%)
Exanthems (0.4%)
Lichenoid eruption
  (1990): Franz CB+, *J Am Acad Dermatol* 22, 128
  (1984): Barnett JH+, *Cutis* 34, 542
Lupus erythematosus
Photosensitivity (1–10%)
Pruritus (0.4%)
Purpura
Rash (sic) (1–10%)
Urticaria (1–10%)

Mucosal/ENT
Dysgeusia
Tongue ulceration
  (1984): Barnett JH+, *Cutis* 34, 542

Other
Hepatotoxicity

(1985): Nakao NL+, *Gastroenterology* 89(1), 192
(1980): Bridges ME+, *South Med J* 73(8), 1072
Paresthesias
Porphyria cutanea tarda

TOLAZOLINE

Trade name: Priscoline (Novartis)
Indications: Pulmonary hypertension in the newborn
Category: Sulfonylurea
Half-life: 3–10 hours (neonates)
Clinically important, potentially hazardous interactions with: cimetidine

Reactions

Skin
Dermatitis
  (1985): Frosch PJ+, *Contact Dermatitis* 13, 272
Edema
Exanthems
  (1989): Cambazard F+, *Ann Dermatol Venereol* (French) 116, 499
Rash (sic)
Urticaria

Other
Injection-site burning (>10%)

TOLBUTAMIDE

Trade names: Abemin; Aglycid; Diaben; Diatol; Dolipol; Mobenol; Novo-Butamid; Orabet; Orinase (Pfizer); Rastinon
Indications: Non-insulin dependent diabetes type II
Category: Sulfonylurea
Half-life: 4–25 hours
Clinically important, potentially hazardous interactions with: aprepitant, phenylbutazones, prednisone

Note: Tolbutamide is a sulfonamide and can be absorbed systemically. Sulfonamides can produce severe, possibly fatal, reactions such as toxic epidermal necrolysis and Stevens–Johnson syndrome

Reactions

Skin
Allergic reactions (sic) (<1%)
Bullous dermatitis (<1%)
Bullous pemphigoid
Dermatitis
  (1982): Fisher AA, *Cutis* 29, 551 (systemic)
Erythema (1.1%)
Erythema multiforme (<1%)
Exanthems (1–5%)
Fixed eruption (<1%)
Lichenoid eruption
Photosensitivity (1–10%)
  (1984): Kar PK+, *J Indian Med Assoc* 82, 289
Poikiloderma
Pruritus (1.1%)
Purpura
Rash (sic) (1–10%)

Side effects (sic) (1%)
Toxic epidermal necrolysis (<1%)
Urticaria (1–10%)

Mucosal/ENT
Dysgeusia
Oral lichenoid eruption

Other
Disulfiram-like reaction
Headache
Hypersensitivity (<1%)
Injection-site thrombophlebitis (<1%)
Paresthesias
Porphyria
Porphyria cutanea tarda
Thrombophlebitis (<1%)

TOLCAPONE

Trade name: Tasmar (Roche)
Indications: Parkinsonism
Category: Catechol-O-methyl transferase inhibitor
Half-life: 2–3 hours

Reactions

Skin
Allergic reactions (sic) (<1%)
Burning (2%)
Cellulitis (<1%)
Diaphoresis (7%)
Eczema (<1%)
Edema (<1%)
Erythema multiforme (<1%)
Facial edema (<1%)
Fungal dermatitis (<1%)
Furunculosis (<1%)
Herpes simplex (<1%)
Herpes zoster (<1%)
Pigmentation (<1%)
Pruritus (<1%)
Rash (sic) (<1%)
Seborrhea (<1%)
Urticaria (<1%)
Vitiligo
  (1999): Sabate M+, *Ann Pharmacother* 33, 1228 (with levodopa)

Mucosal/ENT
Oral ulceration (<1%)
Parosmia (<1%)
Sialorrhea (<1%)
Tongue disorder (<1%)
Vaginitis (<1%)
Xerostomia (5%)

Hair
Hair – alopecia (1%)

Other
Abdominal pain
  (1998): Hauser RA+, *Mov Disord* 13(4), 643 (12%)
Death
  (2006): *Prescrire Int* 15(82), 54
  (2004): Deane KH+, *Cochrane Database Syst Rev* exam(4), CD00
  (2003): Borges N, *Drug Saf* 26(11), 743

(2000): Lambert D+, *Drugs Aging* 16(1), 55
Headache
  (1998): Hauser RA+, *Mov Disord* 13(4), 643 (12%)
Hepatotoxicity
  (2006): *Prescrire Int* 15(82), 54
  (2006): Leegwater-Kim J+, *Expert Opin Pharmacother*
    7(16), 2263
  (2005): Borges N, *Expert Opin Drug Saf* 4(1), 69
  (2005): Korri H+, *Rev Neurol* (Paris) 161(11), 1113
  (2003): Benabou R+, *Expert Opin Drug Saf* 2(3), 263
  (2003): Borges N, *Drug Saf* 26(11), 743
  (2000): Kaakkola S, *Drugs* 59(6), 1233
  (2000): Olanow CW, *Arch Neurol* 57(2), 263
  (2000): Spahr L+, *Dig Dis Sci* 45(9), 1881
  (2000): Watkins P, *Neurology* 55(11), S51
Hypotension
  (1999): Micek ST+, *Am J Health Syst Pharm* 56(21), 2195
Myalgia/Myositis/Myopathy/Myotoxicity (<1%)
Paresthesias (3%)
Rhabdomyolysis
  (2000): Kaakkola S, *Drugs* 59(6), 1233
  (1999): Micek ST+, *Am J Health Sys Pharm* 56(21), 2195
Tumors (1%)
Vertigo
  (1999): Micek ST+, *Am J Health Syst Pharm* 56(21), 2195
  (1998): Hauser RA+, *Mov Disord* 13(4), 643 (12%)

TOLMETIN

Trade names: Donison; Midocil; Novo-Tolmetin; Reutol;
Safitex; Tolectin (Ortho-McNeil)
Indications: Arthritis
Category: Non-steroidal anti-inflammatory
Half-life: 1–2 hours
**Clinically important, potentially hazardous interactions
with:** methotrexate

Reactions

Skin
Angioedema (<1%)
  (1994): Shapiro N, *J Oral Maxillofac Surg* 52, 626
  (1985): Ponte CD+, *Drug Intell Clin Pharm* 19, 479
Bullous dermatitis
Diaphoresis
Edema (3–9%)
Erythema multiforme (<1%)
Exanthems (9%)
  (1985): Bigby M+, *J Am Acad Dermatol* 12, 866
  (1984): Stern RS+, *JAMA* 252, 1433
  (1981): Reimer GW, *S Afr Med J* 60, 843
Photosensitivity
  (1993): Shelley WB+, *Cutis* 52, 201 (observation)
Pruritus (1–10%)
  (1985): Bigby M+, *J Am Acad Dermatol* 12, 866
  (1981): Reimer GW, *S Afr Med J* 60, 843
Purpura
  (1984): Stern RS+, *JAMA* 252, 1433
Rash (sic) (>10%)
Stevens–Johnson syndrome (<1%)
Toxic epidermal necrolysis (<1%)
  (1992): Breathnach SM+, *Adverse Drug Reactions and the Skin*
    Blackwell, Oxford, 191 (passim)
  (1985): Bigby M+, *J Am Acad Dermatol* 12, 866
  (1984): Stern RS+, *JAMA* 252, 1433

Urticaria (1–5%)
  (1985): Bigby M+, *J Am Acad Dermatol* 12, 866
  (1985): Ponte CD+, *Drug Intell Clin Pharm* 19, 479
  (1984): Stern RS+, *JAMA* 252, 1433
  (1980): Ahmad S, *N Engl J Med* 303, 1417

Mucosal/ENT
Aphthous stomatitis
Dysgeusia
Gingival ulceration
Glossitis (<1%)
Oral ulceration
Stomatitis (<1%)
Tinnitus
Xerostomia

Other
Anaphylactoid reactions/Anaphylaxis
  (1985): Bretza JA+, *Western J Med* 143, 55
  (1985): O'Brien WM, *J Rheumatol* 12, 13
  (1983): Paulus HE, *Arthritis Rheum* 26, 1397
  (1982): Rossi AC+, *N Engl J Med* 307, 499
  (1980): Ahmad S, *N Engl J Med* 303, 1417
  (1980): McCall CY+, *JAMA* 243, 1263
Aseptic meningitis
  (1981): Ruppert GB+, *JAMA* 245(1), 67
Gynecomastia
Headache
Hot flashes (<1%)
Myalgia/Myositis/Myopathy/Myotoxicity
Serum sickness (<1%)

TOLTERODINE

Trade name: Detrol (Pfizer)
Indications: Urinary incontinence
Category: Muscarinic antagonist
Half-life: 2–4 hours
**Clinically important, potentially hazardous interactions
with:** ketoconazole, warfarin

Reactions

Skin
Erythema (1.9%)
Fungal dermatitis (1.1%)
Pruritus (1.3%)
Rash (sic) (1.9%)
Xerosis (1.7%)

Mucosal/ENT
Xerostomia (40%)
  (2007): Yang Y+, *Chin Med J* (Engl) 120(5), 370
  (2006): Anderson RU+, *Int Urogynecol J Pelvic Floor Dysfunct*
    17(5), 502
  (2006): Nitti VW+, *BJU Int* 97(6), 1262 (9%)
  (2006): Roehrborn CG+, *BJU Int* 97(5), 1003 (16%)
  (2005): Armstrong RB+, *Int Urol Nephrol* 37(2), 247 (21%)
  (2004): Chapple CR+, *BJU Int* 93(3), 303 (18%)
  (2004): Ethans KD+, *J Spinal Cord Med* 27(3), 214
  (2003): Homma Y+, *BJU Int* 92(7), 741 (33.5%)
  (2002): Zinner NR+, *J Am Geriatr Soc* 50(5), 799
  (2001): Crandall C, *J Womens Health Gend Based Med* 10(8), 735
  (2001): Harvey MA+, *Am J Obstet Gynecol* 185(1), 56
  (2001): Jacquetin B+, *Eur J Obstet Gynecol Reprod Biol* 98(1), 97
  (2001): Layton D+, *Drug Saf* 24(9), 703

(2001): Malone-Lee J+, *J Urol* 165(5), 1452 (37%)
(2001): Olsson B+, *Clin Pharmacokinet* 40(3), 227
(2001): Van Kerrebroeck+, *Urology* 57(3), 414
(1999): Drutz HP+, *Int Urogynecol J Pelvic Floor Dysfunct* 10, 283
(1999): Millard R+, *J Urol* 161, 1551
(1999): Ruscin JM+, *Ann Pharmacother* 33, 1073
(1997): Appell RA, *Urology* 50, 90
(1997): Jonas U+, *World J Urol* 15, 144 (9%)

Other
Abdominal pain
    (2001): Layton D+, *Drug Saf* 24(9), 703
Asthenia
    (2001): Layton D+, *Drug Saf* 24(9), 703
Headache
    (2001): Layton D+, *Drug Saf* 24(9), 703
Paresthesias (1.1%)
Upper respiratory infection (5.9%)
Vertigo
    (2006): Roehrborn CG+, *BJU Int* 97(5), 1003 (5%)

TOPIRAMATE

Trade name: Topamax (Ortho-McNeil)
Indications: Partial onset seizures
Category: Anticonvulsant; Mood stabilizer
Half-life: 21 hours

Reactions

Skin
Acne (>1%)
Basal cell carcinoma (<1%)
Dermatitis (<1%)
Diaphoresis (1.8%)
Eczema (<1%)
Edema (1.8%)
Exanthems (<1%)
    (2003): Warnock JK+, *Am J Clin Dermatol* 4(1), 21
Facial edema (<1%)
    (2002): Nieto-Barrera M+, *Rev Neurol* 34(2), 114
Folliculitis (<1%)
Oligohydrosis
    (2003): Ben-Zeev B+, *J Child Neurol* 18(4), 254
Palmar erythema
    (2007): Serrao R+, *Am J Clin Dermatol* 8(6), 347
    (2004): Scheinfeld N+, *J Drugs Dermatol* 3(3), 321
Photosensitivity (<1%)
Pigmentation (<1%)
Pruritus (1.8%)
    (2003): Ochoa JG, *Seizure* 12(7), 516
Purpura (<1%)
Rash (sic) (4.4%)
    (2007): Arif H+, *Neurology* 68(20), 1701
Seborrhea (<1%)
Urticaria (<1%)
Xerosis (<1%)

Mucosal/ENT
Ageusia (<1%)
Bromhidrosis (1.8%)
Dysgeusia (>1%)
    (2004): Krymchantowski AV+, *Arq Neuropsiquiatr* 62(1), 91
        (12%)
    (2003): Edwards KR+, *CNS Spectr* 8(6), 428
    (2001): Storey JR+, *Headache* 41(10), 968

Gingival hyperplasia/hypertrophy (<1%)
Gingivitis (1.8%)
Parosmia (<1%)
Sialorrhea
    (2001): Buck ML, *Pediatr Pharmacol* 7 (4–5%)
Stomatitis (<1%)
Tongue edema (<1%)
Vaginitis
Xerostomia (2.7%)

Hair
Hair – abnormal texture (<1%)
Hair – alopecia (>1%)
    (2002): Chuang Y-C+, *Dermatology Psychosomatics* 3, 183

Nails
Nails – changes (sic) (<1%)

Eyes
Glaucoma
    (2005): Bhattacharyya KB+, *Neurol India* 253(1), 108
    (2004): Craig JE+, *Am J Ophthalmol* 137(1), 193
    (2004): Fraunfelder FW+, *Ophthalmology* 111(1), 109 (86 cases)
    (2004): Hilton EJ+, *Seizure* 13(2), 113
    (2003): Boentert M+, *Neurology* 61(9), 1306
Myopia
    (2005): Bhattacharyya KB+, *Neurol India* 53(1), 108
    (2004): *Prescrire Int* 13(73), 165
    (2004): Craig JE+, *Am J Ophthalmol* 137(1), 193
    (2004): Fraunfelder FW+, *Ophthalmology* 111(1), 109 (17 cases)
    (2003): Boentert M+, *Neurology* 61(9), 1306
Ocular hypertension
    (2004): *Prescrire Int* 13(73), 165
Periorbital edema
    (2004): Fraunfelder FW+, *Ophthalmology* 111(1), 109 (3 cases)
Scleritis
    (2004): Fraunfelder FW+, *Ophthalmology* 111(1), 109 (4 cases)
Uveitis
    (2005): Cano Parra J+, *Arch Soc Esp Oftalmol* 80(3), 137
Vision blurred
    (2004): Fraunfelder FW+, *Ophthalmology* 111(1), 109

Other
Anhidrosis
    (2005): Grosso S+, *Seizure* 14(3), 183
    (2004): *Prescrire Int* 13(73), 165
Asthenia
    (2008): Zaccara G+, *Seizure* nd, 182
    (2004): Brandes JL+, *JAMA* 291(8), 965
    (2003): Dodson WE+, *Ann Pharmacother* 37(5), 615
Dementia
    (2007): Sommer BR+, *Expert Opin Drug Saf* 6(2), 133
Depression
    (2007): Mula M+, *Drug Saf* 30(7), 555 (~10%)
    (2004): Krymchantowski AV+, *Arq Neuropsiquiatr* 62(1), 91
        (18%)
    (2003): Mula M+, *Epilepsia* 44(12), 1573
    (2001): Klufas A+, *Am J Psychiatry* 158(10), 1736
Gynecomastia (8.3%)
Hot flashes (1–10%)
Myalgia/Myositis/Myopathy/Myotoxicity
Paresthesias (15%)
    (2007): Delpirou-Nouh C+, *Headache*
    (2005): Silberstein SD+, *Clin Ther* 27(2), 154
    (2004): Brandes JL+, *JAMA* 291(8), 965
    (2004): Krymchantowski AV+, *Arq Neuropsiquiatr* 62(1), 91
        (39%)
    (2004): Wilding J+, *Int J Obes Relat Metab Disord* 28(11), 1399
    (2003): Edwards KR+, *CNS Spectr* 8(6), 428

(2002): Appolinario JC+, *Can J Psychiatry* 47(3), 271
(2002): Mathew NT+, *Headache* 42(8), 796 (12%)
(2002): Silberstein SD, *Headache* 42(1), 85
(2002): Young WB+, *Cephalalgia* 22(8), 659
(2001): Chengappa KN+, *Bipolar Disord* 3(5), 215
(2001): Ghaemi SN+, *Ann Clin Psychiatry* 13(4), 185
(2001): Storey JR+, *Headache* 41(10), 968
(1999): Glauser TA, *Epilepsia* 40, S71
Seizures
    (2003): Ben-Zeev B+, *J Child Neurol* 18(4), 254
Somnambulism
    (2003): Varkey BM+, *Indian J Med Sci* 57(11), 508
Somnolence
    (2008): Zaccara G+, *Seizure* nd, 182
Tremor (>10%)
Vertigo (6%)
    (2008): Zaccara G+, *Seizure* nd, 182
    (2003): Dodson WE+, *Ann Pharmacother* 37(5), 615
    (2002): Mathew NT+, *Headache* 42(8), 796 (6%)
Weight loss
    (2007): Ben-Menachem, *Epilepsia* 48, 42
    (2005): Ness-Abramof R+, *Drugs Today* (Barc) 41(8), 547

TOPOTECAN

Synonyms: hycamptamine; SKF 104864; TOPO; TPT
Trade name: Hycamtin (GSK)
Indications: Metastatic ovarian carcinoma
Category: Topoisomerase 1 inhibitor
Half-life: 3 hours

Reactions

Skin
Allergic reactions (sic)
    (2004): Denschlag D+, *Anticancer Res* 24(2C), 1267
Erythema (<1%)
Fixed eruption (cellulitis-like)
    (2002): Senturk N+, *J Eur Acad Dermatol Venereol* 16(4), 414
Neutrophilic eccrine hidradenitis
    (2002): Marini M+, *J Dermatolog Treat* 13(1), 35
Purpura (<1%)
Scleroderma
    (2002): Ene-Stroescu D+, *Arthritis Rheum* 46(3), 844

Mucosal/ENT
Mucositis
    (2001): Seiter K+, *Leuk Lymphoma* 42(5), 963
Stomatitis (24%)
    (2007): Garst J, *Expert Opin Drug Saf* 6(1), 53
    (2004): Daw NC+, *J Clin Oncol* 22(5), 829

Hair
Hair – alopecia (59%)
    (2007): Garst J, *Expert Opin Drug Saf* 6(1), 53
    (2001): Clarke-Pearson DL+, *J Clin Oncol* 19(19), 3967
    (2001): Gore M+, *Br J Cancer* 84(8), 1043
    (2001): Mobus V+, *Anticancer Res* 21(5), 3551
    (1999): Ormrod D+, *Drugs* 58, 533

Nails
Nails – pigmentation
    (2004): Baykal Y+, *J Dermatol* 31(11), 951

Other
Abdominal pain
    (2007): Garst J, *Expert Opin Drug Saf* 6(1), 53

Asthenia
    (2007): Garst J, *Expert Opin Drug Saf* 6(1), 53
Death
    (2004): Anand A+, *Clin Oncol (R Coll Radiol)* 16(8), 543 (1 case)
    (2004): Vaena DA+, *Leuk Res* 28(1), 49 (3 cases)
    (2002): Miller DS+, *Gynecol Oncol* 87(3), 247
    (2001): Seiter K+, *Leuk Lymphoma* 42(5), 963
Fever
    (2007): Garst J, *Expert Opin Drug Saf* 6(1), 53
    (2003): Blaney SM+, *J Clin Oncol* 21(1), 143
Headache
    (2003): Blaney SM+, *J Clin Oncol* 21(1), 143
Infections
    (2004): Vaena DA+, *Leuk Res* 28(1), 49 (4 cases)
Nephrotoxicity
    (2006): Garst J+, *Clin Drug Investig* 26(5), 257 (1 case)
Pain
    (2007): Garst J, *Expert Opin Drug Saf* 6(1), 53
Paresthesias (9%)

TOREMIFENE

Trade name: Fareston (Shire)
Indications: Metastatic breast cancer
Category: Selective estrogen receptor modulator (SERM)
Half-life: ~5 days

Reactions

Skin
Dermatitis
Diaphoresis (20%)
    (1997): Wiseman LR+, *Drugs* 54, 141
    (1990): Valavaara R+, *J Steroid Biochem* 36, 229
Edema (5%)
    (1997): Wiseman LR+, *Drugs* 54, 141
Pigmentation
Pruritus

Eyes
Cataract
    (2003): Parkkari M+, *Acta Ophthalmol Scand* 81(5), 495 (6%)
Maculopathy
    (2003): Parkkari M+, *Acta Ophthalmol Scand* 81(5), 495
Ocular allergy (sic)
    (2003): Parkkari M+, *Acta Ophthalmol Scand* 81(5), 495

Other
Headache
Hot flashes (35%)
    (1997): Wiseman LR+, *Drugs* 54, 141
Thrombophlebitis (1%)

TORSEMIDE

Trade names: Demadex (Roche); Unat
Indications: Edema
Category: Diuretic, loop
Half-life: 2–4 hours
**Clinically important, potentially hazardous interactions
with:** amikacin, aminoglycosides, gentamicin, kanamycin,
neomycin, streptomycin, tobramycin

Note: Torsemide is a sulfonamide and can be absorbed systemically. Sulfonamides can produce severe, possibly fatal, reactions such as toxic epidermal necrolysis and Stevens–Johnson syndrome

Reactions

Skin
Angioedema
Edema (1.1%)
Exanthems
Lichenoid eruption
  (1997): Byrd DR+, *Mayo Clin Proc* 72, 930 (photosensitive)
Photosensitivity (1–10%)
Pruritus
Purpura
  (1998): Sanfelix Genoves J+, *Aten Primaria* (Spanish) 21, 252
Rash (sic) (<1%)
Stevens–Johnson syndrome
  (1997): Billon S, *The Schoch Letter* 47, 32 (obervation)
Urticaria (1–10%)
Vasculitis
  (1998): Palop-Larrea V+, *Lancet* 352, 1909
  (1998): Sanfelix Genoves J+, *Aten Primaria* (Spanish) 21, 252

Mucosal/ENT
Tinnitus
Xerostomia

Other
Abdominal pain
  (2006): Calvo C+, *Med Clin* (Barc) 127(19), 721
Headache
Injection-site erythema (<1%)
Myalgia/Myositis/Myopathy/Myotoxicity (1.6%)
Pseudoporphyria
  (2008): Perez-Bustillo+, *Arch Dermatol* 144(6), 812

TOSITUMOMAB & IODINE131sup

Trade names: Bexxar (Corixa) (GSK); Iodine131sup I-Tositumomab (MDS Nordion); Tositumomab
Indications: Non-Hodgkin lymphoma
Category: Antineoplastic; Monoclonal antibody
Half-life: 8.04 days
Clinically important, potentially hazardous interactions with: None

Reactions

Skin
Allergic reactions (sic)
Angioedema
Carcinoma (skin)
Diaphoresis (8%)
Peripheral edema (9%)
Pruritus
Rash (sic) (17%)

Mucosal/ENT
Rhinitis (10%)

Other
Abdominal pain (15%)
Anaphylactoid reactions/Anaphylaxis
Chest pain (7%)

Chills (29%)
Cough (21%)
Fever (37%)
Headache (16%)
Hypersensitivity
Infections (21%)
Myalgia/Myositis/Myopathy/Myotoxicity (13%)
  (2006): Buchegger F+, *Br J Cancer* 94(12), 1770
  (2006): Visser OJ+, *BioDrugs* 20(4), 201
Pain (19%)
Serum sickness
Vertigo (5%)

TRAGACANTH GUM

Scientific names: *Astragalus gossypinus; Astragalus gummifer*
Family: Fabaceae; Leguminosae
Trade and other common names: E413; Goat's Thorn; Gummi Tragacanthae; Hog Gum
Category: Food additive; Laxative
Purported indications and other uses: Diarrhea. Ingredient in pharmaceuticals, foods, toothpaste, denture adhesives, emulsifier, binding agent, demulcent, stabilizer
Half-life: N/A

Reactions

None

TRAMADOL

Trade names: Contramal; Tadol; Tradol; Tramal; Tramed; Tramol; Tridol; Ultracet (Ortho-McNeil); Ultram (Ortho-McNeil); Zipan
Indications: Pain
Category: Opiate agonist
Half-life: 6–7 hours
Clinically important, potentially hazardous interactions with: citalopram, desflurane, desvenlafaxine, fluoxetine, fluvoxamine, MAO inhibitors, nefazodone, phenelzine, tranylcypromine, venlafaxine

Reactions

Skin
Allergic reactions (sic) (<1%)
Angioedema
  (2005): Hallberg P+, *Eur J Clin Pharmacol* 60(12), 901
  (1996): Kind B+, *Schweiz Med Wochenschr* (German) 85, 567
Diaphoresis (9%)
  (2006): Mattia C+, *Expert Opin Pharmacother* 7(13), 1811
  (2004): Houlihan DJ, *Ann Pharmacother* 38(3), 411
Exanthems
  (1999): Ghislain PD+, *Ann Dermatol Venereol* (French) 126, 38
Nodular eruption
  (2006): Coskun HS+, *J Eur Acad Dermatol Venereol* 20(8), 1008
Pruritus (<10%)
  (2002): Finkel JC+, *Anesth Analg* 94(6), 1469 (7%)
  (1999): Ghislain PD+, *Ann Dermatol Venereol* (French) 126, 38
Rash (sic) (1–5%)
  (2002): Finkel JC+, *Anesth Analg* 94(6), 1469
Shivering

(2004): Houlihan DJ, *Ann Pharmacother* 38(3), 411
Toxic dermatitis (sic)
  (1999): Ghislain PD+, *Ann Dermatol Venereol* (French) 126, 38
Urticaria (1–18%)
  (2003): Asero R, *J Investig Allergol Clin Immunol* 13(1), 56 (18%)

Mucosal/ENT
Dysgeusia (<1%)
Stomatitis
Xerostomia (10%)
  (2004): Gotrick B+, *J Dent Res* 83(5), 393
  (2003): Jarernsiripornkul N+, *Eur J Pain* 7(3), 219

Eyes
Mydriasis
  (2004): Houlihan DJ, *Ann Pharmacother* 38(3), 411
Visual hallucinations
  (2007): Huang SS+, *J Formos Med Assoc* 106(4), 323

Other
Anaphylactoid reactions/Anaphylaxis
  (1999): Moore PA, *J Am Dent Assoc* 130, 1075
Asthenia
  (2007): Rodriguez RF+, *J Palliat Med* 10(1), 56
Death
  (2007): Gholami K+, *Pharmacoepidemiol Drug Saf* 16(2), 229
  (2001): Musshoff F+, *Forensic Sci Int* 116(2), 197
Fever
  (2004): Houlihan DJ, *Ann Pharmacother* 38(3), 411
Headache
  (2006): Gana TJ+, *Curr Med Res* 22(7), 1391
  (2006): Mattia C+, *Expert Opin Pharmacother* 7(13), 1811
Paresthesias (<1%)
Seizures
  (2005): Labate A+, *Med J Aust* 182(1), 42
  (2003): Koussa S+, *Rev Neurol* (Paris) 159(11), 1053
Tremor (5–10%)
Vertigo
  (2007): Rodriguez RF+, *J Palliat Med* 10(1), 56
  (2006): Gana TJ+, *Curr Med Res Opin* 22(7), 1391
  (2006): Hair PI+, *Drugs* 66(15), 2017
  (2006): Mattia C+, *Expert Opin Pharmacother* 7(13), 1811

TRANDOLAPRIL

Trade names: Gopten; Mavik (Abbott); Odrik; Tarka (Abbott); Udrik
Indications: Hypertension
Category: Angiotensin-converting enzyme inhibitor
Half-life: 24 hours
Clinically important, potentially hazardous interactions with: amiloride, spironolactone, triamterene

Note: Tarka is trandolapril and verapamil

Reactions

Skin
Angioedema (0.15%)
  (2001): Cohen EG+, *Ann Otol Rhinol Laryngol* 110(8), 701 (64 cases)
  (1996): *Med Lett Drugs Ther* 38, 104
Edema (>3%)
Pemphigus (<1%)
Pemphigus foliaceus
  (2000): Ong CS+, *Australas J Dermatol* 41(4), 242
Pruritus (>3%)

Rash (sic) (>10%)

Mucosal/ENT
Xerostomia (>3%)

Other
Asthenia
  (2003): Guay DR, *Clin Ther* 25(3), 713 (with verapamil)
Cough
  (2007): Tytus RH+, *Clin Ther* 29(2), 305
  (2003): Guay DR, *Clin Ther* 25(3), 713 (with verapamil)
  (2001): Adigun AQ+, *West Afr J Med* 20(1), 46–7
  (2001): Lee SC+, *Hypertension* 38(2), 166
Headache
  (2007): Tytus RH+, *Clin Ther* 29(2), 305
Myalgia/Myositis/Myopathy/Myotoxicity (>3%)
Paresthesias (>3%)
Rhabdomyolysis
  (2000): Gokel Y+, *Am J Emerg Med* 18(6), 738 (with verapamil)
Vertigo
  (2003): Guay DR, *Clin Ther* 25(3), 713 (with verapamil)

TRANYLCYPROMINE

Trade names: Parnate; Siciton
Indications: Depression
Category: Antidepressant; Monoamine oxidase (MAO) inhibitor
Half-life: 2.5 hours
Clinically important, potentially hazardous interactions with: amitriptyline, amoxapine, amphetamines, bupropion, citalopram, clomipramine, cyproheptadine, desipramine, dextroamphetamine, dextromethorphan, diethylpropion, dopamine, doxepin, entacapone, ephedrine, epinephrine, fluoxetine, fluvoxamine, imipramine, levodopa, mazindol, meperidine, methamphetamine, nefazodone, nortriptyline, paroxetine, phendimetrazine, phentermine, phenylephrine, phenylpropanolamine, protriptyline, pseudoephedrine, rizatriptan, sertraline, sibutramine, sumatriptan, sympathomimetics, tramadol, tricyclic antidepressants, trimipramine, **tryptophan**, **tyramine-containing foods**, venlafaxine, zolmitriptan

Note: Tyramine-containing foods include the following: aged cheeses, avocados, banana skins, bologna and other processed luncheon meats, chicken livers, chocolate, figs, canned pickled herring, meat extracts, pepperoni, raisins, raspberries, soy sauce, vermouth, sherry and red wines

Reactions

Skin
Diaphoresis
Edema (<1%)
Exanthems
Peripheral edema
Photosensitivity (<1%)
Pruritus
Rash (sic) (<1%)
Urticaria

Mucosal/ENT
Tinnitus
Tongue black
Xerostomia (<1%)

Other

Headache

Paresthesias

Rhabdomyolysis

(2002): Lappa A+, *Intensive Care Med* 28(7), 976 (with trifluoperazine)

Tremor

Vertigo

(2004): Birkenhager TK+, *J Clin Psychiatry* 65(11), 1505

TRASTUZUMAB

Trade name: Herceptin (Genentech)
Indications: Metastatic breast cancer
Category: Antineoplastic; HER2 antagonist
Half-life: 5.8 days

Reactions

Skin

Acne (2%)

(2004): Jacot W+, *Br J Dermatol* 151(1), 238

Allergic reactions (sic) (3%)

Angioedema (<1%)

Cellulitis (<1%)

Diaphoresis

(1999): Dillman RO, *Cancer Metastasis Rev* 18(4), 465

Edema (8%)

Hand–foot syndrome

(2007): Bartsch R+, *J Clin Oncol* 25(25), 3853 (with capecitabine)

(2000): Merimsky O+, *Isr Med Assoc* 2(10), 786

Herpes simplex (2%)

Herpes zoster (~1%)

Peripheral edema (10%)

Photosensitivity

(2005): Cohen AD+, *J Dermatolog Treat* 16(1), 19 (with paclitaxel)

Rash (sic) (18%)

(2001): Vogel CL+, *Oncology* 61, 37

(1999): Dillman RO, *Cancer Metastasis Rev* 18(4), 465

Ulcerations (~1%)

Mucosal/ENT

Stomatitis (<1%)

Hair

Hair – alopecia

(2003): Leyland-Jones B+, *J Clin Oncol* 21(21), 3965 (with paclitaxel)

Nails

Nails – dystrophy

(2006): Alexandrescu DT+, *Int J Dermatol* 45(11), 1334 (with docetaxel)

Other

Anaphylactoid reactions/Anaphylaxis (<1%)

(2002): McKeage K+, *Drugs* 62(1), 209

Asthenia

(2005): Baselga J+, *J Clin Oncol* 23(10), 2162

(2003): Leyland-Jones B+, *J Clin Oncol* 21(21), 3965 (with paclitaxel)

Chills (32%)

(2002): McKeage K+, *Drugs* 62(1), 209

(2002): Vogel CL+, *J Clin Oncol* 20(3), 719

(2001): Cook-Bruns N, *Oncology* 61, 58

(2001): Vogel CL+, *Oncology* 61, 37

(2000): Treish I+, *Am J Health Syst Pharm* 57(22), 2063

(1999): Goldenberg MM, *Clin Ther* 21(2), 309

Cough (26%)

(1999): Goldenberg MM, *Clin Ther* 21(2), 309

Death

(2008): Suvarna SK, *J Clin Pathol* 61(1), 143

(2002): McKeage K+, *Drugs* 62(1), 209

Depression (6%)

Fever

(2005): Baselga J+, *J Clin Oncol* 23(10), 2162

(2004): Sawaki M+, *Tumori* 90(1), 40 (11%)

Headache

(2005): Baselga J+, *J Clin Oncol* 23(10), 2162

Infections (20%)

(1999): Goldenberg MM, *Clin Ther* 21(2), 309

Injection-site reactions (sic) (<1%)

(2003): Leyland-Jones B+, *J Clin Oncol* 21(21), 3965 (with paclitaxel)

(2002): Tokuda Y+, *Gan To Kagaku Ryoho* 29(4), 645

(2001): Cook-Bruns N, *Oncology* 61, 58

(2001): Smith IE, *Anticancer Drugs* 12, S3

(2001): Vogel CL+, *Oncology* 61, 37

(2000): Treish I+, *Am J Health Syst Pharm* 57(22), 2063

Myalgia/Myositis/Myopathy/Myotoxicity (~1%)

(2003): Leyland-Jones B+, *J Clin Oncol* 21(21), 3965 (with paclitaxel)

Pain (<47%)

(2002): Vogel CL+, *J Clin Oncol* 20(3), 719 (18%)

(1999): Goldenberg MM, *Clin Ther* 21(2), 309

Paresthesias (9%)

(2003): Leyland-Jones B+, *J Clin Oncol* 21(21), 3965 (with paclitaxel)

TRAVOPROST

Trade name: Travatan (Alcon)
Indications: Open-angle glaucoma, ocular hypertension
Category: Prostaglandin analog
Half-life: N/A

Reactions

Skin

Pruritus

(2001): Goldberg I+, *J Glaucoma* 10(5), 414

Eyes

Blepharitis (1–4%)

Conjunctival hyperemia

(2003): Al-Jazzaf AM+, *Drugs Today* (Barc) 39(1), 61

(2003): Stewart WC+, *Am J Ophthalmol* 135(3), 314

(2002): Eisenberg DL+, *Surv Ophthalmol* 47 Suppl 1, S105

Epiphora

Eyelashes – hypertrichosis

(2003): Al-Jazzaf AM+, *Drugs Today* (Barc) 39(1), 61

(2002): Eisenberg DL+, *Surv Ophthalmol* 47(Suppl 1), S105

Eyelid crusting (1–4%)

Iris pigmentation

(2003): Al-Jazzaf AM+, *Drugs Today* (Barc) 39(1), 61

Ocular burning

(2004): Reis R+, *Clin Ther* 26(12), 2121

Ocular edema

(2005): Arcieri ES+, *Arch Ophthalmol* 123(2), 186

Ocular hemorrhage (35–50%)

Ocular pigmentation (1–5%)

(2002): Novack GD+, *J Am Geriatr Soc* 50(5), 956

(2002): Stjernschantz JW+, *Surv Ophthalmol* 47(Suppl 1), S162
(2001): Goldberg I+, *J Glaucoma* 10(5), 414
(2001): Netland PA+, *Am J Ophthalmol* 132(4), 472 (5%)
Ocular pruritus (5–10%)
(2001): Goldberg I+, *J Glaucoma* 10(5), 414
Ocular stinging (5–10%)
(2001): Goldberg I+, *J Glaucoma* 10(5), 414
Uveitis
(2005): Cano Parra J+, *Arch Soc Esp Oftalmol* 80(3), 137
(2004): Kumarasamy M+, *BMJ* 329(7459), 205
(2003): Faulkner WJ+, *Arch Ophthalmol* 121(7), 1054
(1998): Fechtner RD+, *Am J Ophthalmol* 126(1), 37
(1998): Warwar RE+, *Ophthalmology* 105(2), 263

Other
Abdominal pain
(2005): Lee YC, *Am J Ophthalmol* 139(1), 202
Depression (1–5%)
Headache
Infections
Pain
(2001): Goldberg I+, *J Glaucoma* 10(5), 414

TRAZODONE

Trade names: Alti-Trazodone; Bimaran; Deprax; Desirel;
Desyrel (Bristol-Myers Squibb); Molipaxin; Sideril; Taxagon;
Trazalon
Indications: Depression
Category: Antidepressant, tricyclic; Serotonin reuptake inhibitor
Half-life: 3–6 hours
**Clinically important, potentially hazardous interactions
with:** citalopram, fluoxetine, fluvoxamine, **ginkgo biloba**,
linezolid, nefazodone, paroxetine, sertraline, venlafaxine

Reactions

Skin
Angioedema
(2001): Adson DE+, *Ann Pharmacother* 35(11), 1375
Diaphoresis (>1%)
(1997): Amir I+, *Isr J Psychiatry Relat Sci* 34(2), 119
Edema (1–10%)
Erythema multiforme
(1985): Ford HE+, *J Clin Psychiatry* 46, 294
Exanthems
(1988): Warnock JK+, *Am J Psychiatry* 145, 425
(1986): Rongioletti F+, *J Am Acad Dermatol* 14, 274
(1984): Cohen LE, *J Am Acad Dermatol* 10, 303
(1984): Cohen LE, *J Am Acad Dermatol* 11, 526
(1980): Al-Yassiri MM+, *Neuropharmacology* 19, 1191
Exfoliative dermatitis
(1983): Chu AG+, *Ann Intern Med* 99, 128
Formication
(1987): Peabody CA, *J Clin Psychiatry* 48, 385
Photosensitivity
(1994): Berger TG+, *Arch Dermatol* 130, 609 (in HIV-infected)
(1986): Rongioletti F+, *J Am Acad Dermatol* 14, 274
Pruritus (<1%)
Psoriasis (exacerbation)
(1992): Breathnach SM+, *Adverse Drug Reactions and the Skin*
Blackwell, Oxford, 197 (passim)
(1986): Barth JH+, *Br J Dermatol* 115, 629 (generalized and
pustular)
Purpura
Rash (sic) (<1%)

(1985): Longstreth GF+, *J Am Acad Dermatol* 13, 149
Urticaria
(1988): Warnock JK+, *Am J Psychiatry* 145, 425
(1984): Cohen LE, *J Am Acad Dermatol* 10, 303
(1983): Fabre LF+, *J Clin Psychiatry* 44, 17
Vasculitis
(1984): Mann SC+, *J Am Acad Dermatol* 10, 669

Mucosal/ENT
Dysgeusia (>10%)
Dysphagia
(2004): Passmore MJ+, *Can J Psychiatry* 49(1), 79
Sialorrhea
Xerostomia (>10%)
(1984): Kerr TA+, *Acta Psychiatr Scand* 70(6), 573
(1982): Rawls WN, *Drug Intell Clin Pharm* 16, 7

Hair
Hair – alopecia
(2000): Mercke Y+, *Ann Clin Psychiatry* 12, 35
(1988): Warnock JK+, *Am J Psychiatry* 145, 425

Nails
Nails – leukonychia
(1985): Longstreth GF+, *J Am Acad Dermatol* 13, 149

Other
Gynecomastia
Headache
Hypersensitivity
Myalgia/Myositis/Myopathy/Myotoxicity (1–10%)
Paresthesias (>1%)
Tremor (1–10%)
Vertigo
(2005): Mendelson WB, *J Clin Psychiatry* 66(4), 469

TREPROSTINIL

Trade name: Remodulin (United)
Indications: Pulmonary arterial hypertension
Category: Platelet aggregation inhibitor; Prostaglandin
Half-life: 2–4 hours
**Clinically important, potentially hazardous interactions
with:** anticoagulants, antihypertensives, diuretics, vasodilators

Reactions

Skin
Diaphoresis
Edema (9%)
(2002): Horn EM+, *Expert Opin Investig Drugs* 11(11), 1615
Erythema
Peripheral edema
Pruritus (8%)
Rash (sic) (14%)

Other
Application-site reactions (sic) (83%)
Headache (27%)
(2005): Reisbig KA+, *Ann Pharmacother* 39(4), 739
Injection-site bleeding (33%)
Injection-site erythema
(2002): Horn EM+, *Expert Opin Investig Drugs* 11(11), 1615
Injection-site induration
Injection-site pain (85%)
(2002): Horn EM+, *Expert Opin Investig Drugs* 11(11), 1615
(2002): Simonneau G+, *Am J Respir Crit Care Md* 165(6), 800

(2002): Vachiery JL+, *Chest* 121(5), 1561
Injection-site reactions (sic) (83%)
Pain (13%)
  (2002): Horn EM+, *Expert Opin Investig Drugs* 11(11), 1615
Vertigo (9%)

TRETINOIN

Synonym: All-trans-retinoic acid
Trade names: A-Acido; Aberal; Aberela; Acid A Vit; Acnavit; Acta; Airol; Aknemycin Plus (EM Industries); Alquingel; Alten; ATRA; Atragen; Avita; Avitcid; Avitoin; Cordes VAS; Derm A; Dermairol; Dermojuventus; Epi-Aberel; Eudyna; Relief; Renova (Ortho); Retin-A Micro (Ortho); Retinoic Acid; Retinova; Solage (Galderma); SteiVAA; Stieva-A; Vesanoid (Roche); Vitamin A Acid
Indications: Acne vulgaris, skin aging, facial roughness, fine wrinkles, hyperpigmentation [T], acute promyelocytic leukemia (APL) [O]
Category: Retinoid
Half-life: 0.5–2 hours
Clinically important, potentially hazardous interactions with: aldesleukin, bexarotene

Note: [T] = Topical, [O] = Oral

Note: Oral tretinoin can cause birth defects, and women should avoid Tretinoin when pregnant or trying to conceive. Avoid prolonged exposure to sunlight

Note: The RA-APL syndrome is characterized by fever, dyspnea, weight gain, pulmonary infiltrates and pleural effusions. Some patients have expired due to multiorgan failure

Reactions

Skin

Acne (1%)
  (1996): Shalita A+, *J Am Acad Dermatol* 34, 482
Acute febrile neutrophilic dermatosis (Sweet's syndrome)
  (2007): Jagdeo J+, *J Am Acad Dermatol* 56(4), 690
  (2007): Thompson DF+, *Ann Pharmacother* 41(5), 802
  (2005): Shimizu D+, *Intern Med* 44(5), 480
  (2004): Al-Saad K+, *J Pediatr Hematol Oncol* 26(3), 197
  (2002): Astudillo L+, *Ann Hematol* 81(2), 111
  (2001): Park CJ+, *Korean J Intern Med* 16(3), 218
  (2000): Ueno R+, *Rinsho Ketsueki* 41(9), 718
  (2000): van Der Vliet HJ+, *Am J Hematol* 63(2), 94
  (1999): Levi I+, *Leuk Lymphoma* 34(3–4), 401
  (1999): Takada S+, *Int J Hematol* 70(1), 26
  (1998): Arun B+, *Leuk Lymphoma* 31(5–6), 613
  (1997): Hatake K+, *Int J Hematol* 66(1), 13
  (1996): Christ E+, *Leukemia* 10(4), 731
  (1995): Shirono K+, *Int J Hematol* 62(3), 183
  (1994): Cox NH+, *Clin Exp Dermatol* 19(1), 51
  (1994): Piette WW+, *J Am Acad Dermatol* 30(2 Pt 2), 293
  (1994): Tomas JF+, *Leukemia* 8(9), 1596
Bullous dermatitis
  (1998): Webster GF, *J Am Acad Dermatol* 39, S38–44
  (1997): Cunliffe WJ+, *J Am Acad Dermatol* 36, S126–34
Burning (10–40%) [O][T]
  (2001): Egan N+, *Cutis* 68(4 Suppl), 20
  (2001): Vandana B+, *AAPS PharmSciTech* 2(3), Technical Note 4
  (1998): Ellis CN+, *Br J Dermatol* 139 Suppl 52, 41
  (1998): Webster GF, *J Am Acad Dermatol* 39, S38
  (1997): *Drug Information Handbook* Fifth Ed., American Pharmaceutical Association Hudson, OH
  (1997): Cunliffe WJ+, *J Am Acad Dermatol* 36, S126
  (1997): Gilchrest B, *J Am Acad Dermatol* 36, S27–36

  (1996): Shalita A+, *J Am Acad Dermatol* 34, 482
  (1996): Shroot B, *Presented at Dermatology Update '95 (Montreal) (Canada)*
  (1995): *Package Insert* Hoffman-LaRoche, Inc. Nutley, NJ
  (1995): Hall R, *Inpharma* December, 13
  (1992): Olsen EA+, *J Am Acad Dermatol* 26, 215
  (1991): Weinstein GD+, *Arch Dermatol* 127, 659
  (1989): Goldfarb MT+, *J Am Acad Dermatol* 21, 645
  (1989): Leyden JJ+, *J Am Acad Dermatol* 21, 638
  (1988): Cohen BA+, *Pediatric Dermatology* 1, New York: Churchill Livingstone, 663
Carcinoma [O]
Cellulitis (1–10%) [O]
  (1997): *Drug Information Handbook* Fifth Ed., American Pharmaceutical Association Hudson, OH
  (1995): *Package insert* Hoffman-LaRoche, Inc. Nutley, NJ
  (1995): Gillis JC+, *Drugs* 50(5), 897
Crusting
  (1998): Webster GF, *J Am Acad Dermatol* 39, S38
  (1997): Cunliffe WJ+, *J Am Acad Dermatol* 36, S126
Dermatitis
  (1997): Gilchrest B, *J Am Acad Dermatol* 36, S27
  (1992): Olsen EA+, *J Am Acad Dermatol* 26, 215
  (1991): Weinstein GD+, *Arch Dermatol* 127, 659
  (1989): Goldfarb MT+, *J Am Acad Dermatol* 21, 645
  (1989): Leyden JJ+, *J Am Acad Dermatol* 21, 638
Desquamation (14%)
Diaphoresis (20%)
Edema (29%)
  (1998): Webster GF, *J Am Acad Dermatol* 39, S38
  (1997): *Drug Information Handbook* Fifth Ed. American Pharmaceutical Association, Hudson, OH (29%) ([O])
  (1997): Cunliffe WJ+, *J Am Acad Dermatol* 36, S126
  (1997): Gilchrest BA, *J Am Acad Dermatol* 36, S27
  (1995): *Package insert* Hoffman-LaRoche, Inc., Nutley, NJ (29%) ([O]
  (1992): Olsen EA+, *J Am Acad Dermatol* 26, 215
  (1991): Weinstein GD+, *Arch Dermatol* 127, 659
  (1989): Goldfarb MT+, *J Am Acad Dermatol* 21, 645
  (1989): Leyden JJ+, *J Am Acad Dermatol* 21, 638
Erythema (1–49%) [O][T]
  (2001): Vandana B+, *AAPS PharmSciTech* 2(3), Technical Note 4
  (2000): Kreusch+, *Curr Med Res & Opinion* 16(1), 1
  (1998): Ellis CN+, *Br J Dermatol* 139 Suppl 52, 41
  (1998): Webster GF, *J Am Acad Dermatol* 39(2), S38
  (1997): *Drug Information Handbook* Fifth Ed (American Pharaceutical Association, Hudson, OH)
  (1997): Cunliffe WJ+, *J Am Acad Dermatol* 36(6), S126
  (1997): Gilchrest BA, *J Am Acad Dermatol* 36(3), S27
  (1996): Shalita A+, *J Am Acad Dermatol* 34(3), 482
  (1996): Shroot B, Presented at Dermatology Update '95, Montreal, Canada
  (1995): *Package insert* Hoffman-LaRoche, Inc., Nutley, NJ
  (1995): Hall R, *Inpharma* December, 13
  (1992): Olsen EA+, *J Am Acad Dermatol* 26(2), 215
  (1991): Weinstein GD+, *Arch Dermatol* 127, 659
  (1989): Goldfarb MT+, *J Am Acad Dermatol* 21, 645
  (1989): Leyden JJ+, *J Am Acad Dermatol* 21, 638
  (1988): Cohen BA+, *Pediatric Dermatology* 1. New York: Churchill Livingstone, 663
Erythema nodosum
  (2005): Taguchi A+, *Rinsho Ketsueki* 46(3), 202
  (2004): Kuo MC+, *Ann Hematol* 83(6), 376 (4 cases)
  (1993): Hakimian D+, *Leukemia* 7(5), 758
Exfoliative dermatitis (8.3%) [O]
  (1998): Webster GF, *J Am Acad Dermatol* 39, S38
  (1997): Cunliffe WJ+, *J Am Acad Dermatol* 36, S126
  (1988): Huang ME+, *Blood* 72(2), 567
Facial edema (1–10%) [O]

(1997): *Drug Information Handbook* Fifth Ed. American
     Pharmaceutical Association, Hudson, OH
(1995): *Package insert* Hoffman-LaRoche, Inc., Nutley NJ
Flaking (23%) [O]
Hyperkeratosis (78%) [O]
   (1991): Chen ZX+, *Blood* 78, 1413
Hypomelanosis (5%)
   (1998): Webster GF, *J Am Acad Dermatol* 39, S38
   (1997): Cunliffe WJ+, *J Am Acad Dermatol* 36, S126
Irritation (5%)
   (2003): Greenspan A+, *Cutis* 72(1), 76
   (2001): Vandana B+, *AAPS PharmSciTech* 2(3), Technical Note 4
   (1998): Cohen BA+, *Pediatric Dermatology* 1, New York:
        Churchill Livingstone, 663
   (1997): Clucas A+, *J Am Acad Dermatol* 36, S116
   (1996): Shalita A+, *J Am Acad Dermatol* 34(3), 482
Pallor (1–10%) [O]
   (1997): *Drug Information Handbook* Fifth Ed. American
        Pharmaceutical Association, Hudson, OH
   (1995): *Package insert* Hoffman-LaRoche, Inc., Nutley, NJ
Palmar–plantar desquamation (1–10%) [O]
   (1997): *Drug Information Handbook* Fifth Ed. American
        Pharmaceutical Association, Hudson, OH
   (1995): *Package insert* Hoffman-LaRoche, Inc., Nutley, NJ
Photosensitivity (10%) [O][T]
   (1998): Webster GF, *J Am Acad Dermatol* 39, S38
   (1997): *Drug Information Handbook* Fifth Ed. American
        Pharmaceutical Association, Hudson, OH
   (1997): Cunliffe WJ+, *J Am Acad Dermatol* 36, S126
   (1995): *Package insert* Hoffman-LaRoche, Inc., Nutley, NJ
Pigmentation (5%)
   (1998): Webster GF, *J Am Acad Dermatol* 39, S38
   (1997): Cunliffe WJ+, *J Am Acad Dermatol* 36, S126
Pruritus (10–40%) [O][T]
   (2001): Vandana B+, *AAPS PharmSciTech* 2(3), Technical Note 4
   (2000): Kreusch+, *Curr Med Res & Opinion* 16(1), 1
   (1998): Ellis CN+, *Br J Dermatol* 139 Suppl 52, 41
   (1998): Webster GF, *J Am Acad Dermatol* 39, S38
   (1997): *Drug Information Handbook* Fifth Ed. American
        Pharmaceutical Association, Hudson, OH
   (1997): Cunliffe WJ+, *J Am Acad Dermatol* 36, S126
   (1996): Shalita A+, *J Am Acad Dermatol* 34, 482
   (1995): *Package insert* Hoffman-LaRoche, Inc., Nutley, NJ
   (1995): Gillis JC+, *Drugs* 50(5), 897
   (1988): Cohen BA+, *Pediatric Dermatology* 1, New
        York:Churchill Livingstone, 663
Pyogenic granuloma
   (2004): Teknetzis A+, *J Eur Acad Dermatol Venereol* 18(3), 337 (2
        cases)
   (1998): MacKenzie-Wood AR+, *Australas J Dermatol* 39(4), 248
Rash (sic) (54%) [O][T]
   (1998): Webster GF, *J Am Acad Dermatol* 39, S38
   (1997): *Drug Information Handbook* Fifth Ed American
        Pharmaceutical Association, Hudson, OH
   (1997): Cunliffe WJ+, *J Am Acad Dermatol* 36, S126
   (1995): *Package insert* Hoffman-LaRoche, Inc.,Nutley, NJ
   (1991): Warrell RP+, *N Engl J Med* 324, 1385
Retinoic Acid–APL (RA-APL) syndrome(25%) [O]
   (2003): Paydas S+, *Leuk Lymphoma* 44(3), 547
   (1997): Fenaux P+, *N Engl J Med* 337, 1076
   (1997): Sacchi S+, *Haematologica* 82(1), 106
   (1997): Tallman MS+, *N Engl J Med* 337, 1021
   (1995): *Package insert* Hoffman-LaRoche, Inc., Nutley, NJ
   (1995): Gillis JC+, *Drugs* 50, 897
   (1992): Fenaux P+, *Blood* 80, 2176
Scaling (10–40%)
   (2001): Vandana B+, *AAPS PharmSciTech* 2(3), Technical Note 4
   (2000): Kreusch+, *Curr Med Res & Opinion* 16(1), 1
   (1998): Ellis CN+, *Br J Dermatol* 139 Suppl 52, 41

(1997): Gilchrest BA, *J Am Acad Dermatol* 36, S27–36
(1996): Shalita A+, *J Am Acad Dermatol* 34, 482
(1996): Shroot B, *Presented ar Dermatology Update '95* Montreal,
     Canada
(1995): Hall R, *Inpharma* December, 13
(1992): Olsen EA+, *J Am Acad Dermatol* 26, 215
(1991): Weinstein GD+, *Arch Dermatol* 127, 659
(1989): Goldfarb MT+, *J Am Acad Dermatol* 21, 645
(1988): Cohen BA+, *Pediatric Dermatology* 1 New York:
     Chrurchill Livingstone, 663
Shivering (63%) [O]
   (1997): *Drug Information Handbook* Fifth Ed. American
        Pharmaceutical Association, Hudson, OH
   (1995): *Package insert* Hoffman-LaRoche, Inc., Nutley, NJ
Stinging (1–26%) [O]
   (2001): Egan N+, *Cutis* 68(4 Suppl), 20
   (1997): Gilchrest BA, *J Am Acad Dermatol* 36, S27
   (1996): Shalita A+, *J Am Acad Dermatol* 34, 482
   (1992): Olsen EA+, *J Am Acad Dermatol* 26, 215
   (1991): Weinstein GD+, *Arch Dermatol* 127, 659
   (1989): Goldfarb MT+, *J Am Acad Dermatol* 21, 645
   (1989): Leyden JJ+, *J Am Acad Dermatol* 21, 638
Sunburn (1%)
   (1996): Shalita A+, *J Am Acad Dermatol* 34, 482
Ulcerations (penile)
   (2005): Mourad YA+, *Int J Dermatol* 44(1), 68 (scrotal)
   (2005): Simzar S+, *J Drugs Dermatol* 4(2), 231 (scrotal)
   (2004): Gettinger S+, *J Clin Oncol* 22(22), 4648 (scrotal)
   (2004): Pavithran K+, *Am J Hematol* 75(4), 260 (scrotal)
   (2004): Paydas S, *Am J Hematol* 77(2), 206 (scrotal)
   (2003): Fukuno K+, *Leuk Lymphoma* 44(11), 2009 (scrotal)
   (2000): Esser AC+, *J Am Acad Dermatol* 43(2 Pt 1), 316
   (1995): Gillis JC+, *Drugs* 50, 897
Vasculitis
   (2003): Paydas S+, *Leuk Lymphoma* 44(3), 547
Vesiculobullous eruption
Xerosis (49–100%) [O]
   (2004): Pavithran K+, *Am J Hematol* 75(4), 260
   (2000): Kreusch+, *Curr Med Res & Opinion* 16(1), 1
   (1998): Soignet SL+, *Leukema* 12(10), 1518
   (1997): Gilchrest BA, *J Am Acad Dermatol* 36, S27
   (1996): Shalita A+, *J Am Acad Dermatol* 34, 482
   (1995): Dockx P+, *Br J Dermatol* 133(3), 426
   (1995): Gillis JC+, *Drugs* 50(5), 897
   (1992): Fenaux P+, *Blood* 80(9), 2176
   (1992): Olsen EA+, *J Am Acad Dermatol* 26, 215
   (1991): Chen ZX+, *Blood* 78(6), 1413
   (1991): Weinstein GD+, *Arch Dermatol* 127, 659
   (1989): Leyden JJ+, *J Am Acad Dermatol* 21, 638
   (1988): Huang ME+, *Blood* 72(2), 567

Mucosal/ENT
Cheilitis (10%) [O]
   (2004): Pavithran K+, *Am J Hematol* 75(4), 260
   (1997): *Drug Information Handbook* Fifth Ed. American
        Pharmaceutical Association, Hudson, OH
   (1995): *Package insert* Hoffman-LaRoche, Inc., Nutley, NJ
Gingivitis (<1%) [O]
   (1997): *Drug Information Handbook* Fifth Ed. American
        Pharmaceutical Association, Hudson, OH
   (1995): *Package insert* Hoffman-LaRoche, Inc., Nutley, NJ
Xerostomia (10%) [O]
   (2004): Pavithran K+, *Am J Hematol* 75(4), 260
   (1997): *Drug Information Handbook* Fifth Ed American
        Pharmaceutical Association, Hudson, OH
   (1995): *Package insert* Hoffman-LaRoche, Inc., Nutley, NJ

Hair
Hair – alopecia areata (14%) [O]

(1997): *Drug Information Handbook* Fifth Ed American
    Pharmaceutical Association, Hudson, OH
(1995): *Package insert* Hoffman-LaRoche, Inc., Nutley, NJ

Eyes
Conjunctivitis (<1%) [O]
    (1997): *Drug Information Handbook* Fifth Ed. American
        Pharmaceutical Association, Hudson, OH
    (1995): *Package insert* Hoffman-LaRoche, Inc., Nutley, NJ
Ocular pigmentation (1–10%) [O]
    (1997): *Drug Information Handbook* Fifth Ed. American
        Pharmaceutical Association, Hudson, OH
    (1995): *Package insert* Hoffman-LaRoche, Inc., Nutley, NJ
Ocular pruritus (10%) [O]
    (1997): *Drug Information Handbook* Fifth Ed. American
        Pharmaceutical Association, Hudson, OH
    (1995): *Package insert* Hoffman-LaRoche, Inc., Natley, NJ
Xerophthalmia (1–10%) [O]
    (1997): *Drug Information Handbook* Fifth Ed. American
        Pharmaceutical Association, Hudson, OH
    (1995): *Package insert* Hoffman-LaRoche, Inc., Nutley, NJ

Other
Death [O]
    (1997): Fenaux P+, *N Engl J* 337, 1076
    (1997): Larson RA+ In: Hall JB+, *Principles of Critical Care*
        Second Ed. New York, McGraw-Hill
    (1995): *Package insert* Hoffman-LaRoche, Inc., Nutley, NJ
Depression (14%) [O]
    (1997): *Drug Information Handbook* Fifth Ed, American
        Pharmaceutical Association, Hudson, OH
    (1995): *Package insert* Hoffman-LaRoche, Inc., Nutley, NJ
Fever [O]
    (2004): Kuo MC+, *Ann Hematol* 83(6), 376
    (2003): Datta D+, *Conn Med* 67(9), 541
    (1997): Fenaux P+, *N Engl J Med* 337, 1076
    (1997): Larson RA+ In: Halll JB+, *Principles of Critical Care*
        Second Ed., New York, McGraw
    (1995): *Package insert* Hoffman-LaRoche, Inc., Nutley, NJ
Headache
    (2005): Ganguly S, *Leuk Res* 29(6), 721
Infections (58%) [O]
    (1997): *Drug Information Handbook* Fifth Ed. American
        Pharaceutical Association, Hudson, OH
    (1995): *Package insert* Hoffman-LaRoche, Inc,. Nutley, NJ
    (1991): Chen ZX+, *Blood* 78(6), 1413
Injection-site reactions (sic) (17%)
Myalgia/Myositis/Myopathy/Myotoxicity (14%)
    (2002): Martinez-Chamorro C+, *Haematologica* 87(2), ECR08
    (2000): van Der Vliet HJ+, *Am J Hematol* 63(2), 94
    (1997): *Drug Information Handbook* Fifth Ed. American
        Pharmaceutical Association, Hudson, OH
    (1995): *Package insert* Hoffman-LaRoche, Inc., Nutley, NJ
Pain (37%) [O]
    (1997): *Drug Information Handbook* Fifth Ed. American
        Pharmaceutical Association, Hudson, OH
    (1995): *Package insert* Hoffman-LaRoche, Inc., Nutley, NJ
Paresthesias (17%) [O]
    (1997): *Drug Information Handbook* Fifth Ed. American
        Pharmaceutical Association, Hudson, OH
    (1995): *Package insert* Hoffman-LaRoche, Inc., Nutley, NJ
Phlebitis (11%)
Tremor (1–10%) [O]
    (1997): *Drug Information Handbook* Fifth Ed. American
        Pharmaceutical Association, Hudson, OH
    (1995): *Package insert* Hoffman-LaRoche, Inc., Nutley, NJ

TRIAMCINOLONE

Trade names: Aristocort (Astellas); Aristospan (Sabex);
Azmacort (Kos); Kenacort (Bristol-Myers Squibb); Kenalog
(Apothecon); Nasacort (Aventis); Triacet (Teva)
Indications: Arthralgias, Asthma, Dermatoses, Ophthalmology,
Rhinitis (many others)
Category: Corticosteroid, systemic; Corticosteroid, topical
Half-life: 33 to 5 days
**Clinically important, potentially hazardous interactions
with:** aspirin, diuretics, estrogens, ketoconazole, **live vaccines**,
oral contraceptives, phenobarbital, phenytoin, rifampin

Reactions

Skin
Acne
Adverse effects (sic)
    (2004): Gillies MC+, *Arch Ophthalmol* 122(3), 336
    (2003): Lumry W+, *Allergy Asthma Proc* 24(3), 203
Allergic granulomatous angiitis (Churg–Strauss syndrome)
    (1997): Privat JM+, *Neurochirurgie* 43(4), 212
Allergic reactions (sic)
    (1995): Saff DM+, *Arch Dermatol* s(6), 742
    (1993): Fedler R+, *Hautarzt* 44(2), 91
    (1989): Brambilla L+, *Contact Dermatitis* 21(4), 272
Atrophy
    (2003): Fesq H+, *Br J Dermatol* 149(3), 611
    (2000): Breit W+, *J Rheumatol* 27(11), 2696
    (1996): Ritota PC+, *Ann Plast Surg* 36(5), 508
    (1990): Ford MD+, *Ophthalmic Surg* 21, 215
Bruising
    (2004): Tashkin DP+, *Chest* 126(4), 1123
Cellulitis
    (2004): Chen HM+, *J Oral Pathol* 33(4), 243
Dermatitis
    (2004): Keegel T+, *Contact Dermatitis* 50(1), 6
    (2000): Chew AL+, *Cutis* 65, 307
    (1989): Rivara G+, *Contact Dermatitis* 21(2), 83
Eczema
    (2001): Poon E+, *Australas J Dermatol* 42(1), 36
Erythema
    (1999): Alexiou C+, *Laryngorhinootologie* (German) 78, 573
    (1998): Valsecchi R+, *Contact Dermatitis* 38(6), 362
    (1995): Saff DM+, *Arch Dermatol* 131, 742 (localized)
Exanthems
    (1995): Ijsselmuiden O+, *Acta Derm Venereol* (Stockh) 75, 57
Fixed eruption
    (2001): Sener O+, *Ann Allergy Asthma* 86(3), 335
Necrosis
    (1999): Ostergaard M+, *Ugeskr Laeger* 161(5), 582
Pigmentation
    (2004): Gallardo MJ+, *Am J Ophthalmol* 137(4), 779
    (2002): Evans AV+, *Clin Exp Dermatol* 27(3), 247
    (1998): Kumar P+, *Burns* 24(5), 487
    (1996): Ritota PC+, *Ann Plast Surg* 36(5), 508
Pruritus
    (1995): Saff DM+, *Arch Dermatol* 131, 742 (localized)
Rash (sic)
Thinning
    (2003): Fesq H+, *Br J Dermatol* 149(3), 611
Urticaria
    (1995): Ijsselmuiden OE+, *Acta Derm Venereol* 75, 57

Mucosal/ENT
Mucosal irritation
    (2000): Gawchik SM+, *Drug Saf* 23(4), 309

Xerostomia
(1995): Loesche WJ+, J Am Geriatr Soc 43(4), 401

Eyes
Cataract
(2005): Cekic O+, Am J Ophthalmol 139(6), 993
(2005): Gillies MC+, Ophthalmology 112(1), 139
(2005): Jonas JB+, Eur J Ophthalmol 15(4), 462
(2005): Kuo HK+, Chang Gung Med 28(2), 85 (13%)
(2004): Ciardella AP+, Br J Ophthalmol 88(9), 1131
(2004): Jaissle GB+, Ophthalmologe 101(2), 121
(2004): Jonas JB+, Ophthalmologe 101(2), 113
(2004): Lang GE, Ophthalmologe 101(12), 1165
(2003): Jonas JB+, Klin Monatsbl Augenheilkd 220(6), 384
(2003): Rechtman E+, Am J Ophthalmol 136(4), 739
(2001): Young S+, Clin Experiment Ophthalmol 29(1), 2
(1998): Challa JK+, Aust N Z J Ophthalmol 26(4), 277
Chorioretinopathy
(2005): Imasawa M+, Acta Ophthalmol Scand 83(1), 132
Conjunctival ulceration
(2004): Jaissle GB+, Ophthalmologe 101(2), 121
(2003): Agrawal S+, Am J Ophthalmol 136(3), 539
Endophthalmitis
(2005): Moshfeghi DM+, Ophthalmic Surg Lasers 36(1), 24
(2005): Westfall AC+, Arch Ophthalmol 123(8), 1075 (0.1%)
(2004): Chen SD+, Arch Ophthalmol 122(11), 1733
(2004): Jaissle GB+, Ophthalmologe 101(2), 121
(2004): Jonas JB+, Ophthalmologe 101(2), 113
(2004): Lang GE, Ophthalmologe 101(12), 1165
(2004): Sutter FK+, Ophthalmology 111(11), 2044
(2004): Yamashita T+, Graefes Arch Clin Exp Ophthalmol 242(8), 679
(2003): Benz MS+, Arch Ophthalmol 121(2), 271
(2003): Jonas JB+, Klin Monatsbl Augenheilkd 220(6), 384
(2003): Nelson ML+, Retina 23(5), 686
(2003): Roth DB+, Arch Ophthalmol 121(9), 1279
(2003): Sutter FK+, Br J Ophthalmol 87(8), 972
Eyelid pigmentation
(2004): Gallardo MJ+, Am J Ophthalmol 137(4), 779
Glaucoma
(2005): Agrawal S+, Am J Ophthalmol 139(3), 575
(2005): Kuo HK+, Chang Gung Med J 28(2), 85 (23%)
(2004): Jaissle GB+, Ophthalmologe 101(2), 121
(2004): Kaushik S+, Am J Ophthalmol 137(4), 758
(2004): Levy J+, Can J Ophthalmol 39(6), 672
(2003): Jonas JB+, Arch Ophthalmol 121(5), 729
Ocular edema
(2003): Mackiewicz J+, Ann Univ Mariae Curie Sklodowska [Med] 58(1), 158
Ocular hypertension
(2005): Kuo HK+, Chang Gung Med J 28(2), 85 (77%)
(2004): Degenring RF+, Ophthalmologe 101(3), 251 (31%)
(2004): Detry-Morel M+, Bull Soc Belge Ophtalmol I(292), 45
(2004): Jonas JB+, Ophthalmologe 101(2), 113 (40%)
Ocular pressure
(2005): Jonas JB+, Ophthalmology 112(4), 593
(2005): Kreissig I+, Ophthalmologe 102(2), 153
(2005): Vedantham V, Am J Ophthalmol 139(3), 575
(2004): Agrawal S+, Am J Ophthalmol 138(4), 679
(2004): Ciardella AP+, Br J Ophthalmol 88(9), 1131
(2004): Ferrante P+, Clin Experiment Ophthalmol 32(6), 563
(2004): Gillies MC+, Arch Ophthalmol 122(3), 336
(2004): Lang GE, Ophthalmologe 101(12), 1165
(2004): Lee AC+, Semin Ophthalmol 19(3-4), 119
(2004): Singh IP+, Am J Ophthalmol 138(2), 286
(2004): Smithen LM+, Am J Ophthalmol 138(5), 740
(2003): Bakri SJ+, Ophthalmic Surg Lasers Imaging 34(5), 386
(2003): Jonas JB+, Br J Ophthalmol 87(1), 24
(2003): Jonas JB+, Klin Monatsbl Augenheilkd 220(6), 384 (50%)
(2003): Rechtman E+, Am J Ophthalmol 136(4), 739

(2002): Bui Quoc E+, J Fr Ophtalmol 25(10), 1048
(2001): Young S+, Clin Experiment Ophthalmol 29(1), 2
(1999): Wingate RJ+, Aust N Z Ophthalmol 27(6), 431
(1998): Challa JK+, Aust N Z Ophthalmol 26(4), 277
(1996): Akduman L+, Am J Ophthalmol 122(2), 275
(1995): Helm CJ+, Am J Ophthalmol 120(1), 55
(1995): Kalina PH+, Arch Ophthalmol 113(7), 867
Ptosis
(2005): Dal Canto AJ+, Ophthalmology 112(6), 1092
(2004): Ferrante P+, Clin Experiment Ophthalmol 32(6), 563
Retinal detachment
(2004): Jaissle GB+, Ophthalmologe 101(2), 121
Uveitis
(2005): Cano Parra J+, Arch Soc Esp Oftalmol 80(3), 137
Vision impaired
(2004): Moshfeghi AA+, Am J Ophthalmol 138(3), 489
(2004): Sharma MC+, Cornea 23(4), 398
(2002): Moshfeghi DM+, Am J Ophthalmol 134(1), 132

Other
Anaphylactoid reactions/Anaphylaxis
(2003): Karsh J+, Ann Allergy Asthma Immunol 90(2), 254
(2000): Alexander J, Tulsa, OK (from Internet) (observation)
(2000): Vedamurthy M, Chennai, India (from Internet) (observation)
(1998): Downs AM+, Arch Dermatol 134(9), 1163
Cough
(1998): Berkowitz R+, Chest 114(3), 757
Headache
(2000): Gawchik SM+, Drug Saf 23(4), 309
(1997): Gawchik SM+, Am J Manag 3(7), 1052
(1997): Koepke JW+, Allergy Asthma Proc 18(1), 33 (22%)
(1997): Munk ZM+, Ann Allergy Asthma 78(3), 325
(1997): Russegger L+, Wien Klin Wochenschr 109(20), 808
(1995): Schoenwetter W+, Clin Ther 17(3), 479
Hypersensitivity
(2000): Brancaccio RR+, Cutis 65, 31
Injection-site lipoatrophy
(2002): Cleary JD, Ann Pharmacother 36(4), 726
(2000): Anderson B+, Arch Intern Med 151, 153
(2000): Breit W+, J Rheumatol 27(11), 2696
Injection-site necrosis (avascular)
(2001): Nasser SM+, BMJ 322(7302), 1589
Moon face
(2002): Jansen TL+, Neth J Med 60(3), 151
(2002): Teelucksingh S+, Ann Trop Paediatr 22(1), 89
Myalgia/Myositis/Myopathy/Myotoxicity
(1995): Boonen S+, Br J Rheumatol 34(4), 385
Osteoporosis
(2004): Scanlon PD+, Am J Respir Crit Care Med 170(12), 1302
(2001): Israel E+, N Engl J Med 345(13), 941
(2000): N Engl J Med 343(26), 1902
Pain
(2004): Jirarattanaphochai K+, J Bone Joint Surg Am 86(12), 2700

TRIAMTERENE

Trade names: Amterene; Diarrol; Diuteren; Dyazide (GSK); Dyrenium (Wellspring); Dytac; Maxzide; Reviten; Suloton; Trian
Indications: Edema
Category: Diuretic, potassium-sparing
Half-life: 1–2 hours
Clinically important, potentially hazardous interactions with: ACE inhibitors, benazepril, captopril, cyclosporine, enalapril, fosinopril, indomethacin, **juniper**, lisinopril, moexipril, potassium iodide, potassium salts, quinapril, ramipril, spironolactone, trandolapril

Note: Dyazide is triamterene and hydrochlorothiazide; Maxzide is triamterene and hydrochlorothiazide

Note: Hydrochlorothiazide is a sulfonamide and can be absorbed systemically. Sulfonamides can produce severe, possibly fatal, reactions such as toxic epidermal necrolysis and Stevens–Johnson syndrome

Reactions

Skin
Diaphoresis
Edema (1–10%)
Exanthems
Lupus erythematosus (with hydrochlorothiazide)
  (1991): Wollenberg A+, *Hautarzt* (German) 42, 709
  (1988): Darken M+, *J Am Acad Dermatol* 18, 38
Perleche
Photosensitivity
  (1989): Rosen C, *Semin Dermatol* 8, 149
  (1987): Fernandez de Corres L+, *Contact Dermatitis* 17, 114
Pruritus
Purpura
Rash (sic) (1–10%)
Urticaria
Vasculitis

Mucosal/ENT
Dysgeusia
  (1999): Sorkin M, Denver, CO (from Internet) (observation)
Glossitis
Stomatodynia
  (1999): Sorkin M, Denver, CO (from Internet) (observation)
Xerostomia
  (1987): Fernandez de Corres L+, *Contact Dermatitis* 17, 114

Other
Anaphylactoid reactions/Anaphylaxis
Chills
Gynecomastia (<1%)
Headache
Paresthesias
Pseudoporphyria
  (1990): Motley RJ, *BMJ* 300, 1468

TRIAZOLAM

Trade names: Dumozolam; Halcion (Pfizer); Novo-Triolam; Nu-Triazo; Nuctane; Somese; Somniton; Songar; Trialam
Indications: Insomnia
Category: Benzodiazepine
Half-life: 1.5–5.5 hours
Clinically important, potentially hazardous interactions with: atazanavir, clarithromycin, darunavir, delavirdine, efavirenz, erythromycin, fosamprenavir, indinavir, itraconazole, ketoconazole, rifampin, ritonavir, telithromycin, tipranavir

Reactions

Skin
Dermatitis (1–10%)
  (1984): Greenblatt DJ+, *J Clin Psychiatry* 45, 192
Diaphoresis (>10%)
  (1983): Kroboth PD+, *Drug Intell Clin Pharm* 17, 495
Exanthems
Photosensitivity
  (1984): Hussar DA, *Am Drug* 190, 109
Pruritus
  (1983): Poeldinger W+, *Neuropsychobiology* 9, 135
  (1981): Cobden I+, *Postgrad Med J* 57, 730
Purpura
Rash (sic) (>10%)
  (1985): Jerram TC, *Side Effects Drugs Annu* 9, 39
Urticaria

Mucosal/ENT
Dysgeusia (<1%)
Gingivitis
Glossitis (<1%)
Glossodynia (<1%)
Sialopenia (>10%)
  (1995): Loesche WJ+, *J Am Geriatr Soc* 43, 401
Sialorrhea (1–10%)
Stomatitis (<1%)
Tinnitus
Xerostomia (>10%)
  (1995): Loesche WJ+, *J Am Geriatr Soc* 43, 401
  (1986): Hughes RRL+, *Br J Clin Pract* 40, 279
  (1984): Greenblatt DJ+, *J Clin Psychiatry* 45, 192
  (1983): Cohn JB, *J Clin Psychiatry* 44, 401

Hair
Hair – alopecia
Hair – hirsutism

Other
Headache
Paresthesias (<1%)
Somnambulism
  (1986): Glassman JN+, *J Clin Psychiatry* 47(10), 523 (along with chlorpromazine, benztropine, and lithium)
Tremor (1–10%)

TRICHLORMETHIAZIDE

Trade names: Anatran; Aquacot; Carvacron; Diurese; Doqua; Esmarin; Flute; Iopran; Naqua; Niazide; Trichlon; Trichlorex
Indications: Edema, hypertension
Category: Diuretic, thiazide
Half-life: N/A
Clinically important, potentially hazardous interactions with: digoxin, lithium

Note: Trichlormethiazide is a sulfonamide and can be absorbed systemically. Sulfonamides can produce severe, possibly fatal, reactions such as toxic epidermal necrolysis and Stevens–Johnson syndrome

Reactions

Skin
Exanthems
Lichenoid eruption (<1%)
Lupus erythematosus
Photosensitivity (<1%)
Purpura
Rash (sic)
Urticaria
Vasculitis

Mucosal/ENT
Xerostomia

Other
Anaphylactoid reactions/Anaphylaxis
Hepatotoxicity
Paresthesias

TRIENTINE

Trade name: Syprine (Merck)
Indications: Wilson's disease
Category: Chelator
Half-life: N/A

Reactions

Skin
Dermatitis
  (1980): Rudzki E, *Contact Dermatitis* 6, 235
Desquamation
Lupus erythematosus (<1%)
Thickening (<1%)

Mucosal/ENT
Aphthous stomatitis
Oral lesions

TRIFLUOPERAZINE

Trade names: Calmazine; Domilium; Flupazine; Fluzine; Nerolet; Psyrazine; Sedizine; Stelazine; TFP
Indications: Psychoses, anxiety
Category: Antipsychotic, phenothiazine
Half-life: 10–20 hours
Clinically important, potentially hazardous interactions with: antihistamines, arsenic, chlorpheniramine, dofetilide, piperazine, quinolones, sparfloxacin

Reactions

Skin
Angioedema
Dermatitis
Diaphoresis
Eczema
Erythema
Exanthems
Exfoliative dermatitis
Fixed eruption
  (1987): Kanwar AJ+, *Br J Dermatol* 117, 798
Lupus erythematosus
Peripheral edema
Photosensitivity (1–10%)
Pigmentation (blue-gray) (<1%)
  (1994): Buckley C+, *Clin Exp Dermatol* 19, 149
Pruritus
Purpura
Rash (sic) (1–10%)
Seborrhea
Urticaria
Xerosis

Mucosal/ENT
Dysphagia
  (1996): Bashford G+, *J Geriatr Psychiatry Neurol* 9(3), 133
Oral mucosal eruption
  (1988): Ward DF+, *Postgrad Med* 84, 99
Tongue edema
  (1988): Ward DF+, *Postgrad Med* 84, 99
Xerostomia

Eyes
Blepharospasm
  (1989): Sachdev PS, *Med J Aust* 150(6), 341

Other
Anaphylactoid reactions/Anaphylaxis
Gynecomastia
Headache
Inappropriate secretion of antidiuretic hormone (SIADH)
  (1987): Kennedy MJ+, *Eur J Respir Dis* 71(5), 450
Rhabdomyolysis
  (2002): Lappa A+, *Intensive Care Med* 28(7), 976 (with tranylcypromine)
Tremor

TRIFLURIDINE

Synonyms: F3T; Trifluorothymidine
Trade name: Viroptic (Monarch)
Indications: Keratoconjunctivitis, epithelial keratitis caused by herpes simplex virus
Category: Antiviral
Half-life: N/A

Reactions

Skin
Dermatitis
  (1990): Millan-Parrilla F+, *Contact Dermatitis* 22(5), 289
  (1987): Gailhofer G+, *Wien Klin Wochenschr* 99(6), 192
  (1987): Naito T+, *Curr Eye Res* 6(1), 237 (10.1%)
  (1981): Cirkel PK+, *Contact Dermatitis* 7(1), 49

Eyes
Conjunctivitis
  (1987): Naito T+, *Curr Eye Res* 6(1), 237 (10.1%)
Corneal dysplasia
  (1983): Maudgal PC+, *Graefes Arch Clin Exp Ophthalmol*
Keratitis (<1%)
Keratoconjunctivitis
  (1996): Wilhelmus KR+, *Br J Ophthalmol* 80(11), 969
Ocular burning
Ocular ischemia
  (1997): Jayamanne DG+, *Eye* 11 (PT5), 757
  (1990): Shearer DR+, *Am J Ophthalmol* 109(3), 346
Ocular pressure (<1%)
Ocular stinging (>10%)

TRIHEXYPHENIDYL

Trade names: Acamed; Aparkane; Bentex; Hexinal; Hipokinon; Parkines; Partane; Tridyl; Trihexy; Trihexyphen
Indications: Parkinsonism
Category: Muscarinic antagonist
Half-life: 3–4 hours
Clinically important, potentially hazardous interactions with: anticholinergics, arbutamine

Reactions

Skin
Diaphoresis
Photosensitivity (1–10%)
Rash (sic) (<1%)
Spider angiomas
Urticaria
Xerosis (>10%)

Mucosal/ENT
Glossitis
Glossodynia
Xerostomia (30–50%)

Other
Chills
Paresthesias
  (2005): Funakawa I+, *Rinsho Shinkeigaku* 45(2), 125

TRIMEPRAZINE

Trade names: Nedeltran; Panectyl; Temaril; Theralene; Vallergan; Variargil
Indications: Pruritus, urticaria
Category: Antipsychotic; Histamine H1 receptor antagonist
Half-life: N/A
Duration of action: 3–6 hours

Reactions

Skin
Angioedema (<1%)
Dermatitis
Diaphoresis
Edema (<1%)
Exanthems
Lupus erythematosus
Peripheral edema
Photosensitivity (<1%)
Pruritus
Purpura
Rash (sic) (<1%)
Urticaria

Mucosal/ENT
Stomatitis
Tinnitus
Xerostomia (1–10%)
  (1992): Chambers FA+, *Anaesthesia* 47, 585

Other
Anaphylactoid reactions/Anaphylaxis
Gynecomastia
Myalgia/Myositis/Myopathy/Myotoxicity (<1%)
Paresthesias (<1%)

TRIMETHADIONE

Trade names: Mino Aleviatin; Tridione
Indications: Seizures
Category: Antiepileptic, oxazolidinedione
Half-life: N/A

Note: Withdrawn in the USA

Reactions

Skin
Acne
Bullous dermatitis
Dermatitis
  (1996): Fleming TR+, *Invest New Drugs* 13(4), 363
Erythema multiforme
  (1992): Breathnach SM+, *Adverse Drug Reactions and the Skin*
    Blackwell, Oxford, 210 (passim)
Exanthems
Exfoliative dermatitis
  (1992): Breathnach SM+, *Adverse Drug Reactions and the Skin*
    Blackwell, Oxford, 210 (passim)
Fixed eruption
Lupus erythematosus
  (1993): Drory VE+, *Clin Neuropharmacol* 16, 19
  (1980): Condemi JJ, *Geriatrics* 35(3), 81

Petechiae
Photosensitivity
Pruritus
Purpura
Rash (sic)
  (1992): Fossella FV+, *Invest New Drugs* 10(4), 331
Stevens–Johnson syndrome
Urticaria
  (1992): Breathnach SM+, *Adverse Drug Reactions and the Skin*
    Blackwell, Oxford, 210 (passim)
Vasculitis
  (1993): Drory VE+, *Clin Neuropharmacol* 16, 19
  (1986): Hannedouche T+, *Ann Med Interne Paris* (French)
    137, 57

Mucosal/ENT
Gingivitis
Mucositis (4%)
  (2002): Sarris AH+, *J Clin Oncol* 20(12), 2876 (4%)
  (1996): Fleming TR+, *Invest New Drugs* 13(4), 363

Hair
Hair – alopecia

Other
Fever
  (2002): Sarris AH+, *J Clin Oncol* 20(12), 2876
Infections (3%)
  (2002): Sarris AH+, *J Clin Oncol* 20(12), 2876 (3%)
Paresthesias

TRIMETHOBENZAMIDE

Trade names: Anaus; Arrestin; Benzacot; Bio-Gan; Elen; Ibikin;
Navogan; Stemetic; T-Gene; Tebamide; Tegamide; Ticon; Tigan
(Monarch); Triban; Tribenzagen; Trimazide
Indications: Prevention and treatment of nausea and vomiting
Category: Antiemetic
Half-life: N/A

Reactions

Skin
Allergic reactions (sic) (<1%)

Other
Headache
Hypersensitivity (<1%)
Injection-site reactions (sic)

TRIMETHOPRIM

Trade names: Abaprim; Alprim; Bactin; Bactrim (Women First);
Idotrim; Ipral; Lidaprim; Methoprim; Monotrim; Polytrim;
Primosept; Septra (Monarch); Syraprim; Tiempe; Triprim;
Unitrim
Indications: Various urinary tract infections caused by
susceptible organisms
Category: Antibiotic
Half-life: 8–10 hours
**Clinically important, potentially hazardous interactions
with:** dofetilide, methotrexate

Note: Although trimethoprim has been known to elicit occasional
adverse reactions by itself, it is most commonly used in conjunction

with sulfamethoxazole (co-trimoxazole). The trade names for this
combination are: Bactrim; Cotrim; Septra. Please see co-trimoxazole
for the specific reaction patterns and references

Reactions

Skin
Allergic reactions (sic)
  (2004): Karpman E+, *J Urol* 172(2), 448
Erythema multiforme
Erythema nodosum
  (1983): *Ugeskr Laeger* (Danish) 145, 1070
Exanthems
Exfoliative dermatitis (<1%)
Fixed eruption
  (2007): *Prescrire Int* 16(87), 21 (with sulfamethoxazole)
  (2006): Rasi A+, *Dermatol Online J* 12(6), 12
  (1998): Ozkaya-Bayazit E+, *Contact Dermatitis* 39(2), 87
  (1997): Ozkaya-Bayazit E+, *Br J Dermatol* 137(6), 1028
  (1986): Kanwar AJ+, *Dermatologica* 172(4), 230
  (1982): Gibson JR, *Br Med J* 284(6328), 1529
Linear IgA dermatosis
  (2003): Avci O+, *J Am Acad Dermatol* 48(2), 299 (passim)
Photosensitivity
Pruritus (1–10%)
Rash (sic) (2.9–6.7%)
  (2006): Hemstreet BA+, *Pharmacotherapy* 26(4), 551 (with
    sulfamethoxazole)
Stevens–Johnson syndrome
  (2006): Hemstreet BA+, *Pharmacotherapy* 26(4), 551 (with
    sulfamethoxazole)
Toxic epidermal necrolysis
Urticaria
  (2006): Batioglu F+, *Cutan Ocul Toxicol* 25(4), 281 (with
    sulfamethoxazole)

Mucosal/ENT
Dysgeusia
Glossitis

Eyes
Uveitis
  (1997): Kristinsson JK+, *Acta Ophthalmol Scand* 75(3), 314
Visual disturbances
  (2006): Batioglu F+, *Cutan Ocul Toxicol* 25(4), 281 (with
    sulfamethoxazole)

Other
Abdominal pain
  (2003): Floris-Moore MA+, *Ann Pharmacother* 37(12), 1810
    (with sulfamethoxazole)
Anaphylactoid reactions/Anaphylaxis
  (2006): Hemstreet BA+, *Pharmacotherapy* 26(4), 551 (with
    sulfamethoxazole)
Aseptic meningitis
  (2002): Redman RC 4th+, *Pediatrics* 110(2 Pt 1), e26
Death
  (2005): Mortimer NJ+, *Aust Fam Physician* 34(5), 345
Headache
Hypersensitivity
  (2006): Mohammedi I+, *Rev Med Interne* 27(6), 499 (with
    sulfamethoxazole)
Rhabdomyolysis
  (2006): Walker S+, *Am J Med Sci* 331(6), 339 (with
    sulfamethoxazole)
Tremor
  (2003): Floris-Moore MA+, *Ann Pharmacother* 37(12), 1810
    (with sulfamethoxazole)

TRIMETREXATE

Trade name: Neutrexin (Medimmune)
Indications: *Pneumocystis carinii* pneumonia
Category: Folic acid antagonist
Half-life: 15–17 hours

Reactions

Skin
Angioedema
 (1990): Grem JL+, *Drugs* 8, 211
Exanthems
 (1987): Leiby J+, *Invest New Drugs* 5, 136
Fixed eruption
Photosensitivity
Pruritus (5.5%)
 (1990): Grem JL+, *Drugs* 8, 211
Rash (sic) (1–10%)

Mucosal/ENT
Oral lesions
 (1987): Leiby J+, *Invest New Drugs* 5, 136
Stomatitis (1–10%)

Other
Hypersensitivity (1–10%)

TRIMIPRAMINE

Trade names: Apo-Trimip; Rhotrimine; Stangyl; Sumontil;
Surmontil (Odyssey)
Indications: Major depression
Category: Antidepressant, tricyclic
Half-life: 20–26 hours
**Clinically important, potentially hazardous interactions
with:** amprenavir, arbutamine, bupropion, clonidine,
epinephrine, formoterol, guanethidine, isocarboxazid, linezolid,
MAO inhibitors, phenelzine, quinolones, sparfloxacin,
tranylcypromine, venlafaxine

Reactions

Skin
Allergic reactions (sic) (<1%)
Diaphoresis (1–10%)
 (1991): Eikmeier G+, *Int Clin Psychopharmacol* 6(3), 147
Exanthems
Petechiae
Photosensitivity (<1%)
Pruritus
Purpura
Rash (sic)
Urticaria

Mucosal/ENT
Dysgeusia (>10%)
Glossitis
Sialadenitis
 (1982): Ponte CD, *Drug Intell Clin Pharm* 16(3), 248
Stomatitis
Tinnitus
Xerostomia (>10%)
 (1994): Hohagen F+, *Eur Arch Psychiatry Clin Neurosci* 244(2), 65

(1991): Eikmeier G+, *Int Clin Psychopharmacol* 6(3), 147

Hair
Hair – alopecia (<1%)

Other
Gynecomastia (<1%)
Hypotension
 (2003): Frieboes RM+, *Pharmacopsychiatry* 36(1), 12
Nephrotoxicity
 (1986): Leighton JD+, *N Z Med J* 99(799), 248
Paresthesias
Seizures
 (2001): Enns MW, *J Clin Psychiatry* 62(6), 476 (with bupropion)
 (2000): Schlienger RG+, *Ann Pharmacother* 34(12), 1402 (with
 venlafaxine)
Tremor
 (1991): Eikmeier G+, *Int Clin Psychopharmacol* 6(3), 147
Vertigo
 (1991): Eikmeier G+, *Int Clin Psychopharmacol* 6(3), 147

TRIOXSALEN

Trade names: Neosoralen; Puvadin; Trisoralen (Valeant)
Indications: Vitiligo, hypopigmentation
Category: Psoralen; Repigmenting agent
Half-life: ~2 hours

Reactions

Skin
Acne
Bullous dermatitis (with UVA)
 (1999): Chuan MT+, *J Formos Med Assoc* 98, 335
Eczema
Ephelides
 (1984): Kietzmann E+, *Dermatologica* 168, 306
 (1983): Kanerva L+, *Dermatologica* 166, 281
Granuloma annulare
Herpes simplex
 (1982): Stüttgen G, *Int J Dermatol* 21, 198
Herpes zoster
 (1982): Stüttgen G, *Int J Dermatol* 21, 198
Lupus erythematosus
 (1985): Bruze M+, *Acta Derm Venereol* (Stockh) 65, 31
Melanoma
 (1980): Forrest JB+, *J Surg Oncol* 13, 337
Pemphigus
Photosensitivity
Phototoxicity
 (2001): Snellman E+, *Acta Derm Venereol* 81(3), 171
 (1992): George SA+, *Br J Dermatol* 127, 444
Pigmentation
 (1989): Weiss E+, *Int J Dermatol* 28, 188
 (1987): Bruce DR+, *J Am Acad Dermatol* 16, 1087
 (1986): MacDonald KJS+, *Br J Dermatol* 114, 395
Porokeratosis (actinic)
 (1988): Beiteke U+, *Photodermatology* 5, 274
 (1985): Hazen PG+, *J Am Acad Dermatol* 12, 1077
 (1980): Reymond JL, *Acta Derm Venereol* (Stockh) 60, 539
Pruritus (>10%)
 (1999): Chuan MT+, *J Formos Med Assoc* 98, 335
Scleroderma
Seborrheic dermatitis
 (1983): Tegner E, *Acta Derm Venereol* (Stockh) Suppl 107, 5
Vasculitis

(1981): Barriere H+, *Presse Med* (French) 10, 37
Vitiligo
  (1983): Tegner E, *Acta Derm Venereol* (Stockh) Suppl 107, 5
Xerosis
  (1999): Chuan MT+, *J Formos Med Assoc* 98, 335

Hair
Hair – hypertrichosis
  (1983): Rampen FHJ, *Br J Dermatol* 109, 657

Nails
Nails – photo-onycholysis
  (1987): Baran R+, *J Am Acad Dermatol* 17, 1012
Nails – pigmentation
  (1990): Trattner A+, *Int J Dermatol* 29, 310
  (1989): Weiss E+, *Int J Dermatol* 28, 188
  (1986): MacDonald KJS+, *Br J Dermatol* 114, 395
  (1982): Naik RPC+, *Int J Dermatol* 21, 275

Other
Lymphoproliferative disease
  (1989): Aschinoff R+, *J Am Acad Dermatol* 21, 1134
Pain
  (1987): Norris PG+, *Clin Exp Dermatol* 12, 403
  (1983): Tegner E, *Acta Derm Venereol* (Stockh) Suppl 107, 5
Tumors
  (1995): Halder RM+, *Arch Dermatol* 131, 734
  (1989): Hannuksela M+, *J Am Acad Dermatol* 21, 813
  (1988): Gupta AK+, *J Am Acad Dermatol* 19, 67
  (1987): Henseler T+, *J Am Acad Dermatol* 16, 108
  (1986): Kahn JR+, *Clin Exp Dermatol* 11, 398

TRIPELENNAMINE

Trade names: Azaron; PBZ (Novartis); Pyribenzamine; Triplen
Indications: Allergic rhinitis, urticaria
Category: Histamine H1 receptor antagonist
Half-life: N/A
Clinically important, potentially hazardous interactions with: alcohol, barbiturates, chloral hydrate, ethchlorvynol, paraldehyde, phenothiazines

Note: The intravenous use of a pentazocine/tripelennamine combination (T's and Blues) has become a major drug abuse problem

Reactions

Skin
Angioedema (<1%)
Dermatitis (systemic)
Diaphoresis
Edema (<1%)
Fixed eruption
Lichenoid eruption
Lupus erythematosus
Peripheral edema
Photosensitivity (<1%)
Pityriasis rosea
Purpura
Rash (sic) (<1%)
Urticaria

Mucosal/ENT
Stomatitis
Xerostomia (1–10%)

Other
Anaphylactoid reactions/Anaphylaxis
Hepatotoxicity
  (1982): Caplan LR+, *Neurology* 32(6), 623 (with pentazocine)
Infections
  (1982): Caplan LR+, *Neurology* 32(6), 623 (with pentazocine)
Myalgia/Myositis/Myopathy/Myotoxicity (<1%)
Paresthesias (<1%)
Seizures
  (1982): Caplan LR+, *Neurology* 32(6), 623 (with pentazocine)
  (1980): Lahmeyer HW+, *Int J Addict* 15(8), 1219 (with pentazocine)
Stroke
  (1982): Caplan LR+, *Neurology* 32(6), 623 (with pentazocine)
Tremor (<1%)

TRIPROLIDINE

Trade names: Actagen; Actidil; Actidilon; Actifed; Allerphed; Cenafed; Genac; Myidil; Trifed; Triofed; Triposed
Indications: Allergic rhinitis
Category: Histamine H1 receptor antagonist
Half-life: N/A

Note: Most of the trade name drugs contain pseudoephedrine as well

Reactions

Skin
Angioedema (<1%)
Diaphoresis (1–10%)
Edema (<1%)
Exanthems
Fixed eruption
Lichenoid eruption
Photosensitivity (<1%)
Purpura
Rash (sic) (<1%)
Urticaria

Mucosal/ENT
Xerostomia (1–10%)

Other
Myalgia/Myositis/Myopathy/Myotoxicity (<1%)
Paresthesias (<1%)

TRIPTORELIN

Synonym: Decapeptyl
Trade name: Trelstar (Debiopharma)
Indications: Palliative treatment of advanced prostate carcinoma
Category: Gonadotropin-releasing hormone agonist
Half-life: 2.8–1.2 hours

Reactions

Skin
Angioedema (<1%)
Pruritus (1%)
Vasculitis
  (1993): Amichai B+, *Eur J Obstet Gynecol Reprod Biol* 52, 217

Hair

Hair – alopecia
  (1997): Kauschansky A+, *Acta Derm Venereol* 77, 333

Other

Anaphylactoid reactions/Anaphylaxis (<1%)
Headache
Hot flashes (59%)
  (1996): Choktanasiri W+, *Int J Gynaecol Obstet* 54, 237
  (1994): Neskovic-Konstantinovic ZB+, *Oncology* 51, 95
  (1994): Vercellini P+, *Fertil Steril* 62, 938
Hypersensitivity (<1%)
Injection-site pain (4%)

TROLEANDOMYCIN

Trade name: TAO (Pfizer)
Indications: Various infections caused by susceptible organisms
Category: Antibiotic, macrolide
Half-life: N/A
**Clinically important, potentially hazardous interactions
with:** aprepitant, astemizole, carbamazepine, colchicine,
cyclosporine, dihydroergotamine, ergot alkaloids, ergotamine,
erythromycin, fluoxetine, fluvoxamine, methylprednisolone,
methysergide, oral contraceptives, paroxetine, pimozide,
prednisolone, rifampicin, sertraline, solifenacin, terfenadine,
warfarin

Reactions

Skin

Angioedema
Erythema multiforme
Exanthems
Pruritus
  (1987): Larrey D+, *J Hepatol* 4(3), 327
Rash (sic) (1–10%)
Urticaria (1–10%)

Mucosal/ENT

Oral lesions

Other

Anaphylactoid reactions/Anaphylaxis
Hepatotoxicity
  (1993): Uzzan B+, *Therapie* 48(1), 61
  (1987): Larrey D+, *J Hepatol* 4(3), 327
  (1985): Pessayre D+, *J Antimicrob Chemother* 16, 181 (with
    erythromycin)
  (1983): Fevery J+, *Acta Clin Belg* 38(4), 242 (with oral
    contraceptives)
  (1983): Laburthe-Tolra Y, *Sem Hop* 59(22), 1675
  (1982): Dellas JA+, *Therapie* 37(4), 443 (with oral
    contraceptives)
  (1980): Meyniel D+, *Therapie* 35(6), 754 (with oral
    contraceptives)
  (1980): Miguet JP+, *Ann Intern Med* 92(3), 434 (with oral
    contraceptives)

TROSPIUM

Trade name: Sanctura (Odyssey-Indevus)
Indications: Overactive bladder
Category: Anticholinergic; Antispasmodic
Half-life: 12–18 hours
**Clinically important, potentially hazardous interactions
with:** None

Reactions

Skin

Angioedema (<1%)
Stevens–Johnson syndrome
Xerosis

Mucosal/ENT

Dysgeusia (1–10%)
Xerostomia (20%)
  (2005): *Obstet Gynecol* 105(2), 431
  (2005): Singh-Franco+, *Clin Ther* 27(5), 511
  (2005): Zinner NR, *Expert Opin Pharmacother* 6(8), 1409
  (2004): Sand PK, *J Am Acad Nurs Pract* 16(10), 8
  (2003): Halaska M+, *World J Urol* 20(6), 392

Eyes

Ocular xerosis (1.2%)
Vision blurred

Other

Abdominal pain
Asthenia (2%)
Chest pain (<1%)
Headache (4%)
  (2005): Singh-Franco+, *Clin Ther* 27(5), 511
  (2005): Zinner NR, *Expert Opin Pharmacother* 6(8), 1409
Rhabdomyolysis (<1%)
Vertigo

TROVAFLOXACIN

Trade name: Trovan (Pfizer)
Indications: Various infections caused by susceptible organisms
Category: Antibiotic, quinolone
Half-life: 9.5 hours

Note: Trovafloxacin has been withdrawn in the USA except for
intravenous hospital use

Reactions

Skin

Acne
Allergic reactions (sic) (<1%)
Angioedema (<1%)
Dermatitis (<1%)
Diaphoresis (<1%)
Edema (<1%)
Erythema multiforme
Exanthems
  (1999): Litt JZ, Beachwood, OH (personal case) (observation)
Exfoliative dermatitis (<1%)
  (1999): Triller DM+, *Ann Pharmacother* 33(10), 1122
Facial edema (<1%)
Lichen planus

(1999): Smith KC, Niagara Falls, NY (from Internet)
(observation)
Peripheral edema (<1%)
Photosensitivity (0.03%)
(2000): Ferguson J+, J Antimicrob Chemother 45, 503
Phototoxicity
(2000): Traynor NJ+, Toxicol Vitr 14, 275
Pruritus (2%)
(1999): Litt JZ, Beachwood, OH (personal case) (observation)
(1998): Mayne JT+, J Antimicrob Chemother 39, 67
Pruritus ani et vulvae (<1%)
Rash (sic) (2%)
Seborrhea (<1%)
Stevens–Johnson syndrome (<1%)
Toxic epidermal necrolysis
(1999): Matthews MR+, Arch Intern Med 159, 2225
Ulcerations (<1%)
Urticaria (<1%)
Vasculitis

Mucosal/ENT
Balanitis (<1%)
Cheilitis (<1%)
Dysgeusia (<1%)
Gingivitis (<1%)
Sialorrhea (<1%)
Stomatitis (<1%)
Tongue disorder (<1%)
Tongue edema (<1%)
Vaginitis (<10%)
(1998): Jones RB+, Am J Med 104(1), 28 (4%)
Xerostomia (<1%)

Eyes
Periorbital edema (<1%)

Other
Anaphylactoid reactions/Anaphylaxis (<1%)
Candidiasis (<1%)
Headache
(1999): Alghasham AA+, Ann Pharmacother 33(1), 48
(1998): Williams D+, Eur J Clin Microbiol Infect Dis 17(6), 454
(1998): Williams DJ+, Am J Surg 176(6A), 74S
Hepatotoxicity
(2005): Liguori MJ+, Hepatology 41(1), 177
(2005): Peters TS, Toxicol Pathol 33(1), 146
(2003): Ball P, J Antimicrob Chemother 51, 21
(2002): Zhanel GG+, Drugs 62(1), 13
(2001): Lazarczyk DA+, Dig Dis Sci 46(4), 925
(2000): Bertino J+, Clin Ther 22(7), 798
(2000): Chen HJ+, N Engl J Med 342(5), 359
(2000): Lucena MI+, Clin Infect Dis 30(2), 400
Hypersensitivity
Injection-site edema (<1%)
Injection-site inflammation (<1%)
Injection-site pain (<1%)
Myalgia/Myositis/Myopathy/Myotoxicity (<1%)
Neurotoxicity
(2001): Cohen JS, Ann Pharmacother 35(12), 1540
(1999): Menzies D+, Am J Med 107(3), 298
Paresthesias (<1%)
Serum sickness
Tendinopathy/Tendon rupture
Thrombophlebitis (<1%)
Vertigo
(2003): Klossek JM+, J Laryngol Otol 117(1), 43
(1999): Alghasham AA+, Ann Pharmacother 33(1), 48
(1999): Lipsky BA+, Clin Infect Dis 28(2), 352

(1998): Williams D+, Eur J Clin Microbiol Infect Dis 17(6), 454
(1998): Williams DJ+, Am J Surg 176(6A), 74S

TRYPTOPHAN

Scientific name: L-2-amino-3-(indole-3yl) propionic acid
Family: None
Trade and other common names: 5-HT; 5-HTP; 5-hydroxytryptophan; 5-OHTrp; L-trypt; L-tryptophan
Category: Amino acid; Antidepressant
Purported indications and other uses: Insomnia, depression, myofascial pain, premenstrual syndrome, smoking cessation, bruxism
Half-life: N/A
Clinically important, potentially hazardous interactions with: fluoxetine, fluvoxamine, isocarboxazid, phenelzine, sibutramine, tranylcypromine

Reactions

Skin
Acanthosis nigricans
(1991): Blauvelt A+, Arch Dermatol 127(8), 1159
Diaphoresis (with phenelzine)
(1985): Levy AB+, Can J Psychiatry 30(6), 434 (with phenelzine)
Scleroderma
(2000): Egermayer P, J Intern Med 247(1), 11
(2000): Nietert PJ+, Curr Opin Rheumatol 12(6), 520
(1998): Haustein UF+, Clin Dermatol 16(3), 353
(1993): Morgan JM+, Br J Dermatol 128(5), 581
(1992): Guerin SB+, J Cutan Pathol 19(3), 207
(1991): Joly P+, J Am Acad Dermatol 25(2 Pt 1), 332
(1990): Silver RM+, N Engl J Med 322(13), 874
Shivering (with phenelzine)

Mucosal/ENT
Dysphagia
(1995): Levine B+, Ann Otol Rhinol Laryngol 104(2), 90 (56%)
Xerostomia
(1995): Levine B+, Ann Otol Rhinol Laryngol 104(2), 90 (66%)

Other
Death
(2002): Avarello TP+, Neurol Sci 23, S55 (from contaminants)
Fever
(2002): Avarello TP+, Neurol Sci 23, S55
Myoclonus
(1985): Levy AB+, Can J Psychiatry 30(6), 434 (with phenelzine)

TURMERIC

Scientific names: *Curcuma aromatica; Curcuma domestica; Curcuma longa; Curcuma xanthorrhiza*
Family: Zingiberaceae
Trade and other common names: Calebin-A; Chiang Huang; Curcumin; E100; Haridra; Indian Saffron; Jiang Huang; Yellow Root; Yu Jin; Zedoary
Category: Anti-inflammatory; TNF inhibitor
Purported indications and other uses: Arthritis, anticarcinogen, stimulant, carminative, amenorrhea, angina, asthma, colorectal cancer, delirium, diarrhea, dyspepsia, flatulence, hemorrhage, hepatitis, hypercholesterolemia, hypertension, jaundice, mania, menstrual disorders, ophthalmia, tendonitis. **Topical:** conjuctivitis, skin cancer, smallpox, chickenpox, leg ulcers. Food coloring in cheese, margarine, sweets, snack foods, cosmetics, essential oil in perfumes, culinary spice
Half-life: N/A

Reactions

Skin
Allergic reactions (sic) (rare)
Dermatitis
  (1997): Hata M+, *Contact Dermatitis* 36(2), 107
  (1993): Futrell JM+, *Cutis* 52(5), 288
  (1987): Goh CL+, *Contact Dermatitis* 17(3), 186

Other
Headache
  (2004): Thaler D, Monona, WI (from Internet) (observation)

UNOPROSTONE

Synonym: UF-021
Trade name: Rescula (Novartis)
Indications: Open-angle glaucoma
Category: Prostaglandin
Half-life: 14 minutes

Reactions

Skin
Allergic reactions (sic) (1–10%)
Diaphoresis
Irritation
  (1999): Hejkal TW+, *Semin Ophthalmol* 14, 114
Shivering

Mucosal/ENT
Xerostomia
  (1998): Stewart WC+, *J Glaucoma* 7, 388
  (1996): Haria M+, *Drugs Aging* 9, 213
  (1993): Azuma I+, *Jpn J Ophthalmol* 37, 514

Eyes
Eyelashes – hypertrichosis
  (1999): Hejkal TW+, *Semin Ophthalmol* 14, 114
Eyelid edema
Ocular burning (10–25%)
  (2003): Hommer A+, *Br J Ophthalmol* 87(5), 592 (with timolol)
Ocular edema
  (2005): Arcieri ES+, *Arch Ophthalmol* 123(2), 186
Ocular erythema

  (2001): Aung T+, *Am J Ophthalmol* 131(5), 636
Ocular pigmentation
  (2002): Novack GD+, *J Am Geriatr Soc* 50(5), 956
  (2002): Stjernschantz JW+, *Surv Ophthalmol* 47, S162
  (1999): Hejkal TW+, *Semin Ophthalmol* 14, 114
Ocular pruritus (10–25%)
Ocular stinging (10–25%)
  (2003): Hommer A+, *Br J Ophthalmol* 87(5), 592 (with timolol)

Other
Headache
Myalgia/Myositis/Myopathy/Myotoxicity
Paresthesias (tongue)
  (1998): Stewart WC+, *J Glaucoma* 7, 388
  (1996): Haria M+, *Drugs Aging* 9, 213
  (1993): Azuma I+, *Jpn J Ophthalmol* 37, 514

URACIL/TEGAFUR

Synonyms: UFT; TS-1; Ftorafur
Trade name: Uftoral (Bristol-Myers Squibb)
Indications: Metastatic colorectal cancer
Category: Folic acid antagonist
Half-life: 6.5 hours
Clinically important, potentially hazardous interactions with: allopurinol, cimetidine, clozapine, metronidazole, phenytoin, warfarin

Note: Tegafur is a prodrug of fluorouracil

Reactions

Skin
Acral erythema
  (1997): Bastida J+, *Acta Derm Venereol* 77(1), 72
  (1995): Jucgla A+, *Arch Dermatol* 131(3), 364
Dermatitis
  (1990): Unda Urzaiz M+, *Arch Esp Urol* 43(2), 143
Dermatomyositis
  (1997): Akiyama C+, *Acta Derm Venereol* 77(6), 490
Eczema
  (1986): Horio T+, *Photodermatol* 3(3), 192
Edema
  (1998): Mani S+, *Ann Oncol* 9(9), 1035
Hand–foot syndrome
  (2007): Kanaji N+, *Nihon Kokyuki Gakkai Zasshi* 45(6), 474 (with docetaxel)
  (2000): Lin JK+, *Jpn J Clin Oncol* 30(11), 510 (2 cases)
  (1997): Bastida J+, *Acta Derm Venereol* 77(1), 72
  (1997): Rios-Buceta L+, *Acta Derm Venereol* 77(1), 80
  (1995): Jucgla A+, *Arch Dermatol* 131(3), 364
  (1991): Camps C+, *Rev Clin Esp* 188(3), 165
Keratoderma
  (1998): Won YH+, *Int J Dermatol* 37(4), 315
  (1995): Jucgla A+, *Arch Dermatol* 131(3), 364
Lupus erythematosus
  (2001): Yoshimasu T+, *Eur J Dermatol* 11(1), 54
Mucha–Habermann disease
  (1999): Kawamura K+, *J Dermatol* 26(3), 164
Palmar–plantar pigmentation
  (1991): Llistosella E+, *Cutis* 48(3), 205
Photosensitivity
  (1997): Usuki A+, *Int J Dermatol* 36(8), 604
  (1986): Horio T+, *Photodermatol* 3(3), 192
  (1984): Sun CC+, *Photodermatol* 1(2), 94
Pigmentation

(1990): Del Pozo LJ+, *Med Cutan Ibero Lat Am* 18(1), 78
Rash (sic)
  (1997): Pazdur R+, *Invest New Drugs* 15(2), 123 (with leucovorin)
Raynaud's phenomenon
  (2000): Seishima M+, *Eur J Dermatol* 10(1), 55
Scleroderma
  (2000): Kono T+, *J Am Acad Dermatol* 42(3), 519
Side effects
  (1999): Revenga F, *Int J Dermatol* 38(12), 955
  (1997): Rios-Buceta L+, *Acta Derm Venereol* 77(1), 80
Toxicity (sic)
  (1997): Ribas A+, *Clin Oncol (R Coll Radiol)* 9(4), 269 (with leucovorin)

Mucosal/ENT
Anosmia
  (1995): Nakamura H+, *Eur Arch Otorhinolaryngol* 252(1), 48
  (1986): Majima H+, *Gan To Kagaku Ryoho* 13(6), 2128
Dysgeusia
Hyposmia
  (1986): Majima H+, *Gan To Kagaku Ryoho* 13(6), 2128
Mucositis
  (2004): Nagy B+, *Magy Onkol* 48(2), 145 (56%)
  (2004): Okita J+, *Auris Nasus Larynx* 31(1), 43 (with carboplatin)
  (2001): Wellington K+, *Drugs Aging* 18(12), 935
  (1995): Gonzalez-Baron M+, *Eur J Cancer* 31A(13–14), 2215 (with leucovorin)
Oral mucositis
  (2003): Iwase H+, *Int J Clin Oncol* 8(5), 305 (with cisplatin) (4%)
  (1998): Nogue M+, *Cancer* 83(2), 254 (with leucovorin) (18%)
  (1997): Kim YH+, *Oncology (Williston Park)* 11(9 Suppl 10), 119 (with leucovorin)
Stomatitis
  (2004): Feliu J+, *Br J Cancer* 91(10), 1758 (with oxaliplatin) (1%)
  (1997): Pazdur R+, *Invest New Drugs* 15(2), 123 (with leucovorin)
  (1994): Tanaka K+, *Gan To Kagaku Ryoho* 21(8), 1229 (18%)

Nails
Nails – brittle
Nails – changes
  (1990): Unda Urzaiz M+, *Arch Esp Urol* 43(2), 143
Nails – pigmentation
  (2004): Chen GY+, *Acta Derm Venereol* 84(3), 238
  (1991): Llistosella E+, *Cutis 1991 Sep* 48(3), 205
Nails – ridging

Eyes
Blepharospasm
  (1984): Salminen L+, *Am J Ophthalmol* 97(5), 649
Conjunctivitis

Other
Abdominal pain
  (2001): Wellington K+, *Drugs Aging* 18(12), 935
  (1997): Pazdur R+, *Invest New Drugs* 15(2), 123 (with leucovorin)
Asthenia
  (2004): Feliu J+, *Br J Cancer* 91(10), 1758 (with oxaliplatin) (9%)
  (2002): Feliu J+, *Ann Oncol* 13(11), 1756 (with gemcitabine) (2%)
  (2001): Wellington K+, *Drugs Aging* 18(12), 935
  (1999): Mani S+, *Invest New Drugs* 17(1), 97 (with leucovorin)
  (1998): Nogue M+, *Cancer* 83(2), 254 (with leucovorin) (10%)
  (1997): Pazdur R+, *Invest New Drugs* 15(2), 123 (with leucovorin)
Hypertension
  (1998): Maemondo M+, *Nihon Kokyuki Gakkai Zasshi* 36(9), 823
Infections

(1997): Ribas A+, *Clin Oncol (R Coll Radiol)* 9(4), 269 (with leucovorin)
Neurotoxicity
  (2004): Feliu J+, *Br J Cancer* 91(10), 1758 (with oxaliplatin) (14%)
Pain
  (2003): Iwase H+, *Int J Clin Oncol* 8(5), 305 (with cisplatin) (7%)
  (1998): Mani S+, *Ann Oncol* 9(9), 1035

URAPIDIL

Trade names: Ebrantil; Eupressyl (Altana)
Indications: Hypertension
Category: Adrenergic alpha-receptor antagonist; Serotonin agonist
Half-life: Oral: 4.7 hours; I.V.: 2.7 hours

Reactions

Skin
Allergic reactions (sic)
Pruritus
Psoriasis
  (2007): Takehara Y+, *J Eur Acad Dermatol Venereol* 21(4), 577

Mucosal/ENT
Nasal congestion

Other
Asthenia
  (1990): Liebau H+, *Fortschr Med* 108(16), 325
  (1989): Langtry HD+, *Drugs* 38(6), 900
  (1989): Schook CE+, *Am J Cardiol* 64(7), 30D
  (1988): Rosendorff C, *Drugs* 35, 188
Headache
  (2006): Wacker JR+, *Eur J Obstet Gynecol Reprod Biol.* 127(2), 160
  (1993): Amodeo C+, *Arq Bras Cardiol* 61(2), 127
  (1989): Langtry HD+, *Drugs* 38(6), 900
  (1989): Rosenthal J+, *Am J Cardiol* 64(7), 25D
  (1989): Schook CE+, *Am J Cardiol* 64(7), 30D
  (1989): Stumpe KO+, *Fortschr Med* 107(1), 54
  (1988): Trimarco B+, *Drugs* 35, 173
Hypotension
Somnolence
  (1990): Liebau H+, *Fortschr Med* 108(16), 325
  (1988): Bottorff MB+, *J Clin Pharmacol* 28(5), 420
Vertigo
  (1993): Amodeo C+, *Arq Bras Cardiol* 61(2), 127
  (1990): Liebau H+, *Fortschr Med* 108(16), 325
  (1989): Langtry HD+, *Drugs* 38(6), 900
  (1989): Rosenthal J+, *Am J Cardiol* 64(7), 25D
  (1989): Schook CE+, *Am J Cardiol* 64(7), 30D
  (1989): Stumpe KO+, *Fortschr Med* 107(1), 54
  (1988): Rosendorff C, *Drugs* 35, 188
  (1988): Trimarco B+, *Drugs* 35, 173

UROFOLLITROPIN

Trade names: Bravelle; Fertinex; Fertinorm; Follegon; Follimon; Gonotrop F; Medtrodine HP; Metrodin; Metrodin HP
Indications: Infertility, Polycystic ovary syndrome, Follicle stimulation
Category: Follicle-stimulating hormone
Half-life: N/A
Clinically important, potentially hazardous interactions with: None

Reactions

Skin
Exanthems
Urticaria
Xerosis

Hair
Hair – alopecia

Other
Abdominal pain
Asthenia
Chills
Fever
Hot flashes
Injection-site edema
Injection-site irritation
Injection-site pain
Myalgia/Myositis/Myopathy/Myotoxicity
Thrombophlebitis

UROKINASE

Trade names: Abbokinase (Abbott); Ukidan
Indications: Acute myocardial infarction, coronary artery thrombosis, pulmonary embolism
Category: Fibrinolytic; Plasminogen activator
Half-life: 10–20 minutes
Clinically important, potentially hazardous interactions with: aspirin, bivalirudin, ibuprofen, indomethacin

Reactions

Skin
Angioedema (>10%)
 (2001): Pechlaner C+, *Blood Coagul Fibrinolysis* 12(6), 491
Bullous dermatitis (hemorrhagic)
 (1995): Ejaz AA+, *Am J Nephrol* 15, 178
Diaphoresis (<1%)
Exanthems
Pruritus
Purpura
Rash (sic) (<1%)
Urticaria

Eyes
Periorbital edema (>10%)

Other
Anaphylactoid reactions/Anaphylaxis (>10%)
 (2001): Pechlaner C+, *Blood Coagul Fibrinolysis* 12(6), 491
Chills

Hypersensitivity
 (2001): Pechlaner C+, *Blood Coagul Fibrinolysis* 12(6), 491
Injection-site phlebitis

URSODIOL

Synonym: Ursodeoxycholic Acid
Trade names: Actigall (Watson); Adursall; Arsacol; Biliepar; Cholacid; Cholit-Ursan; Cholofalk; Coledos; Delursan; Desocol; Desoxil; Destolit; Deurcil; Dexo; Estazor; Fraurs; Galmax; Lentorsil; Litanin; Litocure; Litoff; Litursol; Lyeton; Peptaron; Solutrat; UDC; UDC Hexal; Urdafalk; Urdes; Urosofalk; Urso (Axcan); Urso Heumann; Urso Vinas; Ursochol; Ursofal; Ursoflor; Ursolac; Ursolism; Ursolvan; Urson; Ursoproge; Ursosan; Ursotan; USCA
Indications: Cholelithiasis
Category: Urolithic
Half-life: 100 hours

Reactions

Skin
Allergic reactions (sic) (5%)
Dermatitis herpetiformis
 (2001): Stroubou E+, *J Am Acad Dermatol* 45(2), 319
Diaphoresis
Lichen planus
 (1992): Ellul JP+, *Dig Dis Sci* 37, 628
Lichenoid eruption
 (2002): Matsuzaki Y+, *Gastroenterology* 122(5), 1547
 (2001): Horiuchi Y, *Gastroenterology* 121(2), 501
Pruritus (<1%)
Psoriasis
Rash (sic) (1–3%)
Urticaria
Xerosis

Mucosal/ENT
Dysgeusia (<1%) (metallic taste)
Stomatitis

Hair
Hair – alopecia (<1–5%)

Other
Asthenia (<1%)
Depression
Myalgia/Myositis/Myopathy/Myotoxicity
Vertigo (~17%)

VALACYCLOVIR

Trade name: Valtrex (GSK)
Indications: Genital herpes, herpes simplex, herpes zoster
Category: Antiviral; Guanine nucleoside analog
Half-life: 3 hours
Clinically important, potentially hazardous interactions with: immunosuppressants, meperidine

Reactions

Skin
Dermatitis (systemic)

(2001): Lammintausta K+, *Contact Dermatitis* 45(3), 181
Facial edema (3–5%)
  (2000): Colin J+, *Ophthalmology* (107) 1507 (3–5%)
Pruritus (generalized)
  (2004): Danby WF, Manchester, NH (from Internet)
    (observation)
  (2001): Vaughan TK, Tacoma, WA (from Internet) (observation)
Purpura
  (2000): Rivaud E+, *Arch Intern Med* 160, 1705

Eyes
Periorbital edema (3–5%)
  (2000): Colin J+, *Ophthalmology* 107, 1507 (3–5%)

Other
Abdominal pain
  (2004): Sra KK+, *Skin Therapy Lett* 9(8), 1
Aseptic meningitis
  (2003): Olin JL+, *Ann Pharmacother* 37(12), 1814
Chills
  (2004): Danby WF, Manchester, NH (from Internet)
    (observation)
Confusion
  (2006): Das V+, *Nephrol Dial Transplant* 21(5), 1395
Headache
  (2004): Sra KK+, *Skin Therapy Lett* 9(8), 1
Myalgia/Myositis/Myopathy/Myotoxicity
  (2004): Danby WF, Manchester, NH (from Internet)
    (observation)
Neurotoxicity
  (2003): Olin JL+, *Ann Pharmacother* 37(12), 1814
Paresthesias
  (2003): Baker D+, *Cutis* 71(3), 239

VALDECOXIB

Trade name: Bextra (Pfizer)
Indications: Osteoarthritis, adult rheumatoid arthritis,
dysmenorrhea
Category: COX-2 inhibitor; Non-steroidal anti-inflammatory
Half-life: 8–11 hours
**Clinically important, potentially hazardous interactions
with:** aspirin, dextromethorphan, lithium, warfarin

Note: This drug has been withdrawn

Note: Valdecoxib is a sulfonamide and can be absorbed systemically.
Sulfonamides can produce severe, possibly fatal, reactions such as
toxic epidermal necrolysis and Stevens–Johnson syndrome

Reactions

Skin
Acne (<2%)
Acute generalized exanthematous pustulosis
  (2005): Byerly FL+, *Burns* 31(3), 383
Allergic reactions (sic) (<2%)
Basal cell carcinoma
Cellulitis (<2%)
Dermatitis (<2%)
  (2005): Jaeger C+, *Contact Dermatitis* 52, 47
Diaphoresis (<2%)
Eczema (<2%)
Edema (<2%)
Erythema multiforme
  (2003): Sharma R, Aligarh, India (from Internet) (observation)
Exanthems (<2%)

(2002): Litt JZ, Beachwood, OH (personal case)
(2002): Smith JG, Mobile, AL (from Internet) (observation)
Facial edema (<2%)
Hematomas (<2%)
Herpes simplex
Herpes zoster
Malignant melanoma
Peripheral edema (2–3%)
Photosensitivity (<2%)
Pruritus (<2%)
  (2004): Klein AD, Streetsboro, GA (not allergic to celecoxib)
    (from Internet) (observation)
Psoriasis (<2%)
Rash (sic) (1–2)
Stevens–Johnson syndrome
  (2005): La Grenade L+, *Drug Saf* 28(10), 917 (63 cases)
  (2004): Thaler D, Monona, WI (from Internet) (observation)
Toxic epidermal necrolysis
  (2005): La Grenade L+, *Drug Saf* 28(10), 917 (63 cases)
  (2003): Glasser DL+, *Pharmacotherapy* 23(4), 551
Ulcerations (<2%)
Urticaria (<2%)
  (2005): Boehncke S+, *Dtsch Med Wochenschr* 130(40), 2249
  (2005): Sanchez-Borges M+, *Ann Allergy Asthma Immunol*
    94(1), 34
  (2004): Klein AD, Streetsboro, GA (not allergic to celecoxib)
    (from Internet) (observation)
Vesiculobullous eruption
  (2004): Sharma R, Aligarh, India (from Internet) (observation)
Xerosis (<2%)

Mucosal/ENT
Dysgeusia (<2%)
Stomatitis (<2%)
Tinnitus (2–10%)
Vulvovaginal candidiasis
Xerostomia (<2%)

Hair
Hair – alopecia (<2%)

Eyes
Periorbital edema (<2%)

Other
Candidiasis
Chills (<2%)
Cough (<2%)
Depression (<2%)
Headache
Hot flashes (<2%)
Lipomatosis (<2%)
Myalgia/Myositis/Myopathy/Myotoxicity (2%)
Nephrotoxicity
  (2005): Muhlfeld AS+, *Clin Nephrol* 63(3), 221
  (2003): Ott E+, *J Thorac Cardiovasc Surg* 125(6), 1481
Paresthesias (<2%)
Stroke
  (2005): Hersh EV+, *Curr Med Res Opin* 21(8), 1217
  (2005): Nussmeier NA+, *N Engl J Med* 352(11), 1081
Tendinopathy/Tendon rupture (<2%)
Thrombophlebitis (<2%)
Tremor (<2%)
Upper respiratory infection (6–7%)

VALERIAN

Scientific names: *Valeriana edulis; Valeriana jatamansii; Valeriana officinalis; Valeriana sitchensis; Valeriana wallichii*
Family: Valerianaceae
Trade and other common names: All-Heal; Amantilla; Baldrian; Garden Heliotrope
Category: Anxiolytic
Purported indications and other uses: Depression, tremors, epilepsy, attention deficit hyperactivity disorder, rheumatism, nervous asthma, gastric spasms, colic, menstrual cramps, hot flashes. Flavoring in foods and beverages
Half-life: N/A
Clinically important, potentially hazardous interactions with: escitalopram

Reactions

Skin
Adverse effects (sic)
  (2002): Haller CA+, *Adverse Drug React Toxicol Rev* 21(3), 143

Other
Toxicity (sic)
  (2001): Boniel T+, *Harefuah* 140(8), 780
Tremor
  (2001): Boniel T+, *Harefuah* 140(8), 780

VALGANCICLOVIR

Trade name: Valcyte (Roche)
Indications: Cytomegalovirus retinitis (in patients with AIDS)
Category: Antiviral; Guanine nucleoside analog
Half-life: 4 hours (In severe renal impairment up to 68%)
Clinically important, potentially hazardous interactions with: tenofovir

Note: Valganciclovir is rapidly converted to ganciclovir in the body

Reactions

Skin
Allergic reactions (sic) (<5%)
Pruritus
  (2004): Constable S+, *Expert Opin Drug Saf* 3(3), 249
Rash (sic)
  (2004): Constable S+, *Expert Opin Drug Saf* 3(3), 249

Mucosal/ENT
Oral candidiasis
  (2003): *Prescrire Int* 12(66), 133
  (2002): Lalezari J+, *J Acquir Immune Defic Sybdr* 30(4), 392 (17%)

Eyes
Retinal detachment
  (2001): Curran M+, *Drugs* 61(8), 1145

Other
Abdominal pain
  (2001): Curran M+, *Drugs* 61(8), 1145
Asthenia
  (2004): Constable S+, *Expert Opin Drug Saf* 3(3), 249
Fever
  (2004): Constable S+, *Expert Opin Drug Saf* 3(3), 249

  (2002): Lalezari J+, *J Acquir Immune Defic Syndr* 30(4), 392 (18%)
  (2001): Curran M+, *Drugs* 61(8), 1145
Headache
  (2004): Constable S+, *Expert Opin Drug Saf* 3(3), 249
  (2001): Curran M+, *Drugs* 61(8), 1145
Infections (<5%)
  (2004): Constable S+, *Expert Opin Drug Saf* 3(3), 249
Neurotoxicity
  (2006): Peyriere H+, *Ann Pharmacother* 40(1), 143
  (2001): Curran M+, *Drugs* 61(8), 1145
Paresthesias (8%)
  (2001): Curran M+, *Drugs* 61(8), 1145

VALPROIC ACID

Trade names: Depacon (Abbott); Depakene (Abbott); Depakote (Abbott)
Indications: Seizures, migraine
Category: Anticonvulsant; Antipsychotic
Half-life: 6–16 hours
Clinically important, potentially hazardous interactions with: aspirin, cholestyramine, clobazam, doripenem, **ginkgo biloba**, ivermectin, vorinostat

Reactions

Skin
Acne
Allergic reactions (sic) (<5%)
Bullous dermatitis
  (2001): Christ EA+ (poster at meeting of the American Federation for Medical Research)
Dermatitis
Diaphoresis
  (2001): Hebert AA+, *J Clin Psychiatry* 62(suppl 14), 22
Edema
  (2002): Witters I+, *Prenat Diagn* 22(9), 834
Erythema multiforme (<1%)
  (2001): Hebert AA+, *J Clin Psychiatry* 62(suppl 14), 22
  (1990): Chan HL+, *Arch Dermatol* 126, 43
Exanthems (5%)
  (2003): Warnock JK+, *Am J Clin Dermatol* 4(1), 21
Facial edema (>5%)
Fixed eruption
  (1997): Chan HL+, *J Am Acad Dermatol* 36, 259
Furunculosis (<5%)
Hand–foot syndrome
  (2005): Bhasin S+, *J Assoc Physicians India* 53, 155
Lupus erythematosus
  (1996): Gigli GL+, *Epilepsia* 37(6), 587
  (1996): Park-Matsumoto YC+, *J Neurol Sci* 143, 185
  (1994): Fritzler MJ, *Lupus* 3, 455
  (1993): Drory VE+, *Clin Neuropharmacol* 16, 19 (passim)
  (1990): Bleck TP+, *Epilepsia* 31, 343
Morphea
  (1980): Goihman-Yahr M+, *Arch Dermatol* 116, 621
Peripheral edema (<5%)
Petechiae (<5%)
  (2001): Hebert AA+, *J Clin Psychiatry* 62(suppl 14), 22
Photosensitivity
  (2001): Hebert AA+, *J Clin Psychiatry* 62(suppl a4), 22
Pruritus (>5%)
  (2001): Hebert AA+, *J Clin Psychiatry* 62(suppl 14), 22
Psoriasis

Purpura
 (1984): *Drugs Ther Bull* 22, 23
Rash (sic) (>5%)
 (2007): Arif H+, *Neurology* 68(20), 1701
 (2002): Gallagher RM+, *J Am Osteopath Assoc* 102(2), 92
Scleroderma
 (1980): Goihman-Yahr M+, *Arch Dermatol* 116, 621
Seborrhea
Stevens–Johnson syndrome
 (2007): Kocak S+, *Am J Clin Dermatol* 8(2), 107 (with
   lamotrigine)
 (2005): Mockenhaupt M+, *Neurology* 64(7), 1134
 (1999): Rzany B+, *Lancet* 353, 2190
 (1998): Tsai SJ+, *J Clin Psychopharmacol* 18, 420
 (1995): Kuper K+, *Ophthalmologe* 92(6), 823
Toxic epidermal necrolysis
 (2004): Hashim N+, *Acta Derm Venereol* 84(1), 90 (with
   lamotrigine)
 (1999): Rzany B+, *Lancet* 353, 2190
 (1991): Porteous DM+, *Arch Dermatol* 127, 740
Urticaria
Vasculitis
 (2003): Bonnet F+, *J Rheumatol* 30(1), 208
 (1991): Kamper AM+, *Lancet* 1, 497

Mucosal/ENT

Dysgeusia (<5%)
Gingival hyperplasia/hypertrophy
 (2004): Tan H+, *J Child Neurol* 19(12), 958
 (1997): Anderson HH+, *ASDC J Dent Child* 64, 294
 (1991): Behari M, *J Neurol Neurosurg Psychiatry* 54, 279
Glossitis (<5%)
Sialorrhea
Stomatitis (<5%)
Tinnitus
 (2000): Reeves RR+, *South Med J* 93(10), 1030
Vaginitis (<5%)
Xerostomia (<5%)
 (2002): Tohen M+, *Arch Gen Psychiatry* 59(1), 62 (with
   olanzapine)

Hair

Hair – alopecia (7%)
 (2002): Gallagher RM+, *J Am Osteopath Assoc* 102(2), 92
 (2001): Hebert AA+, *J Clin Psychiatry* 62(suppl 14), 22
 (1998): Fetterman M, Miami, FL (from Internet) (observation)
 (1996): McKinney PA+, *Ann Clin Psychiatry* 8, 183
 (1996): Wallace SJ, *Drug Saf* 15, 378
 (1995): Fatemi SH+, *Ann Pharmacother* 29, 1302
 (1981): Herranz JL, *Dev Med Child Neurol* 23, 386
Hair – curly
 (2001): Caneppele S+, *Ann Dermatol Venereol* 128(2), 134
 (1988): Gupta AK, *Br J Clin Pract* 42, 75
 (1986): Bittencourt PR, *Arq Neuropsiquiatr* 44(1), 78
Hair – poliosis
 (1981): Herranz JL+, *Dev Med Child Neurol* 23, 386

Nails

Nails – pigmentation
 (2003): Buka R+, *J Drugs Dermatol* 2(5), 545 (yellow)

Other

Abdominal pain
 (2004): Dutta S+, *Am J Health Syst Pharm* 61(21), 2280
Anticonvulsant hypersensitivity syndrome
 (2004): Papp Z+, *Orv Hetil* 145(32), 1665
 (2003): Arevalo-Lorido JC+, *Br J Clin Pharmacol* 55(4), 415
 (2003): Bin-Nakhi HA+, *Med Princ Pract* 12(3), 197
 (2002): Galindo PA+, *J Investig Allergol Clin Immunol* 12(4), 299
 (2000): Picart N+, *Presse Med* 29(12), 648

Aplasia cutis congenita
Asthenia
 (2004): Dutta S+, *Am J Health Syst Pharm* 61(21), 2280
Coma
 (2005): Meyer S+, *Klin Padiatr* 217(2), 82
Death
 (2003): Huang YL+, *J Am Acad Dermatol* 49(2), 316
 (2002): Yazdani K+, *Medicine* (Baltimore) 81(4), 305
DRESS syndrome
 (2006): Yun SJ+, *Acta Derm Venereol* 86(3), 241 (with
   carbamazepine)
Gynecomastia
 (1983): Kollipara S+, *J Pediatr* 103, 501
Headache
 (2004): Dutta S+, *Am J Health Syst Pharm* 61(21), 2280
Hepatotoxicity
 (2002): Chitturi S+, *Semin Liver Dis* 22(2), 169
Hypersensitivity
 (2003): Huang YL+, *J Am Acad Dermatol* 49(2), 316
 (2000): Moore SJ+, *J Med Genet* 37, 489
 (1999): Conilleau V+, *Contact Dermatitis* 41(3), 141
 (1994): Garcia-Bravo B+, *Contact Dermatitis* 30, 40
Inappropriate secretion of antidiuretic hormone (SIADH)
 (2001): Miyaoka T+, *Int Clin Psychopharmacol* 16(1), 59
 (1998): Branten AJ+, *Ann Neurol* 43(2), 265
 (1994): Ikeda K+, *Rinsho Shinkeigaku* 34(9), 911
Myalgia/Myositis/Myopathy/Myotoxicity
 (2005): Kasturi L+, *Indian J Pediatr* 72(3), 243
Pain
 (2004): Dutta S+, *Am J Health Syst Pharm* 61(21), 2280
Paresthesias (<5%)
Porphyria
 (1991): Jalil P+, *Rev Med Chil* 119, 920
 (1981): Doss M+, *Lancet* 2, 91
Pseudolymphoma
 (2003): Choi TS+, *Br J Dermatol* 148(4), 730
 (2001): Cogrel O+, *Br J Dermatology* 144, 1235
Rhabdomyolysis
 (2001): Kottlors M+, *Neuromuscul Disord* 11(8), 757
 (1997): Chattergoon DS+, *Neurology* 49(5), 1442 (with
   lamotrigine)
Seizures
 (2001): Lerman-Sagie T+, *Epilepsia* 42(7), 941
Somnambulism
 (2003): Sattar SP+, *Ann Pharmacother* 37(10), 1429 (with
   zolpidem)
Tremor
 (2005): Rinnerthaler M+, *Epilepsia* 46(2), 320 (6–45%)
 (2002): Gallagher RM+, *J Am Osteopath Assoc* 102(2), 92
 (2002): Thibault M+, *Epilepsy Res* 50(3), 243
 (2002): Tohen M+, *Arch Gen Psychiatry* 59(1), 62 (with lithium)
Vertigo
 (2005): Kochar DK+, *QJM* 98(1), 29 (1 case)
Weight gain
 (2007): Ben-Menachem, *Epilepsia* 48, 42
 (2005): Ness-Abramof R+, *Drugs Today* (Barc) 41(8), 547
 (1986): Bittencourt PR, *Arq Neuropsiquiatr* 44(1), 78

VALRUBICIN

Trade name: Valstar (Celltech)
Indications: Bladder carcinoma
Category: Antibiotic, anthracycline
Half-life: N/A
**Clinically important, potentially hazardous interactions
with:** None

Reactions

Skin

Irritation (sic) (<1%)
Peripheral edema (1%)
Pruritus (<1%)
Rash (sic) (3%)

Mucosal/ENT

Ageusia (<1%)

Other

Abdominal pain (5%)
  (1996): Markman M+, *Gynecol Oncol* 61(1), 90
Fever (2%)
Myalgia/Myositis/Myopathy/Myotoxicity (1%)
Vertigo (3%)

VALSARTAN

Trade name: Diovan (Novartis)
Indications: Hypertension
Category: Angiotensin II receptor antagonist
Half-life: 9 hours

Reactions

Skin

Allergic reactions (sic) (>2%)
Angioedema (>2%)
  (2003): Irons BK+, *Ann Pharmacother* 37(7–8), 1024
  (2002): Biswas PN I, *J Hum Hypertens* 16(11), 795
  (2000): de la Serna Higuera C, *Med Clin* (Barc) (Spanish)
    114, 599
  (1998): Frye Cb+, *Pharmacotherapy* 18, 866
Bullous pemphigoid
  (2003): Femiano F, *Minerva Stomatol* 52(4), 187
Eczema
  (2006): Selden ST, *Chesapeake VA* (from Internet) (observation)
Edema (>1%)
  (2000): Prat H, *Rev Med Chil* (Spanish) 128, 475
  (1996): Corea L+, *Clin Pharmacol Ther* 60, 341
Facial edema
  (2002): Biswas PN+, *J Hum Hypertens* 16(11), 795
Lupus erythematosus
  (2006): Sontheimer RD, Oklahoma City, OK (from Internet)
    (observation)
Photosensitivity
  (1998): Frye Cb+, *Pharmacotherapy* (18) 866
Pruritus (>2%)
Psoriasis
  (2005): Litt JZ, Beachwood, OH (personal case) (observation)
Rash (sic) (>2%)
Urticaria
  (2000): de la Serna Higuera C, *Med Clin* (Barc) (Spanish)
    114, 599

Mucosal/ENT

Aphthous stomatitis (1–10%)
Dysgeusia (>10%)
Xerostomia (>10%)

Nails

Nails – onychocryptosis
Nails – pigmentation

Other

Cough
  (2002): Biswas PN+, *J Hum Hypertens* 16(11), 795
  (2000): Prat H, *Rev Med Chil* 128, 475
Death
  (2001): Briggs GG+, *Ann Pharmacother* 35(7), 859
Depression
  (2003): Ullrich H+, *Dtsch Med Wochenschr* 128(48), 2534 (with
    hydrochlorothiazide)
Headache
Injection-site extravasation (<1%)
Injection-site pain
Injection-site phlebitis
Injection-site reactions (sic)
Myalgia/Myositis/Myopathy/Myotoxicity (10–29%)
Paresthesias (>2%)
Vertigo
  (2005): Ripley TL, *Ann Pharmacother* 39(3), 460
  (2002): Biswas PN+, *J Hum Hypertens* 16(11), 795 (1%)

VANCOMYCIN

Trade names: Balcoran; Diatracin; Vancocin (Lilly); Vanmicina
Indications: Various infections caused by susceptible organisms
Category: Antibiotic, glycopeptide
Half-life: 5–11 hours
**Clinically important, potentially hazardous interactions
with:** rocuronium, succinylcholine

Note: The vancomycin-induced red man syndrome is characterized
by pruritus, erythema and, in severe cases, angioedema, hypotension,
and cardiovascular collapse

Reactions

Skin

Acute generalized exanthematous pustulosis (AGEP)
  (2006): Davidovici BB+, *Harefuah* 145(7), 477 (with furosemide)
  (1996): Sawhney RA+, *Int J Dermatol* 35, 826
  (1995): Moreau A+, *Int J Dermatol* 34, 263 (passim)
  (1991): Roujeau J-C+, *Arch Dermatol* 127, 1333
Allergic reactions (sic) (<5%)
  (2001): Bernedo N+, *Contact Dermatitis* 45(1), 43
  (1997): Kahata S+, *Bone Marrow Transplant* 20, 1001
  (1997): Korman TM+, *J Antimicrob Chemother* 39(3), 371
  (1992): Breathnach SM+, *Adverse Drug Reactions and the Skin*
    Blackwell, Oxford, 158 (passim)
Angioedema
  (1989): Koestner B+, *Schweiz Med Wochenschr* (German)
    119, 28
Bullous dermatitis
  (1996): Heald PW, *Skin and Allergy News* 27, 18
  (1992): Carpenter S+, *J Am Acad Dermatol* 26, 45
  (1990): Forrence EA+, *Drug Intell Clin Pharm* 24, 369
  (1988): Baden LA+, *Arch Dermatol* 124, 1186
Erythema multiforme
  (2007): Lai MY+, *Allergy* 62(7), 824
  (2001): Hsu SI, *Pharmacotherapy* 21(10), 1233
  (2000): Padial MA+, *Allergy* 55, 1201
  (1992): Laurencin CT, *Ann Pharmacotherapy* 26, 1520
  (1988): Gutfeld MB+, *Drug Intell Clin Pharm* 22, 881
Exanthems
  (2004): Spencer L, Crawfordsville, IN (with daptomycin) (from
    Internet) (observation)
  (1991): McCullough JM+, *Drug Intell Clin Pharm* 25, 1326
  (1991): Valero R+, *J Cardiothorac Vasc Anesth* 5, 574

(1988): Neal D+, *BMJ* 296, 137
(1988): Schlemmer B+, *N Engl J Med* 318, 1127
(1987): Lacouture PG+, *J Pediatr* 111, 615 (35%)
(1987): Longon P+, *Presse Med* (French) 16, 682
(1986): Davis RL+, *Ann Intern Med* 104, 285
(1986): Markman M+, *South Med J* 79, 382 (passim)
(1986): McElrath MJ+, *Lancet* 1, 47
(1985): Schifter S+, *Lancet* 2, 499 (8%)
(1984): Odio C+, *Am J Dis Child* 138, 17
(1984): Rimailho A+, *Presse Med* (French) 13, 567

Exfoliative dermatitis
(1990): Forrence EA+, *Drug Intell Clin Pharm* 24, 369
(1988): Gutfeld MB+, *Drug Intell Clin Pharm* 22, 881
(1988): Neal D+, *BMJ* 296, 137

Fixed eruption
(2004): Gilmore ES+, *Pediatr Dermatol* 21(5), 600

Linear IgA dermatosis
(2006): Coelho S+, *Int J Dermatol* 45(8), 995
(2006): Navi D+, *Dermatol Online J* 12(5), 12
(2005): Onodera H+, *J Dermatol* 32(9), 759
(2004): Armstrong AW+, *J Cutan Pathol* 31(5), 393
(2004): Jones DH+, *J Am Osteopath Assoc* 104(4), 157
(2004): Joshi S+, *Ann Allergy Asthma Immunol* 93(1), 101
(2004): Solky BA+, *Cutis* 73(1), 65
(2004): Waldman MA+, *Clin Exp Dermatol* 29(6), 633
(2003): Avci O+, *J Am Acad Dermatol* 48(2), 299 (passim)
(2003): Brinkmeier T+, *J Dtsch Dermatol Ges* 1(3), 212
(2003): Dellavalle RP+, *J Am Acad Dermatol* 48(5), S56
(2003): Lesueur A+, *Presse Med* 32(23), 1078
(2003): Montagnac R+, *Nephrologie* 24(6), 287
(2002): Cohen LM+, *J Am Acad Dermatol* 46(2), S32
(2002): Neughebauer BI+, *Am J Med Sci* 323(5), 273
(2002): Rocha JL+, *Braz J Infect Dis* 6(4), 196
(2001): Ahkami R+, *Cutis* 67, 423
(2001): Chang A+, *Arch Dermatol* 137, 815
(2001): Palmer RA+, *Br J Dermatol* 145(5), 816 (2 cases)
(2001): Wiadrowski TP+, *Austral J Dermatol* 42, 196 (with ciprofloxacin)
(2000): Klein PA+, *J Am Acad Dermatol* 42, 316
(2000): Mofid MZ+, *J Burn Care Rehabil* 21(3), 246 (with phenytoin)
(1999): Nousari HC+, *Medicine* 78, 1
(1998): Bernstein EF+, *Ann Intern Med* 129, 508
(1998): Nousari HC+, *Ann Intern Med* 129, 507
(1997): Norland A, Minneapolis, American Academy of Dermatology Meeting (SF) (Gross and Microscopic)
(1996): Bitman LM+, *Arch Dermatol* 1289
(1996): Primka E+, *J Cutan Pathol* 58
(1996): Tranvan A+, *J Am Acad Dermatol* 865
(1996): Whitworth JM+, *J Am Acad Dermatol* 890
(1995): Geissmann C+, *J Am Acad Dermatol* 296
(1995): Richards S+, *Arch Dermatol* 1447
(1994): Kuechle MK+, *J Am Acad Dermatol* 187
(1994): Piketty C+, *Br J Dermatol* 130
(1992): Carpenter S+, *J Am Acad Dermatol* 45
(1988): Baden LA+, *Arch Dermatol* 1186

Lupus erythematosus
(1993): Ena J+, *JAMA* 269, 598
(1986): Markman M+, *South Med J* 79, 382

Necrotizing vasculitis
(2002): Rocha JL+, *Braz J Infect Dis* 6(4), 196

Photoallergic reaction
(2001): Zabawski E, Longview, TX (from Internet) (observation)

Pruritus
(2004): Spencer L, Crawfordsville, IN (with daptomycin) (from Internet) (observation)
(1991): Killian AD+, *Ann Intern Med* 115, 410
(1991): McCullough JM+, *Drug Intell Clin Pharm* 25, 1326
(1989): Koestner B+, *Schweiz Med Wochenschr* (German) 119, 28

(1986): Davis RL+, *Ann Intern Med* 104, 285

Purpura
(1998): Michael S+, *Scand J Rheumatol* 27, 233

Rash (sic)
(2001): Hsu SI, *Pharmacotherapy* 21(10), 1233
(1998): Elting LS+, *Cancer* 83(12), 2597 (11%)
(1997): Reis AG+, *Rev Paul Med* 115, 1452
(1993): Ena J+, *JAMA* 269, 598
(1983): Farber BF+, *Antimicrob Agents Chemother* 23, 138

Red man syndrome(1–14%)
(2005): Mitchell D, Thomasville, GA (from Internet) (observation)
(2004): Blumenthal HL, Beachwood, OH (personal case) (observation)
(2002): Cohen E+, *J Antimicrob Chemother* 49(1), 155 (10–14%)
(2002): Hui YL+, *Acta Anaesthesiol Sin* 40(3), 149
(2002): Rocha JL+, *Braz J Infect Dis* 6(4), 196
(2001): Wazny LD+, *Ann Pharmacother* 35(11), 1458
(2000): Wood MJ, *J Chemother* 12, 21
(1999): Khurana C+, *Postgrad Med J* 75, 41
(1998): Polk RE, *Ann Pharmacother* 32, 840
(1998): Wilson AP, *Int J Antimicrob Agents* 10(2), 143
(1997): Kralovicova K+, *J Chemother* 9(6), 420
(1996): Szymusiak-Mutnick BA+, *Am J Health Syst Pharm* 53, 2098
(1995): Lilley LL+, *Am J Nurs* 95, 14
(1994): Bergeron L+, *Ann Pharmacother* 28, 581
(1993): Ena J+, *JAMA* 269, 598
(1993): O'Sullivan TL+, *J Infect Dis* 168, 773
(1993): Polk RE+, *Antimicrob Agents Chemother* 37, 2139
(1992): Levy M+, *Harefuah* (Hebrew) 122, 36
(1992): Rengo C+, *Recenti Prog Med* (Italian) 83, 726
(1991): Killian AD+, *Ann Intern Med* 115, 410
(1991): Maccabruni A+, *Recenti Prog Med* (Italian) 82, 17
(1991): Valero R+, *J Cardiothorac Vasc Anesth* 5, 574
(1991): Wallace MR+, *J Infect Dis* 164, 1180
(1990): Bailie GR+, *Clin Pharm* 9, 671
(1990): Healey DP+, *Antimicrob Agents Chemother* 34, 550
(1990): Levy M+, *Pediatrics* 86, 572
(1990): No Author, *Lancet* 335, 1006
(1990): Sahai J+, *Antimicrob Agents Chemother* 34, 765
(1989): Pearson DA, *J Am Dent Assoc* 118, 59
(1989): Sahai J+, *J Infect Dis* 160, 876
(1988): Polk RE+, *J Infect Dis* 157, 502
(1988): Rubin M+, *Ann Intern Med* 108, 30 (3%)
(1987): Duro JC+, *Med Clin* (Barc) (Spanish) 89, 218
(1986): Daly BM+, *Drug Intell Clin Pharm* 20, 986
(1986): Davis RL+, *Ann Intern Med* 104, 285
(1986): Rolston KV+, *JAMA* 255, 2445
(1986): Wade TP+, *Arch Surg* 121, 859
(1985): Cole DR+, *Lancet* 2, 280
(1985): Garrelts JC+, *N Engl J Med* 312, 245
(1985): Holliman R, *Lancet* 1, 1399

Red neck syndrome
(1985): Ackerman BH+, *Ann Intern Med* 102, 723
(1985): Pau AK+, *N Engl J Med* 313, 756

Stevens–Johnson syndrome (<1%)
(2004): Jones DH+, *J Am Osteopath Assoc* 104(4), 157
(2002): Rocha JL+, *Braz J Infect Dis* 6(4), 196 (2 cases)
(1996): Alexander II+, *Allergy Asthma Proc* 17, 75
(1995): Patterson R+, *Allergy Proc* 16, 115
(1992): Laurencin CT+, *Ann Pharmacother* 26, 1520
(1990): Forrence EA+, *Drug Intell Clin Pharm* 24, 369

Toxic epidermal necrolysis
(2005): Craycraft ME+, *Pharmacotherapy* 25(2), 308
(2002): Rocha JL+, *Braz J Infect Dis* 6(4), 196
(2001): Hsu SI, *Pharmacotherapy* 21(10), 1233
(2000): Chan-Tack K, *Mo Med* 97, 131
(1992): Vidal C+, *Ann Allergy* 68, 345
(1990): Hannah BA+, *South Med J* 83, 720

(1985): Heng MCY, *Br J Dermatol* 113, 597
Urticaria
   (1989): Koestner B+, *Schweiz Med Wochenschr* (German) 119, 28
   (1988): Neal D+, *BMJ* 296, 137
   (1987): Longon P+, *Presse Med* (French) 16, 682
   (1986): Davis RL+, *Ann Intern Med* 104, 285
   (1986): Markman M+, *South Med J* 79, 382 (passim)
Vasculitis (<1%)
   (1987): Rawlinson WD+, *Med J Australia* 147, 470
   (1986): Markman M+, *South Med J* 79, 382

Mucosal/ENT
Dysgeusia (>10%)
Ototoxicity
   (2002): Rocha JL+, *Braz J Infect Dis* 6(4), 196
   (2001): Tanaka M+, *Yakugaku Zasshi* 121(8), 621
   (1998): Elting LS+, *Cancer* 83(12), 2597 (6%)
Tinnitus
   (1985): Mellor JA+, *J Antimicrob Chemother* 15(6), 773
   (1984): Snavely SR+, *Ann Intern Med* 101(1), 92

Eyes
Epiphora
   (2002): Rocha JL+, *Braz J Infect Dis* 6(4), 196

Other
Anaphylactoid reactions/Anaphylaxis
   (2001): Wazny LD+, *Ann Pharmacother* 35(11), 1458
   (2000): Chopra N+, *Ann Allergy Asthma Immunol* 84, 633
   (1992): Breathnach SM+, *Adverse Drug Reactions and the Skin* Blackwell, Oxford, 158 (passim)
   (1988): Rubin M+, *Ann Intern Med* 108, 30 (1 in 63 patients)
   (1987): Longon P+, *Presse Med* (French) 16, 682
   (1986): Markman M+, *Southern Med J* 79, 382 (passim)
Chills (>10%)
Death
   (2001): Hsu SI, *Pharmacotherapy* 21(10), 1233
DRESS syndrome
   (2007): Tamagawa-Mineoka R+, *Int J Dermatol* 46(6), 654 (with teicoplanin)
   (2005): Zuliani E+, *Clin Nephrol* 64(2), 155
Fever
   (2002): Rocha JL+, *Braz J Infect Dis* 6(4), 196
Hypersensitivity
   (2001): Hsu SI, *Pharmacotherapy* 21(10), 1233
   (1997): Marik PE+, *Pharmacotherapy* 17, 1341
Injection-site thrombophlebitis
Nephrotoxicity
   (2001): Tanaka M+, *Yakugaku Zasshi* 121(8), 621
   (1999): Fanos V+, *Drug Saf* 20(3), 245
   (1998): Elting LS+, *Cancer* 83(12), 2597 (17%)
   (1998): Wilson AP, *Int J Antimicrob Agents* 10(2), 143
   (1997): Fanos V+, *Pediatr Med Chir* 19(4), 259
   (1997): Kralovicova K+, *J Chemother* 9(6), 420
Paresthesias
Phlebitis (14–23%)
   (2002): Cohen E+, *J Antimicrob Chemother* 49(1), 155 (14–23%)
   (1998): Elting LS+, *Cancer* 83(12), 2597 (3%)
   (1983): Farber BF+, *Antimicrob Agents Chemother* 23, 138

VARDENAFIL

Trade name: Levitra (GSK) (Schering)
Indications: Erectile dysfunction
Category: Phosphodiesterase type 5 inhibitor
Half-life: 4–5 hours
Clinically important, potentially hazardous interactions with: alpha blockers (alfuzosin), doxazosin, erythromycin, fosamprenavir, indinavir, itraconazole, ketoconazole, nitrates, ritonavir, tamsulosin, terazosin

Reactions

Skin
Diaphoresis (<2%)
Facial edema (<2%)
Photosensitivity (<2%)
Pruritus (<2%)
Rash (sic) (<2%)
Urticaria
   (2004): Minciullo PL+, *J Clin Pharm Ther* 29(5), 483

Mucosal/ENT
Rhinitis (9%)
   (2005): Giuliano F+, *BJU Int* 95(1), 110
   (2005): Nehra A+, *J Urol* 173(6), 2067
   (2004): Markou S+, *Int J Impot Res* 216(6), 470
   (2003): Brock G+, *J Urol* 170(4), 1278
   (2003): Goldstein I+, *Diabetes Care* 26(3), 777 (10%)
   (2003): Hellstrom WJ+, *Urology* 61(4), 8
   (2001): Porst H+, *Int J Impot Res* 13(4), 192 (7%)
Sinusitis (3%)
Tinnitus (<2%)
Xerostomia (<2%)

Eyes
Dyschromatopsia (<2%)

Other
Abdominal pain (<2%)
Anaphylactoid reactions/Anaphylaxis (<2%)
Headache (7–15%)
   (2005): Giuliano F+, *BJU Int* 95(1), 110
   (2005): Nehra A+, *J Urol* 173(6), 2067
   (2004): Markou S+, *Int J Impot Res* 16(6), 470
   (2003): Brock G+, *J Urol* 170(4), 1278
   (2003): Goldstein I+, *Diabetes Care* 26(3), 777 (13%)
   (2003): Hellstrom WJ+, *Urology* 61(4), 8
   (2003): Porst H+, *Urology* 62(3), 519
   (2001): Porst H+, *Int J Impot Res* 13(4), 192 (7–15%)
Myalgia/Myositis/Myopathy/Myotoxicity (<2%)
Pain (<2%)
Paresthesias (<2%)
Vertigo (2%)

VARENICLINE

Trade name: Chantix (Pfizer)
Indications: Smoking deterrent
Category: Nicotinic antagonist
Half-life: 24 hours
Clinically important, potentially hazardous interactions with: None

Reactions

Skin
Acne
Dermatitis
Eczema
Edema
Erythema
Hyperhidrosis
Psoriasis
Urticaria
Xerosis

Mucosal/ENT
Dysgeusia (4%)
Dysphagia
Gingivitis
Nasopharyngitis
  (2007): Nakamura M+, *Clin Ther* 29(6), 1040
Oral ulceration
Parosmia
Tinnitus

Eyes
Cataract
  (2007): Williams KE+, *Curr Med Res Opin* 23(4), 793
Conjunctivitis
Ocular pain
Ocular stinging
Vision blurred

Other
Abdominal pain
  (2007): Lam S+, *Cardiol Rev* 15(3), 154 (7%)
Anxiety
  (2007): Tsai ST+, *Clin Ther* 29(6), 1027
Chest pain
Chills
Depression
Headache (15%)
  (2007): Lam S+, *Cardiol Rev* 15(3), 154
  (2007): Nakamura M+, *Clin Ther* 29(6), 1040
  (2007): van Bronswijk H+, *Ned Tijdschr Geneeskd* 151(45), 2503
Hot flashes
Hypersensitivity
Hypertension
Hypotension
Insomnia
  (2007): Lam S+, *Cardiol Rev* 15(3), 154 (18%)
  (2007): Tsai ST+, *Clin Ther* 29(6), 1027
  (2007): Williams KE+, *Curr Med Res Opin* 23(4), 793
  (2006): *Prescrire Int* 15(86), 210
Mania
  (2007): Kohen I+, *Am J Psychiatry* 164(8), 1269
Myalgia/Myositis/Myopathy/Myotoxicity
Schizophrenia
  (2007): Freedman R, *Am J Psychiatry* 164(8), 1269
Tremor
Vertigo

VARICELLA VACCINE

Trade names: Varilrix (GSK); Varivax (Merck)
Indications: Immunization, varicella
Category: Vaccine
Half-life: N/A
Clinically important, potentially hazardous interactions with: N/A

Reactions

Skin
Allergic reactions (sic) (~1%)
Cellulitis
Dermatitis (~1%)
Diaper rash (~1%)
Eczema (~1%)
Erythema multiforme
Herpes simplex
  (2001): Takayama N+, *Pediatr Infect Dis J* 20(2), 226
Herpes zoster
  (2003): Levin MJ+, *J Infect Dis* 188(7), 954
  (2003): Naseri A+, *Am J Ophthalmol* 135(3), 415
  (2002): Uebe B+, *Eur J Pediatr* 161(8), 442
  (2000): Brunell PA+, *Pediatrics* 106(2), E28
  (1999): Christensen CL+, *Ugeskr Laeger* 161(6), 794
  (1989): Hammerschlag MR+, *J Infect Dis* 160(3), 535
  (1988): Gershon AA+, *J Infect Dis* 158(1), 132
Impetigo
Miliaria (~1%)
Pruritus (~1%)
Purpura
  (1986): Lee SY+, *Am J Pediatr* 8(1), 78
Rash (sic)
  (2005): *Prescrire Int* 14(77), 85
  (2005): Quinlivan M+, *J Med Virol* 75(1), 174
  (2004): Quinlivan ML+, *J Infect Dis* 190(4), 793
  (2000): Wise RP+, *JAMA* 284(10), 1271
  (1986): Arbeter AM+, *Pediatrics* 78(4), 748
  (1986): Gershon AA+, *Pediatrics* 78(4), 757 (in children with leukemia)
  (1985): Gershon AA+, *Postgrad Med J* 61, 73
  (1984): Gershon AA+, *JAMA* 252(3), 355
  (1984): Oka T+, *Biken J* 27, 2
Stevens–Johnson syndrome
Urticaria (~1%)
Vesiculation
  (2000): Sharrar RG+, *Vaccine* 19(7-8), 916
Xerosis (~1%)

Mucosal/ENT
Otitis (~1%)

Eyes
Intraocular pressure increased
  (2003): Naseri A+, *Am J Ophthalmol* 135(3), 415
Keratitis
  (2003): Naseri A+, *Am J Ophthalmol* 135(3), 415
Scleritis
  (2003): Naseri A+, *Am J Ophthalmol* 135(3), 415
Uveitis
  (2003): Naseri A+, *Am J Ophthalmol* 135(3), 415

Other
Abdominal pain (~1%)
Anaphylactoid reactions/Anaphylaxis
  (2000): Wise RP+, *JAMA* 284(10), 1271

Asthenia (~1%)
Chills (~1%)
Cough (~1%)
Death
    (2000): Wise RP+, *JAMA* 284(10), 1271
Fever (15%)
    (2005): *Prescrire Int* 14(77), 85
Headache (~1%)
Injection-site edema (19%)
Injection-site erythema (19%)
Injection-site hematoma (19%)
Injection-site induration (19%)
Injection-site pain (19%)
    (2004): Kosuwon P+, *Southeast Asian J Trop Med Public Health*
        35(3), 697
Injection-site pruritus (19%)
Injection-site reactions
    (2005): Oxman MN+, *N Engl J Med* 352(22), 2271
    (2000): Wise RP+, *JAMA* 284(10), 1271
    (1986): Arbeter AM+, *Pediatrics* 78(4), 748
Myalgia/Myositis/Myopathy/Myotoxicity (~1%)
Paresthesias
Seizures
Upper respiratory infection (~1%)
Vertigo

VASOPRESSIN

Synonyms: ADH; antidiuretic hormone
Trade names: Pitressin (Monarch); Pressyn
Indications: Diabetes insipidus
Category: Antidiuretic hormone
Half-life: 10–20 minutes

Reactions

Skin

Allergic reactions (sic) (<1%)
Angioedema
Bullous dermatitis
    (2002): Kahn JM+, *Crit Care Med* 30(8), 1899
    (1997): Lin RY+, *Dermatology* 195, 271
    (1991): Colemont LJ+, *J Clin Gastroenterol* 13, 91
    (1986): Korenberg RJ+, *J Am Acad Dermatol* 15, 393
Diaphoresis (1–10%)
Exanthems
Pallor (1–10%)
Purpura
    (1996): Lemlich G+, *Cutis* 57, 330
    (1985): Thomas TK, *Am J Gastroenterol* 80, 704
Rash (sic)
Urticaria (1–10%)

Hair

Hair – alopecia
    (1994): Maceyko RD+, *J Am Acad Dermatol* 31, 111

Other

Anaphylactoid reactions/Anaphylaxis
Death
    (2001): Rizzo V+, *J Pediatr Endocrinol Metab* 14(7), 861
Gangrene
    (1997): Lin RY+, *Dermatology* 195, 271
Headache
Injection-site inflammation

(2002): Kahn JM+, *Crit Care Med* 30(8), 1899
(1997): Lin RY+, *Dermatology* 195, 271 (amber-like)
(1996): Lemlich G+, *Cutis* 57, 330
(1991): Colemont LJ+, *J Clin Gastroenterol* 13, 91
(1990): Stump DL+, *Drugs* 39, 38
(1986): Korenberg RJ+, *J Am Acad Dermatol* 15, 393
(1985): Thomas TK, *Am J Gastroenterol* 80, 704
Injection-site necrosis
    (2002): Kahn JM+, *Crit Care Med* 30(8), 1899
Rhabdomyolysis
    (1995): Hino A+, *Rinsho Shinkeigaku* 35(8), 911
    (1993): de Cuenca Moron B+, *Rev Clin Esp* 192(2), 79
    (1993): Pierce ST+, *Am J Gastroenterol* 88(3), 424
    (1991): Moreno-Sanchez D+, *Gastroenterology* 101(2), 529
    (1991): Moreno-Sanchez D+, *Rev Esp Enferm Dig* 79(2), 160
    (1984): Affarah HB I, *South Med J* 77(7), 918
Tremor (1–10%)

VECURONIUM

Trade names: Norcuron; Vecuron
Indications: Adjunct to general anesthesia
Category: Non-depolarizing neuromuscular blocker
Half-life: 65–75 minutes
**Clinically important, potentially hazardous interactions
with:** aminoglycosides, betamethasone, cyclosporine, gentamicin,
halothane, inhalational anesthetics, kanamycin, magnesium salts,
neomycin, quinidine, streptomycin, succinylcholine, tobramycin

Reactions

Other

Anaphylactoid reactions/Anaphylaxis
    (2005): Bhananker SM+, *Anesth Analg* 101(3), 819
    (2005): Karila C+, *Allergy* 60(6), 828
    (1994): Watkins J, *Acta Anaesthesiol Scand Suppl* 102, 6
    (1993): Yagi T+, *Masui* 42(4), 598
    (1990): Treuren BC+, *Br J Anaesth* 64(1), 125
    (1988): Charlton SM, *Anaesthesia* 43(8), 707
    (1988): Farrell AM+, *Anaesthesia* 43(3), 207
    (1988): Holt AW+, *Anaesth Intensive Care* 16(3), 378
    (1988): Thacker MA+, *Anaesth Intensive Care* 16(1), 129
Hypersensitivity
    (2004): Sanchez Palacios A+, *Allergol Immunopathol* (Madr)
        32(6), 352
Hypotension
    (1996): Soukup J+, *Anaesthesist* 45(11), 1024
Injection-site pain
    (2003): Blunk JA+, *Eur J Anaesthesiol* 20(3), 245
    (1998): Ti LK+, *Br J Anaesth* 81(3), 487
    (1995): Chow LH+, *Zhonghua Yi Xue Za Zhi* 55(4), 315
    (1988): Kent AP+, *Anaesthesia* 43(4), 334
Neurotoxicity
    (2001): Geller TJ+, *Neuromuscul Disord* 11(6-7), 579

VENLAFAXINE

Trade name: Effexor (Wyeth)
Indications: Depression
Category: Antidepressant, bicyclic; Serotonin-norepinephrine reuptake inhibitor
Half-life: 3–7 hours
Clinically important, potentially hazardous interactions with: dexibuprofen, isocarboxazid, linezolid, MAO inhibitors, metoclopramide, phenelzine, selegiline, sibutramine, sumatriptan, tramadol, tranylcypromine, trazodone, trimipramine

Reactions

Skin

Acne (<1%)
Allergic reactions (sic) (<1%)
Dermatitis
Diaphoresis
  (2005): Marcy TR+, *Ann Pharmacother* 39(4), 748
  (2004): Montgomery SA+, *Neuropsychobiology* 50(1), 57
  (2003): Denys D+, *J Clin Psychopharmacol* 23(6), 568
  (2000): Pierre JM+, *J Clin Psychopharmacol* 20(2), 269
  (1999): Schwartz TL, *Ann Pharmacother* 33(9), 1009
  (1997): Garber A+, *J Clin Psychiatry* 58(4), 176
Eczema (<1%)
Edema (<1%)
Exanthems (<1%)
Exfoliative dermatitis (<1%)
Facial edema (<1%)
Furunculosis (<1%)
Herpes simplex (<1%)
Herpes zoster (<1%)
Keratoderma
  (2006): Dalle S+, *Br J Dermatol* 154(5), 999
Lichenoid eruption (<1%)
Palmar–plantar hyperkeratosis
  (2006): Dalle S+, *Br J Dermatol* 154(5), 999
Peripheral edema
Photosensitivity (<1%)
Pruritus (1–10%)
  (1999): Schwartz TL, *Ann Pharmacother* 33(9), 1009
Psoriasis (<1%)
Pustules (<1%)
Rash (sic) (3%)
  (2005): Evans ML+, *Obstet Gynecol* 105(1), 161
Stevens–Johnson syndrome
  (2004): Weiss NT+, *J Clin Psychiatry* 65(10), 1431
Urticaria (<1%)
Vesiculobullous eruption (<1%)
Xerosis (<1%)

Mucosal/ENT

Ageusia (<1%)
Bromhidrosis (<1%)
Dysgeusia (2%)
Gingivitis (<1%)
Glossitis (<1%)
Oral ulceration (<1%)
Parosmia (<1%)
Sialorrhea (<1%)
Stomatitis (<1%)
Tinnitus
Tongue edema (<1%)
Tongue pigmentation (<1%)

Vaginitis
Vulvovaginal candidiasis (<1%)
Xerostomia (22%)
  (2005): Evans ML+, *Obstet Gynecol* 105(1), 161
  (2003): Denys D+, *J Clin Psychopharmacol* 23(6), 568
  (2000): Gelenberg AJ+, *JAMA* 283, 3082
  (1998): Joffe RT+, *J Clin Psychiatry* 59(10), 515

Hair

Hair – alopecia (<1%)
  (2001): Pitchot W+, *Am J Psych* 158, 1159
Hair – hirsutism (<1%)
Hair – pigmentation (<1%)

Nails

Nails – subungual hyperkeratosis
  (2006): Dalle S+, *Br J Dermatol* 154(5), 999

Other

Candidiasis
Congestive heart failure
  (2003): Drent M+, *Am J Respir Crit Care Med* 167(7), 958
Gynecomastia (<1%)
Headache
  (1998): Joffe RT+, *J Clin Psychiatry* 59(10), 515
Inappropriate secretion of antidiuretic hormone (SIADH)
  (1998): Masood GR+, *Ann Pharmacother* 32(1), 49
  (1997): Ranieri P+, *J Geriatr Psychiatry Neurol* 10(2), 75
Myalgia/Myositis/Myopathy/Myotoxicity (>1%)
Paresthesias (3%)
Thrombophlebitis (<1%)
Tremor (1–10%)
  (2005): Evans ML+, *Obstet Gynecol* 105(1), 161
Vertigo
  (2005): Evans ML+, *Obstet Gynecol* 105(1), 161

VERAPAMIL

Trade names: APO-Verap; Arpamyl LP; Azupamil; Berkatens; Calan (Pfizer); Chronovera; Cordilox; Covera-HS (Pfizer); Geangin; Isoptin (Abbott); Isoptine; Nu-Verap; Tarka (Abbott); Veraken; Verelan (Schwarz)
Indications: Angina, hypertension
Category: Antiarrhythmic class IV; Calcium channel blocker
Half-life: 2–8 hours
Clinically important, potentially hazardous interactions with: acebutolol, amiodarone, aspirin, atenolol, atorvastatin, betaxolol, carbamazepine, carteolol, celiprolol, clonidine, dantrolene, digoxin, dofetilide, epirubicin, eplerenone, erythromycin, esmolol, **eucalyptus**, everolimus, lovastatin, metoprolol, **mistletoe**, nadolol, penbutolol, pindolol, propranolol, quinidine, ranolazine, sibutramine, simvastatin, timolol

Note: Tarka is trandolapril and verapamil

Reactions

Skin

Acne
  (1989): Stern R+, *Arch Intern Med* 149, 829
Acute febrile neutrophilic dermatosis (Sweet's syndrome)
  (1998): Knowles S+, *J Am Acad Dermatol* 38, 201 (passim)
Angioedema
  (1998): Knowles S+, *J Am Acad Dermatol* 38, 201 (passim)
  (1989): Sadick NS+, *J Am Acad Dermatol* 21, 132

(1989): Stern R+, *Arch Intern Med* 149, 829

Dermatitis

Diaphoresis (<1%)
 (1989): Stern R+, *Arch Intern Med* 149, 829
 (1983): Lewis JG, *Drugs* 25, 196

Edema (1.9%)
 (2003): Ioulios P+, *Dermatol Online J* 9(5), 6 (passim)

Erythema multiforme (<1%)
 (1991): Kürkçüoglu N+, *J Am Acad Dermatol* 24, 511
 (1989): Lin AYF+, *Drug Intell Clin Pharm* 23, 987
 (1989): Stern R+, *Arch Intern Med* 149, 829
 (1987): Naito S+, *Skin Res* (Japanese) 29, 602

Erythema nodosum
 (1998): Knowles S+, *J Am Acad Dermatol* 38, 201 (passim)

Exanthems
 (1998): Knowles S+, *J Am Acad Dermatol* 38, 201 (passim)
 (1989): McTavish D+, *Drugs* 38, 19
 (1989): Sadick NS+, *J Am Acad Dermatol* 21, 132
 (1989): Stern R+, *Arch Intern Med* 149, 829
 (1983): Lewis JG, *Drugs* 25, 196 (3.2%)
 (1982): Anon, *Lakartidningen* (Swedish) 79, 3822
 (1980): Midtbo K+, *Curr Ther Res* 27, 830

Exfoliative dermatitis
 (1998): Knowles S+, *J Am Acad Dermatol* 38, 201 (passim)
 (1989): Stern R+, *Arch Intern Med* 149, 829

Hyperkeratosis (palms) (<1%)
 (1989): Sadick NS+, *J Am Acad Dermatol* 21, 132
 (1983): Major P, *Tidsskr Nor Laegeforen* (Norwegian), 103, 2061

Lichenoid eruption

Lupus erythematosus
 (2005): Kurtis B+, *J Drugs Dermatol* 4(4), 506
 (1998): Callen JP, Academy '98 Meeting (4 patients)
 (1997): Crowson AN+, *Hum Pathol* 28, 67 (subacute cutaneous)

Lymphomatoid papulosis
 (2004): Atridi S+, *J Neurol* 251(4), 473

Peripheral edema (1–10%)
 (2002): No author, *Medscape Primary Care* 4

Photosensitivity
 (1994): Berger TG+, *Arch Dermatol* 130, 609 (in HIV-infected)
 (1989): McTavish D+, *Drugs* 38, 19
 (1983): Lewis JG, *Drugs* 25, 196

Prurigo
 (1983): Lewis JG, *Drugs* 25, 196

Pruritus
 (1998): Knowles S+, *J Am Acad Dermatol* 38, 201 (passim)
 (1989): McTavish D+, *Drugs* 38, 19
 (1989): Stern R+, *Arch Intern Med* 149, 829
 (1988): Burgunder JM+, *Hepatogastroenterology* 35, 169
 (1983): Lewis JG, *Drugs* 25, 196
 (1982): Fischer Hansen J+, *Clin Exp Pharmacol Physiol* 6, 31

Purpura (<1%)
 (1982): *Lakartidningen* (Swedish) 79, 3822

Rash (sic) (1.2%)
 (1989): Stern R+, *Arch Intern Med* 149, 829
 (1987): Johnson BF+, *Clin Pharmacol Ther* 42, 66

Side effects (sic)
 (1993): Kitamura K+, *J Dermatol* 20, 279 (psoriasiform)
 (1989): McTavish D+, *Drugs* 38, 19. (0.6%)

Stevens–Johnson syndrome (<1%)
 (1998): Knowles S+, *J Am Acad Dermatol* 38, 201 (passim)
 (1993): Kitamura K+, *J Dermatol* 20(5), 279
 (1992): Gonski PN, *Med J Aust* 156, 672
 (1989): Lin AYF+, *Drug Intell Clin Pharm* 23, 987
 (1989): Stern R+, *Arch Intern Med* 149, 829

Urticaria (<1%)
 (1998): Knowles S+, *J Am Acad Dermatol* 38, 201 (passim)
 (1989): McTavish D+, *Drugs* 38, 19
 (1989): Sadick NS+, *J Am Acad Dermatol* 21, 132

(1989): Stern R+, *Arch Intern Med* 149, 829
 (1983): Lewis JG, *Drugs* 25, 196

Vasculitis (<1%)
 (1989): Sadick NS+, *J Am Acad Dermatol* 21, 132
 (1983): Lewis JG, *Drugs* 25, 196

Mucosal/ENT

Gingival hyperplasia/hypertrophy (19%)
 (1998): Young PC+, *Cutis* 62(indu), 41
 (1995): Moghadam BKH+, *Cutis* 56, 46 (passim)
 (1993): Steele RM+, *Arch Intern Med* 120, 663
 (1992): Mehta AV+, *Am Heart J* 124(2), 535
 (1992): Miller CS+, *J Periodontol* 63(5), 453
 (1989): Pernu HE+, *J Oral Pathol Med* 18, 422
 (1987): Giustiniani S+, *Int J Cardiol* 15, 247
 (1985): Cucchi G+, *G Ital Cardiol* 15(5), 556
 (1985): Seymour RA+, *J Clin Periodontol* 12(6), 413

Oral ulceration
 (1999): Cohen DM+, *J Am Dent Assoc* 130(11), 1611

Xerostomia (<1%)

Hair

Hair – alopecia (<1%)
 (1994): Litt JZ, Beachwood, OH (personal case) (observation)
 (1991): Shelley WB+, *Cutis* 48, 364 (observation)
 (1989): Sadick NS+, *J Am Acad Dermatol* 21, 132
 (1989): Stern R+, *Arch Intern Med* 149, 829
 (1981): Rosing DR+, *Am J Cardiol* 48, 545
 (1980): Rosing DR+, *Chest* 78 (Suppl), 239

Hair – hypertrichosis
 (1991): Sever PS, *Lancet* 338, 1215

Hair – pigmentation
 (1991): Read GM, *Lancet* 338, 1520

Nails

Nails – dystrophy
 (1989): Stern R+, *Arch Intern Med* 149, 829

Eyes

Eyelid edema
 (2005): Cock JM, Manizales, Colombia (unilateral) (from Internet) (observation)

Other

Asthenia
 (2003): Guay DR, *Clin Ther* 25(3), 713 (with verapamil)

Congestive heart failure
 (2001): Kodama-Takahashi K+, *Nippon Ronen Igakkai Zasshi* 38(4), 544

Cough
 (2003): Guay DR, *Clin Ther* 25(3), 713

Erythromelalgia
 (1992): Drenth JP+, *Br J Dermatol* 127, 292

Gynecomastia (<1%)
 (2000): Hugues FC+, *Ann Med Interne* (Paris) (French) 151, 10 (passim)
 (1994): *BMJ* 308, 503
 (1994): Deniel-Rosanas J, *Med Clin* (Barc) (Spanish) 102, 399
 (1993): Braunstein GD, *N Engl J Med* 328(7), 490
 (1988): Tanner LA+, *Arch Intern Med* 148, 379

Headache

Hypotension
 (1996): Hosl P+, *Geburtshilfe Frauenheilkd* 56(6), 313

Paresthesias (<1%)

Rhabdomyolysis
 (2003): Chiffoleau A+, *Therapie* 58(2), 168 (with simvastatin and cyclosporinee)
 (2000): Gokel Y+, *Am J Emerg Med* 18, 738 (with trandolapril)

Serum sickness
 (1989): Pascual-Velasco F, *Med Clin* (Barc) (Spanish) 92, 719

Vertigo
(2003): Guay DR, *Clin Ther* 25(3), 713

VERTEPORFIN

Trade name: Visudyne (Novartis)
Indications: Wet form of age-related macular degeneration
Category: Photosensitizer
Half-life: 5–6 hours

Reactions

Skin
Diaphoresis
Eczema (1–10%)
Erythema
Pallor
Photosensitivity (<3%)
(2002): Houle JM+, *Retina* 22(6), 691
(2000): Scott LJ+, *Drugs Aging* 16, 139
Pigmentation
Pruritus
Purpura
Rash (sic)
Shivering
Ulcerations
Urticaria
(1998): Mitchell D, Thomasville, GA (generalized) (from Internet) (observation)
Vesiculation
(1998): Mitchell D, Thomasville, GA (from Internet) (observation)

Mucosal/ENT
Burning mouth syndrome (1–10%)
(1998): Mitchell D, Thomasville, GA (from Internet) (observation)
Cheilitis
(1998): Mitchell D, Thomasville, GA (from Internet) (observation)

Eyes
Ocular pruritus

Other
Chest pain
(2003): *Prescrire Int* 12(63), 17
(2002): Cahill MT+, *Am J Ophthalmol* 134(2), 281
Chills
Injection-site pain
(2000): Scott LJ+, *Drugs Aging* 16, 139
Injection-site reactions (sic)
Pain (chest and neck)
(2002): Cahill MT+, *Am J Ophthalmol* 134(2), 281
Paresthesias

VIDARABINE

Synonyms: adenine arabinoside; ara-A
Trade names: Adena a Ungena; Arasena; Vira-A Ophthalmic (Pfizer)
Indications: Herpetic keratoconjunctivitis
Category: Antiviral, nucleoside analog
Half-life: 3.3 hours
Clinically important, potentially hazardous interactions with: allopurinol, insulin

Reactions

Skin
Pruritus
Rash (sic)

Eyes
Ocular burning
Ocular erythema
Ocular flutter
(1990): Gizzi M+, *Am J Ophthalmol* 109(1), 105
Ocular pruritus

Other
Death
(1985): Burdge DR+, *Can Med Assoc J* 132(4), 392 (1 case)
(1981): Van Etta L+, *JAMA* 246(15), 1703
Inappropriate secretion of antidiuretic hormone (SIADH)
Myalgia/Myositis/Myopathy/Myotoxicity
(1990): Mak KH+, *Aust N Z J Med* 20(6), 811
Myoclonus
(1986): Vilter RW, *Antimicrob Agents Chemother* 29(5), 933
Neurotoxicity
(1988): Krause KH+, *Dtsch Med Wochenschr* 113(17), 686
(1986): Feldman S+, *J Infect Dis* 154(5), 889
(1986): Vilter RW, *Antimicrob Agents Chemother* 29(5), 933
(1985): Burdge DR+, *Can Med Assoc J* 132(4), 392
(1985): Chauplannaz G+, *Presse Med* 14(20), 1154
(1985): Shibuya N+, *Rinsho Shinkeigaku* 25(1), 21
(1984): Chauplannaz G+, *Rev Neurol* (Paris) 140(12), 743
(1984): Cullis PA+, *J Neurol Neurosurg Psychiatry* 47(12), 1351
(1983): Collignon PJ+, *Aust N Z J Med* 13(6), 627
Pain
(1985): Burdge DR+, *Can Med Assoc J* 132(4), 392
(1982): Sacks SL+, *Antimicrob Agents Chemother* 21(1), 93
Tremor
(1985): Burdge DR+, *Can Med Assoc J* 132(4), 392
(1982): Sacks SL+, *Antimicrob Agents Chemother* 21(1), 93
(1981): Nadel AM, *Arch Neurol* 38(6), 384

VIGABATRIN

Trade name: Sabril (Ovation)
Indications: Epilepsy, infantile spasms (West's syndrome)
Category: Anticonvulsant
Half-life: 5–8 hours (young adults); 12–13 hours (elderly)
Clinically important, potentially hazardous interactions with: phenytoin

Reactions

Skin
Rash (sic)
(2007): Arif H+, *Neurology* 68(20), 1701

Mucosal/ENT

Gingival hyperplasia/hypertrophy
(2004): Mesa F+, *J Periodontal Res* 39(1), 66
Sialorrhea

Eyes

Dyschromatopsia (blue-yellow)
(2000): Nousiainen I+, *Ophthalmology* 1(5), 884
Ocular pain
Optic atrophy
(2003): Frisen L+, *Acta Ophthalmol Scand* 81(5), 466
(2003): Viestenz A+, *Ophthalmologe* 100(5), 402
Retinal atrophy
(2004): Buncic JR+, *Ophthalmology* 111(10), 1935 (3 cases)
Retinopathy
(2006): Kinirons P+, *Epilepsia* 47(2), 311
(2005): Hadjikoutis S+, *Eur J Neurol* 12(7), 499
(2005): Moraes MH+, *Arq Neuropsiquiatr* 63(2B), 469
(2003): Banin E+, *Arch Ophthalmol* 121(6), 811
(2003): McDonagh J+, *Neurology* 61(12), 1690
(2003): Morong S+, *Doc Ophthalmol* 107(3), 289
(2002): Jensen H+, *Doc Ophthalmol* 104(2), 171
(2001): Coupland SG+, *Ophthalmology* 108(8), 1493
Vision impaired
(2005): Best JL+, *Eye* 19(1), 41
(2005): Moreno MC+, *Can J Neurol Sci* 32(4), 459
(2004): Constable S+, *Expert Opin Drug Saf* 3(3), 249
(2003): Fledelius HC, *Acta Ophthalmol Scand* 81(1), 41
(2003): Hardus P+, *Acta Ophthalmol Scand* 81(5), 459
(2003): Mrugacz M+, *Klin Oczna* 105(5), 326
(2003): Riise P+, *Ugeskr Laeger* 165(10), 1034
(2002): Hilton EJ+, *Epilepsia* 43(11), 1351
(2002): Newman WD+, *Eye* 16(5), 567
(2002): van der Torren K+, *Doc Ophthalmol* 104(2), 181

Other

Abdominal pain (1.4%)
Asthenia (1.1%)
Depression (2.5%)
(2007): Mula M+, *Drug Saf* 30(7), 555 (~10%)
(2002): Paciello N+, *Clin Ter* 153(6), 397
(1999): Levinson DF+, *Neurology* 53(7), 1503
Headache (3.8%)
(1999): Gidal BE+, *Ann Pharmacother* 33(12), 1277
Hepatotoxicity
(2001): Locher C+, *Gastroenterol Clin Biol* 25(5), 556
Myoclonus
(2000): Garcia Pastor+, *Neurologia* 15(8), 370
Paresthesias
Seizures
(2003): Yang MT+, *Brain Dev* 25(1), 51 (absence seizures)
(1997): Shields WD+, *Semin Pediatr Neurol* 4(1), 43
Tremor
Vertigo (3.8%)
Weight gain
(2007): Ben-Menachem, *Epilepsia* 48, 42

VINBLASTINE

Trade names: Velban (Lilly); Velbe (Lilly); Velsar (Lilly)
Indications: Lymphomas, melanoma, carcinomas
Category: Antimitotic; Vinca alkaloid
Half-life: initial phase: 3.7 minutes; terminal phase: 24.8 hours
**Clinically important, potentially hazardous interactions
with:** aldesleukin, aprepitant, erythromycin, fluconazole,
itraconazole, ketoconazole, miconazole

Reactions

Skin

Acne
Acral necrosis
(1998): Reiser M+, *Eur J Clin Microbiol Infect Dis* 17, 58
(1997): Hladunewich M+, *J Rheumatol* 24, 2371
Angioedema
(2003): Haas NB+, *Cancer* 98(9), 1837 (with estramustine)
Bullous dermatitis (<1%)
Cellulitis
(1983): Bronner AK+, *J Am Acad Dermatol* 9, 645
Dermatitis (1–10%)
Erythema
Erythema multiforme
(1991): Arias D+, *J Cutan Pathol* 18, 344
Exanthems
Photo-recall
(1992): Nemechek PM+, *Cancer* 70, 1605
Photosensitivity (1–10%)
(1992): Breathnach SM+, *Adverse Drug Reactions and the Skin*
Blackwell, Oxford, 302 (passim)
Phototoxicity
Pigmentation
(2001): Mutafoglu-Uysal K+, *Turk J Pediatr* 43(2), 172
(1997): Smith KJ+, *J Am Acad Dermatol* 36, 329
(1994): Cecchi R+, *Dermatology* 188, 244
Purpura
Radiodermatitis (reactivation)
Rash (sic) (1–10%)
Raynaud's phenomenon (1–10%)
(1998): Reiser M+, *Eur J Clin Microbiol Infect Dis* 17, 58
(1997): Hladunewich M+, *J Rheumatol* 24, 2371
(1993): von Gunten CF+, *Cancer* 72, 2004
(1992): Doll DC+, *Semin Oncol* 19(5), 580
(1992): Hansen SW, *Dan Med Bull* 39(5), 391 (with bleomycin)
(1991): Heier MS+, *Br J Cancer* 63(4), 550 (with bleomycin &
vinblastine)
(1990): Hansen SW+, *Ann Oncol* 1(4), 289 (with bleomycin &
vinblastine)
(1989): Hansen SW+, *J Clin Oncol* 7(7), 940 (with bleomycin &
vinblastine)
(1988): Stefenelli T+, *Eur Heart J* 9(5), 552 (with bleomycin &
vinblastine)
(1985): Vogelzang NJ+, *Cancer* 56(12), 2765 (with bleomycin &
vinblastine)
(1984): Davis TE+, *Gynecol Oncol* 19(1), 46 (with bleomycin &
vinblastine)
(1982): Scheulen ME+, *Dtsch Med Wochenschr* 107(43), 1640
(with bleomycin)
(1981): Harvey HA+, *Ann Intern Med* 94, 542
(1981): Vogelzang NJ+, *Ann Intern Med* 95, 288
(1980): Paty JG+, *J Rheumatol* 7(6), 927 (with bleomycin)
Ulcerations
Urticaria

Mucosal/ENT

Dysgeusia (>10%) (metallic taste)
Oral lesions (1–5%)
Oral vesiculation
Ototoxicity
(1992): Hansen SW, *Dan Med Bull* 39(5), 391 (with bleomycin &
vinblastine)
Stomatitis (>10%)
Tinnitus
(1999): Moss PE+, *Ann Pharmacother* 33(4), 423

Hair

Hair – alopecia (>10%)
  (1992): Breathnach SM+, *Adverse Drug Reactions and the Skin*
    Blackwell, Oxford, 302 (passim)
Hair – changes (sic)

Other

Headache
Hypersensitivity
  (2001): Mutafoglu-Uysal K+, *Turk J Pediatr* 43(2), 172
Inappropriate secretion of antidiuretic hormone (SIADH)
  (1987): Fraschini G+, *Tumori* 73(5), 513 (3 cases)
  (1983): Ravikumar TS+, *J Surg Oncol* 24(3), 242
  (1982): Stahel RA+, *Cancer Chemother Pharmacol* 8(2), 253
  (1980): Antony A+, *J Urol* 123(5), 783
Injection-site extravasation
  (2000): Kassner E, *J Pediatr Oncon Nurs* 17, 135
Injection-site necrosis
  (1992): Misery L+, *Presse Med* (French) 21, 2153
  (1991): Arias D+, *J Cutan Pathol* 18, 344
Injection-site pain
Myalgia/Myositis/Myopathy/Myotoxicity (1–10%)
Nephrotoxicity
  (1992): Hansen SW, *Dan Med Bull* 39(5), 391 (with bleomycin &
    vinblastine)
Neurotoxicity
  (1992): Hansen SW, *Dan Med Bull* 39(5), 391 (with bleomycin &
    vinblastine)
Paresthesias (1–10%)
Phlebitis
  (1989): Kerker BJ+, *Semin Dermatol* 8, 173
Rhabdomyolysis
  (1995): Anderlini P+, *Cancer* 76(4), 678

VINCRISTINE

Trade name: Vincasar (Gensia)
Indications: Leukemias, lymphomas, neuroblastoma, Wilm's
tumor
Category: Antimitotic; Vinca alkaloid
Half-life: 24 hours
**Clinically important, potentially hazardous interactions
with:** aldesleukin, aprepitant, **bromelain**, fluconazole, **influenza
vaccines**, itraconazole, ketoconazole, miconazole

Reactions

Skin

Acral erythema
  (1995): Komamura H+, *J Dermatol* 22(2), 116 (with
    cyclophosphamide, doxorubicin and GCSF)
Actinic keratoses
  (1987): Johnson TM+, *J Am Dermatol* 17(2 Pt 1), 192
Allergic reactions
  (2005): Nakashima H+, *Br J Dermatol* 153(1), 225
Angioedema
  (1984): Gassel WD+, *Oncology* 41, 403
Dermatitis herpetiformis
  (1986): Gottlieb D+, *Med J Aust* 145, 241 (flare)
Edema
Erythroderma
  (1989): Matsumoto N+, *Gan To Kagaku Ryoho* (Japanese)
    16, 2297
  (1984): Gassel WD+, *Oncology* 41, 403
Exanthems

  (1984): Gassel WD+, *Oncology* 41, 403
Hand–foot syndrome
  (2003): Leighl NB+, *Clin Lung Cancer* 5(2), 107 (with
    doxorubicin and cyclophosphamide)
  (2002): Hussein MA+, *Cancer* 95(10), 2160 (with
    dexamethasone)
Palmar–plantar erythema
  (1990): Pagliuca A+, *Postgrad Med J* 66, 242
Pigmentation
  (2000): Marcoux D+, *J Am Acad Dermatol* 43, 540 (with
    dactinomycin)
Pruritus
Rash (sic) (1–10%)
Raynaud's phenomenon
  (2004): Gottschling S+, *J Pediatr Hematol Oncol* 26(11), 768
  (1998): Reiser M+, *Eur J Clin Microbiol Infect Dis* 17, 58
Urticaria

Mucosal/ENT

Dysgeusia (1–10%) (metallic taste)
Oral lesions (1–10%)
  (1989): Kerker BJ+, *Semin Dermatol* 8, 173 (1–5%)
Oral ulceration (1–10%)
Stomatitis (<1%)
Tinnitus
  (1999): Moss PE+, *Ann Pharmacother* 33(4), 423

Hair

Hair – alopecia (20–70%)
  (2002): Klasa RJ+, *J Clin Oncol* 20(24), 4649 (with
    cyclophosphamide and prednisone)
  (1987): David J+, *Nurs Times* 83, 36

Nails

Nails – Beau's lines (transverse nail bands)
  (2006): Dasanu CA+, *Dermatol Online J* 12(6), 10 (with
    doxorubicin and dexamethasone)
  (1994): Ben-Dayan D+, *Acta Haematol* 91, 89
Nails – leukonychia
  (1990): Bader-Meunier B+, *Ann Pediatr Paris* (French) 37, 337
    (transverse)
Nails – Mees' lines
  (1983): James WD+, *Arch Dermatol* 119, 334
  (1982): Jeanmougin M+, *Ann Dermatol Venereol* (French)
    109, 169
Nails – muehrcke's lines
  (2006): Dasanu CA+, *Dermatol Online J* 12(6), 10 (with
    doxorubicin and dexamethasone)
Nails – onychodermal band
  (1993): Kowal-Vern A+, *Cutis* 52, 43 (plus erythema of proximal
    nail fold)
Nails – pigmentation
  (2006): Dasanu CA+, *Dermatol Online J* 12(6), 10 (with
    doxorubicin and dexamethasone)

Other

Anaphylactoid reactions/Anaphylaxis
Headache
Inappropriate secretion of antidiuretic hormone (SIADH)
  (2000): Nishihori Y+, *Rinsho Ketsueki* 41(11), 1231
  (1998): Tsujita Y+, *Gan To Kagaku Ryoho* 25(5), 757
  (1992): Escuro RS+, *Cleve Clin J Med* 59(6), 643
  (1988): Indiano JM+, *An Esp Pediatr* 29 Suppl 34, 155
  (1986): Nishinarita S+, *Rinsho Ketsueki* 27(10), 1916
Injection-site cellulitis (>10%)
  (1983): Bronner AK+, *J Am Acad Dermatol* 9, 645
Injection-site extravasation
  (2000): Kassner E, *J Pediatr Oncon Nurs* 17, 135
Injection-site necrosis (>10%)

Myalgia/Myositis/Myopathy/Myotoxicity (1–10%)
Neurotoxicity
  (2004): Schiavetti A+, *Pediatr Blood Cancer* 43(5), 606
Paresthesias (1–10%)
Phlebitis (1–10%)
Sjøgren's (Sicca) syndrome
  (1989): Monno S+, *Jpn J Med* 28, 399

VINORELBINE

Trade name: Navelbine (Kyowa)
Indications: Non-small cell lung cancer
Category: Antimitotic; Vinca alkaloid
Half-life: 28–44 hours
**Clinically important, potentially hazardous interactions
with:** aldesleukin

Reactions

Skin

Angioedema
Erythema
Hand–foot syndrome
  (2004): Martin M+, *Clin Breast Cancer* 5(5), 353 (6%) (with
    doxorubicin)
  (2001): Laack E+, *Ann Oncol* 12(12), 1761 (with gemcitabine)
  (1998): Hoff PM+, *Cancer* 82, 965
Pigmentation
  (1994): Cecchi R+, *Dermatology* 188, 244
Pruritus
Rash (sic) (<5%)
Toxic epidermal necrolysis
  (1992): Misery L+, *Presse Med* (French) 21, 2153
Vasculitis
  (2007): Bilku DK+, *Clin Oncol (R Coll Radiol)* 19(5), 363

Mucosal/ENT

Dysgeusia (>10%) (metallic taste)
Mucositis
  (2004): Martin M+, *Clin Breast Cancer* 5(5), 353 (15%) (with
    doxorubicin)
Stomatitis (>10%)
  (2005): Serin D+, *Br J Cancer* 92(11), 1989 (with epirubicin)
  (2002): Bonneterre J+, *Br J Cancer* 87(11), 1210 (40%) (with
    fluorouracil)
  (1989): Marty M+, *Nouv Rev Fr Hematol* (French) 31, 77 (12%)

Hair

Hair – alopecia (12%)
  (2004): Martin M+, *Clin Breast Cancer* 5(5), 353 (53%) (with
    doxorubicin)
  (1994): Gasparini G+, *J Clin Oncol* 12, 2094
  (1989): Marty M+, *Nouv Rev Fr Hematol* (French) 31, 77

Other

Anaphylactoid reactions/Anaphylaxis
Asthenia
  (2005): Lena MD+, *Lung Cancer* 48(1), 129 (with cisplatin)
  (2005): Muggia FM+, *Gynecol Oncol* 96(1), 108
  (2005): Winton T+, *N Engl J Med* 352(25), 2589 (81%) (with
    cisplatin)
Cough
  (2005): Lena MD+, *Lung Cancer* 48(1), 129 (with cisplatin)
Death
  (2005): Winton T+, *N Engl J Med* 352(25), 2589 (%) (with
    cisplatin)

Extravasation
  (2001): Bertelli G+, *Tumori* 87(2), 112
Hypertension
  (2005): Muggia FM+, *Gynecol Oncol* 96(1), 108
Inappropriate secretion of antidiuretic hormone (SIADH)
  (1998): Garrett CA+, *Ann Pharmacother* 32(12), 1306
Infections
  (2002): Bonneterre J+, *Br J Cancer* 87(11), 1210 (with
    fluorouracil)
Injection-site irritation (1–10%)
Injection-site necrosis (1–10%)
Injection-site pain
  (2001): Long TD+, *Am J Clin Oncol* 24(4), 414
Injection-site phlebitis (12%)
  (1998): Sauter C+, *Schweiz Med Wochenschr* (German) 128, 343
  (1989): Marty M+, *Nouv Rev Fr Hematol* (French) 31, 77 (12%)
Myalgia/Myositis/Myopathy/Myotoxicity (<5%)
Neurotoxicity
  (2005): Muggia FM+, *Gynecol Oncol* 96(1), 108
  (2005): Winton T+, *N Engl J Med* 352(25), 2589 (48%) (with
    cisplatin)
Pain
  (2005): Lena MD+, *Lung Cancer* 48(1), 129 (with cisplatin)
Paresthesias (1–10%)
Phlebitis (7%)

VITAMIN A

Trade names: Acaren; Acon; Afaxin; Aquasol A (aaiPharma);
Arovit; Avipur; Avitin; Axerol; Dolce; Palmitate A; Vogan
Indications: Vitamin A deficiency
Category: Vitamin
Half-life: N/A
**Clinically important, potentially hazardous interactions
with:** acitretin, bexarotene, **fish oil supplements**, isotretinoin,
minocycline, prednisone, tetracycline, warfarin

Reactions

Skin

Dermatitis
  (1996): Bazzano C+, *Contact Dermatitis* 35, 261
  (1995): Heidenheim M+, *Contact Dermatitis* 33, 439
  (1994): Manzano A+, *Contact Dermatitis* 31, 324
  (1994): Sanz de Galdeano C+, *Contact Dermatitis* 30, 50
  (1984): Blondeel A, *Contact Dermatitis* 11, 191
Eczema (pellagra-like)
  (1982): Hamann K+, *Hautarzt* (German) 33, 559
Erythema
  (1992): Breathnach SM+, *Adverse Drug Reactions and the Skin*
    Blackwell, Oxford, 254 (passim)
Erythema multiforme (<1%)
Exanthems
Exfoliative dermatitis
Fissures
  (1992): Breathnach SM+, *Adverse Drug Reactions and the Skin*
    Blackwell, Oxford, 254 (passim)
Hyperkeratosis
  (1992): Breathnach SM+, *Adverse Drug Reactions and the Skin*
    Blackwell, Oxford, 254 (passim)
Perleche
Photosensitivity
Pigmentation (yellow-orange)
Pruritus (<1%)

(1992): Breathnach SM+, *Adverse Drug Reactions and the Skin*
  Blackwell, Oxford, 254 (passim)
Stevens–Johnson syndrome
Xerosis (1–10%)

Mucosal/ENT
  Cheilitis
  Gingivitis
  Oral mucosal eruption
  Stomatodynia
  Xerostomia
    (1992): Breathnach SM+, *Adverse Drug Reactions and the Skin*
      Blackwell, Oxford, 254 (passim)

Hair
  Hair – alopecia
    (1992): Breathnach SM+, *Adverse Drug Reactions and the Skin*
      Blackwell, Oxford, 254 (passim)

Eyes
  Ocular adverse effects
    (2004): Fraunfelder FW, *Am J Ophthalmol* 138(4), 639

Other
  Anaphylactoid reactions/Anaphylaxis
  Hypersensitivity
    (1995): Shelley WB+, *BMJ* 311, 232

VITAMIN B₁

(See THIAMINE)

VITAMIN B₁₂

(See CYANOCOBALAMIN)

VITAMIN B₂

(See RIBOFLAVIN)

VITAMIN B₃

(See NIACINAMIDE)

VITAMIN B₅

(See PANTOTHENIC ACID)

VITAMIN B₆

(See PYRIDOXINE)

VITAMIN B₉

(See FOLIC ACID)

VITAMIN C

(See ASCORBIC ACID)

VITAMIN D

(See ERGOCALCIFEROL)

VITAMIN E

Synonym: alpha tocopherol
Trade names: Aquasol E (aaiPharma); Bio E; Davitamon E;
Detulin; E Perle; E-Vitamin Succinate; Ephynal; Eprolin; Optovit-
E; Pheryl-E; Vita Plus E; Vita-E; Vitec
Indications: Vitamin E deficiency
Category: Vitamin
Half-life: N/A
**Clinically important, potentially hazardous interactions
with:** amprenavir, warfarin

Reactions

Skin
  Dermatitis (<1%)
    (2004): Matsumura T+, *Contact Dermatitis* 51(4), 211
    (1997): Parsad D+, *Contact Dermatitis* 37, 294 (xanthomatous)
    (1994): Manzano D+, *Contact Dermatitis* 31, 324
    (1994): Perrenoud D+, *Dermatology* 189, 225
    (1992): Garcia-Bravo B+, *Contact Dermatitis* 26, 280
      (generalized)
    (1991): de Groot AC+, *Contact Dermatitis* 25, 302
    (1991): Fisher AA, *Cutis* 48, 272
    (1991): Hunter D+, *Cutis* 47, 193
    (1986): Goldman MP+, *J Am Acad Dermatol* 14, 133
  Erythema multiforme
    (1994): Spreux A+, *Therapie* (French) 49, 460
    (1986): Fisher AA, *Cutis* 37, 158 and 262 (topical administration)
    (1984): Saperstein H+, *Arch Dermatol* 120, 906
  Exanthems
  Lupus erythematosus
    (1995): Whittam J+, *Am J Clin Nutr* 62, 1025
  Urticaria

Mucosal/ENT
  Gingivitis
    (1998): Liede KE+, *Ann Med* 30, 542

Hair
  Hair – poliosis (at injection sites)

Other
  Gynecomastia
    (1994): Roberts HJ, *Hosp Pract Off Ed* 29, 12
  Sclerosing lipogranuloma
    (1983): Foucar E+, *J Am Acad Dermatol* 9, 103
  Thrombophlebitis

VITAMIN K

(See PHYTONADIONE)

VORICONAZOLE

Synonym: UK109496
Trade name: Vfend (Pfizer)
Indications: Invasive aspergillosis
Category: Antibiotic, triazole
Half-life: 6–24 hours (dose dependent)
Clinically important, potentially hazardous interactions with: astemizole, barbiturates, carbamazepine, ergot alkaloids, ixabepilone, lapatinib, pimozide, quinidine, rifabutin, rifampin, ritonavir, sirolimus, solifenacin, temsirolimus

Reactions

Skin

Adverse effects (sic) (20%)
  (2003): Jeu L+, *Clin Ther* 25(5), 1321 (20%)
Allergic granulomatous angiitis (Churg–Strauss syndrome) (<1%)
Allergic reactions (sic) (<1%)
Angioedema (<1%)
  (2008): Gencer S+, *J Med Microbiol* 57(Pt), 1028
Cellulitis (<1%)
Dermatitis (<1%)
Diaphoresis (<1%)
Eczema (<1%)
Edema (<1%)
Erythema
  (2005): Racette AJ+, *J Am Acad Dermatol* 52(5 Suppl 1), S81
Erythema multiforme
Exfoliative dermatitis (<1%)
Facial edema (<1%)
Facial erythema
  (2001): Denning DW+, *Clin Exp Dermatol* 26(8), 648
Fixed eruption (<1%)
Furunculosis (<1%)
Graft-versus-host reaction (<1%)
Herpes simplex (<1%)
Lupus erythematosus (<1%)
  (2005): Racette AJ+, *J Am Acad Dermatol* 52(5), S81
Peripheral edema (1%)
Petechiae (<1%)
Photosensitivity (8.2%)
  (2007): McCarthy KL+, *Clin Infect Dis* 44(5), e55
  (2006): Auffret N+, *Ann Dermatol Venereol* 133(4), 330 (9 cases)
  (2005): Racette AJ+, *J Am Acad Dermatol* 52(5 Suppl 1), S81
  (2004): Rubenstein M+, *Pediatr Dermatol* 21(6), 675 (2 cases)
  (2004): Vandecasteele SJ+, *Eur J Clin Microbiol Infect Dis* 23(8), 656 (2 cases)
  (2003): Johnson LB+, *Clin Infect Dis* 36(5), 630
  (2002): Herbrecht R+, *N Engl J Med* 347(6), 408 (8.2%)
Pigmentation (<1%)
Pruritus (8.2%)
  (2002): Herbrecht R+, *N Engl J Med* 347(6), 408 (8.2%)
Psoriasis (<1%)
Purpura (<1%)
Rash (sic) (8.2%)
  (2007): Eiden C+, *Ann Pharmacother* 41(5), 755 (17%)
  (2003): Johnson LB+, *Clin Infect Dis* 36(5), 630
  (2002): Herbrecht R+, *N Engl J Med* 347(6), 408 (8.2%)
  (2002): Purkins L+, *Antimicrob Agents Chemother* 46(8), 2546
Scrotal edema (<1%)
Stevens–Johnson syndrome
  (2005): Racette AJ+, *J Am Acad Dermatol* 52(5), S81
Toxic epidermal necrolysis

  (2005): Racette AJ+, *J Am Acad Dermatol* 52(5), S81
  (2004): Huang DB+, *South Med J* 97(11), 1116
Urticaria (<1%)
Xerosis (<1%)
  (2005): Racette AJ+, *J Am Acad Dermatol* 52(5 Suppl 1), S81

Mucosal/ENT

Ageusia (<1%)
Cheilitis (<1%)
  (2005): Racette AJ+, *J Am Acad Dermatol* 52(5 Suppl 1), S81
Dysgeusia (<1%)
Gingival bleeding (<1%)
Gingival hyperplasia/hypertrophy (<1%)
Gingivitis (<1%)
Glossitis (<1%)
Oral ulceration (<1%)
Stomatitis (<1%)
Tongue edema (<1%)
Xerostomia (1%)

Hair

Hair – alopecia (<1%)

Eyes

Visual disturbances
  (2007): Eiden C+, *Ann Pharmacother* 41(5), 755 (18%)
  (2006): Imhof A+, *Swiss Med Wkly* 136(45-46), 739
  (2002): Herbrecht R+, *N Engl J Med* 347(6), 408 (44.8%)
  (2002): Walsh TJ+, *N Engl J Med* 346(4), 225
  (2001): Ally R+, *Clin Infect Dis* 33(9), 1447 (23%)
Visual hallucinations
  (2007): *Prescrire Int* 16(87), 18 (passim)
  (2005): Flox Benitez G+, *Rev Clin Esp* 205(12), 632
  (2004): Boyd AE+, *Clin Infect Dis* 39(8), 1241

Other

Anaphylactoid reactions/Anaphylaxis (<1%)
Chills (3.1%)
  (2002): Herbrecht R+, *N Engl J Med* 347(6), 408
Delirium
  (2007): *Prescrire Int* 16(87), 18 (passim)
Depression (<1%)
Headache
  (2007): Eiden C+, *Ann Pharmacother* 41(5), 755
Hepatotoxicity
  (2007): *Prescrire Int* 16(87), 18 (passim)
  (2007): Eiden C+, *Ann Pharmacother* 41(5), 755 (23%)
Infections (<1%)
Injection-site infection (<1%)
Injection-site inflammation (<1%)
Injection-site pain (<1%)
Myalgia/Myositis/Myopathy/Myotoxicity (<1%)
Nephrotoxicity
  (2007): Eiden C+, *Ann Pharmacother* 41(5), 755 (4%)
Neurotoxicity
  (2007): Eiden C+, *Ann Pharmacother* 41(5), 755 (14%)
Pain (<1%)
Paresthesias (<1%)
Phlebitis (<1%)
Pseudoporphyria
  (2007): Kwong WT+, *J Drugs Dermatol* 6(10), 1042
  (2007): Tolland JP+, *Photodermatol Photoimmunol Photomed* 23(1), 29
  (2005): Sharp MT+, *J Am Acad Dermatol* 53(2), 341
  (2004): Dolan CK+, *Int J Dermatol* 43(10), 768
Thrombophlebitis (<1%)
Tremor (<1%)

VORINOSTAT

Synonym: Suberoylanilide hydroxamic acid (SAHA)
Trade name: Zolinza (Merck)
Indications: Cutaneous T-cell lymphoma
Category: Histone deacetylase (HDAC) inhibitor
Half-life: ~2 hours
Clinically important, potentially hazardous interactions with: valproic acid

Reactions

Skin
Angioedema (9%)
Exfoliative dermatitis (9%)
Peripheral edema (13%)
Pruritus (12%)

Mucosal/ENT
Dysgeusia (28%)
Xerostomia (16%)

Hair
Hair – alopecia (19%)

Other
Asthenia (9%)
Chest pain (9%)
Chills (16%)
Cough (10.5%)
Death (9%)
Fever (10%)
Headache (12%)
Stroke (9%)
Upper respiratory infection (10%)
Vertigo (15%)
Weight loss

WARFARIN

Trade names: Aldocumar; Coumadin (Bristol-Myers Squibb); Coumadine; Marevan; Waran; Warfilone
Indications: Thromboembolic disease, pulmonary embolism
Category: Anticoagulant; Coumarin
Half-life: 1.5–2.5 days (highly variable)
Clinically important, potentially hazardous interactions with: amiodarone, amobarbital, antithyroid agents, aprepitant, aprobarbital, **arnica**, aspirin, azathioprine, azithromycin, barbiturates, beclomethasone, bismuth, bivalirudin, bosentan, butabarbital, **capsicum**, **chamomile**, **chondroitin**, cimetidine, clarithromycin, clofibrate, clopidogrel, clorazepate, co-trimoxazole, **coenzyme Q-10**, cyclosporine, **dan-shen**, danazol, daptomycin, delavirdine, desvenlafaxine, **devil's claw**, dexamethasone, dexibuprofen, dicloxacillin, dirithromycin, disulfiram, **dong quai**, erythromycin, etoricoxib, **evening primrose**, fenofibrate, **feverfew**, fluconazole, flunisolide, fluoxymesterone, fosamprenavir, **garlic**, gemfibrozil, **ginger**, **ginkgo biloba**, ginseng, glucagon, **grapefruit juice**, **green tea**, **guarana**, **horse chestnut (bark, flower, leaf, seed)**, imatinib, **influenza vaccines**, itraconazole, ketoconazole, leflunomide, levothyroxine, liothyronine, **melatonin**, mephobarbital, methimazole, methylprednisolone, methyltestosterone, metronidazole, miconazole, moricizine, nafcillin, nalidixic acid, nilutamide, orlistat, PEG-interferon, penicillin g, penicillin V,

penicillins, pentobarbital, phenobarbital, phenylbutazones, phytonadione, piperacillin, primidone, propoxyphene, propylthiouracil, quinidine, quinine, **red clover**, rifampin, rifapentine, rofecoxib, ropinirole, rosuvastatin, roxithromycin, salicylates, **saw palmetto**, secobarbital, simvastatin, sitaxentan, sorafenib, **St John's wort**, stanozolol, sulfamethoxazole, sulfinpyrazone, sulfisoxazole, sulfonamides, sulindac, telithromycin, testosterone, thyroid, tigecycline, tolterodine, troleandomycin, valdecoxib, vitamin A, vitamin E, zileuton

Note: Alternative remedies, including herbals, may potentially increase the risk of bleeding or potentiate the effects of warfarin therapy. Some of these include the following: angelica root, arnica flower, anise, asafetida, bogbean, borage seed oil, bromelain, dan shen, devil's claw, fenugreek, feverfew, garlic, ginger, ginkgo biloba, ginseng, horse chestnut, lovage root, meadowsweet, onion, parsley, passionflower herb, poplar, quassia, red clover, rue, turmeric and willow bark

Reactions

Skin
Abscess
  (1997): Clayton BD, *J Geriatr Dermatology* 5, 314
Acral purpura
  (1986): Stone MS+, *J Am Acad Dermatol* 14, 796
Angioedema (<1%)
Bullous dermatitis
  (1993): Elis A+, *J Intern Med* 234, 615 (hemorrhagic)
  (1986): Stone MS+, *J Am Acad Dermatol* 14, 796 (passim)
Dermatitis
  (1992): Breathnach SM+, *Adverse Drug Reactions and the Skin* Blackwell, Oxford, 248 (passim)
  (1991): Quintavalla R+, *Int Angiol* 10, 103
Exanthems
  (2003): Spyropoulos AC+, *Pharmacotherapy* 23(4), 533
  (1993): Antony SJ+, *South Med J* 86, 1413
  (1989): Kruis-de Vries MH+, *Dermatologica* 178, 109
  (1988): Cole MS+, *Surgery* 103, 271 (passim)
Exfoliative dermatitis
Hematomas
  (1997): Clayton BD, *J Geriatr Dermatology* 5, 314
Hemorrhage
  (1989): Geoghegan+, *BMJ* 298, 902
  (1988): Cole MS, *Surgery* 103, 271
  (1980): Schleicher SM+, *Arch Dermatol* 116, 444
Livedo reticularis
  (1993): Park S+, *Arch Dermatol* 129, 775
Necrosis (>10%)
  (2004): Khalid K, *J Postgrad Med* 50(4), 268 (breast)
  (2003): Parsi K+, *Australas J Dermatol* 44(1), 57
  (2003): Roche-Nagle G+, *Eur J Vasc Endovasc Surg* 25(5), 481
  (2002): Clark JA+, *J Arthroplasty* 17(8), 1070
  (2002): Francesconi Do Valle F+, *World Congress Dermatol* Poster, 0101 (2 cases)
  (2002): Piccoli GB+, *Med Sci Monit* 8(11), CS83
  (2002): Scarff CE+, *Australas J Dermatol* 43(3), 202
  (2002): Sharkey MP+, *Australas J Dermatol* 43(3), 218
  (2000): Ad-El DD+, *Br J Plast Surg* 53(7), 624
  (2000): Chan YC+, *Br J Surgery* 87, 266
  (2000): Zimbelman J+, *J Pediatr* 137, 266
  (1999): Gailine D+, *Am J Hematol* 60, 231
  (1999): Martin FL, *Am J Nursing* 99, 53
  (1999): Stewart AJ+, *Postgrad Med J* 75, 233
  (1999): Yang Y+, *N Engl J Med* 340, 735
  (1998): Essex DW+, *Am J Hematol* 57, 233
  (1998): Gelwix TJ+, *Am J Emerg Med* 16, 541
  (1998): Sallah S+, *Haemostasis* 28, 25

(1997): English JC+, J Am Acad Dermatol 37, 1 (passim)
(1997): Hermes B+, Acta Derm Venereol 77, 35
(1997): Sallah S+, Thromb Haemost 78, 785
(1997): Wynn SS+, Haemostasis 27, 246
(1996): Jillella AP+, Am J Hematol 52, 117
(1996): Makris M+, Thromb Haemost 75, 523
(1995): DeFranzo AJ+, Ann Plast Surg 34, 203
(1995): Hauben M, N Engl J Med 332, 959
(1995): Sternberg ML+, Ann Emerg Med 26, 94
(1994): Lewandowski K+, Thromb Haemost 69, 311
(1994): Soisson AP+, Mil Med 159, 252
(1993): Bauer KA, Arch Dermatol 129, 766
(1993): Colman RW+, Am J Hematol 43, 300
(1993): Eby CS, Hematol Oncol Clin North Am 7, 1291
(1993): Hiers CL, J Ark Med Soc 89, 443
(1993): LaPrade RF+, Orthopedics 16, 703
(1993): Locht H+, J Intern Med 233, 287
(1993): Schramm W+, Arch Dermatol 129, 753
(1993): Yates P+, Clin Exp Dermatol 18, 138
(1992): Anderson DR+, Haemostasis 22, 124
(1992): McKnight JT+, Arch Fam Med 1, 105
(1992): Sharafuddin MA+, Arch Dermatol 128, 105
(1992): Viegas GV, J Am Podiatr Med Assoc 82, 463
(1991): Berkompas DC, Indiana Med 84, 788
(1991): Brooks LW+, J Am Osteopath Assoc 91, 601
(1991): Humphries JE+, Am J Hematol 37, 197
(1991): Ritchie AJ+, Ulster Med J 60, 248
(1990): Comp PC+, Semin Thromb Hemost 16, 293
(1989): Barkley C+, J Urology 141, 946
(1989): Grimaudo V+, BMJ 289, 233
(1988): Cole MS+, Surgery 103, 271
(1988): Conlan MG+, Am J Hematol 29, 226
(1988): Dominic W+, Burns Incl Therm Inj 14, 139
(1988): Kandrotas RJ+, Pharmacotherapy 8, 351
(1988): Konrad P+, Vasa, 17, 208
(1987): Gladson CL+, Arch Dermatol 123, 1701
(1987): Haimovici H+, J Vasc Surg 5, 655
(1987): Norris PG, Clin Exp Dermatol 12, 370
(1986): Brennan M+, J Tenn Med Assoc 79, 210
(1986): Everett RN+, Postgrad Med 79, 97
(1986): Rowbotham B+, Aust N Z J Med 16, 513
(1986): Sjoberg A+, Lakartidningen (Swedish) 83, 4089
(1986): Zauber NP+, Ann Intern Med 104, 659
(1984): Franson TR+, Arch Dermatol 120, 927
(1984): McGehee WG+, Ann Intern Med 101, 59
(1984): Schwartz RA+, Dermatologica 168, 31 (linear localized)
(1984): Slutzki S+, Int J Dermatol 23, 117
(1983): Caldwell EH+, Plast Reconstr Surg 72, 231
(1983): Leath MC, Tex Med 79, 62
(1983): Papa MA+, Harefuah (Hebrew) 104, 504
(1982): Faraci PA, Int J Dermatol 21, 329
(1982): Torngren S+, Acta Chir Scand 148, 471
(1981): Horn JR+, Am J Hosp Pharm 38, 1763
(1980): Hislop IG+, Aust N Z J Med 10, 51
(1980): Schleicher SM+, Arch Dermatol 116, 444
Pruritus (<1%)
(2003): Spyropoulos AC+, Pharmacotherapy 23(4), 533
Purple toe syndrome
(2003): Talmadge DB+, Pharmacotherapy 23(5), 674
Purplish erythema (feet and toes) (<1%)
(1998): Krahn MJ+, Can J Cardiol 14, 90 (purple toes)
(1997): Sallah S+, Thromb Haemost 78, 785 (purple toes)
(1994): Soisson AP+, Mil Med 159, 252
(1993): Park S+, Arch Dermatol 129, 775
(1982): Lebsack CS+, Postgrad Med 71, 81 (purple toes)
(1981): Akle CA+, J R Soc Med 74, 219 (purple toe syndrome)
Purpura
(2002): Scarff CE+, Australas J Dermatol 43(3), 202
(1988): Cole MS+, Surgery 103, 271 (passim)
Rash (sic) (<1%)

(2003): Spyropoulos AC+, Pharmacotherapy 23(4), 533
Ulcerations
(2002): Scarff CE+, Australas J Dermatol 43(3), 202
Urticaria
(1988): Cole MS+, Surgery 103, 271 (passim)
(1986): Stone MS+, J Am Acad Dermatol 14, 796 (passim)
Vasculitis
(2005): Yaghoubian B+, Cutis 75(6), 329
(1998): Krahn MJ+, Can J Cardiol 14, 90
(1994): Tamir A+, Acta Derm Venereol 74, 138
(1982): Howitt AJ+, Postgrad Med J 58, 233
(1982): Tanay A+, Dermatologica 165, 178
Vesiculation
(1986): Stone MS+, J Am Acad Dermatol 14, 796 (passim)

Mucosal/ENT
Oral ulceration (<1%)
Tongue hemorrhage
(2000): Shojania KG, Am J Med 109, 77

Hair
Hair – alopecia (>10%)
(1995): Nagao T+, Lancet 346, 1004
(1989): Kruis-de Vries MH+, Dermatologica 178, 109 (passim)
(1988): Umlas J+, Cutis 42, 63
(1986): Stone MS+, J Am Acad Dermatol 14, 796 (passim)

Eyes
Ocular hemorrhage
(2002): Mootha VV+, Arch Ophthalmol 120(1), 94 (with fluconazole)
Retinal vein occlusion
(2004): Browning DJ+, Ophthalmology 111(6), 1196

Other
Death
(2002): Clark JA+, J Arthroplasty 17(8), 1070
Gangrene
Hypersensitivity
(2004): Konishi H+, J Clin Pharm Ther 29(5), 485
(2002): Kristensen SR, Blood 100(7), 2676
Hypotension
(2002): Zaidenstein R+, Pharmacoepidemiol Drug Saf 11(3), 235
Rhabdomyolysis
(1999): Mogyorosi A+, J Intern Med 246(6), 599 (with simvastatin)

WILLOW BARK

Scientific names: *Salix alba; Salix fragilis; Salix purpurea*
Family: Salicaceae
Trade and other common names: Basket Willow; Brittle Willow; Crack Willow; White Willow; Willowbark
Category: Anti-inflammatory
Purported indications and other uses: Colds, infections, headaches, pain, muscle and joint aches, influenza, gouty arthritis, ankylosing spondylitis, rheumatoid arthritis, osteoarthritis
Half-life: N/A
Clinically important, potentially hazardous interactions with: NSAIDs, salicylates

Reactions

Skin
Rash (sic)

Other
Anaphylactoid reactions/Anaphylaxis
(2003): Boullata JI+, *Ann Pharmacother* 37(6), 832

YARROW

Scientific name: *Achillea millefolium*
Family: Compositae
Trade and other common names: Angel flower; Bad Man's Plaything; Bloodwort; Carpenter's Weed; Devil's Nettle; Devil's Plaything; Herbe Militaris; Knight's Milfoil; Milfoil; Millefoil; Nose Bleed; Nosebleed; Old Man's Pepper; Sanguinary; Soldier's Woundwort; Staunchgrass; Staunchweed; Thousand Weed; Thousand-leaf; Yarroway
Category: Anti-inflammatory
Purported indications and other uses: Fevers, common cold, essential hypertension, digestive complaints, loss of appetite, amenorrhea, dysentery, diarrhea, cerebral and coronary thromboses, menstrual pain, bleeding piles, toothache, muscle spasms, gastrointestinal disorders. **Topical:** slow-healing wounds, skin inflammations, cosmetics
Half-life: N/A
Clinically important, potentially hazardous interactions with: anticoagulants, antiepileptics, hypertensives, hypotensives

Reactions

Skin
Allergic reactions (sic)
(1996): Hausen BM, *Am J Contact Dermat* 7(2), 94
Dermatitis
(2002): Schempp CM+, *Hautarzt* 53(2), 93
(1991): Hausen BM+, *Contact Dermatitis* 24(4), 274
(1991): Rucker G+, *Arch Pharm* (Weinheim) 324(12), 979
(1983): Hausen BM+, *Acta Derm Venereol* 63(4), 308
Photosensitivity
(2002): Schempp CM+, *Hautarzt* 53(2), 93
Rash (sic)
(2002): Schempp CM+, *Hautarzt* 53(2), 93
Urticaria
(2001): Uter W+, *Am J Contact Dermat* 12(3), 182

Eyes
Rhinoconjunctivitis
(2001): Uter W+, *Am J Contact Dermat* 12(3), 182

YOHIMBINE

Scientific name: *Pausinystalia yohimbe*
Family: Rubiaceae
Trade and other common names: Actibane (Consolidated Midland); Aphrodyne (Star); Yocon (Palisades); Yohimex (Kramer); Yomax
Category: Rauwolfia alkaloid
Purported indications and other uses: Impotence, alpha2-adrenergic blocker, orthostatic hypertension
Half-life: 36 minutes
Clinically important, potentially hazardous interactions with: tricyclic antidepressants

Reactions

Skin
Adverse effects (sic)
(2002): Haller CA+, *Adverse Drug React Toxicol Rev* 21(3), 143
Diaphoresis
Exfoliative dermatitis
(1993): Sandler B+, *Urology* 41, 343
Lupus erythematosus
(1993): Sandler B+, *Urology* 41, 343

Other
Death

ZAFIRLUKAST

Trade name: Accolate (AstraZeneca)
Indications: Asthma
Category: Leukotriene receptor antagonist
Half-life: 10 hours
Clinically important, potentially hazardous interactions with: CYP3A4 substrates, **high protein foods**

Reactions

Skin
Allergic granulomatous angiitis (Churg–Strauss syndrome)
(2007): Guilpain P+, *Presse Med* 36(5 Pt 2), 890
(2006): Reyes-Balaguer J+, *J Investig Allergol Clin Immunol* 16(1), 69
(2003): Cakir B+, *South Med J* 96(7), 677
(2003): Garcia-Marcos L+, *Drug Saf* 26(7), 483
(2002): Soy M+, *Clin Rheumatol* 21(4), 328
Lupus erythematosus
(1999): Finkel TH+, *J Allergy Clin Immunol* 103, 533
Vasculitis
(2002): Soy M+, *Clin Rheumatol* 21(4), 328

Mucosal/ENT
Oral ulceration
(1999): Finkel TH+, *J Allergy Clin Immunol* 103(3), 533
Sinusitis

Other
Asthenia
(1999): Finkel TH+, *J Allergy Clin Immunol* 103(3), 533
Cough
(2001): Spector SL, *Ann Allergy Asthma Immunol* 86(6 Suppl 1), 18
Headache
Myalgia/Myositis/Myopathy/Myotoxicity (1.6%)
(1999): Finkel TH+, *J Allergy Clin Immunol* 103(3), 533

ZALCITABINE

Synonyms: ddC; dideoxycytidine
Trade name: Hivid (Roche)
Indications: Advanced HIV disease
Category: Antiretroviral; Nucleoside analog reverse transcriptase inhibitor
Half-life: 2.9 hours

Reactions

Skin

Acne (<1%)
Angioedema (5%)
  (1988): Yarchoan R+, *Lancet* 1, 76 (5%)
Bullous dermatitis (<1%)
Dermatitis (<1%)
Diaphoresis (<1%)
Edema (1–70%)
  (1991): Pluda JM+, *Hematol Oncol Clin North Am* 5, 229
  (1991): Yarchoan R+, *Blood* 78, 859
  (1989): McNeely MC+, *J Am Acad Dermatol* 21, 1213 (70%)
    (dose-related)
Erythema multiforme
  (1995): Wardropper AG+, *Int J STD AIDS* 6, 450
Erythroderma (10%)
  (1989): McNeely MC+, *J Am Acad Dermatol* 21, 1213 (10%)
Exanthems (1–66%)
  (1991): Fischl MA, *Recent Advances in Antiretroviral Therapy* New York, Triclinica Communications
  (1991): Merigan TC, *Am J Med* 90, 8S
  (1991): Pluda JM+, *Hematol Oncol Clin North Am* 5, 229
  (1990): Pizzo PA+, *J Pediatr* 117, 799
  (1989): McNeely MC+, *J Am Acad Dermatol* 21, 1213 (40%)
  (1989): Merigan TC+, *Ann Intern Med* 110, 189 (66%)
  (1989): Yarchoan R+, *N Engl J Med* 321, 726 (1–5%)
  (1988): Yarchoan R+, *Lancet* 1, 76 (65%)
  (1987): Richman DD+, *N Engl J Med* 317, 192 (1–5%)
Exfoliative dermatitis (<1%)
Folliculitis
Granuloma annulare
  (2001): Peñas PF+, *Arch Dermatol* 137, 964
Penile edema (<1%)
Peripheral edema
  (1989): Jeffries DJ, *J Antimicrob Chemother* 23, 29
Photosensitivity (<1%)
Pruritus (3–5%)
Rash (sic) (2–11%)
  (1990): Bozzette SA+, *Am J Med* 88, 24S
  (1989): Jeffries DJ, *J Antimicrob Chemother* 23, 29
Side effects (sic)
  (1991): Yarchoan R+, *Blood* 78, 859
  (1990): Broder S+, *Am J Med* 88, 31S
Urticaria (3.4%)
  (1992): Roche Laboratories Monograph
Xerosis (<1%)

Mucosal/ENT

Ageusia (<1%)
Aphthous stomatitis
  (1991): Fischl MA, *Recent Advances in Antiretroviral Therapy* . New York, Triclinica Communications
  (1991): Merigan TC, *Am J Med* 90, 8S
  (1991): Pluda JM+, *Hematol Oncol Clin North Am* 5, 229
  (1989): Jeffries DJ, *J Antimicrob Chemother* 23, 29
  (1989): Yarchoan R+, *N Engl J Med* 321, 726
  (1988): Yarchoan R+, *Lancet* 1, 76

Dysgeusia (<1%)
Gingivitis (<1%)
Glossitis (<1%)
Glossodynia (<1%)
Oral lesions (40–73%)
  (1991): Fischl MA, *Recent Advances in Antiretroviral Therapy* . New York, Triclinica Communications
  (1989): Merigan TC+, *Ann Intern Med* 110, 189 (73%)
  (1988): Yarchoan R+, *Lancet* 1, 76 (40%)
Oral ulceration (3–64%)
  (1997): Schiodt M, *Oral Dis* 3 Suppl 1, S208
  (1990): Bozzette SA+, *Am J Med* 88, 24S
  (1990): Pizzo PA+, *J Pediatr* 117, 799 (painful)
  (1989): McNeely MC+, *J Am Acad Dermatol* 21, 1213 (64%)
Parosmia (<1%)
Stomatitis (3%)
  (1991): Yarchoan R+, *Blood* 78, 859
Tinnitus
Tongue disorder (sic) (<1%)
Xerostomia (<1%)

Hair

Hair – alopecia

Nails

Nails – changes (sic)
  (1989): Jeffries DJ, *J Antimicrob Chemother* 23, 29

Other

Anaphylactoid reactions/Anaphylaxis
  (1992): Roche Laboratories Monograph
Headache
Myalgia/Myositis/Myopathy/Myotoxicity (1–6%)
Paresthesias

ZALEPLON

Trade name: Sonata (Wyeth)
Indications: Insomnia
Category: Hypnotic, non-benzodiazepine
Half-life: 1 hour
Clinically important, potentially hazardous interactions with: alcohol, cimetidine, erythromycin, imipramine, ketoconazole, promethazine, rifampicin, rifampin, thioridazine

Reactions

Skin

Pruritus
Rash (sic)

Mucosal/ENT

Xerostomia

Other

Abdominal pain
Anaphylactoid reactions/Anaphylaxis
Chest pain
Depression
Fever
Headache
Myalgia/Myositis/Myopathy/Myotoxicity
Somnambulism
  (2004): Liskow B+, *J Am Acad Child Adolesc Psychiatry* 43(8), 927
Vertigo

ZANAMIVIR

Trade name: Relenza (GSK)
Indications: Influenza A and B
Category: Antiviral; Neuraminidase inhibitor
Half-life: 2.5–5.1 hours

Reactions

Skin
Erythema
(2005): Kaji M+, *J Infect Chemother* 11(1), 41
Urticaria (<1.5%)

Other
Infections (2%)
Myalgia/Myositis/Myopathy/Myotoxicity (<1.5%)
(2001): McNicholl IR+, *Ann Pharmacother* 35(1), 57
Upper respiratory infection
(2001): McNicholl IR+, *Ann Pharmacother* 35(1), 57

ZICONOTIDE

Trade name: Prialt (Elan)
Indications: Analgesic, severe chronic pain
Category: Calcium channel blocker
Half-life: 4.6 hours
**Clinically important, potentially hazardous interactions
with:** CNS depressants

Note: Ziconotide is a synthetic analog of a substance isolated from
the venom of carnivorous oceanic snails that sting their prey with a
cocktail of neurotoxins injected through a harpoon-like tube.
Ziconotide is 100 to 1,000 times more powerful than morphine.

Reactions

Skin
Cellulitis (~2%)
Diaphoresis (~2%)
Edema (~2%)
Peripheral edema
(2008): Webster LR+, *Pain Med* 9(3), 282
Pruritus (~2%)
(2008): Webster LR+, *Pain Med* 9(3), 282
Xerosis (~2%)

Mucosal/ENT
Dysgeusia (~2%)
Tinnitus (~2%)
Xerostomia (~2%)

Eyes
Diplopia (~2%)
Nystagmus (8%)
(2004): Doggrell SA, *Expert Opin Investig Drugs* 13(7), 875
(2000): Atanassoff PG+, *Reg Anesth Pain Med* 25(3), 274
Periorbital edema (~2%)
Photophobia (~2%)
Vision blurred
(2004): Doggrell SA, *Expert Opin Investig Drugs* 13(7), 875
(2000): Atanassoff PG+, *Reg Anesth Pain Med* 25(3), 274
Visual disturbances (10%)

Other
Abdominal pain (~2%)

Asthenia (22%)
Chest pain (~2%)
Chills (~2%)
Confusion
(2008): Wallace MS+, *Anesth Analg* 106(2), 628
Depression (~2%)
Fever
(2004): Doggrell SA, *Expert Opin Investig Drugs* 13(7), 875
Headache (15%)
(2008): Wallace MS+, *Anesth Analg* 106(2), 628
Hypertension (~2%)
Hypotension (~2%)
Infections (~2%)
Myalgia/Myositis/Myopathy/Myotoxicity (~2%)
Pain (11%)
(2008): Wallace MS+, *Anesth Analg* 106(2), 628
Paresthesias (7%)
Rhabdomyolysis (<2%)
Seizures (<2%)
Somnolence
(2008): Wallace MS+, *Anesth Analg* 106(2), 628
Suicidal ideation (<2%)
Tremor (~2%)
Vertigo (47%)
(2008): Wallace MS+, *Anesth Analg* 106(2), 628
(2008): Webster LR+, *Pain Med* 9(3), 282
(2004): Doggrell SA, *Expert Opin Investig Drugs* 13(7), 875
(2000): Atanassoff PG+, *Reg Anesth Pain Med* 25(3), 274

ZIDOVUDINE

Synonyms: azidothymidine; AZT; compound S
Trade names: Combivir (GSK) (Shire); Novo-AZT; Retrovir
(GSK); Retrovis; Trizivir
Indications: HIV infection
Category: Antiretroviral; Nucleoside analog reverse
transcriptase inhibitor
Half-life: 1 hour
**Clinically important, potentially hazardous interactions
with:** clarithromycin, ganciclovir, PEG-interferon, ribavirin

Reactions

Skin
Acne (<5%)
(1988): McEvoy GK, *Am Hosp Formulary Service: Drug Info* 392
Acute generalized exanthematous pustulosis
(1998): Aquilina C+, *Arch Intern Med* 158(19), 2160 (with
lamivudine)
Allergic reactions (sic)
(1988): Diven DG+, *Arch Intern Med* 148, 2296
Bullous dermatitis
(1989): Caumes E+, *Presse Med* (French) 18, 1708 (fatal in
AIDS)
Diaphoresis (5–19%)
(1988): McEvoy GK, *Am Hosp Formulary Service: Drug Info* 392
Edema of lip (<5%)
(1988): McEvoy GK, *Am Hosp Formulary Service: Drug Info* 392
Erythema multiforme
(1989): Langtry HD+, *Drugs* 37, 408
(1989): Yarchoan R+, *N Engl J Med* 321, 726
Erythroderma
(1996): Duque S+, *J Allergy Clin Immunol* 98, 234
Exanthems (1–5%)

(1990): Petty BG+, *Lancet* 335, 1044 (1–5%) (in AIDS patients)
(1989): Gelman K+, *AIDS* 3, 555 (>5%)
(1989): Langtry HD+, *Drugs* 37, 408
(1987): Richman DD+, *N Engl J Med* 317, 192
Neutrophilic eccrine hidradenitis
(1990): Smith KJ+, *J Am Acad Dermatol* 23, 945
Pigmentation
(1993): Hermanns-Le T+, *Ann Pathol* (French) 13, 328
(1992): Baudo F+, *Eur J Dermatol* 2, 448
(1992): Hill DA+, *Hosp Pract Off Ed* 27, 29
(1991): Poizot-Martin I+, *Presse Med* (French) 20, 632
(1991): Tal A+, *Cutis* 48, 153
(1990): Greenberg RG+, *J Am Acad Dermatol* 22, 327
(1989): Bendick C+, *Arch Dermatol* 125, 1285 (palms and soles)
(1989): Merenich JA+, *Am J Med* 86, 469
(1989): Valencia ME+, *Med Clin* (Barc) (Spanish) 92, 357
Pruritus
(1989): Gelman K+, *AIDS* 3, 555 (>5%)
(1988): McEvoy GK, *Am Hosp Formulary Service: Drug Info* 392
Purpura
Rash (sic) (17%)
(1996): Henry K+, *Ann Intern Med* 124, 855
(1987): Richman DD+, *N Engl J Med* 317, 192
Stevens–Johnson syndrome
(2003): Rotunda A+, *Acta Derm Venereol* 83(1), 1
(1989): Langtry HD+, *Drugs* 37, 408
(1989): Yarchoan R+, *N Engl J Med* 321, 726
Toxic epidermal necrolysis
(2003): Rotunda A+, *Acta Derm Venereol* 83(1), 1
(1996): Murri R+, *Clin Infect Dis* 23, 640
Urticaria (<5%)
(1990): McKinley GF+, *Lancet* 336, 384
(1988): McEvoy GK, *Am Hosp Formulary Service: Drug Info* 392
Vasculitis
(1992): Torres RA+, *Arch Intern Med* 152, 850
(1990): Lee MH+, *Int Conf AIDS* 6, 360 (leukocytoclastic)
Vitiligo
(1994): Ivker R+, *J Am Acad Dermatol* 30, 829

Mucosal/ENT

Bromhidrosis (<5%)
(1988): McEvoy GK, *Am Hosp Formulary Service: Drug Info* 392
Dysgeusia (5–19%)
(1988): McEvoy GK, *Am Hosp Formulary Service: Drug Info* 392
(1987): Richman DD+, *N Engl J Med* 317, 192
Gingivitis
Oral lichenoid eruption
(2001): Scully C+, *Oral Dis* 7(4), 205 (passim)
(1993): Ficarra G+, *Oral Surg Oral Med Oral Pathol* 76, 460
Oral mucosal eruption (>5%)
(1989): Gelman K+, *AIDS* 3, 555 (>5%)
Oral pigmentation
(1991): Poizot-Martin I+, *Presse Med* (French) 20, 632
(1991): Tadini G+, *Arch Dermatol* 127, 267
(1990): Ficarra G+, *Oral Surg Oral Med Oral Pathol* 70, 748
(1990): Grau-Massanes M+, *J Am Acad Dermatol* 22, 687
(1990): Greenberg RG+, *J Am Acad Dermatol* 22, 327
(1990): Poizot-Martin I+, *Int Conf AIDS* 6, 357
(1989): Merenich JA+, *Am J Med* 86, 469
Oral ulceration (<5%)
(1988): McEvoy GK, *Am Hosp Formulary Service: Drug Info* 392
Stomatopyrosis
(2008): Moura MD+, *J Contemp Dent Pract* 9(1), 84 (with nevirapine and lamivudine)
Tongue edema (<5%)
(1988): McEvoy GK, *Am Hosp Formulary Service: Drug Info* 392
Tongue pigmentation
(1991): Tadini G+, *Arch Dermatol* 127, 267
(1991): Tal A+, *Cutis* 48, 153

(1990): Grau-Massanes M+, *J Am Acad Dermatol* 22, 687
(1990): Greenberg RG+, *J Am Acad Dermatol* 22, 327
Tongue ulceration
(1993): Schwander S+, *Med Klin* (German) 88, 60

Hair

Hair – alopecia
(1996): Geletko SM+, *Pharmacotherapy* 16, 69
Hair – hypertrichosis (eyelashes)
(1991): Klutman NE+, *N Engl J Med* 324, 1896
(1991): Sahai J+, *AIDS* 5, 1395

Nails

Nails – paronychia
(1999): Russo F+, *J Am Acad Dermatol* 40, 322
Nails – pigmentation (42%)
(1992): Rahav G+, *Scand J Infect Dis* 24, 557
(1991): Sahai J+, *AIDS* 5, 1395
(1991): Tadini G+, *Arch Dermatol* 127, 267
(1990): Don PC+, *Ann Intern Med* 112, 145 (42%) (bluish)
(1990): Grau-Massanes M+, *J Am Acad Dermatol* 22, 687
(1990): Greenberg RG+, *J Am Acad Dermatol* 22, 327
(1990): Poizot-Martin I+, *Int Conf AIDS* 6, 357
(1990): Ramos C+, *Rev Clin Esp* (Spanish) 187, 94
(1990): Tosti A+, *Dermatologica* 180, 217 (longitudinal)
(1989): Anders KH+, *J Am Acad Dermatol* 21, 792
(1989): Bendick C+, *Arch Dermatol* 125, 1285
(1989): Bendick C+, *Z Hautkr* (German) 64, 91
(1989): Depaoli MA+, *G Ital Dermatol Venereol* (Italian) 124, 71
(1989): Dupon M+, *Scand J Infect Dis* 21, 237
(1989): Fisher CA+, *Cutis* 43, 552
(1989): Groark SP+, *J Am Acad Dermatol* 21, 1032
(1989): Langtry HD+, *Drugs* 37, 408
(1989): Merenich JA+, *Am J Med* 86, 469
(1989): Valencia ME+, *Rev Clin Esp* (Spanish) 185, 167 (blue striae)
(1989): Yarchoan R+, *N Engl J Med* 321, 726
(1988): Azon-Masoliver A+, *Arch Dermatol* 124, 1570
(1988): Gonzalez-Lahoz JM+, *Rev Clin Esp* (Spanish) 183, 278 (bluish)
(1988): Vaiopoulos G+, *Ann Intern Med* 108, 777
(1987): Furth PA+, *Ann Intern Med* 107, 350

Other

Abdominal pain
(2007): McMahon DK+, *HIV Clin Trials* 8(5), 269 (28%) (with indinavir and lamivudine)
Asthenia
(2007): McMahon DK+, *HIV Clin Trials* 8(5), 269 (49%) (with indinavir and lamivudine)
Death
Headache
(2007): McMahon DK+, *HIV Clin Trials* 8(5), 269 (28%) (with indinavir and lamivudine)
Hypersensitivity
Lipoatrophy
(2004): McComsey GA+, *Clin Infect Dis* 38(2), 263
Lipodystrophy
(2001): Bogner JR+, *J Acquir Immune Defic Syndr* 27(3), 237
Myalgia/Myositis/Myopathy/Myotoxicity (<1%)
(1993): Simpson DM+, *Neurology* 43, 971
(1989): Gertner E+, *Am J Medicine* 86, 814
(1988): Helbert M+, *Lancet* 2, 689
Paresthesias (<8%)
(1988): McEvoy GK, *Am Hosp Formulary Service: Drug Info* 392
Polymyositis
(1988): Bessen LJ+, *N Engl J Med* 318, 708 (4 patients)
Porphyria cutanea tarda
(1988): Ong EL+, *Postgrad Med J* 64, 956

ZILEUTON

Trade name: Zyflo (Abbott)
Indications: Asthma
Category: Leukotriene receptor antagonist
Half-life: 2.5 hours
Clinically important, potentially hazardous interactions
with: anisindione, anticoagulants, astemizole, dicumarol, pimozide, warfarin

Reactions

Skin

Allergic granulomatous angiitis (Churg–Strauss syndrome)
  (2000): Dellaripa PF+, *Mayo Clin Proc* 75(6), 643
Eosinophilic fasciitis
  (2000): Dellaripa PF+, *Mayo Clin Proc* 75(6), 643
Erythema nodosum
  (2000): Dellaripa PF+, *Mayo Clin Proc* 75, 643
Morphea
  (2000): Dellaripa PF+, *Mayo Clin Proc* 75(6), 643
Pruritus (>1%)
Scleroderma
  (2000): Dellaripa PF+, *Mayo Clin Proc* 75(6), 643

Mucosal/ENT

Vaginitis (>1%)

Other

Cough
  (2001): Spector SL, *Ann Allergy Asthma Immunol* 86(6 Suppl 1), 18
Hepatotoxicity
  (2007): Li F+, *Chem Res Toxicol* 20(12), 1854
Myalgia/Myositis/Myopathy/Myotoxicity (3.2%)
Paresthesias (1%)

ZINC

Trade names: Calamine; Cold-Eeze (The Quigley Corp); Galzin; Zicam
Category: Food supplement; Trace element
Half-life: N/A
Clinically important, potentially hazardous interactions
with: chlorothiazide, chlorthalidone, ciprofloxacin, cisplatin, deferoxamine, demeclocycline, ethambutol, gatifloxacin, hydrochlorothiazide, indapamide, levofloxacin, metolozone, minocycline, moxifloxacin, ofloxacin, propofol, valproic acid

Note: Zinc is found in meats, seafood, dairy products, legumes, nuts, whole grains. Zinc oxide and zinc sulfate are used to fortify wheat products

Reactions

Skin

Allergic granulomatous angiitis (Churg–Strauss syndrome)
  (1989): Jordaan HF+, *Clin Exp Dermatol* 14(3), 227
  (1989): Sandler M+, *S Afr Med J* 75(7), 342
Burning
Dermatitis
  (2003): Shimizu T+, *Clin Exp Dermatol* 28(6), 675 (dental fillings)
  (1997): Nielsen NH+, *Am J Contact Dermat* 8(3), 170 (zinc pyrithione shampoo)
  (1988): Nigam PK+, *Contact Dermatitis* 19(3), 219 (zinc pyrithione)

Erythroderma
Itching
Lupus erythematosus
Palmoplantar pustulosis
  (2005): Yanagi T+, *Lancet* 366(9490), 1050 (dental fillings)
Pigmentation
  (2002): Greenberg JE+, *J Cutan Pathol* 29(10), 613

Mucosal/ENT

Anosmia
  (2006): Davidson TM, *Laryngoscope* 116(9), 1721 (intranasal)
  (2006): Seidman MD, *Laryngoscope* 116(9), 1720 (intranasal)
Dysgeusia
  (1998): Garland ML+, *Ann Pharmacother* 32(1), 63 (zinc gluconate)
  (1996): Mossad SB+, *Ann Intern Med* 125(2), 81 (zinc gluconate)
  (1984): Eby GA+, *Antimicrob Agents Chemother* 25(1), 20 (zinc gluconate)
  (1982): Rasker JJ+, *Scand J Rheumatol* 11(3), 168 (zinc sulfate)
  (1980): Zetin M+, *Clin Nephrol* 13(1), 20
Oral lichen planus
  (2002): Ido T+, *Contact Dermatitis* 47(1), 51
Oral mucosal irritation
  (1998): Garland ML+, *Ann Pharmacother* 32(1), 63 (zinc gluconate)
  (1984): Eby GA+, *Antimicrob Agents Chemother* 25(1), 20 (zinc gluconate)
Xerostomia

Other

Abdominal pain
  (1987): Samman S+, *Med J Aust* 146(5), 246
Asthenia
  (2002): Igic PG+, *Mayo Clin Proc* 77(7), 713
Cancer
  (2007): Gallus S+, *Eur Urol* 52(4), 1052 (prostate)
Candidiasis
  (1993): Schlesinger L+, *Acta Paediatr* 82(9), 734
Headache
  (1987): Samman S+, *Med J Aust* 146(5), 246
Nephrotoxicity
  (1999): Barceloux DG, *J Toxicol Clin Toxicol* 37(2), 279
Toxicity (sic)
  (2002): Igic PG+, *Mayo Clin Proc* 77(7), 713

ZIPRASIDONE

Synonym: Zeldox
Trade name: Geodon (Pfizer)
Indications: Schizophrenia
Category: Antipsychotic, benzothiazolylpiperazine
Half-life: 4–5 hours
Clinically important, potentially hazardous interactions
with: astemizole, moxifloxacin, pimozide, ranolazine

Reactions

Skin

Angioedema
  (2007): Akkaya C+, *J Psychopharmacol* 21(5), 550
Dermatitis
Diaphoresis
  (2006): Borovicka MC+, *Ann Pharmacother* 40(1), 139
Eczema (<1%)
Exanthems (<1%)
Exfoliative dermatitis (<1%)

Facial edema (<1%)
Fungal dermatitis (2%)
Lupus erythematosus
  (2004): Swensen E+, *Can J Psychiatry* 49(6), 413
Peripheral edema (<1%)
Photosensitivity (<1%)
Rash (sic) (4%)
Urticaria (5%)
  (2007): Akkaya C+, *J Psychopharmacol* 21(5), 550
Vesiculobullous eruption (<1%)

Mucosal/ENT
Gingival bleeding (<1%)
Sialorrhea
Tinnitus (<1%)
Tongue edema (<1%)
Xerostomia (4%)

Hair
Hair – alopecia (<1%)

Other
Chills (<1%)
Death
  (2005): Scahill L+, *J Psychopharmacol* 19(2), 205
Depression
  (2007): Kaptsan A+, *Clin Neuropharmacol* 30(6), 357 (3 cases)
Gynecomastia (<1%)
Headache
  (2007): Ratner Y+, *Prog Neuropsychopharmacol Biol Psychiatry* 31(7), 1401
Mania
  (2007): Wickham R+, *CNS Spectr* 12(8), 578
Myalgia/Myositis/Myopathy/Myotoxicity (1%)
Paresthesias (<1%)
Rhabdomyolysis
  (2002): Yang SH+, *Am J Psychiatry* 159(8), 1435
Somnolence
  (2007): Barzman DH+, *J Child Adolesc Psychopharmacol* 17(4), 503
  (2007): Klein-Schwartz+, *Clin Toxicol (Phila)* 45(7), 782
  (2007): Ratner Y+, *Prog Neuropsychopharmacol Biol Psychiatry* 31(7), 1401
Thrombophlebitis (<1%)
Tremor (<1%)
Upper respiratory infection (8%)

ZOLEDRONIC ACID

Trade name: Zometa (Novartis)
Indications: Hypercalcemia of malignancy, Paget's disease
Category: Bisphosphonate
Half-life: 7 days

Reactions

Skin
Rash (sic)
  (2006): Rizos EC+, *Clin Exp Rheumatol* 24(4), 455

Eyes
Conjunctivitis
  (2005): Durnian JM+, *Eye* 19(2), 221
Scleritis
  (2008): Moore MM+, *Med J Aust* 188(6), 370
  (2006): Benderson D+, *Clin Lymphoma Myeloma* 7(2), 145

Uveitis
  (2008): Moore MM+, *Med J Aust* 188(6), 370
  (2005): Durnian JM+, *Eye* 19(2), 221

Other
Asthenia
  (2003): Rosen LS+, *Cancer* 98(8), 1735
Candidiasis
Fever
  (2007): Body JJ+, *Ann Oncol* 18(7), 1165
  (2007): Lyles KW+, *N Engl J Med* 357(18), 1799
  (2006): Carteni G+, *Oncologist* 11(7), 841
  (2006): Rizos EC+, *Clin Exp Rheumatol* 24(4), 455
Headache
  (2007): McClung M+, *Bone* 41(1), 122
Myalgia/Myositis/Myopathy/Myotoxicity
  (2007): Lyles KW+, *N Engl J Med* 357(18), 1799
Nephrotoxicity
  (2007): Diel IJ+, *J Support Oncol* 5(10), 475
  (2006): Bergner R+, *Onkologie* 29(11), 534
  (2005): Munier A+, *Ann Pharmacother* 39(7–8), 1194
  (2005): von Moos R, *Oncologist* 10 Suppl 1, 19
  (2003): Markowitz GS+, *Kidney Int* 64(1), 281
Pain
  (2007): Lyles KW+, *N Engl J Med* 357(18), 1799
Seizures
  (2007): Navarro M+, *J Palliat Med* 10(6), 1226
Upper respiratory infection
  (2001): Berenson JR+, *Clin Cancer Res* (10%)

ZOLMITRIPTAN

Trade name: Zomig (AstraZeneca)
Indications: Migraine attacks
Category: 5-HT1 agonist; Serotonin receptor agonist; Triptan
Half-life: 3 hours
Clinically important, potentially hazardous interactions with: cimetidine, dihydroergotamine, ergot, fluoxetine, fluvoxamine, isocarboxazid, MAO inhibitors, methysergide, moclobemide, naratriptan, oral contraceptives, phenelzine, rizatriptan, sertraline, sibutramine, **St John's wort**, sumatriptan, tranylcypromine

Reactions

Skin
Allergic reactions (sic) (<1%)
Diaphoresis (2%)
Edema (<1%)
Facial edema (<1%)
Fixed eruption
  (2004): Baykal Y+, *Dermatology* 208(3), 235
Photosensitivity (<1%)
Pruritus (<1%)
Rash (sic) (<1%)
Urticaria (<1%)

Mucosal/ENT
Dysgeusia
  (2005): Dowson AJ+, *Headache* 45(1), 17 (19%)
  (2002): Yates R+, *J Clin Pharmacol* 42(11), 1244
Parosmia (<1%)
Tongue edema (<1%)
Xerostomia (3%)
  (1997): Edmeads JG+, *Cephalalgia* 17, 41

Other

Headache
(2002): Yates R+, *J Clin Pharmacol* 42(11), 1244
Hepatotoxicity
(2003): Redondo Cerezo E+, *Gastroenterol Hepatol* 26(10), 664
Hot flashes (>10%)
Myalgia/Myositis/Myopathy/Myotoxicity (2%)
(2007): Fernandez-Diaz A+, *Rev Neurol* 45(10), 639
(2005): Alonso-Navarro H+, *Clin Neuropharmacol* 28(5), 241
Nephrotoxicity
(2006): Fulton JA+, *Clin Toxicol (Phila)* 44(2), 177
Paresthesias (11%)
(2005): Dowson AJ+, *Headache* 45(1), 17 (6.8%)
(2004): Spierings EL+, *CNS Drugs* 18(15), 1133 (7%)
(2002): Yates R+, *J Clin Pharmacol* 42(11), 1244
(1998): Multiple Authors, *Headache* 38, 173 (11%)
Thrombophlebitis (<1%)
Vertigo
(2004): Spierings EL+, *CNS Drugs* 18(15), 1133 (7%)

ZOLPIDEM

Trade names: Ambien (Sanofi-Aventis); Niotal; Stilnoct; Stilnox
Indications: Insomnia
Category: Hypnotic, non-benzodiazepine
Half-life: 2.6 hours
Clinically important, potentially hazardous interactions with: alcohol, antihistamines, azatadine, azelastine, brompheniramine, buclizine, chlorpheniramine, cimetidine, clemastine, dexchlorpheniramine, erythromycin, ketoconazole, meclizine, rifampicin, ritonavir

Reactions

Skin

Acne (<1%)
Allergic reactions (sic) (4%)
Bullous dermatitis (<1%)
Dermatitis (<1%)
Diaphoresis (<1%)
Edema (<1%)
Facial edema (<1%)
Furunculosis (<1%)
Herpes simplex (<1%)
Herpes zoster (<1%)
Photosensitivity (<1%)
Pruritus
(1994): Litt JZ, Beachwood, OH (personal case) (observation)
Purpura (<1%)
Rash (sic) (2%)
Urticaria (<1%)

Mucosal/ENT

Dysgeusia (<1%)
(2001): Tsutsui S, *J Int Med Res* 29(3), 163
(1999): Hajak G, *Drug Saf* 21(6), 457
(1998): Noble S+, *Drugs* 55(2), 277
(1993): Wadworth AN+, *Drugs Aging* 3(5), 441
Tinnitus
Vaginitis (<1%)
Xerostomia (3%)
(1993): Wadworth AN+, *Drugs Aging* 3(5), 441

Eyes

Periorbital edema (<1%)

Visual hallucinations
(2006): Kito S+, *Int Psychogeriatr* 18(4), 749 (with fluvoxamine)
(2003): Huang CL+, *Ann Pharmacother* 37(5), 683
(2003): Tsai MJ+, *J Toxicol Clin Toxicol* 41(6), 869
(2000): Toner LC+, *Clin Neuropharmacol* 23(1), 54
(1998): Elko CJ+, *J Toxicol Clin Toxicol* 36(3), 195 (with antidepressants)
(1996): Markowitz JS+, *Ann Clin Psychiatry* 8(2), 89
(1996): van Puijenbroek EP+, *Int J Clin Pharmacol Ther* 34(7), 318

Other

Anaphylactoid reactions/Anaphylaxis (<1%)
Anxiety
(2008): Krystal AD+, *Sleep* 31(1), 79
Asthenia
(1998): Hajak G+, *Int Clin Psychopharmacol* 13(4), 157
Delirium
(2007): Sharan P+, *Natl Med J India* 20(4), 180
(2001): Brodeur MR+, *Ann Pharmacother* 35(12), 1562
(2000): Toner LC+, *Clin Neuropharmacol* 23(1), 54
Headache
(2008): Krystal AD+, *Sleep* 31(1), 79
(1999): Ganzoni E+, *Schweiz Rundsch Med Prax* 88(25-2), 1120
(1998): Hajak G+, *Int Clin Psychopharmacol* 13(4), 157
Hepatotoxicity
(1999): Karsenti D+, *BMJ* 318(7192), 1179
Hot flashes (<1%)
Injection-site inflammation (<1%)
Myalgia/Myositis/Myopathy/Myotoxicity (7%)
Paresthesias (<1%)
Seizures
(2007): Cubala WJ+, *Prog Neuropsychopharmacol Biol Psychiatry* 31(2), 539 (withdrawal)
(2003): Tavakoli SA+, *Psychosomatics* 44(3), 262
(2003): Tripodianakis J+, *Eur Psychiatry* 18(3), 140
(2000): Aragona M, *Clin Neuropharmacol* 23(5), 281 (withdrawal)
Somnambulism
(2008): Sansone RA+, *Gen Hosp Psychiatry* 30(1), 90
(2007): *Prescrire Int* 16(91), 200
(2006): *Lakartidningen* 103(37), 2661
(2005): Yang W+, *Arch Phys Med Rehabil* 86(6), 1265
(2003): Sattar SP+, *Ann Pharmacother* 37(10), 1429 (with valproic acid)
(2003): Yanes Baonza M+, *Aten Primaria* 32(7), 438
(1999): Harazin J+, *Mil Med* 164(9), 669
(1994): Mendelson WB, *J Clin Psychopharmacol* 14(2), 150
Somnolence
(2008): Krystal AD+, *Sleep* 31(1), 79
Tremor (<1%)
Vertigo
(2000): Holm KJ+, *Drugs* 59(4), 865
(1999): Ganzoni E+, *Schweiz Rundsch Med Prax* 88(25-2), 1120
(1998): Hajak G+, *Int Clin Psychopharmacol* 13(4), 157

ZONISAMIDE

Trade name: Zonegran (Eisai)
Indications: Epilepsy
Category: Antiepileptic, sulfonamide
Half-life: 63 hours
Clinically important, potentially hazardous interactions with: caffeine

Note: Zonisamide is a sulfonamide and can be absorbed systemically. Sulfonamides can produce severe, possibly fatal, reactions such as toxic epidermal necrolysis and Stevens–Johnson syndrome

Reactions

Skin
Acne (<1%)
Allergic reactions (sic) (<1%)
Diaphoresis (<1%)
Eczema (<1%)
Edema (<1%)
Exanthems (<1%)
Facial edema (<1%)
Lupus erythematosus (<1%)
  (2001): Mutoh K+, *Pediatr Neurol* 25(4), 340
Oligohydrosis
  (2007): *Prescrire Int* 16(89), 95
  (2007): Ohtahara S+, *Seizure* 16(1), 87
  (2004): Low PA+, *Epilepsy Res* 62(1), 27
  (2003): Knudsen JF+, *Pediatr Neurol* 28(3), 184 (6 cases)
  (1999): Isumi H+, *No To Hattatsu* (Japanese) 31, 468
  (1997): Shimizu T+, *Brain Dev* 19, 366
  (1996): Okumura A+, *No To Hattatsu* (Japanese) 28, 44
Peripheral edema (<1%)
Petechiae (<1%)
Pruritus (<1%)
Purpura (2%)
Pustules (<1%)
Rash (sic) (3%)
  (2007): *Prescrire Int* 16(89), 95
  (2007): Arif H+, *Neurology* 68(20), 1701
Stevens–Johnson syndrome
  (2002): Yoshioka M+, *Digestion* 65(4), 234
  (1985): Wilensky AJ+, *Epilepsia* 26, 212
Toxic epidermal necrolysis
  (2008): Teraki Y+, *Arch Dermatol* 144(2), 232
Urticaria (<1%)
Vesiculobullous eruption (<1%)
Xerosis (<1%)

Mucosal/ENT
Dysgeusia (2%)
Gingival hyperplasia/hypertrophy (<1%)
Gingivitis (<1%)
Glossitis (<1%)
Oral ulceration (<1%)
Parosmia (<1%)
Stomatitis (<1%)
Ulcerative stomatitis (<1%)
Xerostomia (2%)

Hair
Hair – alopecia (<1%)
Hair – hirsutism (<1%)

Other
Asthenia
  (2006): Ashkenazi A+, *Cephalalgia* 26(10), 1199
  (2006): Tosches WA+, *Epilepsy Behav* 8(3), 522
Depression
  (2007): Mula M+, *Drug Saf* 30(7), 555 (7%)
Gynecomastia (<1%)
  (1998): Ikeda A+, *J Neurol Neurosurg Psychiatry* 65, 803
Headache
  (2005): Brodie MJ+, *Epilepsia* 46(1), 31
  (2004): Kothare SV+, *Epileptic Disord* 6(4), 267
Hypersensitivity
Mania
  (2006): Sullivan KL+, *J Clin Psychopharmacol* 26(4), 439
Myalgia/Myositis/Myopathy/Myotoxicity (<1%)

Paresthesias (4%)
Somnolence
  (2008): Ghaemi SN+, *J Affect Disord* 105(1-3), 311
  (2008): Zaccara G+, *Seizure*
  (2006): Arzimanoglou A+, *Expert Rev Neurother* 6(9), 1283
  (2006): Kothare SV+, *Pediatr Neurol* 34(5), 351
  (2006): Tosches WA+, *Epilepsy Behav* 8(3), 522
Suicidal ideation
  (2006): Mago R+, *Psychosomatics* 47(1), 68
Thrombophlebitis (<1%)
Tremor (<1%)
  (1992): Taira T, *No To Shinkei* (Japanese) 44, 61
Vertigo
  (2006): Arzimanoglou A+, *Expert Rev Neurother* 6(9), 1283
  (2006): Kothare SV+, *Pediatr Neurol* 34(5), 351
  (2005): Brodie MJ+, *Epilepsia* 46(1), 31
  (2004): Faught E, *Seizure* 13 Suppl 1, S59
  (2004): Kothare SV+, *Epileptic Disord* 6(4), 267
Weight loss
  (2007): Ben-Menachem E, *Epilepsia* 48(Suppl 9), 42
  (2006): Kothare SV+, *Pediatr Neurol* 34(5), 351
  (2006): Post RM+, *Curr Psychiatry Rep* 8(6), 489
  (2006): Tosches WA+, *Epilepsy Behav* 8(3), 522
  (2005): Ness-Abramof R+, *Drugs Today* (Barc) 41(8), 547

ZOSTER VACCINE

Trade name: Zostavax (Oka/Merck)
Indications: Reactivation, varicella zoster (in people over 60), shingles
Category: Vaccine
Half-life: N/A
Clinically important, potentially hazardous interactions with: N/A

Reactions

Skin
Herpes zoster
  (2006): Holcomb K+, *J Drugs Dermatol* 5(9), 863 (7cases)
Rash (sic)
  (2008): Curtis KK+, *J Gen Intern Med* 23(5), 648 (in immunocompromised)
Skin reactions (sic)

Mucosal/ENT
Rhinitis
  (2007): Kockler DR+, *Pharmacotherapy* 27(7), 1013

Other
Anaphylactoid reactions/Anaphylaxis
Asthenia (1%)
  (2007): Kockler DR+, *Pharmacotherapy* 27(7), 1013
Fever (<2%)
  (2007): Kockler DR+, *Pharmacotherapy* 27(7), 1013
Headache (1%)
  (2007): Kockler DR+, *Pharmacotherapy* 27(7), 1013
  (2006): Robinson DM+, *Drugs Aging* 23(6), 525
Injection-site edema (25%)
  (2006): Holcomb K+, *J Drugs Dermatol* 5(9), 863 (26.2%)
Injection-site erythema (34%)
  (2006): Holcomb K+, *J Drugs Dermatol* 5(9), 863
Injection-site pain (33%)
  (2006): Holcomb K+, *J Drugs Dermatol* 5(9), 863
Injection-site pruritus (7%)
  (2006): Holcomb K+, *J Drugs Dermatol* 5(9), 863 (7.1%)

Injection-site reactions
  (2007): Kockler DR+, *Pharmacotherapy* 27(7), 1013
  (2007): Tyring SK+, *Vaccine* 25(10), 1877
  (2006): Robinson DM+, *Drugs Aging* 23(6), 525

ZUCLOPENTIXOL ACETATE

Trade name: Clopixol–Acuphase (Lundbeck Pharmaceutical)
Indications: Schizophrenia
Category: Antipsychotic
Half-life: 32 hours
Clinically important, potentially hazardous interactions with: guanethidine, levodopa, metoclopramide, piperazine

Reactions

Skin
  Allergic reactions (sic)
  Dermatitis
  Photosensitivity
  Pigmentation
  Pruritus
  Purpura
  Rash (sic)

Mucosal/ENT
  Pharyngitis
  Rhinitis
  Tinnitus
  Xerostomia

Eyes
  Conjunctivitis
  Lens opacities

Other
  Abdominal pain
  Agitation
  Amnesia
  Anxiety
  Asthenia
  Chest pain
  Confusion
  Depression
  Fever
  Gynecomastia
  Headache
  Hypotension
  Insomnia
  Migraine
  Paresthesias
  Seizures
  Somnolence
  Tremor
  Vertigo

ZUCLOPENTIXOL DECANOATE

Trade name: Clopixol Depot (Lundbeck Pharmaceutical)
Indications: Schizophrenia
Category: Antipsychotic
Half-life: 19 days
Clinically important, potentially hazardous interactions with: guanethidine, levodopa, metoclopramide, piperazine

Reactions

Skin
  Allergic reactions (sic)
  Dermatitis
  Photosensitivity
  Pigmentation
  Pruritus
  Purpura
  Rash (sic)

Mucosal/ENT
  Pharyngitis
  Rhinitis
  Tinnitus
  Xerostomia

Eyes
  Conjunctivitis
  Lens opacities
  Visual disturbances

Other
  Abdominal pain
  Agitation
  Amnesia
  Anxiety
  Asthenia
  Chest pain
  Confusion
  Depression
  Fever
  Gynecomastia
  Headache
  Hypotension
  Insomnia
  Migraine
  Myalgia/Myositis/Myopathy/Myotoxicity
  Paresthesias
  Seizures
  Somnolence
  Tremor
  Vertigo
  Weight gain
  Weight loss

ZUCLOPENTIXOL DIHYDROCHLORIDE

Trade name: Clopixol tablets (Lundbeck Pharmaceutical)
Indications: Schizophrenia
Category: Antipsychotic
Half-life: 20 hours
Clinically important, potentially hazardous interactions with: guanethidine, levodopa, metoclopramide, piperazine

Reactions

Skin
Allergic reactions (sic)
Dermatitis
Photosensitivity
Pigmentation
Purpura
Rash (sic)

Mucosal/ENT
Pharyngitis
Rhinitis
Tinnitus
Xerostomia

Eyes
Conjunctivitis
Lens opacities
Visual disturbances
Visual hallucinations

Other
Abdominal pain
Agitation
Amnesia
Anxiety
Asthenia
Chest pain
Confusion
Depression
Fever
Gynecomastia
Headache
Hypotension
Insomnia
Migraine
Paresthesias
Seizures
Somnolence
Tremor
Vertigo

Drugs responsible for common reaction patterns

Acanthosis Nigricans
Amprenavir
Azathioprine
Diethylstilbestrol
Estrogens
Fusidic acid
Gemfibrozil
Heroin
Mechlorethamine
Methsuximide
Methyltestosterone
Niacin
Niacinamide
Oral contraceptives
Prednisolone
Prednisone
Somatropin
Thioridazine
Tryptophan

Acneform Lesions
Acamprosate
Acyclovir
Adalimumab
Adapalene
Alosetron
Alprazolam
Amcinonide
Amitriptyline
Amobarbital
Amoxapine
Androstenedione
Aprepitant
Aripiprazole
Atorvastatin
Azathioprine
Basiliximab
Beclomethasone
Betamethasone
Betaxolol
Bexarotene
Bisoprolol
Botulinum toxin (A & B)
Budesonide
Bupropion
Buspirone
Butabarbital
Cabergoline
Carbamazepine
Carteolol
Cefamandole
Cefpodoxime
Ceftazidime
Cetirizine
Cetuximab
Chasteberry
Chloral hydrate
Chlorotrianisene
Cidofovir
Cimetidine
Ciprofloxacin
Clobetasol
Clofazimine
Clomiphene
Clomipramine

Creatine
Cyanocobalamin
Cyclosporine
Daclizumab
Dactinomycin
Danazol
Dantrolene
Dasatinib
Deferoxamine
Demeclocycline
Desipramine
Dexamethasone
Diazepam
Diethylstilbestrol
Diltiazem
Disulfiram
Duloxetine
Efalizumab
Eflornithine
Epoetin alfa
Erlotinib
Erythromycin
Escitalopram
Esmolol
Esomeprazole
Estazolam
Estramustine
Estrogens
Eszopiclone
Ethambutol
Ethionamide
Everolimus
Famotidine
Felbamate
Fenoprofen
Fexofenadine
Floxuridine
Fluconazole
Fluocinonide
Fluorides
Fluoxetine
Fluoxymesterone
Fluticasone
Fluvoxamine
Folic acid
Foscarnet
Fosphenytoin
Gabapentin
Ganciclovir
Gefitinib
Glatiramer
Gold and gold compounds
Granulocyte colony-
  stimulating factor (GCSF)
Grepafloxacin
Halcinonide
Haloperidol
Halothane
Heroin
Histrelin
Hyaluronic acid
Hydrocortisone
Imatinib
Imipramine

Infliximab
Interferon alfa
Isoniazid
Isotretinoin
Lamotrigine
Lansoprazole
Leflunomide
Leuprolide
Levothyroxine
Lithium
Maprotiline
MDMA
Medroxyprogesterone
Mephenytoin
Mesalamine
Methotrexate
Methoxsalen
Methyltestosterone
Minoxidil
Mirtazapine
Mometasone
Mycophenolate
Nabumetone
Nafarelin
Naltrexone
Naratriptan
Nefazodone
Nimodipine
Nisoldipine
Nizatidine
Nortriptyline
Olsalazine
Oral contraceptives
Oxcarbazepine
Panitumumab
Pantoprazole
Paramethadione
Paroxetine
Pentobarbital
Pentostatin
Pergolide
Phenobarbital
Phenylbutazone
Phenytoin
Potassium iodide
Prednisolone
Prednisone
Primidone
Progestins
Propafenone
Propranolol
Propylthiouracil
Protriptyline
Psoralens
Pyrazinamide
Pyridoxine
Quinidine
Quinine
Ramipril
Riboflavin
Rifampin
Rifapentine
Risperidone
Ritonavir

Saquinavir
Sertraline
Sibutramine
Sirolimus
Smallpox vaccine
Sorafenib
Sparfloxacin
Stanozolol
Tacrine
Temsirolimus
Testosterone
Tetracycline
Tiagabine
Tizanidine
Topiramate
Trastuzumab
Tretinoin
Triamcinolone
Trimethadione
Trioxsalen
Trovafloxacin
Valdecoxib
Valproic acid
Varenicline
Venlafaxine
Verapamil
Vinblastine
Zalcitabine
Zidovudine
Zolpidem
Zonisamide

Acral Erythema
Bleomycin
Capecitabine
Cisplatin
Clofarabine
Cyclophosphamide
Cytarabine
Didanosine
Doxorubicin
Etoposide
Fluorouracil
Granulocyte colony-
  stimulating factor (GCSF)
Hydroxyurea
Idarubicin
Lomustine
Mercaptopurine
Methotrexate
Mitotane
Paclitaxel
Quinine
Uracil/tegafur
Vincristine

Acute Febrile Neutrophilic Dermatosis
Abacavir
Amoxapine
Arnica
Azathioprine
BCG vaccine
Bortezomib
Capsicum
Celecoxib

Citalopram
Clindamycin
Clofazimine
Clozapine
Co-trimoxazole
Cytarabine
Diazepam
Furosemide
Gabapentin
Glucagon
Granulocyte colony-
    stimulating factor (GCSF)
Hydralazine
Hydroxyurea
Imatinib
Infliximab
Influenza vaccines
Isotretinoin
Lenalidomide
Minocycline
Nitrofurantoin
Norfloxacin
Ofloxacin
Oral contraceptives
Pegfilgrastim
Perphenazine
Phenylbutazone
Piperacillin
Propylthiouracil
Quinupristin/dalfopristin
Sulfamethoxazole
Tretinoin
Verapamil

Acute Generalized
Exanthematous Pustulosis
Abciximab
Acarbose
Acetaminophen
Acetazolamide
Allopurinol
Amoxapine
Amoxicillin
Amphotericin B
Ampicillin
Aspirin
Azathioprine
Bacampicillin
Carbamazepine
Carbimazole
Cefaclor
Cefazolin
Ceftazidime
Ceftriaxone
Cefuroxime
Celecoxib
Cephalexin
Cephradine
Chloramphenicol
Chloroquine
Chlorzoxazone
Ciprofloxacin
Clindamycin
Clozapine
Co-trimoxazole
Codeine
Cytarabine
Dexamethasone
Diltiazem
Doxycycline
Erlotinib

Erythromycin
Famotidine
Fluconazole
Furosemide
Galantamine
Gefitinib
Ginkgo biloba
Hydrochlorothiazide
Hydroxychloroquine
Hydroxyzine
Ibuprofen
Icodextrin
Imatinib
Imipenem/cilastatin
Infliximab
Isoniazid
Itraconazole
Lamivudine
Lamotrigine
Lansoprazole
Levofloxacin
Lincomycin
Lindane
Meropenem
Metamizole
Methoxsalen
Methylprednisolone
Metronidazole
Mexiletine
Minocycline
Morphine
Nifedipine
Nimesulide
Nimodipine
Nystatin
Olanzapine
Phenobarbital
Phenytoin
Piperacillin
Prednisolone
Progestins
Propafenone
Propoxyphene
Pseudoephedrine
Pyrimethamine
Quinidine
Ranitidine
Rifampin
Senna
Sertraline
Simvastatin
Streptomycin
Sulfamethoxazole
Sulfasalazine
Terbinafine
Thallium
Ticlopidine
Valdecoxib
Vancomycin
Zidovudine

Ageusia
Acarbose
Acetazolamide
Amitriptyline
Aspirin
Atorvastatin
Azelastine
Benazepril
Betaxolol
Candesartan

Captopril
Carbamazepine
Cetirizine
Chlorhexidine
Cisplatin
Clidinium
Clomipramine
Clopidogrel
Cocaine
Cyclobenzaprine
Diazoxide
Dicyclomine
Doxorubicin
Enalapril
Etidronate
Feverfew
Fluoxetine
Fluvoxamine
Fosinopril
Gadofosveset
Glatiramer
Grepafloxacin
Hyoscyamine
Indomethacin
Interferon alfa
Interferon beta
Isotretinoin
Levodopa
Losartan
Mepenzolate
Methantheline
Methimazole
Mirtazapine
Nefazodone
Nitroglycerin
Paroxetine
Penicillamine
Pentamidine
Phenytoin
Pregabalin
Propantheline
Propylthiouracil
Ramipril
Rifabutin
Rifaximin
Rimantadine
Ritonavir
Rivastigmine
Spironolactone
Sulfadoxine
Sulindac
Terbinafine
Tiagabine
Tiopronin
Topiramate
Valrubicin
Venlafaxine
Voriconazole
Zalcitabine

Alopecia
Acamprosate
Acebutolol
Acenocoumarol
Acetaminophen
Acetohexamide
Acitretin
Acyclovir
Adalimumab
Albendazole
Aldesleukin

Alitretinoin
Allopurinol
Altretamine
Amantadine
Amiloride
Aminolevulinic acid
Aminophylline
Aminosalicylate sodium
Amiodarone
Amitriptyline
Amlodipine
Amoxapine
Amphotericin B
Anagrelide
Anastrozole
Androstenedione
Anisindione
Anthrax vaccine
Aprepitant
Aripiprazole
Arsenic
Asparaginase
Aspirin
Astemizole
Atazanavir
Atenolol
Atorvastatin
Atovaquone/proguanil
Azathioprine
Balsalazide
Bendamustine
Bendroflumethiazide
Benzphetamine
Betaxolol
Bevacizumab
Bexarotene
Bicalutamide
Bismuth
Bisoprolol
Bleomycin
Brinzolamide
Bromocriptine
Bupropion
Buspirone
Busulfan
Cabergoline
Capecitabine
Captopril
Carbamazepine
Carbimazole
Carboplatin
Carmustine
Carteolol
Carvedilol
Celecoxib
Certolizumab pegol
Cetirizine
Cetuximab
Cevimeline
Chlorambucil
Chloramphenicol
Chlordiazepoxide
Chloroquine
Chlorothiazide
Chlorotrianisene
Chlorpropamide
Chlorthalidone
Chondroitin
Cidofovir
Cimetidine

Ciprofibrate
Cisplatin
Citalopram
Clarithromycin
Clofibrate
Clomiphene
Clomipramine
Clonazepam
Clonidine
Colchicine
Cyclobenzaprine
Cyclophosphamide
Cyclosporine
Cytarabine
Dacarbazine
Dactinomycin
Dalteparin
Danazol
Darunavir
Dasatinib
Daunorubicin
Decitabine
Delavirdine
Desipramine
Dexamethasone
Dexibuprofen
Dexmethylphenidate
Dexrazoxane
Diazoxide
Diclofenac
Dicumarol
Didanosine
Diethylpropion
Diethylstilbestrol
Diflunisal
Digoxin
Diltiazem
Disopyramide
Docetaxel
Donepezil
Dopamine
Doxazosin
Doxepin
Doxorubicin
Duloxetine
Efavirenz
Eflornithine
Eletriptan
Enalapril
Enoxaparin
Epinephrine
Epirubicin
Epoetin alfa
Erlotinib
Erythromycin
Escitalopram
Esmolol
Estramustine
Estrogens
Eszopiclone
Etanercept
Ethambutol
Ethionamide
Ethosuximide
Etidronate
Etodolac
Etoposide
Exemestane
Ezetimibe
Famotidine

Felbamate
Fenofibrate
Fenoprofen
Finasteride
Flecainide
Floxuridine
Fluconazole
Fludarabine
Fluorouracil
Fluoxetine
Fluoxymesterone
Flurbiprofen
Fluvastatin
Fluvoxamine
Foscarnet
Gabapentin
Ganciclovir
Gefitinib
Gemcitabine
Gemfibrozil
Gentamicin
Glatiramer
Goserelin
Granisetron
Granulocyte colony-
    stimulating factor (GCSF)
Grepafloxacin
Guanethidine
Guanfacine
Haloperidol
Halothane
Heparin
Hepatitis B vaccine
Hydromorphone
Hydroxychloroquine
Hydroxyurea
Hyoscyamine
Ibritumomab
Ibuprofen
Idarubicin
Ifosfamide
Imipramine
Immune globulin I.V.
Indinavir
Indomethacin
Interferon alfa
Interferon beta
Ipratropium
Irinotecan
Isoniazid
Isotretinoin
Itraconazole
Ixabepilone
Ketoconazole
Ketoprofen
Labetalol
Lamivudine
Lamotrigine
Lanreotide
Lansoprazole
Leflunomide
Letrozole
Leucovorin
Leuprolide
Levamisole
Levobetaxolol
Levobunolol
Levodopa
Levothyroxine

Liothyronine
Lisinopril
Lithium
Lomustine
Loperamide
Loratadine
Lorazepam
Losartan
Lovastatin
Loxapine
Lutropin alfa
Maprotiline
Mebendazole
Mechlorethamine
Meclofenamate
Medroxyprogesterone
Mefloquine
Melphalan
Memantine
Mephenytoin
Mercaptopurine
Mesalamine
Mesoridazine
Metformin
Methimazole
Methotrexate
Methsuximide
Methyldopa
Methylphenidate
Methyltestosterone
Methysergide
Metoprolol
Mexiletine
Minocycline
Minoxidil
Misoprostol
Mitomycin
Mitotane
Mitoxantrone
Mizoribine
Moexipril
Mycophenolate
Nabumetone
Nadolol
Nalidixic acid
Naltrexone
Naproxen
Naratriptan
Nefazodone
Neomycin
Nifedipine
Nilutamide
Nimodipine
Nisoldipine
Nitisinone
Nitrofurantoin
Nortriptyline
Octreotide
Olanzapine
Omeprazole
Ondansetron
Oral contraceptives
Oxaliplatin
Oxaprozin
Oxcarbazepine
Paclitaxel
Pantoprazole
Paramethadione
Paroxetine
PEG-interferon

Pegfilgrastim
Penbutolol
Penicillamine
Pentosan
Pentostatin
Peplomycin
Pergolide
Phensuximide
Phentermine
Phenytoin
Pindolol
Pirbuterol
Piroxicam
Pramipexole
Pravastatin
Prazepam
Prazosin
Pregabalin
Probenecid
Procarbazine
Progestins
Propafenone
Propranolol
Propylthiouracil
Protriptyline
Pyrimethamine
Quazepam
Quinacrine
Quinapril
Quinidine
Rabeprazole
Raltitrexed
Ramipril
Ranitidine
Rasagiline
Ribavirin
Riluzole
Risperidone
Ritonavir
Rivastigmine
Rofecoxib
Ropinirole
Saquinavir
Selegiline
Selenium
Sertraline
Simvastatin
Sorafenib
Sotalol
Sparfloxacin
Spironolactone
St John's wort
Stanozolol
Sulfasalazine
Sulfisoxazole
Sulindac
Sunitinib
Tacrine
Tacrolimus
Tamoxifen
Temozolomide
Teniposide
Terbinafine
Terfenadine
Testolactone
Testosterone
Thalidomide
Thallium
Thioguanine
Thioridazine

Thiotepa
Thiothixene
Tiagabine
Timolol
Tinzaparin
Tiopronin
Tizanidine
Tocainide
Tolcapone
Topiramate
Topotecan
Trastuzumab
Trazodone
Triazolam
Trimethadione
Trimipramine
Triptorelin
Urofollitropin
Ursodiol
Valdecoxib
Valproic acid
Vasopressin
Venlafaxine
Verapamil
Vinblastine
Vincristine
Vinorelbine
Vitamin A
Voriconazole
Vorinostat
Warfarin
Zalcitabine
Zidovudine
Ziprasidone
Zonisamide

Angioedema
Acetaminophen
Acetylcysteine
Adalimumab
Albendazole
Albuterol
Aldesleukin
Alefacept
Alemtuzumab
Alendronate
Alfuzosin
Alglucerase
Alglucosidase alfa
Aliskiren
Allopurinol
Alprazolam
Alteplase
Aminoglutethimide
Aminosalicylate sodium
Amiodarone
Amitriptyline
Amlodipine
Amobarbital
Amoxicillin
Amphotericin B
Ampicillin
Anastrozole
Anidulafungin
Anistreplase
Anthrax vaccine
Aprepitant
Aprobarbital
Aprotinin
Arformoterol
Aripiprazole

Armodafinil
Ascorbic acid
Asparaginase
Aspartame
Aspirin
Astemizole
Atomoxetine
Atorvastatin
Atovaquone/proguanil
Azatadine
Azathioprine
Azithromycin
Aztreonam
Bacampicillin
Beclomethasone
Benactyzine
Benazepril
Betaxolol
Bicalutamide
Bismuth
Bisoprolol
Bleomycin
Bortezomib
Bosentan
Brompheniramine
Budesonide
Bupivacaine
Bupropion
Butabarbital
Caffeine
Candesartan
Captopril
Carbamazepine
Carbenicillin
Carisoprodol
Carteolol
Carvedilol
Cefaclor
Cefadroxil
Cefepime
Cefixime
Cefoxitin
Cefprozil
Ceftazidime
Ceftriaxone
Cefuroxime
Celecoxib
Cephalexin
Certolizumab pegol
Cetirizine
Chloral hydrate
Chlorambucil
Chloramphenicol
Chlordiazepoxide
Chloroquine
Chlorpheniramine
Chlorpromazine
Chlorpropamide
Chlorthalidone
Chlorzoxazone
Ciclesonide
Cilazapril
Cimetidine
Cinoxacin
Ciprofloxacin
Cisplatin
Citalopram
Clemastine
Clonazepam
Clonidine

Clopidogrel
Cloxacillin
Clozapine
Co-trimoxazole
Cocaine
Codeine
Colchicine
Cromolyn
Cyanocobalamin
Cyclamate
Cyclobenzaprine
Cyclophosphamide
Cyclosporine
Cyproheptadine
Dacarbazine
Danazol
Daunorubicin
Deferoxamine
Delavirdine
Demeclocycline
Desipramine
Dexchlorpheniramine
Dexibuprofen
Diazepam
Diclofenac
Dicloxacillin
Dicumarol
Diethylstilbestrol
Diflunisal
Digoxin
Diltiazem
Dimenhydrinate
Diphenhydramine
Diphenoxylate
Dipyridamole
Disopyramide
Docetaxel
Dofetilide
Doxazosin
Doxorubicin
Doxycycline
Droperidol
Echinacea
Efalizumab
Enalapril
Enoxaparin
Epoetin alfa
Eprosartan
Esomeprazole
Estramustine
Estrogens
Eszopiclone
Etanercept
Ethambutol
Etidronate
Etodolac
Etoricoxib
Ezetimibe
Famotidine
Fenoprofen
Feverfew
Fluconazole
Fluorouracil
Fluoxetine
Fluphenazine
Flurbiprofen
Fluvastatin
Fluvoxamine
Formoterol
Fosfomycin

Fosinopril
Galsulfase
Gatifloxacin
Gemfibrozil
Gemifloxacin
Glatiramer
Glucagon
Glyburide
Gold and gold compounds
Griseofulvin
Halothane
Hemophilus B vaccine
Henna
Heparin
Hepatitis B vaccine
Heroin
Histrelin
Hyaluronic acid
Hydralazine
Hydrochlorothiazide
Hydrocortisone
Hydroxychloroquine
Hydroxyzine
Ibritumomab
Ibuprofen
Imidapril
Imiglucerase
Imipenem/cilastatin
Imipramine
Imiquimod
Indapamide
Indomethacin
Influenza vaccines
Insulin
Interferon alfa
Iopromide
Irbesartan
Isoniazid
Isotretinoin
Itraconazole
Ivermectin
Ketoconazole
Ketoprofen
Ketorolac
Labetalol
Lamivudine
Lamotrigine
Levamisole
Levobupivacaine
Levothyroxine
Lidocaine
Lincomycin
Lisdexamfetamine
Lisinopril
Lithium
Loratadine
Losartan
Lumiracoxib
Mebendazole
Mecamylamine
Mechlorethamine
Meclizine
Meclofenamate
Medroxyprogesterone
Mefenamic acid
Meloxicam
Melphalan
Meperidine
Mephenytoin
Mephobarbital

Meprobamate
Meropenem
Mesna
Mesoridazine
Methadone
Methicillin
Methohexital
Methylphenidate
Metoclopramide
Metoprolol
Metronidazole
Mezlocillin
Miconazole
Midazolam
Minocycline
Mitomycin
Mitotane
Moclobemide
Moexipril
Monosodium glutamate
Montelukast
Nabumetone
Nafcillin
Nalidixic acid
Naloxone
Naproxen
Neomycin
Nifedipine
Nimesulide
Nisoldipine
Nitrofurantoin
Nitroglycerin
Norfloxacin
Ofloxacin
Olanzapine
Olmesartan
Omeprazole
Ondansetron
Oral contraceptives
Oxacillin
Oxaliplatin
Oxaprozin
Oxcarbazepine
Oxytetracycline
Paclitaxel
Paliperidone
Pamidronate
Pantoprazole
Paroxetine
PEG-interferon
Pegaptanib
Pegaspargase
Penicillin G
Penicillin V
Pentagastrin
Pentobarbital
Pentoxifylline
Perindopril
Perphenazine
Phenelzine
Phenindamine
Phenobarbital
Phenolphthalein
Phenylbutazone
Phenytoin
Pioglitazone
Piperacillin
Piroxicam
Potassium iodide
Pravastatin

Praziquantel
Prazosin
Pregabalin
Primaquine
Procainamide
Procarbazine
Progestins
Promethazine
Propranolol
Propylthiouracil
Protamine sulfate
Protein C concentrate
   (human)
Protriptyline
Pseudoephedrine
Pyrilamine
Pyrimethamine
Quetiapine
Quinapril
Quinestrol
Quinidine
Quinine
Ramipril
Ranitidine
Riboflavin
Rifampin
Rifaximin
Risperidone
Ritonavir
Rituximab
Rofecoxib
Roxithromycin
Salmeterol
Salsalate
Secobarbital
Sertraline
Simvastatin
Sirolimus
Sparfloxacin
Streptokinase
Streptomycin
Sucralfate
Sulfamethoxazole
Sulfasalazine
Sulfisoxazole
Sulfites
Sulindac
Sumatriptan
Tacrolimus
Tamsulosin
Tartrazine
Telithromycin
Telmisartan
Tenecteplase
Terbinafine
Terfenadine
Testolactone
Tetracycline
Thiabendazole
Thiamine
Thiopental
Thioridazine
Thiotepa
Ticarcillin
Ticlopidine
Timolol
Tinidazole
Tinzaparin
Tiopronin
Tiotropium

Tolmetin
Torsemide
Tositumomab & iodine[131]
Tramadol
Trandolapril
Trastuzumab
Trazodone
Trifluoperazine
Trimeprazine
Trimetrexate
Tripelennamine
Triprolidine
Triptorelin
Troleandomycin
Trospium
Trovafloxacin
Urokinase
Valsartan
Vancomycin
Vasopressin
Verapamil
Vinblastine
Vincristine
Vinorelbine
Voriconazole
Vorinostat
Warfarin
Zalcitabine
Ziprasidone

Anosmia
   Acetazolamide
   Amikacin
   Aspirin
   Ciprofloxacin
   Cocaine
   Cromolyn
   Dorzolamide
   Doxycycline
   Enalapril
   Ganciclovir
   Interferon alfa
   Levodopa
   Methazolamide
   Methoxsalen
   Minoxidil
   Nifedipine
   Paroxetine
   Pentamidine
   Sparfloxacin
   Terbinafine
   Uracil/tegafur
   Zinc

Aphthous Stomatitis
   Aldesleukin
   Anagrelide
   Asparaginase
   Aspirin
   Atazanavir
   Azathioprine
   Azelastine
   Aztreonam
   Candesartan
   Captopril
   Certolizumab pegol
   Cetuximab
   Cidofovir
   Co-trimoxazole
   Cyclosporine
   Delavirdine
   Diclofenac

Diflunisal
Doxepin
Erlotinib
Fenoprofen
Fluorides
Fluoxetine
Flurbiprofen
Gold and gold compounds
Hepatitis B vaccine
Ibuprofen
Imiquimod
Indinavir
Indomethacin
Interferon alfa
Interferon beta
Ketoprofen
Ketorolac
Losartan
Meclofenamate
Methotrexate
Midodrine
Mirtazapine
Naproxen
Nicorandil
Olanzapine
Pantoprazole
Paroxetine
Pemetrexed
Penicillamine
Piroxicam
Pregabalin
Rifabutin
Rofecoxib
Sertraline
Sirolimus
Sulfamethoxazole
Sulfasalazine
Sulfisoxazole
Sulindac
Terbinafine
Tolmetin
Trientine
Valsartan
Zalcitabine

Baboon Syndrome
   Aminophylline
   Amoxicillin
   Ampicillin
   Aspirin
   Betamethasone
   Cefuroxime
   Cephalexin
   Cimetidine
   Clarithromycin
   Erythromycin
   Heparin
   Hydroxyurea
   Immune globulin I.V.
   Iopromide
   Mesalamine
   Naproxen
   Omeprazole
   Oxycodone
   Pseudoephedrine
   Roxithromycin
   Terbinafine

Black Tongue
   Amitriptyline
   Amoxapine
   Amoxicillin

Ampicillin
Bacampicillin
Benztropine
Carbenicillin
Ceftriaxone
Chloramphenicol
Clarithromycin
Clomipramine
Clonazepam
Cloxacillin
Co-trimoxazole
Cocaine
Desipramine
Dicloxacillin
Doxycycline
Fluoxetine
Griseofulvin
Imipramine
Isocarboxazid
Lansoprazole
Maprotiline
Methicillin
Methyldopa
Mezlocillin
Minocycline
Nafcillin
Nicotine
Nortriptyline
Olanzapine
Oxacillin
Oxytetracycline
PEG-interferon
Penicillin G
Penicillin V
Phenelzine
Protriptyline
Ribavirin
Streptomycin
Sulfamethoxazole
Tetracycline
Thiothixene
Ticarcillin
Tranylcypromine

Bullous Dermatitis
Acetazolamide
Acitretin
Aldesleukin
Alemtuzumab
Alitretinoin
Amifostine
Aminocaproic acid
Aminophylline
Aminosalicylate sodium
Amitriptyline
Amobarbital
Amoxicillin
Ampicillin
Anthrax vaccine
Argatroban
Arsenic
Aspirin
Atropine sulfate
Benactyzine
Bergamot
Bleomycin
Bumetanide
Buspirone
Busulfan
Butabarbital
Butalbital

Caffeine
Capsicum
Captopril
Carbamazepine
Carbenicillin
Celecoxib
Cetirizine
Cevimeline
Chloral hydrate
Chloramphenicol
Chlorothiazide
Chlorpromazine
Chlorpropamide
Ciprofloxacin
Clopidogrel
Co-trimoxazole
Cocaine
Codeine
Colchicine
Cyanocobalamin
Cyclamate
Cyclosporine
Cytarabine
Dalteparin
Dapsone
Demeclocycline
Denileukin
Dextromethorphan
Diazepam
Diclofenac
Dicloxacillin
Dicumarol
Diethylstilbestrol
Diflunisal
Digoxin
Dirithromycin
Disulfiram
Entacapone
Ephedrine
Estrogens
Ethambutol
Ethchlorvynol
Ethotoin
Etodolac
Felbamate
Fenoprofen
Floxuridine
Fluconazole
Fluorouracil
Fluoxetine
Flutamide
Fluvoxamine
Fondaparinux
Fosphenytoin
Frovatriptan
Furosemide
Ganciclovir
Garlic
Glyburide
Gold and gold compounds
Griseofulvin
Henna
Hydralazine
Hydrochlorothiazide
Hydroxychloroquine
Ibritumomab
Ibuprofen
Ibutilide
Idarubicin
Imipramine

Imiquimod
Indapamide
Indomethacin
Infliximab
Influenza vaccines
Insulin
Interferon alfa
Isoniazid
Ivermectin
Ketoprofen
Lamotrigine
Leflunomide
Lidocaine
Lindane
Lisinopril
Lithium
Mafenide
Mechlorethamine
Meclofenamate
Meloxicam
Mephenytoin
Meprobamate
Methicillin
Methotrexate
Methoxsalen
Mezlocillin
Miconazole
Minoxidil
Mitomycin
Moxifloxacin
Mycophenolate
Nabumetone
Nafcillin
Nalidixic acid
Naproxen
Neomycin
Nifedipine
Nitrofurantoin
Norfloxacin
Ofloxacin
Omeprazole
Oral contraceptives
Oxacillin
Penicillamine
Pentamidine
Pentobarbital
Pentostatin
Phenobarbital
Phenolphthalein
Phenytoin
Piperacillin
Piroxicam
Prednicarbate
Promethazine
Propranolol
Pyridoxine
Pyrimethamine
Quinapril
Quinethazone
Quinidine
Quinine
Reserpine
Rifampin
Risperidone
Ritonavir
Rivastigmine
Rofecoxib
Rue
Saquinavir
Senna

Sertraline
Smallpox vaccine
Sparfloxacin
Streptomycin
Sulfadoxine
Sulfamethoxazole
Sulfasalazine
Sulfisoxazole
Sunitinib
Tacrine
Temazepam
Tetracycline
Thalidomide
Thiopental
Ticarcillin
Tinzaparin
Tolbutamide
Tolmetin
Tretinoin
Trimethadione
Trioxsalen
Urokinase
Valproic acid
Vancomycin
Vasopressin
Vinblastine
Warfarin
Zalcitabine
Zidovudine
Zolpidem

Dress Syndrome
Acetaminophen
Allopurinol
Amitriptyline
Amoxicillin
Armodafinil
Bupropion
Carbamazepine
Ceftriaxone
Dapsone
Efalizumab
Ibuprofen
Imatinib
Minocycline
Naproxen
Nelfinavir
Nevirapine
Oxazepam
Oxcarbazepine
Phenobarbital
Phenytoin
Piperacillin
Quinine
Spironolactone
Streptomycin
Sulfadiazine
Sulfasalazine
Terbinafine
Thiamine
Valproic acid
Vancomycin

Erythema Multiforme
Abacavir
Acamprosate
Acarbose
Acebutolol
Acetaminophen
Acetazolamide
Adalimumab
Albuterol

Aldesleukin
Alendronate
Allopurinol
Amantadine
Amifostine
Aminosalicylate sodium
Amiodarone
Amlodipine
Amoxapine
Amoxicillin
Amphotericin B
Ampicillin
Anastrozole
Anisindione
Anthrax vaccine
Arsenic
Aspirin
Atazanavir
Atenolol
Atorvastatin
Atovaquone
Atovaquone/proguanil
Atropine sulfate
Azathioprine
Azithromycin
Aztreonam
Bacampicillin
Benactyzine
Botulinum toxin (A & B)
Bumetanide
Bupropion
Busulfan
Butabarbital
Butalbital
Candesartan
Capsicum
Captopril
Carbamazepine
Carbenicillin
Carisoprodol
Carvedilol
Cefaclor
Cefadroxil
Cefamandole
Cefazolin
Cefdinir
Cefditoren
Cefepime
Cefixime
Cefonicid
Cefoperazone
Cefotaxime
Cefotetan
Cefpodoxime
Cefprozil
Ceftazidime
Ceftriaxone
Cefuroxime
Celecoxib
Cephalexin
Cephalothin
Cephapirin
Cephradine
Chloral hydrate
Chlorambucil
Chloramphenicol
Chlordiazepoxide
Chlormezanone
Chloroquine
Chlorothiazide

Chlorotrianisene
Chlorpromazine
Chlorpropamide
Chlorthalidone
Chlorzoxazone
Cimetidine
Cinoxacin
Ciprofloxacin
Citalopram
Clindamycin
Clofibrate
Clomiphene
Clonazepam
Clopidogrel
Cloxacillin
Clozapine
Co-trimoxazole
Codeine
Collagen
Cyclophosphamide
Dactinomycin
Danazol
Dapsone
Darunavir
Deferoxamine
Delavirdine
Demeclocycline
Desoximetasone
Dexamethasone
Dexibuprofen
Dexmethylphenidate
Diclofenac
Dicloxacillin
Didanosine
Diethylpropion
Diethylstilbestrol
Diflunisal
Diltiazem
Dipyridamole
Dorzolamide
Doxycycline
Efalizumab
Enalapril
Enoxacin
Enoxaparin
Erythromycin
Esomeprazole
Estrogens
Eszopiclone
Ethambutol
Ethosuximide
Etodolac
Etoposide
Etoricoxib
Etravirine
Famotidine
Fenbufen
Fenoprofen
Fluconazole
Fluorouracil
Fluoxetine
Flurbiprofen
Fluvastatin
Fosphenytoin
Furazolidone
Furosemide
Gemfibrozil
Glucagon
Gold and gold compounds
Griseofulvin

Hemophilus B vaccine
Henna
Hepatitis B vaccine
Hyaluronic acid
Hydrochlorothiazide
Hydrocodone
Hydroxychloroquine
Hydroxyurea
Hydroxyzine
Ibritumomab
Ibuprofen
Icodextrin
Imipenem/cilastatin
Indapamide
Indinavir
Indomethacin
Isoniazid
Isotretinoin
Itraconazole
Ixabepilone
Ketoprofen
Lamotrigine
Lansoprazole
Leflunomide
Levamisole
Levofloxacin
Lidocaine
Lincomycin
Lithium
Loracarbef
Loratadine
Lorazepam
Lovastatin
Maprotiline
Mechlorethamine
Meclofenamate
Mefenamic acid
Mefloquine
Meloxicam
Mephenytoin
Meprobamate
Meropenem
Metamizole
Methenamine
Methicillin
Methotrexate
Methsuximide
Methyclothiazide
Methyldopa
Methylphenidate
Metoprolol
Mezlocillin
Midodrine
Minocycline
Minoxidil
Mitomycin
Mitotane
Nabumetone
Nadolol
Nafcillin
Nalidixic acid
Naproxen
Neomycin
Nifedipine
Nitrofurantoin
Nitroglycerin
Norfloxacin
Nystatin
Ofloxacin
Omeprazole

Oral contraceptives
Oxacillin
Oxaprozin
Oxazepam
Oxcarbazepine
Oxybutynin
Pantoprazole
Paramethadione
Paroxetine
Penicillamine
Pentobarbital
Phenobarbital
Phenolphthalein
Phensuximide
Phenylbutazone
Phenytoin
Pindolol
Piroxicam
Pravastatin
Prednicarbate
Prednisolone
Primidone
Probenecid
Progestins
Promethazine
Propranolol
Pseudoephedrine
Pyrazinamide
Pyrimethamine
Quetiapine
Quinidine
Quinine
Ramipril
Ranitidine
Ribavirin
Rifampin
Ritodrine
Roxatidine
Saquinavir
Scopolamine
Senna
Sertraline
Simvastatin
Smallpox vaccine
Sorafenib
Spironolactone
Streptomycin
Sulfacetamide
Sulfadiazine
Sulfadoxine
Sulfamethoxazole
Sulfasalazine
Sulfisoxazole
Sulindac
Tadalafil
Tamsulosin
Tea tree
Telithromycin
Terbinafine
Tetracycline
Thalidomide
Thiabendazole
Thiopental
Thioridazine
Ticarcillin
Ticlopidine
Timolol
Tiopronin
Tobramycin
Tocainide

Tolbutamide
Tolcapone
Tolmetin
Trazodone
Trimethadione
Trimethoprim
Troleandomycin
Trovafloxacin
Valdecoxib
Valproic acid
Vancomycin
Varicella vaccine
Verapamil
Vinblastine
Vitamin A
Vitamin E
Voriconazole
Zalcitabine
Zidovudine

Erythema Nodosum
Acetaminophen
Acyclovir
Aldesleukin
Amiodarone
Arsenic
Aspartame
Aspirin
Azathioprine
Busulfan
Carbamazepine
Carbenicillin
Carbimazole
Cefdinir
Certolizumab pegol
Chlordiazepoxide
Chlorotrianisene
Chlorpropamide
Ciprofloxacin
Clomiphene
Co-trimoxazole
Codeine
Colchicine
Dapsone
Diclofenac
Dicloxacillin
Diethylstilbestrol
Disopyramide
Echinacea
Enoxacin
Estrogens
Fluoxetine
Furosemide
Glatiramer
Glucagon
Gold and gold compounds
Granulocyte colony-
    stimulating factor (GCSF)
Heparin
Hepatitis B vaccine
Hydralazine
Hydroxychloroquine
Ibuprofen
Indomethacin
Interferon alfa
Interferon beta
Isotretinoin
Levofloxacin
Lidocaine
Loperamide
Meclofenamate

Medroxyprogesterone
Meprobamate
Mesalamine
Metamizole
Methicillin
Methimazole
Methyldopa
Mezlocillin
Minocycline
Montelukast
Naproxen
Nifedipine
Nitrofurantoin
Ofloxacin
Omeprazole
Oral contraceptives
Oxacillin
Paroxetine
Penicillamine
Piperacillin
Progestins
Propylthiouracil
Quinacrine
Simvastatin
Smallpox vaccine
Sparfloxacin
Streptomycin
Sulfamethoxazole
Sulfasalazine
Sulfisoxazole
Thalidomide
Ticarcillin
Ticlopidine
Tretinoin
Trimethoprim
Verapamil
Zileuton

Exanthems
Abacavir
Acamprosate
Acebutolol
Acenocoumarol
Acetaminophen
Acetazolamide
Acetohexamide
Acitretin
Acyclovir
Albuterol
Aldesleukin
Alendronate
Allopurinol
Alprazolam
Altretamine
Amantadine
Amcinonide
Amikacin
Amiloride
Aminocaproic acid
Aminoglutethimide
Aminophylline
Aminosalicylate sodium
Amiodarone
Amitriptyline
Amlodipine
Amobarbital
Amoxapine
Amoxicillin
Amphotericin B
Ampicillin
Amprenavir

Anidulafungin
Anisindione
Anistreplase
Anthrax vaccine
Aprobarbital
Aprotinin
Aripiprazole
Arsenic
Asparaginase
Aspartame
Aspirin
Astemizole
Atazanavir
Atenolol
Atorvastatin
Atovaquone
Atovaquone/proguanil
Atropine sulfate
Azatadine
Azathioprine
Azelastine
Azithromycin
Aztreonam
Bacampicillin
Baclofen
Benactyzine
Benazepril
Bendamustine
Bendroflumethiazide
Benztropine
Betamethasone
Betaxolol
Bexarotene
Bicalutamide
Biperiden
Bisacodyl
Bismuth
Bisoprolol
Bleomycin
Bromocriptine
Brompheniramine
Budesonide
Bumetanide
Bupropion
Buspirone
Busulfan
Butabarbital
Butalbital
Butorphanol
Calcitonin
Candesartan
Capreomycin
Captopril
Carbamazepine
Carbenicillin
Carboplatin
Carisoprodol
Carmustine
Carteolol
Carvedilol
Cefaclor
Cefadroxil
Cefamandole
Cefazolin
Cefdinir
Cefepime
Cefoperazone
Cefotaxime
Cefotetan
Cefoxitin

Cefprozil
Ceftazidime
Ceftriaxone
Cefuroxime
Celecoxib
Cephalexin
Cephalothin
Cephapirin
Cephradine
Cetirizine
Cetuximab
Cevimeline
Chloral hydrate
Chlorambucil
Chloramphenicol
Chlordiazepoxide
Chlormezanone
Chloroquine
Chlorothiazide
Chlorpromazine
Chlorpropamide
Chlorthalidone
Chlorzoxazone
Cholestyramine
Cimetidine
Ciprofloxacin
Cisplatin
Citalopram
Cladribine
Clarithromycin
Clemastine
Clindamycin
Clofazimine
Clofibrate
Clomiphene
Clomipramine
Clonazepam
Clonidine
Clopidogrel
Clorazepate
Cloxacillin
Clozapine
Co-trimoxazole
Codeine
Colchicine
Colestipol
Cromolyn
Cyanocobalamin
Cyclamate
Cyclophosphamide
Cycloserine
Cyclosporine
Cyclothiazide
Cyproheptadine
Cytarabine
Dacarbazine
Dactinomycin
Dalteparin
Danazol
Dantrolene
Dapsone
Darunavir
Daunorubicin
Deferoxamine
Delavirdine
Demeclocycline
Denileukin
Desipramine
Dexamethasone
Diazepam

Diazoxide
Diclofenac
Dicloxacillin
Dicumarol
Dicyclomine
Didanosine
Diethylpropion
Diethylstilbestrol
Diflunisal
Digoxin
Dihydrotachysterol
Diltiazem
Dimenhydrinate
Diphenhydramine
Dipyridamole
Disopyramide
Disulfiram
Docetaxel
Docusate
Dopamine
Doxazosin
Doxepin
Doxorubicin
Doxycycline
Efalizumab
Efavirenz
Eletriptan
Emtricitabine
Enalapril
Enfuvirtide
Enoxacin
Enoxaparin
Ephedrine
Epinephrine
Epoetin alfa
Eprosartan
Erythromycin
Esomeprazole
Estramustine
Estrogens
Eszopiclone
Etanercept
Ethacrynic acid
Ethambutol
Ethionamide
Ethosuximide
Etidronate
Etodolac
Etoposide
Etoricoxib
Famotidine
Felodipine
Fenofibrate
Fenoprofen
Fentanyl
Flavoxate
Flecainide
Floxuridine
Fluconazole
Flucytosine
Fludarabine
Fluorouracil
Fluoxetine
Fluoxymesterone
Fluphenazine
Flurazepam
Flurbiprofen
Flutamide
Fluvoxamine
Folic acid

Fosamprenavir
Foscarnet
Fosfomycin
Fosphenytoin
Furazolidone
Furosemide
Gabapentin
Gadodiamide
Ganciclovir
Gatifloxacin
Gefitinib
Gemcitabine
Gemfibrozil
Gemifloxacin
Gentamicin
Ginkgo biloba
Glatiramer
Glimepiride
Glipizide
Glucagon
Glyburide
Gold and gold compounds
Granisetron
Granulocyte colony-
    stimulating factor (GCSF)
Grepafloxacin
Griseofulvin
Guanethidine
Guanfacine
Haloperidol
Halothane
Heparin
Heroin
Hydralazine
Hydrochlorothiazide
Hydrocodone
Hydromorphone
Hydroxychloroquine
Hydroxyurea
Hydroxyzine
Ibuprofen
Icodextrin
Idarubicin
Imatinib
Imipenem/cilastatin
Imipramine
Indapamide
Indinavir
Indomethacin
Infliximab
Insulin
Interferon alfa
Interferon beta
Ipodate
Ipratropium
Irbesartan
Irinotecan
Isocarboxazid
Isoniazid
Isosorbide dinitrate
Isotretinoin
Isradipine
Itraconazole
Ivermectin
Kanamycin
Ketamine
Ketoconazole
Ketoprofen
Ketorolac
Labetalol

Lamivudine
Lamotrigine
Lansoprazole
Letrozole
Leuprolide
Levamisole
Levodopa
Levofloxacin
Lidocaine
Lincomycin
Linezolid
Lisinopril
Lithium
Lomefloxacin
Loperamide
Loracarbef
Loratadine
Lorazepam
Losartan
Lovastatin
Loxapine
Maprotiline
Marihuana
Mazindol
Mebendazole
Mechlorethamine
Meclizine
Meclofenamate
Medroxyprogesterone
Mefenamic acid
Mefloquine
Meloxicam
Melphalan
Memantine
Mephenytoin
Mephobarbital
Meprobamate
Mercaptopurine
Mesalamine
Mesna
Metamizole
Metformin
Methadone
Methantheline
Methazolamide
Methenamine
Methicillin
Methimazole
Methocarbamol
Methohexital
Methotrexate
Methoxsalen
Methsuximide
Methyclothiazide
Methyldopa
Methylphenidate
Methyltestosterone
Methysergide
Metoclopramide
Metolazone
Metoprolol
Metronidazole
Mexiletine
Mezlocillin
Miconazole
Midazolam
Minocycline
Minoxidil
Misoprostol
Mitomycin

Mitotane
Moexipril
Moricizine
Morphine
Moxifloxacin
Nabumetone
Nadolol
Nafarelin
Nafcillin
Nalidixic acid
Naloxone
Naltrexone
Naproxen
Naratriptan
Nateglinide
Nefazodone
Nelfinavir
Neomycin
Nevirapine
Niacin
Nicardipine
Nifedipine
Nimodipine
Nisoldipine
Nitisinone
Nitrofurantoin
Nitroglycerin
Nizatidine
Norfloxacin
Nortriptyline
Nystatin
Octreotide
Ofloxacin
Olanzapine
Olsalazine
Omeprazole
Ondansetron
Oral contraceptives
Orphenadrine
Oxacillin
Oxaliplatin
Oxaprozin
Oxazepam
Oxcarbazepine
Oxytetracycline
Paclitaxel
Pamidronate
Pantoprazole
Pantothenic acid
Papaverine
Paramethadione
Paromomycin
Paroxetine
PEG-interferon
Pemoline
Penbutolol
Penicillamine
Penicillin V
Pentagastrin
Pentamidine
Pentazocine
Pentobarbital
Pentostatin
Pentoxifylline
Perflutren
Pergolide
Perindopril
Perphenazine
Phenazopyridine
Phenelzine

Phenobarbital
Phenolphthalein
Phenylbutazone
Phenytoin
Phytonadione
Pimozide
Pindolol
Piperacillin
Piroxicam
Plicamycin
Polythiazide
Potassium iodide
Pravastatin
Prazepam
Prazosin
Prednisolone
Primaquine
Primidone
Probenecid
Procainamide
Procarbazine
Prochlorperazine
Progestins
Promazine
Promethazine
Propafenone
Propantheline
Propofol
Propoxyphene
Propranolol
Propylthiouracil
Protamine sulfate
Protriptyline
Pseudoephedrine
Pyrazinamide
Pyrimethamine
Quinacrine
Quinapril
Quinethazone
Quinidine
Quinine
Quinupristin/dalfopristin
Ramipril
Ranitidine
Rapacuronium
Reserpine
Ribavirin
Rifampin
Ritodrine
Ritonavir
Rituximab
Rivastigmine
Rofecoxib
Ropinirole
Rosiglitazone
Rotigotine
Saccharin
Salmeterol
Salsalate
Saquinavir
Scopolamine
Secobarbital
Sertraline
Simvastatin
Smallpox vaccine
Sotalol
Sparfloxacin
Spectinomycin
Spironolactone
Stanozolol

Streptokinase
Streptomycin
Streptozocin
Succimer
Succinylcholine
Sucralfate
Sulfadiazine
Sulfadoxine
Sulfamethoxazole
Sulfasalazine
Sulfinpyrazone
Sulfisoxazole
Sulindac
Sumatriptan
Tacrine
Tacrolimus
Tamoxifen
Temazepam
Temsirolimus
Terazosin
Terbinafine
Terbutaline
Terfenadine
Testolactone
Testosterone
Tetracycline
Thalidomide
Thiabendazole
Thiamine
Thimerosal
Thioguanine
Thiopental
Thioridazine
Thiothixene
Tiagabine
Ticarcillin
Ticlopidine
Timolol
Tinzaparin
Tiopronin
Tipranavir
Tizanidine
Tobramycin
Tocainide
Tolazamide
Tolazoline
Tolbutamide
Tolmetin
Topiramate
Torsemide
Tramadol
Tranylcypromine
Trazodone
Triamcinolone
Triamterene
Triazolam
Trichlormethiazide
Trifluoperazine
Trimeprazine
Trimethadione
Trimethoprim
Trimetrexate
Trimipramine
Triprolidine
Troleandomycin
Trovafloxacin
Urofollitropin
Urokinase
Valdecoxib
Valproic acid

Vancomycin
Vasopressin
Venlafaxine
Verapamil
Vinblastine
Vincristine
Vitamin A
Vitamin E
Warfarin
Zalcitabine
Zidovudine
Ziprasidone
Zonisamide

Exfoliative Dermatitis
Acamprosate
Acebutolol
Acetaminophen
Acitretin
Aldesleukin
Alitretinoin
Allopurinol
Amifostine
Aminoglutethimide
Aminolevulinic acid
Aminophylline
Aminosalicylate sodium
Amiodarone
Amitriptyline
Amlodipine
Amobarbital
Amoxicillin
Amphotericin B
Ampicillin
Anisindione
Aprobarbital
Aripiprazole
Arsenic
Aspirin
Atropine sulfate
Azathioprine
Aztreonam
Bacampicillin
Benactyzine
Bendroflumethiazide
Betaxolol
Bevacizumab
Bexarotene
Bismuth
Bisoprolol
Bumetanide
Bupropion
Butabarbital
Butalbital
Caffeine
Capecitabine
Captopril
Carbamazepine
Carbenicillin
Carteolol
Carvedilol
Cefdinir
Cefoxitin
Cefpodoxime
Celecoxib
Chlorambucil
Chloroquine
Chlorothiazide
Chlorpromazine
Chlorpropamide
Chlorthalidone

Cimetidine
Ciprofloxacin
Cisplatin
Clofazimine
Clofibrate
Clotrimazole
Cloxacillin
Co-trimoxazole
Codeine
Cromolyn
Cytarabine
Dapsone
Daunorubicin
Demeclocycline
Desipramine
Dexamethasone
Dexmethylphenidate
Diazepam
Diclofenac
Dicloxacillin
Diethylstilbestrol
Diflunisal
Diltiazem
Doxorubicin
Doxycycline
Efavirenz
Eletriptan
Enalapril
Enoxacin
Ephedrine
Epirubicin
Esmolol
Estrogens
Ethambutol
Ethosuximide
Etodolac
Fenoprofen
Fentanyl
Flecainide
Fluconazole
Fluoxetine
Fluphenazine
Flurbiprofen
Fluvoxamine
Fosinopril
Fosphenytoin
Furosemide
Ganciclovir
Gefitinib
Gemfibrozil
Gentamicin
Glimepiride
Glipizide
Glyburide
Gold and gold compounds
Granulocyte colony-
   stimulating factor (GCSF)
Grepafloxacin
Griseofulvin
Guanfacine
Haloperidol
Hydrochlorothiazide
Hydroxychloroquine
Ibritumomab
Icodextrin
Imatinib
Imipramine
Indomethacin
Interferon beta
Isoniazid

Isotretinoin
Ixabepilone
Ketoconazole
Ketoprofen
Ketorolac
Labetalol
Leflunomide
Levamisole
Levofloxacin
Lidocaine
Lincomycin
Lithium
Lomefloxacin
Lumiracoxib
Meclofenamate
Mefenamic acid
Mefloquine
Mephenytoin
Mephobarbital
Meprobamate
Mesoridazine
Methantheline
Methicillin
Methimazole
Methoxsalen
Methsuximide
Methylphenidate
Metolazone
Metoprolol
Mexiletine
Mezlocillin
Minocycline
Mirtazapine
Mitomycin
Nadolol
Nafcillin
Nalidixic acid
Naproxen
Nifedipine
Nisoldipine
Nitisinone
Nitrofurantoin
Nitroglycerin
Nizatidine
Norfloxacin
Ofloxacin
Omeprazole
Oxacillin
Oxaprozin
Oxytetracycline
Panitumumab
Paramethadione
Penicillamine
Penicillin G
Penicillin V
Pentobarbital
Pentostatin
Perphenazine
Phenobarbital
Phenolphthalein
Phenylbutazone
Phenytoin
Pindolol
Piperacillin
Piroxicam
Pregabalin
Primidone
Procarbazine
Prochlorperazine
Propranolol

Propylthiouracil
Pseudoephedrine
Pyrimethamine
Quinacrine
Quinapril
Quinidine
Quinine
Raltitrexed
Rifampin
Riluzole
Risperidone
Rivastigmine
Rosiglitazone
Secobarbital
Senna
Sildenafil
Smallpox vaccine
Sorafenib
Sparfloxacin
Streptomycin
Sulfacetamide
Sulfadiazine
Sulfadoxine
Sulfamethoxazole
Sulfasalazine
Sulfisoxazole
Sulindac
Tacrolimus
Terfenadine
Tetracycline
Thalidomide
Thiopental
Thioridazine
Tiagabine
Ticarcillin
Ticlopidine
Timolol
Tizanidine
Tobramycin
Tocainide
Trazodone
Tretinoin
Trifluoperazine
Trimethadione
Trimethoprim
Trovafloxacin
Vancomycin
Venlafaxine
Verapamil
Vitamin A
Voriconazole
Vorinostat
Warfarin
Yohimbine
Zalcitabine
Ziprasidone

Fixed Eruptions
Aceclofenac
Acetaminophen
Acyclovir
Adalimumab
Albendazole
Alendronate
Allopurinol
Aminosalicylate sodium
Amitriptyline
Amlexanox
Amoxicillin
Amphotericin B
Ampicillin

Arsenic
Aspirin
Atenolol
Atropine sulfate
Azathioprine
Azithromycin
Bacampicillin
BCG vaccine
Benactyzine
Bisacodyl
Bismuth
Bleomycin
Bucillamine
Butabarbital
Butalbital
Cabergoline
Carbamazepine
Carisoprodol
Cefaclor
Cefazolin
Celecoxib
Cephalexin
Cetirizine
Chloral hydrate
Chloramphenicol
Chlordiazepoxide
Chlorhexidine
Chlormezanone
Chloroquine
Chlorothiazide
Chlorpromazine
Chlorpropamide
Cimetidine
Ciprofloxacin
Clarithromycin
Clindamycin
Clioquinol
Co-trimoxazole
Codeine
Colchicine
Cyclosporine
Dacarbazine
Dapsone
Demeclocycline
Dextromethorphan
Diazepam
Diclofenac
Diflunisal
Dimenhydrinate
Diphenhydramine
Disulfiram
Docetaxel
Doxorubicin
Doxycycline
Ephedrine
Epinephrine
Erythromycin
Estrogens
Ethchlorvynol
Ethotoin
Etodolac
Etoricoxib
Fentanyl
Flavoxate
Fluconazole
Flurbiprofen
Foscarnet
Furosemide
Ganciclovir
Gatifloxacin

Glipizide
Gold and gold compounds
Griseofulvin
Guanethidine
Heparin
Heroin
Hydralazine
Hydrochlorothiazide
Hydroxychloroquine
Hydroxyurea
Hydroxyzine
Ibuprofen
Imipramine
Indapamide
Indomethacin
Influenza vaccines
Isotretinoin
Itraconazole
Ketoconazole
Lamotrigine
Levamisole
Levocetirizine
Lidocaine
Loperamide
Loratadine
Lorazepam
Meclofenamate
Mefenamic acid
Melatonin
Meprobamate
Mesna
Metamizole
Metaxalone
Methenamine
Methimazole
Methyldopa
Methylphenidate
Metronidazole
Minocycline
Moxifloxacin
Mycophenolate
Naproxen
Neomycin
Niacin
Nifedipine
Nimesulide
Nitrofurantoin
Norfloxacin
Nystatin
Ofloxacin
Omeprazole
Ondansetron
Oral contraceptives
Orphenadrine
Oxaprozin
Oxazepam
Oxytetracycline
Paclitaxel
Papaverine
PEG-interferon
Pentobarbital
Phenobarbital
Phenolphthalein
Phenylbutazone
Phenylpropanolamine
Phenytoin
Piroxicam
Procarbazine
Prochlorperazine
Promethazine

Propofol
Propranolol
Pseudoephedrine
Pyrazinamide
Pyridoxine
Pyrimethamine
Quinacrine
Quinidine
Quinine
Ranitidine
Ribavirin
Rifampin
Rofecoxib
Roxithromycin
Saccharin
Saquinavir
Scopolamine
Sertraline
Sildenafil
Sparfloxacin
Streptomycin
Sulfadiazine
Sulfadoxine
Sulfamethoxazole
Sulfasalazine
Sulfisoxazole
Sulindac
Tartrazine
Temazepam
Terbinafine
Terfenadine
Tetracycline
Thiabendazole
Thiopental
Ticlopidine
Tinidazole
Tolbutamide
Topotecan
Triamcinolone
Trifluoperazine
Trimethadione
Trimethoprim
Trimetrexate
Tripelennamine
Triprolidine
Valproic acid
Vancomycin
Voriconazole
Zolmitriptan

Gingival Hyperplasia
Amlodipine
Basiliximab
Cevimeline
Co-trimoxazole
Cycloserine
Cyclosporine
Diltiazem
Erythromycin
Estrogens
Ethosuximide
Ethotoin
Felodipine
Fosphenytoin
Ganciclovir
Isradipine
Ketoconazole
Lamotrigine
Lithium
Mephenytoin
Methsuximide

Mycophenolate
Nicardipine
Nifedipine
Nisoldipine
Oral contraceptives
Oxcarbazepine
Palifermin
Phenobarbital
Phensuximide
Phenytoin
Primidone
Sertraline
Sirolimus
Tacrolimus
Tartrazine
Tiagabine
Topiramate
Valproic acid
Verapamil
Vigabatrin
Voriconazole
Zonisamide

Lichenoid (Lichen Planus-Like) Eruptions
Acebutolol
Acetohexamide
Acyclovir
Aminosalicylate sodium
Amlodipine
Anakinra
Aspirin
Atenolol
Atorvastatin
Azathioprine
BCG vaccine
Captopril
Carbamazepine
Chloral hydrate
Chloroquine
Chlorothiazide
Chlorpromazine
Chlorpropamide
Cinnarizine
Clopidogrel
Co-trimoxazole
Colchicine
Cycloserine
Cyclosporine
Cyproheptadine
Dactinomycin
Dapsone
Demeclocycline
Diazoxide
Diclofenac
Diflunisal
Diltiazem
Dorzolamide
Doxazosin
Enalapril
Epoetin alfa
Ethambutol
Fluoxetine
Fluoxymesterone
Flurbiprofen
Fluvastatin
Furosemide
Glimepiride
Glipizide
Glyburide
Gold and gold compounds

Granulocyte colony-
stimulating factor (GCSF)
Griseofulvin
Henna
Hepatitis B vaccine
Hydrochlorothiazide
Hydroxychloroquine
Hydroxyurea
Ibuprofen
Imatinib
Immune globulin I.V.
Indomethacin
Infliximab
Interferon alfa
Interferon beta
Irbesartan
Isoniazid
Isotretinoin
Ketoconazole
Ketorolac
Labetalol
Lansoprazole
Leflunomide
Levamisole
Lisinopril
Lorazepam
Losartan
Lovastatin
Mercaptopurine
Mesalamine
Metformin
Methamphetamine
Methyldopa
Methyltestosterone
Metoprolol
Minocycline
Nadolol
Naproxen
Nebivolol
Nelfinavir
Nifedipine
Olmesartan
Omeprazole
Oral contraceptives
Orlistat
Pantoprazole
Penicillamine
Peppermint
Phenytoin
Pindolol
Piroxicam
Pravastatin
Prazosin
Pregabalin
Propranolol
Propylthiouracil
Pyrimethamine
Quinacrine
Quinidine
Quinine
Ranitidine
Ribavirin
Risperidone
Roxatidine
Salsalate
Sildenafil
Simvastatin
Solifenacin
Sotalol
Sparfloxacin

Spironolactone
Streptomycin
Sulfadoxine
Sulfamethoxazole
Sulindac
Temazepam
Tenofovir
Terazosin
Terbinafine
Testosterone
Tetracycline
Thimerosal
Thioridazine
Timolol
Tiopronin
Tiotropium
Tolazamide
Tolbutamide
Torsemide
Trichlormethiazide
Tripelennamine
Triprolidine
Ursodiol
Venlafaxine
Verapamil
Zidovudine

Lupus Erythematosus
Acebutolol
Acetazolamide
Adalimumab
Albuterol
Allopurinol
Aminoglutethimide
Aminosalicylate sodium
Amiodarone
Amitriptyline
Amlodipine
Anastrozole
Anthrax vaccine
Atenolol
Benazepril
Betaxolol
Bisoprolol
Bupropion
Butabarbital
Butalbital
Capecitabine
Captopril
Carbamazepine
Carteolol
Cefuroxime
Celecoxib
Celiprolol
Chlorambucil
Chlordiazepoxide
Chlorothiazide
Chlorpromazine
Chlorpropamide
Chlorthalidone
Cilazapril
Cimetidine
Cinnarizine
Clobazam
Clofibrate
Clonidine
Clozapine
Co-trimoxazole
Cyclophosphamide
Cyclosporine
Cyproheptadine

Danazol
Dapsone
Demeclocycline
Dexibuprofen
Diclofenac
Diethylstilbestrol
Diltiazem
Disopyramide
Docetaxel
Domperidone
Doxazosin
Doxycycline
Efalizumab
Enalapril
Estrogens
Etanercept
Ethambutol
Ethionamide
Ethosuximide
Ethotoin
Felbamate
Fluorouracil
Fluoxetine
Fluoxymesterone
Fluphenazine
Flutamide
Fluvastatin
Fosphenytoin
Furosemide
Gemfibrozil
Glatiramer
Gold and gold compounds
Granulocyte colony
    stimulating factor (GCSF)
Griseofulvin
Guanethidine
Hepatitis B vaccine
Hydralazine
Hydrochlorothiazide
Hydroxyurea
Ibuprofen
Imipramine
Infliximab
Interferon alfa
Interferon beta
Isoniazid
Labetalol
Lamotrigine
Lansoprazole
Leflunomide
Leuprolide
Levodopa
Lidocaine
Lisinopril
Lithium
Lovastatin
Meclofenamate
Mephenytoin
Meprobamate
Mercaptopurine
Mesalamine
Mesoridazine
Methimazole
Methoxsalen
Methsuximide
Methyldopa
Methyltestosterone
Methysergide
Metoprolol
Mexiletine

Minocycline
Minoxidil
Nadolol
Nafcillin
Nalidixic acid
Naproxen
Nifedipine
Nitrofurantoin
Olsalazine
Omeprazole
Oral contraceptives
Oxcarbazepine
Oxytetracycline
Paclitaxel
Pantoprazole
Paramethadione
Penicillamine
Pentobarbital
Perphenazine
Phenelzine
Phenindamine
Phenobarbital
Phenolphthalein
Phensuximide
Phenylbutazone
Phenytoin
Pindolol
Piroxicam
Potassium iodide
Pravastatin
Prazosin
Prednicarbate
Primidone
Procainamide
Prochlorperazine
Promethazine
Propafenone
Propranolol
Propylthiouracil
Psoralens
Pyrilamine
Quinidine
Quinine
Ranitidine
Reserpine
Rifabutin
Rifampin
Selenium
Sertraline
Simvastatin
Smallpox vaccine
Somatropin
Spironolactone
Streptomycin
Sulfadiazine
Sulfadoxine
Sulfamethoxazole
Sulfasalazine
Sulfisoxazole
Tamoxifen
Terbinafine
Terfenadine
Testosterone
Tetracycline
Thioridazine
Ticlopidine
Timolol
Tiopronin
Tiotropium
Tocainide

Tolazamide
Triamterene
Trichlormethiazide
Trientine
Trifluoperazine
Trimeprazine
Trimethadione
Trioxsalen
Tripelennamine
Uracil/tegafur
Valproic acid
Valsartan
Vancomycin
Verapamil
Vitamin E
Voriconazole
Yohimbine
Zafirlukast
Zinc
Ziprasidone
Zonisamide
Onycholysis
Acebutolol
Adalimumab
Allopurinol
Atenolol
Bleomycin
Capecitabine
Captopril
Chloramphenicol
Chlorpromazine
Clofazimine
Clorazepate
Cloxacillin
Demeclocycline
Diflunisal
Docetaxel
Doxorubicin
Doxycycline
Estrogens
Etoposide
Fluorouracil
Gold and gold compounds
Hydroxyurea
Ibuprofen
Indapamide
Indomethacin
Irinotecan
Isoniazid
Isotretinoin
Ketoprofen
Methotrexate
Methoxsalen
Metoprolol
Minocycline
Mycophenolate
Nadolol
Nitrofurantoin
Norfloxacin
Ofloxacin
Oral contraceptives
Paclitaxel
Pindolol
Piroxicam
Propranolol
Psoralens
Quinine
Roxithromycin
Sparfloxacin
Tetracycline

Timolol
Trioxsalen
Paresthesias
Abacavir
Acamprosate
Acetazolamide
Acetohexamide
Acitretin
Acyclovir
Adalimumab
Adenosine
Agalsidase
Alitretinoin
Allopurinol
Almotriptan
Alprazolam
Altretamine
Amikacin
Amiloride
Amiodarone
Amitriptyline
Amlodipine
Amoxapine
Amphotericin B
Amprenavir
Anagrelide
Anastrozole
Anthrax vaccine
Apraclonidine
Arbutamine
Arformoterol
Aripiprazole
Armodafinil
Aspirin
Astemizole
Atorvastatin
Azatadine
Azithromycin
Aztreonam
Baclofen
Basiliximab
Benactyzine
Benazepril
Bendroflumethiazide
Benzthiazide
Benztropine
Bepridil
Betaxolol
Bicalutamide
Biperiden
Bisoprolol
Bleomycin
Bortezomib
Bromocriptine
Brompheniramine
Bupivacaine
Bupropion
Buspirone
Butorphanol
Cabergoline
Caffeine
Calcitonin
Candesartan
Capecitabine
Captopril
Carisoprodol
Carteolol
Carvedilol
Caspofungin
Cefaclor

Cefamandole
Cefotaxime
Cefpodoxime
Cefprozil
Ceftazidime
Ceftibuten
Ceftizoxime
Celecoxib
Celiprolol
Cephapirin
Cetirizine
Cevimeline
Chloramphenicol
Chlordiazepoxide
Chlorothiazide
Chlorpheniramine
Chlorpropamide
Chlorthalidone
Cholestyramine
Cidofovir
Cilostazol
Cinoxacin
Ciprofloxacin
Citalopram
Clemastine
Clomipramine
Clonazepam
Clopidogrel
Clorazepate
Codeine
Colistin
Cromolyn
Cyanocobalamin
Cyclamate
Cyclobenzaprine
Cycloserine
Cyclosporine
Cyclothiazide
Cyproheptadine
Dacarbazine
Danaparoid
Danazol
Daptomycin
Darifenacin
Darunavir
Delavirdine
Demeclocycline
Denileukin
Desipramine
Desvenlafaxine
Dexamethasone
Dexchlorpheniramine
Diazepam
Diazoxide
Diclofenac
Didanosine
Diflunisal
Dihydroergotamine
Diltiazem
Dimenhydrinate
Dimercaprol
Dinoprostone
Diphenhydramine
Diphenoxylate
Dipyridamole
Dirithromycin
Disopyramide
Disulfiram
Dobutamine
Docetaxel

Dofetilide
Dolasetron
Donepezil
Doxapram
Doxazosin
Doxepin
Doxycycline
Dronabinol
Echinacea
Efavirenz
Eflornithine
Eletriptan
Emtricitabine
Enalapril
Enfuvirtide
Enoxacin
Epoetin alfa
Epoprostenol
Eprosartan
Ertapenem
Escitalopram
Esmolol
Esomeprazole
Estazolam
Eszopiclone
Ethambutol
Ethchlorvynol
Etidronate
Etodolac
Etoposide
Etravirine
Exemestane
Famciclovir
Famotidine
Felbamate
Felodipine
Fenofibrate
Fentanyl
Flecainide
Floxuridine
Fluconazole
Flucytosine
Fludarabine
Flumazenil
Flumetasone
Flunisolide
Fluorouracil
Fluoxetine
Fluoxymesterone
Flurazepam
Flurbiprofen
Flutamide
Fluticasone
Fluvastatin
Fluvoxamine
Fosamprenavir
Foscarnet
Fosfomycin
Fosinopril
Fosphenytoin
Frovatriptan
Fulvestrant
Furosemide
Gabapentin
Gadobutrol
Gadodiamide
Gadofosveset
Galantamine
Ganciclovir
Gatifloxacin

Gemcitabine
Gemfibrozil
Gentamicin
Glatiramer
Glipizide
Glyburide
Grepafloxacin
Griseofulvin
Guanadrel
Guanethidine
Guanfacine
Hepatitis B vaccine
Histrelin
Hydralazine
Hydrochlorothiazide
Hydroflumethiazide
Hydromorphone
Ibuprofen
Imipenem/cilastatin
Imipramine
Indapamide
Indinavir
Indomethacin
Infliximab
Insulin
Interferon alfa
Interferon beta
Iodixanol
Iohexol
Iopromide
Ipratropium
Irbesartan
Isoniazid
Isradipine
Kanamycin
Ketoconazole
Ketoprofen
Ketorolac
Labetalol
Lamivudine
Lamotrigine
Lansoprazole
Laronidase
Leflunomide
Leuprolide
Levalbuterol
Levamisole
Levetiracetam
Levobupivacaine
Levodopa
Levofloxacin
Lidocaine
Lindane
Lisinopril
Lomefloxacin
Loratadine
Lorazepam
Lorcainide
Losartan
Lovastatin
Loxapine
Lubiprostone
Lutropin alfa
Maraviroc
Mazindol
MDMA
Mecamylamine
Meclizine
Meclofenamate
Medroxyprogesterone

Meloxicam
Meprobamate
Meropenem
Mesalamine
Mesoridazine
Methazolamide
Methimazole
Methyclothiazide
Methyldopa
Methyltestosterone
Methysergide
Metoclopramide
Metolazone
Metoprolol
Metronidazole
Mexiletine
Midazolam
Midodrine
Miglustat
Minocycline
Minoxidil
Mirtazapine
Mitomycin
Modafinil
Monosodium glutamate
Moricizine
Moxifloxacin
Mycophenolate
Nabumetone
Nadolol
Nafarelin
Nalbuphine
Nalidixic acid
Naratriptan
Nebivolol
Nefazodone
Nelarabine
Nelfinavir
Nesiritide
Nevirapine
Niacin
Niacinamide
Nicardipine
Nicotine
Nifedipine
Nilutamide
Nisoldipine
Nitrofurantoin
Nizatidine
Norfloxacin
Nortriptyline
Ofloxacin
Omeprazole
Ondansetron
Orphenadrine
Oxaliplatin
Oxazepam
Oxilan
Oxytetracycline
Paclitaxel
Palifermin
Palonosetron
Pantoprazole
Paramethadione
Paroxetine
Pegaspargase
Pegvisomant
Pemetrexed
Penbutolol
Penciclovir

Pentagastrin
Pentazocine
Pentostatin
Pentoxifylline
Perflutren
Pergolide
Perindopril
Phenylephrine
Phenytoin
Pindolol
Piperacillin
Pirbuterol
Piroxicam
Pneumococcal vaccine
Polythiazide
Potassium iodide
Pramipexole
Pravastatin
Prazepam
Prazosin
Prednicarbate
Pregabalin
Procarbazine
Promethazine
Propafenone
Propranolol
Propylthiouracil
Protriptyline
Pyridoxine
Pyrilamine
Quazepam
Quetiapine
Quinapril
Quinethazone
Quinupristin/dalfopristin
Rabeprazole
Ramipril
Ranolazine
Rasburicase
Reboxetine
Repaglinide
Rifabutin
Riluzole
Rimonabant
Risedronate
Risperidone
Ritonavir
Rivastigmine
Rizatriptan
Rofecoxib
Romiplostim
Ropinirole
Rosuvastatin
Rotigotine
Roxithromycin
Salmeterol
Saquinavir
Selegiline
Selenium
Sertraline
Sibutramine
Sildenafil
Simvastatin
Sincalide
Sirolimus
Smallpox vaccine
Somatropin
Sotalol
Sparfloxacin
Spironolactone

St John's wort
Stavudine
Streptomycin
Succimer
Sulindac
Sumatriptan
Tacrine
Tacrolimus
Tadalafil
Tartrazine
Telithromycin
Telmisartan
Temazepam
Temozolomide
Tenofovir
Terazosin
Terfenadine
Teriparatide
Testolactone
Testosterone
Tetrabenazine
Tetracycline
Thalidomide
Thallium
Thiabendazole
Thiamine
Thioridazine
Thiothixene
Tiagabine
Tiludronate
Timolol
Tinidazole
Tiotropium
Tizanidine
Tobramycin
Tocainide
Tolazamide
Tolbutamide
Tolcapone
Tolterodine
Topiramate
Topotecan
Tramadol
Trandolapril
Tranylcypromine
Trastuzumab
Trazodone
Tretinoin
Triamterene
Triazolam
Trichlormethiazide
Trihexyphenidyl
Trimeprazine
Trimethadione
Trimipramine
Tripelennamine
Triprolidine
Trovafloxacin
Unoprostone
Valacyclovir
Valdecoxib
Valganciclovir
Valproic acid
Valsartan
Vancomycin
Vardenafil
Varicella vaccine
Venlafaxine
Verapamil
Verteporfin

Vigabatrin
Vinblastine
Vincristine
Vinorelbine
Voriconazole
Zalcitabine
Ziconotide
Zidovudine
Zileuton
Ziprasidone
Zolmitriptan
Zolpidem
Zonisamide
Zuclopentixol acetate
Zuclopentixol decanoate
Zuclopentixol
   dihydrochloride

Pemphigus Vulgaris
Acetaminophen
Aldesleukin
Amoxicillin
Ampicillin
Aspirin
Bendroflumethiazide
Bucillamine
Caffeine
Captopril
Carbamazepine
Cefadroxil
Cefazolin
Ceftazidime
Ceftriaxone
Cefuroxime
Cephalexin
Cilazapril
Clonidine
Cyclophosphamide
Diclofenac
Enalapril
Epinephrine
Fludarabine
Fosinopril
Garlic
Glyburide
Gold and gold compounds
Heroin
Ibuprofen
Imiquimod
Indomethacin
Influenza vaccines
Interferon alfa
Isotretinoin
Ketoprofen
Levamisole
Levodopa
Lisinopril
Metamizole
Methoxsalen
Moexipril
Montelukast
Mycophenolate
Nifedipine
Omeprazole
Penicillamine
Phenobarbital
Phenylbutazone
Phenytoin
Piroxicam
Propranolol
Psoralens

Quinapril
Ramipril
Rifampin
Rituximab
Spironolactone
Timolol
Tiopronin
Trandolapril
Trioxsalen

Peyronie's Disease
Acebutolol
Atenolol
Betaxolol
Bisoprolol
Carteolol
Interferon beta
Labetalol
Methotrexate
Metoprolol
Nadolol
Penbutolol
Phenytoin
Pindolol
Propranolol
Ropinirole
Timolol

Photosensitivity
Acamprosate
Aceclofenac
Acetaminophen
Acetazolamide
Acetohexamide
Acyclovir
Aldesleukin
Alendronate
Alitretinoin
Allopurinol
Almotriptan
Aloe vera (gel, juice, leaf)
Alprazolam
Amantadine
Amiloride
Aminolevulinic acid
Aminosalicylate sodium
Amiodarone
Amitriptyline
Amobarbital
Amoxapine
Anagrelide
Anthrax vaccine
Arsenic
Astemizole
Atazanavir
Atenolol
Atorvastatin
Atovaquone/proguanil
Atropine sulfate
Azatadine
Azathioprine
Azithromycin
Benazepril
Bendroflumethiazide
Benzthiazide
Benztropine
Bergamot
Betaxolol
Bexarotene
Bisoprolol
Brompheniramine
Bumetanide

Bupropion
Butabarbital
Butalbital
Calcipotriol
Capecitabine
Captopril
Carbamazepine
Carisoprodol
Carteolol
Carvedilol
Cefazolin
Ceftazidime
Celecoxib
Cetirizine
Cevimeline
Chlorambucil
Chlordiazepoxide
Chlorhexidine
Chloroquine
Chlorothiazide
Chlorotrianisene
Chlorpheniramine
Chlorpromazine
Chlorpropamide
Chlortetracycline
Chlorthalidone
Cidofovir
Cinoxacin
Ciprofloxacin
Citalopram
Clemastine
Clofazimine
Clofibrate
Clomipramine
Clopidogrel
Clorazepate
Clozapine
Co-trimoxazole
Colchicine
Cromolyn
Cyclamate
Cyclobenzaprine
Cyclothiazide
Cyproheptadine
Dacarbazine
Danazol
Dantrolene
Dapsone
Dasatinib
Demeclocycline
Desipramine
Desoximetasone
Dexamethasone
Dexchlorpheniramine
Dexibuprofen
Diazoxide
Diclofenac
Diflunisal
Diltiazem
Dimenhydrinate
Diphenhydramine
Disopyramide
Docetaxel
Dong quai
Doxepin
Doxycycline
Duloxetine
Efavirenz
Enalapril
Enoxacin

Epirubicin
Epoetin alfa
Erlotinib
Esomeprazole
Estazolam
Estrogens
Eszopiclone
Ethacrynic acid
Ethambutol
Ethionamide
Etodolac
Felbamate
Fenofibrate
Floxuridine
Flucytosine
Fluorouracil
Fluoxetine
Fluphenazine
Flurbiprofen
Flutamide
Fluvastatin
Fluvoxamine
Fosinopril
Furazolidone
Furosemide
Ganciclovir
Gatifloxacin
Gemifloxacin
Gentamicin
Glatiramer
Glimepiride
Glipizide
Glyburide
Glycopyrrolate
Gold and gold compounds
Goldenseal
Grepafloxacin
Griseofulvin
Haloperidol
Henna
Heroin
Hydralazine
Hydrochlorothiazide
Hydroflumethiazide
Hydroxychloroquine
Hydroxyurea
Hydroxyzine
Hyoscyamine
Ibuprofen
Imatinib
Imipramine
Indapamide
Indomethacin
Infliximab
Interferon alfa
Interferon beta
Irinotecan
Isocarboxazid
Isoniazid
Isotretinoin
Itraconazole
Kanamycin
Kava
Ketoconazole
Ketoprofen
Ketotifen
Lamotrigine
Leuprolide
Levofloxacin
Lincomycin

Lisinopril
Lomefloxacin
Loratadine
Losartan
Loxapine
Maprotiline
Meclizine
Meclofenamate
Medroxyprogesterone
Mefenamic acid
Melatonin
Meloxicam
Meprobamate
Mercaptopurine
Mesalamine
Mesoridazine
Metformin
Methazolamide
Methenamine
Methotrexate
Methoxsalen
Methyclothiazide
Methyldopa
Methylphenidate
Metolazone
Minocycline
Mirtazapine
Mitomycin
Moexipril
Molindone
Moxifloxacin
Nabumetone
Nalidixic acid
Naproxen
Naratriptan
Nefazodone
Nifedipine
Nimesulide
Nisoldipine
Nitrofurantoin
Norfloxacin
Nortriptyline
Ofloxacin
Olanzapine
Oral contraceptives
Oxaprozin
Oxcarbazepine
Oxytetracycline
Paclitaxel
Panitumumab
Pantoprazole
Paroxetine
Pentobarbital
Pentosan
Pentostatin
Perphenazine
Phenelzine
Phenindamine
Phenobarbital
Phenylbutazone
Pilocarpine
Pimozide
Piroxicam
Polythiazide
Porfimer
Pravastatin
Pregabalin
Procarbazine
Prochlorperazine
Procyclidine

Promazine
Promethazine
Propranolol
Propylthiouracil
Protriptyline
Psoralens
Pyrazinamide
Pyridoxine
Pyrilamine
Pyrimethamine
Quetiapine
Quinacrine
Quinapril
Quinestrol
Quinethazone
Quinidine
Quinine
Rabeprazole
Ramipril
Ranitidine
Ribavirin
Riluzole
Risperidone
Ritonavir
Rofecoxib
Ropinirole
Rosemary
Rue
Saccharin
Saquinavir
Scopolamine
Selegiline
Selenium
Sertraline
Sildenafil
Simvastatin
Smallpox vaccine
Sotalol
Sparfloxacin
Spironolactone
St John's wort
Streptomycin
Sulfacetamide
Sulfadiazine
Sulfadoxine
Sulfamethoxazole
Sulfasalazine
Sulfisoxazole
Sulindac
Sumatriptan
Tacrolimus
Tartrazine
Terbinafine
Terfenadine
Tetracycline
Thimerosal
Thioguanine
Thioridazine
Thiothixene
Tiagabine
Timolol
Tiopronin
Tiotropium
Tolazamide
Tolbutamide
Tolmetin
Topiramate
Torsemide
Tranylcypromine
Trastuzumab

Trazodone
Tretinoin
Triamterene
Triazolam
Trichlormethiazide
Trifluoperazine
Trihexyphenidyl
Trimeprazine
Trimethadione
Trimethoprim
Trimetrexate
Trimipramine
Trioxsalen
Tripelennamine
Triprolidine
Trovafloxacin
Uracil/tegafur
Valdecoxib
Valproic acid
Valsartan
Vardenafil
Venlafaxine
Verapamil
Verteporfin
Vinblastine
Vitamin A
Voriconazole
Yarrow
Zalcitabine
Ziprasidone
Zolmitriptan
Zolpidem
Zuclopentixol acetate
Zuclopentixol decanoate
Zuclopentixol
    dihydrochloride

Pigmentation
Acebutolol
Alitretinoin
Amantadine
Aminolevulinic acid
Amiodarone
Amitriptyline
Amlodipine
Amoxicillin
Amphotericin B
Apomorphine
Arformoterol
Arsenic
Azacitidine
Azathioprine
Bergamot
Betamethasone
Betaxolol
Bevacizumab
Bimatoprost
Bismuth
Bisoprolol
Bleomycin
Bupropion
Busulfan
Calcipotriol
Capecitabine
Captopril
Carbamazepine
Carboplatin
Carmustine
Carteolol
Ceftriaxone
Cetirizine

Cevimeline
Chlorhexidine
Chloroquine
Chlorotrianisene
Chlorpromazine
Cidofovir
Ciprofloxacin
Cisplatin
Citalopram
Clobetasol
Clofazimine
Clomipramine
Clonazepam
Clonidine
Collagen
Cyclobenzaprine
Cyclophosphamide
Cyclosporine
Dactinomycin
Dapsone
Dasatinib
Daunorubicin
Deferoxamine
Demeclocycline
Desipramine
Diazepam
Dicumarol
Diethylstilbestrol
Diltiazem
Dinoprostone
Docetaxel
Dolasetron
Donepezil
Doxorubicin
Doxycycline
Eletriptan
Emtricitabine
Enoxacin
Epirubicin
Esmolol
Estramustine
Estrogens
Eszopiclone
Etodolac
Etoposide
Floxuridine
Fluocinolone
Fluocinonide
Fluorouracil
Fluoxetine
Fluphenazine
Flurbiprofen
Fluvastatin
Fluvoxamine
Foscarnet
Gadodiamide
Ganciclovir
Gefitinib
Glatiramer
Gold and gold compounds
Grepafloxacin
Griseofulvin
Halcinonide
Haloperidol
Hemophilus B vaccine
Henna
Heroin
Hydroxychloroquine
Hydroxyurea
Ifosfamide

Imatinib
Imipramine
Imiquimod
Indapamide
Indinavir
Insulin
Interferon alfa
Interferon beta
Irinotecan
Isotretinoin
Ixabepilone
Kava
Ketoconazole
Ketoprofen
Labetalol
Latanoprost
Leflunomide
Leuprolide
Levobupivacaine
Levodopa
Levofloxacin
Lidocaine
Linezolid
Lithium
Lomefloxacin
Loxapine
Lycopene
Mechlorethamine
Medroxyprogesterone
Mephenytoin
Mercaptopurine
Mesoridazine
Methamphetamine
Methimazole
Methotrexate
Methoxsalen
Methyldopa
Methysergide
Metoclopramide
Metoprolol
Minocycline
Minoxidil
Mirtazapine
Mitomycin
Mitotane
Mitoxantrone
Molindone
Mometasone
Naratriptan
Niacin
Nicotine
Nifedipine
Nisoldipine
Nitazoxanide
Ofloxacin
Olanzapine
Omeprazole
Oral contraceptives
Orphenadrine
Oxytetracycline
Paclitaxel
Palifermin
Panitumumab
Pantoprazole
Paroxetine
Penciclovir
Pentazocine
Pentostatin
Pergolide
Perphenazine

Phenazopyridine
Phenobarbital
Phenolphthalein
Phenytoin
Pimozide
Porfimer
Pregabalin
Procarbazine
Prochlorperazine
Progestins
Promazine
Promethazine
Propofol
Propranolol
Propylthiouracil
Psoralens
Pyridoxine
Pyrimethamine
Quinacrine
Quinestrol
Quinidine
Quinine
Rabeprazole
Ribavirin
Rifabutin
Rifapentine
Riluzole
Risperidone
Ropinirole
Saquinavir
Selenium
Sertaconazole
Sertraline
Sildenafil
Smallpox vaccine
Sparfloxacin
Spironolactone
Stanozolol
Sulfadiazine
Sulfasalazine
Sunitinib
Tacrolimus
Tamoxifen
Terbinafine
Tetracycline
Thioridazine
Thiotepa
Thiothixene
Tiagabine
Timolol
Tinidazole
Tolcapone
Topiramate
Toremifene
Travoprost
Tretinoin
Triamcinolone
Trifluoperazine
Trioxsalen
Unoprostone
Uracil/tegafur
Venlafaxine
Verapamil
Verteporfin
Vinblastine
Vincristine
Vinorelbine
Vitamin A
Voriconazole
Zidovudine

Zinc
Zuclopentixol acetate
Zuclopentixol decanoate
Zuclopentixol
    dihydrochloride
Pityriasis Rosea
Acetaminophen
Acyclovir
Allopurinol
Ampicillin
Arsenic
Aspirin
BCG vaccine
Bismuth
Captopril
Clonidine
Codeine
Gold and gold compounds
Griseofulvin
Hydrochlorothiazide
Imatinib
Isotretinoin
Ketotifen
Lisinopril
Meprobamate
Metronidazole
Mitomycin
Naproxen
Nimesulide
Omeprazole
Pneumococcal vaccine
Terbinafine
Tiopronin
Tripelennamine
Pruritus
Abacavir
Abarelix
Abatacept
Abciximab
Acamprosate
Acebutolol
Aceclofenac
Acetaminophen
Acetazolamide
Acetohexamide
Acetylcysteine
Acitretin
Acyclovir
Adalimumab
Adapalene
Adefovir
Agalsidase
Albendazole
Albuterol
Alclometasone
Aldesleukin
Alefacept
Alemtuzumab
Alendronate
Alfentanil
Alglucerase
Alglucosidase alfa
Alitretinoin
Allopurinol
Almotriptan
Alpha-lipoic acid
Alprazolam
Alprostadil
Altretamine
Amantadine

Amcinonide
Amifostine
Amikacin
Amiloride
Aminocaproic acid
Aminoglutethimide
Aminolevulinic acid
Aminophylline
Aminosalicylate sodium
Amiodarone
Amitriptyline
Amlodipine
Amoxapine
Amoxicillin
Amphotericin B
Ampicillin
Amprenavir
Anagrelide
Anastrozole
Anidulafungin
Anthrax vaccine
Apraclonidine
Aprotinin
Aripiprazole
Arsenic
Artemisia
Asparaginase
Aspartame
Aspirin
Astemizole
Atazanavir
Atenolol
Atomoxetine
Atorvastatin
Atovaquone
Atovaquone/proguanil
Atracurium
Atropine sulfate
Azacitidine
Azathioprine
Azelastine
Azithromycin
Aztreonam
Bacampicillin
Baclofen
Balsalazide
Basiliximab
Beclomethasone
Benactyzine
Benazepril
Bendamustine
Bendroflumethiazide
Benzonatate
Benztropine
Betaxolol
Bexarotene
Bicalutamide
Bimatoprost
Bismuth
Bisoprolol
Black cohosh
Bleomycin
Bortezomib
Bosentan
Botulinum toxin (A & B)
Brimonidine
Brinzolamide
Budesonide
Bumetanide
Bupivacaine

Buprenorphine
Bupropion
Buspirone
Butabarbital
Butalbital
Butorphanol
Butterbur
Cabergoline
Caffeine
Calcipotriol
Calcitonin
Calcium hydroxylapatite
Candesartan
Capecitabine
Capreomycin
Captopril
Carbamazepine
Carbenicillin
Carbimazole
Carboplatin
Carisoprodol
Carteolol
Carvedilol
Caspofungin
Cefaclor
Cefadroxil
Cefamandole
Cefazolin
Cefdinir
Cefditoren
Cefepime
Cefixime
Cefmetazole
Cefonicid
Cefoperazone
Cefotaxime
Cefotetan
Cefoxitin
Cefpodoxime
Cefprozil
Ceftazidime
Ceftibuten
Ceftizoxime
Ceftobiprole
Ceftriaxone
Cefuroxime
Celecoxib
Cephalexin
Cephalothin
Cephapirin
Cephradine
Cetirizine
Cetrorelix
Cetuximab
Cevimeline
Chasteberry
Chloral hydrate
Chlorambucil
Chloramphenicol
Chlordiazepoxide
Chlorhexidine
Chlormezanone
Chloroquine
Chlorothiazide
Chlorpheniramine
Chlorpromazine
Chlorpropamide
Chlortetracycline
Chlorzoxazone
Cholestyramine

Cidofovir
Cilostazol
Cimetidine
Cinoxacin
Ciprofibrate
Ciprofloxacin
Cisatracurium
Cisplatin
Citalopram
Cladribine
Clarithromycin
Clindamycin
Clioquinol
Clobazam
Clofarabine
Clofazimine
Clofibrate
Clomiphene
Clomipramine
Clonazepam
Clonidine
Clopidogrel
Clorazepate
Clotrimazole
Cloxacillin
Clozapine
Co-trimoxazole
Cocaine
Cocoa
Codeine
Colchicine
Colistin
Collagen
Cromolyn
Cyanocobalamin
Cyclamate
Cyclobenzaprine
Cyclophosphamide
Cycloserine
Cyclosporine
Cytarabine
Daclizumab
Dactinomycin
Dalteparin
Dan-shen
Danaparoid
Danazol
Dantrolene
Dapsone
Daptomycin
Darbepoetin alfa
Darifenacin
Dasatinib
Daunorubicin
Decitabine
Deferoxamine
Delavirdine
Demeclocycline
Denileukin
Desflurane
Desipramine
Desloratadine
Desonide
Dexamethasone
Dexibuprofen
Diatrizoate
Diazepam
Diazoxide
Diclofenac
Dicloxacillin

Dicumarol	Fluconazole	Hydroxychloroquine	Lithium
Dicyclomine	Flucytosine	Hydroxyurea	Lodoxamide
Didanosine	Flumetasone	Ibritumomab	Lomefloxacin
Diethylpropion	Fluocinolone	Ibuprofen	Loperamide
Diethylstilbestrol	Fluocinonide	Icodextrin	Loracarbef
Diflunisal	Fluorides	Idursulfase	Loratadine
Digoxin	Fluorouracil	Imatinib	Lorazepam
Dihydroergotamine	Fluoxetine	Imidapril	Losartan
Dihydrotachysterol	Fluoxymesterone	Imiglucerase	Lovastatin
Diltiazem	Fluphenazine	Imipenem/cilastatin	Loxapine
Diphenhydramine	Flurazepam	Imipramine	Lutropin alfa
Diphenoxylate	Flurbiprofen	Imiquimod	Mafenide
Diphtheria antitoxin	Fluticasone	Immune globulin I.V.	Maprotiline
Dipyridamole	Fluvastatin	Indapamide	Maraviroc
Dirithromycin	Fluvoxamine	Indinavir	Marihuana
Disopyramide	Folic acid	Indomethacin	Mebendazole
Dobutamine	Fondaparinux	Infliximab	Mechlorethamine
Docetaxel	Formoterol	Insulin	Meclofenamate
Dolasetron	Fosamprenavir	Insulin detemir	Medroxyprogesterone
Domperidone	Foscarnet	Insulin glargine	Mefenamic acid
Donepezil	Fosfomycin	Insulin glulisine	Mefloquine
Dopamine	Fosinopril	Interferon alfa	Meloxicam
Doxapram	Fosphenytoin	Interferon beta	Melphalan
Doxazosin	Frovatriptan	Iodixanol	Memantine
Doxepin	Furazolidone	Iohexol	Meperidine
Doxercalciferol	Furosemide	Iopromide	Mephenytoin
Doxorubicin	Gabapentin	Ipodate	Meprobamate
Doxycycline	Gadobutrol	Ipratropium	Mercaptopurine
Droperidol	Gadodiamide	Irbesartan	Meropenem
Duloxetine	Gadofosveset	Irinotecan	Mesalamine
Efavirenz	Ganciclovir	Isocarboxazid	Mesna
Eflornithine	Ganirelix	Isoniazid	Mesoridazine
Eletriptan	Gatifloxacin	Isoproterenol	Metaxalone
Emtricitabine	Gefitinib	Isosorbide mononitrate	Metformin
Enalapril	Gemcitabine	Isotretinoin	Methadone
Enfuvirtide	Gemfibrozil	Isradipine	Methazolamide
Enoxacin	Gentamicin	Itraconazole	Methenamine
Enoxaparin	Ginkgo biloba	Ivermectin	Methicillin
Epinastine	Ginseng	Ixabepilone	Methimazole
Epirubicin	Glatiramer	Kanamycin	Methocarbamol
Epoetin alfa	Glimepiride	Kava	Methotrexate
Epoprostenol	Glipizide	Ketamine	Methoxsalen
Eprosartan	Glucosamine	Ketoconazole	Methsuximide
Ergocalciferol	Glyburide	Ketoprofen	Methyldopa
Erlotinib	Gold and gold compounds	Ketorolac	Methylphenidate
Ertapenem	Granulocyte colony-	Ketotifen	Methylprednisolone
Erythromycin	stimulating factor (GCSF)	Labetalol	Methyltestosterone
Escitalopram	Grepafloxacin	Lamivudine	Methysergide
Esomeprazole	Griseofulvin	Lamotrigine	Metolazone
Estazolam	Guanabenz	Lanreotide	Metoprolol
Estramustine	Guanfacine	Lansoprazole	Metronidazole
Estrogens	Halcinonide	Latanoprost	Mexiletine
Eszopiclone	Halobetasol	Leflunomide	Mezlocillin
Etanercept	Halometasone	Lenalidomide	Miconazole
Ethambutol	Haloperidol	Letrozole	Midazolam
Ethchlorvynol	Hemophilus B vaccine	Leucovorin	Midodrine
Ethosuximide	Henna	Leuprolide	Minocycline
Etidronate	Heparin	Levalbuterol	Minoxidil
Etodolac	Hepatitis A vaccine	Levamisole	Mirtazapine
Etoposide	Hepatitis B vaccine	Levobunolol	Mistletoe
Exemestane	Heroin	Levobupivacaine	Mitomycin
Famciclovir	Histrelin	Levocetirizine	Mitotane
Famotidine	Human papillomavirus	Levofloxacin	Moclobemide
Felbamate	vaccine	Levoleucovorin	Modafinil
Felodipine	Hyaluronic acid	Levothyroxine	Moexipril
Fenofibrate	Hydralazine	Lidocaine	Molindone
Fenoprofen	Hydrochlorothiazide	Lincomycin	Mometasone
Fentanyl	Hydrocodone	Lindane	Moricizine
Flecainide	Hydrocortisone	Linezolid	Morphine
Floxuridine	Hydromorphone	Lisinopril	Moxifloxacin

Mupirocin
Muromonab-CD3
Mycophenolate
Myrrh
Nabumetone
Nadolol
Nafarelin
Nafcillin
Nalbuphine
Nalidixic acid
Nalmefene
Naloxone
Naltrexone
Naproxen
Natalizumab
Nefazodone
Nelfinavir
Neomycin
Nepafenac
Nesiritide
Nevirapine
Niacin
Niacinamide
Nicotine
Nifedipine
Nilutamide
Nimesulide
Nimodipine
Nisoldipine
Nitazoxanide
Nitisinone
Nitrofurantoin
Nitrofurazone
Nizatidine
Norfloxacin
Nortriptyline
Nystatin
Octreotide
Ofloxacin
Olanzapine
Olopatadine
Olsalazine
Omalizumab
Omeprazole
Ondansetron
Oral contraceptives
Orphenadrine
Oxacillin
Oxaliplatin
Oxaprozin
Oxazepam
Oxcarbazepine
Oxilan
Oxybutynin
Oxycodone
Oxymorphone
Oxytetracycline
Paclitaxel
Palifermin
Palonosetron
Pancuronium
Panitumumab
Pantoprazole
Pantothenic acid
Papaverine
Paramethadione
Paromomycin
Paroxetine
PEG-interferon
Pegaspargase

Pegvisomant
Pemetrexed
Penbutolol
Penciclovir
Penicillamine
Pentagastrin
Pentamidine
Pentazocine
Pentobarbital
Pentosan
Pentostatin
Pentoxifylline
Perflutren
Pergolide
Perindopril
Perphenazine
Phenazopyridine
Phenelzine
Phenobarbital
Phenolphthalein
Phensuximide
Phenylbutazone
Phenytoin
Pilocarpine
Pimecrolimus
Pimozide
Pindolol
Piperacillin
Pirbuterol
Piroxicam
Pneumococcal vaccine
Polypodium leucotomos
Posaconazole
Pramipexole
Pramlintide
Pravastatin
Prazepam
Praziquantel
Prazosin
Prednicarbate
Prednisolone
Prednisone
Pregabalin
Primaquine
Probenecid
Procainamide
Procarbazine
Prochlorperazine
Progestins
Propafenone
Propofol
Propoxyphene
Propranolol
Propylthiouracil
Protein C concentrate
   (human)
Protriptyline
Psoralens
Pyrazinamide
Pyrimethamine
Quazepam
Quinacrine
Quinapril
Quinethazone
Quinidine
Quinine
Quinupristin/dalfopristin
Rabeprazole
Raltegravir
Raltitrexed

Ramipril
Ranibizumab
Ranitidine
Rapacuronium
Reserpine
Retapamulin
Ribavirin
Rifampin
Rifapentine
Rifaximin
Riluzole
Rimonabant
Risedronate
Risperidone
Ritonavir
Rituximab
Rizatriptan
Rocuronium
Rofecoxib
Ropinirole
Rosuvastatin
Rotigotine
Roxatidine
Roxithromycin
Saccharin
Salmeterol
Salsalate
Saquinavir
Selenium
Senna
Sermorelin
Sertaconazole
Sertraline
Sevoflurane
Sibutramine
Sildenafil
Simvastatin
Sinecatechins
Sirolimus
Smallpox vaccine
Somatropin
Sorafenib
Sotalol
Sparfloxacin
Spectinomycin
Spironolactone
St John's wort
Streptokinase
Streptomycin
Streptozocin
Succimer
Succinylcholine
Sucralfate
Sufentanil
Sulfacetamide
Sulfadiazine
Sulfadoxine
Sulfamethoxazole
Sulfasalazine
Sulfisoxazole
Sulfites
Sulindac
Sumatriptan
Tacrine
Tacrolimus
Tadalafil
Tamoxifen
Tamsulosin
Tartrazine
Tea tree

Tegaserod
Telithromycin
Telmisartan
Temazepam
Temozolomide
Temsirolimus
Terazosin
Terbinafine
Terbutaline
Terconazole
Terfenadine
Testosterone
Tetracycline
Thalidomide
Thallium
Thiabendazole
Thiamine
Thioguanine
Thiopental
Thiotepa
Thiothixene
Tiagabine
Ticarcillin
Ticlopidine
Tigecycline
Tiludronate
Timolol
Tinidazole
Tinzaparin
Tiopronin
Tiotropium
Tipranavir
Tizanidine
Tobramycin
Tocainide
Tolazamide
Tolbutamide
Tolcapone
Tolmetin
Tolterodine
Topiramate
Toremifene
Torsemide
Tositumomab & iodine[131]
Tramadol
Trandolapril
Tranylcypromine
Travoprost
Trazodone
Treprostinil
Tretinoin
Triamcinolone
Triamterene
Triazolam
Trifluoperazine
Trimeprazine
Trimethadione
Trimethoprim
Trimetrexate
Trimipramine
Trioxsalen
Triptorelin
Troleandomycin
Trovafloxacin
Unoprostone
Urapidil
Urokinase
Ursodiol
Valacyclovir
Valdecoxib

Valganciclovir
Valproic acid
Valrubicin
Valsartan
Vancomycin
Vardenafil
Varicella vaccine
Venlafaxine
Verapamil
Verteporfin
Vidarabine
Vincristine
Vinorelbine
Vitamin A
Voriconazole
Vorinostat
Warfarin
Zalcitabine
Zaleplon
Ziconotide
Zidovudine
Zileuton
Zolmitriptan
Zolpidem
Zonisamide
Zoster vaccine
Zuclopentixol acetate
Zuclopentixol decanoate

Pseudoporphyria
Acetohexamide
Amiodarone
Ampicillin
Aspirin
Bismuth
Bumetanide
Busulfan
Butabarbital
Butalbital
Carbamazepine
Carisoprodol
Cefepime
Celecoxib
Chloramphenicol
Chlordiazepoxide
Chloroquine
Chlorotrianisene
Chlorpropamide
Chlorthalidone
Cimetidine
Ciprofloxacin
Cisplatin
Clorazepate
Cocaine
Colchicine
Cyanocobalamin
Cyclophosphamide
Cyclosporine
Dapsone
Demeclocycline
Diazepam
Diethylstilbestrol
Diflunisal
Duloxetine
Epoetin alfa
Estrogens
Fluorouracil
Flutamide
Furosemide
Gemifloxacin
Glimepiride

Glipizide
Glyburide
Griseofulvin
Hydrochlorothiazide
Hydroxychloroquine
Hydroxyurea
Ibuprofen
Imatinib
Indinavir
Indomethacin
Isotretinoin
Ketoprofen
Lamotrigine
Mafenide
Meclofenamate
Mefenamic acid
Meprobamate
Methotrexate
Metoclopramide
Nabumetone
Nalidixic acid
Naproxen
Nitisinone
Ondansetron
Oral contraceptives
Oxaprozin
Oxytetracycline
Pentobarbital
Phenobarbital
Phenytoin
Piroxicam
Pravastatin
Pyrazinamide
Pyridoxine
Quinidine
Quinine
Ranitidine
Rifampin
Rofecoxib
Simvastatin
Sodium oxybate
Tetracycline
Thiopental
Thioridazine
Tolazamide
Tolbutamide
Torsemide
Triamterene
Valproic acid
Voriconazole
Zidovudine

Psoriasis
Acebutolol
Aceclofenac
Acetazolamide
Acitretin
Adalimumab
Aldesleukin
Alefacept
Aminoglutethimide
Amiodarone
Amoxicillin
Ampicillin
Aripiprazole
Arsenic
Aspirin
Atenolol
BCG vaccine
Betamethasone
Betaxolol

Bisoprolol
Botulinum toxin (A & B)
Bupropion
Calcipotriol
Candesartan
Captopril
Carbamazepine
Carteolol
Carvedilol
Celecoxib
Chlorambucil
Chloroquine
Chlorthalidone
Cimetidine
Citalopram
Clarithromycin
Clomipramine
Clonidine
Clopidogrel
Co-trimoxazole
Cyclosporine
Diclofenac
Digoxin
Diltiazem
Dipyridamole
Doxorubicin
Doxycycline
Efalizumab
Eletriptan
Enalapril
Esmolol
Etanercept
Fexofenadine
Flecainide
Fluorouracil
Fluoxetine
Fluoxymesterone
Foscarnet
Ganciclovir
Gemfibrozil
Glatiramer
Glimepiride
Glipizide
Glyburide
Gold and gold compounds
Granulocyte colony-
   stimulating factor (GCSF)
Henna
Hydroxychloroquine
Hydroxyurea
Ibuprofen
Imatinib
Imiquimod
Indomethacin
Infliximab
Interferon alfa
Interferon beta
Ketoprofen
Labetalol
Letrozole
Levamisole
Levobetaxolol
Lithium
MDMA
Meclofenamate
Mefloquine
Meloxicam
Mesalamine
Methicillin
Methotrexate

Methyltestosterone
Metipranolol
Metoprolol
Modafinil
Morphine
Nadolol
Olanzapine
Omeprazole
Oral contraceptives
Paroxetine
PEG-interferon
Penbutolol
Penicillamine
Pentostatin
Perindopril
Phenylbutazone
Pindolol
Potassium iodide
Prednisolone
Primaquine
Propafenone
Propranolol
Psoralens
Quinidine
Quinine
Rabeprazole
Ranitidine
Ribavirin
Risperidone
Ritonavir
Rivastigmine
Rofecoxib
Ropinirole
Saquinavir
Sotalol
Sulfamethoxazole
Sulfasalazine
Sulfisoxazole
Tacrine
Terbinafine
Terfenadine
Testosterone
Tetracycline
Thalidomide
Thiabendazole
Thioguanine
Tiagabine
Timolol
Trazodone
Urapidil
Ursodiol
Valdecoxib
Valproic acid
Valsartan
Varenicline
Venlafaxine
Voriconazole

Purpura
Aceclofenac
Acenocoumarol
Acetaminophen
Acetazolamide
Acitretin
Aldesleukin
Alemtuzumab
Allopurinol
Alprazolam
Alteplase
Alvimopan
Amiloride

Aminocaproic acid	Citalopram	Etanercept	Lamotrigine
Aminoglutethimide	Cladribine	Ethacrynic acid	Leflunomide
Aminosalicylate sodium	Clarithromycin	Ethambutol	Leuprolide
Amiodarone	Clemastine	Ethchlorvynol	Levamisole
Amitriptyline	Clidinium	Ethionamide	Levobupivacaine
Amlodipine	Clindamycin	Ethosuximide	Levodopa
Amobarbital	Clofibrate	Ethotoin	Levofloxacin
Amoxapine	Clomiphene	Etodolac	Lidocaine
Amoxicillin	Clomipramine	Etoposide	Lincomycin
Amphotericin B	Clonazepam	Famotidine	Lindane
Ampicillin	Clopidogrel	Felbamate	Lisinopril
Anistreplase	Clorazepate	Felodipine	Lithium
Anthrax vaccine	Clozapine	Fenoprofen	Lomefloxacin
Aprobarbital	Co-trimoxazole	Fentanyl	Loratadine
Aripiprazole	Codeine	Floxuridine	Lorazepam
Arsenic	Colchicine	Fluconazole	Losartan
Aspartame	Creatine	Flucytosine	Lovastatin
Aspirin	Cromolyn	Fluoxetine	Loxapine
Atazanavir	Cyclobenzaprine	Fluoxymesterone	Maprotiline
Atenolol	Cyclophosphamide	Fluphenazine	Mecasermin
Azacitidine	Cycloserine	Flurazepam	Mechlorethamine
Azatadine	Cyclosporine	Flurbiprofen	Meclofenamate
Azathioprine	Cyclothiazide	Fluvastatin	Medroxyprogesterone
Aztreonam	Cyproheptadine	Fluvoxamine	Mefenamic acid
Beclomethasone	Danaparoid	Fondaparinux	Meloxicam
Bendroflumethiazide	Danazol	Frovatriptan	Melphalan
Benzthiazide	Dapsone	Furosemide	Mephenytoin
Beta-carotene	Decitabine	Gabapentin	Mephobarbital
Betaxolol	Deferasirox	Gadodiamide	Meprobamate
Bisoprolol	Deferoxamine	Galantamine	Mercaptopurine
Bortezomib	Delavirdine	Ganciclovir	Metformin
Botulinum toxin (A & B)	Demeclocycline	Gentamicin	Methadone
Bromocriptine	Denileukin	Glatiramer	Methazolamide
Bumetanide	Desipramine	Glipizide	Methicillin
Buspirone	Dexibuprofen	Glyburide	Methimazole
Busulfan	Dexmethylphenidate	Gold and gold compounds	Methotrexate
Butabarbital	Diazepam	Griseofulvin	Methoxsalen
Butalbital	Diazoxide	Guanethidine	Methsuximide
Caffeine	Diclofenac	Guanfacine	Methyclothiazide
Capecitabine	Dicloxacillin	Haloperidol	Methyldopa
Captopril	Dicumarol	Heparin	Methylphenidate
Carbamazepine	Didanosine	Hepatitis B vaccine	Methyltestosterone
Carbenicillin	Diethylpropion	Heroin	Metolazone
Carteolol	Diethylstilbestrol	Histrelin	Metoprolol
Carvedilol	Diflunisal	Horse chestnut (bark, flower,	Mexiletine
Cefaclor	Digoxin	leaf, seed)	Miconazole
Cefamandole	Diltiazem	Hydralazine	Minocycline
Cefdinir	Diphenhydramine	Hydrochlorothiazide	Mitomycin
Cefmetazole	Dipyridamole	Hydrocortisone	Mitoxantrone
Cefonicid	Disopyramide	Hydroflumethiazide	Montelukast
Cefoxitin	Disulfiram	Hydroxychloroquine	Nalidixic acid
Ceftriaxone	Dolasetron	Hydroxyurea	Naltrexone
Cefuroxime	Donepezil	Hydroxyzine	Naproxen
Celecoxib	Doxazosin	Ibritumomab	Naratriptan
Cephalexin	Doxepin	Ibuprofen	Nifedipine
Cephalothin	Doxorubicin	Imipramine	Nimesulide
Cephradine	Doxycycline	Indapamide	Nimodipine
Cetirizine	Drotrecogin alfa	Indomethacin	Nitrofurantoin
Cetrorelix	Duloxetine	Influenza vaccines	Nitroglycerin
Chloral hydrate	Enalapril	Insulin	Nortriptyline
Chlorambucil	Enoxacin	Interferon alfa	Octreotide
Chloramphenicol	Enoxaparin	Interferon beta	Ofloxacin
Chlordiazepoxide	Entacapone	Iohexol	Omalizumab
Chlorothiazide	Ephedrine	Ipodate	Omeprazole
Chlorpromazine	Eprosartan	Isoniazid	Oral contraceptives
Chlorpropamide	Escitalopram	Itraconazole	Oxaliplatin
Chlorthalidone	Esmolol	Ketoconazole	Oxaprozin
Cilostazol	Estazolam	Ketoprofen	Oxazepam
Cimetidine	Estramustine	Ketorolac	Oxcarbazepine
Ciprofloxacin	Estrogens	Labetalol	Oxytetracycline

Paclitaxel
Paroxetine
PEG-interferon
Pegaspargase
Pemetrexed
Penbutolol
Penicillamine
Pentagastrin
Pentamidine
Pentobarbital
Pentosan
Pentostatin
Pentoxifylline
Perindopril
Perphenazine
Phenindamine
Phenobarbital
Phensuximide
Phentermine
Phenylbutazone
Phenytoin
Pindolol
Piperacillin
Pirbuterol
Piroxicam
Plicamycin
Polythiazide
Potassium iodide
Pravastatin
Prazepam
Prednisone
Pregabalin
Procainamide
Procarbazine
Prochlorperazine
Promazine
Promethazine
Propafenone
Propranolol
Propylthiouracil
Protriptyline
Pyrazinamide
Pyridoxine
Pyrilamine
Pyrimethamine
Quazepam
Quinethazone
Quinidine
Quinine
Rabeprazole
Ramipril
Ranitidine
Rapacuronium
Reserpine
Reteplase
Rifampin
Rifapentine
Riluzole
Risperidone
Rivastigmine
Rofecoxib
Ropinirole
Rotigotine
Roxithromycin
Salsalate
Secobarbital
Sertraline
Simvastatin
Sirolimus
Smallpox vaccine

Sparfloxacin
Spironolactone
Streptokinase
Streptomycin
Streptozocin
Sulfadiazine
Sulfadoxine
Sulfamethoxazole
Sulfasalazine
Sulfinpyrazone
Sulfisoxazole
Sulindac
Tacrine
Tacrolimus
Tamoxifen
Tartrazine
Temazepam
Tenecteplase
Tenofovir
Terfenadine
Tetracycline
Thalidomide
Thiamine
Thioguanine
Thiopental
Thioridazine
Ticarcillin
Ticlopidine
Timolol
Tinzaparin
Tizanidine
Tobramycin
Tolazamide
Tolbutamide
Tolmetin
Topiramate
Topotecan
Torsemide
Trazodone
Triamterene
Triazolam
Trichlormethiazide
Trifluoperazine
Trimeprazine
Trimethadione
Trimipramine
Tripelennamine
Triprolidine
Urokinase
Valacyclovir
Valproic acid
Vancomycin
Varicella vaccine
Vasopressin
Verapamil
Verteporfin
Vinblastine
Voriconazole
Warfarin
Zidovudine
Zolpidem
Zonisamide
Zuclopentixol acetate
Zuclopentixol decanoate
Zuclopentixol
  dihydrochloride

Raynaud's Phenomenon
Acebutolol
Amphotericin B
Arsenic

Atenolol
Azathioprine
Betaxolol
Bisoprolol
Bleomycin
Bromocriptine
Carboplatin
Carteolol
Celiprolol
Cisplatin
Clonidine
Cocaine
Cyclosporine
Dopamine
Doxorubicin
Estrogens
Ethosuximide
Fluoxetine
Gemcitabine
Gemfibrozil
Hepatitis B vaccine
Interferon alfa
Interferon beta
Labetalol
Lamotrigine
Methotrexate
Methysergide
Metoprolol
Minocycline
Nadolol
Octreotide
Phentermine
Pindolol
Propofol
Propranolol
Quinine
Sotalol
Spironolactone
Sulfasalazine
Sulindac
Sumatriptan
Tegaserod
Thiothixene
Timolol
Uracil/tegafur
Vinblastine
Vincristine

Rhabdomyolysis
Abacavir
Acetaminophen
Aldesleukin
Aminocaproic acid
Aminophylline
Amiodarone
Amitriptyline
Amobarbital
Amoxicillin
Amphotericin B
Aprobarbital
Aripiprazole
Atorvastatin
Azacitidine
Azathioprine
Baclofen
Benztropine
Buprenorphine
Bupropion
Butabarbital
Butalbital
Caffeine

Carbamazepine
Chlorpromazine
Cholestyramine
Ciprofibrate
Cisplatin
Citalopram
Clarithromycin
Clofibrate
Clopidogrel
Clozapine
Co-trimoxazole
Cocaine
Colchicine
Creatine
Cyclophosphamide
Cyclosporine
Cytarabine
Dacarbazine
Danazol
Daptomycin
Delavirdine
Desipramine
Dextroamphetamine
Diatrizoate
Diazepam
Diclofenac
Didanosine
Diltiazem
Diphenhydramine
Domperidone
Doxepin
Droperidol
Enflurane
Enoxacin
Erythromycin
Esomeprazole
Fenbufen
Fenofibrate
Fluconazole
Fluorouracil
Fluoxetine
Fluphenazine
Fluvastatin
Fusidic acid
Gemfibrozil
Grapefruit juice
Haloperidol
Halothane
Heroin
Hydroxychloroquine
Ibuprofen
Influenza vaccines
Interferon alfa
Interferon beta
Isoniazid
Isotretinoin
Itraconazole
Ketoconazole
Labetalol
Lamivudine
Lamotrigine
Leflunomide
Levofloxacin
Licorice
Lindane
Lithium
Lorazepam
Lovastatin
Loxapine
MDMA

Melphalan
Mephobarbital
Meprobamate
Methadone
Methamphetamine
Methohexital
Minocycline
Mirtazapine
Mizoribine
Molindone
Morphine
Myrrh
Naltrexone
Nefazodone
Nelfinavir
Nitrazepam
Norfloxacin
Ofloxacin
Olanzapine
Pancuronium
Pemetrexed
Pemoline
Pentamidine
Pentobarbital
Perphenazine
Phendimetrazine
Phenelzine
Phenobarbital
Phenylpropanolamine
Phenytoin
Pravastatin
Primidone
Propofol
Protamine sulfate
Protriptyline
Pyrazinamide
Quetiapine
Quinacrine
Quinine
Rabeprazole
Rasagiline
Red rice yeast
Risperidone
Ritodrine
Ritonavir
Rosuvastatin
Secobarbital
Sevoflurane
Simvastatin
Sodium oxybate
Streptokinase
Streptomycin
Succinylcholine
Sulfamethoxazole
Tenecteplase
Tenofovir
Terbinafine
Terbutaline
Thiopental
Tolcapone
Trandolapril
Tranylcypromine
Trifluoperazine
Trimethoprim
Trospium
Valproic acid
Vasopressin
Verapamil
Vinblastine
Warfarin

Ziconotide
Ziprasidone
Tinnitus
Acamprosate
Acetazolamide
Albuterol
Allopurinol
Almotriptan
Alprazolam
Amikacin
Amiloride
Aminocaproic acid
Amitriptyline
Amlodipine
Amoxapine
Amphotericin B
Anagrelide
Anthrax vaccine
Aprepitant
Aripiprazole
Artemisia
Aspirin
Atazanavir
Azatadine
Azithromycin
Aztreonam
Baclofen
Benazepril
Bendroflumethiazide
Benztropine
Bepridil
Betaxolol
Bismuth
Bisoprolol
Bleomycin
Botulinum toxin (A & B)
Bupivacaine
Buprenorphine
Bupropion
Buspirone
Butorphanol
Capreomycin
Carbamazepine
Carbimazole
Carboplatin
Carisoprodol
Carteolol
Cefpodoxime
Chlorambucil
Chloramphenicol
Chloroquine
Chlorpheniramine
Cholestyramine
Cinoxacin
Ciprofloxacin
Cisplatin
Clarithromycin
Clemastine
Clindamycin
Clomipramine
Co-trimoxazole
Colistin
Cyclobenzaprine
Cyclosporine
Cyproheptadine
Dapsone
Dasatinib
Deferoxamine
Desipramine
Devil's claw

Dexibuprofen
Diazoxide
Diclofenac
Diflunisal
Diltiazem
Diphenhydramine
Doxazosin
Doxepin
Dronabinol
Eletriptan
Enalapril
Enoxacin
Erythromycin
Escitalopram
Esomeprazole
Estramustine
Eszopiclone
Etanercept
Ethacrynic acid
Ethambutol
Etodolac
Etoposide
Famotidine
Felodipine
Fenoprofen
Flecainide
Flumazenil
Fluoxetine
Flurbiprofen
Foscarnet
Fosinopril
Frovatriptan
Furosemide
Gabapentin
Gadodiamide
Gentamicin
Glatiramer
Guanfacine
Guarana
Hepatitis B vaccine
Hydroxychloroquine
Ibuprofen
Imipenem/cilastatin
Imipramine
Indomethacin
Interferon alfa
Iohexol
Isoniazid
Isosorbide
Isotretinoin
Itraconazole
Ketoprofen
Ketorolac
Lapatinib
Levobetaxolol
Levobupivacaine
Lidocaine
Lincomycin
Lisinopril
Lithium
Lomefloxacin
Loratadine
Maprotiline
Mechlorethamine
Meclofenamate
Mefloquine
Memantine
Mesalamine
Methazolamide
Methotrexate

Metolazone
Metoprolol
Metronidazole
Mexiletine
Misoprostol
Moricizine
Muromonab-CD3
Nabumetone
Nadolol
Naltrexone
Naproxen
Nicardipine
Nicotine
Nifedipine
Nitroprusside
Norfloxacin
Nortriptyline
Ofloxacin
Olsalazine
Omeprazole
Oxaprozin
Pamidronate
Paroxetine
PEG-interferon
Penicillamine
Pentazocine
Pentostatin
Pergolide
Perphenazine
Phenelzine
Piperacillin
Piroxicam
Prazosin
Pregabalin
Promethazine
Propafenone
Propofol
Propylthiouracil
Protriptyline
Pseudoephedrine
Pyrazinamide
Pyrilamine
Pyrimethamine
Quinidine
Quinine
Ramipril
Ranolazine
Ribavirin
Rifaximin
Risperidone
Rofecoxib
Rotigotine
Salsalate
Selegiline
Sertraline
Sildenafil
Sirolimus
Sorafenib
Streptomycin
Sulfadiazine
Sulfadoxine
Sulfisoxazole
Sulindac
Tacrolimus
Terazosin
Tetracycline
Thiabendazole
Ticlopidine
Timolol
Tobramycin

Tocainide
Tolmetin
Torsemide
Tranylcypromine
Triazolam
Trimeprazine
Trimipramine
Valdecoxib
Valproic acid
Vancomycin
Vardenafil
Varenicline
Venlafaxine
Vinblastine
Vincristine
Zalcitabine
Ziconotide
Ziprasidone
Zolpidem
Zuclopentixol acetate
Zuclopentixol decanoate
Zuclopentixol
    dihydrochloride

Toxic Epidermal Necrolysis (Ten)

Abacavir
Acebutolol
Aceclofenac
Acetaminophen
Acetazolamide
Aldesleukin
Alendronate
Alfuzosin
Allopurinol
Alprostadil
Amifostine
Aminosalicylate sodium
Amiodarone
Amobarbital
Amoxapine
Amoxicillin
Ampicillin
Anthrax vaccine
Armodafinil
Asparaginase
Aspirin
Atenolol
Atorvastatin
Atovaquone
Azathioprine
Aztreonam
BCG vaccine
Betaxolol
Bortezomib
Bucillamine
Butabarbital
Butalbital
Captopril
Carbamazepine
Carbenicillin
Carvedilol
Cefaclor
Cefadroxil
Cefamandole
Cefazolin
Cefdinir
Cefditoren
Cefepime
Cefixime
Cefmetazole

Cefonicid
Cefoperazone
Cefotaxime
Cefotetan
Cefoxitin
Cefpodoxime
Cefprozil
Ceftazidime
Ceftibuten
Ceftizoxime
Ceftriaxone
Cefuroxime
Celecoxib
Cephalexin
Cephalothin
Cephapirin
Cephradine
Chlorambucil
Chloramphenicol
Chlormezanone
Chloroquine
Chlorothiazide
Chlorpromazine
Chlorpropamide
Chlorthalidone
Cimetidine
Cinoxacin
Ciprofloxacin
Cladribine
Clarithromycin
Clindamycin
Clobazam
Clofibrate
Clopidogrel
Co-trimoxazole
Codeine
Colchicine
Cyclophosphamide
Cyclosporine
Cytarabine
Dactinomycin
Dapsone
Deferoxamine
Demeclocycline
Denileukin
Dexamethasone
Dexibuprofen
Dextroamphetamine
Diatrizoate
Diclofenac
Dicloxacillin
Diflunisal
Diltiazem
Diphenhydramine
Dipyridamole
Disulfiram
Docetaxel
Doripenem
Dorzolamide
Doxycycline
Enalapril
Enoxacin
Ephedrine
Erythromycin
Esomeprazole
Ethambutol
Etidronate
Etodolac
Famotidine
Felbamate

Fenbufen
Fenofibrate
Fenoprofen
Fluconazole
Fluoxetine
Fluphenazine
Flurazepam
Flurbiprofen
Flutamide
Fluvastatin
Fluvoxamine
Foscarnet
Fosphenytoin
Furosemide
Gatifloxacin
Gemcitabine
Gentamicin
Gold and gold compounds
Grepafloxacin
Griseofulvin
Heparin
Heroin
Hydrochlorothiazide
Hydrocodone
Hydroxychloroquine
Ibritumomab
Ibuprofen
Imatinib
Imipenem/cilastatin
Immune globulin I.V.
Indapamide
Indomethacin
Infliximab
Isoniazid
Isotretinoin
Ketoprofen
Ketorolac
Lamotrigine
Lansoprazole
Latanoprost
Leflunomide
Letrozole
Levofloxacin
Lincomycin
Lisdexamfetamine
Lisinopril
Lomefloxacin
Lovastatin
Lumiracoxib
Meclofenamate
Mefenamic acid
Mefloquine
Meloxicam
Meperidine
Mephenytoin
Meprobamate
Mercaptopurine
Meropenem
Metamizole
Methamphetamine
Methazolamide
Methicillin
Methimazole
Methotrexate
Methyldopa
Metolazone
Metoprolol
Metronidazole
Mezlocillin
Moxifloxacin

Nabumetone
Nadolol
Nafcillin
Nalidixic acid
Naproxen
Neomycin
Nevirapine
Nifedipine
Nitrofurantoin
Norfloxacin
Ofloxacin
Omeprazole
Oseltamivir
Oxacillin
Oxaprozin
Oxazepam
Oxcarbazepine
Pantoprazole
Papaverine
Paroxetine
Penicillamine
Penicillin V
Pentamidine
Pentazocine
Pentobarbital
Phenobarbital
Phenolphthalein
Phenylbutazone
Phenytoin
Pindolol
Piperacillin
Piroxicam
Plicamycin
Pravastatin
Primidone
Procarbazine
Prochlorperazine
Promethazine
Propranolol
Pyridoxine
Pyrimethamine
Quinidine
Quinine
Ranitidine
Reserpine
Rifampin
Ritodrine
Rituximab
Rofecoxib
Simvastatin
Smallpox vaccine
Sparfloxacin
Streptomycin
Streptozocin
Sulfacetamide
Sulfadiazine
Sulfadoxine
Sulfamethoxazole
Sulfasalazine
Sulfisoxazole
Sulindac
Terbinafine
Terconazole
Tetracycline
Thalidomide
Thiabendazole
Thiopental
Thioridazine
Ticarcillin
Timolol

Tiopronin
Tolbutamide
Tolmetin
Trimethoprim
Trovafloxacin
Valdecoxib
Valproic acid
Vancomycin
Vinorelbine
Voriconazole
Zidovudine
Zonisamide
Urticaria
Abarelix
Abatacept
Acamprosate
Acarbose
Acebutolol
Aceclofenac
Acenocoumarol
Acetaminophen
Acetazolamide
Acetohexamide
Acetylcysteine
Acitretin
Acyclovir
Adalimumab
Agalsidase
Albendazole
Albuterol
Alclometasone
Aldesleukin
Alefacept
Alemtuzumab
Alendronate
Alfentanil
Alglucerase
Alglucosidase alfa
Allopurinol
Alpha-lipoic acid
Alprazolam
Alprostadil
Alteplase
Amantadine
Amcinonide
Amifostine
Amikacin
Amiloride
Aminocaproic acid
Aminoglutethimide
Aminolevulinic acid
Aminophylline
Aminosalicylate sodium
Amiodarone
Amitriptyline
Amlodipine
Amobarbital
Amoxapine
Amoxicillin
Amphotericin B
Ampicillin
Anagrelide
Anastrozole
Anidulafungin
Anisindione
Anistreplase
Anthrax vaccine
Aprepitant
Aprobarbital
Aprotinin

Arformoterol
Aripiprazole
Arsenic
Artichoke
Asparaginase
Aspartame
Aspirin
Astemizole
Atazanavir
Atenolol
Atomoxetine
Atorvastatin
Atovaquone/proguanil
Atracurium
Atropine sulfate
Azacitidine
Azatadine
Azathioprine
Azithromycin
Aztreonam
Bacampicillin
Bacitracin
Baclofen
Basiliximab
BCG vaccine
Beclomethasone
Benactyzine
Benazepril
Bendroflumethiazide
Benzphetamine
Benzthiazide
Benztropine
Betaxolol
Bicalutamide
Biperiden
Bisacodyl
Bisoprolol
Bleomycin
Bortezomib
Botulinum toxin (A & B)
Brinzolamide
Bromocriptine
Bumetanide
Bupivacaine
Buprenorphine
Bupropion
Buspirone
Busulfan
Butabarbital
Butalbital
Butorphanol
Caffeine
Calcitonin
Candesartan
Capreomycin
Capsicum
Captopril
Caraway
Carbamazepine
Carbenicillin
Carbimazole
Carboplatin
Carisoprodol
Cefaclor
Cefadroxil
Cefamandole
Cefazolin
Cefdinir
Cefditoren
Cefepime

Cefixime
Cefmetazole
Cefonicid
Cefoperazone
Cefotaxime
Cefotetan
Cefoxitin
Cefpodoxime
Cefprozil
Ceftazidime
Ceftibuten
Ceftizoxime
Ceftriaxone
Cefuroxime
Celecoxib
Cephalexin
Cephalothin
Cephapirin
Cephradine
Certolizumab pegol
Cetirizine
Chasteberry
Chloral hydrate
Chlorambucil
Chloramphenicol
Chlordiazepoxide
Chlorhexidine
Chlormezanone
Chloroquine
Chlorothiazide
Chlorotrianisene
Chlorpromazine
Chlorpropamide
Chlorthalidone
Chlorzoxazone
Cholestyramine
Cidofovir
Cilostazol
Cimetidine
Cinoxacin
Ciprofibrate
Ciprofloxacin
Cisplatin
Citalopram
Cladribine
Clarithromycin
Clemastine
Clidinium
Clindamycin
Clioquinol
Clobazam
Clofazimine
Clofibrate
Clomiphene
Clomipramine
Clonazepam
Clonidine
Clopidogrel
Clorazepate
Clotrimazole
Cloxacillin
Clozapine
Co-trimoxazole
Cocaine
Codeine
Colchicine
Colestipol
Collagen
Cromolyn
Cyanocobalamin

Cyclamate
Cyclobenzaprine
Cyclophosphamide
Cycloserine
Cyclosporine
Cyclothiazide
Cyproheptadine
Cytarabine
Dacarbazine
Daclizumab
Dactinomycin
Danazol
Dantrolene
Dapsone
Darbepoetin alfa
Dasatinib
Daunorubicin
Decitabine
Deferasirox
Deferoxamine
Delavirdine
Demeclocycline
Denileukin
Desipramine
Desloratadine
Dexchlorpheniramine
Dexibuprofen
Dexmethylphenidate
Dexrazoxane
Dextroamphetamine
Diatrizoate
Diazepam
Diazoxide
Diclofenac
Dicloxacillin
Dicumarol
Dicyclomine
Didanosine
Diethylpropion
Diethylstilbestrol
Diflunisal
Digoxin
Diltiazem
Dimenhydrinate
Diphenhydramine
Diphenoxylate
Dipyridamole
Dirithromycin
Disopyramide
Disulfiram
Docetaxel
Dolasetron
Domperidone
Donepezil
Dopamine
Dornase alfa
Doxacurium
Doxazosin
Doxepin
Doxorubicin
Doxycycline
Echinacea
Edrophonium
Efalizumab
Efavirenz
Eletriptan
Emtricitabine
Enalapril
Enfuvirtide
Enoxacin

Enoxaparin
Ephedrine
Epinephrine
Epirubicin
Epoetin alfa
Epoprostenol
Erdosteine
Ertapenem
Erythromycin
Esmolol
Esomeprazole
Estazolam
Estramustine
Estrogens
Eszopiclone
Etanercept
Ethacrynic acid
Ethambutol
Ethchlorvynol
Ethionamide
Ethosuximide
Etidronate
Etodolac
Etoposide
Etoricoxib
Ezetimibe
Famotidine
Felbamate
Felodipine
Fenofibrate
Fenoprofen
Fentanyl
Finasteride
Flavoxate
Flecainide
Fluconazole
Flucytosine
Flumazenil
Fluorides
Fluorouracil
Fluoxetine
Fluoxymesterone
Fluphenazine
Flurazepam
Flurbiprofen
Flutamide
Fluvastatin
Fluvoxamine
Folic acid
Formoterol
Foscarnet
Fosinopril
Furazolidone
Furosemide
Gabapentin
Gadobutrol
Gadodiamide
Gadofosveset
Galsulfase
Ganciclovir
Garlic
Gatifloxacin
Gefitinib
Gemfibrozil
Gemifloxacin
Gentamicin
Glatiramer
Glimepiride
Glipizide
Glucagon

Glyburide
Glycopyrrolate
Gold and gold compounds
Goserelin
Granisetron
Granulocyte colony-
    stimulating factor (GCSF)
Grapefruit juice
Grepafloxacin
Griseofulvin
Guanethidine
Guanfacine
Haloperidol
Halothane
Hemophilus B vaccine
Henna
Heparin
Hepatitis B vaccine
Heroin
Histrelin
Hops
Hydralazine
Hydrochlorothiazide
Hydrocodone
Hydrocortisone
Hydroflumethiazide
Hydromorphone
Hydroxychloroquine
Hydroxyurea
Hydroxyzine
Hyoscyamine
Ibritumomab
Ibuprofen
Idarubicin
Idursulfase
Imatinib
Imiglucerase
Imipenem/cilastatin
Imipramine
Immune globulin I.V.
Indapamide
Indinavir
Indomethacin
Infliximab
Insulin
Insulin detemir
Insulin glulisine
Interferon alfa
Interferon beta
Iodixanol
Iohexol
Iopromide
Ipodate
Ipratropium
Irbesartan
Isoniazid
Isoproterenol
Isotretinoin
Isradipine
Itraconazole
Ivermectin
Kanamycin
Kava
Ketoconazole
Ketoprofen
Ketorolac
Labetalol
Lamivudine
Lamotrigine
Lansoprazole

Laronidase
Leflunomide
Leucovorin
Leuprolide
Levamisole
Levobunolol
Levobupivacaine
Levocetirizine
Levodopa
Levofloxacin
Levoleucovorin
Levothyroxine
Lidocaine
Lincomycin
Lindane
Liothyronine
Lisdexamfetamine
Lisinopril
Lithium
Lomefloxacin
Loperamide
Loracarbef
Loratadine
Lorazepam
Losartan
Lovastatin
Loxapine
Lubiprostone
Lutropin alfa
Maprotiline
Marihuana
Mazindol
Mebendazole
Mechlorethamine
Meclizine
Meclofenamate
Medroxyprogesterone
Mefenamic acid
Mefloquine
Meloxicam
Melphalan
Memantine
Mepenzolate
Meperidine
Mephenytoin
Mephobarbital
Meprobamate
Mercaptopurine
Meropenem
Mesalamine
Mesna
Mesoridazine
Metamizole
Metaxalone
Metformin
Methadone
Methamphetamine
Methantheline
Methazolamide
Methenamine
Methicillin
Methimazole
Methocarbamol
Methohexital
Methotrexate
Methoxsalen
Methsuximide
Methyclothiazide
Methyldopa
Methylphenidate

Methylprednisolone
Methyltestosterone
Methysergide
Metoclopramide
Metolazone
Metoprolol
Metronidazole
Mexiletine
Mezlocillin
Miconazole
Midazolam
Milk thistle
Minocycline
Minoxidil
Mitomycin
Mitotane
Mitoxantrone
Moclobemide
Moexipril
Monosodium glutamate
Montelukast
Moricizine
Moxifloxacin
Mycophenolate
Nabumetone
Nadolol
Nafarelin
Nafcillin
Nalbuphine
Nalidixic acid
Naloxone
Naproxen
Naratriptan
Nefazodone
Nelfinavir
Neomycin
Niacin
Nicardipine
Nicotine
Nifedipine
Nilutamide
Nimesulide
Nisoldipine
Nitrofurantoin
Nitroglycerin
Nizatidine
Norfloxacin
Nortriptyline
Nystatin
Octreotide
Ofloxacin
Olanzapine
Olsalazine
Omalizumab
Omeprazole
Ondansetron
Oral contraceptives
Orphenadrine
Oxacillin
Oxaliplatin
Oxaprozin
Oxazepam
Oxilan
Oxybutynin
Oxycodone
Oxymorphone
Oxytetracycline
Paclitaxel
Pantoprazole
Pantothenic acid

Papaverine
Paroxetine
PEG-interferon
Pegaptanib
Pegaspargase
Pegfilgrastim
Penciclovir
Penicillamine
Penicillin G
Penicillin V
Pentagastrin
Pentamidine
Pentazocine
Pentobarbital
Pentosan
Pentostatin
Pentoxifylline
Perflutren
Pergolide
Perphenazine
Phendimetrazine
Phenelzine
Phenindamine
Phenobarbital
Phenolphthalein
Phentermine
Phenylbutazone
Phenytoin
Phytonadione
Pilocarpine
Pimozide
Pindolol
Pipecuronium
Piperacillin
Piroxicam
Pneumococcal vaccine
Polythiazide
Porfimer
Potassium iodide
Pravastatin
Prazepam
Praziquantel
Prazosin
Prednicarbate
Prednisolone
Prednisone
Pregabalin
Primaquine
Primidone
Probenecid
Procainamide
Procarbazine
Prochlorperazine
Procyclidine
Progestins
Promazine
Promethazine
Propafenone
Propantheline
Propofol
Propoxyphene
Propranolol
Propylthiouracil
Protamine sulfate
Protein C concentrate
  (human)
Protriptyline
Pseudoephedrine
Psoralens
Pyrazinamide

Pyrilamine
Pyrimethamine
Quazepam
Quinacrine
Quinapril
Quinestrol
Quinethazone
Quinidine
Quinine
Quinupristin/dalfopristin
Rabeprazole
Ramipril
Ranitidine
Rapacuronium
Rasburicase
Reserpine
Ribavirin
Riboflavin
Rifabutin
Rifampin
Rifapentine
Rifaximin
Risedronate
Risperidone
Ritodrine
Ritonavir
Rituximab
Rivastigmine
Rofecoxib
Ropinirole
Roxithromycin
Saccharin
Salmeterol
Salsalate
Saquinavir
Scopolamine
Secobarbital
Secretin
Sermorelin
Sertraline
Sildenafil
Simvastatin
Smallpox vaccine
Somatropin
Sorafenib
Sotalol
Sparfloxacin
Spectinomycin
Spironolactone
Squill
Stanozolol
Streptokinase
Streptomycin
Succinylcholine
Sucralfate
Sufentanil
Sulfadiazine
Sulfadoxine
Sulfamethoxazole
Sulfasalazine
Sulfisoxazole
Sulfites
Sulindac
Sumatriptan
Tacrine
Tacrolimus
Tamoxifen
Tartrazine
Telithromycin
Temazepam

Tenecteplase
Teniposide
Terbinafine
Terbutaline
Terfenadine
Testosterone
Tetracycline
Thalidomide
Thiabendazole
Thiamine
Thimerosal
Thiopental
Thioridazine
Thiotepa
Thiothixene
Tiagabine
Ticarcillin
Ticlopidine
Tigecycline
Timolol
Tinidazole
Tinzaparin
Tiopronin
Tiotropium
Tirofiban
Tizanidine
Tobramycin
Tolazamide
Tolazoline
Tolbutamide
Tolcapone
Tolmetin
Topiramate
Torsemide
Tramadol
Tranylcypromine
Trazodone
Triamcinolone
Triamterene
Triazolam
Trichlormethiazide
Trifluoperazine
Trihexyphenidyl
Trimeprazine
Trimethadione
Trimethoprim
Trimipramine
Tripelennamine
Triprolidine
Troleandomycin
Trovafloxacin
Urofollitropin
Urokinase
Ursodiol
Valdecoxib
Valproic acid
Valsartan
Vancomycin
Vardenafil
Varenicline
Varicella vaccine
Vasopressin
Venlafaxine
Verapamil
Verteporfin
Vinblastine
Vincristine
Vitamin E
Voriconazole
Warfarin

Yarrow
Zalcitabine
Zanamivir
Zidovudine
Ziprasidone
Zolmitriptan
Zolpidem
Zonisamide

Vasculitis
Acebutolol
Aceclofenac
Acenocoumarol
Acetaminophen
Acyclovir
Adalimumab
Aldesleukin
Allopurinol
Amiloride
Aminosalicylate sodium
Amiodarone
Amitriptyline
Amlodipine
Amoxapine
Amoxicillin
Amphotericin B
Ampicillin
Anistreplase
Anthrax vaccine
Aspartame
Aspirin
Atenolol
Azatadine
Azathioprine
Azithromycin
Basiliximab
BCG vaccine
Benazepril
Bendroflumethiazide
Benzthiazide
Bexarotene
Bismuth
Bisoprolol
Bortezomib
Bosentan
Bromocriptine
Bumetanide
Busulfan
Butabarbital
Butalbital
Captopril
Carbamazepine
Carbenicillin
Carbimazole
Caspofungin
Cefdinir
Celecoxib
Certolizumab pegol
Cevimeline
Chloramphenicol
Chlordiazepoxide
Chloroquine
Chlorothiazide
Chlorpromazine
Chlorpropamide
Chlorthalidone
Chlorzoxazone
Cimetidine
Ciprofloxacin
Citalopram
Cladribine

Clarithromycin
Clindamycin
Clomipramine
Clopidogrel
Clorazepate
Clozapine
Co-trimoxazole
Cocaine
Colchicine
Cromolyn
Cyclophosphamide
Cyclosporine
Cyclothiazide
Cyproheptadine
Cytarabine
Dacarbazine
Delavirdine
Desipramine
Dexibuprofen
Diazepam
Diclofenac
Dicloxacillin
Didanosine
Diflunisal
Digoxin
Diltiazem
Diphenhydramine
Disulfiram
Doxepin
Doxycycline
Efavirenz
Enalapril
Enfuvirtide
Ephedrine
Epirubicin
Erythromycin
Estrogens
Etanercept
Ethacrynic acid
Etodolac
Famciclovir
Famotidine
Fenbufen
Fluoxetine
Flurbiprofen
Fluticasone
Fluvastatin
Fosinopril
Furosemide
Gabapentin
Gatifloxacin
Gemcitabine
Gemfibrozil
Gentamicin
Ginkgo biloba
Glucagon
Glyburide
Gold and gold compounds
Granulocyte colony-
  stimulating factor (GCSF)
Griseofulvin
Guanethidine
Heparin
Hepatitis B vaccine
Heroin
Hydralazine
Hydrochlorothiazide
Hydroflumethiazide
Hydroxychloroquine
Hydroxyurea

Ibuprofen
Imatinib
Imipenem/cilastatin
Imipramine
Immune globulin I.V.
Indapamide
Indinavir
Indomethacin
Infliximab
Influenza vaccines
Insulin
Interferon alfa
Interferon beta
Isoniazid
Isotretinoin
Itraconazole
Ixabepilone
Ketoconazole
Leflunomide
Levamisole
Levofloxacin
Lisinopril
Lithium
Lomefloxacin
Lovastatin
Maprotiline
Meclofenamate
Mefenamic acid
Mefloquine
Meloxicam
Melphalan
Meperidine
Meprobamate
Mercaptopurine
Mesalamine
Metformin
Methazolamide
Methicillin
Methimazole
Methotrexate
Methoxsalen
Methyldopa
Methylphenidate
Metolazone
Metronidazole
Mezlocillin
Minocycline
Mitotane
Nabumetone
Nafcillin
Naproxen
Nelfinavir
Nicotine
Nifedipine
Nimesulide
Nizatidine
Norfloxacin
Nortriptyline
Ofloxacin
Olanzapine
Omeprazole
Oxacillin
Oxaprozin
Oxytetracycline
Pantoprazole
Paroxetine
Pemetrexed
Penicillamine
Penicillin V
Pentamidine

Pentobarbital
Pergolide
Phenobarbital
Phentermine
Phenylbutazone
Phenytoin
Phytonadione
Piperacillin
Piroxicam
Polythiazide
Potassium iodide
Pramipexole
Pravastatin
Procainamide
Propylthiouracil
Protriptyline
Psoralens
Pyridoxine
Pyrimethamine
Quinapril
Quinethazone
Quinidine
Quinine
Ramipril
Ranitidine
Rifampin
Ritodrine
Rofecoxib
Simvastatin
Sirolimus
Sorafenib
Sotalol
Sparfloxacin
Spironolactone
Streptokinase
Streptomycin
Sulfamethoxazole
Sulfasalazine
Sulfisoxazole
Sulfites
Sulindac
Tamoxifen
Tartrazine
Telithromycin
Terbutaline
Tetracycline
Thalidomide
Thiamine
Thioridazine
Ticarcillin
Ticlopidine
Tinidazole
Tocainide
Torsemide
Trazodone
Tretinoin
Triamterene
Trichlormethiazide
Trimethadione
Trioxsalen
Triptorelin
Trovafloxacin
Valproic acid
Vancomycin
Verapamil
Vinorelbine
Warfarin
Zafirlukast
Zidovudine

Vertigo
Abacavir
Abarelix
Abatacept
Acamprosate
Aceclofenac
Acenocoumarol
Adenosine
Agalsidase
Alefacept
Alfuzosin
Aliskiren
Almotriptan
Alpha-lipoic acid
Amlodipine
Anidulafungin
Apomorphine
Aprepitant
Armodafinil
Artemisia
Atazanavir
Atomoxetine
Atovaquone/proguanil
Azacitidine
Baclofen
Benzphetamine
Bepridil
Bevacizumab
Biperiden
Black cohosh
Bortezomib
Bosentan
Botulinum toxin (A & B)
Buprenorphine
Bupropion
Butorphanol
Cabergoline
Candesartan
Capecitabine
Capreomycin
Carbamazepine
Carbinoxamine
Carvedilol
Ceftobiprole
Celiprolol
Certolizumab pegol
Cilazapril
Cilostazol
Cinacalcet
Cinnarizine
Ciprofibrate
Citalopram
Clevidipine
Clobazam
Clofarabine
Clozapine
Colistin
Cyclobenzaprine
Dantrolene
Daptomycin
Darbepoetin alfa
Darifenacin
Darunavir
Dasatinib
Decitabine
Desvenlafaxine
Dexibuprofen
Dexmethylphenidate
Dexrazoxane
Dextromethorphan

Diatrizoate
Diazepam
Dihydroergotamine
Diltiazem
Dinoprostone
Dolasetron
Donepezil
Doxazosin
Dronabinol
Duloxetine
Dutasteride
Echinacea
Eculizumab
Edrophonium
Efavirenz
Emtricitabine
Enfuvirtide
Entacapone
Entecavir
Eplerenone
Epoprostenol
Eprosartan
Escitalopram
Eszopiclone
Etanercept
Etravirine
Eucalyptus
Fenoldopam
Fentanyl
Floxuridine
Flumazenil
Fluticasone
Fomepizole
Fomivirsen
Frovatriptan
Gabapentin
Gadobutrol
Gadodiamide
Gadofosveset
Galantamine
Gatifloxacin
Gemifloxacin
Gentamicin
Glatiramer
Glimepiride
Granulocyte colony-
    stimulating factor (GCSF)
Guanabenz
Guanadrel
Guanethidine
Guarana
Hawthorn (fruit, leaf, flower
    extract)
Histrelin
Hydralazine
Hydrocortisone
Hydromorphone
Hyoscyamine
Ibandronate
Icodextrin
Iloprost
Imidapril
Imiglucerase
Imiquimod
Immune globulin I.V.
Infliximab
Influenza vaccines
Insulin detemir
Interferon beta
Iodixanol

Iohexol
Iopromide
Irinotecan
Isocarboxazid
Isradipine
Ivabradine
Ixabepilone
Kava
Ketorolac
Lamivudine
Lamotrigine
Lenalidomide
Levetiracetam
Liothyronine
Lisdexamfetamine
Lithium
Lodoxamide
Lorcainide
Lubiprostone
Lumiracoxib
Lutropin alfa
Maraviroc
Mazindol
Mebendazole
Mecamylamine
Mecasermin
Mefloquine
Memantine
Mepenzolate
Meperidine
Meropenem
Metaxalone
Methotrexate
Methylprednisolone
Metipranolol
Mianserin
Miglustat
Moclobemide
Modafinil
Morphine
Moxifloxacin
Mupirocin
Muromonab-CD3
Mycophenolate
Nabilone
Nalbuphine
Nalmefene
Naltrexone
Naratriptan
Nateglinide
Nebivolol
Nefazodone
Nelarabine
Nelfinavir
Nicorandil
Nilutamide
Nimesulide
Nisoldipine
Nitazoxanide
Nitrazepam
Norfloxacin
Nortriptyline
Olanzapine
Olmesartan
Omalizumab
Oxaliplatin
Oxcarbazepine
Oxilan
Oxymorphone
Paclitaxel

Palonosetron
Paricalcitol
Pegaptanib
Pegaspargase
Pegvisomant
Pemetrexed
Perflutren
Pergolide
Phenelzine
Phenoxybenzamine
Posaconazole
Pramipexole
Pramlintide
Pranlukast
Praziquantel
Prednicarbate
Prednisolone
Prednisone
Pregabalin
Promazine
Propoxyphene
Protein C concentrate
    (human)
Pyrimethamine
Quetiapine
Ramelteon
Ramipril
Ranolazine
Rasagiline
Reboxetine
Red rice yeast
Regadenoson
Rifampin
Rifaximin
Riluzole
Rimantadine
Rimonabant
Rivastigmine
Rizatriptan
Rofecoxib
Romiplostim
Ropinirole
Rosuvastatin
Rotigotine
Roxatidine
Scopolamine
Sermorelin
Sibutramine
Sincalide
Sitaxentan
Solifenacin
Spectinomycin
Succimer
Sulfadoxine
Sumatriptan
Sunitinib
Tadalafil
Tamsulosin
Tegaserod
Telbivudine
Telithromycin
Telmisartan
Teriparatide
Tetrabenazine
Thalidomide
Tiagabine
Tigecycline
Tiludronate
Tinidazole
Tipranavir

Tizanidine
Tolcapone
Tolterodine
Topiramate
Tositumomab & iodine[Protein C concentrate]
Tramadol
Trandolapril
Tranylcypromine
Trazodone
Treprostinil
Trimipramine
Trospium
Trovafloxacin
Urapidil
Ursodiol
Valproic acid
Valrubicin
Valsartan
Vardenafil
Varenicline
Varicella vaccine
Venlafaxine
Verapamil
Vigabatrin
Vorinostat
Zaleplon
Ziconotide
Zolmitriptan
Zolpidem
Zonisamide
Zuclopentixol acetate
Zuclopentixol decanoate
Zuclopentixol
    dihydrochloride

Xerostomia
Acamprosate
Acebutolol
Acetazolamide
Acitretin
Albendazole
Albuterol
Aldesleukin
Almotriptan
Alprazolam
Alprostadil
Amantadine
Amifostine
Amiloride
Amisulpride
Amitriptyline
Amlodipine
Amoxapine
Amoxicillin
Amphotericin B
Anastrozole
Apraclonidine
Arbutamine
Aripiprazole
Armodafinil
Astemizole
Atomoxetine
Atropine sulfate
Azatadine
Azathioprine
Azelastine
Bacampicillin
Baclofen
Balsalazide
Benactyzine

Bendamustine
Bendroflumethiazide
Benzphetamine
Benztropine
Bepridil
Betaxolol
Bevacizumab
Bexarotene
Bicalutamide
Biperiden
Bismuth
Bisoprolol
Botulinum toxin (A & B)
Brimonidine
Brinzolamide
Bromocriptine
Brompheniramine
Buclizine
Bumetanide
Buprenorphine
Bupropion
Buspirone
Butorphanol
Cabergoline
Caffeine
Captopril
Carbamazepine
Carbenicillin
Carbinoxamine
Carisoprodol
Carteolol
Carvedilol
Cefditoren
Cefixime
Ceftibuten
Celecoxib
Cetirizine
Cevimeline
Chloramphenicol
Chlordiazepoxide
Chlormezanone
Chlorpheniramine
Chlorpromazine
Chlortetracycline
Ciclesonide
Cidofovir
Cimetidine
Cinnarizine
Ciprofloxacin
Citalopram
Clarithromycin
Clemastine
Clidinium
Clobazam
Clomipramine
Clonazepam
Clonidine
Clorazepate
Clozapine
Codeine
Conivaptan
Cromolyn
Cyclobenzaprine
Cyproheptadine
Darifenacin
Darunavir
Delavirdine
Desipramine
Desloratadine
Desvenlafaxine

Dexchlorpheniramine
Dextroamphetamine
Diazepam
Diazoxide
Diclofenac
Dicloxacillin
Dicyclomine
Didanosine
Diethylpropion
Diflunisal
Dihydroergotamine
Dihydrotachysterol
Diltiazem
Dimenhydrinate
Diphenhydramine
Diphenoxylate
Dirithromycin
Disopyramide
Donepezil
Doxazosin
Doxepin
Dronabinol
Duloxetine
Efavirenz
Enalapril
Enoxacin
Entacapone
Ephedra
Ephedrine
Epinephrine
Eprosartan
Ergocalciferol
Escitalopram
Esmolol
Esomeprazole
Estazolam
Eszopiclone
Ethacrynic acid
Ethionamide
Etodolac
Etravirine
Famotidine
Felbamate
Felodipine
Fenoprofen
Fentanyl
Flavoxate
Flecainide
Fluconazole
Flucytosine
Flumazenil
Fluorides
Fluoxetine
Fluphenazine
Flurazepam
Flurbiprofen
Fluvoxamine
Formoterol
Foscarnet
Fosfomycin
Fosinopril
Fosphenytoin
Frovatriptan
Furosemide
Gabapentin
Gadobutrol
Gadodiamide
Gadofosveset
Galantamine
Ganciclovir

Gemifloxacin
Glatiramer
Glycopyrrolate
Granisetron
Grepafloxacin
Griseofulvin
Guanabenz
Guanadrel
Guanethidine
Guanfacine
Haloperidol
Hydrochlorothiazide
Hydrocodone
Hydromorphone
Hydroxyzine
Hyoscyamine
Ibuprofen
Imipramine
Indapamide
Indinavir
Indomethacin
Insulin
Interferon alfa
Interferon beta
Ipratropium
Isocarboxazid
Isoetharine
Isoniazid
Isoproterenol
Isosorbide dinitrate
Isotretinoin
Isradipine
Itraconazole
Ketoprofen
Ketorolac
Ketotifen
Labetalol
Lamotrigine
Lansoprazole
Leflunomide
Lenalidomide
Levocetirizine
Levodopa
Levofloxacin
Lisdexamfetamine
Lisinopril
Lithium
Lomefloxacin
Loperamide
Loratadine
Lorazepam
Losartan
Lovastatin
Loxapine
Lubiprostone
Maprotiline
Marihuana
Mazindol
MDMA
Mebendazole
Mecamylamine
Meclizine
Meclofenamate
Mefenamic acid
Meloxicam
Mepenzolate
Meperidine
Meprobamate
Mesoridazine
Metamizole

Methadone
Methamphetamine
Methantheline
Methazolamide
Methicillin
Methyldopa
Methylphenidate
Metoclopramide
Metolazone
Metronidazole
Mexiletine
Mezlocillin
Mianserin
Midodrine
Miglustat
Mirtazapine
Moclobemide
Modafinil
Moexipril
Molindone
Moricizine
Morphine
Moxifloxacin
Mupirocin
Nabilone
Nabumetone
Nadolol
Nafcillin
Nalbuphine
Nalmefene
Naloxone
Naltrexone
Naproxen
Nedocromil
Nefazodone
Nevirapine
Niacin
Nicardipine
Nicotine
Nifedipine
Nilutamide
Nisoldipine
Nitrofurantoin
Nitroglycerin
Nizatidine
Norfloxacin
Nortriptyline
Octreotide
Ofloxacin
Olanzapine
Omeprazole
Ondansetron
Orphenadrine
Oxacillin
Oxaliplatin
Oxazepam
Oxcarbazepine
Oxybutynin
Oxycodone
Oxymorphone
Paliperidone
Palonosetron
Pantoprazole
Papaverine
Paricalcitol
Paroxetine
Pentamidine
Pentazocine
Pentoxifylline
Perflutren

Pergolide
Perindopril
Perphenazine
Phendimetrazine
Phenelzine
Phenindamine
Phenobarbital
Phenoxybenzamine
Phentermine
Phenylbutazone
Phenylpropanolamine
Pimozide
Pirbuterol
Piroxicam
Pramipexole
Prazepam
Prazosin
Pregabalin
Procarbazine
Prochlorperazine
Procyclidine
Promazine
Promethazine
Propafenone
Propantheline
Propofol
Propoxyphene
Propranolol
Protriptyline
Pseudoephedrine
Pyrilamine
Pyrimethamine
Quazepam
Quetiapine
Quinapril

Quinethazone
Rabeprazole
Raltitrexed
Ramipril
Ranolazine
Rasagiline
Reboxetine
Reserpine
Riluzole
Rimantadine
Risperidone
Ritonavir
Rivastigmine
Rizatriptan
Rofecoxib
Ropinirole
Rotigotine
Saquinavir
Scopolamine
Selegiline
Sertraline
Sevoflurane
Sibutramine
Sildenafil
Solifenacin
Sorafenib
Sotalol
Sparfloxacin
Spironolactone
St John's wort
Sucralfate
Sulfasalazine
Sulindac
Sumatriptan
Tacrine

Tadalafil
Tamoxifen
Telithromycin
Telmisartan
Temazepam
Terazosin
Terbutaline
Terfenadine
Thalidomide
Thiabendazole
Thioguanine
Thioridazine
Thiothixene
Tiagabine
Ticarcillin
Tigecycline
Tiludronate
Timolol
Tinidazole
Tiopronin
Tiotropium
Tizanidine
Tocainide
Tolcapone
Tolmetin
Tolterodine
Topiramate
Torsemide
Tramadol
Trandolapril
Tranylcypromine
Trazodone
Tretinoin
Triamcinolone
Triamterene

Triazolam
Trichlormethiazide
Trifluoperazine
Trihexyphenidyl
Trimeprazine
Trimipramine
Tripelennamine
Triprolidine
Trospium
Trovafloxacin
Tryptophan
Unoprostone
Valdecoxib
Valproic acid
Valsartan
Vardenafil
Venlafaxine
Verapamil
Vitamin A
Voriconazole
Vorinostat
Zalcitabine
Zaleplon
Ziconotide
Zinc
Ziprasidone
Zolmitriptan
Zolpidem
Zonisamide
Zuclopentixol acetate
Zuclopentixol decanoate
Zuclopentixol
    dihydrochloride

DESCRIPTION OF THE 41 MOST COMMON REACTION PATTERNS

Acanthosis nigricans

Acanthosis nigricans (AN) is a process characterized by a soft, velvety, brown or grayish-black thickening of the skin that is symmetrically distributed over the axillae, neck, inguinal areas and other body folds.

While most cases of AN are seen in obese and prepubertal children, it can occur as a marker for various endocrinopathies as well as in female patients with elevated testosterone levels, irregular menses, and hirsutism.

It is frequently a concomitant of an underlying malignant condition, principally an adenocarcinoma of the intestinal tract.

Acneform lesions

Acneform eruptions are inflammatory follicular reactions that resemble acne vulgaris and that are manifested clinically as papules or pustules. They are monomorphic reactions, have a monomorphic appearance, and are found primarily on the upper parts of the body. Unlike acne vulgaris, there are rarely comedones present. Consider a drug-induced acneform eruption if:

- The onset is sudden

- There is a worsening of existing acne lesions

- The extent is considerable from the outset

- The appearance is monomorphic

- The localization is unusual for acne as, for example, when the distal extremities are involved

- The patient's age is unusual for regular acne

- There is an exposure to a potentially responsible drug.

The most common drugs responsible for acneform eruptions are: ACTH, androgenic hormones, anticonvulsants (hydantoin derivatives, phenobarbital, trimethadione), corticosteroids, danazol, disulfiram, halogens (bromides, chlorides, iodides), lithium, oral contraceptives, tuberculostatics (ethionamide, isoniazid, rifampin), vitamins B2, B6, and B12.

Acral erythema

Chemotherapy-induced acral erythema (CIAE), a toxic reaction to a number of different chemotherapeutic agents, causes a symmetrical, painful erythema of the palms and soles, often culminating in the formation of vesicles or bullae. Some of the well known chemotherapeutic agents responsible are cytarabine, fluorouracil and methotrexate.

Acute febrile neutrophilic dermatosis

Acute febrile neutrophilic dermatosis, also known as Sweet syndrome, is a reactive process characterized by the abrupt onset of tender, red-to-purple papules, and nodules that coalesce to form plaques. The plaques usually occur on the upper extremities, face, or neck and are typically accompanied by fever and peripheral neutrophilia. Common causes of this disorder are Granulocyte Colony-Stimulating Factor (35 references), hydralazine and co-trimoxazole.

Acute generalized exanthematous pustulosis

Arising on the face or intertriginous areas, acute generalized exanthematous pustulosis (AGEP) is characterized by a rapidly evolving, widespread, scarlatiniform eruption covered with hundreds of small superficial pustules.

Often accompanied by a high fever, AGEP is most frequently associated with acetaminophen, carbamazepine, penicillin and macrolide antibiotics, and usually occurs within 24 hours of the drug exposure.

Ageusia

Ageusia is the loss of taste functions of the tongue, particularly the inability to detect sweetness, sourness, bitterness, saltiness, and umami (the taste of monosodium glutamate). It is sometimes confused for anosmia - a loss of the sense of smell. True aguesia is relatively rare compared to hypogeusia – a partial loss of taste – and dysgeusia – a distortion or alteration of taste.

Atorvastatin, captopril, enalapril, indomethacin, and paroxetine are some of the drugs that can occasion ageusia.

Alopecia

Many drugs have been reported to occasion hair loss. Commonly appearing as a diffuse alopecia, it affects women more frequently than men and is limited in most instances to the scalp. Axillary and pubic hairs are rarely affected except with anticoagulants.

The hair loss from cytostatic agents, which is dose-dependent and begins about 2 weeks after the onset of therapy, is a result of the interruption of the anagen (growing) cycle of hair. With other drugs the hair loss does not begin until 2–5 months after the medication has been begun. With cholesterol-lowering drugs, diffuse alopecia is a result of interference with normal keratinization.

The scalp is normal and the drug-induced alopecia is almost always reversible within 1–3 months after the therapy has been discontinued. The regrown hair is frequently depigmented and occasionally curlier.

The most frequent offenders are cytostatic agents and anticoagulants, but hair loss can occur with a variety of common drugs, including hormones, anticonvulsants, amantadine, amiodarone, captopril, cholesterol-lowering drugs, cimetidine, colchicine, etretinate, isotretinoin, ketoconazole, heavy metals, lithium, penicillamine, valproic acid, and propranolol.

Angioedema

Angioedema is a term applied to a variant of urticaria in which the subcutaneous tissues, rather than the dermis, are mainly involved.

Also known as Quincke's edema, giant urticaria, and angioneurotic edema, this acute, evanescent, skin-colored, circumscribed edema usually affects the most distensible tissues: the lips, eyelids, earlobes, and genitalia. It can also affect the mucous membranes of the tongue, mouth, and larynx.

Symptoms of angioedema, frequently unilateral, asymmetrical and non-pruritic, last for an hour or two but can persist for 2–5 days.

The etiological factors associated with angioedema are as varied as that of urticaria (which see).

Anosmia

Anosmia is the loss of the sense of smell. While termed as a disability, anosmia is often viewed in the medical field as a trivial problem. The loss of the sense of smell, however, can have profound psychological and somatic consequences. It has been estimated that two million Americans suffer with smell and taste disorders, but because this disorder is not life threatening, its importance is frequently underestimated.

Drugs that have been reported to cause anosmia are cocaine (10%), terbinafine, interferon alfa-2, doxycycline, enalapril, and others.

The various types of olfactory disorders can be listed as anosmia (loss of smell), hyposmia (partial loss of smell), hyperosmia (enhanced smell sensitivity), and dysosmia (distortion in odor perception.) Dysosmia can further be divided into parosmia (distortion of perception of external stimuli) and phantosmia (smell perception with no external stimuli).

Aphthous stomatitis

Aphthous stomatitis – also known as canker sores – is a common disease of the oral mucous membranes.

Arising as tiny, discrete or grouped, papules or vesicles, these painful lesions develop into small (2–5 mm in diameter), round, shallow ulcerations having a grayish, yellow base surrounded by a thin red border.

Located predominantly over the labial and buccal mucosae, these aphthae heal without scarring in 10–14 days. Recurrences are common.

Baboon syndrome

The Baboon Syndrome is an unusual presentation of a drug eruption with a characteristic intertriginous distribution pattern. Several drugs have been implicated, notably mercury, nickel, heparin, aminophylline, pseudoephedrine, terbinafine, IVIG, various antibiotics (amoxicillin, ampicillin), and food additives.

Originally described as a type of systemic contact dermatitis characterized by a pruritic exanthem involving the buttocks and major flexures – groins and axillae, some investigators believe that this entity is a form of recall phenomenon. In children, it is important in the differential diagnosis of viral exanthems.

Black tongue (lingua villosa nigra)

Black hairy tongue (BHT) represents a benign hyperplasia of the filiform papillae of the anterior two-thirds of the tongue.

These papillary elongations, usually associated with black, brown, or yellow pigmentation attributed to the overgrowth of pigment-producing bacteria, may be as long as 2 cm.

Occurring only in adults, BHT has been associated with the administration of oral antibiotics, poor dental hygiene, and excessive smoking.

Bullous dermatitis

Bullous and vesicular drug eruptions are diseases in which blisters and vesicles occur as a complication of the administration of drugs. Blisters are a well-known manifestation of cutaneous reactions to drugs.

In many types of drug reactions, bullae and vesicles may be found in addition to other manifestations. Bullae are usually noted in erythema multiforme, Stevens–Johnson syndrome, toxic epidermal necrolysis, fixed eruptions when very intense, urticaria, vasculitis, porphyria cutanea tarda, and phototoxic reactions (from furosemide and nalidixic acid). Tense, thick-walled bullae can be seen in bromoderma and iododerma as well as in barbiturate overdosage.

Common drugs that cause bullous eruptions and bullous pemphigoid are: nadalol, penicillamine, piroxicam, psoralens, rifampin, clonidine, furosemide, diclofenac, mefenamic acid, bleomycin, and others.

DRESS syndrome

The DRESS syndrome is an acronym for Drug Rash with Eosinophilia and Systemic Symptoms. It is also known as the Drug-Induced Pseudolymphoma and Drug Hypersensitivity Syndrome. The symptoms of DRESS syndrome usually begin 1 to 8 weeks after exposure to the offending drug. Common causes include carbamazepine, phenobarbital, phenytoin, terbinafine, and valproic acid.

Erythema multiforme and Stevens–Johnson syndrome

Erythema multiforme is a relatively common, acute, self-limited, inflammatory reaction pattern that is often associated with a preceding herpes simplex or mycoplasma infection. Other causes are associated with connective tissue disease, physical agents, X-ray therapy, pregnancy and internal malignancies, to mention a few. In 50% of the cases, no cause can be found. In a recent prospective study of erythema multiforme, only 10% were drug related.

The eruption rapidly occurs over a period of 12 to 24 hours. In about half the cases there are prodromal symptoms of an upper respiratory infection accompanied by fever, malaise, and varying degrees of muscular and joint pains.

Clinically, bluish-red, well-demarcated, macular, papular, or urticarial lesions, as well as the classical 'iris' or 'target lesions', sometimes with central vesicles, bullae, or purpura, are distributed preferentially over the distal extremities, especially over the dorsa of the hands and extensor aspects of the forearms. Lesions tend to spread peripherally and may involve the palms and trunk as well as the mucous membranes of the mouth and genitalia. Central healing and overlapping lesions often lead to arciform, annular and gyrate patterns. Lesions appear over the course of a week or 10 days and resolve over the next 2 weeks.

The Stevens–Johnson syndrome (erythema multiforme major), a severe and occasionally fatal variety of erythema multiforme, has an abrupt onset and is accompanied by any or all of the following: fever, myalgia, malaise, headache, arthralgia, ocular involvement, with occasional bullae and erosions covering less than 10% of the body surface. Painful stomatitis is an early and conspicuous symptom. Hemorrhagic bullae may appear over the lips, mouth and genital mucous membranes. Patients are often acutely ill with high fever. The course from eruption to the healing of the lesions may extend up to 6 weeks.

The following drugs have been most often associated with erythema multiforme and Stevens–Johnson syndrome: allopurinol, lamotrigine phenytoin, barbiturates, carbamazepine, estrogens/progestins, gold, NSAIDs, penicillamine, sulfonamides, tetracycline, and tolbutamide.

Erythema nodosum

Erythema nodosum is a cutaneous reaction pattern characterized by erythematous, tender or painful subcutaneous nodules commonly distributed over the anterior aspect of the lower legs, and occasionally elsewhere.

More common in young women, erythema nodosum is often associated with increased estrogen levels as occurs during pregnancy and with the ingestion of oral contraceptives. It is also an occasional manifestation of streptococcal infection, sarcoidosis, secondary syphilis, tuberculosis, certain deep fungal infections, Hodgkin's disease, leukemia, ulcerative colitis, and radiation therapy and is often preceded by fever, fatigue, arthralgia, vomiting, and diarrhea.

The incidence of erythema nodosum due to drugs is low and it is impossible to distinguish clinically between erythema nodosum due to drugs and that caused by other factors.

Some of the drugs that are known to occasion erythema nodosum are: antibiotics, estrogens, amiodarone, gold, NSAIDs, oral contraceptives, sulfonamides, and opiates.

Exanthems

Exanthems, commonly resembling viral rashes, represent the most common type of cutaneous drug eruption. Described as maculopapular or morbilliform eruptions, these flat, barely raised, erythematous patches, from one to several millimeters in diameter, are usually bilateral and symmetrical. They commonly begin on the head and neck or upper torso and progress downward to the limbs. They may present or develop into confluent areas and may be accompanied by pruritus and a mild fever.

The exanthems caused by drugs can be classified as either:

• Morbilliform eruptions: fingernail-sized erythematous patches

• Scarlatiniform eruptions: punctate, pinpoint, or pinhead-sized lesions in erythematous areas that have a tendency to coalesce. Circumoral pallor and the subsequent appearance of scaling may also be noted.

Maculopapular drug eruptions usually fade with desquamation and, occasionally, postinflammatory hyperpigmentation, in about 2 weeks. They invariably recur on rechallenge.

Exanthems often have a sudden onset during the first 2 weeks of administration, except for semisynthetic penicillins that frequently develop after the first 2 weeks following the initial dose.

The drugs most commonly associated with exanthems are: amoxicillin, ampicillin, bleomycin, captopril, carbamazepine, chlorpromazine, co-trimoxazole, gold, nalidixic acid, naproxen, phenytoin, penicillamine, and piroxicam.

Exfoliative dermatitis

Exfoliative dermatitis is a rare but serious reaction pattern that is characterized by erythema, pruritus and scaling over the entire body (erythroderma).

Drug-induced exfoliative dermatitis usually begins a few weeks or longer following the administration of a culpable drug. Beginning as erythematous, edematous patches, often on the face, it spreads to involve the entire integument. The skin becomes swollen and scarlet and may ooze a straw-colored fluid; this is followed in a few days by desquamation.

High fever, severe malaise and chills, along with enlargement of lymph nodes, often coexist with the cutaneous changes.

One of the most dangerous of all reaction patterns, exfoliative dermatitis can be accompanied by any or all of the following: hypothermia, fluid and electrolyte loss, cardiac failure, and gastrointestinal hemorrhage. Death may supervene if the drug is continued after the onset of the eruption. Secondary infection often complicates the course of the disease. Once the active dermatitis has receded, hyperpigmentation as well as loss of hair and nails may ensue. The following drugs, among others, can bring about exfoliative dermatitis: barbiturates, captopril, carbamazepine, cimetidine, furosemide, gold, isoniazid, lithium, nitrofurantoin, NSAIDs, penicillamine, phenytoin, pyrazolons, quinidine, streptomycin, sulfonamides, and thiazides.

Fixed eruptions

A fixed eruption is an unusual hypersensitivity reaction, characterized by one or more well demarcated erythematous plaques, that recur at the same cutaneous (or mucosal) site or sites each time exposure to the offending agent occurs. The sizes of the lesions vary from a few millimeters to as much as 20 centimeters in diameter. Almost any drug that is ingested, injected, inhaled, or inserted into the body can trigger this skin reaction.

The eruption typically begins as a sharply marginated, solitary edematous papule or plaque – occasionally surmounted by a large bulla – which usually develops 30 minutes to 8 hours following the administration of a drug. If the offending agent is not promptly eliminated, the inflammation intensifies, producing a dusky red, violaceous or brown patch that may crust, desquamate, or blister within 7 to 10 days. The lesions are rarely pruritic. Favored sites are the hands, feet, face, and genitalia – especially the glans penis.

The reason for the specific localization of the skin lesions in a fixed drug eruption is unknown. The offending drug cannot be detected at the skin site. Certain drugs cause a fixed eruption at specific sites, for example, tetracycline and ampicillin often elicit a fixed eruption on the penis, whereas aspirin usually causes skin lesions on the face, limbs and trunk.

Common causes of fixed eruptions are: ampicillin, aspirin, barbiturates, dapsone, metronidazole, NSAIDs, oral contraceptives, phenolphthalein, phenytoin, quinine, sulfonamides, and tetracyclines.

Gingival hyperplasia

Gingival hyperplasia, a common, undesirable, non-allergic drug reaction begins as a diffuse swelling of the interdental papillae.

Particularly prevalent with phenytoin therapy, gingival hyperplasia begins about 3 months after the onset of therapy, and occurs in 30 to 70% of patients receiving it. The severity of the reaction is dose-dependent and children and young adults are more frequently affected. The most severe cases are noted in young women.

In many cases, gingival hyperplasia is accompanied by painful and bleeding gums. There is often superimposed secondary bacterial gingivitis. This can be so extensive that the teeth of the maxilla and mandible are completely overgrown.

While it is characteristically a side effect of hydantoin derivatives, it may occur during the administration of phenobarbital, nifedipine, diltiazem and other medications.

Lichenoid (lichen planus-like) eruptions

Lichenoid eruptions are so called because of their resemblance to lichen planus, a papulosquamous disorder that characteristically presents as multiple, discrete, violaceous, flat-topped papules, often polygonal in shape and which are extremely pruritic.

Not infrequently, lichenoid lesions appear weeks or months following exposure to the responsible drug. As a rule, the symptoms begin to recede a few weeks following the discontinuation of the drug.

Common drug causes of lichenoid eruptions are: antimalarials, beta-blockers, chlorpropamide, furosemide, gold, methyldopa, phenothiazines, quinidine, thiazides, and tolazamide.

Lupus erythematosus

A reaction, clinically and pathologically resembling idiopathic systemic lupus erythematosus (SLE), has been reported in association with a large variety of drugs. There is some evidence that drug-induced SLE, invariably accompanied by a positive ANA reaction with 90% having antihistone antibodies, may have a genetically determined basis. These symptoms of SLE, a relatively benign form of lupus, recede within days or weeks following the discontinuation of the responsible drug. Skin lesions occur in about 20% of cases. Drugs cause fewer than 8% of all cases of systemic LE.

The following drugs have been commonly associated with inducing, aggravating or unmasking SLE: beta-blockers, carbamazepine, chlorpromazine, estrogens, griseofulvin, hydralazine, isoniazid (INH), lithium, methyldopa, minoxidil, oral contraceptives, penicillamine, phenytoin (diphenylhydantoin), procainamide, propylthiouracil, quinidine, and testosterone.

Onycholysis

Onycholysis, the painless separation of the nail plate from the nail bed, is one of the most common nail disorders.

The unattached portion, which is white and opaque, usually begins at the free margin and proceeds proximally, causing part or most of the nail plate to become separated. The attached, healthy portion of the nail, by contrast, is pink and translucent.

Paresthesia

Paresthesias are abnormal neurological sensations such as burning, prickling, numbness, itching, formication, or tingling, often described as "pins and needles" or of a limb being "asleep." It is a symptom of partial damage of a peripheral nerve (e.g. from a head or spinal injury), lack of blood supply to a nerve, or in many cases medications. Paresthesias can affect various parts of the body. Hands, fingers, and feet are common sites but all areas are possibilities. Afflictions of specific nerves or spinal nerves can also cause paresthesias in particular skin areas of the body.

Scores of generic drugs have been reported to occasion paresthesias including alprazolam, allopurinol, amitriptyline, bupropion, buspirone, celecoxib, ciprofloxacin, cyclosporine, enalapril, glipizide, glyburide and many others.

Pemphigus vulgaris

Pemphigus vulgaris (PV) is a rare, serious, acute or chronic, blistering disease involving the skin and mucous membranes.

Characterized by thin-walled, easily ruptured, flaccid bullae that are seen to arise on normal or erythematous skin and over mucous membranes, the lesions of PV appear initially in the mouth (in about 60% of the cases) and then spread, after weeks or months, to involve the axillae and groin, scalp, face and neck. The lesions may become generalized.

Because of their fragile roofs, the bullae rupture leaving painful erosions and crusts may develop principally over the scalp.

Peyronie's disease

First described in 1743 by the French surgeon, François de la Peyronie, Peyronie's disease is a rare, benign connective tissue disorder involving the growth of fibrous plaques in the soft tissue of the penis. Beginning as a localized inflammation, it often develops into a hardened scar. Affecting as much as 1% of men, it may cause deformity, pain, cord-like lesions, or abnormal curvature of the penis when erect.

It has been associated with several drugs, including all the adrenergic blocking agents (beta-blockers), methotrexate, colchicine and others.

Photosensitivity

A photosensitive reaction is a chemically induced change in the skin that makes an individual unusually sensitive to electromagnetic radiation (light). On absorbing light of a specific wavelength, an oral, injected or topical drug may be chemically altered to produce a reaction ranging from macules and papules, vesicles and bullae, edema, urticaria, or an acute eczematous reaction.

Any eruption that is prominent on the face, the dorsa of the hands, the 'V' of the neck, and the presternal area should suggest an adverse reaction to light. The distribution is the key to the diagnosis.

Initially the eruption, which consists of erythema, edema, blisters, weeping and desquamation, involves the forehead, rims of the ears, the nose, the malar eminences and cheeks, the sides and back of the neck, the extensor surfaces of the forearms and the dorsa of the hands. These reactions commonly spare the shaded areas: those under the chin, under the nose, behind the ears and inside the fold of the upper eyelids. There is usually a sharp cut-off at the site of jewelry and at clothing margins. All light-exposed areas need not be affected equally.

There are two main types of photosensitive reactions: the phototoxic and the photoallergic reaction.

Phototoxic reactions, the most common type of drug-induced photosensitivity, resemble exaggerated sunburn and occur within 5 to 20 hours after the skin has been exposed to a photosensitizing substance and light of the proper wavelength and intensity. It is not a form of allergy – prior sensitization is not required – and, theoretically, could occur in anyone given enough drug and light. Phototoxic reactions are dose-dependent both for drug and sunlight. Patients with phototoxicity reactions are commonly sensitive to ultraviolet A (UVA radiation), the so-called 'tanning rays' at 320–400 nm. Phototoxic reactions may cause onycholysis, as the nail bed is particularly susceptible because of its lack of melanin protection.

Patients with a true photoallergy (the interaction of drug, light and the immune system), a less common form of drug-induced photosensitivity, are often sensitive to UVB radiation, the so-called 'burning rays' at 290–320 nm. Photoallergic reactions, unlike phototoxic responses, represent an immunologic change and require a latent period of from 24 to 48 hours during which sensitization occurs. They are not dose-related.

If the photosensitizer acts internally, it is a photodrug reaction; if it acts externally, it is photocontact dermatitis.

Drugs that are likely to cause phototoxic reactions are: amiodarone, nalidixic acid, various NSAIDs, phenothiazines (especially chlorpromazine), and tetracyclines (particularly demeclocycline).

Photoallergic reactions may occur as a result of exposure to systemically administered drugs such as griseofulvin, NSAIDs, phenothiazines, quinidine, sulfonamides, sulfonylureas, and thiazide diuretics as well as to external agents such as para-aminobenzoic acid (found in sunscreens), bithionol (used in soaps and cosmetics), paraphenylenediamine, and others.

Pigmentation

Drug-induced pigmentation on the skin, hair, nails, and mucous membranes is a result of melanin synthesis, increased lipofuscin synthesis, or post-inflammatory pigmentation.

Color changes, which can be localized or widespread, can also be a result of a deposition of bile pigments (jaundice), exogenous metal compounds, and direct deposition of elements such as carotene or quinacrine.

Post-inflammatory pigmentation can follow a variety of drug-induced inflammatory cutaneous reactions; fixed eruptions are known to leave a residual pigmentation that can persist for months.

The following is a partial list of those drugs that can cause various pigmentary changes: anticonvulsants, antimalarials, cytostatics, hormones, metals, tetracyclines, phenothiazine tranquilizers, psoralens, amiodarone, etc.

Pityriasis rosea-like eruptions

Pityriasis rosea, commonly mistaken for ringworm, is a unique disorder that usually begins as a single, large, round or oval pinkish patch known as the 'mother' or 'herald' patch. The most common sites for this solitary lesion are the chest, the back, or the abdomen. This is followed in about 2 weeks by a blossoming of small, flat, round or oval, scaly patches of similar color, each with a central collarette scale, usually distributed in a Christmas tree pattern over the trunk and, to a lesser degree, the extremities. This eruption seldom itches and usually limits itself to areas from the neck to the knees.

While the etiology of idiopathic pityriasis rosea is unknown, we do know that various medications have been reported to give rise to this disorder. These are: barbiturates, beta-blockers, bismuth, captopril, clonidine, gold, griseofulvin, isotretinoin, labetalol, meprobamate, metronidazole, penicillin, and tripelennamine.

In drug-induced pityriasis rosea, the 'herald patch' is usually absent, and the eruption will often not follow the classic pattern.

Pruritus

Generalized itching, without any visible signs, is one of the least common adverse reactions to drugs. More frequently than not, drug-induced itching – moderate or severe – is fairly generalized.

For most drugs it is not known in what way they elicit pruritus; some drugs can cause itching directly or indirectly through cholestasis. Pruritus may develop by different pathogenetic mechanisms: allergic, pseudoallergic (histamine release), neurogenic, by vasodilatation, cholestatic effect, and others.

A partial list of those drugs that can cause pruritus are as follows: aspirin, NSAIDs, penicillins, sulfonamides, chloroquine, ACE inhibitors, amiodarone, nicotinic acid derivatives, lithium, bleomycin, tamoxifen, interferons, gold, penicillamine, methoxsalen, isotretinoin, etc.

Pseudoporphyria

Pseudoporphyria is an uncommon, reversible, photo-induced, cutaneous bullous disorder with clinical, histologic and immunofluorescent similarities to porphyria cutanea tarda but without the accompanying biochemical porphyrin abnormalities. It is commonly seen as localized bullae and skin fragility on sun-exposed skin, often on the dorsum of the hands and fingers. While pseudoporphyria has been linked with numerous causes, including chronic renal failure, dialysis, and ultraviolet radiation, several medications, primarily naproxen and other nonsteroidal inflammatory drugs, have been reported to trigger this reaction pattern. Blue/gray eye color appears to be an independent risk factor for the development of pseudoporphyria.

Psoriasis

Many drugs, as a result of their pharmacological action, have been implicated in the precipitation or exacerbation of psoriasis or psoriasiform eruptions.

Psoriasis is a common, chronic, papulosquamous disorder of unknown etiology with characteristic histopathological features and many biochemical, physiological, and immunological abnormalities.

Drugs that can precipitate psoriasis are, among others, beta-blockers and lithium. Drugs that are reported to aggravate psoriasis are antimalarials, beta-blockers, lithium, NSAIDs, quinidine, and photosensitizing drugs. The effect and extent of these drug-induced psoriatic eruptions are dose-dependent.

Purpura

Purpura, a result of hemorrhage into the skin, can be divided into thrombocytopenic purpura and non-thrombocytopenic purpura (vascular purpura). Both thrombocytopenic and vascular purpura may be due to drugs, and most of the drugs producing purpura may do so by giving rise to vascular damage and thrombocytopenia. In both types of purpura, allergic or toxic (nonallergic) mechanisms may be involved.

Some drugs combine with platelets to form an antigen, stimulating formation of antibody to the platelet–drug combination. Thus, the drug appears to act as a hapten; subsequent antigen–antibody reaction causes platelet destruction leading to thrombocytopenia.

The purpuric lesions are usually more marked over the lower portions of the body, notably the legs and dorsal aspects of the feet in ambulatory patients.

Other drug-induced cutaneous reactions – erythema multiforme, erythema nodosum, fixed eruption, necrotizing vasculitis, and others – can have a prominent purpuric component.

A whole host of drugs can give rise to purpura, the most common being: NSAIDs, thiazide diuretics, phenothiazines, cytostatics, gold, penicillamine, hydantoins, thiouracils, and sulfonamides.

Raynaud's phenomenon

Raynaud's phenomenon is the paroxysmal, cold-induced constriction of small arteries and arterioles of the fingers and, less often, the toes.

Although estimates vary, recent surveys show that Raynaud's phenomenon may affect 5 to 10 percent of the general population in the United States. Occurring more frequently in women, Raynaud's phenomenon is characterized by blanching, pallor, and cyanosis. In severe cases, secondary changes may occur: thinning and ridging of the nails, telangiectases of the nail folds, and, in the later stages, sclerosis and atrophy of the digits.

Rhabdomyolysis

Rhabdomyolysis is the breakdown of muscle fibers, the result of skeletal muscle injury, which leads to the release of potentially toxic intracellular contents into the plasma. The causes are diverse: muscle trauma from vigorous exercise, electrolyte imbalance, extensive thermal burns, crush injuries, infections, various toxins and drugs, and a host of other factors.

Rhabdomyolysis can result from direct muscle injury by myotoxic drugs such as cocaine, heroin and alcohol. About 10 to 40 percent of patients with rhabdomyolysis develop acute renal failure.

The classic triad of symptoms of rhabdomyolysis is muscle pain, weakness and dark urine. Most frequently, the involved muscle groups are those of the back and lower calves. The primary diagnostic indicator of this syndrome is significantly elevated serum creatine phosphokinase.

Some of the drugs that have been reported to cause rhabdomyolysis are salicylates, amphotericin, quinine, statin drugs, SSRIs, theophylline, amphetamines, and others.

Tinnitus

Tinnitus is a sound or noise in one or both ears that has been described as a buzzing, ringing, swishing, clicking, pulsations, or whistling – even thumping or roaring – in one or both ears as a result of an ear infection, a head injury, a blocked auditory canal or following the use of certain drugs. Nearly 40 million Americans suffer from this disorder.

There are over 200 generic drugs listed in this Manual that have been reported to cause tinnitus and the more common ones are aspirin, quinine, aminoglycoside antibiotics, cytotoxic drugs, diuretics and NSAIDs.

Toxic epidermal necrolysis (TEN)

Also known as Lyell's syndrome, toxic epidermal necrolysis is a rare, serious, acute exfoliative, bullous eruption of the skin and mucous membranes that usually develops as a reaction to diverse drugs. TEN can also be a result of a bacterial or viral infection and can develop after radiation therapy or vaccinations.

In the drug-induced form of TEN, a morbilliform eruption accompanied by large red, tender areas of the skin will develop shortly after the drug has been administered. This progresses rapidly to blistering, and a widespread exfoliation of the epidermis develops dramatically over a very short period accompanied by high fever. The hairy parts of the body are usually spared. The mucous membranes and eyes are often involved.

The clinical picture resembles an extensive second-degree burn; the patient is acutely ill. Fatigue, vomiting, diarrhea and angina are prodromal symptoms. In a few hours the condition becomes grave.

TEN is a medical emergency and unless the offending agent is discontinued immediately, the outcome may be fatal in the course of a few days.

Drugs that are the most common cause of TEN are: allopurinol, ampicillin, amoxicillin, carbamazepine, NSAIDs, phenobarbital, pentamidine, phenytoin (diphenylhydantoin), pyrazolones, and sulfonamides.

Urticaria

Urticaria induced by drugs is, after exanthems, the second most common type of drug reaction. Urticaria, or hives, is a vascular reaction of the skin characterized by pruritic, erythematous wheals. These welts – or wheals – caused by localized edema, can vary in size from one millimeter in diameter to large palm-sized swellings, favor the covered areas (trunk, buttocks, chest), and are, more often than not, generalized. Urticaria usually develops within 36 hours following the administration of the responsible drug. Individual lesions rarely persist for more than 24 hours.

Urticaria may be the only symptom of drug sensitivity, or it may be a concomitant or followed by the manifestations of serum sickness. Urticaria may be accompanied by angioedema of the lips or eyelids. It may, on rare occasions, progress to anaphylactoid reactions or to anaphylaxis.

The following are the most common causes of drug-induced urticaria: antibiotics, notably penicillin (more following parenteral administration than by ingestion), barbiturates, captopril, levamisole, NSAIDs, quinine, rifampin, sulfonamides, thiopental, and vancomycin.

Vasculitis

Drug-induced cutaneous necrotizing vasculitis, a clinicopathologic process characterized by inflammation and necrosis of blood vessels, often presents with a variety of small, palpable purpuric lesions most frequently distributed over the lower extremities: urticaria-like lesions, small ulcerations, and occasional hemorrhagic vesicles and pustules. The basic process involves an immunologically mediated response to antigens that result in vessel wall damage.

Beginning as small macules and papules, they ultimately eventuate into purpuric lesions and, in the more severe cases, into hemorrhagic blisters and frank ulcerations. A polymorphonuclear infiltrate and fibrinoid changes in the small dermal vessels characterize the vasculitic reaction.

Drugs that are commonly associated with vasculitis are: ACE inhibitors, amiodarone, ampicillin, cimetidine, coumadin, furosemide, hydantoins, hydralazine, NSAIDs, pyrazolons, quinidine, sulfonamides, thiazides, and thiouracils.

Vertigo

Vertigo, a specific type of dizziness, is a feeling of unsteadiness. It is the sensation of spinning or swaying while the body is actually stationary with respect to the surroundings, and is commonly caused by either motion sickness, a viral infection of the organs of balance, low blood sugar, low blood pressure, or medications. It is a symptom of multiple sclerosis, carbon monoxide poisoning, and Meniere's disease.

Vertigo is one of the most common health problems in adults. According to the National Institutes of Health (NIH), about 40% of people in the United States experience feeling dizzy at least once during their lifetime. Prevalence is slightly higher in women and increases with age.

Classes of drugs that have been reported to cause vertigo include: aminoglycosides, antihypertensives, diuretics, vasodilators, phenothiazines, tranquilizers, antidepressants, anticonvulsants, hypnotics, analgesics, alcohol, caffeine, and tobacco.

Xerostomia

Xerostomia is a dryness of the oral cavity that makes speaking, chewing and swallowing difficult. Some people also experience salivary gland enlargement or changes in taste. Resulting from a partial or complete absence of saliva production, xerostomia can be caused by a variety of medications. Lack of saliva may predispose one to oral infections, such as candidiasis, and increase the risk of dental caries.

ALPHABETICAL INDEX

711

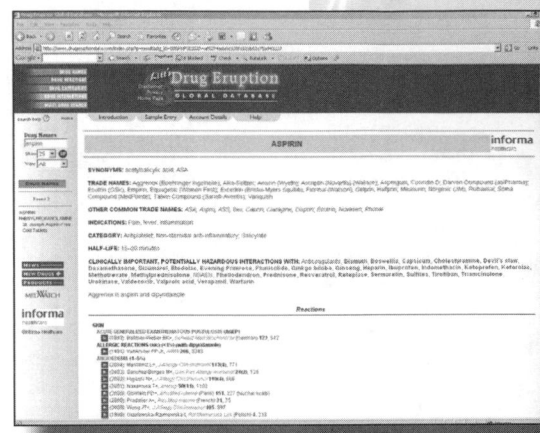